Burns' Pediatric Primary Care

Burns' Pediatric Primary Care

EIGHTH EDITION

Editors

Dawn Lee Garzon, PhD, RN, CPNP-PC, PMHS, FAANP, FAAN

Nurse Practitioner
Department of Child and Adolescent Psychiatry
Washington University School of Medicine
St. Louis, Missouri

Mary Dirks, DNP, RN, ARNP, CPNP-PC, FAANP, ELAN Fellow

Co-Lead Editor
Clinical Professor
College of Nursing
The University of Iowa
Iowa City, Iowa

Martha Driessnack, PhD, RN, PNP

Emerita Faculty
School of Nursing
Oregon Health & Science University
Portland, Oregon

Karen G. Duderstadt, PhD, RN, CPNP-PC, FAAN

Clinical Professor Emerita
Department of Family Health Care Nursing
School of Nursing
University of California San Francisco
San Francisco, California

Nan M. Gaylord PhD, RN, CPNP-PC, PMHS, FAANP, FAAN

Professor
College of Nursing
University of Tennessee
Knoxville, Tennessee

Associate Editors

Jaime Panton, DNP, CPNP-AC/PC

Associate Professor
School of Nursing
Columbia University
New York, New York

Daniel Crawford, DNP, ARNP, CPNP-PC, CNE, FAANP

Clinical Associate Professor
College of Nursing
The University of Iowa
Iowa City, Iowa

ELSEVIER

ELSEVIER
3251 Riverport Lane
St. Louis, Missouri 63043

BURNS' PEDIATRIC PRIMARY CARE, EIGHTH EDITION

ISBN: 978-0-323-88231-6

Notices

Knowledge and best practice in this field are constantly changing. As new research and experience broaden our understanding, changes in research methods, professional practices, or medical treatment may become necessary.

Practitioners and researchers must always rely on their own experience and knowledge in evaluating and using any information, methods, compounds, or experiments described herein. In using such information or methods they should be mindful of their own safety and the safety of others, including parties for whom they have a professional responsibility.

With respect to any drug or pharmaceutical products identified, readers are advised to check the most current information provided (i) on procedures featured or (ii) by the manufacturer of each product to be administered, to verify the recommended dose or formula, the method and duration of administration, and contraindications. It is the responsibility of practitioners, relying on their own experience and knowledge of their patients, to make diagnoses, to determine dosages and the best treatment for each individual patient, and to take all appropriate safety precautions.

To the fullest extent of the law, neither the Publisher nor the authors, contributors, or editors, assume any liability for any injury and/or damage to persons or property as a matter of products liability, negligence or otherwise, or from any use or operation of any methods, products, instructions, or ideas contained in the material herein.

Senior Content Strategist: Sandra Clark
Senior Content Development Specialist: Laura Selkirk
Publishing Services Manager: Catherine Jackson
Senior Project Manager/Specialist: Carrie Stetz
Book Design: Maggie Reid

Printed in India

Last digit is the print number: 9 8 7 6 5 4 3 2 1

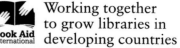

Working together
to grow libraries in
developing countries

www.elsevier.com • www.bookaid.org

Contributors

Andrea Achenbach, DNP, ARNP, FNP-C
Clinical Assistant Professor
College of Nursing
The University of Iowa
Iowa City, Iowa

Britta G. Beblavi, RDN, CD, LD
Owner, Registered Dietitian
Grow Well Nutrition LLC
Greenwood Village, Colorado

Tami B. Bland, DNP, CPNP-PC
Clinical Associate Professor
College of Nursing
University of Tennessee
Knoxville, Tennessee

Jodi Bloxham, DNP, ARNP, CPNP-AC, CPNP-PC
Assistant Professor (Clinical) and Director
Pediatric Acute Care Nurse Practitioner Program
The University of Iowa College of Nursing
Pediatric Critical Care Nurse Practitioner
Pediatric Intensive Care Unit
Stead Family Children's Hospital
The University of Iowa Hospitals and Clinics
Iowa City, Iowa

Eliza Buyers, MD
Pediatric and Adolescent Gynecology
Children's Hospital Colorado
Assistant Professor
Department of Obstetrics and Gynecology
University of Colorado
Aurora, Colorado

Donald L. Chi, DDS, PhD
Professor
Oral Health Sciences
University of Washington School of Dentistry
Professor
Health Systems and Population Health
University of Washington School of Public Health
Seattle, Washington

Hana Conlon, BSN, MSN, CPNP
Nurse Practitioner
Columbia University Irving Medical Center
New York, New York

Daniel Crawford, DNP, ARNP, CPNP-PC, CNE, FAANP
Clinical Associate Professor
College of Nursing
The University of Iowa
Iowa City, Iowa

Sandra Daack-Hirsch, PhD, RN, FAAN
Professor
College of Nursing
The University of Iowa
Iowa City, Iowa

Renée L. Davis, DNP, APRN, CPNP-PC
Associate Professor, Traditional BSN Coordinator, Level II
Trudy Busch Valentine School of Nursing
Saint Louis University
St. Louis, Missouri;
Dr. Norman Pediatrics
Belleville, Illinois

Sara D. DeGolier, MS, RN, CPNP AC/PC
Pediatric Intensive Care Unit
Children's Hospital Colorado
Aurora, Colorado

Anne L. Derouin, DNP, APRN, CPNP, PMHS, FAANP
Assistant Dean, MSN Program
Clinical Professor
Duke Community and Family Medicine
Duke Global Health Institute
Duke University
Durham, North Carolina

Mary Dirks, DNP, RN, ARNP, CPNP-PC, FAANP, ELAN Fellow
Clinical Professor
College of Nursing
The University of Iowa
Iowa City, Iowa

Martha Driessnack, PhD, RN, PNP
Emerita Faculty
School of Nursing
Oregon Health & Science University
Portland, Oregon

Karen G. Duderstadt, PhD, RN, CPNP-PC, FAAN
Clinical Professor Emerita
Department of Family Health Care Nursing
School of Nursing
University of California San Francisco
San Francisco, California

Martha G. Fuller, PhD, RN, PPCNP-BC
Associate Professor of Nursing
University of San Diego
Nurse Practitioner
Developmental Services
Rady Children's Hospital
San Diego, California

Dawn Lee Garzon, PhD, CPNP-PC, PMHS, FAANP, FAAN
Nurse Practitioner
Department of Child and Adolescent Psychiatry
Washington University School of Medicine
St. Louis, Missouri

Nan M. Gaylord, PhD, RN, CPNP-PC, PMHS, FAANP, FAAN
Professor
College of Nursing
University of Tennessee
Knoxville, Tennessee

Valerie Griffin, DNP, PPCNP-BC, FNP-BC, PMHS, FAANP
Associate Professor, Director NP Specializations
School of Nursing
Southern Illinois University Edwardsville
Edwardsville, Illinois

Beth Heuer, DNP, CRNP, CPNP-PC, PMHS
Associate Professor of Clinical Instruction
Department of Nursing
College of Public Health
Temple University
Aston, Pennsylvania

Gail A. Hornor, DNP, CPNP, SANE-P
Forensic Nursing Specialist, Education
International Association of Forensic Nurses
Elkridge, Maryland

Mary Koslap-Petraco, DNP, PPCNP-BC, CPNP, FAANP
Clinical Assistant Professor
Parent Child Health
Stony Brook University School of Nursing
Stony Brook, New York;
Nurse Consultant
Immunize.org
St. Paul, Minnesota;
Owner/Nurse Practitioner
Pediatric Nurse Practitioner House Calls
Massapequa Park, New York

Tasha Lowery, MSN, FNP-C, ENP-C, CPNP-AC
Assistant Professor, APRN Programs
Azusa Pacific University
Azusa, California;
Nurse Practitioner, CARES Center
General Pediatrics
Children's Hospital of Los Angeles
Los Angles, California

Jennifer Newcombe, DNP, MSN, BSN
Nurse Practitioner
Pediatric Cardiothoracic Surgery
Loma Linda Children's Hospital
Assistant Professor
Loma Linda School of Nursing
Loma Linda, California

Katherine M. Newnam, PhD, CPNP-PC, NNP-BC, FAAN, FAANP
Associate Professor
College of Nursing
University of Tennessee
Knoxville, Tennessee

Sarah Obermeyer, PhD, CNM, WHNP, IBCLC, CNE
Associate Professor
Nurse Midwifery and Women's Health
Frontier Nursing University
Versailles, Kentucky;
Certified Nurse Midwife
Women's Health Center
Eisner Pediatric and Family Medicinal Center
Los Angeles, California

Adebola M. Olarewaju, PhD, MS
Pediatric Nurse Practitioner
Otolaryngology–Head and Neck Surgery
University of California Davis Health
Sacramento, California

Jaime Panton, DNP, CPNP-AC/PC
Associate Professor
School of Nursing
Columbia University
New York, New York

Jessica Peck, DNP, APRN, CPNP-PC, CNE, CNL, FAANP, FAAN
Clinical Professor
Louise Herrington School of Nursing
Baylor University
Dallas, Texas;
Past President
National Association of Pediatric Nurse Practitioners
New York, New York

Michele L. Polfuss, PhD, RN, APNP-AC/PC, FAAN
Professor, College of Nursing
University of Wisconsin–Milwaukee
Joint Research Chair in the Nursing of Children
Nursing Research and Evidence-Based Practice
Children's Wisconsin
Milwaukee, Wisconsin

Leslie N. Rhodes, DNP, PPCNP-BC
Pediatric Nurse Practitioner
Orthopaedics
Le Bonheur Children's Hospital
Assistant Professor
College of Nursing, Health Promotion and Disease Prevention
University of Tennessee Health Science Center
Memphis, Tennessee

Deanna Schneider, DNP, CPNP-PC/AC
Assistant Professor
Pediatric Nurse Practitioner Program
Columbia University School of Nursing
New York, New York

Danielle Sebbens, DNP, CPNP-AC/PC
Associate Director DNP Program
Associate Professor
Coordinator Acute Care Pediatric Nurse Practitioner Program
Edson College of Nursing and Health Innovation
Arizona State University
Pediatric Critical Care Nurse Practitioner
Pediatric Intensive Care Unit
Phoenix Children's Hospital
Phoenix, Arizona

Jennifer Sonney, PhD, APRN, PPCNP-BC, FAANP, FAAN
Joanne Montgomery Endowed Professor
Child, Family, and Population Health Nursing
University of Washington School of Nursing
Seattle, Washington

Jessica L. Spruit, DNP, RN, CPNP-AC, CPHON, BMTCN
Certified Pediatric Nurse Practitioner, Acute Care
Pediatric Palliative Care
Pediatric Blood and Marrow Transplant
C.S. Mott Children's Hospital
Ann Arbor, Michigan

Nancy Barber Starr, MS, RN, CPNP
Pediatric Nurse Practitioner
Advanced Pediatric Associates
Aurora, Colorado

Helen N. Turner, DNP, APRN, PCNS-BC, AP-PMN, FAAN
Associate Professor
School of Nursing
Oregon Health & Science University
Portland, Oregon

Amber Wetherington, MSN, BSN, CPNP-PC
Pediatric Nurse Practitioner
Pediatric Urology
East Tennessee Children's Hospital
Knoxville, Tennessee

Lauren Siebrase-Wilkes, MSN, FNP-C
Advanced Practice Provider Supervisor
Co-Director, New Onset Seizure Clinic
Department of Pediatrics
The University of Iowa
Iowa City, Iowa;
Managing Clinical Director
Chapter Aesthetics Studios
Coralville, Iowa

Teri Moser Woo, PhD, ARNP, CPNP-PC, FAANP
Professor and Director of Nursing
Department of Nursing
Saint Martin's University
Lacey, Washington;
ARNP, Pediatric Urgent Care
Mary Bridge Children's Hospital
Puyallup, Washington

We thank the previous edition contributors for their efforts in the Seventh Edition and whose work and ideas influenced this edition's content:

Sandra Ann Banta-Wright, PhD, RN, NNP-BC
Assistant Clinical Professor
Pediatric Nurse Practitioner Program
Oregon Health & Science University
Portland, Oregon

Jennifer Bevacqua, RN, MS, CPNP-AC, CPNP-PC
Instructor, Pediatric Nurse Practitioner
    Program
Oregon Health & Science University
Portland, Oregon

Catherine G. Blosser, MPA, HA, RN, PNP
Pediatric Nurse Practitioner (Retired)
Multnomah County Health Department
Portland, Oregon

Cris Ann Bowman-Harvey, RN, MSN, CPNP-PC, CPNP-AC
Emergency Department
Children's Hospital Colorado
Aurora, Colorado;
Faculty, Department of Pediatrics
University of Colorado
Denver, Colorado

Jennifer Chauvin, MA, BSN, RN-BC
DNP Candidate, College of Nursing
Washington State University, Vancouver
Vancouver, Washington

Cynthia M. Claytor, RN, MSN, PNP, FNP-C, CCRN
Faculty, Graduate Nursing
Azusa Pacific University
Azusa, California

Ardys Dunn, PhD, RN, PNP
Associate Professor Emeritus
University of Portland School of Nursing
Portland, Oregon;
Professor (Retired)
Samuel Merritt College School of Nursing
Oakland, California

Terea Giannetta, DNP, CPNP, FAANP
Chief Nurse Practitioner, Hematology
Valley Children's Hospital
Madera, California;
Professor Emeritus, School of Nursing
California State University, Fresno
Fresno, California

Emily Gutierrez, DNP, C-PNP, PMHS, IFM-CP
Practice Owner
Neuronutrition Associates
Austin, Texas;
Adjunct Faculty, School of Nursing
Johns Hopkins University
Baltimore, Texas

Susan Hines, RN, BSN, MSN, CPNP
Pediatric Pulmonary Medicine
Children's Hospital Colorado
Aurora, Colorado

Jennifer Michele Huson, MS, RN, CPNP, CNS
Nurse Practitioner
Pediatric Intensive Care
Children's Hospital Los Angeles
Los Angeles, California

Belinda James-Petersen, BS, MS, DNP, CPNP
Gastroenterology
Children's Hospital of The Kings Daughters
Norfolk, Virginia

Rita Marie M. John, EdD, DNP, CPNP, PMHS, FAANP
Associate Professor of Nursing at CUMC, PNP Program
Columbia University School of Nursing
Hillsborough, New Jersey

Victoria Keeton, PhD, RN, CPNP-PC, CNS
Assistant Professor
Betty Irene Moore School of Nursing
University of California Davis
Sacramento, California

Sharon Norman, DNP, RN, CPNP, CNS, CCRN
School of Nursing
Oregon Health & Science University
Randall Children's Hospital at Legacy Emanuel
Portland, Oregon

Catherine O'Keefe, DNP, CPNP-PC
Adjunct Associate Professor Emerita
College of Nursing
Creighton University
Omaha, Nebraska

Sarah Elizabeth Romer, DNP, FNP
Assistant Professor, Adolescent Medicine, Pediatrics
University of Colorado, Denver School of Medicine
Medical Director, BC4U Clinic
Children's Hospital Colorado
Aurora, Colorado

Ruth K. Rosenblum, DNP, RN, PNP-BC, CNS
Assistant Professor
School of Nursing
San Jose State University
San Jose, California

Susan K. Sanderson, DNP, MSN FNP
Assistant Professor of Pediatrics
University of Utah
Salt Lake City, Utah

Kathryn Schartz, BA, BSN, MSN
Pediatric Nurse Practitioner
General Academic Pediatrics
The Children's Mercy Hospital
Kansas City, Missouri

Alan T. Schultz, MSN, CPNP
Pediatric Nurse Practitioner
Pediatric, Adolescent, and Young Adult Section
Joslin Diabetes Center
Boston, Massachusetts

Isabelle Soulé, PhD, RN
Human Resources for Health Rwanda
University of Maryland
Baltimore, Maryland

Asma Ali Taha, PhD, RN, CPNP-PC/AC, PCNS-BC, CCRN
Professor and Director
Pediatric Nurse Practitioner Program
School of Nursing
Oregon Health & Science University
Doernbecher Children's Hospital
Portland, Oregon

Becky Whittemore, MN, MPH, BSN
Nurse Practitioner
Metabolic Clinic
Oregon Health & Science University
Portland, Oregon

Elizabeth Willer, BA, BSN, MSN
Pediatric Nurse Practitioner (Retired)
Kaiser Permanente
Walnut Creek, California

Robert J. Yetman, MD
Professor of Pediatrics
Director of Division of Community and General Pediatrics
University of Texas Houston Medical School
Houston, Texas

Reviewers

Jacqueline Costello, DNP, MSN Ed, APRN, CPNP-PC
Advanced Practice Provider
Brody School of Medicine
East Carolina University
Greenville, North Carolina

Patricia Dempsey, DNP, APN-BC, PPCPNP-BC
Adjunct Faculty
Monmouth University
West Long Branch, New Jersey

Jennifer Klimek-Yingling, PhD, RN, FNP-BC
Associate Professor of Nursing
Utica College
Utica, New York

Laura Roettger, BS, MS, PhD, APRN, CPNP-PC
Assistant Professor
Director of the Pediatric Nurse Practitioner Program
Thomas Jefferson University College of Nursing
Philadelphia, Pennsylvania;
Pediatric Nurse Practitioner
CompleteCare Health Network
New Jersey

Preface

We are delighted to introduce the eighth edition of *Burns' Pediatric Primary Care*. Maintaining the clinical relevancy of a book of this size requires frequent updates and intentional thought about how pediatric primary care practice evolves in an ever-changing healthcare environment. We reorganized content into three distinct units: health promotion, health supervision, and disease management. The editorial team consists of actively practicing pediatric nurse practitioners who understand the challenges of practicing in post-pandemic healthcare settings and the increasing complexities and responsibilities placed on the primary care healthcare system. This text's success over the last two decades is largely attributable to the contributions of the chapter authors, each of whom is an expert in their field and actively is in their specialty and actively relevant for contemporary clinicians.

Burns' Pediatric Primary Care is a complete reference for anyone who provides primary care to infants, children, and adolescents. Pediatric nurse practitioners (PNPs) and family nurse practitioners (FNPs) are the primary audiences for this textbook. However, physicians, physician assistants, and nurses who care for children in a variety of settings also find this book to be a valuable resource. The textbook emphasizes health promotion, disease prevention, and problem management from the primary care provider's point of view. Each chapter introduces key concepts and provides an evidence-based and theoretical care foundation. Content is designed to allow experienced clinicians to easily navigate or jump to the topic or diagnosis in question, while the novice clinician or learner can read the entire chapter for immersion into the topic. Additional resources for each chapter include websites to access organizations and printed materials that may be useful for clinicians and their patients and families.

Special Features of the Eighth Edition

Some features of the eighth edition about which we are particularly excited include:

- Content reorganization that aligns our health supervision section with Bright Futures[1] and other national health guidelines. We made this change to reflect the current understanding of the continuum of health and illness and to ensure that the flow and classification of information are intuitive to students and providers.
- An introductory **Pediatric Primary Care** chapter helps set the tone for the book, focusing on the role of and influences on pediatric primary care.
- The **Global and National Influences on Child Health Status** chapter highlights selected topics, including adverse childhood experiences (ACEs) and the global effects of the COVID-19 pandemic.
- The **Environmental Influences on Pediatric Health** chapter focuses on the effects of climate change and its impact on health, as well as pediatric social, cultural, and physical environments. The chapter was redesigned to have less emphasis on specific environmental toxins.

- The **NEW Justice, Equity, Inclusion, and Diversity** chapter is completely redesigned to reflect a contemporary understanding of the roles of inequity and racism and their impact on pediatric health care and outcomes.
- The **Sexuality and Gender Identity** chapter was modified to include a discussion of gender identity and an expanded discussion of lesbian, gay, bisexual, transgender, queer, intersex, and asexual (LGBTQIA+) health.
- A **NEW Child Maltreatment** chapter, separating this content from the Injury Prevention chapter to emphasize the importance of its diagnosis and management in pediatric care.
- The impact of the COVID-19 pandemic on child physical and mental health was incorporated throughout the text, and the **Immunizations** chapter was updated with information about novel immunization technologies pioneered to develop the COVID-19 vaccines.
- The **Prescribing Traditional and Complementary Therapies** chapter is restructured with evidence-based treatments most likely to be helpful for the pediatric primary care provider.
- A **NEW Pediatric Palliative Care** chapter. This subspecialty has grown substantially in the last 2 to 3 years, and the chapter serves as a guide for primary care providers who manage and provide care coordination for pediatric patients at the end of life or who need palliative care.

Organization of the Book

Infants, children, and adolescents are a unique population. Pediatric primary healthcare requires unique perspective grounded in a fundamental understanding of the complexities of pediatric development, unique epidemiologic health influences, varied social determinants and environmental influences of health, and each child's unique genetic influences. These themes are incorporated throughout this book, along with the influence of telehealth and nontraditional appointment types in primary care.

The book is now reorganized into three units: Pediatric Primary Care, Pediatric Health Supervision, and Pediatric Diseases and Disorders. Unit I, Pediatric Primary Care, provides an overview of pediatric health care and influences that affect child health. Unit II, Pediatric Health Supervision, begins with overviews of pediatric/family assessment, behavioral/mental health, and sexuality/gender identity, followed by three subsections: Growth and Development, Health Promotion, and Health Protection. Unit III, Pediatric Diseases and Disorders, has two subsections: General Management and Specific Management. Special care was taken to ensure each chapter has the same organizational format to assist readers in locating information in busy clinical settings. Standards and guidelines for care are clearly identified, relevant child development is described, the physiologic and assessment parameters are discussed, management strategies are identified, and the management of common problems is presented in a problem-oriented format. The scope of practice of the primary care provider is emphasized with appropriate referral and consultation strategies identified.

It is our hope that this book continues in the tradition of the prior editions. It is our aim to support the primary care provider with the highest quality, evidence-based care strategies and foster improved health and wellness of pediatric patients and their families.

Reference

[1]Hagan JF, Shaw JS, Duncan PM. *Bright Futures: Guidelines for Health Supervision of Infants, Children and Adolescents*. 4th ed. American Academy of Pediatrics; 2017.

Acknowledgments

A book of this size and complexity cannot be completed without considerable help—the work of the chapter authors who researched, wrote, and revised content; the various specialty expert consultations and reviews that critiqued drafts and provided important perspectives and guidance; and the essential technical support from those who managed the production of the manuscript and the final product. We are particularly grateful to Laura Selkirk, Carrie Stetz, and Sandra Clark at Elsevier for their tireless support and advocacy during the development of this book.

Our Thanks to Family and Friends

- To my amazing daughters, Rachel and Elizabeth, whom I admire and respect and who give my life meaning, you are my heroes; to my dearest friend, Michelle Lowe, who is my person and who always has my back; and to Amy DiMaggio, friends, and family for loving me and giving me wings. Gracias y bendicciones. *Dawn Lee Garzon*
- With sincere gratitude and love to my amazing husband Chuck for his endless support and understanding during the extended time dedicated toward work on this edition. To my family and friends for their steadfast love, support, and encouragement, particularly my children Taylor and Jack and grandson Henry, my pride, joy, and true blessings. *Mary Dirks*
- I dedicate this new edition to my family, as they have supported me and allowed time for me to write and edit. To my parents, who passed on during my involvement with the text but who always encouraged my professional endeavors and taught me the importance of family, good health, and love. To my children, who have tolerated my busyness and still choose health care professions for themselves while producing wonderful grandchildren. And, finally, to my husband, who encouraged my involvement and provided the time and space to write by assuming additional home responsibilities. My love and appreciation to all of you. *Nan Gaylord*
- To my children and their children and their children who, along with children everywhere, are the living messages we send to a time we will not see. Here's hoping we have done well by them. *Martha Driessnack*
- The health of our nation's children is our most important resource. My hope is that this edition will contribute to that critical mission of improving the health and well-being of our children and families. Further, to my ever-patient husband who has sustained and bolstered me through the work on this edition! *Karen Duderstadt*
- To my husband Theo for his constant love and support, and to our children, who give my life so much joy and meaning. To my mentors, who have guided me along my professional path, and to God, for opening life-changing doors. *Jaime Panton*
- My deepest gratitude to my favorite people on earth, my wife Tina and children Madison, Nolan, Kaitlin, and Calvin, for your support in this work and all that I do. I love you so much and am so glad that we get to do life together. To my parents, family, friends, and colleagues (past and present), thank you for all you have taught me and for making life a great adventure! *Dan Crawford*

Contents

1

Pediatric Primary Care

MARTHA DRIESSNACK

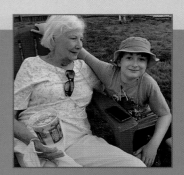

This chapter provides a brief review of the history and core concepts of pediatric primary care, including health promotion and protection, disease and/or disability prevention, the pediatric medical home, and the distinction between primary care versus prevention. It also draws attention to some of the many unique challenges in pediatrics, including caring for a two-generation or dual patient (parent/child), the importance of early influences and protective factors, children and youth with special healthcare needs, and facilitating transitions within/across pediatric healthcare specialists and from pediatric to adult health care. The chapter concludes by introducing Bright Futures, a national health promotion and preventive care initiative from the American Academy of Pediatrics (AAP), along with a list of other professional resources for pediatric primary care providers (PCPs). Subsequent chapters focus on global, national, and local issues; environmental influences; justice, equity, diversity, and inclusion; behavioral mental health promotion; and sexuality amidst emerging gender identity.

Pediatric Primary Care

Primary care represents one level of care within the larger health system. Subsequent levels of healthcare involve increased complexity, additional specialists, and specialized equipment. Accordingly, *primary* care is generalist care; *secondary* care requires specialized expertise; *tertiary* care requires both specialized expertise and equipment; and *quaternary* care requires highly specialized expertise and highly unusual or specialized equipment. Primary care is not site specific; however, it is often incorrectly used synonymously with *outpatient* or ambulatory care, while subsequent levels of care are typically associated with *inpatient* or acute care.

Primary care is conceptualized as being more *person* rather than *disease* centered and makes prevention as important as cure by addressing the root causes of poor health and focusing on threats to health. It includes the provision of continuous, relationship-oriented care over time, rather than being a series of limited disease-based interactions. Pediatric primary care serves as the primary interface between the child/family and the health system, except in the case of serious emergencies. The emphasis is on health promotion and protection, and disease and/or disability prevention. It is designed to be a first contact point, not simply a point of entry into the health system, and the "hub" of coordination (Fig. 1.1). In this central position, the PCP provides continuity as well as integrates subsequent or specialty care, regardless of where the care is delivered and who provides it. Decades of experience tell us that primary healthcare produces better outcomes, at lower costs, and with higher user satisfaction.[1,2] Because it is comprehensive,

continuous, and person-centered care, primary care is also the ideal place for the establishment of the medical home.

The pediatric *medical home* is a care model that delivers patient- and family-centered care, coordinated, and tracked by a PCP within a community-based system, or *medical neighborhood*.

The AAP introduced the medical home concept over 50 years ago as a central location for archiving a child's medical record. In its 2002 policy statement (https://publications.aap.org/pediatrics/article-abstract/110/1/184/64107/The-Medical-Home?redirectedFrom=fulltext), the AAP expanded the medical home concept to include operational characteristics, such as accessible, continuous, comprehensive, family-centered, coordinated, compassionate, and culturally effective care. At the core of the medical home is the PCP whose provision of high-quality, developmentally appropriate healthcare services needs to continue uninterrupted as the child moves within/across the healthcare system and later when transitioning from pediatric to adult care.

Primary Care Versus Primary Prevention

While primary care represents one of four levels of *care* within the larger health system, these levels are sometimes confused with levels of [disease] *prevention*. Disease prevention covers measures that not only prevent the occurrence of disease, but also arrest its progress and reduce its consequences once established. Preventive measures can be applied at any stage along the natural history of a disease, with the goal of preventing further progression of the condition. First described by Leavell and Clark,[3] primary, secondary, and tertiary levels of prevention are best understood in terms of the natural history of disease (Fig. 1.2).

All healthcare providers aim to favorably influence the natural history of disease, but the anticipatory preventive actions they take differ based on the disease, disease stage, and the provider's role in the health system. Preventive care is an important task that is assigned principally to PCPs.

Primary prevention includes efforts that keep disease processes from becoming established by either eliminating the causes or increasing individual resistance to disease. Preventive actions are taken before the onset of disease to remove the possibility that a disease ever occurs. There are two subcategories in primary prevention: (1) health promotion and (2) specific protection. *Health promotion* involves health maintenance and education efforts, including lifestyle changes/choices, nutrition, and maintenance of safe environments. *Specific protection* involves actions targeted at specific diseases, such as immunizations, antimalarial prophylaxis, and environmental modifications (such as fluoride).

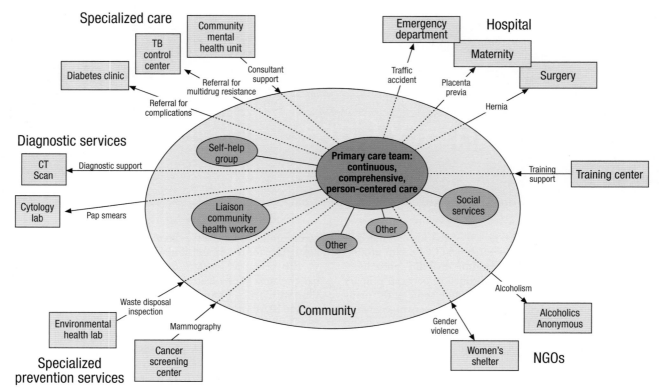

• **Fig 1.1** Primary Care as a Hub of Coordination: Networking Within the Community Served and With Outside Partners. (From Van Lerberghe W. *World Health Organization. Primary Health Care: Now More Than Ever.* World Health Organization; 2008: 55.)

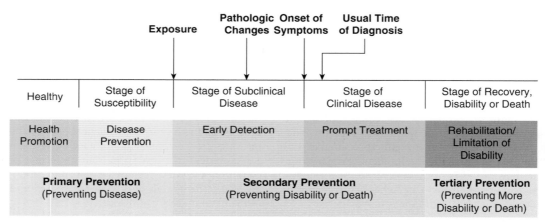

• **Fig 1.2** The Natural History of Disease Aligned With Levels of Prevention. (From Health Beyond Hospitals. Lecture for Ramathibodi Clinical Fellows. https://www.slideshare.net/nawanan/health-beyond-hospitals-lecture-for-ramathibodi-clinical-fellows/.)

Secondary prevention involves early diagnosis and prompt treatment, focusing on efforts that interrupt the disease process before it becomes symptomatic or halting the disease process at its incipient stage to prevent complications. The goal of secondary prevention efforts, including screening, early detection, and prompt treatment, is to cure the disease at the earliest stage, delay disease onset and/or duration, and reduce or reverse the transmission of disease.

Tertiary prevention efforts limit the physical and social consequences of symptomatic disease. The goal is to improve survival and/or quality of life. As with primary prevention, there are two subcategories: (1) disability limitation and (2) rehabilitation. *Disability limitation* focuses on early symptomatic disease and includes measures aimed at correcting the anatomic and/or physiologic components of disease, thus preventing or limiting the impairment or disability caused by the disease. *Rehabilitation* focuses on late symptomatic disease. The goal is to mitigate the ultimate effects of the disease by preventing total social and/or functional disability or by restoring persons with disabilities to a self-sufficient role in society through psychosocial, medical, and/or vocational services.

Pediatric Primary Care Providers

There are several different pediatric PCPs, including pediatric and family nurse practitioners, pediatric and family physicians, and physician assistants. All are important and all are needed. It has been almost 10 years since the Children's Health Fund (CHF) shared that more than 20 million children (~28%) in the United States lacked sufficient access to essential healthcare. These statistics have only worsened as the CHF recently (2022) reported a 40% decrease in health screenings and a 44% decrease in outpatient mental health (see https://www.childrenshealthfund.org/covid-19-has-kept-kids-from-primary-care/). The fact that so many children are not receiving the care they need is a call to action for all who care for children.

> *Not only does failing to address healthcare access barriers threaten and undermine the health and wellbeing of children, but it also may have a direct impact on a child's ability to succeed academically and enter the workforce at their full potential. Loss of later productivity and the extraordinary costs of remediation will clearly have deleterious consequences for the future economic strength and vibrancy of the United States. The stakes could not be higher.[4]*

This call to action is particularly timely as pediatric health concerns take on new issues and importance. For example, gun violence became the leading cause of death of youth under age 20 in the United States in 2020, surpassing deaths from car accidents, cancer, and even COVID-19 (see https://www.childrenshealthfund.org/a-public-health-crisis-gun-violence-and-child-health-and-well-being/).

Pediatric Nurse Practitioners Then and Now

In 1965 Dr. Loretta Ford and Dr. Henry Silver started the nation's first nurse practitioner (NP) program at the University of Colorado. As a result, Dr. Ford is often referred to as the mother of the NP movement and remains one of its greatest champions. One important piece of history is that this first NP program was pediatric, and its focus was on primary care. The emphasis in those early years was to expand public health nurses' roles, integrating the traditional role of the nurse with advanced training and authority in the delivery of primary care to children and families. This early focus on health promotion, protection, and disease prevention remains the mainstay of primary care pediatric nurse practitioner (PNP) programs across the country.

Today, the PNP role continues to evolve. The key difference between a primary care PNP and an acute care PNP is not the site where they practice, but the acuity of the patient for whom they are caring.[5] Primary care PNPs, much like those in the early days with Dr. Ford, provide primary care, which includes well-child care and the prevention and/or management of both common pediatric acute illnesses and chronic conditions. In contrast, acute care PNPs provide care for acutely, critically, and chronically ill children who are unstable, experiencing life-threatening illness, are medically fragile, and/or are technologically dependent.

Unique Issues in Pediatrics

In this section, some of unique issues in pediatrics are introduced along with the inherent challenges that accompany them.

The Two-Generation or Dual Patient

One of the unique challenges in pediatrics is the two-generation or dual patient. Although the primary focus in pediatrics is the patient, each pediatric patient comes with at least one parent or caregiver, if not three or four. Taking the time to understand and work with parents is essential to caring for the child; however, there are some distinctions with patient- and family-centered care (PFCC) and shared decision-making that are unique to pediatrics. When providing PFCC in adult care, providers acknowledge that it is the patient who has ultimate control over health-related decisions, while also knowing these decisions are contextualized within each patient's broader life experiences and family (see Chapter 5). The challenge of using a PFCC model in pediatrics is that there is not one patient, but two, and while the child is the focus, the parent is considered the authority in terms of decisions. For pediatric PCPs, one of the ongoing challenges is how to access, acknowledge, and include the child's voice in care decisions, as it is often lost and/or overridden in health care.

This ongoing tendency to lose track of children's voices is rooted in the long-standing tradition of looking at children across the pediatric lifespan through a deficit-based or developmental lens (see Chapter 8). For example, when it comes to children and adolescents, there is a presumption of decisional incapacity and therefore deference to parental authority. In contrast, adult patients get a presumption of decisional capacity, with familial insight serving only as adjunctive. While most parents make decisions in the best interests of their children most of the time, balancing the needs and wishes within the context of the dual patient can create difficult and challenging care decisions, especially as children's cognitive and executive function mature. Children's needs, and more often their wishes, do not take priority, especially when they differ from their parents. While parents are clearly authorities and caregivers, they are not complete surrogates. PCPs need to remember that, ultimately, they are the child's advocate and need to seek out their voices, actively engaging them in care and health-related decision making, and work to ensure that their voices are heard.

Lifelong Impact of Protective and Adverse Childhood Experiences

Science continues to highlight that early exposure to protective and adverse experiences can promote or disrupt healthy development. This awareness is fueling a new way of looking at life itself, not as disconnected stages, but as an integrated process across time. This *life course perspective* highlights that an individual's physical, mental, socioemotional, and spiritual health results from multiple risk and protective factors that operate throughout the lifespan, and the impact of those factors varies based on the life stage and context.[6] As the science continues to develop, the scope of adverse experiences is evolving to include new factors (e.g., racism, weight stigma). It also focuses attention on the long-term effect of health-related interventions, such as the danger of ionizing radiation exposure from diagnostic medical radiation. *Image Gently* is a long-standing campaign to reduce pediatric risk for cancer during adulthood by increasing awareness and advocating for the protection of children from unnecessary radiation.[7]

In other words, what happens in childhood does not stay in childhood.[8] Instead, what children experience in their earliest days and years of life shapes and defines their future, as early experiences shape the architecture of the developing brain and lay a foundation for long-term health (See Professional Resources, Center for the Developing Child). The World Health Organization (WHO), World Bank, and the United Nations International Children's Emergency Fund (UNICEF) have all drawn attention to the First 1000 Days of Life (https://www.unicef-irc.org/article/958-the-first-1000-days-of-life-the-brains-window-of-opportunity.html) as the brain's "window of opportunity" or unique period when the foundations of health, growth, and neurodevelopment across the life span are established. Equally intriguing is the science behind Developmental Origins of Health and Disease (DOHaD), which suggests that harmful exposures early in life may increase the risk of disease (e.g., obesity, type 2 diabetes, insulin resistance, asthma, cardiovascular diseases, behavioral disorders, neurodegenerative diseases, reproductive disorders, some cancers) later in life.[9] Further, some of these risks carry over into future generations. The link between early-life environmental factors and later-life disease was originally called the *Barker hypothesis,* a proposal that low birth weight predisposes to higher death rates in adult life.[10]

British epidemiologist David Barker's early work highlighting the influences of adverse events that occur during early phases of human development on the patterns of an individual's health and disease throughout life provided the foundation for the identification and study of adverse childhood experiences (ACEs). ACEs are linked to risky health behaviors (e.g., smoking, alcohol use, drug use), chronic health conditions (e.g., obesity, diabetes, depression, heart disease, cancer, stroke, chronic obstructive pulmonary disease), low life potential (graduation rates, academic achievement, lost time from work), and early death (see https://www.cdc.gov/violenceprevention/aces/). As the number of ACEs increases, so does the risk for adverse outcomes, which highlights the call for all pediatric PCPs to screen for and identify adversity in early life (See Professional Resources, The Resilience Project). Paralleling the work on adverse experiences and exposures is the science that identifies and promotes protective factors and ensuring that children flourish despite adversity.[8] At the core of this research is seeking out and ensuring that children are exposed to safe, stable, and nurturing relationships (SSNRs), which can buffer adversity and build resilience. These efforts are particularly evident in the attachment and biobehavioral catch-up (ABC) interventions being introduced in foster care.[11] The PCP is well positioned to seek out, assess, and support protective factors at each well-child visit.

One additional protective factor for PCPs to consider is children's exposure to nature and/or green space, as there is continuing evidence that shows a positive relationship between nature contact and children's health.[12] In his now classic book, *Last Child in the Woods,*[13] Louv wrote about what he called *nature-deficit disorder,* citing studies looking at the benefits of nature and calling attention to the problems that can come from being too isolated from the natural world. PCPs need to continue to emphasize, and perhaps even write prescriptions, for children to go outside and play in nature, limit screen time, and read stories about nature (or have them read to them). At the same time, they need to advocate for equitable nature contact for children in neighborhoods, schools, and communities.[12]

Transition to Adult Care

One of the core responsibilities of pediatric PCPs is coordinating transitions in care within/across the healthcare system as well as preparing all youth for the smooth transition to adulthood, to being responsible for their own health and decisions, and to adult care.[14] The transition from pediatric to adult primary care is critical for all children, but especially for children and youth with special healthcare needs and those with congenital and/or inherited conditions. As advances in neonatal and pediatric medicine continue to improve the prognosis for many childhood conditions, transitioning care is increasingly identified as a critical process for ongoing wellbeing. The AAP and the National Center for Medical Home Implementation created practice-based quality improvement guidelines that include specific activities, decision points, and a clear timeline for transition planning, transfer, and integration into adult care.[15]

Caring for Children and Youth With Special Healthcare Needs

In the United States, the federal government maintains a special responsibility to serve children living with complex and chronic medical conditions beginning with the early "crippled children's programs," which then evolved with the establishment of the Title V Maternal and Child Health Services Block Grant program.[16] More recently, the Health Resources and Services Administration's Maternal and Child Health Bureau (HRSA-MCHB) established the term Children and Youth With Special Health Care Needs (CYSHCN) as "those who have or are at increased risk for a chronic physical, developmental, behavioral, or emotional condition and who also require health and related services of a type or amount beyond that required by children generally," such as asthma, cerebral palsy, and inherited conditions.[17] A subset of CYSHCN is children with medical complexity, a fraction of the overall CYSHCN population, that require the most intensive services including home nursing care, respite, and palliative care.[18]

The proportion of CYSHCN increased over the past few decades, creating new challenges for the healthcare system as their care spans inpatient, outpatient, and community-based settings. These children and youth make up a sizable, yet diverse, population. While the overall prevalence of CYSHCN is approximately 19% of the pediatric population, the majority (85.1%) of these families report their child's care is poorly coordinated.[16] Also of note are the inequities experienced by CYSHCN and their families, particularly those in under-resourced communities.[16] One effort to address these issues is the HRSA-MCHB Blueprint for Change,[18] which identifies four critical, yet interconnected, areas: health equity, family and child wellbeing and quality of life, access to services, and financing of services. Addressing these critical areas requires a concerted, holistic, and integrated approach so that CYSHCN can enjoy a full life from childhood through adulthood; thrive in a system that supports their families and their social, health, and emotional needs; and be assured that their dignity, autonomy, independence, and active participation in their communities will be supported.[18]

The role of the PCP in the care of CYSHCN cannot be overstated, as these children and youth also require ongoing health maintenance, illness prevention, and developmental surveillance. As noted earlier, primary care is designed to be a first contact point, not simply a point of entry into the health system, and the "hub" of coordination (see Fig. 1.1). For CYSHCN, the PCP provides much needed continuity and coordination of care as these children and youth grow and develop. In this role, the PCP reviews subspecialty notes and recommendations, looks for areas of duplication or contradictions, and helps understand recommendations, treatments, and federal and state programs [e.g., Section 504 Plan, Individualize Education Plan (IEP)]. For some CYSHCN, an interdisciplinary specialty clinic (e.g., spina bifida) may be the preferred care coordinator, reaching out to the PCP as a consultant on primary care issues.

All families with a CYSHCN need to be prepared for acute and/or emergency care from those not familiar with their child's condition. The AAP and the American College of Emergency Physicians created an Emergency Information Form (EIF) that ensures a CYSHCN's complicated medical history, as well as special needs and/or considerations, are concisely summarized. This form can be used to transfer relevant information when the CYSHCN has an acute health problem and their parent, caregiver, or familiar PCP is not immediately available, as well as shared with unfamiliar emergency departments and/or personnel (e.g., EMS professionals). A downloadable version is available at: https://www.acep.org/by-medical-focus/pediatrics/medical-forms/emergency-information-form-for-children-with-special-health-care-needs/. Other resources for these families include:

- Centers for Medicare and Medicaid Services Forms: https://www.cms.gov/Medicare/CMS-Forms/CMS-Forms/CMS-Forms-List.html
- Child Care Aware: state-by-state resources. Includes childcare, health and social services, financial assistance, children with special needs, additional resources available in each US state. https://www.childcareaware.org/resources/map/
- Children and Youth with Special Health Care Needs (CYSHCN): https://mchb.hrsa.gov/programs-impact/focus-areas/children-youth-special-health-care-needs-cyshcn
- Family Voices: National Center for Family Professional Partnerships (NCFPP): www.fv-ncfpp.org
- Medical Home Portal: https://www.medicalhomeportal.org/issue/writing-letters-of-medical-necessity

Additional Resources

Bright Futures: Health Promotion and Preventive Care Initiative

While there are many resources for primary care, Bright Futures (https://www.brightfutures.org/) is a key resource for all pediatric PCPs. It provides theory-based and evidence-driven guidance for well-child care and preventive care screenings. The resource emphasizes the family as the child's primary source of strength and support and recognizes the importance of the child's and family's perspectives in clinical decision-making. This patient- and family-centered approach captures the importance of engaging both the family and the patient in a developmentally supportive manner as essential members of the primary healthcare team.

Bright Futures is led by the AAP and supported by the Maternal and Child Health Bureau, Health Resources and Services Administration (HRSA). It identifies 12 key health promotion themes, including healthy development, family support, mental health and emotional wellbeing, nutritional health, physical activity, healthy weight, lifelong health for families and communities, oral health, healthy adolescent development, safety and injury prevention, healthy and safe use of social media, and children and youth with special health needs. These themes align with the content of this textbook, providing a parallel resource for pediatric PCPs.

Other Resources for Primary Care Providers

- Bright Futures for Families: https://familyvoices.org/projects/
- Center for the Developing Child: https://developingchild.harvard.edu/
- National Resource Center for Patient/Family-Centered Medical Home: https://www.aap.org/en/practice-management/medical-home/
- The Resilience Project: https://www.acesaware.org/resource/american-academy-of-pediatrics-the-resilience-project-related-aap-policy/

References

1. Mold JW. How primary care produces better outcomes: a logic model. *Ann Fam Med.* 2014;12(5):483–484.
2. *Primary Health Care Measurement Framework and Indicators: Monitoring Health Systems through a Primary Care Lens.* Geneva: World Health Organization and the United Nations Children's Fund (UNICEF); 2022.
3. Leavell H, Clark AE. *Preventive Medicine for Doctors in the Community.* New York: McGraw-Hill; 1965.
4. Children's Health Fund Children's Health Fund. *Unfinished Business. 20 Million Children in U.S. Still Lack Sufficient Access to Essential Health Care*; 2016. https://www.childrenshealthfund.org/advocacy-publications/.
5. American Nurses Association. *Pediatric Nursing: Scope and Standards of Practice.* American Nurses Association; 2015.
6. Russ SA, Hotez E, Berghaus M, et al. Building a life course intervention research framework. *Pediatrics.* 2022;149(suppl 5).
7. Applegate KE, Cost NG. Image gently: a campaign to reduce children's and adolescents' risk for cancer during adulthood. *J Adolesc Health.* 2013;52(5 Suppl):S93–S97.
8. Garner A, Yogman M. Preventing childhood toxic stress: partnering with families and communities to promote relational health. *Pediatrics.* 2021;148(2):e2021052582.
9. Heindel JJ, Vandenberg LN. Developmental origins of health and disease: a paradigm for understanding disease cause and prevention. *Curr Opin Pediatr.* 2015;27(2):248–253.
10. Bianchi ME, Restrepo JM. Low birthweight as a risk factor for non-communicable diseases in adults. *Front Med (Lausanne).* 2022;8:793990.
11. Grube WA, Liming KW. Attachment and biobehavioral catch-up: a systematic review. *Infant Ment Health J.* 2018;39(6):656–673.
12. Fyfe-Johnson AL, Hazlehurst MF, Perrins SP, et al. Nature and children's health: a systematic review. *Pediatrics.* 2021;148(4):e2020049155.
13. Louv R. *Last Child in the Woods.* Algonquin Books; 2008.
14. Davidson LF, Doyle MH. Healthcare transition: a vital part of care, growth, and change for pediatric patients. *Pediatr Rev.* 2021;42(12):684–693.
15. White PH, Cooley WC, Transitions Clinical Report Authoring Group; American Academy of Pediatrics; American Academy of Family Physicians; American College of Physicians. Supporting the health care transition from adolescence to adulthood in the medical home. *Pediatrics.* 2018;142(5):e20182587. Erratum in *Pediatrics.* 2019;143(2).
16. Ghandour RM, Hirai AH, Kenney MK. Children and youth with special health care needs: a profile. *Pediatrics.* 2022;149(suppl 7).
17. McPherson M, Arango P, Fox H, et al. A new definition of children with special health care needs. *Pediatrics.* 1998;102(1 Pt 1):137–140.
18. McLellan SE, Mann MY, Scott JA, Brown TW. A blueprint for change: guiding principles for a system of services for children and youth with special health care needs and their families. *Pediatrics.* 2022;149(suppl 7):e2021056150c.

2

Global and National Influences on Child Health Status

KAREN G. DUDERSTADT

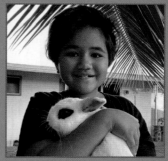

The health of all children is interconnected worldwide, and each child's health must be viewed through a global lens. Whether considering pandemic infectious diseases or global migration, child health status inequities globally and nationally are largely determined by socioeconomic status, which affects overall pediatric health and child development. Biosocial circumstances, or social determinants of child health, are shaped by economics, social policies, politics, and climate change at local, regional, national, and global levels. This social health gradient that runs from the top to the bottom of the socioeconomic spectrum creates health inequities that affect low-, middle-, and high-income countries (HICs) disproportionately.

Significant global progress had been made to reduce childhood morbidity and mortality before the onset of the COVID-19 global pandemic. Although there was a low risk of severe illness or death in children who contracted COVID-19, the pandemic had a profound effect on the physical and mental health of the pediatric population nationally and globally.

This chapter presents an overview of the global health status of infants, children, and adolescents. It describes the effects of the COVID-19 pandemic on pediatric health, the impact of climate change on child health inequality, the progress towards achieving the United Nations (UN) Sustainable Development Goals (SDGs) and Healthy People 2030 targets, and the factors that affect child health in the Unites States, including food and housing insecurity. The chapter also discusses the important role pediatric primary care providers (PCPs) have in advocating for policies that foster health equity and access to quality healthcare services for all children and families.

COVID-19 and the Global Health Status of Children

The launch of the 2030 Agenda for the UN SDGs a decade ago heralded a period of dramatic improvements in most countries in maternal and child survival rates (Fig. 2.1). The global maternal mortality rate (MMR) declined 38% from 2000 to 2017 and the mortality rate for children younger than 5 years declined by more than half.[1] However, the global crises of the COVID-19 pandemic, climate change, and warring conflicts are all affecting the likelihood of reaching the 2030 SDGs.

The recent indicators for the 17 UN SDGs reflect the impact of a reversal of progress towards achieving improving maternal and child health status globally.[2] Findings include[1,2]:

- The COVID-19 pandemic erased previous progress on poverty eradication and pushed 93 million more people into extreme poverty in 2020.
- Twenty-five percent of the global population lives in conflict-affected countries. A record 100 million people were forcibly displaced worldwide.
- More than 24 million learners from primary school to university are at risk of never returning to school.
- Childhood immunization coverage dropped for the first time in a decade, and a global rise in deaths from tuberculosis and malaria occurred. Coverage for the third dose of diphtheria-tetanus-pertussis (DTP) declined from 86% to 81% globally during the first 2 years of the pandemic.
- Global administration of the first dose of the human papillomavirus (HPV) vaccine declined from 20% (2019) to 15% (2021), leaving millions of adolescents at risk for cervical, genital, and oral cancers later in life.

Around 40% of the global population forcibly displaced worldwide are children, and this disruption to their lives and development results in adverse stress and childhood trauma, which is linked to later impairments in learning, behavior, and physical and mental wellbeing.[3] Anxiety and depression among adolescents and young adults increased significantly during the pandemic, particularly in females, and highlighted the lack of available counseling and psychiatric services in health system structures globally and nationally.

Since the onset of the COVID-19 pandemic, international data regarding pediatric mortality were published and the recent UN Inter-Agency Group for Child Mortality Estimation (UNIGME) reported on data from 77 countries. This organization found that the youngest children were the least vulnerable to COVID-19 variants. UNIGME defines pediatric deaths as those that occur in individuals under the age of 24 years. Twenty-seven percent of the COVID-19 pediatric deaths occurred in children from birth to 9 years of age, while 42% occurred in youth 20 to 24 years of

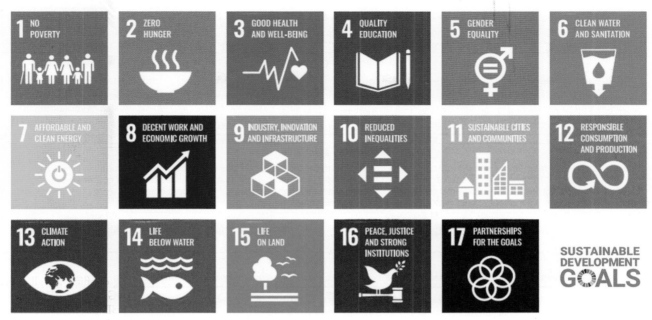

• **Fig 2.1** United Nations Development Program (UNDP) Sustainable Development Goals (SDGs) for 2030. (From United Nations. *The Sustainable Development Goals Report 2022.* https://www.un.org/sustainabledevelopment/. The content of this publication has not been approved by the United Nations and does not reflect the views of the United Nations or its officials or Member States.)

age.[4] Overall child mortality remains high, and the COVID-19 pandemic exacerbated the burden of pediatric loss of life. In 2020 alone, 5 million children died from all causes before reaching their third birthday.[4] Children born in sub-Saharan Africa had the highest mortality rate at 74 deaths per 1000, 14 times higher than in the HICs. Sub-Saharan Africa has the highest rate of neonatal mortality at 27 per 1000 live births, followed by Southeastern Asia at 23 per 1000 live births.[4] If the current trend continues, 54 countries will not meet the 2030 UN SDGs.

It became evident during the pandemic that the COVID-19 crisis was an extraordinary challenge for national statistical systems and a wake-up call for the need for stronger information and communication technology (ICT) infrastructure foundations.[2] It also became an opportunity for countries to experiment with innovative data collection methods, explore new data sources, and modernize ICT infrastructures to meet data demands for global and national policymaking to guide healthcare decisions.

In 2022 the UN General Assembly adopted a resolution that codified the human right to a clean, healthy, and sustainable environment on the 75th anniversary of the Universal Declaration of Human Rights.[5] The confirmation of this human right gives global activists a new tool for advocacy on the effects of climate change and the loss of biodiversity. Reigniting optimism and collective action are required as the impact of the global pandemic eases to strengthen healthcare systems and social and political protective systems to create a more resilient and secure world for our children and families.[1]

Pediatric Mortality Globally

The UN SDGs called for an end to preventable deaths of newborns and children under 5 years old, set the goal of a neonatal mortality rate of 12 or fewer deaths per 1000 live births and an under-5 years mortality rate of 25 or fewer deaths per 1000 live

births. However, 54 countries will not meet the under-5 mortality target by 2030, and 61 countries will miss the neonatal mortality target.[4] Of further concern, neonatal and infant mortality remains highest in sub-Saharan Africa, Central Asia, and Southeast Asia.

About 43% of pediatric deaths globally occurred among those 5 to 24 years old. Although adolescent mortality declined by nearly 40% since 1990, almost 1 million adolescents died in 2020.[4] Over 70% of all pediatric deaths occurred in sub-Saharan Africa (45%) and Central and Southern Asia (27%). The global pandemic contributed to a significant setback in recent progress on each of these health indicators.

Food Insecurity

Hunger and undernutrition are often associated with *food insecurity,* which exists when individuals, families, and/or whole populations do not have physical and economic access to sufficient, safe, nutritious, and culturally acceptable food to meet nutritional needs. Food insecurity may occur in impoverished populations in developing countries and in industrialized nations, particularly among immigrant populations. Children affected by migration and family separation are at the highest risk for food insecurity and are also vulnerable to adverse health consequences such as exposure to exploitation and child trafficking.

Growing evidence indicates the dramatic effect of climate change on food crop production and distribution issues globally and subsequent contributions to human migration patterns and food insecurity. Globally, undernutrition is an important determinant of maternal and child health and accounts for 45% of deaths in children younger than 5 years.[6] Children who are exclusively breastfed for the first 6 months of life are 14 times more likely to survive than nonbreastfed infants, yet the lowest breastfeeding rates are in nations with the lowest per capita incomes.

Climate Change
Indicated by extreme weather events, heat waves, floods, droughts, rising temperatures, natural disasters, rising sea levels, etc.

Dimensions of Inequality

Within-country inequality	**Between-country inequality**	**Geographic inequality**	**Intergenerational inequality**
Income, education, socioeconomic position, indigenous populations	High-, middle-, and low-income countries or regions	Proximity to high-risk areas, such as coastal areas, glaciers, and climate zone	Differential probability to experience severe effects of climate change in the future

Explanatory Mechanisms
- Financial and social resources on individual and group levels determine access to protective factors within countries
- Poor sanitation, poor infrastructure, weak economy, and poor political leadership determine inequalities between countries
- Double burden of high exposure to extreme weather events and low mitigation capacity in low-income countries
- Direct effect on health vs indirect effects mediated by social determinants of health

Child Health Inequalities
Malnutrition, vector-borne diseases, respiratory diseases, diarrhea, perinatal health, mental health, mortality, etc.

• **Fig 2.2** Relationship Between Climate Change and Child Health Inequalities. (From Arpin E, Gauffin K, Kerr M, et al. Climate change and child health inequality: a review of reviews. *Int J Environ Res Public Health.* 2021;18[20]:10896.)

Climate Change and Global Child Health Inequality

Climate change is an urgent problem that impacts the global pediatric population disproportionately. Many children living in low- and middle-income countries (LMICs) lack the essential determinants of health, including clean air, adequate shelter, nutrition, safe water, and sanitation, which contributes to the higher risk of malnutrition and growth stunting. These factors are exacerbated by the direct and indirect effects of climate change, which include vector-, water-, and food-borne infectious diseases.[7] Inequalities also exist within HICs, as many children in low-income households experience high levels of air pollution, food insecurity, and poor housing conditions (Fig. 2.2).[7] Even with recent improvements in childhood survival rates in LMICs, the mortality rate of children under 5 years of age remains twice as high for children born in the poorest countries compared to the highest per-capita income countries.[1]

The mental health of children and adolescents globally is impacted by immigration, social, and economic environments including loss of native lands due to crop failures resulting in food insecurities, exposure to violence, and disruption in learning and teaching as well as the COVID-19 pandemic (Fig. 2.3).[8] The overall prevalence of pediatric posttraumatic stress (PTS) increased globally, with the highest prevalence in regions impacted by natural disasters. In a recent study in the United States, more than 80% of children 10 to 12 years of age revealed fear, sadness, and anger when discussing their feelings about environmental problems.[8] As the pandemic eased, many 10- to 19-year-olds globally moved to environmental advocacy, despite adversity, and established "Fridays for Future" to put moral pressure on policymakers to take forceful action to address climate change (https://fridaysforfuture.org/).

The recent Intergovernmental Panel on Climate Change (IPCC) Report illustrated the urgent need for interventions to mitigate the effects of climate change and echoed editorials published in 200 medical journals calling for urgent action to address

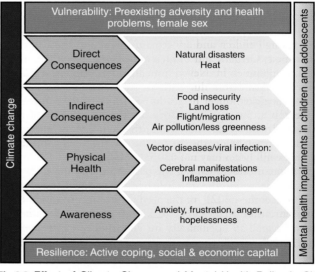

• **Fig 2.3** Effect of Climate Change and Mental Health Policy in Children and Adolescents. (From Clemens V, von Hirschhausen E, Fegert J. Report of the intergovernmental panel on climate change: implications for the mental health policy of children and adolescents in Europe—a scoping review. *Eur Child Adolesc Psychiatry.* 2022;31:701–713.)

climate change, restore biodiversity, and protect health.[9] LMICs have limited capacity to mitigate the effects of climate change with current economic structures and prevailing political forces. Enhanced interventions by HICs are necessary to promote and fund mitigation and adaptation in LMICs to address climate change.[7]

Despite the recognition of the health-related inequities due to climate change, quantitative data are lacking on the direct consequences of extreme heat events, hurricanes, and subsequent flooding and infrastructure damage on child health outcomes.[7] Global greenhouse gas emissions must decline 43% by 2030 to stave off the worst climate-related impacts.[2] Current national commitments point to a nearly 14% increase by 2030, and greater engagement in policy action and behavior change is urgently needed to meet the 1.5°C target.[2]

Health Status of Children in the United States

The COVID-19 pandemic disrupted data collection for the key child health indicators—economic wellbeing, education, health, and family and community—resulting in some data in the latest report reflecting 2020 estimates. As a result, the child health indicators do not fully reflect the effect of the pandemic on children and families. In 2020 fewer children were living in poverty, with one in six children living in poor families.[10] Massachusetts continues to rank first in overall child wellbeing, followed by New Hampshire and Minnesota. Three states including Mississippi (48th), Louisiana (49th), and New Mexico (50th) ranked the lowest nationally.[10] Children living in the Southwest have the lowest rating in child wellbeing indicators. California ranks seventh in child health indicators but 45th in family economic wellbeing.[10]

The United States has significant gaps in educational achievement and graduation outcome by race and income among all pediatric age groups.[10] High-school graduation rates dipped in 20 of 26 states reporting in 2021, ending two decades of national progress. Home confinement and learning remotely during the pandemic disrupted teaching and learning, with greater impacts seen among children and adolescents living in low-income families. Illinois, Oregon, and North Dakota dropped 2% in 2021.[11] In some counties in Nevada, graduation rates dropped 2.6% during the pandemic due to adolescents living in low-income families working longer hours and caring for younger siblings.[11] In Oregon and Nevada, the share of high-school freshmen who completed their last school year on track to graduate was about 10% lower than before the pandemic.[11] Students contending with mental health issues may not be able to focus in the classroom, fall behind in core areas such as math and reading, and often struggle to graduate.[10]

In December 2021 the US Surgeon General and leaders in pediatric health policy declared a child mental health emergency.[12] The 2019 National Survey on Drug Use report indicated in the year before the onset of the pandemic, 3.5 million adolescents had a major depressive episode, about one in seven youths aged 12 to 17 years (15.7%).[13] Between March and October 2020, emergency department (ED) visits for mental health issues rose by 24% for children ages 5 to 11 years and 31% for those ages 12 to 17 years. Compared to the same period in 2019, in early 2021, ED visits for suspected suicide attempts increased by nearly 51% among girls ages 12 to 17 years.[14] Suicidal behaviors increased among youth with 19% seriously considering suicide (33% increase from 2009 to 2019).[15] Pediatric deaths nationally reflect increased suicide rates and include victims of gun violence, which surged ahead of motor vehicle deaths to become the leading cause of death for young people ages 1 to 19 years in 2020.[15]

The pandemic contributed significantly to the youth mental health crisis. More than 140,000 children in the United States lost a primary and/or secondary caregiver, with youth of color disproportionately impacted.[16] This family crisis compounded the already increasing rates of depression, anxiety, trauma, loneliness, and suicidality among youth in the United States. The current challenges facing children and adolescents are so widespread that urgent action is needed at all levels of government and by PCPs and advocates for children and adolescents for increased policy action nationally.[12]

Infant Mortality

Infant mortality in the United States remains higher than other HICs. The United States ranks 21st among the other higher per-capita income countries. In 2020 the overall infant mortality rate in the United States was 5.4 deaths per 1000 live births. Almost 20,000 infants died in the United States in 2020 from causes including preterm birth and low birth weight, birth defects, maternal pregnancy and neonatal complications, and sudden infant death syndrome (SIDS).[17] Inequality in infant mortality rates remains, with Black infants having the highest mortality rate at 10.38 per 100,000, followed by Native American and Alaskan Native infants at 7.68 per 100,000. Hispanic infant mortality rates improved slightly in 2020 at 4.69 per 100,000 and non-Hispanic White infants at 4.40 per 100,000.[18]

Childhood Obesity

One of the most concerning pediatric health indicators is the percentage of overweight and obese children in the United States. In 2020 the prevalence of pediatric obesity was 19.7%, with about 14.7 million children and adolescents.[19] Children gained weight at a faster rate during the pandemic compared to prepandemic, with younger school-aged children (6–11 years) experiencing a body mass index change rate that was 2.5 times higher than before the pandemic.[20] Schools contribute to obesity prevention efforts for school-aged youth by providing regularly scheduled opportunities for physical activity and offering nutritious foods through school meal programs. This approach does not single out students according to their weight status or body size but aims to support the health and wellbeing of all students. With the prevalence of pediatric obesity, there is a significant increase in the prevalence of type 2 diabetes, metabolic syndrome, and hypertension. Of all the pediatric health indicators, overweight and obesity significantly directly affect public health costs and the cost of providing healthcare services nationally.

Food and Housing Insecurity

Despite many government food assistance programs in the United States, 10.2% (13.5 million) of US households were food insecure at some time during 2021.[21] Children who are food insecure are more likely to have poor general health, higher hospitalization rates, experience more behavioral problems, and have increased incidence of overweight, asthma, and anemia. Factors other than income impact whether a household is food insecure. Lower maternal education, single-parent households, intimate partner violence, and parental substance abuse all contribute to food-insecure households. Maternal depression increases the likelihood that young children experience food insecurity by 23% to 79%, depending on enrollment in public programs, which play an important role in buffering the effects of food insecurity nationally.[22]

Three-quarters of children spend some portion of their preschool years being cared for outside of the home. Depending on childcare arrangements, the care contributes to or ameliorates the effects of food insecurity for children. Those who attend a preschool or childcare center have lower food insecurity, whereas children cared for at home by an unrelated adult are at higher risk for food insecurity. The Supplemental Nutritional Assistance Program (SNAP), the Special Supplemental Nutrition Program for Women, Infants, and Children (WIC), and the School Breakfast Program (SBP) are federally funded programs established to address childhood hunger. WIC provides an average of $56.90 per participant per month for purchasing healthy food.[23] Recent WIC data indicate the proportion of infant formula distributed to enrollees declined during the pandemic, which may reflect the trends of increased rates of breastfeeding in the United States.

Children living in poverty are significantly affected by access to affordable housing, particularly immigrant children and families living in large metropolitan areas. The affordable housing crisis is one of the primary reasons so many families are homeless. Children made up 107,069—nearly one in five—of the nearly 568,000 people who were homeless on a single night in January 2019.[24] Although many children who are homeless are reportedly in shelter programs, experiencing this lack of family financial stability, the limited housing supply in inner cities, and the high eviction rates during the pandemic negatively combined to impact the education and physical and mental health of the children in these families.

Healthy People 2030

Healthy People (HP) 2030 is the fifth national initiative focused on improving healthcare services and health outcomes for children, adolescents, and families. The initiative monitors the national data trends on 23 specific leading health indicators (LHIs) on child and adolescent health status and includes foci specific to the social determinants of health and health-related quality of life objectives. The HP 2020 initiative met five of the target objectives in the LHIs[25]:

- 36% of children aged 9 to 35 months were screened for autism spectrum disorder and other developmental delays in the past 12 months.
- 46% of children and adolescents accessed oral health care.
- 95% of children entering kindergarten had received two doses of MMR vaccine.
- Reduced the proportion of children who get no recommended vaccines by 2 years of age to less than 2%.
- Reduced the number of children who experience child abuse and neglect (8.4 per 1000 children).

Reporting on HP 2020 initiative found that progress declined in seven of the target areas, including[24]:

- The percentage of fourth-grade students attending public and private schools with reading skills at or above their grade level fell to 35%.
- The proportion of children 6 to 13 years of age who have sufficient aerobic physical activity declined to 25.6%.
- The proportion of students participating in the School Breakfast Program declined to 21%.
- The rate of deaths in children and adolescents aged 1 to 19 years of age increased to 27.6 deaths per 1000.
- The percentage of children and adolescents under 18 years of age with special healthcare needs who received care in family-centered, comprehensive health care declined to 14%.

To meet the target objectives for HP 2030, strong advocacy is needed by PCPs and policymakers to move the national focus to improve healthcare and educational systems that better address the needs of children and adolescents to improve overall pediatric healthcare status.

Advocacy for Improved Child Health Status

Pediatric PCPs have a key role in advocating for child health locally, nationally, and globally. They provide continuity of care in the ambulatory care setting for underserved children with health conditions such as asthma, pneumonia, and vaccine-preventable conditions that might otherwise lead to greater use of costly emergency departments and hospitalizations. Increasing access to pediatric PCPs who deliver comprehensive primary care services reduces healthcare costs, improves health outcomes, and produces healthcare savings—all steps that would allow the United States to lead rather than trail the other economically developed countries in child health indicators. In addition, pediatric PCPs can advocate for children and influence economic and political decisions to ameliorate health disparities and increase health equality among populations and communities to build a healthier generation of adults. A sustained effort is required globally and nationally to build better health systems to continue to positively impact child health outcomes. The framework of the UN Millennium Development Goals and Healthy People 2030 goals sets the mark for improving child health status globally and nationally.

References

1. World Health Organization (WHO) and United Nations Children's Fund (UNICEF). *Protect the Promise: 2022 Progress Report on the Every Woman Every Child Global Strategy for Women's, Children's, and Adolescents' Health (2016–2030)*; 2022. https://data.unicef.org/resources/protect-the-progress-every-woman-every-child-report-2022/#.
2. United Nations (UN). *The Sustainable Development Goals Report*; 2022. https://unstats.un.org/sdgs/report/2022/The-Sustainable-Development-Goals-Report-2022.pdf.
3. Shonkoff J, Garner A, et al. The lifelong effects of early childhood adversity and toxic stress. *Pediatrics*. 2012;129(1):e232–e246.
4. United Nations Inter-Agency Group on Child Mortality Estimation (UNIGME). *Levels & Trends in Child Mortality: Report*; 2021. https://www.who.int/publications/m/item/levels-and-trends-in-child-mortality-report-2021.
5. United Nations Development Programme. UN General Assembly Resolution July 28th 2022. https://news.un.org/en/story/2022/07/1123482
6. World Health Organization (WHO). *Child Mortality (under 5 years)*; 2020. https://www.who.int/news-room/fact-sheets/detail/levels-and-trends-in-child-under-5-mortality-in-2020.
7. Arpin E, Gauffin K, Kerr M, et al. Climate change and child health inequality: a review of reviews. *Int J Environ Res Publ Health*. 2021;18(20):10896.
8. Clemens V, von Hirschhausen E, Fegert J. Report of the intergovernmental panel on climate change: implications for the mental health policy of children and adolescents in Europe—a scoping review. *Eur Child Adolesc Psychiatr*. 2022;31:701–713.
9. Masson-Delmotte V, Zhai P, Pirani A, et al. *Climate Change 2021: The Physical Science Basis*; 2021.
10. A.E. Casey Foundation. An annual report on how children are faring in the United States. The 2022 KIDS COUNT Data Book: State Trends in Child Well-Being. https://assets.aecf.org/m/resourcedoc/aecf-2022kidscountdatabook-2022.pdf.
11. Barnum M, Belsha K, Wilburn T. *Graduation Rates Dip across U.S. As Pandemic Stalls Progress*; 2022. https://www.chalkbeat.org/2022/1/24/22895461/2021-graduation-rates-decrease-pandemic.
12. American Academy of Pediatrics (AAP). *American Academy of Child and Adolescent Psychiatry (AACAP) AAoCaAP, Children's Hospital Network (CHN). A Declaration from the American Academy of*

Pediatrics. American Academy of Child and Adolescent Psychiatry and Children's Hospital Association; 2021. https://www.aap.org/en/advocacy/child-and-adolescent-healthy-mental-development/aap-aacap-cha-declaration-of-a-national-emergency-in-child-and-adolescent-mental-health/.

13. Substance Abuse and Mental Health Services Administration. *Key Substance Use and Mental Health Indicators in the United States: Results from the 2019 National Survey on Drug Use and Health*; 2020. https://store.samhsa.gov/sites/default/files/SAMHSA_Digital_Download/PEP20-07-01-001-PDF.pdf.

14. Leeb R, Bitsko R, Radhakrishnan L, et al. Mental health-related emergency department visits among children aged <18 years during the COVID-19 pandemic—United States, January 1–October 17. *Morb Mortal Wkly Rep*. 2020;69:1675–1680.

15. Centers for Disease Prevention and Control. Youth risk behavior survey data: Summary and trend Reports 2009-2019. https://www.cdc.gov/healthyyouth/data/yrbs/.

16. Hillis S, Blenkinsop A, Villaveces A, et al. COVID-19–Associated orphanhood and caregiver death in the United States. *Pediatrics*. 2021;148(6):31–43.

17. Center for Disease Prevention and Control. Infant Mortality. https://www.cdc.gov/reproductivehealth/maternalinfanthealth/infantmortality.htm.

18. Ely D, Driscoll A. Infant mortality in the United States, 2020: data from the period linked birth/infant death file. *Natl Vital Stat Rep*. 2022;71(5):1–18.

19. Center for Disease Prevention and Control. Prevalence of Childhood Obesity in the United States. https://www.cdc.gov/obesity/data/childhood.html.

20. Center for Disease Prevention and Control. Obesity. https://www.cdc.gov/healthyschools/obesity/.

21. US Department of Agriculture. Food Insecurity in the U.S. https://www.ers.usda.gov/topics/food-nutrition-assistance/food-security-in-the-u-s/key-statistics-graphics/.

22. Noonan K, Corman H, Reichman N. Effects of maternal depression on family food insecurity. *Econom Hum Biol*. 2016;22:201–215.

23. Center on Budget and Policy Priorities. *Policy Basics: Special Supplemental Nutrition Program for Women, Infants, and Children*; 2022. https://www.cbpp.org/research/food-assistance/special-supplemental-nutrition-program-for-women-infants-and-children.

24. Children's Defense Fund. *The State of America's Children*; 2021. https://www.childrensdefense.org/wp-content/uploads/2021/04/The-State-of-Americas-Children-2021.pdf.

25. US Department of Health and Human Services. Healthy People 2030. Children. https://health.gov/healthypeople/objectives-and-data/browse-objectives/children.

3

Environmental Influences on Pediatric Health

MARTHA G. FULLER AND KAREN G. DUDERSTADT

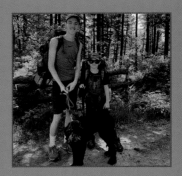

The environment is a basic determinant of human health and illness. The World Health Organization (WHO)[1] credits environmental concerns—including climate change, indoor and outdoor air pollution, second-hand smoke, unsafe water, lack of sanitation, and inadequate hygiene—to be responsible for 22% of the global burden of disease. Children are particularly vulnerable to environmental risks due to their rapid growth and development in early childhood. Worldwide, one in four deaths of children younger than 5 years old can be attributed to unhealthy environments.[2] Children living in poverty are disproportionately affected by pollution.[3]

Climate change is also associated with increased levels of pollen. Asthma is now the most common chronic disease in pediatrics in the United States and is increasing in prevalence.[4] This, combined with increased carbon dioxide and other air pollutants, will lead to increased frequency and severity of pediatric asthma attacks.[5]

Principles for Understanding Children's Environmental Health

Children go through critical developmental periods or *windows of vulnerability* both prenatally and during early childhood due to rapid brain development in the first 2 years of life. There are sensitive periods throughout childhood when rapid growth occurs and during which exposure to toxic or other harmful substances affects growth or damages organs or body systems.[6] Table 3.1 presents environmental risk factors for children at different stages of development.

The lungs, skin, and gastrointestinal (GI) tract of newborns are highly permeable. At the same time, the newborn's immature organ systems metabolize more slowly and make it difficult for infants to detoxify and excrete harmful substances. Children's rapidly developing tissues readily absorb environmental toxins, and they have a higher metabolic rates, breathing more pollutants than adults, increasing exposure to pesticides and other chemicals.[7,8] Children also consume more fresh fruit, water, milk, and juice per pound of body weight than adults. Infants and toddlers crawl on floors and engage in oral behaviors that can result in more absorption of toxicants, including lead. Children engage in more outdoor activities than adults and are physically closer to harmful substances such as fertilizers and chemicals applied to yards and fields. Playing outside and having contact with pets and domestic animals increase exposures to pesticides and are associated with both short- and long-term health risks, including neurodevelopmental problems.[9]

Children in low-income communities face higher exposures to environmental toxins, including lead, and in many communities have limited access to protective factors such as quality healthcare services.[10] Exposure to endocrine-disrupting chemicals in childhood is associated with changes in the onset of puberty.[11] Adolescents face increased risks to toxicants and pollutants due to short-term direct exposure through employment or recreation and long-term exposures.[7]

Principles of Toxicology

Toxicology is the science dealing with detection, interpretation, and treatment of toxins or poisons. Toxicologic principles assess the exposure, absorption, distribution, metabolism, tissue sensitivity, and therapeutic or toxic effects related to the exposure to environmental toxins. Toxic substances are those chemicals in the environment capable of causing harm. *Toxicants* are environmental hazards from chemical pollutants, and *toxins* are environmental hazards from biologic sources. Toxicants that cross the placenta (e.g., drugs, carbon monoxide [CO], mercury, lead, and cotinine [from environmental tobacco smoke]) can contribute to low birth weight, spontaneous abortion, and birth defects. Exposure to higher temperatures in utero is associated with preterm birth and intrauterine growth restriction (IUGR), and Black and Latinx mothers are disproportionately impacted by exposure to heat and pollution.[7] Exposure to pollutants in air, water, and soil cause a high burden of disease in pediatrics, including childhood cancers, autism, intellectual and learning disabilities, and attention-deficit disorder.[3]

Exposure

The extent to which exposure creates a health problem depends on factors such as frequency and duration of exposure, concentration of the agent at the point of contact, and the susceptibility of the organism (e.g., an infant's skin burns much more easily than an adult's). Contact of a biologic, chemical, or physical agent with the skin, lungs, or GI tract constitutes an exposure.

Absorption

Absorption is the process by which an agent is taken into the organism. It occurs through the skin, mucous membranes, lungs,

TABLE 3.1	Pediatric Environmental Risk Factors and Role of Primary Care Providers			
Developmental Stage	**Biologic Characteristics**	**Selected Primary Care Provider Responsibilities**		
Preconception	• Maternal and paternal health • Epigenetic changes from exposure to toxins • Compromise of reproductive organs, ova, or sperm, risk of infertility • Adverse adult health	At all ages and stages to improve population health: • Local, state, federal environmental advocacy • Advocacy for environmental equity and justice • Counseling re: hazards of tobacco use and exposure • Handwashing before eating • Dietary counsel: encourage fresh or frozen fruits and vegetables, limit or avoid processed meats, avoid microwaving food or beverages in plastic, limit consumption of seafood high in mercury • Home safety: carbon monoxide monitors, asbestos, radon levels, ventilation, lead • Consider risks of personal care products • Determine chemical exposures in environment/employment/activities • History/assessment of patient specific environmental risks		
Developmental Stage	**Biologic Characteristics**	**Developmental Characteristics**	**Selected Child (Fetal) Exposures**	**Selected Primary Care Provider Responsibilities**
Prenatal	• Dependent on in utero environment • All body systems rapidly developing, exquisitely sensitive to toxin exposures		• Environmental heat or radiation • Transplacental toxin exposures from food, water, drugs, chemical exposures from work or leisure activities • Environmental tobacco smoke (ETS)	As above for all ages and: • Counseling re: hazards of tobacco use and exposure • Limit heat exposure • Attend to outdoor air quality alerts and limit outdoor activity
• Newborn: Birth to 1 mo • Infant: 1–2 mo	• High metabolic rate • Rapid growth of all organs • Skin very permeable • High respiratory rate and immature lungs with developing alveoli • Rapid neurologic development, cell migration, synapse development Immature metabolism of toxins • High fluid intake for body weight	• Dependent, no mobility	• ETS • Indoor air pollution • Contaminated water • Breastmilk if mother exposed to toxins • Contaminated infant formula • Chemicals in clothing and bedding • Chemicals in personal care products • Heat	As above for all ages and: • Dietary counsel for breastfeeding mothers • Appropriate formula preparation: what is water source? Use water from cold water tap, boil only if necessary and if so for only 1 min to prevent over concentration of toxins • Ask re: mold in environment • How is home heated?
• Infant: 2–12 mo • Early childhood: 12–24 mo	• High metabolic rate • Rapid growth of all organs • Skin permeable • High respiratory rate and developing alveoli • Rapid neurologic development, synapse development • Immature metabolism of toxins • High fluid intake for body weight • Diet high in fruits, vegetables, grains	• Exploratory mouthing behavior • Mobility develops and plays on the floor (at a lower level than adults, increasing exposure to some toxins)	• ETS • Indoor and outdoor air pollution • Contaminated food and water • Breastmilk if mother exposed to toxins • Contaminated infant formula • Chemicals in clothing and bedding • Chemicals in personal care products • Heat • Lead	As above for all ages and: • Dietary counseling: arsenic in rice products • Sun protection • Universal blood lead testing as per guidelines • Anticipatory guidance regarding risks with increasing mobility: safety of household chemicals and products

Continued

TABLE 3.1	Pediatric Environmental Risk Factors and Role of Primary Care Providers—Cont'd			
Developmental Stage	Biologic Characteristics	Developmental Characteristics	Selected Child (Fetal) Exposures	Selected Primary Care Provider Responsibilities
Preschool: 3–5 yr	• High metabolic rate • Higher respiratory rate and developing alveoli • Rapid neurologic changes synapse pruning • High fluid intake for body weight • Diet high in fruits, vegetables, grains	• Floor play continues • Increasing outdoor play • Oral behaviors continue • Poor hand hygiene can expose to toxins on hands • Arts and crafts	• ETS • Indoor and outdoor air pollution • Contaminated food and water • Heat • Lead • Chemicals from arts and crafts • Chemicals in the soil	As above for all ages and: • History/assessment of patient-specific environmental risks • Assess for risk of exposure and blood lead testing as per guidelines • Discuss potential exposures from age-appropriate activities, choose nontoxic products as alternatives • Safety of household chemicals and products • Assess childcare or school environmental risks
Middle childhood: 6–11 yr	• Continued lung growth • Continued synapse pruning • Improved liver and kidney function	• Improved motor skills • More outdoor and playground play • Use of personal electronics • Arts and crafts • School activities	• ETS • Indoor and outdoor air pollution • Contaminated food and water • Heat • Lead • Chemicals from arts and crafts • Chemicals in the soil	As above for all ages and: • Assess childcare or school environmental risks • Discuss potential exposures in outdoor environments
Adolescence: 12–21 yr	• Rapid physical growth, maturation and development of gonads	• Striving for independence, more time with peers and at school • May have a job • Risk taking behaviors may occur	• ETS • Substance use and exposures • Indoor and outdoor air pollution • Contaminated food and water • Heat • Chemicals from activities and jobs • Electronic cigarette use • Mental health impacts of climate change	As above for all ages and: • Assess employment or school environmental risks • Tobacco and electronic cigarette counseling • Substance use/exposure counseling • Assess mental health, refer as needed

From Etzel RA. The special vulnerability of children. *Int J Hyg Environ Health*. 2020;227:113516; AAP Committee on Environmental Health. 4th ed. *Pediatric Environmental Health American Academy of Pediatrics*; 2019; Pediatric Environmental Health Toolkit. UC San Francisco Pediatric Environmental Health Specialty Unit. https://peht.ucsf.edu/index.php; and Trasande L, Shaffer RM, Sathyanarayana S. Food additives and child health. *Pediatrics*. 2018;142(2).

or GI tract, and involves active or passive transport. For example, lead is taken up through active transport in the GI tract (at higher rates for children than adults) or through the respiratory system and stored in bone or other tissues.[12]

Distribution

Toxic agents are spread through the body via the blood and lymph systems. The ability of an agent to cross the blood-brain barrier, the amount of blood flow, and the tissue uptake of a particular agent influence the degree to which a toxicant will be distributed throughout the body.

Metabolism

Metabolic enzymes in the body interact with toxic agents through oxidation, reduction, and hydrolysis of the agent or through conjugation and breakdown to promote elimination or excretion. Metabolism is influenced by the individual's age, sex, nutritional status, genetic makeup, presence of other agents or medications, and disease or illness.

Tissue Sensitivity

Susceptibility and reaction of tissue to a particular agent varies with increased tissue susceptibility during critical periods of gestation and early child development.

Toxic Effects

Toxic effects result in a wide range of pathologic conditions. Prenatal exposures to toxins such as endocrine disrupters can result in abnormalities in timing of puberty, infertility, miscarriage, stillbirth, congenital malformations, fetal growth restriction, prematurity, and chronic illnesses.[11,13] Prenatal exposure to air pollution impacts the methylation and telomere length of the infant's DNA.[14] Currently, most chemicals used commercially have had minimal to no testing for pediatric toxicity.[3]

Epidemiologic Model of Environmental Health Hazards: Assessment of Risk

Using principles of epidemiologic relationships and toxicology, providers can better understand and explain to their patients and families the intersection between the environment and health.

The first step using an epidemiologic approach identifies the interactive factors in the environment, including *receptors* (hosts that are susceptible or exposed to environmental agents); *toxins* or the agents (harmful substances that might cause damage); and the environmental *medium* or route (air, soil, water, or food) by which exposure could occur.

The second step of risk assessment uses a standardized approach to determine if harm could occur.[6] A number of questions are asked when making this determination:

- *Hazard:* source of risk; any substance or action that can cause harm to health under certain conditions. How susceptible is the receptor to the agent (e.g., age, sex, genetics, diet, and general health)?
- *Dose-response relationship:* increasing levels of exposure (either amount, intensity, or length of exposure time) are associated with either an increasing or a decreasing risk. At what exposure level (i.e., dose) will the hazard present a problem or cause a response in this receptor?
- *Risk:* likelihood (probability) and magnitude (severity) of an adverse event. What is the concentration of the hazard? How much is there? How potent is it? What is the extent of contact of the exposure with the receptor?
- *Risk characterization:* Compare facts about the hazard and population exposure to determine the risk for an adverse health outcome in those most at risk. How long will it stay around? With the amount of exposure present, is an individual or population at risk for health problems?

In addition to considering hazards, it is important to identify protective factors such as diet, support from caregivers, and an environment that supports development.[7]

Assessing Risk for Environment-Related Illness

Environmental Health History

Assessment of environmental health hazards should be integrated into primary care visits and illness visits. The WHO recommends documentation in the electronic health record (EHR) of specific exposures and known risks the child or adolescent faces.[15] Fig. 3.1 presents an environmental health history guide for use in primary care, and Fig. 3.2 an environmental health history form for pediatric asthma patients. The environmental health history forms are available at https://www.neefusa.org/resource/pediatric-environmental-history. When obtaining a health history, be alert for subtle, nonspecific complaints such as fatigue and headaches and ask if others in the home or school have similar symptoms.

Physical Examination and Clinical Findings

The physical examination should be detailed and cover all body systems. If there is a known exposure, evaluate agent-specific findings such as skin findings or abnormal developmental or neurologic findings. The provider should maintain a high index of suspicion to avoid missing physical or neurologic manifestations of toxicant exposure. The effects of toxicants on the body are often indistinct or subclinical. Effects can occur immediately or a long time after exposure.

Diagnostic Studies

Laboratory studies should be considered for suspicion of exposure to toxicants, overt signs of exposure, and/or physical findings, and the availability of local or state laboratories testing for toxicants. Box 3.1 presents laboratory tests available for screening for environmental toxins.

Before ordering tests, the primary care provider (PCP) should understand that very few pediatric exposures can be accurately identified, much less quantified and definitively linked to symptoms. Many agents have no defined reference or toxic ranges. Laboratories may report urine test results using a creatinine-corrected process to assess dilution, which may be inaccurate for pediatrics.[16] Offending agents are metabolized and stored in the body in different ways, affecting the validity of serum testing. Many factors affect the outcome of exposure: dose, child's age, nutritional status, psychosocial and socioeconomic status, and developmental delay or genetic predisposition. Different children may respond differently to the same exposure, complicating assessment of exposures and their effects in children. Regional Pediatric Environmental Health Specialty Units (PEHSUs; www.pehsu.net) are a valuable resource and can recommend appropriate testing.

If the PCP has suspicion for an uncommon exposure, the regional PEHSU will provide expert advice on whether and how to test. Before ordering any tests, key questions for the PCP to consider include[16]:

- Could the health problem be related to an environmental exposure? What are the possible exposures in the child's environment?
- Did the potential exposure clearly occur before the onset of the health problem?
- Are laboratory tests available to document the exposure? Will the laboratory measurements accurately reflect toxicity if present? What is required to perform the testing? What is the cost of testing? What is the timeline from testing to receive results?
- Will the results change the treatment plan for the child and family? Will it inform care?

The diagnostic testing of hair, nails, or teeth is not recommended for clinical use. Toxins and toxicants are ubiquitous in our environment (e.g., air pollution, personal care products, processed foods), and hair is often contaminated with a multitude of chemicals, so hair levels may not accurately reflect serum levels of a toxicant or substance. Capillary finger sticks are not recommended due to the variety of chemicals used daily.

Pediatric environmental history (0–18 years of age)

The screening environmental history

For all of the questions below, most are often asked about the child's primary residence. Although some questions may specify certain locations, one should always consider all places where the child spends time, such as daycare centers, schools, and relative's houses.

Where does your child live and spend most of his/her time?	_____
What are the age, condition, and location of your home?	_____
Does anyone in the family smoke?	❑ Yes ❑ No ❑ Not sure
Do you have a carbon monoxide detector?	❑ Yes ❑ No ❑ Not sure
Do you have any indoor furry pets?	❑ Yes ❑ No ❑ Not sure

What type of heating/air system does your home have?
❑ Radiator   ❑ Forced air   ❑ Gas stove   ❑ Wood stove   ❑ Other_____

What is the source of your drinking water?
❑ Well water   ❑ City water   ❑ Bottled water

Is your child protected from excessive sun exposure?	❑ Yes ❑ No ❑ Not sure
Is your child exposed to any toxic chemicals of which you are aware?	❑ Yes ❑ No ❑ Not sure
What are the occupations of all adults in the household?	_____
Have you tested your home for radon?	❑ Yes ❑ No ❑ Not sure
Does your child watch TV, or use a computer or video game system more than two hours a day?	❑ Yes ❑ No ❑ Not sure
How many times a week does your child have unstructured, free play outside for at least 60 minutes?	_____
Do you have any other questions or concerns about your child's home environment or symptoms that may be a result of his or her environment?	_____

Follow-up/Notes

_____

_____

_____

The screening environmental history is taken in part from the following sources:

- American academy of pediatrics committee on environmental health. Pediatric environmental Health, 2nd ed. Etzel RA, Balk SJ, Eds. American Academy of Pediatrics; 2003. Chapter 4: How to take an environmental history.
- Balk SJ. The environmental history: asking the right questions. *Contemp Pediatr.* 1996;13:19–36.
- Frank A, Balk S, Carter W, et al. Case Studies in Environmental Medicine: Taking an Exposure History. Agency for Toxic Substances and Disease Registry; 2000.

This screening environmental history is designed to capture most of the common environmental exposures to children. The screening history can be administered regularly during well-child exams as well as to assess whether an environmental exposure plays a role in a child's symptoms. If a positive response is given to one or more of the screening questions, the primary care provider can consider asking questions on the topic provided in the additional categories and questions to supplement the screening environmental history, accessible at www.neefusa.org/pdf/PEHIhistory.pdf.

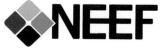

Additional resources and Spanish language materials avilable at www.neefusa.org/health
health@neefusa.org

• **Fig 3.1** Pediatric Environmental History (0–18 Years of Age). (From the National Environmental Education Foundation, Washington, DC. https://www.neefusa.org/resource/pediatric-environmental-history.)

Pediatric environmental history (0–18 years of age)

Additional categories and questions to supplement
The screening environmental history

For all of the questions below, most are often asked about the child's primary residence.
Although some questions may specify certain locations, one should always consider all places
where the child spends time, such as daycare centers, schools, and relative's houses.

General housing characteristics (For lead poisoning, refer to Table 3.2 in CDC managing elevated blood lead levels among young children 1.usa.gov/KAL9Yc)

Do you own or rent your home?	_____
What year was your home built? (Or: Was your home built before 1978? 1950?)	_____
Has your child been tested for lead?	❏ Yes ❏ No ❏ Not sure
Is there a family member or playmate with an elevated blood lead level?	❏ Yes ❏ No ❏ Not sure
Does your child spend significant time at another location? (e.g. baby sitters, school, daycare?)	_____

Indoor home environment (For asthma, refer to environmental history form for pediatric asthma patient goo.gl/4JdUIs)

If a family member smokes, does this person want to quit smoking?	❏ Yes ❏ No ❏ Not sure
Is your child exposed to smoke at the baby sitters, school, or daycare center?	❏ Yes ❏ No ❏ Not sure
Do regular visitors to your home smoke?	❏ Yes ❏ No ❏ Not sure
Have there been renovations or new carpet or furniture in the home during the past year?	❏ Yes ❏ No ❏ Not sure
Does your home have carpet?	❏ Yes ❏ No ❏ Not sure
Is the room where your child sleeps carpeted?	❏ Yes ❏ No ❏ Not sure
Do you use a wood stove or fire place?	❏ Yes ❏ No ❏ Not sure
Have you had water damage, leaks, or a flood in your home?	❏ Yes ❏ No ❏ Not sure
Do you see cockroaches in your home daily or weekly?	❏ Yes ❏ No ❏ Not sure
Do you see rats and/or mice in your home weekly?	❏ Yes ❏ No ❏ Not sure
Do you have smoke detectors in your home?	❏ Yes ❏ No ❏ Not sure

Air pollution/Outdoor environment (For asthma, refer to environmental history form for pediatric asthma patient goo.g1/4JdUIs)

Is your home near an industrial site, hazardous waste site, or landfill?	❏ Yes ❏ No ❏ Not sure
Is your home near major highways or other high traffic roads?	❏ Yes ❏ No ❏ Not sure
Are you aware of air quality alerts in your community?	❏ Yes ❏ No ❏ Not sure
Do you change your child's activity when an air quality alert is issued?	❏ Yes ❏ No ❏ Not sure
Do you live on or near a farm where pesticides are used frequently?	❏ Yes ❏ No ❏ Not sure

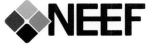

• **Fig 3.1, cont'd**

Food and water contamination

If you use well water for drinking, when was the last time the water was tested?
Coliform bacteria_____Other microbials_____ Nitrites/nitrates_____ Arsenic_____ Pesticides_____

For all types of water sources:

Have you tested your water for lead?	❑ Yes ❑ No ❑ Not sure
Do you mix infant formula with tap water?	❑ Yes ❑ No ❑ Not sure

Which types of seafood do you normally eat? _____

How many times per month do you eat that particular fish or shellfish?

How many times a week do you eat any of the following types of fish?
Shark_____ Swordfish_____ Tile fish_____ King mackerel_____Albacore tuna_____Other_____

How often do you wash fruits and vegetables before giving them to your child? _____

What type of produce do you buy? ❑ Organic❑ Local❑ Grocery store❑ Other

Toxic chemical exposures (also refer to taking an environmental history and environmental and occupational history in recognition and management of pesticide poisonings)

Consider this set of questions for patients with seizures, frequent headaches, or other unusual or chronic symptoms

How often are pesticides applied inside your home?	_____
How often are pesticides applied outside your home?	_____
Where do you store chemicals/pesticides?	_____
Do you often use solvents or other cleaning or disinfectant chemicals?	_____
Do you have a deck or play structure made from pressure treated wood?	❑ Yes ❑ No ❑ Not sure
Have you applied a sealant to the wood in the past year?	❑ Yes ❑ No ❑ Not sure
What do you use to prevent mosquito bites to your children?	_____
How often do you apply that product?	_____

Occupations and hobbies

What type of work does your child/teenager do?	_____
Do any adults work around toxic chemicals?	❑ Yes ❑ No ❑ Not sure
If so, do they shower and change clothes before returning home from work?	❑ Yes ❑ No ❑ Not sure
Does the child or any family member have arts, crafts, ceramics, stained glass work or similar hobbies?	❑ Yes ❑ No ❑ Not sure

Health related questions

Have you ever relocated due to concerns about an environmental exposure?	❑ Yes ❑ No ❑ Not sure
Do symptoms seem to occur at the same time of day?	❑ Yes ❑ No ❑ Not sure
Do symptoms seem to occur after being at the same place every day?	❑ Yes ❑ No ❑ Not sure
Do symptoms seem to occur during a certain season?	❑ Yes ❑ No ❑ Not sure
Are family members/neighbors/co-workers experiencing similar symptoms?	❑ Yes ❑ No ❑ Not sure
Are there environmental concerns in your neighborhood, child's school, or day care?	❑ Yes ❑ No ❑ Not sure

Has any family member had a diagnosis of any of the following?
❑Asthma ❑ Autism ❑ Cancer ❑ Learning disability

Does your child suffer from any of the following recurrent symptoms?
❑Cough ❑Headaches ❑ Fatigue ❑ Unexplained pain_____

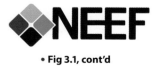

• Fig 3.1, cont'd

PEDIATRIC ASTHMA

Environmental history form for pediatric asthma patient

Specify that questions related to the child's home also apply to other indoor environments where the child spends time, including school, daycare, car, school bus, work, and recreational facilities.

	Follow-up/Notes
Is your child's asthma worse at night?	❏ Yes ❏ No ❏ Not sure
Is your child's asthma worse at specific locations? If so, where? _____	❏ Yes ❏ No ❏ Not sure
Is your child's asthma worse during a particular season? If so, which one? _____	❏ Yes ❏ No ❏ Not sure
Is your child's asthma worse with a particular change in climate? If so, which?_____	❏ Yes ❏ No ❏ Not sure
Can you identify any specific trigger(s) that makes your child's asthma worse? If so, what? _____	❏ Yes ❏ No ❏ Not sure
Have you noticed whether dust exposure makes your child's asthma worse?	❏ Yes ❏ No ❏ Not sure
Does your child sleep with stuffed animals?	❏ Yes ❏ No ❏ Not sure
Is there wall-to-wall carpet in your child's bedroom?	❏ Yes ❏ No ❏ Not sure
Have you used any means for dust mite control? If so, which ones? _____	❏ Yes ❏ No ❏ Not sure
Do you have any furry pets?	❏ Yes ❏ No ❏ Not sure
Do you see evidence of rats or mice in your home weekly?	❏ Yes ❏ No ❏ Not sure
Do you see cockroaches in your home daily?	❏ Yes ❏ No ❏ Not sure
Do any family members, caregivers or friends smoke?	❏ Yes ❏ No ❏ Not sure
Does this person(s) have an interest or desire to quit?	❏ Yes ❏ No ❏ Not sure
Does your child/teenager smoke?	❏ Yes ❏ No ❏ Not sure
Do you see or smell mold/mildew in your home?	❏ Yes ❏ No ❏ Not sure
Is there evidence of water damage in your home?	❏ Yes ❏ No ❏ Not sure
Do you use a humidifier or swamp cooler?	❏ Yes ❏ No ❏ Not sure
Have you had new carpets, paint, floor refinishing, or other changes at your house in the past year?	❏ Yes ❏ No ❏ Not sure
Does your child or another family member have a hobby that uses materials that are toxic or give off fumes?	❏ Yes ❏ No ❏ Not sure
Has outdoor air pollution ever made your child's asthma worse?	❏ Yes ❏ No ❏ Not sure
Does your child limit outdoor activities during a Code Orange or Code Red air quality alert for ozone or particle pollution?	❏ Yes ❏ No ❏ Not sure
Do you use a wood burning fireplace or stove?	❏ Yes ❏ No ❏ Not sure
Do you use unvented appliances such as a gas stove for heating your home?	❏ Yes ❏ No ❏ Not sure
Does your child have contact with other irritants (e.g., perfumes, cleaning agents, or sprays)?	❏ Yes ❏ No ❏ Not sure

What other concerns do you have regarding your child's asthma that have not yet been discussed?

Reference: Environmental Management of Pediatric Asthma: Guidelines for Health Care Providers
www.neefusa.org/resource/environmental-management-pediatric-asthma-guidelines-health-care-providers

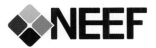

Additional resources and Spanish language materials available at www.neefusa.org/health/asthma
health@neefusa.org

• **Fig 3.2** Environmental History Form for the Pediatric Asthma Patient. (From the National Environmental Education Foundation, Washington, DC. www.neefusa.org/resource/asthma-environmental-history-form.)

- Plasma lead levels
- Gas-liquid chromatography (for polychlorinated biphenyls)
- Atomic absorption spectrometry (for mercury)
- Carboxyhemoglobin (for carbon monoxide poisoning)
- 24-h urine (for heavy metals)
- Plasma cholinesterase levels (for pesticide metabolites, organophosphates)
- Urinary cotinine assays (for tobacco metabolites)

Etzel RA, Balk SJ, editors. *Pediatric Environmental Health*. 4th Edition. American Academy of Pediatrics Council on Environmental Health; 2018.

Federal Regulation of Environmental Health Risks

In 2016 the Frank R. Lautenberg Chemical Safety for the 21st Century Act was passed in Congress, which modernized the Toxic Substances Control Act (TSCA) passed in 1976, the nation's primary chemicals management law. Provisions of the new law include (1) a mandatory requirement for the Environmental Protection Agency (EPA) to evaluate existing chemicals with clear and enforceable deadlines, (2) new risk-based safety standards, (3) increased public transparency for chemical information, and (4) a consistent source of funding for EPA to carry out the responsibilities under the new law. The EPA oversees management of approximately 85,000 chemicals in the United States, with a current pace of 2000 new substances annually. Only a small percentage of these chemicals have been tested for safety and risk in pediatrics due to the TSCA provision that "grandfathered in" many chemicals in existence before 1976. The new law has an improved process for monitoring safety of existing chemicals: prioritization, risk evaluation, and risk management.[17] The law was enacted to minimize those populations and communities most at risk for environmental hazards and to look more comprehensively at risk through enacting risk assessment of chemicals coming to market. The EPA is currently in the process of prioritizing existing chemicals for risk evaluation and implementing a more comprehensive framework of testing and surveillance for newly marketed chemical substances.

Regulation of air pollution has been primarily through the Clean Air Act that was revised and expanded in 1990, providing the EPA broader authority to implement and enforce public protections to reduce outdoor air pollutants.[18] The EPA has been charged with regulating emissions of 180 more pollutants, many of which have adverse impacts on health.

There is currently inadequate knowledge about the effects of human exposure to the numerous toxins and toxicants used in daily life and in the environment for parents and caregivers to make definitive decisions regarding protection of human health.[16] Many leading health organizations in the United States and abroad recommend use of the "precautionary principle" for controlling environmental health risks. This states that scientific uncertainty should not be used as a reason to postpone preventive measures. Invoking this principle allows action to be taken when there is valid concern that an exposure to a substance, product, or a process could be toxic. In effect, this moves the burden of proof of safety to the manufacturer when a valid concern has been raised, instead of recipients needing to prove harm before action can be taken. Many scientists, organizations, and governments favor and have adopted the precautionary principle, and it is enshrined in the laws of the European Union,[19] yet the precautionary principle is not currently applied to environmental policy and has not been adopted by the United States.

Environmental Equity

Low-income and minority populations are at higher risk for exposure to and adverse effects from environmental toxins and toxicants.[16] They are more likely to be exposed to air pollution, pesticides, and lead from a variety of sources. The 2018 crisis in Flint, Michigan, highlights the dangers stemming from unacceptable levels of lead in the water system. A change in the community water supply allowed lead from aging pipes to leach into the city drinking water. Increased lead levels in the children in Flint more than doubled in the 2 years following the change in the water supply, with those residing in the poorest neighborhoods being most affected.[20] Activism by healthcare providers, members of the community, and environmental advocates was required to address this emergency and demonstrate the importance of local advocacy in responding to environmental crises.[21]

The historic practice of redlining (in which banks did not make home loans available in neighborhoods that were predominantly populated by Black people or immigrants) led to limited home ownership and increased poverty in neighborhoods that persist today. There are more oil and gas wells located in these formerly redlined neighborhoods, exposing the residents to hazardous levels of pollution.[22] These communities have higher rates of asthma than nonredlined neighborhoods in the same city.[23]

Entire communities, both urban and rural, can be threatened by environmental hazards ranging from wildfires and floods to exposure to lead and toxins found in aging housing and infrastructure. PCPs can use awareness of current inequities in their communities to advocate for environmental justice. The environmental justice movement aims to rectify inequities. The Office of Environmental Justice (OEJ), is housed within the EPA[24] and provides multiple resources to address issues of environmental inequities.

Climate Change

The WHO calls climate change "the biggest health threat facing humanity."[25] The human population has grown from 2.54 billion in 1950 to 7.9 billion in 2022.[26] This increase in population and industrialization has been accompanied by marked increase in use and production of fossil fuels, leading to greenhouse gases blocking heat from escaping the atmosphere. Carbon dioxide emissions have increased dramatically from the production of and burning of fossil fuels.[27] This has led to an increase in air pollution and has resulted in climate change, with the average surface temperature of the earth increasing 1.1°C (2°F) since the preindustrial era.[28] Other gases including methane (from animal/agricultural sources), nitrous oxide, and chlorofluorocarbons also play roles in warming our planet as does widespread removal of trees. Deforestation of tropical forests has led to the release of carbon dioxide due to fewer trees to process and sequester carbon dioxide.[29]

Climate change is associated with increased frequency and severity of natural disasters including wildfires, hurricanes, floods, and droughts, leading to adverse impacts on health.[30] Wildfires lead to increased air pollution and increased asthma attacks and emergency department visits.[31] These natural disasters cause immediate- and long-term morbidity and mortality impacting both physical and mental health; healthcare providers must prepare to respond to reduce adverse health outcomes.[32] The consequences of climate change on pediatric health are exacerbated in poor and disadvantaged communities. Those living in formerly redlined communities have less green space and are more severely affected by heat events.[33]

The pediatric health consequences of climate change include[34-36]:

- Exposure to waterborne illness
- Acute heat-related illnesses
- Adverse learning due to heat
- Negative mental health impacts, including anxiety and depression
- Increased asthma and allergy exacerbations due to increases in particulate matter, pollen, and mold
- Increased risk for vector borne illnesses including those previously seen only in tropical climates, such as malaria and dengue

Ambient Air Pollution

Outdoor Air. Despite the achievements of the Clean Air Act, the American Lung Association (ALA) notes that over 40% of the US population lives in areas that exceed safe levels of ozone or particulate pollution, mostly due to burning of fossil fuels.[37] Ozone exposure has been found to lead to decreased lung function in children.[38] Exposure to both ozone or particulate matter is associated with preterm birth and low birth weight.[39] In addition to ozone and particulate matter, fossil fuels emit multiple chemicals including silver dioxide, mercury, and nitrogen dioxide, all of which have adverse impacts on health.[40] Particle pollution is defined by size, coarse PM10 (2.5–10 μm in diameter) such as dust and pollen, and fine PM2.5 (less than 2.5 μm in diameter) such as combustion particles and organic compounds. Worldwide, there are approximately 4.2 million premature deaths per year due to air pollution, primarily exposure to PM2.5 pollution.[41]

Updated outdoor air quality information and recommendations for participation in outdoor activities for anywhere in the United States is available at https://airnow.gov/. When air quality is poor, outdoor activity participation particularly for children may need to be avoided.

Indoor Air. Indoor air pollution is associated with 4 million deaths each year worldwide. The EPA does not have regulatory power over indoor air quality. Indoor air is often polluted by the same pollutants as outdoor air, but there are additional activities and sources that create hazardous air indoors.[42] These include exposure to volatile organic compounds (VOCs), sulfur dioxide, carbon dioxide, and particulate matter from cooking or heating. The most significant source of indoor particulate matter is tobacco smoking. Electronic cigarettes release fine and ultrafine particulate matter.[43] Exposure to household marijuana smoke has been associated with increased respiratory infections.[44] Animals, including pets and pests such as mice, produce allergens that contribute to particulate matter and worsen atopic illnesses.[42] Radon, a ubiquitous gas, is associated with development of lung cancer later in life, and there is some concern that high levels of exposure may be associated with development of leukemia in childhood.[45] See Table 3.2 for more information on the health effects and prevention strategies for selected air pollutants.

Effects of exposure to indoor and outdoor toxicants can be acute, subacute, or chronic. The likelihood of acute effects from air pollutants depends on the amount of the exposure, and individual susceptibility factors including age, preexisting medical conditions, genetics, and nutritional status. During temperature inversions, there are high concentrations of pollutants at ground level leading to an increase in acute respiratory illnesses.[46] In addition to worsening preexisting conditions such as asthma, some pollutant exposures mimic respiratory infections and illnesses causing wheezing, pneumonitis, rhinitis, sinusitis, and recurrent hoarseness.[16] It is important for the PCP to take a careful exposure history noting when and where symptoms occur and advise families on monitoring air quality in their communities at https://www2.purpleair.com/ or other sources available to the public.

Tobacco Smoke. Tobacco smoke is an indoor air pollutant and is harmful to pediatric health. Over 40% of young children in the United States are exposed to secondhand smoke. Of further concern is the early initiation of e-cigarette use in middle childhood. Recent studies have shown that over 28% of e-cigarette use is initiated at 14 years of age or younger, and 90% of adult smokers begin smoking by 18 years of age.[17] It is imperative that PCPs discuss with their patients, parents, and caregivers the risks of secondhand smoke in the home and the risks of early initiation of smoking and vaping in adolescence.

Endocrine Disruptors

Endocrine-disrupting chemicals (EDCs) are varied types of chemicals that mimic or disrupt naturally occurring hormones in the body, such as estrogens, androgens, and thyroid hormones. EDCs alter the function of endogenous hormones through a variety of mechanisms: binding to hormone receptors to mimic natural hormones (potentially producing overstimulation), blocking/antagonizing hormone receptors, or altering the production or metabolism of endogenous hormones. These chemicals are ubiquitous and present in multiple sources including food packaging, clothing, pesticides, foods, toys, and materials used in electronics and buildings. Ingestion is the primary means of exposure, although inhalation and exposure through the skin also occur.[16] They have a high degree of stability and do not degrade rapidly once discarded, continuing to pollute the environment. As fat-soluble substances, they accumulate in the body and have a very long half-life.[47] Developing tissues are more vulnerable to endocrine disruption than are mature tissues. Transplacental transfer to the developing fetus is of great concern, and exposure to phthalates is associated with higher risk for preterm birth.[48] Humans are exposed to multiple different endocrine disrupters. Children born to women who were exposed to a mixture of EDCs are more likely to have language delays.[49]

EDCs interfere with gene expression, changing developing tissues in permanent ways that can be passed to offspring.[50] The incidence of endocrine disruption is difficult, if not impossible, to quantify. Endocrine disruption generally does not result in acute illness for which the patient or caregiver would seek care, but rather is insidious with a long latent period. Many effects will manifest years after exposure, often in adulthood. One example is that of diethylstilbestrol, a potent endocrine disrupter that was prescribed to millions of pregnant women to prevent miscarriage. Their daughters had an unusually high incidence of malignancy (clear cell adenocarcinoma of the vagina and/or cervix) in adolescence and adulthood. Exposures to EDCs has also been associated with changes in pubertal timing, obesity, and neurodevelopmental disabilities.[47] Building on animal research and epidemiologic studies, researchers are seeking to refine our understanding of the impact of EDCs and developing assays to test for exposures. Extremely low doses and extremely high doses may have adverse effects; the toxicologic concepts of "dose response" may not apply

TABLE 3.2 **Air Pollutants and Health Effects**

Substance	Source	Health Effects/ Systems Affected	Signs and Symptoms	Prevention Strategies
Environmental tobacco smoke	• First-, second-, or thirdhand smoke from multiple sources: cigarettes, hookahs, e-cigarettes, etc.	• Respiratory • Cardiac • Growth • Neurologic	• Bronchitis • Bronchiolitis • Pneumonia • Asthma • Otitis media • Premature coronary artery disease • Low birth weight • Sudden infant death syndrome • Cognitive delays	• Educate on smoking cessation and limiting smoking to outdoor areas • Enroll child in smoke-free childcare center • Anticipatory guidance in middle childhood and adolescent on risks of vaping/nicotine use
Radon	• Air • Water • Generally concentrated in basements and underground	• Respiratory • Hematologic	• Lung cancer • Emerging evidence of leukemias	• Test air in basements and first floor of home for radon levels • Avoid having children play in basements of homes with radon exposure • Advise parent on mitigation of radon exposure in home
Particulate matter	Outdoor: • Industrial pollution • Agricultural pollution • Gasoline and diesel exhaust • Pollens • Natural phenomena (e.g., forest fires, volcanic activity) Indoor: • Wood stoves • Dust mites • Animal dander • Cockroach particles • Gas stove and furnace use	• Respiratory • Cardiovascular	• Bronchitis • Pneumonia • Wheezing • Chronic cough • Decreased lung function • Asthma • Lung cancer • Cardiovascular conditions	• When outdoor air pollution is high, keep children indoors • Use high-efficiency particulate air filters for heating/air conditioning, vacuuming • Evaluate heating system for filtration of outdoor air • Cover mattresses, wash bedding frequently, launder or discard stuffed animals • Assess exposures in school and childcare settings
Molds	• Damp areas (leaking roofs/walls/floors, wet basements, backed-up sewers) • Humidifiers • Steam from shower, bath, or cooking • Wet clothes • House plants • Dry leaves	• Respiratory • Dermatologic • Central nervous system	• Cough • Wheezing, dyspnea • Sinus congestion • Watery, itchy, light-sensitive eyes • Sore throat • Skin rash • Headaches, memory loss, mood changes • Myalgias, pain • Fever	• Maintain dry, clean environment • Affected areas can be cleaned with hot water and detergent; may require deep scrubbing • Bleach solutions are not routinely recommended; diluted bleach solution is recommended for immunocompromised children or adolescents • Discard moldy materials to prevent airborne mold spores • Use dehumidifiers and air conditioners as necessary • Fix leaks promptly • Use exhaust fans in kitchens and bathrooms • Ensure carpets do not stay damp
Asbestos	• Construction materials: • Insulation • Ceiling and floor tiles • Shingles	• Respiratory	• Lung irritation • Lung disease later in life with repeated exposure	• If buildings that contain asbestos are in good repair, leave asbestos in place • Contact a certified asbestos professional to evaluate home or building • Use asbestos abatement measures as appropriate when renovating

Modified from Etzel RA, Balk SJ, editors. *Pediatric Environmental Health*. 4th Edition. American Academy of Pediatrics Council on Environmental Health; 2018; and Raju S, Siddharthan T, McCormack MC. Indoor air pollution and respiratory health. *Clin Chest Med*. 2020;41(4):825–843.

to exposure to endocrine disruptors. Table 3.3 presents specific chemicals or groups of chemicals, common sources of exposure, and health effects of EDCs in pediatrics.

Primary Care Educational Strategies for Outdoor and Indoor Air Pollution

There are strategies that can be used to prevent or reduce individual exposure to air pollution. Staying indoors when outdoor air pollution levels are high and limiting outdoor activity (to reduce respiratory volumes), using portable or central air cleaning systems, avoiding areas with high levels of pollution (e.g., traffic), and using a well-fitting N-95 or equivalent respirator mask when air quality is poor[51] may be helpful. Efforts to mitigate climate change will also reduce air pollution by decreasing emissions from fossil fuels. Source control is key to address indoor air pollution, remove toxins from the home, improve ventilation, and mitigate by use of air filtration systems to improve air quality. CO detectors should be in every home and building. Homes or buildings with poorly vented heating appliances are most at risk for elevated CO levels. Children and adolescents are exposed to indoor air pollution

in schools and on school buses. In the United States, regulations regarding in-school exposure to radon vary by state.[52] The PCP should identify local risks associated with school attendance as part of the environmental risk assessment. PCPs need to advocate and work to reduce or mitigate the impacts of climate change in their communities to reduce the impact on children and families.[53] It is important to assess environmental risks when obtaining a health history, discuss climate change, and assist families in preparing for extreme weather events in their community.[7,54]

As PCPs, it is our aim to care for the health of children. Although our focus is often on individual treatment strategies and relief of symptoms, our patients and families are embedded in the larger community context and impacted by multiple environmental issues. Assessing for exposures in the context of excellent clinical care and advocating for a healthy environment for children are well within the providers scope of practice. Significant environmental threats, including climate change, air pollution, and exposure to endocrine disruptors, will require national and global governmental policy shifts to prevent and address urgent health issues.

TABLE 3.3 Selected Endocrine Disruptors Including Pesticides

Chemical Group	Selected Sources	Known Toxic Effects[a]	Alternatives
BPA	• Hard, polycarbonate plastics (e.g., some water bottles) • Aluminum can linings • Thermal/carbonless receipts • Dental sealants • Plastic baby products (e.g., toys)	• BPA acts as a weak estrogen • Delayed onset of breast development in girls; adverse effect on oocytes and implantation • Externalizing behaviors (hyperactivity and aggression); abnormal neuronal circuit formation (those under thyroid hormone control) • Association with obesity and asthma, cardiovascular diagnoses, abnormal liver enzymes and diabetes	• Avoid canned and processed foods • When purchasing items, choose ones labeled phthalate free and BPA free • Use organic personal care products • Choose glass, stainless steel, ceramic, or wood instead of plastics for food storage • If using hard polycarbonate plastics, do not use warm/hot liquids in them (BPA/phthalates leach out of warmed plastics)
Phthalates	• Flexible, soft plastics and polyvinyl chloride products • Medical products: IV tubing, IV fluid bags, catheters, some medications (as excipient) • Food processing: plastics used in factory conveyor belts, jar lids, gloves, packaging, storage • Processed foods • High-fat dairy and meats	• Phthalates are anti-androgenic • Decreased anogenital distance (a marker of androgenization) • Altered sex hormone levels (e.g., luteinizing hormone, testosterone, sex hormone binding globulin) • Externalizing behaviors (hyperactivity and aggression) and declines in executive functioning • Abnormal sperm morphology in postpubescents • Preterm birth	• Encourage frequent handwashing • Minimize handling of receipts • Take shoes off at home to avoid tracking in dust that may contain these chemicals • Keep carpets and windowsills clean to minimize chemical-containing dust
Pesticides	• Residue on/in foods (often leaches into foods and cannot be "washed off") • Large-scale agricultural exposure (e.g., farm workers) • Small-scale garden and yard exposure • Contaminated drinking water • Pesticide-laden dust or residue that has settled on clothes, surfaces, floors, etc.	• Central nervous system dysfunction (neurologic and neurodevelopmental problems, polyneuropathy specifically) • Endocrine disruption (precocious puberty, thyroid dysfunction, hormone-mediated congenital defects (e.g., hypospadias), micropenis, poorly organized testis, abnormal ovarian morphology) • Cancer (specifically leukemias, lymphomas, neuroblastoma, Wilms and brain tumors) • Dermatologic problems • Respiratory problems including asthma exacerbations and pulmonary fibrosis	• Use integrated pest management principles (see text) indoors and outdoors • Consider tolerating low levels of nonharmful pests (e.g., ants, weeds) • Buy organic foods when possible; buy local when possible (increased travel time often necessitates pesticide use) • Keep children away from recently treated outdoor or indoor areas • Do not wear shoes or clothing that has been exposed to pesticides indoors • Store any pesticides out of reach of children

Continued

TABLE 3.3   Selected Endocrine Disruptors Including Pesticides—Cont'd

Chemical Group	Selected Sources	Known Toxic Effects[a]	Alternatives
Perfluorinated compounds	• Industrial and consumer products that need surface protection (stain-, water-, and oil-resistant coatings for cookware, sofas, carpets, mattresses, clothes [e.g., raincoats], shoes, food packaging, firefighting materials) and friction reduction (used in aerospace, automotive, construction and electronic industries) are persistent pollutants (degrade very slowly) • Contaminated drinking water • Animal fats (e.g., certain types of fish)	• Antiandrogenic; decreased thyroid hormone levels • High cholesterol; elevated liver enzymes • Link to ulcerative colitis • Link to cancer (kidney, testicular) • Preeclampsia • Adverse developmental outcomes	• Avoid stain-resistance treatments • Choose clothing that does not carry Teflon or Scotchgard tags • Use stainless steel cookware instead of nonstick cookware • Avoid greasy packaged foods (packages often contain grease-repellent coatings) (e.g., microwave popcorn bags, French fry boxes)
PBDEs	• Flame retardants found in a wide range of products, including electronics, plastics, paint, furniture, synthetic textiles[b] • Animal fat (from bioaccumulating through the food chain) • Contaminated drinking water	• Associated with cryptorchidism; decrease thyroid hormone levels • Abnormal neuronal circuit formation (those under thyroid hormone control)	• Choose PBDE-free electronics and furniture • Avoid contact with decaying or crumbling foam • Use a high-efficiency particulate air vacuum frequently • Use caution when replacing carpet (foam padding often contains PBDEs) • Buy products made with natural fibers (cotton, wool) that are naturally fire resistant • Avoid high-fat meat and certain fish (generally the larger the fish, the more contaminated)
Polychlorinated biphenyls	• Industrial, lipophilic chemicals that have been banned for decades in most countries. Unfortunately, they are persistent pollutants (degrade very slowly) still found in the environment and in humans, including fetuses. • Animal fat (from bioaccumulating through the food chain) • Contaminated drinking water	• Lower sperm count, abnormal sperm morphology, reduced ability of sperm to penetrate oocyte; reduced anogenital distance; decrease thyroid levels (T4). Studies equivocal on pubertal timing alterations. • Abnormal neuronal circuit formation (those under thyroid hormone control)	• Children should avoid playing with old appliances, electrical equipment, or transformers. • Avoid high-fat meat and certain fish (generally the larger the fish, the more contaminated)

[a]Not exhaustive lists. See Additional Resources for more information.

[b]Products made before 2005 may be the most hazardous. Seek out products made without flame retardants (this will be challenging).

BPA, Bisphenol A; *IV*, intravenous; *PBDE*, polybrominated diphenyl ethers.

Modified from Etzel RA, Balk SJ, editors. *Pediatric Environmental Health*. 4th Edition. American Academy of Pediatrics Council on Environmental Health; 2018; Yilmaz B, Terekeci H, Sandal S, Kelestimur F. Endocrine disrupting chemicals: exposure, effects on human health, mechanism of action, models for testing and strategies for prevention. *Rev Endocr Metab Disord*. 2020;21(1):127–147; and Welch BM, Keil AP, Buckley JP, et al. Associations between prenatal urinary biomarkers of phthalate exposure and preterm birth: a pooled study of 16 US cohorts. *JAMA Pediatr*. 2022;176(9):895–905.

Additional Resources

Agency for Healthcare Research and Quality (AHRQ): www.ahrq.gov

Agency for Toxic Substances and Disease Registry (ATSDR): www.atsdr.cdc.gov

Centers for Disease Control and Prevention (CDC): National Center for Environmental Health: www.cdc.gov/nceh

Center for Disease Control and Prevention (CDC): Environmental Health Infographics Air Quality & Asthma: https://www.cdc.gov/nceh/multimedia/air_pollution_asthma_infographics.html

Children's Environmental Health Network: www.cehn.org

Clean Water Action: www.cleanwateraction.org

Collaborative on Health and the Environment: CHE Toxicant and Disease Database: www.healthandenvironment.org/tddb

Environmental Working Group (EWG): www.ewg.org

Green Guide for Health Care: www.gghc.org

Haz-Map: Information on Hazardous Chemicals: www. https://haz-map.com/ Health Care Without Harm: www.noharm.org

Material Safety Data Sheets: www.ilpi.com/msds

National Environmental Education Foundation (NEEF): www.neefusa.org

National Environmental Health Association (NEHA): www.neha.org

National Institute of Environmental Health Sciences: www.niehs.nih.gov

National Safety Council: www.nsc.org

Pediatric Environmental Health Specialty Units (PEHSUs): www.pehsu.net

US Environmental Protection Agency (EPA): www.epa.gov

World Health Organization (WHO) Environmental Health: https://www.who.int/health-topics/environmental-health#tab=tab_1

References

1. World Health Organization, Wolf J, Corvalán C, Bos R, Neira M, Organization WH, eds. *Preventing Disease through Healthy Environments: A Global Assessment of the burden of Disease from Environmental Risks*. Vol. 176. World Health Organization; 2016. https://www.who.int/publications/i/item/9789241565196.

2. WHO. The cost of a polluted environment: 1.7 million child deaths a year, says WHO. News Release. https://www.who.int/news/item/06-03-2017-the-cost-of-a-polluted-environment-1-7-million-child-deaths-a-year-says-who.

3. Landrigan PJ, Fuller R, Fisher S, et al. Pollution and children's health. *Sci Total Environ*. 2019;650(Pt 2):2389–2394.

4. Serebrisky D, Wiznia A. Pediatric asthma: a global epidemic. *Ann Glob Health*. 2019;85(1).

5. Poole JA, Barnes CS, Demain JG, et al. Impact of weather and climate change with indoor and outdoor air quality in asthma: a work group report of the AAAAI environmental exposure and respiratory health committee. *J Allergy Clin Immunol Pract*. 2019;143(5):1702–1710.

6. Chartres N, Bero LA, Norris SL. A review of methods used for hazard identification and risk assessment of environmental hazards. *Environ Int*. 2019;123:231–239.

7. Mastorci F, Linzalone N, Ait-Ali L, Pingitore A. Environment in children's health: a new challenge for risk assessment. *Int J Environ Res Publ Health*. 2021;18(19).

8. Etzel RA. The special vulnerability of children. *Int J Hyg Environ Health*. 2020;227:113516.

9. Pascale A, Laborde A. Impact of pesticide exposure in childhood. *Rev Environ Health*. 2020;35(3):221–227.

10. Philipsborn RP, Chan K. Climate change and global child health. *Pediatrics*. 2018;141(6).

11. Lopez-Rodriguez D, Franssen D, Heger S, Parent AS. Endocrine-disrupting chemicals and their effects on puberty. *Best Pract Res Clin Endocrinol Metab*. 2021;35(5):101579.

12. US Department of Health and Human Services. Toxicological Profile for Lead. 2020. https://www.atsdr.cdc.gov/toxprofiles/tp13.pdf

13. Nidens N, Krönke A, Jurkutat A, et al. Associations of prenatal exposure to phthalates and one phthalate substitute with anthropometric measures in early life: results from the German LIFE Child cohort study. *Best Pract Res Clin Endocrinol Metab*. 2021;35(5):101532.

14. Isaevska E, Moccia C, Asta F, et al. Exposure to ambient air pollution in the first 1000 days of life and alterations in the DNA methylome and telomere length in children: a systematic review. *Environ Res*. 2021;193:110504.

15. WHO. Children's environmental record: Green page. https://www.who.int/publications/m/item/children-s-environmental-record–green-page.

16. Etzel RA, Balk SJ, editors. *Pediatric Environmental Health*. 4th Edition. American Academy of Pediatrics Council on Environmental Health; 2018.

17. Aoyama B, McGrath-Morrow S. Vaping and electronic cigarette use in the pediatric population. *Contemp Pediatr*. 2020;37(4).

18. EPA. Overview of the Clean Air and Air Pollution. https://www.epa.gov/clean-air-act-overview.

19. EUR-Lex. The precautionary principle. EUR-Lex. https://eur-lex.europa.eu/EN/legal-content/summary/the-precautionary-principle.html.

20. Hanna-Attisha M, LaChance J, Sadler RC, Champney Schnepp A. Elevated blood lead levels in children associated with the flint drinking water crisis: a spatial analysis of risk and public health response. *Am J Publ Health*. 2016;106(2):283–290.

21. Abbasi A. Lead, mistrust, and trauma-whistleblowing pediatrician discusses the legacy of Flint's water crisis. *JAMA*. 2021;325(21):2136–2139.

22. Gonzalez DJX, Nardone A, Nguyen AV, Morello-Frosch R, Casey JA. Historic redlining and the siting of oil and gas wells in the United States. *J Expo Sci Environ Epidemiol*. 2022.

23. Nardone A, Chiang J, Corburn J. Historic redlining and urban health today in U.S. Cities. *Environ Justice*. 2020;13(4):109–119.

24. EPA. EPA Office of Environmental Justice. https://www.epa.gov/environmentaljustice.

25. WHO. Climate change and health. https://www.who.int/news-room/fact-sheets/detail/climate-change-and-health#:~:text=Climate%20change%20is%20already%20impacting,diseases%2C%20and%20mental%20health%20issues.

26. Roser M, Ritchie H, Ortiz-Ospina E. World population growth. *Our World in Data*. 2019. https://ourworldindata.org/world-population-growth.

27. Perera F, Nadeau K. Climate change, fossil-fuel pollution, and children's health. *N Engl J Med*. 2022;386(24):2303–2314.

28. Portner HO, Roberts DC, Tignor M, et al, editors. *Climate Change 2022: Impacts, Adaptation, and Vulnerability. Contribution of Working Group II to the Sixth Assessment Report of the Intergovernmental Panel on Climate Change*. Cambridge University Press; 2022.

29. UCS. Tropical deforestation and global warming. Union of Concerned Scientists. https://www.ucsusa.org/resources/tropical-deforestation-and-global-warming.

30. Tong S, Ebi K. Preventing and mitigating health risks of climate change. *Environ Res*. 2019;174:9–13.

31. Xu R, Yu P, Abramson MJ, et al. Wildfires, global climate change, and human health. *N Engl J Med*. 2020.

32. Ebi KL, Vanos J, Baldwin JW, et al. Extreme weather and climate change: population health and health system implications. *Annu Rev Public Health*. Apr 1 2021;42:293–315.

33. Nardone A, Rudolph KE, Morello-Frosch R, Casey JA. Redlines and greenspace: the relationship between historical redlining and 2010 greenspace across the United States. *Environ Health Perspect*. 2021;129(1):17006.

34. Ebi KL, Hess JJ. Health risks due to climate change: inequity in causes and consequences. *Health Aff*. 2020;39(12):2056–2062.

35. Park RJ, Goodman J, Behrer AP. Learning Is Inhibited by Heat Exposure, Both Internationally and within the United States. *Nat Hum Behav*. 2020/10/05 2020.

36. Burke SEL, Sanson AV, Van Hoorn J. The psychological effects of climate change on children. *Curr Psychiatr Rep*. 2018;20(5):35.

37. ALA. *American Lung Association State of the Air 2022*; 2022. Lung.org/sota.

38. Dimakopoulou K, Douros J, Samoli E, et al. Long-term exposure to ozone and children's respiratory health: results from the RESPOZE study. *Environ Res*. 2020;182:109002.

39. Bekkar B, Pacheco S, Basu R, DeNicola N. Association of air pollution and heat exposure with preterm birth, low birth weight, and stillbirth in the US: a systematic review. *JAMA Netw Open*. 2020;3(6):e208243.

40. Perera FP. Multiple threats to child health from fossil fuel combustion: impacts of air pollution and climate change. *Environ Health Perspect*. 2017;125(2):141–148.

41. WHO. Ambient (outdoor) air pollution. WHO. https://www.who.int/news-room/fact-sheets/detail/ambient-(outdoor)-air-quality-and-health.

42. Raju S, Siddharthan T, McCormack MC. Indoor air pollution and respiratory health. *Clin Chest Med*. 2020;41(4):825–843.

43. Destaillats H, Singer B, Salthammer T. Does vaping affect indoor air quality? *Indoor Air*. 2020;30(5):793–794.

44. Johnson AB, Wang GS, Wilson K, et al. Association between secondhand marijuana smoke and respiratory infections in children. *Pediatr Res*. 2022;91(7):1769–1774.

45. Moon J, Yoo H. Residential radon exposure and leukemia: a meta-analysis and dose-response meta-analyses for ecological, case-control, and cohort studies. *Environ Res*. 2021;202:111714.

46. Jans J, Johansson P, Nilsson JP. Economic status, air quality, and child health: evidence from inversion episodes. *J Health Econ.* 2018;61:220–232.

47. Yilmaz B, Terekeci H, Sandal S, Kelestimur F. Endocrine disrupting chemicals: exposure, effects on human health, mechanism of action, models for testing and strategies for prevention. *Rev Endocr Metab Disord.* 2020;21(1):127–147.

48. Welch BM, Keil AP, Buckley JP, et al. Associations between prenatal urinary biomarkers of phthalate exposure and preterm birth: a pooled study of 16 US cohorts. *JAMA Pediatr.* 2022.

49. Caporale N, Leemans M, Birgersson L, et al. From cohorts to molecules: adverse impacts of endocrine disrupting mixtures. *Science.* 2022;375(6582):eabe8244.

50. Montjean D, Neyroud AS, Yefimova MG, Benkhalifa M, Cabry R, Ravel C. Impact of endocrine disruptors upon non-genetic inheritance. *Int J Mol Sci.* 2022;23(6).

51. Schraufnagel DE, Balmes JR, De Matteis S, et al. Health benefits of air pollution reduction. *Ann Am Thorac Soc.* 2019;16(12):1478–1487.

52. Gordon K, Terry PD, Liu X, et al. Radon in schools: a brief review of state laws and regulations in the United States. *Int J Environ Res Publ Health.* 2018;15(10).

53. Council on Environmental Health. Global climate change and children's health. *Pediatrics.* 2015;136(5):992–997. https://doi.org/10.1542/peds.2015-3232.

54. Wellbery CE, Lewandowski A, Holder C. Climate change and the local environment: communicating with your patients about health impacts. *Am Fam Physician.* 2021;104(5):526–530.

4

Justice, Equity, Inclusion, and Diversity

JAIME PANTON AND DAWN LEE GARZON

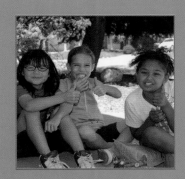

Justice, equity, inclusion, and diversity are foundational pillars that a just and equitable healthcare system must strive to achieve. Unfortunately, health disparities, health inequity, and institutional racism often plague the healthcare system. While many healthcare professional organizations issued a call to action in the elimination of race-based medicine and actively address health disparities and inequity,[1–4] there is still much work to be done (Fig. 4.1). Adherence to principles of social justice, such as access to resources, equity, participation, diversity, and human rights,[5,6] is the primary method to reduce disparities and inequities that lead to poor health outcomes.[7] It is important to address these issues as primary care providers (PCPs), as there is significant evidence that racism and discrimination are substantive contributors to health inequities and disparities.[8] Inequity, inequality, and lack of respect for diversity contribute to social determinants of health that are significant "upstream" issues, which influence and exacerbate underlying health states. Much of the chronic pathology providers see on a daily basis in patients is preventable when equity and the social determinants of health are addressed.[9]

Healthcare systems should be designed to provide care that respects and values the individual's beliefs while understanding that systems are stronger when multiple worldviews are present. This chapter begins with meaningful definitions of justice, equity, inclusion, and diversity as language is important as it provides insight into understanding critical concepts. *Justice* in healthcare is the creation of a caring environment through innovation and directed policy that includes compassion to dismantle structures of inequity. Structural inequities create differential access to healthcare and result in disparate health outcomes for individuals from different societally defined groups. *Equity* in healthcare recognizes that all pediatric patients, regardless of age, sex, race, sexual orientation, socioeconomic status, or another societal-defined status, deserve equal access to health-promoting and health-restoring services and care. Equity to access does not negate the fact that some individuals may need more additional resources (e.g., access to early childhood intervention programs, subsidized health insurance premiums, improved nutrition programs) than others to overcome negative social determinants of health. *Inclusivity* in healthcare is different, in a nuanced way. It holds that all children and youth and their families should have systems developed that allow them to have a voice in healthcare decisions and access to the highest quality of pediatric healthcare. *Diversity* recognizes that each individual defines and experiences health through their own personal lens that is influenced by culture, religion, gender, sexual orientation, health education, and socioeconomic status, to name a few.

PCPs must be aware of structural racism to be able to identify and advocate for patients and families who are adversely affected by its effects. When discussing race within the context of healthcare, it is important to reiterate that race is a social, not a biological, construct.[1] Racism is the power system that affords opportunity and attributes value based on the social interpretation of how one looks (i.e., race). Racism creates a systemic disadvantage for some groups. It is at the core of racial health disparities and was pervasive in the systems that were developed generations ago. The insidious institutionalization of racism and inequities are ubiquitous and often invisible to those not affected. Structural racism occurs when societies develop systems that are reinforced through policy, such as housing, healthcare, employment, criminal justice, and education, to control, segregate, and/or discriminate and affect resource allocation. Structural racism is linked to disparities in birth outcomes, increased risk of chronic illness, and increased interaction with the justice system.[10]

History of Racism in Healthcare

Understanding the history of the US healthcare system is important to understand its connection to racism and how that shapes individuals' trust or mistrust of healthcare providers, institutions, and organizations. Modern healthcare systems were developed after the Civil War, as medical schools defined the standards for health and healthcare delivery. At that time, only White males with financial means were admitted to medical schools.[11] Similarly, nursing education was largely limited to White women who could afford nursing training and education.[12] Before that time, most healing occurred in communities, largely provided by women who were known healers and midwives. The early hospital systems that were developed did not serve Black and indigenous people of color (BIPOC), and racially integrated hospitals did not exist until the passage of the Hill-Burton Act in 1946.[11] The founder of gynecology, Dr. James Marlon Sims, conducted experiments on freed and enslaved Black women to learn about female anatomy and physiologic function. In addition, he sterilized them against their will and without anesthesia.[12] During the same time, the eugenics movement institutionalized and sterilized individuals with disabilities, those who were poor, and Black and Native American individuals, many by departments of the federal government such as the Indian Health Services.[12]

Equality

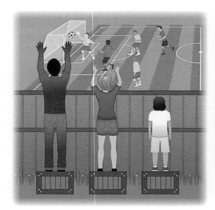

The assumption is that **everyone benefits from the same supports.**This is equal treatment.

Equity

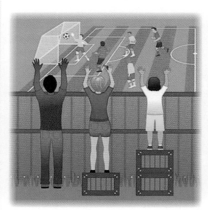

Everyone gets the supports they need (this is the concept of "affirmative action"), thus producing equity.

Justice

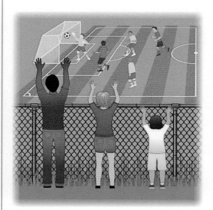

All 3 can see the game without supports or accommodations because the cause(s) of the inequity was addressed. The systemic barrier has been removed.

• **Fig. 4.1** Comparison of Equality, Equity, and Justice.

Distrust in the medical and scientific systems runs deep in some BIPOC communities due to a long history of unethical investigations that used BIPOC subjects in ways that would be unlikely to pass human subjects review boards today. Conducted from 1932 to 1972 by the US Public Health Service, the Tuskegee syphilis study involved monitoring Black Americans who had syphilis to establish the natural course of illness; subjects were allowed to progress to tertiary syphilis even after treatment was readily available.[11] An extension of the Manhattan Project involved injecting 18 Black males with plutonium between 1945 and 1947 to determine how this radioactive isotope is excreted and metabolized in the human body with the aim of determining the effect of plutonium exposure in causing illnesses such as leukemia.[11] All subjects had numerous tissue and blood samples taken, bone biopsies, and tooth extractions to measure how plutonium is deposited in various tissues. Unfortunately, mistreatment of BIPOC individuals in the healthcare setting continues.

In the 1800s scientists believed there were significant anatomic, physiologic, and functional differences between races, and these differences were often used to justify different social policies.[13] Decades of research that attributes differences in health and disease states between races can now be understood to be largely influenced by economic, environmental, and healthcare access differences between groups, and to a lesser extent biological differences between groups.[1,13] The American Academy of Pediatrics, in their *Eliminating Race-Based Medicine* statement (2022), notes the importance of recognizing that differences in race-based clinical care is a direct result of structural and systemic inequities and disparities in marginalized populations and, as such, these should be removed from use. For example, the current clinical practice guidelines listing race-based differences for spirometry in asthmatic youth should be removed in future recommendations, as differences between groups are not believed to be genetic but rather due to differences in social determinants, such as crowded living conditions or poor air quality, that affect pulmonary function.[1]

Adverse Childhood Experiences

Adverse childhood experiences (ACEs), such as emotional, physical, and sexual abuse; homelessness; divorce; parental drug use; family mental health concerns and parental incarceration, have been shown to impact the lives of children well into their adulthood years. The original ACEs study included mostly White adults, many of whom had attended college; therefore a new framework has been proposed to include ACEs and adverse community events to include factors such as violence, poor housing, discrimination, and lack of opportunity.[14,15] ACEs, as well as community factors, have been shown to disproportionately affect historically marginalized communities.[14]

The COVID-19 pandemic highlighted the effect ACEs and community factors have on health disparities. Poor quality and often overcrowded, racial, segregated housing led to challenges and the inability to practice social distancing. In addition, racial and ethnic minority adults are more likely to be employed in places where they are considered "essential workers" and therefore had less opportunity to work from home and social distance.[14]

Health Equity

The US Department of Health and Human Services (HSS)[16] defines health equity as achieving the highest level of health for everyone. Health equity must include societal efforts to mitigate the inequalities and injustices that contribute to inequity. HSS also defines racial and ethnic disparities as "a particular type of health difference that is closely linked with social, economic, and/or environmental disadvantage."

Current State

The impact of racism, especially in healthcare, has been highlighted in recent years. The news media has brought much needed attention to systemic racism, both in and out of the healthcare system with the treatment, or lack thereof, provided to Black Americans and immigrants.[10]

Health Indicators

Health indicators, such as receiving preventive care and accessing primary and subspecialty care, reveal disparities in care based on race/ethnicity, socioeconomic status, and geography. For instance, Hispanic, Black, and Asian youth were less likely to have received medical care in the past year compared to White youth. Black and Hispanic youth were more likely to have cost as a factor in not having a healthcare need met and were less likely to have accessed mental healthcare services in the past 12 months compared to White peers.[17]

Mental Health Disparities

Racially and ethnically diverse children and adolescents have higher rates of mental health and behavioral disorders, yet access services less frequently for these disorders compared to their White peers.[18] Black and Hispanic youth are less likely to be prescribed medication for mental health disorders and are less likely to be treated utilizing evidence-based care. Suboptimal care and lack of access to high-quality mental health services have led to poor outcomes among these children and adolescents.[18]

Infant Mortality and Premature Births

The Centers for Disease Control and Prevention (CDC) data indicate infant mortality rates are twice as high in Black infants compared to White infants. Black and Hispanic infants are at risk of receiving care at lower quality neonatal intensive care units (NICUs) and worse care within a NICU compared to White infants.[19–21] One small qualitative study also found Black and Latinx mothers whose infants were in the NICU reported feeling disrespected and receiving disparaging treatment.[22]

Low socioeconomic status is not always a contributing factor to disproportionate rates of prematurity among Black infants, as Black women with high socioeconomic status also face higher rates of prematurity and low birth weight.[17] Some studies suggest stress, related to racism and discrimination, as a potential factor for this disparity. Segregation in residential areas is also thought to lead to decreased access to prenatal care, and increased exposure to environmental hazards such as pollution are also hypothesized to impact prematurity and low birth weight.[17]

Asthma

The CDC reports that Native Americans, Alaskan Natives, Mainland Puerto Ricans, and Black children have higher rates of asthma compared to White children.[23] One study also showed that Black children had statistically significant higher rates of emergency department visits for asthma compared to Hispanic/Latinx and White youth.[24]

Future Directions

Healthcare provider professional organizations are making strides to mitigate racism in healthcare. There is a call to eliminate race-based medicine, especially within clinical algorithms. For example, the American Academy of Pediatrics retired the clinical practice guideline on urinary tract infections (UTIs), which had included race as a decision-making factor, asserting that Black children were at lower risk for UTI.[1]

At the local level, pediatric providers must be willing to have conversations about the impact of racism on the young person experiencing racism and those who witness racism. PCPs must also be aware of their own biases, both conscious and unconscious, that could potentially impact the care they provide. Pediatric practices should create welcoming environments where all patients are treated with dignity and respect.[25] Incorporating health equity concepts into daily clinical practice is a crucial step in addressing organizational and systemic inequities that contribute to health disparities among marginalized groups.[1]

Other strategies to consider include[25]:
- Create a medical home in which providers are sensitive to the impacts of racism on children and families.
- Educate staff to provide culturally sensitive care and provide appropriate linguistic services.
- Assess for social determinants of health that are linked to racism (environmental safety, food insecurity, housing insecurity).
- For patients disclosing that they have experienced racism, assess for mental health concerns such as anxiety and posttraumatic stress.
- Incorporate positive approaches to youth development to identify strengths and protective factors.
- In early literacy efforts, ensure stories include characters and other images that reflect diversity.

Additional Resources

National Association of Pediatric Nurse Practitioners Statement on Discrimination: https://www.napnap.org/napnap-statement-on-discrimination-and-child-health/.

American Academic of Pediatrics: Racism and Its Effect on Pediatric Health: https://publications.aap.org/journals/collection/655/Pediatric-Collections-Racism-and-Its-Effect-on/.

Academic Pediatric Association: Anti-Racism and Equity Toolkit: https://www.academicpeds.org/publications-resources/apa-anti-racism-equity-toolkit/.

American Association of Child and Adolescent Psychiatry: Anti-Racism Resource Library https://www.aacap.org/AACAP/Families_and_Youth/Resource_Libraries/Racism_Resource_Library.aspx.

References

1. Wright JL, Davis WS, Joseph MM, et al. Eliminating race-based medicine. *Pediatrics*. 2022;150(1):e2022057998.
2. American Psychiatric Association. *APA's Apology to Black, Indigenous and People of Color for its Support of Structural Racism in Psychiatry*; 2021. https://www.psychiatry.org/news-room/apa-apology-for-its-support-of-structural-racism.

3. American Medical Association. Organizational Strategic Plan to Embed Racial Justice and Advance Health Equity: 2021-2023. https://www.ama-assn.org/system/files/2021-05/ama-equity-strategic-plan.pdf.

4. National Association of Pediatric Nurse Practitioners. *NAPNAP Statement on Discrimination and Child Health*; 2020. https://www.napnap.org/napnap-statement-on-discrimination-and-child-health/.

5. Human Rights Careers. Four Principles of Social Justice. https://www.humanrightscareers.com/issues/four-principles-of-social-justice/.

6. Kent State MPA Online. *Five Principles of Social Justice*; 2020. https://onlinedegrees.kent.edu/political-science/master-of-public-administration/community/five-principles-of-social-justice.

7. Moss MP, Phillips JM. *Health Equity and Nursing: Achieving Equity through Policy, Population Health, and Interprofessional Collaboration*. Springer; 2021.

8. Gee CG, Ford CL. Structural racism and health inequities: old issues, new directions. *Du Bois Rev*. 2011;8(1):115–132.

9. Stringer Smith C. History of racism in healthcare: from medical mistrust to Black African-American dentists as moral exemplar and organizational ethics—a bioethical synergy awaits. *Am J Bioeth*. 2022:1–3.

10. Jindal M, Trent M, Mistry KB. The intersection of race, racism, and child and adolescent health. *Pediatr Rev*. 2022;43(8):415–425.

11. Washington HA. *Medical Apartheid: The Dark History of Medical Experimentation on Black Americans from Colonial Times to the Present*; 2008. Anchor.

12. Moore SS, Drake D. *We are the solution to our problem. A brief review of the history of nursing and racism*; 2021. https://www.npwomenshealthcare.com/we-are-the-solution-toour-problem-a-brief-review-%E2%80%A8of-the-history-of-racism-%E2%80%A8and-nursing/.

13. Bhopal R. Spectre of racism in health and health care: lessons from history and the United States. *BMJ*. 1998;316(7149):1970–1973.

14. Sonu S, Marvin D, Moore C. The intersection and dynamics between COVID-19, health disparities, and adverse childhood experiences. *J Child Adolesc Trauma*. 2021;14(4):517–526.

15. Ellis W, Dietz W. A new framework for addressing adverse childhood and community experiences: the Building Community Resilience (BCR) Model. *Acad Pediatr*. 2017;17(2017):S86–S93.

16. US Department of Health and Human Services. Healthy People 2030: Questions and answers. https://health.gov/our-work/national-health-initiatives/healthy-people/healthy-people-2030/questions-answers#:~:text=Healthy%20People%20defines%20a%20health,%2C%20and%2For%20environmental%20disadvantage.

17. Prachter L. Child health disparities. In: Kliegman RM, Geme J S, eds. *Nelson Textbook of Pediatrics*. 21st ed. Elsevier; 2020:9–21.

18. Hoffmann JA, Alegría M, Alvarez K, et al. Disparities in pediatric mental and behavioral health conditions. *Pediatrics*. 2022;150(4):e2022058227.

19. Ravi D, Iacob A, Profit J. Unequal care: racial/ethnic disparities in neonatal intensive care delivery. *Semin Perinatol*. 2021;45(4):151411.

20. Howell EA, Egorova NN, Balbierz A, et al. Site of delivery contribution to black-white severe maternal morbidity disparity. *Am J Obstet Gynecol*. 2016;215(2):143–152.

21. Fanta M, Ladzekpo D, Unaka N. Racism and pediatric health outcomes. *Curr Probl Pediatr Adolesc Health Care*. 2021;51(10):101087.

22. Glazer KB, Shoshanna S, Balbierz A, et al. Perinatal care experiences among racially and ethnically diverse mothers whose infants required a NICU stay. *J Perinatol*. 2021;41(3):413–421.

23. Centers for Disease Control and Prevention. *Most Recent National Asthma Data*; 2022. https://www.cdc.gov/asthma/most_recent_national_asthma_data.htm.

24. Kaufmann J, Marino M, Lucas J, et al. Racial and ethnic disparities in acute care use for pediatric asthma. *Ann Fam Med*. 2022;20(2):116–122.

25. Trent M, Dooley DG, Dougé J. Section on adolescent health; council on community pediatrics; committee on adolescence. The impact of racism on child and adolescent health. *Pediatr syst*. 2019;144(2):e20191765.

5

Pediatric and Family Assessment

MARTHA DRIESSNACK AND DANIEL CRAWFORD

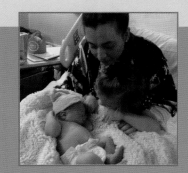

One of the unique challenges in pediatric primary care is that there is not one patient, but two, as pediatric primary care providers (PCPs) cannot care for their patients without also caring for their families. It is essential that PCPs move from child to family and back again during the assessment, although this process is not always easy, especially when the priorities and/or needs of the two conflict. Over a decade ago, the American Academy of Pediatrics (AAP) issued a policy statement that introduced a shift away from "family-centered care" to "patient- and family-centered care" (PFCC) as it captures the importance of engaging pediatric patients as essential members of the healthcare team, while acknowledging the key role and voice of their families. This chapter provides an overview of the foundational knowledge needed for the delivery of PFCC, covering pediatric and family assessment basics. The chapter concludes with a review of shared decision-making (SDM), which is central to PFCC, some additional resources, and a brief reflection as virtual interactions become increasingly integrated into all levels of care.

Pediatric Assessment

Understanding how children develop from conception through adolescence is foundational to pediatric primary care, not only because it prioritizes *what* to assess at different ages, but it also informs *how* to approach and engage children at different developmental stages. Although the principles of examining children are very similar to adult examination, there are important differences in terms of approach, content, and patterns of disease. The following section highlights some of these important differences, or more specifically, the unique issues to consider when assessing patients across the pediatric lifespan.

Basic Principles

Understanding the principles of growth, development, and maturation are key to assessing children over time. *Growth* refers to an increase in number and size of cells, as well as the increased size and weight of the whole or any of its parts. *Development* is a gradual change and expansion in capabilities, which represents advancement from lower to more advanced stages of complexity. *Maturation* represents an increase in competence and adaptability. Growth and development have a *cephalocaudal* (i.e., head-to-toe)

and *proximodistal* (i.e., midline-to-periphery) progression. There is also a distinct pace and focus to growth, with the infant experiencing *rapid* growth (primarily head); toddler and preschooler experiencing *slow* growth (primarily trunk); school-age child experiencing *slow* growth (primarily limbs); and adolescents returning to *rapid* growth (primarily sexual maturation).

Each child progresses at their own pace, which means growth and development occur on a spectrum. This knowledge means there are *ranges* for typical physical, social, emotional, and cognitive growth during infancy, childhood, and adolescence. One child will gain weight quickly but be slower to speak, whereas another will acquire speech early but be slower to walk. Many children progress smoothly, whereas others do so in fits and starts. It is important to view any deviations in the context of the whole child.

Measurement

A variety of measurements can be obtained, recorded, and plotted to assist PCPs in assessing growth, development, and maturation. The most common measurements during pediatric encounters include vital signs, length/height, weight, body mass index, occipital frontal (head) circumference (OFC), and assessment of sexual maturity. Other types of body measurements are also used depending on the context. For example, obtaining crown-rump length and sitting height can be used as a proxy for length and height for an older child who cannot stand but is able to sit. In other situations, a PCP may need to measure leg length, arm span, a single body part (e.g., testicular volume, interpupillary distance), circumferences (e.g., chest, waist), and/or skinfold thickness, to name a few (Appendix A). The most important piece to remember is that reliable and reproducible measurements are required to obtain meaningful data.

Growth Charts

Growth measurements are the gold standard by which PCPs assess the health and wellbeing of a child; they must know what to measure, how to measure, and what growth charts are best suited for each child. Growth charts are tools that contribute to forming an overall clinical impression of the child being measured; however, they are not intended to be used as a sole diagnostic instrument. Serial measurements are used to assess patterns and identify aberrations. The Centers for Disease Control and Prevention (CDC) recommend that providers use the World Health Organization

(WHO) growth charts to monitor growth in infants and children from birth until 2 years of age and the CDC growth charts for children aged 2 years and older. Of note, the WHO growth charts are for *length* (*supine* measurement), whereas the CDC growth charts are for *height* (*standing* measurement). The OFC are for measurements in an upright position. Complete sets of WHO and CDC age- and sex-specific pediatric growth charts, along with a set of self-directed, interactive training courses, are available from the CDC (https://www.cdc.gov/growthcharts/index.htm). For those children with disorders that alter the growth pattern (e.g., Down syndrome, Turner syndrome), a number of specialized growth charts should be used in place of standardized growth charts (see Chapter 27).

Health Supervision, Surveillance, and Screening

Health supervision (routine well-child) visits are a core component of pediatric primary care because they allow for comprehensive assessment of the individual patient and family environment, and the opportunity for further evaluation if abnormalities are detected. Each visit typically includes a complete history, a head-to-toe physical examination, screenings, immunization review and updates, and sharing of anticipatory guidance. Unlike focused or ill-child encounters, during which the primary aim is to attend to the presenting concern, health supervision visits are multifaceted, focusing on health promotion and protection as well as disease prevention and detection. Each visit is guided by knowledge of growth patterns, developmental milestones, individual and age-related disease and environmental risks, as well as protective factors, family history and function, and family and cultural priorities and needs. Through ongoing assessment, each patient's health and developmental trajectory can be tracked, compared with normative data, evaluated, and managed in the context of their family and environment, so any variation can be quickly attended to.

The timing and focus of health supervision visits typically align with AAP Periodicity Schedule (https://downloads.aap.org/AAP/PDF/periodicity_schedule.pdf?_ga=2.56067563.194872493.1687402697-1772658741.1687402697), which serves as a roadmap. Embedded in each health supervision visit is ongoing disease detection, which involves two techniques: surveillance and screening. *Surveillance* is the systematic collection, analysis, and interpretation of data for the purpose of prevention, because findings from health surveillance guide *primary* prevention measures. Surveillance is a continuous, long-term process, which may or may not include screenings. *Screenings* are targeted systematic actions at a single point in time that are designed to identify a preclinical condition or disease in individuals suspected of having or being at risk for the specific health impairment. Screening is recommended when the individual will benefit from early treatment or intervention and is a secondary prevention measure. *Universal* screening is conducted on all children at defined time intervals or ages, whereas *selective* screening is conducted only on those children for whom a risk assessment suggests follow-up. Health supervision, surveillance, and screening priorities for each pediatric age group are included in Chapters 9–13.

History and Physical Examination

It is important to distinguish between the different types of primary care encounters, including the *routine well-child* encounter focused on screening for abnormalities of growth and/or development, the *ill-child* encounter focused on establishing the nature, cause, and extent of an acute or chronic illness/injury, and the *focused, single-purpose* encounter, such as to establish fitness for

school or sports, or a forensic examination performed in sexual or maltreatment cases. However, there is not always a clear distinction between visit types, as single-purpose sports physicals can be completed within well-child encounters, problems with growth, development, and/or behavior may be noted during an ill-child visit, and recognition and documentation of child maltreatment can occur during any encounter and is an ever-present concern. What is important across all types of encounters is that PCPs have a good working knowledge of growth, developmental milestones, age-related risk factors, and routine physical findings at different ages.

History

Obtaining a history begins with the establishment of trust. Remember that in any pediatric encounter there are at least two historians in the room: the parent and the child. Seek out and listen to both whenever possible, paying close attention to any differences. A thorough, thoughtful health history is the first and often most critical step because it helps to focus the clinician's diagnostic reasoning and guides the physical examination. However, in pediatrics, it is important to remember that the history and physical examination often occur simultaneously. As children grow and develop, the emphasis changes. Although each history needs to be individualized, be developmentally appropriate, and consider the child's family, health status, and physical/social environment, having a practical approach that encompasses key aspects of children's ongoing growth and developmental needs and progress is helpful. The typical elements of a routine well-child and ill-child health history are presented in Boxes 5.1 and 5.2, respectively. However, it is important to note that ill-child encounters also provide an opportunity to assess a child's growth and development, as well as complete missed or scheduled surveillance, and/or screening.

Of particular note in pediatrics is actively seeking out any evidence of adverse childhood experiences (ACEs), as these experiences can have profound near- and long-term effects on mental and physical health across the pediatric lifespan and into adulthood. A number of evidence-based tools, including the ACES Family Health History and Health Appraisal Questionnaire (https://www.cdc.gov/violenceprevention/aces/about.html), can be included in every pediatric encounter.

Physical Examination

The best path to an accurate and complete physical examination is to secure the cooperation of the child; however, predictable, developmentally related fears or previous frightening experiences can impact a potentially positive encounter before it ever begins. Although the physical examination is traditionally conducted following the history, the reality of pediatric primary care often means moving back and forth from subjective data gathering to objective assessment. Content and priorities for the physical exam vary depending on the child's age, cues from the history, and the various problems being considered, including patient and family queries. A list of principal findings PCPs are expected to identify is presented in Box 5.3, while Box 5.4 includes tips for developmental modification during physical examinations. Additional physical examination techniques and findings, such as a completing a sports exam, neurologic examination, or screening for inherited disorders, are found in later chapters, and Box 5.5 draws attention to the challenges of virtual assessment. It is also recommended that PCPs have access to pediatric physical examination resources, such as the *Pediatric Physical Exam: An Illustrated Handbook*[1] and the *Atlas of Pediatric Physical Diagnosis*.[2]

• BOX 5.1 Well-Child History (Comprehensive, Ongoing)

- Patient-identifying information/statement
  - Identify if this is a new or established patient/family
  - Child age, sex/gender
  - Accompanying adult(s)
- Reason for the visit
  - Highlight parental (and child) concerns and priorities
- Date of last visit
  - Interval history (with an established patient/family, seek an update of the comprehensive history on record)
- Past health and medical history
  - Prenatal, birth, and neonatal history
  - Childhood illness/injury
  - Hospitalization, surgery, and procedures
  - Allergies (food, medication, environment)
  - Immunizations
  - Medications (prescription, OTC, folk or herb, complementary and alternative therapies)
- Prior screening/results
- Review of systems: begin with global questions in each system; pursue areas of concern in further detail
- Current health
  - Daily activities: nutrition, sleep, activity, elimination
  - Development surveillance/milestones: affective, cognitive, language, physical
  - Preventive health history: screenings, immunizations, health protection activities
- Family assessment and history
  - Family structure and function
    - Parenting skills/history
  - Family health history, three-generation pedigree
  - Family ethnic and cultural beliefs and practices
  - Family health habits (e.g., literacy, smoking, seatbelts, helmets)
- Household and environment
  - Protective factors and strengths: parental resilience, social connections, knowledge of parenting/child development, concreate support in times of need, social and emotional competence of children
  - Safety and risks: access to firearms, exposure to violence, adverse childhood experiences, toxic exposures, social determinants of health, housing, and food security
  - Nature exposure and access

OTC, Over the counter.

• BOX 5.2 Ill-Child History (Episodic, Problem Focused)

- Patient-identifying information or statement
  - Identify if this is a new or established patient/family
  - Child age, sex/gender
  - Accompanying adult(s)
- Reason for the visit
  - Highlight parental (and child) concerns and priorities
- Date child was last well
- Interval/history of the present illness: chronologic description for each concern
  - Symptom analysis (onset, duration, course, symptom characteristics, aggravating or alleviating factors, exposure to illnesses or other causative factors, similar problems in close contacts, previous episodes of similar illnesses and symptoms, previous diagnostic measures, pertinent negative data, and the meaning of the concern for the family and child)
- Focused past health and medical history
  - Prenatal, birth, and neonatal history
  - Illness or injury
  - Radiographs, laboratory tests, procedures
  - Hospitalizations or surgery
  - Allergies (food, medication, environment)
  - Immunizations
  - Medications (prescription, OTC, folk or herb, complementary and alternative therapies)
- Review of systems
- Focused family history
  - ACEs
  - Family disease history, genetic risk
  - Family ethnic and cultural beliefs and practices
- Environment
  - Family structure and function, caregiver strain
  - Social determinants of health
  - Environmental exposures

ACEs, Adverse childhood experiences; *OTC,* over the counter.

Family Assessment

The composition and context of a "typical" family unit have changed significantly. For example, fewer children are residing in homes with both of their biological parents, and more children are living in homes where both parents are working. Further, children can be part of a married, cohabitating, or kinship family; a single-parent, blended, or stepfamily; an intergenerational and/or grandparent-led household; a family with same-gender parents; parental gamete-donators or surrogates; as well as foster, adoptive, and/or large, community-led families. Regardless of the family structure, the ability of the family to meet the needs and support the growth and development of its members (especially children) is particularly important. Whatever their composition, children's family environments are integral to their wellbeing and unless the family is healthy, the child may be at risk. Childhood experiences—the good, bad, and ugly—can have a dramatic impact on children that stays with them for the rest of their lives. Assessing children's strengths, protective factors, and risks involves ongoing family assessment.

Family assessment begins with the assumption that families are central to and inseparable from the health of children. The basic elements of family assessment include its (1) composition or structure, (2) lifecycle or developmental stage, (3) functioning, and (4) presence of protective factors.

Family Composition or Structure

The current standard for assessing family composition or structure is to construct a three-generation pedigree, which provides a valuable visual record of family structure, genetic links, and health-related information. Insights about families are gained, not only because families share genes but also because they also often share environments, behaviors, and culture—all of which contribute to shared health problems. However, it is also important to note the pedigree includes genetically linked individuals, and many families are composed of individuals who are not genetically linked. These individuals need to be included when documenting structure but are noted differently. Details about how to construct the three-generation pedigree, along with genetic red flags, are found in Chapter 27.

Although the three-generation pedigree and genogram include biological or genetically linked relatives, a *genogram* expands the

• BOX 5.3 Essential Pediatric Physical Examination Data

- **General appearance:** Note the child's general state (e.g., Is the child alert? Active or interactive? Ill appearing?). Note general appearance (e.g., overall nutrition, color, respiratory effort, general body positions and movements). Does the child appear congruent with the stated age? How is the parent-child interaction? Are there any physical signs that may indicate the presence of a syndrome?
- **Head:** Assess size and shape (e.g., micro- or macrocephaly, craniosynostosis, positional plagiocephaly), note size and appearance of fontanels, approximation or closure of suture lines.
- **Eyes:** PERRLA, EOMs, red reflex, cover/uncover, abnormal and/or asymmetric eye shape, movements, or color are standard elements. Vision screening begins early, beginning with whether or not the infant can fixate and follow and respond to visual stimulation and later to formal vision screening beginning in early childhood.
- **Ears:** Shape and placement of the ear, response to auditory stimuli, and the presence of preauricular sinus/tags should be noted. Check that newborn hearing testing was done. Hearing screening also continues with assessment of an infant's response to voices and noises and language development. Formal audiometric evaluation begins in early childhood and continues through adolescence. Examination of TM, using a soft tip (Fig. 5.1), which is gentle and provides better occlusion when assessing for TM mobility.
- **Nose:** Newborns are obligate nose breathers. Assess for patency, septum position, deviation, and flaring. Note discharge. Infants and young children may place foreign bodies in nasal passages.
- **Mouth:** Assess tooth eruption and shedding sequences, early or overt caries, abnormal mucosal color, lesions, uvula, intact palate, tonsil size and appearance, and tongue tie.
- **Neck:** Note ROM, noting any abnormalities (e.g., nuchal rigidity, webbed neck, torticollis) in motion. Palpate thyroid. Note presence of thyroglossal or branchial cleft cysts or sinus, Delphian node.
- **Skin:** Note color and texture of skin, describe color and texture and distribution (e.g., dermatomal, flexural, extensor) of congenital or other lesions or rashes. Attend to lesions that might indicate the presence or risk of disease (e.g., hemangiomas, café-au-lait spots, acanthosis nigricans) or injury (e.g., color, shape, location of bruises) or are atypical for age (e.g., acne, secondary sexual characteristics).
- **Lymph nodes:** Note size, mobility, pain or tenderness, and warmth. Remember drainage paths and look for related issues or source if enlarged or tender.
- **Chest:** Assess overall shape, congenital malformations (e.g., shield chest), and thoracic cage variations (e.g., pectus carinatum or excavatum). Note any dyspnea, retractions, and use of accessory muscles.
- **Breasts:** Note placement, discharge, and SMR.
- **Lungs:** Assess for symmetric expansion, air movement, and lung sounds.
- **Cardiovascular:** Assess heart sounds, noting abnormalities or presence of murmurs. Note presence and nature of femoral pulses. Check peripheral perfusion and circumoral cyanosis.
- **Abdomen:** Assess for age-appropriate contour, distention, tenderness, organ position size, masses, umbilicus for hernia, erythema, or leakage, inguinal bulging or hernia, and congenital malformations. Most umbilical hernias resolve by 2 years of age, whereas all inguinal hernias require surgical intervention.
- **Genitalia:** Note SMR, including orchidometer (males) and chart (Fig. 5.2). Assess for congenital or acquired variations, defects, or malformations (e.g., ambiguous genitalia, hypospadias, cryptorchidism, fused labia, vaginal discharge).
- **Anus:** Assess for patency and placement. Note abnormalities (e.g., bleeding, fissures, rectal prolapse).
- **Musculoskeletal:** Assess full and symmetric ROM, presence of abnormal movements, joint laxity, abnormal or asymmetric tone and strength, extremity position or symmetry, gross and fine motor development, and presence of congenital or acquired abnormalities (e.g., tibial torsion, equinovarus, pes planus, metatarsus adductus, genu varum or valgum, femoral anteversion). All infants require hip evaluation (e.g., Barlow, Ortolani). Gait progression evaluation is standard. Careful attention to spine curvatures until growth is complete.
- **Neurologic:** Note presence or persistence of primitive reflexes. Assess overall alertness and interaction with others; cranial nerves, overall tone and abnormalities (e.g., spasticity, hypotonicity), tics, and seizure activity or abnormal movements. Assess for sacral dimple or spinal deformity, modifications for younger children.

EOM, Extraocular movement; *PERRLA,* pupils equal round reactive to light accommodation; *SMR,* sexual maturity rating; *TM,* tympanic membrane.

---

pedigree to include information about the sociocultural context of the family's relationships, much like the ecomap. In addition, the Colored Eco-Genetic Relationship Map is an interactive approach adapted for use with children.[3]

Family Development or Life Cycle Stage

Just as children can be described in terms of their individual developmental stage, it is also possible to describe socioemotional stages that occur throughout the life of a family unit. Special attention is given to families in several overlapping stages, as well as to those in transition from or to different stages, because each stage has its unique issues and tasks. In any given family, each member is in a developmental stage, while the family unit is simultaneously going through various stages in the family life cycle.

Family Functioning

A number of tools are available to assess family functioning, including the family ecomap, Family APGAR, and SCREEM mnemonic. A family *ecomap* is a graphic portrayal of the type, number, and quality of relationships or connections individuals have within their family and their community. It provides a snapshot of an individual's personal and social relationships, as well as how much energy the relationships use, by identifying each relationship as close/distant, strong/weak, mutual/one-sided, positive/negative, nurturing/damaging, and/or secure/plagued by conflict. It is a valuable tool in determining a family's strengths, resources, needs, and deficits. The long-standing Family APGAR[4] is used to assess a family's *A*daptation, *P*artnership, *G*rowth, *A*ffection, and *R*esolve. It consists of five questions, which make it easy and quick to administer and a popular choice for evaluating family function in busy primary care settings (http://www.stritch.luc.edu/lumen/MedEd/family/apgar1.pdf). The SCREEM mnemonic is also used to identify a family's *S*ocial, *C*ultural, *R*eligious, *E*conomic, *E*ducation, and *M*edical resources, as well as their absence. For example, social interaction may be evident among family members, or the family may be socially isolated.

Protective Factors

Protective factors are attributes of families, as well as the larger community and society, that promote optimal development and resiliency across the pediatric lifespan. The goal is to focus on positive ways to engage families, emphasizing their strengths while identifying areas where they have room to grow with support. The Strengthening Families movement is an evidence-based approach supporting the concept that children are more likely to thrive when their families have the support they need (https://cssp.org/our-work/project/strengthening-families/). The Parents' Assessment of Protective Factors (PAPF)[5] measures the presence, strength, and growth of five key protective factors: parental resilience, social connections, concrete support in times of need, children's social and emotional competence, and knowledge of parenting and child development.

Shared Decision Making

Although the elements, principles, and positive health outcomes of SDM are well documented, there has been a lack of guidance for PCPs as to how to apply them in clinical practice. At its core, SDM is a process in which decisions are made in a collaborative way, trustworthy information is provided in accessible formats about a set of options, typically in situations where the concerns, personal circumstances, and contexts of patients/families play a major role in decisions.[6] The very practical *three-talk model* of SDM (Fig. 5.3) offers a clear pathway to application of SDM in

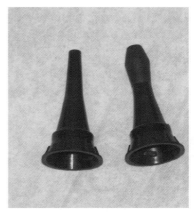

• **Fig. 5.1** Ear Specula Designed to Facilitate Pneumatic Otoscopy. A comfortable but tight seal in the ear canal is important for insufflation to be effective. Both of these specula have the same internal diameter. Note that the soft-tip speculum on the right is flared at the tip (with a coating of soft rubber) to provide a seal without traumatizing the ear canal. (From Swartz MH. *Textbook of Physical Diagnosis: History and Examination*. 7th ed. Elsevier; 2014.)

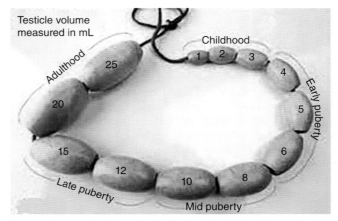

• **Fig. 5.2** Prader Orchidometer to Assess Testicular Volume (in milliliters). Charts for assessing testicular volume can be found here at https://www.academia.edu/24168091/Charts_for_testicular_volume_development_orchidometer_. (From Mathew KG, Aggarwal P. *Medicine: Prep Manual for Undergraduates*. 7th ed. Elsevier; 2023.)

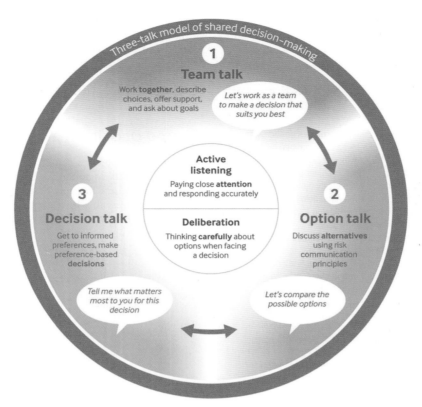

• **Fig. 5.3** Three-Talk Model of Shared Decision-Making. (From Elwyn G, Durand MA, Song J, et al. A three-talk model for shared decision-making: multistage consultation process. *BMJ.* 2017;359:j4891.)

practice. *Team talk* emphasizes the need to provide support to patients/families as they are made aware of choices, as well as eliciting their goals as a means of guiding decision-making processes. *Option talk* refers to the task of comparing alternatives, using risk-communication principles. *Decision talk* refers to the task of arriving at decisions that reflect the informed preferences of patients/families, guided by the experience and expertise of the PCP. The three-talk model holds space open for collaboration and deliberation as the patient/family moves from *initial* to *informed* preferences to decision-making. The PCP role is one of active listening and decision support.

Tailoring discussion with families also needs to address health literacy levels. Using the principles of universal precautions, the Agency for Healthcare Research and Quality developed the Health Literacy Universal Precautions Toolkit (https://www.ahrq.gov/health-literacy/improve/precautions/index.html), which instructs PCPs to assume all families may have difficulty comprehending health information and access services. The toolkit helps PCPs minimize the risk of miscommunication and make their office environment easier to navigate, while supporting pediatric patients/families' efforts to improve their health.

When assessing household literacy, one approach is to use a simple screening question that can identify households in need of further support. The question posed to children is, "How many children's books do you have at home?" Any household with less than 10 children's books at home warrants further exploration.[7]

Additional Resources

Bright Futures

Bright Futures is a national health promotion and prevention initiative that provides age-specific guidelines, tools, and recommendations for health supervision visits. It is led by the AAP and supported, in part, by the U.S. Department of Health and Human Services (HHS), Health Resources and Services Administration (HRSA), and Maternal and Child Health Bureau (MCHB). The Bright Futures website (https://brightfutures.aap.org) houses multiple resources, such as *Building Positive Parenting Skills Across Ages*, which is an online course that guides PCPs as to how to provide developmentally appropriate parenting advice and reinforce parenting skills during health supervision visits.

Strengthening Families

Strengthening Families is a protective factors framework that summarizes best practices to achieve positive outcomes for all families. It is based on five protective factors: parental resilience, social connections, knowledge of parenting and child development, concrete support in times of need, and social and emotional competence for children. Each factor has been shown to protect against risk factors and poor outcomes for both children and families, as well as promote strong families and optimal development for children. Strengthening Families is one of

TABLE 6.2	Level of Stress, Response, and Outcome			
Level of Stress	Example	Response	Outcome	
Positive = brief duration, mild to moderate severity, infrequent, normal, and essential	Receiving an injection, beginning daycare or school, big test or project in middle or high school	Brief increase in heart rate with mild elevation in stress hormones Socioemotional buffers (responding to nonverbal cues, consolation, reassurance, assistance in planning) allow a return to baseline stress response	Quickly returns to normal Builds resiliency and motivation	
Tolerable = sustained duration, moderate/severe severity, more frequently occurring	Car accident, death in family, natural disaster, frightening injury	Greater activation of stress response Socioemotional buffers (above) allow a return to baseline stress response	A single major, negative event does not mean long-lasting problems	
Toxic = severe intensity, frequent or prolonged duration	Physical, sexual, emotional abuse or neglect; parent substance abuse or mental illness; household or environmental dysfunction	Insufficient social-emotional buffers (deficient levels of emotional coaching, reprocessing, reassurance, and support) cause changes in baseline stress response	Changes in brain architecture and function (hyperresponsive stress response with decreased calm/coping) that can affect learning and development and impact long-term health	

Concept 2: Adversity Disrupts the Foundations of Learning, Behavior, and Health (One Principle)

Stress is a normal response to life's challenges. By itself, it is a bad thing; however, the degree or level of stress influences its likely impact or outcome (Table 6.2). The experience of stress is variable, depending on the individual's (subjective) perception of and reaction (objective) to the stress. When assessing stress/stressors, it is important to consider its frequency, duration, and severity.

Principle 1: Toxic stress responses can impair development and have lifelong effects on learning, behavior, and health. Stress reaches a toxic level due to the repetition of stress or an accumulation of different stressors (i.e., dose response). Significant hardship or ongoing and/or prolonged toxic stress leads to chronic and/or continuous activation of the fight-or-flight response, which can disrupt the development of the brain architecture, contribute to a hyperresponsive stress response, and a lessened ability to calm and/or cope. The science behind the developmental origins of health and disease (DOHaD) and ACEs (see Chapter 1) points to the strong association between toxic stress, brain development disruption, functional learning differences, behavior and mental health, and the immediate and long-term impacts on health, prosperity, and life-course trajectory.

Concept 3: Protective Factors in Early Years Strengthen Resilience (Three Principles)

Principle 1: Providing the right environment from the start produces better outcomes than trying to fix problems later. It has been said that "it is easier to raise a healthy child than to fix a broken one." Although it is possible to change established brain pathways later in life, it takes more effort from the individual and more resources from society to facilitate change once dysfunctional pathways have been established.

Principle 2: Positive early experiences, support from adults, and the early development of adaptive skills can counterbalance the lifelong consequences of adversity. Not all children who experience adverse events have negative sequelae later in life. Those at particular risk are individuals who come from families who experience poverty, have low education levels, and experience systemic racism that results in changes in individual, family, and community sustained stressors.[7] Even one SSNR supports

and provides a framework that not only prevents developmental disruption but also allows a child opportunity to regulate during periods of stress and build protective capabilities against future stress. The combination of positive experiences, supportive relationships and adaptive skills can lead to individual *resilience*, which provides neuroprotection that offsets and/or prevents any epigenetic changes.[7] Strategies for promoting resilience are highlighted in Box 6.1.

Principle 3: Children and adults need core capabilities to respond to and/or avoid adversity, and these capabilities can be strengthened through coaching and practice. Using a brain development perspective, the following core capabilities (i.e., life skills) help adults deal effectively with life, work, and parenting:

- Focus—concentrating on what is most important at any given time
- Awareness—noticing people and situations and one's place in their world
- Planning—being able to make concrete plans, carry them out, and set and meet goals
- Flexibility—adapting to changing situations
- Self-control—controlling one's response to emotions and stressful situations

These same core capabilities are needed across the pediatric lifespan to learn, as well as manage school, outside interests, and social relationships successfully. They require communication between the prefrontal cortex and other parts of the brain (e.g., hippocampal structures, including the amygdala). The interaction between/across these capabilities allows the individual to focus on goals, resist distractions, and find alternate approaches (Fig. 6.3).

Protective, Promotive, and Risk Factors

Children, as well as their families, can experience protective and promotive factors alongside risk factors. *Protective factors* (i.e., strengths, assets) are individual, family, neighborhood, or community level characteristics that moderate or buffer the negative effect of stress on development (Table 6.3). *Promotive factors*, often combined with protective factors, are those that encourage healthy development. *Risk factors* (i.e., vulnerabilities, problems) are measurable characteristics that undermine healthy development (Table 6.4). These factors interact in complicated ways. For

• BOX 6.1 Evidence-Based Strategies for Protecting Early Childhood Resiliency

1. Promote healthy pregnancy and normative child development through:
   - Programs supporting maternal and child nutrition and health
   - Early child intervention programs including home visitations programs
   - Quality prenatal and episodic pediatric care
   - Quality universal early child education beginning at age 3 years
   - Head Start and Early Head Start to support low-income families, children in foster care, and children with disabilities and other special needs
2. Promote protective factors that foster resiliency including a belief in one's self-efficacy, personal motivation to mastery, and the ability to self-regulate including:
   - Sensitive and responsive caregiving
   - Close emotional relationships that provide a sense of belonging and security
   - Opportunities to practice problem solving and self-efficacy in an environment that allows for safe failure
   - Caregiving that includes routines, rituals, and structure
   - Opportunities to practice emotional skills and emotional skill building
   - Opportunities to interact with a greater community and to create a self-narrative and self-identity
3. Access to trauma-informed care for those who experience adversity—includes parent-child psychotherapy, parent-child interaction therapy (PCIT)
4. Social policies that support economically healthy families and promote family functioning, including paid family leave and support for economically disadvantaged families to help ensure access to quality childcare

Modified from Bartlett JD, Halle T, Thomson D. Promoting resilience in early childhood. *Resilient Children.* 2021:165–190; and National Association of Pediatric Nurse Practitioners, Spratling R, Cavanaugh N, et al. Building resilience in childhood and adolescence. *J Pediatr Health Care.* 2019;33:A11–A13.

TABLE 6.3 Protective/Promotive Factors for Child Wellbeing

Relational/family	• Family support for children's executive functioning • Parent/adult responsiveness • Parent/adult warmth • Shared family activities • Parent/parent engagement with school and community • Safe and supportive home environment • Family routines • Stimulating home environment • Parenting skills and attributes (e.g., authoritative style) • Religious involvement • Enduring presence and positive support of caring adults and kin • Control over number and timing of children in the family
Contextual/community	• Relevant, high-quality, culturally appropriate available local services • Safe and healthy school environment • Safe and cohesive neighborhood, safe housing • Access to nutritious food • Access to jobs and transportation for the job • Access to medical care including wellness and behavioral health

From Kristin Anderson Moore et al. *Child Wellbeing: Constructs to Measure Child Wellbeing and Risk and Protective Factors that Affect the Development of Young Children;* 2016. Copyright Child Trends.

TABLE 6.4 Risk Factors for Child Wellbeing

Relational/family	• Economic downturns and material hardship • Parental depression/mental health problems • Parental substance abuse • Parental unemployment • Parental social isolation • Parental rigidity, harshness, or inconsistent discipline • Conflict/domestic violence • Parental history or maltreatment • Family stress • Family instability/turbulence • Toxic trauma, high level of adverse childhood experiences, accumulation of stresses • Younger child age at maltreatment, type of maltreatment • Removal from parents, placement with kin, placement stability • Inconsistent medical care
Community/contextual	• Exposure to violence/unsafe environment • Unavailable, inconsistent, poor-quality childcare and other services • Negative peers • Unsupportive, negative child welfare service providers • Absence of foster care families • Lack of emergency housing • Inadequate recreational opportunities

From Kristin Anderson Moore et al. *Child Wellbeing: Constructs to Measure Child Wellbeing and Risk and Protective Factors that Affect the Development of Young Children;* 2016. Copyright Child Trends.

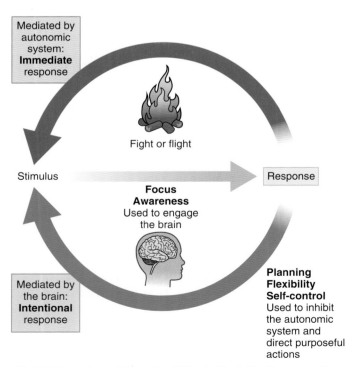

• **Fig 6.3** Interactions of Core Capabilities in Mediating Response. (From Building Core Capabilities for Life, The Science Behind the Skills Adults Need to succeed in Parenting and the Workplace, 2016. http://www.ddcf.org/globalassets/child-wellbeing/16-0304-core-capabilities-for-life.pdf.)

example, child temperament can be a protective or a risk factor depending on the situation and the interactions that result.

Relationships and Attachment

The ability to form relationships is a critical human trait that provides the glue for family, community, and society. Relationships range from transient and superficial to deep and enduring. Because the brain is designed to derive pleasure from human interaction, early relationships result in attachment bonds that establish maps or neural templates for future relationships.

Safe, Stable, Nurturing Relationships

SSNRs provide neural protection against the effects of toxic stress, foster individual resilience, and provide a deep sense of emotional wellbeing and interconnectedness, which is a driving need of the mammalian brain.[8] A competent, caring, positively attuned, engaged parent addresses the child's physiologic and safety needs (i.e., protects), promotes healthy relationships and attachment (i.e., relates), and encourages foundational and advancing coping skills (i.e., nurtures). Strategies that reflect a healthy parent-child relationship include the use of loving verbal and nonverbal communication, consistent routines, frequent "fun" and playtime, as well as accurately reading child signals and providing timely responses to the child's needs. Positive caregiving is critical to children's ability to learn, self-regulate, and get along with others, and is a precursor to positive mental health. Emerging science indicates that high levels of family resilience, strong family connection, and parent-child interactions not only provide positive relational experiences and opportunities for children and adolescents to develop, thrive, and even flourish, but they also provide protection from high levels of adversity.[8]

Patterns of Attachment

Healthy attachment provides attention, approval, and recognition of success, which are critical to the development of healthy, happy, and self-confident children. Infants and young children with healthy attachment experiences learn to cope and deal with adversity, develop the confidence to explore their world, and obtain cognitive and social skills. While parent-child attachment is influenced by parent, child, and environmental factors, it is categorized into patterns (Table 6.5). Observing the pattern

(e.g., secure, insecure/avoidant, ambivalent/resistant) and helping insecure families move toward secure attachment build the child's trust, comfort, and sense of self-worth.

Temperament

Temperament is defined as inborn characteristics that describe an individual's emotional and behavioral response style across situations. Although biologic in origin, its characteristics evolve and develop over time and are shaped by the social environment (Box 6.2). Every characteristic is normal, even at extremes, but each predisposes the individual to behavioral, emotional, and/or functional difficulties by causing parental distress when there is a poor fit with expectations and values. While different from personality, which influences motivation, interest, and drive, temperament is crucial to understanding how children and adolescents interact with their environment, including their peers and families. For example, temperament influences an individual's social-emotional adjustment by affecting parent-child interactions, which has given rise to temperament types:

- *Difficult*: intense, slow to adapt, withdrawing, negative mood, and irregular rhythmicity
- *Slow to warm up*: low activity level, low intensity, withdrawing, slow adaptability, negative mood
- *Easy*: moderate to low intensity, fast adapting, approaching, positive mood, regular or high rhythmicity

The *goodness of fit* is the congruence between the child's temperament and the expectations, demands, and opportunities of the social environment, including those of parents, family, and daycare or schools or other community settings. Short- and long-term social-emotional adjustments are shaped by the goodness of fit between the individual's temperament and the social environment.

Family Assets

The Search Institute has identified relationships, interactions, opportunities, and values that provide SSNRs and help families thrive (Table 6.6). Children with these assets are more likely to have good mental health, regardless of family structure, income, education, immigrant status, community type, or other demographic factors. Importantly, these factors can be intentionally nurtured within a family and included in anticipatory guidance plans by PCPs.

TABLE 6.5	Attachment Patterns	
Pattern	**Parent**	**Child**
Secure	Is sensitive responsive, and available	Feels valued and worthwhile; has a secure base; able to explore and master, knows parent is available; becomes autonomous Engages with PCP, seeks and receives reassurance and comfort from parent
Insecure and avoidant	Is insensitive to child's cues, avoids contact, and rejects child	Feels no one is there for them, cannot rely on adults to get needs met, feels they will be rejected if needs for attachment and closeness are shown; asks for little to maintain connection and learns not to recognize their need for closeness and connectedness. May act fearful or angry with parent, may seek contact, then arch away and struggle, or may act extremely helpless or sad but not seek comfort or protection
Insecure Characterized by ambivalence and resistance	Shows inconsistent patterns of care, is unpredictable, may be excessively close or intrusive but then push away (seen frequently in depressed parent)	Feels they should keep the adult engaged because they never know when they will get attention back; is anxious, dependent, and clingy

• BOX 6.2 Characteristics of Temperament

- Activity level
- Intensity of reaction
- Adaptability or flexibility tolerance
- Persistence and attention span
- Distractibility
- Rhythmicity
- Threshold of response
- Approach/withdrawal
- Mood

TABLE 6.6 Family Assets

Types of Family Assets	Examples
Nurturing Relationships Healthy relationships begin and grow as family members show each other they care about each other's thoughts, feelings, statements, and value each other's unique and shared interests.	• Positive communication • Affection • Emotional openness • Support for sparks
Establishing Routines Shared routine, traditions, and activities give a dependable rhythm to family life.	• Family meals • Shared activities • Meaningful traditions • Dependability
Maintaining Expectations Expectations make it clear how each person participates in and contributes to family life	• Openness about tough topics • Fair rules • Defined boundaries • Clear expectations • Contributions to family
Adapting to Challenges Every family faces challenges, large and small. The ways families face and adapt to those changes together help them through the ups and downs of life.	• Management of daily commitments • Adaptability • Problem-solving • Democratic decision-making
Connecting to the Community Community connections, relationships, and participation sustain, shape, and enrich how families live their lives together.	• Neighborhood cohesion • Relationship with others • Enriching activities • Supportive resources

Modified from the Framework of Family Assets. Copyright 2012 by Search Institute, Minneapolis, MN. https://www.search-institute.org/wp-content/uploads/2018/02/Family_Assets_Framework.pdf.

Connectedness and Developmental Relationships

As an individual develops during childhood and adolescence, connections with others in schools, neighborhoods, and through religious or community activities can offer further attachment opportunities. These developmental relationships are close connections through which young people discover who they are, cultivate abilities, and learn how to engage with and contribute to the work around them. Relationships and experiences based on the individual's cultural identity, race, and ethnicity also help

TABLE 6.7 Developmental Relationships Framework

Element	Action
Express care: "Show me that you care."	Be dependable, listen, believe in me, be warm, encourage
Challenge growth: "Push me to keep getting better."	Expect my best, stretch my limits, hold me accountable, reflect on my failures
Provide support: "Help me complete tasks and achieve goals."	Navigate, empower, advocate, set boundaries
Share power: "Treat me with respect and give me a say."	Respect me, include me, collaborate, let me lead
Expand possibilities: "Connect me with people and places that broaden my world."	Inspire, broaden horizons, connect

Modified from the Framework of Developmental Relationships. Copyright 2012 by Search Institute, Minneapolis, MN. https://info.searchinstitute.org/developmental-relationships-framework-download.

form identity and add to a sense of meaning and purpose. The Search Institute draws attention to those relationships with an adult (e.g., teacher, coach), friend/peer, or sibling, in which both persons are fully engaged, experience, contribute to, and benefit from the interaction. Essential elements and associated actions of these relationships are found in Table 6.7.

Social-Emotional and Spiritual Development

Social development enables children to contribute in positive ways to family, school, and community, leading to awareness of social values and expectations, and building a sense of who they are and where they fit in society. *Emotional development* helps children understand what feelings and emotions are, gain emotional awareness of self and others, and learn how to manage emotions. *Spiritual development* provides inner resources and identity, interconnectedness, purpose or meaning to life, and transcendence; it is different from religion. Children and adolescents with positive social-emotional skills share feelings, manage themselves, relate and connect to others effectively (e.g., develop friendships), resolve conflict, and feel positive about themselves and the world. Critical skills include emotional regulation, tolerance of distress, control of impulses, flexibility of thought, ability to plan and work towards a goal, language development, abstract thought, working memory, and problem solving.[8] These skills also serve as a buffer against toxic stress by turning off the physiologic stress response and lead to improved cognitive, linguistic, self-regulation, and executive functioning skills, and improved moral outcomes.[8] Social-emotional skills are learned through modeling, nurturing, and practicing, and mastered through the complex interplay of developmental domains. For example, character traits, such as empathy and honesty (emotional domain) influence successful interaction with others (social domain) and contribute to a strong foundation for learning and problem-solving (cognitive domain).

Bright Futures identifies the key *components* of social-emotional development as[9]:

- *Empathy.* Being able to understand how others feel leads to empathy, which is also expressed in the generosity of action toward family and friends and volunteer activities.

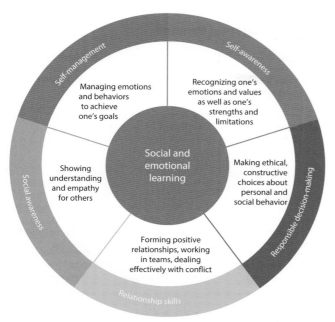

• **Fig 6.4** Social Emotional Learning Competencies. (From KidsMatter www.kidsmatter.edu.au. Adapted from The Collaborative for Academics, Social, and Emotional Learning [CASEL]. *Sustainable Schoolwide Social and Emotional Learning [SEL]: Implementation Guide*; 2006.)

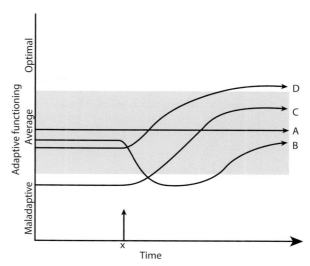

• **Fig 6.5** Pathways to Resilience. *Path A:* relatively steady course even with acute trauma or chronic adversity. *Path B:* normal course with overwhelming adversity and eventual recovery. *Path C:* normalization, or a major shift in the quality of adaptation from poor functioning to good functioning over time. *Path D:* posttraumatic growth with improved adaptive function following trauma or adversity. (From Masten AS. *Ordinary Magic: Resilience in Development.* Guilford Press; 2014.)

- *Competence and mastery.* In a safe relationship and environment, children explore and gain skills and knowledge that result in a sense of competence and a feeling of mastery. Accomplishments in school, arts, athletics, and community service contribute to the child/adolescent's identity and self-concept.
- *Autonomy and independence.* As children grow, their interests and abilities expand, and they are required to make more decisions. In this process, the parent role transitions to one of coach, giving guidance and helping youth build self-advocacy and self-care, leading to independence and autonomy.

The Collaborative for Academic, Social, and Emotional Learning identifies key *competencies*, which include self-awareness, social awareness, responsible decision-making, self-management, and relationship skills (Fig. 6.4). Two areas of assessment include resilience and self-regulation skills.

Resilience and Self-Regulation

Resilience is broadly defined as the ability to overcome difficulty and succeed in life. It can be learned, promoted, and supported through protective relationships, skills, and experiences. Children who are resilient have healthy social-emotional skills, specifically the intrapersonal skills of self-regulation, self-reflection, creating, and nurturing a sense of self and confidence, as well as interpersonal skills in which they can establish SSNRs. Assessing resiliency in children requires looking at both the supportive elements in the child's life as well as the threats to child development and adaptation (i.e., the level of stress and degree to which stress is cumulative or allostatic). Four patterns or pathways of resilience are identified in Fig. 6.5.[10]

Self-regulation involves a transition from reflexive responses in the newborn period to the ability to recognize and control one's thoughts and actions. Actions can either be automatic responses useful for threatening situations (e.g., fight or fight) or intentional responses that are conscious, proactive, and goal directed. When the brain recognizes a situation that requires a response, the automatic self-regulation system initially responds. As conscious self-regulation develops, the individual focuses and prioritizes action

and then modifies or controls the automatic self-regulation system (see Fig. 6.3). Self-regulation is influenced by the individual's abilities (e.g., attention, cognition, and impulsivity), temperament, genetics, and characteristics of their environment. People best learn to self-regulate when they experience loving and nurturing caregiving, are provided consistent and appropriate discipline, and have opportunities to learn and experience safe failure, or the opportunity to fail without fear of negative repercussions.

Spiritual and Moral Development

Social-emotional development includes matters of the spirit and mind. Spiritual integrity is fundamentally a sense of meaning and purpose: one has direction, control, and promise for the future. Morality is the quality that encompasses that which is right (justice or fairness) and that which is good (empathy or kindness). Faith, which is closely linked to spirituality, is the basis for developing beliefs, values, and meaning. Empathy, a fundamental moral emotion, is the ability to understand the condition of another and to experience a visceral or emotional reaction to that condition (i.e., to take the perspective of another). Mature morality is built through social interactions in which individuals mutually "reverse" their thinking: each strives to understand and feel how the other thinks and feels, and as a result, each deepens their own understanding and emotions. As children mature and experience life events, the foundation of their moral system is laid, and their values and beliefs are reflected in different behaviors at different ages as they gain greater cognitive and social skills. As moral integrity and spiritual values develop, healthy individuals achieve a positive sense of self, learn to value themselves and their contribution to the family and larger social system, and feel a sense of understanding and belonging.

Family and Community Influences on Mental Health of Children

SSNRs and environments are essential to children's wellbeing. Social determinants of health (SDoH) are conditions in which people live, learn, work, play, worship, and develop that affect a wide range of health, functioning, and quality-of-life outcomes and risks. For example, place (i.e., physical conditions), race, and social-economic status (e.g., poverty) significantly impact the connectedness a child, adolescent, or family feels to the neighborhood where they live and the community in which they participate. SDoH either supports the development of wellbeing or adds to the challenges faced by children and families. *Healthy People 2030* identifies improvements in economic stability (reducing poverty), social and community context, neighborhood, and environment as objectives for the decade.[11]

Parent Wellbeing and Caregiving Style

The largest factor that influences child mental health is family health and parent wellbeing. As such, the most effective strategies for promoting pediatric mental health are promoting family health and assisting parents to take care of their own mental health needs.[12] Parenting behavior may reflect efforts to "be like my parents were" or "not do things wrong, as my parents did with me." PCPs should acknowledge that parents are trying to do the best that they can and encourage them to relax and discover how to best interact with their child. However, parents come with their own life experience, stressors and changes, fund of knowledge (e.g., beliefs, education, strategies), temperament, perceptions (e.g., expectations, needs, desires related to other people's reactions), and degree of physical and emotional health. Research confirms that parents' personal history of being cared for significantly affects the quality of care provided to their children, as well as the powerful influence it has on their perceptions of child behavior, beliefs about children and childrearing, and ultimately their parenting behaviors.

Identifying parenting styles can be useful when working with parents. *Authoritative* parents are present, set limits but still listen to the child, and provide warmth and support, resulting in children who are friendly, self-reliant, and self-controlled. *Authoritarian* parents establish strict rules and expect the child to follow them ("Because I said so"), often punishing the child for not obeying, resulting in youth who may appear to follow the rules but stuff anger inside, resulting in lower social competence, self-regulation, and self-esteem. *Permissive* parents are warm and want to be their child's friend but are lax with rules, leading to youth who have difficulty with self-regulation, tend to be aggressive and impulsive, and have more social issues. Finally, *uninvolved* parents fulfill a youth's basic needs, but demand little of them and are not present or responsive, resulting in youth who lack self-control and have low self-esteem and confidence.

Newer parenting labels include the helicopter, snowplow/lawnmower parent, and the free-range parent. The *helicopter* parent is overly protective and thus controlling, wanting to protect the child from any danger and provide ultimate success. This parent micromanages everything about the child's life, wanting to be constantly aware of where the child is, and is intimately involved in every detail. The *snowplow* or *lawnmower* parent likewise desires the very best for their child and will go to any length to clear the path, removing any obstacle to future success. Though the motivation behind both of these is positive, children emerge with low confidence and feelings of inadequacy, often fearful as they see life through an overly protective lens, and sometimes harboring negativity toward the parent. *Free-range* parents believe that children are smart and capable, and do not need constant supervision. For example, their motto "Fail! It is the new success!" encourages parents to let youth go out into the world, giving them independence, free time, and self-directed play.

TABLE 6.8	Indicators of Mindset		
Indicator	**Growth Mindset**	**Fixed Mindset**
What does the individual think it takes to succeed?	Effort, practice	Intelligence, talent
What does the individual think makes a genius?	Hard work	Innate ability
What is the individual's typical response to new challenges?	Yes, please	No, thank you
How does the individual respond to setbacks?	Looks for new approaches and strategies	Blames others, becomes defensive, or gives up
What might you see if the individual experiences failure?	Tries again with a new approach	Lies about performance, makes excuses
What might you expect if you know the test is very difficult?	Sustained effort at studying	Cheating, procrastination

Growth Mindset. *Mindset* is an important part of a child's wellbeing, as it develops and stabilizes mental health, but also repairs previous damage. Families who encourage a *growth mindset* teach a child that hard work is at the crux of success and that effort and practice are contributing factors that lead to continued or expanded growth. Receiving praise for the process (i.e., effort, concentration, approach, patience) allows children to focus on learning rather than performing and develop an expandable mindset, which provides resiliency when dealing with failure. With a growth mindset, challenges are opportunities for growth, not fearful experiences of failure.

In contrast, children who are approached with a *fixed mindset* learn that success is due to a certain trait or talent, and when failure or challenge occurs, it is due to the lack of that trait or talent. These children often receive praise in the form of appreciation for a certain talent or trait (e.g., intelligence, musical/athletic ability) and their performance is their measure of worth. When they experience a failure, they have nowhere to turn, believing that talent is all they have, so they expend their energy trying to bolster their own self-perception by looking for an excuse, blaming someone, or comparing themselves to someone who did not do as well as they did. Table 6.8 shows indicators of a growth versus fixed mindset.

Family Functioning and Dynamics

The foundation of mental health lies in ongoing safe, stable, nurturing environments, but the initial groundwork is laid in families. The family is a dynamic social system that is usually the most powerful and constant influence shaping an individual's development and socialization. The family provides emotional connections, behavioral constraints, and modeling that affect the development of self-regulation, emotional expression, and expectations regarding behaviors and relationships. Parent satisfaction with parenting is an important outcome measure of how well the family is functioning as a family unit. Common themes exist within all families, and six key dimensions (Box 6.3) have a significant effect

Resources available to the family (e.g., social support network of extended family members, friends, and community), and financial and other material assets. Families with limited resources or social support networks are more vulnerable to stressful life events than are families with resources and support systems in place.

Transitions and stresses (e.g., financial strains, illness, marital strain, family transitions, losses, and lack of effective coping strategies) necessitate change. Some are normal, some anticipated, and others unexpected; all can have a significant effect.

Childrearing styles (e.g., caregiving behaviors, beliefs, and actions) influence the environmental milieu in which the child learns about the world. Certain childrearing styles (e.g., an uninvolved, permissive, or strict authoritarian caregiving style) are ineffective and have dire consequences for the child's emotional health.

Values (e.g., spiritual, religious, cultural) provide a framework to find comfort, joy, and solace, and to guide, explain, and understand events being experienced.

Roles and structures vary from one family to another, within an individual family, and as family members grow and develop in response to external demands; shifts in the role of one family member affect other family members.

Coping style of the family speaks to the ways that demands are met, transitions handled, and concerns resolved. Positive or effective coping is characterized as a creative response to a change or stressor that results in a new behavior or attitude. Coping styles reflect habitual patterns of action. Over time, coping effort develops into a coping style.

on family functioning, contributing to cohesiveness, adaptability, and positive communication. To assist parents and children across the family life cycle, especially during times of stress, the PCP must carefully assess these elements.

Family Routines, Rituals, and Celebrations. *Family routines* are activities done over and over in the same way that provides a dependable rhythm to life. By providing comfort and safety, they create a chance for trust and relationships and help individuals learn to deal with stress and transition by making everything appear normal. Routines help people know what comes next and provide organization, giving individuals the confidence to try new things and gain competence. They can decrease anxiety, lower resistance to tedious tasks, and send messages about values. Common routines include bedtime and wake-up, mealtimes, reading times, and playtime. Family *rituals* are routines with a symbolic value and are often linked to cultural or spiritual meaning. Rituals help people learn to work together and provide social support. Family *celebrations* that acknowledge even little milestones provide positive time and bring joy.

Family Communication. Communication is one of the most critical elements in any relationship. Healthy families demonstrate positive communication patterns, family cohesion, and adaptability. Family *cohesion* is an indication of the strength of the emotional bonding between family members, while *family adaptability* is the ability of a family to change its power structure, role relationships, and relationship rules in response to situational and/or developmental stress. Family communication patterns range from positive, respectful communication that conveys positive messages (e.g., empathy, reflective listening, supportive comments) to negative communication (e.g., double messages, double binds, criticism) that minimizes opportunities to share feelings. Family cohesion and adaptability are threatened and/or thwarted by

negative communication patterns, which can then result in a chaotic household marked by high family distress levels.

Listening attentively, showing interest, and taking time are critical to helping children identify, handle, and express feelings by accepting and acknowledging what is said. Emotional openness and warmth with affection allow family members to share feelings. Maintaining a strength-based approach, looking for what a child does well but not being afraid to talk about disappointment, is key. Family communication when facing problems includes talking about what to do, working together to solve problems, knowing there are strengths to draw on, and staying hopeful even in difficult times.

Assessment of Mental Health

The assessment of mental health status covers a broad range of dimensions, including social, emotional, and behavioral variables. Mental health assessment focuses on the child's behavior and on the protective, promotive, and risk factors in the child's environment (see Tables 6.3 and 6.4). Correctly pinpointing these factors requires a thorough history. The comprehensive child and family assessment model found in Chapter 5 gives the PCP a foundation, screening tools assist in collecting information, and the physical examination helps detect underlying physical conditions that may contribute to behavioral or emotional changes. Every primary care visit provides an opportunity to assess the quality of the verbal and nonverbal exchanges between children and their parents, giving specific attention to the child's emotions and energy, and the presence or absence of interaction among those present in the examination room. The PCP should also ask parents if they have any concerns or worries about their child's mental/emotional health or behavior or if they have seen a change in how they behave at home or at school. If a positive response is received, further symptoms analysis is warranted, including the degree of impairment, distress, severity of symptoms, frequency, intensity, duration, what is being done, and how helpful it is.

Underlying Principles

The way the PCP conducts the history and physical examination is as important as the information obtained. Many parents and children, especially adolescents, only share concerns after a long period of trying to solve the problem themselves. They may be upset, worried, or frustrated. Many are already reluctant to discuss symptoms because of the social stigmas surrounding mental illness. PCPs are more likely to get a clear picture of what is happening and gain the family's trust if they take the time to sit down and actively listen to the parent's and child's concerns. It is critical to avoid rapidly firing questions, restricting the history to a preprinted schedule of questions, searching the electronic health record, or taking notes that detract from giving full attention to the child and family. If a potentially significant but nonemergent problem is uncovered during an episodic visit, a lengthier appointment should be scheduled to avoid hurrying the assessment and potentially missing important data. While parental data is important, the PCP also needs to obtain the child's perspective using age-appropriate strategies.

To assess mental health, the PCP should[13]:
1. Remember the important role trust plays in interactions with families and providers.
2. Consider time when taking histories; set a return appointment to expand on clues/concerns.

3. View all family members as agents of change for the patient, the parent, and others around them.
4. Empower parents/children—help them become active problem solvers, rather than simply providing them with specific answers.
5. Listen with curiosity, empathy, and support.
6. Associate or connect ideas that emerge as concerns.
7. Record the individual's affect in responses, as well as specific answers.
8. Assess who the real patient is; parents often think it is the child or adolescent, but often it is the parent or other family members.
9. Identify family secrets—problems often stem from a family history of other issues (e.g., alcoholism, incarceration, mental illness, abuse).

Approaches to Behavioral Assessment of Pediatric Patients of Different Ages

Observations of infants and toddlers with their parents offer valuable clues to individual and interactional strengths and limitations. Structured and unstructured situations allow the observer to appreciate emotional exchanges and the quality of interactions. Unstructured play with dolls and/or toys provides a way for children to spontaneously express their feelings and emotions, offers the PCP an opportunity to ask questions within a nonthreatening context, and can help evaluate the history provided by parents. For example, if the concerning behaviors began shortly after the birth of a new sibling, providing a set of dolls (parent, child, infant) may help the child spontaneously express their emotional state).

Offer children in early and middle childhood the opportunity to draw a picture of themselves and their family and ask them to tell you about their picture. This process allows the time and space for children to collect and represent their thoughts as well as the opportunity for the PCP to evaluate the child's feelings and emotions. If problems and concerns become apparent, clarify details from the child's perspective in a nonthreatening and familiar way. The child in late middle childhood and adolescence should be interviewed separately from their parents. Most children and adolescents are comfortable talking about their feelings and experiences if they have a supportive listener.

It is important to clarify issues related to confidentiality with both the patient and the parent before initiating a mental health assessment. Tailor questions to the child's or adolescent's level of understanding, keeping questions simple and providing examples to younger children. Sample questions include:
1. "Tell me some of the things you do very well. What types of things do you have a hard time doing?"
2. "How are things going at home?" "What do you like to do with your family?"
3. "How is school going?" "Do you ever feel scared?"
4. "Many children have things they worry about. What worries you most?"
5. "Everyone feels angry at times. What makes you angry? What do you do when you are angry?"
6. "Tell me what you think the problem is from your point of view."
7. "You look very sad to me. Is there something that is making you sad?"
8. "If you could change one thing in your life, what would it be?"

History

Clarifying developmental milestones, including social, emotional, and cognitive skills, is crucial. It can be helpful to ask about prior

---

• BOX 6.4 Symptom Analysis

- Describe your child's behavior.
- What seems to make it better or worse?
- How have you tried to help your child?
- How does the behavior make you feel?
- How do think your child feels?

---

physical, occupational, and speech therapy as sometimes parents do not realize their child had a developmental delay. When collecting family health history, it is critical to check for any mental and developmental disorders in family members, including school failure, delinquency, substance abuse, learning disorders, reading problems, mood disorders, personality disorders, schizophrenia, attention-deficit/hyperactivity disorder (ADHD), autism, genetic syndromes, and birth defects. Beyond this initial data, symptom analysis, family, and additional stress histories can offer further insight.

Relationship as a Vital Sign

The AAP suggests that relationships be considered a *vital sign* and should be assessed and supported at every well-child visit. The vital sign concept emphasizes its importance in health promotion but also paves the way for secondary and tertiary interventions when needed. The acronym PRN (protect, relate, and nurture), provides a framework for evaluating each relationship (e.g., Does the parent protect, relate, and nurture the child during the visit?).

Symptom Analysis: Behavioral Manifestations

Parents are keen observers of their children, so it is wise to listen carefully to their observations and concerns. They may be troubled by behaviors that are developmentally normal, extremes of normal child behavior, and/or abnormal. By obtaining a clear idea of the concern (Box 6.4), the PCP assesses the parent's knowledge level about typical child development and behavior, clarifies which behaviors are developmentally normal but distressing to the parent, and/or confirms which behaviors fall outside the range of normal. With this information, the PCP can develop a mutually agreeable plan of care with the parent/child. Eliciting information from the child, as well as from teachers and others, can reinforce and/or compete with parent reports. It is important to obtain the big picture or contextual understanding of the child's behavior. For parents, underlying many behavioral concerns are:
- A lack of knowledge about healthy development and behavior
- Unrealistic parental expectations for child behavior
- Parental hurt or an inability to empathize with how the child feels
- A situational context that elicits or maintains problem behavior
- A behavior that negatively affects relationships or patient functioning
- Negative peer and/or teacher responses to and consequences of problem behavior
- A recent escalation, increasing frequency or severity of the behavior

Family Stress History

All parents face stress and feel overwhelmed from time to time. It is important to assist them to identify times or situations in which stress is greatest (Table 6.9). For example, certain developmental stages can be more taxing than others, and children often have

TABLE 6.9	Additional Stress History		
Topic	**Sample Questions**		**Potential Stressors**
Recent changes in the family, work, school, and other settings	What events or changes occurred in your family in the past year?		Job promotion (more travel or time away) Move or parent deployment
Recent changes in life circumstances, for better or worse, which provoke changes in the youth's perception of self, family, or feelings of relationship security resulting in self-blame or a sense of betrayal	Who lives in your home? Have there been any recent changes at home or changes in family relationships? Any new health issues or deaths? Have parents separated or divorced or remarried? Has an older sibling moved away?		Changes in household composition (e.g., births, expansion to include elders) Risk of loss or loss of attachment figure(s) New role or responsibilities presenting a psychological challenge Child or sibling with special healthcare needs
Recurring experiences that a youth may deal with	Tell me about the things you find difficult or stressful as a parent, especially in caring for this child? What is overwhelming? Who do you have to help you with childrearing?		Parent overprotection, lack of supervision, restrictive or over permissive caregiving Control struggles, ineffective limit-setting strategies, harsh discipline practices
Parents' personal history of being cared for: it is important to have the parents share memories, good and bad, of their childhood and what they liked and disliked about the caregiving they experienced	Tell me about your most favorite and least favorite memories of growing up. How is your caregiving similar to and different from the caregiving you received as a child? What are your expectations for your child?		Unhappy childhood, poor role models, unrealistic academic, athletic, or social expectations for the child, harsh discipline, poor family communication Reliance on the child by the parents for emotional comfort and support

an increase in behavioral problems in the late afternoon hours as fatigue (for child and parent) increases and energy levels lag. Anticipatory guidance helps parents predict and minimize these "at-risk" times or situations. Parents with mental illness have an increased risk of role strain and parenting difficulties depending on how the illness affects their perceptions and coping skills. It is helpful to ask about potential and actual family-related stressors or changes because parents may not perceive these as sources of stress for their child. For example, a parent may welcome a job promotion that includes travel; however, this change may stress the child who worries how that travel will impact their life. Further, routine screening of mothers for symptoms of postpartum depression is merited during health visits, especially in early infancy (see Chapter 9).

Social-Emotional Development and Behavioral Screening

Routine social-emotional and behavioral screening should be a part of all health maintenance or well-child visits.[9] PCPs can incorporate age-appropriate screening efforts, which are discussed in Chapters 9 through 13, but there are also specific social-emotional screening tools available to PCPs (Table 6.10). When assessing behavioral concerns, a behavioral diary or log informs the PCP about the situational context and severity of the behavior, especially if it includes input from the child, parent, and teachers. With all screening efforts, attention must be paid to scores, problem behavior witnessed over time, and attenuating circumstances. Suspicious or ambiguous findings may warrant a referral for a more thorough evaluation by a skilled psychologist or multidisciplinary developmental assessment team.

Physical Examination and Diagnostic Studies

The PCP should complete a thorough physical examination with particular attention to mental status, physical anomalies, and the neurologic system. Documenting mental status includes:

- Appearance (groomed?)
- Attitude/interaction (cooperative, guarded, avoidant?)

- Activity level/behavior (calm, active, restless?)
- Psychomotor activity (abnormal movements, tics?)
- Speech (loud or quiet; flat in tone, or full of intonation; slow or rushed; does the child understand and express appropriately?)
- Thought processes (coherent, disorganized, flight of ideas, blocking [inability to fill in memory gaps], loosening associations [shifting of topics quickly though unrelated], echolalia, perseveration?)
- Thought content (delusions, obsessions, perceptual disorders, phobias, hypochondriasis?)
- Impulse control (aggressive, oppositional?)
- Mood/affect (depressed, anxious, flat, guarded, fearful, irritable, elated, euphoric?)

If exam findings suggest problems, laboratory tests (e.g., hemoglobin, thyroid screen, antistreptolysin O titer, serum lead level, serum electrolytes, serum/urine screen for alcohol/illicit substances) should be considered. At times, the family history, developmental, and neurologic findings may warrant the need for specialized imaging (e.g., magnetic resonance imaging, computed tomography, positron-emission tomography scan) and/or referral to specialists (e.g., endocrinology, genetic testing/counseling).

Mental Health Management Strategies

Management of mental health in pediatrics is two-pronged: (1) promoting thriving, while (2) preventing and mitigating toxic stress. The most effective approach within the limited time constraints of the pediatric visit is for PCPs to (1) use a strengths-based, eco-biodevelopmental framework that examines how life-course and developmental trajectories affect normative development, (2) identify biological health threats and address environmental risks early, and (3) proactively build wellness, buffer adversity, and foster resiliency.[14] As in all encounters, the PCP must focus on both the child and family. Strategies discussed here are also relevant to many pediatric developmental problems and are applicable to the management of neurodevelopmental and mental health problems, as discussed in Chapter 29. Key components of mental health promotion include strengthening relationships, supporting family

<table>
<tr><td colspan="2">**TABLE 6.10**</td><td colspan="3">**Screening Tools for Social-Emotional Development**</td></tr>
</table>

Screening Tool	Age Group	Time/What Screens	Cost
Ages and Stages Social Emotional, ed 2: https://www.brookespublishing.com/product/asqse-2/.	1–72 months	10–15 min to complete; 1–3 min to score Social-emotional development	Cost; Brookes Publishing
Pediatric Symptom Checklist 17 and 35 items: https://www.brightfutures.org/mentalhealth/pdf/professionals/ped_sympton_chklst.pdf	4–16 years; Youth version; multiple languages	<5 min to complete; 2 min to score General psychosocial screening of externalizing, internalizing, and attention behaviors	Free
Survey of Wellness in Young Children: www.floatinghospital.org/The-Survey-of-Wellbeing-of-Young-Children/Overview.aspx	<5 years	15 min to complete Developmental milestones, behavioral/emotional development, family risk factors	Free; Tufts Medical Center
Strengths and Difficulties (SDQ): sdqinfo.org	Parent report 4–10 years and 11–17 years Youth report 11–17 years Teacher report 4–10 years and 11–17 years Baseline and follow-up	Five scales: Emotional symptoms, conduct problems, hyperactivity/inattention, peer relationship problems, prosocial behavior; and total difficulties score	Copyrighted, not in public domain
Child Behavior Checklist 2 (CBCL): https://aseba.org/	Preschool (18 months–5 years) School age (6–18 years) for parent and teacher Youth (11–18 years)	Emotional and behavioral	Cost; requires training
Temperament: www.preventiveoz.org	4 months–6 years	Temperament questionnaire and profile Behavioral advice	Cost ($10 annual membership)
Temperament and Atypical Screening (TABS): www.brookespublishing.com	11–71 months	15 question screener takes 5–10 min to complete 55 question assessment takes 15–20 min to complete Detects detached, hypersensitive and hyperactive, reactive, and dysregulated behaviors	Cost; Brookes Publishing
Sensory Processing Disorder Checklist: www.spdstar.org/basic/symptoms-checklist	Infant/toddler, preschool, school age, adolescent, adult	10–15 min to complete; interpretive	Free; Star Institute
Adverse Childhood Questionnaire (ASE-Q): https://centerforyouthwellness.org/cyw-aceq/	Child, teen, and teen self-response	2–5 min to complete	Free; Center for Youth Wellness

functioning and caregiving, and providing strategies to facilitate social, emotional, and cognitive growth.

Strategies to Build Relationships

Relationships are so key to child health and the future of the world that there are several national and international approaches recommended that can be incorporated in the PCP's mental health management. The following examples are well known.

Essentials for Parenting

The Centers for Disease Control and Prevention (CDC) Essentials for Parenting program (https://www.cdc.gov/parents/essentials/index.html) identifies three key components, along with tips, videos, and resources for each.[15]

- Communicate—interact with your child by taking time to listen, let your child know when they have done something good, read with your child, make time to laugh, and avoid distractions.

- Create structure and rules—these provide consistency and predictability, and follow-through by providing choices, establishing routines, and preventing temper tantrums.
- Give directions—get your child's attention, give the direction, check compliance, and use discipline and consequences by rewarding, praising, and paying attention to the positive; or ignoring, distracting, using time-out, and natural and logical consequences.

The First 1000 Days

The First 1000 Days initiative (https://thousanddays.org/) is an international movement focused on healthy nutrition as an essential building block for brain development. This initiative is grounded in the science that neural pathways were formed in utero and neuronal growth in the first 2 years of life are the foundation of human behavior and function across the lifespan. It is aimed at creating a strong start to life by optimizing nutrition, supporting SSNRs, and incorporating an eco-biodevelopmental framework to optimize brain development. This action framework provides general principles for assessing and teaching by *exploring* the socioemotional home environment, *building* relationships (reciprocity), *cultivating* development, and *developing* parent confidence and competence.

Additional Strategies

Two additional strategies to build relationships are easily adapted in PCP practice. The first is *Serve and Return* (https://developingchild. harvard.edu/resources/5-steps-for-brain-building-serve-and-return/). Just as sports players serve the ball and it is returned, this strategy applies this concept to relationships to build healthier brains and social interaction. It involves five steps: (1) notice the serve and share the child's focus of attention, (2) return the serve by supporting and encouraging, (3) give it a name, (4) take turns and then wait, keeping the interaction going back and forth, and (5) practice endings and beginnings. In summary, a response that is sensitive, responsive, and attentive to the child's action provides a rich environment for continued interaction that becomes increasingly complex as a child grows.

The Circle of Security model illustrates the ongoing process of attachment, coregulation, and learning, where a child ventures out from a secure base to explore the world, growing in independence. Once things become difficult, the child returns to their safe haven for security, seeking help in regulating their distress. The model (Fig. 6.6) applies to children and adolescents of any age and is available in several languages and formats (www.circleofsecurityinternational.com).

Strategies to Promote Family Functioning and Parenting

By and large, parents want to do a good job and primarily need education and skills that support them, while providing help managing stress. These supports can easily be interwoven into routine anticipatory guidance provided at well-child visits or be introduced as a brief intervention. There are many options to choose from when working with families, and selecting two or three favorites as mainstays works well for PCPs (Box 6.5).

The Parenting Pyramid from the Incredible Years Parenting Program illustrates positive caregiving with a focus on both the parent (skills and strategies) and the child.[16] The base and foundation of the pyramid, where most time should be spent, centers on connecting, teaching, and celebrating the individual child. From the base upward, clear and consistent limits, rules, and follow-through help direct pediatric behaviors. The top layers of the pyramid address correcting behaviors a child or adolescent knows but did not adhere to. If there is a problem at one layer of the pyramid, the solution is often in the layer below.

The *Five R's of Early Childhood Education*[17] include (1) reading together every day; (2) rhyming, playing, and cuddling every day; (3) developing routines around meals, sleep, and family fun; (4) rewarding children with praise for successes to build self-esteem and promote positive behavior; and (5) developing relationships that are strong and nurturing. These activities are easy for parents to engage in while building skills and minimizing stress. The *Reach Out and Read* (www.reachoutandread. org) program provides parents of infants from 6 months to the start of school with a book at clinic well visits and guidance to promote reading together. The *Imagination Library* (www. imaginationlibrary.com) similarly provides free books through affiliate organizations for children until 5 years of age, regardless of socioeconomic status. The aim is fostering a love of reading in all children.

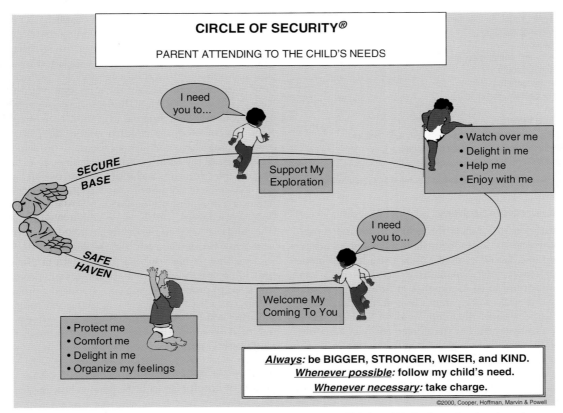

• **Fig 6.6** Circle of Security. (From Circle of Security Network; 2000. http://circleofsecuritynetwork.org/ the_circle_of_security.html.)

• BOX 6.5 Positive Caregiving Strategies

Attend to the Child Individually

- Respond to child's bids for attention with eye contact, smiles, and physical contact.
- Provide guaranteed child led special time daily: No interruptions, no directions, and no interrogations.
- Allow the child to make reasonable choices. Believe in the ability to learn, improve, and grow.
- Comment on child's appropriate and desirable behavior frequently and positively throughout the day.
- Be available both physically and emotionally to teach and model behavior.
- Do things with them, not just for them.
- Know your child's personality, temperament, dreams, and value your child's thoughts and opinions.
- Know your child's friends and encourage positive involvement with friends and activities.
- Prevent secondary gains for the child's minor transgressions by having no discussion, physical contact, perhaps even eye contact; be neutral and simply state the preferred behavior.
- Show up at their concerts, games, and events. Visit their schools.

Listen Actively

- Paraphrase or describe what the child is saying.
- Reflect the child's feelings.
- Share the child's affect by matching the child's body posture and tone of voice.
- Avoid giving commands, judging, or editorializing.
- Follow the child's lead in the interaction.
- Insist on family meals, especially as a child gets older.

Convey Positive Regard

- Communicate positive feelings (e.g., love) directly.
- Give directions positively, firmly, and specifically.
- Provide notice before requiring the child to change activities.
- Label the behavior, not the child.
- Strive for consistency.
- Praise competency and compliance; say thank you.
- Celebrate accomplishments.
- Apologize when appropriate.
- Avoid shaming or belittling the child.

Know Yourself as a Parent

- Understand and accept yourself, be aware of your own feelings.
- Acknowledge your strengths and accept uniqueness.
- Take care of yourself and treat yourself with respect.

Discipline as a Parenting Strategy

Discipline is education that molds the behavior, mental capacities, or moral character of an individual. It is related to behavioral expectations and should be used to teach youth appropriate behavior and to ensure safety. In contrast, *punishment* is loss, pain, or suffering administered in response to behavior; it should never include withdrawal of the parent's love or affection. Based on appropriate expectations, discipline modifies and structures behavior using positive behavior reinforcement (catching the child being good) more than negative reinforcement of undesirable behavior (time-out). Discipline reinforces social norms, helps a child fit into daily family and school routine, and makes childrearing fun.[9] Parents' abilities to discipline appropriately are determined not only by their knowledge of appropriate ways to discipline, but also by their responsibilities and stressors, their "fit" with the child, and their past experiences. The manner and intent

of providing discipline are as important as the techniques used. When coming from an SSNR, children and adolescents learn to choose acceptable behaviors and develop self-control.

Expectations must be appropriate to the age, development, personality, temperament, strengths, and weaknesses of the individual. If expectations are too high, children feel pressured and may feel shame or guilt or internalize failure even when they are doing their best. Expecting a child to do their "best" can be overly demanding because no one can "do their best" all the time. In contrast, expectations that are too low diminish an individual's value and make them feel as if the parent has no faith in them. Knowing where expectations begin (parent-driven or child-driven) and how they fit the individual youth and family is important. Clearly stating expectations and identifying limits and consequences so both the child and the parent understand provide security for the child and prevent frustration, distrust, and further problems. When mistakes and failures are accepted and expected, resilience develops by helping children learn to view them as opportunities to learn. A realistic assessment of the child's performance, emphasizing strengths and discussing strategies that lead to success, prepares children to approach future obstacles and disappointments constructively.

One of the easiest ways to provide discipline is by establishing structure, including family routines, which is simply information about how the family does things. Parents teach skills by modeling the desired behavior, but often, especially with younger children, by simply stating exactly what is desired followed by immediate reinforcement. As children mature, they can learn to negotiate with their parents to help set the rules. Praise, with a specific description of what was accomplished, paired with the social values, is good reinforcement (e.g., "Great job sharing with your sister. It makes me proud that you know how to get along."). In these situations, children should move toward behavior ownership, now self-rewarded by the satisfaction of doing something well.

Consequences help youth learn to socialize. Appropriate planned consequences are timely, logically related to the behavior, appropriate to the child's age and developmental capabilities, and meet the significance of the infraction. Natural consequences (e.g., "You want to sleep in, but you are going to miss the bus, so I guess you wear your pajamas to school.") are often more accepted (and remembered). As children mature, they can be involved in determining the consequences for their misbehavior. Time-out, being sent to the child's room, restricting a favorite activity, turning off the television, and losing phone or video game privileges are examples of commonly used consequences. The basic principles for discipline are outlined in Box 6.6. One example is the loss of privilege(s), which, along with a brief explanation, teaches the child the "why" of the discipline (e.g., "You can't ride your bike tomorrow because you left it in the street.").

Teaching problem-solving is also a part of discipline. Begin by providing opportunities to make choices and decisions, then teach the steps to problem-solving (i.e., stating the problem, expressing needs, considering alternatives, agreeing on a solution, and implementing and following through with the agreed-on solution). By taking time and letting the child work through the process, the child's self-confidence is built.

Managing Temperament

The PCP can discuss with the parents how they view their child's temperament, how it fits with the parent's temperament or that of other family members, and what parent-child strategies can be used if conflicts emerge. The intent of these strategies is to alleviate guilt and frustration, support the parenting role, and assist parents to develop skills that enhance positive behaviors rather than exaggerate difficult temperamental characteristics. Supporting both the parents and child can prevent significant problems in the future. Understanding a child's unique temperament helps parents better understand the child's behavior, especially when behaviors are perceived as confusing or problematic. As parents identify traits in their child's temperament, they gain a tool for understanding their child and for managing responses to a variety of situations. In addition, parents benefit from understanding their own temperaments since goodness of fit between the child and parent is crucial (e.g., to a parent with a high activity level, an adolescent with an average or low activity level might seem lazy or dull). It is important to remind parents (and children) that no temperament characteristic is bad. For example, the persistent individual may be "stubborn" when faced with discipline but may work for an extended period to understand a math problem or to master a technique for sports or musical performance.

Temperamental traits that parents find difficult to manage tend to engender parent criticism and irritability, power struggles, and restrictive caregiving, and may be associated with behavior disorders, although temperament alone is not a risk factor for maladjustment. Parent psychological functioning, marital adjustment, childrearing attitudes and practices, and social support factors all influence the role temperament plays in the development of behavioral disorders.

The goal for the PCP is to reframe temperament traits in such a way that they become more understandable and workable, enabling the parent-child duo to achieve goodness of fit. Helpful strategies for parents, teachers, and others include (1) recognizing the child's innate behavioral qualities as temperament expressions, (2) understanding how temperament relates to behavior and that temperament does not change but can be worked with and reframed, and (3) encouraging parents to express their feelings and learn to develop strategies to work with the traits they find most challenging. Specific strategies for different temperament traits are found in Table 6.11.

• BOX 6.6 Additional Principles of Discipline

- Parents should talk with each other and agree on how to handle discipline and their child's misbehavior. They should distinguish between discipline and punishment.
- Interactions with children should focus on discipline or teaching, rather than punishment.
- Treat children with respect and empathy, even when being reprimanded for misbehavior.
- Misbehavior can often be prevented. When a child appears willful, bored, or out-of-sorts, distraction and active engagement with the parent (e.g., giving the child something to do; talking to, playing with, dancing with the child) can stop misbehavior before it starts.
- Be alert to when children reach their limits (i.e., are nearing "meltdown" because they are tired, hungry, or overstimulated) and intervene to prevent problems. Children in a meltdown stage are not able to relate rationally to a parent's reasoned explanation or request; the underlying problem—hunger, lack of sleep, and so on—must be dealt with first.
- Parents may also need a "time-out" from the child to cool down and regain self-control and they should have a plan for help when they need respite.
- Use flexible limit setting ("You have to wear a coat, but you may choose the blue or red one.").

Corporal punishment is unnecessary and has the potential to cause physical and/or psychologic damage.

TABLE 6.11 Strategies to Help Children With Different Temperaments

Temperament Characteristic	Strategy
Activity level—amount of child movement across different situations	Recognize activity level and plan high-energy activities (long walks, family outings). Plan activities to keep children busy in situations when quiet is required (such as during religious services).
Intensity of reaction—amount of reactive energy shown in response to both positive and negative events	Help children recognize their responses to positive and negative emotions. When an overresponse occurs, teach children how to modify their behavioral response to their feelings.
Adaptability/frustration tolerance—how quickly the initial response pattern can be modified in desired direction	Provide reassurance when things don't go as planned. Teach how to deal with disappointment. Do not avoid situations in which frustrations may occur as part of developing emotional maturity is experiential.
Persistence and attention span—how long a child pursues activity especially in face of obstacles	Teach strategies to help stay on track. Help parents set realistic expectations of the child's attention span.
Distractibility—how easily external events or stimulation interfere or divert from ongoing activity	Take development and distractibility into consideration when doing tasks that require concentration (i.e., homework, quiet time).
Rhythmicity—regularity and predictability of sleep, feeding, and daily activity patterns	Keep normal sleep (including nap), wake, and feeding schedule in mind when planning activities and outings. Use normal elimination patterns as a guide during toilet training.
Threshold of response—sensitivity or amount of stimulation needed to evoke a discernible response	Recognize that not all children use the same strategies for calming and adapt to the child (i.e., use care not to overrespond to more mild situations such as when juice spills or things break).
Approach or withdrawal—response to anything new (e.g., food, people, places, toys, etc.)	Recognize that new situations may be stressful Teach skills and provide opportunities to deal with discomfort in a supporting and loving environment.
Mood—amount of pleasant, joyful, and friendly behavior typically shown in contrast to unpleasant, crying, and unfriendly behavior	Use positive reinforcement for good mood responses to situations. Ignore negative mood responses.

Social and Emotional Strategies

Helping infants, children, and adolescents develop healthy social-emotional skills comes easily to some parents, while others require direction and guidance. Some basic approaches include:

- Early infancy—help parents be attentive to their baby's likes and dislikes, sensitivities, and signals
- Older infancy/early childhood—allow the child to express and recognize the full spectrum of human emotion, from good to bad, and to develop skills to cope with negative emotions
- Middle childhood—support the child's self-esteem and help them explore a wide range of interests; avoid overscheduling, provide plenty of "downtime" and relaxation
- Adolescence—provide clear expectations, sensitive support, pride in achievements, and positive affect toward the adolescent

Self-Regulation, Resilience, and Executive Function Skills

Three skills that all children need to develop are self-regulation, resilience, and executive function. These skills are learned in stages. *Skill acquisition*, or show-and-tell, occurs as the child has the skill explained, then demonstrated, receives positive feedback with effort, and then practices it. *Skill fluency*, or "practice makes perfect," comes as the child practices the skill in various settings, links it to similar situations, and is reminded of when to use the skill. *Skill maintenance and generalization*, "You've got it!", comes as the parent reinforces use of the skill.

Self-regulation is the ability to manage emotions and behavior. Remaining calm in the face of changes, challenges, and frustrations is at the heart of self-regulation, which is also called *self-control*. In contrast, emotional dysregulation occurs when the child "melts down" and is unable to handle strong emotions and can be instantaneous, intense, and immediate, or build over time and lead to an outburst. An individual's temperament and environment contribute to the ability to self-regulate. Self-regulation is taught by skill isolation and practicing the encouraged behavior in a supportive environment, as well as practice runs, or breaking things into smaller steps (i.e., scaffolding). Staying calm and taking time to help the child evaluate what went wrong and why, and how it can be better next time, are other effective strategies. (See https://child-mind.org/article/can-help-kids-self-regulation/; https://nurture-andthriveblog.com/how-to-teach-your-child-self-regulation/.)

Resilience is defined and understood within the context of stress, as it is the child's response to it. Therefore PCPs need to assess the stresses the child has experienced and how the child is doing in response. Resilience is fostered by having SSNRs that allow choices, skill mastery, and safe opportunities for failure, as well as having chores and responsibilities, learning to show appreciation, building friendships, working as a team, learning to ask for help, and developing self-esteem and a sense of control.

Core life skills, which are developed and fine-tuned in adolescence, require advances in *executive function*. There are three areas of executive function, including working memory, cognitive flexibility (flexible thinking), and inhibitory control, which includes self-control or regulation. The Center for the Developing Child[18] identifies five ways to help build core skills: (1) practice with real-life situations (focus and flexibility), (2) spot and plan for triggers (awareness and self-control), (3) take another's view of stressors (awareness, flexibility, self-control), (4) focus on personally motivating goals (planning, flexibility), and (5) build on positive memories and small successes (focus, planning).

Promoting Strengths

A *strength-based approach* allows both the PCP and parent to work together to optimize child outcomes and minimize the effects of toxic stress. At times, parents may need help to identify strengths in their child, especially if parent/child goodness of fit is poor or parents are too stressed themselves. Strengths can be classified as *general* (e.g., independent, works well with others, creative, and curious), *social* (e.g., comforts others, follows routines, has a good sense of humor), *language* (e.g., expresses needs, participates in discussions, asks who, what, where), *literacy* (e.g., enjoys reading, tells stories, connects stories to life), and *math* (e.g., understands patterns in nature, thinks logically, remembers math facts). Additional information about each of these strengths is available from Understood.org (https://www.understood.org/en/friends-feelings/empowering-your-child/building-on-strengths/types-of-strengths-in-kids).

Developmental assets are another approach to identifying strengths in the child or family. Backed by evidence from the Search Institute,[19] 40 assets are identified and serve as building blocks that help children become healthy, happy, and contributing members of society. Assets are applicable regardless of sex or gender, culture, socioeconomic situation, or environment. The more assets a child has, the more likely the child is to make wise decisions and choose positive lifestyles while avoiding harmful or unhealthy choices. Developmental asset lists for adolescents (12–18 years of age), middle childhood (ages 5–9 and 8–12 years of age), and early childhood (3–5 years of age) are available and have been translated into 14 different languages.[19]

Sparks, also identified by the Search Institute,[20] are interests, talents, and passions that motivate children to grow, learn, contribute, and make positive choices about their activities and time, while leading them to express their unique personalities and contribute to the world. Children who thrive or flourish have knowledge of their sparks and are surrounded by adults who support the development of these sparks. The 10 most common sparks identified by American adolescents are creative arts, athletics, learning (e.g., languages, science, history), reading, volunteering (e.g., helping, serving), spirituality or religion, nature, ecology, and environment, living a quality life (e.g., joy, tolerance, caring), animal welfare, and leading.

Prevent and Mitigate Effects of Toxic Stress

Because PCPs typically have established ongoing relationships with children and their families, they are able to integrate their knowledge of brain development, the child and family, and assessment skills to promote mental health by: (1) helping children figure out how to turn off or minimize their stress response (primary prevention) and (2) intervening early if unable to turn off the stress response (secondary and tertiary prevention).[14] PCPs are ideally positioned to help identify family issues, prepare families and children for developmental changes/challenges, understand temperament issues, and prepare for predictable life events that impact children (e.g., school readiness).

For PCPs, early detection, intervention, and addressing unanticipated life events are the main components of secondary prevention. Social, emotional, or behavioral problems may emerge, even in the context of healthy families and positive childrearing approaches. Early recognition of pediatric stress and mental illness is facilitated when parents have a realistic understanding of their child's development and PCPs actively screen for developmental red flags. Secondary prevention also involves working collaboratively to identify and implement appropriate management strategies or to explain and reinforce the value of mental health recommendations. For example, children with a known adversity but no actual symptoms and families with multiple SDoH can benefit from early referral to programs like Healthy Steps and other community networks.[14]

Tertiary prevention addresses major losses and trauma (e.g., sexual or physical abuse, parent marital problems/divorce, substance abuse, parent psychiatric conditions) and/or significant behavioral symptoms that impair daily functioning. In addition, any child who experiences trauma should be referred to a mental health specialist for further assessment and intervention, even in the absence of behavioral manifestations of distress. For parents, especially those who may not understand the need for referral, it is helpful to frame the child's behavior as a "normal response" to a stress and/or trauma, with the goal of referral being to minimize harm and maximize the child's growth and development.

Violence Prevention

Across the pediatric lifespan, the prevention of violence requires use of a public health model that addresses the intersection and complexity of causes and risk factors. Primary prevention of violence begins with strengthening parenting skills and creating SSNRs within families. PCPs can teach families how to incorporate protective factors (Box 6.7) and minimize risk factors (Box 6.8) by encouraging parents to be actively involved with their children, supervising youth and their activities, and monitoring the child's peer group (having friends who engage in conventional, nonviolent behaviors). Parents may need additional information about the effects of indirect violence (media and technology) and ways to minimize exposure. Working to strengthen the developmental competencies includes educating children at an early age about violence and its prevention, teaching anger management and strategies for fight prevention (role-playing), promoting self-defense strategies (learning a martial art), and discussing ways to manage difficult or potentially violent and/or dangerous situations (Boxes 6.9 and 6.10). All PCPs should be particularly attentive, as gun violence became the leading cause of death of youth under age 20 in the United States in 2020, surpassing deaths from car accidents, cancer, and even COVID-19 (see Chapter 1).

Efforts should also focus on helping improve the environment for youth in schools and communities. Strategies include supporting diversity training and bullying prevention programs in schools, supporting after-school and community programs, working to make neighborhoods and schools safe places, involving the community in a commitment to prevent violence, and addressing the issues of media violence and of condoning violence as a way of life. Advocacy efforts focused on enforcing current and encouraging additional sale regulations of consciousness-altering substances to youth and supporting legislation that aims to decrease firearm violence are needed.

Secondary prevention is focused on screening for potential problems, including assessing for violence risk factors at all visits, screening for drug and alcohol abuse problems, asking about firearms/weapons in the home (their presence, use, storage, and access), and caring for children exposed to or threatened by violence by addressing any violence-related physical or emotional problems in the primary care setting. Other effective interventions include community programs that make home visits to mothers of new babies, especially those in low-income and/or adolescent

parent families; support groups for children who have suffered trauma or loss or witnessed violence (e.g., school counseling for traumatic experiences); and referral of families to community support programs, such as Big Brothers/Big Sisters of America.

Tertiary prevention focuses on treatment and rehabilitation programs for offenders and treatment for victims and their families. This can be difficult and costly and yield only mixed results.

The CDC's Comprehensive Technical Package for the Prevention of Youth Violence and Associated Risk Behaviors[21] identifies six key strategies to help communities focus on successful violence prevention. It remains the gold standard for the prevention of youth violence. The strategies are to promote family environments that support healthy development, provide quality education early in life, strengthen youth's skills, connect youth to caring adults and activities, create protective community environments, and intervene to lessen harms and prevent future risk. PCPs are especially helpful in promoting SSNRs, but they are increasingly becoming involved outside their practices to ensure protective environments through community engagement, advocacy, and policy development.

• BOX 6.7 Protective Factors Against Youth Violence

Individual Protective Factors
- Intolerant attitude toward deviance
- High intelligence quotient
- High-grade point average (as an indicator of high academic achievement)
- High educational aspirations
- Positive social orientation
- Popularity acknowledged by peers
- Highly developed social skills/competencies
- Highly developed skills for realistic planning
- Religiosity

Family Protective Factors
- Connectedness to family or adults outside the family
- Ability to discuss problems with parents
- Perceived parent expectations about school performance are high
- Frequent shared activities with parents
- Consistent presence of parent during at least one of the following: when awakening, when arriving home from school, at evening mealtime or going to bed
- Involvement in social activities
- Parent/family use of constructive strategies for coping with problems (provision of models of constructive coping)

Peer and Social Protective Factors
- Affective relationships at school that are strong, close, and pro-socially oriented
- Commitment to school (invested in school and in doing well at school)
- Close relationships with nondeviant peers
- Membership in peer groups that do not condone antisocial behavior
- Involvement in prosocial activities
- Exposure to school climates characterized by:
  - Intensive supervision
  - Clear behavior rules
  - Consistent negative reinforcement of aggression
  - Engagement of parents and teachers

From Centers for Disease Control and Prevention, Injury Prevention & Control Division of Violence Prevention. *Understanding and Preventing Violence: Summary of Research Activities Summer*, CDC; 2013. https://www.cdc.gov/violenceprevention/youthviolence/riskprotectivefactors.html.

• BOX 6.8 Risk Factors for Serious Youth Violence

Individual Risk Factors

- History of violent victimization
- Attention deficits, hyperactivity, or learning disorders
- Deficits in social cognitive or information-processing abilities
- Poor behavioral control
- History of early aggressive behavior
- Low intelligence quotient
- High emotional distress
- History of treatment for emotional problems
- Antisocial beliefs and attitudes
- Involvement with drugs, alcohol, or tobacco
- Exposure to violence and conflict in the family

Family Risk Factors

- Authoritarian childrearing attitudes
- Harsh, lax, or inconsistent disciplinary practices
- Low parent involvement
- Poor monitoring and supervision of children
- Low emotional attachment to parents or parents
- Poor family functioning
- Low parent education and income
- Parent substance abuse or criminality

Peer and Social Risk Factors

- Association with delinquent peers
- Involvement in gangs
- Social rejection by peers
- Lack of involvement in conventional activities
- Poor academic performance
- Low commitment to school and school failure

Community Risk Factors

- Diminished economic opportunities
- High concentrations of poor residents
- High level of transiency
- High level of family disruption
- Low levels of community participation
- Socially disorganized neighborhoods

Modified from Centers for Disease Control and Prevention (CDC). *Youth Violence: Risk and Protective Factors.* CDC. www.cdc.gov/violenceprevention/youthviolence/riskprotectivefactors.html.

• BOX 6.9 Talking With Teens About How to Keep Out of Trouble

- Do not carry a weapon; instead, "fight clean" (i.e., discuss the issue in conflict). Carrying weapons only makes one less safe; pulling out a weapon begins a cycle of retaliation.
- Do not go into harm's way. Avoid being around fights because the cycle of escalation and retaliation often involves innocent people.
- Avoid being caught alone; stay with friends.
- Do not be provoked into fighting. Words are said, and names are called, not because the names are true, but to provoke anger and a fight.
- If one becomes involved in a fight, try to end the incident on equal ground; that way anger is more likely to be diffused. The person who wins often takes on the aggressor role; the loser then becomes the scapegoat. Thus, violence continues and becomes cyclic.
- Suggest discussions with friends about ways to handle potential situations in which a gun or knife might be brandished.
- Do not join gangs or associate with individuals who turn to violence as a way of settling differences.
- Report threats of school violence to adults.

• BOX 6.10 Talking With Teens About Sexual Abuse/Assault

- Males as well as females can be victimized.
- Alcohol intoxication or the use of drugs is a major factor in sexual assault. Prevention includes not placing oneself in harm's way by using such substances.
- Manipulative verbal threats and physically trapping the victim are common tactics used by perpetrators.
- Reluctance to report gang or date rape is common. However, keeping the rape a secret only leads to self-doubt and delays healing. The teen should report the rape immediately and seek professional counseling.

Counseling and Brief Interventions

In addition to providing anticipatory guidance and assistance in developing healthy coping strategies, the PCP can provide a variety of services that assist families in need of mental health services. Many PCPs work in collaboration with mental health providers in integrated care models. Community services, such as home visits, strengthen families and are often aimed at a high-risk population (premature babies, adolescent mothers, low-income families). Referrals for art, music, or movement therapy allow a child/teen self-expression, which improves wellbeing and confidence, and the opportunity to work with intense emotions, poor social skills, and low self-esteem. These therapies often use physical activity and sensory integration to engage different parts of the brain, leading to relaxation and improved mood. Their focus is on the process, not the product of these therapies, with the parent or adult asking the youth questions (without directing or judging) and talking about feelings that emerge.

The PCP can schedule brief or very brief interventions as billable office visits to provide effective counseling strategies accomplished in 5- to 15-minute (maximum 30) time periods. These interventions serve as interim treatment while awaiting specialist care. For example, active monitoring and follow-up, behavioral approaches (e.g., checklists, reward charts, logical consequences, special times with parents [time-in] as well as time-out), and supportive counseling can all be effective brief interventions.

Mindfulness

Mindfulness is defined as paying attention, being intentional, staying in the present moment, and being nonjudgmental. The goal of mindfulness is to take negative thoughts about one's past or future fears and listen to these emotions and thoughts, recognizing that feelings rise and subside, and thoughts are just thoughts. This process allows one to wait out the emotional over-reactions (e.g., fight or flight) and return to a calm state (i.e., intentional regulation). Among other benefits, mindfulness helps social and academic performance; improves sleep, self-confidence, and immune function; changes maladaptive stress coping; and reduces anxiety and depression. It can be prescribed for parents and/or children during healthcare visits or taught to parents to help them cope and in turn set them up to teach their children. Helpful techniques include taking "awareness walks" around the block, noticing sounds, sights, feelings, and smells; abdominal breathing; or focusing on a snow globe and watching the chaos of the snowflakes settle down. Multiple initiatives, websites, classes, and apps (e.g., Calm, Breethe, Insight Timer) are also available to help learn this technique.

Parent-Focused Interventions

One of the most effective ways to help the parent-child relationship is to reframe the parent's perception of their child by identifying the child's strengths and avoiding comparison with other children. This approach can be used at any age, is easy to begin, and can be used proactively at every visit, as it starts by identifying child and parent strengths as contributors to child skill development. For example, a PCP can reframe a parent's negative perception of their child as destructive of everything in the house to a positive lens by identifying the child as curious and investigative, like many inventors or scientists. Such reframing allows an opening for next steps, rather than a dead-end label.

Collaborative Problem-Solving: The Nurtured Heart

The nurtured heart approach holds that difficult behaviors are red flags for *lagging skills* and the inability of children to move forward as they struggle to meet parent or adult expectations.[22] There are six collaborative problem-solving (CPS) tenets: (1) emphasize (solving) problems rather than (modifying) behavior; (2) work together (bi-directional) with the child, not unilaterally or imposed by the parent; (3) use *pro*active not *re*active problem-solving (timing is key); (4) understanding precedes helping (children need skills to meet expectations before behavior can be corrected); (5) children do well if they can, rather than if they want to; and (6) children prefer doing well. Lives in the Balance (https://www.livesinthebalance.org) has a wealth of resources (e.g., Assessment of Lagging Skills, worksheets, FAQs, Bill of Rights) for PCPs interested in learning more about this approach.

Motivational Interviewing

Motivational interviewing (MI) establishes a solid base for counseling, even in brief time periods, and especially when there is an established partnership between the PCP and family. Using open, respectful, encouraging communication, and nonjudgmental questions and reflective listening, MI provides information and then guides the child/family to identify beliefs, values, strengths, and readiness to change, followed by self-guided behavioral change strategies. Taking a difficult situation, identifying strengths, and working with the child and/or family to problem solve not only helps at the moment but also models problem-solving for other difficult or challenging times. The stages of change are identified in Table 6.12. Other MI tools include agenda setting (client determines priorities), getting permission, using open-ended questions to start, reflective listening, summarizing, eliciting self-motivational statements (i.e., change talk), and upfront clarifications of willingness, importance, and/or confidence. Additional resources for MI can be found at https://case.edu/socialwork/centerforebp/practices/motivational-interviewing/motivational-interviewing-resources.

Common Factors Intervention

Common factors are aspects that positively influence the patient-provider relationship's ability to change patient behavior.[23] The factors are considered common, as they are effective across mental health issues, settings, and providers, as well as across the life span. They can be used in brief interventions and/or to close difficult conversations and maintain the provider-patient therapeutic relationship. The eight common factors include alliance, empathy, shared goals, positive regard, affirmation, and optimism, genuineness, and a skilled, experienced clinician. The *HELP* mnemonic highlights the factors in this approach:

TABLE 6.12	How People Change	
Stages of Change	**Intervention by Healthcare Provider**
Precontemplation: not considering change	Increase awareness
Contemplation: considering change, but ambivalent	Facilitate the resolution of ambivalence
Preparation: willing to accept direction, anxious about change	Help the client develop an action plan
Action: learning the new behavior	Solve problems related to new behavior
Maintenance: stable in new behavior	Review successes and reinforce healthy behavior
Relapse: reappearance of old behavior (a process, not an event)	Move into action once again

*H*ope (provide realistic expectations based on strengths and assets)
*E*mpathy (in communication)
*L*anguage (using the family's words to show their perspective is understood)
*L*oyalty (through support and commitment)
*P*ermission (to go more in-depth); *P*artnership (working together to overcome); *P*lan (make measurable goals with clear follow-up planned)

Cognitive Behavioral Therapy

Cognitive behavioral therapy (CBT) is an interactive, short-term, problem-oriented therapy focused on how one's thoughts, feelings, and behaviors interact. The goal in CBT is to modify unrealistic assumptions and change them by correcting cognitive distortions, reframing negative expectations, improving social skills, and improving problem-solving. This process of cognitive restructuring includes five steps:
1. Identify the situation—What made me upset?
2. Name the feeling—What was my response (usually fear and anxiety, sadness and depression, anger, or guilt and shame)?
3. Determine the thought—What am I thinking that is making me feel this way? How is this a thought problem (all-or-nothing, emotional reasoning, overgeneralizing, overestimation of risk, must/should/never, self-blame, catastrophizing)?
4. Challenge the thought—What evidence do I have for this thought? Is there an alternate way to look at the situation? What would someone else think?
5. Make a decision—Do things mostly support my thought or not?

Parent Training Models/Behavioral Therapies

Basic behavioral principles underlying parent training are to (1) implement positive reinforcement to promote positive behaviors; (2) ignore low-level provocative behaviors; and (3) respond in a clear, safe, consistent manner to unacceptable behaviors. The same principles inform behavioral therapies used in the classroom. The Substance Abuse and Mental Health Service Administration (SAMHSA) maintains a national registry of evidence-based programs and practices based on behavioral therapies, limit setting, and problem-solving (https://www.samhsa.gov), some of which are listed in Additional Resources.

Mental Health: Referral and Follow-up

While the PCP is ideally suited to work with families on promoting and developing mental health and helping families deal with concerns, a mental health referral is sometimes needed. The degree of impairment and the persistence of the problem are key concepts in determining if a referral is indicated (see Chapter 29). Bright Futures identified situations that may be appropriate for referral, including (1) emotional dysfunction in more than one area (home, school, peers, activities, mood), (2) acutely suicidal or signs of psychosis, (3) diagnostic uncertainty, (4) poor response to treatment, (5) parent request for referral, (6) behavior creating discomfort for the PCP, and/or (7) a previous difficult social relationship with the PCP.[9] Communicating about the referral in positive terms (e.g., an opportunity to grow/improve oneself), rather than in negative terms, helps overcome barriers some people feel when approaching mental health intervention. Because specialized mental health services are in such shortage, the PCP needs to facilitate the process, helping the family find appropriate care and secure an appointment.

The PCP not only monitors mental health during well-child visits, but also initiates follow-up when issues arise, with the type and frequency dependent on the issue and the family. When referrals are made, follow-up with the PCP is essential to ensure the child/family followed through and are comfortable with the consultant and/or plan of care. Maintaining a central and ongoing, supportive relationship between the PCP and the child/family is critical when managing social and emotional issues. In this position, the PCP provides continuity, as well as integrates subsequent care, regardless of where the care is delivered and who provides it (see Chapter 1).

Behavioral Issues

It is common for behaviors exhibited by children or adolescents to concern parents, relatives, teachers, or other adults. The issues of concern are often developmental or variations of normal for which the PCP can provide education and reassurance, either through anticipatory guidance given during well-child visits or during brief intervention visits. Newborn sleep, crying and colic, postpartum depression, toilet training, temper tantrums, breath holding, learning challenges, school refusal, risk behavior, tobacco use, self-injury, and social media are just a few examples. Common developmental issues are discussed by age group in Chapters 9 through 13, while specific mental health issues as well as neurodevelopmental and inherited vulnerabilities are discussed in Chapter 29.

Behavioral issues can emerge from issues of nature and/or nurture. Behaviors that emerge from issues surrounding *nature* include temperament and goodness of fit, neurodevelopmental and inherited vulnerabilities (e.g., autism spectrum disorder [ASD]), and medical conditions (e.g., brain injury, premature birth, auditory or visual disorders, medication effects). Behaviors that emerge from issues surrounding *nurture* include caregiving that is either too lenient or too controlling, disruptions in parent-child relationships/attachment affecting how the child views the world and/or self, and serious life stressors (e.g., ACEs).

It is helpful to remember that all behavior has meaning and is often based on a need. Behaviors may be indicative of stress that is greater than the child's ability to cope at that moment, or it may indicate a maladaptive response. The goal for the PCP is to understand the behavior not only from the perspective of the parent but

also from the child. The antecedent-behavior-consequence (ABC) technique is helpful in analyzing and understanding any behavioral situation, but it can also be helpful in teaching the parents how to handle the behavior (Table 6.13). This allows an assessment to be made and a plan to be formulated.

The PCP can also use a four-visit approach, where the *first visit* focuses on the complete mental health assessment, identifying strengths, as well as using the ABC method to identify the problems or issues that need to be addressed. If extended time is available, work can begin on deciding what strategies to be used. If not, the family should be asked to return within the week for a *second visit* to establish a clear approach. The child/family are involved in determining the issues and the management strategies, but the PCP bears the responsibility of guiding the discussion. During the first or second visit, the PCP should also acknowledge the effort it requires to be a good parent, and the fact that children instinctually want to do well if they have the skills to do so. In addition, it is often helpful to provide a brief intervention, such as reframing the behavior and/or pointing out skills that the child lacks that are contributing to the problem (e.g., it is not laziness; it is that she has not yet learned how to get dressed). Providing a skills acquisition framework or "basic training" can give the parent a focus and the child an area in which to succeed (Box 6.11). These strategies can be used for a variety of behaviors, but work well in developing self-calming, social, and anger management skills. The *third visit*, after a week or two, focuses on progress and addressing difficulties. If needed, further visits can be scheduled, but a final visit 6 to 8 weeks after the initial visit is important to ensure that progress has been made. If it has not, or there are other red flags (Box 6.12), a referral should take place.

TABLE 6.13	ABC Strategy for Assessing and Managing Behavioral Difficulties	
	For Assessing Behavior	**For Management**
Antecedents	*What led up to this?* The events, actions or circumstances that happen immediately before the behavior (when, where, who, what)	Avoid or prepare for situations that are likely to cause behavior, and, as possible, give cues
Behavior	*What did the child do?* The observed behavior in detail, what need is not getting met	Interpret, ignore, teach, or manage behavior—give it meaning and modify response
Consequences	*What did you do?* The action or response that immediately follows the behavior, including feelings	Remain calm, not reactive, and consistent; model or show what to do, rather than tell what not to do

• **BOX 6.11** Basic Skills Training

Step 1: Provide practice of the appropriate behavior with feedback
Step 2: Praise and reinforce effort
Step 3: Model or point out others doing that skill
Step 4: Prompt the child to use the behavior when the situation arises

The behavior is:
- Frequent
- Persistent over time
- Uncommon for child's age
- Maladaptive: causes serious changes in emotional maturation or social or cognitive functioning
- Turned inward (e.g., depression, self-destruction)
- Turned outward (e.g., complaints, aggression)
- Disruptive
- Distancing (e.g., withdrawal, denial, somatization)

The following section organizes common behavioral issues/concerns using the following framework: (1) difficulties in parental or interpersonal relationships, (2) social difficulties, (3) emotional difficulties, (4) bereavement, (5) difficulties with sensory perception, (6) recurrent physical symptoms, and (7) bullying.

Relationship Difficulties: Parental/Family

As noted earlier, SSNRs are key to child wellbeing. When they are missing, disrupted patterns of attachment emerge along with unexplained withdrawal, fear, sadness, or irritability; a sad and listless appearance; no seeking of comfort or response to comfort; failure to smile; watching others closely but not engaging in social interaction; and failure to ask for support or assistance. If any of these symptoms are evident, it is critical to intervene as soon as possible.

The relationship between parent and child is influenced by parenting knowledge and style as well as the child's development and temperament. Impaired parenting occurs when there is a mismatch between the two that results in inappropriate stimulation, inconsistent care, inappropriate supervision, developmentally inappropriate behavioral expectations, harsh words, child rejection, child abuse, or neglect. Parents often face challenges when trying to adapt their parenting skills to the developmental needs and behaviors of their children. This mismatch may surface as verbal dissatisfaction with their role, exacerbation of tensions between the parent and child, or inappropriate communication with the child. Child behaviors that may indicate impaired parenting include acting out, developmental regression, and other aberrant behaviors. Because of the unique characteristics of each person in a family, parenting strategies may be less successful with one child than with another, or the entire family unit may be dysfunctional due to parent and or larger family stressors or problems.

Management

Using the relationship as a vital sign (assessed at every visit) and offering strategies that build relationships and promote family and parent functioning help prevent problems, while also allowing the PCP to get to know the family. When relationship concerns are evident or expressed, a thorough mental health assessment is the first step to help identify some of the more specific issues. Once issues are identified, the PCP may use counseling and brief interventions based on parent-focused training or refer the parent and patient to more intense programs and therapy.

Social Difficulties: The Shy Child, the Fearful Child, the Child With Lack of Moral Integrity

Children who struggle socially may lack social skills, may be shy or fearful, or may lack a moral conscience or integrity. Some children are by nature outgoing and therefore more social, while others are quiet, reserved, deep thinkers, and cautious. Others may only be lacking the skills to help them become more social. Helping parents know and understand their child's strengths and temperament allows the parent to help facilitate their child's acquisition of missing or underdeveloped social skills. Age-related social skills are discussed in Chapters 9 to 13.

Shyness is a common pattern of social inhibition with unfamiliar people or novel objects, or in unfamiliar situations, and is related to a temperamental disposition toward withdrawal and often linked to family factors. Children with *social withdrawal* (vs. shyness) have a lower rate of social interaction overall and do not warm up to social situations. Shy children are slower to approach peers or initiate play with an unfamiliar peer; they often spend more time observing the situation and others before engaging. Infants have an inborn inhibition bias, as they respond to unfamiliar events with anxiety, distress, or disorganization and socially withdraw. During early childhood, the inhibition bias persists (e.g., irritability, withdrawal, and clinging to the parent in new situations), but it diminishes by middle childhood. Elementary school children who are shy are often viewed by their peers as likable but shy; these children continue to make fewer social approaches and may be ignored or neglected by their peers. Behavioral inhibition in social situations can be adaptive and also indicate optimal self-regulation and conscience development. Although most shy children do not develop internalizing disorders later, extremely shy toddlers may be at risk for social withdrawal in later childhood and for developing an adolescent anxiety disorder.

Fears and phobias can also create social difficulties. *Fear* is the occurrence of various avoidance responses triggered by the anticipation or exposure to particular stimuli (e.g., person, object) or a state of apprehension in response to a threatening situation. Fears are considered a normal part of development; they also have a developmental function. Infants typically react fearfully to loss of physical support, heights, and unexpected stimuli. Toddlers experience separation anxiety and fear physical injury and strangers. Preschoolers fear imaginary creatures, animals, darkness, and being alone, and may demonstrate some persistent separation anxiety. Fear of animals and darkness extends into middle childhood, but safety, natural events, and school- and health-related fears dominate. In preadolescence and adolescence, fears of bodily injury, economic and political catastrophes, and social fears are central. In contrast, *phobias* are persistent, extreme, and irrational fears often distinguished from fears by their magnitude and maladaptiveness. They are determined by multiple factors, including genetic influences, temperament, parental mental health problems, and individual conditioning histories. Fear is an evolutionary protective trait in that it allows individuals to identify and avoid threats; however, it becomes problematic when it impacts daily living and social functioning. True phobias occur in only 5% of the population, yet they are seen in 15% of children referred for anxiety-related problems. Fear and phobic reactions typically involve symptoms of autonomic arousal. The symptoms of autonomic arousal in those with phobias may evolve into panic attacks or phobic-avoidant reactions.

A *lack of moral integrity* or conscience is not a clinically defined condition; however, some children lack an age-appropriate capacity to respect others or the environment, judge behavior as right or wrong, and express empathy or remorse. These children frequently engage in antisocial behaviors (e.g., social aggression, conduct disorder, oppositional defiant disorder). Contributing factors include temperament, negative experiences in infancy and childhood (e.g., parental depression, unresponsive parenting, abuse), and environmental damage to neurologic systems. While all children demonstrate negative behaviors at some point (e.g., lying, hitting, refusing to share), the child who lacks moral integrity, or a conscience, expresses little or no remorse for the behavior; demonstrates a callous demeanor; lacks internalization of a sense of justice, fairness, or right and wrong; fails to develop an ability to self-regulate behavior; and continues antisocial behaviors beyond the expected developmental age. The lack of moral integrity is a key component of antisocial behavior and delinquency.

Management

Parenting the shy child with warmth, sensitivity, and responsiveness fosters security in attachment and social competence. Social-emotional strategies help build much-needed skills. Some examples include focusing on strengths and building confidence, preparing shy children for new situations (e.g., visiting new settings), identifying a sensitive adult to whom they may turn with requests or concerns, and negotiating time to watch and observe before having to engage in play or other activities. Parents can praise brave behavior but should avoid over comforting, as it reinforces the fear. In middle childhood, playdates, practicing show-and-tell, and extracurricular activities help children learn the skills to overcome the urge to remain shy. In contrast, parent insensitivity and a lack of responsiveness foster a sense of insecurity in the child as well as predict social withdrawal and associated internalizing disorders (e.g., depression, anxiety).

Most fears are short lived, not serious, and have no association with adult mental health problems. Warmth, sensitivity, and responsiveness foster a sense of security for the fearful child. Strategies that are helpful include acknowledging the child's fear as real while remaining calm, without belittling the child or the fear. Children's fears are contextual in that fears emerge when children perceive they are alone, unsupported, and/or taken off guard. When a child is afraid, it is important to let them know they are not alone and that you can work together to be more prepared in the future. PCPs should point out that fears can be protective and reassure the child about measures that are in place to provide security. Helping the child express their fears and rate the fear (e.g., up to my knees, my stomach, or my head) and using one-sentence self-statements, like "I can do this; it is not a big deal," help the child develop coping skills. Treatment of fears and phobias may focus on improving parent mental health, parent-child behavior management skills, and parent role satisfaction and self-efficacy. Parents should be careful to model behaviors that do not emphasize fear avoidance. Parents must be cautioned against using fears as a form of behavioral control (e.g., threats of abandonment during early childhood, threatening a child with a "shot") or as a discipline strategy (e.g., leaving a 3- or 4-year-old alone in a dark room or with a dog). When the fear negatively affects a child's (over the age of 5 years) functioning, developmental progress, learning experiences, or level of comfort, treatment can include contingency management, CBT, and family interventions.

Early and assertive intervention for the child with lack of moral integrity can help the child develop a healthier moral self and decrease antisocial behaviors, especially if treatment emphasizes developing moral judgment and a conscience. Storytelling, especially the child's personal narrative, can be used to explore issues. Interaction with older children who demonstrate more mature moral reasoning may be helpful. Discussing books or watching shows or films together allows for discussion of moral dilemmas and behaviors. Encourage parents to monitor the child's access to internet and computer games. Assist in clarifying values (e.g., ask the child or adolescent to talk about what is most important

to them, or to describe what characteristics of other people [and themselves] they see as being the "best" or most desirable). However, if these baseline strategies are unsuccessful, referral to a psychiatric/mental health provider is needed.

Emotional Difficulties: The Upset, Angry Child With Underdeveloped Coping Skills

Children who are upset often respond in anger to a perceived threat (e.g., fear, hurt, embarrassment). Small disappointments (e.g., broken toy) can become overwhelming as they do not have context or developed coping skills. Children may be frustrated and have difficulty expressing themselves, or they may be frustrated by a problem that is beyond their capabilities. Young children act out, expressing themselves physically (e.g., hitting, kicking, biting) when they do not have the words to say what they want or how they are feeling about minor events. Frequent episodes of emotional dysregulation are often found in children who are inflexible and/or prone to have poor adaptation, frustration tolerance, and problem-solving skills. Learning to name, understand, and process emotions takes time and requires opportunities to observe and practice, especially with adults with whom the child has positive, nurturing relationships. It is also important to remind parents that children who are tired, hungry, out of sorts, uncertain, overwhelmed, or anxious are more likely to have difficulty handling emotions, even though they are otherwise able.

Management

Early intervention is essential for children having difficulty coping or self-regulating. Teaching parents to use positive strategies and supporting them in the process is a basic but effective approach. Having the family keep a log or diary noting patterns (e.g., place, time of day, people, events, behaviors before/warnings the child is about to or actually loses control) is also helpful. The long-term goal is for the child to learn to develop the skills that are lacking. In general, encourage collaborative problem-solving and remind parents:

1. Not to take their child's emotions personally (as the emotion is not typically being directed at them).
2. Stay calm and patient. Structure and routine give predictability and help children remain calm.
3. Be present, stay connected, and focus on what is going well, not what is wrong.
4. Avoid being hurried, especially during times of transition.
5. Schedule times to be together to play and inject life with positive daily activities.
6. Do not expect the worst; this self-fulfilling prophecy can prove true.
7. Have realistic expectations for the child's developmental stage and individual skills. Just like you would never expect someone to run a marathon on their first day, putting a child in a situation beyond their capacity is a recipe for disaster.
8. Communicate clearly and emphasize positive choices rather than prohibitions.
9. Give the child tasks that can be accomplished, and do not put them in situations that outstrip their ability, even if it means breaking a task down into small, attainable parts. Remember that humans need to practice new skills and children work at slower speeds than adults.
10. Eliminate trigger buttons. Putting away a favorite toy when friends come over or attempting to get one more thing done during nap time or lunchtime may make the child feel overwhelmed or trigger an outburst.

11. De-escalate. Remove the child from an environment when escalating behavior happens to allow the child to calm down and regroup. This may mean physically removing them from a location or negotiating social space between peers during a disagreement. By allowing distance and time to reset, the youth can return to the activity less frustrated and aggressive and can experience success.

To help children develop lacking skills, parents are encouraged to use the following strategies, liberally reinforced with praise for calm behaviors and any progress that is seen. *First*, make a CALM plan. Determine activities (e.g., LEGOs, coloring) and teaching strategies that are calming (e.g., deep breaths, blow bubbles, count to 10). Create a safe spot for the child, using "time-in" to help the child learn to regulate and identify a cue/phrase to communicate when calming is needed (e.g., "I think I need to do LEGOs"). *Second*, talk about feelings/emotions and work to figure out not only what was upsetting but also how to handle it. With young children, starting with familiar emotions, such as mad, sad, happy, and scared is helpful. Then create an anger thermometer (e.g., level 1 = happy; 5 = getting angry;10 = ready to explode) and identify how the child's body is feeling at each level. With older children and adolescents, ask them to identify where in their body they feel or house their emotion. Both help to ground and associate emotions with their physical experience and may even counter a sympathetic nervous response. *Third*, teach empathy and kindness through understanding the situation. Practice seeing the other side or experiencing the world from another's perspective. This is emotional exercise. When periods of dysregulation occur, it can be challenging to understand how others are experiencing the situation; however, parents can go back and debrief, perhaps helping the child revise negative assumptions and be more flexible, optimistic, and relaxed toward others. *Last*, take time to brainstorm solutions to problems and negotiate conflicts. Then practice what the child needs to say. The bottom line—insist on making amends, which is distinct from punishment. Instead, it is making things right. However, if behaviors are severe or become more frequent or self-directed, causing injury to self or others, pets, or property, referral is needed.

Bereavement: Loss and Grief

Grief is a feeling of distress, sorrow, and loss, whereas *bereavement* is the process of dealing with loss. Many people use the terms grief and bereavement interchangeably. *Mourning* is the psychological process set in motion by loss of a loved one. The death of someone important to a child is one of the most stressful life events, and for children and adolescents, the death of a parent or sibling is a significant, often life-changing loss. A cast of losses occur across the pediatric lifespan, including the death of a pet, loss of a friend, parent separation/divorce, deployment, or deportation, as well as losing one's home (e.g., financial, moving, or natural disaster). Most children experience at least one significant loss before they reach adulthood, with an estimated 5% losing one or both parents to death before they are 15 years old.

The clinical picture of bereavement and grief depends in part on how one understands death. In the first 2 years of life, death is perceived as separation or abandonment, with no real cognitive understanding of death or ability to use the emotional resources to deal with loss. The central issue is the sense of loss or abandonment due to temporary causes (e.g., parent travel, sibling hospitalization, natural disaster), long-term causes (e.g., parent separation, foster care placement), or permanent causes (e.g., death). Loss of a family member is particularly difficult because it results in the loss of love and support from that person, and often has a significant effect on family routines, functioning, and resources. In early childhood, children perceive death as a continuation of life under different circumstances, with death personified and often perceived as a punishment. By age 5 years, children begin to grasp the irreversibility of death, although they struggle to understand the specific loss of the loved one. Adolescents become more abstract and philosophical about death; however, they may not fully grasp the social and cultural beliefs that adults attribute to death and dying. Children understand and process death at their developmental capacity; however, bereavement resurfaces, and the significance of the loss is reworked at each subsequent developmental stage. For example, a child who loses a parent at age 4 years codifies memories of that loss, carrying those 4-year-old memories with them, which continue to shape their understanding of loss as they mature.

Grieving infants and 1-year-olds cry out or search for the absent parent, refuse the attempts of others to soothe them, withdraw emotionally, appear sad, and no longer engage in age-appropriate activities. Sleep and feeding are often disturbed, and they may display developmental regression and react to reminders of the missing parent with apathy, anger, or crying. For the older child, grief is a process that unfolds over time. Initially, children may seem emotionally unmoved, but the initial shock and denial give way to depressive symptoms that can last for weeks or months. Depressive symptoms include sadness, feeling depressed, vomiting, bed-wetting, poor appetite, weight loss, insomnia, crying, internalizing symptoms (e.g., headache, stomachache), anxiety, guilt, and idealization of the person who died. Anger and even rage are common reactions to the death of a parent, typically directed at the surviving parent and others in the immediate family as well as peers. Identification with the deceased is common and needs to be assessed to determine whether it furthers or inhibits development. Similarly, a fantasy connection to a dead parent can develop and may be helpful. Guilt and responsibility are typical issues in early and middle childhood but are less problematic in adolescence. In contrast, adolescents often manifest a sudden "maturity," along with numbness, regrets, disorganization, and despair before closure and reorganization are achieved. It is not unusual for adolescents to develop stronger ties with friends and to distance from family while grieving.

In general, children at higher risk for pathologic bereavement or depression have a previous history of individual and family problems. Symptoms of bereavement that should concern the PCP and merit referral to a mental health specialist include long-term denial and avoidance of feelings, suicidal wishes and preoccupation with death, distressing guilt about actions taken or not taken, preoccupation with worthlessness, persistent anger, decline in school performance; social withdrawal, persistent sleep problems, or hallucinations beyond transitory experience of hearing the voice of, or seeing the image of, the deceased.

Management

It is critical for children to have an adult who can be an effective source of support and involvement, as well as a focus for reactions to loss. There are several ways to support youth through bereavement:
1. Be honest. They need to know what happened even if they do not ask. Considering their age, tell them as simply and honestly as you can. Do not use words like "asleep" or "lost," as young children may understand that literally.
2. Know that grief takes time.

3. Involve children in funerals or ceremonies. They need to see/ participate in the rituals around death as much as they can, as these activities provide even young children with an important way to grieve, especially if such involvement is supportive, appropriately explained, and congruent with the family's values.

4. Help children express their feelings. They need to work through thoughts and feelings related to the loss. Be available to talk and answer questions. Find ways for them to express feelings (play, writing a letter, drawing, music). If they are old enough, it is helpful for them to anticipate a range of difficult feelings. Books about death, loss, and grieving geared to various developmental levels may be helpful.

5. Share your feelings. Parents often need to be reassured that showing their own feelings (e.g., disbelief, guilt, sadness, anger) is normal after a loss; it is also helpful to the youth to let them know how the adults in their world are feeling and coping. Sharing feelings about and memories of the family member who died is helpful.

6. Provide routine and support. Maintain family routines as much as possible to provide security. Extra "time in" for closeness and comfort is essential. Prepare them for and minimize any changes if possible.

7. Remember that grief resurfaces. Because bereavement resurfaces at subsequent developmental phases, prepare families about the need to deal with grief at each subsequent developmental level. Grief can come in unpredictable waves and times ("grief bursts"). The PCP must assess the child's symptoms over time as a possible manifestation of a new stage of bereavement.

8. Get extra help if needed. Any child who loses a parent before age 5 years warrants referral. Those children who become overly preoccupied with death, have persistent grief, persistent loss of performance, or feel like they would be better off dead should also be referred for further counseling.

Difficulties With Sensory Processing

Sensory input comes from our primary senses (i.e., vision, hearing, touch, taste, smell), from position (proprioception), and through movement (vestibular). Sensory modulation describes the individual's ability to regulate and organize the intensity and nature of response to sensory input. Children with sensory difficulties often respond inappropriately to input, perceiving sensations that most individuals sense as pleasurable or positive to be painful, irritating, or unpleasant, and who may demonstrate extreme behaviors (e.g., dysregulations in reaction to overwhelming physical sensations, or being overly aggressive in seeking stimulation). This inappropriate response affects the individual's ability to appropriately adapt to daily life situations, learn, regulate attention and mood, and function in many social situations. The child who is *sensory overresponsive* responds too much, for too long, or to stimuli of weak intensity. The child who is *sensory underresponsive* responds too little or needs extremely strong stimulation to become aware of stimuli. The *sensory seeking/craving* child responds with intense searching for more frequent or intense stimulation.

Children with sensory processing disorder (SPD) face many everyday challenges. They may be sensitive to touch, pulling away from hugs and cuddling; have trouble with transitions, family gatherings, parties, and vacations (things considered fun by most people); do best in an environment that is predictable and routine; have rigid control in an attempt to manage sensory input; and, although able to perform developmentally typically tasks, require

substantially more effort than their peers and/or not be able to sustain function or perform at 100% for developmentally typical time periods.

Children who are overresponders have difficulties with clothing, physical contact, light, sound, and/or food. Children who are underresponders may have little or no reaction to stimulation, pain, or extreme hot or cold and have higher injury risks. Children who are sensory seekers are on perpetual overdrive and often in trouble at home, in school, and in structured settings because of their need for sensory stimulation. In addition, muscle and joint impairments affect posture and motor skills and can result in decreased tone, poor muscle control, and frequent unintentional injuries. Children with dyspraxia have difficulty recognizing and distinguishing shapes and textures, may have poor handwriting, or may have an altered ability to perform tasks such as tying shoes, using buttons, or dressing themselves.

Infants with sensory processing issues may be colicky or fussy, have eating and sleeping difficulties, be fearful of movement, and resist being held or comforted. In early childhood, they may not engage in purposeful interactive play; have delayed development; be defiant, irritable, and stubborn; resist transitions and certain activities; and have feeding, dressing, and sleep issues. By middle childhood, they may have trouble with handwriting, understanding steps in a game, or organizing schoolwork; may be able to perform in school but may come home and experience dysregulation because they exhausted their coping skills earlier in the day; have difficulty with transitions; and be easily frustrated. Adolescence can bring trouble with social interactions, learning in the classroom, and physical skill development. They are at risk for difficulty making friends, poor self-concept, or academic failure and being labeled as clumsy, uncooperative, or disruptive; they may have poor impulse control, as well as anxiety, depression, aggression, or other behavior problems.

There is not a distinct diagnosis of sensory processing disorder in the Diagnostic and Statistical Manual of Mental Disorders (DSM-5-TR), though sensory overresponsiveness is acknowledged in ASD.[24] Sensory processing issues can exist independently, comorbidly, or as part of other diagnoses. For example, issues are frequently found in premature children, gifted children, those with neurodevelopmental disorders (e.g., ASD, ADHD), and fragile X syndrome. In addition, sensory issues occur with toxic stress from environmental factors, such as institutionalization (e.g., international adoptions), severe physical and/or sexual abuse, poverty, lead poisoning, and alcohol or drug exposure.

Neurobiology related to SPD centers on the child's ability to individually or collectively process sensory stimuli (i.e., ability of the central nervous system [CNS] to receive and respond to external stimuli); neuronal gating, which is the ability to ignore unnecessary stimuli; and neuronal habituation, which occurs when nerves have a decreasing response to repetitive stimuli.[25] Of note, the failure of the CNS to regulate sensory input has been implicated in multiple behavioral health conditions, including ASD, depression, and schizophrenia, and is a significant contributor to the experience of chronic pain.[25]

Management

Individuals with SPD need early identification, psychoeducation, and referral for treatment. The PCP can screen, assess motor tone and planning, and determine if symptoms are part of another neurodevelopmental disorder. Red flags for sensory processing issues are found in Box 6.13. Screening tools can be found at www.spd-star.org. If screening or assessment results are concerning, the PCP

• BOX 6.13 Red Flags for Sensory Processing Difficulties

Infants and Toddlers
- Problems eating or sleeping
- Refuses to go to anyone but a specific person
- Irritable when being dressed, uncomfortable in clothes
- Rarely plays with toys
- Resists cuddling, arches away when held
- Cannot calm self
- Floppy or stiff body, motor delays

Early Childhood
- Overly sensitive to touch, noises, smells, other people
- Difficulty making friends
- Difficulty dressing, eating, sleeping, and/or toilet training
- Clumsy; poor motor skills; weakness
- In constant motion; in everyone else's face and space
- Frequent or long temper tantrums

Middle Childhood
- Overly sensitive to touch, noise, smells, other people
- Easily distracted, fidgety, craves movement; aggressive
- Easily overwhelmed
- Difficulty with handwriting or motor activities
- Difficulty making friends
- Unaware of pain and/or other people

Adolescents and Adults
- Overly sensitive to touch, noise, smells, and other people
- Poor self-esteem; afraid of failing at new tasks
- Lethargic and slow
- Always on the go; impulsive; distractible
- Leaves tasks uncompleted
- Clumsy, slow, poor motor skills or handwriting
- Difficulty staying focused at work and in meetings

When children have more than two symptoms, refer for evaluation.

should initiate a referral to a specially trained occupational therapist (OT) for further evaluation and treatment, although it can be expensive and is not always covered by insurance.

For the hyporesponsive child, active play (e.g., trampolines, swinging, swimming) is encouraged. In contrast, the hyperresponsive child needs calming activities (cozy corner with soft beanbag chair, decreased lighting/noise). The goal of therapy is to develop appropriate and automatic responses to sensations so that the child can function competently in play, at school, and in activities of daily living. It typically includes the use of sensory stimuli in a sensory-rich environment, providing what is called *sensory nourishment* or a *sensory diet*. This fosters new neurologic connections, arousal and attention regulation, and social relationships. Counseling with families is essential, as they are often blamed or criticized for the child's behavior. Books and websites provide additional information. A school-based OT can often provide adaptations to help the child deal with specific challenges at school.

Recurrent Physical Symptoms

Children may experience emotional stress as physical symptoms, which differ by age groups. Stomachaches are a common symptom in early/middle childhood, followed by headaches. By adolescence, trouble sleeping and fatigue also emerge. Physical symptoms are often accompanied by a body sensation, heightened emotional response, poor coping skills, anger, and difficulty verbally expressing emotional distress. Before adolescence, the incidence is equal in males and females, but after adolescence physical symptoms are twice as frequent in females. History may reveal overprotective families or stressors, such as parental separation or divorce. Difficulties at school, either academically or socially, can also be at the root of the physical complaints, especially for those from high-achieving families. At times, the PCP may also uncover another family member with similar symptoms. The presence of maltreatment and/or other trauma must be considered. A thorough history and physical exam, and lab studies as indicated, are done to ensure there is no medical disorder. The parent and/or child should keep a pain/symptom diary, recording the sensation, intensity, location, timing, and circumstances surrounding the pain/symptom. Daily entries should include a summary of the daily stressors (positive/negative) and emotions felt during the day. Screening tools such as the Children's Somatization Inventory (CSI) for the child and parent and the Functional Disability Inventory (FDI), which assesses the severity of symptoms, may be helpful in discerning the underlying issue.

Management

The PCP can begin working with the family to help them understand that physical symptoms are often a coping strategy for the child who has emotional discomfort that the child is not aware of; however, the pain is real, and the goal is to help the child identify stress and learn how to cope to minimize the distress. Parents should respond briefly and then help the child shift focus elsewhere, trying not to give attention to the pain/symptom. Strategies such as deep breaths, mindfulness, progressive relaxation, distraction, and guided imagery may be helpful. If the pain/symptoms are disruptive of normal routine, progressive, or not improving, referral for mental health intervention is necessary. Cognitive-behavioral techniques and family interventions to treat underlying stressors may provide effective coping strategies and improve overall functioning. Referral is necessary for children who have experienced maltreatment or trauma, or who are at risk for functional disorders, as evidenced by intense worry about mild physical symptoms, acute anxiety, and interference with school performance and relationships with family and friends.

Bullying

Bullying is any unwanted aggressive behavior(s) by another youth or group of youths that involves a power imbalance and is repeated or likely to be repeated multiple times. Bullying includes physical (hitting, tripping), verbal (name calling, teasing), or relational/social aggression (e.g., spreading rumors, leaving one out of a group). *Cyberbullying*, another form of bullying over digital devices, includes sending, posting, or sharing harmful, false, or negative content about someone. It occurs 24 hours a day, is harder to detect, and is more likely to become part of a permanent online profile. All states have legislation regarding bullying, but not all states extend protections to include protection against cyberbullying.

Youth rarely report bullying because the incidents typically occur when adults are not present or have not witnessed it. Seen or unseen, bullying impacts the sense of safety of schools, neighborhoods, and society. In 2019 25% of US high school students reported being bullied in the previous 12 months.[26] Females experience bullying at higher rates than males (30% vs. 19%) and LGBTQ+ youth at higher rates than heterosexual youth (40% vs.

22%).[26] Youth involved in bullying behaviors can be a bully, a victim, or a bully/victim. Bullying behaviors cause direct and indirect harm or distress to those who are targeted, including physical injury, social and emotional distress, depression, anxiety, sleep difficulties, and lower academic achievement, as well as increased risk for depression, anxiety, eating disorders, health issues, and other academic issues. The stress of bullying also presents an increased risk of suicide and self-harming behaviors in some young people. It is also important to realize that those who bully are also at risk for problems, including substance abuse, academic problems, as well as criminal activity and mental health disorders later in life. The bully/victim is at the greatest risk for mental health disorders.

Management

Bullying results in injury at many levels, and the PCP is likely to become involved only when that injury is reported, when there are mental health concerns, or during a routine social-emotional assessment. It is ideal to interview the child separately from the parent; however, it is necessary to gather the history from both to obtain a complete picture. It is also necessary to determine if the child is the perpetrator, a victim, or a bully/victim, as well as if any weapons were used or threatened during the event. Assess for drug or alcohol use and obtain details of any previous incidences. In addition, the PCP is responsible to report to both CPS and/or law enforcement when indicated.

The ideal goal is to stop bullying before it starts. There are many school-based bullying and violence prevention programs, as well as community intervention programs (see Additional Resources). The PCP needs to be familiar with the resources in the schools and community in which they practice, advocate for antibullying policies and bystander intervention training, and integrate violence prevention efforts into routine well-child care.

Caregiving Challenges and Special Circumstances

Separation, Divorce, and Remarriage

Parental separation, divorce, and remarriage are emotionally stressful, complex family events that often lead to significant emotional disruption and disequilibrium for parents and children. Children can experience the transition as a dramatic and painful time, including the experience of grief over the loss of family as they know it. Children and parents tend to adjust better when there is a stable parenting foundation in the child's early years, if parents maintain a civil relationship with each other that focuses on what is best for the children in the home, if parents each provide warmth and praise for the children throughout the process, and if the children know or sense that both parents will remain in their lives. The goal for the PCP is to determine the family's needs and strengths, assist them with healthy coping, and share specific developmental stages of the children and common psychosocial reactions to divorce that typically occur at that stage. The social-emotional effects of the divorce on the parents and the economic consequences of divorce on the family unit must also be considered (Box 6.14).

Remarriage creates a reorganized and/or blended family that introduces a stepparent, possibly stepsiblings, and the potential for half-siblings going forward. The majority of children in blended families adjust to their new family situations; however, the children's age and developmental stage will affect their

BOX 6.14   Assessment Factors in Divorce

Common Reactions of Children by Developmental Stage to Divorce by Age Group
- 2–5 years: Regression, irritability, sleep disturbances, aggression
- 6–8 years: Open grieving and feelings of rejection or being replaced; whiny, immature behavior; sadness; fearfulness
- 9–12 years: Fear and intense anger at one or both parents
- >13 years: Worried about own future, depressed, or acting-out behaviors (e.g., truancy, sexual activity, alcohol or drug use, suicide attempts)

Economic Consequence of Divorce
- Devastating economic hardships and decline in living standards (especially for women because of nonpayment or delinquency in payment of child support)

Common Issues for Children of Divorcing Parents
- Continued tension, conflict, and fighting between parents
- Litigation over custody and visitation arrangements
- Abandonment by one parent or sporadic visitation (decreased availability) vs. denial of visitation
- Diminished caregiving resulting from availability issues or emotional inaccessibility, distress, or instability
- Limited social support system outside nuclear family
- Feelings of loneliness or emotional abandonment, or both

response and coping skills. Early adolescence is often a time of greatest difficulty in adjustment to remarriage, and a mother's subsequent pregnancy is a time of increased frequency and intensity of problems for young children. Common issues in newly blended families include complex relationships with new family members; altered relationships with established family members; possible feelings of betraying a biological parent or being torn between parents; possible relocation and separation from family members and friends; continued or new tensions between parents; rivalries between parents and stepparents; jealousy among stepsiblings; the establishment of new family traditions and values, while continuing to respect earlier family history, traditions, and loyalties that may be in conflict; unrealistic expectations by the child or stepparent (e.g., instant love, respect, obedience from child); and tensions within a blended-family household, creating anxiety and fear of another family breakup. The PCP's role includes assessing how the child is coping with these significant life changes and realignment of the family roles (see Box 6.10), carefully considering any behavioral concerns. This information helps both the PCP and the parents decide how to best focus their attention.

Management

Anticipatory guidance given to parents who are in the process of separating and divorcing is outlined in Table 6.14. Custodial and visitation arrangements for children vary and may change as the child matures. Joint custody is an option that allows both parents the opportunity to participate in mutual decision-making about their child's life and welfare. Various living arrangements and visitation rights are possible with joint custody. In some instances, however, single custody is in the best interest of the child, and the noncustodial parent may have limited or no contact and involvement with the child. Custody disputes and exposure to parental conflict place additional stress on children and can increase their feelings of insecurity.

TABLE 6.14	Anticipatory Guidance for Families Experiencing Separation or Divorce

Anticipatory Guidance	Discussion Points With Parents
Advise parents to prepare the child for the impending breakup	• If possible, tell the child in advance of the breakup. Children who are appropriately prepared may cope better with the separation and change in family structure. • Discussions should focus on supporting the child's needs for reassurance and stability, not on blame, recriminations, or the parent's needs.
Explain to parents the need to discuss these key issues with their children	• Discuss what arrangements have been made for the children to see departing parent unless visitation is not possible or problematic. Consider whether the children will be best served by continuing to see the departing parent when possible. • Explain what divorce means in language appropriate to the child's cognitive and developmental level; explain reasons for the divorce in the same terms. • Reassure children that they did not cause the divorce or separation that they cannot correct their parents' unhappiness in the marriage, and that the divorce is the parents' decision. • Explain what the family structure will look like afterward and what changes will be necessary in the way the family functions. • Explain the visitation arrangements as soon as they are established. • Reassure children that they will be cared for, and they are not being abandoned by either parent, unless a parent disappeared or refuses involvement. • Tell children that feelings of sadness, anger, and disappointment are normal; encourage them not to "take sides," but love both parents. • Discuss how to handle special circumstances, such as when the "other parent" does not visit or simply leaves.
Discuss the need for consistency	• Parents should strive to maintain consistent daily routines between the two households; encourage the use of security items that the child may depend on or carry familiar items between the homes during the transitional period. • Be consistent in disciplinary practices.
Suggest self-help measures	• Children and parents may benefit from attending divorce recovery workshops, classes about families in transition, or peer support groups. • School counselors, religious groups, or community and social service agencies may be helpful resources.
Acknowledge grief	• PCPs should acknowledge the grief that both the parent and child are experiencing and provide support.
Discuss when referral for mental health counseling might be indicated	• Children often demonstrate internalized or externalized psychosocial problems in response to divorce. Counseling may be indicated for the family members.

PCPs, Primary care providers.

• BOX 6.15 Factors Affecting a Child's Ability to Achieve Healthy Adjustment to Separation and Divorce

• The opportunity for continued participation of the noncustodial or visiting parent in the child's life on a regular basis
• Custodial parent attempts to make visits with the other parent a routine event so that there is consistent contact (phone, visiting, email)
• The ability of the custodial parent to handle and successfully care for the child
• The ability of parents to separate their own feelings of anger and conflict and resolve their own hostility toward each other so that the child's need for a relationship with both parents is met
• The child does not become involved in parent conflict and does not feel rejected; the child should not be put in the middle
• The availability of a social support network
• The ability of parents to meet the child's developmental needs and to help the child master developmental tasks
• The child's overall personality, temperament, personal assets, and deficits

---

• BOX 6.16 Six Psychological Tasks Children of Divorce Must Master

1. Acknowledge the reality of the marital breakup.
2. Disengage from parent conflict and distress and resume customary pursuits.
3. Resolve loss of familiar daily routine, traditions, and symbols and the physical presence of two parents.
4. Resolve anger and self-blame.
5. Accept the permanence of the divorce.
6. Achieve realistic hope regarding relationships—the capacity to love and be loved.

The goal for parents experiencing changes in the family unit is to help them restore a sense of wholeness and integrity in their children's lives. Factors that have been shown to significantly affect whether the child will experience a healthy adjustment to the divorce are found in Box 6.15. Successful efforts implemented during initial

periods of disequilibrium and reorganization strengthen normal development and prevent future psychological trauma. A classic research study[27] identified six mental tasks that children of divorce must master, beginning at the time of parental separation and culminating in young adulthood (Box 6.16). Support can also be provided with additional visits or telephone contacts and by focusing on the family's positive strengths and resilience.

The goal in remarriage is to foster positive parenting behaviors, protect child development, and enhance family functioning. Before remarriage, PCPs can counsel parents regarding strategies for healthy transitions. Many children and adolescents develop strong and meaningful attachments to their stepparents if the relationship is cultivated over time with careful sensitivity to the needs of the child, parent, and family. Some tips for families include:

- Discuss upcoming changes with your child before remarriage and address fears, feelings, and expectations.
- Keep the adult relationship strong by nurturing the marital relationship.
- Blended-family parents need to agree on discipline issues, how to set limits, and type of discipline, remembering to be consistent between homes.
- Start new family traditions, such as weekly family meetings.
- Be patient and as flexible as possible; do not expect your child to have an immediate positive relationship with the new stepparent.
- Spend quiet, alone time with your child as much as possible and preferably every day.
- Do not force your child to align with the new stepparent, and remember that a stepparent does not replace the first parent; support and help maintain the relationship of your child with the other birth parent.

Military Deployment

In 2022 there were 1.8 million children belonging to a military family, with 40% of them being under 5 years of age.[28] A full-time military family moves, on average, every 2 years. The average military child will change schools six to nine times, and military spouses face unemployment that is three times greater than the national average.[29] These children face a multitude of stressors, and yet many manage remarkably well. In addition to these many moves, a deployment separates the military parent(s) from the family for up to 1 year. The Deployment Life Study (https://www.rand.org/nsrd/ndri/centers/frp/deployment-life.html), a longitudinal study over a deployment cycle, assessed child emotional, behavioral, social, and academic functioning, and no significant effects were found. This may be due to the larger military support network; however, understanding of the stressors of the deployment cycle helps the PCP prepare military families.[30] These stressors begin predeployment, 3 to 6 months before departure, as the departing parent may begin to have duties away from the family in preparation and the remaining parent needs to be preparing for handling all family responsibilities. It can be overwhelming for the family, who may begin to experience conflict, stress, and fear in anticipation of the separation. The period of deployment may be stable once a new routine is established; however, depending on the assignment, families also worry about the safety of the deployed parent. One of the most stressful parts of deployment is that the family must move off the military base, losing their familiar neighborhood and support network. Postdeployment involves family reintegration and, while it is exciting, it is always stressful as, once again, family routines and roles readjust. Among many variables, successful reintegration is influenced by the age of the children. For example, the critical first 1000 days of life is impacted by both the absent parent and the stress experienced by the remaining one, or grandparents, who often take children when both parents are deployed. In early childhood, the changes can be disorienting, and the level of parent stress may be the most critical factor in determining the child's reactions. In middle childhood, multiple changes are disruptive as children switch schools, say goodbye to friends, and face new ones; adolescents dealing with identity often struggle as they are put in the position of carrying some of the responsibilities during deployment.

Management

Children with a parent in the military have unique needs that should be addressed in primary care settings. PCPs must recognize them, anticipate needed coping strategies specific to their situation, screen for potential stressors, and be alert to the need for mental health referral. Having a parent sent to an active combat zone may rank as one of the most stressful events for children and their parents. Children may be especially vulnerable, as the coping resources of the remaining parent (or guardian) are already challenged. While no significant differences have been found in overall wellbeing, children with a deployed parent often have more emotional difficulties compared with their peers.[30] Older youth and females of all ages report more school, family, and peer-related difficulties if a parent was deployed.[30] The longer the parent deployment and the poorer the nondeployed parent's mental health, the more likely the children will experience role-shifting and behavior problems during deployment and reintegration. Additional family risk factors include a history of rigid coping styles, family dysfunction, young families (especially first military separation), families recently moved to a new duty station, foreign-born spouses, families with young children, families without unit affiliation, pregnancy, and dual-career or single parents. Equally important is the presence of protective factors, including resilience, family preparedness, active coping style, and positive psychological and mental health status of the at-home parent. Indications for referral include ineffective intervention after two to three visits, worsening symptoms or symptoms that continue for 3 months after redeployment, academic declines, situations where an at-home parent is having difficulty coping, or situations where the deployed parent is injured or fatally wounded.[30]

Adolescent Parent(s)

In the United States, the adolescent or teen birth rate for ages 15 to 19 years was 15.4 per 1000 in 2020, down 8% from 2019, and down 75% from 61.8 per 1000 births in 1991.[31] However, the United States has a significantly higher teen birth rate than other developed countries, and adolescent parents and their children continue to be at high risk for medical, socioemotional, and developmental issues.[32] Predictors of adolescent motherhood are listed in Box 6.17.

Adolescents who become parents often face problems because they are not developmentally ready to assume the parenting role and their developmental needs frequently conflict with the needs of their children, which sets them up to be isolated, exhausted, and depressed. Further, children of adolescent mothers are more

---

• BOX 6.17   Predictors of Adolescent Motherhood

- Victim of sexual abuse as a child
- Adverse events in childhood
- Being a child of an addicted parent
- Family history of mental illness
- Lack of family involvement; an intolerable home situation as defined by the adolescent
- Poor academic achievement or school dropout
- Loss of a parent by death, separation, divorce, or foster placement
- Living in an impoverished social environment where adolescent pregnancy is commonplace and accepted
- Confusion about own sexual orientation

likely to have a low birth weight, experience ongoing health problems, grow up without active fathers or father involvement, and be raised in poverty or near poverty. There are adolescents who successfully parent their infant; however, the same factors that lead to becoming an adolescent parent are relevant predictors of successful parenting. To better understand the environment in which a child will be raised, PCPs should ask about the adolescent parent's support system, their attitudes toward caregiving, and sources of caregiving advice. In addition, PCPs should determine the adolescent's school status, childcare arrangements, financial situation, and future plans. Assessment of at-risk status varies depending on the stage of the adolescent (Box 6.18). Addressing issues on an ongoing basis contributes to more successful parenting and prevention of problems later in the child's or adolescent parent's life. As their child gets older, adolescent mothers transition to the "young mother" role; however, as children enter early childhood, it can be particularly challenging for mothers who are survivors of abuse or neglectful caregiving. In general, children of adolescent/young mothers, especially those who are poor and living in urban settings, are more likely than their peers to have behavioral problems. Of note, adolescent mothers may later become young grandparents, and the adolescent pregnancy cycle repeats.

Management

Management strategies for the adolescent parent include:
- Maintain regular and frequent contact during the child's infancy and early childhood as both the adolescent mother and infant/child need health supervision and guidance.
- Provide a supportive environment for the adolescent parent(s). Have a plan for follow-up so that the adolescent parent(s) do not get lost in the system. Emphasize the strengths of the adolescent mother, praise positive efforts, and encourage engagement of other family members (e.g., father, grandparents) in discussions about childrearing issues.
- Facilitate education and identify resources to minimize the effects of poverty.

• BOX 6.18 Assessing Adolescent Parenting

What to assess for when adolescent parents have an:

Infant
- Parent-infant attachment: Is there evidence of healthy attachment or emotional or physical neglect?
- Confidence and ability of adolescent parent(s) to care for their infant
- Conflicts between the adolescent's needs and those of their infant: Is the adolescent more interested in reestablishing an adolescent lifestyle or caring for the infant?
- Living arrangements: With whom and where are the adolescent parent(s) and baby living?
- Degree of involvement of the social support network in the adolescent's and infant's life: Is the baby's other parent invested in the child? Support from extended family?
- Return to school or the workforce: What are the childcare arrangements?
- Adequacy of financial resources

Older Child
- How well do they understand child development and cope with the variety of toddler or older child behaviors
- How well the family unit is functioning
- Progress made by the adolescent parent(s) toward reaching their life goals

---

- Refer to a community health nurse for home visits early in pregnancy and postpartum. This intervention has been successful in delaying subsequent pregnancy and improving healthy caregiving and family life.
- Provide referrals for resources and community agencies that assist adolescent mothers (e.g., parenting classes, support groups, special clinic programs that see both infants and teen mothers; Woman, Infants, and Children [WIC] program; early child intervention programs provided by school districts/Head Start).
- Intervene early with warning signs of child maltreatment and refer as necessary.

Premature or Multiple Gestational Birth

Premature infants present special issues for all parents, especially when there is an extended time between the birth and when parents can bring their infant home. The infant's physiologic vulnerability is always a concern, along with the cost and time commitment, both of which are in addition to the concerns of all new parents with a newborn, but their fears and anxieties may be magnified and the care responsibilities may be significantly increased.

A family caring for new twins, triplets, or more can be quickly overwhelmed by the added responsibility and amount of work involved. Behavioral issues and the children's own unique relationships can be a challenge. For example, multiples often develop a special relationship marked by loyalty and cooperative play, function more independently, need less parental attention, and develop their own language among themselves during early childhood.

Management

PCPs need to be particularly alert to parents' attachment, fatigue levels, ability to seek access and accept support, and plans for ongoing care. Role strain or difficulties should be identified early, and interventions implemented for parent mental health and role difficulties.

Adoption

Adoption is the legal process that gives individuals who are not birth parents legal and permanent parental responsibility for a nonbiological child. Adoptions occur in a variety of different family types—married couples, single parents, gay and lesbian parents, grandparents, or other extended family members. Examples of types of adoptions include independent, identified, and international adoptions; surrogacy arrangements; intrafamily adoption; subsidized adoption of children with special healthcare needs; and open adoptions. Public and private agencies, independent adoption through attorneys, and foreign adoption services are potential avenues to assist in child placement.

Adoptive family assessment includes:
- Legal status, arrangements, and circumstances surrounding the adoption process.
- What, if any, contact will the biological parent(s) and family have with the child?
- Timing of the adoption finalization and length of waiting period; how old was the child when the child was adopted?
- Decisions about how and when to tell the child about being adopted (their adoption story).
- Support services available for the adoptive family.
- Any known or suspected medical (including growth and development) problems with the child.

- Thorough history of the birth parents and family medical, genetic, or psychosocial concerns.
- Information about the pregnancy, delivery, and neonatal period or subsequent medical problems.

Management

Schedule a preadoption consultation, if possible, to review any issues or concerns. Parents often have many questions about the initial adoption period and the establishment of a family relationship. Issues that the PCP should address include:

1. Disclosure of the adoption to the child is best done earlier rather than later, and children should always be told the truth about where they came from and why they were adopted.
2. Discussion about adoption should be open, keeping in mind the child's developmental stage, cognitive abilities, and emotional needs, reassuring the child in words and actions.
3. Addressing any myths, concerns, or fears that parents might have about adoption.
4. If or when a child wishes to learn more about, seek out, and/or meet their biological parents, it should not be seen as a rejection of their adoptive parents.
5. Adolescence can be difficult for adoptive children as they seek their own identity and explore what being adopted means to them.
6. Adoption of an older child may present an extra challenge, especially if the child shuffled between homes or was emotionally scarred by abuse or neglect. Telling parents about such challenges can help them better prepare to handle some of the difficulties that may lie ahead for their family and seek counseling early if needed.

Once the adoption is finalized, close monitoring and support during the initial adoption period are important. All adopted children need a comprehensive medical evaluation immediately after their adoptive placement, and ongoing additional health supervision visits even when all appears to be going well. The medical evaluation should include age-appropriate physical, dental, and behavioral/developmental screenings and vaccination review. The presence of a social support network is important for adoptive families and often provides preventive resources, reassurance of competence, and encouragement. Families adopting older children and children with special needs may require extra assistance with family bonding and behavioral, mental health, and physical needs.

Foster Care

Children in family foster care or group home settings are often there because of suspected or reported child maltreatment. Some children are placed in foster care because their parents are either unable to care for them or they needed specialized medical, psychiatric, or developmental assistance beyond the ability of their parents. Other children may need to be removed due to a chaotic and unsafe family environment or being abandoned or orphaned. These children are at high risk for deep-seated feelings of insecurity, loss, and anger. In 2021 the US Department of Health and Human Services reported that 407,000 children were in foster care.[33] Half of these children lived in foster homes with nonrelatives, a third lived with relatives, and the remainder were in group homes, institutions, and other locations.[33]

A complete assessment needs to be completed by the PCP and should include exploring the reason for the child's placement in foster care, physical or mental health issues that precipitated or resulted from separation from their parents, and evaluation of the foster parent(s) and home environment. Information that is critical for the PCP to assess includes the history of chronic stress, hardship, and emotional trauma in their original family/successive placements; multiple placements; separation from siblings; and current or pending family reunification efforts and plans for visitation or placement back with biological parents. Foster children do best when they receive care in homes that mirror their ethnic, racial, and cultural identity as much as possible. PCPs need to be aware that these children often have a history of disjointed care, and a disproportionate number will have weight problems, medical issues, or developmental delays.

Separation from foster care is a major life change requiring preparation, which includes the transition from pediatric to adult primary care. Formal emancipation from the foster care system happens between 18 and 21 years of age, depending on the child's needs and state statutes.

Management

Foster parents have a challenging role in society, and they often need assistance to provide the best care possible to the children in their care. Healthy Foster Care America (https://www.aap.org/en-us/advocacy-and-policy/aap-health-initiatives/healthy-foster-care-america/Pages/default.aspx) is an AAP initiative to improve health and wellbeing in foster families, with multiple resources for the PCP. The Child Welfare League of America (https://www.cwla.org/) and the National Foster Parent Association (https://nfpaonline.org/) are other resources providing support and caregiving information for foster families.

Additional Resources

American Academy of Child & Adolescent Psychiatry Facts for Families: AACAP/Families_and_Youth/Facts_for_Families/Layout/FFF_Guide-01.aspx?hkey=fd45e409-3c3c-44ae-b5d4-39ba12e644b7

Bright Futures in Practice: Mental Health: http://www.brightfutures.org/mentalhealth

Center for the Study of Social Policy Strengthening Families: A Protective Factors Framework: https://www.cssp.org/young-children-their-families/strengtheningfamilies

Centers for Disease Control Essentials for Childhood Framework: https://www.cdc.gov/violenceprevention/childabuseandneglect/essentials.html

Child Mind Institute: https://childmind.org/

Child Trends Social and Emotional Development: https://www.childtrends.org/research-topic/social-and-emotional-developmentCommittee on Psychosocial Aspects of Child and Family Health, American Academy of Pediatrics: https://www.aap.org/en-us/about-the-aap/Committees-Councils-Sections/Pages/Committee-on-Psychosocial-Aspects-of-Child-and-Family-Health.aspx

Community Resilience Initiative: https://resiliencetrumpsaces.org

Family Voices: http://www.familyvoices.org

Harvard Center on the Developing Child: https://developingchild.harvard.edu/

Imagination Library: https://imaginationlibrary.com/

Incredible Years: http://www.incredibleyears.com

Lives in the Balance (collaborative and proactive solutions): https://www.livesinthebalance.org

National Alliance on Mental Illness (NAMI): Child and Adolescent Action Center: https://www.nami.org/Find-Support/Teens-and-Young-Adults

National Association of Pediatric Nurse Practitioners Developmental Behavioral Mental Health Special Interest Group Resource Page: http://www.dbmhresource.org/

Parent Child Interaction Therapy (PCIT): http://www.pcit.org

Reach Institute: http://www.thereachinstitute.org

Reach Out and Read: http://www.reachoutandread.org/

Resilience Project: https://www.resilienceproject.com/

Society for Developmental and Behavioral Pediatrics: http://www.sdbp.org

Star Institute for Sensory Processing: https://sensoryhealth.org/

Substance Abuse and Mental Health Services Administration (SAMHSA): http://www.samhsa.gov/children

References

1. Cree RA, Bitsko RH, Robinson LR, et al. Health care, family, and community factors associated with mental, behavioral, and developmental disorders and poverty among children aged 2–8 years — United States, 2016. *MMWR Morb Mortal Wkly Rep.* 2018;67(50):1377–1383.

2. Bethell C, Health JBS of P. Rethinking: The New Science of Thriving. Johns Hopkins Bloomberg School of Public Health. https://magazine.jhsph.edu/2016/spring/forum/rethinking-the-new-science-of-thriving/.

3. Robert Wood Johnson Foundation. *An Update on Building and Measuring a Culture of Health Moving Forward Together*; 2018. https://www.rwjf.org/content/dam/COH/PDFs/MovingForwardTogether-FullReportFinal.pdf.

4. Sege RD, Harper Browne C. Responding to ACEs with HOPE: health outcomes from positive experiences. *Acad Pediatr.* 2017;17(7):S79–S85.

5. Luby JL, Baram TZ, Rogers CE, Barch DM. Neurodevelopmental optimization after early-life adversity: cross-species studies to elucidate sensitive periods and brain mechanisms to inform early intervention. *Trends Neurosci.* 2020;43(10):744–751.

6. Center on the Developing Child at Harvard University. *From Best Practices to Breakthrough Impacts*; 2016. https://developingchild.harvard.edu/resources/from-best-practices-to-breakthrough-impacts/.

7. Bartlett JD, Halle T, Thomson D. Promoting resilience in early childhood. *Resilient Children.* 2021;165–190.

8. Garner A, Yogman M. Preventing childhood toxic stress: partnering with families and communities to promote relational health. *Pediatrics.* 2021;148(2):e2021052582.

9. Hagan J, Shaw JS, Duncan PM. *Bright Futures: Guidelines for Health Supervision of Infants, Children, and Adolescents.* Bright Futures/American Academy of Pediatrics; 2017.

10. Masten AS. *Ordinary Magic: Resilience in Development.* The Guilford Press; 2014.

11. U.S. Department of Health and Human Services Office of Disease Prevention and Health Promotion. Healthy People 2030. https://health.gov/healthypeople.

12. Buka SL, Beers LS, Biel MG, et al. The Family is the patient: promoting early childhood mental health in pediatric care. *Pediatrics.* 2022;149(suppl 5).

13. King H. Learning to care for mental health. *Contemporary Pediatrics.* Published online June 2016. https://www.contemporarypediatrics.com/view/learning-care-mental-health.

14. Garner A, Yogman M. Preventing childhood toxic stress: partnering with families and communities to promote relational health. *Pediatrics.* 2021;148(2):e2021052582.

15. Centers for Disease Control and Prevention. *Essentials for Parenting Toddlers and Preschoolers*; 2019. https://www.cdc.gov/parents/essentials/index.html.

16. What is the Incredible Years? Incredible Parents. http://www.incredibleparents.org/our-methods.

17. Early Childhood Learning & Knowledge Center. *5Rs of Early Learning Leadership: Building a Foundation of Responsive Relationships*; 2021. https://eclkc.ohs.acf.hhs.gov/video/5rs-early-learning-leadership-building-foundation-responsive-relationships.

18. Center on the Developing Child at Harvard University. *Building the Core Skills Youth Need for Life: A Guide for Practitioners.* https://developingchild.harvard.edu/resources/building-core-skills-youth/.

19. Search Institute. The developmental assets framework. Published 2018. https://www.search-institute.org/our-research/development-assets/developmental-assets-framework.

20. Search Institute. Understanding sparks and thriving. https://www.search-institute.org/our-research/youth-development-research/sparks-and-thriving/.

21. David-Ferdon C, Vivolo-Kantor AM, Dahlberg L, et al. *A Comprehensive Technical Package for the Prevention of Youth Violence and Associated Risk Behaviors.* National Center for Injury Prevention and Control, Centers for Disease Control and Prevention; 2016. https://www.cdc.gov/violenceprevention/pdf/yv-technicalpackage.pdf.

22. Hektner JM, Brennan AL, Brotherson SE. A review of the nurtured heart approach to parenting: evaluation of its theoretical and empirical foundations. *Fam Process.* 2013;52(3):425–439.

23. Foy JM, Green CM, Earls MF. Mental health competencies for pediatric practice. *Pediatrics.* 2019;144(5):e20192757.

24. American Psychiatric Association. *Diagnostic and Statistical Manual of Mental Disorders: DSM-5-TR.* 5th ed. American Psychiatric Association Publishing; 2022.

25. Harrison LA, Kats A, Williams ME, et al. The importance of sensory processing in mental health: a proposed addition to the Research Domain Criteria (RdoC) and suggestions for RdoC 2.0. *Front Psychol.* 2019;10.

26. Basile KC, Clayton HB, DeGue S, et al. Interpersonal violence victimization among high school students — youth risk behavior survey, United States, 2019. *MMWR Suppl.* 2020;69(1):28–37.

27. Wallerstein JS. Children of divorce: the psychological tasks of the child. *Am J Orthopsychiatry.* 1983;53(2):230–243.

28. Military Active-Duty Personnel, Civilians by State. Department of Defense. https://dwp.dmdc.osd.mil/dwp/api/download?fileName=DMDC_Website_Location_Report_2203.xlsx&groupName=milRegionCountry.

29. Walters JM. *12 Things You Didn't Know about Military Families. Care.Com Resources*; 2022. https://www.care.com/c/12-things-you-didnt-know-about-military-fami/.

30. Panton J. Caring for military children: implications for nurse practitioners. *J Pediatr Health Care.* 2018;32(5):435–444.

31. Osterman M, Hamilton B, Martin J, et al. *Births: Final Data for*; 2020.

32. Centers for Disease Control. *About Teen Pregnancy*; 2019. http://www.cdc.gov/teenpregnancy/about/index.htm.

33. www.acf.hhs.gov. *AFCARS Report #28*; 2021. https://www.acf.hhs.gov/cb/report/afcars-report-28.

7

Sexuality and Gender Identity

MARY DIRKS

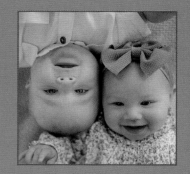

S exuality is influenced by biological, ethical, spiritual, cultural, and moral issues and includes an individual's beliefs, attitudes, values, and behaviors. Sex refers to the biological characteristics that define individuals as male or female and is assigned at birth based on the appearance of the external genitalia, chromosomes, reproductive organs, and their functions. Achieving a sense of one's sexuality in its broadest context begins at birth and continues throughout life during various behavioral, relational, and normative transition periods, including adolescence. During puberty, hormonal changes accelerate physical sexual development. Knowledge of anatomy, physiology, and biochemistry of the sexual response system is important at various developmental stages. During childhood and adolescence, individuals gradually develop their gender identity, sexual orientation, and experiment with romantic roles, relationships, and intimacy. Theoretically, healthy sexuality development is highly correlated to empowerment and the ability to understand and navigate feelings of desire and attraction. Fig. 7.1 details a conceptual framework for sexual wellbeing in adolescents that is multifactorial and situational and includes six key competencies for healthy sexual development: sexual literacy, gender-equitable attitudes, respect for human rights and understanding consent, critical reflection skills, coping skills and stress management, and interpersonal relationship skills.[1] The World Health Organization (WHO) affirms that sexual health is essential to the overall wellbeing of individuals and is reliant on[2]:

- Access to high-quality, comprehensive information about sex and sexuality
- Understanding of the risks and adverse consequences related to sexual activity
- Access to appropriate sexual healthcare
- Exposure to an environment that is affirming and promotes their sexual health development

Sexual literacy includes a developmentally appropriate understanding of the human body, reproduction, and relationships. The sexual literacy model demonstrates that sexual wellbeing is fostered through accepting different gender roles and relationships, understanding consent and privacy, and demonstrating respect for others' sexual choices. Finally, sexual wellbeing grows as individuals develop interpersonal social coping skills and a positive sense of their own gender and sexuality.[1] Strengthening child and adolescent knowledge, skills, and attitudes about sexuality using a positive, developmentally grounded approach, rather than presenting the topic only by addressing negative physical and psychological consequences, promotes healthy sexual wellbeing.

The primary care provider (PCP) plays a crucial part in educating parents to anticipate, recognize, and guide their children through the stages of sexual development and gender identity. The primary care visit gives parents a chance to ask questions and solicit advice from the child's provider. Also, at age-appropriate times, the primary care visit provides children and adolescents with opportunities to explore questions they have about their sexuality. Current societal norms create a challenging environment for children and adolescents who experience same-sex attraction, who question their assigned gender identity, or who have reservations about their developing bodies and feelings. The American Academy of Pediatrics[3] and the National Association of Pediatric Nurse Practitioners[3a] reaffirm that pediatric health clinicians play an important role in supporting and expanding access to sexual and reproductive healthcare for all adolescents and young adults.[3] This chapter focuses on sexual health promotion and gender identity, emphasizing that sexual development is a normal and healthy part of human growth.

Patterns of Sexuality

Cultural Context of Sexuality

In most Western cultures, gender is based on the sex assigned at birth, endures for life, and defines the individual's personality and identity. Since the beginning of the 21st century, and with global Internet technology changing the way world views are disseminated, individuals have more opportunities to communicate their social realities regarding their sexual values, norms, relationships, and behaviors. Some cultures are more accepting of those whose gender identity does not match the sex assigned at birth or whose sexual orientation does not fit within a heteronormative narrative. There are also cultures that have strict laws (cultural or religious) against the practice of anything other than heterosexuality. Providers must understand gender development concepts and standards of care for youth in this evolving environment.

Contemporary Definitions

Approaching sexual health as a paradigm of intersecting but distinctly separate factors between sexuality, sex, and gender identity

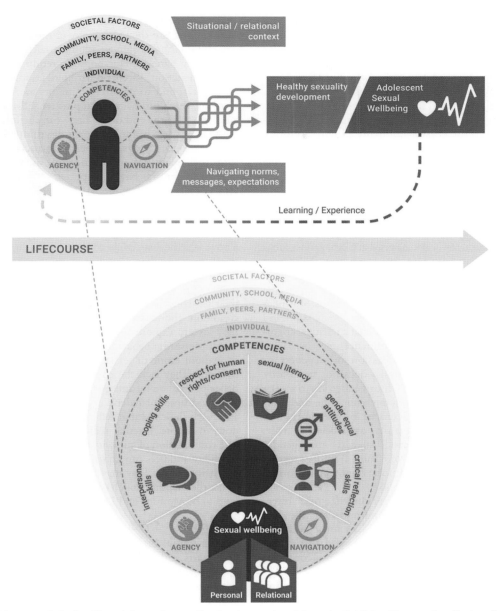

• **Fig 7.1** Conceptual framework for healthy adolescent sexuality development and its potential link with sexual wellbeing. (From Kågesten A, van Reeuwijk M. Healthy sexuality developed in adolescence: proposing a competency-based framework to inform programmes and research. *Sex Reprod Health Matters*. 2021;29(1):104–120.)

enables providers to appreciate the complexities of the child and adolescent's developing sexual wellbeing. PCPs provide more appropriate and effective patient care by understanding terminology and distinctions between seemingly similar constructs. The complexity of sexuality hinges on the key notion of gender. The following are contemporary definitions:

- *Sexual health* is "a state of physical, emotional, mental, and social wellbeing in relation to sexuality and requires a positive and respectful approach to sexuality and sexual relationships, as well as the possibility of having pleasurable and safe sexual experiences, free of coercion, discrimination, and violence.[2] For sexual health to be attained and maintained, the sexual rights of all persons must be respected, protected, and fulfilled.
- *Sexual function* incorporates the biological component of the human sexual response cycle and refers to the ability to give and receive sexual pleasure.

- *Sexual self-concept* is the psychological component of sexuality, the image one has of oneself, and the evaluation of one's satisfaction with masculine and feminine roles.
- *Sexual relationships* are the social domain of sexuality and include the interpersonal relationships in which one's sexuality is shared with others.
- *Sexual orientation* is an individual's feelings of sexual attraction and erotic potential to a male, female, or someone else on the gender continuum. Sexual orientation is not dichotomous, and individuals tend to fall along a continuum of sexual expression and desires rather than into exclusive categories. The phrase *sexual preference* implies choice and should not be used in reference to, or confused with, sexual orientation. Heterosexuality, homosexuality, bisexuality, pansexuality, and asexuality are part of the spectrum of human sexuality and will be discussed further in this chapter. There are genetic (neuroanatomic),

hormonal (neurophysiologic), developmental, social, and cultural influences of sexual orientation, but none have been definitively identified. Adolescents typically express different sexual behaviors, including short-term same-sex experiences. It is common for teens to not be sexually active but label themselves with a sexual orientation because of whom they are physically or emotionally attracted to.

- *Sex or gender assignment* generally occurs at birth based on genital appearance and is the keystone in many societies to future gender socialization (i.e., gender identity). In most cases, genital appearance is based on the 46XX and 46XY chromosome karyotypes and the appropriate masculinization effect of prenatal steroid exposure (testosterone and dihydrotestosterone).
- *Gender identity:* Gender identity is the internal perception of one's gender. Common identity labels include man, woman, gender nonbinary, transgender, or gender nonconforming. Often confused with biological sex or sex assigned at birth, gender identity is self-determined and can exist on a continuum. Numerous studies illuminate that one's gender identity develops over time in a transactional manner according to personal and interpersonal social and biological ongoing interactions.[4] Elements of gender development theory, known as the gender web, are dynamic and incorporate chromosomes, hormones, sex characteristics, cognitive function, and social and cultural influences.[5]
- *Gender expression:* The outward expression of maleness or femaleness—that is, gender expression—does not necessarily correlate with the sex assigned at birth or gender identity. The expression of one's gender begins at preschool age and continues into adulthood. It is characterized by the emergence of behaviors, attitudes, and feelings that are labeled as male, female, or neutral. Previous research suggests that gender expression is dependent on testosterone and estradiol exposure. Testosterone levels, measured in amniotic fluid, appear to predict male-typical behavior in childhood.[6]

Sex, gender, and sexual orientation are multifactorial interdependent constructs that may be evolving and dynamic in a child or adolescent's sexual development. PCPs must be aware and sensitive to appropriate gender pronouns and sexual orientation terminology when working with gender nonconforming children or adolescents and their parents. (See Table 7.1 for developmental considerations and Box 7.8 for more detailed definitions of terms.)

Sexuality Developmental Stages

The PCP is in a unique position to incrementally educate parents about their child's sexual maturation starting in infancy, as well as to help parents distinguish between typical and potentially problematic sexual behaviors. Anticipatory guidance not only enables parents to accurately understand their child's typical sexual development but also provides a structure for healthy parent-child sexual discussions in an ongoing open manner throughout the child's life. Table 7.2 discusses the components of development and behavior related to sexuality.

Infancy (Birth–1 Year Old)

Infants are reflexive beings, responding to their physical environment without hesitation or cognition. Sexual reflexes are present prenatally and are easily stimulated in the infant. It is not uncommon to observe a penile erection in prenatal ultrasounds or in the nursing child. Just as infants are fascinated by and explore their hands and feet, they explore their genitalia. Touching the genitalia is pleasurable and soothing, is a natural part of exploring their

environment, and begins as early as 3 to 5 months old. The PCP should point out the spontaneity of this reflexive behavior so that a parent does not assign an adult sexuality intent to it.

Healthy parent-infant bonding requires physical contact and social interaction. Parents must hold, cuddle, stroke, talk to, look at, and respond to children if infants are to develop a sense of trust on which intimacy and a positive self-image will be based in later years. By the end of the first year, the infant can differentiate between genders; some may even discriminate between culturally gender-associated toys. As society furthers its influence, infants form their identities and learn about their gender roles from the reinforcement of behaviors expected of males, females, or all individuals regardless of gender.

Early Childhood (1–2 Years Old)

Toddlers recognize and pronounce themselves "I'm a girl" or "I'm a boy," but they can easily confuse gender in others and sometimes in themselves. Changing one's clothing style, for example, can be perceived as a gender change. The traditional model of gender development proports that children cannot integrate gender identity into their self-concept until they understand that gender is a permanent condition. Toddlers are extremely curious about their environment; they love to explore and experiment. Children this age are aware of self-pleasuring behaviors and frequently masturbate, but they do so without erotic or sexual intent but rather because it feels good to them. They lack the concept of personal space and how their behavior may be misinterpreted as being sexual or improper. This is a good time for parents to discuss the notion of "private parts" and teach the child that self-pleasuring is acceptable but should be done in private. Parental redirection is usually all that is required. The combination of curiosity and lack of self-consciousness characteristic of toddlers can contribute to embarrassing social incidents for their parents. They may be curious about what others look like under their clothes, touch other children's bodies, "play doctor," pretend to be Mommy and Daddy, and enjoy running around naked.

Preschool (3–5 Years Old)

Parents should be encouraged to use the appropriate names for body parts and bodily functions, even though they may also use slang words. This enables children to better comprehend discussions with health providers, teachers, or health educators when the anatomic and physiologic terms are used.

Because preschool children at this age interpret statements literally and have "magical" thinking, their understanding of the physical self can be distorted, and lengthy explanations about body functions can be misunderstood. Parents should help children understand that their bodies come in different shapes, sizes, and colors; that all of these are equally important; that boys and girls share many of the same parts, but different genital parts; and that having things in common and respecting differences are important aspects for developing friendships. It is appropriate for parents to introduce the notion of germs and hygiene, such as when washing hands. Situational factors can induce an increase in observed sexual behaviors in this age group, such as the birth of a new sibling, watching their mother breastfeed, and viewing another child's or adult's nudity. By the end of the early childhood stage, questions often arise about how babies are made. This helps establish a framework for parents to discuss contraception, pregnancy prevention, and prevention of sexually transmitted infections (STIs) later in life.

Middle Childhood (6–10 Years Old)

School-age children have a high level of curiosity about sexuality, their bodies, and their environment. They are aware of the

TABLE 7.1   Binary and Gender-Neutral Pronouns

	Nominative (Subject)	Objective (Object)	Possessive Adjective	Possessive Pronoun	Reflexive
He	He	Him	His	His	Himself
She	She	Her	Her	Hers	Herself
They	They	Them	Their	Theirs	Themself
Ze	Ze	Hir	Hir	Hirs	Hirself
Ey	Ey	Em	Eir	Eirs	Eirself

Modified from Trans Student Educational Resources: *Gender Pronouns*; 2022. https://transstudent.org/graphics/pronouns101/.

TABLE 7.2   Sexual Behaviors, Self-Concept, and Relationship Milestones From Infancy Through Late Adolescence

Developmental Age	Typical Sexual Behaviors	Sexual Self-Concept Development	Sexual Role and Relationship Development
Infancy (birth to year)	Erectile function present; May explore genital area during diaper changes	Gender identity reinforced	Reflexive response; Parent-infant bonding
Early childhood (1–2 years)	Genital pleasuring and exploration; Sensual activity (e.g., hugging, stroking mother's breasts or other body parts)	Association of sexuality and good and bad; Distinction between self and others	Sex role differences developing; Permanence of male and female genders unclear; Sexual vocabulary developing
Preschool (3–5 years)	Sex play—exploration of own body and those of playmates; taking clothes off; showing genitals to other children or adults; Self-pleasuring (masturbation) especially when tired	Gender identity understood as a permanent condition; Understanding of cultural and physical differences in bodies	Sex roles learned; Parental attachment and identification; Sexual vocabulary learned; Understanding of germs and hygiene
Middle childhood (6–10 years)	Sex play between peers (playing "house" or "doctor"); exploration through looking at and touching genitals; Masturbation (may occur more in public); Asking questions and talking about sex; Dressing up as the opposite sex as part of dramatic play	Curiosity about sex; Sexual fears and fantasies; Interest in aspects of sexual development; Self-awareness as a sexual being	Same-sex friends; Understands gender permanency; Attempts at humor related to sexuality; often aimed as insults or to appear smart to friends
Early adolescence (11–14 years)	Menarche (female); Seminal emissions (male); Increased interest in sexual anatomy	Concerns about body image; Anxieties and questions about pubertal changes	Same-sex friends; Sexual experiences as part of friendship; Limited capacity for intimacy
Middle adolescence (15–17 years)	Testing ability to attract a partner; Masturbation, petting; May or may not be sexually active; May be aware of or question sexual orientation; Awkwardness in the first sexual encounter	Anxiety over inadequacy, lack of partner, virginity; Exploration of sexual identity	Initiation of sexual friendships; Dating; Sexual debut
Late adolescence (18–24 years)	May or may not be sexually active; May be aware of or question sexual orientation; Experimentation with sexual expressions; Awkwardness in the first sexual encounter	Responsibility for sexual activity; Responsibility for sexual health (e.g., contraception, STI prevention); Develop personal sexual values and tolerance for others	Intimacy in relationships learned; Long-term relationship commitments

STI, Sexually transmitted infection.

Modified from Hagan, JF, Shaw, JS, Duncan, PM. *Bright Futures: Guidelines for Health Supervision of Infants, Children and Adolescents*. 4th ed. American Academy of Pediatrics, 2017; and Holland-Hall, C. Adolescent physical and social development. In: Kliegman R, St. Geme J, eds. *Nelson Textbook of Pediatrics*, 21st ed. Elsevier; 2020;1014–1020.

pleasure stimulation gives and they continue to actively seek and enjoy autoerotic arousal. Contact with other children may give them new ideas about sex, and exploration games are typical (e.g., playing house or doctor) between same-age children, either of the same or opposite sex. This is typical behavior if a child is not emotionally distraught by the encounter and if it involves children who are of similar ages. Parents should avoid being overly alarmed if they witness this play. It is appropriate for parents to redirect the play to other activities, and they should discuss the situation later with their child to explore the experience, ascertain if the child was uncomfortable, and emphasize the notion of privacy and respect for one's body. Box 7.1 discusses sexual actions beyond self-pleasuring and sexual play that may indicate possible sexual abuse.

By 6 to 7 years old, the use of sexual or "potty" language becomes evident—often to test parental reaction. Children at this age understand gender identity permanence and tend to identify more with their same-sex parent and cluster into same-sex peer groups if given the opportunity.

By the time children are about 8 years old, they begin to understand the significance of their sexuality. They learn more about their body and body functions and "giggle" with children of their same sex when talking about sexuality, perhaps because they conceive that sex is a secretive topic. Unless parents actively communicate with their children, sexual lessons are learned from peers, the media, jokes, and movies.

Parents and teachers are in key positions to teach children that their sexual curiosity and feelings are normal, to help boys and girls better understand how sexual development is an integral part of growing up, to use respectful language, and to reinforce that they are always available for questions. Simple discussions about the body can introduce further discussions about hormones and reproductive systems. Establishing a good communication history about sexuality and other subjects lays the groundwork for being accessible to update information as the child matures. This is also a good time for parents and others to reinforce the notion that there is diversity in families within which parents and adults love and care for children. This may include families with same-sex parents, families with racial or ethnic diversity, and single parent households, to name a few.

Some children begin pubertal changes during this time and may be embarrassed by them. As their bodies change, they become curious and want to see others' bodies. Masturbation is still a way for them to explore their bodies. Sexual language is often used more to insult others or to appear smart in front of their friends.

Early Adolescence (11–14 Years Old)

Early adolescence is typically marked by the onset of pubertal changes. At this stage, youth understand sexuality as a normal part of life. Both males and females understand the changes that occur in each other's bodies and by 11 to 12 years old are ready to discuss sexual behavior and reproduction. Self-pleasuring because of sexual reflexes may now become connected to sexual fantasies, sexual behavior, and sexual relationships. It is still common for preadolescents to socialize and develop close relationships, mostly with members of the same sex. Both sexes often become uncomfortable or embarrassed about the changes in their bodies, particularly girls because breast development is more obvious to others. Privacy becomes more important.

Parents should discuss menstruation before menarche to avoid unnecessary alarm. Being mindful of their values and beliefs, parents should discuss abstinence, STIs (including human immunodeficiency virus [HIV]), birth control, the human papilloma virus

• **BOX 7.1** **Signs That Sexual Play Is Not Typical**

- The behavior is not age appropriate.
- The behavior is prolonged.
- The child looks anxious or guilty or becomes extremely aroused.
- Child is being forced into sexual play through bribes, name-calling, and/or physical force.
- Child knows more about sex/sexual acts than is appropriate for his or her age.

immunization for both sexes, consequences of early sexual activity (including teen pregnancy), and the influence of peer pressure. This is also a good time to discuss sexual orientation.

Middle Adolescence (15–17 Years Old)

Middle adolescence is a period of rapid physical, emotional, and social change that presents a developmental challenge to both teens and parents. In terms of sexuality, adolescents fit their sense of sexual being into their evolving self-image and personal identity; they learn about their bodies' (sometimes unexpected and embarrassing) sensual and sexual responses to stimulation, and they develop a sense of the moral significance of sexuality. The Guttmacher Institute (2019) reports that 65% of adolescents have sexual intercourse by the time they reach their 18th birthday.[7] Activities such as group social functions, dating, sports participation, and interactions at work and school provide opportunities to learn the social and interpersonal skills of intimacy.

Late Adolescence (18–24 Years Old)

Learning how to communicate about sex, how to set limits, how to prevent misunderstandings, and how to say yes or no are important skills for older adolescents. Equally important is the process of developing a set of sexual values. Whether the older adolescent practices abstinence or is sexually active, if they have healthy emotional and/or physical boundaries in their intimate relationships, and how they respond to the risks inherent to expressing their sexuality reflect the adolescent's sexual values and how well they learned accountability for sexual behaviors. Older adolescents seek the autonomy to independently assume responsibility for their sexual health, and the PCP can foster informed decision-making and assist with transition to adult preventative health services.

Assessment of Sexual Development

Sexual development, questions, and concerns are present throughout childhood and adolescence; therefore assessment of sexuality and sexual maturation should be integrated into the health history, interview and discussion, and physical examination at *all* health maintenance visits. Creating a safe environment for the discussion of sensitive topics when taking a sexual history is critical to establishing trust and open communication. Minimizing charting during the visit and maintaining eye contact also help build rapport. A useful tool for the clinician is the Child Sexual Behavior Inventory (CSBI; see Additional Resources). This tool is completed by parents and helps evaluate normal and age-appropriate sexual behaviors for those 2 to 12 years old. Developed to evaluate whether a child has a history of sexual abuse, the CSBI assists the PCP working with a parent who is concerned about their child's sexual behavior.

Confidentiality

Leading national healthcare associations endorse confidential healthcare for adolescents in accordance with state consent law regulations for minors.[7] The provision of confidential care includes the adolescent spending time alone with the provider to discuss sexual and reproductive health issues. One-on-one time with teens is the standard of practice; it provides teens with regular opportunities to raise sexuality concerns and allows providers to give personalized information aimed at risk reduction. Despite these guidelines, many adolescents do not seek healthcare due to concerns about confidentiality, especially due to concerns that their parents will be informed of discussions. Studies show that the odds of avoiding medical care due to confidentiality concerns increase in the presence of poor parental communication, high depressive symptoms, and suicidal ideation and/or attempt in the past year for both sexes.[8] Females are more likely to forgo medical care due to confidentiality concerns when they have a history of sexual intercourse, not using birth control with their last sexual encounter, having prior STI, or using alcohol in the past year. With this information in mind, PCPs need to be clear about their policy of confidentiality with both the youth and parents before the need arises. This discussion needs to include confidentiality boundaries (i.e., severe mental health issues and safety) and how information is communicated with parents (i.e., office discussion, explanation of benefits sent to parents).

History

Obtaining a sexual history achieves several purposes. In addition to collecting information, the process itself gives permission to the child, adolescent, or parent to ask questions and receive reliable information regarding issues of sexual concern. It sets the stage to incorporate accurate, sexuality-specific education as an essential component of anticipatory guidance.

Types of Sexual Histories

The sexual history can be either comprehensive or problem-focused. The comprehensive sexual history (Box 7.2) is detailed and encompasses all aspects of sexuality from the youth, their family of origin, siblings, and peer relationships. A comprehensive history is lengthy and may not be accomplished at the first visit or in a single interview; it can be anxiety producing to have the child or adolescent disclose detailed sensitive information during early visits, and individuals may become fatigued by one lengthy interview.

In contrast, the problem-focused sexual history (Box 7.3) usually centers on the current complaint or assessment of specific behaviors, such as pregnancy or STI risk. Problem-focused sexual histories are shorter, direct, and specific to the presenting issue.

Approach to Taking a Sexual History

The interviewer should do the following when taking a sexual history:

- Reassure the youth that asking sexual questions is a normal part of clinical practice: "I'm going to ask you a few personal questions about your life and wellbeing that I ask all my patients."
- Give appropriate, factual information; use medical-sexual terminology rather than slang, unless the child or adolescent cannot relate to medical terms.

- Use language that validates the youth's understanding of terms and concepts. For example, when talking with adolescents, the question "Are you sexually active?" seeks information regarding current sexual activity on a planned and regular basis. The adolescent who has concrete cognitive abilities or who does not anticipate having sex in the immediate future may respond negatively. However, the question "Have you ever had a romantic relationship with a boy or a girl?" allows for a more inclusive description of sexual activity. Ask the youth what they think sex is. Define "sex" as oral, vaginal, or anal.
- Use open-ended questions. Questions that contain "why" can require a level of analysis beyond the capabilities of teens operating at a cognitive concrete level.
- Avoid assumptions of heteronormativity. Instead, ask questions such as "Are you attracted to males, females, both, neither, or are you not sure yet?"
- Phrase questions that may be emotionally laden in a way that lets clients know that their experience may not be exceptional (e.g., "I often hear of people who have been touched sexually in a way that made them feel uncomfortable; has this happened to you?").

When asking sensitive questions, phrase the question in a way that normalizes it to make it easier to answer: "If you masturbate, how often?" is better than "Do you masturbate?"

Physical Examination

The physical examination identifies normal sexual anatomy variations, the sexual maturity rating (SMR) stage, and any pathologic condition present. The physical examination should include an examination of the breasts, body hair growth patterns, and external genitalia (see Chapter 13). Current recommendations do not recommend pelvic examinations for asymptomatic, nonpregnant adolescents.[9] Perform noninvasive laboratory studies only as indicated for STI screening beginning with highly sensitive first pass urine-based nucleic acid amplification test (NAAT) or self-collected vaginal swab[10] (see Chapter 43).

The physical examination should be performed with care and sensitivity. Very young children and toddlers make no distinction between the examination of the external genitalia and other body parts. Young school-age children can be extremely modest, act embarrassed, and resist taking off their clothes for the examination. Older school-age children and adolescents can misinterpret the examination procedures and may feel violated or abused. The child needs to feel an element of control during the examination. PCPs should clearly explain procedures before the exam begins, use straightforward techniques, and involve the child in the examination (e.g., ask if they wish to have the parent or another adult present), to give the youth autonomy while performing a thorough, respectful examination.

Fostering Healthy Sexuality

The health provider has two primary goals related to the management of pediatric sexual development: first, to help youth achieve a healthy sexual identity and function, and second, to provide support for parents as they guide their children through the process. Counseling parents about children's sexual development achieves both goals. Age-appropriate anticipatory guidance about sexual development and maturation should be provided to parents and their children. In particular, the provider must:

• BOX 7.2 Comprehensive Adolescent Sexual and Reproductive History

Background Data
- Adolescent's name, age (birth date), and sex
- History of risk behaviors (e.g., drug history: onset, duration, and frequency of use of cigarettes, alcohol, and/or other illicit drugs)
- Access to sexual social media (e.g., pornography), sexting
- Parents:
  - Age:
  - Religion:
  - Education levels:
  - Occupations:
  - Parent's marital status:
- Youth's feelings toward parent(s)

Sexuality
- What were your parents' attitudes about sexuality when you were growing up?
- How did your parents handle nudity?
- When do you first recall seeing a nude person of the same sex? Opposite sex?
- Who taught you about sex, sex play, pregnancy, intercourse, masturbation, homosexuality, sexually transmitted infections (STIs), birth?
- How often did you play doctor or nurse or have other sex play with another child?
- Tell me about any other sexual activity (e.g., sexting) or experience that had a strong effect on you.

Puberty
Females
- Onset of breast development?
- When did pubic hair appear?
- Onset of menstruation (age, regularity of periods [initially, now])?
- When was your last normal menstrual period (LNMP)?
- What hygienic methods are used (pads, tampons)?
- How were you prepared for menstruation? By whom?
- What were your feelings about early periods? Later periods?
- Have you had unusual bleeding or pains?

Males
- How were you prepared for adolescence? By whom?
- Age of first orgasm (ejaculation)?
- What were "wet dreams" like? How did they make you feel?
- When did pubic hair appear?

Body Image
- How do you feel about your body? Breasts? Genitals?
- How much time do you spend nude in front of a mirror?
- Have you ever texted a picture of yourself nude?

Masturbation
- How old were you when you began?
- What are others' reactions to your masturbation?
- What methods do you use?
- What are your feelings about it?

Kissing and Caressing
- How old were you when you began? How often?
- How many partners do you currently have?

Intercourse
- How often have you had intercourse?
- How many partners?
- How often do you initiate sex?
- How often do you currently have sex?
- How often have you had oral sex?
- Are your partners male, female, or both?
- Type of intercourse: Penile-vaginal, orogenital, penile-anal, oral-anal

Contraceptive Use
- What kinds of contraceptives have you used?
- What are you using now?
- Do you have any problems with contraceptives?
- Do you use condoms?
- How do you communicate about contraception with your partner?

Gender Identity
- What is your gender?
- What are your pronouns? (e.g., he, him, she, her, ze, hir)
- How long have you identified as transgender? (If applicable)

Sexual Orientation
- What does it mean to you to be straight, lesbian, gay, or bisexual, queer, questioning, or asexual?
- What is your sexual orientation?
- How long have you known your sexual orientation?
- How often have you had sexual experiences? What kinds of experiences? What were the circumstances?

Seduction and Rape
- When have you seduced someone sexually?
- When has someone seduced you?
- Have you participated in sexting?
- Have you been touched in a way sexually that made you feel uncomfortable? Can you tell me about it?
- Have you ever touched someone without their consent? How often have you forced someone to have sex?
- Have you ever accepted money for sex?

Incest and Abuse
- Did anyone in your family touch you in a way that made you feel uncomfortable? Has anyone else? Can you tell me about it?
- Was it your mother? Father? Brother(s)? Sister(s)? Other relatives? Others?

Sexually Transmitted Infections
- How old were you when you learned about STIs?
- Have you ever had an STI? Gonorrhea? Syphilis? Chlamydia?
- Do you have any signs or symptoms of STIs now such as discomfort, sores, or drainage?

Pregnancy
- Have you ever been pregnant? At what age?
- Tell me about the pregnancy—did you have a miscarriage, abortion, adoption, live birth- was it vaginal or caesarean section?
- Do you think there is a chance you are pregnant now?
- Have you caused a pregnancy?

- Assess the parent's level of understanding regarding typical physical and psychosocial sexual development in children and adolescents.
- Provide or clarify information, as needed.
- Provide strategies and support for teaching about pediatric sexuality.
- Assist the parent to connect to community-based resources.

"Typical sexual behavior" is not always clear, and the range is especially wide in 2- to 6-year-old children. Tables 7.2 and 7.3 provide information to help distinguish between the common, uncommon, and atypical displays of sexual behavior.

When working with children and adolescents, the PCP must focus on establishing and maintaining a positive relationship based on mutual trust and respect to feel validated and comfortable

• BOX 7.3 Problem-Focused Adolescent Sexual History

Describe the sexual concern, problem, issue, or difficulty that you have. Include the following history:

- Type of sex: oral, anal, and/or vaginal
- Condoms: consistency of use, for which sexual practices
- Previous sexually transmitted infections (STIs); medication allergies
- Most recent sexual encounter; number of partners in past 2 months
- Use of illegal drugs and alcohol by self and partner (include which drugs, frequency, route)
- Does patient and/or partner have sex with men, women, or both?
- Recent travel and location
- Any symptoms of dysuria, frequency, hematuria; adenopathy; fatigue; weight loss; night sweats; unexplained diarrhea; fever; rectal discharge, bleeding, constipation, pain?
- *Females only:* Additional symptoms of:
  - Vaginal discharge, bleeding, color of discharge; skin rashes, lesions, sores, and location; pruritus (vulvar, anal, oral, other); pain (abdominal, vaginal, vulvar, anal, headache, joints)
  - Last normal menstrual period (LNMP), description, changes
  - Birth control method(s), consistency of use
- *Males only:* Symptoms of:
  - Penile discharge; lesions and/or pruritus (penis, scrotum, urethra, oral cavity); pain or lumps in testes, difficulty with penis becoming erect/aroused?
  - How do you feel about discussing this problem?
  - How long have you had it? When did this problem begin?
  - What do you think caused you to have this problem?
  - What might be contributing to this problem?
  - What kinds of things have you done to treat or solve this problem?
  - What health professionals have you seen?
  - What, if any, medication have you taken or are you taking?
  - Have you talked to anyone (e.g., friend, relative, provider)?
  - Have you read any books to solve this problem? What books?

revealing concerns and asking questions. In addition to using a constructive approach to taking a sexual history, a positive relationship can be achieved by:

- Asking questions that give the message that the child is expected to change and be aware of and curious about those changes (e.g., "How are you feeling?" "How's your body?" "Do you notice that you're getting taller?" "Have you noticed your breasts getting any bigger?" "Boys' penises begin to get longer and wider as they become teenagers. Have you noticed any changes in yours?").
- Listening thoughtfully and carefully to the child's or adolescent's responses.
- Responding positively by answering the youth's questions as fully as possible, being nonjudgmental, calm, friendly, and open. Have a sense of humor but take them seriously.
- Using appropriate teachable moments during the health visit (e.g., when examining a 3-year-old child for inguinal hernia, the PCP can discuss appropriate and inappropriate touching with the child and his or her parent).
- Providing accurate information and referral resources.
- Respecting the youth's need for privacy (e.g., knocking before entering the examination room, providing appropriate gowns, examining the child semi-clothed).
- Maintaining confidentiality as appropriate, especially with an adolescent. Youth of any age may voice concerns about typical sexual development that do not need to be shared with the parent.

Sexuality Education

For a child or adolescent, developing healthy sexuality means gaining knowledge about physical changes; shaping a positive gender identity; clarifying one's sexual identity; establishing close, intimate relationships with others; and demonstrating the ability to make healthy judgments about sexuality and sexual activity. The questions a child or adolescent asks and the behaviors they display may embarrass some parents, who may respond in a manner that frightens, shames, or confuses the youth. Parents who are engaged and comfortable talking about sexual health with their children have children who are more knowledgeable and proactive in seeking reproductive healthcare. Infants are born as sexual beings, and parents, whether or not they are aware of it, constantly provide sex education lessons. The ways parents respond to a child's innate sexuality (innocent curiosity about sex, gender, and body parts and functions) and how they allow their sexuality to evolve are the core of a child's sex education.

Parents should be encouraged to take advantage of teaching opportunities about typical childhood sexual play and to answer questions simply and directly at the child's level of understanding (Box 7.4). Box 7.5 outlines what children should know about sexuality at different ages.

Research demonstrates that comprehensive sexuality education contributes to improved sexual health knowledge, skills, and attitudes and a subsequent reduction in risky sexual behaviors, adolescent pregnancy, STIs, sexual abuse, and interpersonal violence.[11] A comprehensive sexuality education program should include information about sexual anatomy, reproduction, STIs, sexual orientation, gender identity, abstinence, contraception, and reproductive rights and responsibilities. This information should be provided to parents, religious and community groups, healthcare professionals, and educators. Sex education in schools remains political and content is subject to federal, state, and local mandates. With the passage of the Patient Protection and Affordable Care Act, there are funds available for comprehensive sex education. States may apply for grants from the State Personal Responsibility Education Program but must use evidence-based elements in the curriculum (see Administration for Children and Families in Additional Resources). Box 7.6 lists the criteria for effective curriculum-based comprehensive programs.

Several national organizations, including Sex Ed for Social Change (SIECUS), Advocates for Youth, and Answer partnered to create the Future of Sex Education (FoSE) Initiative and published the National Sexuality Education Standards.[12] These standards are organized around seven key topics (anatomy and physiology, puberty and adolescent development, identity, pregnancy and reproduction, sexually transmitted diseases and HIV, healthy relationships, and personal safety), and these concepts are discussed at five developmental/grade levels. Quality evidence-based sex education provides comprehensive foundational content as well as allows for the exploration of personal identity, values, and beliefs (see Additional Resources).

Many professional nursing and medical organizations have policy statements or position papers that support comprehensive sex education in schools and at home.[13] They encourage abstinence as the adolescents' best choice to prevent pregnancy and STIs, and they encourage parental involvement in sexuality education.

TABLE 7.3	Red Flags Related to Sexual Behavior of Children and Adolescents	
Age	**Can Occur in All Children but Assess Child's Environment for Violence, Abuse, Neglect**	**Red Flags**
12 years or younger	Asking peer/adult to engage in sexual act(s) Simulating foreplay with dolls/peers (e.g., petting, French kissing) Inserting objects into genitals Imitating intercourse Touching animal genitalia	Preoccupied with sexual play Engaging in sexual play with children who are 4 or more years apart Attempting to expose others' genitals (e.g., pulling another's pants down) Precocious sexual knowledge Sexually explicit proposals or behaviors that induce fear/threats of force or that are physically aggressive (including written notes, graffiti) Compulsive masturbation; interrupts tasks to masturbate Chronic peeping/accessing pornography, exposing self/revealing postings, using obscenities, exhibiting pornographic interests Simulating intercourse with dolls/peers/animals with clothing on or off Oral, vaginal, anal penetration of dolls, peers, animals Sexual behaviors that are persistent and cause anger in child if they are distracted
Older than 12 years	Pornographic interest Sexually aggressive themes/obscenities; may embarrass others with these interests Sexual preoccupation/anxiety interferes with daily activities Single occurrences of peeping, exposing self, simulating intercourse with clothes on	Chronic, public masturbation Degrading or humiliating self or others with sexual themes Grabbing or trying to expose others' genitals Chronic occupation with sexually aggressive pornography Sexually explicit talk or sexual behaviors with children 4 or more years younger (sexual abuse) Making sexually explicit threats (including written) Obscene phone calls, voyeurism, exhibitionism, sexual harassment Performing rape or bestiality Genital injury to others

aUncommon but can occur in children 2 to 6 years.

Modified from Hagan, JF, Shaw, JS, Duncan, PM. *Bright Futures: Guidelines for Health Supervision of Infants, Children and Adolescents*. 4th edAmerican Academy of Pediatrics, 2017; Holland-Hall C. Adolescent physical and social development. In: Kliegman R, St. Geme J, eds. *Nelson Textbook of Pediatrics*, 21st ed. Elsevier; 2020; and Sege RD, Amaya-Jackson L. Clinical considerations related to the behavioral manifestations of child maltreatment. *Pediatrics*. 2017;139(4):e1–13.

However, all statements agree that counseling and education on contraception, STIs, and HIV/acquired immune deficiency syndrome (AIDS) are essential.

Counseling of the Adolescent

Today's adolescents are influenced by multiple conflicting sources, including societal expectations; the media's portrayal of sexuality; the family of origin's cultural norms, beliefs, and attitudes; peer group pressure; and the individual's own values and belief system. All these influences need to be considered and addressed when providing sexuality counseling.

The PCP ideally uses the answers given by the adolescent in the sexual history to further guide the counseling and educational needs of that individual. It may take several visits for the trust relationship to grow before the adolescent is willing to divulge certain aspects of his or her sexual self. The provider's job is to assure the adolescent of the confidential nature of the relationship and provide opportunities for trust to develop.

Adolescents should be counseled that abstinence is the most effective strategy for the prevention of pregnancy, STIs, and HIV/AIDS. Further, they need to know that it is a choice to remain abstinent and a choice to become sexually active, not just something that happens, and with each choice comes responsibilities. Open communication and respect for self and their partner leads to choices that should include STI and pregnancy protection.

When counseling adolescents, the provider's approach needs to be appropriate for the teen's psychosocial developmental stage. Early adolescents (12–14 years old) are concrete thinkers and cannot comprehend the abstract thought of "what if." Counseling language should be in simple, concrete terms. Using pictures, direct questions, and statements helps facilitate this. Middle adolescents (15–17 years old) understand abstract concepts but may often regress to concrete thinking in stressful situations. An adolescent at this age may demonstrate mature thought processes at one point in time yet revert to concrete thinking at another. The PCP needs to adjust the approach to middle adolescents accordingly to help them identify the inconsistencies in their thought processes and guide them through to the logical consequences. Late adolescents (18–21 years old) typically think abstractly and are future oriented. However, this ability varies, as with the general adult population.

Contraceptive and Safer Sex Counseling

It is important to use gender-neutral phrasing when discussing safer sex and contraception and to not assume heterosexuality. Providers who provide contraceptive and safer sex counseling to adolescents should understand that the successful use of any method requires a complex process of knowledge acquisition, decision-making skills, and public behaviors. To use contraceptives and/or protective barriers successfully, an individual must master the following:

• BOX 7.4 Approaches to Teaching Your Child About Sex

- Find out what your child already knows. Make sure you understand what your child is asking before you answer the question. Do not make assumptions. Check to be sure your answer is understood. Make sure you answer the question that is asked and give your child a chance to ask more questions.
- If your child asks a question about sexuality at an inconvenient time, set a time and place as soon as possible to answer the question.
- Discuss sex in a matter-of-fact way.
- Use correct terminology when talking about body parts; use dolls and books as guides.
- Keep the topics short and to the point. Keep the child's attention span in mind.
- Do not worry about telling children too much about sex. They tune out what they do not understand.
- Encourage questions. Never embarrass children or tell them they are too young to understand or that they will learn that when they grow up.
- Include values, emotions, feelings, and decision-making in your discussion. Do not focus only on biological facts.
- Let your child know that people have different beliefs about sexuality.
- Bring up topics of STIs, including HIV/AIDS.
- Discuss anticipated puberty changes before they occur. Do not wait until your child is a teenager. Discuss menstruation with both girls and boys.
- If you do not know the answer to your child's question, say so, and then look it up. Ask your pediatric PCP.
- If your child is masturbating in public or engaging in sex play, redirect him or her to other activities. Later, discuss where a more appropriate private place is for the child to masturbate.
- When your child uses obscene or derogatory words, calmly explain what they mean, why it is not appropriate to use them, and that use of certain words can be insulting (e.g., "gay"). Do not laugh or joke about your child's use of such words, because this can serve as encouragement.

AIDS, Acquired immune deficiency syndrome; *HIV,* human immunodeficiency virus; *PCP,* primary care provider; *STI,* sexually transmitted infection.

- *Knowledge.* For most adolescents, this means mastery of the use of a barrier method (e.g., male or female condoms) to prevent an STI and a secondary contraceptive method (e.g., oral contraceptive, intrauterine device).
- *Ability to plan for the future.* Planning for the future requires self-admission that the adolescent will have sex in the future and the ability to take the steps necessary to use a method consistently and correctly.
- *Willingness to acquire needed contraceptive and/or barrier methods.* The adolescent must be willing and able to be public with requests for contraceptive and/or protective devices (e.g., to purchase condoms at a local pharmacy or to seek services at the local clinic, school-based health facility, or private practice; see Chapter 43 for more in-depth information on contraceptive methods).
- *Communication skills.* Adolescents must have the ability to communicate with another person, such as their partner, healthcare provider, school nurse, or pharmacist, about their individual contraceptive and/or protective barrier needs.

Sexuality in Individuals With Intellectual and Physical Developmental Disabilities

The sexual development of youth with intellectual and physical developmental disabilities or youth with disabilities (YWD) is the

• BOX 7.5 Sexual Development: Content Children Should Know

By 5 Years Old
- Use correct words for all sexual body parts.
- Understand what it means to be male or female.
- Understand that their bodies belong to themselves, and they should say "no" to unwanted touch. However, having their private parts touched (for hygiene purposes by a parent) and during physical examinations by their healthcare provider when accompanied by a parent are normal.
- Know where babies come from; how they "get in" and "get out."
- Be able to talk about body parts without feeling "naughty."
- Be able to ask trusted adults questions about sexuality.
- Know that "sex talk" is for private times at home.

By 6–9 Years Old
- Be aware that all creatures grow and reproduce.
- Be aware that sexuality is important at all ages, including at their parents' and grandparents' ages, and that it changes over time.
- Know and use proper words for body parts—their own and those of the opposite sex.
- Understand that there are many kinds of caring family types so that they do not see a sole family model as the only valid one.
- Be aware that sexual identity includes sexual orientation: lesbian, gay, heterosexual, bisexual, transgender, questioning, queer, and asexual.
- Understand the basic facts about how an individual acquires HIV/AIDS.
- Take an active role in managing their body's health and safety.

By 9–13 Years Old/Young Teens[a]
- Be informed about human reproduction.
- Be aware of changes they can expect in their bodies before puberty (by 9–11 years old).
- Know how normal developmental changes begin, including normal differences and when those events occur for males and females.
- Know how male and female bodies grow and differ.
- Understand the general stages of the body's growth.
- Understand the facts about menstruation and wet dreams.
- Know that emotional changes are very common during this time.
- Understand that human sexuality is a natural part of life (by 12–13 years old).
- Be aware of how behavior can be seen as sexual and how to deal with sexual behavior (by 12–13 years old).
- Be aware that sexual feelings are normal and okay.
- Know how to recognize and protect themselves against potential sexual abuse and how to react to such dangers.
- Be able to recognize male and female prostitution and its dangers.
- Know how babies are made and what behaviors are likely to lead to pregnancy.
- Know that it is possible to plan parenthood.
- Understand that having a child is a long-term responsibility and that every child deserves mature, responsible, loving parents.
- Be aware that contraceptives (birth control methods) exist (and be able to name some).
- Know what abortion is.
- Know what STIs are.
- Understand how a person can get STIs.
- Be aware of how a person can protect himself or herself from STIs.
- Know how STIs are treated.

[a]See www.plannedparenthood.org/parents/talking-to-kids-about-sex-and-sexuality for more detailed information and information about what older teens should know and understand about sexuality.
AIDS, Acquired immune deficiency syndrome; *HIV,* human immunodeficiency virus; *STI,* sexually transmitted infection.

• BOX 7.6	Criteria of Effective Curriculum-Based Comprehensive Sexuality Education Program

- Focus on clear health goals.
- Focus narrowly on specific types of behavior leading to the health goals.
- Address sexual psychosocial risk and protective factors that affect sexual behavior.
- Create a safe social environment.
- Include multiple activities to change each of the targeted risk and protective factors.
- Use instructionally sound teaching methods that actively involve participants, help them personalize information, target risk and protective factors.
- Use activities, methods, and messages that are appropriate to the teens' culture, developmental age, and sexual experience.
- Cover topics in a logical sequence.
- Select educators with the ability to relate to young people and then train and support them.

• BOX 7.7	Sexual Education Topics for the Individual With Intellectual and Physical Developmental Disabilities

- Body parts
- Concepts of privacy and choice
- Masturbation
- Sexual abuse prevention
- Menstruation
- Homosexuality
- Marriage
- Sexual interaction
- Dating and intimacy
- Appropriate social behaviors
- Birth control, pregnancy
- Sexually transmitted infections
- Self-esteem
- Attitudes and values
- Sexual responsibility, privileges, and consent

same as those without such physical or cognitive limitations. The PCP should focus on the youth's developmental level rather than chronological age when determining the appropriateness of sexual behavior. For example, an individual with a cognitive level of a preschooler will normally exhibit sexual behaviors consistent with that developmental level.

YWD individuals have the same desires to make decisions and foster fulfilling relationships with others as do their nonaffected peers. Their abilities to develop healthy sexual identities and engage in sexual behaviors often largely hinge on society's comfort and proactive support concerning their right to healthy sexual expression, rather than on their disability itself. YWD may be viewed by society (including health providers, teachers, and parents) as being childlike, asexual, sexually inappropriate, or having uncontrollable sexual urges. Institutional isolation, overprotection, lack of awareness by others of their sexual needs, and pessimism about their potential often end up inhibiting the healthy sexual and psychosocial development of these individuals. Consequently, many people with disabilities are vulnerable to sexual abuse and exploitation by those who house, employ, and care for them. A person with a disability is three times more likely to be a victim of physical and sexual abuse; those with intellectual and mental disabilities are even more vulnerable.[14] Sexual abuse victimization can lead to posttraumatic stress, low self-esteem, anxiety, depression, dissociation, eating disorders, sleep disorders, externalizing symptoms, adjustment disorders, and suicidal ideation.[2]

YWD are less likely to acquire sex education from parents, peers, PCPs, or school-based programming than through misguided navigation via virtual outlets.[15] YWD may be less likely to share their thoughts, feelings, and experiences with family and friends. Unless healthy sexuality is taught and supported, unhealthy choices and vulnerability to sexual victimization can occur.[16] Effective sex education curricula topics for YWD should include those listed in Box 7.7. Excellent resources and books for parents, teachers, and clinicians can be accessed from Parent Advocacy Coalition for Educational Rights, SIECUS, and the Center for Parent Information and Resources (CPIR; see Additional Resources).

Factors That Can Alter Sexual Behaviors

Many factors influence the frequency and number of sexual behaviors children and adolescents exhibit. These include exposure to family nudity, co-bathing, limited privacy, exposure to pornographic materials, exposure to sexual acts (including in the media), the extent of adult supervision, stressors (e.g., violence, parental absence, criminal activity, death, illness), sexual and physical abuse, neglect (can result in indiscriminate affection-seeking or interpersonal boundary problems), and psychiatric diagnoses (e.g., conduct disorder, attention-deficit/hyperactivity disorder, oppositional defiant disorder)[17] (see Chapter 22).

Children's sense of self; personality; relationship to others and to the physical world; cognitive, emotional, and spiritual abilities; perceptions; and expressions are all influenced by and, in turn, influence their sexual development. If children experience challenges with sexuality, all other aspects of development are affected. Issues of major concern include child sexual abuse (see Chapter 22) and adolescent pregnancy (see Chapter 43).

Lesbian, Gay, Bisexual, Transgender, and Questioning Youth

Sexual orientation includes at least three distinctive components: (1) sexual imagery (fantasies or attraction); (2) sexual behavior responsiveness; and (3) the person's self-identification as straight, lesbian, gay, bisexual, or other. Transgender is an umbrella term that describes individuals whose sex assigned at birth is incongruent with their gender identity. Sexual orientation, the attraction to one or both genders, is not synonymous with one's gender identity.

Adolescent-specific data on sexual orientation are sparse due to difficulty in surveying, social stigma, and lack of personal awareness as to whom they are attracted. Approximately 10% of the adolescent population self-identify as non-heterosexual or bisexual.[18] These data suggest that today's adolescents self-identify earlier than in the past and spend less time feeling unsure as to their sexual orientation.

Approach and Management

The goal of the PCP working with adolescents who are LGBTQ+ is the same as with any adolescent: promote healthy sexual development, assess social and emotional wellbeing, and encourage physical health through healthy lifestyle choices. It is important to support and validate the adolescent throughout the process of developing his or her awareness of and commitment to both sexual orientation and gender identity and to provide a safe healthcare environment. See Box 7.8 for LGBTQ+ terms and definitions.

The counseling needs of LGBTQ+ youth are much the same as those with any adolescent. Specific interventions include the following: ensuring confidentiality, using correct gender pronouns (see Table 7.1) and nonjudgmental language, displaying information that is important to LGBTQ+ youth, and providing information about available resources for support. Encourage abstinence, promote safer sex for those who are sexually active, and counsel about the association between substance abuse and unsafe sexual practices.

For many LGBTQ+ youth, adolescence unfolds without event, especially for those with family support, whereas others have a rockier transition and engage in risky behaviors and experience complications. Family support and acceptance are associated with increased levels of self-esteem, social support, and overall health and are protective against depression, substance abuse, and suicidal ideation and attempts.[19] Maturity, access to accurate information, positive role models, and social support influence the LGBTQ+ youth's self-acceptance and success with intimate relationships.

LGBTQ+ youth tend to engage in high-risk behaviors and face stress and victimization at a higher rate than their heterosexual peers, which may lead to poor health outcomes for these adolescents.[20] Providers need to be aware of the increased risks surrounding LGBTQ+ youth and address these needs through education and counseling at every health visit (Box 7.9).

• BOX 7.8 Glossary of LGBTQ+ Terms for Healthcare Providers

Agender (adj.)—Describes a person who identifies as having no gender.
Ally (noun)—A person who supports and stands up for the rights of LGBTQ+ people.
Asexual (adj.)—Describes a person who experiences little or no sexual attraction to others. Asexuality is not the same as celibacy.
Bigender (adj.)—Describes a person whose gender identity is a combination of two genders.
Biphobia (noun)—The fear of, discrimination against, or hatred of bisexual people or those who are perceived as such.
Bisexual (adj.)—Describes a person who is emotionally and sexually attracted to people of their own gender and people of other genders.
Bottom surgery (noun)—Colloquial way of describing gender-affirming genital surgery.
Cisgender (adj.)—Describes a person whose gender identity is consistent with sex assigned birth.
Gay (adj.)—Describes those who are emotionally and sexually attracted to people of their own gender. It can be used regardless of gender identity but is more commonly used to describe males.
Gender (noun)—The characteristics and roles of women and men according to social norms. Can be described as feminine, masculine, androgynous, bigender, cisgender, misgender, transgender, polygender, and two spirit.
Gender-affirming hormone therapy (noun)—Feminizing and masculinizing hormone treatment to align secondary sex characteristics with gender identity.
Gender binary (noun)—The idea that there are only two genders, male and female, and that a person must strictly fit into one category or the other.
Gender dysphoria (noun)—Distress experienced by some individuals whose gender identity does not correspond with their assigned sex at birth.
Gender expression (noun)—The way a person acts, dresses, speaks, and behaves (i.e., feminine, masculine, androgynous).
Gender fluid (adj.)—Describes a person whose gender identity is not fixed and may feel more one gender some days, and another gender other days.
Gender identity (noun)—A person's internal sense of being a man/male, woman/female, both, neither, or another gender.
Gender nonconforming (adj.)—Describes a gender expression that differs from a given society's norms for males and females.
Intersex (adj.)—Can be used as an identity term for those with sexual anatomy development differences.
Lesbian (adj., noun)—A female who is emotionally and sexually attracted to other females.

Nonbinary (adj.)—Describes a person whose gender identity fall outside of the traditional male and female gender structure.
Outing (verb)—Involuntary or unwanted disclosure of another person's sexual orientation or gender identity.
Pangender (adj.)—Describes a person whose gender identity is comprised of many genders.
Pansexual (adj.)—Describes a person who is emotionally and sexually attracted to people regardless of gender.
Queer (adj.)—An umbrella term used by some to describe people who think of their sexual orientation or gender identity as outside of societal norms; not embraced or used by all members of the LGBTQ+ community and offensive to some.
Questioning (adj.)—Describes individuals who are unsure about or are exploring their own sexual orientation and/or gender identity.
Sex- (noun)—Assigned (male or female) at birth, most often based on external anatomic and biological characteristics.
Sexual orientation (noun)—How a person characterizes their emotional and sexual attraction to others.
Top surgery (noun)—Colloquial way of describing gender-affirming surgery on the chest.
Transgender (adj.)—Describes a person whose gender identity and assigned sex at birth do not correspond. Also used as an umbrella term to include gender identities outside of male and female.
Trans man/transgender man/female-to-male (FTM) (noun)—Transgender persons whose gender identity is male may use these terms to describe themselves.
Trans woman/transgender woman/male-to-female (MTF) (noun)—Transgender persons whose gender identity is female may use these terms to describe themselves.
Two spirit (adj.)—A contemporary term that connects today's experiences of LGBT Native American and American Indian people with the traditions from their cultures.
Outdated terms to avoid:
- Biological male/female
- Gender nonconforming
- Hormone replacement therapy
- Homosexual
- Preferred pronouns
- Sexual preference
- Sex change
- Transgendered
- Transsexual

From National LGBTQIA+ Health Education Center: A program of the Fenway Institute (SIECUS). https://www.lgbtqiahealtheducation.org/wp-content/uploads/2020/02/Glossary-2022.02.22-1.pdf.

• BOX 7.9   Stressors and Potential High-Risk Behaviors of LGBTQ+ Youth

- Stigma and harassment
- Bullying and victimization
- Depression/anxiety
- Substance abuse
- Suicidal thoughts and attempts
- Academic underachievement/school truancy/dropping out
- Running away/homelessness
- Sexual risk-taking/STIs
- Obesity and disordered eating
- Avoidance of healthcare services

From Adelson S, Schuster M. Gay, Lesbian and bisexual adolescents. In: Kliegman R, St. Geme J, eds, *Nelson Textbook of Pediatrics*, 21st ed. Elsevier; 2020;1024–1026.

Additional Resources

Administration, Administration for Children and Families, US Department of Health and Human Services (HHS): State Personal Responsibility Education Program, Family and Youth Services Bureau (FYSB): https://www.acf.hhs.gov/fysb/adolescent-pregnancy-prevention

American Academy of Pediatrics: Adolescent Health Care Campaign Toolkit. https://www.aap.org/en/news-room/campaigns-and-toolkits/adolescent-health-care/

Center for Parent Information and Resources (CPIR), Center for Parent Information and Resources (CPIR): www.parentcenterhub.org

Child Sexual Behavior Inventory (CSBI): https://www.nctsn.org/measures/child-sexual-behavior-inventory

Comprehensive Sex Education for Youth with Disabilities (SIECUS): https://siecus.org/wp-content/uploads/2021/03/SIECUS-2021-Youth-with-Disabilities-CTA-1.pdf

ETR Associates: www.etr.org

Family Equality Council: www.familyequality.org

Future of Sex Education (FoSE), Future of Sex Education (FoSE) Initiative: www.advocatesforyouth.org/wp-content/uploads/2021/11/NSES-2020-web-updated2.pdf

Guttmacher Institute: www.guttmacher.org

National LGBTQIA+ Health Education Center. Gender-Affirming Pediatric Care Toolkit: https://www.lgbtqiahealtheducation.org/collection/trans-pediatric-care-toolkit/

Parent Advocacy Coalition for Educational Rights: www.pacer.org

Parents, Families, and Friends of Lesbians and Gays, Inc. (PFLAG): http://community.pflag.org

Physicians for Reproductive Health: https://prh.org/arshep-ppts/#sexual-health

Planned Parenthood Federation of America: www.plannedparenthood.org

ReproLine: www.reprolineplus.org

Sexuality Information and Education Council of the United States (SIECUS), Sexuality Information and Education Council of the United States (SIECUS): https://siecus.org/

Society for Adolescent Health and Medicine (SAHM), Society for Adolescent Health and Medicine (SAHM): www.adolescenthealth.org

World Health Organization (WHO), Sexual Health: www.who.int/health-topics/sexual-health#tab_1

References

1. Kågesten A, van Reeuwijk M. Healthy sexuality development in adolescence: proposing a competency-based framework to inform programs and research. *Sex Reprod Health Matters*. 2021;29(1):104–120.
2. World Health Organization (WHO): Sexual Health 2022. https://www.who.int/health-topics/sexual-health#tab=tab_1.
3. American Academy of Pediatrics. *Equitable Access to Sexual and Reproductive Health Care for All Youth*; 2022. aap.org/AAP/PDF/FINAL_Equitable%20Youth%20Access%20to%20SRH%20Care.pdf.
3a. National Assocation of Pediatric Nurse Practitioners. NAPNAP strongly opposes actions by Texas leaders. https://www.napnap.org/napnap-strongly-opposes-actions-by-texas-leaders/#:~:text=NAPNAP%20strongly%20urges%20Texas%20leaders,youth%20and%20improve%20health%20equity.
4. Fausto-Sterling A. Gender/sex, sexual orientation, and identity are in the body: how did they get there? *J Sex Res*. 2019;56(405):529–555.
5. Ehrensaft D. Gender nonconforming youth: current perspectives. *Adolesc Health Med Ther*. 2017;8:57–67.
6. Korpaisarn S, Safer JD. Etiology of gender identity. *Endocrinol Metabol Clin North Am*. 2019;48(2):323–329.
7. Guttmacher Institute. *Fact Sheet: Adolescent Sexual and Reproductive Health in the United States*; 2022. Available at: https://www.guttmacher.org/fact-sheet/american-teens-sexual-and-reproductive-health.
8. Fuentes L, Ingerick M, Jones R, et al. Adolescents' and young adults' reports of barriers to confidential health care and receipt of contraceptive services. *J Adolesc Health*. 2018;62(1):36–43.
9. American College of Obstetrics and Gynecology. ACOG Committee opinion No. 754: the utility of and indications for routine pelvic examination. *Obstet Gynecol*. 2018;132(4):e174–e180.
10. Qin J, Saraiya M, Martinez G, Sawaya G. Prevalence of potentially unnecessary bimanual pelvic examinations and papanicolaou tests among adolescent girls and young women aged 15-20 years in the United States. *JAMA Intern Med*. 2020;180(2):274–280.
11. Goldfarb ES, Lieberman LD. Three decades of research: the case for comprehensive sex education. *J Adolesc Health*. 2021;68:13–27.
12. Future of Sex Education Initiative (FoSE). *National Sexuality Education Standards: Core Content and Skills*. 2nd ed. 2020. *K-12*. https://www.advocatesforyouth.org/wp-content/uploads/2021/11/NSES-2020-web-updated2.pdf.
13. Guttmacher Institute. *An Overview of Minor's Consent Law*; 2022. https://www.guttmacher.org/state-policy/explore/overview-minors-consent-law.
14. Fang Z, Cerna-Turoff C, Zhang C, Lu M, Lachman J, Barlow J. Global estimates of violence against children with disabilities: an updated systematic review and meta-analysis. *Lancet Child Adolescent Health*. 2022;6(5):313–323.
15. Sexuality Information and Education Council of the Unites States (SIECUS). *Guidelines for Comprehensive Sexuality Education*. 3rd ed. Fulton Press; 2021. https://siecus.org/wp-content/uploads/2018/07/Guidelines-CSE.pdf.
16. Sexuality Information and Education Council of the United States (SIECUS). *Comprehensive Sex Education for Youth with Disabilities; A Call to Action*; 2021. From: https://siecus.org/wp-content/uploads/2021/03/SIECUS-2021-Youth-with-Disabilities-CTA-1.pdf.
17. Sege RD, Amaya-Jackson L. Clinical considerations related to the behavioral manifestations of child maltreatment. *Pediatrics*. 2017;139(4):e1–e13.
18. Conron KJ. *LGBT Youth Population in the United States*. The Williams Institute; 2020.
19. McConnell EA, Birkett M, Mustanski B. Families matter: social support and mental health trajectories among lesbian, gay, bisexual, and transgender youth. *J Adolesc Health*. 2016;59(6):674–680.
20. Lapinski J, Covas T, Perkins JM, et al. Transgender health; a clinician's guide. *Prim Care Clin Office Pract*. 2018;45:687–703.

8

Developmental Principles and Theories

MARTHA DRIESSNACK AND DANIEL CRAWFORD

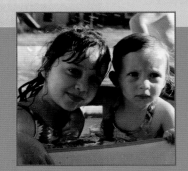

This chapter introduces basic developmental principles and theories, with an emphasis on the vital intersection between development and health. The concept of developmental surveillance is introduced, highlighting recent changes, followed by a brief overview of parent/family development and theories. This introductory chapter is followed by five chapters, each of which highlights age-specific development/surveillance, health supervision issues, screening tools, red flags, and family resources. The five age groups include neonate (0–1 month), infant (1–12 months), early childhood (1–5 years), middle childhood (6–10 years), and adolescence (11–21 years). Collectively, these six chapters serve as foundational knowledge for primary care providers (PCPs) tasked with understanding the dynamic nature of development, as well as integrating and applying it into pediatric primary care in the midst of an ever-changing environment and society.

Understanding developmental concepts and principles, the evolving contexts in which newborns, infants, children, and adolescents live and learn, and how they all interact is foundational knowledge for pediatric PCPs. A number of theories have contributed to our understanding of child development over the past century but have come under criticism over time, especially in terms of contemporary understanding of gender and contemporary lenses of diversity, equity, and inclusion. Alternative theories, as well as theories from other disciplines, are now used to examine the impact of modern societal contexts, advances in science and technology, and the expanding use of media. Underlying all of these theories are basic developmental principles, each of which is introduced and briefly discussed.

Development Is a Dynamic and Lifelong Process

Development reflects gradual changes and expanding capabilities, each of which allows for simple skills and behaviors to be mastered and integrated into more complex skills and behaviors. Milestone achievements at early levels set the stage for achievement in later levels. Simple behaviors (e.g., self-feeding) are often taken for granted; yet each milestone is the result of the acquisition of numerous small changes and skills. While pediatric PCPs closely monitor the developmental changes during the pediatric lifespan, we all continue to develop throughout our lives, with each advancing level marked by subtle changes and advancing integration.

There Are Different Aspects of Development, and Each Is Dynamically Related to the Others

Development can be examined as a whole and/or by its individual aspects or domains. *Biophysical* development focuses on organ development, including the brain, sensory abilities, and advancing motor skills. *Cognitive* development focuses on information processing, including language acquisition, problem solving, and other learning abilities and skills, with an emphasis on the sociocultural environment in which the child learns. *Psychosocial* development focuses on personality, including temperament, emotional regulation, attachment, and relationships with others. While each aspect can be studied separately, they do not present independently and most often need to work together. For example, the ability of a child to walk involves both brain organization and muscle strength.

Development Is Systematic, Organized, and Successive

Developmental progression is predictable, which makes it easier to assess for deviations from the typical. Developmental changes occur in an orderly and predictable way, with specific changes occurring together to support specific skills and behaviors. Each successive change relies on successful attainment of earlier changes, resulting in skills and behaviors that are increasingly regulated, organized, and differentiated. Much like growth patterns, development follows a *cephalocaudal* (i.e., head-to-toe) and *proximodistal* (i.e., midline-to-periphery) progression. A child needs head control before they can sit; they need to be able to sit, as well as grasp and release, to be able to bring two hands together to examine and transfer or learn about different objects.

The Pace of Development Is Not Universal

Each child progresses at their own pace, which means development occurs on a spectrum. Accordingly, there are *ranges* for attaining biophysical, cognitive, and psychosocial milestones. For example, one child will walk early but be slower to speak, while another will speak early but be slower to walk. Some children will progress smoothly, while others do so in fits and starts.

There Can Be Critical and/or Sensitive Periods for Development

The early pediatric environment is formative and its effects on development are important. *Critical* periods are points in time when it is thought that something *must* occur (e.g., biological or environmental event) to ensure normal development. These periods reflect times when new skills or abilities develop but only with specific exposures or experiences; however, if specific exposures and experiences are not available during that time, it becomes much harder or even impossible to develop or acquire the skill or ability after the window of opportunity closes. While critical periods are most often associated with fetal development, there are also infant and childhood critical periods surrounding vision, hearing, language, and psychosocial development. In contrast, *sensitive* periods are points in time when a development is most likely but does not have to occur. These times are often referred to as *windows of opportunity* and are times when the brain is most likely to strengthen important connections and eliminate unneeded ones; however, new synapses still form outside of this optimal period, despite it being more difficult.

Both Nature and Nurture Shape Development

The term "nature" refers to our biological processes, including our genome, which have the potential to influence every aspect of development. In contrast, nurture refers to our immediate and expanding environments, from the womb to home to school to community, and the people in those environments. Past conversations about nature versus nurture shifted to understanding how nature and nurture work together to shape development. While our individual genomes include our unique DNA, which is fixed, they also include proteins that regulate gene expression, turning gene activity on or off, and these proteins can change in response to our experience and exposures. This discovery led to the field of epigenetics, exploring how gene expression is mediated and moderated by our internal and external environments.

Developmental Theories

Developmental theories provide different lenses for understanding emerging behaviors, personality, and abilities. They attempt to account for how children's development is affected by who and what are around them. Being familiar with a number of different theories helps pediatric PCPs to understand the various developmental aspects to consider as they care for newborns, infants, children, and adolescents. In this section, a subset of theories is introduced, beginning with well-known psychoanalytic, cognitive, and learning theorists, while also including less familiar information processing, ethologic, and system theorists. Individually and collectively, these theories, along with others, help to provide insight into the increasingly complex intersection between development and health (Table 8.1). Each theory has valuable insights to offer.

TABLE 8.1	Cross-Section of Developmental Theorists	
Theory, Major Theorists	**Focus, Key Concepts**
Psychodynamic • Psychosexual: Freud • Psychosocial: Erikson	Personality *How personalities are formed*
Cognitive • Constructivist, discontinuous: Piaget • Constructivist, continuous: Vygotsky • Information processing • Social cognition: Theory of Mind	Thinking *Different ways of acquiring knowledge*
Learning • Classical conditioning: Watson • Operant conditioning: Skinner • Self-efficacy: Bandura	Learning *How experience affects learning and behavior*
Ethologic • Bowlby (attachment) • Lorenz	Biology *The role of experience during specific times*
System • Bronfenbrenner • Gottlerb • Lerner • Sameroff	Interaction *How interacting systems shape development*
Ethics • Moral development: Kohlberg, Gilligan, Coles • Spiritual: Fowler	Moral/spiritual *How moral reasoning and spirituality develop*

Psychodynamic Theories

Psychodynamic theorists focus on personality and emotions. They view development through the lens of conflict resolution, with different ages facing unique conflicts that need to be resolved for successful or adaptive development. They also view development as discontinuous, or staged, with each conflict or stage viewed as qualitatively different from the others.

Psychosexual: Sigmund Freud

Freud proposed that an individual's personality is made up of three conflicting forces, and healthy development is the ability to balance them as children pass through a series of stages, during which maturing biological instincts interact with different erogenous or pleasure zones. The *id*, which is present from birth, operates on the pleasure principle, constantly seeking to satisfy basic impulses/urges and as quickly as possible. During the first year of life, the infant is in Freud's first, or *oral* stage, when pleasure is centered around the mouth, including sucking, chewing, and biting. Later in the first year, the ego begins to emerge. The *ego* operates in reality, seeking to find a way to satisfy the id's need for immediate gratification in socially acceptable ways. During the second year of life, biological maturation gives rise to the *anal* stage, shifting the pleasure zone to bowel/urine elimination. This stage lasts until the child is approximately 3 years of age, at which time the focus of pleasure migrates to the genitalia. This is the *phallic* stage, which lasts throughout early childhood until the child enters school at age 5 to 6 years. At the beginning of this stage, children theoretically desire the opposite-sex parent and compete with their same-sex parent for the other parent's attention. This ongoing conflict gives rise to the *superego*, or conscience, which enables children to control their behavior based on what they internalize from their parents or caregivers as right and wrong or acceptable versus unacceptable behavior. Resolution occurs when the child aligns, rather than competes, with the same-sex parent. This is also referred to as *resolving the Oedipus complex* for males, or less-known *Electra complex* for females. The fourth, or *latent* stage, occurs during the school-age years, during which sexual impulses are suppressed and pleasure is redirected to intellectual and social activities. These activities further develop the superego. The final, or genital, stage occurs during puberty. During this stage, sexual impulses reemerge and the adolescent must learn to satisfy their sexual needs in socially appropriate ways.

Freud's psychosexual theory has fewer and fewer followers over time, as there is much less emphasis on internal urges in later psychoanalytic theories. However, both Freud and his daughter Anna are credited with introducing the idea that early childhood experiences are important. Neo-Freudian, as well as other contemporary theorists, clinicians, and researchers, continue to learn about the effects of early experiences, both positive and negative, on children's immediate and long-term behaviors, beliefs, and health.

Psychosocial: Erik Erikson

Erikson was influenced by Freud but widened the scope beyond biological urges to include social factors (e.g., cultural influences) and the larger social world (e.g., contemporary issues). His theory is also different in that its eight stages extend across the lifespan, while Freud's ended with adolescence. Each of Erikson's age-related stages focuses on a developmental task or conflict set up by biological maturation and expanding social demands. Erikson believed that if the developmental tasks and conflicts were not resolved, the individual would continue to struggle, with the unresolved conflicts surfacing during, and at times interfering with, future stages. Six of these stages occur during the pediatric lifespan, each of which is presented in Table 8.2. Of note are the parallels with Freud, as Erikson's first stage parallels Freud's oral stage; the second stage parallels Freud's anal stage; and the third stage parallels Freud's idea of a superego.

Other Psychoanalytic Theorists

There are many other psychoanalytic and neo-Freudian theorists.[1] In this section, we highlight a few whose theories continue to impact pediatric practice.

Anna Freud. Anna Freud expanded on her father's work, focusing exclusively on children and calling attention to the important role developmental processes play as a child (and their id, ego, and superego) grows. She is credited with introducing the idea of defense mechanisms, and the idea that personality depends on the overall process of these defense mechanisms (e.g., repression, regression, denial, projection, reaction-formation) throughout development.

Melanie Klein. Melanie Klein is recognized as the first *object relations* theorist and the first to use *play analysis*. She believed that by watching children at play, an analyst can gain a deep understanding of the psychodynamic processes taking place in the child's mind.

Harry Sullivan. Harry Sullivan introduced the idea that *interpersonal* interactions, or what goes on *between* people, are more important in personality development than intrapersonal interactions, or what goes on *inside* people. He believed our developing sense of self (e.g., *good* me, *bad* me, and *not* me) is enhanced and/or inhibited by and through the reflected appraisals of others. As a result, a child's early (e.g., parents) and evolving (e.g., peers, other adults) exposures are seen as crucial.

Margaret Mahler. Margaret Mahler was a pediatrician turned psychoanalyst whose understanding of child development centered around the concept of separation-individuation. She emphasized the importance of mothers and the need for infants to separate from their mothers on their journey to developing their own individuality. Mahler created and taught the *Tripartite Treatment Model*, a therapeutic approach involving both the child and mother.

Donald Winnicott. Donald Winnicott was a pediatrician turned psychoanalyst who introduced the idea that for children to develop a healthy personality and realize their true self, they needed to move from *subjective omnipotence* to *objective reality* with the aid of a *good enough* mother (e.g., one who learns to step in only when needed), not a perfect one (e.g., one who is always present and doing for the child). He is also credited with

TABLE 8.2	Erikson's First Six (6) Developmental Stages		
Developmental Crisis	**Age**	**Theme**	**Outcome if Unresolved**
Basic trust vs. mistrust	Birth–1 year	To get/to give in return Developing confidence in/reliance on others	View others as unreliable and/or untrustworthy
Autonomy vs. doubt	1–3 years	To hold on/to let go Developing a sense of self-reliance and will	Doubt one's abilities and/or feel shame
Initiative vs. guilt	4–6 years	To make things/to play Developing courage, independence, and a sense of purpose	Trouble balancing or resolving conflict between self and others
Industry vs. inferiority	6–puberty	To make things/To complete developing confidence, work ethic, and responsibility	Feelings of incompetence and inferiority
Identity vs. role confusion	Puberty–20 years	To be oneself/to share oneself/not oneself with others Developing one's sense of self/identity	Remain confused about who they are/role in society
Intimacy vs. isolation	21–40 years	To lose/to find oneself in another Developing how to be intimately involved with others without losing one's sense of self	Failure to form close friendships/intimate relationships, leading to isolation

understanding that transitional experiences children must go through may be facilitated by transitional objects (e.g., blanket, stuffed animal). Winnicott introduced the *Squiggle Game*, a therapeutic technique that allows children to draw pictures to represent their thoughts and feelings.

Cognitive Theories

Cognitive theorists focus on the way children think and how thinking evolves over time to influence development. The three most influential cognitive theories are Piaget's stage theory, Vygotsky's sociocultural theory, and, more recently, information processing theories and Theory of Mind (ToM). Both Piaget and Vygotsky are considered constructivists, in that they focus on the way children construct knowledge. Information processing theories are broad and focus on how children attend to and store information, while ToM is specific to processing information about others. They are similar in that they all recognize children as active participants in their own development, while Piaget's stage approach supports discontinuous development and information processing and ToM support the notion of continuous development. Vygotsky acknowledges both continuous and discontinuous development but is primarily continuous.

Constructivists

Jean Piaget: Stage Theory of Cognitive Development. Piaget's theory focuses on children's progressive creation of mental structures, or *schema*, which are the ways children make sense of their experiences. *Adaptation* refers to the process of building schemas, which occurs by *assimilation* and *accommodation*. Children can assimilate new experiences into existing schemas, or they can adjust existing schemas or create new ones when existing schemas cannot accommodate their new experiences. During times when children are not being exposed to new information, assimilation dominates. Piaget referred to this state as *cognitive equilibrium*. During periods of cognitive stimulation and change, children experience *cognitive disequilibrium* and rely more on accommodation. Children can also build schemas through organization, which is when children link and organize existing schemas into new interconnected systems. Piaget proposed that the organization of schemas proceeded through four universal stages that occurred in a fixed order. Each of these stages represents a period when schemas are qualitatively similar (Table 8.3). Piaget's stage theory of cognitive development is widely known and referenced, and it was influential to the work of his contemporaries in the fields of moral reasoning (Kohlberg) and spiritual development (Fowler). However, Piaget has also been criticized for his tendency to underestimate the capabilities of the child.

Lev Vygotsky: Sociocultural Theory. Vygotsky was a contemporary of Piaget but took a totally different approach. While Piaget believed development preceded learning, Vygotsky proposed the opposite, that learning precedes development. It is a subtle but important distinction. Vygotsky stressed social interaction, viewing development in terms of what children could achieve with help of others, rather than what they could achieve on their own. He also focused on an endpoint, rather than stages, and the social processes that impact getting there. Core to Vygotsky's theory is the *zone of proximal development* (ZPD),

TABLE 8.3	Piaget's Stages of Cognitive Development	
Stage	**Age**	**Major Developments**
Sensorimotor	0–2 years	Understands the world through actions Moves from simple reflective behavior to acquiring mental representations
Reflexive schemas	0–1 month	Innate infant reflexes dominate
Primary circular reactions	1–4 months	Repetitive behaviors that lead to satisfying responses
Secondary circular reactions	4–8 months	Outward directed behaviors; events caused by their actions
Coordination of secondary circular reactions	8–12 months	Goal-directed behavior begins; combining schemas into larger action sequences Appearance of object permanence
Tertiary circular reactions	12–18 months	Repeat, vary, and combine schemas in explorations Acquisition of object permanence
Inventions of new means through mental combinations	18–24 months	Ability to think using mental images; memory used for problem solving Pretend play emerges
Preoperational	2–7 years	Starting to use representations (e.g., words, pictures) rather than actions to understand the world Egocentric/animistic thinking; able to focus on only one part of a problem (e.g., centration)
Concrete operations	7–11 years	Able to reason about concrete objects Increasingly logical and organized; uses mental operations Able to solve conservation problems, classify hierarchies, order objects by size (e.g., classification, seriation) Can solve transitive inference problems
Formal operations	11+ years	Able to progressively use abstract thinking and reasoning with more complex symbols Able to think logically; uses hypothetico-deductive reasoning Able to engage in propositional thought; work with abstract ideas

Modified from Crowley K. *Child Development: A Practical Introduction.* 2nd ed. Sage Publications; 2017; and Hauser-Cram P, Nugent JK, Thies KM, Travers JF. *The Development of Children and Adolescents.* John Wiley & Sons; 2014.

which is the space between children's actual developmental level and what they learn on their own through independent problem solving versus the next or higher developmental level, or what they can do with guidance from adults and more capable peers. In the ZPD, others provide *scaffolding* (e.g., guidance, support) until children achieve stand-alone competence in the task or skill being mastered. Vygotsky is known for his *strength*-based lens, pointing to what children can do, which is often contrasted with Piaget, who used a *deficit*-based lens, pointing to what children are not yet able to do at each stage.

Information Processing Theories

Information processing theories present another way of examining and understanding how children develop cognitively. They first emerged in the late 1960s to early 1970s and had an enormous impact on the study of cognition.[2] At their core, these theories conceptualize the human brain using the metaphor of a computer processing, encoding, storing, and decoding data. Unlike Piaget, there are no stages, and unlike Vygotsky, there is little focus on social interaction. Instead, these theories concentrate on cognitive processes, beginning with what information children attend to, how that information is encoded, how and if it moves from their working to their long-term memory, and how it is retrieved and returned to the working memory for relearning as new information is processed. Infants and toddlers learn primarily through sensory input from their surroundings; however, during childhood and adolescence, there is increased attention and ability to focus the attention, faster processing, increased working memory, and more efficient information processing.[3]

Social Cognition: Theory of Mind

Theory of Mind (ToM) refers to children's developing ability to understand the mental states of others. At first, it is recognizing humans as mental beings who have minds "full" of mental processes (e.g., intentions, beliefs, perceptions, emotions) that influence behavior and actions. Around the age of 3 years, children begin to learn that others are also "mind-full" and that their thoughts and beliefs may be different than theirs and, even when similar, may lead to different behaviors and actions. In some ways, ToM is better understood as a social-cognitive skill than as a theory. It is referred to as a theory because one person's beliefs about what might be going on in another person's head is just that—a theory. Children's ToM abilities progress sequentially, with most children able to pass ToM tasks by age 4 to 5 years (Box 8.1). However, ToM is relatively unstable, as children may understand mental states in some situations but struggle in others.[4] ToM

abilities continue to improve and develop through late adolescence and into adulthood.[5] Of note is that children's ToM abilities align with their social competence, as those children who are more adept at understanding what other people are thinking tend to have stronger social abilities.

Learning Theories

Learning theories focus on how experience affects learning and the importance of learned behavior. Accordingly, the emphasis is on children's exposures and experiences (e.g., nurture), and development is seen as continuous. This group of theories is typically divided into two categories: (1) behaviorists, who emphasize observable *behavior*, and (2) social learning theorists, who emphasize observable *learning*.

Behaviorists

John Watson. John Watson was an American psychologist who built on the work of Russian physiologist, Ivan Pavlov, who first documented the concept of *classical conditioning*. Classical conditioning is a type of learning in which a particular *stimulus* becomes associated with a particular *response*. He felt that learning occurred through ongoing stimulus-response associations and that children's environments were the main factor influencing how children developed, based on the stimuli they received. While highlighting the importance of children's environment is one of the strengths of Watson's theory, the main critique is that Watson saw children as passive.

B.F. Skinner. B.F. Skinner distinguished himself from Watson in a number of ways. First, he viewed children as active participants, or *operators,* interacting with and having an impact on their environments. He was particularly focused on how the consequences of actions influenced subsequent behavior, introducing the concept of *operant conditioning*. Operant conditioning proposes that actions followed by reinforcement will be strengthened and more likely to occur again in the future. *Positive reinforcers* are favorable outcomes or events (e.g., praise, reward) presented after a positive behavior, while *negative reinforcers* involve the removal of unfavorable (e.g., unpleasant) outcomes after a positive behavior; both are directed at having the positive behavior repeat itself in the future. Reinforcers are distinct from *punishment*. Punishment involves administering an *adverse* outcome or event after an undesired behavior with the aim of stopping the undesired behavior. Table 8.4 provides a visual schematic differentiating reinforcement from punishment. Skinner's concepts form the basis of therapy using behavioral modification.

Social Learning

Albert Bandura. Albert Bandura said learning was inherently social and that children played an active role in their own development. He emphasized observation and imitation, rather than reinforcement, as key mechanisms in child development. He stressed that children can and do learn in the absence of reinforcements and punishments through *observational learning* (e.g., *modelling*) by watching and/or imitating others, both real (e.g., adults, parents, caregivers, siblings, peers) and symbolic (e.g., book characters, TV or movie actors). He emphasized the role of cognitive processes in observational learning (e.g., attention, encoding, storing and retrieving information), which parallels contemporary information processing theories. Later in his career, he introduced the concept of *self-efficacy*, which is the belief that individuals manage (e.g., behaviors, thoughts, emotions) or are successful in

---

• BOX 8.1   Theory of Mind: Progressive/Sequential Tasks

Children progress through the following sequence or levels of understanding:
- Reasons why others want (desire) something may differ from one person to another.
- Others can have different ideas (feeling/beliefs) about the same thing.
- Others may not comprehend (or have the knowledge) that something is true.
- Others can have false beliefs about the world (and others).
- Others can have hidden emotions; they may act one way while feeling another way.

Modified from Wellman HM, Fuxi F, Peterson CC. Sequential progressions in a theory-of-mind scale: longitudinal perspectives. *Child Dev.* 2012;82(3):780–792.

TABLE 8.4	Operant Conditioning: Reinforcement vs. Punishment		
		ACTION ENCOURAGES THE CHILD/INDIVIDUAL'S BEHAVIOR TO…	
		Increase	Decrease
A child/individual engages in or demonstrates a certain behavior Afterward, an ACTION is…	Added	Positive (+) Reinforcement	Positive (+) punishment
	Removed	Negative (–) Reinforcement	Negative (–) punishment

Modified from Hauser-Cram et al. *The Development of Children and Adolescents.* John Wiley & Sons; 2014.

a given situation. He perceived self-efficacy as also influenced and learned by observing how others succeed.

Ethologic Theories

Ethology focuses on evolutionary behaviors by exploring their ongoing adaptive or survival value. Konrad Lorenz, a zoologist, is often referred to as its founder, while John Bowlby, a psychologist, is known for one of its more influential applications.

Konrad Lorenz

Konrad Lorenz introduced the concept of *imprinting*, an instinctual behavior in birds that keeps their young near, protected, and fed. It occurs during what Lorenz called *critical periods* of development, which are points in time when it is thought that something *must* occur to ensure normal development.

John Bowlby

John Bowlby built on Lorenz's work, shifting from animal to infant attachment. He also introduced *sensitive periods* of development, which are points in time when a development is most likely, but does not have to occur at that time. Bowlby argued that infants need to develop a primary attachment bond with a specific figure during infancy and early childhood. He also argued that infants needed their mothers in particular, and the absence of a specific and consistent mother figure during infancy would have long-term detrimental effects on the child's mental health.[6] Bowlby's work has been amended, noting bonding with at least one parent figure is sufficient for optimal development.

System Theories

System theories introduce an interactionist view of child development, including the idea of *intersectionality*. Interest in intersectionality is also used to understand how aspects of an individual's different identities (e.g., race, class, gender) interact and/or combine to create discrimination, social inequality and injustice, and privilege. While there are a number of systems theorists, Bronfenbrenner's ecological theory is highlighted, as it focuses specifically on children and provides an ideal example of the complexity involved with a systems lens and integration of intersectionality.

Urie Bronfenbrenner

Urie Bronfenbrenner saw development as occurring in an environment of nested, interacting layers of systems with the child at the center (Fig. 8.1). He viewed children as active agents bringing their own complex, interacting constellation of characteristics (e.g., genome, sex, gender, age, temperament, health, cognitive

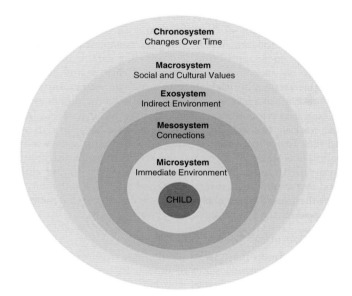

• **Fig. 8.1** Bronfenbrenner's Ecologic Systems Theory. (From Benson JB. *Encyclopedia of Infant and Early Childhood Development*, ed 2. Elsevier; 2020.)

capabilities). His interactionist view of child development draws attention to how different layers of systems affect how a child develops within as a result of their interactions, as well as how a change in one system can affect the others. The nested layers include the *microsystem*, which is the child's immediate environment, including *who* the child directly interacts with (e.g., family, peers, daycare, school, extended family) and the settings in which they are nurtured and learn; the *mesosystem*, which are the relationships/connections among microsystems (e.g., home–school); the *exosystem*, those social contexts/settings that the child is not a part of but that affect the children's development (e.g., parents' workplace, mass media, school board, community health services); the *macrosystem*, the broader sociocultural and political context in which the child and all the other systems are embedded (e.g., laws, attitudes, values, culture, social class); and the *chronosystem,* which represents how time affects the child and their environment.

Developmental Surveillance/Milestones

Developmental *surveillance*, or monitoring, is an integral part of every pediatric visit as it provides insight into children's ongoing developmental progression, parental concerns, and/or which children might be at risk for developmental delays. A developmental *delay* is a *quantitative* departure from typical developmental progression in that development is proceeding but slowed. Developmental delays that persist beyond 6 years of age are typically considered a developmental *disability*, as these delays are more likely to persist in some capacity. Other quantitative departures include *asynchrony*, which occurs when different aspects of development proceed, but are out of step; *regression*, when there is a loss of earlier progress and skills; and *precocity*, when development is accelerated. A *qualitative* departure or *deviation* is said to occur when a behavior appears that would not be expected.

Developmental *surveillance* typically involves the use of developmental milestone lists and charts that are reviewed collaboratively by PCPs and parents. In contrast, developmental *screening*, while also integrated into health supervision visits, typically involves the use of specific tools completed at specific ages (e.g., autism). Screening is also done when ongoing developmental surveillance reveals a concern. *Diagnostic evaluations* are done for children with concerns or risks identified through surveillance and screening.

In 2019 the American Academy of Pediatrics revised the Learn the Signs, Act Early checklists used for pediatric developmental surveillance according to evidenced-based criteria.[7] The resulting universal checklists are updated and easy for families of different social, cultural, and ethnic backgrounds to understand and use. Two major changes were to (1) add new checklists for the 15- and 30-month visit, and (2) shift the milestone achievement time to the point at which 75% versus 50% of children should have achieved the milestone. The final product highlights 159 milestones and 12 checklists. These checklists include what information should be included when providing anticipatory guidance.

Anticipatory Guidance

The goal of anticipatory guidance is to help parents and caregivers plan for and cope with upcoming or anticipated developmental changes and challenges. It is age specific, highlighting information about developmental changes as well as related practices that promote health and prevent injury and disease. Anticipatory guidance is typically provided during well-child visits to parents, beginning with the first infant visit and extending across the pediatric lifespan. As children age, should be increasingly included in the conversation so they too can be prepared for what is coming next.

Anticipatory guidance is an ongoing conversation that includes information that reinforces positive health behaviors, minimizes or eliminates health risks, and facilitates optimal family functioning. Being open to, listening to, and engaging caregivers in these conversations helps build their confidence, creates a trusting relationship, and establishes comfort for bringing forth more difficult concerns when necessary. The various components of anticipatory guidance include:
- Assessing caregivers':
  - Knowledge of child development
  - Level of comfort with current/emerging caregiving role
  - Past experiences of caregiving (e.g., adverse childhood experiences [ACEs])
- Providing age-specific information about:
  - Child development/upcoming milestones
  - Strategies to provide a developmentally supportive environment
  - Age-appropriate resources (e.g., Reach Out and Read; https://reachoutandread.org/)

- Continuous evaluation and reinforcement of positive caregiving styles and strategies to foster healthy caregiver role development, including caregivers':
  - Problem-solving and coping skills, support, and resources

Talking With Caregivers About Developmental Delays

Having an established relationship that includes ongoing discussions about development makes talking with caregivers about their child's development easier if developmental delays or issues appear. Caregivers are often the first to suspect or notice differences. PCPs need to listen and be sensitive to their concerns as they seek reassurance or confirmation. However, some may choose to wait until the PCP notices or initiates the conversation. Either way, when a developmental concern arises, a strength-based approach is advised, as focusing on strengths first provides parents with a framework for understanding their child's unique strengths along with any particular developmental challenges. Above all, it is important to be honest, positive, and realistic. Caregivers want to know what they can do and, specifically, how they can assist their child. They also need support and time to cope with their own feelings. Different families have different expectations for their children, so a child with mild delay may be more devastating to one family than a child with severe developmental delays may be to another.

Caregiver Role

Understanding developmental concepts and principles, as well as the evolving contexts in which our pediatric patients live and learn, is not only foundational knowledge for pediatric practice, but it is also foundational knowledge for parents and caregivers in terms of how best to approach childrearing. In fact, knowledge of caregiving and child development is a protective factor in the prevention of child maltreatment (see Chapters 9–13). Understanding that children benefit from close and dependable relationships that provide love, nurturance, and security also points to why caregivers are key aspects of pediatric practice (See Additional Resources, Center on the Developing Child at Harvard University). Taking the time to learn about their backgrounds, experiences, and current environmental influences is critical to understanding what individuals bring to their caregiving journey (e.g., intergenerational transmission). Collectively, this information can help PCPs tailor the information and support they provide to caregivers, individualizing developmental knowledge and skills for each family.

Behavioral Economics

Behavioral economics combines the field of psychology with economic theory to leverage predictable patterns in decision-making to explore how to move individuals in the direction of better decision-making and overcome barriers to behavior change.[8] This emerging field offers both insights and tools to help PCPs develop novel approaches to supporting parental decision-making while improving child health. PCP efforts to impact caregiver behavioral change are influenced by caregivers' cultural influences and beliefs, economic status, and social views, each of which presents challenges to behavior change.

The shift to behavioral economics draws attention to the ways in which individual, family, community, and cultural contexts affect caregiver decision making (https://www.behavioraleconomics.com/). Behavioral economic strategies, or nudges, focus

Action bias	Tendency to act to gain a sense of control over a situation and eliminate a problem
Present bias	Tendency to overemphasize the present and discount the future
Availability heuristic	Tendency to lean in or understand an event or example based on how easily it is imagined or comes to mind
Optimism bias	Tendency to overestimate the likelihood of positive events and underestimate the likelihood of negative events
In-group/out-group bias	Tendency to trust individuals within one's social group/communities as opposed to outsiders
Hot/cold empathy gap	Tendency to underestimate the influence of one's visceral state(s) on one's behavior/ preferences (e.g., anger, fear)
Choice overload	Tendency to defer the choice as the number or complexity of choices increases

Modified from the Behavioral Economic Guide; 2022. https://www.behavioraleconomics.com/.

on influencing behavior predictably without restricting choice using message framing, defaults, and enhanced active choice and leveraging social forces, implementation prompts, and in-group messengers as effective strategies.[8,9] For example, when discussing actions targeting prevention, it is important to emphasize the potential benefits of the actions; when discussing screening interventions, the emphasis should be on the potential harms of inaction.

Each of these strategies is grounded in an understanding of cognitive biases and behavioral constructs, or levers, that impact or leverage decision making (Box 8.2). Some examples of these constructs include present bias, availability heuristic, optimism bias, information avoidance, hot/cold empathy gaps, and choice overload, among others.[9] By better understanding behavioral levers, PCPs can increase the salience of their messaging by designing tailored interventions specific to the most prominent biases within relevant subgroups. One of the best examples of using behavioral economics is the focused effort to enhance safe firearm storage.[9]

Family

There is a continuing shift away from focusing solely on caregiving to looking at families as a complex social system. The family systems approach acknowledges individual (e.g., mother-child, father-child, sibling-sibling) and collective interactions (e.g., family dynamics, functioning) as well as the direct and indirect influences from outside the family. *Direct* influences include the family's culture (e.g., customs, values, traditions), immediate neighborhood, and larger community. *Indirect* influences include the impact of local and government policies on food insecurity,

availability of and access to greenspaces, and access to high-speed internet. Chapter 5 provides information about assessing family composition and structure, family development or life-cycle stage, and family functioning.

Additional Resources

Child Development

Crowley K. *Child Development: A Practical Introduction* 2e. Sage Publications; 2017.
Hauser-Cram P, Nugent JK, Thies KM, Travers JF. *The Development of Children and Adolescents*. John Wiley & Sons; 2014.

Professional/Parent Resources

American Academy of Pediatrics (AAP), Section on Developmental and Behavioral Pediatrics (SODBP): https://www.aap.org/en-us/about-the-aap/Sections/Section-on-Developmental-and-Behavioral-Pediatrics/Pages/SODBP.aspx
Brazelton Touchpoints Center: www.touchpoints.org
Bright Futures: www.brightfutures.org
Center on the Developing Child at Harvard University: https://developingchild.harvard.edu/
Hawaii Early Learning Program (HELP): www.vort.com
Parents as Teachers: www.parentsasteachers.org
Zero to Three: www.zerotothree.org

Acknowledgment

We acknowledge Dawn Lee Garzon, the chapter author in the previous edition.

References

1. Mitchell SA, Black MJ. *Freud and Beyond: A History of Modern Psychoanalytic Thought*. Basic Books; 1995.
2. Kail R, Bisanz J. Information processing and cognitive development. *Adv Child Dev Behav*. 1982;17:45–81.
3. McDevitt TM, Ormrod JE. *Child Development: Educating and Working with Children and Adolescents*. 2nd ed. Prentice Hall Pearson Education; 2004.
4. Thompson RB, Thornton B. Gender and theory of mind in preschoolers' group effort: evidence for timing differences behind children's earliest social loafing. *J Soc Psychol*. 2014;154(6):475–479.
5. Scott RM, Baillargeon R. Early false-belief understanding. *Trends Cogn Sc*. 2017;21(4):237–249.
6. Crowley K. *Child Development: A Practical Introduction*. 2nd ed. Sage Publications, Inc; 2017.
7. Zubler JM, Wiggins LD, Macias MM, et al. Evidence-informed milestones for developmental surveillance tools. *Pediatrics*. 2022;49(3): e2021052138.
8. Jenssen BP, Buttenheim AM, Fiks AG. Using behavioral economics to encourage parent behavior change: opportunities to improve clinical effectiveness. *Acad Pediatr*. 2019;19(1):4–10.
9. Hoskins K, Paladhi UR, McDonald C, Buttenheim AM. Applying behavioral economics to enhance safe firearm storage. *Pediatrics*. 2020;145(3):e20192268.

9

Developmental Management of Newborns and Neonates

NAN M. GAYLORD AND KATHERINE M. NEWNAM

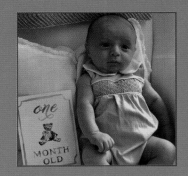

The newborn, or neonatal period, includes the first 28 days of extrauterine life. It is a period of multiple transitions, both for the newborn and for the parents. This chapter focuses primarily on the extraordinary transitions that occur following birth, with intermittent attention to the transitions associated with becoming a parent. Healthy People 2030 includes specific objectives for newborns that focus on keeping newborns safe and healthy through the first 28 days, which can only be accomplished by ensuring high-quality care during pregnancy, increasing breastfeeding rates, promoting vaccinations, providing developmental screenings, encouraging safety interventions, and, consequently, improve the general health and wellbeing of women, newborns, children, and families in the United States.[1]

Transition to Parenthood

The transition to parenthood is a significant life change whether it be the birth or addition of a first child or new sibling. It can be especially challenging if the parent is without a partner or supportive environment. Accordingly, how parents are adjusting should be assessed prenatally and at every well-child visit, especially during the newborn period. Bright Futures: Guidelines for Health Supervision of Infants, Children, and Adolescents and the American Academy of Pediatrics (AAP)[2,3] details the components of a prenatal visit with parents. At this visit, whether in the office, by telehealth, or by telephone, the goal is the same—developing a positive relationship with the primary care provider (PCP). Along with parental adjustment, other topics include a prenatal and family health history and anticipatory guidance related to feedings and the encouragement of breastfeeding, safety, circumcision, delivery and newborn care, and newborn office visits.

Transition From Intrauterine to Extrauterine Life

The intrauterine to extrauterine transition requires an extraordinary number of biochemical and physiologic changes. In utero, the placenta provides metabolic functions for the fetus. Oxygenated blood from the placenta arrives in the fetus through the umbilical vein. Because of high fetal pulmonary vascular pressure, this blood is shunted from the right to the left side of the fetus' heart through the foramen ovale and to the systemic circulation through the ductus arteriosus. At birth, the umbilical cord is clamped and severed, the newborn begins to breathe, and the high pulmonary vascular pressure drops, allowing blood to flow from the heart to the lungs for oxygenation. The foramen ovale and ductus arteriosus close. The newborn undergoes other physiologic transformations, including the gastrointestinal tract now being responsible for absorbing nutrients and excreting waste, the renal system taking over the excretion of waste and maintaining chemical balance, the liver metabolizing and excreting toxins, and the immunologic system now protecting against infection.

A predictable series of changes in vital signs, reactivity, and clinical appearance takes place after the delivery in most newborns (Fig. 9.1). The first period of reactivity includes sympathetic nervous system changes, including tachycardia, rapid respirations, transient rales, grunting, flaring and retractions, falling body temperature, hypertonus, and alertness. Parasympathetic nervous system changes during this first period of reactivity include the initiation of bowel sounds and the production of oral mucus. After an interval of sleep, the newborn will enter the second period of reactivity. During the second period, oral mucus production becomes evident, the heart rate becomes labile, the newborn becomes more responsive to endogenous and exogenous stimuli, and meconium is often passed.

Newborn Assessment

History

- Maternal health history
  - Past hospitalizations, surgeries, illnesses, accidents, and injuries
  - Past and current medications, ongoing and chronic diseases, last OBGYN and/or PCP visit
  - Past obstetric history
    - Number of previous pregnancies; number of newborns born alive or stillborn
    - Number of elective or spontaneous abortions; number of preterm and term deliveries
    - Cesarean birth(s) and indications

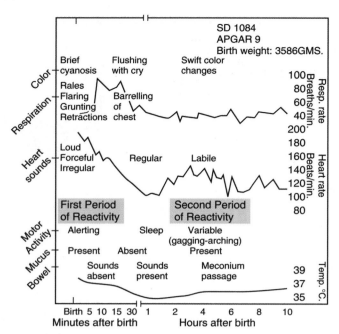

• **Fig. 9.1** Summary of Normal Transition. *SD,* Standard deviation. (From Desmond MM, Rudolph AJ, Phitaksphraiwan P. The transitional care nursery. *Pediatr Clin North Am.* 1966;13:651–668.)

TABLE 9.1	APGAR Scores		
	SCORE		
Sign	**0**	**1**	**2**
Activity (muscle tone)	Limp	Some flexion of extremities	Well flexed
Pulse: heart rate (beats/min)	Absent	Slow (<100)	>100
Grimace: reflex irritability (response of skin stimulation to feet)	No response	Some motion	Cry
Appearance: skin color	Blue; pale	Body pink; extremities blue	Completely pink
Respiration: respiratory effort	Absent	Weak cry; hypoventilation	Good; strong cry

- Family history
  - Three-generation pedigree (shared genetics).
    - Focus on history of fetal demise/stillborn, inherited conditions, congenital defects or disorders, intellectual disability, and other diseases and conditions such as hypertension, hyperlipidemias, heart disease, and familial cancers (see Chapter 27).
    - Age and health status of living relatives and/or age at death and cause
  - Kin or other significant household members (not genetically linked)
- Obstetric history
  - Current physical and mental health
  - Maternal age
  - Prenatal care—timing of initial and ongoing visits
  - Medications during pregnancy, including prescription, over-the-counter therapeutics, and natural or other health products
  - Use of fertility or pregnancy support medication and/or reproductive technology
  - Infections (including group B streptococcus status and results of other screening tests)
  - Immunization status and vaccinations received during pregnancy
  - Illnesses and related treatment and interventions
  - Alcohol, tobacco, or other drugs used during pregnancy
  - Environmental exposure to heavy metals (e.g., mercury, lead) or bacteria (e.g., *Listeria*)
  - Hypertension or glucose intolerance
  - Duration of labor, duration of ruptured membranes, analgesia, anesthesia, presentation and route of delivery, use of forceps or vacuum assist
  - Polyhydramnios (excessive fluid) or oligohydramnios (reduced fluid)
  - Meconium stained or foul-smelling amniotic fluid
  - Fever and/or tachycardia

- Social history
  - Emotional stressors during pregnancy (e.g., death of partner or family member, deployment of spouse, homelessness, intimate partner abuse)
  - Planned or unplanned pregnancy
  - Employment and work conditions
  - Financial and emotional support
  - Dietary considerations (e.g., vegan diet)
  - Educational background and health literacy of parent(s)
  - Cultural or religious practices
  - Partner's anticipated involvement in childrearing and support of breastfeeding
  - Other people in the home, including ages of other children in the home

Physical Examination: Immediately After Birth

Appearance, Pulse, Grimace, Activity, and Respiration (APGAR) Score

The evaluation of the newborn at 1 and 5 minutes of age is a valuable practice (Table 9.1). The 1-minute score reflects how well the newborn tolerated the birthing process, while the 5-minute score reflects how well the newborn is transitioning to extrauterine life as well as the impact of any resuscitation effort.
- APGAR score: 8 to 10
  - Vigorous, pink, and crying
  - Requires only warming, drying, gentle stimulation
  - Occasionally requires oxygen for a short period
- APGAR score: 5 to 7
  - Cyanotic
  - Slow, irregular respirations
  - Good muscle tone and reflexes
  - Responds to positive pressure ventilation (PPV) by bag and mask or T-piece resuscitator (e.g., Neopuff)
- APGAR score: 4 or less
  - Limp, pale, or blue
  - Apneic, slow heart rate
  - Maximal resuscitative efforts with bag and mask, chest compressions, intravenous volume expansion, and drug therapy may be needed.

The APGAR score does not predict long-term mortality and developmental outcomes, but it is useful in determining long-term health outcomes when combined with other factors, such as fetal status, umbilical cord or scalp blood pH, evidence of organ injury, or seizures.[4] The decision for neonatal resuscitation is based on a structured assessment completed within the first minute, which includes heart rate, color, and respiratory rate. This decision is not based on the 1-minute APGAR score, unless resuscitative decisions have been made before delivery when fetal anomalies are known (see Chapter 28).

Gestational Age

Maturational assessment of a newborn's gestational age is based on the physical examination (Fig. 9.2)[5] completed within 2 hours after birth. It is interpreted with information on the mother's menstrual history, obstetric milestones achieved during pregnancy, and prenatal ultrasonograms. A newborn's length, weight, and occipital-frontal (head) circumference (OFC) are then measured and plotted on growth curves (Fig. 9.3) based on sex and gestational age to assess growth.[6] Newborns, whose weight exceeds the 90th percentile for age, are classified as large for gestational age (LGA), and infants whose weights fall below the 10th percentile for age are classified as small for gestational age (SGA). Those whose weight measurements fall between the 10th and 90th percentiles are classified as appropriate for gestational age (AGA) (Fig. 9.4).[7]

Temperature Regulation

Newborn body surface area relative to weight is approximately three times that of an adult and their estimated heat loss rate is four times that of an adult. The newborn's body temperature falls precipitously in cool and/or drafty environments unless adequate precautions are taken. Warm towels are used to dry the newborn after birth to prevent evaporative heat loss, and newborns are preferably placed skin-to-skin with the mother in stable situations. Alternatively, using a radiant warmer or wrapping the newborn in warm blankets, with the head covered, reduces heat loss when the newborn is held.

Lungs

During labor, maternal hormonal influences activate epithelial sodium (Na^+) channels (ENaC) in the fetal lung, which is necessary to begin the active transport of amniotic fluid to interstitial spaces in preparation for the newborn's first breath. The squeezing action on a newborn's chest during vaginal delivery contributes to the expulsion of amniotic fluid from the lungs. The first spontaneous breath begins the process of decreasing pulmonary vascular resistance supporting the respiratory process.[8] Gentle bulb suctioning can assist in clearing the amniotic fluid from the naso-/oropharynx. A newborn from a cesarean birth (CB) may not experience labor and/or reduced hormonal activation of ENaC and does not experience the thoracic action of a vaginal birth; therefore CB increases the risk for respiratory distress and requires close respiratory assessment and appropriate bulb suctioning. Auscultation of all newborns' lungs reveals bronchovesicular or bronchial breath sounds. Fine crackles can be present during the first few hours of life and are a normal variant.

Umbilical Cord

The umbilical cord contains two thick-walled arteries and a single thin-walled vein. Rarely, newborns will have a single umbilical artery (SUA), which can be associated with chromosomal aberrations and/or congenital malformations. There is increasing evidence to support delayed umbilical cord clamping for 30 to 60 seconds as it improves newborn iron stores, thus helping to prevent anemia. In preterm newborns, this practice also appears to decrease the risk of intracerebral hemorrhage and necrotizing enterocolitis.[9] It is important to note that delayed clamping does decrease umbilical cord blood volume available for banking; families who are considering umbilical cord blood banking should be informed about this tradeoff.

Developmental Overview

Physical Examination: Following Stabilization

After a quick initial assessment immediately after birth, a more complete physical examination is performed within the next 24 hours (Table 9.2). When performing the physical examination, the newborn's gestational age, age in hours, and stage of transition must be considered.

Physical Growth and Development

Organ and System Maturation

The most significant changes occur in the cardiovascular and pulmonary systems as the newborn transitions to the extrauterine environment (see Chapters 32 and 33). Renal function initiated in utero continues in the newborn period with urine concentration increasing with time. Hearing is fully developed; however, visual acuity is 20/200 to 20/400 in the newborn and will not mature until 6 years of age.

Motor

The newborn is assessed for symmetry and equality of movement in all extremities. Newborn (primitive) reflexes dominate, including the Moro, rooting, sucking, Galant (i.e., trunk incurvation), stepping, placing, cremasteric, and anal wink. The asymmetric tonic neck reflex (ATNR) is rare in newborns but typically appears by 1 month of age.

Social and Emotional

Newborns respond to voice by turning and trying to locate the sound, especially if the voice is higher pitched (often mothers). They also prefer en face (i.e., face-to-face) interactions. Newborns thrive in a secure, safe, and predictable environment so they can develop trust in their surroundings and caretakers. The Ages and Stages questionnaire[10] assists in assessing the newborn's social and emotional development and is typically completed at the end of the newborn period (e.g., 1 month of age).

Communication

Newborns communicate their needs through vocalization (e.g., crying). Newborns who have their needs quickly attended to are often easily consoled. Parents are encouraged to tend to their newborns in a consistent and timely fashion and need to be reminded that newborns cannot be "spoiled." In contrast, quick attention is assuring and helps the newborn feel secure.

Common Issues

Circumcision

The decision to circumcise male infants rests with the parents. In 2012 the AAP issued a policy statement stating that there is no evidence to support routine circumcision. They also highlighted that the benefits of the procedure are greater than its risks, and circumcision access should be provided for all families desiring the procedure.[11] Proponents of routine male circumcision claim

MATURATIONAL ASSESSMENT OF GESTATIONAL AGE (New Ballard Score)

NAME ______________________ SEX ______________________

HOSPITAL NO. ______________________ BIRTH WEIGHT ______________________

RACE ______________________ LENGTH ______________________

DATE/TIME OF BIRTH ______________________ HEAD CIRC. ______________________

DATE/TIME OF EXAM ______________________ EXAMINER ______________________

AGE WHEN EXAMINED ______________________

APGAR SCORE: 1 MINUTE __________ 5 MINUTES __________ 10 MINUTES __________

NEUROMUSCULAR MATURITY

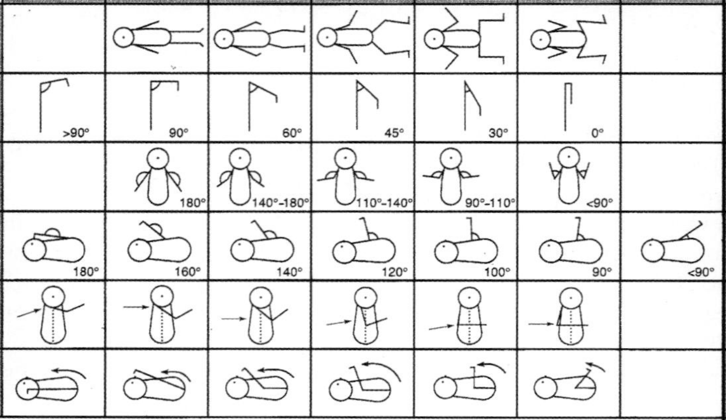

NEUROMUSCULAR MATURITY SIGN	SCORE -1	0	1	2	3	4	5	RECORD SCORE HERE
POSTURE								
SQUARE WINDOW (Wrist)	>90°	90°	60°	45°	30°	0°		
ARM RECOIL		180°	140°-180°	110°-140°	90°-110°	<90°		
POPLITEAL ANGLE	180°	160°	140°	120°	100°	90°	<90°	
SCARF SIGN								
HEEL TO EAR								

TOTAL NEUROMUSCULAR MATURITY SCORE

PHYSICAL MATURITY

PHYSICAL MATURITY SIGN	SCORE -1	0	1	2	3	4	5	RECORD SCORE HERE
SKIN	sticky friable transparent	gelatinous red translucent	smooth pink visible veins	superficial peeling &/or rash, few veins	cracking pale areas rare veins	parchment deep cracking no vessels	leathery cracked wrinkled	
LANUGO	none	sparse	abundant	thinning	bald areas	mostly bald		
PLANTAR SURFACE	heel-toe 40-50 mm:-1 <40 mm:-2	>50 mm no crease	faint red marks	anterior transverse crease only	creases ant. 2/3	creases over entire sole		
BREAST	imperceptible	barely perceptible	flat areola no bud	stippled areola 1-2 mm bud	raised areola 3-4 mm bud	full areola 5-10 mm bud		
EYE/EAR	lids fused loosely: -1 tightly: -2	lids open pinna flat stays folded	sl. curved pinna; soft; slow recoil	well-curved pinna; soft but ready recoil	formed & firm instant recoil	thick cartilage ear stiff		
GENITALS (Male)	scrotum flat, smooth	scrotum empty faint rugae	testes in upper canal rare rugae	testes descending few rugae	testes down good rugae	testes pendulous deep rugae		
GENITALS (Female)	clitoris prominent & labia flat	prominent clitoris & small labia minora	prominent clitoris & enlarging minora	majora & minora equally prominent	majora large minora small	majora cover clitoris & minora		

TOTAL PHYSICAL MATURITY SCORE

Reference
Ballard JL, Khoury JC, Wedig K, et al: New Ballard Score, expanded to include extremely premature infants. *J Pediatr* 1991; 119:417-423. Reprinted by permission of Dr Ballard and Mosby-Year Book, Inc.

SCORE

Neuromuscular __________

Physical __________

Total __________

MATURITY RATING

score	weeks
-10	20
-5	22
0	24
5	26
10	28
15	30
20	32
25	34
30	36
35	38
40	40
45	42
50	44

GESTATIONAL AGE (weeks)

By dates __________

By ultrasound __________

By exam __________

• **Fig. 9.2** Classification of Newborns by Intrauterine Growth and Gestational Age. (From Ballard JL, Khoury JC, Wedig K, et al. New Ballard score, expanded to include extremely premature infants. *J Pediatrics.* 1991;119:417–423.)

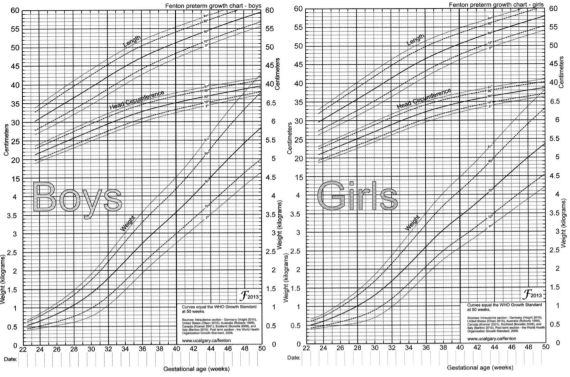

• **Fig. 9.3** Fenton Prematurity Growth Chart to 50 Weeks of Age. (From Fenton TR, Kim JH. A systematic review and meta-analysis to revise the Fenton growth chart for preterm infants. *BMC Pediatr*. 2013;13:59.)

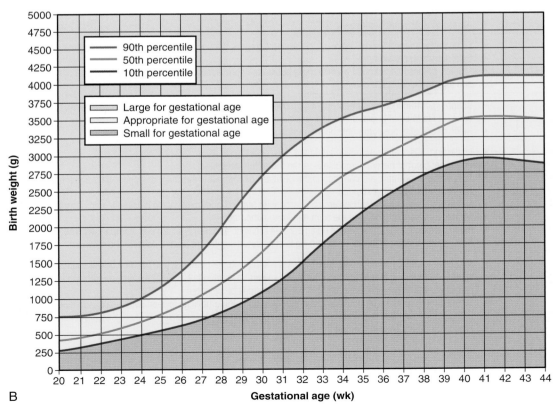

• **Fig. 9.4** Assignment of Size for Gestational Age (Small, Large, Appropriate) at Birth. (Data from Alexander GR, Himes JH, Kaufman RB, et al. A United States national reference for fetal growth. *Obstet Gynecol*. 1996;87(2):163–168; and Lowdermilk DL, Cashion K, Alden KR, et al. *Maternity & Women's Health Care*. 13th ed. Elsevier; 2024.)

TABLE 9.2   Newborn Physical Examination Findings

System	Findings
Measurements	• Vital signs: check frequently in the first hours, then every 6–8 h when stable • Evaluate temperature stability (97.7°F–99.3°F [36.5°C–37.4°C]) in open crib after birth • Respiratory rate = 30–60 breaths/min • Heart rate = 100–190 beats/min • Baseline weight, length, OFC (head) circumference • Daily weight measurement: losses of up to 10% in the first 2–3 days are normal
Skin	• Lanugo, vernix, dry and cracked skin are common. • See Table 9.3
Head	• Vaginal delivery: newborns may have molding, overriding suture lines • Anterior fontanel about 2–3 cm in diameter; posterior fontanel about 1 cm in diameter • Note presence of cephalohematoma/caput succedaneum
Face	• Symmetric facial structures/grimace • Note any dysmorphic findings
Eyes	• Check symmetry, size, and angle of palpebral fissures • Intermittent uncoordinated eye movements (disconjugate gaze) during the first weeks after birth are common, improving by 2–4 months old and resolving by 6 months old • Conjunctivae may be reddened due to the ocular prophylaxis agent • Note presence of red reflex bilaterally
Ears	• Identify size, shape, position, skin tags or pits • Establish patency of the external auditory canal • Evaluate for low-set and/or posterior rotated ears • Complete initial universal hearing screening
Nose	• Nasal passage patency tested by obstructing one nostril at a time
Mouth	• Evaluate size and symmetry of the lips, time spent with the mouth closed, appearance with movement • Evaluate palate to assure its intact • Presence of tight tongue/lip frenulum
Neck	• Assess for full range of motion
Thorax	• Evaluate for shape: rounded appearance (about 2 cm less than occipitofrontal head circumference) • Symmetrical expansion • Nipples: fullness/secretion of a white milky substance normal, secondary to maternal hormonal stimulation; Supernumerary and inverted nipples are common
Lungs	• Coughing, retractions, and intermittent increases in respiratory rate occur immediately after birth, transitioning by about 12 hours of life to smooth and unlabored respirations • Rales or crackles are commonly heard immediately after birth as lung fluid is resorbed
Heart	• Inspection: observe for perfusion adequacy • Palpation: point of maximal impulse is at the fourth left intercostal space • Auscultation: murmurs are common in the newborn period; many murmurs disappear after a few hours or days. Significant murmurs should be investigated • Pulses: brachial or radial pulses are compared with femoral or dorsalis pedis pulses for symmetry of impulse and strength • Measure oxygen saturation of the right hand and either foot • Blood pressure: by Doppler device using a 2.5–4 cm wide and 5–9 cm long cuff, compare with normal for age and gestation. Note: Systolic blood pressure > 96 mm Hg is considered significant hypertension in the newborn.
Abdomen	• Abdomen is slightly protuberant, soft, moves smoothly with respirations, and has fine bowel sounds scattered throughout • Liver is 1–2 cm below the right costal margin; spleen tip is often felt at the left costal margin; kidneys, deep within lateral aspects of the abdomen measuring 3–4 cm in size, may be palpated • Diastasis recti: midline outpouching from the sternum to the umbilicus is seen with weak abdominal musculature • Umbilical hernia: large opening with protuberant umbilicus • First stool should pass in the first 24–48 hours of life

TABLE 9.2	Newborn Physical Examination Findings—Cont'd
System	**Findings**

• Genitalia	• Male:
	  • The urethral opening should be at the tip of the penis; foreskin should be completely developed
	  • Note presence or absence of rugae; testes not located in the scrotal sac but retrievable from the inguinal canal to the scrotum are normal
	  • Hydrocele is identified by transilluminating scrotal fluid collection and is normal unless it is associated with inguinal hernia, or it lasts >12 months
	• Female:
	  • Labia majora are large and surround the labia minora
	  • Labia and vagina should be patent, often with a white discharge
	  • Blood-tinged fluid in small amounts by day 2–3 is normal
	• Anus and rectum:
	  • Patency and placement of the anus should be noted

• Extremities, back, hip	• Intrauterine constraint and resultant molding cause mild curvatures of the feet and legs • Fractures can occur anywhere because of the delivery process; note crepitus and range of motion in all extremities; clavicles are particularly vulnerable • Note dimples, hemangiomas, tufts of hair, or other lesions along the spine • Perform Ortolani and Barlow maneuvers to assess for dislocated or dislocatable hips
• Neurologic examination	• Observe tone, movement, and symmetry of the extremities while the newborn is awake • Elicit the following reflexes: rooting, suck/swallow, palmar grasp, Moro, ankle clonus, stepping/placing response, Galant (truncal incurvation), and later (~1 month of age) asymmetric tonic neck

OFC, Occipital-frontal (head) circumference.

that it keeps the glans penis cleaner; it lowers the chance of developing urinary tract infections (although the chance of urinary tract infections in uncircumcised males is only 1%); it reduces the incidence of penile cancer, phimosis, balanitis, adhesions, and occlusion of the urethral meatus; and it may be preferred to allow the male child to look more like his father or peers. The opponents of circumcision claim that it does not prevent sexually transmitted infections; that good hygiene prevents penile cancer; that circumcision leaves the glans open to the chance of cautery burns and meatal stenosis; and that because fewer males are being circumcised, they will not be different from many of their peers.

Contraindications to circumcision include the presence of epispadias or hypospadias, ambiguous genitalia, exstrophy of the bladder, a familial bleeding disorder, and illness. *Complications* of circumcision are rare but include infections, bleeding, gangrene, scarring, meatal stenosis, cautery burns, urethral fistula, amputation or trauma to the glans, and pain. For newborns who undergo circumcision, local anesthesia is recommended, such as the application of topical anesthetics (eutectic mixture of local anesthetics [EMLA] cream), dorsal penile nerve block, or subcutaneous ring block.[11] Other comforting measures include providing a sucrose pacifier, acetaminophen, soft music, and physiologic positioning in a supported, semirecumbent position on a padded surface.

Birth Trauma Involving Head

The two most common disorders involving the head from birth trauma are caput succedaneum and cephalohematoma. *Caput succedaneum* is a diffuse, superficial swelling of the soft tissue of the scalp with possible underlying bruising. It is the result of trauma as the baby descends through the birth canal. Clinical findings include obvious swelling and bruising in the parietal regions of the scalp and superficial swelling that crosses suture lines. No treatment is necessary as swelling resolves spontaneously over the first few days after birth. If there is associated bruising, the newborn should be observed for the development of jaundice as the blood from bruising is reabsorbed. *Cephalohematoma* is a deep collection of blood in the subperiosteal area of the scalp. Surface bruising is rare. It results from trauma, most often from a difficult delivery. The swelling appears hours to days after delivery. Clinical findings include swelling in the parietal area that does not cross suture lines. No treatment is indicated as it resolves in a few weeks to months. Calcification of the hematoma can occur, which is felt as bony prominences on the cranium; resolution of a calcified hematoma may require months. It is important to monitor the newborn for the development of jaundice as the blood is resorbed.

Infant Jaundice

Infant jaundice, a yellow discoloration of a newborn's skin and eyes, occurs because of an excess of bilirubin. It is common, particularly in premature and breastfed newborns; however, most infants born between 35 weeks' gestation and full term need no treatment. The newborn's bilirubin levels are checked in the hospital until discharge and again at the 3- to 5-day visit. This first visit is important as bilirubin levels typically peak between 3 and 7 days. Rarely, an unusually high blood level of bilirubin can place a newborn at risk of brain damage, particularly in the presence of certain risk factors for severe jaundice. Pathologic jaundice is discussed in more detail in Chapter 28, and breastfeeding jaundice is discussed in Chapter 15.

Skin Conditions

Parents may discover several skin conditions as they observe their newborns, some of which can be alarming. For example, *harlequin color change* (or *harlequin sign*) is the sudden change in skin color that appears to divide the body into erythemic and pallor halves along a straight line from the newborn's forehead to the pubis. The cause is unknown, but it occurs in up to 10% of newborns, usually between days 2 and 5 of life, but has been reported as late as 3 weeks following birth. While no treatment is indicated for this transient and benign condition (Fig. 9.5), it is alarming.

Congenital dermal melanocytosis (previously referred to as *Mongolian spots*), café-au-lait macules ("spots"), nevus simplex ("salmon patch," "stork bite," "angel kiss"), and nevus flammeus (i.e., port-wine stain, port-wine nevus) are other skin discolorations that present in the newborn period. These skin conditions are not transient. Further discussion, including associated disorders, is found in Chapter 37.

Common skin conditions are outlined in Table 9.3.

Preauricular Skin Tags and Pits

Preauricular skin tags (fleshy bumps) and pits (sinus tracts) are minor anomalies; however, these newborns should be evaluated for hearing loss and other congenital anomalies (e.g., branchio-oto-renal syndrome).[12] Pits occur anterior to the pinna and can be unilateral or bilateral. They result from imperfect fusion of the tubercles of the first and second branchial arches during gestational development and are often familial.

Supernumerary Nipples

Solitary or multiple accessory nipples occur in unilateral or bilateral distribution along a line from the mid-axilla to the inguinal area. The cause is unknown; however, the newborn should be evaluated for urinary tract anomalies, as they can occur in conjunction with the finding.

Discharge and Follow-up

The Newborns' and Mothers' Health Protection Act of 1996, with final rules issued in 2008, prevents insurers from requiring hospital discharge before 48 hours for a vaginal delivery and 96 hours for a cesarean birth.[13] All parents leaving the hospital with a newborn should have a confirmed provider, time, place for follow-up,

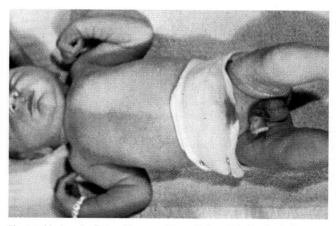

• Fig 9.5 Harlequin Color Change. (From Cohen BA. *Pediatric Dermatology.* 5th ed. Elsevier; 2022.)

and contact in case of an emergency or questions. Guidelines for discharge of healthy newborns are listed in Box 9.1.[14] Before discharge, it is important to confirm plans for follow-up care and the need for ongoing health maintenance visits (Box 9.2).[14] Some newborns may need follow-up care within the first few days of life (e.g., jaundice), but the first visit is recommended to occur at 3 to 5 days.

Health Supervision

Primary care begins immediately after birth, as newborns undergo repeated assessments to ensure they are successfully transitioning to their new extrauterine environment. Additional care includes prophylaxis for ophthalmia neonatorum with antibiotic ointment and vitamin K injection intramuscularly for the prevention of classic and late-onset hemorrhagic disease. Before discharge, all newborns should also undergo newborn screening (Baby's First Test: https://babysfirsttest.org/), a newborn hearing test, and pulse oximetry to rule out critical congenital heart disease, and bilirubin screening (see Screenings, below). In addition, they should begin the vaccination schedule with the first dose of Hepatitis B.

Health Visits

During the newborn period, the Bright Futures/American Academy of Pediatrics Recommendations for Preventive Pediatric Health Care outlines health visits should occur at birth, at 3 to 5 days, and at 1 month of age. [15] Each visit should include an interim history, an unclothed physical examination, measurement of weight, length, and OFC, developmental surveillance, assigned screenings and immunizations, and anticipatory guidance.

Screenings

In the United States, each state requires newborn screening (i.e., Baby's First Test) for a variety of congenital and inherited disorders, although the number and types of the Recommended Uniform Screening Panel screening tests performed vary by state.[16,17] Newborns are typically screened before hospital discharge; however, if the test was done before 24 hours of life, rescreening should be done before the newborn is 2 weeks of age.

All newborns should undergo universal hearing screening. The Centers for Disease Control and Prevention recommend the first screening should occur no later than 1 month of age. Most hospitals and birthing centers complete the first screening using otoacoustic emissions (OAE) or auditory brainstem response (ABS) before the newborn is discharged. If the newborn does not pass the initial screening, a full hearing test should be completed no later than 3 months of age. Special attention is paid to any newborn at higher risk for hearing loss, including those with low birth weight, exposure to rubella or other infections (e.g., cytomegalovirus), congenital and/or inherited disorders, physical malformation of the ear, trauma, asphyxia, prematurity, extended intensive care unit stay, or antibiotic use..

Another newborn screening to be completed before discharge is for critical congenital heart disease (CCHD), such as coarctation of the aorta, pulmonary atresia, and Tetralogy of Fallot, to

TABLE 9.3	Comparison of Common Newborn Skin Conditions			
Rash	Significant Maternal or Newborn History	Rash Description	Diagnostics	Management/Treatment
Milia	None	Firm, pearly, white papules over cheeks, nose, and forehead	None	Superficial inclusion cysts will spontaneously resolve
Sebaceous hyperplasia	None	Prominent, yellow-white papules over cheeks, nose, and forehead	None	Overgrowth of sebaceous glands will spontaneously resolve in first few weeks
Erythema toxicum	None Presents at 24–48 hours	Yellow-white papules with an erythematous base over cheeks, nose, and forehead	Wright stain demonstrates large number of eosinophils Cultures are sterile	Clears within 2 weeks, completely gone in 4 months
Transient neonatal pustular melanosis	None More common in darker skinned newborns	Vesico-pustules that rupture easily and leave a halo of white scales around a central macule of hyperpigmentation on trunk, limbs, palms, and soles	None	Spontaneous resolution in 2–3 days although hyperpigmentation can persist for up to 3 months
Sucking blisters	Results from vigorous sucking in utero on the affected part	Scattered superficial bullae on the upper arms and lips of newborns at birth	None	Will resolve without additional intervention
Cutis marmorata	Accentuated physiologic response to cold	Lacy, reticulated, red or blue vascular pattern	None	Transient and will resolve with warming
Harlequin color change	None	Half of the baby's coloring is red and the other pale	None	Transient and will resolve
Nevus sebaceous	None	Yellow, hairless smooth plaque on head or neck	None	Total excision before adolescence; refer to dermatologist
Herpes simplex virus (HSV) (see Chapter 35)	Mother may have active lesions or a history of disease	Grouped vesicles on erythematous base	DFA or ELISA detection of HSV antigens	Acyclovir

DFA, Direct fluorescent antibody; ELISA, enzyme-linked immunosorbent assay.

name a few. CCHD screening is completed using pulse oximetry (right hand and/or foot) after the first 24 hours of life. Any infant who fails the screen should have an evaluation for causes of hypoxemia.

Screening newborns for hyperbilirubinemia is done using bilirubin levels obtained transcutaneously or via serum analysis (see Chapter 28).

Some newborns are at higher risk for predictable complications. For example, newborns born to mothers with poorly controlled diabetes and those deemed LGA or SGA have a higher risk for hypoglycemia and usually require serum glucose level screening. Similarly, newborns with Coombs test positivity secondary to maternal-child blood incompatibility need follow up screening for evidence of hemolysis. Some nurseries opt to screen both mothers and newborns for syphilis; however, all mothers should be screened for HIV and hepatitis B, unless it was done prenatally.

Mothers also need to be screened for depression, as a newborn's ability to thrive depends on the ability of primary caretakers to care for them. The Edinburgh Postpartum Depression Scale (EPDS)[18] inventory or other assessment of the mother's mental status (e.g., PHQ-9 or PHQ-2) is considered a component of each newborn health visit, as the consequences of depression on both parent and newborn can have significant short- and long-term impacts on both if not treated.[19] Further, PCPs have early and ongoing contact with mothers, as most mothers are not seen by their obstetric providers until 6 weeks postpartum.

All newborns need to complete these screenings, including those born outside the hospital (e.g., home birth, birthing center). Midwives and PCPs are often able to complete newborn screening; however, sometimes arrangements need to be made with the local health department or the hospital. The important detail is for the newborn to undergo screening at the recommended time.

Anticipatory Guidance

Anticipatory guidance is an essential element of pediatric health supervision as it ensures parents/caregivers understand expected growth and development issues. It is tailored to the age of the child and includes information about practices that promote health as

---

• BOX 9.1 Guidelines for Discharge of Healthy Newborns

- No ongoing medical issues that require continued hospitalization
- Term newborn
- Stable vital signs for at least 12 hours before discharge:
  - Rectal temperature of 97.7°F–99.3°F (36.5°C–37.4°C) in open crib
  - Heart rate 100–190 beats/min
  - Respiratory rate <60 breaths/min
- Passage of urine and at least one stool
- Two successful feedings
- Normal physical examination
- Vitamin K received; no bleeding at circumcision site or umbilicus
- Baseline bilirubin: clinical significance of jaundice determined and appropriate follow-up plans made
- Evaluation and monitoring for sepsis based on maternal risk factors
- Newborn laboratory data, including maternal syphilis, maternal hepatitis B status, and human immunodeficiency virus (HIV), and newborn blood type and Coombs testing (as indicated) completed
- Appropriately timed newborn screenings completed (including Baby's First Test, CCHD, hearing)
- First dose of hepatitis B administered
- Mother has received (if needed) tetanus toxoid, reduced diphtheria toxoid, and acellular pertussis, influenza, or other vaccines (e.g., COVID-19) as indicated[20,21]
- Social support identified
- Social situation adequate: screen for drug abuse, previous child abuse, mental illness, lack of social support, lack of permanent home, history of domestic violence, communicable diseases in the household, teenage mother, inadequate transportation, communication abilities
- Appropriate medical home/primary care provider identified with early follow-up care achievable within 3–5 days
- Mother knowledgeable in the care of the newborn, including:
  - Feeding, with breastfeeding encouraged
  - Stool and urine elimination and frequency
  - Skin, genital, and cord care
  - Ability to identify illness (especially jaundice)
  - Proper safety ensured (e.g., car seat, sleeping position, tobacco-free environment, room vs. bed sharing)
  - Smoke/carbon monoxide alarms in the home

CCHD, Critical congenital heart disease.
Modified from Benitz WE. Hospital stay for healthy term newborn infants. *Pediatrics.* 2015;135(5):948–953.

• BOX 9.2 Guidelines for 3-to 5-Day Follow-up Visit of the Healthy Newborn

- Review the delivery and discharge summary for any identified follow-up needs (e.g., hearing screening, specialty referrals).
- Assess the newborn's general health, weight, hydration, and jaundice; identify any new problems; review feeding, stooling, and urination; consider lactation consultation if needed.
- Assess the quality of mother-infant bonding and maternal assessment of infant cues.
- Assess home environment/safety (e.g., tobacco-free, safe sleep environment).
- Evaluate maternal/family support and education needs.
- Review outstanding laboratory data.
- Perform/repeat neonatal screen and/or other tests (e.g., bilirubin) if indicated.
- Develop plan for healthcare maintenance, including emergency care, preventive care, immunizations, and periodic screenings.
- Evaluate mother for postpartum depression.
- Refer to Women, Infants, and Children (WIC) and Supplemental Nutritional Assistance Program (SNAP) programs as appropriate.

Modified from Benitz WE. Hospital stay for healthy term newborn infants. *Pediatrics.* 2015;135(5):948–953.

---

well as prevent injury and disease. For parents of newborns, there is much to learn.

Establishing Feeding

PCPs must ensure that the mother/parent and newborn begin to establish a feeding pattern before discharge. Follow-up care is scheduled at 3 to 5 days to assess feeding and adequate intake. Later chapters provide additional information on breastfeeding (Chapter 15) and infant formulas, as well as the addition of solids (Chapter 14).

Physical Care

Umbilical Cord. Bright Futures Guidelines for cord care include leaving the cord to air dry and placing the diaper below the cord until it separates on its own.[2] Alcohol application is no longer recommended. After cord separation, which usually occurs after 10 to 14 days, a slight bloody discharge can be seen for 1 to 2 days. If a foul-smelling discharge or rapidly expanding erythema appears around the umbilicus, the newborn (i.e., omphalitis) should be

evaluated immediately. If an umbilical granuloma appears after the cord separates, an application of silver nitrate can help to heal it. Parents should be instructed to avoid bellybands or coins covering the umbilicus because of an increased risk of infection.

Foreskin and Circumcision Care. Care of the uncircumcised male infant includes gentle cleaning around the genital area. The skin normally adheres to the penis and is not retractable at birth but loosens gradually. Counsel parents not to forcefully retract the foreskin. If the newborn is circumcised, the penis should be cleansed daily with cotton balls dipped in tap water followed by the application of a small amount of petroleum jelly to the tip of the penis with each diaper change for the first 2 to 3 days after the procedure to prevent any discharge from sticking to the diaper.

Bathing. Newborns do not require daily baths and should not be immersed in water until the umbilical cord separates and the umbilicus is healed. Parents should be encouraged to sponge bathe their newborn using mild cleansing agents (e.g., Dove, Caress, Neutrogena, Basis) that are gentle enough for newborn skin. Oils and greasy substances are not recommended as they tend to clog pores and lead to rashes. Powders should be avoided, as inhaling talc can lead to respiratory problems and increased cancer risk. For dry skin, lotion (e.g., Keri, Eucerin, Aveeno, Cetaphil) is recommended.

Elimination and Diapers. While there is ongoing controversy as to whether disposable or cloth diapers are the better choice for the newborn (and the environment), emphasis should be on what works best for each family situation. The primary focus should be on keeping the newborn clean and dry through frequent changing and proper cleansing.

Safety. All newborns need to be transported in an appropriate, backward-facing car seat located in the back seat of the car, even as they leave the hospital. Before discharge, parents need to be comfortable to provide safe newborn care basics (e.g., supporting the neck when handling the newborn, keeping a hand on newborn when changing diaper). The other major safety concern is ensuring the sleep environment is safe (Fig. 9.6).

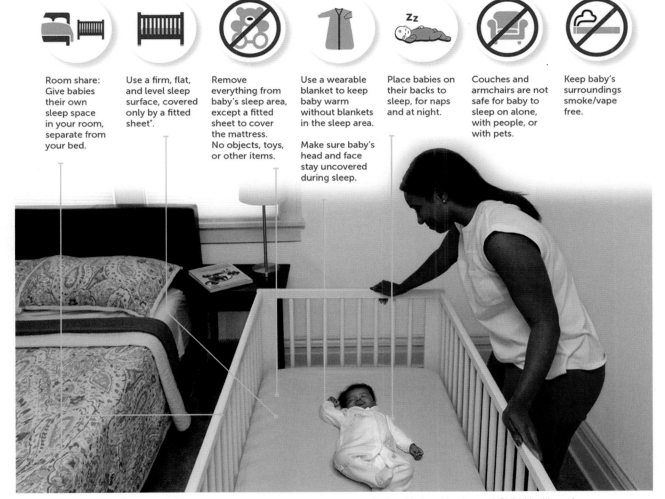

Room share: Give babies their own sleep space in your room, separate from your bed.

Use a firm, flat, and level sleep surface, covered only by a fitted sheet*.

Remove everything from baby's sleep area, except a fitted sheet to cover the mattress. No objects, toys, or other items.

Use a wearable blanket to keep baby warm without blankets in the sleep area.

Make sure baby's head and face stay uncovered during sleep.

Place babies on their backs to sleep, for naps and at night.

Couches and armchairs are not safe for baby to sleep on alone, with people, or with pets.

Keep baby's surroundings smoke/vape free.

• **Fig. 9.6** Safe Sleep Environment. (From Eunice Kennedy Shriver National Institute of Child Health and Human Development. What does a safe sleep environment look like? https://safetosleep.nichd.nih.gov/resources/caregivers/environment/look.)

Additional Resources

University of Calgary. Fenton premature growth charts: https://ucalgary.ca/resource/preterm-growth-chart/preterm-growth-chart

References

1. Healthy people 2030: Building a healthier future for all. http://health.gov/healthypeople.
2. Hagan JF, Shaw JS, Duncan PM, eds. *Bright Futures: Guidelines for Health Supervision of Infants, Children and Adolescents*. 4th ed. American Academy of Pediatrics; 2017.
3. Yogman M, Lavin A, Cohen G. The prenatal visit. *Pediatrics*. 2018;142(1).
4. Simon LV, Hashmi MF, Bragg BN. APGAR score. https://www.ncbi.nlm.nih.gov/books/NBK470569/.
5. Ballard J. The Ballard Score Maturational Assessment of Gestational Age in Newly Born Infants. https://www.ballardscore.com/.
6. Fenton Tanis R, Kim Jae H. A systematic review and meta-analysis to revise the fenton growth chart for preterm infants. *BMC Pediatr*. 2013;13:59.
7. University of Calgary. Table for the assignment of size for gestational age (small, large, appropriate) at birth. https://live-ucalgary.ucalgary.ca/sites/default/files/teams/418/Tablefortheassignmentofsizeforgestationalagesmalllargeappropriateatbirthv3.pdf.
8. Jain L, Eaton DC. Physiology of fetal lung fluid clearance and the effect of labor. *Semin Perinatol*. 2006;30(1):34–43.
9. ACOG Committee Opinion No. 814. American College of Obstetricians and Gynecologists. Delayed umbilical cord clamping after birth. *Obstet Gynecol*. 2020;136:e100–106.
10. Ages & Stages Questionnaires: Social-Emotional, Second Edition (ASQ:SE-2) Age range: 1–72 months. https://publications.aap.org/toolkits/resources/15625/.
11. American Academy of Pediatrics. Task force on circumcision: circumcision policy statement. *Pediatrics*. 2012;130(3).
12. American Academy of Pediatrics, Joint Committee on Infant Hearing Year 2007 Position Statement. Principles and guidelines for early hearing detection and intervention programs. *Pediatrics*. 2007;120(4):898–921.
13. Department of the Treasury, Department of Labor, US Department of Health and Human Services. Final rules for group health plans and health insurance issuers under the Newborns' and Mothers' Health Protection Act. *Fed Register*. 2008;73(203):62410–62429.

14. Benitz WE. Hospital stay for healthy term newborn infants. *Pediatrics*. 2015;135(5):948–953.

15. Bright Futures/American Academy of Pediatrics. Recommendations for preventative pediatric health care. https://downloads.aap.org/AAP/PDF/periodicity_schedule.pdf.

16. Center for Disease Control. Newborn screening. https://www.cdc.gov/newbornscreening/Page.

17. HRSA Advisory Committee on Heritable Disorders in Newborns and Children Recommended uniform screening panel. https://www.hrsa.gov/advisory-committees/heritable-disorders/rusp.

18. American Academy of Pediatrics. Edinburgh Postpartum Depression Scale (EPDS). https://publications.aap.org/toolkits/resources/15625/.

19. Slomian J, Honvo G, Patrick E, et al. Consequences of maternal postpartum depression: a systematic review of maternal and infant outcomes. *Women Health*. 2019;15(1):1–55.

20. Centers for Disease Control and Prevention. Vaccines During Pregnancy FAQs. https://www.cdc.gov/vaccinesafety/concerns/vaccines-during-pregnancy.html.

21. Centers for Disease Control and Prevention. COVID-19 Vaccines While Pregnant or Breastfeeding. https://www.cdc.gov/coronavirus/2019-ncov/vaccines/recommendations/pregnancy.html.

10
Developmental Management of Infants

MARY DIRKS

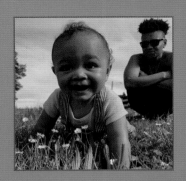

The infant stage spans the period from 1 to 12 months (1 year) of age. It is a time of dramatic developmental changes and evolving skills. All body systems mature, giving rise to a sequential and coordinated expansion of abilities that allow the infant to respond to, cope, and potentially flourish within their new environment. Understanding infant growth and development is essential for the primary care provider (PCP) as it provides the basis for health assessment and surveillance, anticipatory guidance, and the identification of variations requiring additional management or referral.

Developmental Overview

Physical Growth and Development: Measurement

Physical growth is monitored through the frequent, careful measurement and recording of key growth parameters, including weight, length (supine), occipital frontal (head) circumference (OFC), chest circumference, and vital signs. The Centers for Disease Control and Prevention (CDC) recommend that providers use the World Health Organization (WHO) growth charts (https://www.cdc.gov/growthcharts/who_charts.htm) to monitor growth in infants and children from birth until 2 years of age. Length is measured with the infant in the supine position, while the OFC is measured with the infant in an upright position (see Chapter 5).

Weight

Infants gain 150 to 210 g (approximately 5–7 ounces) weekly during the first 6 months of life. By 6 months, the birth weight has typically doubled. During the next 6 months, weight gain slows; however, by 1 year of age, the infant's weight has typically tripled the birth weight. The average weight at 1 year is 9.75 kg, or 21.5 pounds.

Length

Infant length increases an average of 2.5 cm (1 inch) a month during the first 6 months but slows during the next 6 months to 1.25 cm (0.5 inch) per month. While weight gain is steady and gradual, length increases occur in spurts. By 6 months of age, infants average 65 cm (25.5 inches) in length, increasing to 72 cm (29 inches) by 12 months of age—a 50% increase from birth. This increase is primarily due to head and truncal growth.

Occipital Frontal (Head) Circumference

Like the rest of the growing infant, OFC growth is rapid. During the first 6 months of life, the OFC increases approximately 1.5 cm (0.6 inches) per month, slowing to only 0.5 cm (0.2 inches) per month in the second 6 months. On average, the OFC is 43 cm (17 inches) at 6 months and 46 cm (18 inches) by 12 months. The 33% increase in OFC in the first year of life accompanies the doubling in size of the brain during the same period. Cranial sutures begin to close, with the posterior fontanel closing between 6 and 8 weeks of age, followed by the anterior fontanel, closing around 14 months, with a range between 12 and 18 months of age.

Chest Circumference

At birth, the chest circumference is approximately 2 cm (0.7 inches) smaller than the OFC; however, it gradually increases and is approximately equal to the OFC by age 12 months, primarily due to an increase in the chest's lateral versus anteroposterior diameter.

Vital Signs

Vital signs stabilize early in infancy. The typical infant heart rate is 80 to 160 beats/min. Sinus arrhythmias are common, causing increased heart rates during inspiration and decreasing rates with expiration. The respiratory rate slows to 30 to 50 breaths/min. Infants use their diaphragms to breathe but abdominal respiratory movements are normal. Fluctuations in blood pressure can be observed during the various states of activity (e.g., feeding, sleeping) and emotions. The normal infant temperature (37°C/98.6°F) typically refers to the rectal temperature as it offers a truer reflection of the infant's basal body temperature.

Organ/System Maturation

While external focus is on the progressive, coordinated neurologic and musculoskeletal maturation which results in the decrease of primitive reflexes and the development of purposeful movements, internal organs/body systems also mature during infancy, with changes in the immune, hematologic, digestive, and fluid/renal systems are most notable.

Immune System

A full-term newborn receives a significant amount of maternal immunoglobulin G (mIgG); however, mIgG level begins to decrease right away, disappearing by 9 months of age. Between 1

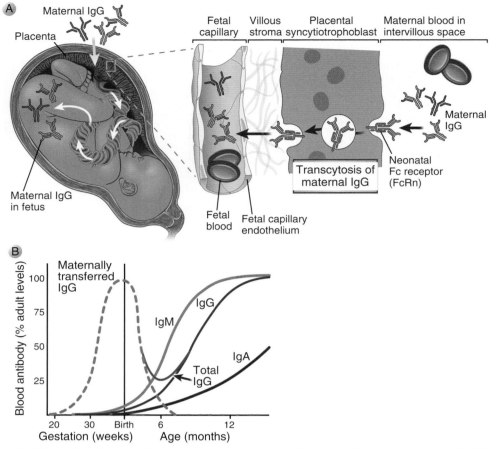

• **Fig. 10.1** Fetal and Neonatal Immunity Mediated by Passive Transfer of Maternal Immunoglobulin (Ig) G. (A) IgG is transported from maternal blood in the intervillous spaces of the placenta across the placental syncytial trophoblast cells by the neonatal Fc receptor (FcRn) and is then transported across fetal vessel endothelial cells into the fetal circulation. (B) Serum Ig levels in the fetus and neonate. The neonate starts making IgG soon after birth, but the loss of maternal IgG and the slow increase in neonatally derived IgG results in a nadir of blood IgG concentration at about 6 months of age. The fetus starts making IgM late in pregnancy, and the IgM concentrations approach adult levels more quickly in the baby than IgG. Nonetheless, these IgMs will not be specific for the wide range of microbes that the maternal IgGs will recognize, and the baby has a heightened risk for infection at the time of the IgG nadir. IgA levels in the baby take longer to reach adult levels than either IgM or IgG, but maternal IgA in breast milk can provide passive intestinal immunity in nursing babies. (From Abbas AK, Lichtman AH, Pillai S. *Cellular and Molecular Immunology*, 10th ed. Elsevier; 2022.)

and 3 months, infants begin to synthesize their own IgG, which increases to 40% of adult levels by 1 year of age but creates a transient period of low IgG levels (Fig. 10.1). Infants produce IgM, which will reach adult levels by 9 months of age. Secretory IgA is present in saliva and tears by 5 weeks. The function and quality of T-lymphocytes, lymphokines, interferon-γ, interleukins, tumor necrosis factor, and complement are reduced throughout the infant period, affecting the infant's ability to respond efficiently to infectious bacteria and viruses.

Hematologic System

After birth, the neonate begins the transition from predominantly fetal hemoglobin (Hgb F) to the adult distribution of Hgb A1, Hgb A2, and Hgb F. This transition begins soon after birth, with a major crossover around 3 to 4 months of age, which is the same time that Fe (iron) stores received in utero begin to run out. The combination of hematologic events makes the infant vulnerable for iron-deficiency anemia. It is also the key period to identify

hemoglobinopathies, such as thalassemia and sickle cell disease, all of which are critical for the PCP to understand and facilitate management (see Chapter 38).

Digestive System

At birth, the digestive system is immature with decreased enzymatic activity. Saliva is present in minimal amounts but begins to reach adult levels and function by 3 months of age, peaking between 4 and 6 months, at which time drooling becomes prominent. This drooling is due to poor coordination of the swallow reflex; however, it also often coincides with the eruption of the infant's first teeth. Gastric digestion is controlled by hydrochloric acid and rennin, an enzyme that acts on milk casein to cause curd formation, which facilitates milk retention and digestion. Pancreatic amylase, which is needed for the metabolism of complex carbohydrates, is deficient until approximately 4 to 6 months of age. In contrast, trypsin is present from birth in adequate amounts to catabolize proteins into polypeptides and amino acids. During infancy, the stomach enlarges to accommodate an increasing volume of food. By the end of the first year, the infant's stomach tolerates three meals, two to three snacks, plus supplemental oral intake of breastmilk and/or infant formula. Stool appearance shifts from a soft yellow, cottage cheese consistency to the passage of one to two stools a day by 1 year of age. The liver begins gluconeogenesis, bilirubin conjugation, and bile secretion in the first few weeks after birth alongside the establishment of the intra- and extrahepatic regulatory systems controlling ketone body metabolism.

Fluid/Renal System

The two water compartments, intra- and extracellular, undergo changes throughout infancy, with an increase in intracellular space and a decrease in extracellular space as the child grows. The total body water is higher in infants (70%) as compared to children (65%) and adults (60%), which predisposes infants to fluid loss and dehydration, aggravated by an immature renal system. While nephrogenesis is considered complete in the term infant, there are significant functional changes that take place as the infant matures, such as the ability to concentrate urine (at around 2 months of age).

Physical Growth and Development

The infant experiences many physical and developmental changes during this time. These changes are summarized by age in the following paragraphs and presented in a detailed, month-by-month visual in Table 10.1.

1 to 3 Months

Length increases by 2.5 cm (1 inch) and OFC increases by 1.5 cm (0.6 inch) per month. The young infant gains 15 to 30 g (0.5–1 ounce) per day and eats 8 to 10 times in a 24-hour period. Feedings vary in length from 20 to 30 minutes. At 6 to 8 weeks, the infant experiences a growth spurt and eat more frequently. Weight checks and growth chart recordings help parents and caregivers understand if their infant is gaining weight appropriately.

Wet diapers tend to occur after each feeding; however, there is a change in stool elimination patterns, moving from stooling with each feeding to having one to two bowel movements a day or every other day. By 6 weeks of age, an infant may not have a bowel movement every day. The stools of breastfed infants tend to be more yellow, seedier, and pasty than those infants fed infant formula. Regardless of feeding type, the stool is soft, loose, or even runny. Stool texture and frequency can help identify a problem; for example, a hard or dry bowel movement may reflect inadequate fluid intake.

Infants sleep 15 to 17 hours a day. As sleep periods consolidate into consistent nap times, the infant may benefits from organized periods of play. Typically, infants have a fussy period in the late afternoon into the evening that should subside by 3 to 4 months of age. It is vital for the PCP to discuss with parents plans to cope with the increased fussiness and crying before this time is upon them and *Shaken baby syndrome* and the *Period of PURPLE crying* should be discussed (see "Crying"). Parents need a repertoire of coping skills, such as knowing how to respond when they are feeling overwhelmed and frustrated by their infant's increased demands and should be encouraged to take a "parent time-out," such as putting the infant in the crib and calling a support person, to allow the infant to cry in a safe environment.

4 to 5 Months

At this age, infants have regular feeding, sleeping, and playing patterns. Some infants sleep through the night. By 6 months of age,

the infant typically doubles their birth weight. Growth continues with a gain of 150 to 210 g (5–7 ounces) per week, and length increases by 2.5 cm (1 in) per month and OFC by 1.5 cm (0.6 in) per month. This growth period may be in spurts, yet growth occurs along a steadily upward curve.

6 to 8 Months

As the extrusion reflex fades, infants can manage intake of pureed solid foods in their diets, which decreases their intake of breastmilk or infant formula. Growth rate declines as the weight gain decreases to 90 to 150 g (3–5 ounces) per week over the next 6 months. In addition, height growth rate declines to 1.25 cm (0.5 inch) per month over the next 6 months. Most infants experience symptoms as their first teeth erupt, beginning with lower central incisors. While timing of eruption varies widely, the sequence does not (see Ch. 20).

9 to 12 Months (1 Year)

Infants continue to have growth spurts and lags. Between 11 and 12 months of age, they gain about 0.5 kg (1 pound) per month. They typically eat three meals a day along with two snacks, one midmorning and one in the afternoon. Most infants transition to solid foods and increasingly demand to self-feed, yet not consistently eating the same amount from meal to meal even as they develop food likes and dislikes. The older infant begins to have regular bowel and bladder elimination patterns. Sleeping through the night becomes more consistent, but infants may fear being left alone; having a routine, with a favorite toy or security object can help with transitions.

Gross and Fine Motor Skill Development

1 to 3 Months

As primitive reflexes begin to fade, voluntary actions emerge. This process of reflex integration is important to monitor as persistent reflexes interfere with developing motor and cognitive skills. The PCP should observe increasing head control and assess that all body movements are symmetrical. As the primitive grasp reflex fades, hands are increasingly open. When a rattle or similar object is offered, the infant will hold it but will not yet reach for it. As infants practice their new voluntary grasp, they hold their own hands and pull at blankets and clothing. The infant Landau reflex emerges around 3 months, typically disappearing by 12 months. This reflex is elicited by holding the infant horizontally in the air in the prone position. The infant should spontaneously extend the head, looking forward; however, when the head is flexed, the legs will drop, flexing responsively. When the head is extended again, the legs will extend out again.

4 to 5 Months

As the Moro and asymmetric tonic neck reflexes go away, the infant begins to roll from back to side first, then prone to supine. Prone ("tummy") floor time is encouraged as infants learn to lift their head for increasing amounts of time. They sit in an auto-supported tripod position at first, progressing to unsupported, straight back as they become stronger. When pulled to sit, there is no head lag and when standing and held by their hands, they can bear full weight and enjoy bouncing on the floor or parental lap. Fine motor skills are evident as infants play with their hands and reach for clothing, earrings, hair, and eyeglasses. They grasp toys and attempt to hold the breast or bottle. Eventually, they grasp objects with both hands and bring them to the mouth to feel, taste, and differentiate.

TABLE 10.1   Infant Growth and Development

Age	Physical	Gross Motor	Fine Motor	Communication and Language	Cognitive and Sensory	Social and Emotional	Sleep
1 month	Gains 150–210 g (5–7 oz)/week (first 6 months); grows 2.5 cm (1 in)/month (first 6 months); OFC increases by 1.5 cm (0.6 in)/month (first 6 months); primitive reflexes present; doll's eye and dance reflexes fading; obligate nose breathing	Turns head from side to side when prone; lifts head briefly when prone; marked head lag; sits with back rounded; when held standing, hips downward are limp	Hands mostly closed with nondirectional hand swipes; strong grasp reflex; clenches objects on contact	Primarily crying	Fixates eyes on an object 20–25 cm (8–10 inches) away; quiets to voices	Intently watches faces when talked to; fixes on colors; calms when spoken to	Sleeps 16–17 h/day; active sleep 50% of time
2 months	Posterior fontanel closes; crawling reflex disappears	Decreasing head lag when pulled to sit; lifts head and chest while prone; holds head upright but forward when sitting	Hands frequently open; fading grasp reflex	Vocalizes more than crying; cooing and vocalizes vowel sounds (ah, ooh), responds to familiar voices	Follows object side to side when supine; searches for sounds; turns head to sounds	Has social smile; is more alert when awake during the day	Sleeps more at night (8.5–10 h), and 6–7 h during the day; takes 3–4 naps
3 months	Primitive reflexes fading	Holds head erect when sitting, but bobs forward; minimal head lag when pulled to sit; body symmetric when prone; raises head and shoulders to a 45- to 90-degree angle when prone; begins to bear weight when standing; regards hand; Landau reflex emerges	Holds rattle, but will not reach for it; absent grasp reflex; hands kept loosely open; clutches own hand; pulls at blankets and clothes	Squeals to show pleasure; begins babbling; vocalizes when smiling and when spoken to	Looks at mirrors, pictures of faces, shapes, and colors; follows object 180 degrees; turns head to locate sound	Shows interest in surroundings; stops crying when parent(s) enter the room; recognizes familiar objects and faces; begins to be aware of strange stimuli or situations	Sleeps 15–17 hours/day
4 months	Begins drooling; Moro and ASTN reflexes disappear	Minimal to no head lag when pulled to sit; balances head well in sitting position; sits upright if propped; raises head and chest 90 degrees off surface when prone; begins to roll prone to supine	Plays with own hands; reaches for items (e.g., eyeglasses, hair, earrings, etc.); grasps with both hands; grasps rattle when placed in hand, but cannot pick it up; mouths most objects	Vocalizations show mood; laughs out aloud; makes d, b, g, k, n, and p sounds (da, ba, etc.)	Focuses on objects; begins to develop binocular vision/depth perception and eye–hand control	Enjoys interacting with others; fusses to demand attention; anticipates feedings when sees bottle or mother if breastfeeding (shows the beginning of memory); prefers certain toys	Develops regular sleep and wake pattern; self-soothes briefly; usually settles back to sleep; may sleep through the night without feeding; sleeps 12–15 h/day

Age	Physical	Gross Motor	Fine Motor	Communication and Language	Cognitive and Sensory	Social and Emotional	Sleep
5 months	Birth weight doubles by the end of this month	Rolls supine to prone; inserts toes in mouth when supine; keeps back straight without head lag when pulled to sit; holds erect when sitting; sits well with support	Uses palmar grasp to pull objects to mouth; holds one cube; plays with toes	Squeals in delight; vocalizes displeasure when objects taken away	Visually follows dropped object; localizes sound made below ear	Recognizes family members; smiles at mirror image; pats bottle or breast with hands; plays enthusiastically; may have rapid mood swings; discovers body parts	Sleeps for 10–11 hours at night, with 3 naps/day
6 months	Growth rate declines, gains 90–150 g (3–5 oz)/week Height increases by 1.25 cm (0.5 in)/month, OFC rate slows to 0.5 cm (0.2 in)/month, Chewing and biting begins as eruption of lower central incisors occurs	Rolls from supine to prone, lifts chest and upper abdomen and bears weight on hands when prone, sits in highchair with back straight; bears weight on legs when supported	Grasps, manipulates, and bangs small objects, releases one object when offered another; grasps feet and pulls to mouth; holds bottle if bottle feeding	Begins to imitate sounds, has one-syllable utterances, vocalizes to toys and mirror image; face brightens to own sounds	Adjusts posture to see an object; localizes sound made above ear	Recognizes parents; fears strangers; extends arms to be picked up; imitates sticking out tongue or coughing, definite likes and dislikes; searches briefly for dropped objects	Sleeps 13–14 h/day; uninterrupted night sleep with 2–3 naps
7 months		Lifts head off surface when supine; bears weight on hands when prone; sits erect momentarily then leans forward to tripod position; bounces when held standing	Grasps with one hand; holds two objects; bangs objects on table; transfers objects from one hand to the other	Vocalizes 4 distinct vowels; combines vowel sounds with consonants to produce syllables (e.g., baba and dada) without meaning	Responds to own name; turns head to localize sound; has definite taste preferences; gaze fixates on very small objects	Imitates simple acts and noises; attracts attention by coughing or snorting; increasing stranger anxiety; worries when parent disappears from sight; plays peek-a-boo; refuses foods by keeping lips closed; bites in frustration	
8 months	Starts regular bladder and bowel patterns; parachute reflex emerges; eruption of upper central incisors	Sits steadily unsupported for short periods of time; bears weight on legs when standing; may stand holding onto furniture; readily adjusts position to reach an object	Develops pincer grasp, releases objects at will ("dropping game"); shakes rattle or bell; holds two cubes while eyeing a third; reaches for out of reach objects	Listens selectively to familiar words; consonant sounds include t and w; begins to have vocalizations with emphasis and emotion		Increased anxiety when parent is unseen; increased stranger anxiety; understands the word "no"; dislikes dressing or diaper changes	Can sleep through the night without a feeding; sleeps 11–12 h/night plus takes 2–3 naps daily
9 months	Eruptions of upper lateral incisors	Steadily sits on floor for up to 10 min; recovers if leans forward but may still fall over if leans sideways; pulls to stand when holds unto furniture; crawls	Hand dominance emerges; refines pincer grasp; compares cubes by bringing them together; grasps a third cube	Comprehends "no"; responds to simple verbal commands	Localizes sounds by turning head	Shows increased interest to please parent; fights having face washed by putting hands in front of face; fears of bedtime/being left alone begin	Sleeps 11–12 h/night plus 2 naps/day

Continued

TABLE 10.1   Infant Growth and Development—Cont'd

Age	Physical	Gross Motor	Fine Motor	Communication and Language	Cognitive and Sensory	Social and Emotional	Sleep
10 months	Eruption of lower lateral incisors may begin	Walks and begins to stand and walk holding on to furniture; changes from standing to sitting by falling down; begins to lift one foot as if taking a step; changes from prone to sitting position	Mature pincer grasp Begins to grasp objects (e.g., chew toy, rattle) by handle	Says "mama" and "dada" with meaning; comprehends "bye-bye"; may say one-syllable words such as "hi" or "bye"		Develops object permanence; repeats actions that attract attention and cause laughter; plays interactively with others (e.g., as with pat-a-cake); stops behavior when told "no"; reacts to scolding or anger with crying; looks at and follows along with picture books; attempts to feed self; helps to dress by extending a leg or arm	Sleeps through the night for 11–12 hours without a feeding; takes 2 naps
11 months		Pivots while sitting to reach toward back to pick up an object; walks while holding on to furniture or with both hands held	Explores objects more intently; offers objects to others and then intentionally drops object for them to be picked up ("the dropping game"); places one object into a container (sequential play); manipulates object to remove from a container	Continues to imitate speech sounds		When task is completed, experiences delight; rolls ball forward when requested; anticipates body gestures in games and songs plays games such as "peek-a-boo"; shakes head sideways for "no"	Sleeps 11–12 h/night without a feeding and takes 2 naps for a total of 2–2.5 h/day
12 months	Triples birth weight; increased birth length by 50%; has equal head and chest circumference; anterior fontanel starts closing; Landau reflex fading; lordosis when walking	Walks holding one hand; attempts to stand without holding on to furniture; may take first steps; sits from standing position	Easily releases cubes into cup; builds two-cube towers; tries to release pellet into narrow-necked bottle; begins using spoon and cup; easily turns book pages	Says "mama" and "dada" and 3–5 other words; receptive language > expressive language; knows object names (e.g., ball, blanket); imitates animal noises; understands one-step commands	Follows rapidly moving objects; listens for sounds to return	Enjoys familiar settings of home and day care; begins to explore away from parent; shows joy and delight; gives affection by hugging or kissing when asked; gets angry when jealous; may cling to parent when unsure; may have a favorite object, such as a security blanket; searches for unseen objects (object permanence)	Sleeps 8–11 hours/night with 1–2 naps

ASTN, Asymmetric tonic neck; *OFC,* occipital frontal (head) circumference.

From Kliegman RM, St Geme J, et al, eds. *Nelson Textbook of Pediatrics.* 21st ed. Elsevier; 2020.

6 to 8 Months

When prone, infants lift their head, chest and upper abdomen off surfaces, bear weight on hands, easily roll from front to back, and begin rolling from back to abdomen. Infants begin to sit erect and progress to sitting unsupported. The infant may begin to scoot while sitting, crawl, and rock in place when on the hands and knees. Some infants crawl, while others push with their arms using frog-like leg movements while their abdomen remains on the floor. They eventually pull themselves to a stand and bounce when standing or holding on to furniture.

Infants typically hold and drop objects to take another that is offered. They begin to transfer objects from hand to hand and then hold more than one object without dropping one. They bang objects on surfaces and rake objects to grasp them. The pincer grasp (using the index finger against the thumb) develops. Although it can be entertaining to watch the infant release objects at will and laugh in delight (i.e., "dropping game"), the infant is fine tuning depth perception. This is further evidenced by the emergence of the protective parachute reflex.

9 to 12 Months (1 Year)

By 9 to 10 months, infants crawl and some will pull to stand or cruise (i.e., walking while holding onto furniture). They eventually take a few steps and progress from momentarily standing alone and walking with the support of adult hands, to taking cautious steps.

By 12 months, advancing fine motor skills infants, especially as the pincer grasp matures. Infants delight in putting objects into containers and taking them out again. As they are read to, they easily turn the pages.

Social and Emotional Development

1 to 3 Months

Infants become more social over this time, imitating parental expressions, visually following others, as well as attending to sounds by quieting body movements or demonstrating visual responses. By 3 months, the infant has a social smile, smiling in response to their parent's voice as well as to others who engage them. With the increase in activity, alertness, and responsiveness, parents need to continue to observe for cues the infant needs to rest or decrease stimulation, rather than assume the infant is always ready for more stimulation.

4 to 5 Months

Infants delight in social interaction while taking in more of their environment. They smile spontaneously and turn their heads to follow others' movements. They look at and grab objects placed in front of them and vocalize displeasure when objects are taken away. Distraction can be used to offset an upset infant. Infants at this age can discriminate between family members and strangers. This reciprocal recognition is an important aspect of attachment, and parents begin to recognize their child's unique, developing personality.

6 to 8 Months

Infants express frustration or reject being spoon fed, preferring to feed themselves. They try to communicate needs by pointing at objects, tugging on clothing, and/or vocalizing with varied pitch and tone. Issues surrounding the infant's desire to control begin to emerge. Understanding and engaging with the infant and learning their cues assist parents, especially when dealing with a determined, strong-willed infant. The PCP can remind parents that this newly found control is a positive quality.

9 to 12 Months (1 Year)

Infants become selective, attach to one person, and exhibit less friendliness to others. They fear strangers, and may cry, turn away, and cling to their parent. They like to please parents and repeat actions that attract attention and cause laughter. They are also learning to say no. They often stop behavior and cry in response to a stern voice or firm verbal command. They love to interact and anticipate body gestures in games, such as "peek-a-boo," and songs, such as "pat-a-cake." They also delight in mastering new skills and want others to notice their skills.

Cognitive Development

1 to 3 Months

Infants become more aware of their environment as they visually track faces and respond to sounds by turning their head. They also attempt to imitate facial expressions and sounds. By 3 months, infants enjoy toys and may wave their arms when a toy is brought into sight.

4 to 5 Months

Infants actively seek out objects, their hands, and toys. They smile, have improved eye-hand control, and bring objects to their mouth to learn about them.

6 to 8 Months

The infant is increasingly aware of their surroundings and expresses individual preferences. Toys that introduce the concept of cause-and-effect (e.g., pull on a string and a bell rings or toy comes closer) encourage learning. They enjoy dropping items; their delight reflects their learning about the objects (e.g., how they sound when they hit the ground and/or how long it takes till they hear the sound). Around 8 months, infants begin to search for objects, especially those that were recently within their sight. This behavior is a sign of developing object permanence, which continues through interactions, such as hide-and-seek and peek-a-boo.

9 to 12 Months (1 Year)

Older infants attempt more complicated tasks, such as stacking blocks. They start to do things on their own, remember learned cause and effect, and follow simple commands, such as "put the toy in the box." They now understand object permanence and enjoy peek-a-boo and hide-and-seek without worry that the items or individuals are gone forever. Their play is often spontaneous and self-directed. They enjoy simple household objects, such as pots and pans, spoons, and measuring cups, as well as toys.

Communication and Language Development

1 to 3 Months

When the infant is in a quiet alert state, parents are encouraged to connect and engage with them in face-to-face quiet verbal interactions. As parents talk, infants begin to learn different sounds and will start to coo (vowel sounds) and later babble (adding consonants) in return. Infants' body movements continue to be a form of communication, from snuggling, to turning the head, or arching the back.

4 to 5 Months

Vocalization increases as the infant squeals in delight, coos/babbles more purposively, and laughs. Infants actively search out sounds, whether incidental, such as a dog's bark or doorbell, or purposeful, such as a bell or rattle, pairing the sound to the item.

6 to 8 Months

Vocalizations continue to increase sound imitation, using pitch and tone, and including "raspberries" and coughing. Babbling (one-syllable utterances combining a consonant and vowel, such as "da") progresses to chained syllables, including "ba-ba" and "da-da" without connecting meaning to them. Infants delight in hearing their own voice and begin to "talk" with emphasis and emotion. Their receptive language increases as they listen to those around them and begin to associate facial expressions and gestures. As noted earlier, infants tend to quiet when a stern voice is used, and they often cry. Reading to infants introduces new words, sounds, and rhythms. Engaging books with simple illustrations introduce associated visuals. The American Academy of Pediatrics (AAP) recommends that infants not watch television or other forms of passive media such as videos before 2 years of age.[1] Instead, the infant should be exposed to language via human interaction, which does include video chatting.

9 to 12 Months

Growing receptive language is reflected as infants begin to understand and follow simple commands. They learn to mimic new sounds, including animal sounds. They comprehend the question "what does a dog say?" and can respond correctly. They enjoy toys that make noise and participating in simple interactive games. Their receptive language is greater than their expressive language, which typically includes around five words, which may not always be easily understood.

Common Developmental Issues

Parents' concerns during the first year of life are often related to inexperience or lack of knowledge about infant growth and development. Anticipating and sharing information about growth and development is an important component of pediatric primary care. Parents' questions and concerns need to be acknowledged and responded to by the PCP. When parents understand the sequence and complexity of growth and development, as well as certain benchmarks, they are better able to parent and make decisions. Two of the more common issues for parents are infant crying/colic and postpartum depression/psychiatric disorders.

Crying/Colic

Crying infants trigger parental concern that something is wrong with their infant. When parents cannot determine the cause of the irritability, it is stressful. It is helpful to be proactive with parents, reminding them that crying is their infant's primary mode of communication. While it is normal for infants to cry up to 5 to 6 hours a day (Table 10.2), there is a fussy period beginning when around 2 weeks of age and continuing until about 3 to 5 months of age. During this time, crying can start and stop for no apparent reason and is often unrelated to anything that a parent does or does not do. Increased, hard-to-soothe crying may signal discomfort or illness, but it may also reflect their infant's temperament (e.g., easy, slow-to-warm, difficult—see Chapter 6). Referring to

TABLE 10.2	Types of Infant Cries and Possible Causes	
Type of Cry	**Possible Cause**
Vigorous and lusty	Healthy, infant
Specific sound	High-pitched, shrieking: central nervous system, such as Cornelia de Lange syndrome
	Like a bleating sheep: cri-du-cat syndrome
	Like a cat meowing: cerebral irritability, such as meningitis
Grunting	Sepsis
	Respiratory distress
Hoarseness	Hypothyroidism
Stridorous	Infection, such as croup or epiglottis
	Tracheal abnormalities
	Foreign bodies
Weak	Overall muscle weakness (e.g., ill, specific disease/syndrome, such as muscular dystrophy, myasthenia gravis)

hard-to-soothe crying as "colic" may relieve some parents from worry, but for others it may feed a belief that something is wrong.

Colic is often defined as excessive crying of more than 3 hours a day in infants between 1 and 4 months old, for longer than 3 weeks. Not all crying infants have colic; however, all infants go through a period of increased fussiness. The Period of PURPLE Crying Initiative (www.purplecrying.info) is a resource for parents during this fussy period. The acronym PURPLE is used to describe specific characteristics of an infant's cry. It also provides parents with knowledge that it could be a temporary developmental phenomenon (Fig. 10.2). However, the PCP must attend to any parent who reports an infant who is difficult to soothe. A careful history and physical examination including a thorough gastrointestinal and neurological assessment should be performed along with an assessment of parent coping skills and resources. If the infant is gaining weight appropriately and has a normal physical examination, laboratory and radiographic studies are unnecessary. There is no evidence to support changing infant formulas or using medications to manage crying. Herbal remedies and/or supplements should be used with caution; however, external interventions, such as the use of white noise (noise that contains many frequencies with equal intensities) may calm infants. Other parents find that their infants calm when the vacuum, blender, or ceiling fan is on, while others notice a car ride breaks up the crying. It is important that whatever distraction is used is safe. For example, parents should be cautioned about putting the infant in a car seat on top of the dryer as it introduces a fall risk, much like a nearby hair dryer introduces a burn risk. In summary, the crying infant as well as the parent(s) need to be assessed and supported with the development of an individualized plan.

Postpartum Psychiatric Disorders

Identification of postpartum psychiatric disorders is important for the mother, family, and infant. Maternal depression can negatively impact cognitive development of infants, interfere with attachment, feeding, and sleep, and contributes to developmental delay and behavior issues.[2] Mild depressive symptoms, often referred

THE LETTERS IN "PURPLE" STAND FOR:					
P	**U**	**R**	**P**	**L**	**E**
PEAK OF CRYING	UNEXPECTED	RESISTS SOOTHING	PAIN-LIKE FACE	LONG LASTING	EVENING
Your baby may cry more each week, the most in month 2, then less in months 3–5.	Crying can come and go and you don't know why.	Your baby may not stop crying no matter what you try.	Crying babies may look like they are in pain even when they are not.	Crying can last as much as 5 h a day or more.	Your baby may cry more in the late afternoon and evening.

• **Fig. 10.2** The PURPLE Acronym for the Period of Infant Crying. (From National Center on Shaken Baby Syndrome: The Period of Purple Crying. http://purplecrying.info/what-is-the-period-of-purple-crying.php.)

to as *postpartum or "baby" blues*, occur in 50% to 80% of mothers. Maternal symptoms include crying, confusion, mood lability, anxiety, and a depressed mood,[3] which appear during the first week postpartum, typically last a few hours to a few days, and have no negative sequelae. These mothers may also report feelings of inadequacy, unhappiness, and fatigue, all of which should resolve.

Postpartum depression is more serious. Unlike baby blues, postpartum depression does not resolve by itself, can appear days to months after the birth, and last for weeks to months. Ongoing depression makes getting through the day difficult due to periods of sadness, anxiety, and loss of interest in activities and affects maternal ability to care for herself and her new infant. Postpartum depression occurs more often in new mothers who are:

- Less than 24 years of age
- American Indian or Alaska Native, Asian, or Native Hawaiian and/or Other Pacific Islander
- Not a high school graduate
- Single
- Postpartum smoker
- Have three or more stressful life events in the year before the infant's birth
- Have a term, low-birth-weight infant (<2500 g)
- Have newborns admitted to a neonatal intensive care unit

Screen all mothers for depression. Pediatric PCPs have ongoing contact with them. The 10-question Edinburgh Postnatal Depression Scale is an easy to administer screening tool and a valuable and efficient way to identify mothers at risk for perinatal depression (Fig. 10.3). Mothers who score 13 or more should be referred for further evaluation with an appropriate mental health professional. Intervention should be individualized. Mothers need to know that postpartum depression is important to recognize, that it is treatable, and that treatment is available. Treatment from a licensed provider should be arranged.

Postpartum psychosis is a severe disorder that includes delusions, paranoia, hallucinations, and gross functional impairment that begins within 4 weeks postpartum. Maternal thoughts of harming herself and/or her newborn may occur. Postpartum psychosis is far less common than postpartum depression and postpartum blues. In addition, mothers with a history of bipolar disorder, schizoaffective disorder, and those with a history or family history of postpartum psychosis are at an increased risk. The cognitive lapses that occur with postpartum psychosis result in the mother's inability to care for herself, neglecting her infant's needs, and proving unsafe caregiving.

In the first year after childbirth, maternal suicide risk increases dramatically, becoming the leading cause of maternal death up to 1 year after delivery. PCPs must inquire about maternal mental health. Each pediatric well-child check is an opportunity to screen mothers and assess families for risk factors that affect infant safety as well as growth and development.

Health Supervision

Monitoring infant growth and development is critical because of the rapid changes that occur. Delays or concerns need to be promptly evaluated rather than using the "wait and see" approach. Referrals for early intervention can make a tremendous difference in quality of life, learning, and later development. Sharing a concern about an infant's growth and/or development with a parent is never easy, but it is important to ensure that the infant receives the help they need. Having a consistent PCP enhances the ability to evaluate the infant and strengthens the provider–parent relationship to allow for providing anticipatory guidance, validating parental efforts, and reinforcing parental success. See Table 10.3 for standardized screening tools for infants.

Periodic Wellness Visits

Routine well-child checks are recommended during infancy at 1, 2, 4, 6, 9, and 12 months of age. Each visit includes a comprehensive history and physical examination (see Chapter 5), appropriate screening, immunizations, and anticipatory guidance according to the AAP and Bright Futures periodicity schedule (https://downloads.aap.org/AAP/PDF/periodicity_schedule.pdf). Table 10.4 summarizes anticipatory guidance topics during infancy and Table 10.5 highlights red flags. Age-related discussion points about infant regulation and sleep/wake patterns, strength and motor coordination, nutrition, communication and language, social and emotional growth, and cognitive and environmental stimulation are highlighted in the following paragraphs.

1 to 3 Months
Regulation and Sleep-Awake Patterns
- *Safe sleep.* Infants should be placed on their backs to sleep. Remind parents to remove stuffed animals, comforters, and bumpers from cribs and bassinets. Review the dangers of cosleeping, especially on soft surfaces (e.g., couch, reclining chair).

Edinburgh Postnatal Depression Scale (EPDS)

Name: _____   Address: _____

Your date of birth: _____

Baby's date of birth: _____   Phone: _____

As you are pregnant or have recently had a baby, we would like to know how you are feeling. Please check the answer that comes closest to how you have felt IN THE PAST 7 DAYS, not just how you feel today.

Here is an example, already completed.

I have felt happy:
- ○ Yes, all the time
- X Yes, most of the time
- ○ No, not very often
- ○ No, not at all

This would mean: "I have felt happy most of the time" during the past week.

Please complete the other questions in the same way.

In the past 7 days:

1. I have been able to laugh and see the funny side of things
   - ○ As much as I always could
   - ○ Not quite so much now
   - ○ Definitely not so much now
   - ○ Not at all

2. I have looked forward with enjoyment to things
   - ○ As much as I ever did
   - ○ Rather less than I used to
   - ○ Definitely less than I used to
   - ○ Hardly at all

*3. I have blamed myself unnecessarily when things went wrong
   - ○ Yes, most of the time
   - ○ Yes, some of the time
   - ○ Not very often
   - ○ No, never

4. I have been anxious or worried for no good reason
   - ○ No, not at all
   - ○ Hardly ever
   - ○ Yes, sometimes
   - ○ Yes, very often

*5. I have felt scared or panicky for no very good reason
   - ○ Yes, quite a lot
   - ○ Yes, sometimes
   - ○ No, not much
   - ○ No, not at all

*6. Things have been getting on top of me
   - ○ Yes, most of the time I haven't been able to cope at all
   - ○ Yes, sometimes I haven't been coping as well as usual
   - ○ No, most of the time I have coped quite well
   - ○ No, I have been coping as well as ever

*7. I have been so unhappy that I have had difficulty sleeping
   - ○ Yes, most of the time
   - ○ Yes, sometimes
   - ○ Not very often
   - ○ No, not at all

*8. I have felt sad or miserable
   - ○ Yes, most of the time
   - ○ Yes, quite often
   - ○ Only occasionally
   - ○ No, never

*9. I have been so unhappy that I have been crying
   - ○ Yes, most of the time
   - ○ Yes, quite often
   - ○ Only occasionally
   - ○ No, never

*10. The thought of harming myself has occurred to me
   - ○ Yes, quite often
   - ○ Sometimes
   - ○ Hardly ever
   - ○ Never

Administered/reviewed by _____   Date _____

SCORING

QUESTIONS 1, 2, and 4 (without an *) are scored 0, 1, 2 or 3 with top box scored as 0
QUESTIONS 3, 5, 6, 7, 8, 9, and 10 (marked with an *) are reverse scored, with the top box scored as a 3
   Maximum score: 30
   Possible depression: 10 or greater
   Always look at item 10 (suicidal thoughts)

Instructions for using the Edinburgh Postnatal Depression Scale:
1. The mother is asked to check the response that comes closest to how she has been feeling in the previous 7 days.
2. All the items must be completed.
3. Care should be taken to avoid the possibility of the mother discussing her answers with others. (Answers come from the mother or pregnant woman.)
4. The mother should complete the scale herself, unless she has limited English or has difficulty with reading.

Users may reproduce the scale without further permission providing they respect copyright by quoting the names of the authors, the title and the source of the paper in all reproduced copies.

• **Fig. 10.3** Edinburgh Postnatal Depression Scale (EPDS). (Modified from Cox JL, Holden JM, Sagovsky R. Detection of postnatal depression: development of the 10-item Edinburgh Postnatal Depression Scale. *Br J Psychiatry.* 1987;150:782–786; and Wisner KL, Parry BL, Piontek CM. Postpartum depression. *N Engl J Med.* 2002; 347[3]:194–199.)

TABLE 10.3	Standardized Screening Tools		
Screening Tool/Ages	**Purpose/Description**	**Number of Items**	**Time Frame**
Ages and Stages Questionnaires (ASQ-3) 1 month–5.5 years www.brookespublishing.com	Developmental milestones Measures communication, gross and fine motor, problem-solving, social, and overall development Written at the 4th–6th grade level	30 items plus overall concerns	10–15 min to complete
Bright Futures 2 days–21 years https://www.healthychildren.org	Age-appropriate child questionnaire that focuses on developmental milestones, nutrition, safety, and child and family's emotional wellbeing	14 items plus overall concerns	
Child Development Inventory 1-6 years of age https://childdevrev.com/specialiststools/ child-development-inventory	Measures gross and fine motor, language, social, and comprehension skills	60 yes/no questions	Less than 10 min
Parents' Evaluations of Developmental Status (PEDS) Birth–8 years www.pedstest.com	Screening/surveillance of development/social- emotional/behavior/mental health. Written at the 4th–5th grade level	10 items	2–10 min
Survey of Wellbeing of Young Children (SWYC) 2–60 months https://www.floatinghospital.org/The- Survey-of-Wellbeing-of-Young-Children/ Overview.aspx	Age specific, based on the Pediatric Symptom Checklist (PSC). Every form contains sections on developmental milestones, behavioral/emotional development, and family risk factors Written at 6th grade level	12–18 items with 1–3 subscales based upon age	<15 min
Battelle Developmental Inventory (BDI-2) Birth–8 years www.riversidepublishing.com/products/ bdi2/	Screening for early childhood developmental milestones Measures personal-social, adaptive, motor, communication, and cognitive ability	100 items	Takes 10–30 min; complete test in 1–2 hours
Infant-Toddler and Family Instrument (ITFI) 6–36 months www.brookespublishing.com	Assesses infant, family, and home environment Includes gross and fine motor, social and emotional development, language, coping, and self-help		Parent interview: takes two 45- to 60-min interviews
Ages and Stages Questionnaire: Social- Emotional (ASQ:SE) 3–60 months www.brookespublishing.com	Screening of social-emotional development	34 items	10–20 min or less to administer
Temperament and Atypical Behavior Scale (TABS) Birth–6 years www.brookespublishing.com	Screening for behavioral concerns Measures detached, hypersensitive and hyperactive, underreactive, and dysregulated behaviors Written at 3rd grade level	55 items	15–20 min to complete
www.pearsonclinical.com	Screens for sensory processing patterns Measures tactile sensitive, taste-smell sensitivity, movement, underresponsiveness, auditory filtering, low energy and weakness, visual and auditory processing	25 items	15–20 min
Oral Health Risk Assessment 6 months–6 years aap.org/AAP/PDF/oralhealth_ RiskAssessmentTool.pdf	Screens for risk of oral caries. Endorsed by the National Interprofessional Initiative on Oral Health	17 items	Provider interview and exam 10 min

- Place drowsy infants in the crib or bassinet to help them learn to self-soothe and go to sleep on their own.
- Help parents identify how family work routines, childcare, breastfeeding patterns, and infant and parental temperament influence family sleep patterns and nighttime routines.
- Establish nap/sleep routines.

Strength and Motor Coordination
- *Tummy time* allows the infant to develop core strength and head, neck, and arm control. Parents can enhance this time with engaging mats, mirrors, and toys/objects placed on the floor within sight, but out of reach.

- Encourage parents to offer/supervise easy-to-hold toys, such as rings or rattles.

Nutrition
- Infants have a strong need to suck, especially *nonnutritive* sucking on fingers, pacifiers, and toys/objects as well as on the breast long after it has emptied.
- Feedings are important to meet nutritional and developmental needs, but they also offer the opportunity for close, affectionate communication between parent and infant.
- Infants often provide readiness to eat and satiation cues. For example, they may vocalize and increase their movements as

TABLE 10.4	Anticipatory Guidance Topics: 1, 2, 4, 6, 9, and 12 Months of Age			
Age	Injury Prevention	Violence Prevention	Nutritional Counselling	Fostering Optimal Development
1 month	Falls Safe sleep Care seat Emergency care	Assess bonding and attachment Discuss sibling rivalry Assess if guns in the home	Breastfeeding or infant formula guidance/ problem-solving	Recognize and manage postpartum blues Childcare options
2 months	Burns/drownings/falls Safe sleep Car seat Appropriate toys	Reassess firearm safety Understanding infant cues/ temperament	Breastfeeding or infant formula guidance/ problem-solving	Parent getting enough rest and managing return to work Reading and interacting
4 months	Infant walkers/falls Choking/suffocation Oral health Safe sleep Car seat	Reassess firearm safety Understanding infant cues/ temperament	Breastfeeding or infant formula guidance/problem-solving Delaying solids	Discuss central to peripheral motor development Reading and interacting
6 months	Burns/hot surfaces Childproofing Infant walkers/falls Choking/suffocation Oral health/fluoride Safe sleep Car seat Sun exposure	Reassess firearm safety Family relationships and support	Breastfeeding or infant formula guidance Introduction of solid foods/ allergen food introduction	Consistent limit setting Praise good behavior Reading and interacting
9 months	Water safety Fall prevention Home safety review Ingestions/poisoning Car seat safety Heatstroke prevention	Assess parents' ideas on discipline Caregiver time away	Avoid juice Encourage practice with cup drinking	Assist infant to sleep through the night if not accomplished Praise good behavior Reading and interacting
12 months	Firearm and water hazards Auto-pedestrian safety Care seat safety Pet safety Poisoning Oral care	Discuss time out vs. corporal punishment Avoiding media violence Review firearm safety	Introduction of whole milk Discuss iron-rich foods Self-feeding Weaning from bottle	Safe exploration Proper shoes Praise good behavior Media exposure

Modified from Marcdante KJ, Kliegman RM, and Schuh AM. *Nelson Essentials of Pediatrics*, 9th ed. Elsevier; 2023:22; and American Academy of Pediatrics Bright Futures Tool and Resource Kit; 2022. https://www.aap.org/en/practice-management/bright-futures/bright-futures-materials-and-tools/bright-futures-tool-and-resource-kit/.

they see the parents prepare for a feeding, and seal their lips, turn their head, or slow or stop sucking when they are satiated. Overfeeding can occur when cues are not recognized or ignored.

- Positive reinforcement for continued breastfeeding is essential and proactive strategies for the mother who is returning to work are beneficial (see Chapter 15); however, not all mothers are able/choose to continue or breastfeed at all. All mothers need to be encouraged to be comfortable with their choices about feeding.
- Some infants will require further evaluation, especially if they show little interest in feeding or are not growing. A detailed feeding history including a minimum 3-day diet history, and caloric analysis is a great starting point (see Chapter 14).
- Assess the infant's mouth, oral motor skills, and general development because feeding difficulties may indicate a physical abnormality (e.g., tight frenulum, subglottal cleft) or a neuromuscular issue.
- Use a standard feeding assessment tool (e.g., NCAST Feeding Scale) to assess the parent–child relationship and develop

individualized recommendations. If needed, refer to a comprehensive infant feeding disorders clinic, nutritionist, gastroenterology specialist, speech and language therapist, or psychologist.

Communication and Language. Parents should be encouraged to talk and sing to the infant during everyday activities. The words/tunes do not necessarily matter; it is important for them to hear their parent's voice. Reading is another great way to encourage communication and language development. Encourage parents to read with their infant, especially books with bright-colored pictures or smiling faces. Parents should continue to talk to their infant, even when supine, to help get and keep the infant's attention.

Social and Emotional Growth

- Relationship development begins at birth and continues throughout childhood. Infants are social and desire to interact with others. Infants with limited social interaction can present as "fussy."
- Infant temperament influences how the child approaches and reacts to the world. When parents understand their infant's

TABLE 10.5 Developmental Red Flags: Infants 3, 6, 9, and 12 Months of Age						
Age	Physical Development, Sleep and Temperament	Gross Motor, Strength and Coordination	Fine Motor, Feeding and Self-Care	Language and Hearing	Social and Emotional	Cognition and Vision
3 months	Weight gain <1 lb (0.5 kg)/month OFC not increasing or increasing >2 standard deviations on growth curve Problems with suck-swallow Difficulty with sleep-wake cycle Fussy baby	Asymmetrical movements Hypertonia or hypotonia No attempt to raise head when prone No Landau reflex	Hands fisted with oppositional thumb No hand-to-mouth activity Feedings taking longer than 45 min Consistently waking hourly for feeding	Does not turn to voice, rattle, or bell No verbalizations, coos, squeals	Lacks social smile Withdrawn or flat affect Lack of consistent, safe childcare Lack of eye contact	No visual tracking Does not fix on face or object
6 months	Has not doubled birth weight OFC not increasing or too large Poor feeding or sleep regulation Poor self-calming	Persistent primitive reflexes Unable to sit with support Head lag with pull to sit	Not reaching for objects Does not hold rattle Does not hold hands together Does not grasp at clothes	No babbling Does not respond to voice, bell, rattle, or loud noise Parent concern about hearing	No smiles No response to play Withdrawn or flat affect Lack of eye contact	Parental concerns about vision No reach for objects Does not look at caregiver
9 months	Parent concerns about feeding or sleep Persistent night awakening Poor self-calming, self-regulation	Does not sit even in tripod position Asymmetric crawl or other movements	No self-feeding No highchair sitting No solid foods Does not pick up toy with one hand	No single- or double-consonant sounds Does not respond to name or voice Lacks reciprocal vocalizations	Intense or absent stranger anxiety Does not seek comfort from caregiver Poor eye contact	Parent concern about vision No visual awareness Does not reach out for toys Does not explore toys visually or orally
12 months	Has not tripled birth weight Change of >2 standard deviation on growth curve for weight, length, or OFC Poor sleep-wake cycles Extreme separation anxiety	Not pulling self to stand Not exploring environment	Persistently mouths objects Does not attempt to feed self or hold cup Cannot hold toy in each hand or transfer objects	Does not localize to sound Does not imitate speech sounds Does not use two or three words Uses only gestures or pointing	No response to games, reading, or other interactive activities Withdrawn or flat affect Poor eye contact	Not visually following activities in the environment

OFC, Occipital frontal (head) circumference.

temperament, they can anticipate and understand how their infant reacts and relates to the world around them. Parent–child temperament mismatch can be challenging (see Chapter 6).
- Happy, healthy parents help make for happy, healthy babies. Infants react to their parent's emotional states. Accordingly, parents need to develop strategies to have time together as a couple and do activities they find enjoyable. PCPs can identify criteria for parents seeking childcare resources and how to locate those resources.

Cognitive and Environmental Stimulation
- Provide a stimulating environment for infants. Some parents may be stressed or have limited time to spend with their infants. Use of short, daily activities, such as singing a nursery rhyme or song, dancing with the infant in their arms, blowing bubbles toward the infant, looking at pictures in the house and explaining who the people in the pictures are great examples.

Parents can also visit the local public library to borrow board books with high contrast/brightly colored pictures.
- Select toys that are safe and developmentally appropriate. Use caution with small toys that pose choking hazards (e.g., those with small pieces or that are smaller than the size of the infant's fist), and painted toys. Good choices include toys that squeak or rattle, or an unbreakable mirror to look at themselves.

4 to 5 Months
Regulation and Sleep-Awake Patterns. Infants can differentiate between day and night and usually sleep 14 hours a day, including 8 hours at night without a feeding. By 5 months, most infants sleep 10 to 11 hours straight. During the day, they nap from 4 to 5 hours usually spread out over two to three naps.
- Infants outgrow the bassinet and need to move to a crib.
- Bedtimes rituals are important to signal what is going to happen next, which builds a sense of security.

- Parents should modify routines to fit the infant's temperament.

Strength and Motor Coordination

- Increasing infant mobility means childproofing the home and the homes of close relatives and friends. Measures include safety latches on drawers and cabinets, wrapping appliance cords, covering electrical outlets, and using gates for stairs or rooms. Avoid placing the crib near windows because of the presence of drapery and blind cords.
- Floor time encourages motor strength and coordination. A few bright toys just beyond their infant's reach encourages rolling over to reach them. Time spent in playpens should be minimal.
- Movable walkers should be avoided as they allow mobility beyond an infant's natural ability and are faster than a parent's reaction time. Stationary activity centers are safer; however, their use should be limited to avoid undue stress on the infant's developing hips.

Nutrition

- Drooling is common. It is often aligned with teething but primarily occurs because of salivary gland maturation. The infant gradually develops the ability to swallow excessive saliva.
- Infants only need breastmilk or infant formula for the first 6 months of life, though many parents desire to start solid foods earlier. Infants are ready for solids when they have good head control, can sit upright alone, and have a diminished tongue thrust reflex. All infants are different and develop at their own pace, so parents need to understand infant readiness cues.
- There is evidence that introducing allergenic foods by 6 months can decrease the risk of developing a food allergy. All infants should be evaluated for the introduction to peanuts between 4 and 11 months of age. Current guidelines suggest infants with severe eczema undergo allergy testing, and those with moderate to no eczema be introduced to peanut-containing food at 6 months depending on parent preference.[4]
- Spoon feeding helps the infant develop new oral-motor skills including tongue, lip, and cheek control. Infant cereal is typically one of the first solid foods offered and should be offered on a spoon, not mixed in a bottle or cup.

Communication and Language

- Parents should talk and sing to their infant and encourage back-and-forth communication.
- Infants start to babble using many of the characteristics of their native language. Although babbling may sound like nonsense, encourage parents to listen for changes in the infant's pitch.
- Daily reading time develops the habits of quiet time, reading time, and parent-infant time together. Parents should explore colorful books with their infants describing the pictures, colors, and actions. The *Imagination Library* is a great resource; families can sign up to receive a new developmentally appropriate book for the child every month.

Social and Emotional Growth

- Nonnutritive sucking is a means of infant self-regulation. Sucking on fingers, toes, and toys uses different oral-motor movements from those needed to suck on a nipple or pacifier.
- Information about infant development and strategies to deal with difficult behaviors is important. Parents should understand their child's behavior in terms of infant development. Encourage parents to change gears to change behavior. Because infants have very short attention spans, it is easy to distract them. For example, if the infant is determined to rip up the paper or book pages, encourage parents to offer a favorite toy to change his or her focus. Modeling desired behavior and redirecting behavior should be discussed before it is needed. Some

parents may benefit from parenting classes or parent support groups that provide information on developmental milestones and anticipated changes. Healthy Steps and Bright Futures have one-page downloadable handouts that provide anticipatory guidance.
- Communication between parents about their roles, responsibilities, expectations, and differences is crucial, as is finding couple time. This time provides emotional wellbeing and allows them to better care for their infant.

Cognitive and Emotional Stimulation

- Infants this age are awake more and parents need strategies to provide more attention and play activities. Infants seek their parents' attention by cooing, babbling, smiling, or crying. Providing the infant one or two toys then adding others when their focus wanes stretches the activity out. Not all activities need to involve toys, as infants enjoy common household objects such as pots, pans, plastic containers, and lids to stack, shake, or roll.
- Time spent outside in nature can be an adventure. Explore environments through walks to the neighborhood park/playground or farmer's market, as well as the small/local grocery store, and library.

6 to 8 Months

Regulation and Sleep-Wake Patterns

- Encourage a sleep routine (e.g., Brush, Book, Bed) to help the infant anticipate sleep. Put infants in their cribs when they are drowsy and awake, but not asleep.
- Allow infants who awaken at night to return to sleep on their own. If the infant does not return to sleep, encourage parents to intrude as little as possible, using only a soft voice, then gently touching, and finally holding the infant if other attempts fail.

Strength and Motor Coordination

- *Floor time* is essential at this stage as infants learn to scoot, crawl, and stand.
- Toys provide the infant with enticement to reach and to move with the result of rolling, scooting, or crawling over to reach it.
- Parents must balance safety versus exploration. Childproofing needs to occur with the focus on the infant's view. Getting down to the infant's level can identify hazards. Be aware of things that can be pulled down (e.g., electrical cords, tablecloths, curtains, pot and pan handles), anything that can topple over (e.g., floor lamps), and electrical sockets. Padding sharp corners of coffee tables and fireplace hearths, removing small objects from the infant's reach including pet food bowls, and keeping window covering cords out of reach and toilet seat lids closed are essential.
- Active supervision is the best way to prevent injuries as the infant becomes more mobile. An adult needs to be within reach and free of distractions while watching the infant. Infants should never be left unattended during baths.

Nutrition

- Many 6-month-old infants can go for 6 to 12 hours without feeding. If the infant is still waking for feedings at night, this is most likely a learned behavior. If not already started, solids should begin at 6 months. Breastfed infants now need iron-fortified foods.
- The ideal highchair is sturdy and stable and stands up to heavy use, spills, and frequent cleaning. It makes feedings more enjoyable for both the infant and parents.
- There is no evidence to wait to introduce highly allergic foods, such as eggs, soy, peanuts, or fish, to prevent food allergy.

All infants should be considered for peanut introduction between 4 and 11 months of age to prevent serious peanut allergy.[4]

- Allow the infant to hold a spoon or cup to encourage self-feeding.
- It is important for infants to eat with their family at least once a day. The likelihood that infants will try new foods increases as they observe others eat. Distractions, such as toys and television, should be avoided. Mealtime conversation should be pleasant, helping all family members enjoy their time together.

Communication and Language

- Continue talking and singing to the infant using facial expressions and gestures. Name body parts while bathing the infant or changing a diaper.
- Read to the infant daily using a variety of brightly colored, age-appropriate books. Name family members in pictures around the home.

Social and Emotional Growth

- Many infants attach to a favorite toy or security blanket, which can ease separation anxiety.
- Infants begin to express feelings of discomfort, anxiety, pleasure, hunger, and being tired. In new or different situations, infants may seek comfort from parents or familiar caregivers and act anxious around less familiar people.

Cognitive and Environmental Stimulation

- Toys and objects that stack or involve a cause-and-effect reaction, and container play are ideal as are interactive games including "peek-a-boo" and "this little piggy."
- Objects smaller than 2.25 inches (5.7 cm) long by 1.25 inches (3.2 cm) wide are choking hazards for children younger than 3 years, and toys with small pieces that can break off should be avoided.

9 to 12 Months (1 Year)

Regulation and Sleep-Wake Patterns

- Predictability in the daily routine allows the infant to gain mastery over new situations.
- A daily schedule of mealtimes, snack times, and playtimes, a nighttime routine, and consistent caregivers increases the infant's sense of security during transitions. As infants enjoy the freedom that their increased mobility brings, they also start to experience separation anxiety.
- Many infants latch on to a "comfort" object, such as a stuffed animal or blanket, which provides continuity and eases stressful situations. This love affair often lasts through toddlerhood or longer. A second, identical spare is vital in case the "favorite" gets lost; trade the spare with the original so that both feel and smell the same.
- Infant temperament becomes more evident in activity and curiosity levels and in adjustment to new situations. Help parents identify strategies and creative solutions for temperament-based concerns.

Strength and Motor Coordination

- Infants refine old and achieve new motor skills. Parents should cheer on their infant to build on cause-and-effect actions with positive reinforcement.
- Childproofing continues as the mobile and curious infant explores the surrounding environment. Medications and potentially hazardous items should not be stored in purses or other areas the infant can reach. Firearms should be in a locked cabinet and not just out of reach. Ammunition must be locked and stored separate from firearms. In addition, small objects, plastic grocery bags, and balloons must be kept away from the ever-curious infant. Making the home child-safe allows parents to spend more time playing and less time saying "no."
- Infants should never be left alone in the tub. Discourage standing up to prevent a slippery fall.

Nutrition

- Food varies from pureed to blended, finger foods, and soft solids to a wide range of table foods. Regardless of the type, self-feeding should be encouraged even though many parents struggle due to the "messiness" and mealtime taking longer.
- Talk with parents about strategies to encourage self-feeding using fingers, spoons, and cups. Using hands and trying to use a spoon are important aspects of how an infant learns to self-feed and regulate oral intake. Start out with one meal and snack for self-feeding with the goal to build up to full self-feeding.
- Hunger is inconsistent for infants. Three meals and two to three snacks a day are usually sufficient. It is important to continue family meals and avoid distracted eating.
- By 12 months, infants should be weaned from the bottle and pacifier and transitioned to a cup.

Communication and Language

- This is a fun time with infants as they are more interactive.
- Reinforce the infant's efforts to communicate through gestures, pointing, and rather unclear vocalizations. Encourage the infant to "ask" for the item or the need. This provides groundwork for future speech development and socialization.
- While reading a book, parents can say "point to the cat" and ask "where is the red car?" Imitating animal sounds while reading and allowing infants to turn the page are encouraged.
- While bathing, dressing, or diapering the infant, encourage naming body parts such as "this is your nose!" Name utensils during meals or when cooking, and describe food colors, smells, and taste, ("this is sour"; "this is sweet").

Social and Emotional Growth

- Degrees of independence and autonomy emerge in infants as they distinguish themselves from their parents.
- Discipline is a process to teach positive behaviors, rather than a punishment for negative behavior. It is easy to distract infants at this age by guiding their curiosity to other activities or objects.
- Parents may struggle to find the energy to deal with busy, on-the-go infants. Suggestions on how to cope with exhaustion and a busy infant may be needed (parents having a simple dinner out together or letting the infant stay with someone for a few hours while the parents take a much-needed nap).
- Stranger anxiety can be challenging, but establishing a separation routine helps infants to understand that the parent is leaving but will return. Eventually, parents may feel sad or disappointed when their infant easily separates and enjoys time away from them.

Cognitive and Environmental Stimulation

- Play is the work of infants. When parents participate in playing with their infant, the parent–child bond is strengthened while simultaneously stimulating cognitive development of the infant.
- Taking command during play fosters the infant's emerging independence and facilitates parents being able to model new activities and skills with interactive games such as a couch cushion obstacle course or singing "itsy, bitsy spider" and "wheels on the bus."
- A container of toys prevents toy boredom; rotate toys in and out of the box.

- A mixture of board books, blocks, and stacking, pull, and pretend toys, such a spoons and cups, helps develop the infant's dexterity skills and promote self-feeding.
- "Messy" play provides further exploration and allows creativity (e.g., sandboxes, water tables, gelatin).

Screening

Developmental *screening* is more in-depth than simple assessment and observation and involves the use of an appropriate, validated developmental and behavioral screening tool. Universal developmental, behavioral, and social screening and surveillance of infants is recommended throughout infancy with formal norm-validated developmental screening at age 9 months.[6] Developmental *surveillance* includes acknowledging the parental concerns, obtaining a developmental and behavioral history, and completing a thorough examination of the infant's development.

Routine well-child checks are recommended at 1, 2, 4, 6, 9, and 12 months, or whenever there are concerns. Table 10.3 includes evidence-based screening tools for use during infancy. The AAP and Bright Futures have Medical Screening Reference Tables available as well (see https://downloads.aap.org/AAP/PDF/Bright%20Futures/MSRTable_InfancyVisits_BF4.pdf). They provide guidance for infants who meet at-risk criteria for further relevant assessments, such as blood pressure measurement, vision and hearing referrals, tuberculosis, Hgb, hematocrit, lead level testing, and oral fluoride supplementation. Further prompt evaluation is critical when screening identifies a potential developmental, behavioral, or social concern. A positive screen does not indicate a diagnosis. The prevalence of American children with a developmental, behavioral, or social delays or disability is one in six.[5] Early intervention programs are great community resources for infants with developmental delays.

Red Flags

Developmental delay in infants involves disorders that manifest as motor problems (e.g., cerebral palsy), communication problems (e.g., receptive or expressive), and/or cognitive problems (e.g., problem solving, cognitive delay, specific deficits in processing information). Processing disorders include peripheral problems (e.g., deafness and blindness) and/or central processing that results in motor, language, and perceptual dysfunction; and behavioral problems. Disorders may be degenerative (e.g., muscular dystrophy) or static (e.g., brachial plexus injury, cerebral palsy). Signs and symptoms of developmental delay may also be a function of the disorder itself (e.g., progressive neurologic loss) or secondary to the disorder (e.g., contractures with cerebral palsy).

All children develop at their own pace, so it is difficult to predict when they will learn a specific skill. Infant developmental delays can be difficult to identify, but the PCP must be alert to red flags that place the infant at risk or indicate a potential problem. Parents may be the first to notice that their infant is lagging behind other infants of similar age and should be encouraged to discuss their concerns with their PCP. Pediatric providers need to listen carefully to parental concerns and be aware of the infant's history. The following are examples of specific risk factors for developmental delay or disorder:

- Maternal infections during pregnancy, such as cytomegalovirus infections

- Genetics, such as Angelman, Fragile X, and Prader-Willi syndromes (see Chapter 27)
- Maternal use of alcohol, tobacco, and drugs, both prescription and illicit
- Infants who were low birth weight (<2500 g), premature (born before 37 weeks' gestation), small for gestational age or had symmetrical intrauterine growth restriction, or part of multiple gestations such as twins and triplets
- Infants with an older sibling with a developmental delay
- Infants admitted to the neonatal intensive care unit and required long-term hospitalization
- Infants who experienced birth trauma

Infants at risk need closer developmental surveillance and more frequent screening. They often require referral to developmental centers for more in-depth assessments and intervention. Table 10.5 outlines red flags, or developmental findings that are indications for referral to a child development center, a state's early child development identification program, or a child development specialist. When indicators are present, referral should be made rather than waiting some months to validate observations. If a genetic condition is suspected, a referral to a pediatric genetic specialist may be indicated.

Additional Resources

Brazelton TB, Sparrow JD. *Touchpoints—Birth to Three: Your Child's Emotional and Behavioral Development.* Perseus; 2006.

Bright Futures: www.brightfutures.org.

Bright Futures Tool and Resource Kit: http://brightfutures.aap.org/tool_and_resource_kit.html.

Bright Futures Medical Screening Reference Table for Infancy: https://downloads.aap.org/AAP/PDF/Bright%20Futures/MSRTable_InfancyVisits_BF4.pdf.

Bright Futures Oral Health Risk Assessment Tool: https://downloads.aap.org/AAP/PDF/oralhealth_RiskAssessmentTool.pdf

Brush, Book, Bed: https://www.healthychildren.org/English/healthy-living/oral-health/Pages/Brush-Book-Bed.aspx.

Centers for Disease Control and Prevention growth charts: www.cdc.gov/growthcharts/who_charts.htm#The%20WHO%20Growth%20Charts.

Duderstadt K. *Pediatric Physical Examination.* 4th ed. Elsevier; 2023.

Hagan JF, Shaw JS, Duncan PM, eds. *Bright Futures: Guidelines for Health Supervision of Infants, Children, and Adolescents.* 4th ed. American Academy of Pediatrics; 2017.

Healthy Steps for Young Children: A National Initiative to Foster Healthy Growth and Development: www.healthysteps.org.

Imagination Library: https://imaginationlibrary.com/.

National Capital Poison Center (800-222-1222): www.poison.org/actFast/1800.asp.

National Center on Shaken Baby Syndrome/Period of PURPLE Crying: www.clickforbabies.org/.

Nursing Child Assessment Satellite Training (NCAST): http://www.ncast.org/.

Zero to Three: www.zerotothree.org.

Acknowledgment

The author acknowledges the contributions of Sandra Banta-Wright, author of this chapter in the previous edition.

References

1. American Academy of Pediatrics Council on Communications and Media. *Media and Children*; 2021. https://www.aap.org/en/patient-care/media-and-children/.
2. Oyetunji A, Chandra P. Postpartum stress and infant outcome: a review of current literature. *Psychiatr Res.* 2020;284:112769.
3. National Institutes of Mental Health. Postpartum Depression Facts. https://www.nimh.nih.gov/health/publications/postpartum-depression-facts/index.shtml.
4. Greer FR, Sicherer SH, Burks AW, AAP Committee on Nutrition, AAP Section On Allergy And Immunology. The effects of early nutritional interventions on the development of atopic disease in infants and children: the role of maternal dietary restriction, breastfeeding, hydrolyzed formulas, and timing of introduction of allergenic complementary foods. *Pediatrics.* 2019;143(4):e20190281.
5. Zablotsky B, Black LI, Maenner MJ, et al. Prevalence and trends of developmental disabilities among children in the United States: 2009–2017. *Pediatrics.* 2019;144(4):e20190811–e20190816.
6. Hagan JF, Shaw JS, Duncan B. *Bright Futures: Guidelines for Health Supervision of Infants, Children and Adolescents.* 4th ed. Elk Grove, IL: American Academy of Pediatrics; 2018.

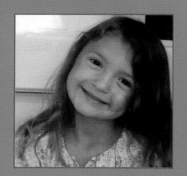

11

Developmental Management of Early Childhood

VALERIE GRIFFIN

Developmental changes in early childhood (1–5 years old) are more subtle than those seen in the first year of life, yet they are highly significant. Early childhood is especially marked by rapidly developing psychosocial skills. Children enter this stage as toddlers, very dependent on parents and caregivers for their survival, and leave as accomplished preschoolers with skills to enter the social world of school and community and a sense of self that shapes the quality of their character for the rest of their lives. This chapter reviews many of the changes that occur in early childhood, the common issues encountered, and the role of primary care provider (PCP) when working with these children and their families.

Developmental Overview of Early Childhood

Physical Growth and Development

PCPs use the World Health Organization growth charts to monitor growth up until 2 years of age, then shift to the Centers for Disease Control and Prevention (CDC) growth charts for children 2 years of age and older. Around the time of this shift, the average 2-year-old weighs approximately 28 pounds (12.7 kg), is approximately 34 inches (86 cm) tall, and has a head circumference of approximately 18.5 inches (47 cm). There may be a small discrepancy in percentiles as children are now measured standing (height) rather than supine (length). The anterior fontanelle should completely close by 18 to 19 months, while the body's skeletal growth continues, especially during the fourth and fifth year, as additional ossification centers appear in the wrist and ankle and additional epiphyses develop in some of the long bones.

Organ and System Maturation

Specific changes in body systems during early childhood are highlighted in Table 11.1.

Motor Development

Advances in gross motor skills (use of the large muscles) and fine motor skills (hand/finger and oral-motor development) are

summarized in Table 11.2. Hand dominance usually develops between 2 and 4 years but may not be evident until 4 to 6 years.

Social and Emotional Development

These are years of intense learning about identifying and managing feelings (e.g., love, happiness, anger, frustration, aggression, and jealousy) and developing social skills (e.g., sharing, giving and receiving affection). Emotions and cognition are interconnected, as this age group learns the words that go with their feelings and, with guidance, the appropriate corresponding actions and behaviors. A major developmental milestone for this age is the achievement of a sense of independence and autonomy. The road from depending on parents/caregivers for everything to doing some things for themselves can be rocky and uneven. A child's ability to achieve independence is influenced by the positive (e.g., strengths, protective factors) and negative influences (e.g., adversity) in their environment. For example, adverse childhood experiences and household dysfunction can cause short- and long-term impacts on childhood development, disease risk, and social problems.[1]

Feelings and Emotions

Children in early childhood need a great deal of love, warmth, and comfort, primarily from their parents. *One- to 2-year-olds* learn to give love and find satisfaction in pleasing their parents. They learn to respond to kisses, hugs, and cuddles they receive by giving kisses, hugs, and cuddles in return. Children who attempt giving love and are rejected or ignored soon stop trying and learn to find pleasure elsewhere. However, children with sensory issues avoid some gestures unless they are in control and decide that they can handle the tactile or sensory feelings. Some 1- to 2-year-olds find that thumb sucking, rhythmic body movements, and body manipulation are more pleasurable and reliable than person-to-person contact. *Three- to 5-year-olds* gradually develop more sophisticated ideas about feeling, giving, and sharing as they move away from the self-centered attitude of toddlerhood and focus more on pleasing behaviors. At this stage, parents are (and should model) the epitome of wisdom, power, integrity, and goodness. Children who do not feel loved often respond with an increase in fears, inhibitions, explosive behavior, and demands for attention.

TABLE 11.1	Changes in Body Systems in Early Childhood	
Body System	Developmental Changes
Dental	By 1 year of age, the child usually has 2–4 primary teeth. Calcification begins for the first premolars at 18–24 months, second premolars at 24–30 months, and second molars at 30–36 months. By 3 years of age, the child has a complete set of 20 primary teeth, including second molars. By 4–5 years of age, central and lateral incisor enamel is complete.
Neurologic	Myelinization increases and cortical development occurs. Gross motor skills are smoother and more coordinated; fine motor movements are more detailed and sustained. Visual acuity improves to 20/40 by 4 to 5 years of age. Portions of the brain that respond to complex sounds connect what is heard to meaning; this continues until approximately age 10 years.
Cardiovascular	Little change occurs in the second and third years. By the fifth year, heart size has quadrupled since birth; heart rate is 70–110 beats/min; and innocent murmurs and sinus arrhythmia are common. Hemoglobin level for children 1–6 years ranges from 9.5–14; adult distribution of Hgb A1, A2, and F is already established (6–9 months).
Pulmonary	Respiratory rate slows to about 20–30 breaths/min. As the diaphragm matures, abdominal respiration movement decreases; by the end of the fifth year, respiratory movement is primary diaphragmatic.
Gastrointestinal	By 2 years, the salivary glands reach adult size. The stomach becomes more bowed and increases its capacity to about 500 mL. Many children still require a nutritious snack between meals because of small stomach size. During the second year, the liver matures and becomes more efficient in vitamin storage, glycogenesis, amino acid changes, and ketone body formation. The lower edge of the liver may still be palpable. By age 5 years, the gastrointestinal system is mature, allowing the child to eat a full range of foods. Stools are more like those of adults.
Renal	Urine characteristics are similar to adults. Kidneys are well developed and begin descending deeper into the pelvic area and grow in size; ureters remain short and relatively straight. A 2-year-old child may excrete as much as 500–600 mL of urine a day. A 4- to 5-year-old child excretes between 600 and 750 mL daily.
Endocrine	Quiescent time for sexual growth, with few hormonal changes. Growth hormone (primarily secreted during sleep) stimulates body growth.

Social Competence

Children gradually increase their ability to follow commands as they work to gain and maintain adult approval and to behave the way they learn "good" children are expected to. By 3 to 5 years, children begin to show interest in table manners, being polite, saying "thank you" without a reminder, sharing, saying (and meaning) "I'm sorry," and taking turns. These social skills are learned through daily interactions at home, as well as other social exposures (e.g., preschool, church) and through those around them, including parents, caregivers, siblings, peers, relatives, teachers, and neighbors. Children begin to realize that others have feelings, fears, and doubts. They learn to read others' social cues (e.g., the voice tone, facial expression, posture) and to self-correct their own behavior. Some children find interpreting others' cues challenging (i.e., empathetic recognition), and parents can help by modeling, explaining, and discussing cues with them.

Self-Control and Autonomy

Throughout early childhood, children vacillate between being a "big" boy or girl and being mommy's or daddy's baby—taking pride in doing as many things as possible for themselves, yet still needing to feel totally secure in their parent's care. On some days, 1- to 2-year-olds cling to their parents' side, not letting them out of sight; on other days, the child can play for short periods in the next room, trotting back every so often to see, touch, and hear the parent and be reassured by their presence. The child who feels secure uses the parent as a base from which to go out and safely explore the world. Gradually, the periods of separation lengthen, and the child needs only to hear the parent's voice or to check occasionally for security. Separation anxiety occurs during these years and can be traumatic for both parent and child. Having a choice and learning the power of the word "no" emerge early on. Younger children can become extremely negative, practicing the power of "no" every day for months, even when their answer is actually "yes." They practice making choices, but they are clumsy, awkward, and frequently wrong. This can be frustrating for them, and their outraged responses can be equally frustrating for parents. One- to 2-year-olds discover the delights of control over others and themselves. This control not only increases their sense of power but also leads to misunderstandings and hurt feelings if their parents do not read their moods properly. During early childhood, children become

TABLE 11.2 Fine and Gross Motor Development Milestones for Early Childhood

Age	Fine Motor	Gross Motor
12 months	• Uses pincer grasp • Points at objects • Stacks two blocks • Clasps hands together	• Pulls to stand • Stands alone for 3–5 seconds • Walks holding on to furniture • Lowers self from standing to sitting without falling • Rolls a ball
15 months	• Puts blocks in a cup • Drinks from a cup • Holds utensils, some attempt to use • Stacks two blocks	• Stands alone well • Walks forward and backward • Stoops and recovers • Climbs up stairs without alternating feet • Pulls a pull toy
18 months	• Builds tower of four cubes • Scribbles spontaneously • Puts blocks in large holes • Drinks from cup with little spilling • Removes socks • Stacks 4–6 blocks	• Throws while aiming • Walks well independently • Pushes and pulls toys • Pulls toy while walking backward
24 months	• Builds tower of seven cubes • Circular scribbling • Imitates folding paper once • Turns doorknob • Turns pages one at a time • Unbuttons or unzips clothing • Washes hands with assistance • Uses a spoon	• Throws overhand • Runs well • Climbs up on furniture • Kicks ball • Walks up and down stairs, may not alternate feet • Walks with control • Runs • Jumps up • Assists with dressing • Able to pull pants down with assist
30 months	• Builds tower of nine cubes • Draws vertical and horizontal lines • Imitates circle • Buttons large buttons • Holds fork in fist and attempts to use • Dresses self with assistance	• Jumps with both feet • Climbs stairs alternating feet • Stands on one foot for 1 second • Walks on tiptoes
36 months	• Builds tower of 9–10 cubes • Imitates three-cube bridge • Copies circle • Uses scissors • Brushes teeth but not well • Puts on shoes • Feeds self with utensils • Plays with 1- to 3-piece puzzle • Puts on shoes and socks • Brushes hair • Imitates drawing a cross • Twists jar lids	• Jumps with both feet • Climbs ladders • May pedal tricycle • Balances on one foot for 2–3 seconds • Kicks ball with direction • Catches a ball
48 months	• Copies bridge from model • Cuts curved line with scissors • Dresses self independently • Strings small beads • Demonstrates hand preference • Imitates a square • Undresses self • Buttons • Strings beads • Pours from small pitcher	• Tries to skip using alternate feet • Catches a bouncing ball • Runs around corners lightly on toes and stops voluntarily • Stands on one foot for 5 seconds • Walks down stairs with alternating feet • Throws ball underhand

Children develop at their own rate and often concentrate on one area of development and not necessarily on another. This chart provides general information and is not specific to any one child. To screen for developmental delays and concerns in early childhood, a validated screening tool must be used.

more skilled, make better choices, have more successes, and feel more powerful. They no longer have to work so hard to show others their power, and the dominantly negative phase passes. *Three- to 5-year-olds* are much less dependent on their parents and frequently tolerate physical separation for several hours. As their sense of separateness increases, children are more aware that they are different from their surroundings, families, and friends. Learning about how to have and be friends is challenging but significant. Interactions become easier and more enjoyable as the child learns to verbally express needs and feelings. They are also able to perform increasingly more self-care tasks (e.g., feed themselves using appropriate utensils, blow their own noses, and go to the bathroom unassisted).

Play and Peer Relationships

One- to 2-year-olds may be fascinated by children their own age and demonstrate curiosity by physically examining the other child closely, poking, and probing; however, they generally do not engage in an interactive way. Parallel play is the norm. Three- to 5-year-olds learn to interact with peers, especially as symbolic language develops. As their social world grows, play is more interactive, cooperative, and shared. Play offers more than cherished memories of growing up; it allows children to develop creativity and imagination while developing physical, cognitive, and emotional strengths. Fantasy and make-believe are also important during these years. Imaginary play leads to "pretend play," role-playing, and creation of imaginary friends, all of which allow children to work through challenges. Play is the major mechanism through which children in early childhood practice social roles, such as housekeeping, caring for baby dolls, "fixing" household items, going to work or school, cooking, practicing religious or cultural rituals and practices, and doing garden or yard work. Children need both structured and free play. Shared or cooperative play makes simple games of hide-and-seek and tag possible. Games with complicated rules can be frustrating for the 3- to 5-year-old child, who prefers simple games with the option of making up the rules as the game proceeds. Cheating is common because the boundaries of acceptable play are not yet clear, and the earliest stages of moral behavior are beginning to emerge.

Environmental factors can affect a child's ability to make healthy play choices.[2] Children today spend less time playing outside than previous generations and they are more likely to play in their yard (if they have one) than any other location. Larger neighborhood environments can impact children's access to the natural world, outdoor play, and physical activity. Creating environments with easy access to nature trails or outdoor play equipment increases exposure to the natural world and different types of physical activity. Safe spaces occur when there are fewer connecting streets and more visually appealing play areas are attractive to children and parents; however, any outdoor activity exposes children to the natural world and its unique form of stimulation.

Moral Development

The ability to know right from wrong is based on evolving external controls as well as from children's evolving desire to please those they love. One- to 2-year-olds cannot be expected to make correct choices if left alone in potentially dangerous situations because their conscience is rudimentary, and judgment is absent. For example, any room with electrical sockets, knobs for technical equipment, guns, open windows, unsecured television and furniture, or hot food represents a risk. As children gain language skills, they begin to echo their parent's firm "no," but they do not fully understand its meaning. By age 2 years, children show beginning internalization, often saying "no" to themselves as they proceed with or stop the act. As they develop, 3- to 5-year-olds establish a moral foundation that is more internally controlled. Instead of basing all decisions on their knowledge of and consequences of an act (e.g., "If I take a cookie, I will be sent to my room"), children begin to show an elementary understanding of justice, which includes what is right and wrong, as well as what is fair or unfair. They recognize others' needs and can help or comfort others. They begin to think ahead as well as plan and control their urges, thus avoiding punishment. By age 4 years, most children internalize some demands from their parents, and feelings of guilt can be elicited after some transgressions. In the long term, children's successes and failures at controlling their worlds will impact their immediate and future behaviors. Parents often worry about how to help children develop decision making skills; the recommendation is to focus more on helping the child to make safe decisions first, the moral ones will follow.

Body Image

One- to 2-year-olds realize that they are separate persons and begin to notice their own bodies. They are fascinated with body function and may also become fascinated with sex and gendered differences. Bodily injury becomes a concern, and cuts and bruises elicit much discussion and often warrant attention (e.g., Band-Aids). Two- to 3-year-olds increasingly notice the inner signals (e.g., the urge to move the bowels, the release and relaxation resulting from going to the bathroom, the discomfort of hunger, the sense of feeling full). Three- to 5-year-olds' curiosity about their bodies continues as they learn to understand and express themselves. Curiosity about their bodies and those of others generates a wealth of innocent questions. They frequently examine and reexamine themselves, sharing worries over a skinned knee, cut, bruise/discoloration, as well as their first loose or lost tooth. Masturbation is a continuation of discovering parts of their body and the pleasurable feelings it elicits and is a very typical behavior during early childhood.

Cognitive Development

Cognitively, *1- to 2-year-olds' thinking* is highly concrete. According to Piaget, 18- to 24-month-old children use mental imagery and infer causality when they can see only the effect. For example, if they see a puddle of milk on the floor, they might say "uh-oh" because they assume it was spilled by someone. By age 3 years, children enter the preoperational stage with preconceptual and intuitive thinking. Primitive conceptualization processes begin with the development of symbolic thinking. For example, a block becomes a car; words become symbols for ideas. They develop symbolic thinking, which manifests through drawing and acting out elaborate play scenarios. However, children at this age generally are unable to take another's perspective, instead continuing to view the world egocentrically. Attending to one characteristic at a time is another feature of 3- to 5-year-old thinking. For example, the child will try to fit a jigsaw puzzle piece using either color or shape, but not both.

Parents may have difficulty understanding a *3- to 5-year-old's* thoughts. On the surface, preoperational thinking has many characteristics of adult thinking, and parents may misinterpret this and believe children are now able to think as adults do. For example, as children develop their use of language and the ability to symbolize concepts mentally, some of their verbalizations appear quite precocious, as evidenced by the child who stares out the window and then states, "Look, Mommy, the trees are saying yes and no." Table 11.3 identifies major characteristics and examples of children's thinking in early childhood.

One of the most sensitive indicators of cognitive development is language development, and many assessment tools plot language ability as a way of measuring cognitive levels. As noted earlier regarding social and emotional development, assessment of any one developmental area is somewhat arbitrary. For example, social development and adaptive skills are major indicators of cognitive abilities. Differentiation of the self from others, with increasing sensitivity to the rules and norms for social interaction and the perspectives and feelings of others, requires ever increasing cognitive capability. In addition, play quality is an indicator of cognitive development as children manipulate and learn to control their environment in safe yet stimulating ways.

Communication

Language and communication development during early childhood is fundamental to social, cognitive, and academic growth.[3] At 15 months, children speak few words but understand many; thus, their *receptive* language is considerably greater than their *expressive* language. During Piaget's preoperational stage, children typically think symbolically, and language becomes more mature. Beginning around 2 years of age, children use words to convey their thoughts and feelings. Rich reciprocal communication may be the most important speech development factor throughout early childhood.[4] It is important to remember that hearing is vital to speech development and should be monitored. While each child develops speech at different rates, Table 11.4 lists common speech and language milestones.

Cognitive development is required for language development because the child must decipher language rules independently, problem solve to understand others' communication, and create symbols so their ideas and emotions that can be understood by others. Literacy programs, including Reach Out and Read, as well as informal efforts through parental reading aloud, foster language growth.[3]

Language development requires mastery of the following:
- Oral fine motor ability to articulate sounds
- Auditory perception to distinguish words and sentences
- Cognitive ability to understand syntax, semantics, and pragmatics
- Psychosocial-cultural environment providing opportunity and exposure to engage in language use

Language milestones occur in two general categories: receptive and expressive. Understanding these milestones includes taking a closer look at the development of speech, including articulation, lexicon, syntax, semantics, and bilingualism.

Articulation

Young children practice articulation skills daily, and by age 2 years sounds are 50% intelligible to a stranger. The intelligibility rate jumps to about 75% by 3 years of age. By age 4 years, speech should be completely intelligible with the exception of particularly difficult consonants; however, these tongue-contact sounds of "t," "d," "k," "g," "y," and "ng" become more intelligible by age 5 years and school entrance. Some sounds, such as the "zh," are not added until the child is older. Children usually progress through a

TABLE 11.3	Preoperational Stage, Characteristics and Examples of 3- to 5-Year-Old Thinking
Characteristic	**Example**
Egocentrism	"It's snowing because I want to play in it"
Unable to see another's viewpoint	If John is holding a doll with its face toward Ann, Ann thinks Trey can also see the doll's face
Incomplete understanding of sequence of time	Knows names of time components (today, tomorrow, yesterday, minutes, days, weeks, etc.), but uses them inconsistently: "I'm not going to take a nap yesterday" Yesterday means any time before now; tomorrow means any time in the future Historical events are conceptualized in terms of the present: "Mommy, do you know George Washington?"
Developing sense of space and position: from experiencing them as a part of their activity, and to understanding them in detail and direction	Frequently used words: *in, on, up, down, at, under*
Evolving ability to categorize or order objects and phenomena	*Early preschooler:* No understanding of concept of class or groups; undisturbed to see a new Santa Claus on every corner *Cluster phenomena:* When asked to sort a series of blocks, the child may cluster a small, medium, and large block as a "baby," "mommy," and "daddy" block By age 4–5 years, child consistently use one or two categories to arrange objects in some order (color, number, form, or size)
Developing ability to establish causality (e.g., realism, animism, artificialism)	*Realism:* Intellectual (dreams are actually real) and nominal (a horse can only be called a horse, not a stallion or filly) *Animism:* 2- to 3-year-olds think objects possess innate person-like qualities that cause results: "The chair made me fall down" *Artificialism:* 3- to 4-year-olds think things are caused by some controlling force that controls the world
Transductive reasoning: from particular to particular	If the child does not like one particular vegetable, they will not like another particular fruit: "I can't eat my banana because my potatoes are burned"
Developing sense of conservation of quantity, weight, mass	By 3 to 5 years, children are usually unable to conceptualize that change in shape does not affect quantity, weight, or mass of an object In general, 50% of 5-year-olds have mastered conservation of quantity, and 50% of 6-year-olds have mastered conservation of weight or mass
Rigidity	Most children in the preoperational stage are very rigid in their thinking

CHAPTER 11 Developmental Management of Early Childhood   125

TABLE 11.4 Language Development of Early Childhood

Age	Receptive Language	Expressive Language
12–18 months	• Follows one-step commands • Each week understands new words • Increased interest in naming pictures • Differentiates environmental sounds • Points to familiar objects and body parts when named • Understands simple questions • Begins to distinguish "you" from "me"	• Uses all vowels, many consonants • Increased use of real words • Jargon is sentence-like • Likes to use negatives (i.e., says "no" often) • Names a few pictures • By 18 months old, articulates 15–20 words and understands 50 • Imitates nonspeech sounds (e.g., cough, tongue click) • Identifies body parts
18–24 months	• Follows two-step commands without visual cues • Vocabulary increases rapidly • Enjoys simple stories and songs • Recognizes pronouns	• Imitates two-word combinations • Dramatic increase in vocabulary, 200+ words • Speech combines jargon and words • Names self • Answers some questions • Begins to combine words • Begins to use pronouns, such as my, me, and mine
24–30 months	• Understands prepositions *in* and *on* • Seems to understand most of what is said • Understands more reasoning ("when you are finished, then …") • Identifies object when given function (wear on feet, cook on)	• Babbles less • Two- to three-word sentences • Repeats two numbers • Increased use of pronouns • Asks simple questions • Joins in songs and nursery rhymes • Can repeat simple phrases and sentences
30–36 months	• Listens to adult conversations • Understands preposition *under* • Can categorize items by function • Begins to recognize colors • Begins to take turns • Understands descriptive concepts, such as "big" and "little"	• Three- to four-word sentences • Answers questions ("wear on feet," "to bed") • Repeats three numbers • Use of plurals • Can help tell simple story
36–42 months	• Understands *fast* • Understands prepositions *behind* and *in front* • Responds to simple three-part commands • Increasing understanding of adjectives and plurals • Understands "just one"	• Understands and answers ("cold," "tired," "hungry") • Mostly three- to four-word sentences • Appropriate use of pronouns • Gives full name when asked • Begins rote counting • Begins to relate events • Lots of questions, some beginning prepositions (on, in)
42–48 months	• Recognizes coins • Begins to understand future and past tenses • Understands number concepts—more than one	• Uses prepositions • Tells stories • Can give function of objects • Repeats longer than six-word sentences • Repeats four numbers • Gives age • Good intelligibility • Can explain what, who, where, and why
48–60 months	• Responds to three-step commands	• Asks "how" questions • Answers verbally to questions, such as "How are you?" • Uses past and future tenses • Can use conjunctions to combine words and phrases

regular sequence of mispronunciations as they learn new articulation skills. At first, they omit the new sound, and they try to substitute a more familiar sound for the new one (e.g., the "w" for "r" substitution, as in "wabbit" for "rabbit"). Distortion is followed by "addition" as the child adds an extra sound (e.g., "gulad" for "glad"). Knowing each of these steps allows the examiner to assure the parent whether the child is developing appropriately or needs

additional monitoring. Fig. 11.1 identifies sounds articulated at specific ages.

Related to specific sounds are pitch, hesitancy and stuttering, and disfluencies. The 2-year-old practices playful changes in pitch and loudness; 3- and 4-year-olds show typical hesitance in speech or stuttering. Stuttering may occur as a child develops language skills. They "stutter" by repeating words, especially those at the

Age of Customary Consonant Production

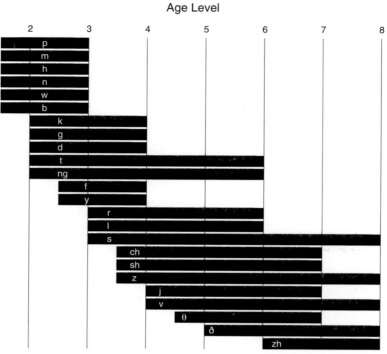

• **Fig. 11.1** Average Age Estimates and Upper Age Limits of Consonant Production. The solid bar corresponding to each sound starts at the median age of customary articulation; it stops at an age level at which 90% of all children are customarily producing the sound. θ, th(umb); δ, th(at). (Data from Sander EK. When are speech sounds learned? *J Speech Hear Disord.* 1972;37(1):55–63; Templin M. *Certain Language Skills in Children: Their Development and Interrelationships.* University of Minnesota Press; 1957; and Wellman B, Case I, Mengert I, and Bradbury D. Speech sounds of young children. *University of Iowa Study, Child Welfare.* 1931;5[2]:1–82.) θ = th(umb), δ = th(at).

start of a sentence, or when excited, such as when they want to convey an important message (e.g., "Mommy, I... Mommy, I... Mommy, I want to tell you I hear the ice cream truck"). This speech variant is notable in that it does not include syllable repetition. While developmental disfluencies are typically temporary, they are concerning if they cause significant stress for the child, last longer than 6 months, occur in children over 5 years old, or if they involve syllable instead of word repetition.

Lexicon

A child's vocabulary, or lexicon, is influenced by many factors, including environment, stimulation, intelligence, multilingualism, culture, and personality. As noted earlier, in early childhood children's receptive language is far greater than their expressive language. The addition of words to their expressive vocabulary comes with ongoing exposure and practice. Female children typically say their first word(s) between 8 and 11 months, and males by about 14 months. Most 2-year-olds have more than 200 words in their vocabulary; with 4- to 5-year-olds adding approximately 50 words a month to their vocabulary. In addition, 5-year-olds can define some words using other words (e.g., "cup" is "you drink with it," or "chair" is "to sit on").

Syntax

Syntax, or grammar, refers to the word structure in sentences or phrases. The ability to construct sentences that convey meaning

is a complex skill, proceeding through several stages, including receptive, holophrastic, and telegraphic speech. Syntax skills begin to develop in late infancy and continue through early childhood. At the beginning of early childhood (12–18 months), children use holophrases, or single words, to express a complete sentence or complex idea. For example, a child will say "milk," to convey "I want a glass of milk." These holophrastic sentences are typically denominative (labeling) or imperative (commanding). Around 18 months, children begin using telegraphic speech, or phrases that have many words omitted and sound like a telegram (e.g., "get milk," "go bye-bye"); by age 2 years, children begin to expand their vocabulary and to form short phrases, involving adjectives, like "my big ball" and "the yummy cookie." Children will mimic phrases and gestures used by caregivers, like "Oh, my goodness." Their sentence structure continues to become more complex as they move from active sentences, to questions, passive/negative constructions, and adding plurals (~3 years) and past tense (~4 years). Three- or four-word sentences should be evident by 3 years; syntax is close to adult style by 5 years. By the end of early childhood, they also use future tense and complete sentences five to six words in length.

Semantics

Semantic development, the understanding that words have specific meaning and the child's use of words to convey specific meaning, is an ongoing process that extends into adulthood. It occurs in stages, moving from global to more specific, and requires interaction through conversation, listening, and reading. Words have both denotative (the specific, concrete referent of the word) and connotative (a broader range of feelings aroused by the word) meanings. Even though children may be adept at using words correctly, they may have only a vague, diffuse connotative understanding of these words. For example, the child who drops a toy and uses an expletive that she heard when her father dropped a dish does not understand the connotative meaning. As a child's overall language progresses from simple to more complex, semantic (meaning) and cognitive understanding evolve.

Bilingualism

Raising children to be bilingual helps preserve the family culture and heritage, and studies suggest that bilingual children have greater mental flexibility and enhanced employment and lifestyle opportunities. Parents who ask PCPs how to best introduce two languages to children are often told to use the "one parent, one language" approach, where parents speak in their native language when conversing with their child. While this approach has some supportive evidence, the number of families who follow this advice has not been documented.

Children who learn two languages at the same time may have smaller vocabularies in each of their languages, but the sum total for both languages should be equal to that of children who are monolingual.[5] For example, children from bilingual homes may show mild delays in initial spoken words and a mixing of words and phrases from the two languages. However, most children are able to proficiently sort one language from the other, although they may "code switch" to the other language for clarity. They become flexible, switching languages depending on the circumstances and the person with whom they are speaking. Some children even translate for others, understanding that not everyone speaks or understands both languages. Ultimately, whether a second, third, or even more languages are learned simultaneously or sequentially, most children have one dominant language. The challenge for PCPs is diagnosing true speech and/or language delays in bilingual children. To date, there is no evidence that links bilingualism to language delay. Instead, speech delays are more typically related to factors including multiple ear infections, hearing loss, anatomic abnormalities, neurologic impairment, injuries, and more. If the PCP suspects a language delay, further exploration is warranted.

Common Developmental Issues in Early Childhood

Sibling Rivalry

Sibling rivalry involves the realization by one child that they must share their parents' attention and affection with their siblings. It can continue in varying degrees over time, but at each age, the child may feel threatened or displaced. Interaction patterns between siblings vary and are affected by individual and family characteristics, such as sex and gender, age, temperament, degree of attachment, nature of family interactions, discipline used in the family, and the child's perception of the equality of a parent's treatment of each child. When siblings argue or fight amongst themselves, parents need to stop the activity, describe the situation, and provide even-handed direction while providing options or compromise actions. Blaming one child, except in a clear-cut instance of misbehavior, is usually nonproductive. Instead, the focus should be on promoting sibling support, loyalty, and friendship. To assess sibling rivalry, ask parents to:

- Describe sibling behaviors of concern: fighting, verbal abuse, bickering.
- Identify precipitating events or situations that elicit negative behaviors.
- Reflect on how sibling rivalry behaviors between siblings were handled in the past and encourage the siblings to resolve the issues between them rather than the parents.
- Describe how they reacted to the behaviors or verbal comments and if and how they have disciplined the child.

The introduction of a new sibling by birth or adoption is a life-changing experience for the older sibling. The developmental stage of the older sibling is an important consideration in helping parents prepare. Some children in early childhood regress when a new infant arrives, while others experience excitement, love, and enhanced self-esteem. Parents must address any aggression expressed by the older child, and at the same time provide love, attention, and opportunities to talk about their feelings. To assess sibling rivalry after the arrival of a new infant, ask the parent whether the older child has:

- Regressive behaviors since the new sibling arrived (e.g., bedwetting, return to the bottle, temper tantrums, separation issues).
- Made negative comments about the new sibling or has demonstrated verbal or physical aggression toward the parents or new sibling.
- Voiced psychosomatic complaints.

The cornerstone of sibling rivalry management is anticipatory guidance and prevention. The PCP needs to prepare parents before the arrival of the new sibling for the possibility of sibling rivalry and guide them in managing this situation.

Before delivery or adoption:

- Explain to parents that at the time of the arrival of the new baby, the other sibling(s) may exhibit regressive behaviors.
- Encourage parents to do the following:
  - Tell the child about the pregnancy or adoption of the new baby, using a time frame and language appropriate to the child's developmental stage.
  - Investigate the possibility of sibling preparation classes for older siblings.
  - Prepare the child for a change in daily routines and change in the amount of time they will have with the parents.
  - Give children realistic expectations of their interactions with the baby.
  - Include an older child in preparations for the new baby and in the excitement of the event (e.g., have the child visit the mother and baby in the hospital if possible).

After the infant or child comes home:

- Encourage parents to consistently spend "alone time" each day with the older sibling.
- Have parents include the older sibling in the care of the new baby as appropriate (e.g., the toddler can help by bringing Mommy a diaper).
- Reinforce the older sibling's efforts to be a "big brother or sister"; praise the child for helping.
- Explain the need for tolerance when a child exhibits regressive behaviors, knowing the behaviors are not permanent.
- Educate parents about teaching children to distinguish between acceptable and unacceptable behaviors as well as accountability for negative behaviors.

As siblings grow, parents should avoid intervening for minor squabbles; rather they should encourage child-centered articulation of more significant arguments and intervene primarily if physical or verbal abuse occurs. Box 11.1 has other strategies to help siblings develop healthy relationships.

Temper Tantrums

All parents struggle when a child has a temper tantrum. These unplanned outbursts of anger and frustration can be physical, verbal, or both; however, they are always disruptive and include unpleasant behavior. One way to approach tantrums is to tell parents their children are acting this way because they need or want something, but cannot express themselves with words, so they get frustrated, then angry, and ultimately lose control of their feelings. Temper tantrums and disruptive behaviors are discussed in in more depth in Chapter 6.

Toilet Training

Toilet training occurs in early childhood. It is typically complete by the time the child is 4 years old, with a variation of up to 1 year for individual children. Children typically first learn nocturnal bowel control, then daytime bowel control, daytime bladder control, and finally nocturnal bladder control. Successful toilet training requires sensitivity, understanding of development, good communication, hope, humor, and patience. In addition to becoming self-sufficient in their toileting, children should also learn that elimination is a natural and necessary process. As self-toileting is mastered, both parents and children should experience pride and satisfaction in having worked together to accomplish an important developmental task.

The PCP plays an important role in providing anticipatory guidance to parents. Introducing the topic of toilet training by the 15- or 18-month visit is common, along with assessing parents' expectations and plans. This provides ample opportunity for discussion and possible development of realistic toileting outcomes. It can also be useful to remind parents that toilet training is not related to or indicative of their child's intelligence.

When parents ask about the best time is to start toilet training, the PCP should emphasize that every child is unique, and readiness cues should ultimately be used to decide when to begin training. Physiologic readiness develops by about 18 months. True voluntary sphincter control is a function of psychological and social development as well, so most children are not ready for independent toilet training until 24 months of age or older. Guidelines for assessing toilet-training readiness include physical, cognitive, interpersonal or psychological, and parental skills (Table 11.5). It is also essential that parents understand and can express to children that the goal is to use the toilet, not to hold in urine or stool. This is an important distinction, as holding of urine and stool can lead to bowel and bladder dysfunction.

PCPs need to understand family practices and be open to developing mutually agreed-upon approaches to toilet training. Many cultures start toilet training earlier or later than what is typically practiced in the United States, and toilet training strategies vary widely. As such, it is critical to understanding parents' expectations for the process. If begun too early, toilet training can be very stressful for both parents and children and can contribute to family dysfunction. Further, starting independent toilet training too early (e.g., before 24 months) may contribute to holding urine and stool, which can lead to daytime wetting, incontinence, and constipation, while starting too late may lead to dysfunctional voiding.[6]

There is little evidence regarding which, if any, toilet training strategy (e.g., child-oriented approach; operant conditioning) is most effective. When children and parents are ready to begin toilet training, several management techniques can be helpful (Box 11.2).In general, it appears that a structured yet flexible approach that is responsive to the child's cues is likely to be most successful. Reassure parents that this needs to be individualized to each parent/child dyad and may be different for siblings.

TABLE 11.5	Toilet Training Readiness Assessment L: Skills and Description
Skill Type	Description
Child's physical skills	Has voluntary sphincter control Stays dry for 2 hours; may wake from naps still dry Is able to sit, walk, and squat Assists in dressing self
Child's cognitive skills	Recognizes urge to urinate or defecate Understands meaning of words used by family in toileting Understands what the toilet is for Understands connection between dry pants and toilet Is able to follow directions Is able to communicate needs
Child's interpersonal skills	Demonstrates desire to please parent Expresses curiosity about use of toilet Expresses desire to be dry and clean
Parental skills	Expresses desire to assist child with training Recognizes child's cues of readiness Has no compelling factor that will interfere with training (e.g., new job, move, newborn, and/or family loss or gain)

• BOX 11.1   Managing Sibling Rivalry

DO
- Allow children to vent negative feelings.
- Encourage children to develop solutions for problems with siblings.
- Anticipate problem situations.
- Foster individuality in each child.
- Spend time with children individually.
- Compliment children when they are playing together well.
- Tell children about the conflict you had with your siblings when you were a child.
- Define acceptable and unacceptable behaviors for sibling interactions.

DO NOT
- Take sides.
- Serve as a referee.
- Foster rivalry by comparing siblings or their accomplishments.
- Use derogatory names.
- Permit physical or verbal abuse between siblings.

Management of Toilet Training

- Keep child as clean and dry as possible:
  - Change diapers frequently.
  - Use training pants or underwear when child stays dry for several hours during the day; use diaper at night.
- Talk to child about toilet training:
  - Praise child for asking to have diaper changed.
  - Explain connection between being clean and dry and using toilet.
  - Emphasize that the goal is to eliminate in the toilet, not to hold to stay clean and dry.
  - Provide opportunity for child to use toilet, especially before going out to play, going on a trip, before naps, and at bedtime; set an example with adult behavior.
  - Do not ask child if they need to go, rather set up a time schedule of every 1.5 hours for voiding, and state matter-of-factly it is time to go.
- Teach child how to use toilet:
  - Allow child to observe while parents or older siblings use toilet.
  - Demonstrate how to sit on toilet with feet supported and knees spread with forward pelvic tilt, use toilet paper, flush, and wash hands.
- Provide practice time for child:
  - Provide a potty chair or portable toilet seat.
  - Allow child to sit on potty chair with clothes or diaper on.
  - Encourage child to use potty chair while parent uses regular toilet.
  - Have child sit on potty chair without diapers for 5–10 min at a time.
  - Practice at times the child usually urinates or defecates.
- Provide a comfortable, safe-feeling environment:
  - Seat child facing backward on a regular toilet or provide a footstool to rest the feet on with knees wide and forward pelvic tilt.
  - Never flush the toilet when child is sitting on it. Use sticky notes to stop automatic flush on public toilets.
  - Stay with child for safety reasons.
- Give consistent, positive feedback:
  - Praise child for trying and for success.
  - Be understanding of child's refusal to use toilet.
  - Never demand performance.
  - Never make child sit on toilet if child resists.
  - Ignore or minimize undesired behavior.
  - Never scold or punish if a child wets or soils.
  - Use star chart or other reward for success or effort; consider having the reward the child is working toward in the bathroom so that the job and reward are clearly connected for the child.
  - Do not praise excessively.

Parents can become extremely frustrated if their expectations do not match the abilities and performance of their children, and child abuse related to toilet training may occur. PCPs play a crucial role in making the experience a positive one and preventing abuse by giving parents information about child development, techniques for managing the training process, and support and encouragement for their efforts. This includes proactively doing follow-up with families who express frustration or appear to be having difficulty with the toilet training process.

If children resist training, the effort should be put on hold for a few weeks before trying again. It is important to stress to parents that none of these "holds" should be viewed as a failure for either parent or child. If a child is toilet trained for a brief period and suddenly regresses to wetting and soiling consistently, they should be placed back in diapers and the process begun again within a few weeks. It is extremely important that parents and children do not become engaged in a battle for control over toilet training. The PCP should emphasize to parents that they should never ask the child, "Do you need to go potty, pee?" and so on. The answer will always be "No," and thus an immediate battle ensues that is not even about the actual toileting. It is important to remember that it is the child's responsibility to control their bowel and urinary function, and toilet training is only one of the many tasks children master on their way to independence. Parents have the responsibility to assist in the process by providing a positive environment and opportunities, teaching the techniques, and setting a positive example.

Childcare and Preschool

Either or both parents often have to return to work during the first few months or years of their child's life. In 2019, 59% of children under 5 years old attended at least one weekly nonparental care arrangement with a reported 62% attending a daycare center, preschool, or prekindergarten setting.[7] In 2021, 65.6% of mothers with children younger than 6 years were employed, and 75.5% of women with children between 6 and 17 years old were employed.[8]

Childcare issues can be a source of significant parental concern. Parents are challenged with evaluating and selecting a qualified childcare provider who provides a safe, nurturing, and developmentally appropriate setting. The individual needs of the child together with parental needs for work coverage and flexibility must be matched with the philosophy and constraints of the childcare setting. The PCP is often called on to advise parents about how to select a suitable provider (Box 11.3).

Entering preschool can be stressful for both the children attending the school and their families. Some children have difficulty adapting to the more structured school environment, whereas others are comfortable with limits and rules. Parents may find their child compared with other children, and a child with developmental delays (e.g., speech, motor, physical) may be singled out as different, not fitting in, or as having a behavior problem. Preschool and kindergarten were originally intended to help children learn separation, sharing, listening, paying attention, and simple social skills. Today, kindergarten students are often expected to show preacademic skills, such as writing, counting, and letter and word recognition, in addition to the preschool social skills of paying attention and sitting still. In making their preschool selection, the PCP can remind parents that a play-based learning curriculum is the most comfortable way for children to learn during early childhood.

When selecting a preschool, parents should also consider their children's characteristics, including their:
- Social skills (e.g., ability to separate from parent for several hours)
- Language skills, both expressive and receptive
- Physical size
- Energy level (e.g., ability to actively participate)
- Neurologic maturation required for fine and gross motor activities (e.g., writing, cutting, coloring, climbing, running, walking)
- Neurologic maturation of sensory and cognitive function (e.g., visuospatial perception, tactile maturation, auditory processing, attending skills, memory)

Health Supervision and Surveillance

Health Visits

Developmental assessment is an essential part of each health supervision encounter. Early identification of developmental and behavioral problems is key to providing early intervention. The process begins by establishing rapport with the parents, reviewing parent report tools, and attending to their concerns. Collect data through interviews with parents/caregivers, standardized screening tools, observation of the interactions between the child and parent(s), physical examination, and laboratory or other diagnostic measures. If there are concerns about the child's development or if a child is identified through screening as having a potential problem, a thorough diagnostic assessment is required. Referral to an appropriate specialist should be made to determine the degree of developmental delay and to identify intervention strategies.

Screening

Children require screening for delays in the progression of gross and fine motor skills, communication and language, problem solving, and social, emotional, and cognitive development. Screenings can be conducted at health supervision or at visits for episodic illnesses. Validated screening tools provide quick, inexpensive methods of identifying potential delays or concerns. These tools are generally appropriate for all children, although culture and experience can affect outcomes. Parents can complete a screening tool in the waiting room, or the PCP can directly ask them questions. PCPs should ensure they understand the parents' responses and clarify any concerns. Table 11.6 lists a variety of developmental screening tools. Tables 11.7–11.10 list questions and rationales that PCPs can use to assess behaviors.

Physical Development

Children should have annual anthropometric measurements. They should also have blood pressure readings beginning at age 3 years, or earlier for at-risk children. Hearing screening should continue through the early childhood period, especially if the child has frequent ear infections or language issues. Age-appropriate visual acuity measurement is recommended starting at 3 years of age.[3] Dental screening is ongoing (See Chapter 20).

Motor Skills Development

During early childhood, children develop and refine their motor skills, driven by curiosity, a desire for independence, and endless energy. Asking parents about their child's development is an important part of surveillance. Gross and fine motor skills are best assessed using standardized, validated screening tools, such as the Ages and Stages Questionnaire-3 (ASQ-3). Fine motor skills are evaluated by assessing finger, hand, and oral movements, while gross motor skills are evaluated by assessing large muscle abilities, such as the ability to sit, crawl, walk, run, hop, skip, and climb. The quality of the child's movements during these activities is important to note as well.

Social and Emotional Development

Assessment of social and emotional development includes exploring the child's role in the family, success making friends and interacting with peers, self-esteem, and feelings of contentment and security. The social-emotional section of the ASQ-3 assesses these behaviors, but a more comprehensive screening can be done by using the Ages and Stages Questionnaire: Social-Emotional-2 (ASQ: SE-2) for children 3 months to 5 years-old. The Pediatric Symptom Checklist (PSC) is another validated screening tool that can be used beginning at age 4 years to screen for cognitive, emotional, and behavioral concerns (see Chapter 6).

Cognitive and Intellectual Development

As children's thinking moves into the preconceptual stages, cognitive development is increasingly expressed through symbol systems and language. Children enjoy stories, make believe, and they become masters at games involving pretending and fantasy.

Communication and Language Development

Communication is a vital part of being a happy, functioning human being. A careful history of the child's abilities and learning patterns (e.g., when did the child first articulate words?) provides much of the essential information. Listening to children and talking with their parents are essential, but the PCP should remember that parents may not be fully attuned to speech problems because they are accustomed to hearing their child's speech. Physical examination helps to determine if physical structures necessary for speech are intact (e.g., a cleft uvula may indicate an occult cleft palate that could interfere with the child's ability to shape words). See Table 11.11 for speech and language evaluation tools for use in primary care. Language screening needs to evaluate expressive and receptive language skills. Because language and cognitive skills are intricately interwoven, most intelligence tests have language sections that are also useful. Expressive language screening emphasizes articulation and vocabulary. Receptive language screening focuses on comprehension, repetition, and follow-up after spoken language (e.g., child's ability to follow directions).

Anticipatory Guidance for Early Childhood

Anticipatory guidance during early childhood focuses on facilitating children's transition from being highly dependent to establishing a sense of autonomy with an evolving understanding of the self as a separate, creative, and powerful being. During

TABLE 11.6 Screening Tools During Early Childhood	
Screening Tool/Website	**Use**
Ages and Stages Questionnaires, 3e (ASQ-3) www.brookespublishing.com	• Screening and surveillance of five key developmental areas: communication, gross motor, fine motor, problem solving, and personal-social • For use with 1-month-olds to 5.5-year-olds • Parents report on 30 items plus overall concerns • Written at the 4th- to 6th-grade level; manual includes activity handouts for parents • Available in English, Spanish, and French
Ages and Stages Questionnaire: Social-Emotional, 2e (ASQ: SE-2) www.brookespublishing.com	• Screening and surveillance of social-emotional development: self-regulation, compliance, social-communication, adaptive functioning, autonomy, affect, and interaction with people • Parents report on 32 items • For use with 1- to 72-month-olds • Takes 10–15 minutes or less to administer • Available in English and Spanish
Battelle Developmental Inventory, 2e (BDI-2) www.riversidepublishing.com/products/bdi2/	• Screening for early childhood developmental milestones • Measures personal-social, adaptive, motor, communication, and cognitive abilities • Parents report on 100 items • For use from birth to 8 years old • Takes 10–30 minutes; complete test 1–2 hours
Child Development Inventory (CDI) https://childdevelopmentreview.com/	• Screening for motor, social skills, expressive language, language comprehension, self-help, letters, and numbers • Parents report on 300 items • For use with 15-month-olds to 6-year-olds • Takes 30-40 minutes to administer • Measures fine and gross motor skills
Parents' Evaluation of Developmental Status (PEDS test) www.pedstest.com	• Screening/surveillance of development, behavior, social-emotional, mental health, and autism • Parents complete 10 questions • For use from birth to 8 years old • Test takes 2 minutes to administer • Available in English, Spanish, Vietnamese, and many other languages
Pediatric Symptom Checklist (PSC) www.massgeneral.org/psychiatry/services/psc_forms.aspx	• Psychosocial screen designed to recognize cognitive, emotional, and behavioral problems • Parents complete 35 items • For use with 4- to 11-year-olds • Test takes 5–10 minutes to complete • Available in English and dozens of other languages
Modified Checklist for Autism in Toddlers–Revised; in 1- to 2-year-old children, Revised with Follow-Up (M-CHAT-R/F) (2013) https://mchatscreen.com/	• Screening for autism risk • Parents complete 20 items • For use from 16–30 months • Takes 5 minutes to complete • Available in multiple languages
Survey of Wellbeing of Young Children (SWYC) https://www.floatinghospital.org/The-Survey-of-Wellbeing-of-Young-Children/Overview.aspx	• Screening for developmental milestones, behavioral/emotional development, and family risk factors • For use from 2–60 months • Takes 15 minutes to complete

this process, parents continue to learn new communication and interaction skills with their children. Although the early childhood years can be frustrating at times, the ultimate outcome of good communication and relationships that support the potential of both child and parent is worth the effort. According to the American Academy of Pediatrics (AAP) recommendations for preventive pediatric health care and the Bright Futures Guidelines, PCPs should offer anticipatory guidance in the following areas: family support, child development, mental health, healthy weight, nutrition, physical activity, oral health, healthy sexual

TABLE 11.7   Surveillance of Physical Development and Motor Skills: Questions and Rationale

Question	Rationale
Tell me about your child's health	Invites discussion of somatic issues and complaints
Do you have any concerns about your child's development?	Assesses parental concerns and tailoring of next steps
Does your child appear to be developing similar to other children of the same age?	Assesses parent perceptions of physical development; developmental milestones
Has illness affected your child's daily activities?	Assesses possible chronic medical problem and effects on development
Tell me about your child's daily habits: elimination, toilet training, sleeping, eating	Assesses parent understanding of readiness, child's cues, changing behaviors, and current status
How does your child move from place to place?	Assesses gross motor skills (e.g., walks, climbs, runs, pedals tricycle), and activity level
How does your child feed himself or herself (e.g., cup, bottle, utensils)?	Assesses fine motor skills
Tell me about your child's play activities	Assesses gross and fine motor skills

TABLE 11.8   Surveillance of Communication and Speech Development: Questions and Rationale

Question	Rationale
Do you have any concerns about your child's speech?	Assesses parent/caregiver concerns and allows tailoring of assessment to identify them
How does your child communicate needs and desires?	Assesses verbal and nonverbal communication strategies, vocabulary, and expressive language
How much do you think your child understands?	Evaluates cognitive level and receptive language
How does your child respond to one-step commands? To two- or three-step commands?	Evaluates receptive language; evaluates short-term memory and auditory sequencing
Does your child use plurals, pronouns, phrases, and sentences?	Indicates increased understanding of more complex structures
How well can you understand your child's speech? How well can others?	Indicates increased articulation ability

TABLE 11.9   Surveillance of Social and Emotional Development: Questions and Rationale

Question	Rationale
Do you have any concerns about how your child gets along with others? Do you have any concerns about your child's emotions?	Allows tailoring of assessment to identify them
Is your child able to feed himself/herself, dress, and take care of their own toileting?	Assesses adaptive skills, comfort with own abilities
How does your child behave with family members they live with? How do they behave with other family members?	Assesses child's development of roles within the family system; attachment should be evident
How do you guide or discipline your child without always saying "no"?	Evaluates adaptability, creativity, repertoire of parent's skills in response to child's behaviors
How does your child respond when you set limits?	Assesses child's understanding of limits of appropriate behavior, social rules, and self-control
How does your child react to strangers or new situations?	Evaluates child's ability to deal with increasingly complex social situations
Tell me about any tantrums your child has What causes them? How do they behave? How do you respond?	Evaluates responses to stress, development of independence, and social control
What does your child do for play?	Indicates social and emotional wellbeing
How does your child behave around other children?	Considers social development with peers and development of appropriate play
What is your child's best friend's name? Do they have shared activities with peers?	Indicates child is developing a social circle and increasing opportunities for practicing new social skills
Does your child seem to understand others' feelings?	Assesses empathy
Is your child afraid of anything in particular? How do you handle that fear?	Evaluates parent's responses to child's emotional stresses and understanding of child's view and feelings
Does your child have imaginary friends? Does she or he have a fantasy play time?	Allows child to explore emotions and developing roles in a safe way

Sleep-Wake Patterns/Regulation

- Discuss the need to assist children to transition from one state to another. Consistent sleep and naptime schedules are essential. Use of a comfort or transitional object (e.g., teddy bear) and establishing a bedtime ritual help.
- Explain how children process information, gain control, and how they can be overwhelmed if they have too much stimulation.

development and sexuality, safety and injury prevention, and social determinants of health. They should also provide education, counseling, and support services.[3] Specific topics are discussed below in more detail.

TABLE 11.10	Surveillance of Cognitive Development: Questions and Rationale	
Questions	**Rationale for Questions**	
1- to 3-year-olds		
Tell me about a typical day. What sorts of things does your child do? With whom does she or he play? (Ask parent/caregiver)	Assesses complexity of manipulation of objects, parallel and cooperative play, and role-playing	
Can your child follow simple instructions? (Ask parent/caregiver)	Assesses ability to retain and process instructions and respond to input	
Does your child speak clearly? How much do you understand when your child speaks to you? Can your child understand what you say to him or her? (Ask parent/caregiver)	Assesses progress in decoding, encoding, and using a language system effectively	
How does your child behave with family members and other children? (Ask parent/caregiver)	Indicates understanding of social systems and norms	
What is your name? Are you a boy or girl? How old are you? (Ask child)	Should know these facts by 3 years of age	
4- to 5-year-olds		
Ask child general information questions (e.g., colors, numbering, objects)	Assesses general fund of knowledge	
Ask child what makes the sun come up	Illustrates child's belief about causality	
Ask child about concepts of time (e.g., What time do you have lunch? What time do you go to bed?)	Assesses understanding of a relatively sophisticated concept	
Ask child about spontaneous play (e.g., with puppets or dolls), imaginative use of play materials (e.g., clay, crayons, other toys)	Assesses imagination and magical thinking	
Ask child to draw a person	50% of 4-year-olds draw a three-part person; by 5 years old, child can draw an eight-part person	
How does the child behave in preschool or childcare setting? (Ask parent/caregiver)	Assesses language, social, and play development in relation to peers in a setting where expectations differ from those at home	

- Explain that some children may have sensory integration issues that require environmental structuring and modulation.
- Discuss how to help children identify and name their feelings. This ability will help them organize and integrate the sensations they experience and respond appropriately.
- Encourage parents to provide opportunities for children to have some control and choice in daily activities (e.g., select the

story to be read at bedtime) while maintaining important rituals.
- Discuss common sleep-related issues for this age group, including sleep resistance, bruxism, nightmares, and somnambulism (see Chapter 16).
- Encourage parents to offer naps and opportunities for rest, but not to force them.
- Encourage parents to create consistent and comforting sleep routines for the child, provide positive reinforcement of healthy sleep behavior, and use firm, loving, and consistent discipline when dealing with sleep refusal and other behavioral sleep problems.

Strength and Coordination

- Encourage parents to provide a wide range of safe play opportunities that use both fine and gross motor skills.
- Urge parents to allow children to take the lead during play and to follow and expand on whatever the child is interested in.
- Encourage parents to provide a variety of play activities that expose children to nature:
  - Take children to parks or playgrounds to run, throw balls, swing, and slide.
  - Encourage play with natural materials (e.g., water, sand, grass, leaves).
- Provide age-appropriate play materials: stickers, pencils, crayons, paper, paints, utensils, blocks, cardboard boxes, and building toys.
- Explain how parents can incorporate motor skills practice as part of daily routines (e.g., have child help pour the milk, squeeze the toothpaste, do own buttons, snaps, zippers).
- Emphasize the need for constant adult supervision of children's activities.
- Discuss how parents can make the environment safer for their child: securing doors and using window guards, removing toxic substances and dangerous objects, and providing toys that are developmentally appropriate and safely constructed.
- Reinforce teaching about car seat use and understanding when to transition booster seats as the child grows. Explain to parents the importance of modeling for the child by using their own seat restraint.
- Encourage bicycle helmet use with all riding toys (e.g., scooters, tricycles, bicycles).

Nutrition, Self-Care, and Safety

- Provide parents with information about age-appropriate nutrition(see Chapter 14). Three meals and two nutritious snacks per day are encouraged throughout early childhood.
- Discuss it is the parents' job to provide nutritious foods and the child's job to decide how much they will eat. Starting with small portions of different foods will help the child choose a variety of foods. Discourage parents from making separate meals for their children.
- Young children may go on "food jags," refusing some foods or requesting the same food day after day. Parents need to make sure food that is being eaten is nutritious.
- Explain how changes in eating habits can be due to developmental changes (e.g., child has a decrease in appetite, is easily distracted, demonstrates more curiosity about what is going on around her than in eating, is more interested in using gross motor skills than in sitting still).
- Explain the nonnutritive value of food and eating (e.g., water, fiber, flavor, aroma)

TABLE 11.11 Speech and Language Evaluation Tools

Evaluation Tool	Characteristics	Source
The Capute Scales: Cognitive Adaptive Test and Clinical Linguistic and Auditory Milestone Scale (CAT/CLAMS)	• Use from birth–36 months • Interview • Tests language and problem-solving skills to help clearly identify between the two	https://brookespublishing.com/product/the-capute-scales/
Clinical Evaluation of Language Fundamentals—Preschool (CELF-P)	• Use from 3–6 years • Assesses receptive and expressive language	www.pearsonclinical.com/language/products/100000316/celf-preschool-2-celf-preschool-2.html
Early Language Milestone Scale (ELM Scale-2)	• Use from birth to 36 months • Tests visual and auditory receptive, and auditory expressive abilities History, testing, and observation completed in 1–10 minutes	https://www.proedinc.com/Products/6580/elm-scale2-early-language-milestone-scale.aspx
Goldman-Fristoe Test of Articulation	• Use from 2–22 years old • Assesses articulation skills	pearsonassessments.com
Peabody Picture Vocabulary Test	• Use from 2.5–90+ years old • Screens for receptive vocabulary	pearsonassessments.com
Receptive-Expressive Emergent Language Test, 4e (REEL 4)	• Use from birth to 36 months • Interview or direct observation of expressive and receptive language	pearsonclinical.ca

- Encourage self-feeding to help the child gain new skills (e.g., finger foods stimulate fine motor and cognitive development, in addition to fostering a child's sense of control and independence; eating together as a family can strengthen relationships and develop social skills).
- Encourage parents to structure mealtimes that are pleasant and interactive; this may mean offering foods that can be eaten in short periods of sitting. Avoid making meals a power struggle.
- Discuss plans for weaning (if the child has not already weaned).
- Explain the importance of the child gaining mastery of self-care (e.g., toileting, bathing, dressing, eating) and the role the parent plays as a teacher and role model. Assist parents to cope with the frustration or tensions generated by children wanting to "do it myself." Ask parents how they handle these situations.
- Encourage children to help with their self-care. They can brush their teeth and hair and clean up in the bath, and the parents can follow up to ensure that they did a sufficient job.
- Remind parents that injury is a leading cause of early childhood morbidity and mortality; continued and updated childproofing is needed, and choking foods should be avoided (see Chapter 21).
- Parents should safety-proof all environments their children spend time in. They also need to be reminded that safety-proofing alone is not enough; children need to have adult supervision at all times in this age group.

Behavioral, Social, and Emotional Growth

Socio-emotional growth, development, and behavioral consequences are areas in which parents often need anticipatory guidance and support. In early childhood, children master multiple social tasks, as well as learning how to identify, control, and manage their feelings and emotions around anger, joy, love, and frustration. They learn about making and keeping friends, sharing, cooperative play, and living within a family. They also learn to handle separation from parents, home,

and neighborhood. To help families with this process, PCPs should:
- Emphasize the role of parents as guides of their child's social and emotional growth.
- Encourage parents to give their children opportunities to expand social skills and form important attachments outside the immediate family by:
  - Providing toys and other items that children can use creatively.
  - Allowing children to explore, guiding them to activities that are fun and stimulate their curiosity.
  - Structuring time for children to play in natural settings. Access to green space enhances physical, mental, and emotional health of children.[9]
  - Allowing children to make choices when possible. Do not give children a choice when there really is none (e.g., "Do you want to go to bed?"). Instead, use choices that allow the child to have a say and yet still get toward the final objective (e.g., "Do you want to put your pants or shirt on first? Do you want to take the bunny or the bear with you during your nap?").
  - Discussing similarities and differences among people openly and positively.
  - Helping children identify, name, and express feelings, both positive and negative.
  - Teaching children how to manage anger and resolve conflicts without aggressive behavior or violence.
  - Limiting screen time, while being present to discuss television programs and movies they watch, especially when they need help distinguishing fantasy from reality.
  - Taking children on trips to places of interest in the community.
  - Arranging play times with other children; encourage cooperative play (e.g., tag, hide-and-seek, board games).
  - Reinforcing positive behavior ("catch the child being good").

- Making clear, consistent, and achievable expectations for the child.
- Differentiate discipline and teaching from punishment (see Chapter 6).
- Help parents resolve different expectations and present a united front.
- Provide information related to child development and what parents can expect their child to be able to do. For example, the CDC has development handouts available online at https://www.cdc.gov/ncbddd/childdevelopment/index.html.
- Recommend evidence-based parenting resources that provide information on developmental milestones, anticipated changes, and parenting strategies.
- Encourage parents to show affection in the family.
- Explain that myths or fables can be important ways of teaching children abstract concepts (e.g., love, sharing, giving).
- To provide children a feeling of safety and security, parents should:
  - Encourage comfort or transitional objects to allay fears (e.g., blanket).
  - Consider providing a nightlight.
  - Respond to children's nightmares or fears when they occur. Offer ongoing reassurance.
  - Explain about "good" and "bad" touch.
  - Reinforce that the child can always come to the parent for comfort (e.g., "time-in")

Cognitive and Environmental Stimulation

- Explain to parents that children in early childhood use concrete and preoperational thinking. As a result, parents need to be ready to explain things over and over patiently. Children may use words to convey thoughts and feelings, but many responses are repetitive, and trial-and-error problem solving is usually crude. They frequently attend to only one aspect of a problem, giving partial answers.
- Emphasize that parents should avoid putting their own meaning on the child's behavior or statements. For example, the child's statement, "What if you bought a new house and I had allergies to something in the house? I guess you'd have to get rid of me," should not be interpreted to mean the parents have somehow failed to show the child how much they love him or her. Rather the child may be exploring the concepts of place, ownership, belonging, size, or importance. An appropriate response from the parent might be, "No, we'd probably have to get a new house or take out whatever is making you sick. Even if we just bought it, you are more important than any house, and we wouldn't want to lose you."
- Reassure parents that "Why?" will not continue to be the child's most frequent question. Children in early childhood actively explore meaning in their world and learn that asking "Why?" brings them more information—and attention. As parents provide answers, children will show threads of symbolic and advancing thought processes.

Communication and Language

Children learn and refine communication and language skills best through their interactions with others. When adults listen, talk interactively, and read to children, children's language blossoms. Encourage parents to stimulate their child's language skills by:
- Reading to children daily, using short, simple stories or picture books.

- Modeling appropriate language.
- Explaining in clear, simple language what is happening around the child; this helps increase vocabulary and the child's understanding of the world. Quality reciprocal speech is the best way to help children learn to express themselves.[4]
- Listening with care and responding actively to the child.
- Providing opportunities to interact verbally with other children and adults.
- Keeping screen time to a minimum. Children younger than age 2 years should avoid all screens. After age 2, limit television viewing, smartphone, tablet, and videos to less than 1 hour of developmentally appropriate programs per day. Children should not have screens in their bedrooms.
- Watching programs with children and talking about what is happening.[3]

PCPs should emphasize the following anticipatory guidance:
- Explain that children need constant reinforcement of their speech and language efforts, but remind them that nonverbal language, especially touch, is equally important.
- Give parents an opportunity to share their expectations for their child; discourage parental pressure on the child to perform (e.g., use of flash cards, requirement that child articulate sounds correctly), and point out that daily activities (e.g., meal preparation) provide a wealth of opportunities to practice language skills.
- Reassure parents that early language errors usually disappear as children grow.
- Inform parents that children develop receptive language skills first, then expressive. Children may not fully understand the meaning of what they say, especially connotative meaning (e.g., a child may innocently ask a stranger about their private body parts). Parents should explain clearly, simply, and unemotionally which words are appropriate and in which settings.

Red Flags

Although there is a wide range of typical development, the PCP needs to be alert to red flags—signs of delayed or abnormal development. In addition to obvious abnormalities, minor problems that are left untreated can develop into major concerns; minor signs and symptoms that persist can indicate a more serious underlying problem, or a major problem can occur as a one-time event (e.g., a child who sets a fire). Some children and families are at high risk and need careful monitoring and guidance to detect problems at an early stage or to prevent their occurrence (e.g., families with a history of violence, families with chronic medical or mental health problems,). These warning signs, or red flags, can be found in Table 11.12. Each red flag warrants follow up. Immediate referral is required for children who stop eating, demonstrate cruelty to animals or other people, are self-harmful, start fires, or talk of harming themselves, their peers, or others.

Physical

Children should be monitored for physical growth milestones. Further investigation and referral may be appropriate when children deviate from an established growth pattern or percentile, whether it is an increase or decrease. Some children have overt symptoms—they stop eating, complain of tiredness, are not as active as usual, or the parents state that the child regressed. Growth pattern changes always warrant further investigation.

Cognitive

Cognitive delays are difficult to recognize and categorize. Screening tools help to determine variances from typical development. Some tools rate child development based on a standardized score or against standardized criteria (e.g., word definition). For example, children with scores below 85 on intelligence scales predictably have difficulty in school. Significant discrepancies between test scores taken over time also suggest problems. The causes must be carefully assessed as some children may have a neurologic limitation, whereas others may be delayed because of material or environmental deprivation; however, identifying the cause is necessary to plan effective interventions. When delays are suspected, prompt referral to developmental specialists or early

TABLE 11.12 **Red Flags in Early Childhood**

Age	Growth, Rhythmicity, Sleep, and Temperament	Psychosocial and Emotional Skills	Cognitive Abilities	Gross Motor, Language, and Hearing	Fine Motor, Feeding, and Self-Care	Strength and Coordination
12 months		No smiles or joyful expressions		No babbling Does not recognize own name when called	Does not point or use sounds to get desired object; may just cry	
15 months	Difficulty with transitions, including bedtime Parents express concern about temperament or control issues	Problems with attachment to caregiver(s)	No object permanence	No words or gestures Only single words by 16 months Lack of consonant production, uses mostly vowel sounds Consistent and frequent omission of initial consonants Does not imitate words	No self-feeding	No attempts to walk
18 months	Poor sleep schedule Problems with control and behavior	Does not pull person to show something	Primary play: mouthing of toys/no finger exploration of objects Lack of imitation Not using toys as they were intended	Unable to follow simple directions (e.g., "no," "jump") Excessive, indiscriminate, irrelevant verbalizing	Does not try to scribble spontaneously Unable to use spoon	Not yet walking or frequent falls
24 months	Falling off growth curve Poor sleep schedule Awakens at night; unable to put self back to sleep	Displays destructive behaviors Always clings to parent	Absent symbolic play No evidence of parallel or pretend play	No meaningful 2-word phrases Use of noncommunicative speech (echolalia, rote phrases) Unable to identify 5 pictures Unable to name body parts No jargon History of greater than 10 episodes of otitis media	Unable to stack 4–5 blocks Still eating pureed foods Unable to imitate scribbles on paper Unable to dump pellet from bottle	Unable to walk downstairs holding a rail Persistent waddle walk Persistent toe walking
30 months	Resistance to regular bedtime Beginning behavior issues	Biting, hitting playmates, parents Not able to play with others	Cannot follow 2-step commands	Cannot name self Does not use pronouns	Unable to feed self Unable to build a tower of six blocks Unable to copy a circle shape Unable to imitate vertical stroke	Unable to jump in place Unable to kick ball on request

TABLE 11.12	Red Flags in Early Childhood—cont'd					
Age	Growth, Rhythmicity, Sleep, and Temperament	Psychosocial and Emotional Skills	Cognitive Abilities	Gross Motor, Language, and Hearing	Fine Motor, Feeding, and Self-Care	Strength and Coordination
36 months	Problems with toilet training Unable to calm self	Not able to dress self Does not understand taking turns	No expanded pretend play Unable to name colors or identify common objects Does not understand same/ different	Unable to give full name Unable to match two colors Does not use plurals Does not know 2 or 3 prepositions Unable to tell/recall a story Unclear consonants Unintelligible speech Unable to speak in sentences	Unable to build a tower of 10 blocks Holds crayon with fist Unable to draw circle	Unable to balance on one foot for 1 s Toeing-in causes tripping with running
48 months	No bedtime ritual Behavior concerns: Withdrawn or acting out Stool holding Problems with toilet training	Unable to play games, follow rules Unable to follow limits or rules at home (e.g., put toys away) Cruelty to animals, friends Interest in fires, fire starting Persistent fears or severe shyness Inability to separate from parent	Unable to count 3 objects Unable to recall 4 numbers Unable to identify what to do with danger, fire, and a stranger Consistent poor judgment	Difficulty understanding language Problems understanding prepositions Limited vocabulary Unclear speech	Lack of self-care skills: dressing feeding, Unable to button clothes Unable to copy square	Unable to balance on one foot for 4 s Unable to alternate steps when climbing stairs
60 months	Sleep problems Concerns with night terrors Hair pulling: scalp or eyelashes	Difficulty making/ keeping friends; no friends Difficulty understanding sharing, school rules, organization of daily activities Cruelty to animals/ others Interest in fires/fire starting Bullying or being bullied Prolonged fighting, hitting, hurting Withdrawal, sadness Extreme rituals	Unable to count to 10 Unable to identify colors Unable to follow 3-step commands	Speech pattern not 100% understandable Cannot identify a penny, nickel, or dime Abnormal rate or rhythm of speech	Unable to copy triangle Unable to draw a person with a body	Difficulty hopping, jumping

childhood intervention programs for more detailed assessment and intervention is essential.

Language

Language delays or disorders can affect other areas of development, especially cognitive, behavioral, social, and emotional development. Because language development is the best indicator of cognitive development, language delays may indicate serious issues requiring intervention. Children with language delays can experience problems in receptive or expressive language. They may start talking late, talk very little, or have prolonged stages of stuttering, distortion, and substitution.

Cognitive, familial, environmental, physical, psychological, or cultural factors can lead to language delays. Language delays or disorders may also occur if the child does not hear, is not immersed in a language-rich environment, or has a disorder, such as severe deprivation or autism. Speech disorders (i.e., problems producing sounds) are associated with specific physical problems (e.g., cleft lip, cleft palate, cerebral palsy, hearing impairments), but they can also be idiopathic.

Language evaluation involves assessment of the child's physical, cognitive, social, emotional, and perceptual abilities. Evaluation should include both expressive and receptive language. The inability to use the symbols of language may be characterized by:
- Improper use of words and their meanings
- Inappropriate grammatical patterns
- Improper use of speech sounds

Speech disorders involve problems producing correct speech sounds and may be characterized by difficulty:
- Producing speech sounds (articulation)
- Maintaining speech rhythm (fluent speech)
- Controlling vocal production (voice)

Management of children with language disorders requires a clear understanding of the nature of the problem. Referral to a specialist (e.g., pediatric speech pathologist) to make that determination is often the first step. Deficits identified in Table 11.11 are cause for referral for additional testing. Other criteria that warrant referral include:
- Unusual "connected" speech confusion, reversals, or telescoping.
- A loss of previously acquired language skills.
- The child stops talking.
- The child reacts to their own speech with embarrassment or withdrawal.
- The child's voice is monotone, extremely loud, largely inaudible, or of poor quality.
- Pitch is not appropriate to the child's age and sex.
- Hypernasality or lack of nasal resonance occurs.

Additional Resources

AAP parenting website: https://healthychildren.org/English/Pages/default.aspx.
Bright Futures: https://www.brightfutures.org/wellchildcare/toolkit/family.html.

CDC Essentials for Parenting Toddlers and Preschoolers: https://www.cdc.gov/parents/essentials/toddlersandpreschoolers/index.html.
CDC Learn the Signs, Act Early: https://www.cdc.gov/ncbddd/actearly/index.html.
CDC information for parents of infants and toddlers (ages 0–3): https://www.cdc.gov/parents/infants/index.html.
CDC information for parents of children (ages 4–11): https://www.cdc.gov/parents/children/index.html.
Personal Safety for Children, A Guide for Parents: https://www.ncjrs.gov/html/ojjdp/psc_english_02/index.html.
Zero to Three: https://www.zerotothree.org.

References

1. Centers for Disease Control and Prevention. Risk and Protective Factors. https://cdc.gov/violenceprevention/aces/riskprotectivefactors.html.
2. Goddard A. Adverse childhood experiences and trauma-informed care. *J Pediatr Health Care*. 2021;35(2):145–155.
3. Hagan JF, Shaw JS, Duncan PM, eds. *Bright Futures: Guidelines for Health Supervision of Infants, Children, and Adolescents 4e*. American Academy of Pediatrics; 2017.
4. Head Zauche L, Darcy Mahoney AE, Thul TA, et al. The power of language nutrition for children's brain development, health, and future academic achievement. *J Pediatr Health Care*. 2017;31(4):493–503.
5. Feldman H. How young children learn language and speech. *Pediatr Rev*. 2019;40(8):398–411.
6. Hodges S, Richards K, Gorbachinsky I, Krane LS. The association of age of toilet training and dysfunctional voiding. *Res Rep Urol*. 2014;6:127–130.
7. Cui J and Natzke L. Early Childhood Program Participation: 2019 (NCES 2020-075REV), National Center for Education Statistics, Institute of Education Sciences, US Department of Education. Washington, DC. http://nces.ed.gov/pubsearch/pubsinfo.asp?pubid=2020075REV.
8. Bureau of Labor Statistics. *News Release, Employment Characteristics of Families Summary*; 2021. https://www.bls.gov/news.release/pdf/famee.pdf.
9. McCormick R. Does access to green space impact the mental well-being of children: a systematic review. *J Pediatr Nurs*. 2017;37:3–7.

12

Developmental Management of Middle Childhood

JENNIFER SONNEY

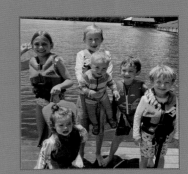

Children in middle childhood are busy, active, curious, and creative. With guidance and encouragement, they eagerly apply the skills they learned in early childhood as they move into structured school environments, home schooling, or community settings. While each child is unique and typical development patterns have broad parameters, the developmental goals for this age group (6–10 years old) include laying the groundwork for lifelong learning, creating a sense of self-worth, developing the ability to contribute to the world around them, and ultimately gaining satisfaction with life.

Primary care providers (PCPs) must be familiar with physical, cognitive, social, and emotional development to provide high-quality, comprehensive care for this age group (see Chapter 8). They support children's successful growth and development through obtaining appropriate health history details, conducting physical assessment, and providing anticipatory guidance and health promotion education.

Developmental Overview

This section discusses the developmental context for the elements of the well-child preventive health visit. It introduces the physical, social, emotional, and cognitive tasks that are mastered during typical middle child development.

Physical Growth and Development

Physical growth velocity in middle childhood is slower than infancy and early childhood. Prepubertal children gain an average of 2.4 to 2.8 inches and 6.5 to 7.5 pounds/year, with growth occurring discontinuously or in spurts several times per year.[1] The occipital frontal (head) circumference (OFC) increases an inch or less and is no longer routinely measured. Physical growth and neurologic maturation give children the ability to master many new skills. The cerebral cortex (responsible for intelligence) and the frontal lobe (responsible for problem-solving and decision-making) are the last to fully develop. Increasing brain maturation allows children to complete increasingly complex motor and cognitive skills and to have greater body control. Visual acuity development is generally complete by 6 years old.[2] Table 12.1 gives an overview of the typical physical development during middle childhood.

Body image and a sense of self begin to develop as young as age 5 to 6 years.[1] Children this age are often curious about changes happening to them as they grow, and they are sensitive to others around them. Highly literal in their thinking, they can be very frank and question people they trust (e.g., "Why do you have a mustache?"). Their achievements and failures help them define who they are and influence their evolving self-image. Social status among children is often based on physical competence; therefore the children's feelings about their physical development can be as important as the physical growth itself. Their body image comes from the experiences they have and feedback from family, peers, teachers, and others in the community. They are also sensitive to opinions they perceive from social media. When positive, this feedback helps clarify their self-understanding and allows the child to gain self-confidence and feelings of worth; however, negative messaging can have the opposite effect.

Children in middle childhood often compare their bodies with friends of the same sex. At the same time, they learn the importance of social politeness (e.g., what is appropriate and how to behave in certain situations) and may be uncomfortable or shy about new or unusual situations. During puberty, children may have mixed feelings ranging from curiosity and excitement to anxiety and shame about the physical changes occurring in their body. These feelings may be amplified for children who are gender nonconforming, as physical body changes may create discomfort or distress. Exploration of one's sexual organs, including masturbation, is common in this period.

Gross and Fine Motor Development

Children in middle childhood gain strength and coordination, leading to more physical capabilities and setting the stage for sports and other physical activity participation. Their gross motor skills are refined, allowing them to run, jump, climb, hop, skip, tandem walk, alternate their foot patterns, and use an overhand motion. Activities that require balance and coordination (e.g., riding a bicycle, swimming, roller skating) demonstrate their expanding skills. Toward the end of middle childhood, gross motor skills

TABLE 12.1   Physical Development in Middle Childhood

Body System	Developmental Change
Skin and lymph	Tonsillar and adenoid size peaks around 6 years. Apocrine sweat glands begin appearing, though they are largely nonfunctional until puberty. Pubertal development can begin as early as 8–10 years old, including increased hair growth in axilla and genital regions.
Head, eyes, ears, nose, mouth, neck	Head size becomes smaller in proportion to body size. Frontal sinuses develop; sinus maturity is reached typically between age 12 and 14 years. By age 6–7 years, the retina is fully developed and visual acuity development is complete. External auditory canal and pinna reach adult size; the eustachian tube lengthens and is more angled. Primary teeth are intermittently shed as permanent teeth erupt. Thyroid approximates adult size and is more readily palpable.
Pulmonary	By age 8 years, alveolar development is complete. Tidal volume increases and normal adult respiratory rate is achieved (18–30 breaths/min). Increased maturation of the macrophagocytic activity of mucus and ciliary function in lungs makes the child more resistant to lower respiratory infections.
Cardiovascular	By age 5 years, the heart is four times larger than at birth. By age 7 years, the left ventricle thickens and is two to three times greater in size than the right; blood pressure increases to 90–108/60 mm Hg; cardiac volume increases; heart rate declines to 60–100 beats/min; and atherosclerosis begins.
Gastrointestinal	Gastrointestinal tract size and function are adult-like.
Genitourinary	By age 6 years, elimination patterns are established; more than 90% of children are toilet trained. Bladder capacity continues to expand. Pubertal changes before age 8 years (females) and before age 9 years (males) may indicate precocious puberty.
Musculoskeletal	Long bones grow along epiphysis until growth plates mature in puberty, leading to the taller, thinner appearance. Exaggerated thoracolumbar curvature and protuberant abdomen of early childhood resolve; spine and legs straighten.
Immune system	The immune system matures rapidly during middle childhood and allergic conditions may appear.

are more controlled and purposeful and are perfected with practice. These children tend to be competitive as they try to outlast or outperform one another, and they often enjoy participating in competitive activities such as sports.

Fine motor skills mastery includes improved dexterity and better control of scissors and writing tools. Their drawings become more recognizable, showing eyes, ears, and other body part details. Technology is part of classroom daily life, and children progress in their mastery of digital devices. In early middle childhood, children become adept at dressing themselves, including being able to tie shoelaces and manage buttons and zippers and self-care skills (e.g., combing hair, brushing teeth) improve. As they mature, hand-eye coordination improves, and they are able to use each hand independently with speed and smoothness. As an example, skill playing musical instruments may emerge.

Social Development

Children this age experience substantial psychosocial development, which includes increasing independence from their home and family, establishing friendships, negotiating with siblings and other family members, and working on developing a sound sense of who they are as unique members of the community.[1] The ability of children to form friendships depends on social cognitive development and is a direct result of parent-child relationships during earlier development. As they increasingly interact within their community, children maintain their role and feelings of belonging

within their family, but they also develop secondary attachments with adults outside the home. Having positive relationships with adults outside the home is especially important for children who come from families with dysfunction or conflict.[3] For parents and PCPs, it is important in this age group to reinforce the recognition and avoidance of predatory adult behavior, both in person and through electronic media.[3]

It is important for children to have the opportunity to engage in social extracurricular activities to facilitate interaction skills development, including how to understand social meaning and interpret others' social cues. They learn to form and engage in relationships through the initiation, maintenance, and termination of peer interactions. Friends are generally chosen because of shared skills, interests, personality, and loyalty. Gaining social acceptance from peers depends on skills, such as being socially responsive, understanding group "rules" and jargon, being appropriately assertive, and being empathetic. Children who do not have those skills can experience a sense of failure when they are compared with their peers who do. Children often view themselves through the eyes of their friends. They develop "best friends" and dress and talk like their peers. A special-friend phase typically occurs around 10 years old. With that friend, the child expands the self, learns altruism, shares feelings, and learns how others manage problems. Talking on the telephone, texting, emailing, using social media, and having sleepovers with friends become more common. These early friendships are the basis for later relationships. Family conflicts arise when peer activities and expectations conflict with family rules and values. Further, the values of the family are challenged as the child learns that other families make decisions and have beliefs that differ from theirs.

Relationships are crucial to biological and behavioral development. Adverse childhood experiences (ACEs) refer to events or experiences that negatively impact child health, particularly social, emotional, and cognitive development; ACEs are also predictive of negative health outcomes in adulthood. The landmark ACE study[4] and subsequent research have affirmed that early identification of ACEs is critical so that early intervention and support services may be initiated.[5] ACEs include physical, verbal, or sexual abuse; household dysfunction such as domestic violence, household substance abuse, mental illness, and criminal activity.[4] Additional ACEs have been suggested to include physical and emotional neglect; parental separation; bullying (including weight stigma), and foster care (see Chapter 6).[5]

Emotional Development

Assessment of emotional development is an important aspect of the well-child examination as an estimated 16.5% of US children have at least one mental health disorder.[6] Attention-deficit/hyperactivity disorder (ADHD) and anxiety are the most common mental health disorders of middle childhood.[7] During this time, children gain the ability to self-regulate, control impulses, and manage emotions. By 7 years of age, children are typically competent, functioning in a variety of settings (e.g., home, school, playground). Emotional problems during these years often follow frustrations, losses, and/or situations in which the child's self-esteem is threatened or the child is faced with adversity.

At this age children tend to be rigid in their views of right and wrong, which is consistent with concrete thinking. They understand the relationship between responsibility and privileges and realize choices between right and wrong behaviors are within their control. Some children are motivated to behave to get a direct reward, whereas others are motivated by their sense of duty, viewing moral behavior as following the rules of higher authority. The ability to reason through difficult situations with a variety of influencing factors is heavily dependent on cognitive development; however, children this age do not have the cognitive maturity to cope with all situations. The school environment, where rules and values may differ from those of their family, must be confronted and negotiated daily. Social pressures, often from peers, may make it even more difficult to choose actions that the child believes are right.

Temperament affects the way in which children interact with peers, teachers, family, and others in their environment. As part of the process of developing relationships with others, they refine their ability to identify, label, and manage their feelings; however, their experiences are limited, and their cognitive abilities are still developing. Therefore children's coping responses are largely dependent upon parent support and modeling and they continue to need help labeling complex emotions, such as sadness, depression, worry, and envy. They also need help to managing feelings in acceptable ways. Maladaptive behaviors may occur when the child's coping responses are overwhelmed.[1]

Entry into school can be emotionally stressful because children must adjust to a new social situation, routine, and a changing relationship dynamic within their family. Some parents feel that they have "lost" their child, watching them move from dependence on the family to participation in a new world of which they are not a part. Other parents anticipate these new opportunities facing their child and family and are ready to help their child cope with challenges that emerge in the school environment. Impulse control is an important coping skill for children to develop. Without impulse control, erratic behavior may occur; conversely, overly controlled children may be perceived as hostile, uncreative, or both. ADHD and disruptive behavioral disorders may emerge during this time. Behavioral challenges may impact a child's school performance, and disruptive behavior often leads to a negative disciplinary consequence pattern that affects the child's self-esteem and motivation.

Of note, children may face a variety of stressors within and outside of the home, including violence, bullying, divorce, family or peer group substance use/abuse, early responsibilities, and/or lack of support in school. Any stressor has the potential to adversely impact child development. Safety is a constant concern for many, in neighborhoods where children live and play, and in their families and schools.

Cognitive Development

In middle childhood, children transition from preoperational thinking (e.g., intuitive problem-solving) to early concrete operational thinking. Magical thinking and egocentric logic are replaced by rule-driven behaviors, including understanding the consequences of breaking rules. The concepts of conservation, transformation, reversibility, decentration, seriation, and classification also emerge. Concrete operational abilities allow effective reading, writing, and thought communication. Learning about the world, people, and the views and values of others is possible. They can focus on more than one aspect of a problem and use logical thinking. New social skills appear with the ability to understand others' viewpoints, and egocentricity declines. *Empathy*, the ability to share and understand another's feelings, emerges, which allows for added depth in peer and family relationships. Empathy also helps children negotiate complex situations, especially when disparity occurs.[3]

Cognitively, children in middle childhood face daunting challenges. They must master the intellectual skills of reading, writing, mathematics, science, and other academic work. They progress from learning to read to reading to learn. Those who fall behind in reading or do not master early reading skills tend to struggle as they face increasing challenges and expectations for reading comprehension. Performance expectations increase progressing from homework and quizzes to examinations, graded papers, and projects. Many schools lack the resources to maintain small class sizes or offer special programs for children with learning difficulties, which increases the risk of children passing from grade to grade without remediation of their fundamental learning problems and, equally important, with the stigma of failure. Unless struggling children are provided with social and remedial support, they may see school as an unpleasant burden, develop feelings of failure, and look for validation through nonacademic experiences. Social supports help children cope with this stress and they are buoyed by interacting with healthy, interested, and caring adults.[3] While support is an important element, children also need interventions that are specific to their learning disorder (see Chapter 29).

Communication and Language Development

During middle childhood, children develop increasingly complex receptive and expressive language skills that are the result of continued brain maturation. Consider the difference in how a

6-year-old expresses themselves versus the conversational ability of the 10-year-old. Children's language patterns provide insight into their neurologic developmental status. They have a well-developed vocabulary and retrieve words quickly; their expressive language should be fully intelligible.[1] Stuttering usually resolves during early childhood but may still be present in early middle childhood, especially when children are overly eager to express themselves. Occasional or brief stuttering (repetition of sounds, syllables, or short words) that does not cause distress is considered normal disfluency at this age.[8] Table 12.2 provides a more detailed summary of the progression of language development in this period.

Multilingualism is increasingly prevalent as societies continue to diversify. Multilingualism proficiency is reported to be associated with improved cognitive functioning performance, though this remains controversial.[9] Children who are learning English as a second language may need additional support as they juggle learning a new language with their other academic competencies. The assessment of communication skills in multilingual children should consider their primary language abilities; this approach also applies to children who are deaf or hearing impaired and use sign language for communication.

Communication disorders affect approximately 9% of children between 7 and 10 years of age.[10] Speech and language impairment may interfere with daily functioning, including the ability to learn, communicate, and interact socially.[11] Language delays related to hearing impairment are associated with a higher risk for emotional and behavioral difficulties during childhood and adolescence.[12] The identification of language delays or issues should ideally occur in early childhood, but many are first identified only after the child is in school. Prompt referral for focused intervention and/or speech therapy is needed to maximize academic potential and success.

Common Developmental Concerns in Middle Childhood

Chronic conditions that impact development may have already been identified by the time children enter school age, or developmental concerns, particularly those related to learning or the school environment, may emerge during this age period. Wide variations in growth and development necessitate evaluations occur in the context of the child's age, developmental trajectory, and peer and family functioning. Common developmental concerns during middle childhood include school adjustment, learning challenges, and school refusal.

School Adjustment

School entrance is based on chronologic rather than developmental age, and generally begins with kindergarten enrollment at 5 years old; however, the process for determining school readiness and preparing children for this transition takes place earlier. School participation requires the ability to perform self-care, interact with a variety of new people, act with a sense of responsibility, and separate emotionally from the family and home base. Likewise, families must also be ready for school and be able to

TABLE 12.2	Progression of Communication Skills in Middle Childhood	
Age	**Communication Skills**
6–7 years	Have basic syntactic abilities and can follow simple directions May not be accustomed to attending to total auditory stimuli (e.g., in the classroom environment) Still mastering *connotative* and *semantic* rules, such as understanding the concepts "before" and "after," relative clauses (e.g., "the cat was chased by the dog"), and the structures of sentences May have difficulty following complicated directions or coping with increased demands to recall information within a specific timeframe Narrative skills are developing; reading may be difficult or challenging Receptive language strengthens; language *decoding* generally mastered; working on *encoding* information Can organize previous knowledge and express it verbally or in writing; can solve word problems Articulation mastery of the "l" and "th" sounds may not be achieved before age 7–8 years
8–9 years	Significant syntactic growth with better use of pronouns and understanding of convoluted sentences *Comparative*s learned; able to distinguish qualities, such as "more or less," "near or far," and "heavy or light" Follow complex directions Begin to tell jokes because they understand different meanings of words Have better narrative and storytelling abilities and summarization skills needed for activities such as explaining a task to other children Vocabulary grows with gradual improvements in grammar
10–12 years	Able to discuss ideas and understand inflections and metaphors Understand ambiguities of sentence structure, word meaning, and language; this contributes to their enjoyment of jokes and riddles Use concrete operational thinking to analyze and interpret language; more aware of the inconsistency in spoken languages Understand that words can mean more than their literal definition Able to answer questions involving sophisticated concepts Sentences mostly grammatically correct; have more detail in their verbal skills Improved ability to verbally express emotion Language becomes a means of socializing with fewer gestures used

support the child to develop new routines and adjust to the school environment.[13]

Children must learn to adapt many of their former behaviors as they adjust to school life. Sleep schedules are often altered to accommodate earlier wake times; such sleep routine changes may negatively impact learning, mood, and behavior. Learning to adjust to structured schedules for school attendance, family and household responsibilities, extracurricular activities, and homework demands are challenging for children and families. Children may choose to bring food or eat meals provided by the school, and thus experience increased independence over their dietary choices and eating habits. Elimination may be affected if a child is reluctant to use the school bathroom, especially for defecation.

Self-regulation of attention, emotion, and behavior is an important predictor of school adjustment.[13] The initial immersion in the academic learning environment is challenging for all children, but those who lack the necessary skills to meet school demands and expectations may experience maladjustment and early school failure. Children with maladjustment may demonstrate *internalizing* behaviors (e.g., low self-esteem, depression, impaired social skills, lower adaptive functioning) or *externalizing* behaviors (e.g., aggression, impulsivity, disruptive behaviors), underachievement, and/or failure.

Parents need to support their children as they adjust to school. Parents may have difficulty adapting to their children's increasing independence and worry about how to appropriately supervise and monitor them now that children spend more time outside the home.[13] Some parents have ambivalent attitudes about their child's school and distrust the school's capacity to meet their children's educational needs, while others get involved with their children's academic and social development. The primary care visit is an optimal time to encourage relationship-building with the school. PCPs have a responsibility to work with children, parents, and communities to promote optimal development for children and their families during the transition and adjustment to school. See Table 12.3 for details on history, physical examination, assessment, and planning related to school adjustment.

Learning Challenges

Learning challenges often present during this age, especially as the child transitions to and progresses through school. Academic success requires the integration of information processing, memory formation and recall, selective attention, expressive and receptive language processing, and beginning problem-solving skills.[1] Knowledge (the sum of what children know) continually expands due to academic gains, experiences at home, activities with friends, and observations in the community. Self-awareness is reflected by a child's ability to predict performance and emerges first in areas in which they have the most knowledge. Children with learning challenges may have difficulties with one or more areas of cognition, including information processing, language, attention, and organizational skills; higher cognitive functions, such as memory and sensory function; motor capacities; visuospatial analysis and neuromotor function; and social awareness and behavior. PCPs need to be alert to comorbid mental health and behavioral conditions, as they may also occur in children with learning challenges (see Chapter 29).

Dysfunction in sensory integration or processing may also interfere with learning. Children with sensory integration dysfunction may require classroom modification and assistance. Sensory integration can be particularly challenging for children with

developmental or behavioral disorders such as autism spectrum disorder or ADHD (see Chapters 6 and 29).

Early identification of learning challenges is important to ensure that children access resources to maximize their potential and facilitate academic success. The PCP must be alert to red flags that indicate school success may be in jeopardy, and they must be ready to intervene with families and school professionals to obtain necessary evaluations and resources to address these problems. See Table 12.3 for details on history, physical examination, assessment, and planning related to learning challenges.

School Refusal

School refusal is a term that was introduced in the 1970s to describe a phenomenon arising from a cluster of heterogeneous causes. The estimated prevalence of school refusal ranges from 1% to 4% in middle childhood.[14] School refusal is characterized by severe difficulty attending school, refusal to attend school, or severe emotional upset when attempting to go to school that occurs in the absence of significant antisocial disorders and involves staying at home with parental knowledge. Children typically request to stay home from school for a variety of physical complaints, including stomachaches, headaches, dizziness, fatigue, or a combination of these. The symptoms gradually improve as the day progresses and often disappear on weekends. School refusal may occur at any age, though unexcused school absences peak during early adolescence, between ages 11 and 13 years old.[14] It is important for providers to be aware that mental health disorders, such as separation anxiety, social anxiety, or depression are common among children with school refusal. See Table 12.3 for details on history, physical examination, assessment, and planning related to school refusal.

Intervention is generally successful when behavioral measures are combined with supportive counseling for the entire family. In mild cases, school refusal can be managed in primary care. The PCP should evaluate somatic symptoms to rule out organic disease, without excessive medical attention or diagnostic testing, which can reinforce the behavior. In addition, the PCP should address environmental factors, such as bullying or home stressors, through communication with the family and school and include referral to community support services as needed. Once there is a plan in place to evaluate organic causes and address environmental contributors, children are encouraged to return to school. In many cases, once the aforementioned concerns are addressed, the child's symptoms resolve.[14] Children with more severe presentations, such as those whose symptoms persist despite intervention or screen positive for underlying psychosocial conditions, should be referred to a mental health specialist. They may benefit from further interventions such as cognitive-behavioral therapy (CBT), counseling, and/or medication.

Health Promotion Topics in Middle Childhood

During middle childhood, parents and caregivers should provide opportunities for children to incorporate their emerging skills and abilities with family expectations and beliefs about health maintenance such as nutrition, oral health, sleep, and safety. For children this age, assuming responsibility for their own health begins with simple goals and tasks, progressing to more complex decision-making strategies with mastery.

Nutrition

Careful attention to nutrition is important given that 36.5% of US school children are overweight or obese.[15] As children become more independent, their food choices and eating habits can significantly impact on their overall health. For example, consumption of sugar-sweetened beverages, high-calorie snacks, and other high-calorie foods contribute to obesity in middle childhood. Nutritional monitoring is necessary throughout childhood, and early intervention must be provided when indicated (see Chapter 14). Choosing nutritious foods while away from home and learning to eat new foods are areas for learning. Children this age progress from simple (e.g., deciding to have a fruit or vegetable at each meal) to more complex nutritional responsibilities (e.g., helping plan some meals and participate in their preparation). PCPs should engage children and parents in discussions about their nutritional habits and provide guidance for healthy eating with a supportive and nonjudgmental approach. The PCP also needs to investigate child statements suggestive of disordered eating or weight modification behaviors. Table 12.4 provides a list of anticipatory guidance for health promotion related to nutrition.

Oral Health

During this age period, children begin shedding their primary (baby) teeth and their permanent (adult) teeth erupt. Oral hygiene, including brushing and flossing, is an essential practice. Children assume increasing responsibility but should only be independent when they have sufficient manual dexterity to perform appropriate brushing and flossing. Even when children are independent, parents should ensure oral hygiene is completed twice daily and periodically ensure the child is using proper technique. Healthy habits to encourage include choosing water over sugar-sweetened beverages and juices and limiting candy and sticky/gummy food consumption. In addition to examining the teeth for caries or other dental concerns, PCPs should obtain an oral health history, assess for oral health risk factors (diet, history of caries, fluoridated water), understand the child's oral hygiene routine, and ensure the child and family have a dental home. For children without a dental home, the PCP should provide resources or referrals as needed. Chapter 20 provides more detailed information regarding oral health needs and management. Table 12.4 provides a list of anticipatory guidance for health promotion related to oral health.

Sleep

Sleep is an important consideration as disrupted sleep negatively impacts a child's cognition, academic performance, emotional regulation, and other health outcomes, such as obesity.[16] The American Academy of Sleep Medicine recommends children this age sleep between 9 and 12 hours per night without naps.[17] Night terrors or sleepwalking may occur (see Chapter 16). PCPs should

TABLE 12.3   Developmental Concerns in Childhood: History, Physical Examination, Assessment, and Planning

	History	Physical Examination	Assessment and Planning
School adjustment	• Ask the child about school, including likes and dislikes, examples of daily activities, who their friends are, and general level of comfort in the environment • Assess the parents' feelings about their child's school, including level of trust in administration and staff, sense of community with other families, and who they might go to for help if they had a concern related to their child's experience • Inquire about family activities, sibling school experiences, traumatic events, or separation of the child or parents/caregivers, which may affect the child's adjustment in school • Investigate any stressors (e.g., chronic illness, economic issues, homelessness, and family disruption) that might compromise regular school attendance or school success	• Neurologic function, including sensory, cognitive, and language abilities • Affect and behavior, including symptoms of anxiety or depression	• Consider psychosocial screening tool (see Table 12.7) • Ensure school adjustment involves collaboration among family, school staff, and PCP • Encourage parents to visit the school, meet the teacher, and discuss their child's characteristics with the teacher • Encourage involvement in the classroom or school, if the parent is able, to become more familiar with the school environment • Urge children to share details of their daily school routines with caregivers, including any changes in eating and elimination habits • Help parents deal with their own stress of separation as their children progress in development and independence • Review expectations for the child and identify what will be new and different with each school transition (e.g., new school year) • Provide parents with available community and school resources to access to meet the developmental needs of their child • Advocate on behalf of parents and child with special needs to ensure the school adequately assesses both child's strengths and struggles and develops a program of study (e.g., an IEP) that maximizes child's strengths • Reassure parents that difficulties in a child's adjustment to school may occur even with the best of parenting/caregiving • Monitor the child's progress throughout the year, advocating as necessary

TABLE 12.3	Developmental Concerns in Childhood: History, Physical Examination, Assessment, and Planning—Cont'd		
	History	**Physical Examination**	**Assessment and Planning**
Learning challenges	• Vision and hearing abilities, either reported by the parents or conveyed during routine school screenings • Progress, interest, and success in school, including any sudden changes in school performance • Changes or differences noted by parents, caregivers, or teachers in vocabulary or language, logical reasoning, or the ability to problem-solve • Hyper- or hyposensitivity to sensory stimuli such as loud noises, bright lights, or specific textures • Difficulty maintaining appropriate boundaries of physical space with others • Reports of frequent fidgeting or inability to meet age-appropriate expectations for seated activities • Concerns with peer interactions, particularly related to learning and progression of social skills • Identification of learning problems by school or other outside professionals • Request results of any educational testing completed as well as any school plans or placements based on identified needs and abilities • Medical history: prenatal history, including in utero exposure to drugs, infection, toxins, and alcohol; neonatal history; recurrent or chronic medical conditions; allergies; medications; hospitalizations; syndromes; congenital, neurologic, metabolic, or endocrine conditions; current illnesses; vision and hearing problems; fetal alcohol spectrum disorder (FASD); history of accidents, concussions, or other brain injury • Neuro/developmental history (see Chapter 29) • Achievement or regression of developmental milestones, especially in language; experiences for achieving developmental skills at home or in preschool; daily routines and preferred play activities; temperament; behavioral concerns of parents/caregivers; ability of the child to handle transitions and change; child's initiation of activities versus parent-guided activities; repetitive behaviors • Family medical history: family history of difficulties in school or school dropout, learning difficulties, ADHD, intellectual disability, or genetic disorders; overall family members' functioning; substance abuse • Family social history: problem-solving and decision-making skills, use of community resources, financial resources, family stressors, substance abuse, homelessness, violence, criminal behavior, ACEs	• General appearance, interaction with parent and examiner, and ability to follow commands • The eye, including maneuvers to assess for nystagmus or strabismus • Neuromuscular function, such as sensation, mobility, tone, and strength in all extremities, and fine motor skills such as writing or drawing • Mental status, including sensory, cognitive, and language abilities	• Explore possible etiologies for the child's learning challenges and consider including in referral to a specialist • Audiometry and visual acuity assessment • Psychosocial screening for emotional or behavioral conditions (see Table 12.7) • Additional testing may be recommended by specialist, such as genetic testing with chromosome studies, brain scans, or endocrine and metabolic testing • Management predominantly focused on support, consultation, and provision of resources to families • Encourage intervention and educational supports, including IEPs and 504 plans

Continued

TABLE 12.3	Developmental Concerns in Childhood: History, Physical Examination, Assessment, and Planning—Cont'd		
	History	**Physical Examination**	**Assessment and Planning**

School refusal	• Patterns and characteristics of potentially somatic complaints (e.g., headache, abdominal or chest pain, or sleep difficulties)
	• School environment and evidence of bullying, violence, mismatch with teacher, academic failure
	• Socialization away from family: friends, involvement with peer group, participation in group activities
	• Child self-concept and self-esteem; suicidal ideation or self-harm behaviors
	• Patterns of isolation or withdrawn behavior; whether described as "shy" or "introverted"
	• Parents' feelings about child's school attendance, evidence of overindulgence or overprotection
	• Other symptoms of anxiety, such as persistent worry or obsessive behavior (see Chapter 29)
	• Recent or anticipated loss or separation from parent/caregiver or other family member, such as death or divorce
	• History of traumatic event, including abuse or neglect
	• Significant home responsibilities (e.g., caring for a caregiver who is chronically ill or has substance use disorder)
	• Social determinants of health: housing status, food security, parent employment
		• General emotional state, including interactions and engagement with PCP and parent	• Laboratory analyses or diagnostic imaging are rarely necessary to differentiate somatic from organic complaints, and PCPs should be judicious and use evidence-based clinical judgment for the appropriate use of these resources
			• Table 12.7 describes validated tools that may be used to screen for psychosocial contributors most relevant to school refusal.
			• Collaborate with school personnel to intervene and address any factors in the school environment related to the child's reasons for refusal
			• Engage with social service agencies such as the local Department of Public Health, if needed, to assess the home situation and identify areas for social support
			• Provide referrals as needed for child or family counseling
			• Notify child protective services in the case of suspected abuse or neglect
			• Criteria for mental health referral include the following:
			  • Symptoms are severe or do not improve within 2 weeks
			  • Out of school for at least 2 months
			  • Symptoms of depression, panic, or psychosis
			  • Parental inability to cooperate with plan

ACEs, Adverse childhood experiences; *ADHD,* attention-deficit/hyperactivity disorder; *IEP,* individualized education plan; *PCP,* primary care provider.

assess for child sleep duration, quality, and hygiene and explore problems related to falling or staying asleep. Parents can support healthy sleep habits by providing an environment conducive to uninterrupted sleep, including a dark sleep space without electronics, and encouraging a consistent and calming bedtime routine. Table 12.4 provides a list of anticipatory guidance for health promotion related to sleep.

Safety

Children this age enjoy increasing capabilities related to their continued physical development. They will often test rules and boundaries, which underscores the importance of safety considerations in this age group. To make safe choices, they need guidance and direction as well as clear family expectations and associated consequences. Increasingly, peers and influences outside the family impact children's decisions related to risk-taking behaviors. The PCP has an important role in providing safety guidance to children and families (see Chapter 21).

Children typically outgrow car safety seats and transition to booster seats before middle childhood; however, they should remain in a booster seat as early as age 8 years or up to age 12 years, depending on the child's height and state child restraint laws.[3] During middle childhood, most children ride bicycles or other wheeled devices; therefore emphasis on consistent helmet usage and rules for riding safely are important. In middle childhood, a high proportion of children engage in organized sports and other extracurricular activities, therefore PCPs need to emphasize proper safety equipment use and adult supervision. Other safety considerations to highlight include crossing streets, sun protection, fire prevention and planning, and activation of emergency services.

PCPs should assess safety within children's homes, neighborhoods, and schools. With the widespread accessibility of the Internet and social media, online safety is also a growing concern in the age group. Families should be counseled on supervised internet use, internet safety tools, and restricted access; access may expand with maturity and demonstrated responsibility.[3] As firearms are a leading cause of death in children,[18] PCPs must also promote firearm safety, which includes screening for firearms in the home and advising on safe firearm storage in the child's home as well as in the homes they visit (e.g., peers, grandparents). Children need to be taught about stranger danger, inappropriate touching, "private" parts, and the potential dangers associated with keeping secrets for and from others. Children who experience physical, emotional, or sexual abuse require immediate referral to Child Protective Services. Further, bullying and ostracism have been shown to interfere with development and academic performance. Therefore the PCP needs to assess for bullying and, if suspected or confirmed, work with the family and school to ensure it is addressed. Table 12.4 provides a list of anticipatory guidance for health promotion related to safety.

TABLE 12.4	Anticipatory Guidance Topics in Middle Childhood	

Nutrition	• Ensure child has three nutritious meals and two nutritious snacks daily • Establish an eating routine, ideally with at least one daily meal together as a family to preserve family time and share interests and experiences from the day's events • Monitor food choices and opportunities to determine best foods and beverages • Teach about the importance of eating healthy foods and drinking water • Encourage participation in meal planning, food shopping and selection, and meal preparation • Discuss nutritious choices for quick meals, school lunches, and when eating out • Model healthy behaviors related to nutrition and other healthy self-care behaviors
Oral health	• Encourage proper oral hygiene habits, including brushing and flossing • Establish a dental home and schedule biannual visits • Limit juice, soda, and candy consumption • Ensure proper hygiene for orthodontic appliances • Wear protective equipment during contact sports, such as mouth guards or helmets
Sleep	• Set clear expectations for sleep, including consistent bedtime and wake time, bedtime routine • Turn off screens at least 1 hour before bedtime • Avoid exposure to violent or scary imagery in books or media, especially before bed • Recognize "nonadherence" with sleep routine as a means of exerting independence; discussions about decision-making and healthy choices may be needed to resolve issues • Model healthy behaviors related physical activity and sleep
Safety	• Discuss safety and help child to think about safety aspects of activities • Help learn "survival skills" (e.g., name, telephone number, address, use of 911, How to say "no," how to ask adults for help, and what to do if lost) • Require protective gear when riding bicycles, skateboards, scooters, or other "wheels" and as appropriate in sports activities • Use booster seats or wear seatbelts; be familiar with and follow state child restraint laws • Use sunscreen consistently (sun protection factor [SPF] of 30 or higher) • Teach to swim; always supervise activities in or near water • Educate about hazards, both physical and social (e.g., pedestrian traffic on busy streets; stranger danger and unwanted touch; what to do if they find a weapon or syringe) • Monitor all digital and social media use. Use security tools to prevent instant messages from strangers. Use parental controls to limit access on all electronic devices • Provide opportunities to ask questions about sexuality, drugs, alcohol, and tobacco; encourage family discussion about these topics • Educate that Internet and technology use is a privilege—not a right • Remove firearms or ensure they are properly stored in a locked cabinet, with ammunition in a different location and the key accessible only to parent • Know child's whereabouts when away from home, and know child's friends

Health Supervision Visits

Middle childhood health supervision (preventive) visits occur annually. PCPs can best assist children and families during these visits by reviewing the child's progress, validating parent efforts, and providing education and guidance. Every health supervision visit should include a history, physical examination, developmental surveillance, and anticipatory guidance.

History

The health history includes a comprehensive summary of the child's physical, nutritional, neurodevelopmental, psychosocial, behavioral, and emotional status. The visit should begin by building rapport with the child and parent/caregiver. During middle childhood, direct questions first to the child, including aspects of daily routines, family experiences, school activities and status, socialization, and any concerns. Invite parents to confirm or expand on the data collected and to provide additional information. In pediatrics, family system assessment is crucial. It is particularly important to evaluate how well the family is nurturing

the child while supporting the child's efforts to become more independent and create a unique sense of self. The PCP should strive to integrate the health history with anticipatory guidance by eliciting information about a topic and providing education and resources within the same discussion (see Table 12.5). Box 12.1 provides a list of topics to address during the annual health supervision visit in middle childhood.

Physical Examination

Physical examination includes a comprehensive assessment of all body systems, including growth and sexual maturity (see Table 12.5). It is also an opportunity for the PCP to elicit child and parent questions or concerns about body changes and to provide education and anticipatory guidance about physical growth and pubertal development. Engaging the parent and child during the examination is important and can be achieved by providing a verbal summary of findings as the examination progresses, with emphasis on expected findings. The PCP should incorporate a developmental assessment within the context of the examination and note any physical manifestations pointing to delayed or

TABLE 12.5   Health Supervision Visits: History, Physical Examination, and Anticipatory Guidance

	History	Physical Examination	Anticipatory Guidance
Growth and development	• Open-ended questions about physical changes • Explore child's feelings about body image and sexual maturation (as appropriate) • Physical capabilities and endurance during peer play or sports	• Review objective height and weight measurements and trends, including body mass index • Respect the child's privacy during examination as physical modesty is characteristic of this age • Sexual maturity rating should be included at every preventive health visit	• Review typical physical changes and average growth expected in following year • Remind that growth and development follow individual trajectories and there is much individual variation • Promote nutrition and physical activity to support healthy growth and development • Discuss increasing independence in self-care and hygiene • Encourage shared decision-making and increased self-care during wellness and illnesses • Teach about pubertal body changes and variations in timing of puberty
Gross and fine motor development	• Discuss school performance, physical activity and self-care • Review participation in physical education or extracurricular physical activity (may elicit gross motor concerns) • Review writing tasks, competence in dressing, grooming, and use of utensils (may elicit fine motor concerns)	• Systematic musculoskeletal and neurologic examination • If child participates in sports or strenuous physical activity, include a full 14-point preparticipation musculoskeletal examination (see Chapter 18) • Ask the child to write or draw to evaluate fine motor abilities	• Encourage physical activities and activities that promote dexterity, such as art or musical instruments • Encourage healthful hobbies and activities fostering fitness and increased motor skills • Encourage activities that require commitment, training, and effort, especially for an older child • Discuss safety equipment, as increased gross and fine motor skills may coincide with more accidents and injuries • Limit recreational screen time to <2 h/day • Motor concerns may qualify the child for a school plan (individualized education plan [IEP] or 504 plan) that outlines accommodations and services, such as physical and/or occupational therapy • For children with physical limitations, explore ways they may participate in activities
Social development	• Explore child's success in making friends and working with peers • Ask child to name one or more friends • Probe into what child does during school recesses or after school (i.e., What is your favorite thing to do with your friend?) • Ask about any bullying experiences • Ask the child to name a trusted adult aside from parent(s) • Consider screening for ACEs via history or with formalized questionnaire	• Social development is difficult to assess outside of child's natural environment • Interaction between child and examiner or others in the room is an indicator of social skills • Pay attention to child's verbal and nonverbal behavior with parent and provider	• Clearly establish home rules and expectations; apply consistently • Provide opportunities at home to build collaboration, empathy, and conflict resolution skills • Establish and recognize traditions or special family activities (e.g., birthday celebrations, afternoon walks, movie nights) • Discuss family values and rules; explain differences child may face when away from home • Review strategies for appropriate behavior when values challenged (e.g., "No, my parent won't let me do that") • Teach respect for authority and help child to learn to communicate with other adults • Provide support and guidance for healthy interactions with peers (how to initiate, sustain, and terminate relationships) • If child is bullying others or being bullied, coach families to intervene and work with the school to address issue • Monitor activity on social networking sites; set and adhere to rules for Internet use and social networking inside and outside the home

TABLE 12.5   Health Supervision Visits: History, Physical Examination, and Anticipatory Guidance—Cont'd

	History	Physical Examination	Anticipatory Guidance
Emotional development	• Table 12.7 provides tools appropriate for screening for emotional and behavior concerns • Routinely assess for stressors, anxiety, depression and suicidality, self-esteem, parent-child relationships • Family history of mental and behavioral health conditions • In late middle childhood, consider interviewing child without parent present	• Assess the child's affect • Explore any signs of sadness, worry, and apathy • Observe parent-child interactions • During skin assessment, observe for signs of self-harm, mutilation, bruising • Significant weight loss or gain warrants further evaluation for possible emotional concerns	• Provide positive expressions of love, concern, and pride to promote self-esteem and sense of belonging • Role model coping skills and self-regulation of emotion • Encourage child to share emotional concern without fear of judgment or stigma • Help child identify and appropriately express emotions, including feelings of aggression and anger • Help child with decision-making and accepting consequences of actions • Help child learn delayed gratification and increased frustration tolerance while remaining sympathetic • Enhance goal setting and motivation with reward charts, calendars, and tally sheets • Provide opportunities to experiment with appropriate healthy behaviors that allow child to develop self-expression (e.g., new hairstyle, temporary tattoos) • Provide opportunities to discuss emerging sexuality and sexual values in a safe and accepting manner
Cognitive development	• Child's performance compared to their peers, grades, and teacher feedback reflect cognitive abilities • Learning difficulties need further exploration, including specialist evaluation • Inquire whether child receives any special education or support services (i.e., tutoring, resource classes)	• Cognitive assessment is difficult in school-age children • Engage in conversation and ask to follow directions with increasing complexity • If new-onset concerns arise, assess vision and hearing • Referral to specialist is often needed for definitive diagnosis	• Stimulate school-age child's thinking about comparisons and differences • Provide opportunities to gain knowledge through reading, outings, classes, and family discussions • Offer experiences with other languages, music, and cultural groups; promote broader understanding of the world • Monitor school assignments and progress; offer encouragement • Establish regular homework time and environment to encourage focus and completion with clearly defined expectations • Provide help with academic challenges • Encourage problem solving efforts • Provide increasingly complex opportunities at home (e.g., household chores, planning and cooking meals, planning family outings, and managing a budget) • Clearly establish expectations, including rewards or consequences to promote problem solving, empathy, and logic • If cognitive delay identified, encourage IEP or 504 plan to outline school services and upload to child's health record

Continued

TABLE
12.5

	History	Physical Examination	Anticipatory Guidance
Communication and language development	• School performance and reports from child's teacher are good indicators of language skills • Inquire whether child receives any support services • Any new concerns should be explored further, including detailed history of hearing or related issues (i.e., frequent ear infections)	• Ongoing surveillance of communication and language development throughout visit • Speak directly with the child and probe child's understanding (e.g., Can the child follow directions? Does the child understand the PCP's explanations?) • Monitor child's articulation, vocabulary, sentence structure, and grammar • Note child's ability to interact socially with examiner, parent, and others • If child speak another language than the examiner, use a certified interpreter to evaluate the child's command of their primary language	• Read stories to child and listen to child read aloud • Model reading and writing often • Encourage the child to keep a journal and write letters to friends and family • Talk with and actively listen to child; play vocabulary and other strategy games • Never punish by removing books or writing materials • Encourage ongoing communication with the teacher to facilitate early identification of concerns • If language delay identified, encourage IEP or 504 plan to outline school services and upload to child's health record

ACEs, Adverse childhood experiences; *PCP,* primary care provider.

• BOX 12.1 Topics for the Health Supervision Visit

• Transitions and progress in school and extracurricular activities
• Peer and family relationships
• Coping skills and problem-solving away from home
• Food choices, eating practices, and body image
• Oral hygiene
• Physical and sedentary activities
• Sleep patterns and hygiene
• Home and community safety
• Internet and social media practices
• Sexual development, gender identity, and sexuality

• BOX 12.2 Common Physical Conditions in Middle Childhood

• Allergic rhinitis
• Asthma
• Constipation/encopresis
• Dental caries
• Orthodontic issues
• Eczema
• Enuresis
• Obesity
• Scoliosis
• Unintentional injuries

asynchronous development. Findings that are atypical should be explored further. Box 12.2 contains information about common conditions that should be screened for during the physical examination in middle childhood.

Screening

Formal screening in middle childhood may include questionnaires, laboratory analysis, or other testing. Universal, annual surveillance of development, overall psychosocial function, and body mass index are important. Table 12.6 provides a summary of health screening recommendations in middle childhood. Selective screening may also be performed in children with specific risk factors or health concerns. Developmental and psychosocial screening tools may be used to facilitate the child, parents, and teachers to provide specific information about a child's development, behaviors, and emotional status (Table 12.7).

Growth and development surveillance is an essential aspect of the visit history because visits occur less frequently than in earlier childhood, and much can change from year to year (see Chapter 5). Surveillance does not entail formalized screening tools, but rather monitoring of growth and development. The PCP should follow up on any concerns raised related to physical growth, and motor, social-emotional, cognitive, or language development. If concerns arise, it is useful to elicit parent, teacher, and child perceptions about the specific issue, as perspectives can vary across environments.

Anticipatory Guidance

The provision of age-appropriate anticipatory guidance should be directed at children and parents because children are increasingly responsibility for self-care as they mature. Table 12.5 includes anticipatory guidance topics that are not intended to be exhaustive, but rather to illustrate how these concepts can be applied to everyday living. Parents typically welcome PCP suggestions and resources that help them understand, respond to, and support various aspects of their child's behavior and development.

<table>
<tr><td colspan="3">TABLE 12.6 Recommended Health Screenings During Middle Childhood</td></tr>
</table>

	Universal	Selective
Anemia	Identify dietary iron sources at every preventive health visit	Risk-based if poor nutrition or other risk factors
Blood pressure	Sphygmomanometry at every preventive health visit; if elevated, perform manually twice and average both results	At any visit if previously elevated
Body mass index	Calculate from weight and height measurements and compare to Centers for Disease Control and Prevention (CDC) growth charts at every preventive health visit	At any visit if overweight or obese
Development	Surveillance at every preventive health visit	At any visit if concerns from home or school
Dyslipidemia	Serum total cholesterol and high-density lipoprotein (HDL) at one preventive health visit between age 9–11 years	Every 2 years if positive family history or other cardiovascular risk factors
Lead toxicity	Serum lead level for new immigrants, refugees, or internationally adopted children upon arrival	Risk-based if concerns for exposure
Oral health	Oral hygiene surveillance: brushing/flossing and fluoride at every preventive health visit. Monitor teeth losses and eruptions	Risk-based if no dental home
Psychosocial/behavior	Surveillance of general socioemotional concerns, parent depression, and social determinants at every preventive health visit	Standardized screening if concerns or risk-based for other mental health and substance abuse beginning at 11 years
Sexually transmitted infection	Surveillance of sexual abuse at every preventive health visit	Standardized screening if concerns or risk-based beginning at 11 years
Tuberculosis	Risk factor questionnaire at every preventive health visit	Tuberculin skin test or serum quantiferon level if concerns for exposure
Vision and hearing	Snellen chart and audiometry at 6, 8, 10, and 12 years	Risk-based if concerns from home or school

From American Academy of Pediatrics. *Recommendations for Preventive Health Care (Periodicity Schedule)*; 2021. www.aap.org/periodicityschedule

<table>
<tr><td colspan="3">TABLE 12.7 Developmental-Behavioral Screening Tools for Middle Childhood</td></tr>
</table>

Screening Tool	Target Population	Purpose
Caregiver's Evaluation of Developmental Status (CEDS)	Birth to 8 years	Elicits parent/caregiver concerns for their child's language, motor, self-help, language, behavioral, and socioemotional abilities
Pediatric Symptom Checklist (PSC)	Children 4–16 years (Y-PSC for youth ≥11 years)	Generalized cognitive, emotional, and behavioral problems
Screen for Child Anxiety-Related Disorders (SCARED)	Children 8–18 years	Childhood anxiety disorders (see Chapter 6)
NICHQ Vanderbilt Assessment Scale	Children 6–12 years	Parent and teacher evaluation of inattention, hyperactivity, conduct disorders, and anxiety or depression (see Chapter 29)

Developmental Red Flags for Middle Childhood

Children this age may present with serious problems. Table 12.8 identifies red flags during middle childhood. PCPs must be alert for indications of more serious concerns and, if needed, assess the child and family more thoroughly. PCPs can address risk factors and provide guidance on prevention of health concerns. In situations where the child is referred to subspecialty care, the PCP has a crucial role in serving as a medical home and collaborating with subspecialty professionals to ensure children and families receive timely, appropriate, and coordinated services.

Acknowledgment

The author acknowledges Victoria F. Keeton, the chapter author in the previous edition.

TABLE 12.8	Developmental Red Flags: Middle Childhood	
Motor skills	**Gross motor** • Unable to catch a ball • Unable to walk a straight line • Poor coordination, endurance, strength • Problems throwing or catching • Frequent falls or accidents **Fine motor** • Unable to print name • Unable to tie shoes • Difficulty holding pencil • Illegible handwriting • School failure related to handwriting skills
Cognition and perception	• School failure related to attention or focus • Unable to state age or days of the week • Unable to perform basic addition or subtraction • Lack of operational thinking: cause and effect, relationships of whole and parts • Persistent difficulty understanding and completing school work • Reports of double vision, blurred vision, or loss of vision • Difficulty or loss of hearing
Communication and language	• Unable to read and write simple words or phrases • Unable to relate a simple story • Unable to follow verbal instructions • Problems with reading comprehension • Speech not 100% intelligible
Social and emotional skills	• Problems developing or maintaining peer relationships; unable to name a friend • Lack of hobbies or interests • Social isolation or withdrawal • Persistently flat, depressed, or withdrawn affect • Unable to sit still in class • Cruelty to animals or people • Illicit behavior such as fire setting, theft, vandalism • Persistent defiance or deliberate disregard for rules • Gang involvement • Risk-taking behaviors: smoking, alcohol, sex

References

1. Finkelstein LH, Feigelman S. Middle childhood. In: Kliegman RM, St Geme JW, Blum NJ, Shah SS, Tasker RC, Wilson KM, eds. *Nelson Textbook of Pediatrics.* 21st ed. Elsevier; 2020.
2. Duderstadt KG. *Pediatric Physical Examination.* 3rd ed. Elsevier; 2016.
3. Hagan JF, Shaw JS, Duncan PM, eds. *Bright Futures Guidelines for Health Supervision of Infants, Children, and Adolescents.* 4th ed. American Academy of Pediatrics; 2017.
4. Felitti VJ, Anda RF, Nordenberg D, et al. Relationship of childhood abuse and household dysfunction to many of the leading causes of death in adults. The Adverse Childhood Experiences (ACE) Study. *Am J Prev Med.* 1998;14(4):245–258.
5. Petruccelli K, Davis J, Berman T. Adverse childhood experiences and associated health outcomes: a systematic review and meta-analysis. *Child Abuse Negl.* 2019;97:104127.
6. Whitney DG, Peterson MD. US national and state-level prevalence of mental health disorders and disparities of mental health care use in children. *JAMA Pediatr.* 2019;173(4):389–391.
7. Bitsko RH, Claussen AH, Lichstein J, et al. Mental health surveillance among children - United States, 2013-2019. *MMWR Suppl.* 2022;71(2):1–42.
8. Sander RW, Osborne CA. Stuttering: understanding and treating a common disability. *Am Fam Physician.* 2019;100(9):556–560.
9. Marton K, Gehebe T, Pazuelo L. Cognitive control along the language spectrum: from the typical bilingual child to language impairment. *Semin Speech Lang.* 2019;40(04):256–271.
10. Black LI, Vahratian A, Hoffman HJ. Communication disorders and use of interventions services among children aged 3-17 years: United States, 2012. *NCHS Data Brief.* 2015;(205):1–8.
11. Feldman HM. How young children learn language and speech. *Pediatr Rev.* 2019;40(8):398–411.
12. Stevenson J, Kreppner J, Pimperton H, et al. Emotional and behavioural difficulties in children and adolescents with hearing impairment: a systematic review and meta-analysis. *Eur Child Adolesc Psychiatr.* 2015;24(5):477–496.
13. Williams PG, Lerner MA, Council on Early Childhood; Council on School Health. School readiness. *Pediatrics.* 2019;144(2):e20191766.
14. Elliott JG, Place M. Practitioner review: school refusal: developments in conceptualisation and treatment since 2000. *J Child Psychol Psychiatr.* 2019;60(1):4–15.
15. Wang Y, Beydoun MA, Min J, et al. Has the prevalence of overweight, obesity and central obesity levelled off in the United States? Trends, patterns, disparities, and future projections for the obesity epidemic. *Int J Epidemiol.* 2020;49(3):810–823.
16. Matricciani L, Paquet C, Galland B, et al. Children's sleep and health: a meta-review. *Sleep Med Rev.* 2019;46:136–150.
17. Paruthi S, Brooks LJ, D'Ambrosio C, et al. Consensus Statement of the American Academy of Sleep Medicine on the recommended amount of sleep for healthy children: methodology and discussion. *J Clin Sleep Med.* 2016;12(11):1549–1561.
18. Goldstick JE, Cunningham RM, Carter PM. Current causes of death in children and adolescents in the United States. *N Engl J Med.* 2022;386(20):1955–1956.

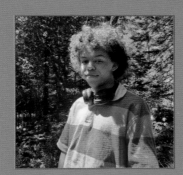

13

Developmental Management of Adolescents

JAIME E. PANTON

A dolescence is a period of significant growth and development, which in many ways rivals the rate and degree of changes seen during infancy. It is separated into three phases: early adolescence (11–14 years), middle adolescence (15–17 years), and late adolescence (18–21 years). Throughout each phase, reassurance, information, and anticipatory guidance about what to expect are among the most valuable services a primary care provider (PCP) can offer the adolescent and family. In addition, acknowledging and respecting gender and sexual identities, as well as using correct pronouns are crucial for developing rapport with teens (see Chapter 7). Successful adolescent development culminates in the achievement of goals that provide the basis for a healthy, productive adult life. This chapter provides an overview of development, focusing specifically on pubertal changes and sexual maturation, along with social, emotional, and cognitive changes. Common issues are then highlighted, assessment and management are emphasized, and the chapter concludes with health supervision content that is organized by adolescent phase. Collectively, this information provides PCPs with a framework for structuring primary care of the adolescent.

Developmental Overview of Adolescence

Adolescence comes from the Latin root *adolescere*, meaning to grow up. This period involves psychological and physical transition from child to adult and is influenced by social, genetic, and environmental factors.[1] Pubertal physical changes are accompanied by significant social, emotional, and cognitive shifts that affect how adolescents view themselves and how others view adolescents. *Puberty* is the development of secondary sexual characteristics and the biological process that ultimately leads to fertility. Pubertal changes occur on a continuum with individual differences in timing or tempo. Our understanding of pubertal timing and progression comes from studies of White participants of European heritage. Research with racially and ethnically diverse children and with sexual and gender minority young people continues to emerge.[2] Also, of note in recent years is the impact of early adversity (e.g., adverse childhood experiences [ACEs]), as it appears to predict earlier pubertal timing, especially for girls; this highlights another important rationale for ACEs screening.[3]

Physical Growth and Development and Organ Maturation

Puberty is characterized by a period of rapid growth, development, and maturation. The hormonal regulatory systems in the hypothalamus, pituitary, gonads, and adrenal glands undergo major changes between prepubertal and adult states. Accompanying these changes are rapid height and weight growth, secondary sex characteristics development, and fertility onset (Fig. 13.1). Typical development can be difficult to define and is, at best, an approximation rather than a precise parameter. Even though the timing of adolescent development varies, the sequence of events is consistent (Fig. 13.2).

Sexual Maturity Rating

Pubertal growth and maturation assessment is completed using the Sexual Maturity Rating (SMR) scales, which are divided into five stages (Figs. 13.3–13.5).

Female Stages. Females tend to enter puberty earlier than males. They progress sequentially in the following pattern:
- Ovaries increase in size; no visible body changes occur.
- *Thelarche* (breast budding) begins as a result of estradiol secretion; it traditionally occurs between age 8 and 13 years, with the average onset at 10.3 years.[4,5] Most females (85%) experience breast bud development approximately 6 months before the appearance of pubic hair. The timing of breast development onset in females has no relationship to adult breast size.
- Rapid linear growth begins shortly after breast budding onset. Most females reach *peak height velocity* (PHV) during SMR 2 and 3, at an average age of 11 or 12 years, which is typically 6 to 12 months before menarche (onset of menses). The growth rate slows, as females typically expect to grow no more than 2 to 3 inches after menarche. By age 15 years, females usually complete their linear growth.[4,6] Final height is determined by the amount of bone growth at the long bone epiphyses. Growth stops when hormonal factors shut down the epiphyseal plates.
- *Adrenarche, or pubarche* (pubic hair) begins around 11.5 years and is due to adrenal development. The pubic patch

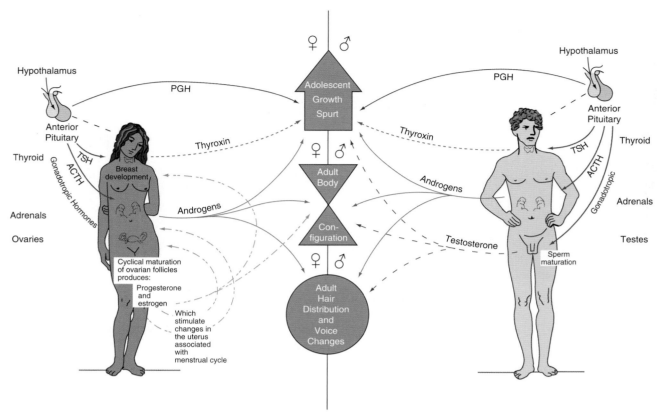

• **Fig. 13.1** The Endocrine System at Puberty. *ACTH,* Adrenocorticotropic hormone; *PGH,* pituitary growth hormone; *TSH,* thyroid-stimulating hormone. (From Valadian I, Porter D. *Physical Growth and Development from Conception to Maturity.* Little, Brown; 1977.)

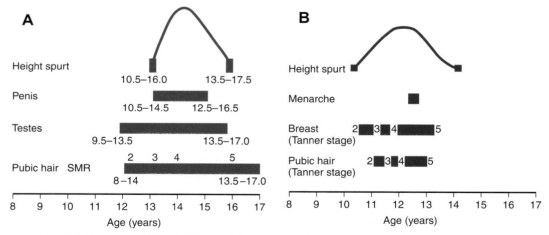

• **Fig. 13.2** Sequence of Pubertal Events. (A) Age at time of physiologic changes during natal female and natal male puberty. (B) Sequence of pubertal events in the average American female. *SMR,* Sexual maturity rating. (A, Modified from Tanner JM. *Growth at Adolescence.* Oxford: Blackwell Scientific Publications; 1962. B, From Tanner JM. Growth and endocrinology of the adolescent. In: Gardner LI, editor. *Endocrine and Genetic Diseases of Childhood and Adolescents.* 2nd ed. WB Saunders; 1975.)

initially grows in a triangular pattern that covers the vulva and mons pubis. Pubic hair is less valid than other secondary sex characteristics when assessing sexual maturation, as some females shave or wax their body hair and there is some familial variation. To accurately assess SMR stage, the PCP should ask where pubic hair would be present if the patient did not shave.[7] In addition to public hair, adrenal changes in puberty

also lead to the development of axillary hair, acne, and adult-type body odor.

• *Menarche* (onset of menses) occurs approximately 2.5 years after thelarche.[4] The mean age of menarche is highly dependent on ethnic, socioeconomic, and nutritional factors and ranges from 9 to 15 years. It can take up to 2 years after menarche before females establish regular ovulatory cycles.

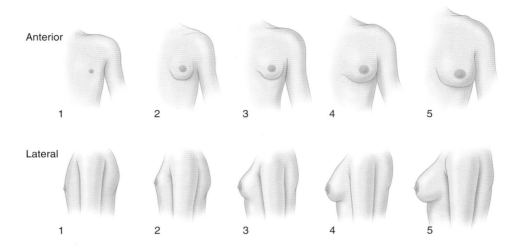

• **Fig. 13.3** Normal Female Breast Development, SMR Stages 1 to 5. *SMR*, Sexual maturity rating. (From Herring JA. *Tachdjian's Pediatric Orthopaedics*. 4th ed. Elsevier; 2008.)

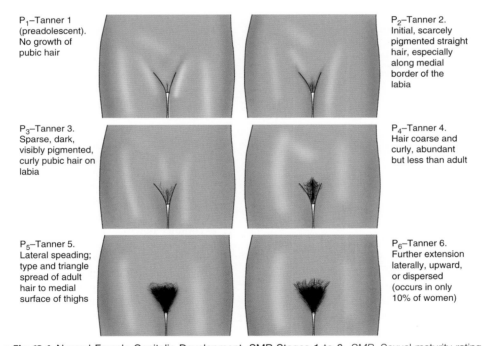

P_1–Tanner 1 (preadolescent). No growth of pubic hair

P_2–Tanner 2. Initial, scarcely pigmented straight hair, especially along medial border of the labia

P_3–Tanner 3. Sparse, dark, visibly pigmented, curly pubic hair on labia

P_4–Tanner 4. Hair coarse and curly, abundant but less than adult

P_5–Tanner 5. Lateral speading; type and triangle spread of adult hair to medial surface of thighs

P_6–Tanner 6. Further extension laterally, upward, or dispersed (occurs in only 10% of women)

• **Fig. 13.4** Normal Female Genitalia Development, SMR Stages 1 to 6. *SMR*, Sexual maturity rating. (From Duderstadt K. *Pediatric Physical Examination: An Illustrated Handbook*. 2nd ed. Elsevier; 2014:245.)

Female pubertal changes occur at earlier ages than in past decades with some notable variations. For example, thelarche occurs earlier in Black females (median age 8.8 years) compared to Latina (9.3 years) and White (9.9 years) females.[8] Understanding racial and ethnic differences in pubertal timing is vital to improving health and reducing disparities.[8] Further, females who develop secondary sex characteristics earlier than their peers are at increased risk for sexual assault, sexual abuse, psychosocial issues, and depression.[9]

There are changes in body composition during puberty, and adolescent girls benefit from the PCP's reassurance that these changes are typical. For example, initial breast development usually begins as a unilateral disk-like subareolar swelling, and many adolescents and parents may initially present with concerns about breast tumors. Girls often have asymmetric breasts and need assurance that breasts become approximately the same size within a few years after breast budding onset. Further, the female body shape changes, with broadening of the shoulders, hips, and thighs, and increases in proportion of fat to total body mass. Girls begin puberty with approximately 80% lean body weight and 20% body fat. By the end of puberty, lean body mass drops to about 75%. Body fat is an important mediator for the onset of menstruation and regular ovulatory cycles. An average of 17% of body fat is needed for menarche, and about 22% is needed to initiate and

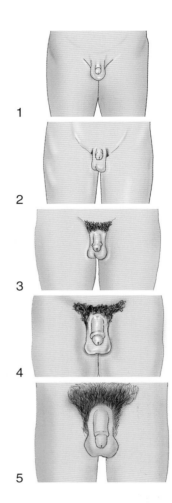

• **Fig. 13.5** Normal Male Genitalia Development, SMR Stages 1 to 5. *SMR,* Sexual maturity rating. (From Duderstadt K. Pediatric *Physical Examination: An Illustrated Handbook.* 2nd ed. Elsevier; 2014:216.)

maintain regular ovulatory cycles, which is particularly relevant when working with extreme athletes or individuals experiencing malnutrition. The American Academy of Pediatrics (AAP) and the American Congress of Obstetricians and Gynecologists recommend that PCPs recognize the menstrual cycle as a "vital sign" because of the need for education regarding normal timing and characteristics of menstruation and other pubertal signs.[10,11]

Acne is extremely common and while it can affect people of all ages, adolescents and young adults between 12 and 24 years tend to be the most affected group. It usually begins during the start of puberty, affecting girls earlier than boys. Both typically outgrow acne but about 12% of females (vs. 3% of males) may continue with acne into middle age.

Male Stages. Pubertal changes occur sequentially in males, as follows:
- The initial male pubertal sign (~11.5 years) is testicular enlargement.[4] Testes growth occurs approximately 6 months before pubic hair development in most males and can be assessed using an orchidometer (see Chapter 5). Once puberty begins, the left testis generally lies lower than the right. If testicular enlargement does not precede other changes, the PCP needs to consider whether the adolescent might be taking exogenous anabolic steroids.

- *Adrenarche,* or pubarche. Pubic hair development timing is similar to females; however, the distribution differs as the pubic patch tapers upward to a line of hair pointing toward the navel (upside-down triangle). Like females, some males shave or wax their body hair. To assess SMR, the PCP should ask where the pubic hair would grow if the patient did not shave (see Fig. 13.5).
- *Spermarche,* the first release of spermatozoa, generally occurs at any development stage from SMR 3 to 5.[6] The first ejaculation marks the potential for reproduction, but fertility is typically reached later, about one year after the first ejaculation.
- Elongation and widening of the penis usually begin in SMR 3 and continues through SMR 5 (see Fig. 13.5).
- Rapid growth in height occurs. The PHV occurs during SMR 4/5 and around age 14 years. Most males complete linear growth by age 17 years,[6] but they can continue to grow well beyond their teenage years. In general, boys generally lag 2 years behind girls and have a higher PHV than females.
- Change (lowering) in the male voice occurs in both males and females, but it is more striking in males, coinciding with the PHV. The increase in testosterone leads to a lengthening of the larynx cartilage as it moves down in the neck. The vocal cords also thicken and enlarge. This process begins with the first signs of testicular enlargement.
- Facial and body hair appears only after SMR 4 pubic hair appears. Facial hair starts at the outer corners of the upper lip and moves inward, then appears on the upper parts of the cheeks and middle of the lower lip, and finally grows along the sides and lower chin border. Body hair distribution is variable, influenced by dominant trait heredity and ethnicity.

Male body composition also changes. In contrast to females, males generally increase muscle mass from approximately 80% to 90% and lose body fat during puberty. Some additional changes associated with puberty may be unwelcome. Between 50% and 75% of males experience *gynecomastia,* a transient benign unilateral or bilateral enlargement of breast tissue, generally occurring mid-puberty (SMR 2–3) right before PHV.[12] Gynecomastia generally regresses in 6 months but can persist for 1 to 2 years. Most cases completely resolve by late puberty. In a small percentage of males, however, some palpable breast tissue persists. Although generally benign, gynecomastia can also occur secondary to anabolic steroid or illicit drug use. As with females, acne may develop in early puberty. By mid-puberty, many males have moderate to severe acne. In cases of persistent gynecomastia and/or severe acne, the PCP should ask if the adolescent is using alcohol, marijuana, or anabolic steroids, all of which can exacerbate these conditions. Other conversations to have with males relate to nocturnal emissions ("wet dreams"), which tend to emerge with puberty, and involuntary erections, which are ongoing but more noticeable with advancing puberty (see Chapter 7).

Motor Development

Changes in motor development plateau in adolescent females, while males continue to improve in skills requiring strength, power, and muscular endurance, which plateau later in adolescence to young adulthood. While overall motor development and abilities are attained, individual fine and gross motor skills vary widely, depending on the teen's body, interests, activity level, and opportunity. The tendency for motor and sports injury also varies, with female athletes having significant more knee injuries (anterior cruciate ligament [ACL]). Stress fractures are also more common among girls with the female athlete triad—a combination of inadequate calorie/nutrient intake, irregular menstrual periods, and bone loss (see Chapters 18 and 40).

Social, Emotional, and Cognitive Development

Adolescents are increasingly independent and self-sufficient, often in pursuit of rewarding experiences while avoiding painful ones; however, their decision-making abilities are still forming.[13] During the transition from childhood to adulthood, specific social, emotional, and cognitive milestones need to be assessed, as achievement helps the adolescent:

- Feel a sense of belonging in a valued group
- Acquire skills and master tasks that are important to the valued group
- Develop a sense of self-worth
- Develop at least one reliable relationship with another individual
- Demonstrate cognitive potential

Biophysical Influences

Although full sized, the adolescent brain continues to develop functional ability along with ongoing pruning and reinforcement, based on stimuli and the teen's activities and experiences. Dopaminergic and noradrenergic receptors become more active and neurotransmitter levels increase during adolescence. There is an increase of dopamine in the prefrontal cortex (PFC) and a decrease of dopamine in the *accumbens*, or "reward center."[14,15] The PFC, which coordinates executive functions of abstract thinking, reasoning, judgment, self-discipline, ethical behavior, personality, behavioral modification and emotions, experiences rapid growth. Emotional, social, and behavioral changes seen during adolescence are influenced by neural reactivity in the brain, particularly within the amygdala and PFC. Neuroimaging studies suggest the PFC also influences emotional regulation.[16] Gonadal hormones also influence pubertal brain development and behavioral responses, although these neurobiological mechanisms are not yet fully understood.[17,18]

The hypothalamic-pituitary-adrenal axis, one of the body's principal stress response systems, changes significantly during adolescence and makes the adolescent brain particularly vulnerable to stressors from adverse experiences, including abuse, maltreatment, racism, discrimination, mental illness, altered social interaction, and chronic illness.[19] In particular, adolescents exposed to adverse experiences are at increased risk of anxiety, depression, and other mental health disorders (see Chapters. 6 and 29).[19,20]

Other brain changes during this time may place adolescents at risk of substance abuse. Dopamine peaks in the frontal region and limbic system lead to enhanced neural sensitivity after reward exposure while they have lower inhibitory control. These two factors combine to increase the potential for adolescent risk-taking behavior.[21] Drugs and alcohol have a significant negative effect on the adolescent brain by damaging the neural circuitry in the "reward" or motivation pathways and shutting down the body's ability to respond to stimuli that normally generate pleasurable feelings. In essence, the drug becomes the only thing that leads to pleasurable feelings; a craving for the drug is "etched" into the brain and thus the individual becomes addicted. Neuroimaging studies in adolescents with alcohol use and/or abuse demonstrate decreased PFC volume, smaller temporal volumes, and decreased cortical thickness.[22] Brain changes resulting from exposure to alcohol, especially binge drinking, can also lead to loss of memory and cognitive function. Some longitudinal studies show adolescent alcohol use is associated with a decrease in frontal gray matter and poor white matter integrity.[21]

Simultaneous Changes

The central issues in adolescent development are summarized in Table 13.1. These issues cannot be understood, however, without an awareness of the simultaneous social, emotional, and cognitive changes.

Social Transitions. Transition from adolescence to adulthood is continuous and generally smooth. A commonly held myth is that adolescence is a period of "storm and stress" (a view originally described by G. Stanley Hall in 1908).[23] Although this characterization was not based on research, it continues to be widely believed. Adolescence is one of life's many transitional phases, and although some teens and families experience significant challenges during these years, others pass through this critical time with relative ease. One of the most significant social changes in late adolescence is gaining the right to vote, which is an external recognition of the transition to adulthood.

Changing Family Relationships. The biological, cognitive, and emotional changes experienced by adolescents require reworking of family relationships. Some degree of adolescent-parent adjustment or conflict is expected, but disruptive family conflict is not the norm. Everyday issues (e.g., clothes, hairstyles, household chores, curfew) are typical sources of conflict and ongoing negotiations between parent and teen are expected and essential. Inexperienced in negotiation, yet shifting to abstract thinking, adolescents can argue a point to excess. For parents, it may help to them that their teen's "arguing" is a way of practicing abstract thinking and that they should be delighted that their teen is at least engaging with them, although it may not seem like it (Box 13.1). When true turmoil exists, it usually represents individual and/or family pathology and is not simply "outgrown." Careful assessment and treatment are required. Behavior that results in negative consequences is especially worrisome. For example, fights over hair color may not be worthwhile because hair color will grow out, but delinquent or destructive behaviors need to be addressed.

Emotional Changes. Adolescent emotions are typically front and center, appearing more often and more intensely than those of adults. Pubertal hormonal changes contribute to this period of emotional changes, but as with the teen's physical growth and development, emotional changes can vary by individual, family norms, and sex, gender identity, and sexual orientation.

Testosterone increases can be associated with sad or anxious feelings, acting out, aggressive behavior, or interest in sexual activity. Males typically develop a positive self-image and mood and tend to be more satisfied with their body and body image than females. Depending on their size, they may want to gain or lose weight, which needs to be monitored, as disordered eating often begins in adolescence (see Chapter 29). Of note, male teens with adult physiques are given more leadership roles, are often more proficient or excel in sports, and are often perceived as more attractive, smarter, and more popular than their peers, and demonstrate higher self-esteem in early adolescence. In contrast, late-maturing boys, who are short and more childlike in appearance at 15 years or older, tend to show more personal and social maladjustment over the entire course of adolescence. They can be insecure, suggestible, and vulnerable to peer pressure and are often the subjects of bullying and seen as weak, immature, and less competent.

TABLE 13.1 Central Issues in Early, Middle, and Late Adolescence

Variable	Early Adolescence (11–14 years)	Middle Adolescence (15–17 years)	Late Adolescence (18–21 years)
Sexual maturity rating (SMR)	1–2	3–5	5
Somatic	• Secondary sex characteristics • Rapid growth begins • Awkward appearance	• Height growth peaks • Body shape and composition change • Acne and odor • Menarche/spermarche	• Physically mature • Slower growth
Cognitive and moral	• Concrete operations • Unable to perceive long-term outcomes of current decision-making • Avoids punishment by following rules	• Emergence of abstract thought (formal operations) • May perceive future implications, but may not apply in decision-making • Sees the perspective of others	• Future-oriented with sense of perspective • idealism • Increased independent thinking
Self-concept/identity formation	• Preoccupied with changing body • Self-conscious about appearance and attractiveness	• Concern with attractiveness • Increasing introspection	• More stable body image • Attractiveness may still be of concern • Firmer self-identity
Family	• Increased need for privacy • Increased bid for independence	• Conflicts over control and independence • Struggle for acceptance of greater authority	• Emotional and physical separation from family • Increased autonomy
Peers	• Seeks same-sex peer affiliation to counter instability	• Intense peer group involvement • Preoccupation with peer culture • Peers provide behavioral example	• Peer group and values recede in importance • Intimacy/possible commitment takes precedence
Sexual	• Increased interest in sexual anatomy • Anxieties and questions about genital changes, size • Limited dating and intimacy	• Testing ability to attract partner • Initiation of relationships and sexual activity • Explores sexual identity	• Consolidation of sexual identity • Focus on intimacy and formation of stable relationships • Planning for future and commitment

From Kleigman RM, St. Geme JW, et al. *Nelson Textbook of Pediatrics.* Elsevier; 2020:1015.

In contrast to males, female teens can feel a diminished sense of attractiveness as their bodies mature and they begin menstruation. While both early-maturing boys and girls demonstrate more risky behaviors than those who are late maturing, girls are at greater risk as a result of romantic liaisons, as these early bloomers often get "bumped up" to an older group of peers and become the objects of sexual attention from older males. Of note, the body of early-maturing females may not match their emotional maturity. This difference influences decision-making and behavior, often placing them at increased risk for sexual activity, dating abuse, depressive symptoms, and antisocial behavior.[24,25]

Cognitive Changes. Adolescents enter what Piaget referred to as *formal operations*, a phase characterized by using propositional thinking and abstract reasoning. The principal difference between concrete and formal operations is the emerging ability to reason using verbal manipulation. In early adolescence, thinking is still very concrete, but most teens acquire increasing sophistication in abstract thought by 14 years of age. What makes things particularly volatile during adolescence is that different parts of the brain change at different times. For example, the frontal lobe, which controls executive function, is one of the last parts of the brain to fully mature. This lag can

lead to lapses in judgment, an increase in risk-taking behavior, and mood swings.

As they learn to conceptualize past and future events and relate actions to consequences, adolescents begin to:
• Question values, often challenging familiar ones.
• Understand the concepts of good and evil and variations in human nature (e.g., not all authority figures are good people).
• Notice contradictions between what is said and what is done (e.g., when parents tell them not to smoke or drink even although the parents do; when parents tell them to wear their seat belts although the parents do not).
• Understand the significance of their existence within the construct of time (past, present, and future) and what they want or will be doing in the future (e.g., college, technical school, job, marriage, and family).

While neurologic changes underlie executive function, memory, social inhibition, intelligence, and cognitive development in adolescence, emerging evidence indicates that a combination of environmental influences (e.g., drugs, alcohol, and stress) and genetic susceptibility can have long-term effects on brain structure, cognitive ability, memory, and higher executive function.[13,26] Up

• BOX 13.1 Tips for Parents

- Start with clear rules and expectations before children are teenagers. Work on good communication with children early and continue through adolescence. State expectations and future consequences before trouble occurs (e.g., identify curfew expectations before the dance, not when the teen comes home late).
- Be firm and consistent with follow through.
- Be flexible and allow teens to negotiate safety-related rules. Do not negotiate rules that are nonnegotiable.
- Fighting and arguing are often used by teens as they practice their developing reasoning skills. If parents are stressed or tired, they should disengage and walk away. Try not to take what teens say too personally.
- Teens want and need their parents to be involved, concerned, and ask questions. They just may not know it or know how to express it.
- Know who their friends are; call those parents from time to time. Compare household rules and risks (e.g., guns, smoking, drinking, supervision) if possible.
- Be involved with their schoolwork and at their school. Try to meet their teachers and stay in contact with them.
- Continue to involve teens in family activities, even when they no longer want to. Encouraging them to include friends helps.
- Keep your promises; it builds trust and respect.
- Model good behavior. Adolescents recognize the hypocrite of saying one thing and doing another.
- Don't forget that teens still need adult supervision at times.
- Keep communication lines open; start conversations. Adolescents sometimes want to talk to adults but are nervous or do not know how to bring up a topic.

to one-third of adolescents never achieve fully developed formal operational thinking, even as adults.

Communication

As with motor development, communication abilities are mature; however, communication skills are variable and particularly challenging for parents. Understanding how our basic information needs are affected by adolescent development can be helpful, especially for parents (Table 13.2).

Common Developmental Issues for Adolescents

Risk-Taking Behaviors

Adolescence is a time of developing autonomy, yet many adolescents encounter situations they are ill-prepared to navigate. Risk-taking behaviors continue to be a major contributor to morbidity and mortality for adolescents.[27] Risk-taking behaviors include drug, alcohol, and nicotine use, as well as risky sexual and physical actions, all of which can have significant long-term health consequences. Consequently, many adolescent healthcare visits are for treatment of preventable conditions or injuries that could have been avoided, especially if a risk behavior assessment had been conducted.[28] In the era of increased technological advances, risk-taking behaviors now include inappropriate use of social media (e.g., cyberbullying, "sexting") and unsafe use of mobile devices (e.g., texting while driving). It is a paradox of adolescence that developmental tasks (i.e., gaining independence, developing one's own values, becoming comfortable with one's body, and establishing meaningful relationships) may be achieved, albeit in negative ways, through risk-taking behavior. Adolescents in need of peer affiliation simultaneously strive for increased autonomy while exploring, experimenting, and otherwise pushing the limits of their personal experience—often in ways that put them at risk for health-compromising outcomes. It is important to recognize that risk-taking is important, as teens learn to test their sense of self and limits, understanding that risk-taking does not always equate to risky behaviors as many adolescents engage in risk-taking behaviors without negative outcomes.

Adolescents vary tremendously in their ability to think abstractly about the consequences of their behavior and/or actions, and often rationalize by thinking "it can't happen to me," especially when it comes to emotionally charged topics (e.g., peer acceptance, sex). An adolescent who drinks may be doing so to feel less inhibited, be accepted by peers and/or feel a sense of independence and maturity. Because the behavior meets important developmental needs, it may be difficult for the adolescent to look at it objectively or use their advancing cognitive skills. In addition, the effect of alcohol and drugs further limits the adolescent's reasoning ability.

Assessment

Environmental factors also influence adolescents' decisions to take risks, including lack of sleep, negative or deviant behavior role models, constructive relationships and support (or their absence), poverty, or a history of or ongoing adversity (e.g., ACEs). At the same time, protective factors can counter these factors and help adolescents make healthier lifestyle choices. It is important for adolescents to have active parental influence during these critical years, as safe, stable, and nurturing relationships buffer adversity and build resilience (see Chapter 6).[29] Adolescents with multiple risk factors and few protective factors are more likely to engage in risky behaviors. These adolescents need prompt attention and ongoing assessment. Conversely, adolescents who do well or are flourishing, despite multiple risk factors, should be acknowledged and applauded, calling attention to the protective factors in their lives.

While the PCP should assess for risky behavior, equal attention should be given to the assessment of protective factors. Examples of protective factors are[11]:
- High self-esteem
- Parental engagement and family connectedness
- Relationships with caring adults
- Community engagement (e.g., school, religious institutions, volunteering)
- Sense of future
- Academic success
- Strong executive functioning and coping skills
- Access to recreation

All adolescents should be assessed for their level of risk-taking behavior. The PCP's approach to discussing sensitive issues should include ensuring confidentiality, providing privacy, using constructive communication strategies, and establishing rapport. The HEEADSSS technique is a method of assessing risk behavior. Areas for assessment include *H*ome, *E*ducation and employment, *E*ating, *A*ctivities, *D*rugs, *S*exuality, *S*uicide/depression, and *S*afety (Box 13.2).[30] PCPs also need to be alert for developmental red flags because inconsistencies and delays in development may contribute to negative behavior (Table 13.3).

The following are considered risky behaviors:
- Tobacco or nicotine use
- Substance use or abuse, including alcohol
- Poor academic performance

TABLE 13.2 Basic Information Needs

Basic Information Needs	As the Adolescent Ventures out Into the Larger World
The Need to Know • Being adequately informed and assured	• Parents have an increased need to know about what is happening in their child's life. • Adolescents have a greater need to know not just about the world but that parents will be there with support should they have need.
The Need to be Known • Being adequately understood and recognized	• Parents have an increased need for their rules and restraints to be understood. • Adolescents have more need for parents to recognize their readiness to make more of their own decisions.
The Need Not to Know • Being spared information that feels disturbing or excessive	• Parents have a need not to know about all the misadventures and misfortunes that happen to other young people who their teenager knows of or personally knows. • Adolescents (with enough fears already) need not to know about the host of worries that are constantly preying on parental minds.
The Need Not to be Known • The need for concealment and privacy	• Parents do not want the adolescent to know how anxious they are about the risks of their increasing worldly freedoms. • Adolescents protect their freedom by becoming more selective about what personal information they choose to disclose to parents.

Modified from Pickhardt CE. How Communication becomes more complicated in adolescence, 2011. https://www.psychologytoday.com/us/blog/surviving-your-childs-adolescence/201108/how-communication-becomes-more-complicated-in#:~:text=With%20onset%20of%20adolescence%20%28around%20ages%209%20-,to%20create%20more%20separation%2C%20usually%20wants%20significantly%20less

- Risky sexual activity (e.g., multiple partners, unprotected sexual intercourse)
- Drinking and driving
- Body dysmorphia or eating disorders (see Chapter 29)
- Behaviors that result in injury or violence
- Delinquency or involvement with gangs
- Violence-related behavior (e.g., carrying weapons, threatening violence)
- Mental or psychiatric disorders
- Signs or symptoms of physical, mental, sexual, or emotional abuse
- Poor nutrition and physical inactivity
- Inappropriate use of social media or technology devices

The consequences of these risky behaviors can include addiction, school failure, pregnancy, sexually transmitted infections (STIs), injuries, conviction for driving under the influence, incarceration, and even death. Of note, half of all STI cases in the United States occur in 15- to 24-year-olds.[31]

• BOX 13.2 HEEADSSS Assessment: Related Questions

The HEEADSSS assessment focuses on adolescent relationships with others, functioning at school and work, self-efficacy, resilience, and independent decision-making.

Home: Who lives with you? How are your relationships with the other people with whom you live? Have there been any changes at home? Do you feel safe at home?

Education/employment: What do you like and dislike about school? How is school going? How are your grades? Have you ever had trouble at school? Do you work? How many hours do you work? Where do you work? Do you have friends at school? At work?

Eating: Are you comfortable with your body? Are you interested in gaining or losing weight? How do you manage your weight? Tell me about how often you exercise. Tell me about what you normally eat every day.

Activities: What do you do for fun? What types of things do you like to do with your friends? What types of things do you like to do with your family? Do you play sports? Are you in clubs or other organizations? How much time do you watch TV? Use the computer? Text? Listen to music? What types of activities do you like to do online? On your phone?

Drugs: Do you, anyone in your family, or your friends use drugs, tobacco, or alcohol? Have you ever used performance-enhancing drugs?

Sexuality: Do you date? Have you ever had a romantic relationship? What do you consider to be sex? Have you ever had sex? How many partners have you had? Are you interested in males or females or both? Have you ever had someone hurt or threaten you sexually? Do you use birth control or condoms? How often?

Suicide/depression: Do you ever feel like you are all alone or no one cares? Do you feel sad most of the time? Have you ever thought of hurting yourself? Do you ever need to use drugs (alcohol, tobacco, street drugs) to make you feel better? Have you lost interest in being with friends or doing things you previously liked to do?

Safety: Have you ever been hurt by or threatened by someone (who)? Have you ever been seriously injured? Do you use sports safety equipment? Do you use seat belts? Do you text/talk when you drive? Do you ever feel unsafe (where)? Have you ever been bullied? Have you ever met (or do you plan on meeting) someone you first met online?

Management

The PCP's role is to give the adolescent information and guidance to facilitate the teen making the best-informed decisions possible. PCPs can advocate for adolescents, involve their families, communities, and schools, and continue to assess whether they have at least one adult in their lives who cares for them. Consider focused interventions with at-risk adolescents when their behavior interferes with attainment of developmental tasks or threatens their health, safety, and/or wellbeing. Adolescents who pierce their noses, shave half of their hair, and opt to spend evenings with friends rather than family may be irritating to parents, but these behaviors are often a reflection of teens establishing their autonomy and identity, as well as learning about relationships outside of their families. Tattooing and body piercing are concerning, especially if they are associated with high-risk behavior(s), and body modification should be differentiated from nonsuicidal self-injury (NSSI).[32]

High-risk teens require numerous services. PCPs need to know their state laws regarding adolescent health issues and decision-making ability, how to access community resources, and how to engage other professionals, as needed. The following list identifies a sample of basic services that at-risk teenagers may need:

- Food resources for teen parents and their children
- Transportation vouchers

TABLE 13.3   Developmental Red Flags: Adolescence

Age	Physical and Sexual Development	Social-Emotional Development	Cognitive Development
All phases of adolescence	*Physical development:* • Poor vision close or distant • Kyphosis or scoliosis • Poor nutrition, poor oral health, caries, malocclusion • Loss of appetite/underweight • Chronic disease, such as heart disease, hypertension, dyslipidemia, diabetes, or a family member with a chronic or lifelong illness • No physical activity; overweight • Sleep disturbance	• Substance abuse; blackouts • Permissive or authoritarian parental style • No participation in home chores • History of family violence • School fights • No close/best friend • No identified peer group • Friends or siblings in gangs • Cruelty to animals • Sexual orientation worries • Pervasive sad mood, feelings of hopelessness, suicidal thoughts or gestures, history of previous suicide attempt • Flattened affect without expressions of joy, sorrow, or excitement • Excessive worrying or rumination • Negative self-concept/worth; describes self as "ugly" or "fat" • Dieting despite normal body size and shape	• Low IQ • Behind in grade or failing classes • Chronic absenteeism or class skipping • Attention problems • Lack of organizational skills for homework • Disruptive behavior • Lack of impulse control • Unable to control own behavior (e.g., anger, impulsivity)
Early adolescence (11–14 years)	• Less than SMR stage 2 • (Female) Short stature/absence of height spurt • Early bloomer • Early sexual experimentation	*Sexuality:* • Fears about emerging sexuality/sexual orientation *Self-concept:* • Does not fantasize or dream about adult career	• Unable to identify feelings
Middle adolescence (15–17 years)	• Kyphosis or scoliosis • Less than SMR stage 4 • (Male) Short stature/absence of height spurt • Male muscular growth without testicular maturation • Male persistent gynecomastia and acne • Female primary or secondary amenorrhea • Risky sexual activity, including unprotected sexual intercourse and multiple sexual partners	• Drinking and driving • Excessively oppositional, defiant with all authority • Abusive dating relationships • Sexual orientation worries	• Unable to differentiate emotional states from physical states • Poor judgment
Late adolescence (18–21 years)	• Less than SMR stage 4 or 5 • Risky sexual activity, including unprotected sexual intercourse and multiple sexual partners	• No life goals • Does not fantasize or dream about adult career • Drinking and driving • Lacks intimate relationships • Unable to separate from peer groups • Unable to separate from parents • Unable to keep a job • Sexual orientation worries	• High school dropout • Persistent egocentrism • Unable to reason or plan based on future and abstract concepts • Consistent/Pattern of poor judgment • Chronic healthcare seeking for psychosomatic complaints

IQ, Intelligence quotient; *SMR,* sexual maturity rating.

• Temporary shelter
• Counseling and mental health services
• Foster care services for teen parents and their children
• Local medical and social work services
• Local juvenile justice system and protective services
• Drug rehabilitation programs specifically designed for adolescents
• Alternative school and vocational education programs
• Sports, fitness, and community activities, including after-school programs
• Community support programs (e.g., Big Brothers/Big Sisters)

Tobacco Use

Tobacco use is a leading cause of preventable death, and adults who smoke often report smoking before the age 18 years. Many adolescents experiment with tobacco use but may stop after a short period before becoming addicted to nicotine. Tobacco dependence (addiction) varies from one individual to another and can appear at any time after initiating tobacco use, so prevention and early intervention are essential. As previously discussed, the adolescent brain is particularly susceptible to the influence of substances (like nicotine), and there is a resulting higher rate of dependence in teenagers than in adults.

Despite decreases in traditional cigarette use, the rates of alternative tobacco product (ATP) use, including hookahs and electronic nicotine delivery systems (ENDS) such as electronic cigarettes (e-cigarettes), continue to increase. E-cigarettes are now the most commonly used tobacco product among youth,[33] with appealing flavors and small and inconspicuous devices. The National Youth Tobacco Survey reported 11.3% of high school students and 2.8% of middle school students currently use e-cigarette products.[33] E-cigarette use is highest in males and Hispanic and non-Hispanic White youth. The US Food and Drug Administration (FDA) issued guidance to address the increased use of ENDS, with strategies to enforce the ban on selling ENDS to minors.[34] According to the 50th Anniversary Surgeon General's Report (https://www.cdc.gov/tobacco/sgr/50th-anniversary/index.htm), over 5 million youth will experience premature death from smoking-related illnesses. E-cigarette use is also associated with the use of alcohol, marijuana, and other risky behaviors.[35]

Assessment

Annual health supervision visits and/or sports/work participation exams serve as an opportunity to screen for substance use (see AAP Periodicity table).[36] Both the Substance Abuse and Mental Health Services Administration and the AAP recommend that PCPs not only screen for substance use, but also use a brief intervention and, if indicated, refer to treatment. One approach is ACT: *A*sk about tobacco use at each visit, *C*ounsel on smoking cessation if screen is positive, and *T*reat by linking youth with behavioral health specialists if indicated.[37] Ask adolescents whether they (or their friends) smoke or use other forms of tobacco and the specific types of use (e-cigarettes, hookahs) at all visits.

Management

The PCP's primary goal is to keep teens from starting use; however, in those teens who do use, the goal is cessation (Table 13.4). The US Public Health Service promotes the use of cognitive-behavioral strategies, motivational interviewing, and examining the effects of social influences on smoking. Interventions need to be tailored to the adolescent's context and readiness to change. One strategy is to provide the adolescent with a quit line referral number such as 800-QUIT-NOW and 800-44U-QUIT. These telephone-based interventions have been shown to help with tobacco cessation.[38] Smokefree is a text-based service where one can text QUIT to IQUIT (47848).[39]

Education should specifically address the avoidance of ATPs and ENDS, as many adolescents view these products as "safer" than traditional cigarettes.[35] Factors associated with adolescent smoking cessation include enforcing public policy that bans smoking in educational and recreational settings, enhancing self-efficacy, and developing plans to manage cravings as they quit smoking.[40] Another important tobacco exposure source is parental tobacco use. Parental tobacco use increases the risk of their child using and becoming tobacco dependent. Anticipatory guidance should address adverse effects of secondhand smoke on the adolescent's health. Evidence shows that even short messages can

TABLE 13.4	Tobacco Use Cessation Strategies for Adolescents: Primary and Secondary Prevention	
Primary Prevention	**Secondary Prevention**
• Provide multimedia, multisite health information, not limited to schools • Use Social Norms Theory to encourage adolescent to forgo tobacco use • Emphasize skills to avoid peer pressure • Focus on adolescents' developmental need to belong to a social group	• Ask at every visit whether adolescent or friends use tobacco • Inform adolescent of health risks of tobacco use and how one becomes addicted to nicotine; emphasize it is easier to stop early • Use brief motivational interviewing to spark interest in tobacco cessation • Determine realistic stop-use date • Help adolescent identify barriers to stopping and ways to overcome those barriers • Provide information about self-help and support groups; encourage adolescent to try to stop smoking with a friend • Provide nicotine pharmacologic cessation therapy, where appropriate • Schedule follow-up visits to monitor progress; reinforce positive efforts • Assess parents' tobacco use patterns; provide information/support to stop use

improve smoking cessation rates in families. Pharmacologic treatments can be offered for those with moderate to severe tobacco dependence, although with caution, as these agents are only FDA approved for use in adults.[41]

Nonsuicidal Self-Injurious Behaviors

NSSI is a group of repetitive behaviors with the intent of causing physical harm to oneself but not with the intent of ending one's own life.[42] Repetition is the key as signs and symptoms must have occurred at least five times within the past year and be associated with at least two of the following[43]:
- Previous negative emotions
- Preoccupation with and a repetitive desire to engage in the activity
- Feelings of relief from negative emotions or a sensation of positive feelings with activity
- Impaired interpersonal relationships.

NSSI behaviors vary widely and include cutting (the most common mechanism), scraping, hitting, burning or ripping of skin, subdermal tissue, or hair; hindering wound healing (does not include scab picking); and head banging.[32,44] Piercings and tattoos are not usually included, as most are seen as socially acceptable.[32] The common factor among NSSI is that they are used to relieve distress, anger, stress, and other negative emotions. Research demonstrates engaging in NSSI causes decrease in negative affect and arousal and an increase in positive emotions. NSSI typically begins in mid- to late adolescence and declines in early adulthood, but at least 20% of those with NSSI behavior recall they began before age 12 years.[43,45] Prevalence rates vary widely across studies, from 2% to 49%; however, rates potentially increased during the COVID-19 pandemic.[46–48]

NSSI is not suicidal behavior; however, individuals who engage in NSSI are more likely to attempt suicide or have an eating disorder, an abuse or trauma history, a mood disorder, or psychological distress than those in the general population and should be assessed for suicide risk. As many as 70% of those with a history of NSSI have had at least one prior suicide attempt. Characteristics of NSSI that are associated with increased risk of suicidality include more frequent NSSI behaviors, NSSI occurring over a longer period, multiple methods of NSSI, more severe methods used (such as burning), history of abuse, and coexisting psychiatric disorders (borderline personality disorder, posttraumatic stress disorder).[44] Although NSSI is a component of borderline personality disorder, it can be present in those without borderline personality disorder.[32,44,47]

Assessment

A mental health assessment is needed when adolescents present with suspected NSSI. History should focus on the type(s) of self-injury, a description of the frequency of these behaviors, and what responses/benefits the adolescent gets by doing self-injury (e.g., The Non-Suicidal Self-Injury Assessment Tool [NSSI-AT]: http://www.selfinjury.bctr.cornell.edu/perch/resources/fnssi.pdf). Although self-injuries decrease emotional pain, they can also result in guilt. Therefore adolescents who engage in NSSI often hide evidence of their activities, mask physical evidence, and will deny or not disclose their NSSI behaviors, thus making diagnosis difficult. Suspicion should be raised if adolescents present with hoodies or heavy clothing on hot days, or when there is resistance to a thorough examination. The most common locations for NSSI injuries are the arms, legs, and front of the torso. There may be scratches or cuts in various stages of healing or that appear to be in patterns or form words. Traction alopecia may be present. The presence of any wounds should be recognized as a call for help. Adolescents should also be assessed for suicidality because NSSI can be a predictive factor for future suicide attempts (see Chapter 29). Further, given the association of NSSI with abuse (see Chapter 22), these adolescents should be assessed for physical and emotional signs of maltreatment.

Management

Those who self-injure will often accept help during acute phases but lose motivation for help when symptoms are not acute. Appropriate therapeutic interventions include cognitive behavioral, dialectical behavioral, and family therapy. The best therapeutic response is usually contingent on the self-injurer feeling emotions, with the goal being the development of positive emotional coping skills. Prompt referral to a mental health professional is needed if symptoms of psychosis or suicide ideation are present[44]; however, not all adolescents with NSSI need a psychiatric referral. Those who are experimenting with self-injury, or who engaged in NSSI because of peer pressure and show no other signs of mental disorder may not require immediate intervention but do need close follow-up.

Technology and Social Media Use

Technology can facilitate connectivity and social interaction, and social media use can be a positive influence when used appropriately. It is no surprise that adolescents spend up to 9 hours a day on different screens, and approximately 66% of adolescents own a smartphone and actively use at least one social media site.[49] Although there are benefits of social media and technology devices (e.g., developing friendships, increased self-esteem, social support), there are also hazards.[50] Cyberbullying includes having negative information reported about them, having personal information made public online; being filmed without consent and the video then being posted online; and/or receiving unwanted emails, messages, or texts. Peer cybervictimization affects millions of US adolescents and increases the risk of substance abuse, depression, and suicidality.[51,52]

Assessment

Parents and PCPs need to have open discussions with adolescents regarding their social media use to identify risky social media usage including:
- Cyberbullying and harassment
- Sexting (e.g., sending nude or provocative photos, and/or sexual messages)
- Depression and social withdrawal
- Problematic use (e.g., obsessive social media use, including avoiding interactions with others to engage online, getting in trouble because of social media use)
- Meeting/engaging with strangers through online profiles
- Using mobile devices while driving

Management

There is often a technology gap between adolescents who have grown up with computers, tablets, and smartphones, and adults (including PCPs) who began technology use later in life. It is common for teens to state that adults do not understand how "everyone" uses social media and how not being able to may have a negative social impact. PCPs can remind adolescents that any posts can, and possibly will be, shared with others and that digital footprints can be accessed years later and negatively impact their future (e.g., university admission, employment). Many adolescents do not realize that the possession of nude or suggestive photos can be considered child pornography, although enforcement of this varies from state to state.[53,54] One rule to share with teens is not to post when they are emotionally upset (e.g., angry, sad, scared), as spur-of-the-moment actions often lead to bad outcomes in the short and long term. Further, while many online profiles are real, there are also some that are complete fabrications, designed to initiate a meeting with others under false pretenses.

Parents need to have frequent, open conversations with adolescents about internet and social media use. The AAP (2018) developed an online family media plan tool that helps families decide how to establish guidelines and set limits on media (www.healthychildren.org/English/media/Pages/default.aspx). In addition, parents should address the issue of devices and distraction, especially the dangers of using mobile devices while driving. One study examining adolescents and motor vehicle crashes found that distractions (using a cell phone, looking for something in the vehicle, grooming, etc.) were a contributing factor almost 60% of the time. Young drivers make up a substantial portion of those involved in fatal car crashes, and 1 in 10 were distracted at the time of the crash.[55,56]

Finally, PCPs and parents need to highlight the negative impact of media devices on sleep. Nearly one-third of adolescents wake up during the night to check their devices, and screen use before sleep interferes with sleep latency and quality.[57] Encourage parents to establish a central location outside of the teen's bedroom to charge and store devices overnight. Parents and PCPs also need to highlight the benefits of adequate sleep, the negative consequences of poor sleep, and how to establish nighttime routines that promote healthy sleep, including avoiding electronic media use before sleep.

Health Supervision and Surveillance

General Guidelines

Primary care visits with adolescents are grounded in good interviewing techniques, which include demonstrating respect, establishing parameters, using appropriate body language, active listening, and communication techniques, and working with the adolescent to develop a realistic, individualized treatment plan. Each encounter needs to underscore that the PCP and teen are a team, that the teen's concerns are important, that no judgments will be made, and that the primary focus is working together to achieve the healthiest outcome possible. It is important to be transparent with the teen, sharing mandated reporting and/or information sharing requirements.

Preserving confidentiality is essential. Adolescents should be reassured that the provider will not share information with their parent or caregiver (*general* confidentiality) unless the adolescent agrees, or unless the health of the child or others may be compromised (e.g., threat of potential suicide, violence, evidence of an eating disorder). Providers must inform the teenager that there are limits to confidentiality (*limited* confidentiality). As mandatory reporters, PCPs are required by law to report information that puts the teen or others in danger (e.g., abuse, homicidal ideation). These mandates vary by state (e.g., some states require reporting teen sexual activity, even if consensual, if an age difference of 3 or more years exists between partners). This proactive approach supports the adolescent while also offering protection from the parent who may be abusive or unsafe. Sharing this approach upfront with the teen and parent not only sets the stage for trust, but also reduces the problem of parents who are upset if they feel they are being denied information.

Establishing trust is paramount, as teens are more likely to disclose sensitive and relevant details about their health concerns, behaviors, and risks. The way confidential care is provided may influence healthcare utilization for the rest of the patient's life.[7] A questionnaire or checklist may be an effective way to collect information for teenagers who are hesitant to discuss sensitive issues. Questionnaires used to identify adolescent strengths were created by the Search Institute (see Chapter 6) and have been used by communities to enhance adolescent self-concept, whereas programs like the Rapid Assessment for Adolescent Preventative Services (RAAPS) help PCPs identify risky adolescent behaviors (see Additional Resources).

Assessment and Screening

Physical Development. Adolescents should have height, weight, body mass index (BMI), and growth trajectory documented at each health maintenance visit. The SMR should be recorded to evaluate progression of pubertal changes. Assess testicular growth by palpation and sizing using a standardized orchidometer. Self-assessment is generally reliable, and adolescent males can be asked to evaluate their own development level if provided with standards against which to compare themselves. Varicocele, or enlarged veins palpable in the scrotum, may develop at sexual maturity and are not cause for alarm unless a discrepancy in testicular size is noted on examination. Gynecomastia in boys

should be noted, especially beyond SMR 3. Scoliosis may develop rapidly during puberty, and assessment should be done annually with careful attention to SMRs and PHV. For example, a female with mild scoliosis, SMR 4, and who had menses 2 years ago is less cause for concern than a female with mild scoliosis, SMR 2 who has not had menarche, as this teen may need close monitoring throughout the growth spurt. Each teen should be asked how they feel about their own physical growth and development. Dissatisfaction with body appearance might warrant further probing to elicit unhealthy behavior (e.g., binging and purging, steroid use; see Chapter 29 for information about eating disorders). The thyroid gland should be palpated, with special attention to the presence of a Delphian node, as autoimmune thyroid disorders (e.g., Hashimoto thyroiditis) can occur in this age group.

Social and Emotional Development. Key areas to assess in social and emotional development include adolescents' emerging independence from family, relationships with peers, and goals for the future, especially as they enter late adolescence. Adolescents need to be interviewed about school, family, and peer relationships; exposure to violence, abuse, or weapons; mental health issues, such as mood, depression, anger problems, or suicidal ideation; sexuality, sexual activity, and sexual orientation; safety (e.g., use of seat belts, driving, drowning); and involvement in risky behaviors, such as tobacco, alcohol, prescription or street drug use; and eating disorders.

Cognitive Development. Cognitive assessment includes the following: questions about school attendance, school performance, and educational or career goals. School connectedness is a significant predictor of adolescent wellbeing; however, the extent to which a teen connects to school depends on characteristics of both the teen and the school. A teen's exposure to a school-based health center is also associated with school connectedness.[58] School connectedness was an important factor with remote learning during the COVID-19 pandemic, as students with more connections to others at school had lower rates of poor mental health outcomes, such as hopelessness and suicidality.[59] Chronic absenteeism, class skipping, and other types of school avoidance indicate a problem that may be related to cognitive ability and should be assessed in depth. Objective assessment of cognitive development, as with school-age children, requires formal psychological testing, which is best done, if needed, through schools. Children who are behind a grade have a much greater risk of dropping out of school, thus leading some to consider school failure as a form of adolescent failure to thrive.

Parent Assessment. Parents of teens need advice, support, and encouragement. Characteristic adolescent mood swings can strain family relationships and lead to arguments. Parents with balanced approaches that include unconditional love, clear boundaries, and consistent discipline are more likely to have adolescents with less depression, less risk-taking, and better academic success than authoritarian parents. It is important to assess parental concerns about their adolescent's health at each visit because their concerns provide additional insight into the teen's physical, socioemotional, and mental health, as well as a glimpse into the family functioning and the parent-teen dynamics. If problems exist in the parent's view, or there is a discrepancy between the parent and teen, or a potential conflict emerges in the interviews, the PCP can facilitate mediation and/or intervention, as needed.

Anticipatory Guidance

Anticipatory guidance should be individualized to help the adolescent understand, respond to, and take responsibility for their own behavior and development (Table 13.5). Separate discussions

TABLE 13.5   Adolescent Area of Development and Related Anticipatory Guidance

Area of Development	Anticipatory Guidance
Physical	
Experience rapid growth and development in transition from prepubescence to sexual maturity	• Teach about emerging body functions (e.g., menstruation, nocturnal emissions, unexpected erections) for both sexes/genders • Teach about the timing and descriptions of primary and secondary sexual characteristics of both genders (e.g., changes in breasts, genitals, and hair) • Discuss masturbation • Discuss sexual orientation/feelings
Reach adult parameters of height/physical growth by late adolescence	• Provide counseling regarding safety and unintentional injuries • Teach and encourage correct and consistent use of helmets, seat belts, and proper sports equipment • Emphasize safety and responsibility regarding access to/use of guns and other weapons
Become comfortable with one's body	• Offer reassurance that physical changes are normal; anticipate what they should expect; listen to concerns; encourage physical activity/exercise, sports participation, and body fitness; encourage healthy nutrition and sleep patterns
Cognitive	
Move from concrete thinking to formal operations and the ability to reason abstractly	• Emphasize value of successful school completion • Discuss how to balance academic responsibilities with other activities • Explain how changes in cognitive abilities may contribute to "overthinking" or a sense of confusion; encourage teen to do "reality checks" with a trusted adult • Engage adolescent in conversation, explain procedures, and answer questions; listen
Develop personal value system and moral integrity	• Encourage discussion of what the adolescent believes is important and finds valuable • Help the adolescent develop skills in conflict resolution and prevention • Discuss how learning to identify feelings is the first step in understanding how feelings influence mental and physical processes • Discuss respect for rights, needs, and opinions of others; teach that maturation involves understanding and appreciating multicultural differences
Move from dependence on others to self for risk reduction	• Provide information about how to manage peer pressure to engage in risky behavior • Discuss injury prevention strategies at home, work, and school; emphasize dangers of weapons
Social and Emotional	
Establish independence from parents	• Explain to parents an adolescent's need for privacy and that not joining in all family activities is not a sign of rejection of the family; some privacy within the home should be expected/provided
Develop sense of self-identity	• Encourage adolescents to take responsibility for their own health care • Encourage adolescents to take on new challenges; discuss future plans (e.g., school, work, and family) • Help adolescents identify their own personal strengths and joys

Create new relationships with peers and adults	• Discuss importance of activities with peers; identify healthy ways to be part of a group
	• Provide counseling on:
	  • Avoiding gang involvement
	  • Bullying, which may be physical, emotional, or sexual
	  • Preventing the use of drugs, cigarettes, and alcohol
	  • Stopping substance use for those who are using
	• Discuss the notion that maturation includes increased independence and increased responsibility at home, school, and in the community
	• Encourage participation in community activities
	• Provide information and opportunity to discuss questions regarding sexuality, sexual responsibilities, and protection from unintended pregnancy and STIs
	• Discuss dating; emphasize that healthy relationships are based on mutual respect and address how to prevent/report date rape or abusive relationships
	• Advocate for safe social media usage/sharing

STI, Sexually transmitted infection.

need to be conducted with parents to help them understand and support their teen's maturation and need for independence. In these discussions, the PCP should clarify which values and expectations parents have for their teen and how the teen perceives those expectations.

In the following sections, specific discussion points are outlined in each of the adolescent phases. While they can be incorporated into the health supervision visit, they are not all-inclusive, and they often cannot be covered exhaustively at each visit. Ideas for assessment and management of specific problems that emerge from these discussions can be found in other chapters (e.g., see Chapter 7—Sexuality Issues).

Early Adolescence (11–14 Years)

Early adolescence is often the most difficult adolescent adjustment period. Rapid physical changes occur simultaneously with changes in all parts of the adolescent's life, yet their cognitive skills may not keep pace with physical changes and their emotions may interfere with or overwhelm their ability to understand and cope. The "early" adolescent is often confused and even frightened by the rate and breadth of change being experienced. Accordingly, they can be difficult to be around; yet, because of this "difficulty," the response(s) from parents and other adults may be exactly the opposite of the support, caring, and understanding they desperately need.

Physical Development

The onset and rate of physical changes in early adolescence varies widely, with some teens exiting early adolescence (at approximately 14 years) still at SMR 2, while others are at SMR 4 and almost their adult height. Close attention to the onset and sequence of changes is a priority for the PCP, while simultaneously monitoring the teen's response to the changes.

Social and Emotional Development

The early adolescent is beginning to renegotiate relationships with parents, other significant adults, and peers. While they may not yet be a part of an adolescent subculture, they can appear to be anti-adult and often find themselves in between the two, feeling lonely. They begin to prefer friends over family, and often report their parents to be an embarrassment. This social behavior pattern is a step toward maturity and independence, as one of the ways of demonstrating independence is to challenge parental authority. Parents may report the early adolescent as more argumentative and disobedient, refusing to do chores, and wanting to renegotiate rules (e.g., curfews, allowance, household responsibilities).

Wide mood swings are characteristically present in the early adolescent. They may shift from euphoria to sadness within a matter of minutes, characterized by their transient nature, commonly measured in hours or days. These emotional fluctuations need to be distinguished from the unremitting, long-standing mood and behavior changes of serious depressive disorders. Further, as they adjust to the physical changes of puberty, they may begin to spend more time in front of the mirror combing their hair, checking their skin, and putting on makeup. Clothes and appearance become more important for most teens, including those with a developmental delay or disability. The onset of secondary sex characteristics typically increases anxieties about menstruation, nocturnal emissions, uncontrolled erections, masturbation, and breast or penis size. This is an opportune time for the PCP to dispel myths (e.g., masturbation causes blindness or acne) and provide focused anticipatory guidance (e.g., a premenarcheal girl often has vaginal leukorrhea, a clear, mucoid discharge); however, they may find these conversations awkward at first. These discussions can be challenging, as early adolescents have a desire for greater privacy, often spending more time in their room alone listening to music, using social media, texting, or talking on the phone. They may magnify their problems and believe that no one could possibly understand what they are feeling.

The development of new types of friendships appears, as a greater number of opportunities become possible. Same-sex friendships occur, usually with one best friend. These strong friendships may lead to fleeting same-sex experimentation as sexual feelings emerge and adolescents develop their sexual identity.

Contact with the opposite sex is usually in groups (e.g., middle school dances with boys on one side of the gym and girls on the opposite side). Other typical sexual behaviors of the early adolescent include masturbating, telling "dirty" jokes, making lewd remarks to others, demonstrating interest in watching explicit sexual scenes in the media, or looking at images of nude individuals. Sexual experimentation may vary greatly, depending on the adolescent's subculture and development. For example, by this age some teenagers have already experienced sexual intercourse or pregnancy, whereas others have not even held hands.

Cognitive Development

As their thinking abilities develop, teens daydream frequently. Parents and teachers need to be reminded that daydreaming is needed cognitive work (and space) for adolescents; it is where they work on and through their identities as well as the changes in and around them. Early adolescents begin developing their own value system, independent from their family of origin. They may try value systems other than the one that they learned from their family, often leaving family members befuddled or even threatened. As they develop, give early adolescents the opportunity to use their growing reasoning skills to actively problem solve, explore values, and examine the principles on which they make decisions. Early adolescents set idealistic goals that change frequently. One day they want to be an engineer and the next day a pilot or a parent who stays home to raise children. Some adolescents at this age experience a drop or rise in academic performance, depending on their current focus.

Health Supervision and Screening

Annual health supervision visits are recommended. Critical components of the visit include growth and developmental surveillance; assessing social and academic progress, including quality of interpersonal relationships and school performance; identifying emotional wellness (e.g., mood, mental health, sexuality); and risk reduction, including injury prevention, substance use prevention, and healthy sexuality. Immunizations for human papillomavirus (HPV), diphtheria and tetanus toxoids and acellular pertussis vaccine (DTaP), influenza, hepatitis A, and meningococcal meningitis are recommended. Blood pressure monitoring should continue and serum lipoprotein analysis should be done if not done earlier in childhood.

Anticipatory Guidance

Anticipatory guidance for the early adolescent focuses on explaining the rapid changes that are occurring; helping the adolescent in the early process of developing self-concept, autonomy, and independence; and providing reassurance that they are "normal." The following should be specifically discussed:

- Physical changes to expect as puberty progresses
- How the adolescent can best manage the rapid physical changes (e.g., engage in physical activity or sports; focus on injury prevention [e.g., bike helmets]; identify strategies to deal with beginning menstruation while at school; eat a well-balanced diet; get enough sleep)
- Nutritional needs: Increased iron and calcium intake is needed after menarche and during periods of rapid growth.
- Coping strategies the teen and family can use during stressful times and building resilience where needed
- What it means to be sexually responsible, both physically and emotionally; can include abstinence counseling or safe-sex practices/education
- Transition to adult health care: Initiate conversations regarding transitioning to adult health care between 12 and 14 years of

age, especially with teens with special healthcare needs. By age 14 to 15 years, a transition plan should be developed with the adolescent and parent.[60,61]

Middle Adolescence (15–17 Years)

Middle adolescence is characterized by continued changes in physical, cognitive, and socioemotional development. Relationships continue to evolve, peers become increasingly influential, and awareness of one's (and others) appearance is accentuated. With increasing cognitive abilities, middle adolescence often provides opportunities to evaluate and develop the skills necessary for adulthood; however, it is also the time when teens are at highest risk for developing mental health disorders, and sexual and risky behavior experimentation begins.[11]

Physical Development

For most teens, especially females, physical development nears completion. Middle adolescents typically have less concerns about body changes, as they have been dealing with them, but have increased interest in making themselves more "attractive," which can be a relative term. Teens spend more time with hair, clothes, and, for some, diet and focused physical activities (e.g., weightlifting). Middle adolescents often try to defy the limits of their bodies, and many have periods of excessive physical activity followed by periods of lethargy.

Social and Emotional Development

School and extracurricular activities outside the family are often the focus of the middle adolescent's life. Peer group involvement is intense and includes the establishment of a dress code, communication style, and code of conduct. Middle adolescents tend to be more non-adult than anti-adult. The need for peer contact is important for all middle adolescents; however, it is especially important for teens with developmental disabilities and/or chronic conditions, although it can be challenging (e.g., due to parental overprotectiveness, social skills deficits, physical constraints). Sexual drive emerges, with physical urges often preceding emotional maturity. While most begin to explore their ability to attract a partner of the opposite gender, same gender, or gender and sexual minority partner, there is often increased peer (and societal) pressure to experiment with sex. Adolescents report that parents are the main influence on the adolescent's decision about sexual behaviors,[11] something parents need to be reminded of, especially as parent/teen conflicts peak over issues such as curfew, allowance, going to parties or movies, and dating. For both the teen and parent, rules and expectations must be clear and consistent.

Cognitive Development

Intellectual sophistication and creativity increase in middle adolescence. Practicing reasoning, logic, and decision-making strengthens the adolescent's ability to establish healthy evaluative and decision-making skills. They may demonstrate increased concern with neighborhood and societal issues, such as racism, poverty, justice, peace, and the environment (e.g., climate change).

Health Supervision and Screening

Annual health supervision visits are recommended, including annual influenza immunization; growth and developmental surveillance; and assessment of social and academic progress, quality of interpersonal relationships, school performance, and emotional wellness (e.g., mood, mental health). Screening for STIs is needed if the adolescent is sexually active. Papanicolaou (Pap) smears are no longer recommended until after age 21 years, regardless of sexual activity. Tuberculosis screening is often needed as teens enter the workforce, but also if risk factors are identified. If a lipid panel was not completed earlier, or if risk factors emerge, it should be completed. Some PCPs order a screening CBC for females after menses begin, although clinical practice guidelines do not support this practice.

Anticipatory Guidance

Anticipatory guidance for the middle adolescent focuses on the teen's expanding physical, cognitive, and socioemotional capabilities; consolidating self-concept; and identifying areas for continued growth and development. The provider should acknowledge and reinforce healthy behaviors and validate the adolescent's physical, intellectual, and social development. Specifically discuss:

- Physical changes that allow for increasing skills; recommend regular, vigorous physical activity, fitness, and engagement in a wide range of activities
- Risks and dangers related to drug, nicotine, performance-enhancing drugs, caffeine, diet pills, and alcohol use and abuse
- Injury prevention (e.g., bike helmets; seat belts and safe driving; safe and responsible handling and use of weapons)
- Risky behaviors (e.g., technology and social media)
- Involvement in extracurricular activities (e.g., clubs, hobbies, volunteer work, community activities)
- Relationship between nutrition, health, and a positive body image (see Chapters 14 and 29)
- Healthy sleep habits (see Chapter 16)
- Importance of completing high school and making plans for the future
- Sex and sexuality:
  - Responsible/safe sexual behavior(s)
  - Prevention of STIs
  - Birth control, including emergency methods
  - Preventing and reporting date rape or intimate partner violence
  - Sexual orientation
  - Breast or testicular self-examination (Note: although the US Preventive Services Task Force [USPSTF] guidelines do not recommend self-examination,[62] this is common practice and is included in the Bright Futures recommendations, but the USPSTF recommendations are challenged by many)[63,64]
- Existence and nature of peer relationships: Are they based on mutual respect and caring? Gang involvement? Bullying?
- Nature of relationship with parents/caregivers. Are reasonable limits set? Do parents show interest and concern for the teenager?
- Emotional maturity: How does the adolescent resolve conflicts? Manage anger and/or frustration? Reduce stress?
- Mental health assessment (e.g., mood, anxiety) (see Chapter 6)
- Potential for self-harm (e.g., cutting, bingeing and purging)

If a plan for transition to adult health care is not already in place, one needs to be developed. These plans must be based on an assessment of the adolescent's ability to provide self-care, and the needs and desires of the teen and their family. Once in place, plans should be reevaluated annually. Adolescents with developmental or intellectual disabilities require additional support to foster the adolescent's ability to participate to the fullest extent possible in their medical decision making.[60,61]

Late Adolescence (18–21 Years)

Late adolescence is a time of behavioral autonomy. It is when most adolescents have a clearer self-concept, life choices are made, and decisions about how they plan to contribute to society as a responsible adult are implemented.

Physical Development

Physical growth and development are typically complete, although some teens, mostly males, will continue to gain height into their early 20s, as PHV occurs later in males.

Social and Emotional Development

Relationships with parents and family are gradually renegotiated during this phase to a more adult-adult pattern of communication and collaborative decision making, even when they disagree. The role of the parent during late adolescence should be one of support as their adolescent evolves toward young adulthood and reengages with their family. Young adults often develop a modified value system, which is very similar to the one with which they grew up. A substantial number of late adolescents have established their sexuality and entered into an intimate, committed partner relationship, including marriage. Partner selection is based more on individual preferences and less on the peer group's values.

Much of the final identity shaping centers on the late adolescents' perceptions of their future options as adults (e.g., college, vocational or technical training, military service). Individuals affected by violence and other traumatic events can experience prolonged stress that jeopardizes their developing identity. As of July 2021, 54% of teens and young adults ages 16 to 24 years were employed, 61% enrolled in colleges and universities, and 33% were working and enrolled in college.[65] For those who are able or choose to attend college, it can offer a "moratorium," or a prolonged adolescence, a time to further clarify one's self-image, as it offers both maximal autonomy and a structured, supportive environment in which to complete developmental tasks. Those who enter the workforce and/or leave home out of high school do not always have the added time and/or supportive structures of the college experience. Adolescents who are unsuccessful in the educational system or the workplace may opt to establish their identity by joining gangs or becoming socially isolated. Some opt to join the military, which provides an alternative structured environment but may lead to them taking on adult responsibilities for which they may not be psychologically or emotionally prepared (e.g., combat).

Cognitive Development

Late adolescents have adult reasoning capabilities and skills but are still gaining experience with both. They are generally capable of understanding the consequences of their actions and behaviors and make complex and sophisticated judgments about human relationships. They no longer base their judgments about people on overt behavior, and have a good understanding of inner motivations, including multiple determinants of an action. Of course, neither teens nor adults consistently use this mature level of thinking, and some never reach this level of cognitive maturity.

Health Supervision and Screening

Annual health supervision visits are recommended, including an annual influenza immunization. Screening for STIs is needed if the adolescent is sexually active, and Pap smears should begin for females at age 21 years, regardless of sexual activity. Tuberculosis screening is indicated if risk factors are identified. A fasting lipoprotein analysis is recommended at least once during late adolescence. A plan for transition to adult care should be clearly developed by this time. Transition involves providing medical records and referring the adolescent to an adult PCP. Many teens benefit from a pretransfer visit with an adult provider.[60] PCPs can also assist the adolescent to learn about health insurance (e.g., access, use), how to use the healthcare system, and to take responsibility for self-care, especially as they may be removed as dependents on their parents' policies.

Anticipatory Guidance

Anticipatory guidance for the late adolescent centers on the transition from being a teen to taking on the responsibility and role of an adult, which includes:

- How physical activity, exercise, nutrition, sleep, and rest are incorporated into their lifestyle and budget
- Strategies to balance responsibilities of school, family, and employment
- Conflict resolution and stress management strategies
- Future goals and plans (e.g., family/children, college/vocational training, military, job options)
- Ways to clarify values and beliefs; identifying talents and interests to be pursued and taking on challenges that increase self-confidence
- Need for and maintaining relationships with family, parents, siblings, friends, significant others, and community
- Injury prevention strategies
- Sex and sexuality:
  - Responsible sexual behaviors, including safe sex
  - Continued exploration and clarification of sexual orientation/management of sexual feelings
  - STI prevention
  - Date rape and intimate partner abuse prevention and reporting
  - Birth control, including emergency methods
  - Childbearing and childrearing consideration
  - Breast or testicular self-examination (see controversy discussed in middle adolescence)

Additional Resources

Adolescent Health Transition Project (AHTP): http://depts.washington.edu/healthtr/

Alliance of Professional Tattooists, Inc. (APT): https://safe-tattoos.com/

American Academy of Family Physicians: www.aafp.org

American Academy of Pediatrics (AAP): www.aap.org

AAP Adolescent Health Care Campaign Toolkit: https://www.aap.org/en/news-room/campaigns-and-toolkits/adolescent-health-care/

AAP Family Media Plan:
https://www.healthychildren.org/English/media/Pages/default.aspx

Centers for Disease Control and Prevention (CDC): www.cdc.gov

Family Acceptance Project: https://familyproject.sfsu.edu

Ginsburg K. *A Parent's Guide to Building Resilience in Children and Teens: Giving Your Child Roots and Wings.* American Academy of Pediatrics; 2006.

8 years (0.76 g/day); 4 to 13 years (0.76 g/day), females 14 to 18 years (0.71 g/day); males 14 to 18 (0.73 g/day); and those over 18 years (0.66 g/day).[5] Protein and amino acid deficiencies rarely appear alone but follow other dietary deficits (e.g., insufficient carbohydrate intake), although young children can be vulnerable to protein deficiency when cow's milk is replaced with low-protein beverages, such as juices or plant-based milk (e.g., rice, almond). Further, stress and disease can deplete nitrogen, a process that contributes to tissue wasting, which creates an increased demand for protein. Adjustments in protein intake may be needed for those building muscle tissue during body conditioning.

Diet trends focusing on lower carbohydrate and higher protein intake can be very dangerous, especially for children and adolescents. Typically, the increased protein comes through supplements and protein powders and bars. The misunderstanding is that more protein will build more muscle; however, excess protein intake can tax the liver and kidneys and increase the risk for dehydration. In addition, protein can only be used to build muscle and synthesize tissue once the body's overall energy (caloric) and carbohydrate needs are met, meaning that before that point, protein will just be used to meet calorie needs. Thus, focusing on overall nutrition is far more important than having high intake of only one component. Spreading one's protein intake throughout the day can help stabilize blood sugar, as well as minimize stress on the liver and kidneys. Further, refocusing on protein intake through lean meats, dairy, nuts and nut butters, beans and legumes, and meat alternatives is far safer and more nutritious.

Carbohydrates

Carbohydrates are the body's primary source of energy, and the brain and nervous system can *only* use carbohydrates as energy. There are two forms of carbohydrates found in fruits, vegetables, milk, and prepared sweets or complex carbohydrates (starches found in whole grains, potatoes, legumes, and other vegetables): (1) simple sugars, or monosaccharides, and (2) disaccharides, namely fructose, lactose, and sucrose. Encouraging the intake of complex carbohydrates increases the nutrient density while not villainizing refined food products. If carbohydrates are extremely limited or absent from the diet, the body uses stored triglycerides, oxidizes fatty acids, and breaks down dietary and tissue protein, leading to an accumulation of ketone bodies. Restrictive eating disorders or other low-carbohydrate/high-protein diets can cause significant health risks; PCPs can ensure good, balanced nutrition by promoting adequate carbohydrate intake despite diet trends in the culture at large. The EAR is 100 g/kg per day across the pediatric lifespan, with 45% to 65% of daily energy requirements being supplied by carbohydrates.[6]

Fats

Lipids, fats, and fatty acids are used by the body to provide energy, to facilitate absorption of the fat-soluble vitamins (A, D, E, K), and to maintain integrity of cell membranes and myelin. The three main omega-3 fatty acids are α-linolenic acid (ALA), eicosapentaenoic acid (EPA), and docosahexaenoic acid (DHA). ALA is found mainly in plant oils such as flaxseed, soybean, and canola oils. DHA and EPA are found in fish and other seafood.[7] Linoleic acid (LA), the precursor to omega-6 fatty acids, is found in soy oil, corn oil, and sunflower, safflower, pumpkin, and sesame seeds. Adequate amounts of omega-3 and omega-6 fatty acids are produced in the body if there is adequate intake of LA and ALA (aka essential fatty acids) and the vitamins (B_3, B_6, C) and minerals (zinc, magnesium) necessary to facilitate their conversion.

Fat intake for children 1 to 3 years old should be 30% to 40% of total caloric intake, while children over 3 years old should gradually adopt a lifelong intake of 25% to 35% of total calories from fats. Saturated fat intake should be less than 10% of total calories, in the form of saturated fat, and trans fatty acids should be excluded from the diet.[6] Numerous studies indicate that diets with high amounts of plant fibers, limited saturated fats, low cholesterol, and zero trans fats reduce serum cholesterol and low-density lipoprotein (LDL) levels without affecting growth and development.[8] However, a diet with less than 20% of the total energy intake from fat can put the child at nutritional risk.

Micronutrients

Vitamins

Fat-Soluble Vitamins. Fat-soluble vitamins (A, D, E, K) require adequate dietary fat for proper absorption and storage. They are absorbed in the small intestines along with fats and lipids in foods and require bile for absorption. Chronic conditions that compromise the hepatobiliary system increase the risk for decreased absorption of fat-soluble vitamins, as do low-fat diets, increased intestinal motility, and malabsorption syndromes. Fat-soluble vitamins are fairly stable when heated in cooking; therefore, food preparation does not typically destroy fat-soluble vitamins as readily, as is the case with water-soluble vitamins. Fat-soluble vitamins can be stored for long periods of time in body tissues, so temporary dietary deficiencies may not affect growth and development. If stores get depleted and nutritional intake is inadequate over time, vitamin deficiencies will appear. In contrast, if the intake of fat-soluble vitamins is excessive (e.g., via supplements), toxic effects can appear. Table 14.1 highlights signs and symptoms of deficient or excess vitamin intake, as well as dietary sources and interactions.

One fat-soluble vitamin, vitamin D, is particularly concerning during the pediatric age when nutritional rickets and impaired bone mass acquisition can occur. While it is agreed that infants need 400 IU/day, with breastfed infants needing supplementation, for children over the age of 1 year, supplementation at doses from 600 IU/day is only considered in the presence of risk factors (e.g., reduced sunlight exposure, obesity, malabsorption syndromes, chronic antiseizure and/or antiretroviral medication use). Vitamin D is also involved in the reduction of inflammation and modulates a variety of processes, including cell growth, neuromuscular function, immune function, and glucose metabolism.[9]

Water-Soluble Vitamins. Water-soluble vitamins (B, C) are primarily absorbed in the jejunum. They can be stored in the body, but only in very small amounts. If water-soluble vitamin intake is more than that needed by the body, absorption decreases and the excess is excreted. As a result, there is a need for daily intake of water-soluble vitamins and, while there is little risk of toxicity from large doses, high-dose supplements have limited benefits. Table 14.1 highlights signs and symptoms of deficient vitamin intake, as well as dietary sources and interactions affecting absorption or use.

Minerals and Elements

The three major elements—calcium, magnesium, and phosphorus—are regulated by cooperative interactions between the kidneys, the gastrointestinal tract, and the bone. While the majority of all three are components of bone, their levels in the plasma are crucial for body function and deviations can lead to serious, even

TABLE 14.1   Vitamins: Function, Dietary Sources, Interactions, Deficiency, and Excess

Function	Dietary Sources	Interactions Affecting Absorption or Utilization	Signs of Deficit	Signs of Excess
Fat-Soluble Vitamins				
Vitamin A				
Vision, cellular differentiation and growth, reproductive and immune system function	Liver, fish liver oils, fortified milk, eggs, red and orange vegetables, dark green leafy vegetables	Facilitated by dietary fat, protein, and vitamin E Absorption of vitamin A is hindered by lack of protein, iron, or zinc	Anorexia, dry skin, keratinization of epithelial cells of respiratory tract, night blindness, corneal lesions, increased susceptibility to infections	Headache, vomiting, double vision, hair loss, dry mucous membranes, peeling skin, liver damage; toxic at 10 times the RDA; excessive intake of carotenoids (e.g., carrots) may cause hypercarotenosis, a benign condition of yellowing of the skin
Vitamin D				
Bone growth and development; regulates intestinal absorption of calcium and phosphorus; reduction of inflammation; modulation of processes, including cell growth, neuromuscular function, immune function, and glucose metabolism	Sunlight, artificial ultraviolet light, fortified food products, especially milk, fish	Utilization compromised in patients with renal failure Increased exposure to sunlight increases synthesis Darker skin and aging skin inhibit synthesis	Inadequate bone mineralization, rickets or skeletal malformations, delayed dentition	Anorexia, nausea, vomiting, diarrhea, weakness, hypercalcemia, hypercalciuria, calcium deposits in soft tissue, permanent renal or cardiovascular damage
Vitamin E				
Antioxidant, traps free radicals, prevents oxidation of polyunsaturated fats	Vegetable oils, margarine, nuts, seeds, wheat germ, green leafy vegetables	Low serum levels have been associated with prematurity and congenital defects of the hepatobiliary system (e.g., cystic fibrosis, biliary atresia)	Macrocytic anemia and dermatitis in infants; neurologic defects in severe malabsorption	None known in dietary doses Supplements may cause hemorrhagic effects, especially if taken long term
Vitamin K				
Forms proteins that regulate blood clotting	Green leafy vegetables, milk, dairy products, liver	Inhibited by long-term antibiotic use, hyperalimentation, chronic biliary obstruction, or lipid malabsorption syndromes	Defective coagulation of blood, hemorrhages, liver injury	Vitamin K–responsive hemorrhagic condition, especially if patient is being treated with anticoagulants
Water-Soluble Vitamins				
Vitamin C				
Essential for collagen formation and function; promotes growth and tissue repair; enhances iron absorption; improves wound healing	Vegetables and fruits, especially citrus fruits, broccoli, collard greens, spinach, tomatoes, potatoes, strawberries, peppers	Vitamin C is easily lost in food storage and preparation with exposure to heat, oxygen, and water Exposure to cigarette smoke increases vitamin C requirement	Scurvy, cracked lips, bleeding gums, slow wound healing, easy bruising	Unknown; excess vitamin is excreted in urine
Thiamin (Vitamin B$_1$)				
Necessary for carbohydrate metabolism; promotes normal appetite and digestion	Whole grains, brewer's yeast, legumes, seeds and nuts, fortified grain products, organ meats, lean cuts of pork	Availability inhibited by presence of thiaminase (found in raw fish); alcohol contributes to thiamine deficiency Rarely, deficiency may follow gastric sleeve surgery for weight loss	Beriberi: muscle weakness, ataxia, confusion, anorexia, tachycardia, heart failure in infants	None by oral intake; excess excreted in urine

TABLE 14.1	Vitamins: Function, Dietary Sources, Interactions, Deficiency, and Excess—Cont'd			
Function	Dietary Sources	Interactions Affecting Absorption or Utilization	Signs of Deficit	Signs of Excess
Riboflavin (Vitamin B_2)				
Necessary for oxidation-reduction reactions; essential for function of vitamin B_6 and niacin; helps to maintain integrity of skin, tongue, and lips	Dairy products, meat, poultry, fish; enriched or fortified grains, cereals, and breads; green vegetables, such as broccoli, spinach, asparagus, turnip greens	Positive nitrogen balance contributes to function of riboflavin	Oral-buccal cavity lesions, generalized seborrheic dermatitis, scrotal and vulva skin changes, normocytic anemia, dimness of vision	None known
Niacin (Vitamin B_3)				
Essential for energy metabolism, glycolysis, fatty acids; maintains nervous system, integrity of skin, mouth, tongue	Meats, fortified grains, cereals, legumes Milk, eggs, and meats contain tryptophan	Requires riboflavin for absorption and utilization Grains treated with lime have more biologically available niacin Dietary tryptophan converts to niacin	Pellagra: dermatitis, diarrhea, inflammation of mucous membranes, indigestion	No known toxicity with dietary doses; heat rush and flushing with excessive doses
Pyridoxine (Vitamin B_6)				
Essential for metabolism of amino acids, lipids, nucleic acids, and glycogen	Chicken, fish, kidney, liver, pork, red meat, eggs, unrefined rice, soybeans, oats, whole wheat, peanuts, walnuts, fortified cereals	Riboflavin enhances function Increased protein intake increases requirements for vitamin B_6	Seen in combination with other B-complex vitamin deficiencies; dermatitis, anemia, convulsions, neurologic symptoms, and abdominal distress in infants	Ataxia, sensory neuropathy when taken in gram quantities for months or years
Folate (Folic Acid, Vitamin B_9)				
Essential for amino acid metabolism and nucleic acid synthesis; red blood cell formation	Liver, fortified grain products, yeast, dark green leafy vegetables, green vegetables, legumes, orange juice, wheat germ	Only about 50% of folate in foods is directly bioavailable for absorption in intestine; more efficiently absorbed if serum levels are low	Megaloblastic anemia in severe cases; macrocytic anemia, glossitis, gastrointestinal disturbances; increased risk of neural tube defects and growth retardation in infants of folate-deficient mothers	None known in dietary doses; excessive folic acid supplementation may reduce serum levels of phenytoin, carbamazepine, and valproate and contribute to seizures in epilepsy controlled by these medications
Vitamin B_{12}				
Essential for neurologic function, adequate red blood cell formation, and DNA synthesis	Animal products: meat, eggs, and milk; shellfish; fortified foods	Absorbed in ileum; intrinsic factor mediated In strict vegetarians, the vitamin excreted in the bile is reabsorbed	Megaloblastic anemia, neurologic symptoms, sore tongue, weakness	None known

DNA, Deoxyribonucleic acid; *RDA*, recommended dietary allowance.

life-threatening, pathologies. Calcium and phosphate are usually discussed together because both their physiologic roles and mechanisms of regulation are intertwined.

Calcium is necessary for bone health, muscle contraction, clot formation, enzyme activation, and neurologic function. Without adequate calcium, bone health can suffer and, if severely deficient, abnormal heart rhythms can occur. Serum levels are not the best reflection of calcium status, as the body needs to maintain constant levels in the blood, and will leach calcium from bones if needed. Peak bone mineral density is directly related to calcium intake throughout the pediatric lifespan; however, bone calcification continues until approximately 25 years of age. Yet, calcium alone is not responsible for bone density, as it is also affected by an individual's weight as well as endogenous estrogen.

Magnesium is a cofactor in more than 300 enzyme systems that regulate protein synthesis, muscle and nerve function, blood glucose control, and blood pressure regulations.[10] The kidneys regulate the excretion of magnesium, making magnesium deficiencies rare in otherwise healthy individuals; however, certain health conditions (gastrointestinal disease, type 2 diabetes, alcohol dependence, etc.) or medications can lead to deficiency. Magnesium deficiency is also related to migraine headaches, and there is some evidence to support magnesium supplementation for migraine prophylaxis even in those without deficiency (see Chapter 41). Magnesium supplements can be used to aid in rest and sleep as well as relieve constipation. Excess magnesium is excreted, so toxic amounts are rare from food sources but possible from supplements or magnesium-containing laxatives and antacids.

Phosphorus also plays key roles in bone health, gene transcription, enzyme activation, and cell membrane structure.[11] Phosphorus homeostasis is regulated by the kidneys, bones, and intestines, as well as several hormones including estrogen and adrenaline. In patients with eating disorders, starvation, vomiting, laxative abuse, and exercise all contribute to a negative phosphate balance. Low phosphorus intake during periods of accelerated growth (puberty) can also lead to phosphate depletion. In addition, preterm newborns may be at risk of phosphorus inadequacy, and those with chronic kidney disease may be at risk of hyperphosphatemia as kidney function declines.

Additional minerals and trace elements include iron, copper, fluoride, iodine, and zinc, among others. Their functions, dietary sources, interactions, and signs of dietary deficit or excess can be found in Table 14.2, and their EARs are available online.[5] Of these, iron is particularly important in pediatrics, as iron-deficiency anemia is the most common nutritional deficiency in children.

Iron has many roles in the body, including hemoglobin synthesis and oxygen transport. Dietary iron is available in two forms: heme and nonheme. Heme iron comes from animal sources, such as meat and fish, and is most bioavailable. Nonheme iron is found in fortified grains, beans and lentils, dried fruit, seeds, soybeans, and soy products. Absorption of nonheme iron can be increased by pairing the food with a food high in vitamin C, whereas calcium inhibits its absorption. The EAR for iron varies by age. There is no EAR for young infants, but the EAR for older infants (6–12 months) is 6.9 mg/day, children 1–3 years (3.0 mg/day), and 4–8 years (4.1 mg/day). The EAR for males (9–13 years) is 5.9 mg/day, increasing to 7.7 mg/day for age 14–18 years, then decreasing to 6 mg/day throughout adulthood. The EAR for females (9–13 years) is 5.7 mg/day, increasing to 7.9 mg/day (14–18 years) and again to 8.1 mg/day throughout adulthood until it decreases to 5 mg/day after menopause.[5] Individuals with iron deficiency typically have other nutrient deficiencies, as iron deficiency is most often associated with poor diet, malabsorptive and gastrointestinal disorders, and/or blood loss.[12] Some athletes are at higher risk for iron deficiency due to an increased demand for oxygen, foot strike hemolysis (i.e., mechanical trauma), and additional loss in sweat. Iron deficiency is associated with immediate outcomes, including anemia, pallor, bruising, mental and physical fatigue, decreased appetite, and slowed growth and development (see Chapter 38). Although some short-term outcomes of iron-deficiency anemia are easily reversible with iron supplementation, there can be negative long-term effects on neurodevelopment and behavior. Iron supplements are also available and can be necessary for iron repletion; however, high doses of supplemental iron can reduce zinc absorption and cause nausea, constipation, and abdominal pain. Taking iron supplements with food can help reduce symptoms, as can focusing on food sources of iron rather than supplementary iron. When using supplements, serum iron levels should be monitored, as toxic levels of iron can be reached. Foods rich in iron are listed in Table 14.3.

Assessment of Nutritional Status

History

Assessment of nutritional status is done to determine variables influencing dietary intake, whether the diet is adequate, and if there is any deviation in growth and development. Much data can be collected in the intake interview or using a 3-day diet recall. Dietary intake data should be combined with clinical, biochemical, and anthropometric data, which collectively provide a more complete picture of nutritional status. Although many children have periods of nonproblematic selective eating, PCPs may diagnose avoidant restrictive food intake disorder (ARFID) when children do not consume enough food to grow and develop properly.[13] In addition, it is important to remember that food and eating are influenced by social, cultural, and economic variables. Box 14.2 outlines the components of a nutrition assessment with examples of related questions. Particular attention should be given to families with limited resources or access. Routine screening for food insecurity (e.g., the Hunger Vital Sign) is recommended. The PCP can also provide resources for families who experience food insecurity, such as Women, Infants, and Children (WIC) Program and Supplemental Nutrition Assistance Program (SNAP). Further, if a child needs more specialized nutrition care, it is appropriate to refer to a registered dietitian (RD). While the title "nutritionist" has no regulation, an RD has completed multiple layers of education, training, accreditation, and continuing education. Within this referral, the PCP can share any pertinent physical examination information, laboratory or diagnostic studies, and growth charts, among other information, to help the dietitian best assist the child.

Physical Examination

A complete physical examination should be done, with particular attention to growth charts (see Chapter 5). A normal growth trajectory is seen when an individual child has stayed on their growth curve, regardless of which percentile. For example, it is not necessarily a problem if a child's weight is in the 95th percentile or the 5th percentile, as body and growth diversity exists within children. Of concern is when a child's pattern of growth changes, such as with rapid weight gain or loss or a shift up or down in height percentiles.

Diagnostic Studies

Helpful studies in the assessment of nutrition issues include:
- Hematologic studies (e.g., complete blood count [CBC] with red blood cell [RBC] indices and peripheral smear)
- Iron, ferritin levels, total iron-binding capacity, and transferrin saturation
- Measures of protein nutritional status (e.g., serum albumin, retinol-binding protein, prealbumin, transferrin, creatinine, blood urea nitrogen [BUN])
- Retinol-binding protein, prealbumin, and transferrin (much better short-term indicators of protein status than albumin)
- Albumin (a better measure of long-term malnutrition because of its longer half-life)
- Urinalysis and stool sample
- Dual-energy x-ray absorptiometry (DEXA) scan for bone density
- Bone radiographs
- Iodine, vitamins C and D, or copper for suspected deficiencies
- Bone age versus height age, the age at which 50% of children reach the current height of the child

TABLE 14.2   Minerals and Trace Elements: Function, Dietary Sources, Interactions, Deficiency, and Excess

Mineral and Function	Dietary Sources	Interactions Affecting Absorption or Utilization	Signs of Deficit	Signs of Excess
Calcium				
Development of bone tissue; vital role in nerve conduction, membrane permeability, blood clotting, and muscle contraction	Milk and milk products, green leafy vegetables, broccoli, kale, and collards, soft bones of fish, sardines, foods processed or fortified with calcium	Absorption enhanced in the presence of vitamin D, adequate protein intake, during periods of rapid growth, and if dietary intake of calcium is low; inhibited by excess sodium or protein	Decreased bone strength, increased risk for fractures, paralysis	Constipation, increased risk for urinary stone formation; risk for decreased renal function
Phosphorus				
Essential for bone integrity and general metabolism; provides essential energy during the metabolic process	Almost all foods, especially meat, poultry, fish, milk, cereal grains; food additives in processed foods	Absorption inhibited by aluminum hydroxide in antacids and by excess iron	Bone loss, weakness, malaise, anorexia, and pain	None known
Magnesium				
Activates enzymes, facilitates cell metabolism, maintains electrical potential of cell membranes, enhances transmission of nerve impulses, assists to maintain adequate serum levels of calcium and potassium	Nuts, legumes, whole (unmilled) grains, green vegetables; bananas provide some magnesium	Absorption reduced with high-fiber diet, excess sodium, calcium, vitamin D, protein, and alcohol	Nausea, muscle weakness, irritability	None in healthy individual; with impaired renal function, excess may contribute to nausea, vomiting, hypotension, bradycardia, central nervous system depression
Iron				
Formation of the heme molecule; used in oxygen transport	Meat, eggs, vegetables, cereals, foods fortified with iron additives; Table 14.3 identifies a number of iron-rich foods	Absorption is enhanced if iron stores or daily intakes are low; presence of ascorbic acid increases absorption Heme iron in meats is more bioavailable than nonheme iron from grains, fruits, and vegetables Absorption inhibited if the iron-rich food is ingested with milk or caffeine or in presence of phytic acid, oxalic acid, or tannic acid	Anemia Children are particularly susceptible to iron deficiency during periods of rapid growth combined with low dietary iron intake: from about 6 months–4 years old and during early adolescence; menstruation puts adolescent girls at risk	Iron poisoning can be fatal; for a 2-year-old, a fatal dose is approximately 3 g; for adolescents and adults, 200–250 mg/kg may be fatal
Zinc				
Cellular metabolism, growth, and repair	Meats, animal products, seafood (especially oysters), eggs	Absorption may be decreased if taken with high-fiber diet, excess iron, copper, folic acid, ascorbic acid	Anorexia, growth retardation, skin changes, immunologic abnormalities	Gastrointestinal disturbances, vomiting, acute toxicity, impaired immune response

Management Strategies for Optimal Nutrition

The foundation of a healthy relationship with food begins with an understanding of responsibility; that is, it is the parents' responsibility to provide healthful foods that meet the child's nutritional needs, in an environment that makes eating enjoyable, and at predictable intervals throughout the day. It is the child's responsibility to decide what and how much of these foods to eat. At times, parents focus on how much their child should eat, rather than allowing the child to choose from a variety of food. Parents may rationalize giving their child the same foods repeatedly because "that's all she will eat, and I know she needs the energy," but this only perpetuates the pattern. There is no substitute for a varied, nutrient-dense diet. Beginning

TABLE 14.3	Iron-Rich Foods[a]		
Food	**High Levels (5 mg/Serving)**	**Moderate Levels (2–4 mg/Serving)**	**Low Levels (<2 mg/Serving)**
Breads, grains, cereals, seeds[b]	• Almonds (1 cup, whole, oil roasted) • Cashews (1 cup, dry roasted) • Pumpkin seed kernels (¼ cup, roasted) • Fortified cereals • Mixed nuts (1 cup, dry roasted with peanuts) • Brown glutinous rice (1 cup, cooked) • Sunflower seeds (1 cup, dry roasted) • Watermelon kernels (1 cup, dried) • Wheat germ (1 cup, toasted)	• Bagel (1, egg or plain) • Bread, Indian fry (1 piece) • Breadstick (10, plain, without salt) • Filberts (1 cup, dried) • Gingerbread (1 piece) • Muffin (1 wheat) • Peanuts (1 cup, dried) • White rice (1 cup, enriched, regular, cooked) • Waffles (2 each) • Walnuts (1 cup, dried)	• Biscuits (1 each) • Bread (1 slice, whole wheat) • Egg noodles (1 cup, cooked) • English muffin (1 each) • Pancakes (1 each) • Peanut butter (2 tbsp) • Oatmeal (1 cup, cooked)
Fruits[b]	• Apricot (1 cup, dried halves)	• Avocado (1 whole) • Currants (1 cup, dried Zante) • Fig (10 each, dried) • Pear (10 each, dried halves) • Prune juice (1 cup) • Raisins (½ cup)	• Apple (1 medium, unpeeled) • Apple juice (1 cup) • Banana (1 medium) • Dried mixed fruit (2 oz) • Orange (1 medium) • Orange juice (1 cup)
Vegetables[b]	• Kidney beans (1 cup, cooked, fresh) • Lentils (1 cup, cooked) • Soybeans (1 cup, cooked) • White beans (1 cup, cooked) • Spinach (1 cup, cooked) • Tofu (½ cup, cooked)	• Black beans (1 cup, cooked) • Garbanzo beans (1 cup, cooked) • Refried beans (1 cup, canned) • Beet greens (1 cup, cooked) • Potatoes (1 medium, with skin, baked) • Peas (1 cup, fresh, cooked) • Snow peas with pods (1 cup, raw or cooked) • Spinach (1 cup, raw) • Molasses (2 tbsp, blackstrap) • Spinach (1 cup, frozen, cooked)	• Kidney beans (1 cup, canned) • Green beans (1 cup, raw or cooked) • Broccoli (1 cup) • Carrots (1 cup) • Corn (½ cup) • Lettuce (1 cup) • Potato (½ cup, baked, with skin) • Sweet potatoes (1 cup, fresh, boiled, mashed) • Tomatoes (1 cup fresh) • Tomato juice (1 cup, canned) • Turnip greens (1 cup, cooked)
Meats poultry, fish, other protein sources[c]	• Clams (3.5 oz, 5 each, or 1 cup) • Oysters (3.5 oz) • Beef heart meat (3.5 oz, cooked) • Beef liver (3.5 oz, simmered) • Veal liver (3 oz, simmered) • Chicken liver (3.5 oz, cooked) • Turkey liver (3.5 oz, cooked)	• Ground beef (3 oz, cooked lean) • Catfish (1 piece, floured, fried) • Tuna (1 cup, canned, water packed) • Lamb (3.5 oz, cooked)	• Roast beef (3 oz, lean) • Chicken (1 cup, dark or light meat) • Egg (1, whole) • Halibut (1 piece, baked or broiled) • Ham (1 cup, roasted) • Bacon (3 pieces, cooked) • Pork (3 oz, lean shoulder roast)

[a]Cooking in cast iron pans increases iron intake, especially with high acid foods (e.g., tomatoes).

[b]Iron in plant foods is better absorbed when eaten with vitamin C.

[c]Iron in meat, poultry, and fish is more bioavailable than iron in other food sources.

Data from Hands ES. *Nutrients in Food.* Lippincott Williams & Wilkins; 2000.

in infancy, parents and caregivers should gently but frequently offer children a wide variety of foods in safe and age-appropriate ways. It can take 10 to 15, or more, introductions of a food before a child will accept it; however, this practice is key to developing a healthy relationship with food, eating autonomy, willingness to try new foods, and ample variety in the diet.

Diet culture, weight stigma, and incessant rules around what to eat and how to eat are pervasive; however, it is important to remember that children's developing relationship with food is just as important as the specific foods they eat. Forbidden foods can lead to increases in children's preferences for those foods, making them more likely to overeat when they do have access to them. Further, children whose parents restrict food or use food as a reward are also more likely to cope with negative emotions by eating.[14,15] For PCPs, it is also important to pay attention to the fact that children today are over 200 times more likely to develop an eating disorder than type 2 diabetes.[16]

Developing Healthy Eating Habits

The early childhood years are critical to establishing lifelong patterns of eating and an openness to exploration. Parents can create

BOX 14.2 Pediatric Nutritional History Guidelines and Questions

Food and Fluid Intake
- Type of feeding used during infancy: Exclusively breastfed? Formula fed? Combination? Any problems? When weaned? When were solids started? Allergies/intolerances?
- Current nutritional intake of child, types/amounts of food/fluids eaten (may use 24-hour recall, 3-day diet history, or length of time/frequency that child is breastfeeding)
- Additional intake (e.g., vitamins, fluoride, iron, supplements)
- Is child's intake different from the rest of the family? How?

Eating Patterns or Behaviors
- Frequency of eating (nursing, bottles, meals, snacks etc.)
- Breastfeeding: On-demand or scheduled? How flexible is mother to demands of infant? Is mother working outside the home? Is mother pumping/expressing milk? If so, how much and how often? Is breast milk frozen and/or fed by someone other than mother? If so, how much and how often?
- Infant Formula: Formula Name? Preparation? Amount per bottle? Any problems?
- Bottle feeding: Is bottle propped? Does the child take the bottle to bed at night/nap time? Who feeds the child? How does the child react to the bottle?
- Describe mealtimes: Does family sit down together? Are meals prepared at home? Does child eat at school? What amount of time is spent eating? How long does it take to feed child? Does the family view TV or other screen time during meals? Is there enjoyable conversation? Tense conversation or fighting?
- How often (times/week) does family eat out? Fast food restaurants?

Reactions to and Attitudes About Food
- Any physical reaction(s) to particular foods (e.g., vomiting, diarrhea, abdominal pain, rash)?
- Food preferences/dislikes? How does child demonstrate likes/dislikes?
- Cultural factors: What beliefs/attitudes does family have about how/what child should eat or family should eat?
- What is child's attitude about food and eating?
- How are conflicts around food and eating handled?

- Has child had any traumatic experiences around food or eating? Family history/experiences around food/eating? Weight stigma?
- Feeding abilities of the child: Does child choke, gag, vomit, have suck/swallow difficulties, refuse certain foods, perhaps because of texture or smell?
- Any dietary restrictions at home or special diets? Gluten? Vegan/vegetarian?
- Parent/child knowledge of foods and nutritional needs

Management of Foods in the Family/Home
- Who plans, purchases, and prepares food/meals?
- What economic or environmental factors influence how food is managed? Are finances adequate to supply nutritious foods? Is there a refrigerator? Does family have transportation to carry larger amounts of food from store? Is there a full-service grocery store in the neighborhood? What is the socioeconomic status of the family? Is food shopping budgeted? Are food stamps or other supplemental programs used?
- Does child receive free/reduced lunch at school?

Health and Nutrition
- Does child have special healthcare needs/condition that requires a special diet, formula, enzymes, or device for feeding?
- Are any medications being taken that must be taken with/without food? Or any medications that will affect the body's ability to digest/process foods?
- Typical elimination patterns. Changes?
- Dental status/care of teeth
- Patterns/history of wound healing issues, infections, and mild illnesses
- Any change in hair, nails, skin, or mucous membranes?
- Tolerance/intolerance of hot or cold weather?
- Typical growth, activity, and exercise patterns: Has child been growing as parent expects? Has there been a history of unusual weight gain/loss? Does child have energy to play? Is the child engaged in strenuous activity, competitive sports, or an athletic training program?
- Family history: Hypertension, diabetes, hyperlipidemia, weight concerns, heart disease, allergies, eating disorders?
- Concerns or diagnoses or eating disorders? Restricting, purging, bingeing, avoidant/restrictive food intake disorder (ARFID), etc.

---

a safe environment for their child to experiment with new tastes, textures, and forms of foods by offering a wide variety of foods on a regular basis, without any expectation that their child has to eat any particular food. Over time, this gentle environment and freedom to explore safely help children broaden their palate.

General guidelines for positive, safe environments for eating include:
- Regular, structured mealtimes during which the family sits down to eat together.
- Developmentally appropriate expectations for children's behavior at mealtimes, access to and instruction in the use of utensils, and opportunities and supervision in planning, preparing, and serving meals.
- Offering a wide variety of food groups and preparations.
- Encouraging mindfulness, checking in for hunger and fullness cues.
- Being positive role models. If children learn early that healthy, nutrient-filled foods are readily available and that their parents enjoy them, they are likely to enjoy them as well.
- Setting limits on "sometimes" foods (e.g., high-sugar, -salt, and -fat foods); however, overzealous restrictions can inadvertently

contribute to unhealthy attitudes and behaviors surrounding these and other foods.
- Encouraging adequate movement, sleep, and rest to stimulate appetites.

Appetite fluctuations and preferences are typical of children, and it may appear that a child is eating less than the parent thinks is sufficient or too much of one particular food to the neglect of others. Remind parents that, if provided with a nutritious variety of foods, children tend to select those necessary for their healthy growth in terms of both number of calories and other nutrients. If parents punish a child for not eating or force a child to eat, they have taken away the child's responsibility to choose. As a result, the child may develop an aversion to certain foods, overeat, or act out in other ways. Mealtimes can become contests of will between parents and children, creating feelings and patterns of interaction that extend far beyond the dinner table.

The introduction of new foods can create tension between parents and children. Children may reject new foods, textures, or tastes as many as 15 to 20 times before they successfully consume and/or enjoy eating them. Parents should not be too concerned if a child refuses a particular food. Rather than force the child to try the new food or give in to the child's demands, the food should be offered along with other foods at the meal and removed without comment when the child is done. The new food can and should be offered again at another meal, as continued exposure will help with acceptance. In the interim, parents should avoid being a "short-order cook," preparing special dishes if the child rejects what has been fixed for the family. If a child chooses not to eat much at a particular meal, they will be hungrier at the next. Between meals, children should be offered intentional age-appropriate snacks, but snacks should not be a substitute for meals; "grazing" or eating whenever food is available tends to override the child's natural sense of satiety and encourages overeating. Strategies that can be used to increase the chances of children accepting a new food include:

- Offering the food when the child is hungry.
- Allowing children to taste the new food, rather than offering a full portion.
- Exposing children to the preparation of the food without expecting them to eat it.
- Being a role model, trying new foods.
- Preparing the food in familiar/enjoyable ways (few spices, lukewarm, recognizable, with familiar dips).

Finally, it is important to remind parents that none of us eat or enjoy all foods, and there are many food options for attaining the same nutrients. Reminding parents that there are foods they dislike helps them afford their child the same courtesy, especially if the child has been offered the food numerous times and repeatedly demonstrates dislike. As children become older, parents can help them to master the social skill of politely trying new foods in new situations (e.g., visiting friends or dining in public places).

Nutrition education includes information tailored to children's ages, abilities and characteristics, family and cultural preferences, and nutritional requirements, as well as an understanding how different foods meet children's nutritional needs, the interaction of diet and health and disease, and a variety of strategies to facilitate the development of healthy eating behaviors. It also involves helping parents to examine their own values and patterns related to eating, identify and reinforce those they would like to foster in their children, and eliminate those they see as negative. MyPlate (https://www.myplate.gov/life-stages/kids) is a useful nutrition education tool with an extensive array of resources and activities that focus on food groups. In addition to a downloadable certificate (Fig. 14.1), there are age-appropriate eBooks (e.g., *The Two-Bite Club, Discover MyPlate*).

Age-Specific Nutritional Considerations

To assist families in creating and following a healthy dietary pattern at every life stage, PCPs should encourage parents to customize foods to reflect personal preferences, cultural traditions, and budgetary considerations; focus on meeting food group needs with nutrient-dense foods; and limit foods and beverages higher in added sugars, saturated fat, and sodium. This section highlights key age-specific needs and considerations, with a focus on energy, vitamins and minerals, and eating habits.

Newborns and Infants

Energy. Rapid growth requires high caloric intake. The American Academy of Pediatrics (AAP) recommends infants be exclusively breastfeeding until age 6 months, then continue breastfeeding along with progressive introduction of solid foods

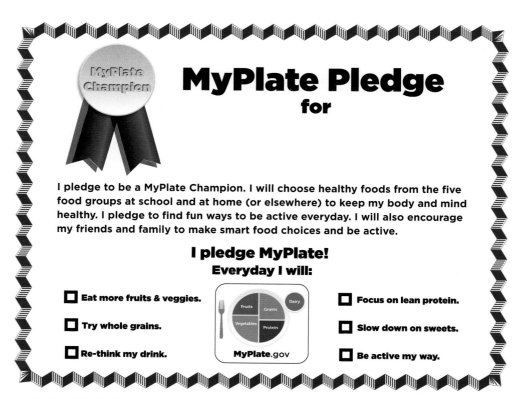

• **Fig 14.1** MyPlate Pledge. (From US Department of Agriculture. https://www.myplate.gov/life-stages/kids.)

for up to 2 years of age. Breast milk is the ideal food for newborns and infants and should be encouraged if it is mutually beneficial for mother and infant. Early introduction (before 12 months old) of cow's milk is not recommended, as it can be too high in sodium and protein for an infant and thus taxing on the kidneys. Most iron-fortified infant formulas (Table 14.4) provide adequate nutrition and, for some families, may be an appropriate alternative to breastfeeding. Some infants demonstrate intolerance to infant formula, showing irritability, weight loss or slow gain, vomiting, diarrhea, constipation, other gastrointestinal problems, or atopic dermatitis. In these situations, the PCP and parents should work closely to identify the best alternatives, being careful to allow sufficient time for the infant to respond. This process can be time and energy consuming, during which parents need support, reassurance, and encouragement. Consultation with or referral to a pediatric RD may be indicated.

Fat is an important source of calories in infancy, and fat restriction is detrimental to neural development. For myelination to occur, infants must have adequate fat intake, which is why fat intake should be 30% to 40% of total caloric intake during the first few years of life. The lipids in breast milk and infant formulas meet these requirements, as does transitioning to whole cow's milk after 12 months old and continuing until 24 months old. For families who are vegetarian, vegan, or prefer plant-based sources of milk, it is important to talk with their child's healthcare team to determine which, if any, alternatives are best for infants in the short term.[17] For example, many plant-based milks are too low in fat to support optimal development in the first 2 years life.

Vitamin and Mineral Supplements. In general, multivitamin supplements are not recommended for healthy children receiving a well-balanced diet; however, vitamin D (400 IU/day) is recommended for all infants until they are 1 year old. Infants should have adequate sources of vitamins A and C once they are 4 to 6 months old, which is typically the focus of early solids (e.g., carrots, apricots). Term infants, whether breastfed or receiving iron-fortified infant formula, should have adequate iron stores to support them until they are 4 to 6 months old, at which time iron-fortified cereals are typically introduced. Premature or low-birth-weight infants who are exclusively breastfed do require iron supplementation for the first 6 to 12 months, depending on the degree of prematurity. Infants who are given cow's milk before they are 12 months old are at high risk for iron deficiency because of its decreased iron density and bioavailability, its interference with absorption of iron from other foods, and the potential for small intestinal bleeding.

The AAP recommends PCPs begin performing oral health risk assessments (Oral Health Risk Assessment Tool)[18] at every routine well-child visit beginning at 6 months of age, which typically coincides with the eruption of the first primary teeth (see Chapter 20). Fluoride supplementation is individualized, beginning at 6 months of age, and is primarily dependent on the child's intake, medical history, and community fluoridation levels.[19]

Eating Habits. Beginning in infancy, feeding relationships can be fostered by feeding on demand and watching for and honoring signs of satiety, and trusting the infant's cues. Parents should be counseled to respond promptly to their infant's cues, allowing the infant to initiate and guide the feeding interaction if possible; however, infants should not be allowed to sleep for long periods of time without feeding. It takes time for parents to recognize the different cries of an infant, but it is also important to reassure parents that they are not creating bad habits by feeding an upset infant. Infants seek emotional comfort in the close contact of being fed

and held. Breastfed infants often continue to suck long after milk flow has ceased (nonnutritive sucking); however, infants fed using a bottle are consequently more at risk for overfeeding.

Introduction of *solid foods* typically begins around 6 months of age when most infants are developmentally able to sit without support, have head control and good swallowing coordination, and show interest (e.g., lean forward) in food, whether it be offered on a spoon or finger, and when the infant had begun to lose their extrusion reflex. There is no strict sequence for introduction of solid foods, which often varies with familial and cultural customs. Iron-fortified infant cereal is often the first choice, as infants have sufficient oral amylase to aid in digestion and they are in need of iron. Cereals are convenient because they can be prepared in small volumes and mixed with infant formula or breastmilk. In recent years, baby-led weaning has gained popularity. Rather than infants being finger- or spoon-fed pureed foods, they are offered foods in strips or chunks when they can safely hold and maneuver them, learning on their own to move the food around in their mouth, including past their gag reflex, and what can be safely swallowed. There are many benefits of baby-led weaning, including exposure to diverse foods and textures and practice with developmental skills, such as fine motor skills, and honoring hunger and fullness cues. Autonomy in early feeding can lead to children who trust their body and are more inclined to follow their intuitive eating cues throughout life. Box 14.3 lists some principles to keep in mind when beginning solids.

Early Childhood

Energy. Growth rate slows in early childhood, resulting in decreased energy needs per unit of body weight; however, because of their increased size and activity, children actually require an increased number of total calories. Further, the addition of muscle mass creates a continued focus on adequate protein intake.

Vitamin and Mineral Supplements. While a multivitamin may be beneficial for some children, it is the exception and should not be encouraged to take the place of encouraging a variety of foods. Children who can tolerate only *extremely* limited food choices or have inconsistent eating behavior may benefit from a multivitamin plus mineral supplement, particularly for adequate daily intake of folate, vitamin A, and zinc. Vitamin D supplementation at doses from 600 IU/day is considered in the presence of risk factors (e.g., reduced sunlight exposure, obesity, malabsorption syndromes, chronic antiseizure and/or antiretroviral therapies).

Eating Habits. In early childhood, children continue to learn how and what to eat by observing those around them and through the variety of foods offered. During these years, children learn to eat and enjoy a variety of foods while becoming skilled using utensils. While they often show an aversion to any new food, taste, or texture, and often become obsessed with their favorite foods (e.g., food jags), parents should continue to offer a variety of foods, be responsive to the child's cues for hunger and satiety, provide age-appropriate portions, and avoid a "clean plate" approach at mealtimes.

Middle Childhood

Energy. Energy needs in middle childhood vary depending on children's sex, body size, growth patterns, and activity levels. Protein needs remain high as children continue to gain muscle mass.

Vitamin and Mineral Supplements. There are no specific supplementation recommendations for this age, except for the ongoing assessment of children with risk factors for low vitamin D, as

TABLE 14.4   Specialized Infant Feeding Guidelines[a]: Formula Selection

Formula	Product	Indications	Contraindications	Main Features
Conventional cow's milk	• Enfamil Infant • Similac Advance • Similac Sensitive	• Healthy infants born >34 week's GA	• Cow's milk protein allergy	• Protein: intact cow's milk proteins (casein and whey)
Partially hydrolyzed	• Enfamil Gentlease • Good Start Gentle • Good Start Soothe • Similac Total Comfort	• Note: marketed as intolerance formulas; not truly hypoallergenic • Good Start Gentle: FDA approved for use in reducing risk of atopic dermatitis in high-risk infants	• Cow's milk protein allergy	• Protein: cow's milk proteins partially hydrolyzed into small peptides • Note: Good Start and Similac: 100% whey
Extensive hydrolyzed	• Alimentum • Nutramigen • Pregestimil	• Hypoallergenic and used in cow's milk and soy protein allergy, protein maldigestion, or fat malabsorption	• Severe cow's milk protein allergy	• Protein: cow's milk proteins extensively hydrolyzed • Increased likelihood of tolerating whole cow's milk at age 1 year
Thickened	• Enfamil A.R. • Similac for Spit Up	• Uncomplicated GERD • Note: decreased efficacy when used with proton-pump inhibitor medications (e.g., Prilosec, Prevacid)	• Premature infants <38 weeks' GA • Do not concentrate above 24 kcal/oz	• Protein: intact cow's milk proteins • Note: contains rice starch, which thickens upon contact with stomach acid • Formulation maintains appropriate nutrient composition as opposed to adding cereal to formula
Soy	• Enfamil • Prosobee • Good Start Soy • Similac Soy • Isomil	• Vegan diet • Family preference • Galactosemia (Isomil and Prosobee powder only)	• Prematurity • Colic • Constipation • Cow's milk protein-induced enteropathy	• Protein: soy protein isolates • Note: all soy formulas are lactose free
Free amino acid	• EleCare Infant • Neocate Infant • PurAmino	• Cow's milk and soy protein allergy • Multiple food protein allergies • GERD • Short bowel syndrome • Malabsorption • Eosinophilic esophagitis • Galactosemia • Note: limited availability and expensive		• Protein: synthetic free amino acids • Fat: EleCare and Neocate: 33% MCT oil • Note: mixing ratios differ from standard formulas; refer to manufacturer's instructions
Low mineral	• Breast milk • Similac PM 60/40	• Impaired renal function • Neonatal hypoglycemia		• Protein: intact cow's milk proteins • Note: breast milk's efficient absorption rate results in a naturally low mineral content • Similac PM 60/40: iron supplementation may be needed
Postdischarge premature	• EnfaCare (Mead Johnson) • Neosure (Abbott)	• Birthweight >2000 g (4.5 lb.) and <34 weeks' GA • Can be used until 1-year corrected age • Contraindications: full-term infants and FTT infants due to the risk of hypervitaminosis and hypercalcemia		• Protein: intact cow's milk proteins • Note: provides 22 kcal/oz at standard dilution

FDA, US Food and Drug Administration; *FTT*, failure to thrive; *GA*, gestational age; *GERD*, gastroesophageal reflux disease; *MCT*, medium-chain triglyceride.

[a]These are general guidelines; not intended for use in the treatment of a specific clinical condition or without medical supervision.

From Oregon Academy of Nutrition and Dietetics. https://www.eatrightoregon.org/opnpg/page/pediatric-nutrition-resources.

- Offer a variety of nutrients, textures, and flavors.
- Introduce one new food (~1 tbsp) at a time, over 3–4 days to assess for any reactions.
- Do not mix foods until you know the infant has tolerated the individual food earlier.
- Prepare and present a variety of foods in developmentally appropriate forms: strained, mashed/pureed, or as a safe finger food (e.g., no gobs of nut butter/whole nuts).
- Include the child in family mealtimes.
- Think about starting with nutrient-dense foods that are a good source of omega-3 fatty acids, zinc, and iron (e.g., cooked pureed meat/fish).
- If there is a family history of allergies or atopy, consider starting with least-allergenic foods, such as oatmeal, root vegetables, avocados, bananas, and sweet potatoes.
- Be observant, responsive, and connected and you will be able to gauge readiness for the next step!

discussed earlier. Children this age are increasingly exposed to and influenced by peers, and their nutritional intake often involves school lunch (or skipping school lunch) and other meals outside direct parental supervision. Supplementation with a daily multivitamin may be recommended for those with *extremely* limited diets or food choices.

Eating Habits. There is great variation in appetite and intake, sometimes paralleling activity levels and/or signaling an impending growth spurt. This is also a time when children begin to exert interest in alternative diets (e.g., vegan) for any number of reasons. Families with hectic schedules or unstructured mealtimes may lean toward reliance on "fast" or packaged and processed foods. Identifying and preparing healthy snacks and foods takes time; engaging children in the process can help them fulfil food group needs using nutrient-dense foods, rather than those high in added sugars, saturated fat, and sodium.

Adolescence

Energy. One of the biggest changes during adolescence is the onset and progression of puberty, including the growth spurt (see Chapter 13). During childhood, average height increases are approximately 6 cm/yr for both males and females, with rates slowing just before puberty. During puberty, the average height increases are 8 cm/yr. Peak height velocity occurs 6 to 12 months before the *menarche* for females, who can then expect to grow 2 to 3 inches more, then stop. Males typically have their spurts approximately 2 years later than females, and the spurt seems to last longer, with their peak growth occurring right before *spermarche*. Accordingly, consuming a balanced diet is extremely important, which is often a challenge as adolescents have increased autonomy and control over dietary intake and habits. For adolescents who express interest in alternative diets (e.g., vegetarian, vegan, paleo), careful planning is needed and consultation with a dietician may be empowering for the adolescent.

Vitamin and Mineral Supplements. Adolescents with irregular eating habits or those who eat a diet with an extremely limited variety of foods may be at risk for vitamin deficiencies. Calcium needs continue, as bone calcification continues until approximately 25 years of age, and assessment of calcium intake is key, along with vitamin D, which assists in its absorption. Adolescent girls are at risk for iron deficiency once menstruation begins. Adolescents who opt for alternative diets may need specific supplements.

Eating Habits. Adolescent eating behaviors and patterns are increasingly independent, influenced by their peers and social life, participation in sports and physical activity, self-perception and body image, and pubertal growth and development timing. Adolescents often appear to have erratic eating patterns (e.g., skipping meals, late-night snacks); however, it is important to monitor and differentiate these behaviors and/or patterns from maladaptive and/or pathologic eating disorders.

Altered Patterns of Nutrition in Children

Altered patterns of nutrition are due to a wide variety of issues, from common short-term pediatric illnesses (e.g., gastroenteritis) to disorders affecting a child's ability to chew or swallow food or absorb specific nutrients (e.g., intestinal atresia, irritable bowel disease), to needed medications that impact nutrients' uptake or needs. Specific nutritional considerations are discussed throughout this book as different diseases and disorders are discussed; however, it is important to note that altered nutritional patterns can also affect the child's family directly (e.g., family meals) and indirectly (e.g., family finances). Accordingly, the family is an integral part of the treatment plan, especially when special dietary needs are required. PCPs can provide additional support when children have altered nutrition by:

- Encouraging parents to express their feelings and acknowledging their feelings.
- Listening without judging.
- Explaining interactions between nutritional patterns and the child's condition, treatments, and prognoses, both short and long term.
- Demonstrating various techniques to increase feeding success.
- Providing guidance as the child ages and treatment progresses and needs change.
- Giving positive reinforcement.

When children and adolescents and their families opt for alternative diets (e.g., vegan/vegetarian, gluten-free), PCPs need to be able to provide nutritional guidance. It is important that PCPs offer advice, counseling, and support within the context of the individual and family's belief system.

Alternative Diets

Vegetarian

Vegetarian diets offer health benefits, as plant-based diets are associated with a lower incidence of hypertension, heart disease, diabetes, and cancer across the lifespan. The different classifications include:

- *Vegan*: Only consume foods of plant origin, including fruits, vegetables, grains, nuts, seeds, tofu, and legumes (e.g., beans, peas, lentils, nuts); no eggs or dairy.
- *Lactovegetarian*: Includes dairy products (e.g., milk) in their plant-based diet.
- *Lacto-ovo-vegetarian*: Includes dairy products and eggs in their plant-based diet.
- *Macrobiotic*: Plant-based diet with increased focus on whole grains, brown rice, vegetables, fruits, legumes, and seaweeds; includes white meats and white fish, but consumed minimally (e.g., 1–2 times/week).
- *Pescatarian*: Includes fish and shellfish in their plant-based diets.
- *"Flex"-itarian*: Primarily plant-based diet, but occasionally eat fish and seafood, chicken, and turkey, but typically avoid or severely limit red meat intake.

When approached intentionally, vegetarian diets can meet the nutritional needs of growing children and adolescents; however, those who decide to merely cut out meat and animal products without thoughtfully replacing them with plant-based alternatives can develop nutritional deficiencies, including iron, calcium, vitamins B_2, B_{12}, and D (Table 14.5).

While children/adolescents and families should be supported in their dietary choices, their PCPs should ensure they also understand potential deficits and alternative sources of nutrients and are assessed regularly to ensure adequate growth and development. As with other diets, consuming a variety of nutrient-dense foods is important, as plant-based sources of protein rarely have all nine essential amino acids; eating foods with complementary proteins (e.g., peanut butter on wheat bread, rice and beans, tofu and almonds) can help provide the missing amino acids (i.e., complementary proteins). Particular attention should be given to vitamin B_{12} intake, as it is sufficiently bioavailable in animal-based foods only.[20] Iron needs of vegetarians are calculated to be 1.8 times greater than nonvegetarians because the nonheme iron in plant-based foods is less bioavailable and phytates in grains and legumes bind with iron to decrease its absorption. Phytates also bind with zinc to inhibit its absorption. As with iron, eating zinc-rich foods (e.g., soy, nuts, cheese, legumes, and grains) with organic acids (e.g., citrus) and processing these foods by soaking, sprouting, or leavening with yeast increases absorption.

Gluten-Free

A gluten-free diet is the primary treatment for celiac disease (see Chapter 34). Outside of this diagnosis, others become gluten-free because they believe it is healthier or will help them lose weight, or to address self-diagnosed gluten sensitivity. For the PCP, it is important to note that gluten-free grain products are often highly processed, have added sugar, and are not enriched with iron or folate.[21] Many gluten-free products are low in protein, which is helpful in selected metabolic diseases, such as phenylketonuria (PKU), with its severely restricted protein allowance. Whether diagnosed with gluten intolerance or sensitivity, it is important to assess product labels. For example, individuals with *nonceliac* wheat sensitivity, who often associate their symptoms (e.g., indigestion, abdominal pain, bloating, fatigue) with wheat consumption, may actually be reacting to dietary fermentable oligo-di-monosaccharides and polyols (e.g., fructose, lactose, fructans, galactans, polyols) and not wheat.[22]

Adverse Reactions to Food

Adverse reactions to food include food allergies, intolerances, and toxicities. A distinction is made between food *allergy*, a hypersensitivity to a food or additive with a reproducible, immediate, or delayed immune system response (e.g., anaphylactic reaction to ingestion of nuts, shellfish), and food *intolerance*, a nonimmunologic inability to process or tolerate the food product (e.g., enzyme

TABLE 14.5 Potential Vitamin, Mineral, and Nutrient Deficits in Vegetarian Diets

Vitamin, Minerals, and Nutrients at Risk for Deficit	Usual Sources	Alternative Sources in Vegan Diet
Vitamin D	Animal products: egg yolk, butter, liver, salmon, sardines, tuna; sunlight	Fortified cereals, milk, or margarine; sunlight (20–30 min/day, 2 or 3 times per week)
Vitamin B_{12}	Animal products only: meat, fish, eggs, dairy products	Fortified soy milk, fortified soy-based meat substitutes, nutritional yeast, fortified cereals, vitamin supplements
Vitamin B_{12} (riboflavin)	Dairy products and meat are best sources; also eggs, dried yeast, grains, dark-green leafy vegetables, avocado, broccoli	Brewer's yeast, wheat germ, fortified cereal, beans, almonds, soybeans, tofu, dark-green leafy vegetables, avocado, broccoli, orange juice
Calcium	Dairy products are best source; also in some fruits, nuts, dark-green leafy vegetables	Fortified soy milk, dried fruits, almonds, sunflower seeds, filberts, whole sesame seeds, green leafy vegetables (at same meal, avoid eating spinach, Swiss chard, beet greens, whose oxalic acid hinders calcium absorption)
Iron	Iron in meat sources is more bioavailable than iron in plants; lentils, beans (cooked black, soy, garbanzo, lima) are good sources	All legumes, almonds, pecans, dates, prunes, raisins, fortified cereals, white or brown rice; absorption is enhanced by ascorbic acid–rich foods
Zinc	Meats, animal products, seafood (especially oysters), eggs; found in whole grains, brown rice, nuts, spinach; however, best plant sources also contain phytic acid, which inhibits zinc absorption	Whole grains, fortified cereal, brown rice, almonds, wheat germ, tofu, pecans, spinach
Omega-3 fatty acids	Fatty fish, eggs	Flax seed, chia seed, walnuts, soybeans
Protein	Animal products (meat, eggs, milk) that have all nine amino acids making them complete proteins	Plant-based foods are considered incomplete proteins because they do not contain all nine amino acids. To remedy this, one can eat a variety of foods such as soy, legumes, nuts seeds, grains, cereals, potatoes, pasta

deficiencies [lactase], PKU [phenylalanine]). Food can also be *toxic* (e.g., food poisoning, toxins in food) or create physiologic effects (e.g., "brain freeze"). Exposure to toxins and chemicals through the food chain contribute to many health problems in children (see Chapters 3 and 25).

Food Allergies

To determine whether an allergic reaction to food has occurred can be extremely challenging and requires engagement of the interprofessional team, including the PCP, dietitian, and allergist to start. Some factors to consider when beginning a food allergy workup include the role of:

- *Heredity:* Children born with metabolic disorders can have adverse reactions to specific foods. Children with a family history of food allergies are more likely to have an allergy themselves.
- *Infant diet:* Breastfeeding may be protective against allergies, although the data about this are mixed. Early introduction of foods considered to be allergenic (e.g., eggs, peanuts) is helpful, as later introduction may actually increase food sensitization.[23]
- *Immature gastrointestinal tract:* In the first 6 months of life, infant gastrointestinal tracts are more permeable to large molecules, including most food proteins. Allergies to milk and eggs are more common in younger infants and often outgrown with age and gastrointestinal maturity.
- *Compromised gastrointestinal tract:* The gastrointestinal system can be more permeable to allergens, such as large proteins, during and after illness or with injury.
- *Type of food:* Some foods are more allergenic than others, and some individuals have greater sensitivity to certain foods. A few foods account for nearly 90% of immunoglobulin (Ig) E–mediated allergic reactions, including cow's milk, eggs, peanuts, tree nuts (e.g., almonds, cashews, hazelnuts, pecans, pistachios, walnuts), soybeans, wheat, fish, and crustaceans. Coconut allergies often occur in those with tree nut allergies, but they are a fruit, not a tree nut. A close reading of food labels is important, including commercial infant foods that feature one fruit or vegetable but have eggs or milk added.
- *Allergic load:* An individual's total allergic load varies by day, week, or through the years. While the number and types of allergies and exposures contribute, there are other contributing factors, including illness, stress, surgery, or trauma, that place excessive metabolic demands and increase vulnerability.

Allergy-Related History and Physical Examination

The *history* needs to include:
- Age of child
- Suspected food or previous exposure
- Route and amount of exposure (e.g., ingested, skin contact, dust inhaled)
- Onset and description of symptoms relative to exposure
- Presence of aggravating or contributing factors (e.g., stress, environment, exercise)
- Treatment given and child's response
- Related symptoms (e.g., atopic disease/disorders, respiratory distress, skin issues, including eczema, urticaria, rashes, colic, vomiting/diarrhea unrelated to illness)
- Family history of allergies, especially a history of reaction to certain foods
- Child's past and current diet history
- Earlier feedings, types, and timing of foods introduced into the diet

- Food diary—foods/fluids ingested for at least 3 days
- Preparation and storage of food (e.g., commercially, at home, fried, baked)
- Current medications, complementary therapies, and supplements
- Food symptom diary—reactions to foods ingested (Note: time-consuming, cumbersome task, especially if more than one food is involved)

The *physical examination* must include an assessment of growth and development, as food elimination and the use of alternative foods can compromise nutrition. Table 14.6 lists possible clinical manifestations of food allergies or intolerances by body system. Chapter 36 reviews the clinical features of an allergic reaction at different levels of severity.

Diagnostic Studies

The double-blind, placebo-controlled food challenge is still considered to be the gold standard in food allergy diagnosis; however, it is not practical for the clinical setting, especially with delayed non–IgE-mediated allergic reactions. Studies that are more common include:

- *Skin prick test* (SPT): The SPT is very sensitive; however, the cutaneous response may not correlate with the clinical systemic

TABLE 14.6	Possible Clinical Manifestations of Food Allergies or Intolerances
System	**Symptoms**
Respiratory system	• Chronic rhinitis • Asthma • Croup • Cough • Serous otitis media • Bronchitis
Gastrointestinal system	• Tingling and swelling of lips, mouth, throat • Nausea, vomiting • Diarrhea • Colic • Protein-losing enteropathy • Bloating, flatulence • Constipation • Gastrointestinal blood loss • Malabsorption
Integumentary system	• Eczema • Pruritus • Atopic dermatitis • Rashes • Urticaria
Central nervous system	• Headaches (sinus, migraine) • Fatigue • Drowsiness, listlessness • Irritability • Depression • Excessive sweating
Circulatory system	• Hypotension • Cardiac dysrhythmias • Anaphylaxis • Pallor

response (Note: antihistamine medications must be discontinued 3–20 days before the test, and the test should be avoided in children who have generalized skin lesions, dermographism, or a severe reaction to food following skin contact or inhalation).

- *Serum IgE and eosinophil count:* This test is done if the child cannot have an SPT done, but it can be expensive, especially if more than one food is suspected. Results must be interpreted carefully by an allergist because findings can reflect exposure to other allergens.
- *Atopy patch tests:* The atopy patch test looks for skin reaction to specific foods but is not as widely used as the SPT in the clinical setting.
- *Food elimination and challenge:* When a food has been identified as a potential source of the problem, elimination and an oral food challenge can be used to confirm the diagnosis. The suspected foods are completely eliminated from the child's diet for at least 3 days and up to 4 weeks and then gradually reintroduced, one at a time. Medical supervision during the challenge is essential. The initial reintroduction dose should be small and then increased until either a reaction recurs or the amount normally eaten is given. If exercise is thought to contribute to the initial allergic reaction, exercise must be part of the challenge. An allergy or intolerance is confirmed if symptoms cease when the food is eliminated and then reappear as it is reintroduced.

Differential diagnoses to consider include other allergens (e.g., environmental), previously undiagnosed diseases or disorders (e.g., asthma, immunodeficiency, malabsorption syndromes), or rare occurrences, such as Heiner syndrome, a milk-induced pulmonary disease.

Management

The goals of managing children with adverse food reactions are to maintain nutrition levels adequate for normal growth and development, prevent nutritional deficits, avoid exposure to offending foods, and respond promptly and appropriately to adverse reactions after exposure. Restricted foods need to be replaced with those of equivalent nutrient value in the context of a well-balanced diet and related physical problems caused by allergies (e.g., diarrhea, vomiting, dehydration, eczema) addressed. Once a child has been assessed as to the cause and severity of the response, a treatment plan can be made. Consultation with a dietitian is recommended.

The standard of practice is to avoid the offending food(s) going forward; however, eliminating food raises different challenges, such as:

- Many allergen-prone foods are nutritious and dietary changes can lead to malnourishment, which is especially true when cross-reacting allergens further limit diets.
- Individuals can be allergic to a food in its raw form but can eat it in a cooked or heat-treated form; eliminating it means unnecessary loss of a good source of nutrients.
- The food may be found in minute amounts in other foods (e.g., processed foods) or contaminate other foods processed in the same area.
- Individuals can still be exposed by skin or inhalant contact (e.g., breathing peanut dust) even if food is not eaten.

Medications

Antihistamines are prescribed for children with mild allergies, unless there is a history of a reaction to trace amounts of the allergen or the child has asthma from another cause; in these cases, epinephrine is appropriate. Self-administered epinephrine is also

prescribed for children with moderate or severe allergies. Children, their parents, and other caregivers should learn how and when to use them. It is often recommended that children at risk for food-related anaphylaxis carry two doses of epinephrine. Children with food allergies should wear a medical-alert bracelet or necklace. School personnel should be informed of the child's allergy, and a medical plan should be implemented in the school.

Focusing on Weight

This discussion of weight begins with an overview of public perceptions and pressure surrounding weight, the current shift toward weight-neutral care, the move toward intuitive eating (IE) and health at every size (HAES), and the impact of weight stigma experiences during childhood. This discussion is followed by a closer look at weight concerns, including the near- and long-term issues, concerns, and consequences related to weight across the pediatric lifespan.[24]

Public Perceptions and Pressure Surrounding Weight

Many providers struggle with *if* and/or *how* to address the issue of weight with their pediatric patients and families. Our current diet- and weight-obsessed culture contributes to an ongoing and often troublesome emphasis on weight. Further, multiple public health initiatives identify and approach obesity as an epidemic; yet the path determining an individual's weight and/or accompanying perceptions is not due to a single pathologic organism, as with most epidemics, but is instead complex and varied. Falling under the banner of "first, do no harm," it is important to understand why weight-neutral care is so critical. The "obesity epidemic" has pressured healthcare providers to recommend weight loss, despite the known risks of weight cycling. Encouragement to "eat fruits and vegetables" or "get exercise" may sound like seemingly harmless interventions, but they inadvertently lay the blame at the feet of children already anxious about the ongoing message: "don't be fat."[25]

Body mass index (BMI) has become a routine screening tool for anthropometric height and weight classification, commonly interpreted to represent an individual's fatness. BMI is used as a risk factor for the development or prevalence of several health issues, and thus weight-based interventions; however, there are many flaws with this approach. For example, the BMI does not take into account muscle mass, bone density, overall body composition, or racial or sex differences. An early warning issued by L.A.J. Quetelet, a 19th century Belgian mathematician, stated that the BMI could not, and should not, be used to indicate the level of health of an individual. PCPs need to be aware that individuals have much less control over their weight than they are led to believe. For example, our individual *set-point* (i.e., the weight range in which the body is programmed to function optimally) is influenced by one's individual genome.

It is important to move away from the idea that higher weight *causes* disease; rather, weight may be a *symptom* of a health problem or of the larger environment or systems in which a child is living. Too often, health-related efforts and policies emphasize weight loss as the treatment and the goal, based on assumptions that higher body weight equals poor health, long-term weight loss is easily achievable, and weight loss results always lead to improvements in physical health. These assumptions are not supported empirically, but instead point to the need to adopt weight-inclusive approaches to health policy and care.[1]

Weight stigma, also known as *weight bias* or *weight-based discrimination*, involves discrimination or stereotyping based on a person's weight. It is a harmful practice. Weight-biased care can contribute to body dissatisfaction and the development of disordered eating patterns in children and adolescents, including dietary restriction, self-induced vomiting, laxative use, or excessive exercise; some go on to develop eating disorders.[26]

For children and adolescents, obesity prevention messaging can easily be misunderstood or internalized, especially when weight loss, rather than healthy eating, is praised and reinforced. Once identified as larger weight, children and adolescents are seen first as their weight—a single number—to the exclusion of their mental health. Weight or BMI alone, isolated from other psychosocial variables and biological markers, is not sufficient to know what is actually going on with the child or teen.

Weight-Neutral Care

The overall message of *weight-neutral care* is that every individual is worthy of dignity, respect, and care regardless of size, and that other measures of health exist besides weight and will be focused on as part of their assessment and treatment plan. Larger weight children and adolescents encounter weight stigma in many places, but they should not encounter it during interactions with their PCPs.[25] For example, office practices that support weight-neutral care have waiting room seating, gowns, and equipment for all body sizes. Although gathering weight and height information may be necessary to plot and assess children's growth and development, it does not have to be done or announced for all to see and hear in hallways or shared spaces. Any health-related weight concerns need to be discussed with parents, but language should center around how to address that actual health concern, rather than defaulting to weight loss.

Mindful eating is one example. It is the practice of slowing down while eating, allowing connection with one's body and focusing on the food. Identifying hunger and fullness can help a child or teen know how much to eat and reduce emotional or boredom eating. The practice of mindful eating is beneficial for physical and emotional health. The PCP can encourage children and families to focus on the following guidelines[27]:

- Eat only when sitting down, ideally at the table, and away from screens.
- Limit eating to the kitchen or dining room; avoid eating in a bedroom or living room.
- Eat with others if possible.
- Focus on slowing down. Take time between bites and chew food thoroughly.
- Monitor hunger and fullness throughout the day, especially before and after meals of snacks.
- Learn to spot eating because of hunger versus boredom, stress, or other emotions.
- Use all senses to really taste food—taste, smell, sight, touch.
- Take time to enjoy the food.

Lastly, PCPs can support children in developing a positive body image. Body image is how a person sees themselves and includes how they feel *about* their body and *in* their body. A person's body image can change over time, and most children start becoming aware of their appearance as they approach puberty. Body image can also be affected by family, peers, and the larger culture. PCPs can support the idea of body diversity—that people come in many different shapes and sizes, and that even if everyone ate exactly the same foods and exercised in exactly the same ways, there would still be different shapes and sizes. They can also discourage the ideas that a certain weight or body shape automatically means someone is healthy or unhealthy, or that size has any correlation with effort, intelligence, capability, or emotions.

Intuitive Eating

IE is defined as having strong connection to physiologic hunger and satiety cues and eating in response to these cues.[28] Since the early 2000s, IE has gained much credibility. For example, a recent meta-analysis (N = 97 studies) found IE eating to be inversely associated with multiple indices of eating pathology, body image disturbances, and psychopathology.[29] Another large, population-based study—Eating and Activity Over Time (EAT)—found that IE predicted better psychological and behavioral health across a range of outcomes and suggested that IE may be a valuable intervention target for improving psychological health and reducing disordered eating behaviors, particularly binge eating.[30]

Health at Every Size

HAES is a framework for care for both providers and individuals that approaches health without a focus on weight or weight loss.[31] Instead, the HAES framework promotes health equity, supports ending weight discrimination, and improves access to quality healthcare, regardless of size. HAES emphasizes *weight inclusivity*, the acceptance and respect for the inherent diversity of body shapes and sizes, and the rejection of idealizing or pathologizing specific weights or body types. They also emphasize *respectful care*: encouraging acknowledgement of our biases; providing information and services that understand that socioeconomic status, race, sex, sexual orientation, age, and other identities impact weight stigma; and supporting environments that address the inequities.

Weight Concerns in Childhood

Larger weight reflects a complex relationship of genetics, environment, and the body's response to environmental factors, including hormonal regulation. The specific moderators of weight gain vary and the interaction within and across biophysical and psychosocial variables is complex.

Biophysical Mechanisms

Insulin and leptin are two major hormones that control satiety and help maintain weight on a long-term basis. Resistance to insulin and/or leptin may contribute to the body's failure to register satiety. Chronic hyperinsulinemia may be the source of insulin and leptin resistance. Leptin stimulates the ventromedial hypothalamus (VMH), sending the message that the body has adequate energy stores; however, insulin and leptin share the same "signaling cascade" in the VMH, and if insulin levels are high, leptin is prevented from signaling its message of satiety.[32,33] Hyperinsulinemia prevents the message from getting through that the body is satiated; thus overeating to satisfy a feeling of hunger can result. Hyperinsulinemia can result from individual genetics, epigenetic influences, and/or environmental dynamics, such as increased stress (increased cortisol production leads to insulin resistance) and diet (e.g., increased fructose and decreased fiber lead to excess insulin secretion).

Decreased physical activity is one contributing factor in the increased prevalence of higher weight. Many schools have discontinued physical education classes, children are increasingly driven to school rather than walking or riding bicycles, and many parents believe their neighborhoods are unsafe for outdoor play. In the

United States, children ages 8 to 12 years spend an average of 4 to 6 hours/day watching or using screens, and teens spend upwards of 9 hours/day in this activity.[34] Increased screen time exposes viewers to snack food and sugar-sweetened beverage advertising. Distracted eating may occur in front of screens, causing children to ignore satiety cues. In addition to weight concerns, excess screen time can also lead to sleep problems, less reading, less time with friends and family, less physical activity, mood problems, poor self-esteem, and body image concerns, to name a few.

Environmental Influences

Food deserts are areas where there is limited or no access to affordable fruits, vegetables, whole grains, low-fat milk, and other nutritious foods that make up the full range of a healthy diet. Access can be limited by family income, location, time, and availability of transportation. Families who have limited or no access to healthy foods, for whatever reason, may turn to unhealthy alternatives, such as fast-food restaurants. Healthier food retail (HFR) initiatives work to improve the quality, variety, and number of healthier foods and beverages at existing stores, as well as developing transportation options to travel to locations with healthy food options.

Assessment When Weight Is a Concern

Assessment of a child or family with a weight concern begins with a careful history, including patterns of eating and activity, and identification of confounding factors and comorbidities (e.g., hypothyroidism, polycystic ovary disease, depression, diabetes). It is also helpful to note the onset of concern. The history should include:

- Dietary and beverage intake, nutrient adequacy, portion sizes, total calories, as well as fat, carbohydrate, and protein percentages of total calories
- Eating patterns and frequency, meals and snacking, fast-food meals per week
- Physical activity and exercise patterns or barriers, hours and type of sedentary activity
- Sleep patterns, comorbid sleep apnea
- Parental weight history
- Child's medical and weight history, including growth charts
- Child's social connections and adjustment, peers, school
- Family medical and weight history
- Readiness and ability to participate in a weight management treatment program based on healthy eating and physical activity

Diagnostic studies are often ordered to assist the PCP. For example:

- Lipid panel
- Thyroid screen: thyroid stimulating hormone (TSH), thyroxine (T_4)
- Liver function studies (e.g., aspartate aminotransferase [AST], alanine aminotransferase [ALT])
- Hemoglobin A_{1c} (HbA_{1c})
- Vitamin D levels

Management. For most children with weight concerns, the primary goal is to slow the rate of weight gain or maintain weight as the child grows. Children and adolescents should not be put on restrictive diets or given weight-loss goals. The PCP should use weight-neutral approaches to care. While higher weight is not the *cause*, children and adolescents may be at risk for hypertension, fatty liver disease, impaired glucose tolerance, diabetes, sleep apnea, orthopedic conditions, decreased energy and mobility, bullying, low self-esteem, depression, and suicide. They should be screened for each at regular intervals and referred as indicated for further evaluation and treatment. Referral to a registered dietitian

---

> **• BOX 14.4** **Parental Guidelines for Managing Childhood Weight Concerns**
>
> - Do not put children on a diet. Instead, gradually modify *the entire family's* eating habits.
> - Respond to children's cues of satiety (e.g., do not force infants to empty the bottle/children to clean their plates). They should eat only until full.
> - Serve age-appropriate portions.
> - Schedule and maintain regular times for meals and snacks. Do not skip meals. Encourage intentional eating instead of grazing throughout the day.
> - Prioritize family meals as often as possible—focus on enjoying the food and time together.
> - Reduce the number of meals eaten outside the home (e.g., in restaurants, fast-food chains).
> - Serve nutritious and satisfying snacks.
> - Increase fiber intake.
> - Do not use food as a reward.
> - Do not overly restrict a child's intake as it can lead to overeating and subsequent weight gain.
> - Promote physical activity. Start slowly, set reasonable goals, and celebrate achieving them. Make joyful movement a priority. Encourage family participation, individual exercise, and team sports with peers as appropriate.
> - Limit daily "screen time" to 1 hour or less for children 2–5 years old and 2 hours or less for children 6 years and older. Replace screen time with family activities, hobbies, or chores. Remove televisions from children's bedrooms.
> - Emphasize the uniqueness of each child, pointing out special talents, abilities, and positive qualities.

and behavioral or mental health specialist may be indicated for some children and adolescents. When lifestyle changes are needed, success is increased when the entire family participates. Box 14.4 outlines suggestions for counseling children and their families.

Acknowledgment

I acknowledge the contributions of Ardys M. Dunn and Karen G. Duderstadt, the authors of this chapter in the previous edition.

Additional Resources

Association for Size Diversity and Health: https://asdah.org/health-at-every-size-haes-approach/
Body Positive: https://thebodypositive.org
Elly Satter Institute: https://www.ellynsatterinstitute.org
Feeding Littles: https://feedinglittles.com
Full Bloom Project: https://www.fullbloomproject.com
Intuitive Eating: https://www.intuitiveeating.org
Kids Health: https://www.kidshealth.org
My Plate for Kids: https://www.myplate.gov/life-stages/kids
National Eating Disorders Association (NEDA): https://www.nationaleatingdisorders.org
University of Connecticut Rudd Center for Food Policy and Obesity: https://uconnruddcenter.org

References

1. Hunger JM, Smith JP, Tomiyama AJ. An evidence–based rationale for adopting weight–inclusive health policy. *Soc Issues Policy Rev*. 2020;14(1):73–107.

2. National Institutes of Health. *Nutrient Recommendations and Databases.* https://ods.od.nih.gov/HealthInformation/nutrientrecommendations.aspx.

3. National Institutes of Health. *Dietary Reference Intakes (DRIs): Recommended Dietary Allowances and Adequate Intakes, Elements.* https://www.ncbi.nlm.nih.gov/books/NBK545442/table/appJ_tab3/?report=objectonly.

4. National Institutes of Health. *Dietary Reference Intakes (DRIs): Acceptable Macronutrient Distribution Ranges.* https://www.ncbi.nlm.nih.gov/books/NBK56068/table/summarytables.t5/?report=objectonly.

5. National Institutes of Health. *Dietary Reference Intakes (DRIs): Estimated Average Requirements.* https://www.ncbi.nlm.nih.gov/books/NBK56068/table/summarytables.t1/?report=objectonly.

6. Dietary Guidelines for Americans. *Current Dietary Guidelines, 2020–2025.* https://www.dietaryguidelines.gov/resources/2020-2025-dietary-guidelines-online-materials.

7. National Institutes of Health. *Omega-3 Fatty Acids: Fact Sheet for Health Professionals.* https://ods.od.nih.gov/factsheets/Omega-3FattyAcids-HealthProfessional/.

8. Raitakari O, Pahkala K, Magnussen CG. Prevention of atherosclerosis from childhood. *Nat Rev Cardiol.* 2022;19(8):543–554.

9. National Institutes of Health. *Vitamin D: Fact Sheet for Health Professionals.* https://ods.od.nih.gov/factsheets/vitamind-healthprofessional/.

10. National Institutes of Health. *Magnesium: Fact Sheet for Health Professionals.* https://ods.od.nih.gov/factsheets/Magnesium-HealthProfessional/.

11. National Institutes of Health. *Phosphorus: Fact Sheet for Health Professionals.* https://ods.od.nih.gov/factsheets/Phosphorus-HealthProfessional/.

12. National Institutes of Health. *Iron: Fact Sheet for Health Professionals.* https://ods.od.nih.gov/factsheets/Iron-HealthProfessional/.

13. Białek-Dratwa A, Szymańska D, Grajek M, Krupa-Kotara K, Szczepańska E, Kowalski O. ARFID—strategies for dietary management in children. *Nutrients.* 2022;14(9):1739.

14. Farrow CV, Haycraft E, Blissett JM. Teaching our children when to eat: how parental feeding practices inform the development of emotional eating—a longitudinal experimental design. *Am J Clin Nutr.* 2015;101(5):908–913.

15. Jansen PW, Derks IPM, Mou Y, et al. Associations of parents. *Pediatr Obes.* 2020;15(11).

16. Rumsey A. *Unapologetic Eating: Make Peace with Food and Transform Your Life.* Victory Belt Publishing; 2021.

17. Wright NS, Smith M. Guidelines suggesting children avoid plant-based milks: a closer examination. *Matern Child Health J.* 2020;24(10):1189–1192.

18. American Academy of Pediatrics, Bright Futures, National Interprofessional Initiative on Oral Health. *Oral Health Risk Assessment Tool.* https://downloads.aap.org/AAP/PDF/oralhealth_RiskAssessmentTool.pdf.

19. Centers for Disease Control and Prevention. *My Water's Fluoride.* https://nccd.cdc.gov/doh_mwf/default/default.aspx.

20. Bivi D, Di Chio T, Geri F, et al. Raising children on a vegan diet: parents' opinion on problems in everyday life. *Nutrients.* 2021;13(6):1796.

21. Elliott C. The nutritional quality of gluten-free products for children. *Pediatrics.* 2018;142(2).

22. Al-Toma A, Volta U, Auricchio R, et al. European Society for the Study of Coeliac Disease (ESsCD) guideline for coeliac disease and other gluten–related disorders. *United European Gastroenterol J.* 2019;7(5):583–613.

23. Sicherer SH, Sampson HA. Food allergy: a review and update on epidemiology, pathogenesis, diagnosis, prevention, and management. *J Allergy Clin Immunol.* 2018;141(1):41–58.

24. Loth KA, Lebow J, Uy MJA, Ngaw SM, Neumark-Sztainer D, Berge JM. First, do no harm: understanding primary care providers' perception of risks associated with discussing weight with pediatric patients. *Global Pediatr Health.* 2021;8.

25. Association for Size Diversity and Health. *Do No Harm: The Importance of Removing Weight Stigma From the Pediatrician's Office.* asdah.org/removing-weight-stigma-from-pediatricians-office/.

26. Montgomery A, Collaboratory for Health Justice. *Public Health Needs to Decouple Weight and Health.* University of Illinois at Chicago; 2021.

27. Seattle Children's Hospital. Mindful Eating. https://www.seattlechildrens.org/globalassets/documents/for-patients-and-families/pfe/pe2976.pdf.

28. Linardon J. Positive body image, intuitive eating, and self–compassion protect against the onset of the core symptoms of eating disorders: a prospective study. *Int J Eat Disord.* 2021;54(11):1967–1977.

29. Linardon J, Tylka TL, Fuller–Tyszkiewicz M. Intuitive eating and its psychological correlates: a meta–analysis. *Int J Eat Disord.* 2021;54(7):1073–1098.

30. Hazzard VM, Telke SE, Simone M, Anderson LM, Larson NI, Neumark-Sztainer D. Intuitive eating longitudinally predicts better psychological health and lower use of disordered eating behaviors: findings from EAT 2010–2018. *Eat Weight Disord.* 2020;26(1):287–294.

31. Association for Size Diversity and Health. Health at Every Size Principles. https://asdah.org/health-at-every-size-haes-approach/.

32. Lustig RH. Which comes first? The obesity or the insulin? The behavior or the biochemistry? *J Pediatr.* 2008;152(5):601–602.

33. Maffei M, Giordano A. Leptin, the brain and energy homeostasis: from an apparently simple to a highly complex neuronal system. *Rev Endocr Metab Disord.* 2021;23(1):87–101.

34. American Academy of Child Adolescent Psychiatry. *Screen Time and Children.* https://www.aacap.org/AACAP/Families_and_Youth/Facts_for_Families/FFF-Guide/Children-And-Watching-TV-054.aspx.

15
Breastfeeding

SARAH OBERMEYER

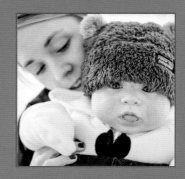

Human milk and breastfeeding are the best choice for newborn and infant nutrition. Breast milk supports infant nutrition and is essential for optimal growth, and breastfeeding can be lifesaving in low-resource countries.[1,2] In addition to healthy nutrients, breast milk contains many immunoglobulins and antibodies that protect against newborn infections. Breastfeeding also offers parents and infants physical, psychological, and emotional benefits that create a lifetime bond. Breastfeeding should be promoted and supported globally.

Promoting breastfeeding is the responsibility of all pediatric primary care providers (PCPs) who are called to promote breastfeeding and engage in breastfeeding assessment, education, support, outreach, and advocacy. Breastfeeding is a learned skill for both the mother and the infant; providers must assess the mother's knowledge and provide information and guidance to increase the skills of the mother-infant dyad as the breastfeeding experience develops. It is important to educate parents and their families about the benefits of breast milk and how to recognize and prevent common breastfeeding problems. This fosters making educated choices about infant feeding practices and quickly seeking professional advice and answers to questions and concerns. Breastfeeding is supported when PCPs take the time to determine the cause of a breastfeeding problem, develop a plan to address the problem, and guide the family through difficulties; early assessment and intervention support a family in the decision to continue breastfeeding. Outreach and advocacy for breastfeeding are demonstrated when PCPs contribute as members of hospital, clinic, and community committees, advisory boards, and establish task forces to develop policies that promote and support breastfeeding. PCPs act as advocates for breastfeeding when they advise and educate colleagues about breastfeeding issues, teach breastfeeding content to students in the health professions, and serve as expert contacts for the media on issues related to breastfeeding. In all these activities, PCPs serve an important leadership duty in promoting and supporting breastfeeding.

Breastfeeding Recommendations

Major health professional organizations, including the National Association of Pediatric Nurse Practitioners (NAPNAP), the American Academy of Pediatrics (AAP), the American Academy of Family Physicians (AAFP), Association of Women's Health, Obstetric and Neonatal Nurses (AWHONN), and the American Dietetic Association (ADA) recommend breastfeeding exclusively for the first 6 months of life and continued breastfeeding in combination with other nutrients for at least the first year.[3–7]

Breastfeeding goals for Healthy People 2030 include the following targets:
- Increase the proportion of infants who are breastfed exclusively through 6 months (target 40.4%).[8]
- Increase the proportion of infants who are breastfed at 1 year (target 51.4%).[8]

There are also efforts to remove the barriers that mothers who are separated from their children (e.g., working mothers) encounter when attempting to breastfeed.[9]

Much work remains to be done, and PCPs are important contributors to the success of efforts to support lactation in the United States and globally. Support of the breastfeeding dyad by family members and education by providers is at the core of breastfeeding success.

Hospital-Based Support

Baby-Friendly Hospital Initiative

The Baby-Friendly Hospital Initiative (BFHI) was developed by the World Health Organization (WHO) and the United Nations International Children's Emergency Fund (UNICEF) to recognize hospitals that provide optimal lactation support. This worldwide initiative trains providers and hospitals to promote breastfeeding internationally. The 10 criteria to meet a "baby-friendly hospital" standard have been revised and are outlined in the joint WHO/UNICEF statement.[10] Every facility that provides maternity services and cares for newborn infants should:
- Key administrative procedures
  1a. Follow all rules from the International Code of Marketing of Breast-milk Substitutes and relevant World Health Assembly resolutions.
  1b. Establish an infant feeding policy that is published and routinely publicized to staff and parents.
  1c. Develop systems to allow for continuous monitoring and data management.
  2. Verify and create systems that support staff knowledge, skills, and abilities to support breastfeeding.
- Key clinical practices
  3. Educate pregnant people and their families about the importance of breastfeeding and provide information about how to breastfeed successfully.
  4. Foster uninterrupted skin-to-skin maternal-newborn contact immediately after birth and help initiate breastfeeding as quickly as can be arranged after birth.
  5. Support lactating mothers as they start and maintain lactation and provide management of common problems.

6. Only give breastfed newborns breast milk; unless medically indicated, do not give them any other fluids or nutrition.
7. Create "rooming-in" policies that allow breastfeeding dyads (mother-infants) to room together 24 hours a day during the postpartum period.
8. Educate parents to identify and respond to the behaviors that indicate their infant is hungry.
9. Educate parents about the use and risks of bottles, artificial nipples, and pacifiers.
10. Ensure that parents and infants have sufficient care, support, and timely follow-up scheduled before newborn discharge.

Currently, there are "baby-friendly" facilities designated in 150 countries internationally.[11] As of 2019, more than 600 hospitals and birthing centers in the United States (including the District of Columbia and the Commonwealth of Puerto Rico) hold a "baby-friendly" designation, and 28% of births in the United States were in "baby-friendly" facilities, greatly exceeding the Healthy People 2030 goal of 8.1%.[11]

Benefits of Breastfeeding

With rare exception, breast milk is the ideal food for the human infant. Each mammalian species provides milk uniquely suited to its offspring, and milk from the human breast is no exception. It is a living fluid rich in vitamins, minerals, fat, proteins (including immunoglobulins and antibodies), and carbohydrates (especially lactose). It contains enzymes and cellular components, including macrophages and lymphocytes, in addition to many other constituents that offer ideal support for growth and maturation of the human infant. Amazingly, as the infant grows and develops, the properties of breast milk change. The sequence of colostrum, transitional milk, and mature milk meets the shifting nutritional needs of the developing newborn and infant. The milk produced by the mother of a newborn contains different concentrations of fat, protein, and carbohydrates and different physical properties, such as pH, compared with the milk produced by the mother of a 1-month-old or 9-month-old infant. Premature infants in particular benefit when receiving colostrum from their own mothers or from a donor with an infant who matches the gestational age of the preemie because of the specific properties of preterm colostrum. In addition, some of the constituent properties in breast milk vary from one time of the day to another. Breast milk has a higher composition of water in the morning when the milk has been in the breast for longer periods of time.

In addition to providing optimal nutrition for growth and development, breastfeeding confers many short- and long-term health benefits to infants. Initiation of breastfeeding at the time of birth allows the growth of protective bacteria necessary for a healthy microbiome. Continuation of breastfeeding promotes further growth of these bacteria, immunoglobulin A (IgA) secretion, and decreased inflammation in the intestinal epithelial cells and underlying tissues. A protective barrier in the intestines is created that prevents penetration of the intestine and may be able to inactivate some viral organisms. An analysis of systematic reviews examining the effect of breastfeeding on infant health revealed a lower risk of respiratory infections and diarrhea, excessive weight gain, type 2 diabetes, and sudden infant death syndrome (SIDS).[2,12] If the WHO goal for Healthy People 2030 were to be reached, more than 190,000 lives of children under the age of 5 years could be saved.[2] Many of the benefits of breastfeeding become more pronounced with breastfeeding duration of at least 6 months.

Maternal benefits of lactation include establishing the strong bond associated with successful nursing and decreased risk for breast and ovarian cancer.[2] In addition, lactation has short-term and long-term benefits that protect against cardiovascular risks associated with metabolic syndrome type, hypertension, and cardiovascular disease.[13]

Contraindications to Lactation

Although rare, there are contraindications to lactation. Certain infections and many drugs or medications can pass to the infant via breast milk. A small number of infant conditions also preclude breastfeeding. Contraindications to breastfeeding include the following[3]:
- Infant with classic galactosemia
- Maternal diagnosis of human T-cell lymphotropic virus type I or II
- Maternal diagnosis of untreated brucellosis
- Mother currently being treated for cancer with chemotherapy or radiation
- Maternal human immunodeficiency virus (HIV) infection (breastfeeding by HIV-infected mothers is not recommended in some countries; see WHO guidelines at www.un.gov)
- Herpetic lesions on the mother's nipples, areolas, or breast (expressed breast milk can be fed to the infant)
- Maternal use of cocaine, phencyclidine, opioids, fentanyl, and cannabis

Many maternal infections do not preclude the mother from breastfeeding. In certain situations where the mother and newborn must be separated because of illness, expressed breast milk may still be fed to the infant. PCPs should consult the Centers for Disease Control and Prevention (CDC) or the AAP for updated guidance on active infections that require separation of the infant from the mother.[3]

There are additional circumstances that affect the advisability or feasibility of breastfeeding, and therefore require special consideration. These circumstances include:
- Significant maternal illness or infant illness affecting the ability to feed
- Invasive breast surgery, in particular breast reduction, in which the areola is removed and reattached
- Documented history of milk supply problems
- Maternal smoking, which increases the risk of low milk supply and poor infant weight gain[3]

There are situations where parents cannot breastfeed but want their infant to be breastfed or when infants can only be fed human milk. For those families, a network of breast milk banks is available. Although it is expensive, the Human Milk Banking Association of North America (HMBANA) provides breast milk at three centers in Canada and 28 in the United States (see Additional Resources). They also accept milk donations from nursing mothers. It is possible to buy breast milk online from other sources; however, this could be hazardous for the infant because many of these donors are unscreened and many samples purchased online have been found to be contaminated, unsuitable for consumption on arrival, or adulterated.[14]

During the COVID-19 pandemic, breastfeeding policies and practices continued to evolve. Infants were initially separated from mothers testing positive for COVID in hospital settings. There are limited data published about the transmission of SARS-CoV-2 virus through breastmilk; however, the benefits of breastfeeding for mother and newborn are sufficient to encourage direct breastfeeding or feeding with extracted breastmilk.[15,16] At the time of this publication, mothers are encouraged to breastfeed regardless of their COVID status.

Induced Lactation and Relactation

Nongestational parents may wish to breastfeed an infant to provide an emotional bond and attachment. A lactation consultant can support the parent to establish and maintain breast milk supply, although there may be insufficient milk supply to solely support the infant's nutritional needs. PCPs should closely follow the infant's weight gain and help the parents to determine the amount and type of supplementation based on the infant's age.

Lactation Consultants

The International Board of Lactation Consultant Examiners (IBLCE) licenses lactation consultants with specialized knowledge and clinical skills to support breastfeeding. These individuals are designated as International Board-Certified Lactation Consultants (IBCLCs) and practice in hospitals, public health or community agencies, or private practice. Consultation with a lactation consultant should be considered when the breastfeeding dyad needs assessment or intervention is required that is outside of the PCP's skillset. Communication between the PCP and lactation consultant is important in supporting the ongoing needs of the breastfeeding family.

Stages of Milk Production

Colostrum

Colostrum production begins at approximately 16 weeks of gestation. The pregnant woman may notice a small amount of yellow discharge on her nipple or clothing. After delivery of the baby, colostrum production increases but is still a low quantity. This thick, rich, yellowish fluid has fewer calories than mature milk (67 vs. 75 kcal/100 mL) and is lower in fat (2% vs. 3.8%). It is rich in immunoglobulins, especially secretory IgA (sIgA), and other antibodies. sIgA is important in the newborn because it coats the gut to protect against invasion of bacteria and decreases overall gut inflammation. In addition, colostrum is higher in sodium, potassium, chloride, protein, fat-soluble vitamins, and cholesterol than mature milk, which facilitates the passage of meconium. Colostrum meets all nutritional needs of a healthy term newborn in the first few days of life. No supplementation is necessary.

Transitional Milk

Transitional milk appears between 32 and 96 hours after birth. The drop in placental hormones and increased prolactin levels trigger the transition of milk. Significant variability is seen in the constituent properties of transitional milk between mothers and within samples from the same mother. Generally, transitional milk has more lactose, calories, and fat and less total protein than colostrum.

Mature Milk

Mature milk gradually replaces transitional milk by the second week after birth and provides, on average, 20 kcal/oz. Ongoing milk production is supported by autocrine, endocrine, and metabolic controls.

Characteristics of Human Milk

The uniqueness of human milk to support the growth and development of the human infant cannot be overestimated. Scientists continue to find new components and to clarify the purposes of known components.

Water

Approximately 90% of human milk is water. Breast milk meets the fluid needs of the infant without water supplementation, even in tropical and desert climates.

Lipid Content

Various lipids make up the second greatest percentage of the constituents of human milk. They are the most variable component, with differences noted within a feeding, between feedings, in feedings over time, and between different mothers. On average, the fat content is approximately 3.8% and contributes 50% of the kilocalories in human milk. During feeding, the fluid contents of the mammary gland mix with droplets of fat in increasing concentration. Thus, the fat content is higher at the end of the feeding than it is at the beginning. The type and amount of fat in the maternal diet affects the type of lipid but not the total amount of fat found in the mother's breast milk. In addition, the fat content in human colostrum is less than in mature milk.[17]

The cholesterol content varies little in human milk and is approximately 240 mg/100 g of fat. Breastfed infants have higher plasma cholesterol levels than do formula-fed infants. Research on naturally occurring fatty acids found in breast milk, such as docosahexaenoic acid and other long-chain polyunsaturated fatty acids, indicates that they play an important role in brain and retinal development.[17,18] Maternal dietary changes to include greater amounts of omega-3 fatty acids can increase the levels found in breast milk.[19]

Protein

Approximately 1% of the content of human milk is protein. Protein levels are higher in colostrum than in mature milk. When milk is heated or exposed to enzymes, as occurs during digestion, a clot, or casein, is formed. The clear portion that remains is known as *whey*. In mature human milk, 60% to 70% of the protein is whey, primarily consists of α-lactalbumin and lactoferrin, and 30% to 40% is casein. The curds of human milk are more easily digested by the infant than other milk types. Lactoferrin is an iron-binding protein, which reduces the available iron for iron-dependent pathogens and promotes growth of the intestinal epithelium. Other proteins include immunoglobulins, non-immunoglobulins, and lysozyme—a nonspecific antibacterial factor. Human breast milk also contains a unique microbiome that contributes to the infant gut colonization.[19]

Carbohydrates

The primary carbohydrate of human milk is lactose, which is synthesized by the mammary gland from glucose. Lactose is highly concentrated in human milk (6.8 vs. 4.9 g/100 mL in cow's milk) and appears to be essential for growth of the human infant. Lactose supports growth of pathogen-competing microflora in the intestines and enhances the absorption of calcium, a potentially important role because of the relatively low level of calcium in human milk.

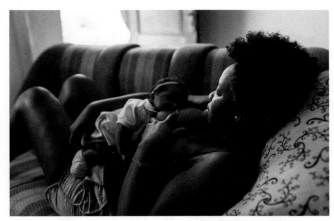

• **Fig 15.9** Laid-Back Position. Also called *biological nurturing*, this position allows the infant to rest against or beside the mother in a prone position. (Copyright Igor Alecsander/iStock.com.)

Physiologic Laid-Back Position

The laid-back position is referred to as the *physiologic* or *biological nurturing position* because it allows the mother to recline and gravity to bring the baby to the breast. In addition, the baby's position is less likely to stimulate the startle (Moro) reflex while it supports the innate feeding reflexes. In the laid-back position, the mother reclines in a position that supports her back and neck, brings her baby to her chest, and allows the baby to rest its cheek against her breast. The baby uses the rooting and sucking reflexes to find the nipple, and the mother supports her breast to help guide the baby. When the baby latches, gravity helps maintain a deeper latch and the mother can relax and enjoy the breastfeeding session (Fig. 15.9).

Ending a Feeding Session

When the feeding session ends, the mother should attend to the way the baby releases the nipple. Suction on the nipple when the baby pulls back from the breast may result in nipple pain or trauma. The mother should insert her finger between the baby's lip and her breast to break the suction before bringing the baby away from the breast.

Breastfeeding Dynamics

Early Feedings

The first breastfeeding should take place as soon as possible after birth. Full-term neonates often have an alert period of 30 to 60 minutes after delivery that is ideal for the first feeding. This first feeding should take place in the delivery area with encouragement by all in attendance. It will not delay, to any significant extent, any procedures required, such as weighing and measuring the infant, instilling ointment in the infant's eyes, and giving a vitamin K injection. These procedures can be done while the baby remains on the mother's abdomen. The mother and infant should remain together as much as possible, with rooming-in preferable. The family's desire to promote close contact and initiate breastfeeding should be clear to and supported by staff.

The infant usually goes into a deep sleep after the initial alertness and is difficult to wake for feeding. Instruct parents to watch for awakening behaviors, such as opening eyes or movement in the bed.

Many newborns will not cry at this point, so parents need to be alert for these signs of feeding readiness. Full-term infants are born with fluid and energy stores to carry them through this early transition to the extrauterine environment, a time of infrequent feedings, and low colostrum volume. During this time, the infant's stomach, liver, and kidneys are gearing up for the larger volumes of higher-fat food that will come in a few days. It is not necessary to provide supplements, including water, to a healthy, full-term neonate.

During this transition time, assistance and support from an individual knowledgeable in breastfeeding is helpful to the mother and infant as they practice latch-on and suckling. The infant should be encouraged to go to each breast for at least 10 to 15 minutes of active suckling, although some infants may spend even longer—up to 20 or 30 minutes. The infant's behavior is much more important during this time than the clock. However, an infant who falls asleep in 5 minutes should be stimulated to continue active suckling. Stimulate the infant to wake and begin sucking by rubbing the infant's back or foot or stroking the cheek or chin. Attention to proper positioning and technique becomes important as the frequency and duration of the suckling behavior increase. A mother is unlikely to get sore or cracked nipples when her infant is latched on correctly. These early feedings are excellent "practice" sessions both for the mother, who gains confidence in her breastfeeding ability, and for the infant, who gets first colostrum and then milk for the efforts at suckling.

The goal of newborn discharge planning is to maintain successful lactation and includes the following:
• Review proper positioning and signs of effective latch-on
• Review signs of infant progress indicating adequate nutrition
• Arrange follow-up for 2 to 3 days after discharge
• Provide a phone contact for questions and concerns
• Encourage the mother to contact lactation resources whenever she has questions

Early efforts to contact and support the nursing dyad during the transition to home support the family and encourages them to maintain lactation. Problems encountered during engorgement, sleep deprivation, times of uncertainty, or lack of confidence should be addressed quickly and directly rather than after a bottle is introduced or the mother's nipples are cracked and bleeding.

Feeding Frequency and Duration

After the first 24 hours, the infant normally goes to the breast 8 to 12 times (or every 2–3 hours) in 24 hours for approximately 20 to 45 minutes at each feeding. Frequent suckling stimulates milk production and establishes a regular routine. Exclusive feeding at the breast for the first 4 to 6 weeks should be encouraged to ensure the establishment of adequate milk supply and prevent nipple preference. During this time, parents need to be on alert if their infant sleeps more than 4 to 5 hours at a time or goes to sleep at the breast within 5 minutes; this infant must be actively awakened and stimulated for feeding.

If the mother and infant must be separated for one or more feedings or supplements are medically necessary, they may be given with a syringe, dropper, a cup, or a 5-Fr feeding tube placed at the breast. Proper instructions, close supervision, and follow-up are needed for each of these methods, and they should not be used routinely.

Hand Expression and Pumping

Routine pumping is unnecessary for mothers who are available for a feeding every 2 to 4 hours. If the mother and infant must be separated for more than one or two feedings, pumping should be part of the plan to assist with milk production. If the mother and infant are separated right after birth, pumping should begin as soon as possible, and within the first 24 hours. The mother should pump 6 to 8 times every 24 hours for 15 minutes if she is using a double-pump setup or 10 minutes per breast if she is using a single-pump setup. This routine mimics the newborn feeding patterns. Instruct the mother to save even the smallest amounts of colostrum to give to her infant.

Hand expression and manual pumps work well for infrequent or short-duration pumping, and some women may choose to hand express exclusively. However, a hospital-grade, piston-style pump that permits pumping both breasts at the same time is ideal for a mother who has to pump for several weeks or months. No pump works as well as an infant in stimulating production, but frequent pumping helps to establish a milk supply and provides the mother with a concrete, healthful contribution to her sick or preterm infant. As the volume of milk goes up over the first few days, the mother can see the success of her efforts. Counsel her about the increase in breast milk production in contrast to the small volume of colostrum produced in the first few days.

Collection and Storage of Breast Milk

Remind mothers to wash hands well before beginning pumping and to use clean containers for collection and storage. The pump parts should be thoroughly cleaned after each use. Many of the pump parts can go through a dishwasher; consult the directions that come with the pump for specific instructions on cleaning.

Store milk collected from pumping in clean plastic bottles or disposable milk bags. It is preferable to store breast milk in small amounts so that only the amount that is needed is defrosted and used. The Academy of Breastfeeding Medicine recommends that saving breast milk from an unfinished bottle for use at another feeding be limited to 2 hours at room temperature.[22] Milk that has been defrosted and not used within 24 hours should be discarded. Pumped breast milk should be refrigerated as soon as possible after pumping and can be stored there for up to 8 days. If a refrigerator is not available, it can be stored with reusable cooler packs in a cooler for approximately 24 hours. All milk that will not be used within 8 days should be frozen. Breast milk can be stored for 3 months in a refrigerator freezer that maintains a steady temperature and can be stored for up to 12 months in a freezer that routinely maintains 0°F. Freezing breast milk has variable effects on its components. After 3 months of freezing, a reduction in calories, fat, protein, and lactoferrin is seen, whereas other bioactive components such as sIgA, cytokines, and growth factors are consistent after 6 months of freezing.[22] The bottles or bags should be labeled with the date of collection and the oldest milk used first. If the milk must be transported to the hospital or day care facility, it should be placed in ice or on a blue ice unit to minimize the amount of warming or thawing.[22]

Growth Spurts

Just when parents begin to think that breastfeeding is well established, the first growth spurt occurs, and they may become concerned. The term *growth spurt* is used to describe those times during breastfeeding when the baby's growth demands exceed the breast milk supply at that moment. For 2 to 4 days, the infant seems to

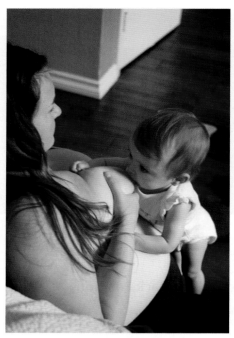

• **Fig 15.10** Breastfeeding Toddlers.

be "hungry all the time" and demands to be fed more frequently. During growth spurts, many babies cluster feed, needing to feed multiple times in a short period of time. The best response is to feed on demand and increase the number of feedings because increased stimulation of the breast increases milk production to the amount needed. However, an inexperienced parent may begin formula supplementation that can lead to a decrease in breast milk production. Once the level of milk production rises, the infant returns to the normal feeding pattern. Growth spurts tend to occur every 3 to 4 weeks, and parents seem to notice them less as time goes on. The behavior becomes an expected part of the breastfeeding experience.

Breastfeeding Toddlers

Many mothers find breastfeeding an enjoyable experience and may continue into the child's second year of life. As the child grows, various changes in feeding position may support the breastfeeding dyad. Children after their first birthday may try various positions of sitting and standing while feeding as they become curious about various ways of moving their bodies (Fig. 15.10). In some cases, a subsequent pregnancy occurs and the mother chooses to breastfeed both the infant and toddler (tandem feeding). There are many benefits to breastfeeding young children who have a wide range of foods in their diet. Breastfeeding provides immunity, strengthens the maternal-child bond, is a source of comfort to the child, and is readily available when the child needs quick nourishment and none other is available.

Considerations for breastfeeding toddlers include:
- Breastfeed after the child eats a meal, not before
- It may not be convenient to breastfeed on demand and mothers may establish times and places when breastfeeding will occur
- If tandem feeding, always feed the infant first
- Have parent consult with the child's dentist regarding risk of caries development with breastfeeding
- Have toddler brush teeth before bedtime but *after* breastfeeding

Weaning

The decision about when to wean is an individual one. Breastfeeding should be encouraged for at least 1 year, but individual circumstances may dictate a different choice for a family. Sometimes weaning is led by the parent and other times by the infant. Typically, a natural weaning process occurs as other foods become a part of the infant's diet and the infant begins to participate in self-feeding. When a family asks about the ideal time to begin weaning, counsel the parent(s) to consider several factors, including the parent's desire, the infant's developmental readiness, and any outside issues affecting the decision (social, environmental, or family). Nutritional replacements for breast milk should be discussed when weaning is anticipated.

Whether weaning occurs as a planned or unplanned activity, it is best to implement it gradually. Some mothers plan a week or so of having three feedings a day, then two, then one either in the morning or at bedtime. If necessary, the mother can use a breast pump to gradually decrease milk production and prevent breast engorgement, blocked ducts, and discomfort. An effective approach is to pump when uncomfortable and to pump only to comfort, not to empty. In situations where weaning is not an anticipated or planned event, the PCP should help the mother to process not only the weaning but also her feelings about it. Some mothers grieve when stopping lactation whether planned or unplanned.

To prevent premature weaning, providers should maintain close communication with families, especially those who are more likely to wean early. Early identification and support of these families may assist them to continue breastfeeding for a longer period.

Clinical Indications of Successful Breastfeeding

Infant Weight Gain

Infant growth rates depend on a variety of factors, including genetics, feeding type, and maternal nutrition and health during pregnancy. Typical newborns lose 5% to 10% of their birth weight in the first few days of life. It is helpful for parents to know both the birth and discharge weights. Once the maternal milk volume increases, the infant gains weight in the range of 0.5 to 1 oz/day or 4 to 7 oz/week. Many breastfed infants regain their birth weight by two weeks, and others may take up to 3 to 4 weeks before return to birth weight is achieved. Breastfed infants usually double their birth weight by the time they are 4 to 6 months old and triple it by 1 year old.

The CDC recommends that PCPs in the United States use the WHO growth standards for children up to 24 months old. WHO standards are based on growth of an international population of healthy infants "predominantly breastfed for at least 4 months and still breastfeeding at 12 months."[23] When growth charts other than WHO charts are used, breastfed infants show a growth decline from 6 to 9 months compared with formula-fed infants, which may lead a provider to falsely conclude that the infant is not growing well. It is essential to assess developmental progress (see Chapters 9 and 10) and other growth measures in all infants, including height, weight, and occipital frontal circumference. Characteristics of a healthy breastfed infant include the following:

- Active and alert state
- Developmentally appropriate progress
- Age-appropriate height and occipital frontal circumference
- Appropriate skin turgor and color
- Sufficient output of at least six wet diapers and several stools per day
- Contented and satisfied behavior after feeding

Urine Output Guidelines

In the first 2 days of life as the volume of breast milk increases, the infant may urinate only 1 to 3 times in 24 hours. By day 3, the infant should have three or more wet diapers in 24 hours; and by day 4, the infant should have 4 to 6 wet diapers per 24 hours. Over time, the infant should have a minimum of 6 to 8 wet diapers in a 24-hour period. The urine should be a light-yellow color with no strong odor. If parents are anxious or have a question about breastfeeding, a diary of wet diapers aids the accurate assessment of progress. However, parents need to be alerted to the difficulty of doing accurate diaper counts with disposable diapers and may elect to insert a tissue liner into the diaper or to use cloth diapers for the first few weeks.

Stool Output Guidelines

In the first 24 hours after delivery, the newborn should have at least one meconium stool followed by another on the second day of life. By the third day, stools begin to transition to the characteristic loose, yellow, seedy stools of the breastfed, and the infant should have two to three stools in 24 hours. That number may increase in the first few weeks of life. Some breastfed infants defecate with every feeding. After the first month, the pattern may change again because some infants begin to stool less frequently and may go several days between stools (see Chapter 17). If the infant is healthy and gaining weight, there is no problem. However, infrequent bowel movements, especially in the first month, should trigger a feeding history and possibly a weight check to make sure that the infant is getting sufficient breast milk.

Maternal Nutritional Needs During Lactation

Maternal nutritional needs change during lactation. The characteristics of an appropriate diet for lactating mothers are similar to those of pregnant women and include[24]:

- Daily caloric intake of 300 extra calories over the prepregnancy recommendations based on weight and activity
- Water intake of 3.4 L/day
- Generous intake of fruits and vegetables, whole grain breads and cereals, calcium-rich dairy products, and protein-rich fish, meats, and legumes
- Rich sources of calcium, zinc, folate, magnesium, and vitamin B_6
- Consider supplementation with calcium if mother is avoiding dairy
- Supplementation of vitamin D

Encourage the mother to eat a well-balanced diet for her own sake to keep herself healthy and to meet the energy demands of nursing. In addition, an adequate fluid intake is necessary, but excessive fluid use does not increase breast milk production. An easy guideline to remember for adequate fluid intake is to drink enough to produce maternal urine that is light yellow and has no strong odor. Refer eligible mothers and infants to the Women, Infants, and Children (WIC) special supplemental food program for nutritional counseling and food supplements; most WIC programs offer food supplements for the lactating mother's diet. Even with a diet adequate in nutrients and calories, a gradual maternal weight loss of 1 to 2 pounds per month usually occurs. In fact, breastfeeding is the ideal way to support a mother in returning to her prepregnancy weight.

No foods need to be routinely excluded from the maternal diet while she breastfeeds unless there is evidence that a particular food bothers the infant. Some mothers of infants with colic wish to reduce or eliminate allergenic foods (e.g., cow's milk, eggs, peanuts, tree nuts, soy, fish, and wheat) from their diet; however, there is little evidence that elimination of foods is protective against colic symptoms (see Chapter 10). Certain foods, such as onions and garlic, may change the flavor and odor of the milk, but they do not negatively affect its quality. Infants begin to have exposure to the foods and flavors of their own culture through breast milk. The nutrient characteristics of breast milk are stable.

The effects of alcohol intake on the breastfeeding infant occur in relation to the amount of alcohol the mother consumes and the timing of breastfeeding. The highest concentration of alcohol in human milk occurs 30 to 60 minutes after alcohol consumption. Alcohol clears from breast milk in the same manner as it does from the mother's plasma and one drink may take 2 to 2.5 hours to be eliminated. Breastfeeding is considered safe for the infant when the mother is feeling neurologically normal.[25]

Moderate caffeine (one to two cups of coffee per day) does not cause concern for the infant. On the other hand, excessive caffeine consumption (>5–10 cups per day) should be avoided as caffeine clearance is poor in infants less than 3 to 5 months of age and may cause jitteriness, tachycardia, and sleep disturbances.[26]

Medications for Lactating Mothers

Frequently, women question whether they can take certain medications while lactating. Concerns relate primarily to two areas: (1) the effect of the drug on maternal milk supply and (2) the effect of the drug on the infant. General guidelines for PCPs related to maternal drug use include the following:

- The best medications for maternal use are those safe for infants or that have been tested in infants.
- Avoid long-acting forms of a drug.
- Schedule feeding at times when the drug level is lowest. For a medication not at steady state, the safest time to breastfeed is immediately after the mother takes the medication.
- Observe the infant for changes in behavior, feeding pattern, fussiness, vomiting or diarrhea, or rash.
- When prescribing medications for the lactating mother, consider all treatment options and select the drug that indicates it is safe for use when breastfeeding.
- Avoid drugs that inhibit prolactin release, such as estrogen, antihistamines, and ergot compounds.
- Be cautious about the use of herbal preparations.
- Avoid medications known to be unsafe for use during lactation.

Not all references available to providers offer adequate up-to-date information. Decisions about drug selection are difficult, especially when considering contraindicated drugs. Always include the consequences of weaning and loss of breast milk for the infant in the deliberations. It is recommended that PCPs maintain a comprehensive drug reference readily available. Two excellent lactation-specific drug references are shown in Box 15.1.

• **BOX 15.1** **Drug References**

Hale TW. *Medications and Mothers' Milk 2021*. 19th ed. New York, NY: Springer Publishing; 2021. Updated and reprinted every other year.
U.S. National Library of Medicine, National Institutes of Health, Health & Human Services. LactMed: Drugs and Lactation Database https://www.ncbi.nlm.nih.gov/books/NBK501922/. Accessed June 11, 2022. Updated weekly.

• **BOX 15.2** **Advice for Mothers on Returning to Work**

Before Delivery
- Discuss plans with employer before maternity leave and gain support of coworkers.
- Provide employer with information to help in planning (see www.usbreastfeeding.org).
- Discuss options with other employees who continued to breastfeed after returning to work.
- Investigate pumps, including rental or purchase.
- Identify a place to pump and to store breast milk at work.

During Maternity Leave
- Practice method of breast milk expression that will be used at work (approximately 2–3 weeks).
- Begin freezing milk. After the baby feeds at each breast, pump each breast and freeze in disposable milk bags. Although the amount will be small initially, the supply will increase with continued pumping.
- Introduce bottle after breastfeeding is well established (usually approximately 4 weeks).

After Return to Work
- If possible, arrange work hours to maximize times to nurse infant (e.g., arrive at work at 8:30 instead of 8:00).
- Have a picture of your baby at the pump.
- Plan on 15–30 minutes to complete pumping.
- Wear clothes with easy access to breasts.
- If possible, have parent bring baby for one feed each day.
- Wash hands before and after pumping.
- Rinse pump parts with cool water, then wash with dish detergent, and rinse well after each use.

Feeding Breast Milk
- Warm or thaw milk in warm water. (Do not use microwave, because milk heats unevenly and presents a risk for burns.)
- Refrigerate thawed milk for no more than 24 hours; do not refreeze.
- Do not add milk to a bottle that has already been used.

Returning to Work

Women who return to work outside the home after initiating lactation should be encouraged to continue lactation and be supported in their decision with accurate information about how to manage both work and lactation. Supporting the family in the mother's return to work includes education on how to best prepare for and make the adjustment back to the work environment (Box 15.2). The ideal work environment provides:
- A location dedicated to pumping breast milk that is private, convenient, has access to a sink for washing up, and a refrigerator for storage.
- Breaks and lunchtime consisting of a reasonable amount of time in which the mother can pump or go to the infant; the

average time needed to set up equipment, express milk, and clean-up is between 20 and 30 minutes.
- Supportive colleagues and supervisors.
- Maximum of 8 hours of work per day, if possible.

In addition to providing support and information to the mother, providers can advocate for community and corporate initiatives that promote these conditions in work settings. Women are more likely to continue lactation if they have workplace support. Moreover, employers benefit from lactating mothers, whose infants tend to be healthier resulting in the mother having fewer work absences because of child illness and increased work productivity.[2] There are many resources available to employers to support lactation programs in their workplaces (see Additional Resources).

The National Conference of State Legislatures (NCSL) maintains a database on laws related to lactation, including lactation in public and lactation in the workplace. Thirty states, the District of Columbia, and Puerto Rico currently have laws specifically related to work and lactation. Individual practitioners can access this website for an update on the laws in their communities (www.ncsl.org/research/health/breastfeeding-state-laws.aspx).[27]

Common Breastfeeding Problems

Flat or Inverted Nipples

A nipple can look as though it is inverted; however, a "pinch test" is necessary to determine the nipple's position during breastfeeding. If the nipple pulls in, it is inverted. If the nipple does not pull in, as happens most often, or everts with compression, it is flat.

Inverted nipples make it more difficult for the infant to latch on in the early days because it is harder to pull the nipple into the mouth when suckling. Over time, as the baby continues to breastfeed, the nipple tissue elongates, and the problem usually lessens making successful breastfeeding possible. Flat nipples do not generally change over time; rather, the infant learns to latch on successfully. Adhesions cause retraction or inversion of the nipples. Flat nipples are often found in women with larger, pendulous breasts.

Differential Diagnosis

The differential diagnosis for flat or inverted nipples is dimpled, fissured, or unusually shaped nipples.

Management

Prenatal. If the patient is not at risk for preterm labor, mothers with inverted nipples can use breast shells during the third trimester. Shells are plastic, dome-shaped devices with small holes for ventilation. An opening in the portion that lies against the skin fits over the nipple, and gentle suction during use helps stretch the nipple tissue. The bra cup holds the shell comfortably in place, and the use of shells during the last trimester generally helps to stretch out adhesions in preparation for lactation.

Postpartum. The provider should stay with the mother during early feeding attempts; give extra praise, reassurance, and support; and emphasize the need for extra patience and persistence. Encourage use of the football-hold position during feedings and have the mother lean slightly forward as she latches the baby on to her nipple.

Helpful suggestions for mothers:
- Wear breast shells between feedings.
- Manually pull or roll the nipple or use a latch assist/nipple extender immediately before latch-on.

- Use a breast pump for 1 or 2 minutes before latch-on.
- Put a cold cloth or ice on the nipple for a few seconds before latch-on to encourage the nipple to become erect before feeding.
- Use a nipple shield to cover the nipple because it provides a rigid nipple that may help the infant to latch.
- Avoid pacifier use until breastfeeding is well established with consistent latch and adequate milk supply.[27]
- If supplementation is medically indicated, use a syringe, dropper, feeding tube, or supplemental nutrition system.

Complications

Complications of flat or inverted nipples include frustration and loss of confidence; inadequate infant nutrition and its sequelae; severe maternal engorgement, plugged ducts, or mastitis related to milk stasis; and discontinued lactation.

Sore Nipples

Nipple soreness is acute pain caused by irritation or trauma to the nipples and areola, often accompanied by a breakdown in skin integrity. Sore nipples have many causes, including:
- Improper latch-on and breast positioning
- Prolonged negative pressure during suckling
- Inappropriate suction release from the breast
- Use of or sensitivity to nipple creams and oils
- Incorrect use of lactation supplies (e.g., pumps, shells, shields)
- Thrush (candidiasis)
- Leaking nipples that are not properly air-dried

Clinical Findings

The nipples, areolae, and breasts are tender, bruised, raw, cracked, bleeding, blistered, discolored, swollen, or traumatized.

Differential Diagnosis

The differential diagnoses for sore nipples include the following:
- Thrush (candidiasis)
- Mastitis/abscess
- Milk blebs at the nipple pores
- Breast or nipple trauma from another cause

Management

Prevention of sore nipples includes the early assessment of breastfeeding and latching, supporting the mother in various breastfeeding positions, and education about the use and maintenance of lactation supplies.

The following measures can be taken to manage sore nipples:
- Assess breastfeeding at an early feeding. Prevent the problem by demonstrating and reinforcing the proper latch-on technique and infant positioning.
- Counsel mothers to seek help early for pain more than mild tenderness. Nipples can be damaged by constant high negative pressure and do not "toughen up" as lactation progresses. Cracking and bleeding are not normal.
- Rub a few drops of colostrum or milk onto the nipple and areola after every feeding, and let it air-dry.
- Expose the nipples to air for short periods several times a day.
- Use breast shells to prevent the bra or clothing from rubbing against the nipple.
- Nurse from the least sore side first and use short, frequent feedings.
- Use a nipple shield during feedings to allow the nipple to heal.

- Pump the affected breast if pain is too severe to allow nursing.
- Use lactation safe mild analgesics (ibuprofen or acetaminophen), as necessary.
- Refer to a lactation specialist as appropriate.

Severe Engorgement

Severe engorgement is characterized by bilateral intense fullness, soreness, and swelling of the breasts beyond the normal fullness experienced as the milk transitions in volume. Engorgement is caused by milk stasis from inadequate emptying of the breast.

Clinical Findings

The following are seen in severe engorgement:
- Painful, hard, lumpy, edematous breasts
- Breasts usually warm to the touch
- Nipples flattened by the edema

Differential Diagnosis

The differential diagnosis for severe engorgement is bilateral mastitis.

Management

The following are strategies to prevent severe engorgement:
- Nurse frequently and make certain that latch-on and position are correct and audible swallowing is present.
- Avoid long stretches between feedings in the early weeks as the milk supply is established. Pump or express the breasts if a feeding is missed.
  If engorgement occurs, the following measures can be taken to manage engorgement:
- Take a hot shower, lean over the sink, and allow the water to run over the breasts, or wrap the breasts with warm, wet compresses for 5 to 10 minutes before nursing.
- Gently massage the entire breast or use an electric pump with intermittent suction on the lowest setting for several minutes after using wet heat to empty the excess milk in the breasts.
- Manually express milk before feeding to soften the areola and make it easier for the infant to latch on properly.

Mastitis

Lactational mastitis is an infection of the breast that can occur at any time during lactation, including pregnancy; *Staphylococcus aureus* is commonly the causative agent.
  Predisposing factors include:
- Stress, fatigue
- Cracked nipples, plugged milk ducts
- Constricting, improperly fitting bra
- Inadequate breast emptying
- Sudden weaning or a significant decrease in the number of feedings

Clinical Findings

The following are commonly noted in mastitis:
- Malaise
- Breast tenderness or pain
- A reddened, warm lump in any quadrant, sometimes associated with red streaking (Fig. 15.11)
- Flulike symptoms, including fever, chills, and body aches. In general, flulike symptoms in a lactating woman are considered mastitis unless proven otherwise.

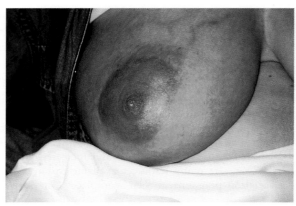

• **Fig 15.11** Lactational Mastitis Characterized by Redness and Streaking Along the Duct. (From Goerke K, Junginger C. Pflege konkret Gynäkologie Geburtshilfe: *Lehrbuch für Pflegeberufe.* Elsevier; 2018.)

Differential Diagnosis

Differential diagnoses for mastitis include plugged ducts, severe engorgement, and breast abscess. Inflammatory breast cancer should be considered when appropriate treatment does not lead to symptom resolution.

Management

Prevention of mastitis includes:
- Frequent breastfeeding
- Attending to cracked or sore nipples immediately
- Treatment of plugged ducts or blocked nipple pore with a warm compress, breast massage, and lecithin supplementation (reducing milk viscosity)
- Oral probiotics taken in late pregnancy or postpartum have a preventative effect on lactational mastitis[28]
  Recommendations for treatment of mastitis include the following:
- Empty the breast. Breast milk is not infected and continue frequent breastfeeding. If the breast is unable to be emptied through feeding at the breast, pump after the feeding has ended.
- Increase fluids and use analgesics as necessary.
- Antibiotic use is considered when conservative management and supportive care are ineffective and symptoms persist beyond 12 to 24 hours. Treatment should be maintained for 10 to 14 days. Dicloxacillin, clindamycin, or trimethoprim-sulfamethoxazole may be used for initial treatment of nonsevere mastitis in the absence of risk factors, such as methicillin-resistant *S. aureus* (MRSA) infection. Mastitis that is not responsive to empiric antibiotic use should be evaluated for possible MRSA and treated appropriately.[28]
- Rest (extremely important for healing).
- Take warm showers or use warm wet compresses.
- Do not wean abruptly because of the possibility of mastitis progressing into an abscess.

Complications

Abscess and septicemia are potential complications of mastitis.

Nipple Preference

Nipple preference (also referred to as *nipple confusion*) occurs when an infant is accustomed to nursing from a bottle and is introduced to the breast. Different oral-motor skills are used in breastfeeding and bottle feeding, and infants given a bottle or pacifier sometimes attempt to breastfeed using the same sucking pattern as with a bottle. This can make it difficult to obtain adequate nourishment and may contribute to maternal sore nipples. The infant may cry, fuss, or push away with their arms during attempts to nurse because they are accustomed to feeding from a synthetic nipple and prefer the ease of sucking from it.

Clinical Findings

The following are seen in nipple preference: ineffective suckling at the breast, breast refusal, or sore, red, or bruised maternal nipples.

Differential Diagnosis

The differential diagnoses for nipple confusion are other causes of fussiness and refusal to feed (e.g., oral thrush, colic, gastroesophageal reflux disease).

Management

The following are recommended to manage nipple confusion:
- Avoid all rubber bottle nipples and pacifiers for the first 4 to 6 weeks or until the infant is breastfeeding successfully unless absolutely necessary.
- Consult with a lactation specialist to retrain the infant to suck correctly at the breast by correct positioning, proper latch-on technique, suck training to repattern tongue movements, and supplementation via alternative methods if required.
- If supplements are medically indicated, give with an eyedropper, spoon, syringe, or cup or through a 5-Fr feeding tube (attached to a 20- or 30-mL syringe) taped to the areola or breast. The end of the tubing protrudes slightly past the end of the nipple so that the tube, nipple, and areola are in the infant's mouth.
- A thin silicone nipple shield may help the infant to successfully latch on. Use the shield with the initial latch and then remove it when the nipple everts, and the infant is sucking well. Cleansing and drying both the shields and breast after feeding are important to prevent skin breakdown and infection.

Complications

The following are complications of ongoing nipple preference: failure to thrive, hyperbilirubinemia, crying, prolonged feedings, sore and cracked nipples, plugged ducts, mastitis, and frustration.

Breast Milk Jaundice

Breast milk physiologic jaundice is an elevated serum indirect bilirubin concentration, with the peak level occurring after the first week of life in an infant drinking an adequate amount of breast milk with no other signs of liver abnormality. The exact cause of breast milk jaundice is unknown; however, it is believed that an enzyme may be present in some mothers' milk that inhibits the action of glucuronyl transferase, an enzyme, in the newborn which causes intestinal reabsorption of bilirubin. While breast milk jaundice is often confused with breastfeeding jaundice, the physiology and timing of these two conditions are distinct. Breastfeeding jaundice (suboptimal intake associated with dehydration) occurs in the first 2 to 7 days of life and is associated with low levels of milk intake, whereas breast milk jaundice occurs after the first week of life and may occur in infants with adequate transfer and consumption of breast milk.[29]

Clinical Findings

Physical Examination. The following are seen with breast milk jaundice:
- Healthy and thriving infant
- Adequate stooling and voiding
- Appropriate weight gain
- Elevated bilirubin levels between days 7 and 10 of life
- Bilirubin peaks at approximately days 10 to 15
- Persistence up to the third month of life

Diagnostic Tests. The following tests are often indicated: initial screening may use transcutaneous bilirubin measurement; total serum bilirubin; and urine and other cultures, which are sometimes necessary to rule out infection.

Differential Diagnosis

The differential diagnosis for breast milk jaundice is pathologic jaundice (see Chapter 28).

Management

Encourage families to continue breastfeeding unless clinical signs of pathologic jaundice are observed. Treatment with phototherapy is commonly required. Rarely does breastfeeding need to be discontinued in an infant with breast milk jaundice.

Oral Candidiasis (Thrush)

When candidiasis is diagnosed in the infant's mouth or found on the mother's nipple or areolae, both members of the dyad should be treated (see Chapter 37).

Poor Weight Gain

Problems associated with poor weight gain occur at two different times and represent different management challenges. During the newborn period, breastfeeding initiation may not proceed normally, and the infant may continue to lose weight or, at best, gain very slowly. After the newborn period, infants may gain weight slower than expected given normal age parameters.[30]

Poor weight gain has several contributing factors, including the following:
- Maternal: infrequent or inadequate feeding because of poorly managed lactation or environmental or social circumstances in the family system. In the first days after birth, this can occur because of the number of visitors the mother receives, making it difficult to breastfeed often enough to establish breast milk supply.
- Inadequate milk production
- Genetic predisposition, infection, organic disease
- Physical anomaly that prevents good suckling or swallowing

Clinical Findings

The following may be seen in poor weight gain:
Infant Factors.
- Continued weight loss after 5 to 7 days old
- Failure to regain birth weight by 2 to 3 weeks old
- Failure to maintain an ongoing weight gain of 0.5 to 1 oz/day
- Weight below the third percentile for age (this finding can be over time or a sudden change)
- Lethargic, sleepy, inactive, unresponsive infant
- Newborn or young infant sleeping longer than 4 hours between feedings
- Dry mucous membranes, poor skin turgor

Breastfeeding Technique Factors.
- Ineffective latch-on or sucking
- Short time at the breast (the infant is removed before nursing is finished, thus reducing access to lipid dense milk and total consumption)
- Infant kept on a preset schedule despite cues for more feeding
- Infant given water between feedings to "get through" to the next feeding
- Infant encouraged or allowed to sleep through the night before 8 to 12 weeks old
- Infant fed in a distracting environment
- Infant in a day care setting that does not facilitate breastfeeding

Maternal Factors.
- Does not initially respond to infant's feeding cues or does not recognize that infant must wake to establish feeding
- Hectic schedule with limited time for breastfeeding
- Recent illness or significant weight loss
- Use of oral contraceptives or other hormones that decrease production of breast milk. Women wishing to use hormonal contraceptives that contain estrogen should wait until 6 months after birth when breast milk supply is well established, and the infant begins to consume solids.

Differential Diagnosis

The differential diagnoses for poor weight gain are a pattern of slower but normal weight gain in healthy breastfed infants and failure to thrive.

Management

The following measures should be taken to manage poor weight gain:
- Complete a thorough history to elicit information regarding infant and maternal factors.
- Conduct a thorough assessment of breastfeeding techniques to accurately determine cause of poor weight gain.
- Use a supplemental system at the breast if supplementation with expressed breast milk or formula is required.
- Provide instruction, encouragement, and reinforcement for correct breastfeeding techniques.
- Be alert for any infant with significant weight loss and poor feeding pattern. Requires consultation, referral, and/or hospitalization.

Complications

Complications of poor weight gain include developmental delay, poor bonding, and severe dehydration. In situations of early failure to establish breastfeeding, an infant who appears dehydrated or septic requires hospitalization for rehydration and further diagnostic evaluation.

Additional Resources

Ameda: www.ameda.com
Australian Breastfeeding Association, breast pumps and breastfeeding products: https://www.breastfeeding.asn.au/
Human Milk Banking Association of North America: www.hmbana.org. (Guidelines and information on human milk banking; a clearinghouse for member milk banks)
International Board of Lactation Consultant Examiners (IBLCE): www.iblce.org
International board certification program for lactation consultants. International Lactation Consultant Association (ILCA): www.ilca.org (annual conference with continuing education programs and peer-reviewed professional journal, *Journal of Human Lactation*)
Kelly Mom Parenting and Breastfeeding: https://kellymom.com/ (Evidence-based information on breastfeeding and parenting)
Lactation Education Resources: www.lactationtraining.com/ (Education materials and training course; parent handouts)
La Leche League International: www.laleleague.org (Educational materials for breastfeeding families; annual workshops for lactation consultants and primary care providers)
March of Dimes: www.marchofdimes.org/hbhb/.
Medela, Inc: www.medela.com (breast pumps and breastfeeding products, referral hotline for consumers, and corporate lactation program)
National Alliance for Breastfeeding Advocacy United States Breastfeeding Committee (USBC): www.usbreastfeeding.org/ (up-to-date information on drugs and breastfeeding)
WHO Global Data Bank on Infant and Young Child Feeding: https://apps.who.int/nutrition/databases/infantfeeding/en/index.html (international information and links on infant, child, and maternal nutrition; links to WHO/UNICEF Baby-Friendly Hospital Initiative)
Work and Pump: www.workandpump.com/

References

1. World Health Organization. *Global Strategy for Infant and Young Child Feeding*; 2003. https://www.globalbreastfeedingcollective.org/global-strategy-infant-and-young-child-feeding.
2. North K, Gao M, Allen G, Lee A. Breastfeeding in a global context: epidemiology, impact and future directions. *Clin Ther.* 2022;44(2):228–244.
3. American Academy of Family Physicians (AAFP). *Breastfeeding, Family Physicians Supporting, Position Paper*; 2021. https://www.aafp.org/about/policies/all/breastfeeding-position-paper.html.
4. American Academy of Pediatrics (AAP). Policy statement: breastfeeding and the use of human milk. *Pediatrics.* 2022;150(1):1–15.
5. American Dietetic Association (ADA). Position of the American Dietetic Association: promoting and supporting breastfeeding. *J Am Diet Assoc.* 2009;109(11):1926–1942.
6. Association of Women's Health, Obstetric and Neonatal Nurses (AWHONN). AWHONN Position statement: breastfeeding and the use of human milk. *J Obstetr Gynecol Neonatal Nurs.* 2022;50(5):e1–e5.
7. National Association of Pediatric Nurse Practitioners. NAP-NAP position statement on breastfeeding. *J Pediatr Health Care.* 2019;33(1):A11–A15.
8. Centers for Disease Control and Prevention (CDC). *Breastfeeding Report Card, United States*; 2020. https://www.cdc.gov/breastfeeding/data/reportcard.htm.
9. US Department of Health and Human Services (HHS). *Policy 990:003 Nursing Mothers Program*; 2019. https://www.hhs.gov/about/agencies/asa/ohr/hr-library/990-003/index.html#:~:text=The%20Fair%20Labor%20Standards%20Act,from%20view%20and%20free%20from.
10. United Nations International Children's Emergency Fund (UNICEF). *Protecting, Promoting and Supporting Breastfeeding in Facilities Providing Maternity and Newborn Services: The Revised Baby-Friendly Hospital Initiative Implementation Guidance*; 2018. https://www.unicef.org/media/95191/file/Baby-friendly-hospital-initiative-implementation-guidance-2018.pdf.
11. *Baby-Friendly USA*; 2022. https://www.babyfriendlyusa.org/about/.
12. Thompson JMD, Tanabe K, Moon TY, et al. Duration of breastfeeding and risk of SIDS an individual participant data meta-analysis. *Child Matern Health News.* 2017;140(5). https://childhealthnews.

wordpress.com/2017/11/10/duration-of-breastfeeding-and-risk-of-sids-an-individual-participant-data-meta-analysis/.

13. Nguyen B, Jin K, Ding D. Breastfeeding and maternal cardiovascular risk factors and outcomes: a systematic review. *PLoS One.* 2017;12(11):e0187923.

14. Palmquist AEI, Perrin M, Cassar-Uhl D, Gribble K, Bond A, Cassidy T. Current trends in research on human milk exchange for infant feeding. *J Hum Lact.* 2019;35(3):433–477.

15. Bhatt H. Should COVID-19 mother breastfeed her newborn child? A literature review on the safety of breastfeeding for pregnant women with COVID-19. *Cur Nutr Rep.* 2021;10:71–75.

16. Groß R, Conzelmann C, Muller J, et al. Detection of SARS-CoV-2 in human breastmilk. *Lancet.* 2020;395(10239):1757–1758.

17. Yi DY, Kim SY. Human breast milk composition and function in human health: from nutritional components to microbiome and microRNAs. *Nutrients.* 2021;(3094):13.

18. Jackson K, Harris W. Should there be a target level of docosahexaenoic acid in breast milk? *Curr Opin Clin Nutr Metab Care.* 2016;19(2):92–96.

19. Ueno H, Higurashi S, Shimomura Y, et al. Associate of DHA concentration in human breast milk with maternal diet and use of supplements: a cross-sectional analysis of data from the Japanese human milk study cohort. *Cur Dev Nutr.* 2020;4(7).

20. Taylor S. ABM clinical protocol #29: iron, zinc, and vitamin D supplementation during breastfeeding. *Breastfeed Med.* 2018;13(6):398–403.

21. Ghaheri B, Lincoln D, Mai T, Mace. Objective improvement after frenotomy for posterior tongue-tie: a prospective randomized trial. *Otolaryngol Head Neck Surg.* 2022;166(5):976–984.

22. Academy of Breastfeeding Medicine Protocol Committee. ABM clinical protocol #8: human milk storage information for home use for full-term infants (original protocol March 2004; revision 2017). *Breastfeeding Med.* 2017;12(5):390–395.

23. Centers for Disease Control and Prevention (CDC). *WHO Growth Standards Are Recommended for Use in the U.S. For Infants and Children to 2 Years of Age;* 2010. https://www.cdc.gov/growthcharts/who_charts.htm.

24. Brown J. *Nutrition through the Life Cycle.* 7th ed. Cengade Learning; 2020.

25. *LactMed Drugs and Lactation Database: Alcohol;* 2022. https://www.ncbi.nlm.nih.gov/books/NBK501469/#:~:text=Effects%20on%20Lactation%20and%20Breastmilk.

26. *LactMed Drugs and Lactation Database: Caffeine;* 2022. https://www.ncbi.nlm.nih.gov/books/NBK501469/#:~:text=Effects%20on%20Lactation%20and%20Breastmilk.

27. National Conference of State Legislatures (NCSL). *Breastfeeding State Laws;* 2021. www.ncsl.org/research/health/breastfeeding-state-laws.aspx.

28. Moon RY, Carlin RF, Hand I. Sleep-related infant deaths: updated 2022 recommendations for reducing infant death in the sleep environment. *Pediatrics.* 2022;150(1):1–22.

29. Academy of Breastfeeding Medicine Protocol Committee. ABM clinical protocol #36: the mastitis spectrum (original protocol 2014; revision 2022). *Breastfeeding Med.* 2022;17(5):360–376.

30. Academy of Breastfeeding Medicine Protocol Committee. ABM clinical protocol #22: guidelines for management of jaundice in the breastfeeding infant 35 weeks or more of gestation – revised 2017. *Breastfeeding Med.* 2017;12(7):250–257.

16
Sleep

ANNE DEROUIN

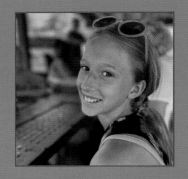

Sleep has a critical role in the health and wellbeing of infants, children, and adolescents. Essential for growth, development, emotional health, and stability, sleep allows the brain to process emotional and physical experiences that occurred during wakefulness, create long-term memories, encode learning, and provide cycles of physiologic rest, healing, and recovery. Sleep for infants, children, and adolescents occurs within a complex psycho-social-environmental system in which adults can hinder or support sleep-related behaviors and sleep health. In addition, sleep patterns and the physiologic need for sleep change across the pediatric lifespan. As the scientific understanding of sleep and the role that technology and socioeconomic influences have on sleep continues to evolve, the value of evidence-based assessment, interventions, and education that promote pediatric sleep health become increasingly important. Pediatric primary care providers (PCPs) must prioritize sleep health, consider implications of poor sleep quality, and be prepared to recommend developmentally appropriate anticipatory guidance to parents, and later to children and adolescents, that promote sleep health.

Sleep health has been defined as "a multidimensional pattern of sleep-wakefulness, adapted to individual, social, and environmental demands, that promotes physical and mental wellbeing. Good sleep health is characterized by subjective satisfaction, appropriate timing, adequate duration, high efficiency, and sustained alertness during waking hours."[1] In pediatrics, sleep health is significantly influenced by a complex myriad of socioecological factors including *proximal* factors, such as individual medical conditions, individual temperament, and family/parenting styles, and *distal* factors, such as sleeping arrangements, light and noise in the bedroom, home and neighborhood, school start times, and cultural norms that influence sleep. A visual representation of socioecological factors that influence pediatric sleep health is shown in Fig. 16.1.

Science of Sleep

Pediatric sleep cycles are regulated by both *intrinsic* factors (e.g., circadian rhythm, homeostatic sleep pressure) and *extrinsic* factors (e.g., environment, family, school). The circadian rhythm is a genetically determined, internal 24-hour sleep/wakefulness cycle influenced by environmental light and darkness. In humans, darkness perceived by a nerve pathway in the retina triggers the suprachiasmatic nucleus (SCN) in the brain. The SCN then signals the secretion of the hormone *melatonin* from the pineal gland, which promotes sleepiness. Melatonin secretion diminishes with exposure to daytime light, promoting wakefulness. The circadian rhythm is not well-established until after the first months of life.

The development of circadian rhythm (i.e., melatonin rhythmicity in response to light) contributes to nighttime sleep consolidation around 3 months of age.[2] The initial phases of sleep-wake cycles are controlled by the homeostatic sleep pressure (i.e., drive), physiologic functions (e.g., hunger, eating, digestion) and cortisol secretion. The homeostatic sleep pressure, or drive for sleep ("feeling sleepy"), is influenced by periods of daytime alertness, physical energy expenditure, diet and nutritional status, and the child's age and developmental phase.

Healthy adults typically require about 16 hours of wakefulness and energy expenditure to build sufficient homeostatic sleep pressure compared to infants and children who require much fewer wakeful hours to expend enough energy to create sleep pressure, accounting for the need for daytime napping. As children mature, their sleep pressure diminishes, resulting in their ability to remain alert without napping during daytime. After puberty, adolescents gain the ability to delay bedtime through natural growth and changes in their circadian rhythms.[3] Recognizing the factors affecting sleep across the pediatric lifespan helps PCPs recommend strategies that are targeted for age and tailored for the individual to promote sleep health, decreased daytime sleep pressure, and increased feelings of alertness and engagement.

Extrinsic factors that influence sleep health include social and cultural behaviors and family systems that children often have no control over, including sleeping arrangements (co-sleeping with parents, "family bed"), sleep location (proximity to siblings/family members, habituating in multiple caregiver homes), family and school schedules, bedtime routines, factors that inhibit sleep health such as diet (e.g., caffeine, sugar, over- or undereating), technology use prior to bedtime, and parent-child interactions. A critical aspect of assessing sleep health is the routine inquiry about extrinsic factors during well-child visits. Evaluation of extrinsic factors and assessment of the regularity of bedtimes and wake times is critical, as consistent routines are essential for maintaining healthy sleep rhythm.[3] Through consistent anticipatory guidance, the PCP can help families anticipate and prevent problematic sleep-wake cycles that result from predictable and modifiable factors including diet, technology usage, and varied bedtime routines among weekdays, weekends, and holidays.

Cycle of Sleep

Although "peaceful slumber" is a phrase often envisioned while an infant or child sleeps, the physiologic process is quite dynamic, consisting of cycles that repeat every 90 to 120 minutes throughout the night (Fig. 16.2). Each cycle has measurable phases of neurologic activity and is important to the overall process of healthy

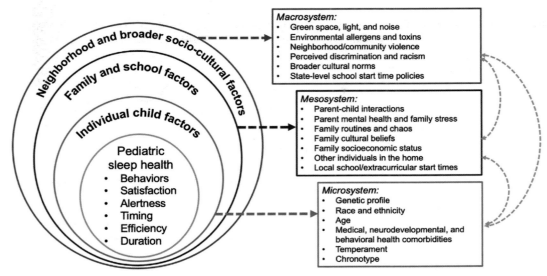

• **Fig 16.1** Socioecological Factors Hypothesized to Contribute to Pediatric Sleep Health Domains. (From Meltzer LJ, Williamson AA, Mindell JA. Pediatric sleep health: it matters, and so does how we define it. *Sleep Med Rev.* 2021;57:101425.)

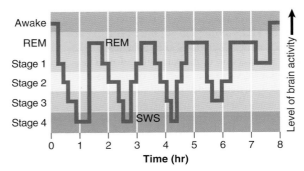

• **Fig 16.2** Sleep Stages. *REM*, Rapid eye movement; *SWS*, slow wave sleep. (From Patton KT, Bell F, Thompson T, et al. *Anatomy & Physiology*. 11th ed. Elsevier; 2022.)

sleep. In each cycle, there are two phases of sleep: (1) rapid eye movement (REM) and (2) non-REM (NREM). NREM sleep is the primary phase of sleep, occurring most of the sleep cycle time; it has three subphases (N1, N2, and N3) that are identifiable by subtle physiologic and electroencephalographic patterns. The typical order for each sleep cycle is N1, N2, N3, and REM, although a greater amount of time is spent in deep sleep (N3) earlier in the night, whereas the amount of REM sleep increases in the last two cycles, just before natural awakening.

NREM Phase 1 (N1)

NREM Phase 1 (N1) is a period of drowsiness that occurs during early transition to sleep. Aside from newborns and children diagnosed with narcolepsy, the average child's sleep stage begins in N1 sleep. It includes slowing body movements, eye rolling, jerky or twitching body movements, and fluttering eyelids. Individuals may even believe they are awake, but they cannot accurately report events that occurred during the time. This first phase of sleep provides the body with musculoskeletal recovery from physical activity and energy expenditure during the day.

NREM Phase 2 (N2)

NREM Phase 2 (N2) is a deeper sleep state in which eye movements, breathing, and heart rate slow and the distal extremities cool. Muscles slacken, although children in N2 are able to reposition their bodies or arouse.

NREM Phase 3 (N3)

NREM Phase 3 (N3) is also known as *deep, delta,* or *slow wave sleep* (SWS). During this stage of sleep, a child is sleeping soundly and difficult to awaken. During N3, sleep occurs in longer periods early in the night, particularly during the first two sleep cycles. It is during N3 that growth hormone is released. It is also when parents note sleep walking (and talking), bed wetting, and night terrors.

REM Sleep

REM sleep is a time of psychological recovery and consolidation of memory and learning from the experiences of the day. It is characterized by increased brainwave activity, dreams/nightmares, and active eye movements that resemble an awakened state. While experiencing vivid dreams (or nightmares), the muscles are slack, which protects the individual from physically acting out their dreams. REM sleep is considered a time for the brain to learn from the experiences of the day. The proportion of REM sleep is highest during infancy but gradually decreases by 5 years of age.

Each phase of sleep is so critical to growth, development, and physiologic wellbeing that when children are deprived of a specific sleep phase, particularly REM or N3, pressure to restore it will mount, a rebound pattern develops in an effort to gain homeostasis, with the body shortening other phases to regain the stage that has been lacking. Discrepancies or imbalances in sleep cycles also affect behavior, mood, and daytime functioning. Those deprived of REM sleep become excitable, irritable, and anxious, while those deprived of N3 sleep experience intense fatigue.

Individuals typically have brief arousals between sleep cycles. Most are so brief that they cannot be recalled; however, the brief

TABLE 16.1	Pediatric Sleep Requirements	
Developmental Age Group	**Hours of Sleep per 24 Hours**
Newborn	14–17
Infant	12–16
Early Childhood	11–14 (1- to 2-year-olds) 10–13 (3- to 5-year-olds)
Middle Childhood	9–12
Adolescence	8–10

Modified from Paruthi S, Brooks LJ, D'Ambrosio C, Hall WA, Kotagal S, Lloyd RM, et al. Recommended amount of sleep for pediatric populations: a consensus statement of the American Academy of Sleep Medicine. *J Clin Sleep Med.* 2016;12(6):785–786.

arousals between cycles in young children may sometimes be misinterpreted by parents and adult caregivers as awakenings that require social engagement or late-night feedings resulting in altered sleeping arrangements and dysregulated sleep for the entire family.

Sleep Patterns

Homeostatic sleep demands change as a child matures, including sleep needs, duration, and cycling. Though individual sleep patterns vary due to instinct and extrinsic factors, the average hours of sleep required for each 24-hour period is well established and can be useful to PCPs when providing anticipatory guidance (Table 16.1).

Developmental Sleep Considerations

Newborns and Infants

Newborns sleep 14 to 17 hours per day, while infants require only 12 to 16 hours (see Table 16.1). Newborns and young infants (<6 months of age) spend 50% of their sleep time in active REM sleep, which gradually decreases to 20% to 25% of sleep time in adults. REM sleep is often evident in newborns with audible suckling, smiling, twitching of arms and legs during sleep. The active REM sleep of infants results in shorter sleep cycles and more frequent arousal; their cycles can last a few minutes to several hours in the first weeks of life. Once the circadian rhythm is established, typically by 3 to 4 months, most infants sleep through the night without need for feeding, while newborn sleep occurs on an irregular schedule with periods of 1 to 3 hours spent awake.

Sudden Unexpected Infant Death. Sudden unexpected infant death (SUID) is an umbrella term used to describe any sudden and unexpected death of an infant (0–12 months of age), explained or unexplained, occurring in the first year of life. SUID includes infant death from suffocation or asphyxia, entrapment, infection, ingestions, metabolic diseases, arrhythmias, and unintentional or nonaccidental trauma. Sudden infant death syndrome (SIDS) is a subcategory of SUID accounting for about half of all SUID cases. It is defined as a death of an infant that is unexplained after a thorough case investigation including autopsy, a scene investigation, and a clinical history analysis.[4]

The pathophysiology of SIDS is multifactorial, with the triple-risk model being the most widely accepted lens for understanding. This model proposes that SIDS occurs when an infant with intrinsic vulnerability (e.g., impaired or immature arousal,

cardiorespiratory, and/or autonomic responses) experiences an exogenous stress trigger (e.g., exposure to unsafe sleeping environment) during a vulnerable period of development.[5] Of note, the risk for SIDS is not linked to infants who have experienced brief (<1 minute) resolved unexplained events (BRUEs) that are witnessed (e.g., apnea, color changes, choking, gagging, decreased muscle tone or limpness).[4]

Infant sleep-related deaths have declined since the American Academy of Pediatrics (AAP) "Back to Sleep" campaign began in 1994; however, SIDS continues to be a leading cause of post-neonatal deaths in infancy. Of note, however, is that infant sleep-related deaths data show notable and persistent racial and ethnic disparitiesjavascript:; that reflect ongoing racial and ethnic societal inequities and health outcomes among populations.[6] Mortality rates for White infants have declined faster when compared to rates in non-Hispanic Black and American Indian/Alaskan Native infants.[7] Low socioeconomic status, unemployment, housing instability, and domestic violence are correlated with higher risk of sleep-related death.[7]

Currently, the occurrence of SIDS remains greater than 3000 deaths/year in the United States, with most occurring before 6 months of age.[5] SIDS deaths are higher among males, those born prematurely or small for gestational age, and among infants with mothers who are less than 20 years of age. While the actual mechanisms for SIDS remain unclear, there are strategies that reduce the risk of SIDS among all infants, bringing attention to modifiable factors. For example, infants who co-sleep or share sleep space in a bed, couch, or chair with adults (i.e., "bed sharing" or "service-sharing"), especially in an overly warm environment (e.g., enhanced by hats, swaddling, or weighted blankets), and in soft bedding are at highest risk for SIDS.[4]

This knowledge gave rise to the Safe to Sleep campaign (formerly known as Back to Sleep), which focuses on multiple ways, other than infant position, to reduce the risk of SIDS and other sleep-related causes of infant death. In 2022 the AAP updated the 2016 SIDS prevention recommendations, enhancing safety recommendations that reduce risk of infant sleep-related mortality (Box 16.1). These recommendations also include a call for pediatric PCPs to offer anticipatory guidance to each new parent and serve as pediatric advocates engaged in policy and industry-safety recommendations.

Early Childhood

The number of hours spent sleeping continues to decrease; however, longer hours are spent sleeping at night, supplemented with two daytime naps. Children 1 to 2 years old require 11 to 14 hours of sleep per day, while those age 3 to 5 years require 10 to 13 hours (see Table 16.1). Sleep difficulties, such as resisting going to bed and nighttime awakenings, are common in children 1 to 2 years of age as part of their seeking independence, paired with increased motor, social, and cognitive abilities. Separation anxiety begins in infancy but can extend to up to 2 years of age, which can contribute to resistance at bedtime. Fears and nightmares are also common in this age group, especially after age 3 years.

Children ages 3 to 5 years often have difficulty with sleep latency or falling asleep. Waking up during the night is also common in this age group. As their daytime imaginations evolve, so do their nighttime fears and nightmares. In addition, somnambulism (i.e., sleepwalking) and night terrors are at their peak, both of which are typically alleviated by ensuring regular daytime routines and sleep patterns. The American Academy of Sleep Medicine (AASM) guidelines for managing

- Supine positioning (Back to Sleep) every time an infant is put down to sleep.
- Firm, flat sleeping surface.
- Breastfeeding.
- Room sharing *without* bed sharing (first 6 months of life).
- Absence of bumper pads, wedges, or loose blankets, bedding, toys in the infant's sleep area.
- Offering an untethered pacifier at sleep (nap, bedtime).
- Parental avoidance of smoking, to eliminate smoke as well as nicotine exposure.
- Parental avoidance of alcohol, marijuana, opioids, and illicit drugs.
- Avoid overheating (e.g., head covering, extra blankets).
- Routine immunizations are up to date.
- Initiating tummy time, to facilitate development. beginning soon after hospital discharge, increasing to at least 15–30 minutes/day by age 7 weeks.
- Avoidance of home cardiorespiratory monitors.

Modified from Moon RY, Carlin RF, Hand I; Task Force on Sudden Infant Death Syndrome and the Committee on Fetus and Newborn. Sleep-related infant deaths: updated 2022 recommendations for reducing infant deaths in the sleep environment. *Pediatrics.* 2022;150(1):e2022057990.

sleep disruptions in early childhood primarily focus on behavioral therapies, including gradual removal of parental presence, positive bedtime routines, and scheduled daytime awakenings as effective therapies.[3]

Middle Childhood

Sleep requirements decrease to 9 to 12 hours a day for this age group (see Table 16.1). Naps are now gone. Sleep disturbances are common, especially when starting school as they adjust to academic routines. Sleep deficiencies are predictive of cognitive, behavioral, emotional, and academic outcomes. Studies show that 5- to 6-year-olds with shorter sleep duration or difficulty settling or staying asleep at night score significantly lower on IQ and other achievement tests,[8] and children who regularly sleep 10 or more hours in a 24-hour period have better social adjustment to academic routines. Social and academic demands (e.g., homework) and extracurricular activities (e.g., sports) also increase during this age. Further, many schools now use computers in the classroom and children also often engage in other screentime activities (e.g., video games, television, virtual devices) with "blue" light, which can affect the child's normal circadian rhythm by fooling the body that it is still light out. Healthy sleep hygiene, which includes an organized, consistent, routine bedtime, limited screen access, especially an hour before bedtime, and avoiding caffeine and sugar after the dinner meal or 4 to 6 hours before sleep initiation, is critical for wellbeing of children.[9]

Adolescence

Up to two-thirds of adolescents in the United States get less than the recommended 8 to 10 hours of sleep per night; they also experience the most sleep disturbances of all pediatric age groups.[10] About one in four teens (25%) report sleep delay, nighttime awakening, or feeling sleepy during the day. This rate nearly doubled (46%) during the SARS-CoV-2 (COVID-19) pandemic, which was mostly attributed to remote learning environments, social isolation, limited outdoor and in-person activities, and poor sleep hygiene.[11] These sleep disturbances have resulted in academic progression delays and increased rates of mental health disorders, especially anxiety, depression, and suicidal thoughts. Coupled with adolescents' risk for sleep disruptions, many had less sleep than recommended for healthy growth and neurocognitive development.

There is a natural circadian shift that occurs around puberty, as circadian rhythm moves forward approximately 2 hours. This shift makes it difficult to fall asleep earlier in the evening and difficult to be awake for the typical early school start times. Even after a call from the AAP to move start time later than 8:30 am, most middle and high schools continue to have early start times.[12] The pubertal circadian rhythm change in sleep cycle, along with a mismatch of school start times, often results in chronic sleep deprivation among many adolescents.[13]

Additional risks include social and school activities that involve screen time technology, after-school activities, employment, homework, and athletic or social obligations, as each contributes to delayed sleep initiation. Many teens report daytime sleepiness, napping, and oversleeping on weekends and school holidays to make up their "sleep debt" from the week. Unfortunately, physical and mental health, safety, and academic outcomes are linked to poor sleep and may have lifelong implications, as adolescents who consistently sleep less than 8 hours/day are more likely to experience greater levels of anxiety, irritability, and other somatic and psychologic symptoms.[14] The results of chronic sleep deprivation and attempts to "catch-up" on weekends are also linked to disordered eating (e.g., overeating, use of caffeine/energy drinks, skipping breakfast), weight gain, hypertension, and abnormal glucose metabolism—all of which have metabolic and cardiovascular implications that extend into adulthood.

Healthy sleep hygiene emphasizes adhering to a routine sleep schedule, eliminating evening caffeine use, turning off blue light–emitting devices at least 1 hour before sleep, promoting exercise during the day, and limiting adolescent school, work, and after-school schedules to ensure adequate rest and sleep habits. There is also evidence to show consistent family mealtimes, occurring even twice a week, have a protective effective that contributes to healthy sleep among adolescents.[15] Family mealtimes promote engagement and offer adolescents opportunity to focus on positive events, attributes, and emotions that occur. Another important role of family meals and engagement is the opportunity to help adolescents gain insight from the information gleaned in their technology and media usage and foster a family commitment to implement agreed-upon boundaries for technology usage.[16] Pediatric sleep experts recommend initiating strategies that promote sleep *before* adolescence, if possible, reiterated during routine adolescent clinical visits, modelled in the home through family engagement, and reinforced in academic settings through education, peer support campaigns, and media reminders. The AAP, AASM, and the Centers for Disease Control and Prevention offer sleep strategies and tool kits for PCPs and families (see Additional Resources).

Impact of Digital Technology. Adolescents are increasingly using digital resources and technology, not only in school for learning, but also to play, entertain, and communicate with each other. This increase in screen time and exposure to the blue light (emitted from most digital devices) has health implications directly related to sleep deprivation. Further, the World Health Organization (WHO) officially recognized Digital Technology Addiction (DTA) in 2020 and identified that digital technology and devices are readily available to most adolescents, placing them at increased risk for addictive behavior.[17] DTA is described as "excessive online activity and internet use resulting in the inability to manage time, energy, and attention during daytime and disturbed sleep patterns or insomnia during nighttime" and has significant implications for adolescent brain development and long-term health outcomes.[18] DTA has been further classified as internet addiction disorder (IAD) or internet gaming addiction (IGA), characterized as uncontrolled internet use and defined by behaviors that include (1) gaming or internet use for long, uninterrupted time periods, (2) skipping school to play, (3) withdrawal from other social activities to use the Internet, (4) resorting to gaming/internet to avoid emotions, and (5) consequential sleep problems.[19] While DTA has been significantly linked to depression and insomnia, studies show that general, nonaddictive use of digital technology is also linked to mental health conditions such as anxiety, isolation, depression, disordered eating, self-harm, substance use disorder, and suicide, all of which have a direct relationship to sleep disruption.[20] Since the use of technology is not likely to diminish in the future, it is critically important for PCPs to educate and empower adolescents and parents with strategies to combat digital technology addiction and ensure adequate sleep.

Assessment of Sleep

Sleep is vital to growth, development, wellbeing, and long-term health outcomes across the pediatric lifespan. Routine assessment of sleep should occur alongside nutrition, safety, activity, and family relationships assessments. The National Sleep Foundation (NSF) advocates that sleep be considered a "vital sign," particularly among adolescents who are notoriously sleep deprived.[21] Routine screening of sleep at each well-child visit should include asking parents broad generalized inquiries, such as:

- Tell me about your child's sleep.
- Does your child have any sleep problems?
- Is there anything you wish to change about your child's sleep?

The PCP should also assess the environment where the child sleeps, the bedtime routine, and if the child snores or experiences other sleep disruptions. It can be challenging in young children who are unable to offer a description of their rest, so PCPs must rely on adult caregivers for accurate history. Once children are old enough, it is important to note any differences between the data from the child versus parent. Parents are often unaware of sleep difficulty, disruptions, or daytime sleepiness in older children and adolescents. Any sleep concerns should be evaluated using a standardized approach, including detailed history, physical examination, and if warranted, special testing or referral to a pediatric sleep specialist.

History

Chief Complaint

Evaluation of sleep concerns or problems involves a comprehensive history of the child's 24-hour routine, focusing on bedtime habits, sleep environment, and daytime behavior. The family medical history and parental attitudes and beliefs about what constitutes normal sleep are also important and can inform the investigation and treatment plan. When sleep difficulties are noted, it is important to conduct a symptom analysis, asking about the age when the problem began, precipitating events, presence of the symptoms on the weekends, holidays, or vacation, and if aggravating or alleviating factors are present. It is also important to assess its effects on the child or adolescent's daily functioning, as well as the impact on other family members.

Past Medical History and Review of Systems

Medical problems are often associated with sleep difficulties, including any associated pain and discomfort. Other areas to assess include:

- Obesity: with associated sleep-disordered breathing (SDB).
- Neurologic disorder: autism spectrum disorder (ASD), attention-deficit/hyperactivity disorder (ADHD), cerebral palsy, and neuromuscular disorders are associated with behavioral sleep problems (BSPs) and/or SDB.
- Respiratory conditions: hypoxemia, asthma, laryngomalacia, allergic rhinitis, obstructive sleep apnea (OSA), and asthma are frequently comorbid conditions.
- Gastroesophageal reflux: may contribute to OSA, especially in newborns and infants.
- Nocturnal enuresis: can be associated with SDB.
- Dermatologic conditions causing discomfort (e.g., itching with eczema).
- Pulmonary hypertension: can be caused by untreated SDB.
- Failure to thrive (FTT): especially when secondary to increased caloric expenditure from increased work of breathing.
- Developmental delays: can affect the child's ability to develop appropriate sleep behaviors.
- Epilepsy: has an increased risk for sleep disorders.
- Depression, anxiety, or other psychiatric problems, such as substance use disorder and internet gaming disorder, can contribute to insomnia.

Family History

- Parental knowledge and expectations about typical sleep patterns.
- Parental ability and willingness to modify sleep hygiene.
- Family history of sleep disorders, including sleep apnea, obesity, substance use, neurodevelopmental or mental health conditions.
- Recent divorce, separation, family or close friend death, changes in living or school arrangements, other family stressors or exposure to trauma, violence, or natural disasters.

Physical Examination

A thorough and complete physical examination is indicated for individuals with sleep issues. Vital signs should be obtained, including occipitofrontal (head) circumference (OFC) for infants, pulse oximetry, weight and length/height, body mass index (BMI), blood pressure, and pain assessment. Adolescents should also be screened for depression using a standardized screening tool. Neurologic evaluation, including the child's muscle tone, range of motion, strength and gait should be completed. Special attention should be paid to obvious tone and strength discrepancies, unstable gait, hyperactivity, rapid speech, jittery or anxious appearance, and symptoms of depression, including self-injury, bruising, or scars. It is important to assess for dermatologic conditions, such as hives, eczema, rashes, acne, and enlarged or multiple hyperpigmented macules that could signal an underlying condition or could be contributing to the sleep concern. Careful assessment of sinuses, nose, mouth, and throat, as well as neck, are also important when assessing risk of snoring. Clinicians may note cough, loud breathing, frequent sniffing/sneezing, clearing of throat, swollen nasal turbinates, dull and/or painful sinuses, a raspy, congested voice or cry of the child with chronic allergic rhinitis, severe asthma, and/or a narrow airway. Findings in children at risk for sleep-related breathing problems may also include deviated nasal septum, nasal polyps, open mouth posture, high-arched palate, adenoid facies (i.e., "long face syndrome"), enlarged tonsils, narrow oropharynx, low-hanging soft palate, and micro- or retrognathia.

Standardized Screening Tools

Sleep assessment tools and questionnaires (Table 16.2) are used to assess the various aspects of sleep domains, including sleep satisfaction, timing, efficiency, duration, and behaviors; however, these tools rely on self-report by either the patient and/or parent. They do not include behaviors observed outside the home (e.g., school, daycare), which may limit an accurate assessment of sleep efficiency and daytime alertness. One tool, the *Pediatric Sleep Practices Questionnaire* (PSPQ), can be used in screening for sleep issues in children 8 to 17 years. It features questions that include assessment of technology use before bedtime and the sleep environment, which have been identified as significant contributors to sleep quality of older children and teens.[22] Importantly, it includes only 15 items, making it useful in busy practices, while still providing the PCP with insight into conditions that impact sleep quality. The findings provide a baseline from which to provide guidance, education, and direct discussions with children, adolescents, and their parents to enhance sleep practices.

Referral and Special Testing

Pediatric sleep specialists typically use an interprofessional approach (pediatric sleep expert, nursing team, social worker, educational specialist) and often collaborate with pediatric developmental specialists, genetics counselors, developmental pediatricians, neurologists, and ENT specialists when children have specific medical conditions. Sleep specialists commonly order a polysomnogram (PSG), a multiparametric test that reports total sleep time, sleep latency, and sleep efficiency (percentage of time in bed spent sleeping).[23] Another test is the actigram, which measures light exposure and activity, typically over 1 week in the child's home environment via a device the child wears like a wristwatch. It is helpful for evaluating the effectiveness of insomnia treatments since the total sleep time is measured through the test. Results offer an objective measurement for children and parents that can dispel sleep misperceptions about length of sleep and the environment that is conducive for quality sleep. For example, adolescents who report "being awake most of the night" gain valuable data on the true length of time they sleep, which can allay concerns about a chronic condition and offer evidence of sleep hygiene. The test also offers clinicians the opportunity to promote or reinforce additional sleep-promoting practices. The PSG is less invasive and less expensive than actigraphy. Other testing (electrocardiogram, electroencephalogram, laboratory values) may be considered depending on the presenting condition, medical history, and examination findings.

Common Sleep-Related Disorders

The most common sleep-related disorder in childhood is *behavioral insomnia*, affecting 10% to 30% of young children. It often results from inconsistent parental limit-setting or inconsistent sleep onset.[24] Other pediatric sleep-related concerns include restless leg syndrome (RLS) and periodic limb movements (PLMs), parasomnias, SDB, OSA, and central sleep apnea (CSA). Children with neurodevelopmental disorders, such as ASD and ADHD, have the highest rates of sleep disorders during childhood.

Insomnia in children is defined as sleep onset delay more than 30 minutes (on average) per night and/or frequent prolonged night waking with impaired daytime functioning. A variety of medications may be considered for insomnia. *Melatonin*, available over the counter, is commonly recommended, though there are currently no treatment guidelines for pediatric dosing; however, it is associated with improved sleep quality among children without significant risk factors or associated side effects.[25] *Antihistamines*, such as diphenhydramine and hydroxyzine, are the most widely prescribed short-acting sedatives in pediatrics, but limited evidence exists to support their use.[26] Guanfacine, an α2-adrenergic agonist, has also been successfully used to promote sleep onset. There is limited evidence to support the use of *α-agonists*, such as clonidine, to improve sleep latency, especially in children with ADHD.[26]

Restless Legs Syndrome and Periodic Limb Movements

RLS is a sensory and motor disorder characterized by irritating sensations in the legs accompanied by an irresistible urge to move the legs, which typically helps. There is an association of RLS and ADHD, which may not be evident to children and parents until after ADHD treatment has been initiated.[24] PLMs are repetitive jerks, typically in the legs, that occur every 5 to 90 seconds. RLS and PLMs usually occur together, but PLMs may occur without RLS. The prevalence of PLMs in school-age children has been estimated to be 1.9% to 3.6%; however, the condition is often unrecognized in younger children or those with delays secondary to communications deficits. The etiology of PLMs remains unclear, but genetic factors, dopaminergic dysfunction, low iron storage status, and side effects of selective serotonin reuptake inhibitors (SSRIs), sedating antihistamines, and dopamine receptor antagonists have been implicated.

Children with RLS and PLMs typically have a history of abruptly awakening during the night following 1 to 3 hours of sleep. Upon waking, affected children cry, kick, and strike their legs, verbally expressing that the legs hurt; the discomfort is often relieved by massage or stretching. Other significant history includes daytime sleepiness and/or hyperactivity and insomnia.[31] Children with RLS often have a normal physical and neurologic examination. Serum ferritin levels are indicated to rule out iron-deficiency anemia, which is associated with RLS. Treatment is typically correction of iron deficiency with oral supplementation of ferrous sulfate (3 mg/kg/day) and removal of any other triggers.[24] Other conditions to rule out include leg cramps and Osgood-Schlatter disease.

Parasomnias

NREM parasomnias include confusional arousals, somnambulism (i.e., sleepwalking), and night terrors. Precipitating factors include sleep deprivation, stress or emotional upset, febrile illnesses, being overheated at night, a full bladder, or use of central nervous system depressant medications such as diphenhydramine. These factors interrupt deep sleep, causing partial awakening, which results in disorientation or fear in young children that they may not recall the following morning.[32]

Confusional arousals typically occur in early childhood and diminish around age 5 years. Often frightening to adult caregivers, the child awakes from a deep sleep early in the sleep cycle night, appears dazed, and is slow to react. It is also described as

TABLE 16.2   Pediatric Sleep Health Questionnaires and Measures

Subjective Measures	Satisfaction	Alertness/ Sleepiness	Timing	Efficiency	Duration	Behaviors	Age	Items	Reporter
Children's Sleep Habits Questionnaire[a]	x	x	x	x	x	x	2–10 y	33/45	Parent
Children's Report of Sleep Patterns[b,c,d]	x	x	x	x	x	x	8–18 y	60	Self
School Sleep Habits Survey[e]	x	x	x	x	x	x	13–19 y	45	Self
Brief Infant Sleep Questionnaire[f,g]	x		x	x	x	x	0–3 y	13/25	Parent
BEARS[h]		x	x		x	x	2–18 y	7–8	Parent/self
PROMIS Pediatric Sleep Disturbance[i]	x						8–18 y 5–18 y	4/8/15 4/8/15	Self Parent proxy
Sleep Disturbance Scale for Children[j]		x		x			6–15 y	27	Parent
Modified Epworth Sleepiness Scale[k]/Epworth Sleepiness Scale for Children and Adolescents[l]		x					12–18 y 2–18 y	8 8	Self Parent proxy
Pediatric Sleep Questionnaire[m]		x					2–18 y	22	Parent
Pediatric Daytime Sleepiness Scale[n]		x					11–15 y	8	Self
PROMIS Pediatric Sleep Related Impairment[o]		x					8–18 y 5–18 y	4/8/15 4/8/15	Self Parent proxy
Morningness-Eveningness Questionnaire for Children[p]			x				11-12 y	10	Self

[a]Owens JA, Spirito A, McGuinn M. The Children's Sleep Habits Questionnaire (CSHQ): psychometric properties of a survey instrument for school-aged children. *Sleep.* 2000;23(8):1043e51.

[b]Meltzer LJ, Avis KT, Biggs S, et al. The Children's Report of Sleep Patterns (CRSP): a self-report measure of sleep for school-aged children. *J Clin Sleep Med.* 2013;9(3):235e45.

[c]Meltzer LJ, Biggs S, Reynolds A, et al. The children's report of sleep patterns—sleepiness scale: a self-report measure for school-aged children. *Sleep Med.* 2012;13(4):385e9.

[d]Meltzer LJ, Brimeyer C, Russell K, et al. The children's report of sleep patterns: validity and reliability of the sleep hygiene index and sleep disturbance scale in adolescents. *Sleep Med.* 2014;15(12):1500e7.

[e]Wolfson AR, Carskadon MA, Acebo C, et al. Evidence for the validity of a sleep habits survey for adolescents. *Sleep* 2003;26(2):213e6.

[f]Sadeh A. A brief screening questionnaire for infant sleep problems: validation and findings for an Internet sample. *Pediatrics* 2004;113(6):e570e7.

[g]Mindell JA, Gould RA, Tikotzy L, et al. Norm-referenced scoring system for the Brief Infant Sleep Questionnaire–Revised (BISQ-R). *Sleep Med.* 2019;63:106e14.

[h]Owens JA, Dalzell V. Use of the 'BEARS' sleep screening tool in a pediatric residents' continuity clinic: a pilot study. *Sleep Med.* 2005;6:63e9.

[i]Forrest CB, Meltzer LJ, Marcus CL, et al. Development and validation of the PROMIS Pediatric Sleep Disturbance and Sleep-Related Impairment item banks. *Sleep.* 2018;41(6).

[j]Bruni O, Ottaviano S, Guidetti V, et al. The Sleep Disturbance Scale for Children (SDSC) Construction and validation of an instrument to evaluate sleep disturbances in childhood and adolescence. *J Sleep Res.* 1996;5(4):251e61.

[k]Melendres MCS, Lutz JM, Rubin ED, et al. Daytime sleepiness and hyperactivity in children with suspected sleep-disordered breathing. *Pediatrics.* 2004;114(3):768e75.

[l]Janssen KC, Phillipson S, O'Connor J, et al. Validation of the Epworth sleepiness scale for children and adolescents using Rasch analysis. *Sleep Med.* 2017;33:30e5.

[m]Chervin RD, Hedger K, Dillon JE, et al. Pediatric sleep questionnaire (PSQ): validity and reliability of scales for sleep-disordered breathing, snoring, sleepiness, and behavioral problems. *Sleep Med.* 2000;1(1):21e32.

[n]Drake C, Nickel C, Burduvali E, et al. The pediatric daytime sleepiness scale (PDSS): sleep habits and school outcomes in middle-school children. *Sleep.* 2003;26(4):455e8.

[o]Forrest CB, Meltzer LJ, Marcus CL, et al. Development and validation of the PROMIS Pediatric Sleep Disturbance and Sleep-Related Impairment item banks. *Sleep.* 2018;41(6).

[p]Carskadon MA, Vieira C, Acebo C. Association between puberty and delayed phase preference. *Sleep.* 1993;16(3):258e62.

From Meltzer LJ, Williamson AA, Mendell JA. Pediatric sleep health: it matters, and so does how we define it. *Sleep Med Rev.* 2021;57:101425.

excessive sleep inertia or "sleep drunkenness."[32] *Somnambulism* occurs in approximately 1% to 15% of children and can pose a safety threat.[33] It begins as confusional arousal characterized by a dazed expression with open eyes and mumbled or slurred speech while they briefly wander, or even run around, their bedroom or home. NREM confusional arousals are typically short lived and benign in young children and best managed by not awakening the child while ensuring safety, especially in a home with stairways. Some parasomnias can be prevented by identifying the stressor, ensuring adequate naptimes, controlling the sleeping environment, or resolving febrile illness.

Night terrors, reported in about 5% of children ages 18 months to 6 years, are an extreme state of agitation characterized by a sudden onset of screaming, dilated pupils, increased heart rate, and sweating during N3 sleep.[34] *Nightmares* are distinct from night terrors, as they occur during REM sleep during the last sleep cycle of the night. They occur in approximately 25% of all children 3 to 6 years of age.[34] Characterized by a sudden arousal from sleep to a fully awake state, nightmare details are often recalled the next day, whereas night terrors are usually not remembered. Occasional nightmares occur throughout life and are more common during times of stress or situational change (e.g., starting school, moving); parental reassurance is generally effective.

Assessment of parasomnias includes a careful history of the event, physical examination, and testing if febrile illness or recurrent nocturnal enuresis is reported. Assessment of parasomnia concerns should include historical data of the event in relation to sleep onset, frequency, and length of the episode; evidence of apnea or limb movements; temperature of sleeping environment and sweating history; family history including consideration of sleepwalking; medications or supplement usage; typical sleep patterns and routines of the child and family; stressors in the environment, including change in school, environment, new siblings, or parental relationships; and the child's memory of the event (if developmentally able). Recurrent nightmares warrant investigation by a healthcare provider including a careful history and physical examination.

Sleep-Disordered Breathing and Obstructive Sleep Apnea

Children with SDB can present with simple snoring, upper airway resistance, and even OSA. Snoring occurs in as many as 17% in children; however, OSA is found in 1% to 5% of infants and children.[24] Untreated OSA can result in various physical problems, including obesity, metabolic disorder, hypertension, and cardiovascular insult, all of which have lifelong implications. OSA is strongly associated with insufficient sleep, which in turn can result in mental health, social issues, and poor academic performance. Risk factors include tonsillar or adenoid hypertrophy, obesity, craniofacial abnormalities, gastroesophageal reflux, neuromuscular disorders, and untreated allergic rhinitis. Children with neuromuscular disorders might not snore but should be evaluated for SDB.

Both SDB and OSA include snoring, gasping, apnea events, increased work of breathing with paradoxical respirations, neck hyperextension, night sweating, tachycardia, and/or restless or disrupted sleep. With SDB, persistent parasomnias and history of insomnia are common. Typically, the child arouses during significant snoring or gasping after an apneic episode, then resumes sleep until another episode occurs during the night. A careful history and physical examination help distinguish snoring from OSA.

A pediatric sleep specialist, evaluation, and positive PSG are typically involved to confirm OSA. Polysomnography identifies the severity of the OSA, provides data to plan for pre- and postoperative care, and offers a baseline for comparison in a postoperative sleep study. Adenotonsillectomy is the first-line treatment for OSA. Other surgical options include partial tonsillectomy, craniofacial surgery (e.g., mandibular distraction for micrognathia), and tracheostomy in severe cases. Additional procedures for the management of OSA may include tongue-base reduction surgery, uvulopalatopharyngoplasty, lingual tonsillectomy, supraglottoplasty, and hypoglossal nerve stimulation.[35]

Surgery is only for children who have tonsillar or adenoid hypertrophy. In those who are a young age or have morbid obesity or family or other risk factors, surgery may be contraindicated. For these children, nasal continuous positive airway pressure (CPAP) may be considered as second-line treatment.[24] Other nonsurgical options may be effective for managing mild to moderate OSA,[36] including nasal steroids and leukotriene receptor antagonists (Montelukast), normal saline rinses, and weight loss. Nasal steroids and Montelukast can be effective in mild to moderate OSA by reducing the lymphoid tissue, especially the adenoids. CPAP provides humidified air pressure via a nasal mask without supplemental oxygen, for SDB treatment. Occasionally, a child with neuromuscular disorders requires extra support with tidal volume, oxygen, high pressure, or a backup respiratory rate. Many children and adolescents do not tolerate or adhere to CPAP treatment, so other treatment alternatives, such as positional therapy, high-flow nasal cannula, and the use of orthodontic procedures, such as rapid maxillary expansion and mandibular advancement devices, are considered.

Central Sleep Apnea

Central sleep apnea (CSA) is a pathologic form of apnea that is rare in children. It typically indicates a significant neurologic condition, such as brainstem lesions, Chiari malformations, or exposure to narcotics that diminish the respiratory drive. Children with CSA have no arousal, snoring, or gasping. The apnea episode frequently results in oxygen desaturation and risk of cardiovascular arrest. Treatment is immediate ventilator support and oxygen via while determining and correcting the underlying cause. CSA occurs among extreme premature infants, who can eventually outgrow apneic events as they mature, with careful monitoring and support.

Sleep Concerns With Neurodevelopmental and Mental Health Disorders

Autism Spectrum Disorder
Children with ASD commonly experience sleep disturbances (50%–80% prevalence), particularly insomnia and maintaining sleep throughout the night. There is evidence of shortened REM cycles in these children along with delayed deep sleep (N3), which contribute to irregular sleep-wake patterns and daytime sleepiness.[27] Sleep disorders, such as parasomnias, PLMs, and SDB, are also common in children with ASD. Decreased muscle tone, which is also common among children with significant ASD, may contribute to apnea during REM sleep, when there is already partial muscle paralysis.

Anxiety
Children with generalized anxiety disorder (GAD) experience high rates of insomnia. Struggling to regulate high-arousal negative

emotions makes sleep onset (i.e., sleep latency) challenging and often impacts the entire family's sleep quality.[23] Approximately 90% of children with GAD have high levels of bedtime fears or worries, difficulty sleeping alone or in a dark room, shorter sleep duration during the night, increased morning anxiety, and greater daytime sleepiness.[28] Poor sleep quality may contribute to persistent or exacerbated symptoms of daytime anxiety and school or social difficulties.

Attention Deficit Hyperactivity Disorder

Children with ADHD commonly have comorbid sleep conditions, including behavioral insomnia, SDB, and RLS.[29] Current guidelines recommend careful assessment of sleep quality and environmental conditions before conducting ADHD evaluation and/or initiating medications.[30] Many ADHD symptoms (e.g., inattention, hyperactivity, social and academic distraction, restlessness, inability to stay on task) resemble those of sleep-deprived children and children with untreated sleep apnea and RLS. Further, insufficient sleep in children without neurologic disorders can mimic symptoms of ADHD.

Sleep difficulties among children with ADHD are thought to be related to shared neurobiological pathways involving areas of the cortex responsible for regulation and arousal, the medication effects of stimulants used, and the presence of comorbid mental health disorders. For example, methylphenidate formulations are first-line stimulant medications used to treat ADHD, but insomnia is a significant side effect. ADHD treatment guidelines recommend starting medication with low doses and titrating slowly to the lowest dose that results in improved outcomes and has the fewest side effects, with the intention that children/family continue long-term treatment.[30] ADHD treatment guidelines emphasize the benefits of sleep hygiene education that involves parent/child participation and integrates cognitive behavioral interventions, positive reinforcement, and use of environmental characteristics that promote and sustain sleep, specifically for children with ADHD taking stimulant medications.[30] As children with ADHD mature, nonstimulant medications are often considered for management of ADHD and to promote sleep (see Chapter 29).

Additional Resources

AASM. Sleep Education for Teens: https://sleepeducation.org/help-your-teen-recharge-sleep/

CDC. Sleep and Sleep Disorders: https://www.cdc.gov/sleep/index.html

Sleep Foundation. Children and Sleep: https://www.sleepfoundation.org/children-and-sleep

Health Children. Sleep: https://www.healthychildren.org/English/healthy-living/sleep/Pages/default.aspx

References

1. Buysee DJ. Sleep health: can we define it? Does it matter? *Sleep.* 2014;37(1):9–17.
2. Rojo-Wissar DM, Bai J, Benjamin-Neelon SE, et al. Development of circadian rest-activity rhythms during the first year of life in a racially diverse cohort. *Sleep.* 2022;45(6):zsac078.
3. Liu A. Sleep training. *Pediatr Ann.* 2020;49(3):e101–e105.
4. Behnam-Terneus M, Clemente M. SIDS, BRUE, and safe sleep guidelines. *Pediatr Rev.* 2019;40(9):443–455.
5. Moon RY, Carlin RF, Hand I, & Task Force on Sudden Infant Death Syndrome. Evidence base for 2022 updated recommendations for a safe infant sleeping environment to reduce the risk of sleep-related infant deaths. *Pediatrics.* 2022;150(1).
6. United States Department of Health and Human Services (US DHHS), Centers for Disease Control and Prevention. CDC WONDER. http://wonder.cdc.gov/.
7. Hirai A, Kortsmith K, Kaplan L, et al. Prevalence and factors associated with safe infant sleep practices. *Pediatrics.* 2019;144(5):e20191286.
8. Teti D, Whitesell C, Mogle J, et al. Sleep duration and kindergarten adjustment. *Pediatrics.* 2022;150(2). e.2021054362.
9. Buxton D, Adams E, Bai L, Teti D. The families' role in sleep health. In: Nieto D, Petersen D, eds. *Foundations of Sleep Health.* 1st ed. San Diego, CA: Academic Press; 2021:149–172.
10. Galván A. The need for sleep in the adolescent brain. *Trends Cogn Sci.* 2020;24(1):79–89.
11. Jahrami HA, Alhaj OA, Humood AM, et al. Sleep disturbances during the COVID-19 pandemic: a systematic review, meta-analysis, and meta-regression. *Sleep Med Rev.* 2022;62:101591.
12. CDC. *Results from School Health Policies and Practices Study (SHIPP)*; 2017. https://www.cdc.gov/healthyyouth/data/shpps/pdf/shpps-results_2016.pdf.
13. Biller AM, Molenda C, Zerbini G, et al. Sleep improvements on days with later school starts persist after 1 year in a flexible start system. *Sci Rep.* 2022;12:2787.
14. Seton C, Fitzgerald DA. Chronic sleep deprivation in teenagers: practical ways to help. *Paediatr Respir Rev.* 2021;40:73–79.
15. Agathão B, Cunha D, Sichieri R, et al. The role of family meal frequency in common mental disorders in children and adolescents over eight months of follow-up. *PLoS One.* 2021;16(2):e0243793.
16. Buxton OM, Chang AM, Spilsbury JC, et al. Sleep in the modern family: protective family routines for child and adolescent sleep. *Sleep Health.* 2015;1(1):15–27.
17. World Health Organization. *International Classification of Diseases for Mortality and Morbidity Statistics (11th Revision)*; 2020. https://icd.who.int/browse11/l-m/en.
18. Dresp-Langley B, Hutt A. Digital addiction and sleep. *Int J Environ Res Publ Health.* 2022;19:6910.
19. American Psychiatric Association. *Diagnostic and Statistical Manual of Mental Disorders.* 5th ed. APA; 2013.
20. Keles B, McCrae N, Grealish A. A systematic review: the influence of social media on depression, anxiety and psychological distress in adolescents. *Int J Adolesc Youth.* 2020;25:79–93.
21. Zhao X, Feng X, Garg R, Kelly K. Reducing late evening bedtime electronic device intention and use among young adults. *Sleep Health.* 2019;5:401–408.
22. Metlzer L, Forrest C, de la Motte A, et al. Development and validation of the pediatric sleep practices questionnaire: a self-report measure for youth ages 8-17 years. *Behav Sleep Med.* 2021;19(1):126–143.
23. Mullin BC, Pyle L, Haraden & Det, et al. A preliminary multimethod comparison of sleep among adolescents with and without generalized anxiety disorder. *J Clin Child Adolesc Psychol.* 2017;46(2):198–210.
24. Deshpande P, Salcedo B, Haq C. Common sleep disorders in children. *Am Fam Physician.* 2022;105(2):168–176.
25. Parker A, Beresford B, Dawson V, et al. Oral melatonin for non-respiratory sleep disturbance in children with neurodisabilities: systematic review and meta-analyses. *Dev Med Child Neurol.* 2019;61(8):880–890.
26. Bruni O, Angriman M, Calisti F, et al. Practitioner review: treatment of chronic insomnia in children and adolescents with neurodevelopmental disabilities. *J Child Psychol Psychiatry.* 2017;59(5):489–508.
27. Cuomo BM, Vaz S, Lim A, Lee E, et al. Effectiveness of sleep-based interventions for children with autism spectrum disorder: a meta-synthesis. *Pharmacother J Hum Pharmacol Drug Ther.* 2017;37(5):555–578.

28. Bai S, Ricketts E, Thamrin H, et al. Longitudinal study of sleep and internalizing problems in youth treated for pediatric anxiety disorders. *J Abn Child Psychol*. 2020;48:67–77.
29. Hobson S, Davie M, Farquhar M. Fifteen-minute consultation: managing sleep problems in children and young people with ADHD. *Arch Dis Child Educ Pract Ed*. 2019;104(6):292–297.
30. Wolraich ML, Hagan JF, Allan C, Subcommittee on Children and Adolescents with Attention-Deficit/Hyperactive Disorder, et al. Clinical practice guideline for the diagnosis, evaluation, and treatment of attention-deficit/hyperactivity disorder in children and adolescents. *Pediatrics*. 2019;144(4). e20192528.
31. Munzer T, Felt B. The role of iron in pediatric restless legs syndrome and periodic limb movements in sleep. *Semin Neurol*. 2017;37(4):439–445.
32. Irfan M, Schenck CH, Howell MJ. Non-rapid eye movement sleep and overlap parasomnias. *Continuum(Minneap Minn)*. 2017;23:1035–1050. 4, Sleep Neurology.
33. American Academy of Sleep Medicine (AASM). Sleep Education for children Resources. https://sleepeducation.org/category/children.
34. Ekambaram V, Maski K. Non-rapid eye movement arousal parasomnias in children. *Pediatr Ann*. 2017;46(9):e327–e331.
35. Rana M, August J, Levi J, et al. Alternative approaches to adenotonsillectomy and continuous positive airway pressure (CPAP) for the management of pediatric obstructive sleep apnea (OSA): a review. *Sleep Disord*. 2020:7987208.
36. Kohn JL, Cohen MB, Patel P, et al. Outcomes of children with mild obstructive sleep apnea treated nonsurgically: a retrospective review. *Otolaryngol Head Neck Surg*. 2019;160(6):1101–1105. Erratum *Otolaryngol Head Neck Surg*. 2019;194599819847684.

17
Elimination

MARY DIRKS

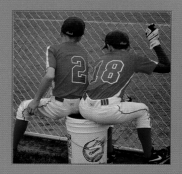

Metabolic by-products and wastes are eliminated from the body via the gastrointestinal (GI), renal, and integumentary systems. Bowel and bladder function in the pediatric population and related typical developmental activities such as toilet training will be discussed in this chapter. Problems that may require additional intervention or are related more directly to GI and genitourinary (GU) pathology are presented in Chapter 34, Gastrointestinal Disorders, and Chapter 42, Nephrology and Genitourinary Disorders. Related dermatologic conditions are discussed in Chapter 37.

Healthy children demonstrate a wide range of elimination patterns, and parents' expectations about elimination vary with culture, social settings, and personal experience. Parents may be unsure whether their child's elimination pattern is problematic or not. The role of the primary care provider (PCP) is to conduct thorough and accurate assessments, provide anticipatory guidance for parents about what to expect as their child develops, and help parents to recognize, understand, and facilitate healthy bowel and bladder function. Ineffective management of toilet training or lack of proper hydration may result in problems such as constipation, stool withholding, decreased appetite, vomiting, and urinary and fecal incontinence (FI). Referral or intervention should be considered when an issue is complicated, out of typical developmental range, or causing distress to the parents and/or child.

Healthy Patterns of Bowel and Urinary Elimination

Elimination patterns are related to age as well as nutrition, fluid intake, activity level, and health-related conditions (e.g., fever). Table 17.1 outlines typical elimination patterns by age of child.

Assessment

Assessment of elimination begins with a thorough health history from the parent and/or child. It is important to seek information from the child or adolescent as parents may not be aware of elimination habits, especially in older children and adolescents.

Health History

Description of Current Status

Current elimination patterns can be assessed with questions related to these topics:

- Description of toileting habits—time of day bowel movements occur and consistency.
- Urination frequency—Urine appearance (e.g., color), smell, and any issues with stream, including discomfort; for infants, number of wet diapers in a 24-hour period; for children, number of urinations a day; frequency of urinations at school; issues with the rules to get permission to go to the bathroom at school.
- Stool—Frequency of bowel movements; description of stool appearance (e.g., color, size; Fig. 17.1), smell, and ease of passage; concerns when having a bowel movement; aversions to using school or public restrooms.
- Elimination habits/rituals, resistance, frequency, or urgency issues.
- Medications, including over-the-counter preparations or home remedies used to aid with bowel movements.
- Infants/early childhood—status or plans for the process of toilet training.
- Early childhood—status of toilet training; when training began, including the process; Frequency of "accidents"; concerns about the process and progression.
- Terms used by the child/family for stool and urine, for body parts, and for the process of using the toilet.

Birth and Early Infancy History

Determine whether any problems with the child's urine or stool were present at birth or within the first month of life. Some questions to consider include: Did the newborn pass a meconium stool within 48 hours after birth? How soon after birth did the newborn urinate? Was the newborn/infant breastfed? When were solids introduced, and did that change stooling patterns or characteristics?

Review of Systems

The review of systems should include the following questions:
- How do you define constipation and diarrhea? Has your child ever been constipated or had diarrhea? Is it persistent or only occasional? Did it start after a particular incident (e.g., illness, during toilet training, with a certain food or change in diet)? Note: PCPs need to remember that diarrhea can be a presenting symptom in constipation due to stool leaking around solid stool.
- Has your child ever had a urinary tract infection (UTI)? At what age? Was there any fever, flank pain, or nausea and vomiting? Any workup (e.g., ultrasonography [US], voiding cystourethrogram [VCUG])? What were the findings, treatment, and follow-up?

| TABLE 17.1 | | Typical Elimination Patterns by Age of Child | | | | | |

TABLE 17.1 Typical Elimination Patterns by Age of Child

Age of Child	Bowel Function	Stool Characteristics	Urinary Function	Urine Characteristics	Signs of Adequate Function	Signs of Concern
Neonate	Meconium stool by 48 h old; then many small stools/day, typically 3–4 times daily	Breastfed infant stool is sticky, light yellow, curdy, with "sour" smell; infant formula-fed infant stool is darker, firmer, and smellier. Iron supplements can darken stool	Minimum of 6 times/day	Pale yellow or colorless	Moist mucous membranes; active; alert Grunting and straining are typical in infants as they pass stool; stool passes easily	Depressed fontanel; dry mucous membranes; fewer than 6 wet diapers a day; fewer than 1–2 stools/week; abdominal distention, vomiting; true constipation (see Rome IV criteria, Box 17.2) requires referral, especially in first month of life
Infant	Stooling typically decreases to one stool/day; breastfed infant may go 8–14 days without stooling Older infants begin to develop a pattern (e.g., first thing after waking in the morning)	Soft, semiformed, color depends on food intake; supplements	6–20 times a day	Pale yellow or colorless	See signs for neonate	
Early childhood	Patterns develop; usually 1 stool/day Most children are toilet trained by 2.5–3.5 years old; bowel control typically precedes urine control	Soft, semiformed, color depends on food intake; supplements	Typically urinate 8–14 times a day; urge to urinate may be stimulated by cold, excitement, or stress	Pale yellow, no odor	Moist mucous membranes, active, alert Bedwetting is common until age 5 or 6 years Stool passes easily	Fewer than 3–5 stools/week; illness or activity that increases need for fluids; vomiting, diarrhea
Middle childhood	Adult function; 1–3 stools/day, 5–7 or more/week	Depends on food intake	Smaller bladder volume than adult; voids 6–8 times/day	Clear yellow; no odor	Increasing independence in toileting; may have poor hygiene	Dysfunctional voiding; daytime incontinence; nocturnal enuresis; encopresis may require referral
Adolescent	Adult function	Depends on food intake, eating patterns	Adult function	Clear yellow; no odor		Sexual activity; eating disorders

- Has your child ever had any illness, injury, or surgery related to the bowel or urinary elimination?
- Is there a history of enuresis (urinary incontinence) and/or encopresis (fecal incontinence)? At what age did it resolve?
- Current:
  - Does your child have a physical condition or chronic illness that affects voiding or bowel movements?
- What medications, including over-the-counter preparations, herbs, or complementary medications, does your child currently take?

Family History

Determine whether any family members have had problems with urinary or bowel elimination (e.g., chronic constipation or

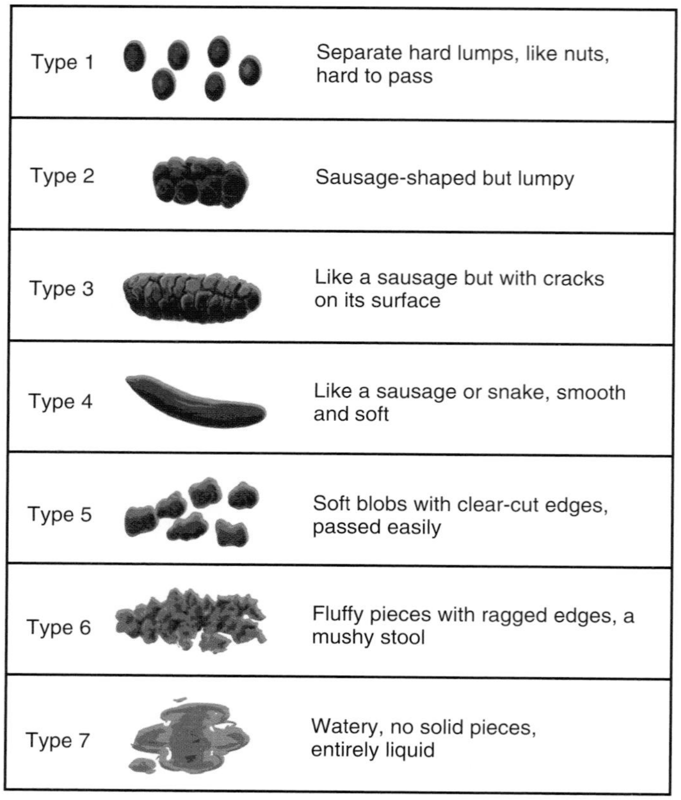

Type 1	Separate hard lumps, like nuts, hard to pass
Type 2	Sausage-shaped but lumpy
Type 3	Like a sausage but with cracks on its surface
Type 4	Like a sausage or snake, smooth and soft
Type 5	Soft blobs with clear-cut edges, passed easily
Type 6	Fluffy pieces with ragged edges, a mushy stool
Type 7	Watery, no solid pieces, entirely liquid

• **Fig. 17.1** Bristol Stool Chart. (From Kliegman RM, Geme JW. *Nelson Textbook of Pediatrics*. 21st ed. Elsevier; 2020.)

diarrhea; enuresis; Hirschsprung disease [HD]). Other questions to consider include: Has the child or family traveled or lived outside the United States? Does the family use well water?

Environmental and Psychosocial Issues

Environmental and psychosocial issues should be assessed, using questions for the parent such as:

- How do you feel about toileting? What do you think are healthy elimination patterns, behaviors, or habits?
- How do you interact with your child around toileting issues?
- How do you deal with toileting "accidents" (including bedwetting)?
- What plans do you have for managing toilet training?
- What are the toileting facilities at your house, day care, and school? How do you think they affect your child's toileting habits?

Physical Examination

The physical examination includes inspection of the perineum, anus, and urinary meatus, foreskin/circumcision, as well as auscultation of the abdomen for bowel sounds and palpation for distention, masses, peristalsis, and tenderness. It should also include an age-appropriate gross motor/neurologic examination and assessing the base of the spine/sacrum for dimples, sinuses, or tufts of hair. A digital examination of the rectum can be helpful to determine constipation, sphincter tone, fissures, hemorrhoids, and presence of stool and its quality and hardness. However, both parents and child need to give consent before the procedure after providing careful explanation and rationale.

TABLE 17.2	Guidelines for Toilet Training Readiness Assessment	
Skill Type	**Description**	
Physical skills	Has voluntary sphincter control	
	Stays dry for 2 h; may wake from naps still dry	
	Is able to sit, walk, and squat	
	Assists in dressing self	
Cognitive skills	Recognizes urge to urinate or defecate	
	Understands meaning of words used by family in toileting	
	Understands what the toilet is for	
	Understands connection between dry pants and toilet	
	Is able to follow directions	
	Is able to communicate needs	
Interpersonal skills	Demonstrates desire to please parent	
	Expresses curiosity about use of toilet	
	Expresses desire to be dry and clean	
Parental skills	Expresses desire to assist child with training	
	Recognizes child's cues of readiness	
	Has no compelling factor that will interfere with training (e.g., new job, move, newborn, and/or family loss or gain)	

Diagnostic Studies

Diagnostic studies may include:

- Urinalysis, urine culture and sensitivity (see Chapter 42)
- Stool specimen for enzymes, reducing substances, occult blood, and ova and parasites, as indicated by history and symptoms (see Chapter 34)
- Diagnostic imaging (see Chapters 34 and 42)

Management Strategies

Toileting Skills

The American Academy of Pediatrics recommends a child-centered approach to toilet training that begins when the child attains physiologic, cognitive, and emotional development, which is typically by 18 to 36 months of age, although anticipatory guidance regarding toilet training readiness begins earlier.[1] PCPs should emphasize that every child is unique, and the child's development, readiness cues, parental expectations, and family circumstances impact when to begin toilet training. Learning to manage elimination for the child can be a stressful (and messy) project. When it is begun too early, it can take longer than the typical 5 to 8 weeks to complete than if it had been started when both the child and the family were ready.[1] In contrast, starting too late can also be problematic because the initiation of toilet training after 32 months of age is associated with constipation and dysfunctional voiding.[2] Guidelines for assessing toilet-training readiness include physical, cognitive, social/emotional, and parental skills (Table 17.2). It is also essential that parents understand and can express to children that the goal is to use the toilet, not to hold in urine or stool. This is an important distinction, as holding urine and/or stool can lead to bowel and bladder dysfunction (BBD).

Children typically experience and learn nocturnal bowel control, followed by daytime bowel control, daytime bladder control, and finally nocturnal bladder control. The average age for being fully toilet trained is 3 to 4 years old, with a normal age variation of up to 1 year. There is little evidence regarding which, if any, toilet training strategy (e.g., child-oriented approach, operant conditioning) is most effective. When children and parents are ready to begin toilet training, several management techniques can be helpful (Box 17.1). If children resist, the effort should be put on hold for a few weeks before trying again. If toddlers seem to be toilet trained for a brief period and suddenly regress to wetting and soiling consistently, they should be placed back in diapers and the process begun again within a few weeks. It is important to stress that none of these "holds" should be viewed as a failure.

It is extremely important that parents and children do not become engaged in a "battle for control" over toilet training, as the parents will lose. If parents ask their child, "Do you need to go potty, pee, etc.?", their answer will most always be "no," even if they have to. Instead of asking *if* the child needs to go, parents should instead say to the child "it's time to go" or something similar that provides a structure cue for the child to attempt using the toilet. As with eating, the child has control over what goes in and out of their bodies. These are some of the many tasks that toddlers master on their way to independence. Parents have the responsibility to assist in the process by providing a positive environment and opportunities, teaching techniques, and setting a positive example. A structured yet flexible approach that is responsive to the child's cues is likely to be most successful. Parents should be reassured that their approach needs to be individualized to each parent/child dyad and may be different for siblings.

Parents can become extremely frustrated if their expectations do not match the abilities and performance of their children, which may escalate to abuse, especially when there are other stressors and/or a lack of support. PCPs play a crucial role in preventing abuse by giving parents information about child development, techniques for managing the training process, and support and encouragement for their efforts. This role includes proactively doing follow-up with families who express frustration or appear to be having difficulty with the toilet training process.

Elimination Communication

There is wide variation in how elimination is viewed and managed. Climate, environment, resources, culture, family structure, and social dynamics play a role in shaping toileting practices and training expectations. In the United States, most infants are diapered until they master self-toileting; however, there are different practices (e.g., assisted infant toilet training [AITT]) and cultural variations (e.g., squat toileting). PCPs need to understand and be open to these practices.

AITT, elimination communication (EC), and natural infant hygiene (NIH) are terms used to describe infant toileting methods that typically begin at 3 to 4 months of age.[3] AITT, EC, and NIH require close caregiver observation of the infant elimination patterns, such as a bowel movement early in the morning or after feeding, or urination immediately after waking from a nap. Attention to infant behavioral cues as to when they are urinating or defecating, such as grunting, straining, or becoming more still, are also used. Parents use these patterns and cues to take the infant to the toilet. They can also introduce other elimination prompts (e.g., the sound of running water, music, a swooshing sound in the infant's ear) when the infant is in position on the "potty," to encourage elimination. The infant is conditioned through practice and repetition to associate these cues with toileting, but the parent is being trained as well to be alert and responsive to the

---

• BOX 17.1   Management of Toilet Training

Keep child as clean and dry as possible:
- Change diapers frequently.
- Use training pants or underwear when child stays dry for several hours during the day; use diaper at night.

Talk with child about toilet training:
- Praise child for asking to have diaper changed.
- Explain connection between being clean and dry and using toilet.
- Emphasize that the goal is to eliminate in the toilet, not to hold to stay clean and dry.
- Provide opportunity for child to use toilet, especially before going out to play, going on a trip, before naps, and at bedtime; set an example with adult behavior.
- Do not ask if child needs to go, rather set up a time schedule of every 1.5 hours for voiding, and state matter-of-factly it is time to go.

Teach child how to use toilet:
- Allow child to observe while parents/siblings use toilet.
- Demonstrate how to sit on toilet with feet supported and knees spread with forward pelvic tilt, use toilet paper, flush, and wash hands.

Provide practice time for child:
- Provide a potty chair or portable toilet seat.
- Allow child to sit on potty chair with clothes or diaper on.
- Encourage child to use potty chair while parent uses regular toilet.
- Have child sit on potty chair without diapers for 5–10 min at a time.
- Practice at times the child usually urinates or defecates.

Provide a comfortable, safe-feeling environment:
- Seat child facing backward on a regular toilet (see Fig. 17.5).
- Provide a footstool to rest the feet on with knees wide and forward pelvic tilt.
- Never flush the toilet when child is sitting on it. Use sticky notes to stop automatic flush on public toilets.
- Stay with child for safety reasons.

Give consistent, positive feedback:
- Praise child for trying and for success.
- Be understanding of child's refusal to use toilet.
- Never demand performance.
- Never make child sit on toilet if child resists.
- Ignore or minimize undesired behavior.
- Never scold or punish if a child wets or soils.
- Use star chart or other reward for success or effort; consider having the reward the child is working toward in the bathroom so that the job and reward are clearly connected for the child.
- Do not praise excessively.

---

infant's signals. Although AITT, EC, and NIH encourage a high level of engagement, success rate for bladder and bowel control by 12 months is only about 12%.[4]

Altered Patterns of Elimination

This section focuses on common alterations in elimination patterns, including bladder/bowel dysfunction, constipation/encopresis, toilet refusal syndrome, dysfunctional voiding, and enuresis. Other GI pathologies, including diarrhea, are discussed in Chapter 34, while GU pathologies are discussed in Chapter 42.

Bladder and Bowel Dysfunction

Bladder and bowel dysfunction (BBD) includes any abnormal pattern in function at an age when an individual is developmentally capable of control. Several factors contribute to the complexity and varied set of BBD dysfunction, including the physical proximity and relationship between bladder and bowel function, due to the function of the pelvic floor. BBD includes children who actively try to prevent bowel movements or urination, such as the school-age child who has restricted access to bathroom facilities, the child who had a painful bowel movement and has decided to hold off so as not to hurt, and the child who is "too busy" to stop and use the bathroom. The cause for each child is likely multifactorial and treatment may be helpful to prevent reoccurrence. However, treatment is not always necessary to resolve the issue.

Urgency, frequency, and nocturnal and diurnal urinary incontinence are common in BBD. The child may have difficulty initiating urination or completely emptying the bladder. Persistent problems with incomplete emptying of the bladder can lead to UTI, vesicoureteral reflux (VUR), and—in severe or long-term situations–kidney damage. Constipation can exacerbate bladder dysfunction by applying direct pressure to the bladder wall or restricting urinary flow. The child with BBD may experience stool incontinence (encopresis), with or without constipation. Lack of bowel and bladder control by 4 years of age has not shown to result in significant psychosocial problems.[5] However, if elimination problems persist, they may contribute to family difficulties, bullying, social isolation, emotional problems, and antisocial behaviors.[6]

Constipation and Encopresis

Constipation is a common condition in pediatric patients with prevalence rates between 12% and 18%.[6] It can be acute or chronic but involves retained, hard, dry, infrequent stools, which can become impacted in the colon. *Functional* constipation is chronic constipation that is idiopathic (Box 17.2).

Encopresis, also known as *fecal soiling,* is defined as repetitive, involuntary passage of stool after an age when the child should be able to control bowel movements. It typically involves FI episodes at least once per month for 3 months before diagnosis.[6] *Primary,* or continuous, encopresis is present in children who have never been toilet trained. *Secondary,* or discontinuous, encopresis is seen in those who were previously trained but who begin to soil. There are two subtypes of encopresis: (1) functional retentive FI (fR-FI), or encopresis with constipation, associated with stool retention, constipation, and incontinence overflow; and (2) functional nonretentive FI (fN-FI), or encopresis without constipation, which is less common.

Children with encopresis *with* constipation (fR-FI) often have a history of an acute stool problem that was not adequately managed (e.g., the child had an illness that caused dehydration and constipation), leading to a cycle of constipation, painful defecation, stool retention, more severe constipation, more painful defecation, more stool retention, and so on. Over time, stool retention leads to distention of the colon and stretching of the rectum, ineffective peristalsis, decreased sensory threshold in the rectum, and weakened rectal and sphincter muscles (Fig. 17.2). Soft, semiformed, or liquid stool from higher in the colon leaks around retained stool and passes uncontrollably through the rectum, causing soiling. The child is almost always unaware of the actual incontinence and may either refuse or be willing to use the toilet.

Children with encopresis *without* constipation (fN-FI) are not constipated but have overflow incontinence or voluntary bowel movements in their clothing or other inappropriate places. These children have a normal physical examination

• BOX 17.2   Rome IV Criteria for Functional Constipation in Infants and Children

Must include two or more of the following occurring at least once per week for a minimum of 1 month with insufficient criteria for a diagnosis of irritable bowel syndrome:

- Two or fewer defecations in the toilet per week in a child of a developmental age of at least 4 years
- At least one episode of fecal incontinence per week
- History of retentive posturing or excessive volitional stool retention
- History of painful or hard bowel movements
- Presence of a large fecal mass in the rectum
- History of large diameter stools that can obstruct the toilet
- After appropriate evaluation, the symptoms cannot be fully explained by another medical condition.

From Hyams J, Di Lorenzo C, Saps M, et al. Functional disorders: child/adolescent. *Gastroenterology.* 2016;150(6):1456-1470.

with no stool retention on examination or radiographic study and no evidence of anorectal sensorimotor function or motility disorder.[6] It is associated with psychological comorbidities, including behavioral and learning disorders, impulsivity, and history of abuse.[6]

Physiologic Factors

Possible physiologic factors related to encopresis with constipation may include the following:

- Inadequate fluid intake
- Dehydration caused by illness and fever or during active play in hot weather
- A change in diet, such as the introduction of solids or increased carbohydrates
- Secondary stool retention and constipation due to:
  - Painful bowel movements
  - Anal fissures
  - Paradoxical constriction of the external anal sphincter during attempted defecation
  - Neurogenic conditions (e.g., HD/aganglionic colon, cerebral palsy, myelomeningocele)
  - Endocrine and metabolic conditions (e.g., hypothyroidism)
  - Medications (e.g., opioids, iron supplements, anticholinergics)

Socioemotional Factors

Possible socioemotional factors related to encopresis with constipation may include the following:

- Major family or life adjustments, such as loss of a parent, sibling, or other significant person; divorce; extended parent absence (e.g., incarceration, deployment).
- Power struggles related to toileting/training; children might rebel/refuse to cooperate.
- Irregular toileting patterns, often caused by travel, unfamiliar or unpleasant bathrooms, or lack of regular routine.
- Children absorbed in play or an activity who do not want to stop to defecate; ignoring cues.
- Behavioral and/or attention problems, including anxiety and depressive symptoms.
- Social boundaries/rules: schools often regulate bathroom use, which affects children's typical attention to cues.
- Physical or sexual abuse.

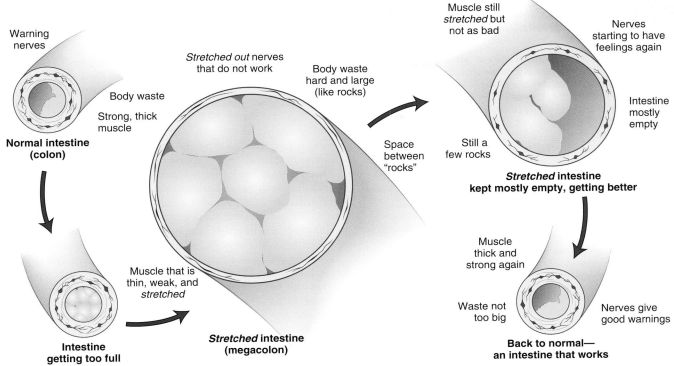

• **Fig. 17.2** Encopresis: Patient Training Diagram. (From Weissman L. Toileting and encopresis. In: Feldman HM, Elias ER, Blum NJ, et al., eds. *Developmental-Behavioral Pediatrics.* 5th ed. Elsevier; 2023.)

Clinical Findings

History. Early detection and treatment are important, so specific and directed questions are needed, such as:

- Is there a significant family or child history related to stooling (e.g., HD? Celiac disease? Cystic fibrosis? Constipation in infancy? Late meconium passage (>48 h)?
- Does the child complain of abdominal pain, bloating, loss of appetite?
- How often does the child have a bowel movement?
- Are there situations when the child refuses to defecate or urinate (e.g., at school, in public bathrooms, when playing)?
- Describe the process of when the child defecates (e.g., Is it painful? Does the child resist using toilet (child hides, defecates outside toilet)?
- What is the quality of stool (e.g., ribbon, hard, large caliber, bloody)?
- Describe any issues with hygiene (e.g., stained underwear, odor, leakage of stool).
- Does the child have enuresis? A history of UTIs?

Box 17.3 outlines specific findings that are red flags for constipation and require further investigation.

Physical Examination. The physical examination should assess for the following:

- Overflow soiling
- Abdominal distention
- Abdominal tenderness on palpation
- Mass felt at the midline in the suprapubic area (descending colon)
- Anal fissures
- Sacral dimple or hair tuft
- Neurologic signs: absent or diminished abdominal, cremasteric, anal wink reflexes, and deep tendon reflexes (DTRs) in lower extremities.

• BOX 17.3 Red Flag Signs and Symptoms in Constipation

- Constipation starting extremely early in life (<1 month)
- Passage of meconium >48 h
- Family history of Hirschsprung disease
- Ribbon stools
- Blood in stools in the absence of anal fissures
- Failure to thrive
- Fever
- Bilious vomiting
- Abnormal thyroid function
- Severe abdominal distension
- Decreased lower extremity strength/tone/reflex
- Perianal fistula
- Abnormal position of anus
- Absent anal or cremasteric reflex
- Tuft of hair on spine, sacral dimple, or gluteal cleft deviation
- Extreme resistance or fear during anal inspection
- Anal scars

Note: The need for a digital examination of the rectum must be carefully evaluated given the level of invasiveness for children.[6]

Diagnostic Studies. Radiographic and laboratory tests to identify structural or organic causes of constipation are not typically recommended unless there are specific or alarming signs that indicate a potential underlying condition (e.g., bowel obstruction, foreign body). For example, a "flat plate" of the abdomen, or KUB (kidney, ureter, and bladder radiograph) can be indicated when fecal impaction is suspected or an abdominal examination cannot be performed or is unreliable. It will show accumulation of stool in the sigmoid colon, which can help parents "see" the problem.

- Monitor diet:
  - Ensure adequate fiber and water intake for age:
  - Recommended water intake is about 1 oz (30 mL)/kg/day.
  - Fiber recommendations vary by age/sex: 1- to 8-year-olds should get about 25 g/day; 9- to 13-year-old females: about 26 g/day, males: about 31 g/day; 14- to 18-year-old females: about 26 g/day, males: about 38 g/day. Legumes, vegetables, and some fruits are good sources of fiber.
  - Decrease milk to 16 oz (475 mL)/day.
  - Do not allow excessive dairy, rice, applesauce, bananas, white flour, or potatoes.
- Give child all responsibility for own toilet habits. Stop parental reminders to use toilet. Stop all encouragement and criticisms.
- Establish a regular toileting routine.
- Avoid use of stool softeners or laxatives.
- Encourage daily physical activity.
- May use incentives or rewards to reinforce positive behavior. Have parent and child agree on reward beforehand so that it can be discussed as a positive, subtle reminder.

Laboratory studies can be done when suspicion for thyroid disease, celiac disease, or hypercalcemia is present.[7]

Differential Diagnosis

The differential diagnosis for encopresis with constipation includes anorectal stenosis, spina bifida occulta, spinal cord dysplasia, HD, intellectual disability, hypothyroidism, hypercalcemia, cerebral palsy, and cystic fibrosis. Parents need to be reminded that the infant exhibiting normal red-faced grunting and straining with defecation is not constipated.

Management

The goals of treatment are to establish a regular bowel routine, "demystify" the problem, alleviate blame, and gain cooperation with treatment. Treatment approaches for children with constipation traditionally include:

- Bowel evacuation—Oral polyethylene glycol (PEG) solutions are as effective as enemas but much less traumatizing to children and families.[6]
- Bowel retraining—To establish a regular pattern of stooling.
- Ongoing maintenance—Medications as needed and regular toileting hygiene.

Additional options include biofeedback and, less often, surgery. Biofeedback is sensory retraining and relaxation of the sphincter muscle during defecation. This approach is used in children with confirmed abnormal sensory threshold and defecation mechanics on anorectal manometry. Surgical treatment is rare (e.g., cecostomy for anterograde colonic enemas).

The emphasis in treating encopresis *without* constipation (fN-FI) is on behavioral therapy, educating the child and parent about normal stooling, and establishing a structured pattern of toileting (Box 17.4). Children who have encopresis *with* constipation (fR-FI) present a greater challenge. Education of parents and children is vital to successful treatment. A clear message should be that the dynamics of encopresis (retention, colon stretching, decreased peristalsis, impaction, leaking) are not voluntary—no one is to blame; however, the dynamics can be reversed through bowel rehabilitation, which takes hard work, cooperation, and time. The PCP works with the family to ensure success. Fig. 17.2 can be used to explain the bowel rehabilitation process and treatment plan. Timed urination may also be helpful, because children who hold their urine activate the pelvic floor and, as a result, hold their stool as well.

In some cases, a pediatric mental health referral may be indicated, but it is considered adjunctive and should not be the first referral because it alone cannot cure the problem.

Specific algorithms for constipation by age group are included in Figs. 17.3 and 17.4, while Table 17.3 provides guidelines to treating a child with encopresis with constipation, including appropriate medications. Although not US Food and Drug Administration (FDA)-approved for use in children, PEG has been proven more effective than other laxatives for children presenting with functional constipation and/or fecal impaction.[8] Enemas are recommended *only* if PEG is not available.

For maintenance management, PEG is recommended as first-line therapy, although lactulose may be given if PEG is not available. Milk of magnesia, mineral oil, and stimulant laxatives may also be considered for maintenance or as second-line treatment. Enemas are not recommended for maintenance therapy. Maintenance medications need to be continued for a minimum of 2 months and should not be stopped until 1 month after resolution of the problem. At this time, medications should be decreased gradually; if any problems recur, the medication should be adjusted back to the last successful dose and given an additional 2 weeks before attempting to decrease again. Throughout the treatment, medications must be adjusted according to the clinical response, so the provider must be readily available for the family to ask questions and make modifications.

Because this condition often occurs in middle childhood, which involves school settings that can discourage children from using the restroom, PCPs should consult with the school nurse to ensure these children have a clear plan in place that allows for restroom access without going through extra steps and without having to draw attention to themselves and hygiene management (e.g., extra underwear). Teamwork and socioemotional support are equally important to a child's success in overcoming encopresis.

Complications

Persistent encopresis is unpleasant, and children with encopresis often experience ridicule and shame from their peers, which can lead to rejection. Teachers and school personnel play a vital role in helping to support the child and family, who have their own anger, guilt, embarrassment, and helplessness. Everyone needs to know that this condition is extremely difficult to manage and will stress social, interpersonal, and family relations.

Some children develop intractable constipation, and even megacolon, especially those with other medical conditions, such as Down syndrome, cerebral palsy, or neuromuscular disorders. When medical management is unsuccessful, surgical intervention (e.g., cecostomy for anterograde colonic enemas) may be necessary.

Patient and Family Education

The PCP must understand the relationship between constipation and encopresis and/or diarrhea, recognize conditions that may contribute to each, and provide parents with anticipatory guidance related to toilet training and healthy elimination habits to prevent problems. The best treatment of constipation or encopresis is prevention. When constipation or encopresis is caused by an underlying anatomic or organic cause (e.g., HD, occult spina bifida, hypothyroidism), early diagnosis and referral are essential. It is equally important for the

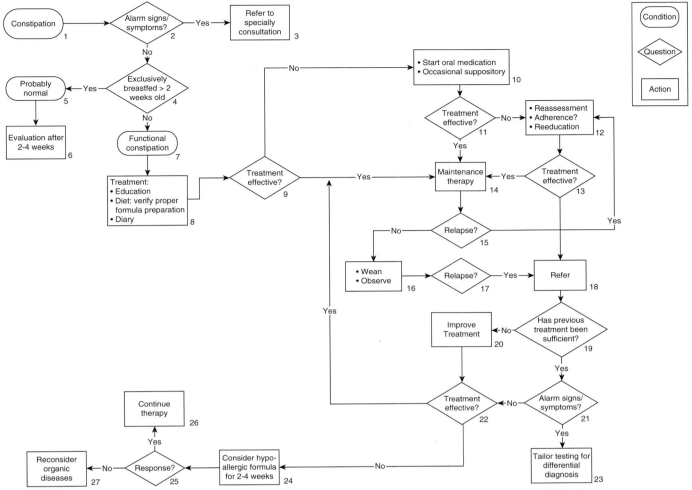

• **Fig. 17.3** Algorithm for the Evaluation and Treatment of Constipated Infants Less Than 6 Months Old. *ACE,* Antegrade continence enema; *MRI,* magnetic resonance imaging; *SNS,* sacral nerve stimulation; T_4, thyroxine; *TENS,* transcutaneous electrical nerve stimulation; *TSH,* thyroid-stimulating hormone. (From Tabbers MM, DiLorenzo C, Berger MY, et al. Evaluation and treatment of functional constipation in infants and children: evidence-based recommendations from ESPGHAN and NASPGHAN. *J Pediatr Gastroenterol Nutr.* 2014;58[2]:258–274.)

PCP to promote consistent, positive, and supportive attitudes during treatment, while removing any negative attributions to soiling. Although parents should be informed that treatment may be required for months or years, providers should emphasize that by following a clear, consistent, aggressive treatment protocol, the condition can be managed. Finally, the PCP and extended care team (e.g., school), parents, and the child must work together to prevent recurrence of symptoms after successful treatment.

Toilet Refusal Syndrome

Toilet refusal syndrome (TRS) is when a child demonstrates a pattern of successfully using the toilet for urine but refuses to use it for bowel movements. Instead, children opt to defecate in a diaper, training pants, or "pull-ups," and in some cases defecate outside the toilet or in a private space (e.g., behind the couch). Encopresis without constipation (fN-FI) is similar in that the child defecates outside the toilet when beyond the age of expected training.

Many healthy children experience TRS for a short time. The cause of TRS is unknown. However, constipation and painful bowel movements appear to precede rather than follow the problem. TRS can persist beyond early into middle childhood and may be associated with comorbid conditions (e.g., behavioral disorders, urinary incontinence).

Clinical Findings

History. Parents/caregivers often report the following:
- Bladder control but refusal to defecate on the toilet
- Regular/irregular pattern of bowel movements
- Consistent child signals and signs that a bowel movement is imminent
- History of hiding when defecating, either before or after toilet training begins

Physical Examination. The physical examination is typically unremarkable but should include the following:
- Examine the anus for fissures or irritation; anal wink.
- Check for signs of stool retention, including abdominal distention or tenderness.
- Palpate for a mass in the sigmoid colon or midline in the suprapubic area (impaction).

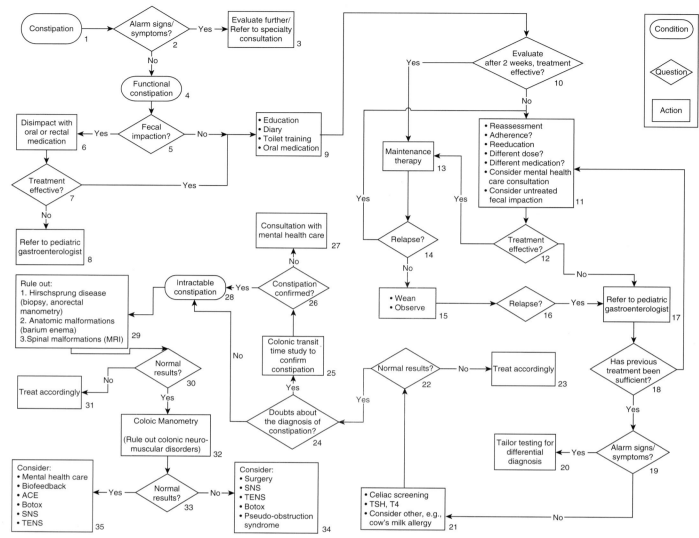

• **Fig. 17.4** Algorithm for the Evaluation and Treatment of Constipated Infants and Children Age 6 Months or Older. (From: Tabbers MM, DiLorenzo C, Berger MY, et al. Evaluation and treatment of functional constipation in infants and children: evidence-based recommendations from ESPGHAN and NASP-GHAN. *J Pediatr Gastroenterol Nutr.* 2014;58[2]:258–274.)

Differential Diagnosis

The differential diagnosis includes stool withholding, constipation, and encopresis.

Management

Return the child to diapers and reintroduce toilet training in about a month or when the child indicates interest. Some children prefer not to wear diapers all the time but ask to have one put on when they feel the urge to defecate. Encourage the child to go into the bathroom for these diaper defecations. After having a bowel movement, the child asks to be changed and returns to wearing training pants. This pattern may continue for several weeks or months. When parents refrain from expressing negative messages and matter-of-factly clean the child after defecating in the diaper, the duration of TRS may shorten. For older children, schedule a daily time for the child to sit on the toilet for 5 to 10 minutes when the child typically has a bowel movement; have these times be positive, never punitive or forced. Never flush the toilet while the child is sitting on it. In public restrooms, parents can cover automatic flush

sensors with "sticky note." Incentives and positive feedback when the child successfully uses the toilet for bowel movements may be effective (e.g., star charts), but excessive praise is not recommended as the child is simply doing what is to be expected. If the child has constipation, fecal impaction, or both, initial bowel cleanout may be necessary, followed by a daily maintenance regimen adjusted to clinical response until toilet training is complete.

Complications

Refusal to use the toilet for bowel movements may lead to stool withholding, constipation, and impaction, which are conditions that result in primary encopresis. Psychological complications include embarrassment or shame, as well as conflict and stress between children and parents, which can escalate to child maltreatment.

Patient and Family Education

Prevention through appropriate toilet training is key. If a child refuses to defecate on the toilet, use of punishment or force can

- Eosinophilic cystitis
- Vaginitis
- Obstructive sleep apnea
- Enterobius vermicularis (pinworms)

Management

The treatment goals are to establish healthy bladder function and prevent physical and socioemotional complications. Self-esteem and social interaction of children are often affected, as sleepovers, camps, and other trips may be avoided due to fear of embarrassment. Intervention involves behavioral modification, medication, treatment of comorbid or organic conditions, or a combination of these modalities. Treatment of daytime urinary dysfunction and constipation should be done before treating nocturnal enuresis. Referral to a pediatric urology specialist may be necessary.

Short-term outcomes are categorized as:
- No response: Less than 50% decrease in enuresis
- Partial response: 50% to 99% reduction
- Complete response: 100% reduction

Long-term outcomes include:
- Relapse: More than one symptom relapse per month
- Continued success: No return of symptoms in 6 months
- Complete success: No return of symptoms after 2 years

Because functional enuresis is largely self-limited, there is consensus to delay aggressive treatment until the child is 6 to 8 years old. Treatment strategies include:

- *Urotherapy:* A nonpharmacologic, nonsurgical intervention (see Box 17.5). Urotherapy increases daytime urination by establishing a regular voiding schedule—not waiting until the micturition urge is felt. It also limits nighttime urine production by regulating fluid intake. The goal is for the bladder to hold urine produced overnight. Children should void before going to bed and again immediately upon waking in the morning. Proper posture while urinating is important to help the child be more sensitive to cues of a full bladder and to control urination. This approach is effective for children with hyperactive bladders and may make medication unnecessary for many children. Urotherapy also involves aggressive treatment of constipation.
- *Enuresis alarms:* The decision to use an alarm should be made after discussion with the child and family. Alarms are more effective in children with "decreased maximal voided volumes" and long-term alarm use is more effective than desmopressin for treatment of primary nocturnal enuresis.[16] An enuresis alarm should be first-line treatment when conditions such as diabetes, kidney disease, or urogenital malformations have been ruled out. Use of an alarm requires commitment and effort on the part of children and parents and support from the PCP.
- *Drug therapy:* Drug therapy (Table 17.4) can be combined with urotherapy and/or alarm therapy, but it is not curative. It usually has high initial success rates. However, it can be expensive and high relapse rates occur when the drug is discontinued. Relapses can be very upsetting to the child, which is a factor that needs to be considered when prescribing. On the positive side, it can be very useful for overnight stays (e.g., camp) when staying dry is important to the child.
  - *Desmopressin* has an antidiuretic effect and appears to be most effective in children with large nocturnal urine production and normal nocturnal bladder capacity. Its effect is immediate and it can be taken only on nights that the child wants to be sure to stay dry, although it may be more effective when combined with urotherapy and titrated slowly to maximal dose. It is available in three forms: nasal spray, oral tablets, or oral lyophilizate preparation (MELT) (sublingual administration).

NOTE: Nasal spray has led to hyponatremia, has a black box warning from the FDA, and is not recommended for routine use.[12]
  - Caution patients to avoid high fluid intake with the oral medication, to give the correct dosage, and to discontinue the medication if headache, nausea, or vomiting occurs.[12]

TABLE 17.4	Drug Therapy for Children 6 Years or Older With Monosymptomatic Nocturnal Enuresis	
Medication	**Dosing**	**Comments**
Desmopressin acetate (DDAVP)	• Oral: 0.2 mg tablet once daily at bedtime; can be adjusted up to maximum of 0.6 mg/day • Oral: 120 mcg Melt (dissolves sublingually) once daily at bedtime; this is the bioequivalent of 0.2 mg tablet; can be adjusted up to 240 mcg/day	• Effective in children with nocturnal polyuria and normal bladder volume • Short-term treatment only (4–8 weeks) • Not recommended in children younger than 6 years • Not recommended to use nasal spray • Caution must be used with patients who are hypertensive or have a potential for fluid-electrolyte imbalance (e.g., children with cystic fibrosis susceptible to hyponatremia) • Use least amount effective • Take on empty stomach; avoid caffeine, chocolate, NutraSweet, and carbonated beverages • Wake children to urinate within 10 h of taking the medication
Oxybutynin chloride, *immediate* release Oxybutynin chloride, *extended* release	• 5 mg once daily at bedtime; increase as tolerated in 5 mg increments to maximum of 20 mg daily	• Effective in children with daytime enuresis • Not recommended in children 5 years old or younger

- Other drugs are not recommended as first-line treatment. These include anticholinergics (antimuscarinic drugs [also used for treatment of overactive bladder], oxybutynin, tolterodine, and solifenacin), which cause constipation and could complicate the problem; botulinum toxin type A, and imipramine, which should only be used by specialists, if at all, due to its cardiotoxic side effects.
- Sacral nerve stimulation for children with severe voiding dysfunction that has not responded to aggressive urotherapy and medical interventions is currently being studied.

Patient and Family Education

Dealing with a child who wets frequently can be frustrating. However, parents need to know that the PCP is committed to working closely with them until the child is dry. A supportive proactive approach and positive reinforcement should be used. For example, in 3- to 5-year-old children, a nonjudgmental attitude of "benign neglect" in the face of accidents is the best approach.

Additional Resources

General Information

National Institute of Diabetes and Digestive and Kidney Diseases: www.niddk.nih.gov/health-information/health-topics/digestive-diseases/Pages/default.aspx
Nemours Foundation: www.kidshealth.org

Constipation/Encopresis

American Gastroenterological Association: www.gastro.org
Journal of Pediatrics. Pediatric constipation action plan with pictograms: https://www.jpeds.com/article/S0022-3476(20)31263-4/fulltext
North American Society for Pediatric Gastroenterology, Hepatology, and Nutrition (NASPGHAN): www.naspghan.org
Pediatric Health Network. Constipation: Cleanout Action Plan: https://pediatrichealthnetwork.org/wp-content/uploads/2020/12/Constipation-Action-Plan-Med-Chart-Revised-1.27.20.pdf

Enuresis

Bedwetting Store: www.bedwettingstore.com
Education and Resources for Improving Childhood Continence (ERIC): www.eric.org.uk
International Children's Continence Society (ICCS): www.i-c-c-s.org
National Association for Continence: www.nafc.org

National Kidney Foundation: www.kidney.org/patients/bw/
Potty MD: www.pottymd.com
Society of Urologic Nurses and Associates: www.suna.org
Urology Care Foundation:. www.urologyhealth.org

References

1. Sejkora EKD, Igler EC, Davies WH. Parent-reported toilet training practices and the role of pediatric primary care providers. *J Am Assoc Nurse Pract.* 2020;33(8):620–629.
2. Li X, Wen JG, Xie H, et al. Delayed in toilet training association with pediatric lower urinary tract dysfunction: a systematic review and meta-analysis. *J Pediatr Urol.* 2020;16(3):352.e1–352.e8.
3. Jordan GJ, Arbeau K, McFarland D, et al. Elimination communication contributes to a reduction in unexplained infant crying. *Med Hypotheses.* 2020;142:109811.
4. Bender J, Lee Y, Hoon Ryoo J, et al. A longitudinal study of assisted infant toilet training during the first year of life. *J Dev Behav Pediatr.* 2021;42:648–655.
5. Axelrod M, Larsen R, Jorgensen K, et al. Psychological differences between toilet trained and non-toilet trained 4-year-old children. *J Spec Pediatr Nurs (JSPN).* 2021;26:1–8.
6. LeLeiko NS, Mayer-Brown S, Cerezo C, et al. Constipation. *Pediatr Rev.* 2020;41(8):379–392.
7. Philichi L. Management of childhood functional constipation. *J Pediatr Health.* 2018;32(1):103–111.
8. Southwell BR. Treatment of childhood constipation: a synthesis of systematic reviews and meta-analyses. *Expert Rev Gastroenterol Hepatol.* 2020;14(3):163–174.
9. Bauer A. Dysfunctional voiding: update on evaluation and treatment. *Curr Opin Pediatr.* 2021;33(2):235–242.
10. Clothier JC, Wright AJ. Dysfunctional voiding: the importance of non-invasive urodynamics in diagnosis and treatment. *Pediatr Nephrol.* 2018;33(3):381–394.
11. Schäfer SK, Niemczyk J, von Gontard A, et al. Standard urotherapy as first-line intervention for daytime incontinence: a meta-analysis. *Eur Child Adolesc Psychiatry.* 2018;27(8):949–964.
12. Kamperis K. Nocturnal enuresis in children: the role of arginine-vasopressin. *Handb Clin Neurol.* 2021;181:289–297.
13. Nevéus T, Fonseca E, Franco I, et al. Management and treatment of nocturnal enuresis-an updated standardization document from the International Children's Continence Society. *J Pediatr Urol.* 2020;16(1):10–19.
14. Chan IHY, Wong KKY. Common urological problems in children: primary nocturnal enuresis. *Hong Kong Med J.* 2019;25(4):305–311.
15. Li Y, Zhang Y, Liu C, et al. Treatment experience of 210 pediatric patients with extraordinary daytime urinary frequency: a prospective study. *Front Pediatr.* 2021;9:713810.
16. Apos E, Schuster S, Reece J, et al. Enuresis management in children: retrospective clinical audit of 2861 cases treated with practitioner-assisted bell-and-pad alarm. *J Pediatr.* 2018;193:211–216.

18

Physical Activity and Sports

MICHELE L. POLFUSS AND RENÉE L. DAVIS

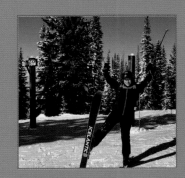

Engaging in physical activity has both immediate and long-term benefits for all children and adolescents, including those with chronic health conditions and special healthcare needs. The benefits of children and adolescents engaging in regular physical activity are broad and include improving bone health and cardiorespiratory fitness, increasing lean mass, decreasing body fat, reducing symptoms of depression, and improving the individual's cognitive skills and ability to concentrate. Achieving a healthy lifestyle in childhood includes participating in physical activity in addition to optimizing nutrition and maintaining healthy body weight. Physical activity is an essential component of overall health and the prevention of overweight, obesity, and the development of chronic health conditions.[1]

Physical Activity: Overview

Physical activity is defined as "any bodily movement produced by skeletal muscles that require energy expenditure."[2] Physical activity in childhood and adolescence can be completed through various mechanisms including free play, games, sports, transportation, chores, recreation, physical education, or planned exercise and can occur in many contexts such as with family, at school, at work, or in the community.[2]

Physical activity recommendations include children and adolescents participating in at least 60 minutes of moderate to vigorous physical activity daily, a timeframe that can be divided into smaller sessions throughout the day. While most of the activities should be aerobic in nature, activities that strengthen muscles and bones should be performed at least three times a week.[3] Currently, children and adolescents in the United States fail to meet the recommended national physical activity goals.[3]

In the United States, the Centers for Disease Control and Prevention (CDC) biannual Youth Risk Behavior Surveillance (YRBS) System monitors priority health risk behaviors of 9th- through 12th-grade students from public and private schools that contribute to leading causes of death, disability, and social problems. Important findings from the 2019 YRBS related to physical activity include[4]:

- 51.6% of the students attended a physical education class on 1 or more days in the average school week.
- 23.2% were physically active at least 60 minutes per day for each of the previous 7 days.
- 16.5% had met both aerobic and muscle-strengthening physical activity guidelines.
- 49.5% of the students participated in muscle-strengthening activities on 3 or more days in 7 days prior to the survey.

- Only 25.9% of the students attended physical education classes on all 5 days of the average school week.
- 57.4% (60% boys and 55% girls) played on at least one sports team related to their school or a community group during the 12 months before taking the survey.

When comparing each of the aforementioned statistics to the 2017 YRBS, no significant change occurred in any of the categories for children and adolescents in this age group.

In 2022, the National Physical Activity Plan Alliance released the US Report Card on Physical Activity for Children and Youth. This document reports on nine key indicators related to physical activity such as overall physical activity levels, sedentary behaviors, active transportation, organized sports participation, active play, health-related fitness, and contexts such as family and peers, schools, and community including the built environment.[5] The grades provided through this document are based on secondary datasets such as the High School Athletics Participation Survey, National Health and Nutrition Examination Survey (NHANES), National Household Travel Survey, National Survey of Children's Health, NHANES National Youth Fitness Survey, School Health Profiles, and YRBS, all which vary in years of origin. The COVID-19 pandemic significantly impacted the health behaviors of children and youth and the rate of body mass index (BMI) approximately doubled during the pandemic and the rate of childhood overweight and obesity increased from 47.3% to 58.8%.[5]

Physical activity has demonstrated a positive impact on mental, cognitive, and physical health in children and adolescents. The benefits of physical activity have been reported on cognitive development, attention span, and academic performance.[6] In addition, young people who exercised regularly had decreased levels of depression and psychological distress and improved self-image and psychological wellbeing. Engaging in physical activity can have a positive impact on self-esteem, building social skills, and relieving stress and anxiety.[6]

The physical inactivity of youth is not only placing them at greater risk of developing chronic diseases such as cardiovascular disease, cancer, and diabetes, but it is dramatically increasing healthcare costs. If a child has obesity, they are more likely to become an adult with obesity with more severe disease risk factors.[7] In the United States, physical inactivity is estimated to cost $117 billion annually in healthcare costs and contributes to 1 in 10 premature deaths.[2,3]

The environment in which an individual lives can influence their engagement in physical activity. For children, activities during the school day and travel to and from school are prominent opportunities for engaging in physical activity. The school environment can also be a mechanism to promote activity as school sports facilities, gymnasiums, or playgrounds can serve the larger community. Children who walk or bike to school tend to have a higher level of engagement in moderate to physical activity. The neighborhood where an individual lives can promote activity by having sidewalks that are walkable, protected bike lanes, streets designed to make crossing safe, access to parks and other activities that are within walking distance are all examples of facilitating physical activity.[8]

Promoting Physical Activity: Guidelines and Standards

In the recent Global Action Plan on Physical Activity, the World Health Organization (WHO) predicts a 15% reduction in the global prevalence of physical inactivity in adolescents and adults by 2030.[2] Globally, more than 80% of the adolescent population is not meeting the guidelines for physical activity.[9] The WHO recommends 60 minutes a day of moderate to vigorous physical activity daily for children 5 to 17 years of age.[9] They further state that sedentary activity should be decreased, with a particular focus on recreational screen time. When promoting moderate to vigorous activity, it is important to understand that the intensity level of physical activity for one individual differs when compared to others based on their baseline level of fitness. General examples of moderate activity include brisk walking, dancing, or some household chores. Examples of vigorous activities include running, fast cycling, swimming, or playing high-intensity sports such as soccer.

The Physical Activity Guidelines for Americans is evidence-based and provides recommendations on improving health through regular participation in physical activity for individuals 3 years and older.[2] The guidelines provide specific clinical recommendations, tested strategies to increase physical activity, the benefits of engaging in activity, and the amount and type of activity recommended by age group. New to this set of guidelines includes guidance for preschool-aged children, 3 to 5 years old, to address and promote physical activity for children from 6 years old through early adulthood. Children and adolescents should engage in a variety of physical activities that are age-appropriate, enjoyable, and encourage sustained interest and participation. Important points include the following[2]:

- Children (ages 3 to 5 years old) should be encouraged to engage in physical activity throughout the day that includes a variety of activities.
- Children and adolescents should strive for a minimum of 60 minutes of physical activity daily; the minutes do not necessarily need to be contiguous.
- Physical activity should be of moderate to vigorous levels and include vigorous-intensity physical activity at least 3 days/week.
- Physical activity should include each of the following on 3 or more days per week: aerobic activity for cardiovascular and respiratory fitness; resistance activities for muscle strengthening; weight loading for bone strengthening.

Health Benefits of Physical Activity

Physical activity plays an integral role and can provide a benefit for children with many chronic health conditions including:
- *Asthma:* Children with asthma may decrease participation in daily physical activity out of concern that the physical activity will trigger symptoms of their asthma, decreasing overall

physical fitness. However, participation in aerobic activity has demonstrated an improvement in the individual's exercise capacity and a reduction in airway inflammation. Asthma should not prevent children from participating in sports or physical activity, as long as symptoms are well controlled.[10] Participation in sports requires their healthcare provider to have the proper asthma plan in place, including medications and techniques for the use of their inhalers prior to vigorous physical activity and daily adherence to the plan including adequate hydration. Additional suggestions include preventative measures, such as gradually increasing their fitness level, performing proper warmups before participation in sports, decreasing exercise in cold weather, or wrapping a scarf around the face to warm up the air prior to participation may be helpful.[10]
- *Hypertension:* For hypertensive youth, recommendations of engaging in moderate to vigorous physical activity (30–60 minutes, 3–5 days/week) along with a DASH (Dietary Approaches to Stop Hypertension) diet should be provided.[11] In general, participation in physical activity should be encouraged and will have a beneficial effect on the adolescent's cardiac status.[11]
- *Metabolic syndrome and type 2 diabetes:* Physical inactivity increases the risk for metabolic syndrome, type 2 diabetes, and cardiovascular disease in adults and is related to increased levels of metabolic syndrome risk factors in children and adolescents. Once diagnosed, each of these risks can be positively impacted through increased physical activity levels.[12] Engagement in aerobic exercise and resistance exercise can improve insulin resistance. Aerobic exercise improves lipid profiles, specifically increasing the high-density lipoprotein cholesterol (HDL-C) and decreasing low-density lipoprotein (LDL)-C and triglycerides.[13]
- *Obesity:* Although obesity is complex and multifactorial in origin, physical activity plays an important role. Decreased physical activity is identified as a risk factor for obesity with higher levels of participation in physical activity being negatively associated with overweight status in school-aged children. Children who engage in physical activity have lower body fat and improved healthcare outcomes. Concurrent with increasing physical activity is the recommendation to reduce time spent on sedentary behaviors, especially screen time, which is in direct competition with physical activity.[14]

Physical Activity and Children With Special Healthcare Needs

Children with intellectual or developmental disabilities are about twice as likely to be overweight or obese when compared to their typically developing peers.[15] Specific to activity, children with disabilities are 4.5 times less likely to engage in regular physical activity than those without a disability.[16] While facing the common risk factors associated with living in an obesogenic society, they can have additional contributing issues specific to or compound by their disability. Examples of these can include difficulty with chewing or swallowing food, texture sensitivities, medications that can influence their appetite and increase weight, physical limitations that can limit or reduce their ability to exercise, pain, environments that are not accessible or create additional challenges, and lack of resources or opportunities that are inclusive to their needs.[17] Barriers at a systems level related to participation in physical activity can be encountered such as the detailed review and need for a student Individualized Educational Plan when planning activities, concern for safety, lack of staff expertise, lack of healthcare provider awareness of resources, cost of special equipment, and decreased access to accessible facilities.[15]

Beyond the typical physical and mental benefits of participating in physical activity, children with special healthcare needs can have additional benefits such as the facilitation of life skill competencies, enhancing socialization, mediating the psychological and social impact of their disability, and the promotion of independence.[15] The 2nd edition of the Physical Activity Guidelines recommends that the child should work with their healthcare professional or physical activity specialist to individualize a plan for engaging in physical activity that is appropriate for their needs and abilities and to avoid or reduce inactivity when possible.[2] Similarly, the WHO recommends that children and adolescents with a disability should engage in an average of 60 minutes a day of moderate to vigorous physical activity at least 3 days a week that is mostly aerobic with a goal to add bone building and muscle strengthening activities and to decrease or limit the amount of time in sedentary activity, particularly recreational screen time.[9]

Many children and adolescents with intellectual and developmental disabilities are capable of performing exercise or strenuous activities. Factors that facilitate participation in physical activity can be integrated within multiple environmental contexts starting within the home and family and extending to the medical home, school, and community. Similar to typically developing children, families should role model and support participation in physical activity. The healthcare provider should assess body mass index regularly and provide guidance on physical activity and decreasing sedentary activity as needed with specific knowledge of opportunities to meet the needs of that individual child. Recognizing unique characteristics that accompany different conditions can be useful when recommending activities. Examples include a child with cerebral palsy who may have decreased flexibility with joint contractures and a lack of motor control, coordination, and balance. This may place them at risk of an increased risk of overuse injuries, particularly to their lower extremities.[18] A child who uses a wheelchair for mobility may have a higher risk of upper extremity overuse injuries and pressure sores on their bony prominences. Awareness and consideration of appropriate adaptive or medical equipment are needed. Having a network of exercise-related experts (e.g., physical therapists, physical medicine and rehabilitation physician, and sports medicine providers) can be an asset to the provider and family.[18]

Schools have a unique opportunity to promote physical activity for all children. Federal law requires states, districts, and schools to provide all children with and without disabilities the equal opportunity to engage in physical activity and physical education. Awareness and compliance with federal policies including the Americans with Disabilities Act (ADA), Section 504 of the Rehabilitation Act, and Title II of the ADA are a priority to support equal opportunity provided.[19] The primary care provider (PCP) is in a unique position as they often have an ongoing relationship with the child and family and have built a level of trust within this collaboration and are a respected member of the community. The provider can facilitate participation by assessing current levels of engagement in moderate to vigorous levels of physical activity. Setting goals and implementing motivational activity strategies, providing resources, and understanding how activities can be adapted can be useful in providing a foundation that can translate to an increased level of physical activity for the child and family.[18] When encouraging physical activity, the age, developmental level,

physical limitations, and factors such as accessibility, socialization, and play should be integrated into the physical activity plan.

More programs that encourage participation in sports and physical activity for children with special needs are needed. Some examples of available programs include the National Center on Health Physical Activity and Disability (NCHPAD), Special Olympics, and the Paralympics.[18] NCHPAD is a public health practice resource center that promotes the health of individuals with disabilities. Their website has information for individuals from health care, public health, education, fitness professionals, and individuals with disabilities. In addition to news items and resources, they provide links to adapted physical activity opportunities that can serve as models to be replicated within other communities. In addition, they offer home workouts and video series that are free and provide adapted physical activity opportunities. Special Olympics has a focus to educate those with disabilities to make healthy lifestyle choices to improve their overall long-term health. The Special Olympics organization provides guidelines for healthy nutrition, lifestyle choices, and ways to increase one's level of physical fitness and holds sports health screening clinics. It also serves as a resource for community and healthcare professionals to learn about athletic participation and how to address healthcare disparities of children with special needs. Visit https://www.nchpad.org/and https://www.specialolympics.org/ for more information and see the Additional Resources at the end of this chapter.

Children with Down syndrome are known to have low tone and looser ligaments that place them at greater risk of having a compression of the spinal cord causing nerve damage, referred to as *atlantoaxial instability.*[20] The exact numbers of individuals with atlantoaxial instability are unknown, but it is thought that one or two in 100 children may exhibit symptoms. Diagnosis includes a radiograph obtained with the child's or adolescent's neck in a neutral position with forward flexion of the cervical spine. If any abnormalities are noted on the radiograph, additional testing such as a magnetic resonance imaging (MRI) or computed tomography (CT) scan should occur. Individuals with atlantoaxial instability may exhibit changes in their ambulation, the ability to use upper extremities, complaints of neck pain, a new fixed head tilt, bowel or bladder dysfunction, or new unexplained weakness.[20] Select physical activities that are contraindicated with atlantoaxial and atlantooccipital joint instabilities include gymnastics, diving, pentathlon, butterfly stroke, swimming that includes a diving start, high jump, certain warm-up exercises, and soccer. They may, however, engage in most noncontact sports. Parents/guardians can consent if the athlete is permitted to perform alternate activities.

During annual visits and preparticipation physicals, the provider should evaluate for signs of atlantoaxial instability and obtain a radiograph. Symptoms of possible spinal cord compression or atlantoaxial instability can include neck pain, localized neurologic pain, weakness, numbness, spasticity (unusual "tightness" of certain muscles) or change in muscle tone, gait difficulties, hyperreflexia, change in bowel or bladder function, or other signs or symptoms of injury to the spinal cord.[21] If abnormalities are present on a radiograph, the child should be referred to a pediatric neurosurgeon or orthopedic surgeon for evaluation and treatment. If there are symptoms suggestive of spinal cord compression and/or atlantoaxial instability, clearance for Special Olympics requires an additional thorough neurologic examination by a qualified licensed healthcare provider. If certified to participate, the athlete (or parent/guardian of a minor) must sign a waiver provided by Special Olympics and may choose to participate in the sport of their choice.[21]

Strategies to Support Physical Activity for Children and Adolescents

Children and adolescents face a variety of barriers daily that influence their ability and choice to be physically active. Table 18.1 presents findings from a systematic review that provide strategies to promote physical activity participation in children and adolescents framed with a socioecological perspective.[22] When promoting physical activity, it is critical to individualize the

TABLE 18.1	Socioecological Model for Effective Promotion of Physical Activity by Healthcare Providers
Level of Intervention	**Examples**
Individual Level	
Using the opportunity of the one-on-one interaction with the child and family members to understand their knowledge, attributions, and beliefs and to promote a positive outlook toward physical activity.	• Assess the child's baseline physical activity level at all patient visits. • Take interest in learning the interests of the child and family. • Discuss physical activity recommendations as part of a healthy lifestyle. • Include recommendations on physical activity when providing obesity prevention, education, or obesity treatment. • Use motivational interviewing techniques to promote behavioral change by increasing physical activity. Base intervention on "stages of change" theory as a collaborative patient/provider model. • Role-model a healthy lifestyle.
Interpersonal Level	
Identify the child's relationships and whom they interact with within their social networks, such as families, peer groups, and friendship-based social networks.	• Recommend social interactions when participating in physical activity as a mechanism to encourage accountability of the group and increase the enjoyment of the activity. • Initiate family goals to participate in physical activity regularly and together. • Role-model a healthy lifestyle and promote engagement in physical activities among clinic staff. • Be aware and provide suggestions for activities within the community that is oriented to youth and families.
Organizational Level	
Participate and be a leader on an institutional level by encouraging physical activity through policies and rules specific to assemblies of individuals. Common examples of assemblies include schools, religious or faith-based institutions, and the workplace.	Support activities that encourage organizational physical activity promotion, for example: • School programs, such as walk or bike to school days (e.g., International Walk to School Day that occurs yearly in October; see www.walkbiketoschool.org/). • Screen time awareness week. • Intramural programs. • Advise childcare centers about ways to increase physical activity for children and staff. • Advise schools and parents about the importance of recess and physical education (PE). • Encourage schools *not* to withhold recess as a punishment for misbehavior.
Community Level	
Communities include individuals who participate in interpersonal relationships within various local groups of institutions and organizations. Communities may be defined geographically, politically, culturally, or by other common characteristics.	Advocate for activities that help communities structure public space and promote physical activity: • Ensure safe and easily accessible park and playground space. • Promote affordable organized activities (e.g., scholarships to pay for team sports, after-school activities for low-income youth, and local recreation department or YMCA offerings). • Advocate for bike lanes and walking trails in the community. • Advocate for vehicular speed control along major routes to schools to encourage walking/cycling safety. • Promote programs that teach bike safety and distribute low-cost helmets. • Advocate for keeping school buildings open after school for supervised physical activities. • Volunteer to sit on school boards or be a part of school parent teaching associations to advocate for physical activity within the realm of school.
Structure, Policy, and Systems Level	
Represents the local, state, and federal structures and systems that affect the built environment, surrounding communities, and individuals.	Advocate for changes in public policy: • Testify at hearings on the importance of maintaining PE in schools. • Address zoning issues to maintain or increase green spaces, such as parks, bike trails, and walking trails. • Work with planners to ensure that communities are designed to promote family-friendly physical activity (e.g., adequate sidewalks/crosswalks, residential areas within walking distance to neighborhood schools, and adequate lighting at playfields and parks).

Data from Hu D, Zhou S, Crowley-McHattan ZJ, Liu Z. Factors that influence participation in physical activity in school-aged children and adolescents: a systematic review from the social ecological model perspective. *Int J Environ Res Public Health.* 2021;18(6); Centers for Disease Control and Prevention. Youth Risk Behavior Surveillance System Results; 2020. https://www.cdc.gov/healthyyouth/data/yrbs/results.htm; and US Department of Health and Human Services Office of Disease Prevention and Health Promotion. Reduce the proportion of children and adolescents with obesity-NWS-04; 2022. https://health.gov/healthypeople/objectives-and-data/browse-objectives/overweight-and-obesity/reduce-proportion-children-and-adolescents-obesity-nws-04.

Healthcare Providers Influence on Lifestyle Behaviors

Healthcare providers have the unique opportunity to impact the health habits of the child and family through regular routine primary care visits. Acknowledging that physical activity is a behavior, the provider should be familiar with theories of change, motivation, and motivational interviewing to support behavioral change (see Chapter 6). If these techniques are used appropriately, the provider can support patient-centered care, educate the child and family, and increase motivation for improved health habits.

Counseling Families About Organized Sports Participation

Unstructured play from early childhood builds creativity and dexterity and should be encouraged; however, parents, schools, and organizations often recommend and offer focused structured, and goal-oriented activities. In the United States, there is a heavy emphasis on organized sports participation for youth as demonstrated by how schools are heavily involved in competitive organized sports. Participating in organized sports has many benefits, including developing physical skills, creating friendships, learning to work as part of a team, following rules and fairness, and improving self-esteem.

The potential negative issues surrounding organized sports participation come when the context of the sport changes from fun to "win at all costs," which increases the level of stress and competition related to the sport. Behaviors and attitudes developed during sports participation, positive and/or negative, are engrained and carried into adulthood. While coaches are instrumental in the development of these attitudes and behaviors, families play a key role in supporting the child by being actively involved and developing good sportsmanship. Specific examples include providing positive feedback and emotional support, having realistic expectations of their child's skills and abilities, keeping an open dialogue about the child's experiences with their coach and team, role-modeling respectful behavior as a fan, and assisting the child to develop skills to handle losses and frustrations with the sport.[23] Structured sports that promote developmentally age-appropriate participation support a child's physical, cognitive, and emotional health.

Early Specialization in Sports

Participating in sports provides benefits that include mental, physical, and social health. Sports participation has been associated with the development of life skills (e.g., goal setting, time management, and negotiation) and social skills, teamwork, and higher academic achievement.[24] As organized sports gain popularity, recreational games, and unstructured activities have decreased. Organized sports have different levels of commitment and expectations and are heavily influenced by coaches and parents. This shift often places an increased emphasis on winning and promotes year-round opportunities to play one sport versus changing sport participation based on the season. Early specialization in one sport has been discouraged and may have potentially negative effects on the young athlete. The National Athletic Trainer's Association published an official statement regarding sport specialization.[25] Recommendations include:

- Delay specializing in a single sport or training for a single sport year-round for as long as possible. This promotes athleticism and reduces injury risk.
- Work with one team or organized sport per season. Participating with multiple teams concurrently increases the volume of activity and can increase the risk of injury.
- Young athletes should diversify sports interests and not participate in one organized sport for more than 8 months of a year.
- Limit hours of participation per week to age in years or less.
- Have a minimum of 2 days of rest weekly from organized training or competition.
- Take a break after each competitive season. This allows for physical and mental recovery, minimizes the risk of injury, promotes wellbeing, and reduces the risk of burnout. If youth decide to specialize in one sport, it is recommended they wait until after puberty to minimize injury risk and have the cognitive, physical, social, emotional, and motor skills to support their success with specialized training. Participation in multiple sports provides additional benefits for the athlete such as increased agility, balance, coordination, and speed that can transfer from sport to sport. Box 18.1 provides guidance for the clinician on sports specialization in youth athletes.

Strength Training

Strength training, or resistance training, uses free weights, weight machines, resistance bands, or the individual's own body weight to allow the individual to build strength or increase conditioning as they progressively exert force against the object of resistance.[26] Plyometric exercises, such as side-to-side hops and squat jumps, use a combination of body weight and rapid movements to enhance power and explosiveness. Strength training can be used for several reasons: to enhance performance in a particular sport, increase stamina and endurance, improve cardiovascular fitness and body composition, reduce the risk of injury or as a component of rehabilitation after some injuries, and enhance muscle mass for appearance. Resistance training can be beneficial for almost all children and adolescents with proper supervision and instruction.[26] A strength training program should be supervised and designed to fit the needs, goals, and abilities of the child or adolescent. Supervision includes monitoring the use of low-weight and high repetitions while taking into consideration the ability to listen and follow directions, existing motor skills and

> **• BOX 18.1 Guidance for Clinicians on Sports Specialization**
>
> - The primary focus of sports participation in youth is to have fun and foster lifelong physical activity skills and thus, it is recommended to only participating in one sport at a time.
> - Recommending less than 8 months per year in a single sport in a year with time away for rest and recovery.
> - During specialized sport participation, recommending a minimum of 2 days off per week decreases the athlete's risk of injury.
> - Athletes' age in years equals the maximum recommended time in sport a week (e.g., a 10-year-old should not participate in more than 10 hours a week in their organized sport)
>
> Data from National Athletic Trainers' Association. NATA Official Statement in support of sports specialization recommendations for adolescent and young athletes; 2019. https://www.nata.org/blog/beth-sitzler/youth-sports-specialization-recommendations

muscle strength, and technical proficiency in combination with biological age and psychosocial maturity. Increases in strength can be evident in programs or training that occur 2 to 3 times a week for a minimum duration of 8 weeks.[26] Resistance training can begin as young as 5 years of age or when they begin participating in sports activities. Examples of strength-building exercises for younger age groups include frog jumps, bear crawls, and hopping on one foot.[26] Box 18.2 lists general guidelines for youth strength training.

If a strength training program is supervised and individualized to the child or adolescent, the risk of injury is low. Potential injuries can occur with prolonged training with heavy loads and engagement in resistance training without adequate rest and recovery between sessions. When resistance training programs are appropriate for the child or adolescent, no negative outcomes on linear growth, physical health, or the cardiovascular system are evident.[26] Until skeletal maturity, the risk of avulsion fracture may occur with explosive contractions of the muscle-tendon attachment at the apophyseal areas during weightlifting. Pediatric data are lacking on the specific prevalence of injuries associated with intensive metabolic conditional or training programs that include a combination of resistance training, running intervals, and repetitive body weight exercises (e.g., plyometrics). As with any physical activity program, proper technique, instruction, and adequate fluid and recovery or rest time between sessions are recommended.

While the potential for injury is present, the current consensus is that strength training is advantageous, even for young athletes,

• BOX 18.2 Recommendations for Strength Training Program for Youth Athletes

- Youth with uncontrolled hypertension, uncontrolled seizure disorders, certain cardiovascular conditions, or a history of being treated with an anthracycline chemotherapeutic agent should consult with a medical professional for clearance prior to starting a strength training program.
- Integrating aerobic conditioning with resistance training along with other skill-related fitness with developmentally appropriate activities is recommended for a comprehensive program.
- Include dynamic warm-up exercises and cool down with less intense stretching for each training session.
- If overweight or obesity is present, begin with basic resistance exercises to increase the sustainability of successful engagement in physical activity.
- Focus on proper technique and begin with a low resistance training intensity of 1–2 sets of 8–12 repetitions. As competence is gained, increase weight in 5%–10% increments and reduce the repetitions to 2–4 sets of 6–12 repetitions.
- Include all muscle groups in a strength training program.
- Recommend following a sequence of working large muscle groups before small muscle groups and complex, multijoint exercises before single-joint exercises.
- Focus on technique and maintain consistency with the needs, abilities, and maturity level of the youth athlete.
- Monitor for signs of injury, illness, or overuse from the strength training program and evaluate prior to returning or continuation of the strength training program.
- Educate youth athletes about the risks associated with the use of performance-enhancing substances and discourage use or experimentation.
- Advise athletes and families of the dangers of using performance-enhancing drugs.

Modified from Stricker PR, Faigenbaum AD, McCambridge TM, et al. Resistance training for children and adolescents. Pediatrics. 2020;145(6).

provided that it is done in a safe and supervised manner. Benefits of strength training include improved cardiovascular fitness, strength, flexibility, bone mineral density, blood lipid profile, and mental health.[26] Furthermore, strength training when combined with aerobic training is a beneficial tool in weight management as it improves body composition by reducing total body fat.[26]

Strength training is not recommended for children or adolescents with certain health conditions. Youths with a complex cardiac congenital cardiac condition such as, but not limited to, hypertrophic cardiomyopathy, pulmonary hypertension, and Marfan syndrome are recommended to avoid resistance training due to the risk for worsening ventricular hypertrophy, a sudden change in hemodynamics, or hemodynamic decompensation secondary to an acute increase in pulmonary hypertension. Consultation with a healthcare provider is recommended prior to beginning a resistance training program for youth with uncontrolled seizure disorders or for those with poorly controlled, preexisting hypertension. Resistance training is acceptable for children with a seizure disorder that is well controlled on medication.[26] Youths previously diagnosed with cancer and treated with anthracycline chemotherapy are at an increased risk for cardiotoxicity and acute congestive heart failure and should consult with a healthcare provider prior to participating in a resistance training program.[26]

Preseason Conditioning and Injury Prevention

A variety of strategies can be used to reduce the incidence and severity of injuries (see Chapter 40). Some of the more typical injury conditions that can be avoided with simple prevention strategies are included in Table 18.2. Readiness can be addressed from two perspectives: developmental readiness as discussed previously and preseason conditioning readiness.

Preseason conditioning and strength training prepare the central nervous system (CNS) to react quickly to muscular stretching and shortening, which decreases overuse injuries (e.g., stress fractures, bursitis, and tendinopathies). Proper preseason conditioning should focus on enhancing strength, flexibility, and endurance, and improving natural sport-specific movements and agility. Conditioning helps to strengthen bone, facilitates weight control, improves balance and coordination, adds muscle mass, improves performance, and decreases the amount of time needed for rehabilitation with injury. Players as young as 10 to 12 years old benefit from establishing overall motion patterns when they participate in warm-up programs. Coaches and fitness instructors should be certified and knowledgeable about age-specific training techniques and safety; adult training techniques should never be applied to children.

Intentional Weight Loss and Weight Gain

Intentional weight loss and weight gain by adolescent athletes can be dangerous practices if they engage in unhealthy weight-control practices. Weight loss through severe restriction of energy intake while participating in high levels of exercise is particularly harmful to young athletes who are still growing and can put the athlete at increased risk for injury during the season.[27] Weight loss may originate from the desire to improve performance, for aesthetic purposes (e.g., figure skaters, gymnasts, or synchronized swimmers), or to meet mandatory weight requirements on the day of competition for certain sports (e.g., wrestlers, lightweight rowers, or jockeys). Use of extreme diets, dehydration, or unsafe weight-loss supplements should be identified and avoided. Intentional

TABLE 18.2 Common Injuries and Prevention Strategies

Medical Condition	Prevention Strategies	Comments
Muscle soreness	• Warm up the body with a mix of static and dynamic stretching that prepares muscles for activity. Holding the stretch for a timeframe (i.e., toe touches and stretches) are static and activities that allow the body to continue to move are dynamic (i.e., jumping jacks). • Start with lighter weights and fewer repetitions when starting a new regimen.	• Soreness should be minor, resulting from microscopic muscle or connective tissue damage; it is a normal result of muscles that are adapting to a new exercise program. • Clinicians should explain this soreness ahead of time so that new exercisers do not use this condition as an excuse to stop their fitness regimen.
Strains and sprains	• Participate in a preseason conditioning program. • Tape site of the previous injury. • Warm up body temperature before stretching. • Maintain playing surfaces. • Use proper footwear. • Limit practice time.	• Injuries are mostly related to pivoting sports, such as basketball, football, and volleyball. • Knee braces should not replace adequate conditioning specific to the sport. Use only after a formal diagnosis and management plan is in place following consultation with a provider or athletic trainer; braces should be only one aspect of acute or overuse injury treatment. Categories of knee braces include sleeves (help with swelling and support but infer no real stability; may have extra knee padding that helps with prevention in sports at high risk for blows to the knee); PTO brace or patellar strap/bands for added patellar stability; and hinged-knee braces (include prophylactic braces [protection of knee ligaments during contact sports]; and functional or rehabilitative [intended to prevent reinjury after torn knee ligaments or postoperatively]). Braces should not replace rehabilitation and surgery if required.
Fractures	• Do strength-conditioning exercises. • Use proper techniques. • Take safety precautions. • Use protective gear that fits well, such as wrist guards.	• Most common fractures are of the elbow and femur. Depending on the age of the child, the growth plate may be open, which places the child at risk of injury to the growth plate and subsequent abnormal healing limitations to the future bone growth. Most fractures heal appropriately, with proper casting and observation since the bone is still remodeling.
Stress fractures	• Use soft running and playing surfaces • Use proper footgear • Do strengthening exercises • Stop activity when pain occurs	• Stress fractures occur after the repetitive force is placed on the musculoskeletal system without adequate time for healing to occur between activities. Children are at an increased risk because of weaker osteochondral junctions, decreased bone mineralization, thinner cortices, and variations in hormone levels.
Lacerations, contusions, abrasions (see Chapter 21)	• Protective equipment is essential.	• Injuries are mostly related to baseball (contusion/abrasion), soccer, cycling, and ice hockey (lacerations).
Anterior leg pain syndrome or medial tibial stress syndrome (shin splints)	• Confirm proper body mechanics for the activity being performed. • Do not increase the duration, frequency, or intensity of an activity too quickly. • Promote bone strength and density by including enough calcium and vitamin D in the diet. • Use a soft playing surface. • Use proper footwear (proper fit, impact-absorbing sole, insert for shoe). • When a shin splint is present, take adequate time to rest and heal or the athlete will risk progression to a stress fracture.	• Improper body mechanics can increase the risk of injury. • Do not increase the duration, frequency, or intensity of an activity too quickly. • During rest periods, the athlete can cross-train with nonimpact activities such as biking, swimming, and weights.

Continued

TABLE 18.2	Common Injuries and Prevention Strategies—Cont'd	
Medical Condition	**Prevention Strategies**	**Comments**
Plantar fasciitis	• Use proper footwear (cushioned with fitted heel counters or lifts). • Stretch calf and Achilles tendon. • Do ice and massage after the event. • Correct biomechanical errors. • Limit hills and speed work; increase soft-surface running.	• When plantar fasciitis is present, avoid activities such as running, jumping, or long periods of standing. • Roll a tennis ball in the arch of the foot to increase circulation and improve healing.
Blisters	• Wear socks. • Wear properly fitted shoes. • Use powder, petroleum jelly, an antifriction product (highly recommended), or Second Skin on at-risk or reddened area(s).	
Head and neck injuries	• Have appropriate supervision and coaching that teaches proper skills, such as tackling. • Adhere to the safety rules of the game. • Strengthen neck muscles. • Use appropriate equipment: helmets and face and mouth gear. • Follow concussion guidelines for RTP after injury (see Table 18.9).	• Greatest risks for these injuries are from cycling, diving, equestrian sports, football, gymnastics, ice hockey, wrestling, trampolines, football, rugby, and cheerleading. • Risks increase with age.
Eye trauma	• Although not required for most sports leagues, parents and coaches should mandate that children wear safety glasses or goggles when they play.	• Protective eyewear is made of ultra-strong polycarbonate that is 10 times more impact resistant and does not decrease the vision for the athlete.

PTO, Patellar tracking orthosis; *RTP,* return-to-play.

Data from Bishop ME, Ahlmen A, Rosendorf J, Erickson BJ, Cohen S. Bone stress injuries in female athletes. *Ann Joint.* 2021;6; National Institute of Health National Eye Institute. Sports and Your Eyes; 2021. https://www.nei.nih.gov/learn-about-eye-health/nei-for-kids/sports-and-your-eyes/; American Academy of Pediatrics. Knee Pain: How to Choose the Right Knee Brace for Your Child; 2019. https://www.healthychildren.org/English/health-issues/injuries-emergencies/sports-injuries/Pages/Knee-Pain-and-braces.aspx. American Academy of Pediatrics. Shin Pain and Athletes. Pediatric Patient Education. 2021; https://publications.aap.org/patiented/article-abstract/doi/10.1542/peo_document573/82203/Shin-Pain-and-Athletes?redirectedFrom=fulltext; and Shelat NH, El-Khoury GY. Pediatric stress fractures: a pictorial essay. *Iowa Orthop J.* 2016;36:138.

weight gain can be encountered when the youth participate in sports such as football, powerlifting, or bodybuilding. Methods of unhealthy weight gain can include rapid weight gain, the use of anabolic compounds, the use of supplements, and weight gain that results in excess body fat.[27] Caloric requirements for youth athletes will differ based on age, developmental growth, gender, and activity level. See resources for an interactive tool to calculate an individual's caloric needs based on their gender, age, and activity level created by the US Department of Agriculture.[27]

Considerations of Climate and Environment

Heat and Humidity

Core body temperature is a balance of heat generation and heat dissipation (see Chapter 24). A major contributor to core body temperature is the heat generated by muscle contractions. Exercising muscle generates up to 20% to 25% of metabolic energy times the amount of heat of resting muscle, and sweating is the main mechanism that is used to rid the body of excess heat.[28] If the body is unable to rid itself of the excessive heat, body temperature will rise. When environmental heat or humidity excesses are added to the equation, the body must dissipate the heat at increased rates. Unless the usual heat dissipation mechanisms are properly working, heat stroke can result within 15 to 20 minutes. Exercise heat illness can begin with exercise-associated muscle

cramps and progress to heat syncope, exhaustion, and stroke, which can be fatal if not recognized and treated promptly. Recognition of heat stroke can be challenging as early symptoms can be nonspecific and can include disorientation, tachycardia, vomiting, and seizures. If not treated, systemic dysfunction can occur including rhabdomyolysis, multiorgan failure, circulatory failure, and disseminated intravascular coagulation.[28] Heat is dissipated through sensible losses such as convection, conduction, and radiation and insensible losses through evaporation. Heat exchange can vary based on factors such as metabolic heat production, clothing, body surface area, body mass, sex, age, and aerobic fitness.[28]

Previously, it had been thought that children were less effective at regulating their body temperature during episodes of exercising in the heat when compared to adults. This was thought to be related to a higher body surface area-to-mass ratio, a decreased capacity to sweat, and lower cardiac output.[28] The research on the perceived disadvantage has changed and is now thought that children are primarily at a higher risk of severe hyperthermia in extreme conditions.[28] With these new findings, there is now a greater focus placed on modifying internal and external risk factors related to heat illness. Internal factors include the individual's metabolic heat production, body surface area, fitness level, lack of heat acclimatization, and excess or inappropriate clothing including protective equipment.

Lifestyle can play an important role in exertional heat illness with greater susceptibility occurring with atypical situations such as a combination of mild illness, lack of sleep, and heat stress from the previous day.[28] External factors such as high heat stress; high humidity that reduces the efficacy of sweating in releasing body heat; air velocity or lack of air movement; solar radiation and individual exercise intensity can further increase risk.[28] Coaches and athletic trainers can prevent or minimize the risk of heat-related illness. This can include helping the student athlete to acclimate to the heat in a structured manner, ensuring adequate hydration, recommending loose-fitting and light-colored clothing, and decreasing or avoiding exercise during extreme temperatures. If engaging in physical activity in extreme temperatures, providing frequent water breaks, periods of rest, and closely monitoring each athlete for signs or symptoms of heat-related illness can prevent heat stroke.[29]

Risk factors for heat illness include obesity, deconditioning, inadequate sleep, large muscle mass, recent or acute illness, sickle cell trait (SCT), skin abnormalities, uncontrolled diabetes mellitus (DM), cardiovascular disease, congenital disorders (e.g., idiopathic anhidrosis), previous heat illness, or preexisting dehydration.[29] Medication use can predispose the athlete to heat illness. Examples include stimulants, anticholinergics, antihistamines, antiseizure medications, angiotensin-converting enzyme inhibitors, angiotensin II receptor blockers, decongestants, tricyclic antidepressants, phenothiazines, amphetamines, ergogenic stimulants, lithium, diuretics, β-blockers, and alcohol.[30] Individuals with these predisposing risk factors need particular supervision because they might not recognize early warning signs of heat effects and may not hydrate adequately.

Dehydration

Dehydration is the imbalance of fluid between the intracellular and extracellular components. When the intra- and extracellular compartments are in balance, the body maintains blood volume through regulation by the kidneys, hormones (antidiuretic hormone and aldosterone), and solutes such as sodium, potassium, proteins, and glucose.[31] The intake of water and electrolytes maintains hydration and regulates the fluid shifts between the intracellular and extracellular compartments. As athletes exert energy, their active muscles generate heat, which raises their core temperature. The body responds by dissipating heat through circulation (warm blood sent to the skin; flushed face), evaporation (sweating), and hormonal adjustment (adjusting to the loss of electrolytes and water through sweat).[29] The amount of fluid lost can vary based on the intensity and time engaged in an activity, the temperature, humidity, the individual's loss of water due to sweat, and wearing of additional clothes, or equipment such as a uniform or pads.[32] Hydration strategies are particularly important for children and adolescents as they get distracted and may forget about drinking fluids or they may be restricted due to logistics related to their activity (i.e., decreased breaks offered during their practice). The use of a sports drink during exercise may be useful for the athlete and provides an easy source of carbohydrates, fluids, and electrolytes.[33]

The coaching staff should play a role in educating, monitoring, and supporting the athlete's ability to maintain hydration and should be proactive in providing drink breaks, having water bottles accessible, and reminding players to drink.[34] Children 9 to 12 years old should replace lost fluids with 3 to 5 ounces every 20 minutes and up to 34 to 50 ounces every hour for adolescents.[32] Fluid options may vary depending on the duration of exercise. For ≤1 hour of exercise, water is ideal. For ≥1 hour of exercise, a sports drink that contains some carbohydrates and replaces nutrients lost in sweat is useful.[32] Recommendations on drinking fluids with caffeine have evolved. While previously thought to avoid their use as it may increase urine output, causing further dehydration, recent reports have documented improvement in performance based on the type of exercise, the timing of drinking the caffeinated beverage, and the amount of caffeine ingested.[35]

For monitoring hydration status, a sense of thirst is usually a late indicator of dehydration and should not be solely relied upon. On a scale of 1 to 9, with 1 being not thirsty and 9 being extremely thirsty, a score between 3 and 5 is related to a 1% to 2% dehydration level. Urine color can be monitored with a goal of pale yellow indicating adequate hydration and any darker colors indicating dehydration. Urine color check charts can be ordered to post in locker rooms to assist athletes to prevent dehydration at http://www.hydrationcheck.com/about.php.

Sports Training Acclimatization for Prevention of Heat-Related Illnesses

Exertional health stroke is the third leading cause of death in US athletes after cardiac disorders and head and neck trauma.[28] Heat-related illness occurs on a spectrum from cramps, exhaustion, and heat stroke being the most severe. The risk is higher for sports that require the athlete to wear heavy equipment such as football, which has an 11.4 times higher incidence of the development of a heat-related illness than all other sports combined.[36] According to the National Center for Catastrophic Sport Injury Research, 28 high school football players died from exertional health stroke between 2008 and 2017 and an increased number of emergency room visits and hospitalizations can be attributed to heat illness.[37] Heat-related illnesses are totally preventable. *Heat acclimatization* is the training process that gradually allows the athlete to physiologically adapt to exercising in high-temperature environmental conditions.[34] This training typically occurs over 10 to 14 days with exercise sessions that last 60 to 90 minutes per day allowing the body to adapt by increasing plasma volume and sweat rates, adjusting kidney function by decreasing urinary sodium excretion, and increasing aldosterone production, sodium excretion, sweat threshold, sweat electrolyte content, and heart rate during a workout.[38] For that reason, many sports associations at both the high school and collegiate levels require heat-acclimatization periods in their initial training schedules.[38] Specific heat-acclimatization guidelines for athletic training are available at https://www.nsca.com/about-us/position-statements/safe-return-to-training/.[38]

Recreational Activities

Safety Issues

Recreational activities play a key role in maintaining and promoting physical activity and health. Activities that are recreational in nature can often be performed independently, may be performed as the youth's mode of transportation (e.g., cycling, skateboarding), or done for purely social reasons (e.g., pick-up game of basketball or playing at the park). Recreational activities are often relatively inexpensive when compared to organized sports. Although recreational in nature, these activities can still place the youth at risk for mild to serious injury (e.g., general body trauma, fractures, torn ligaments, or concussions) and should be reviewed with proper safety precautions identified. Table 18.3 identifies hazards linked to various

TABLE 18.3   Recreational Activities: Hazards and Safety Recommendations

Activity and Hazards	Safety Measures
All-terrain vehicles (ATVs) • Loss of control	• No one <16 years should drive or ride on ATVs. • Those ≥16 years should take a hands-on training course offered by certified instructors. • Wear protective clothing (boots, goggles, helmet, long pants, and reflective outerwear). • Have flags, reflectors, and lights on ATVs. • Never carry passengers. • Never ride on public or paved roads or at night.
Motorcycles, motor scooters, mopeds, minibikes, minicycles, trail bikes • Collisions: inability to accelerate when mixing with other traffic; inadequate brakes	• Wear a helmet at all times. • Teenage motorcyclists should receive at least 30 h of professional instruction, including 10 h of driving in moderate to heavy traffic. • Discourage motorcycles for youth transportation. • Off-road vehicles (minibikes, minicycles, trail bikes) should not be used on the street.
Riding lawnmowers • Collisions or falling off when a passenger or operating; playing in the vicinity of an operating mower	• Be at least 16 years old and take an ATV course prior to operating riding mowers.
Snowmobiles • Collisions, rollovers (teenage boys and young males account for 75% of all collisions)	• The AAP recommends that no one under the age of 16 years should operate. The minimum age to operate a snowmobile varies by state. All youth should obtain a state-certified safety certificate. Adequate instruction/supervision by an adult is paramount. • Do not travel alone. • Wear protective clothing (boots, goggles, helmet, insulated outwear, and reflective clothing). • Travel only on designated trails, and avoid roads, railroads, waterways, and pedestrians.
Personal watercraft (PWC; jet skis/water scooters) • Collisions, turnovers, ejections (some models can carry up to three passengers and reach speeds up to 60 mph)	• No one <16 years should operate a PWC. • Wear a US Coast Guard–approved flotation device • Do not jump waves. • Complete a safe boater course that includes instruction on personal watercraft (i.e., jet skis). • Do not operate a PWC if under the influence of alcohol. • Never operate in swimming areas or after sunset.
Golf carts • Collisions, loss of control, turnovers	• Restrict drivers to those ≥16 years. • Limit the number of riders. • Drive only at safe speeds; wear seat belts; use helmets. • Limit use to designated areas.
Community/school playgrounds • Falls, collisions	• Equipment and surfaces should be regularly inspected (including sharp protrusions, detached matting, exposed concrete footings, and tripping hazards) and maintained by schools and cities; all equipment should meet US Consumer Product Safety Commission guidelines. • Maintain good sight lines for supervision of the child, based upon child's height. • Maintain barriers between playground and street. • Instruct children in the proper use of equipment; monitor and enforce playground rules. • Surfaces should be constructed of shock-absorbing, single-unit materials (double-shredded bark mulch, shredded tires, or sand). Asphalt and concrete are unsuitable. • Separate areas for active and quieter play (e.g., swings from sandboxes) and by age. Have an adequate entry and exit space around equipment so that children do not collide with each other or equipment. • Avoid metal or wood seats (best plastic or rubber); ensure equipment has no sharp edges and no openings that could entrap a child's head.
Roller sports (skateboards, scooters) • Falls, collisions (boys injured more than girls)	• Wear a helmet and other protective gear (e.g., wrist guards, elbow and knee pads). • Do not ride in or near traffic; utilize and promote skateboarding parks. • Check the skating area for holes, bumps, and rocks; do not ride on uneven surfaces. • Limit skateboarding to daylight hours. • Children <5 years should not use skateboards; 5- to 10-year-olds should be under an adult's supervision.

TABLE 18.3	Recreational Activities: Hazards and Safety Recommendations—Cont'd	
Activity and Hazards	**Safety Measures**
Swimming • Drowning (due to drain entrapment/ entanglement; lack of swimming skills; inadequate supervision; lack of cardiopulmonary resuscitation [CPR] training by bystanders)	• Swimming pools should have drain covers, safety vacuum-release systems, filter pumps with multiple drains, or other pressure-venting filters. Home pools should have pool alarms, fences, and covers. • All children should get swimming lessons and demonstrate proficiency. Nonswimmers require constant "arms-length" and "touch supervision." • Never swim alone or in the dark. • Face the waves versus turning your back on them. • Wear protective footwear if surfaces are jagged. • If possible, swim where there are stationed lifeguards. • Parents, caregivers, and swim instructors should have CPR training.
Trampoline • Falls; doing acrobatic maneuvers (somersaults, flips); colliding with others using the trampoline	The AAP does not recommend trampolines for home use. If there is a trampoline at home, general recommendations include: • Adult supervision at all times. • Extend padding to the frame, hooks, and springs. • Prohibit ladders; install netting and monitor the condition of the trampoline and parts frequently. • Prohibit somersaulting, multiple jumpers, and jumping onto a trampoline from a higher surface. • Frequently inspect and replace protective elements; discard trampoline if parts are worn or damaged and replacement parts are unavailable. • Actively supervise children and enforce guidelines; adults should be ready to respond to medical emergencies. • Check homeowner insurance for coverage of trampoline-related injuries; if not covered, obtain a rider for trampoline-related injuries.
Winter sports (skiing, snowboarding) • Falls, collisions	• Dress warmly (insulated outerwear, hat, gloves, and slip-resistant snow boots); wear safety goggles when skiing, snowboarding, or snowmobiling. Wear sunscreen. • Wear special helmets made for skiers, snowboarders, and snowmobilers. When ice skating or sledding, wear a multisport or bicycle helmet if a ski helmet is unavailable. • Receive instruction from certified ski and snowboarding schools. • Use proper equipment, wear knee and elbow pads when ice skating and wrist guards when snowboarding. • Children <5 years should only sled with an adult; children <7 years should not snowboard; children <6 years should not ride on snowmobiles without an adult. • Do not sled in or near streets or in areas with trees, fences, ponds, or light poles. Do not skate on river ice or ice that has thawed and refrozen. • Only one person should ride on a sled unless the child is riding with an adult. • Sit up and face forward; avoid sledding headfirst. • Steerable sleds are safer than snow disks or inner tubes. • Never ride a sled being pulled by a car, ATV, snowmobile, or another motorized vehicle. • Ice skating in designated skating areas.
Bicycle riding	• Always wear a bicycle helmet when riding a bicycle. • Wear fluorescent clothing that can increase the rider's visibility. • Do not allow the child to ride at dusk or after dark. • Use lighting on the bike and/or the bicyclist including front white lights, and rear red lights. • Follow the rules of the road.

AAP, American Academy of Pediatrics.

Data from National Safety Council. Staying safe on playgrounds. https://www.nsc.org/community-safety/safety-topics/child-safety/playground-safety; Centers for Disease Control and Prevention. Bicycle safety. https://www.cdc.gov/transportationsafety/bicycle/index.html?CDC_AA_refVal=https%3A%2F%2Fwww.cdc.gov%2Fmotorvehiclesafety%2Fbicycle%2Findex.html; and Schimelpfenig SS. Skiing and snowboarding: safety on bunny hills and beyond. https://www.healthychildren.org/English/healthy-living/sports/Pages/Skiing-and-Snowboarding.aspx?_gl=1*qnawyt*_ga*MTMxOTYzMDMxNC4xN jAxMzI3NTQ1*_ga_FD9D3XZVQQ*MTY0NjA4ODgxOS43LjEuMTY0NjA4OTA3My4w&_ga=2.100958663.750905837.1646088820-1319630314.1601327545.

recreational activities and related safety measures that providers can discuss with parents and children. Many recreational activities take place outdoors, encouraging children to engage actively with the environment, and environmental health and safety concerns must be considered. The healthcare provider should discuss environmental safety including exposure to toxic compounds, use of protective equipment, traffic and pedestrian safety, and guidelines for lightning safety and sports that can be accessed.[39,40]

Use of Helmets for Cycling and Winter Sports

In the United States, there were more than 1000 deaths attributed to bicycle accidents annually and greater than 450,000 bicycle-related injuries.[41] States that have helmet laws have significantly lower crash-related injuries and deaths.[41] Helmets are also recommended for winter activities such as skiing, snowmobiling, snowboarding, sledding, and ice skating.[42] See Box 18.3 for Proper Helmet Fitting Techniques.

- Helmets should carry a US Consumer Product Safety Commission (USCPSC) sticker. Additional certification labels to look for include American Society for Testing and Materials (ASTM), Snell, or American National Standards Institute (ANSI). Adults should wear a helmet every time they ride to be good role models for their children and others.
- Measure the child's head to have an indication of size. Using a soft tape measure or a string measure just above the eyebrows and ears while keeping the measure level.
- Bring the child along when purchasing the helmet and try on several sizes and models to find the best fit:
  - Position of the helmet should sit level and low on the forehead with 1–2 finger widths above the eyebrow to the helmet.
  - The straps should create a "V" under and slightly in front of the ears.
  - The left buckle should be centered under the chin.
  - When buckled, the helmet should be snug with no more than 1–2 fingers fitting under the strap and the chin.
  - Position the brim so that it is parallel to the ground when the head is upright: the child should be able to see the brim when looking up. This may require removing or installing inside pads to enable a snug fit, or it may require adjusting the sizing ring.
  - Securely fasten the chin strap to the point where the helmet will not shift over the eyes, rock side to side, or come off when the child shakes his or her head.
- Always replace a helmet after a crash, even if the damage is not able to be visualized.
- Do not buy a helmet that you will grow into, it should fit at the time of purchase.
- Ensure the helmet is comfortable to increase the likelihood of wearing it.

Data from Centers for Disease Control and Prevention. Bicycle safety; 2020. https://www.cdc.gov/transportationsafety/bicycle/index.html?CDC_AA_refVal=https%3A%2F%2Fwww.cdc.gov%2Fmotorvehiclesafety%2Fbicycle%2Findex.html/; Schimelpfenig SS. Skiing and snowboarding: safety on bunny hills and beyond; 2019. https://www.healthychildren.org/English/healthy-living/sports/Pages/Skiing-and-Snowboarding.aspx?_gl=1*qnawyt*_ga*MTMxOTYzMDMxNC4xNjAxMzI3NTQ1*_ga_FD9D3XZVQQ*MTY0NjA4ODgxOS43LjEuMTY0NjA4OTA3Ny4w*_ga=2.100958663.750905837.1646088820-1319630314.1601327545/; and Bicycle Helmet Safety Institute. How to fit a bicycle helmet; 2022. https://helmets.org/fit.htm.

Performance Enhancing Nutrition and Supplements

Proper nutrition is a critical component to optimize an athlete's growth and ability to perform. Before puberty, basic nutritional and energy requirements are comparable for boys and girls. Post puberty energy requirements vary depending on age, activity level, rate of growth, and physical maturation stage. If an imbalance exists in the form of an energy deficit, consequences such as short stature, delayed puberty, menstrual irregularity, loss of muscle mass, increased risk for injury, or decreased sports performance may occur. Excess energy can result in overweight or obesity, which also increases the risk of injury or decreases the athlete's ability to perform.

Youth athletes should be able to meet 100% of their dietary needs from a balanced nutrition plan that includes a focus on the athlete's performance, hydration, and recovery. When discussing nutrition, the healthcare provider can play an important role in identifying concerning nutritional practices, dispelling myths about fad diets, and referring to specialists (e.g., registered dietitians) when appropriate.[33] It is important to provide a holistic assessment when assessing food intake and making recommendations. Factors that may influence dietary intake can include convenience, time to prepare, access and cost of food, daily schedules, family members, peers, and their own skillset and ability for food preparation.[33] Nutrition recommendations are summarized in Table 18.4. For additional information about certain metabolic requirements during exercise, see Chapter 14.

Macronutrients: Important for Sports Participation

Carbohydrates

Short-term, high-intensity activities (e.g., anaerobic activity, such as high jumping or diving) exclusively use carbohydrates (glucose) as a fuel source, whereas longer-duration activities (e.g., aerobic activity, such as running or cross-country skiing) use all three sources: carbohydrates, fats, and proteins. Complex carbohydrates (e.g., fruits, nuts, cereals, grains, pasta, and dried beans) are preferable to simple carbohydrates (e.g., bakery items, ice cream, and some crackers) because, although providing readily available energy, they do not cause the rapid spike in blood glucose levels with resultant insulin rebound that simple carbohydrates do. Hypoglycemia can result from insulin excess, which is counterproductive to the energy needed for sports participation. Each gram of carbohydrate contains approximately 4 kilocalories of energy. The glucose is stored as glycogen in muscles and the liver. General recommendations for adolescent athletes based on adult athlete recommendations include daily carbohydrate intake of 3 to 10 g/kg of body weight per day.[33] Too low of intake of carbohydrates for the athlete can result in reduced energy levels due to decreased glycogen stores and dehydration and cramping as carbohydrates store water in the muscle.[33] Carbohydrates should make up 45% to 65% of total calorie intake for youth 4 to 18 years of age. Recommendations for 1 to 4 g/kg of carbohydrates with a low-glycemic index 1 to 4 hours before exercise may improve performance.[43] During exercise, the benefits of carbohydrate ingestion are well supported with the amount and type dependent on the activity.[43] Finally, postexercise, ingestion of a high-glycemic index carbohydrate at 1 g/kg/h in the first 2 to 4 hours to replenish glycogen is suggested.[43]

Protein

Protein is not an initial source of energy but is useful for a longer duration to maintain blood glucose through liver gluconeogenesis and assists in the building and repairing of muscle. The recommended daily intake of protein is 1.2 to 2.0 g/kg of body weight per day.[33] Protein should equal approximately 10% to 30% of total caloric intake for youth 4 to 18 years of age. Adequate protein assists in preserving skeletal muscle integrity in the athlete who is physically active.[44] In general, the athlete needs higher protein daily (1.4–1.7 g/protein/kg) as compared to those who are not physically active (0.8 g/protein/kg).[44] Excessive protein may lead to an underconsumption of adequate carbohydrates and fats, causing the excess protein to be stored as fat and increasing the risk of hypercalciuria with calcium loss and dehydration. Sources of protein should be from food versus a supplement and be spread throughout the day in smaller servings of 20 to 30 grams 3 to 5 times a day.[33] After the workout, it is recommended to have a serving of protein combined with a carbohydrate to prevent further muscle breakdown and to stimulate muscle repair.[33]

Fats

Dietary fats provide necessary essential fatty acids, absorb fat-soluble vitamins (A, D, E, K), protect organs, and provide a

TABLE 18.4   Nutrition Recommendations for Athletes

Nutrient	Recommendations
Recommended daily caloric intake (from carbohydrates, fat, protein)	• When participating in vigorous physical activity, may need 1650–3925 kcal (depending on sex and age) daily to maintain growth and development • Allow appropriate vegetarian diets, and work with a registered dietitian to ensure adequate micronutrients
Vitamins and minerals: for energy production, hemoglobin synthesis, maintenance of bone health, immune function, and antioxidant protection	• Vitamins and minerals (with the exception of fluoride in unfluoridated regions) should be obtained from whole food vs. supplements • Highest likelihood for deficiencies includes iron and calcium (especially in females after the onset of menses) • Iron intake for boys and girls 9–13 years is 18 mg daily and increases to 11 mg and 15 mg for boys and girls, respectively, ages 14–18 years • Iron-rich foods include meats, beans, and green leafy vegetables. Other sources include peanuts and iron-fortified cereals and dried fruits. • Calcium requirements of 1300 mg daily optimize bone loading prior to skeletal maturation, which aids in osteoporosis prevention later in life • Sources of calcium include milk, fortified orange juice, almonds, and broccoli. To absorb calcium, vitamin D needs to be present—many calcium sources are now fortified with vitamin D.
Carbohydrates: help maintain blood glucose levels and replenish muscle glycogen stores	• 50% of the daily caloric intake for youth athletes should be from carbohydrate intake or between 3 and 8 g/kg body weight per day • Use nutritious foods, such as fruits, vegetables, grains, and milk • No specific guidelines for youth regarding ingesting carbohydrates during exercise exist. Suggestions to trial 30–60 g/h for exercise that lasts 60 min or longer and modify as needed. • Ingest 1–1.5 g/kg of body weight in carbohydrates in the 30 min post prolonged exercise
Protein and/or amino acid supplements: needed for normal cellular functioning and to facilitate muscle synthesis and repair	• 15%–20% of daily caloric intake should be from protein. No protein supplements are needed; preference should be toward whole foods vs. supplements • Depending on the level of physical activity athletes may need more protein (1.4–1.7 g/kg/day) than their noncompeting counterparts who need (0.8–1.2 g/kg/day). • Ingest 20 g of protein following exercise to maintain positive protein balance
Fats: for energy and to aid vitamin absorption	• Fats are essential for the absorption of fat-soluble vitamins A, D, E, and K and aid in the synthesis of cholesterol and other hormones • Limit intake of fats to 25%–30% of total caloric daily intake • Low fat or diets with <15% of calories coming from fat have no documented health benefits and >30% can lead to excessive weight gain • Fish oil (containing EPA and DHA) and CLA found in beef, lamb, and dairy products or in over-the-counter supplement form may benefit the athlete's performance. No research has documented the ergogenic effects of EPA, DHA, or CLA or improvements in performance from taking these supplements.
Fluids with/without carbohydates: for hydration, thermoregulation, may provide calories	• Plain water before, during, and after activity if physical exertion lasts no more than an hour • Before exercise consume 5–7 mL/kg 4 h prior to exercise; during exercise continue hydration based on sweat loss (consider fluids with sodium to replace loss by sweat); after exercise consume 450–675 mL/0.5 kg (consider fluids with added sodium to account for loss by sweating) • If exertion lasts more than an hour, fluids should contain carbohydrates; if exertion lasts more than several hours, fluids should also contain added sodium to maintain hydration and performance • Avoid carbonated drinks because of delayed gastric emptying and intestinal absorption

CLA, Conjugated linoleic acid; *DHA*, docosahexaenoic acid; *EPA*, eicosapentaenoic acid; *RDA*, recommended daily allowance.

Data from Berg EK. Performance nutrition for the adolescent athlete: a realistic approach. *Clin J Sport Med.* 2019;29(5):345–352; Mata F, Valenzuela PL, Gimenez J, et al. Carbohydrate availability and physical performance: physiological overview and practical recommendations. *Nutrients.* 2019;11(5); and Manore MM. Weight management for athletes and active individuals: a brief review. *Sports Med.* 2015;45 Suppl 1(Suppl 1):S83–S92.

sense of satiety. Fats should equal 25% to 35% of the total daily calories for athletes while limiting the intake of saturated fats to <10% per day.[33]

Nutritional Supplements. Nutritional supplements are readily available to aspiring athletes who believe use of supplements will improve performance. Supplements generally are composed of one or more of the following: a vitamin, a mineral, an herb or other botanical, an amino acid, a dietary supplement that raises the total daily intake; a concentrate, metabolite, constituent, or extract; or a combination of the last four ingredients. Nutritional supplements are not well regulated, and advertisements tend to target young adults or adolescents. Often, there are inaccuracies in the labeling and amount of the ingredients included in the product, as well as contamination, and the inclusion of dangerous substances.[33] Nutritional supplements in children and adolescents should be discouraged unless taken under the direction of a healthcare provider or registered dietician; vitamins and minerals are best gained through a healthy, well-balanced diet.

Sports Drinks Versus Energy Drinks

Sports drinks and energy drinks should not be confused with each other. Sports drinks typically provide carbohydrates, minerals, electrolytes, and possibly other vitamins.[33] A sports drink can provide benefits for athletes in certain circumstances such as prolonged duration of physical activity (see dehydration). Sports drinks are flavored beverages that often contain carbohydrates, minerals, electrolytes, and sometimes vitamins or other nutrients. However, sports drinks often contain sugar and, when consumed in place of water or low-fat milk, can lead to weight gain or tooth decay.[33]

Energy drinks contain substances that are nonnutritive stimulants, such as caffeine, guarana, taurine, ginseng, or L-carnitine, as well as sugar, carbohydrates, minerals, and electrolytes.[33] They are marketed to improve energy, weight loss, stamina, athletic performance, and concentration. Since energy drinks are not regulated by the US Food and Drug Administration (FDA), the exact amount of caffeine is often unclear, but it can be 10 to 15 times the amount of caffeine in a can of soda.

The medical concerns regarding energy drinks are numerous, including the fact that the excess sugar found in these drinks can result in an increase in calories, obesity, and dental caries. The amount of caffeine present in an energy drink may be over the amount deemed safe by the FDA. The caffeine is readily absorbed with effects notable within 15 to 60 minutes depending on the individual's sensitivity to caffeine.[45] Side effects of consistent and/or high consumption of energy drinks can range from mild (e.g., insomnia, headache, mood swings) to cardiovascular problems (e.g., arrhythmias, palpitations) seizures, and renal and liver disease.[45] The FDA regulates the amount of caffeine in food and drink, but does not have control over energy drinks as they are considered a supplement.[46] Increased bone demineralization may occur based on either caffeine interfering with intestinal calcium absorption or less calcium being ingested if milk is being replaced by energy drinks. When consumed in combination with alcohol, the depressant effects of the alcohol can be masked by the stimulating effect of the energy drink; users may feel wide awake and possibly underestimate their level of intoxication or impairment.[47]

Use of Ergogenic Drugs and Supplements

Ergogenic drugs refer to any legal and illicit substance used to enhance athletic performance, nutritional muscle building, or sports supplements. Athletes use these substances as they are purported to increase energy (prolonging sports endurance), increase lean body mass, decrease adipose tissue, increase, or decrease weight, improve cardiovascular function, and enhance overall sports performance. Steroid precursors, growth hormone, and ephedra substances have not been proven to enhance performance, and can have serious, long-term side effects of elevated blood pressure and cholesterol, blood clotting and liver problems, mood swings, and reduced sperm production.[48]

Many steroid precursors can be sold over the counter without stringent regulation by the FDA.[49] Dietary supplements are regulated differently than foods and drugs. Manufacturers are not required to prove that a product works or that it is safe before it is sold. Once on the market, if it can be proven to be unsafe, the FDA has the ability to remove it.

Young athletes can also be misled by advertising and messages from professional athletes and sports icons who use ergogenic drugs. Young athletes may use performance-enhancing drugs as a mechanism to cope with their own insecurities related to their body image, peer pressure or pressure from others, or the need to increase weight and/or muscles.[48] Adolescents at higher risk of using performance-enhancing drugs include males who are involved in sports that demand strength, power, and speed, such as football, wrestling, gymnastics, baseball, basketball, and weight training.

All high school and collegiate sports associations have strongly worded policies prohibiting the use of performance-enhancing substances, actively enforce no-tolerance policies, and endorse the US Anti-Doping Agency regulations and world antidoping code. "Clean" team members can provide leadership by disavowing performance-enhancing drugs and emphasizing the integrity (fair play) of sports competition. The education of young athletes needs to include both benefits and risks.

Given the prevalence of these drugs on the market, providers need to assess for use of supplements when taking patient histories and during their physical examination. Any potential signs or symptoms of ergogenic drug and supplement use such as rapid changes in body build; behavioral, emotional, or psychological changes; increased acne; or needle marks in the buttocks or thighs in females and males should be noted. Males may have enlarged breasts, male pattern baldness, and/or shrinking of testicles, and females may have smaller breasts, deepening of the voice, and excess body hair growth.[48] Screening for substance use should be incorporated within the developmentally appropriate comprehensive history or the Preparticipation Physical Evaluation (PPE). Additional questions should be open ended and specify different contexts (home, school, peer groups) before discussing the athlete's personal use. The American Academy of Pediatrics (AAP) has guidelines for drug testing when there is a high suspicion of use.[49] Box 18.4 provides screening questions for performance-enhancing drug or supplement use and Box 18.5 has information for parents.

• BOX 18.4 Screening Youth for the Use of Bodybuilding and Other Performance-Enhancing Substances

1. Are you using any substances or supplements to improve your performance in your sports(s)?
2. Do you use any substance to improve your body's appearance, weight, or strength?
3. How do you feel you are doing at your sport? Is your performance where you would like it to be? Are you satisfied with how you are doing? If not, how are you planning to improve?
4. What are your goals regarding your sport?
5. Are there people in your life (coaches, parents, self) who are pressuring you to improve your performance?
6. Do you know of any athletes or other peers who are using performance-enhancing substances?
7. What questions do you have about drugs or supplements, or other things athletes might use to enhance performance?

Be sure to include questions about all drugs, bodybuilding and other nutritional supplements, alcohol use, and needle use as per general adolescent health guidelines.

Modified from Stricker PR, Faigenbaum AD, McCambridge TM, et al. Resistance training for children and adolescents. *Pediatrics.* 2020;145(6); Holland-Hall C. Performance-enhancing substances: is your adolescent patient using? *Pediatr Clin North Am.* 2007;54(4):651-662.

Anabolic-Androgenic Steroids

Anabolic-androgenic steroids (AASs) are equated with increasing muscle mass, speed, and agility.[50] The term *anabolic* refers to the drug's ability to stimulate protein synthesis; *androgenic* refers to the stimulation of male secondary sexual characteristics. AASs react with a variety of receptors in the body, including glucocorticoids, progestin, estrogen, and androgen. Endogenous anabolic steroid production starts in adolescence in the prepubertal male. The exogenous drug used by each gender for performance enhancement or appearance is derived from testosterone and produces changes in the endocrine/reproductive, cardiovascular, hepatic, musculoskeletal, and neurologic systems. The AAS drugs are Class III controlled substances. AASs are available in oral, injectable, buccal, and transdermal forms and can be taken in "stacks" over 6- to 12-week cycles.[49]

Clinical effects can be irreversible and extremely serious. With sustained use, some of the more serious side effects include cardiac failure, impotence, testicular atrophy, hepatic dysfunction suppression of the hypothalamic-pituitary-gonadal axis, neurologic changes (aggression and mania), premature closure of the epiphyseal plates of the long bones, possible malignancy, and tendon or muscle injuries (due to disorganized collagen fibril alignment). In females, AAS use can cause irreversible menstrual irregularities and breast atrophy, virilization-enlargement of the clitoris, hirsutism, male pattern baldness, deepening of the voice with larynx changes, and amenorrhea. Mortality or life-threatening event statistics attributed to steroid use may be inaccurate as they can be masked by the diagnoses of cardiac arrest, liver, or kidney failure.[49]

Androstenedione and Dehydroepiandrosterone

Androstenedione ("andro") and related dehydroepiandrosterone (DHEA) are prohormones that are converted to either testosterone or estrone.[48] Androstenedione is a Class III controlled drug and DHEA may be purchased over the counter.[48] These steroid precursors are used because of the mistaken belief that they will increase testosterone and produce the same effects on muscles and performance as seen with anabolic steroids. Rather than show increases in testosterone levels, steroid precursors can significantly increase androstenedione and estradiol levels, causing the adverse changes seen with anabolic steroids. Changes include androgenizing effects in females, such as virilization; in males, the side effects can include testicular cancer, infertility, stroke, and increased risk of heart disease. Similar to anabolic steroids, if used while the athlete is still growing, height can be stunted.[48]

Growth Hormone

Human growth hormone (HGH) is available in a biosynthetic, injectable form and is banned by sporting leagues.[51] It is often used one or more times a month, and youth use it to enhance athletic performance through anabolic mechanisms of increasing lean body mass and decreasing fat mass. However, it appears to worsen exercise capacity by increasing exercise-induced lactate levels. Potential negative effects related to high-dose HGH use include diabetes, cardiomyopathy, hepatitis, and renal failure. Athletes who take it report a "feel-good" sensation (probably caused by fluid shifts within tissues) and decreases in subcutaneous fat for a fit appearance.

Creatine and Other Supplements

Creatine is involved in the production of energy for muscular contraction and is found in fish, meat, milk, and other foods in small amounts. Creatine is made by the body naturally in the liver, kidneys, and pancreas. Synthetic creatine is an over-the-counter supplement used in the belief that it enhances athletic endurance by improving muscular contraction, strength, and performance. In 2020, the FDA classified creatine generally recognized as safe under the conditions of its intended use. This would not apply to younger children but would cover older children and adolescents. Limited evidence supports that creatine supplementation is likely safe for children and adolescents.[52] Continued work examining creatine safety, efficacy, and dosing in youth is warranted.[53]

Ephedra

Ephedra is a naturally occurring herb known as *ma huang*, and ephedrine is the main active ingredient. It has a chemical structure similar to amphetamine, enhances the release of norepinephrine, and stimulates the CNS. Ephedra was banned as an energy enhancer and diet aid in 2004 by the FDA, and in 2006, the retail sale of pseudoephedrine was regulated. Since the ban, ephedra has been replaced by other sympathomimetics that act similarly. Traditional Chinese herbal medicines, herbal teas, and medications that contain chemically synthesized ephedra are among the products not banned. Dietary supplements for bodybuilding and weight loss are readily available over the Internet and can include ephedra as a listed or unlisted ingredient. Many of these products also contain caffeine or caffeine sources.[54]

Adverse reactions include insomnia, tachycardia, seizures, anxiety, dysrhythmias, dry mouth, headache, abdominal discomfort, tremors, or other life-threatening side effects.[54] The active ingredients in ephedra are known to have serious interactions with amphetamines, antidepressants (tricyclics and monoamine oxidase inhibitors [MAOIs]), blood-thinning medications, blood pressure medication, caffeine, and narcotics.

Preparticipation Physical Examination (PPE) for Sports

Almost 8 million youth participate in competitive high school athletics annually in the United States, and many more participate in recreational sports in school and community programs.[55] There is not a standardized method or use of the PPE, and the provider should check with their state for any special requirements. The AAP has classified the most common sports activities into three types: contact and collision, limited contact, and noncontact (Table 18.5). Table 18.6 provides recommendations and guidance on safe sports for various medical conditions and can be a useful reference for complex decision-making and making specific recommendations as to which sports are appropriate for youth with identified health problems.

The PPE historically served to detect cardiovascular risks for sudden death and inguinal hernias and provide liability protection and satisfy insurance regulations. Over the years, other objectives have been identified including:

- Evaluating health status (primary care prevention), including fitness level and preparticipation physical conditioning, grade-level eligibility, and emotional maturity level
- Detecting injuries, conditions, and illnesses from either inherited or acquired conditions that might limit competition and lead to significant injury, morbidity, or life-threatening medical emergencies
- Recommending alternative sports activities, as appropriate, or recommending the exclusion of the child or youth from certain sports
- Providing anticipatory guidance about safety equipment for athletic participation

- Initiating further evaluation, referral, treatment, and follow-up of conditions impacting sports performance
- Promoting healthy choices while identifying lifestyle risk factors
- Recommending ways to improve athletic performance

For many adolescents, this requirement serves as an entry into the healthcare system and the PPE may be the only opportunity for pediatric healthcare providers to assess the health and health behaviors during the adolescent years. However, PPEs are not required for many recreational or club activities. To encounter these children, it has been recommended that *all* children (not just those in competitive or structured sports programs) be encouraged to have a PPE when they visit their PCP.

The completion of the PPE includes a prescreening health questionnaire targeting previous sports injuries; respiratory, neurologic, and cardiac health history; and the completion of standard PPE forms. The PPE monograph contains the recommended questionnaire, PPE, and clearance forms as well as guidelines for clinicians evaluating children with special needs and female athletes (see Boxes 18.12 and 18.13).[56] The PPE History form can be accessed at https://downloads.aap.org/AAP/PDF/PPE_History_Form_1-18-22-rev.pdf and the Provider PPE Physical Examination form can be accessed at https://downloads.aap.org/AAP/PDF/PPE_Physical_Exam_Form_1-24-22-rev.pdf. Estimates vary but reports indicate that more than 98% of athletes are qualified for participation based on the findings of the PPE and up to

---

TABLE 18.5 Classification of Sports According to Contact

Contact	Limited Contact	Noncontact
Basketball	Adventure racing[a]	Badminton
Boxing[b]	Baseball	Bodybuilding[c]
Cheerleading	Bicycling	Bowling
Diving	Canoeing or kayaking (whitewater)	Canoeing or kayaking (flat water)
Extreme sports[d]	Fencing	Crew or rowing
Field hockey	Field events	Curling
Football, tackle	Floor hockey	Dance
Gymnastics	Football, flag, or touch	Field events: discus, javelin, shotput
Ice hockey[e]	Handball	Golf
Lacrosse	High jump	Orienteering[g]
Martial arts[f]	Horseback riding	Powerlifting[c]
Rodeo	Martial arts[f]	Race walking
Rugby	Pole vault	Riflery
Skiing, downhill	Racquetball	Rope jumping
Ski-jumping	Skateboarding	Running
Snowboarding	Skating: ice, inline, roller	Sailing
Soccer	Skiing: cross-country, water	Scuba diving
Team handball	Softball	Swimming
Ultimate frisbee	Squash	Table tennis
Water polo	Volleyball	Tennis
Wrestling	Weightlifting	Track
	Windsurfing or surfing	

[a]Adventure racing is defined as a combination of two or more disciplines, including orienteering and navigation, cross-country running, mountain biking, paddling, and climbing and rope skills.
[b]The American Academy of Pediatrics (AAP) opposes participation in boxing for children, adolescents, and young adults.
[c]The AAP recommends limiting bodybuilding and powerlifting until the adolescent achieves a sexual maturity rating of 5 (Tanner stage V).
[d]Extreme sports with recent updates.
[e]The AAP recommends limiting the amount of body checking allowed for hockey players 15 years old and younger to reduce injuries.
[f]Martial arts can be subclassified as judo, jujitsu, karate, kung fu, and tae kwon do; some forms are contact sports and others are limited-contact sports.
[g]Orienteering is a race (contest) in which competitors use a map and a compass to find their way through unfamiliar territory.

From American Academy of Family Physicians, American Academy of Pediatrics, American College of Sports Medicine, American Medical Society for Sports Medicine, American Orthopaedic Society for Sports Medicine, American Osteopathic Academy of Sports Medicine. *Preparticipation Physical Evaluation*, 5th ed. American Academy of Pediatrics; 2019.

TABLE 18.6 Medical Conditions and Sports Participation

Condition	May Participate
Atlantoaxial Instability (Instability of the Joint Between C1 and C2)	Qualified yes
Explanation: Athlete (particularly with Down syndrome or juvenile rheumatoid arthritis with cervical involvement) needs evaluation; assess risk of spinal cord injury during sports especially with trampoline use.	
Bleeding Disorder	Qualified yes
Explanation: Athlete needs evaluation.	
Cardiovascular Disease	
• Carditis (inflammation of the heart)	No
Explanation: Carditis may result in sudden death with exertion.	
• Hypertension (high blood pressure) >13 years	Qualified yes
• Elevated BP (120/<80 to 128/<80 mm Hg)	No limitations
• Stage 1 HTN (130/80–139/89 mm Hg) with no end-organ damage, including LVH or concomitant heart disease	No limitations or restrictions
• Stage 2 HTN (≥140/90 mm Hg) with no end-organ damage, including LVH or concomitant heart disease	Restrict from sports with high static or dynamic components until blood pressure is in the normal range.
• Hypertensive with concomitant cardiovascular disease	Eligibility is usually based on the type and severity of the underlying cardiovascular disease.
• Congenital heart disease	Qualified yes
Explanation: Consultation with a cardiologist. Children with mild forms may participate fully in most cases; those with moderate or severe forms or who have undergone surgery need evaluation.	
• Dysrhythmia (irregular heart rhythm) • Long QT syndrome • Malignant ventricular arrhythmias • Symptomatic Wolff-Parkinson-White syndrome • Advanced heart block • Family history of sudden death or previous sudden cardiac event • Implantation of a cardioverter-defibrillator	Qualified yes
Explanation: Consult with a cardiologist. If symptoms (chest pain, syncope, near-syncope, dizziness, shortness of breath, or other symptoms of possible dysrhythmia) or evidence of mitral regurgitation on physical examination, refer for evaluation. All others may participate fully.	
• Heart murmur	Qualified yes
Explanation: If the murmur is innocent, full participation is permitted. Otherwise, refer for evaluation (see structural/acquired heart disease, especially hypertrophic cardiomyopathy and mitral valve prolapse).	
• Structural/acquired heart disease	Qualified no
• Hypertrophic cardiomyopathy	Qualified no
• Coronary artery anomalies	Qualified no
• Arrhythmogenic right ventricular cardiomyopathy	Qualified no
• Acute rheumatic fever with carditis	Qualified no
• Ehlers-Danlos syndrome, vascular form	Qualified yes
• Marfan syndrome	Qualified yes
• Mitral valve prolapse	Qualified yes
• Anthracycline use	Qualified yes
Explanation: Consult with a cardiologist because most of these conditions carry a significant risk of sudden cardiac death (SCD) associated with intense physical exercise.	

• Vasculitis/vascular disease
  • Kawasaki disease (coronary artery vasculitis)
  • Pulmonary hypertension
	Qualified yes

Explanation: Consult with a cardiologist. Risk on the basis of disease activity, pathologic changes, and medical regimen.	

Continued

<table>
<tr><td>TABLE
18.6</td><td>**Medical Conditions and Sports Participation—Cont'd**</td></tr>
</table>

Condition	May Participate
Cerebral Palsy	
Explanation: Evaluate to assess functional capacity to perform the sports-specific activity.	Qualified yes
Diabetes Mellitus	
Explanation: All sports can be played with proper attention and appropriate adjustments to diet (particularly carbohydrate intake), blood glucose concentrations, hydration, and insulin therapy. Monitor before exercise, every 30 min during continuous exercise, 15 min after completion of the exercise, and at bedtime.	Yes
Diarrhea, Infectious	
Explanation: Unless symptoms are mild and the athlete is fully hydrated, no participation is permitted (risk of dehydration and heat illness) (see fever).	Qualified no
Eating Disorders	
Explanation: If an eating disorder is present, the athlete needs medical and psychiatric assessment before participation.	Qualified yes
Eyes	
• Functionally one-eyed athlete • Loss of an eye • Detached retina or family history of retinal detachment at a young age • High myopia • Connective tissue disorder, such as Marfan or Stickler syndrome • Previous intraocular eye surgery or serious eye injury *Explanation:* Boxing and full-contact martial arts are not recommended for functionally one-eyed athletes, because eye protection is impractical and/or not permitted. Some athletes who previously underwent intraocular surgery or had a serious eye injury may have an increased risk of injury because of weakened eye tissue. The availability of eye guards approved by the American Society for Testing and Materials must be judged on an individual basis.	Qualified yes
• Conjunctivitis, infectious *Explanation:* If active infection, exclude from swimming.	Qualified no
Fever	
Explanation: Elevated core temperature may indicate a pathologic medical condition (infection or disease).	No
Gastrointestinal	
• Malabsorption syndromes (celiac disease or cystic fibrosis) *Explanation:* Individual assessment for malnutrition or specific deficits; if treated adequately, may permit full activity.	Qualified yes
• Short-bowel syndrome or disorders requiring specialized nutritional support *Explanation:* Individual assessment for collision, contact, or limited-contact sports. The presence of a central or peripheral, indwelling, venous catheter may require special considerations for activities and emergency preparedness for unexpected trauma to the device.	Qualified yes
Heat illness, History of	
Explanation: With the likelihood of recurrence, needs assessment for the presence of predisposing conditions; develop a prevention strategy for sufficient acclimatization, conditioning, hydration, and salt intake, as well as protective equipment and uniform configurations.	Qualified yes
Hepatitis, Infectious (Primarily Hepatitis C)	
Explanation: Ensure protection with hepatitis B vaccination before participation; cover skin lesions; use universal precautions.	Yes
HIV Infection	
Explanation: As the athlete's state of health allows (especially if viral load is undetectable or very low); cover skin lesions, use universal precautions; avoid sports likely to cause skin breaks/bleeding (e.g., wrestling and boxing). If the viral load is detectable, avoid high-contact sports.	Yes
Kidney, Absence of One	
Explanation: Assess for contact, collision, and limited-contact sports; protective equipment may allow participation in most sports.	Qualified yes
Liver, Enlarged	
Explanation: Acutely enlarged liver: no participation because of risk of rupture; chronically enlarged or liver function compromised: individual assessment and sport dependent.	Qualified yes

TABLE 18.6   Medical Conditions and Sports Participation—Cont'd

Condition	May Participate
Malignant Neoplasm *Explanation:* Individual assessment	Qualified yes
Musculoskeletal Disorders *Explanation:* Individual assessment	Qualified yes
Neurologic Disorders	
• History of serious head or spine trauma or abnormality *Explanation:* Individual assessment for collision, contact, or limited-contact sports	Qualified yes
• History of simple concussion (mild traumatic brain injury), multiple simple concussions, and/or complex concussion *Explanation:* Individual assessment; no athletic participation while symptomatic and/or exhibiting deficits in judgment or cognition; graduated return to full activity.	Qualified yes
• Myopathies *Explanation:* Individual assessment	Qualified yes
• Recurrent headaches *Explanation:* Individual assessment	Yes
• Recurrent plexopathy (burner or stinger) and cervical cord neurapraxia with persistent defects *Explanation:* Individual assessment for collision, contact, or limited-contact sports; regaining normal strength is the benchmark for return to play.	Qualified yes
• Seizure disorder, well-controlled *Explanation:* The risk of seizure during participation is minimal.	Yes
• Seizure disorder, poorly controlled *Explanation:* Individual assessment for collision, contact, or limited-contact sports. Avoid archery, riflery, swimming, weightlifting, powerlifting, strength training, and sports involving heights.	Qualified yes
Obesity *Explanation:* Increased risk of heat illness and cardiovascular strain; needs acclimatization, hydration, and potential activity and recovery modifications during competition and training.	Yes
Organ Transplant Recipients (and Those Taking Immunosuppressive Medications) *Explanation:* Individual assessment	Qualified yes
Ovary, Absence of One *Explanation:* Risk is minimal.	Yes
Pregnancy/Postpartum *Explanation:* Individual assessment with modifications to usual exercise routines in later stages. Avoid fall risk activities and scuba diving. After birth, physiologic changes of pregnancy take 4–6 weeks to return to baseline.	Qualified yes
Respiratory Conditions	
• Pulmonary compromise, including cystic fibrosis *Explanation:* Individual assessment; sports may be played if oxygenation remains satisfactory during graded exercise test; need acclimatization and hydration with cystic fibrosis.	Qualified yes
• Asthma *Explanation:* If controlled and with education, only those with severe asthma need to modify their participation. If using inhalers, have written action plan and use peak flowmeter daily. Scuba diving is a high-risk activity.	Yes
• Acute upper respiratory infection *Explanation:* Individual assessment for all except mild disease (see fever).	Qualified yes
Rheumatologic Diseases	
• Juvenile rheumatoid arthritis *Explanation:* Individual assessment depends on involvement: cervical spine C1 and C2, risk of spinal cord injury; HLA-B27-associated arthritis; cardiovascular assessment for possible complications during exercise; if micrognathia, mouth guards; if uveitis, risk of eye damage from trauma	Qualified yes

Continued

TABLE 18.6	**Medical Conditions and Sports Participation—Cont'd**

Condition	May Participate
• Juvenile dermatomyositis, idiopathic myositis • Systemic lupus erythematosus • Raynaud phenomenon *Explanation:* If cardiac involvement, cardiology assessment is required; if on systemic corticosteroid therapy, at higher risk of fractures and avascular necrosis; if on immunosuppressive medications, risk of serious infection; if myositis, active risk of rhabdomyolysis during intensive exercise with renal injury; photosensitivity with the need for sun protection; if Raynaud phenomenon, the risk to hands and feet with exposure to cold.	Qualified yes
Sickle Cell Disease	
Explanation: Individual assessment; as illness status permits, all sports may be played; avoid sport or activity that entails overexertion, overheating, dehydration, or chilling, or takes place at high altitude, especially when not acclimatized.	Qualified yes
Sickle Cell Trait	
Explanation: Generally no increased risk of sudden death or other medical problems; if the high exertional activity is performed under extreme conditions of heat and humidity or increased altitude, complications can occur; need to progressively acclimatize.	Yes
Skin Infections	
• Herpes simplex, molluscum contagiosum, verrucae (warts), staphylococcal and streptococcal infections (furuncles [boils], carbuncles, impetigo, methicillin-resistant Staphylococcus aureus [cellulitis and/or abscesses]), scabies, and tinea *Explanation:* During contagious periods, gymnastics or cheerleading with mats, martial arts, wrestling, or other collision, contact, or limited-contact sports are not allowed.	Qualified yes
Spleen, Enlarged	
Explanation: If acutely enlarged spleen, participation is avoided due to the risk of rupture; if chronically enlarged, individual assessment is needed.	Qualified yes
Testicle, Undescended or Absent	
Explanation: May require a protective cup depending upon the sport.	Yes

aThis table is designed for use by medical and nonmedical personnel. "Needs evaluation" means that the provider with appropriate knowledge and experience should assess the safety of a given sport for an athlete with the listed medical condition. Unless otherwise noted, this need for special consideration is because of variability in the severity of the disease, the risk of injury for the specific sports, or both.

BP, Blood pressure; *HIV,* human immunodeficiency virus; *HTN,* hypertension; *LVH,* left ventricular hypertrophy.

Data from American Academy of Family Physicians, American Academy of Pediatrics, American College of Sports Medicine, American Medical Society for Sports Medicine, American Orthopaedic Society for Sports Medicine, American Osteopathic Academy of Sports Medicine. *Preparticipation Physical Evaluation,* 5th ed. American Academy of Pediatrics; 2019; and Flynn JT, Kaelber DC, Baker-Smith CM, et al. clinical practice guideline for screening and management of high blood pressure in children and adolescents. *Pediatrics.* 2017;140(3).

14% require further evaluation.[56] The potential need for further evaluation before clearance is supported by the recommendation to have the athlete undergo the PPE a minimum of 6 weeks before the start of the preseason training to allow the additional evaluation to occur as needed.[56]

Mass PPE screenings are common in many school districts as an efficiency measure or because some youth may not have access to regular health care or who may have difficulty making an appointment. However, mass screenings are a missed opportunity for building a trusted continuity patient-provider relationship and the ability to follow up on healthcare needs identified during the examination can be compromised. PCPs provide communication with parents, coaches, and trainers following the PPE, and can be involved in the care of the athlete if issues arise during participation.

Medical Clearance and Liability Issues

The PPE, including all health history and physical examination findings, must be fully documented in the medical record. Recommendations based on the PPE include unconditional clearance; cleared with recommendation for follow-up; not cleared until further evaluation, treatment, or rehabilitation; or not cleared for any sport or level of participation in competitive sports. Counseling

about more appropriate alternative sports should occur and be documented. In addition, the athlete and parents should be counseled that:

- Even though the examination appears "normal," data on the exact risks of a known sport are often limited and sudden cardiac death (SCD) is rare.
- Safety and conditioning are imperative for prevention; injury is a more common cause of morbidity and mortality in sports than medical causes.

Should the athlete, athlete's family, or guardian disagree with the provider's advice against participation in a certain chosen sport or activity, the provider needs to obtain the athlete's, parent's, or guardian's signed informed consent statement acknowledging understanding of the advice and potential dangers of participation and releasing the provider and organization from liability.

Components of the Preparticipation Physical Examination

Health History

The health history is the foundation of the PPE and may reveal 88% of medical conditions and 67% of muscular-skeletal problems.[56] See Box 18.6 for the routine recommended American

• BOX 18.6 Health History for Preparticipation Physical Examination

The AAFP PPE history form is recommended and seeks information about the following:

- Thorough past medical history and family history
- Prior surgeries and any sequelae
- Previous trauma, especially musculoskeletal or central nervous system injuries (notably head injuries)
- Family history of cardiac risk factors, including unexplained drowning or unwitnessed car accidents (these can indicate an undiagnosed heart problem)
- Specific cardiovascular disease questions (see Box 18.7) including uncontrolled hypertension
- Prior heat-intolerance episodes
- Asthma, excessive dyspnea, fatigue associated with exercise, activity intolerance, or other allergic reactions
- Loss of function or absence of any paired organs (eyes, testes, kidneys)
- Seizure disorder or any other unexplained loss of consciousness
- Infectious mononucleosis
- Skin infection or recurrent skin infections, with a concern of MRSA
- Anatomic abnormalities, Down or Marfan syndrome, or history of Marfan syndrome in the family
- Obesity
- Medications, including supplement use, herbal remedies
- Immunization status
- Nutritional history: rapid weight changes, dieting, body perception
- History of sickle cell
- In females: menstrual history (see Box 18.12 regarding screening questions for the female athlete triad)

AAFP PPE, American Academy of Family Physicians Preparticipation Physical Examination; *MRSA,* methicillin-resistant *Staphylococcus aureus.*
Data from American Academy of Family Physicians, American Academy of Pediatrics, American College of Sports Medicine, American Medical Society for Sports Medicine, American Orthopaedic Society for Sports Medicine, American Osteopathic Academy of Sports Medicine. *Preparticipation Physical Evaluation,* 5th ed. American Academy of Pediatrics; 2019.

Academy of Family Physicians PPE health history information. When performing the history portion of the PPE, healthcare providers should also obtain the following history to better understand the scope of sports participation before clearance:

- The particular sports activity planned, the extent of participation, level of competition, and training schedule
- Coaching and supervision: what are the levels of certification of the trainers and coaches?
- Hazardous playing and field conditions
- Injury prevention strategies, including the level of preparticipation conditioning
- Nutritional changes needed for participation
- Risk behaviors present such as sexual history, use of drugs or performance-enhancing substances, and smoking, including e-cigarette use
- Family involvement, stress management during the competitive season, and how success will be measured
- Strategies to maintain schoolwork
- History of COVID-19 illness and severity of symptoms
- History of COVID-19 vaccination

Physical Examination

The PPE should be a comprehensive head-to-toe physical examination including vital signs (heart rate, blood pressure, height, and weight) and vision and hearing screenings with a particular focus on thorough cardiovascular, musculoskeletal, and neurologic examinations. The 90-second musculoskeletal screening examination is recommended for all youth participating in sports (Fig. 18.1). The examination focuses on musculoskeletal alignment, flexibility, and proprioception, which are effective measures of abnormalities and injury sequelae. Table 18.7 describes the components that should be included for examining different organ systems, including elements of the cardiovascular system. See Box 18.7 examination the cardiovascular screening examination for congenital and genetic cardiac disease. In addition, the provider should include a genital examination in males. This examination provides information with regard to sexual maturity (Tanner stage or sexual maturity rating [SMR]; see Chapter 13) and provides an opportunity for counseling about general development; how to do a self-testicular examination, including the risk of testicular cancer; issues of reproductive health; and risks of sexually transmitted infections. The SMR level reflects muscle and spine maturity and is important in contact sports participation and weight and strength training. As the adolescent achieves greater sexual maturity, the risk of participation in high-contact sports decreases although athletic injury remains a concern.

Diagnostic Studies

The use of echocardiographic (ECG) screening has been proposed by cardiologists and others concerned about sickle cell disease and the risk for youths who have a predisposition to this condition, and liability in sports participation. Despite the merits of augmenting the health history and physical examination with an ECG and echocardiogram, their use as universal screening tools for youth participating in competitive sports is not recommended for asymptomatic, low-risk athletes.[56] In the United States, the ECG, echocardiogram, or exercise stress tests are not recommended as a requirement for all PPEs; however, ECG may be recommended based on severity and symptoms of past COVID-19 infection before clearance.[56,57]

Other diagnostic tests that may be indicated or mandated as part of the PPE health screening include hematocrit or hemoglobin recommended for adolescent females with heavy menstrual cycles, a history of iron-deficiency anemia, or a history of iron supplementation or medications that could affect blood count; human immunodeficiency virus (HIV) testing for athletes with risk factors; sickle cell testing to confirm sickle cell trait in high-risk groups; lipid or cholesterol for overweight or obese athletes and those with a personal history of elevated lipid or cholesterol or positive cardiovascular risk factors. Urinalysis is not routinely recommended or supported by research.[56] However, certain amateur recreational or professional organizations may require it as part of a drug screening policy.

Evaluation and Management of Sports Participation for Athletes With Chronic Health Conditions

Several high-risk conditions (chronic and acute) and diagnostic symptoms are discussed in the following sections in terms of their influence on decision-making and for the purposes of counseling and health management (see Table 18.6).

Asthma

Asthma is one of the most common respiratory conditions that impacts children. Documentation of the child's history of symptoms, triggers, treatments, and interventions should be maintained and shared with the teacher and coach. As previously discussed, asthma or exercise-induced bronchospasm (EIB) should not prevent children from participating in

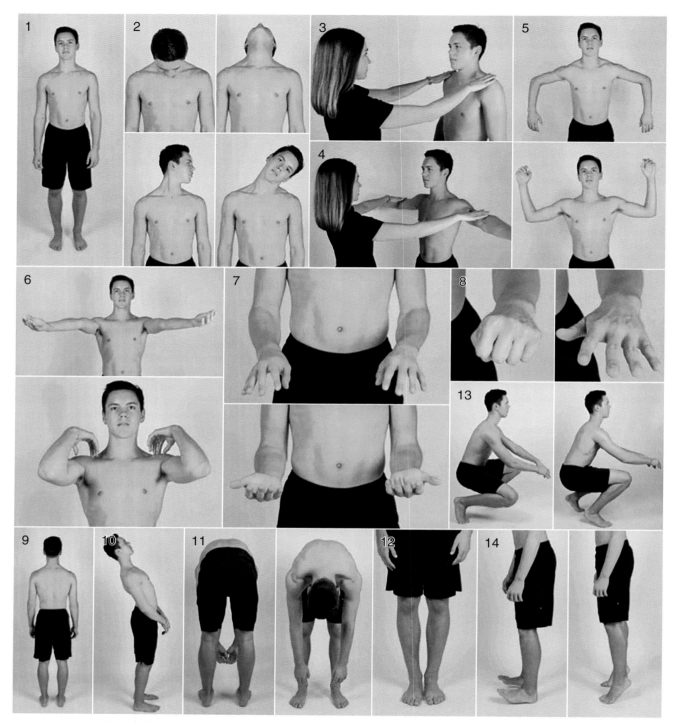

• **Fig 18.1** General Musculoskeletal Screening Examination. (From American Academy of Pediatrics, American Academy of Family Physicians, American College of Sports Medicine, American Medical Society for Sports Medicine, American Medical Society for Sports Medicine, American Orthopaedic Society for Sports Medicine, and American Osteopathic Academy of Sports Medicine. Preparticipation Physical Evaluation (PPE). 2019 (5th ed). https://publications.aap.org/aapbooks/book/656/chapter-split/5834090/Systems-Based-Examination.)

physical activity. The one exception is scuba diving, in which those with asthma should have an evaluation of their pulmonary function test, adherence to their treatment plan, and the number of exacerbations before learning to dive.[58] For other sports and general physical activity, the focus should be on the child's asthma control and having a plan that incorporates preventive measures and proper use of medications and inhalers. Exercise can act as an additional trigger for bronchospasm in those with underlying reactive airway disease, or exercise may serve as the only trigger for bronchospasm. Comprehensive management of intermittent and persistent asthma and EIB is discussed in Chapters 32 and 36.

TABLE 18.7 Components of Preparticipation Physical Examination

Examination Feature	Comments
Height and weight, BMI	Establish a baseline and monitor for eating disorders, steroid abuse, and obesity.
Blood pressure, pulse	Assess in the context of the participant's age, height, and sex.
General appearance	Excessive height and excessive long-bone growth (arachnodactyly, arm span greater than height, pectus excavatum) are suggestive of Marfan syndrome.
Eyes	Important to detect vision defects; one of the eyes should have greater than 20/40 corrected vision. Lens subluxations, severe myopia, retinal detachments, and strabismus are associated with Marfan syndrome. Document anisometropia; the absence of one eye can limit sports choices.
Cardiovascular (see Box 18.7)	Increased intensity and displacement at PMI suggest hypertrophy and CHF, respectively; murmur that intensifies with standing or Valsalva maneuver suggests hypertrophic cardiomyopathy; simultaneous delay between femoral and radial pulses or femoral pulse diminishment suggests aortic coarctation.
Respiratory	Observe for accessory muscle use or prolonged expiration and auscultate for wheezing. EIB requires exercise testing for diagnosis.
Abdominal	Assess for masses, tenderness, or organomegaly (especially liver, spleen, and kidneys). In females, assess for any pain, or enlargement over the hypogastric area or pelvis that might suggest pregnancy or gynecologic problem; proceed with further workup as indicated.
Genitourinary	Hernias and varicoceles do not usually preclude sports participation. Check for single, undescended testicles, and/or masses.
Musculoskeletal	Use the 90-s orthopedic examination (see Fig. 18.1). Consider supplemental shoulder, knee, and ankle examinations as indicated specifically to the chosen sport's injury-prone areas.
Skin	Evidence of molluscum contagiosum, herpes simplex, impetigo, or lesions suggestive of MRSA, tinea corporis, or scabies would temporarily prohibit participation in sports where direct skin-to-skin competitor contact occurs (e.g., wrestling, martial arts).
Neurologic	Gross motor assessment with attention to equality of strength, especially with a history of recurrent stingers/burners, and head injury. Usually sufficiently assessed during the 90-second musculoskeletal examination.

BMI, Body mass index; *CHF*, congestive heart failure; *EIB*, exercise-induced bronchospasm; *MRSA*, methicillin-resistant *Staphylococcus aureus*; *PMI*, point of maximal impulse.

Data from American Academy of Family Physicians, American College of Sports Medicine, American Academy of Pediatrics, American Medical Society for Sports Medicine, American Orthopaedic Society for Sports Medicine, American Osteopathic Academy of Sports Medicine. *Preparticipation Physical Evaluation*, 5th ed. American Academy of Pediatrics; 2019; and Miller SM, Peterson AR. The sports preparticipation evaluation. *Pediatr Rev.* 2019;40(3):108–128.

• BOX 18.7 Cardiovascular Screening History and Examination Checklist for Congenital and Genetic Heart Disease

A thorough medical history with parental verification is recommended for high school and middle school athletes.

Personal History

- Chest pain/discomfort/tightness/pressure related to exertion
- Unexplained syncope/near-syncope (judged not to be of neurocardiogenic [vasovagal] origin; of particular concern when occurs during or after exertion)
- Excessive exertional and unexplained dyspnea/fatigue or palpitations associated with exercise
- Prior recognition of a heart murmur
- Elevated systemic blood pressure
- Prior restriction from participation in sports
- Prior testing for the heart, ordered by a physician

Family History

- Premature death (sudden and unexpected, or otherwise) before age 50 years attributable to heart disease in one or more relatives
- Disability from heart disease in a close relative <50 years
- Hypertrophic or dilated cardiomyopathy, long QT syndrome, or other ion channelopathies, Marfan syndrome, or clinically significant arrhythmias; specific knowledge of certain cardiac conditions in family members

Physical Examination

- Heart murmur (likely to be organic and unlikely to be innocent) auscultation should be with the patient in both supine and standing positions (or with Valsalva maneuver), specifically to identify murmurs of dynamic left ventricular outflow tract obstruction
- Femoral pulses to exclude aortic coarctation
- Physical stigmata of Marfan syndrome
- Brachial artery blood pressure (sitting position); preferably taken from both arms

Data from Maron BJ, Friedman RA, Kligfield P, et al. Assessment of the 12-lead electrocardiogram as a screening test for detection of cardiovascular disease in healthy general populations of young people (12–25 years of age): a scientific statement from the American Heart Association and the American College of Cardiology. *J Am Coll Cardiol.* 2014;64(14): 1479–1514.

Cardiac Conditions

Congenital heart disease encompasses a wide spectrum of cardiovascular problems or abnormalities from basic to complex. The ultimate goal for the healthcare provider performing the PPE is to recognize athletes who are at risk of significant morbidity or mortality from preexisting cardiac conditions that may or may not be diagnosed. The need for increased cardiac output and oxygen demands varies by sport and the child's ability to meet these demands will vary by the underlying condition, history of previous surgical repair, and final anatomical structure. Regardless of the cardiac defect, participation in physical activity and athletics in some capacity is encouraged for most children and youth.

The American Heart Association (AHA) and American College of Cardiology (ACC) published a scientific statement on the eligibility and disqualification criteria for high school and college-age athletes with cardiovascular abnormalities.[59] The criteria provide guidelines on the ability of the athlete to participate in competitive sports in middle school, high school, and college. The guidelines are not meant to be used for basic recreational physical activity participation or as rigid mandates.[59] A key takeaway is that the athlete's health and safety are the priority when determining eligibility to participate and personal motivation or interest in the sport on behalf of the athlete should not be a deciding factor.[59] The ability to auscultate an organic murmur or detect warning signs (e.g., history of chest pain, excessive exertional dyspnea, or syncope) or a positive family history of sudden death due to an unknown cause or heart disease can raise suspicion, and further testing is required to properly clear an athlete for participation. A 12-lead ECG or echocardiogram would be the initial recommended screening. The AHA/ACC document was updated to provide new recommendations that include counseling during the decision process and allowing consideration of participation in competitive sports for athletes with implantable cardioverter-defibrillators and with long QT syndrome.[60]

Cardiac Murmurs

Because cardiac murmurs are common in children, it is important to distinguish between benign and pathologic murmurs. It is important that a cardiovascular examination includes more than auscultation. Inclusion of the athlete's birth history, past medical history, growth chart assessment, and detailed family history will provide important context.[61] For the PPE, evaluate heart sounds and listen for murmurs in each of the four areas of the heart. A systolic murmur of grade 3 or higher, a murmur that disrupts normal heart sounds, radiation of the murmur, wide or fixed splitting of S_2, a murmur heard during diastole, or a murmur that increases in intensity with the different positions or maneuvers should be further evaluated.[61] See Chapter 33 for a thorough discussion on the cardiac examination and interpretation of findings on the physical examination.

Diabetes Mellitus

The goal for youth with both type 1 and type 2 DM is to support athletic participation and physical activity in a safe and supportive manner. Type 1 and type 2 DM are discussed in Chapter 39, including the management and monitoring issues for both type 1 and type 2 DM in terms of participation in sports. In general, youth with DM should follow the same physical activity recommendations of participating in 60 minutes of physical activity daily that is recommended for all youth. While full participation based on the youth's capabilities and interest level is encouraged, acknowledging the risks of glucose variability that is possible with DM and the impact that physical activity can have on the individual's insulin needs is critical. The type of exercise, timing, and duration of the activity will all influence blood glucose control and need to be planned for accordingly.[62] Each athlete should share their DM care plan with their coach and athletic trainer and confirm their comfort level in aspects of care associated with DM (Box 18.8).[63] In addition, sharing the athlete's diagnosis with teammates and having them aware of general guidelines and treatment can increase the safety of the athlete and comfort with the necessary insulin checks and self-management performed by the athlete during practice and events. This is particularly important in children with type 1 DM, because athletic activity can increase short-term complications of hypoglycemia or significant hyperglycemia.

Hypertension

Hypertension is the most common cardiovascular condition seen in competitive athletes. While physical activity is beneficial to cardiovascular health, further evaluation should be conducted before

---

> **• BOX 18.8   Recommendations for the Athlete With Type 1 Diabetes Mellitus**
>
> - The diagnosis of type 1 diabetes should not limit the athlete's ability to participate in sports.
> - Recognize that the muscles need more energy during exercise so the muscles will release glucose, which will influence the individuals' blood sugar and the insulin needed.
> - The duration and type of activity will also alter diabetes management.
> - Your provider may need to adjust the blood testing schedule, insulin dosing, and general recommendations for safe participation in sports.
> - Athletes should frequently test, and record blood sugars as recommended and as needed (often before, during, and after training or competition). Note conditions present during different training or competition sessions.
> - Follow the insulin dosing schedule but be prepared for adjustments depending on the level of physical activity. Avoid injecting insulin into the limb that is most active in the exercise performed (i.e., injecting your leg before soccer) to avoid overly rapid insulin absorption.
> - Plan snacks appropriately. May need to increase snacks before, during, or after activity.
> - Pack extra testing supplies, pump supplies (if using a pump), snacks, and water. Have these items packed in a special bag so you do not have to pack and repack with every activity.
> - Wear a MedicAlert bracelet.
> - Have emergency contact information readily available.
> - Have a copy of the diabetes management plan available.
> - Take control and put diabetes first, take breaks, or ask for help if needed.
> - Monitor for any cuts, scrapes, or blisters and alert a healthcare professional if signs of infection occur (i.e., red, swollen, or oozing).
> - Tell coaches about diabetes diagnosis. Educate coaches and teammates of signs and symptoms of hypoglycemia-sweating, light-headedness, shaking, weakness, anxiety, hunger, headaches, problems concentrating, and/or confusion. If severe, watch for fainting or seizures. Hyperglycemia symptoms include increased urination, dehydration, increased thirst, fatigue, weakness, and/or blurry vision.
>
> Data from Riddell MC, Gallen IW, Smart CE, et al. Exercise management in type 1 diabetes: a consensus statement. *Lancet Diabetes Endocrinol.* 2017;5(5):377–390; Colberg SH, L. Helping a Student-Athlete with Type 1 Diabetes; 2020. https://www.diabetesselfmanagement.com/about-diabetes/diabetes-kids/helping-student-athlete-with-type-1-diabetes/. Pujalte G, Alhumaidi HM, Ligaray KPL, et al. Considerations in the care of athletes with type 1 diabetes mellitus. *Cureus.* 2022;14(2); and Dowshen S. Sports, Exercise, and Diabetes; 2018. https://kidshealth.org/en/teens/sports-diabetes.html.

---

releasing an athlete to competitive, strenuous, intense training or activity. Recent AAP guidelines simplified hypertension classification categories for adolescents. Athletes should be allowed to participate in competitive sports once the hypertensive and cardiovascular risk has been evaluated and/or if stage 2 hypertension with treatment has lowered blood pressure.[11] PCPs should also ask about the use of pharmacologic agents that can be associated with elevated blood pressures including but not limited to (1) over-the-counter drugs such as decongestants, caffeine, and nonsteroidal antiinflammatories; (2) prescription drugs such as stimulants, hormonal contraception, steroids, and tricyclic antidepressants; and (3) illicit drugs such as amphetamines or cocaine. See Chapter 33 for assessment, management, and treatment of hypertension.

Seizures

Children and adolescents with seizure disorders should be encouraged to participate in regular physical activity or sports (with a few exceptions) as physical activity has been associated with a positive quality of life and benefits mental, physical, and emotional health. Exercise rarely triggers seizures, and being physically fit and participating in exercise may reduce seizure activity.[64]

Participation clearance for a specific sport should be based on the type and frequency of seizures, antiseizure medication adherence, and the presence of any comorbid conditions. The athlete, parents, coaches or trainers, and neurology provider should be part of the discussion and plan for physical activity clearance and sports activities. In addition, consideration must be given to possible side effects (e.g., cognitive or behavioral changes, diplopia, dizziness, general fatigue, sedation, ataxia, tremors, hypohidrosis, dyskinesis, weight changes, decreased bone density) from antiseizure medication that could influence physical activity participation.[65]

If the seizures are well controlled, few restrictions are placed on sports participation, including supervised contact sports, such as football, hockey, and wrestling. Youths participating in some cycling and those involving heights should weigh the risk and benefits of participating and follow recommendations given to them after considerable discussion about safety risks. Exclusion from sports or physical activities should be based on the risk of harm to self or others if a seizure occurred while participating. Activities such as water or water-based sports or high-altitude activities, such as scuba diving or skydiving, should be considered based on how well controlled the seizures are and if adequate supervision or use of a buddy system is provided. If the seizures are poorly controlled, an individualized assessment, discussion, and medical decision is needed. The athlete with poorly controlled seizure activity should be excluded from dangerous activities that, if a loss of consciousness occurred, may result in injury or death.[64] When considering contact sports, it is important to remember that the risk of injury is the same for the person with a seizure disorder as others on the team. Taking precautions and wearing appropriate protective gear are important.

Sickle Cell Trait

SCT is generally benign and should not be a barrier to participation in sports, but in rare circumstances, it can place the athlete at higher risk of an exertional sickle cell event or crisis that can be fatal.[66] These events are associated with intense exertion, severe heat, severe hypoxemia increased in high altitudes, acidosis, and red cell dehydration.[67] These conditions can lead to the blockage of the small vessels that supply the vital organs leading to ischemia and muscle breakdown (rhabdomyolysis), the athlete collapses, and death can occur unless treatment is begun immediately. Persons with SCT appear to be at the greatest risk when they are in a deconditioned state and perform short bursts of repetitive, high-intensity activity (e.g., sprints).

Athletes with SCT can participate in all sports, but they need to self-identify to ensure safety in training and in all aspects of participation. Precautions for the athlete include setting their own pace; performing gradual acclimatization to heat, humidity, and altitude; resting as needed; decreasing intense exertional activities to short bursts of less than 2 to 3 minutes; being aware and stopping activities if symptoms (e.g., fatigue, intense pain, swelling, muscle cramps, inability to catch breath) occur; not participating when ill; and staying well hydrated at all times.[66] Educating families about the risks of SCT and providing the option of SCT screening so that youths are aware of their SCT status are considered optimal practices. Working with the coach and athletic trainer on a proactive plan includes support for the athlete to moderate activity as needed, proper heat and humidity acclimation, adequate

hydration, and understanding the conditions that increase the risk of a sickling crisis. If a sickle cell crisis occurs, it is a medical emergency that warrants calling 911. While waiting, the athlete should be cooled if overheated, receive oxygen, and receive respiratory and cardiac support as needed. Sickle cell disease and SCT are discussed in Chapter 38.

Acute Infectious Conditions

Infectious Mononucleosis

Infectious mononucleosis (IM) is a viral illness caused by the Epstein-Barr virus and more commonly affects adolescents and young adults. IM is covered in Chapter 35. Fever, pharyngitis, and lymphadenitis are common initial clinical manifestations, but splenomegaly (which occurs in about 50% of cases of IM) is the most concerning clinical issue for an athlete.[68] There is a 0.1% to 0.5% risk of splenic rupture in those playing sports with this condition.[68] Splenic rupture can occur spontaneously (rare), but the risk of rupture increases when participating in a contact or collision sport or a sport in which there is an increase in intraabdominal pressure (e.g., rowing and weightlifting that require Valsalva maneuvers); the risk is at its highest within the first 3 weeks. Diagnosing splenomegaly can be a challenge as athletes often have well-defined and firm abdominal musculature, making palpation of the spleen difficult and unreliable as a diagnostic tool. The only way to accurately diagnose splenomegaly is to obtain a baseline ultrasound and serial images over time. However, imaging is not recommended as a routine diagnostic measure or in return-to-play (RTP) decisions because there is a great variance in normal spleen size along with the variance based on imaging.[68] Recommendations for RTP for the athlete with IM are as follows:

- Advise the athlete to avoid any form of exertion, including all sports during the first 2 to 3 weeks (minimum) after the onset of symptoms, when the spleen is more likely to enlarge.
- At 3 weeks after symptom onset, if afebrile and symptom free, the athlete may return to light noncontact physical activities. No sport or activity is recommended if there is a risk of chest or abdominal contact or trauma or if it involves increased intraabdominal pressure or Valsalva maneuvers.
- Full RTP should be made on a case-by-case basis based on clinical symptoms and physical examination as there is not a specific guideline or protocol. RTP is generally considered safe at 4 weeks after symptom onset, assuming the patient's physical stamina has returned and all clinical and physical symptoms have resolved. However, if the sport involved increases intraabdominal pressure, a longer recovery time may be suggested.[68]

Skin Infections

Communicable dermatologic conditions are a common concern in sports, especially wrestling and football. Some of the most common skin infections seen in athletes who play contact sports include bacterial skin infections caused by *Staphylococcus* and *Streptococcus*, with impetigo being the most common.[69] Typical treatment of bacterial skin infections include antibiotics, but treatment has been complicated by an increased prevalence of community-acquired methicillin-resistant *Staphylococcus aureus* (CA-MRSA). Of the sports, wrestling has one of the highest rates of being a carrier of CA-MRSA and other dermatologic conditions.[69] The National Federation of High School Associations has published guidelines and recommendations for wrestlers and RTP available at https://nfhs.org/activities-sports/wrestling/. Clinicians should be aware of their own local and regional rules and regulations, recognizing that they may vary.[69]

Utilizing this information reinforces the importance of prevention of infection. Athletes should be educated on proper personal hygiene, avoidance of sharing water bottles and towels, and thorough cleaning of equipment.[70] Box 18.9 lists the most effective measures to prevent transmission of common skin infections among athletes through personal care and care of facilities. Table 18.8 outlines RTP recommendations for athletes with several of the more common communicable skin infections.

Human Immunodeficiency Virus and Other Blood-Borne Viral Pathogens

Physical activity and exercise should be encouraged for children and athletes with HIV, hepatitis B virus (HBV), and hepatitis C virus (HCV). When discussing sports participation clearance for those with an infectious blood-borne pathogen, the risk and

---

• BOX 18.9 **Prevention of Transmission of Communicable Skin Infections Among Athletes**

Prevention at an Individual Level

- Perform frequent hand washing using good technique (with soap or nonwater alcohol hand sanitizer with an ethanol content of at least 60%) by all athletes and trainers. Shower immediately after practice and game (preferably with antimicrobial soap, especially if doing a body contact sport such as wrestling, rugby, or football); do not share soap or towels.
- Wash clothing and uniforms after each use (completely dry in a dryer).
- Regularly clean all personal equipment (e.g., helmets, body pads, knee/ankle sleeves, and braces).
- Wear protective clothing or gear designed to prevent skin abrasions or cuts.
- Keep cuts and abrasions covered with clean dry bandages or other dressings until healed. Do not use whirlpools or therapy pools that are not cleaned after each use until infections and wounds are healed.
- Do not share personal care items (e.g., bar soap, ointments from open containers, razors, towels, and/or cosmetics).
- Place a barrier (such as clothing or a towel) between the skin and shared equipment such as weight-training equipment, saunas, and steam-room benches.

Prevention at an Institutional or Sports Organization Level

- Institutions and sports clubs must follow guidelines for cleaning and disinfecting all commonly used equipment. See "Cleaning and Disinfecting Athletic Facilities for MRSA" at www.cdc.gov/mrsa/community/environment/athletic-facilities.html for information about cleaning common equipment.
- Coaches and training staff must be knowledgeable about communicable disease issues for their sport.
- Coaches should educate athletes about infectious disease guidelines and expectations, including exclusion from play, return to play, hand washing and showering, and bagging up and uniform laundering.
- Refer students to appropriate resources (e.g., team physician, athletic trainer, school nurse, or PCP) when an infection is suspected.

MRSA, Methicillin-resistant *Staphylococcus aureus*; *PCP*, primary care provider.
Data from Davies HD, Jackson MA, Rice SG. Infectious diseases associated with organized sports and outbreak control. *Pediatrics.* 2017;140(4); Centers for Disease Control and Prevention. Methicillin-resistant *Staphylococcus aureus* (MRSA) infections: athletic facilities cleaning and disinfecting; 2019. https://www.cdc.gov/mrsa/community/environment/athletic-facilities.html/; and Centers for Disease Control and Prevention. Methicillin-resistant *Staphylococcus aureus* (MRSA): for athletes, if you think you have MRSA; 2019. https://www.cdc.gov/mrsa/community/team-hc-providers/advice-for-athletes.html.

TABLE 18.8 **Recommendations for Return to Play for Athletes With Communicable Skin Conditions**

Condition	Return-to-Play Guidelines
Tinea corporis	• Minimum 72 h on a topical fungicide • Extensive or active lesions lead to disqualification • Lesions must be covered with either bio-occlusive or gas-permeable dressing followed by under wrap and stretch tape
Tinea capitis	• Minimum 2 weeks of systemic antifungal therapy
Herpes simplex virus (primary)	• Free of systemic symptoms of viral infection, fever, malaise, etc. • No new lesions for at least 72 h • No moist lesions; all lesions covered with a firm, adherent crust • Minimum 120 h on systemic antiviral therapy, if prescribed (fully formed, ruptured, crusted-over lesions will not be affected by antiviral therapy) • Active lesions cannot be covered to allow participation
Herpes simplex (recurrent)	• No moist lesions; all lesions covered with a firm, dry, adherent crust • Minimum 120 h on systemic antiviral therapy, if prescribed (fully formed, ruptured, crusted-over lesions will not be affected by antiviral therapy) • Active lesions cannot be covered to allow participation in practice or competition
Molluscum contagiosum	• Lesions must be curetted or removed • Localized or solitary lesions may be covered with a gas-permeable dressing followed by under wrap and stretch tape
Furuncles, carbuncles, folliculitis, impetigo, cellulitis, *Staphylococcus aureus* including MRSA	• No new lesions for at least 48 h • Minimum 72 h of antibiotic therapy (see also Chapter 37) • No moist, exudative, or draining lesions • Active lesions cannot be covered to allow participation
Scabies	• Negative microscopic skin prep before returning to practice or competition

MRSA, Methicillin-resistant *Staphylococcus aureus*.
Modified from Peterson, Nash E, Anderson BJ. Infectious disease in contact sports. *Sports Health.* 2018;11(1):47–58; Davies HD, Jackson MA, Rice SG. Infectious diseases associated with organized sports and outbreak control. *Pediatrics.* 2017;140(4).

benefits for the athlete participating and for those that could come into contact with the infected athlete should be discussed and considered. Coaches and trainers should be trained on universal precautions and transmission risks.[69] Education for youth and adolescents in and out of sports should be on the prevention of HBV through vaccinations, good personal hygiene tips such as not sharing razors or other personal items, as well as discussion about lifestyle behaviors and infection transmission routes that increase the risk of infection. Mandatory screening for HIV or HBV is not recommended but should be decided on an individual basis based on risk factors.

Although the transmission of HIV through contact sports is very low, importance of universal blood-borne pathogen precautions remains a high priority.[69] This includes coverage of bleeding wounds, cleaning of mats and equipment with appropriate antiviral properties, and the use of gloves for those coming in contact with bodily fluids. There is no evidence that moderate-intensity physical activity or the stresses of athletics are detrimental to the athlete with HIV. If the athlete is asymptomatic and without evidence of deficiencies in immunologic function, then the presence of HIV infection alone does not preclude participation. The highest risk for an athlete becoming positive for HIV occurs off the field.

HBV has a higher risk of transmission than HIV and HCV because of its ability to survive outside the body for longer periods of time and its resistance to many detergents, alcohol, drying, and temperature fluctuations. The high rates of vaccination have reduced the incidence of HBV but, similar to HIV, it is still important to follow universal precautions.[69] Nonetheless, the chance of transmission in sports is considered extremely low, and no exclusion for asymptomatic carriers is recommended. Sustained, close physical contact sports (e.g., wrestling) carry some risk, although minimal, of transmitting HBV. Some sports organizations differ on their policies concerning athletes' HBV status or titers, and current recommendations should be verified before exclusion as the National Collegiate Athletic Association (NCAA), National Federation of State High School Associations, and AAP do not recommend exclusion based on this status.[56]

HCV has the highest likelihood of being transmitted through blood or blood products, injecting drugs, or needle stick exposures. There have been no documented cases of sports-transmitted HCV infection.[69] Athletes with acute HCV infection are not restricted from sports participation by any governing bodies.[69] Refer to Box 18.10 for a summary of standard blood-borne pathogen infection control measures for trainers and coaches.

Exercise-Induced Dyspnea

Exercise-induced dyspnea (EID) is one of the most common symptoms that can limit an athlete's performance or participation in physical activity both at a recreational and at structured sports level. There is a similarity of subjective symptoms to asthma or EIB that are often reported during the history (i.e., coughing, cannot catch their breath or take a deep breath, or breathlessness).[71] During exercise, there is an increase in ventilation and cardiac output, so both systems need to be evaluated to reach a diagnosis. Cardiac conditions causing EID include pulmonary hypertension, exercise-induced arrhythmia, and intracardiac shunting secondary to a cardiac defect. Noncardiac conditions (besides asthma and EIB) include dysfunctional breathing that may be functional (i.e., thoracic dysfunctional breathing secondary to pulmonary disease) or structural in nature (e.g., phrenic nerve palsy, significant

> ### • BOX 18.10 Recommendations for Trainers and Coaches to Prevent the Transmission of Blood-Borne Pathogens in the Sports Environment
>
> - The health status of all athletes with regard to HIV and hepatitis should be held in confidence (as in all other health-related information).
> - Individuals who care for injured or bleeding athletes should be trained in first aid and standard precautions.
> - Standard precautions (blood, body fluids, secretions, and excretions regardless of whether visible blood is present) with the exception of sweat have replaced universal precautions (blood and body fluid). Standard precautions with basic hygiene are appropriate for all athletic settings.
> - Have appropriate supplies and equipment that comply with standard precautions available (e.g., gloves, goggles, masks, bandages, appropriate waste containers, and disinfectants). Any "sharps" or contaminated bandages, dressings, equipment, or clothing should be properly handled and disposed of consistent with facility guidelines. Have a 1:10 dilution of bleach to tap water prepared.
> - Athletes need to be instructed to report any bleeding wound obtained during an athletic event. If bleeding, the athlete should cease playing until the bleeding has stopped, and only return to play when the wound is covered with an activity-resistant covering. A contaminated uniform must be replaced before returning to play.
> - Any equipment or playing surfaces that were in contact with blood or potentially infectious body fluids should be cleaned immediately with disposable cloths or paper towels and disinfected with the 1:10 bleach preparation or EPA-approved germicide by individuals wearing appropriate personal protective equipment. The area should be allowed to dry before reuse.
> - Postexposure evaluation by a licensed healthcare professional should occur after any incident involving the athlete having nonintact skin, eye, mouth, mucous membrane, or parenteral (under the skin) contact with blood or other potentially infectious material.
> - All athletes should be fully immunized against HBV.
> - Educate about all the routes of transmission, particularly risky behaviors practiced when off the field of competition.
>
> *EPA,* US Environmental Protection Agency; *HBV,* hepatitis B virus; *HIV,* human immunodeficiency virus.
> Data from McGrew C, MacCallum D-S, Narducci D, et al. AMSSM position statement update: blood-borne pathogens in the context of sports participation. *Br J Sports Med.* 2020;54(4): 200–207.

bronchomalacia, subglottic stenosis), gastric reflux, vocal cord dysfunction, physical deconditioning, anemia, subclinical pulmonary embolism, and hyperventilation syndrome. To assist the clinician with diagnosis, in addition to a thorough history and examination, spirometry and/or cardiopulmonary exercise testing can be useful tools.[71]

High-Risk Conditions for Sports Participation

Sudden Cardiac Death in Young Athletes

The ACC defines SCD as "nontraumatic and unexpected death that may occur from a cardiac arrest, within 6 hours of a previously normal state of health."[72] The incidence rate can vary depending on varied definitions for SCD. According to the NCAA, there is an increased incidence of SCD in males and non-White athletes (mostly African American).[72] In a 4-year prospective study, the sports with the highest incidence rates of SCD for males included ice hockey, basketball, and football; the highest incident in females is in soccer.[73]

Causes of SCD in youth athletes vary. In college and professional athletes, cardiomyopathies are more prevalent while coronary artery anomalies accounted for almost one-third of the cases reported for middle school athletes.[73] Coronary artery anomalies will not be evident on an ECG but are often associated with symptoms of exertional chest pain or syncope and can be identified by echocardiography in almost 90% of the cases.[73] A cardiac MRI or CT scan is used when the echocardiogram is nondiagnostic, but concerns are still present. For cardiomyopathies, abnormalities are typically present on a resting ECG.[73] The AAP recommends that healthcare providers consider the athlete's clinical and family history, and their clinical examination at all regular physicals to provide ongoing screening for SCD.[74] When evaluating a patient, prioritize four questions, including (1) if the child has ever fainted, (2) has had an unexplained seizure, (3) has had chest pain or shortness of breath, and (4) if family members have a history of cardiac conditions or death before age 50 years. If a concern is present, an ECG is the initial test recommended and should be interpreted by a trained provider with expertise in heart disease. From a policy and advocacy perspective, it is recommended to support community-wide cardiopulmonary resuscitation (CPR) training and the placement of automated external defibrillators (AEDs).[74] For clearance to participate in sports, the AHA and ACC advise against the use of the 12-lead ECG as a universal screening tool with recommendations to provide a focused history and physical examination with the addition of an ECG if concerns are present.[75] Limitations to the use of ECG as a universal screening tool are associated with cost, the inexperience of ECG readers, and some concerns with diagnostic performance in certain populations.[75] The ECG or other tests, such as echocardiograms, are indicated if the youth is at higher risk based on the 14-element questionnaire (see Box 18.6).[75] See Chapter 33 for a discussion about the major underlying cardiac conditions that increase the risk for SCD. Other causes of SCD include:

- Anabolic steroids. The use of anabolic steroids in athletes has been linked to an increased risk of life-threatening cardiac arrhythmias and pathophysiologic cardiac hypertrophy.[76]
- Commotio cordis. A rare occurrence in which an athlete suffers a direct blow to the precordium by a projectile object, such as a baseball or softball, hockey puck, or lacrosse ball. If this happens at a vulnerable period of the cardiac cycle, it can trigger ventricular fibrillation.[77]
- EIB. Although EIB may produce symptoms described as chest pain or chest discomfort, death from EIB is avoidable with appropriate treatment.[78]
- Premature coronary artery disease. Although acquired, it can contribute to disorders of the coronary circulation.[79,80]

Although SCD often occurs without warning, secondary preventive measures are advocated in school districts and community settings. These measures include increasing awareness of the incidence of SCD in youth in competitive sports, recognition of early symptoms of SCD, athletic personnel trained to provide effective CPR, and access to an AED in school, sports fields, and community settings.[74]

Hernia

In male athletes, an examination for inguinal hernias is traditionally performed while the youth is standing. If an inguinal hernia is detected or suspicion is present, further evaluation is recommended.[81] With inguinal or femoral hernias, athletes should be aware of potential complications including incarceration or strangulation. Depending on the type and size of hernia, individual recommendations will be made on the need for repair. The assessment and treatment of umbilical hernias can vary depending on the size of the hernia. The athlete does not warrant being restricted from participation if an asymptomatic inguinal canal hernia is present.[56]

Absence of Paired Organs

When a youth has an impairment or absence of one of the paired organs and wishes to participate in a sport, the PCP should take several factors into consideration.[56] These include the quality and function of the organ; probability of injury to that organ by participation in the sport; and what, if any, protective equipment is available and its effectiveness.[56] Currently, there is no policy or consensus for sports clearance for those with one kidney, but discussion and research for policy updates are occurring.[82] Athletes with a single kidney should be evaluated for functionality, the likelihood of injury, and type of contact and counseled on the benefits and risks of physical activity.[56,81,82] A letter written by the parents or athlete of informed consent of risks involved for the athlete's record is indicated.[56]

Sports that involve hard objects, sticks, racquets, or aggressive play (e.g., football or basketball) have greater risks for eye injuries. High school sports with the highest rate of eye injury or danger are baseball, followed by boys' basketball, girls' field hockey, and boys' wrestling. Studies have found at least a 90% decreased risk of significant eye injuries with protective eyewear.[56] All youth participating in organized sports should wear appropriate protective eyewear that is specified by the American Society for Testing and Materials (ASTM) or other organization with standards specific to football and lacrosse. Streetwear glasses and industrial education safety protective lenses are not appropriate substitutes. Contact lenses afford no protection.

The child who has one eye or best-corrected vision in one eye worse than 20/40 *and* a small face to fit should be required to wear molded polycarbonate sports frames (American National Standards Institute [ANSI] Z87.1 frames).[56] It is better for the parent and child to choose a sport less likely to endanger the child's eye(s). For other functional one-eyed individuals, only participation in sports in which the use of eye protection is possible should be approved. For collision sports involving headgear (e.g., football, hockey, or lacrosse) the same safety ASTM-approved eyewear should be worn under the cage shield or mask with a chin strap on a helmet. A history of a detached retina is significant, and participation should be limited to nonstrenuous sports until consultation with an ophthalmologist is complete (see Table 18.6).

Young men with a single testicle can be adequately protected with the use of a hard-cup athletic supporter for contact and collision sports and those sports in which objects are projected at high speed.[56] Young women with one ovary should not be restricted.

Musculoskeletal and Overuse or Traumatic Injuries

Overuse injuries are becoming more common in young athletes because of early sport specialization, year-round sports participation in multiple sports in the same season, and the increased demands put on young athletes by parents, coaches, and school settings. A common overuse injury unique to the skeletally immature athlete is apophysitis. Apophysitis is an injury caused by inflammation or stress, which results from repetitive irritation, inflammation, and microtrauma at the growth plate. Overuse is associated with a significant proportion of musculoskeletal complaints in youth involved in competitive sports. An avulsion fracture can occur in youth with apophysitis as a result of a forceful muscle contraction displacing a small piece of bone from its origin. Apophysitis may present as a persistent or worsening pain symptom after a specific history of injury or with gradual onset of pain without a specific injury. Persistent pain indicates the need for further diagnostics and referral.

Understanding the demands of a specific sport enables the PCP to thoroughly consider differential diagnoses, management, and a RTP plan for each athlete. Successful RTP includes regaining strength and conditioning of the injured area. A program of gradual RTP with a trial of sports activities may be necessary before full RTP is accomplished. See Chapter 40 for further discussion on overuse injuries and trauma.

Overuse Injuries in Baseball/Softball

Young baseball and softball throwers and pitchers are at particular risk of overuse injury or apophysitis. There are specific guidelines that address this issue for pitchers by age group.[83] General information includes[84]:

- Do not pitch more than 100 innings in any calendar year.
- Refrain from throwing overhead for 2 to 3 months/year (4 months is preferred); no competitive pitching for at least 4 months/year.
- Watch and respond to signs of fatigue.
- Do not play in both pitcher and catcher positions.
- Follow daily and weekly pitch limits based on age; do not pitch on 3 consecutive days.
- Do not use radar guns.
- Pitchers should not pitch for more than one team at a time.

Neck Injury

If there is a neck injury, consideration for a severe condition such as spinal cord injury or neck fracture should be considered. The athlete should undergo medical clearance including a full neurologic examination including a complete neck evaluation, demonstration of a full range of motion, adequate strength in neck flexion and extension, and symmetric strength during lateral flexion along with the absence of neurologic symptoms. If symptoms or concerns are present, radiologic tests should be performed based on the incident, symptoms, and physical examination. This may include a CT scan, radiography, and or MRI.[85]

Burners and Stingers

"Burners and stingers" (neurapraxia) are nerve root or brachial plexus compression or traction injuries that generally cause unilateral symptoms. This is a common injury in contact or collision sports, notably football and wrestling. Neurapraxia is derived from the sensation of a burn, stinging, electric, or "lightning bolt" sensation down an arm to the hand. The sensation can last seconds to minutes; up to 10% can last hours, days, or longer. Athletes can be cleared to return to their sport if they do not have any residual neck or radicular pain and demonstrate a full range of motion and strength. If a history of transient or recurrent quadriplegia has occurred, cervical radiographs are required before the athlete can be cleared for participation. The athlete may require additional evaluation if the weakness lasts more than a few days, there are complaints of neck pain, the burners or stingers occur in both arms, or there is a prior history of burners or stingers.

Head Injury and Concussion

An estimated 1.7 to 3.8 million concussions occur each year in the United States, with 10% occurring as a result of sports and physical activity. Of all traumatic brain injuries, 21% of injuries annually occur in children and adolescents in the United States.[86] The activities posing the highest risk for head injuries include playground equipment, football, basketball, cycling, baseball and softball, and soccer.[86] All 50 states have enacted concussion laws that cover education, assessment, and emergency plans, athlete removal from play, and expert medical evaluation with RTP guidelines.

Less emphasis is now placed on the loss of consciousness, posttraumatic amnesia, and retrograde amnesia as ways to diagnose and classify the severity of the concussion, as these only appear in a minority of injured athletes. Key points for sideline personnel and healthcare providers in assessing young athletes for head injury include (Box 18.11)[87]:

- Baseline (preseason) neurocognitive testing should be done on all athletes and used to compare any sideline assessments after an injury to avoid erroneous conclusions. In addition to

---

• BOX 18.11 Concussion Physical Examination and Tool Resources

- Obtain details about the injury:
  - When did it occur?
  - How did it happen?
  - What were the initial symptoms?
  - What are the current symptoms?
  - Any initial evaluation by a healthcare provider
- Sleep impairment or changes
- School attendance since injury and performance prior to injury
- Medical and family history, does the individual or family have:
  - History of attention-deficit/hyperactivity disorder, dyslexia, and learning disabilities (may complicate the recovery)
  - Have visual disturbances or need corrective lenses
  - History of lazy eye, amblyopia, or strabismus
  - History of anxiety, depression, or migraines
  - Receive special accommodations in school (e.g., reading, speech therapy)
  - History of experiencing motion sickness (may increase after concussion)
- Physical examination to include eye tracking and balance (e.g., https://www.chop.edu/video/pediatric-exams-concussion-evaluation)

Concussion Assessment Tool Resources

SCAT5: a standardized evaluation tool designed for use by licensed healthcare professionals. To be used in children 13 years and older. For children 12 years and younger, use the Child SCAT5 available at https://scat5.cattonline.com/.

Concussion Recognition Tool 5: to be used to identify a suspected concussion and can be used by nonhealthcare providers in children, adolescents, and adults. Includes 4 steps: Step 1: Assess for red flags or concerning symptoms, Step 2: Observe for any visual clues, Step 3: Review symptoms, and Step 4: Assess memory (for 12 years and older). https://bjsm.bmj.com/content/bjsports/early/2017/04/26/bjsports-2017-097508CRT5.full.pdf

Acute Concussion Evaluation (ACE): Evidence-based clinical protocol used to evaluate and diagnose children and adults with a concussion. Reviews details surrounding the injury, provide a symptom checklist, risk factors for a complicated recovery, and red flags that require acute emergency management and a diagnosis with follow-up plan. https://www.cdc.gov/headsup/pdfs/providers/ace-a.pdf

Data from McCrory P, Meeuwisse W, Dvorak J, et al. Consensus statement on concussion in sport—the 5th international conference on concussion in sport held in Berlin, October 2016. *Br J Sports Med.* 2017;51(11):838–847.

the initial sideline assessment, serial assessments postinjury are necessary.

- Recognize that a concussion may have occurred, as most athletes show no obvious indications of a concussion.
- Remove the player from play and do not allow RTP on the day of injury.
- Sideline assessment is imperative for any athlete who receives a significant head blow or is not "acting themselves" no matter the degree of impact to the head.
- Concussion assessment and reassessment must be carried out by a certified trainer or healthcare provider who has been trained to evaluate and manage concussions. The Sport Concussion Assessment Tool 5 (SCAT5), the Concussion Recognition Tool version 5 (CRT5), and/or the Child SCAT5 are recommended by the 5th International Conference on Concussion in Sport as a sideline concussion assessment tool and are available at http://bjsm.bmj.com/content/bjsports/early/2017/04/26/bjsports-2017-097506SCAT5.full.pdf. This tool includes physical examination findings and reassessment.

Both physical and cognitive rest is recommended after the diagnosis of a concussion. Cognitive recovery, which is a key factor in RTP decisions, may lag behind physical symptom resolution. The athlete should rest for 24 to 48 hours, then slowly and progressively become more active and begin progression through the Return to Sport strategy steps (Table 18.9). There should be at least 24 hours (or longer) for each step of the progression. If any symptoms worsen during exercise, the athlete should go back to the previous step. Resistance training should be added only in the later stages (stage 3 or 4 at the earliest). If symptoms are persistent (e.g., more than 10–14 days in adults or more than 1 month in children) or if the adolescent has two or three concussions without loss of consciousness or one to two concussions with loss of consciousness, referral to a specialist is indicated for further evaluation.[87] Chapter 41 discusses the evaluation and management of traumatic brain injury and concussion.

Special Considerations for the Female Athlete

Injuries and the Female Athlete

With the rise in number of elite female athletes, the provider should be cognizant to injuries that are more prevalent in girls and female adolescents because of structural and growth differences, skeletal immaturity, hormonal changes, and nutrition.[56] Intensive sports training does not appear to delay the growth and sexual maturation of young female athletes.

The increased prevalence of knee injuries in female athletes is caused by several factors, including biomechanical factors, greater joint laxity in females, and hormonal effects on connective tissue. Estrogen plays an important role and affects the female athlete's ligaments, influencing the joint laxity. In addition, physical variations such as having less space in the knee region and having wider hips can increase the stress put on the knee when landing after a jump. Sports with increased risk for females include basketball, soccer, field hockey, cheerleading, singles tennis, lacrosse, and skiing. Anterior cruciate ligament (ACL) injuries occur 1.6 times more often in the female high school athlete compared to the male high school athlete.[88] ACL injury typically occurs during deceleration, landing, pivoting, or contact with another athlete. It is recommended that prevention programs use trained coaches who target younger athletes and incorporate strength training for the lower body along with a focus on landing stabilization.[89]

Other injuries common in the female athlete include those of the patellofemoral joint and shoulder (sustained during diving, gymnastics, swimming, throwing, and volleyball) and stress fractures.[90] Stress fractures occur in 9.7% of female athletes compared with 6.5% of males.[91] Risk factors of stress fractures can be related to inherent characteristics of the athlete, including demographics, hormone levels, bone quality, muscle strength, anatomical alignment, and muscle fatigue. External factors that include training schedule, equipment, and diet can play a role and contribute to low bone mineral content,

TABLE 18.9	Graduated Return-to-Play Strategy After a Concussion	
Stage and Aim[a]	**Activity**	**Goal of Each Step**
1. Symptom limited activity	• Daily activities that do not provoke symptoms • High school-aged and younger youth should not return to sports until they have successfully returned to academics	Gradual reintroduction of work/school activities
2. Light aerobic exercise	• Walking or stationary cycling at a slow to medium pace; no resistance training	Increase heart rate
3. Sport-specific exercise	• Running or skating drills • No head impact activities	Add movement
4. Noncontact training drills	• Harder training drills (e.g., passing drills); may start progressive resistance training	Exercise, coordination, and increased thinking
5. Full-contact practice	• Following medical clearance, participate in normal training activities	Restore confidence and assess functional skills by coaching staff
6. Return to play	• Normal gameplay	

[a]An initial period of 24 to 48 hours of both relative physical rest and cognitive rest is recommended before beginning the return-to-sport progression. There should be at least 24 hours (or longer) for each step of the progression. If any symptoms worsen during exercise, the athlete should go back to the previous step. Resistance training should be added only in the later stages (stage 3 or 4 at the earliest). If symptoms are persistent (e.g., more than 10–14 days in adults or more than 1 month in children), the athlete should be referred to a healthcare professional who is an expert in the management of concussion.

Data from McCrory P, Meeuwisse W, Dvorak J, et al. Consensus statement on concussion in sport—the 5th international conference on concussion in sport held in Berlin, October 2016. *Br J Sports Med.* 2017;51(11):838–847.

decreased bone density, and bone diameters, increasing the risk of a stress injury.[91]

Female Athlete Triad and Relative Energy Deficiency in Sports

The female athlete triad consists of three entities: (1) energy availability (optimal energy availability to low energy availability with or without eating disorder), (2) menstrual function (eumenorrhea to functional hypothalamic amenorrhea), and (3) bone mineral density (optimal bone health to osteoporosis).[92] Each of the entities can affect the other entities within the triad. The athlete can be anywhere along the spectrum for each of the three entities and may present with one or any combination of the three.[92] The female athlete triad is associated with sports that emphasize a lean body mass, low weight maintenance, or retaining one's prepubertal physique. Disordered eating patterns can be caused by either intentional caloric restriction (an eating disorder that may or may not encompass all the criteria for an anorexia or bulimia diagnosis) or an unintentional insufficient intake of calories that does not meet the athlete's metabolic demands.[93] Insufficient calories related to their activity and metabolic requirements cause low energy availability. Low energy negatively affects bone remodeling and mineralization and causes menstrual dysfunction (amenorrhea or oligomenorrhea). Inadequate bone mineralization during the critical adolescent years puts the teen at lifelong risk of osteoporosis, which increases the risk of stress fractures during adolescence and throughout life as well as skeletal problems at menopause.

As further understanding of the athlete triad has evolved, it is understood that the concerns secondary to the low energy availability that are insufficient to cover physiological processes are broader than the three symptoms of the triad and that both sexes are affected. For this reason, the term relative energy deficiency in sport (RED-S) has been implemented.[94] Similar to the female athlete triad, important points of RED-S include the recognition that low energy may result from both intentional and unintentional lack of caloric input from an individual's diet or excessive energy. The decreased energy begins a cascade of hormonal changes beginning with a reduction of gonadotropin-releasing hormone, which results in an impairment of anterior pituitary release of gonadotropins. In females, decreased follicle stimulating hormone (FSH) and luteinizing hormone (LH) lead to hypoestrogenism causing functional amenorrhea and decreased bone mass. In males, a decreased level of testosterone and a secondary effect on bone mass occurs. Additional hormonal deviations include thyroid hormone insufficiency, leptin levels, the metabolism of carbohydrates, insulin-like growth factor-1, and sympathetic and parasympathetic tone.[94]

There is also an increased risk for those with sports specialization at an early age and in abusive or unhealthy families.[95] Girls who participate in sports that emphasize leanness are at the greatest risk of the triad of disorders, including distance running, gymnastics, dance/dance team, figure skating, cheerleading, wrestling, lightweight rowing, and pole vaulting.[95] It is estimated that the incidence of the female athlete triad with all three components in female high school athletes is 0%–16% and those having one component of the triad range from 16%–54%, although the true prevalence is hard to determine because of challenges with diagnosing each of the components.[92] The identification of the early existence of an eating disorder, weight loss, or menstrual irregularities from a PPE history and examination should alert the provider to take a more thorough history, provide testing, and initiate early treatment. The symptoms of the triad occur along a continuum rather than in unison, and if one symptom is present, the athlete is at risk of developing additional components of the triad.

Screening questions using the AAP's PPE health history and physical form can direct the provider to provide further screening or testing (Box 18.12). Box 18.13 lists recommendations for the

---

• BOX 18.12 Screening Questions for Female Athlete Triad

Menstrual History
- Have you had a menstrual period?
- What was your age when you had your first period?
- When was your last period? How often do you have your periods?
- How many menstrual periods have you had in the past year?

Medications
- Are you taking hormones (estrogen, progesterone, birth control pills)?
- What is your current weight?
- Are you concerned about your weight or body composition?
- Are you trying to or has anyone recommended that you lose or gain weight?
- Are you on a diet or do you avoid certain foods or food groups?
- Have you done anything to try to control your weight (purging, binging, fasting, diet pills, or other botanicals)? Have you ever had an eating disorder?

Musculoskeletal
- Have you ever had a stress fracture?
- Have you been told that you have low bone density?

Data from Weiss Kelly AK, Hecht S. The female athlete triad. *Ann Joint.* 2022;7; and Hornberger LL, Lane MA, Adolescence TCO, et al. Identification and management of eating disorders in children and adolescents. *Pediatrics.* 2021;147(1).

• BOX 18.13 Female Athlete Triad: Recommendations for the Clinician

- Perform a complete history that includes a physical, daily nutrition intake, exercise, and menstrual function.
  - Menstrual history should document any history of abnormal menses in the previous 12 months.
  - Assess for low body mass index, orthostatic hypotension, bradycardia, signs of an eating disorder (parotid gland swelling, callus of proximal interphalangeal joint, cold/discolored hands or feet, lanugo).
- Screen for all elements of the triad at the PPE and at annual physicals.
- If one component of the triad exists, screen for others.
- If an eating disorder is suspected, refer the athlete to a nutrition professional and a mental health professional for screening/treatment if indicated.
- Consider the use of DEXA, bioelectrical impedance, water or air displacement plethysmography, and or skin fold measures to document fat free mass.
- Diagnosis of amenorrhea: screen for other causes (see Chapter 43). Functional hypothalamic amenorrhea is a diagnosis of exclusion.
  - Obtain an ultrasound if signs of PCOS are present (acne, hirsutism).
- Screen for bone mineral density after a stress or low-impact fracture, 6 months of amenorrhea or oligomenorrhea, or as part of assessment for disordered eating pattern.

DEXA, Dual-energy x-ray absorptiometry; *PCOS,* polycystic ovary syndrome; *PPE,* preparticipation physical examination.
Data from Weiss Kelly AK, Hecht S. The female athlete triad. *Ann Joint.* 2022;7.

clinician evaluating an individual identified as having the female triad.[56] The initial goal of treatment is to increase energy intake and decrease energy expenditure. Therapy, participation, and return to play should be based on the risk categories and reassessed throughout treatment. Preventive counseling for all athletes should include nutritional energy needs for sports; the importance of bone mineralization during child and adolescent years; bone health throughout life; the importance of physical activity, calcium, and vitamin D; and educating female athletes and families about this disorder.

Additional Resources

Academy of Nutrition and Dietetics: Sports, Cardiovascular, and Wellness Nutrition: https://www.scandpg.org/

American Academy of Family Physicians (AAFP): www.aafp.org

American Academy of Family Physicians (AAFP) and American Academy of Pediatrics (AAP) sports injury prevention and downloadable PPE forms: https://downloads.aap.org/AAP/PDF/PPE_History_Form_1-18-22-rev.pdf, https://downloads.aap.org/AAP/PDF/PPE_Physical_Exam_Form_1-24-22-rev.pdf

AAP: www.aap.org

AAP COVID-19 Interim Guidance: Return to Sports and Physical Activity: https://www.aap.org/en/pages/2019-novel-coronavirus-covid-19-infections/clinical-guidance/covid-19-interim-guidance-return-to-sports/

American College of Sports Medicine (ACSM): www.acsm.org

American Orthopaedic Society for Sports Medicine (AOSSM): www.sportsmed.org

BAM! Body and Mind: www.cdc.gov/bam (focused on tweens)

Centers for Disease Control and Prevention (CDC): www.cdc.gov

CDC: Athletic Facilities, Cleaning & Disinfecting for MRSA: https://www.cdc.gov/mrsa/community/environment/athletic-facilities.html

CDC: Physical Education and Physical Activity: https://www.cdc.gov/healthyschools/physicalactivity/index.htm

Easter Seals: https://www.easterseals.com/

Equity Toolkit: https://www.cdc.gov/nccdphp/dnpao/state-local-programs/health-equity/index.html

Healthy People 2030: https://health.gov/healthypeople

International Society of Sports Nutrition (ISSN): www.sportsnutritionsociety.org

Lids on Kids: A Helmet—It's a Smart Idea: www.lidsonkids.org

Little League Pitching Rules: http://www.littleleague.org/learn/rules/pitch-count.htm

Miracle League: http://www.themiracleleague.net

National Athletic Trainers' Association (NATA): www.nata.org

National Center on Health, Physical Activity and Disability: https://www.nchpad.org

National Highway Traffic Safety Administration Bicycle Safety: https://www.nhtsa.gov/road-safety/bicycle-safety

National Lightning Safety Institute: lightningsafety.com

Paralympics: https://www.paralympic.org

Personal Watercraft Industry Association: http://www.pwia.org/rules (rules and regulations listed by state)

Physical Activity Guidelines for Americans:. https://health.gov/sites/default/files/2019-10/PAG_ExecutiveSummary.pdf

Physical Activity Guidelines for Americans for School Aged Children and Adolescents: www.cdc.gov/healthyschools/physicalactivity/guidelines.htm

President's Council on Fitness, Sports & Nutrition (PCFSN): www.hhs.gov/fitness/index.html

Safe Kids Worldwide: www.safekids.org

Special Olympics: www.specialolympics.org

Sport Concussion Assessment Tool (SCAT5): http://bjsm.bmj.com/content/bjsports/early/2017/04/26/bjsports-2017-097506SCAT5.full.pdf

US Anti-Doping Agency: True Sport Parent Handbook: A guidebook to developing young athletes and the role parents play: http://www.truesport.org/library/documents/resources/parent/parent_handbook.pdf

US Youth Soccer Federation: www.usyouthsoccer.org

Walk & Bike to School: http://www.walkbiketoschool.org/

We Can! Ways to Enhance Childhood Nutrition and Physical Activity: www.nhlbi.nih.gov/health/educational/wecan

World Health Organization (WHO): www.who.int/dietphysicalactivity/en/

US Department of Agriculture: Calculate an individual's caloric needs based on their sex, age, and activity level: https://www.nal.usda.gov/human-nutrition-and-food-safety/dri-calculator

US Department of Agriculture MyPlate: https://www.choosemyplate.gov/MyPlatePlan (provides an easy way for athletes to estimate energy requirements)

References

1. Office of Disease Prevention and Health Promotion. Nutrition, Physical Activity, and Obesity. https://www.healthypeople.gov/2020/leading-health-indicators/2020-lhi-topics/Nutrition-Physical-Activity-and-Obesity.
2. World Health Organization (WHO). *Global Action Plan on Physical Activity 2018-2030: More Active People for a Healthier World.* WHO; 2018.
3. US Department of Health and Human Services (USDHHS). *Physical Activity Guidelines for Americans.* 2nd ed. USDHHS; 2018.
4. Merlo CL, Jones SE, Michael SL, et al. Dietary and physical activity behaviors among high school students - youth risk behavior survey, United States, 2019. *MMWR Suppl.* 2020;69(1):64–76.
5. National Physical Activity Plan Alliance. *United States Report Card on Physical Activity for Children and Youth.* NPAPA; 2022.
6. Centers for Disease Control and Prevention. Physical Activity Facts. https://www.cdc.gov/healthyschools/physicalactivity/facts.htm.
7. Centers for Disease Control and Prevention. Childhood Obesity Causes & Consequences. https://www.cdc.gov/obesity/childhood/causes.html.
8. Centers for Disease Control and Prevention. Overcoming barriers to physical activity. https://www.cdc.gov/physicalactivity/basics/adding-pa/barriers.html.
9. World Health Organization. Physical Activity Fact Sheet. https://www.who.int/news-room/fact-sheets/detail/physical-activity#:~:text=Children%20and%20adolescents%20aged%205,least%203%20days%20a%20week.
10. American Academy of Pediatrics. Exercise and Asthma. https://www.healthychildren.org/English/health-issues/conditions/allergies-asthma/pages/Exercise-and-Asthma.aspx.
11. Flynn JT, Kaelber DC, Baker-Smith CM, et al. Clinical practice guideline for screening and management of high blood pressure in children and adolescents. *Pediatrics.* 2017;140(3).
12. Myers J, Kokkinos P, Nyelin E. Physical activity, cardiorespiratory fitness, and the metabolic syndrome. *Nutrients.* 2019;11(7).
13. Fornari E, Maffeis C. Treatment of metabolic syndrome in children. *Front Endocrinol.* 2019;10.
14. Wyszyńska J, Ring-Dimitriou S, Thivel D, et al. Physical activity in the prevention of childhood obesity: the position of the European

and the intervals between antibody-containing blood products and live attenuated vaccines (particularly measles- and varicella-containing vaccines).[5]

Interval Between Doses of the Same Vaccine

Most vaccines in the immunization schedule require two or more doses for the development of an adequate and persistent antibody response. Studies have demonstrated that following the recommended ages and intervals between doses of the same antigen(s) provides optimal protection. In general, decreasing the interval between doses in a multiple-dose vaccine series may interfere with antibody response and protection. For routine vaccination, vaccine doses should not be administered earlier than the minimum age or at less than the minimum intervals. However, exceptions may occasionally be necessary. One exception involves administering a dose up to 4 days before the minimum age or interval to avoid missing an opportunity to vaccinate. However, if the provider has confidence that the patient will return for a later visit, it is preferable to reschedule vaccination on or after the recommended minimum age or interval. If the patient is new to the provider or habitually misses appointments, it may be preferable to administer the vaccine early. These early doses administered within 4 days of the minimum age or interval are considered valid. In certain situations, state or local requirements might mandate doses of selected vaccines be administered on or after specific ages, superseding this 4-day grace period. Doses administered 5 days or more before the minimum age or interval should not be counted as valid and should be repeated as age appropriate.

Other exceptions are administering doses in a vaccine series at shorter intervals than recommended when a person is behind schedule and needs to be brought up to date quickly or when international travel is pending. In these cases, an accelerated schedule using the minimum age or minimum interval criteria can be used. In some cases, a scheduled dose of vaccine may be administered late. A late dose should be administered at the next visit. Available data indicate intervals between doses that are longer than those routinely recommended do not affect seroconversion rates or titers when the schedule is completed. Therefore it is not necessary to restart a series or add doses of any vaccine because of an extended interval between doses.[5]

Simultaneous and Nonsimultaneous Vaccine Administration

Simultaneous Administration of Different Vaccines

Simultaneous administration (i.e., administration of two or more vaccines on the same day) of all recommended vaccines is important because it increases the probability that an individual will be fully vaccinated at the appropriate age. It is also an important part of immunization practice when a PCP is uncertain that a patient will return for additional doses of vaccine. In general, almost all vaccines can be administered at the same visit.[5]

Exceptions to this include:
- Pneumococcal conjugate vaccine 13 (PCV13; Prevnar 13) and MenACWY-D (Menactra) vaccine should not be administered simultaneously to persons with functional or anatomic asplenia or HIV. Menactra brand meningococcal conjugate vaccine is thought to interfere with the antibody response to Prevnar 13. When both Prevnar 13 and Menactra are indicated, Prevnar 13 should be administered first, followed by Menactra at least 4 weeks later.[5]

- PCV13 (Prevnar 13) vaccine and the pneumococcal polysaccharide vaccine (PPSV23; Pneumovax 23) should not be administered at the same visit; studies show a better immune response when Prevnar 13 is administered before Pneumovax 23. When both Prevnar 13 and Pneumovax 23 are indicated, Prevnar 13 should be administered first, and Pneumovax 23 should be administered either at least 8 weeks later or at least 1 year later, depending on the age and health conditions of the vaccine recipient.[5]

- Combination vaccines are generally preferred over the simultaneous administration of single-component vaccines. Combination vaccines contain components that can be divided into independently available routine vaccines and can reduce the number of injections needed. Considerations for using combination vaccines should include an assessment of the number of injections, availability of the vaccine, the likelihood of improved vaccination coverage, the likelihood of patient return, and issues regarding storage and cost. Considerations should also include patient choice and the potential for adverse events.[5]

Nonsimultaneous Administration of Live Vaccines

If any combination of live injected vaccines (MMR-II, ProQuad, Varivax) or live attenuated influenza vaccine (LAIV [FluMist]) is not administered simultaneously, the vaccine doses should be separated by at least 4 weeks. This interval is intended to reduce or eliminate interference from the vaccine administered first with the vaccine administered later. If any two of these vaccines are administered at an interval of less than 4 weeks, then the vaccine administered second should be repeated in 4 weeks or serologic testing should be performed following MMR-II and ProQuad to confirm their effectiveness (serologic testing is not recommended following FluMist or Varivax vaccines). Live vaccines administered by the oral route (e.g., rotavirus) are not believed to interfere with parenteral or intranasal live vaccines or with each other. Therefore they may be administered simultaneously with or at any time before or after other live vaccines.[5]

Vaccines and Antibody-Containing Products

Antibodies, in the form of immune globulin, might be administered simultaneously with or around the same time as certain vaccines; for example, as postexposure prophylaxis for certain diseases, such as hepatitis B, rabies, and tetanus. Immune response to some live attenuated vaccines can be affected by receipt of immune globulin, depending on the type of vaccine, amount of antibody, and timing of administration. Immune response to inactivated vaccines is generally not affected by antibody-containing products. Inactivated vaccines can be administered before, after, or at the same time as the antibody products. The vaccine antigen should be administered at a site distant from where the immune globulin was injected.[5] Refer to Chapter 35, Infectious Diseases, for immunoglobulin administration in children.

Live Attenuated Injectable Vaccines

Live attenuated vaccines must replicate to produce an immune response. Antibodies against injected live vaccine antigens may interfere with replication. If MMR (MMR-II), varicella (VAR [Varivax]), or combination measles, mumps, rubella, and varicella (MMRV [ProQuad]) vaccines must be administered around the same time as an antibody (immunoglobulin, etc.), the two must be separated by enough time to prevent the antibody from interfering with viral replication. If these live vaccines are administered first, it is necessary to wait at least 2 weeks before administering the antibody. If the interval between the vaccine and antibody is less than 2 weeks, the recipient should be tested for immunity, or the vaccine dose should be repeated. If the antibody is administered first, it is necessary to wait until the antibody has waned before administering the vaccine. This will reduce the chance of interference by the antibody.[5]

An exception to the waiting period for an antibody to wane before vaccination is a low dose of RhoGam or Rhophylac (anti-Rho(D) globulin) or any other blood product administered to women who do not have evidence of immunity to rubella or varicella during the last trimester of pregnancy or at delivery. Although passively acquired antibodies can interfere with the response to the rubella vaccine, the low dose of anti-Rho(D) globulin has not been demonstrated to reduce the response to the rubella vaccine. These women should receive MMR-II, Varivax, or ProQuad as indicated immediately after delivery and, if possible, be tested 3 or more months later to ensure immunity to rubella and, if necessary, to measles.

Live Attenuated Oral and Intranasal Vaccines

Rotavirus vaccines (RV; RV1 [Rotarix] and RV5 [RotaTeq]) and LAIV (FluMist) are not known to be affected by the administration of immune globulin or blood products. They may be administered simultaneously with blood products or separated from them by any interval.[5]

Doses

Many factors influence the number of doses recommended in a vaccine series, including the type of vaccine, epidemiology of the disease, and host factors (e.g., age, presence of underlying diseases). For live injected vaccines, the first dose administered at the recommended age usually provides protection. An additional dose is administered to provide another opportunity for vaccine response in the small proportion of recipients who do not respond to the first dose. The second dose is administered to ensure that nearly 100% of persons are immune. Immunity following live vaccines is long-lasting, and booster doses are usually not necessary.[5]

For inactivated vaccines, the first dose administered at the recommended age usually does not provide protection (the hepatitis A vaccine is an exception). A protective immune response may not develop until after dose 2 or 3. For inactivated vaccines, antibody titers may decrease below protective levels after a few years. This phenomenon is most notable with the pertussis vaccine. Tetanus and diphtheria vaccine-induced immunity also wane. For these vaccines, a booster dose is administered to raise antibodies back to protective levels.[5]

Not all inactivated vaccines require boosting throughout the lifetime. For example, additional doses of Hib vaccine is not required after completion of the infant primary series and booster dose because Hib disease is rare in persons older than age 5 years. The Hepatitis B vaccine does not require boosting in immunocompetent persons because of the immunologic memory of the vaccine and the long incubation period for hepatitis B. Immunologic memory produces an "auto boost," which means exposure to the virus causes the established immune memory to respond faster than the virus can cause disease.[5]

Adverse Reactions Following Vaccination

An adverse reaction or side effect is an untoward effect caused by a vaccine. An adverse reaction is different from a vaccine adverse event. A vaccine adverse event refers to any medical event that occurs following vaccination. An adverse event could be a true adverse reaction or a coincidental event, with further investigation needed to distinguish between them. Healthcare providers are required by law to report certain adverse events after vaccination.[5]

Allergic reactions may be caused by the vaccine antigen itself or some other vaccine component, such as cell culture material or a stabilizer, preservative, or antibiotic used to inhibit bacterial growth. Severe allergic reactions (e.g., anaphylaxis) may be life-threatening but fortunately are very rare. The risk of an allergic reaction can be decreased by effective screening before vaccination. All providers who administer vaccines must have an emergency protocol, supplies, and training to treat anaphylaxis.[5]

Local adverse reactions (e.g., pain, swelling, and redness at the injection site) are the most common adverse reactions following vaccination. They generally occur within a few hours of the injection and are usually mild and self-limited. Local reactions may occur with up to 80% of vaccine doses, depending on the type of vaccine. On rare occasions, local reactions may be severe. These reactions, referred to as *Arthus reactions,* are most frequently seen with diphtheria and tetanus toxoids.[5]

Systemic adverse reactions (e.g., fever, myalgia, rash, headache) may occur following vaccination. Adverse reactions such as fever or rash following live attenuated vaccines may be similar to a mild form of the natural disease, with symptoms produced from viral replication. Systemic adverse reactions are usually mild and occur 3 through 21 days after the vaccine was administered. Systemic adverse reactions from live attenuated vaccines are seen at longer intervals following vaccine administration because they are caused by the replication of the vaccine virus in the body, which occurs over several days.[5]

Contraindications and Precautions to Vaccination

Contraindications and precautions to vaccination generally dictate circumstances when vaccines should not be administered. Some contraindications and precautions are temporary, and the vaccine can be administered later.[5]

Contraindications

A contraindication is a health condition in the recipient that increases the likelihood of a serious adverse reaction to a vaccine. In general, vaccines should not be administered when a contraindication is present. A severe allergic reaction (e.g., anaphylaxis) to a vaccine component is a contraindication to any vaccine containing that component, and a severe allergy following a dose of vaccine is a contraindication to subsequent doses of that vaccine. Use of aerosolized steroids, such as inhalers for asthma, is not a contraindication to vaccination; nor are alternate-day, rapidly tapering, and short (<14 days) high-dose steroid schedules, topical formulations, and physiologic replacement steroid dose schedules.[5]

Precautions

A precaution is a health condition in the recipient that might increase the chance or severity of a serious adverse reaction, might compromise the ability of the vaccine to produce immunity, or might cause diagnostic confusion. Injury could result, but the chance of this happening is less than with a contraindication. In general, vaccines should be deferred when a precaution is present. However, situations may arise when the benefit of protection from the vaccine outweighs the risk of an adverse reaction, and a provider may decide to administer the vaccine. Moderate or severe acute illness, with or without fever, is a precaution for all vaccines. With few exceptions, family medical history is not a contraindication or precaution to vaccines.[5]

Contraindications and Precautions in Persons With Specific Health Conditions

History of Allergic Reactions

A severe allergic reaction (e.g., anaphylaxis) following a dose of vaccine is a contraindication for a subsequent dose of that vaccine and is a medical emergency. Anaphylaxis involves two or more organ systems (dermatologic, cardiovascular, respiratory, and/or gastrointestinal) simultaneously. Symptoms and signs of anaphylactic reactions include generalized urticaria (hives), swelling of the mouth and throat, difficulty breathing, wheezing, hypotension, or shock. Anaphylaxis after vaccination occurs rarely and can often be prevented by appropriate screening. Persons may be allergic to a vaccine antigen or to a vaccine component such as an animal protein, antibiotic, preservative, or stabilizer. The most common animal protein allergen is egg protein found in influenza vaccines prepared using embryonated chicken eggs. Asking persons whether they can eat eggs without adverse effects is a reasonable way to screen for those who might be at risk if they receive egg-containing influenza vaccines. Persons with a history of egg allergy who have experienced only hives after exposure to eggs should receive the influenza vaccine. Influenza vaccine may also be administered to persons who report having had reactions to eggs involving symptoms other than hives (such as swelling of the throat and mouth, difficulty breathing, lightheadedness, or recurrent emesis) or who required epinephrine or another emergency medical intervention. If egg-containing influenza vaccine is administered to persons who report having had reactions to eggs involving symptoms other than hives, it should be administered in an inpatient or outpatient medical setting and supervised by a healthcare provider able to recognize and manage severe allergic conditions. A previous severe allergic reaction to the influenza vaccine, regardless of the component suspected of being responsible for the reaction, is a contraindication to the future receipt of the vaccine.[5]

Studies show that children who have a history of a severe allergy to eggs rarely have reactions to MMR-II and MMRV (ProQuad) vaccines. This is probably because measles and mumps vaccine viruses are both grown in chick embryo fibroblasts, not actually in eggs. It appears gelatin, not egg, might be the cause of allergic reactions to MMR-II. Children with egg allergies may be vaccinated with MMR-II or ProQuad without prior skin testing.[5]

Certain vaccines contain trace amounts of neomycin. Persons who have experienced an anaphylactic reaction to neomycin should not receive these vaccines. Most often, neomycin allergy presents as contact dermatitis, a manifestation of a delayed-type (cell-mediated) immune response, rather than anaphylaxis. A history of delayed-type reactions is not a contraindication for the administration of neomycin-containing vaccines.[5]

Latex, which is sap from the commercial rubber tree, contains naturally occurring impurities (e.g., plant proteins and peptides), which are believed to be responsible for allergic reactions. The most common type of latex sensitivity is contact-type (type 4) allergy, usually resulting from prolonged contact with latex-containing gloves. Latex-related allergic reactions after vaccination are rare. If a person reports a severe allergic reaction to latex, vaccines supplied in vials or syringes containing natural rubber should not be administered unless the benefit of vaccination clearly outweighs the risk of an allergic reaction to the vaccine. For latex allergies other than anaphylactic allergies (e.g., a history of contact allergy to latex gloves), vaccines supplied in vials or syringes containing latex can be administered.[5]

Pregnancy

Inactivated influenza and tetanus, diphtheria, and pertussis (Tdap) vaccines are recommended during pregnancy. Live attenuated viral vaccines (e.g., MMR-II, Varivax, FluMist) are contraindicated during pregnancy because of the theoretical risk of virus transmission to the fetus. Sexually active females who receive MMR-II or Varivax should be instructed to practice careful contraception for 1 month following receipt of either vaccine. On theoretical grounds, inactivated poliovirus (IPV) vaccine should not be administered during pregnancy; however, it may be administered if the risk of exposure (e.g., during travel to endemic disease areas) is imminent and immediate protection is needed. HPV vaccine should not be administered to pregnant women. There is no recommendation to administer Hib vaccine (ActHIB, Hiberix, PedvaxHIB), pneumococcal conjugate vaccine (Prevnar 13), or serogroup B meningococcal vaccine (Bexsero, Trumenba) to a pregnant female. Hepatitis A vaccine (Havrix, Vaqta), hepatitis B vaccine (Engerix-B, Recombivax HB), and meningococcal conjugate vaccine (Menactra, Menveo) can be administered to a pregnant female in some circumstances. Data on the use of HepB-CpG (Heplisav-B), MenACWY-TT (MenQuadfi), and the pneumococcal polysaccharide (PPSV23 [Pneumovax 23]) vaccines during pregnancy are limited.[5] (See CDC guidance for vaccination during pregnancy: https://www.cdc.gov/vaccines/pregnancy/hcp-toolkit/guidelines.html/.)

Immunosuppression

Live attenuated vaccines can cause severe or fatal reactions in immunosuppressed persons due to uncontrolled replication of the vaccine virus. Live vaccines should usually not be administered to severely immunosuppressed persons with congenital immunodeficiency, leukemia, lymphoma, or generalized malignancy. However, persons with isolated B-cell deficiency may receive the varicella vaccine. In general, the provider treating an immunosuppressed patient should determine the severity of that patient's immunosuppression.[5]

Certain drugs can also cause immunosuppression. For instance, persons receiving cancer treatment with alkylating agents, antimetabolites, or radiation therapy should not receive live vaccines. Live vaccines can be administered after chemotherapy or radiation therapy has been discontinued for at least 3 months. In addition, persons receiving large doses of corticosteroids should not receive live vaccines. This includes persons receiving 20 mg or more of prednisone daily or 2 mg or more of prednisone per kilogram of body weight per day for 14 days or longer.[5]

The safety and efficacy of live attenuated vaccines administered concurrently with recombinant human immune mediators and immune modulators are not known. There is evidence that the use of therapeutic monoclonal antibodies, especially the anti–tumor necrosis factor agents (e.g., adalimumab, infliximab, etanercept, golimumab, and certolizumab pegol), may lead to reactivation of latent tuberculosis infection and disease. These agents might also predispose persons to other opportunistic infections. Because these drugs vary dramatically in the scope and number of immune-system-targeted components, it is prudent to avoid administering live attenuated vaccines while patients are taking these drugs. For vaccination against seasonal influenza, inactivated injectable alternatives are available.[5]

The time PCPs should wait to administer a live virus vaccine after immune modulator drugs have been discontinued is not specified by the ACIP or other authoritative guidelines. No basis exists for interpreting laboratory studies of immune parameters with vaccines' safety or efficacy. Lymphocyte-depleting agents such as alemtuzumab and rituximab may cause prolonged immunosuppression. Both inactivated and live vaccines should be withheld for at least 6 months following therapy with anti-B cell antibodies. Some experts recommend longer than 6 months following anti-B cell antibodies. The optimal time for restarting immunosuppressive therapy after vaccination with live vaccines has not been studied, but the Infectious Diseases Society of America (IDSA) recommends waiting at least 1 month. Consultation with the prescribing physician (and possibly a hospital pharmacist) is recommended for the management of individual patients and guidance in estimating a patient's degree of immunosuppression.[5]

Inactivated vaccines cannot replicate, so they are safe to use in immunosuppressed persons. Certain vaccines are recommended or specifically encouraged because immunosuppression is a risk factor for complications from certain vaccine-preventable diseases (i.e., influenza, invasive pneumococcal disease, invasive meningococcal disease, invasive Hib disease, and hepatitis B). However, because a relatively functional immune system is required to develop an immune response to a vaccine, the immune response may be poor, depending on the degree of immunosuppression present.[5]

Human Immunodeficiency Virus Infection

Persons infected with HIV may not manifest the disease, or they may be severely immunosuppressed. In general, the same vaccination recommendations apply to other types of immunosuppression. Live virus vaccines are usually contraindicated in those with severe immunosuppression, but inactivated vaccines may be administered if indicated. FluMist should not be administered, but an age-appropriate inactivated or recombinant influenza vaccine (RIV) should be administered.[5]

Hematopoietic Cell Transplant

Hematopoietic cell transplant (HCT) results in immunosuppression due to ablative therapy administered before the transplant and therapies to prevent or treat graft-versus-host disease. In addition, HCT recipients are at increased risk for vaccine-preventable diseases because antibody titers decline 1 to 4 years after HCT if the recipient is not revaccinated. HCT recipients at increased risk should be routinely vaccinated after HCT against tetanus, poliovirus, MMR, *Streptococcus pneumoniae*, and Hib, regardless of the source of the transplanted cells. MMR and varicella-containing vaccines should be administered 24 months after transplantation if the HCT recipient is presumed to be immunocompetent. Revaccination with inactivated vaccines, including influenza vaccine, should begin 6 months after HCT. However, the influenza vaccine may be administered as early as 4 months after HCT, if needed. Three doses of Prevnar 13 should be administered 3 to

6 months after HCT, followed by a dose of PPSV23. A dose of MenACWY should also be administered 6 months after HCT.[5]

Invalid Contraindications and Precautions to Vaccination

Sometimes certain conditions or circumstances are inappropriately considered to be contraindications or precautions to vaccination. Such conditions or circumstances are known as *invalid contraindications* and these misperceptions result in missed opportunities to administer needed vaccines. Some of the most common invalid contraindications are mild illnesses, pregnancy, breastfeeding, allergies that are not anaphylactic in nature, and certain aspects of the patient's family history.[5]

Mild Illness

Children with a mild acute illness, such as a low-grade fever, an upper respiratory infection (URI), otitis media, or mild diarrhea, should be vaccinated on schedule. A low-grade fever is not a contraindication to vaccination. Measuring temperature is not necessary before vaccination if the patient does not appear ill and does not report currently being ill. ACIP has not defined a body temperature above which vaccines should not be administered. The decision to vaccinate should be based on the overall evaluation of the child rather than an arbitrary body temperature.[5]

Nonanaphylactic Allergy

If an allergy to a vaccine component is not severe (e.g., is not anaphylaxis), it is not a contraindication to that vaccine. Only a severe allergic reaction (e.g., anaphylaxis) to a vaccine component is a true contraindication to vaccination.[5]

Allergy to Products Not Present in Vaccines

There is no contraindication or precaution for persons with nonspecific allergies, duck or feather allergies, or penicillin allergies, or for persons who have relatives with allergies or those taking allergy shots. Anyone with these allergies can and should be vaccinated. No vaccine available in the United States contains duck antigen or penicillin.[5]

Antimicrobial Therapy

Antimicrobials do not influence the immune response to most vaccines. However, antiviral drugs may affect vaccine replication in some circumstances. FluMist should not be administered until 48 hours after cessation of oseltamivir and zanamivir, 5 days after cessation of peramivir, and 17 days after baloxavir. If possible, antiviral drugs (acyclovir, famciclovir) that are active against herpes viruses should be discontinued 24 hours before the administration of a varicella-containing vaccine.[5]

Breastfeeding

Breastfeeding does not decrease the response to any routinely recommended childhood vaccine and is not a contraindication to vaccination. Breastfeeding also does not extend or improve the passive immunity to vaccine-preventable disease that is provided by maternal antibodies.[5]

Household Contacts of Pregnant or Immunosuppressed Persons

Being a household contact of a pregnant person or immunosuppressed person is usually not a contraindication to vaccination. It is critical that healthy household contacts of pregnant people and immunosuppressed people be vaccinated. Vaccination of healthy contacts reduces the chance that pregnant people and immuno-suppressed people will be exposed to vaccine-preventable diseases.

Most routinely recommended vaccines, including live vaccines (MMR-II, Varivax, RotaTeq/Rotarix, and FluMist), can be administered to persons who are household contacts of pregnant or immunosuppressed persons. If a varicella vaccine recipient has a rash after vaccination, direct contact with susceptible household contacts with altered immunocompetence should be avoided until the rash resolves. All members of the household should wash their hands after changing the diaper of an infant who received the RV. This minimizes rotavirus transmission, as shedding may occur up to 1 month after the last dose. FluMist should not be administered to close contacts and caregivers of severely immunosuppressed persons who require a protected environment.[5]

Preterm Birth

Vaccines should be started on a schedule based on the child's chronological age. Preterm infants have been shown to respond adequately to vaccines used in infancy. Studies demonstrate that decreased seroprotection rates might occur among infants with low birth weight (<2000 g) after the administration of the hepatitis B vaccine at birth. However, by the chronological age of 1 month, all preterm infants, regardless of initial birth weight or gestational age, are likely to respond as adequately as older and larger infants.[5]

Tuberculin Skin Test

Persons who need a tuberculin skin test (TST) can and should be vaccinated. All vaccines can be administered on the same day as a TST or at any time after a TST is administered. For most vaccines, there are no TST timing restrictions. An MMR-containing vaccine may decrease the response to a TST, potentially causing a false-negative response in someone who has a tuberculosis infection. MMR-II can be administered the same day as a TST, but if MMR-II has been administered and 1 or more days have elapsed, it is recommended in most situations to wait at least 4 weeks before administering a routine TST. There is no information available on the effect of varicella-containing vaccine or FluMist on a TST. Until such information is available, it is prudent to apply the same rules for spacing a measles-containing vaccine and TST to a varicella-containing vaccine and FluMist.[5] An interferon-gamma release assay (IGRA) tuberculosis test may be affected by live vaccines, so it is prudent to apply the same spacing rules as for TST and live vaccines.[5]

Screening for Contraindications and Precautions to Vaccination

The key to preventing serious adverse reactions after vaccination is effective screening. Every patient should be screened for contraindications and precautions before administering any vaccine dose. Effective screening can be accomplished by asking a few questions:

- Is the patient sick today?

  There is no evidence that acute illness reduces vaccine efficacy or increases vaccine adverse events. However, as a precaution, if there is a moderate or severe acute illness, all vaccines should be deferred until the illness has improved. Mild illnesses (such as otitis media, URIs, and diarrhea) are not contraindications or precautions to vaccination, and recommended vaccines should be administered on time.[5]

- Does the patient have allergies to medications, food, a vaccine component, or latex?

  It may be more efficient to inquire about allergies in a generic way (i.e., allergies to any food or medication) rather than to inquire about allergies to specific vaccine components. Most persons will not be familiar with minor components of vaccines, but they should know if they or their child have had an allergic reaction to a food or medication that was severe enough to require medical attention. If a person reports anaphylaxis after eating eggs, a specific protocol should be followed that includes determining the symptoms experienced.[5] For information on egg allergies and influenza vaccination, refer to the most recent ACIP influenza vaccination recommendations https://www.cdc.gov/flu/prevent/egg-allergies.htm#:~:text=For%20persons%20who%20report%20a,egg%20should%20receive%20influenza%20vaccine).

- Has the patient experienced any reaction after receiving a vaccination?

  A history of severe allergic reactions such as urticaria, wheezing or difficulty breathing, or circulatory collapse or shock (not fainting) following a previous dose of vaccine or to a vaccine component is a contraindication to further doses, however, it is extremely rare. A local adverse reaction (redness or swelling at the injection site) is not a contraindication to subsequent doses. Some reactions after vaccination (e.g., Arthus reactions after a previous dose of diphtheria toxoid-containing or tetanus toxoid-containing vaccine) are considered as precautions to receiving further vaccine doses. ACIP recommends for persons with a history of Arthus-type hypersensitivity reactions after a previous dose of tetanus or diphtheria toxoid-containing vaccines should defer vaccination until at least 10 years have elapsed since the last tetanus toxoid-containing vaccine. Usually, vaccines are deferred when a precaution is present. However, situations may arise when the benefit outweighs the risk (e.g., during a community pertussis outbreak).[5]

- Has the patient experienced a brain or other nervous system problem including seizures?

  Diphtheria-tetanus-acellular pertussis (DTaP) and Tdap are contraindicated for persons who have a history of encephalopathy not attributed to an identifiable cause within 7 days following DTaP, DTP, or Tdap vaccination. An unstable or progressive neurologic problem is a precaution for the use of DTaP and Tdap. Children with stable neurologic disorders (including seizures) unrelated to vaccination may be vaccinated as usual. A history of Guillain-Barré syndrome (GBS) is a precaution for tetanus toxoid-containing and influenza vaccines if it occurred within 6 weeks following a dose of the specific vaccine. A personal or family history of febrile or afebrile seizures is a precaution for ProQuad (MMRV) vaccine. Simultaneous administration of MMR-II and Varivax is not associated with an increased risk of fever or seizures and is therefore preferred to ProQuad in children aged 12 through 47 months.[5]

- Does the patient have a long-term health problem with heart, lung, kidney, or metabolic disease (e.g., diabetes), asthma, a blood disorder, no spleen, complement component deficiency, a cochlear implant, or a cerebrospinal fluid leak? Is the patient on long-term aspirin therapy?

  These conditions are contraindications or precautions to LAIV. Age-appropriate inactivated or RIV is preferred for patients with these conditions.[5]

- Does the patient have cancer, leukemia, HIV/AIDS, or any other immune system problem?

  Live virus vaccines (e.g., MMR-II, Varivax, MMRV, Rotarix and RotaTeq, and FluMist) are usually contraindicated in severely immunocompromised persons. However, there are exceptions to consider in consultation with the hematology/oncology or ID specialist. For example, MMR-II and Varivax are recommended for HIV-infected children who do not have evidence of severe immunosuppression.[5]

- Does the patient have a parent or sibling with an immune system problem?

  MMR, VAR, and MMRV vaccines should not be given to a person with a family history of congenital or hereditary immunodeficiency in first-degree relatives (i.e., parents, siblings) unless the immune competence of the potential vaccine recipient has been clinically substantiated or verified by a laboratory.[5]

- Has the patient taken medications that affect the immune system, such as prednisone, other steroids, or anticancer drugs; drugs for the treatment of rheumatoid arthritis, Crohn disease, or psoriasis? Has the patient had radiation treatment?

  Live virus vaccines (e.g., MMR-II, Varivax, FluMist) should be postponed until after chemotherapy or long-term, high-dose steroid therapy has ended.[5]

- Has the patient received a transfusion of blood or blood products, immune (gamma) globulin, or an antiviral drug in the past year?

  Certain live virus vaccines (i.e., MMR-II, ProQuad, and Varivax) may need to be deferred following the administration of blood products, depending on the type of blood product and the interval since the blood product was administered.[5]

- Is the person pregnant or is there a chance the person could become pregnant during the next month?

  Live virus vaccines (e.g., MMR-II, Varivax, FluMist) are contraindicated during pregnancy because of the theoretical risk of virus transmission to the fetus. Sexually active persons who receive MMR-II or Varivax should be instructed to practice careful contraception for 1 month following receipt of either vaccine. On theoretical grounds, inactivated poliovirus vaccine should not be administered during pregnancy; however, it may be administered if the risk of exposure (e.g., during travel to endemic disease areas) is imminent and immediate protection is needed. HPV vaccine should not be administered to pregnant persons. There is no recommendation to administer Hib vaccine (ActHIB, Hiberix, PedvaxHIB), or serogroup B meningococcal vaccine (Bexsero, Trumenba) to a pregnant person. Hepatitis A vaccine (Havrix, Vaqta), hepatitis B vaccine (Engerix-B, Recombivax HB), and meningococcal conjugate vaccine (Menactra, Menveo) should be administered to pregnant females if routinely recommended or indicated. Data on the use of HepB-CpG (Heplisav-B), MenACWY-TT (MenQuadfi), and the pneumococcal polysaccharide (Pneumovax 23) pneumococcal conjugate vaccine during pregnancy are limited.[5]

- Has the patient received vaccinations in the past 4 weeks?

A person who received either Flumist or a live injectable vaccine (e.g., MMR-II, Varivax) in the past 4 weeks should wait 28 days before receiving another live vaccine. Inactivated vaccines may be administered at the same time or at any time before or after a live vaccine.[5]

- For infants, has the patient ever had intussusception? Intussusception is a contraindication for the RV.[5]

  See the CDC guidelines regarding specific recommendations for contraindications (https://www.cdc.gov/vaccines/hcp/acip-recs/general-recs/contraindications.html).

Adverse Events Following Immunization and Assessment of Causality

An adverse event following immunization may or may not be related to the immunization. Further assessment is needed to determine if an adverse event is caused by a vaccine. A vaccine adverse reaction or side effect is an untoward effect caused by a vaccine.[6]

Adverse events following immunization can be classified by frequency (common, rare), extent (local, systemic), severity (mild, moderate, severe), seriousness (e.g., life-threatening, requiring hospitalization, or causing disability or death), causality, and preventability (intrinsic to the vaccine, production challenges, administration error). Adverse events following immunization may be coincidental, or the vaccine may have increased the risk of the adverse event. Many adverse events following vaccination are coincidental; they are temporally related to vaccination but occur by chance without a causal relationship.[6]

To assess the causality of an adverse event following immunization, a great deal of information is generally needed. An adverse health event can be causally attributed to a vaccine more readily under the following conditions:

- The health problem occurs during a plausible time period following vaccination.
- The adverse event corresponds to adverse events previously associated with the vaccine.
- The event is consistent with a specific clinical syndrome where the association with vaccination has strong biologic plausibility (e.g., anaphylaxis) or where the syndrome is known to occur following the natural disease.
- A laboratory result confirms the association (e.g., isolation of vaccine strain varicella virus from skin lesions of a patient with rash).
- The event recurs with readministration of the vaccine in the same patient.
- A controlled clinical trial or epidemiologic study shows a greater risk of a specific adverse event among vaccinated versus unvaccinated groups.
- A finding linking an adverse event to a vaccine has been confirmed by other studies.[6]

Importance of Vaccine Safety Programs

Like any medical product, no vaccine is completely without risk. While most vaccine adverse reactions are minor and self-limited, some vaccines have been associated with extremely rare but serious health effects. The following key considerations underscore the need for an active and ongoing vaccine safety program.[6]

Decreases in Disease Risks

Most vaccine-preventable diseases are at or near record lows. Many people no longer see reminders of the severity and potentially life-threatening complications of these diseases. Parents and providers in the United States may be more likely to know someone who has experienced an adverse event (an event that may or may not be related to vaccination) following vaccination than they are to know someone who has experienced a vaccine-preventable disease. The success of vaccination has led to increased public attention on potential health risks associated with vaccines.[6]

Public Confidence

Maintaining public confidence in vaccines is critical to prevent a decline in vaccination coverage that can result in outbreaks of disease. While most parents understand the benefits of vaccination and have their children vaccinated, some parents have concerns about the safety of vaccines. Despite high national vaccination coverage, there are local areas of low coverage that allow outbreaks of vaccine-preventable diseases to occur, often the result of parents refusing or delaying their children's vaccinations because of concerns about vaccine safety.[6]

A higher standard of safety is generally expected of vaccines than of other medical interventions because, in contrast to most pharmaceutical products that are administered to ill persons for treatment purposes, vaccines are generally administered to healthy persons to prevent disease. Public tolerance for adverse reactions related to products given to healthy persons, especially healthy infants, and children, is substantially less than for reactions to products administered to persons who are already sick. Less tolerance of risk associated with vaccines requires close monitoring and timely assessment of vaccine adverse events to help distinguish true vaccine adverse reactions from coincidental unrelated events and to help maintain public confidence in vaccination.[6] The federal government has several systems in place to ensure public confidence in vaccines.

Vaccine Adverse Event Reporting System

The National Childhood Vaccine Injury Act of 1986 mandates that vaccine providers and vaccine manufacturers report certain adverse events following vaccinations. This led to the creation of the Vaccine Adverse Event Reporting System (VAERS) in 1990. VAERS is a national, spontaneous surveillance system, jointly administered by CDC and the US Food and Drug Administration (FDA). It receives about 30,000 reports per year, a seemingly large number, but relatively small considering that millions of doses of vaccines are administered yearly to adults and children in the United States.[6]

Vaccine providers are required by law to report:
- Any adverse event listed by the vaccine manufacturer as a contraindication to further doses of the vaccine.
- Any adverse event listed in the VAERS Table of Reportable Events Following Vaccination https://vaers.hhs.gov/docs/VAERS_Table_of_Reportable_Events_Following_Vaccination.pdf

Vaccine providers are encouraged to report:
- Any adverse event that occurs after the administration of a US licensed vaccine, whether it is or is not clear a vaccine caused the adverse event.
- Vaccine administration errors.
  Vaccine manufacturers are required to report all adverse events that come to their attention.[6]

VAERS collects information about the patient, the vaccine(s) administered, the adverse event, and the person reporting the event. All reports are coded using the Medical Dictionary for Regulatory Activities (MedDRA) terms and entered into the VAERS database. Attempts are made to obtain additional medical information for all reports classified as a serious adverse event, including hospitalization or prolongation of hospitalization (if a vaccine

was administered in the hospital), life-threatening illness, permanent disability, congenital deformity, or death. For these reports, letters to obtain information about recovery status are also sent to the persons reporting the events. All patient-identifying information submitted to VAERS, directly or as part of follow-up activities, is protected by strict confidentiality requirements. VAERS has limitations inherent to spontaneous reporting systems.

Also, VAERS is not designed to determine if a vaccine caused an adverse event, and additional studies are required to confirm possible safety signals detected by VAERS. Despite these limitations, VAERS has been able to fulfill its primary purpose of detecting new or rare vaccine adverse events, increases in rates of known adverse reactions, and patient risk factors for types of adverse reactions. In addition, VAERS often provides early safety data after a vaccine is licensed or during a public health emergency.[6]

Vaccine Safety Datalink

CDC established the Vaccine Safety Datalink (VSD) to address gaps in the scientific knowledge of rare and serious adverse events following vaccination. This project involves partnerships with large, integrated health plans to monitor vaccine safety. Each participating plan uses its electronic health records and immunization information systems to contribute to a large, linked database. These participating health plans serve more than 10 million people annually, representing nearly 3% of the U.S. population, and contain records for more than 180 million vaccinations, enabling the VSD to study possible rare adverse events. The VSD allows for planned immunization safety studies, as well as timely investigations of hypotheses arising from reviews of medical literature, reports to VAERS, changes in immunization schedules, or the introduction of new vaccines.[6]

Clinical Immunization Safety Assessment Project

The Clinical Immunization Safety Assessment (CISA) Project's mission is to improve the understanding of adverse events following immunization at the individual patient level. The CISA Project provides consultation to public health partners in the United States and conducts high-quality clinical research, including clinical trials across life stages, on the safety of influenza vaccines and the safety of vaccines in special populations.[6]

Postlicensure Rapid Immunization Safety Monitoring System

FDA's Postlicensure Rapid Immunization Safety Monitoring System (PRISM) uses a computer algorithm to conduct active vaccine safety surveillance. A cooperative effort between FDA's Center for Biologics Evaluation and Research and four healthcare and medical insurance organizations, PRISM analyzes health insurance claims data for potential vaccine safety signals. PRISM is also used to evaluate safety issues in targeted groups and to evaluate specific health conditions or outcomes. PRISM is part of the FDA's Sentinel Initiative, a national electronic system for medical product safety surveillance.[6]

Vaccine Injury Compensation Program

The main impact of the National Childhood Vaccine Injury Act (NCVIA) was the creation of the Vaccine Injury Compensation Program (VICP). This program, administered by the Health

Resources and Services Administration, provides financial compensation to persons who are found to have been injured by a vaccine covered by the program. VICP provides liability protection for vaccine manufacturers and administrators. Compensation is provided to persons who experience certain vaccine adverse reactions on a no-fault basis. No fault means persons filing claims are not required to prove negligence on the part of either the healthcare provider or manufacturer to receive compensation. The program covers most vaccines routinely given in the United States. During the 2009 H1N1 influenza pandemic, the federal government implemented another compensation program, the Countermeasures Injury Compensation Program. This program provides compensation for certain persons who are seriously injured by countermeasures as specified in a declaration by the Secretary of the US Department of Health and Human Services. Both bioterrorism and pandemic countermeasures are covered.[6]

Benefit and Risk Communication

Patients and parents should be informed of the benefits and risks of vaccines in understandable language. An opportunity for questions should be provided before each vaccination. Discussion of the benefits and risks of vaccination is sound medical practice and is required by law. The NCVIA legally requires vaccine information statements (VISs) to be provided to the patient, parent, guardian, or legal representative by vaccine providers before each dose of vaccine. Documentation that the VIS was provided is also required. Copies of VISs are available from state and local immunization programs or can be downloaded. Translations of VISs into languages other than English are available from some immunization programs and from Immunize.org. Vaccine providers should anticipate questions parents or patients may have regarding the need for or safety of vaccination.

Some people may refuse certain vaccines or even reject all vaccinations. Some people might have religious or personal objections to vaccination. It is essential that PCPs have a basic understanding of how patients view vaccine risk and develop effective approaches to deal with vaccine safety concerns when they arise. When a parent or patient initiates a discussion of a vaccine concern, the provider should discuss the specific concern and use appropriate language to provide facts. Effective, empathic vaccine risk communication is essential in responding to misinformation and concerns. It is important to remind parents that state laws for school or childcare entry might require unvaccinated children to stay home from school during outbreaks. For patients who question or refuse vaccination, identifying common ground and discussing measures for deferring vaccination are more effective public health strategies than excluding these patients from a practice.[6]

Documentation of VISs distribution is required, and they provide an outline for discussing vaccine benefits and risks. Additional information about discussions should be documented in the patient's record, including the refusal to receive certain vaccines (i.e., informed refusal). Such documentation might reduce any potential liability if a vaccine-preventable disease occurs in the unvaccinated patient.[6]

Managing Adverse Reactions After Vaccination

PCPs should be familiar with identifying immediate-type allergic reactions, including anaphylaxis, and be competent in treating

these events at the time of vaccine administration. While severe allergic reactions to vaccines are rare, occurring at an approximate rate of 1 to 2 for every 1 million doses of vaccine administered, all vaccine providers should have emergency procedures in place and be prepared to provide emergency care for a person who experiences an anaphylactic reaction. This includes the ability to administer epinephrine and certification in cardiopulmonary resuscitation (CPR). Equipment for maintaining an airway should be available for immediate use. All healthcare personnel should be familiar with their office emergency plan.[6]

Vaccine Storage and Handling

Vaccine providers are responsible for proper vaccine storage, handling, and administration; timing and spacing of vaccine doses; observation of contraindications and precautions; and reporting of adverse events following vaccination to VAERS. Providers must discuss the vaccine benefits and risks and for management of vaccine adverse reactions with patients and parents. Vaccines need to be stored according to manufacturers' recommendations following CDC guidelines to prevent the loss of vaccines.[7] The CDC provides the Vaccine Storage and Handling Tool Kit to safely store vaccines (https://www.cdc.gov/vaccines/hcp/admin/storage/toolkit/index.html).

Vaccine Cold Chain

A cold chain is a temperature-controlled supply chain that includes all vaccine-related equipment and procedures. The cold chain begins with the cold storage unit at the manufacturing plant, extends to the transport and delivery of the vaccine and proper storage at the provider facility, and ends with the administration of the vaccine to the patient. Manufacturers, distributors, public health staff, and healthcare providers share the responsibility to ensure the vaccine cold chain is maintained from the time vaccines are manufactured until they are administered.[7]

Vaccine Storage and Handling Standard Operating Procedures

Facilities should develop and maintain clearly written, detailed, and up-to-date storage and handling standard operating procedures (SOPs). SOPs should be reviewed by all staff and updated by the vaccine coordinator annually.

SOPs should contain plans and information for three major areas:

- General information—include contact information for vaccine manufacturers, equipment service providers, and important facility staff, as well as job descriptions, regularly used forms, and staff training requirements.
- Routine storage and handling—include information for all aspects of vaccine inventory management, from ordering to monitoring expiration dates and storage conditions.
- Emergency vaccine storage, handling, and transport—outline steps to be taken in the event of equipment malfunctions, power failures, natural disasters, or other emergencies that might compromise vaccine storage conditions.[7]

Vaccine Administration

Vaccine administration is a key factor in ensuring vaccination is as safe and effective as possible. Administration involves a series of actions: assessing patient vaccination status and determining needed vaccines, screening for contraindications and precautions, educating patients, preparing, and administering vaccines properly, and documenting the vaccines administered. Professional standards for medication administration, manufacturer instructions, and organizational policies and procedures should always be followed.[8]

Assess for Needed Vaccines

The patient's immunization status should be reviewed at every healthcare visit. Using the patient's immunization history, PCPs should assess for all routinely recommended vaccines as well as any vaccines that are indicated based on existing medical condition(s), occupation, or other risk factors. To obtain a patient's immunization history, information from immunization information systems (IISs), current and historical medical records, and personal shot record cards may be used. In most cases, PCPs should only accept written, dated records as evidence of vaccination; however, self-reported doses of influenza vaccine or PPSV23 are acceptable. Missed opportunities to vaccinate should be avoided. If a documented immunization history is not available, administer the vaccines that are indicated based on the patient's age, medical condition(s), and other risk factors, such as planned travel.[8]

Screen for Contraindications and Precautions

Before administering any vaccine, patients should be screened for contraindications and precautions, even if the patient has previously received that vaccine. The patient's health condition or recommendations regarding contraindications and precautions for vaccination may change from one visit to the next. To assess patients correctly and consistently, PCPs should use a standardized, comprehensive screening tool. To save time, some facilities ask patients to answer screening questions before seeing the provider, either electronically via an online healthcare portal or on a paper form while in the waiting or examination room.[8] Immunize.org is an excellent source for screening tools for children, adolescents, and adults.

Educate Patients and/or Parents About Needed Vaccines

Vaccines are one of the safest and most effective ways to prevent diseases. All healthcare personnel, including nonclinical staff, play an important role in promoting vaccination and creating a culture of immunization within a clinical practice. Inconsistent messages from healthcare personnel about the need for and safety of vaccines may cause confusion about the importance of vaccines. Studies[9] show healthcare providers are the most trusted source of vaccine information. Research[10] also shows when a strong recommendation is given by a healthcare provider, a patient is 4 to 5 times more likely to be vaccinated. When providers use presumptive language to initiate vaccine discussions, significantly more parents choose to vaccinate their children, especially at first-time visits. Instead of asking "What do you want to do about shots today?", an approach using presumptive language would be to state "Your child needs three vaccines today." Some patients and parents may have questions or concerns about vaccination. This does not necessarily mean they will not accept vaccines. Sometimes they simply want to hear their provider's answers to their questions (Fig. 19.1).[8]

Aftercare Instructions

Patient and parent education should also include a discussion of comfort and care strategies after vaccination. After-care instructions should include information for dealing with common side effects such as injection site pain, fever, and fussiness (especially in infants) such as cold compresses. Instructions should also provide information about when to seek medical attention and when to notify the healthcare provider about concerns that arise following vaccination. After-care information can be given to patients or parents before vaccines are administered, leaving the parent free to comfort the child immediately after the injection. Pain relievers can be used to treat fever and injection-site pain that might occur after vaccination. In children and adolescents, a non–aspirin-containing pain reliever should be used. Aspirin is not recommended for children and adolescents.[8] Immunize.org has excellent 'After the Shots' patient/parent handouts.

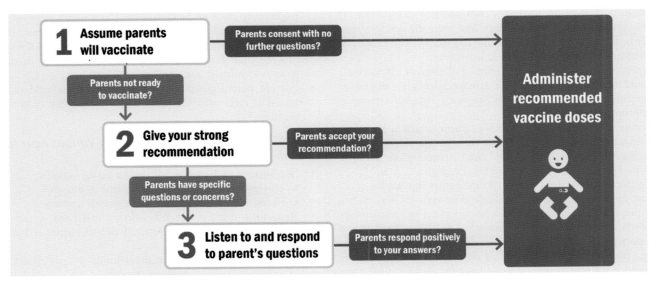

• **Fig 19.1** Talking With Parents About Vaccines for Infants. (Courtesy Centers for Disease Control and Prevention. https://www.cdc.gov/vaccines/pubs/pinkbook/vac-admin.html.)

Vaccine Administration Safety

Occupational Safety and Health Administration (OSHA) regulations have not typically required gloves to be worn when administering vaccines unless the person administering the vaccine is likely to come in contact with potentially infectious body fluids or has open lesions on the hands. In the setting of the COVID-19 pandemic, gloves should be worn when administering intranasal or oral vaccines. If gloves are worn, they should be changed, and hand hygiene should be performed between patients.[8]

Several critical factors are indicated for vaccine preparation and administration. All indicators must be carefully followed to ensure safe and appropriate immunizations.

- Ensure that the vaccine and diluent (if needed) are corrected. Reconstitution is the process of adding a diluent to a dry ingredient to make it a liquid. Lyophilized vaccine (powder or pellet form) and its diluent are packaged together from the manufacturer. Vaccines should be reconstituted according to manufacturer guidelines using only the diluent supplied for a specific vaccine. Diluents vary in volume and composition and are specifically designed to meet the volume, pH balance, and chemical requirements of their corresponding vaccines. A different diluent, a stock vial of sterile water, or normal saline should never be used to reconstitute vaccines. If the wrong diluent is used, the vaccine dose is not valid and must be repeated using the correct diluent. Vaccines should be reconstituted just before administering by following the instructions in the vaccine package insert.
- Once reconstituted, the vaccine should be administered within the time frame specified for use in the manufacturer's package insert; otherwise, the vaccine should be discarded. Changing the needle between preparing and administering the vaccine is not necessary unless the needle is contaminated or damaged.
- Confirm that the expiration date has not passed. An expired vaccine or diluent should never be used. Determining when a vaccine or diluent expires is an essential step in the vaccine preparation process. The expiration date printed on the vial or box should be checked before preparing the vaccine. When the expiration date has only a month and a year, the product may be used up to and including the last day of that month unless the vaccine was contaminated or compromised in some way. If a day is included with the month and year, the product may only be used through the end of that day unless the vaccine was contaminated or compromised in some way.
- Inspect the vaccine. Each vaccine and diluent (if needed) should be carefully inspected for damage, particulate matter, or contamination before use. Verify the vaccine has been stored at the proper temperatures.
- Vaccines should be drawn just before administration. However, while manufacturer-filled syringes are recommended for large vaccination clinics, there may be rare instances when the only option is to predraw vaccines for off-site clinics.
- In general, administer the oral vaccine before injectables.
- Most vaccines are available in single-dose vials (SDVs). SDVs do not contain preservatives to help prevent microorganism growth. Therefore vaccines packaged as SDVs are intended to be punctured once for use in one patient and for one injection. Even if the SDV appears to contain more vaccine than is needed for one patient, it should not be used for more than one patient. Once the appropriate dosage has been withdrawn, the vial and any leftover contents should be discarded

appropriately. SDVs with any leftover vaccine should never be saved to combine leftover contents for later use.
- Manufacturer-filled syringes (MFSs) are prepared with a single dose of vaccine and sealed under sterile conditions by the manufacturer. Like SDVs, MFSs do not contain a preservative to help prevent the growth of microorganisms. MFSs are intended for one patient for one injection. Once the sterile seal has been broken, the vaccine should be used or discarded by the end of the workday.
- Multidose vials (MDVs) contain more than one dose of vaccine. MDVs are labeled by the manufacturer and typically contain an antimicrobial preservative to help prevent the growth of microorganisms. Because MDVs contain a preservative, they can be punctured more than once. Only the number of doses indicated in the manufacturer's package insert should be withdrawn from the vial. Partial doses from two or more vials should never be combined to obtain a dose of vaccine.
- An oral applicator is for use with oral vaccines and contains only one dose of medication. Oral vaccines do not contain a preservative. RV is administered using an oral applicator.
- Intranasal sprayer (nasal sprayer) is used for the LAIV.
- A separate needle and syringe must be used for each vaccine administered. Vaccines should be drawn just before administration. However, while MFSs are recommended for large vaccination clinics, there may be rare instances when the only option is to predraw vaccines for off-site clinics.
- In some instances, a vaccine must be used by a date earlier than the expiration date on the label. This time frame is referred to as the *beyond use date* (BUD). The BUD supersedes but should never exceed the manufacturer's expiration date. Vaccines should not be used after the BUD. The BUD should be noted on the label, along with the initials of the person making the calculation.
- If multiple vaccines are administered at a single visit, administer each preparation at a different anatomic site. Separate all vaccines given in the same limb by at least 1 inch.[8]
- Follow age-appropriate positioning best practices. Parent participation has been shown to increase a child's comfort and reduce the child's perception of pain. Holding infants during vaccination reduces acute distress. A parent's embrace during vaccination offers several benefits. A comforting hold avoids frightening children by embracing them rather than overpowering them. It allows the healthcare professional steady control of the limb and the injection site. It prevents children from moving their arms and legs during injections. It encourages parents to nurture and comfort their children.
- Provide parent/guardian with a copy of the updated shot record at each visit. This can be a written record or computer printout.[8]

Needle Lengths and Injection Sites for Various Ages for Intramuscular Injections

- Newborn: ⅝ to 1-inch needle in the vastus lateralis
  - If ⅝ inch needle is used, do not bunch muscle
- 1–36 months: 1-inch needle in the vastus lateralis
- 36 months–6 years: 1-inch needle in the deltoid
  - Vastus lateralis is the preferred site (decreases redness and swelling)
- 3–10 years: 1-inch needle in the deltoid
- 11–21 years: 1-inch needle in the deltoid
  - If the vastus lateralis is used, a 1.5-inch needle may be needed[11]

Needle Lengths and Injection Sites for Various Ages for Subcutaneous Injections

- Anterolateral thigh is recommended for subcutaneous (SC) vaccines for infants until at least age 12 months.
- Deltoid ⅝ inch needle is recommended for all ages >12 months, using a 45-degree angle.[11]

Pain Relief for Vaccines

Vaccinations are the most common source of procedural pain for healthy children and can be a stressful experience for persons of any age. It has been estimated that up to 25% of adults have a fear of needles, with most needle fears developing during childhood. If not addressed, these fears can have long-term effects such as preprocedural anxiety and avoidance of needed health care throughout a person's lifetime. Fear of injections and needlestick pain are often cited as reasons why children and adults refuse vaccines.[8]

Several techniques can be employed to decrease injection pain. Breastfeed children 2 years of age and younger while vaccines are administered. Give a sweet-tasting fluid such as sucrose to children who are not breastfed. Offer topical analgesics and pain relievers. These medications must be applied either before the child leaves home or while the child is waiting in the waiting room. Inject vaccines quickly and administer vaccines that cause the most pain last such as HPV and MMR.[8] Forms of distraction such as blowing bubbles or watching videos can also be employed.[12]

Managing Acute Reactions After Vaccination

Severe, life-threatening anaphylactic reactions following vaccination are rare. Potential life-threatening adverse reactions that can occur immediately after vaccination are severe allergic reactions and syncope (fainting). Symptoms of immediate-type allergic reactions can include local or generalized urticaria (hives), angioedema, respiratory compromise due to wheezing or swelling of the throat, hypotension, and shock. All vaccine providers should be certified in CPR and be skilled in administering epinephrine. Equipment needed for maintaining an airway should be available for immediate use and the provider should be skilled in using the equipment.[8]

All PCPs who administer vaccines to older children, adolescents, and adults should be aware of the potential for syncope after vaccination and the related risk of injury caused by falls. Appropriate measures should be taken to prevent injuries if a patient becomes weak or dizzy or loses consciousness. Have the patient seated or lying down for vaccination. Be aware of symptoms that precede fainting (e.g., weakness, dizziness, pallor). Provide supportive care and take appropriate measures to prevent injuries if such symptoms occur. Strongly consider observing patients (seated or lying down) for 15 minutes after vaccination to decrease the risk of injury should they faint.[8]

Documenting Immunizations

Accurate and timely documentation can help prevent administration errors and curtail the number and cost of excess vaccine doses. Date of administration, vaccine manufacturer, vaccine lot number, name and title of the person who administered the vaccine, the address of the facility where the permanent record will reside, edition date of the VIS distributed, and the date it was provided to the patient, and the route, dosage, and site all must be documented in the patient's permanent record. Any adverse events after vaccination and any serologic test results related to vaccine-preventable diseases must also be noted. It is also important to document when parents refuse vaccines despite the vaccine provider's recommendation.[8]

Inactivated Vaccines

DTaP Vaccines for Ages 6 Weeks to 6 Years

The only effective prevention of DTP is vaccination, and the vaccines are inactivated. DTaP vaccine is indicated for children ages 6 weeks to 6 years. The routine schedule is a primary series of 3 doses at ages 2, 4, and 6 months, a booster dose between ages 15 through 18 months, and another booster dose between ages 4 through 6 years (a total of 5 doses). See the footnotes on the current ACIP schedule for full dosing and spacing instructions. Infanrix and Daptacel are the single antigen brand names, and although there is a preference for using the same brand for all doses, interchanging is acceptable. If a child has a valid contraindication to the pertussis vaccine, DT should be used to complete the vaccination series. Several tetanus, diphtheria, and pertussis-containing combination vaccines are available for children 6 weeks to 6 years of age. Refer to the current ACIP vaccine schedule footnotes for DTaP for use of these combination vaccines: Pediarix, Pentacel, Daptacel, Quadracel, Vaxelis, and Kinrix. Precautions for any pertussis-containing vaccine include fever 40.5°C (105°F) or higher within 48 hours, continuous inconsolable crying lasting >3 hours within 48 hours, pale or limp episodes or collapse within 48 hours, or seizure within 3 days of dose. Delay administration until moderate to severe febrile illness is resolved. Pertussis-containing vaccine should be deferred for children with a progressive neurologic problem until the condition is stable. Contraindications for any pertussis-containing vaccine are previous encephalopathy within 7 days after DTaP and/or a progressive neurologic disorder (e.g., epilepsy). All DTP vaccines are administered as IM injection.[13]

Diphtheria Tetanus Pertussis Vaccines for Ages 7 Years Through Adulthood

Tdap (Boostrix and Adacel) vaccines are approved for booster doses for persons who have completed the recommended childhood DTP/DTaP vaccination series. A Tdap dose for tetanus prophylaxis is indicated for wound management if at least 5 years have elapsed since the last dose of the tetanus-containing vaccine. Both Tdap vaccines are approved for use in persons 7 years or older. A single Tdap dose is recommended for adolescents 11 through 18 years of age who have completed the recommended childhood DTP/DTaP vaccination series, preferably at ages 11 through 12 years. Individuals who do not have documentation of at least 3 doses of DTaP should receive a series of 3 doses of tetanus- and diphtheria-containing vaccines. One of these doses, preferably the first, should be Tdap. The remaining 2 doses should be either Td or Tdap. To reduce the burden of pertussis in infants, a dose of Tdap has been recommended during each pregnancy since 2012, although this practice is an off-label use. For persons 7 to 9 years of age who receive a dose of Tdap as part of the catch-up series, an adolescent Tdap dose should be administered at 11 through 12 years of age. If a Tdap dose is administered at age 10 years or older, the Tdap dose may count as the adolescent Tdap dose. Td brand names are Tenivac and Tdvax and they can be used interchangeably. After receipt of Tdap, persons should continue to receive a dose of Td or Tdap for routine booster immunization against tetanus and diphtheria with a preference for Tdap. GBS occurring 6 weeks or less after a previous dose of a tetanus toxoid-containing vaccine is a precaution for tetanus toxoid-containing vaccines. Any DTaP or Tdap vaccine can cause redness or swelling at the site or fever. These symptoms can be managed with cool compresses and acetaminophen.[13] Arthus reactions (whole limb swelling) can also occur following immunization but are not common and are not allergic reactions.[14]

Polio Vaccine

The only effective prevention for poliomyelitis is vaccination. The United States has been polio-free since 1979. In 1999 the ACIP recommended an all inactivated polio vaccine (IPV) schedule to eliminate the risk of vaccine-preventable polio. The first dose of IPV vaccine may be administered as early as age 6 weeks but is usually administered at age 2 months, with a second dose at age 4 months. The third dose should be given at ages 6 through 18 months of age. The recommended interval between the doses in the primary series is 2 months. However, if accelerated protection is needed, the minimum interval between each of the first 3 doses of IPV vaccine is 4 weeks. The final dose in the IPV series should be administered at age 4 through 6 years and at least 6 months after the previous dose. A dose of IPV vaccine on or after age 4 years is recommended (regardless of the number of previous doses). IPV is contraindicated if there is an allergy to any component of the vaccine, which may include neomycin, streptomycin, or polymixin B and is very rare. The polio vaccine is administered either SC or IM. The precaution is a moderate or severe illness.[15]

Haemophilus Influenzae Vaccine

Hib disease was the leading cause of meningitis in children under 5 years of age until the introduction of the vaccine. The only prevention is vaccination. The vaccine is inactivated, with a number of doses dependent on the brand administered, and the Hib component is contained in some combination vaccines. Hib vaccine is not given to children 5 years or older. Three monovalent Hib polysaccharide-protein conjugate vaccines (ActHIB, PedvaxHIB, and Hiberix) are currently licensed for use in the United States. Pentacel and Vaxelis are Hib-containing combination vaccines. Consult the current ACIP schedule for dosing schedules and indications. The contraindication includes an allergic reaction to any component of the vaccine and is very rare. Precautions include a moderate or severe acute illness.[16]

Hepatitis B Vaccine

Hepatitis B disease is a leading cause of cirrhosis, liver cancer, and death. Before the introduction of the vaccine, the only prevention was hand washing, avoidance of blood and body fluids, and immune globulin. Hepatitis B vaccination is recommended for all medically stable infants weighing at least 2000 g within 24 hours of birth. Only single-component vaccines should be used for the birth dose and doses administered before age 6 weeks. Single-component vaccines are Engerix-b and Recombivax HB. The usual schedule is 0, 1 through 2, and 6 through 18 months. The hepatitis B vaccine is inactivated and is given IM. The final

dose should be administered no earlier than the 6-month birthday. Hepatitis B is included in Pediatrix and Vaxelis. See the ACIP schedule for use and indications for the combination vaccines. If the mother is hepatitis B+ (Hep Bs Ag+), the neonate must receive Hep B vaccine within 12 hours of life and hepatitis B immune globulin. The second dose is given at age 1 to 2 months and third dose completes the series at age 6 months with serology testing at age 9 months. The hepatitis B vaccine is a component in the combination vaccines Pediarix and Vaxelis. See the ACIP immunization schedule for indications and schedules for these vaccines. All children and adolescents who did not receive the hepatitis B vaccine as infants should receive the vaccine following the 0-, 1-, and 6-month schedule. Recombivax and Engerix-B are single antigens. The contraindication is an allergy to the vaccine, which is very rare. A moderate or severe illness is a precaution.[17]

Hepatitis A Vaccine

In the prevaccine era, the primary methods used for preventing hepatitis A were hand washing and passive protection with immune globulin. Before 2004, hepatitis A was the most frequently reported type of hepatitis in the United States. Single-antigen HepA vaccines (Havrix and Vaqta) are available in pediatric and adult formulations and is an inactivated vaccine. HepA-HepB (Twinrix) is licensed for persons 18 years of age or older and administered as a 3-dose series at 0, 1, and 6 months. Routine HepA vaccine is given at 12 months and 18 months of age OR 2 doses, 6 months apart for all other age groups as catch-up. If children are traveling to high-risk areas the vaccine can be administered at 6 months of age or older. Revaccination would then be required once the child was 12 months of age with 2 doses separated by 6 months. The contraindication is an allergy to the vaccine, which is very rare. The precaution is a moderate or severe illness.[18]

Pneumococcal Vaccine

With the decline of invasive Hib disease, *S. pneumoniae* has become the leading cause of bacterial meningitis among children younger than age 5 years in the United States. All children 2 through 59 months of age should routinely receive a three-dose primary series of PCV13 at age 2, 4, and 6 months, and dose 4 (booster) at age 12 through 15 months. It is an inactivated conjugated vaccine. Unvaccinated children 7 months or older do not require a full series of four doses. The number of doses depends on the child's current age and the age at which the first dose of PCV13 was administered. See the footnotes on the current ACIP schedule for the appropriate number of doses and spacing. Children 2 years of age or older with certain conditions should receive both PCV13 and PPSV23, or PPSV23 alone (Box 19.1). PPSV23 is not recommended for children younger than age 2 years. Children who have a condition for which PCV13 is indicated should receive PCV13 first, followed by PPSV23 at least 8 weeks later.[19] The recently licensed PCV15 may be used as an option to PCV13 for children aged <19 years according to currently recommended PCV13 dosing and schedules.[20] The contraindication is a severe allergic reaction to a vaccine component or following a prior dose, which is very rare. The precaution is moderate to severe illnesses. Local reactions of redness and swelling are common and can be managed with cool compresses.[19]

Human Papillomavirus Vaccine

HPV is the most common sexually transmitted infection in the United States.[21] Although the majority of HPV infections are asymptomatic and resolve spontaneously, persistent infections can develop into anogenital warts, precancers, and cervical, anogenital, or oropharyngeal cancers in women and men. HPV vaccine prevents the two most common strains, HPV types 16 and 18, in addition to five additional high-risk types and types 6 and 11, which cause warts. HPV vaccine should be initiated at age 9 to 11 years with catch-up for all older adolescents and young adults through 26 years of age. Younger-aged children have the most robust immune response. The schedule for ages 9 to 14 at initiation is a two-dose series at 0 and 6 months. If the vaccine is started at age 15 years and older at initiation, the schedule is a three-dose series at 0, 1 to 2 months, and 6 months. Immune-compromised individuals should receive the three-dose series. The contraindication is a severe allergic reaction to a vaccine component or following a prior dose or history of immediate hypersensitivity to yeast. Pregnant people should not receive the vaccine, but there have been no documented birth defects related to accidental administration. Moderate or severe illness is a precaution. Local reactions of redness and swelling are common and can be managed with cool compresses.[22]

Meningococcal Vaccines

Serogroups B and C are the major causes of meningococcal disease in the United States, each being responsible for approximately 25% to 40% of cases; serogroups W and Y, along with non groupable meningococci, are each responsible for another 5% to 15%.[23] The proportion of cases caused by each serogroup varies by age group. Approximately 60% of disease among children and young adults under 24 years of age is caused by serogroup B.[23] In particular, among individuals 18 to 24 years of age, college students have more than 3 times the risk of serogroup B meningococcal disease as similarly aged individuals. Before vaccination, there was no effective prevention. Three quadrivalent meningococcal conjugate vaccines are licensed for use in the United States: MenACWY-D (Menactra), MenACWY-CRM (Menveo), and MenACWY-TT (MenQuadfi). Menactra is approved for use in persons ages 9 months through 55 years, Menveo is approved for use in persons ages 2 months through 55 years, and MenQuadfi is approved for use in persons ages 2 years or older. All are administered IM. Routine dosing is at 11 years of age with a booster at age 16 years. See the current ACIP schedule for specific recommendations for each brand of vaccine and for indicated high-risk conditions. Contraindication is a severe allergic reaction to the vaccine or to any component. The precaution is a moderate or severe illness.[24] Redness and swelling can follow immunization and can be managed with cool compresses and acetaminophen.

Two recombinant serogroup B meningococcal (MenB) vaccines are licensed for use in the United States: MenB-FHbp (Trumenba) and MenB-4C (Bexsero). See the current ACIP schedule for high-risk conditions. These vaccines are not interchangeable, and the series must be restarted if the brand of vaccine used for the previous dose is not available. Adolescents 16 through 23 years of age can receive the MenB vaccine for short-term protection against most strains of serogroup B meningococcal disease based on shared clinical decision-making. The preferred age for vaccination is 16 through 18 years of age. The vaccines are contraindicated if there has been a severe allergic reaction to either the vaccine or a component and such reactions are very rare. See the footnotes on the current ACIP schedule for details. Moderate or severe acute illness are precautions along with latex sensitivity (Bexsero only).[24]

Dengue Vaccine

Dengue is common in the US territories of American Samoa, Puerto Rico, and the US Virgin Islands, and the freely associated states, including the Federated States of Micronesia, the Republic of Marshall Islands, and the Republic of Palau. For this reason, ACIP has added the Dengue vaccine (Dengvaxia) to the ACIP annual schedule. Contraindications include children under 9 years of age since these children are less likely to have had a prior dengue infection, people over 16 years of age because there is not enough data to show how well the vaccine works in that population, children who have not had a prior dengue infection, children with weakened immune systems (immunocompromised), children who have had a severe (life-threatening) allergic reaction to a previous dose of the vaccine, children who have a severe (life-threatening) allergy to any ingredient in this vaccine, travelers and nonresidents of areas where dengue is common since the FDA has not approved dengue vaccine for use in travelers. Dengue vaccine is administered subcutaneously at 0, 6, and 12 months. The most common side effects are soreness, itchiness, or pain in the injection site, headaches, lack of energy, and general discomfort. Syncope is a precaution since recent data suggest that adolescents are more likely to experience syncope following vaccination.[25]

Inactivated and Live Vaccines

Influenza Vaccine

Influenza vaccine composition is reviewed and updated each year since the influenza virus is constantly changing. Considerations include which influenza viruses are causing illness, the extent to which viruses are spreading, and how well the previous season's vaccine protects against those viruses. Three types of influenza vaccine are available in the United States: inactivated influenza vaccine (IIV), LAIV, and RIV. The trivalent vaccine contains three inactivated viruses: type A(H1N1), type A(H3N2), and type B. Quadrivalent influenza vaccines were first introduced during the 2013 to 2014 season. They contain the same antigens as trivalent vaccines, with an additional type B strain. Influenza vaccination is recommended annually for persons 6 months of age and older who do not have contraindications. Vaccination is particularly important for persons at increased risk for severe illness and complications from influenza. All influenza vaccines, with the exception of LAIV, are administered IM. LAIV is administered via the intranasal route. Persons 9 years of age or older should receive 1 dose of a licensed age-appropriate vaccine each influenza season. Children 6 months through 8 years of age who do not have documentation showing receipt of 2 or more doses of any influenza vaccine before July 1 should receive 2 doses of a licensed age-appropriate vaccine. The purpose of the initial two-dose series is to prime the immune system in vaccine-naive infants. This two-dose series should be administered at least 4 weeks apart. The contraindication to any formulation of influenza vaccine is severe allergy following a previous dose. Moderate or severe acute illness and a history of GBS within 6 weeks of receipt of the influenza vaccine are the precautions.[26] See the footnotes for the influenza vaccine on the current ACIP Immunization schedule. Local reactions of redness and swelling are common and can be managed with cool compresses.[26]

Live Attenuated Vaccines

Rotavirus Vaccine

In the prevaccine era, the majority of children were infected by 5 years of age, and rotavirus was responsible for up to 500,000 deaths among children annually worldwide.[27] The RV is a live oral vaccine. It is routinely recommended for infants. ACIP developed age recommendations that vary from those of the manufacturers. The vaccine should be administered orally as a series of either 2 doses (at age 2 and 4 months) for the RV1 vaccine or 3 doses (at age 2, 4, and 6 months) for the RV5 vaccine. The vaccination series for both vaccines may be started as early as age 6 weeks. This is an off-label recommendation for both vaccines because the labeled maximum age for the RV1 vaccine is 24 weeks, and the labeled maximum age for the RV5 vaccine is 32 weeks. Do not start the series on or after 15 weeks, 0 days. The maximum age for the final dose is 8 months, 0 days. If any dose in the series was RV5 vaccine or the vaccine brand used for any prior dose in the series is not known, a total of 3 doses of RV should be administered. Contraindications include hypersensitivity/allergic reaction, severe combined immunodeficiency syndrome, history of intussusception, and latex allergy (stopper contains latex). Spina bifida or bladder exstrophy are precautions for Rotarix (RV1) but not for RotaTeq (RV5) vaccine. Additional precautions are moderate or severe acute illnesses, including gastroenteritis (defer until symptoms improve), and altered immunocompetence. Limited data do not indicate a different safety profile in HIV-infected versus HIV-uninfected infants, or with chronic gastrointestinal disease (data regarding the safety of the RV for infants with preexisting chronic gastrointestinal conditions are lacking).[28]

Measles Mumps and Rubella Vaccines

Before a vaccine was available, infection with the measles virus was nearly universal during childhood, and more than 90% of persons were immune due to past infection by age 15 years.[29] Measles is still a common and often fatal disease in developing countries. In the United States, there have been recent outbreaks; the largest occurring in 2019 primarily among people who were not vaccinated.[30] A successful mumps vaccination program in the United States led to a greater than 99% reduction in the number of mumps cases reported annually. However, starting in 2006, there has been an increase in mumps cases and outbreaks, particularly in close-contact settings, with many occurring among fully vaccinated persons. Mumps is a weaker vaccine and when a case of mumps enters the community, the risk of vaccine breakthrough rises.[31] Rubella used to be a worldwide infection. Due to the vaccine, endemic rubella and congenital rubella syndrome were eliminated in the United States in 2004 and in the region of the Americas in 2009.[32] The MMR vaccine is a live attenuated vaccine and is administered by the SC route. All three antigens are contained in the same vaccine presentation in the United States. There is no single antigen for any of these antigens. A new MMR vaccine, Priorix, was recently licensed and ACIP has determined that it is generically equivalent to the current brand MMR-II and is interchangeable.[20] MMR is a two-dose series administered at ages 12 months and 4 years. MMR can be given at age 6 months for children who are traveling to endemic areas. These children then need to repeat the dose on or after age 12 months and complete the series at age 4 years. Refer to the current ACIP schedule for information on catch-up schedules. ProQuad MMRV can be administered when both MMR and VAR are indicated. CDC expresses a preference for separate MMR and VAR for infants because of the increased risk of fevers and the potential for accompanying febrile seizures. Adverse reactions include fever, rash, seizure due to fever, encephalopathy (primarily in immune-compromised individuals), thrombocytopenia, arthralgias, and very rarely anaphylaxis. The most common are fever and rash while adolescents and adults are more likely to develop arthralgias. Contraindications are severe allergic reaction to a vaccine component or following a prior dose, severe immunocompromise, systemic high-dose corticosteroid therapy for 14 days or more, HIV infection regardless of immunocompetence status (MMRV only), family history of congenital or heredity immunodeficiency in first-degree relatives, and pregnancy. Precautions include moderate or severe acute illness, alpha-gal allergy (consult with a physician), receipt of antibody-containing blood products (wait for 3–11 months to vaccinate), history of thrombocytopenic purpura or thrombocytopenia, need for TST or interferon-gamma release assay testing. MMR-II vaccine should be administered to persons who are not severely immunocompromised. Please see the current CDC schedule footnotes for specific information regarding CD4$^+$ counts under Special Conditions. Simultaneous use of aspirin or aspirin-containing products, personal or family history of seizures of any etiology, and receipt of specific antiviral drugs 24 hours before vaccination are precautions only for MMRV.[30]

Varicella Vaccine

The incidence of varicella, as well as varicella-related hospitalizations, has decreased significantly since the implementation of the national varicella vaccination program in 1995. Varicella infections are generally not life-threatening and the clinical course in healthy children is generally mild with fever (up to 102°F) and other systemic symptoms (e.g., malaise, headache). The infection usually resolves within 2 to 4 days after the onset of the rash. The symptoms are nonetheless very uncomfortable for those affected and severe complications can occur. Varicella is no longer a "rite of passage" for children thanks to the vaccine. VAR (Varivax) is a live virus vaccine and is administered as a two-dose series at ages 12 to 15 months and 4 years and administered SC. See the current ACIP schedule footnotes for catch-up and scheduling information. Adverse reactions include fever, rash, seizure due to fever, encephalopathy (rare), and thrombocytopenia. Contraindications are high-dose/long-term corticosteroids, chemotherapy, severe allergic reaction to a vaccine component or following a prior dose, immunosuppression due to leukemia, lymphoma, generalized malignancy, immune deficiency disease, or immunosuppressive therapy family history of congenital or heredity immunodeficiency in first-degree relatives, HCT (wait 24 months), pregnancy, and HIV infection (only for MMRV, contraindicated for MMRV and for VAR depending on CD4 count).[33]

mRNA Vaccines

COVID-19 Vaccine

The COVID-19 pandemic has caused the loss of over 1 million American lives.[34] Since the advent of the COVID-19 vaccine, case counts have drastically reduced infections in the United States. COVID-19 vaccines for children and adolescents are mRNA vaccines that are designed to provoke the body to remember the antigen and mount an immune response to the spike protein when it is encountered. While the vaccines may be new, the technology has been available for over 10 years. COVID-19 vaccines by Pfizer and BioNTech are now recommended for all children beginning at 6 months of age under an Emergency Use Authorization and are administered IM. The doses vary in both vaccines for the age of children. Consult the CDC immunization website (www.cdc.gov/vaccines) for the latest updates regarding dosage and administration of the vaccine. Vaccine side effects include pain, redness, and swelling at the injection site. Additional side effects may include tiredness, headache, muscle pain and chills, fever, and nausea. Children 3 years and younger can also experience enlarged lymph nodes, irritability, crying, sleepiness, and loss of appetite. Contraindications are a history of a severe allergic reaction (e.g., anaphylaxis) after a previous dose or to a component of the COVID-19 vaccine and a history of a known diagnosed allergy to a component of the COVID-19 vaccine.[35] Rare cases of myocarditis or pericarditis are identified as side effects following mRNA COVID-19 vaccines. This reaction has occurred most frequently in adolescent and young adult males within the first week after receiving the second dose of an mRNA COVID-19 vaccine.[36]

Additional Resources

ACIP schedules: https://www.cdc.gov/vaccines/schedules/hcp/imz/child-adolescent.html.

CDC mobile app: https://www.cdc.gov/digital-social-media-tools/mobile/applications/cdcgeneral/promos/cdcmobileapp.html.

CDC National Center for Immunizations and Respiratory Diseases (NCIRD): http://cdc.gov/vaccines

CDC Vaccine Schedule app: https://www.cdc.gov/vaccines/schedules/hcp/schedule-app.html

Children's Hospital of Philadelphia Vaccine Education Center: http://chop.edu/centers-programs/vaccine-education-center

Families Fighting Flu: http://familiesfightingflu.org

Immunize.org: http://www.immunize.org
- https://www.immunize.org/standing-orders
- www.vaccineinformation.org

National Adult Influenza Immunization Summit: www.izsummitpartners.org

National Network of Immunization Coalitions: www.izcoalitions.org

Nurses Who Vaccinate: http://nurseswhovaccinate.org

Vaccinate Your Family: http://vaccinateyourfamily.org

Voices for Vaccines: http://voicesforvaccines.org

References

1. CDC. Ten Great Public Health Achievements—United States, 1900-1999. *MMWR (Morb Mortal Wkly Rep)*. 1999;48(12):241–243. https://www.cdc.gov/mmwr/preview/mmwrhtml/00056796.htm.
2. Ozawa S, Mirelman A, Stack ML, Walker DG, Levine OS. Cost-effectiveness and economic benefits of vaccines in low- and middle-income countries: a systematic review. *Vaccine*. 2012;31(Issue 1):96–108. https://www.sciencedirect.com/science/article/pii/S02644.
3. Wodi AP, Morelli V. Principles of vaccination. In: Wodi AP, Hall E, Hamborsky J, et al., eds. *Epidemiology and Prevention of Vaccine-Preventable Diseases*. 14th ed. Public Health Foundation; 2021. https://www.cdc.gov/vaccines/pubs/pinkbook/prinvac.html.
4. Hubaud A. *RNA vaccines: a novel technology to prevent and treat disease*; 2015. http://sitn.hms.harvard.edu/flash/2015/rna-vaccines-a-novel-technology-to-prevent-and-treat-disease/.
5. Miller E, Wodi AP. General best practice guidance for immunization. In: Hall E, Wodi AP, Hamborsky J, et al., eds. *Epidemiology and Prevention of Vaccine-Preventable Diseases*. 14th ed. Public Health Foundation; 2021. https://www.cdc.gov/vaccines/pubs/pinkbook/genrec.html.
6. Wodi AP, Shimabukuro T. Vaccine safety. In: Hall E, Wodi AP, Hamborsky J, et al., eds. *Epidemiology and Prevention of Vaccine-Preventable Diseases*. 14th ed. Washington, D.C: Public Health Foundation; 2021. https://www.cdc.gov/vaccines/pubs/pinkbook/safety.html.
7. Objio T, Morelli V, Trimble S. Storage and handling. In: Hall E, Wodi AP, Hamborsky J, et al., eds. *Epidemiology and Prevention of Vaccine-Preventable Diseases*. 14th ed. Public Health Foundation; 2021. https://www.cdc.gov/vaccines/pubs/pinkbook/vac-storage.html.
8. Wolicki J, Miller E. Vaccine administration. In: Hall E, Wodi AP, Hamborsky J, et al., eds. *Epidemiology and Prevention of Vaccine-Preventable Diseases*. 14th ed. Public Health Foundation; 2021. https://www.cdc.gov/vaccines/pubs/pinkbook/vac-admin.html.
9. Brauer E, Choi K, Chang J, et al. Health care providers' trusted sources for information about COVID-19 vaccines: mixed methods study. *JMIR Infodemiol*. 2021;1(1):e33330.
10. Jacobson RM, St Sauver JL, Griffin JM, MacLaughlin KL, Finney Rutten LJ. How health care providers should address vaccine hesitancy in the clinical setting: evidence for presumptive language in making a strong recommendation. *Hum Vaccin Immunother*. 2020;16(9):2131–2135.
11. Kroger A, Bahta L, Hunter P. General Best Practice Guidelines for Immunization. Best Practices Guidance of the Advisory Committee on Immunization Practices (ACIP); 2021. https://www.cdc.gov/vaccines/hcp/acip-recs/general-recs/index.html.

12. Eden L, Macintosh JE, Luthy KE, Beckstrand RL. Minimizing pain during childhood vaccination injections: improving adherence to vaccination schedules. *BYU J Undergrad Res*. 2016. http://jur.byu.edu/?p=20354.

13. Acosta AM, Moro PL, Hariri S, Tiwari TSP. Tetanus. In: Hall E, Wodi AP, Hamborsky J, et al., eds. *Epidemiology and Prevention of Vaccine-Preventable Diseases*. 14th ed. Public Health Foundation; 2021.

14. Peng B, Wei M, Zhu FC, Li JX. The vaccines-associated Arthus reaction. *Hum Vaccin Immunother*. 2019;15(11):2769–2777. https://pubmed.ncbi.nlm.nih.gov/30945978/.

15. Concepcion FE, Link-Gelles R, Shimabukuro T. Poliomyelitis. In: Hall E, Wodi AP, Hamborsky J, et al., eds. *Epidemiology and Prevention of Vaccine-Preventable Diseases*. 14th ed. Public Health Foundation; 2021. https://www.cdc.gov/vaccines/pubs/pinkbook/polio.html.

16. Oliver S, Moro P, Blain AE. Haemophilus influenzae. In: Hall E, Wodi AP, Hamborsky J, et al., eds. *Epidemiology and Prevention of Vaccine-Preventable Diseases*. 14th ed. Public Health Foundation; 2021. https://www.cdc.gov/vaccines/pubs/pinkbook/hib.html.

17. Haber P, Schillie S. Hepatitis b. In: Hall E, Wodi AP, Hamborsky J, et al., eds. *Epidemiology and Prevention of Vaccine-Preventable Diseases*. 14th ed. Public Health Foundation; 2021. https://www.cdc.gov/vaccines/pubs/pinkbook/hepb.html.

18. Foster M, Haber P, Nelson N. Hepatitis A. In: Hall E, Wodi AP, Hamborsky J, et al., eds. *Epidemiology and Prevention of Vaccine-Preventable Diseases*. 14th ed. Public Health Foundation; 2021. https://www.cdc.gov/vaccines/pubs/pinkbook/hepa.html.

19. Gierke R, Wodi AP, Kobayashi M. Pneumococcal disease. In: Hall E, Wodi AP, Hamborsky J, et al., eds. *Epidemiology and Prevention of Vaccine-Preventable Diseases*. 14th ed. Public Health Foundation; 2021. https://www.cdc.gov/vaccines/pubs/pinkbook/pneumo.html.

20. Advisory Committee on Immunization Practices. Meeting recommendations; 2022. https://www.cdc.gov/vaccines/acip/index.html.

21. CDC. *Genital hpv infection-basic fact sheet*; 2022. https://www.cdc.gov/std/hpv/stdfact-hpv.htm.

22. Meites E, Gee J, Unger E, Markowitz L. Human papillomavirus. In: Hall E, Wodi AP, Hamborsky J, et al., eds. *Epidemiology and Prevention of Vaccine-Preventable Diseases*. 14th ed. Public Health Foundation; 2021. https://www.cdc.gov/vaccines/pubs/pinkbook/hpv.html.

23. CDC. Meningococcal disease surveillance. 2022. https://www.cdc.gov/meningococcal/surveillance/index.html.

24. Mbaeyi S, Duffy J, McNamara L. Meningococcal disease. In: Hall E, Wodi AP, Hamborsky J, et al., eds. *Epidemiology and Prevention of Vaccine-Preventable Diseases*. 14th ed. Public Health Foundation; 2021. https://www.cdc.gov/vaccines/pubs/pinkbook/mening.html.

25. CDC. *Dengue Vaccination: What Everyone Should Know*; 2022. https://www.cdc.gov/vaccines/vpd/dengue/public/index.html#:~:text=CDC%20recommends%20dengue%20vaccination%20for,be%20confirmed%20by%20laboratory%20testing.

26. Hall E. Influenza. In: Hall E, Wodi P, Hamborsky J, et al., eds. *Epidemiology and Prevention of Vaccine-Preventable Diseases*. 14th ed. Public Health Foundation; 2021. https://www.cdc.gov/vaccines/pubs/pinkbook/flu.html.

27. Parashar UD, Hummelman EG, Bresee JS, Miller MA, Glass RI. Global illness and deaths caused by rotavirus disease in children. *Emerg Infect Dis*. 2003;9(5):565–572. https://doi.org/10.3201/eid0905.020562.

28. Cortese M, Haber P. Rotavirus. In: Hall E, Wodi AP, Hamborsky J, et al., eds. *Epidemiology and Prevention of Vaccine-Preventable Diseases*. 14th ed. Public Health Foundation; 2021. https://www.cdc.gov/vaccines/pubs/pinkbook/rota.html.

29. CDC. *History of measles*; 2020. https://www.cdc.gov/measles/about/history.html#:~:text=In%20the%20decade%20before%201963,States%20were%20infected%20each%20year.

30. Gastanaduy P, Haber P, Rota PA, Patel M. Measles. In: Hall E, Wodi AP, Hamborsky J, et al., eds. *Epidemiology and Prevention of Vaccine-Preventable Diseases*. 14th ed. Public Health Foundation; 2021. https://www.cdc.gov/vaccines/pubs/pinkbook/meas.html.

31. Marlow M, Haber P, Hickman C, Patel M. Mumps. In: Hall E, Wodi AP, Hamborsky J, et al., eds. *Epidemiology and Prevention of Vaccine-Preventable Diseases*. 14th ed. Public Health Foundation; 2021. https://www.cdc.gov/vaccines/pubs/pinkbook/mumps.html.

32. Lanzieri T, Haber P, Icenogle JP, Patel M. Rubella. In: Hall E, Wodi AP, Hamborsky J, et al., eds. *Epidemiology and Prevention of Vaccine-Preventable Diseases*. 14th ed. Public Health Foundation; 2021. https://www.cdc.gov/vaccines/pubs/pinkbook/rubella.html.

33. Lopez A, Harrington T, Marin M. Varicella. In: Hall E, Wodi AP, Hamborsky J, et al., eds. *Epidemiology and Prevention of Vaccine-Preventable Diseases*. 14th ed. Public Health Foundation; 2021. https://www.cdc.gov/vaccines/pubs/pinkbook/varicella.html.

34. *Usa facts. Us COVID-19 cases and deaths by state*; 2022. https://usafacts.org/visualizations/coronavirus-covid-19-spread-map.

35. CDC. Interim Clinical Considerations for Use of COVID-19 Vaccines Currently Approved or Authorized in the United States; 2022. https://www.cdc.gov/vaccines/covid-19/clinical-considerations/interim-considerations-us.html#not-immunocompromised.

36. CDC. Clinical Considerations: Myocarditis and Pericarditis after Receipt of mRNA COVID-19 Vaccines Among Adolescents and Young Adults; 2022. https://www.cdc.gov/vaccines/covid-19/clinical-considerations/myocarditis.html.

20
Dental and Oral Health

DONALD L. CHI

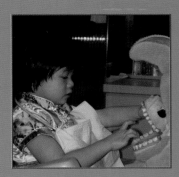

Oral health is increasingly recognized as a barometer of general health and wellbeing across the life span. The current goal is to advance effective and sustainable integrated healthcare systems that include oral health as an essential component of overall health and wellbeing. In fact, the Affordable Care Act named dental care as one of the 10 Essential Health Benefits for children.[1] However, dental benefits remained optional for adults. Many adults currently lack dental coverage through public programs like Medicaid or Medicare, which is relevant because many of these vulnerable adults are caregivers for children and are in a position to influence their oral health.

Pediatric primary care providers (PCPs) are an essential part of the oral health team because they have early and ongoing contact with children and families, which provides opportunities for early identification of oral disease, anticipatory guidance, and specific prevention interventions. Accordingly, the American Academy of Pediatrics (AAP) Section on Oral Health provides education and training, including Smiles For Life (https://cme.aapa.org/local/catalog/view/product.php?productid=214), practice tools, such as the Oral Health Risk Assessment Tool, and Oral Health Flip Chart, and family resources such as Brush, Book, Bed[2] (https://www.aap.org/en-us/advocacy-and-policy/aap-health-initiatives/Oral-Health/Pages/Oral-Health.aspx).

This chapter offers information and practical answers for PCPs to ensure they have basic examination competencies; the ability to distinguish between normal and abnormal structures, pathology, and common oral diseases; provide oral health education; prescribe and apply preventive treatment (e.g., fluoride varnish); and recognize when to engage other members of the oral health team.

Oral Health Care Standards and Guidelines

Healthy People 2030 identified oral health as a priority, including 15 objectives that address the prevention and control of oral and craniofacial disease, conditions, injuries, and improvements in accessing preventive dental services and care. The US Department of Health and Human Services (HHS) launched a cross-agency initiative to improve oral health nationwide among children with Medicaid and the Children's Health Insurance Program (CHIP).[3] Referred to as the New Oral Health Initiative, it set both short- and long-term goals, calling for increasing accountability, expanding research and data collection, emphasizing disease prevention and oral health promotion, and reducing health disparities. They also introduced the concept of oral health care teams, including dentists, dental hygienists, dental therapists, and community dental health practitioners, as well as nondental professionals (e.g., PCPs). Their expanded view included a provision to reimburse

PCPs for preventive dental services (e.g., oral examinations, risk assessment, fluoride varnish).[4]

The US Preventive Services Task Force (USPSTF) subsequently issued two recommendations for preventing caries in children from birth to 5 years old: namely, PCPs should: (1) prescribe oral fluoride supplementation starting at 6 months old if the water supply is fluoride deficient, and (2) fluoride varnish should be applied to the primary teeth of high-risk infants and children beginning at the onset of primary tooth eruption.

The American Academy of Pediatric Dentistry (AAPD) recommends that pediatric PCPs encourage parents to establish a "dental home" for their children at no later than 12 months old. Ideally, referral to a dentist should be considered as early as 6 months old or at the eruption of the first primary tooth.[5] Two additional factors are important to optimize oral health for children: (1) regular exposure to fluoride, mainly through tooth brushing with fluoridated toothpaste and drinking optimally fluoridated water, and (2) minimizing sugary food and beverage intake. Sugar-sweetened beverages are particularly harmful to the teeth, and US children consume high volumes.[6] Social factors, such as poverty, structural racism and implicit bias, and neighborhood environments can constrain whether a child or family is able to engage in optimal oral health behaviors.[7]

Normal Growth and Development

The structures of the mouth include the mucosa (buccal and gingival), palate, salivary glands, frenula, tongue, and teeth. Primary and permanent teeth have similar anatomy, differing primarily in the size and external shape of each tooth. Teeth are encased in mandibular and maxillary bone. A small opening at the root apex allows blood vessels and nerves to pass into the tooth. There are three layers: the outer enamel, dentin (softer than enamel), and pulp (inner most layer containing nerves and blood vessels).

Pattern of Tooth Eruption

The eruption of primary teeth typically begins with the lower central incisors and ends with the maxillary second molars (Fig. 20.1). The sequence of eruption and the timing of eruption for each tooth are similar for boys and girls. Although there is some age variability in timing, the eruption sequence is important to document. In most children, the 20 primary teeth are fully erupted by age 2 years. Each primary tooth has a designated letter (A–T) (Fig. 20.2). Tooth lettering begins at the second molar (tooth A) in the child's upper right quadrant, proceeds to the upper left quadrant

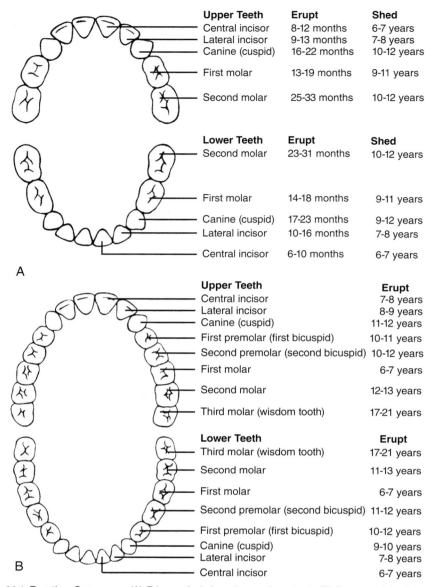

Upper Teeth	Erupt	Shed
Central incisor	8-12 months	6-7 years
Lateral incisor	9-13 months	7-8 years
Canine (cuspid)	16-22 months	10-12 years
First molar	13-19 months	9-11 years
Second molar	25-33 months	10-12 years

Lower Teeth	Erupt	Shed
Second molar	23-31 months	10-12 years
First molar	14-18 months	9-11 years
Canine (cuspid)	17-23 months	9-12 years
Lateral incisor	10-16 months	7-8 years
Central incisor	6-10 months	6-7 years

A

Upper Teeth	Erupt
Central incisor	7-8 years
Lateral incisor	8-9 years
Canine (cuspid)	11-12 years
First premolar (first bicuspid)	10-11 years
Second premolar (second bicuspid)	10-12 years
First molar	6-7 years
Second molar	12-13 years
Third molar (wisdom tooth)	17-21 years

Lower Teeth	Erupt
Third molar (wisdom tooth)	17-21 years
Second molar	11-13 years
First molar	6-7 years
Second premolar (second bicuspid)	11-12 years
First premolar (first bicuspid)	10-12 years
Canine (cuspid)	9-10 years
Lateral incisor	7-8 years
Central incisor	6-7 years

B

• **Fig. 20.1** Eruption Sequence. (A) Primary (baby) teeth eruption chart. (B) Permanent teeth eruption chart. (Courtesy American Dental Association. Copyright 2012; all rights reserved.)

(tooth J), continues down to the lower left quadrant (tooth K), and ends with the lower right mandibular second molar (tooth T).

The permanent teeth begin erupting as children reach school age (~5–6 years old) and the jaw begins to grow. A total of 32 permanent teeth are distributed among four tooth classes: 8 incisors, 4 canines, 8 premolars, and 12 molars. Permanent dentition eruption begins with the mandibular central incisors and ends with the maxillary third molars (i.e., wisdom teeth). The primary teeth shed as the permanent teeth erupt. The shedding and replacement of the primary molars by permanent premolars is usually complete by age 12 years. This period, when both primary and permanent teeth are present, is called *mixed dentition.*

Delayed tooth eruption (DTE) is when eruption of a tooth or multiple teeth is overdue, according to population norms based on chronologic age. Timely screening and recognition of DTE can minimize medical, developmental, functional, and esthetic problems resulting from untreated underlying local and systemic causes. Providers should also make note of children who have congenitally missing teeth (hypodontia) and extra teeth (hyperdontia).

Teething

Teeth typically erupt through the gums without causing any serious symptoms. However, it is important to note teething is not the cause of a report of *systemic* symptoms, such as diarrhea, high fever, vomiting, and cough, which should be addressed separately. Local gum irritation, irritability, and drooling are the most frequent symptoms of teething in infants and toddlers, peaking during the emergence of a child's primary incisors or front teeth.[8] A slight rise in body temperature is often reported but most often is not high enough to be considered a fever. This distinction is important. If a child develops a true fever, generally considered to be greater than 38°C (100.4°F), the inadvertent assumption that

A. Upper occlusal surfaces

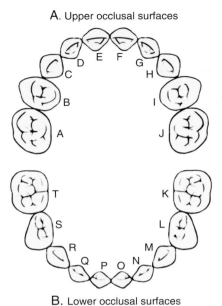

B. Lower occlusal surfaces

• **Fig. 20.2** Lettering of Primary Teeth. (A) Upper occlusal surfaces. (B) Lower occlusal surfaces. (Courtesy Jaemi Yoo, University of Washington School of Dentistry RIDE.)

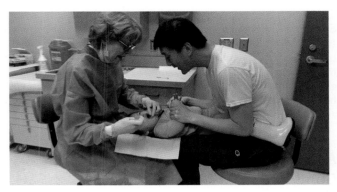

• **Fig. 20.3** Knee-to-Knee Position. (Courtesy Dr. Alaa Alkhateeb.)

the cause is teething may lead parents and/or providers to miss an illness or infection that requires treatment. It is also important to remember other systemic symptoms, such as diarrhea, vomiting, and cough should not be attributed to teething.

The recommended treatment for teething discomfort is to offer a *chilled* rubber teething ring or a wet, *chilled* washcloth for gumming; massaging the gums; or allowing infants older than 6 months old to chew on a *chilled* hard food under supervision. Frozen objects (including those with a liquid component) should not be used because of the potential for trauma to the gums. For example, rubbing an alcoholic beverage (e.g., whiskey) on the gums, tying a penny on a string around the child's neck (creating a potential risk of strangulation), and using a honey-coated pacifier, which could cause tooth decay or introduce botulism, are discouraged. Topical application of salicylates (aspirin) can cause burns and should not be used. Topical anesthetic gels, especially those containing benzocaine, are not recommended because of the rare potential for methemoglobinemia.[9] Silicone teething necklaces, worn by the adult, are becoming popular; however, the use of *amber* necklaces in particular, or any necklace worn by the child, is discouraged.

Performing the Oral Examination

Most important is that an oral examination should be systematic. Take the opportunity to note and point out normal development (e.g., erupted teeth, eruption patterns) and abnormalities (e.g., bloody or inflamed gums, tooth decay) to the parent(s). For an infant, have the parent immobilize the arms. With a tongue blade or toothbrush as a mouth prop, use a penlight and intraoral mirror for optimal visualization. Tip the head back to see the upper teeth. An alternative for examining a young child is for the provider and parent to sit across from each other knee to knee. The child faces the parent, and the child's head is then lowered into the provider's lap. The child's legs can be wrapped around the parent's waist if needed (Fig. 20.3).

Clinical Findings

Oral Mucosa

The soft mucosal tissues are examined before the teeth. This examination should include an assessment of the tonsils for size and the presence of inflammation or exudate. Start the examination with the inside of the lips and continue to the buccal mucosa, including the mucosal surfaces that connect and surround each tooth. Inspect the palate directly by tipping the child's head backward. Examine the dorsal and ventral mucosal surfaces of the tongue and floor of the mouth by retracting the tongue with a tongue blade or a dental mirror or by holding the tongue with cotton gauze. Note ulcerations, changes in color and surface texture, swelling, or fistulae of any of these tissues. When examining the gums, give special attention to any gingival swelling or recession. The gums may exhibit hyperpigmentation, which is normal variation. Note the presence and attachment of both frenula, noting the presence of "tongue tie" (ankyloglossia) and/or "lip tie." In infants, it is important to ask about difficulties latching onto the breast. Abnormal attachment of the frenula can impact feeding in infants and speech development in older children, and early referral for ankyloglossia surgical intervention may be warranted.

Saliva

Note the quantity and quality of the saliva. Decreased salivary flow and changes in sensation around the facial nerve can result from infection or tumor in the parotid space or facial musculature or can be a side effect of dehydration or medications that cause xerostomia (dry mouth). Drooling commonly refers to *anterior* drooling, which peaks between 3 and 6 months of life. It should be distinguished from *posterior* drooling, which entails saliva spilling over the tongue through the facial isthmus. Drooling can be a significant and ongoing disability for a large number of pediatric patients with cerebral palsy and for a smaller number of patients with other types of neurologic or cognitive impairment.

Teeth

The number and types of teeth erupted, discoloration, irregularities, and asymmetries should be noted. Retract or lift the lips so that the teeth can be examined systematically. Beginning with tooth A and moving around to the left, ending with tooth J, examine the lingual surfaces of the upper teeth and the biting surfaces before repeating this examination on the lower teeth K through T (Fig. 20.2). Teeth are best evaluated when dry. Variations in number, morphology, color, and surface structure should be noted, along with the presence of early caries, overt tooth decay, and/or the presence of previous dental work. Primary teeth may be malformed, incompletely formed, or chalky or have pitted enamel due to other systematic conditions, such as ectodermal dysplasia. In the case of traumatically previously injured teeth, the color and translucency of the injured tooth or teeth may be altered. Primary teeth that are discolored from trauma or injury but asymptomatic and nonabscessed can be monitored. In addition, preterm infants have an increased risk of developing early childhood caries (ECC), and prevention of ECC is key in this population.[10]

Aberrations in Primary Tooth Eruption and Gums

Natal and Neonatal Teeth

The prevalence of natal or neonatal teeth is estimated to be 1 out of 2000 to 3000 births and is equally common in boys and girls. The teeth usually erupt in pairs. Natal and neonatal teeth occur in approximately 50 different syndromes, of which approximately 10 are associated with chromosomal aberrations. More than 90% of these prematurely erupting teeth are mandibular central incisors with normal shape and color. Supernumerary teeth or hyperdontia may be abnormal in shape and color and only loosely attached to the gingiva. Natal or neonatal teeth can lead to gingivitis, self-mutilation of the tongue, and trauma to the mother during breastfeeding; however, they should be extracted only if they are loose enough to involve risk of aspiration or sublingual ulceration or if feeding is severely disturbed. Most will develop normally with normal root structure.[11]

Atypical Tooth Eruption

Atypical tooth eruption can result from either *systemic* factors, such as prematurity, low birth weight, or genetic syndromes (e.g., Down, Turner), or local factors, such as a low-protein diet, adjacent supernumeraries, and dental tissue tumors. In general, children with chronic health conditions, who have delays in physical development, experience delayed but otherwise normal tooth eruption.

Preeruption Cysts

When a tooth starts erupting through the gingival tissue, a blood-filled cyst may precede it and alarmed parents may report a purple, reddish, black, or blue bump or bruise on their child's gums. If the enlargement is on the thickened ridge or alveolar ridge just behind the teeth, no treatment is indicated. The cyst will resolve as the tooth erupts.

Bohn Nodules

Bohn nodules are present at birth and appear as firm nonpainful nodules on the buccal surface of the alveolar ridge (Fig. 20.4). They are remnants of dental lamina connecting the developing tooth bud to the epithelium of the oral cavity. No treatment is required because they will resolve spontaneously. If they appear in the midline of the palate, they are referred to as *Epstein pearls*.

Professional Dental Care

Fear of the Dentist

There is a significant relationship between parental and child dental fear, particularly in children 8 years old and younger.[12] Many parents of children with whom PCPs interact may have this fear and consequently avoid dental visits themselves. Approaching these parents using a calm, caring approach is important to help allay anxiety and fears. Early and consistent primary prevention is the best way to avoid the development of fear and dental care avoidance. Allowing tooth decay to go untreated until a child needs extensive restorative intervention is not only costly, but it can also be traumatic.

Choosing a Dentist

The choice of a dentist and identification of a dental home is critical, especially for children who have had negative experiences with dentists. Many general dentists are highly skilled at working with children, so the absence of a pediatric dentist should not be a barrier to care; however, a dentist who is new to the child should be told about any prior dental experiences. Parents should be cautious about dentists with laser-based or other electronic diagnostic devices because these devices are often marketed as being capable of detecting "invisible" cavities and justify unnecessary fillings.[13] The standard method of examination of the teeth is visual, using strong light and transillumination. Most tooth decay in permanent teeth in children occurs on the biting surface, and x-rays are of limited diagnostic value in such cases. When parents report excessive, new, or experimental dental treatments, PCPs, as a member of the oral health team, can query the dental provider regarding approach to diagnosis of dental caries.

First Dental Visit

The child's first dental visit should occur before the child's first birthday (12 months old) or within 6 months of the first tooth eruption. This first visit allows a dentist to begin to establish an ongoing relationship (dental home) for the child, provide education and anticipatory guidance, and deliver preventive care, such as topical fluoride if not performed by the PCP. Establishment of a dental home gives parents a familiar place to take their child for dental checkups and emergencies (e.g., dental/oral trauma, avulsion, dislodged filling). The first dental visit commonly involves

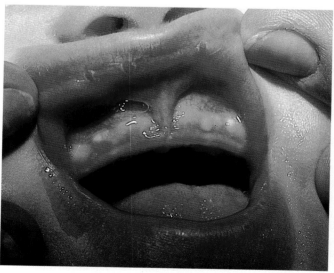

• **Fig. 20.4** Bohn Nodules. (From Eichenfield LF, Frieden IJ, Esterly NB. *Neonatal Dermatology.* 4th ed. Elsevier; 2011.)

a cleaning, dental examination, and topical fluoride treatment in the presence of the parent. For children younger than 3 years old, the parent may be asked to help position the child.

Dental Health Education

Dental health education is a crucial preventive strategy, and PCPs, with their ongoing and early contact with children and families, are ideally situated to introduce and reinforce proper oral hygiene/brushing techniques, emphasize the importance of fluoride, facilitate dental care access, and address nutritional intake, including the use of pacifiers, bottles, and no-spill cups. The PCP should review all materials for readability levels and inconsistencies. For example, the amount of toothpaste to use can be described as "pea sized," but accompanying photos often show a long ribbon of toothpaste on the toothbrush. In addition, PCPs can address and dispel common oral health myths, such as tooth decay in baby teeth is not important because these teeth eventually fall out.

Well-child care is the ideal time to integrate dental health education and prevention. As noted earlier, the AAP has a number of educational resources and interventions. PCPs should introduce oral health–related education and anticipatory guidance, especially during early well-baby visits, to ensure that children have their first visit to the dentist by 12 months old. Earlier studies revealed that young children with a greater number of well-child visits between 1 and 3 years old were significantly more likely to have earlier first dental visits.[14] Furthermore, studies have found that children 2 to 5 years old who received a recommendation by a PCP to see a dentist were more likely to have a dental examination.[15]

Bacterial Diseases of the Mouth

Tooth Decay

Tooth decay is a bacterial disease. The decay is caused by acid demineralization of the tooth's subsurface enamel. The acid is produced by bacteria (e.g., *Streptococcus mutans*) after metabolism of carbohydrates in the diet. Unless neutralized and buffered by saliva or remineralized with fluorides, the demineralization process leads to cavitation of the tooth surface. Although not involved in the initiation of cavities, lactobacilli are frequently found in cavities and contribute to their progression.[16]

In infants, prolonged exposure to infant formula, sugary beverages such as juice, or breast milk is especially impactful when the infant is put to sleep with the nipple in the mouth or when allowed to "graze" on sweet fluids throughout the day. Frequent carbohydrate exposure from continuous snacking and frequent sugary beverages keeps the pH of the mouth fluid less than 5 near the tooth surface and results in an acidic environment conducive to demineralization. The neutralization process does not have enough time to increase the mouth pH to a level that would allow remineralization. In children undergoing chemotherapy or radiation to the head and neck and/or who are immunocompromised, normal salivary flow and salivary buffering of acids can also be disrupted, putting them at further risk for cavities.

The main risk factors in the development of cavities can be categorized as microbiologic, dietary, and environmental. Even though it is largely a preventable condition, tooth decay remains one of the most common childhood diseases. The major contributing factors for the high prevalence are improper feeding practices, familial socioeconomic background, lack of parental education, and lack of access to dental care, as well as the presence of tooth

decay in other family members.[16] Primary teeth are needed for proper nutrition and mastication, esthetics, phonetics, and maintaining space for permanent teeth.

Clinical Findings

- *Early tooth decay.* Early caries appear as white or brown horizontal lines or spots along the central gum line or gingival margin (Fig. 20.5). When white lesions occur, the dentin is initially damaged. Then, as the lesion progresses, the hard enamel breaks, and a clinical cavity is evident.
- *Advanced tooth decay.* Advanced decay appears as cavitations in the teeth. Nearly all cavities in children's permanent teeth begin on the biting surface of the molars. The initial lesion appears as a pinhole surrounded by a white, opaque halo. As the lesion enlarges, greater damage to the enamel becomes apparent.
- Associated signs and symptoms:
  - Sensitivity: cavities can be hot, cold, or sweet sensitive
  - Localized dental or facial pain
  - Abscesses on the gums due to bacterial invasion of the pulpal tissue
  - Gingival inflammation
  - Possible lymphadenopathy or fever

PCPs should know that cavities may spontaneously arrest. This arrest is thought to occur when cavities are exposed to saliva high in fluoride or with changes in dietary and/or feeding practices. Arrested caries appear as open cavities that are black or dark brown. If the child has such open cavities in a primary tooth/teeth, is asymptomatic, and access to dental care is problematic, these teeth can be left alone and allowed to shed normally.

Prevention Strategies

Diet. Sugar-sweetened beverages with energy-containing sweeteners, such as fruit juice concentrates, sucrose, or high-fructose corn syrup, are the primary source of sugars in Western diets. Fruit juice is not recommended for children younger than age 1 year. For children ages 1 to 3 years, juice should be limited to no more than 4 ounces per day and restricted to mealtimes. Because juices contain high concentrations of sugar, diluting juice with water will likely not prevent tooth decay. For children ages 4 to 6 years, juice intake should be limited to 4 to 6 ounces. For children ages 7 years and older, intake should be limited to 8 ounces.

Bottles should be used only for milk, infant formula, or water. Nursing mothers should not allow their infants to sleep attached to the nipple, and bottles should never be propped during naps or bedtime. Some Women, Infants, and Children (WIC) centers

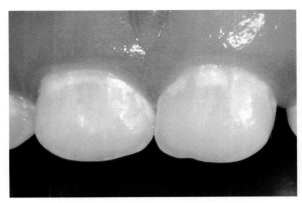

• **Fig. 20.5** White Spots. (From Cameron AC, Widmer RP, eds. *Handbook of Pediatric Dentistry.* 2nd ed. Mosby; 2003.)

in the United States distribute no-spill training cups to promote appropriate eating behaviors and prevent tooth decay. However, personnel may not be aware of the potential danger of the cups themselves if sugar-sweetened beverages are available ad lib. It is ideal for parents to set established snack and mealtimes and avoid allowing their child to graze on foods and beverages all day. Use of vitamins containing table sugar (sucrose) and/or gummy vitamins that are sticky should be discouraged.

Toothbrushing. Parents should be taught to clean a child's teeth with a small toothbrush as soon as teeth erupt, using the "lift the lip" method. The technique involves having a parent lift the child's upper lip and use a soft toothbrush to cleanse each tooth surface. Parents should check regularly to see if dental problems are beginning, looking closely for the signs of demineralization. A demonstration by the PCP during a well-child visit is ideal. By making this an enjoyable routine, the child will become comfortable, and any resistance should decrease (e.g., Brush, Book, Bed).

Toothpaste. Fluoridated toothpaste works by creating a reservoir of fluoride in the fluid layer of the plaque and saliva that are potentially being damaged by bacterial acids. Although fluoridated toothpastes sold in the United States have similar fluoride levels, the PCP also needs to know the fluoride content level in the community drinking water, other sources of fluoride the child might be consuming, and risk factors for tooth decay before recommending the use of fluoride toothpaste in all children.[17]

Child-flavored toothpastes are easier to introduce. Toothpastes containing whitening or bleaching agents are contraindicated. A small amount of toothpaste should be used. Small is defined as a smear or "rice sized" for children less than 3 years old and "pea sized" for children 3 years old and older. The child should not rinse after brushing with fluoridated toothpaste. Swallowing these small amounts of toothpaste twice daily is not harmful; however, the amount of toothpaste used should be controlled by an adult because young children swallow approximately 35% of what is brushed on. It is important to remember that added systemic intake of fluoride can lead to an increased risk of enamel fluorosis, which is particularly important before complete enamel maturation. In children at very high risk for tooth decay, parents should begin brushing teeth with fluoridated toothpaste with the eruption of the first tooth at 6 to 9 months old. Toothpastes and fluoride supplements should be stored out of reach of younger children. If a child ingests a large dose of fluoride, the caregiver must contact 911 immediately if the child is symptomatic or call Poison Control at 800-222-1222.

Sealants. Pit and fissure (occlusal) plastic or glass-ionomer cement sealants are effective in preventing tooth decay in high-risk children.[18] High-risk children are those who have experienced decay in their primary teeth and/or have ongoing exposure to diets with high amounts of refined carbohydrates and sugar-sweetened beverages. Sealants are polymerizing resin or glass ionomer coatings placed on the biting surfaces of primary molars at 2 to 3 years old and permanent molars at about 6 to 7 years old and 13 to 14 years old (Fig. 20.6). Resin sealants are technique sensitive because they require the tooth to be completely dry when they are being placed, which requires cooperation from the child. Glass ionomer sealants do not require the teeth to be dry, making them easier to apply.

Fluoride Varnish. Early white spot lesions in primary and/or permanent teeth can be remineralized using topical fluoride varnish. Fluoride varnish is the agent of choice for young children. Fluoride gels are not recommended because of the risk of acute toxicity. In many states, PCPs are permitted to apply fluoride varnish and are reimbursed by insurance plans, including the Affordable Care Act

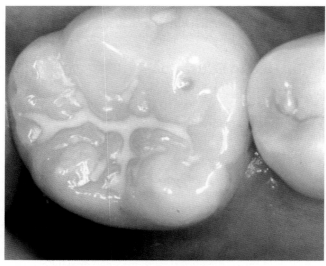

• **Fig. 20.6** Sealant. (From Robinson D. *Essentials of Dental Assisting.* 7th ed. Elsevier; 2023.)

(ACA), Medicaid, and CHIP programs. Twice-yearly applications have been shown to reduce tooth decay by approximately one-third. More frequent applications may be needed in high-risk children (every 3–6 months). The decision to place fluoride on a child's teeth should be based on the child's underlying risk for tooth decay.[17] Plasma fluoride levels following applications of varnish are low and are not associated with toxicity or fluorosis.

To apply fluoride varnish:

1. Dispense approximately 0.25 mL of fluoride varnish into a small well. Prepackaged individual-dose systems come with their own well that is filled with varnish. To avoid risk of overexposure, use only the size package recommended for the age of the child.
2. Dry the teeth with air or gauze to remove excess moisture.
3. While keeping the teeth isolated from further moisture contamination, paint the varnish onto the teeth with a brush or applicator. Only a light coat is required. The varnish sets on contact with the slightly moist teeth.
4. Children can eat immediately after placement of the varnish.

PCPs are in a key position to have discussions with concerned parents about the safety of fluoride varnish as well as other sources of topical fluoride (drinking water, toothpastes, silver diamine fluoride) important in cavity prevention.[19] Opposition to water fluoridation has become increasingly common in communities, which underscores the role that PCPs have in advocating for continued water fluoridation from both a public health and health equity perspective.

Fluoride in Water, Infant Formulas, and Fluoride Supplementation. The most effective preventive measure against dental caries is optimizing community water fluoridation levels to no more than 0.7 mg of fluoride per liter of water (this recommended level updates and replaces the previously recommended range of 0.7–1.2 mg/L). The fluoride level of public water supplies can be ascertained by calling the local health department. Children who consume fluoride-deficient water are at risk for caries and will benefit from dietary fluoride supplementation.[20]

Providers should be aware of the status of fluoride in the community and routinely ask new families about fluoride in their water source. If the child is on a private water supply, the naturally occurring fluoride level should be tested before prescribing

TABLE 20.1	Recommended Fluoride Supplementation Based on Drinking Water Fluoride Concentration[a]		
	FLUORIDE ION LEVEL IN DRINKING WATER (ppm)[b]		
Age	<0.3 ppm	0.3–0.6 ppm	>0.6 ppm
Birth to 6 months	None	None	None
6 months to 3 years	0.25 mg/day[c]	None	None
3–6 years	0.50 mg/day	0.25 mg/day	None
6–16 years	1 mg/day	0.50 mg/day	None

[a]Take all sources of fluoride into consideration: water (including bottled) and amount and frequency of fluoridated toothpaste used in brushing.

[b]Optimal concentration of fluoride in water supply in mg/L or parts per million (ppm).

[c]2.2 mg sodium fluoride contains 1 mg fluoride ion.

From American Academy of Pediatric Dentistry (AAPD). Policy on the use of fluoride. *Pediatr Dent.* 2017;39(6):29–30.

fluoride supplements. To prevent overdose, no prescription should be written for more than a total of 120 mg of fluoride. See Table 20.1 for adjusting the dose of fluoride supplements in relation to that found in the community/well water supply.

Current US Food and Drug Administration (FDA) regulations require that fluoride be listed on the bottled water or infant formula label only if fluoride is added during processing, but the concentration does not have to be stated. A child who uses bottled water instead of fluoridated community water may need fluoride supplementation. On the other hand, powdered infant formulas reconstituted with fluoridated water may pose an increased risk of fluorosis because of the prolonged accumulative effect of fluoride on enamel development. The CDC maintains My Water's Fluoride, where links to available information on fluoride from local water systems available (https://nccd.cdc.gov/doh_mwf/default/default.aspx).[21]

Topical Iodine. Polyvinylpyrrolidone (PVP) iodine (10% PVP-I or povidone-iodine [betadine solution]) can be painted on the teeth before the application of fluoride varnish for an additive effect to depress the bacteria causing tooth decay in high-risk children.[22,23] The teeth are dried with cotton gauze or air, and the povidone iodine is painted onto the teeth and gums with a cotton-tipped applicator and then immediately wiped off with gauze or rinsed with air and water.

Disease Identification and Management Strategies

Active Decay

When tooth decay is present, it can be arrested painlessly by topically treating the decayed surfaces with 38% silver diamine fluoride (SDF). (Note: a side effect is black staining of the lesion.) This treatment was cleared by the FDA in 2014.[24] SDF is a clear liquid that is brushed onto cavities directly and stops them from getting larger.[25] Numerous systematic reviews demonstrate the effectiveness of SDF in preventing cavities.[26,27] SDF can prevent dental pain and abscess formation and is used to manage tooth decay that allows dental treatment to be delayed or avoided completely. SDF may also allow children to forgo dental treatment under conscious sedation or general anesthesia. Even though cavities treated with SDF turn dark, parent acceptance is high.[28]

Studies demonstrate that nondentists can successfully use SDF in clinical settings.[29] SDF is indicated for cavities on primary or permanent teeth that are asymptomatic and where there is no abscess present. It can be applied to cavities on smooth tooth surfaces and those present in between teeth. One or two drops is enough to treat multiple teeth. The affected teeth are isolated with gauze or cotton rolls. A small microbrush is used to apply SDF directly onto the cavitated tooth surfaces. SDF should be left undisturbed for 30 to 60 seconds. Patients can be asked to return for a second SDF application in 1 to 2 weeks and SDF can be reapplied every 3 to 4 months as needed. SDF is part of the Smiles for Life curriculum in management of tooth decay in children.[30]

The American Medical Association now has a category III CPT billing code (X115T) that can be used by PCPs to bill for SDF. A decision to repair or remove teeth depends on the extent of damage and the length of time until the tooth would be normally exfoliated. Retention of primary molars is important because they hold space to allow the normal eruption of permanent successors. Larger cavities in primary teeth can be repaired atraumatically with plastic fillings or with steel or plastic crowns.[24,25] Teeth with deep cavities and draining abscesses are generally extracted. Young children may need to be sedated or receive treatment under a general anesthetic to meet extensive treatment needs, making tooth decay arrest with topical treatment and interim restorative care—at least until they get older to allow conventional dental treatment—is a noteworthy option. In some cases, arresting decay will allow the space to be maintained and the tooth to be shed normally.

Cavities in permanent teeth are typically repaired with tooth-colored composite resin (plastic) fillings. Approximately half of a silver amalgam filling is composed of liquid mercury, a binder for the other amalgam components (silver, copper, and other metals). Although mercury releases low levels of vapor, the FDA, based on scientific evidence, considers silver amalgams safe for children. The FDA recommends that high-risk populations and children younger than 6 years of age avoid dental amalgam, if possible.[9] If a filling is in good condition, the FDA recommends not to have amalgam filling removed, unless medically necessary. The mercury levels from amalgams have been determined by the Environmental Protection Agency (EPA) and the Centers for Disease Control and Prevention (CDC) to be below the lowest levels associated with brain and kidney toxicity. However, amalgams are less commonly used currently, having been replaced by composite fillings. Severe cavities resulting in abscess formation in permanent teeth are treated with root canal therapy. Permanent molars either need to be capped after root canal therapy (e.g., crown) or treated with large amalgam fillings to avoid fracture.

Abscesses

Abscesses may appear as swelling on the buccal or palatal gingival mucosa and frequently present with purulent drainage. A child with an abscessed tooth may not always report pain or sensitivity. Untreated abscesses require urgent dental referral because they may develop into life-threatening bony facial space infections, requiring surgical drainage and parenteral antibiotic treatment. If a dentist or oral surgeon is not immediately available for drainage and the abscess is uncomplicated, antibiotics and pain medication may be appropriate interventions prior to further consultation.[26]

Periodontal Diseases

Gingivitis

Gingivitis is the presence of gingival inflammation without noticeable loss of alveolar bone or clinical attachment of structures that help to anchor the teeth. This condition is caused by plaque and is present in some degree in nearly all children and adolescents. Hormonal fluctuations inherent in puberty may be a determinant of altered inflammatory response to plaque in this age group.[27] The gingiva will present with localized or generalized bleeding when brushed or flossed. The teeth will be covered in varying degrees of plaque and calculus secondary to poor or irregular hygiene. The teeth will not be loose. The treatment is brushing and flossing. It can take several days for the gingiva to respond to the improved hygiene. Gingivitis is reversible. There is also one case report in which SDF was applied to demineralized teeth and improvements in gingivitis were observed.[28]

Aggressive Periodontitis

Aggressive periodontitis is a bacterial infection involving the gums and bone. It results in rapid loss of periodontal attachment and supporting bone around the primary or permanent teeth. The primary infection is by *Actinobacillus* and *Bacteroides* species in younger children and by *Treponema* species and other gram-negative rods in older children. Aggressive periodontitis is the most common type of periodontitis in children and adolescents.[27] Children with a familial history of periodontitis are at higher risk, and frequent dental examinations and radiographs during the peripubertal period are essential.

The disease may be localized, involving the surrounding gums and bone around primary incisors and molars, or generalized, involving all teeth. Teeth may become loose, but in the localized form there is generally no inflammatory response, suppuration, or fever. Children with suspected periodontitis should be referred to a dentist for local debridement (deep cleanings) and coordinated management with systemic antibiotics. The major complication of aggressive periodontitis is loss of bone and tooth attachment, resulting in the loss of teeth. Individuals should be counseled that tobacco products increase the risk of periodontal disease and should be avoided.

Necrotizing Periodontal Disease

Necrotizing periodontal disease is an aggressive disease resulting in damage to the gum tissue between the teeth. Children typically have severe gingival pain and fever and require immediate referral to a dentist or periodontist. The triangular area of gums between the teeth is ulcerated and necrotic and covered with a gray film.

There may be a fetid mouth odor. The gum tissues harbor high levels of spirochetes, and invasion of the tissues has been demonstrated. Predisposing factors are viral infections (including human immunodeficiency virus [HIV] and other systemic diseases), malnutrition, emotional stress, and lack of sleep. Careful oral hygiene and a bland diet are recommended.

Pyogenic Granuloma

Pyogenic granuloma is an inflammatory hyperplasia usually caused by low-grade localized infection, trauma, or hormonal factors. It is usually a small exophytic (i.e., outward growing) lesion that can be smooth, lobulated, and/or hemorrhagic. It typically occurs on the gingiva, lips, tongue, buccal mucosa, and hard plate. The surface color ranges from pink to red to deep purple, depending on how long the lesion has been present in the oral cavity. Pyogenic granulomas can occur after 4 years of age but are more common in pregnant women, including teens. Possible treatments include improved oral hygiene, 0.12% chlorhexidine gluconate rinses, surgical excision, cryosurgery, or intralesional injections of corticosteroids. PCPs can begin with prescribing improved oral hygiene efforts and chlorhexidine rinses followed by a referral to a dentist or periodontist.

Viral Diseases of the Mouth

Herpes Stomatitis

Herpes gingivostomatitis is a viral disease that results in oral and circumoral ulcers. It is usually caused by herpes simplex virus type 1 (HSV-1) (Fig. 20.7) and most commonly affects children 6 months to 5 years old. Antimicrobials are not appropriate because lesions heal without treatment in 7 to 14 days; however, supportive therapy, such as cold liquids and analgesics, is appropriate. Topical treatment with an equal mixture of diphenhydramine and Maalox may also provide symptomatic relief. It is recommended to remove the child from day care or school during the drooling phase of the illness. Encourage parents to clean the teeth with a soft toothbrush or cloth. Oral acyclovir can reduce the degree and length of symptoms if initiated within 3 days of the onset of the initial episode, while topical antiviral agents are ineffective.[29]

Herpes stomatitis/labialis may be confused with aphthous ulcers (canker sores), ulcerative gingivitis, hand-foot-and-mouth disease, trauma, herpangina, or chemical burns. Rare conditions

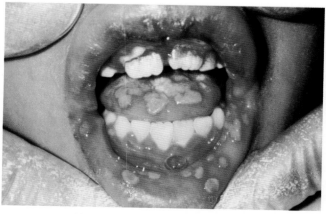

• **Fig. 20.7** Herpes Stomatitis in a Child.

that may also cause similar lesions are neutrophil defects, systemic lupus erythematosus (SLE), Behçet syndrome, and Crohn disease. It is also important to remember that children with herpes are at increased risk for dehydration. Parents should be instructed to watch for signs and symptoms and seek medical care. Careful handwashing should be recommended to the child and the caregivers to prevent autoinnoculation or transmission of infection to the eyes. An urgent referral to ophthalmology is needed if ocular spread is suspected.

Idiopathic Oral Conditions

Ankyloglossia (Tongue-Tie)

Ankyloglossia, or "tongue-tie," is caused by a short *lingual* frenulum that hinders tongue movement beyond the edge of the lips.[30] The frenulum may lengthen as the child gets older and not require intervention. If the extent of the ankyloglossia is severe, breastfeeding may be difficult and a minor surgical incision, called a *frenotomy*, may improve feeding.[31] If speech is affected later in life, referral is also indicated. The evidence supporting frenotomy continues to vacillate about intervening for "tongue-tie," and for "lip-tie," caused by a short *labial* frenulum, when an infant is struggling to latch in breastfeeding.[32]

Aphthous Ulcers (Canker Sores)

The etiology of these recurrent, painful oral ulcers is not well understood. Infectious agents, such as *Helicobacter pylori,* HSV-1, and measles, have been implicated, as well as alterations of cell-mediated immunity. Emotional and physical stress, local trauma (e.g., orthodontic braces, toothbrush abrasion), hormonal factors, genetics, food hypersensitivity, and the presence of sodium lauryl sulfate (SLS) in toothpaste have also been implicated. Vitamin and mineral deficiencies contribute to recurrent oral aphthae, particularly deficiencies in several B vitamins (1, 2, 6, and 12), iron, folic acid, and zinc.

Lesions are present on alveolar or buccal mucosa, tongue, soft palate, or the floor of the mouth. The ulcers are shallow, surrounded with an erythematous halo, and covered by gray, yellow, or white plaques. There are three forms: *minor* (the most common), *major,* and *herpetiform.* Minor lesions are less than 10 mm in diameter, whereas major lesions (i.e., Sutton disease) are generally more than 1 cm in diameter and may take a month or more to heal and leave residual scarring. Herpetiform lesions are clusters of 1- to 2-mm lesions that may coalesce. Healing should be complete in approximately 7 to 10 days. Prodromal symptoms may occur, including localized tingling or burning. Aphthous lesions may be seen with inflammatory bowel disease, Behçet disease, gluten-sensitive enteropathy, HIV infection, and neutropenia.

The goal of treatment is to decrease the ulcers, relieve pain, and reduce frequency of occurrence. Maintaining good oral hygiene is essential. Minor lesions generally resolve spontaneously in 10 to 14 days and heal without treatment or scarring. A bland diet and oral analgesics may be appropriate. Vitamin or mineral replacement may prevent recurrence if dietary history suggests a deficiency. Over-the-counter treatments, such as triamcinolone hexacetonide in Orabase paste, fluocinonide gel covered by Orabase paste, or amlexanox 5% oral paste, may be applied 4 times per day for 3 to 4 days for pain relief and to promote healing. Consider additional diagnostic testing should

symptoms and history suggest an infectious agent or gastrointestinal etiology.

Benign Migratory Glossitis (Geographic Tongue)

Benign migratory glossitis (BMG) usually presents as asymptomatic, yellowish-white, circular, or serpentine-bordered lesions with atrophic red centers varying in intensity. The lesions appear on the anterior two-thirds of the dorsum of the tongue (Fig. 20.8). The lesions may heal spontaneously and reappear on other areas of the tongue. The etiology is unknown. Occasionally, BMG is associated with localized discomfort, especially when eating hot or spicy foods. Proposed risk factors for BMG include immunologic factors, hormonal changes, use of oral contraceptives, diabetes mellitus, and stress. Patients can be reassured that the lesions are benign and do not generally require treatment.

Bruxism/Grinding

Bruxism is a condition of excessive grinding of the teeth that occurs when awake and/or during sleep. Children 12 years old or younger are more likely to report sleep-related bruxism, whereas those 13 years old or older experience more wake-time tooth clenching. Underlying stressors may be a contributing factor. An increase in bruxism has also been found in children exposed to high or moderate amounts of second-hand smoke.[33]

Primary teeth show marked wear.[34] However, parents can be told that tooth grinding of primary teeth is not associated with damage to permanent dentition. Studies have found that both children with sleep-related bruxism and wake-time tooth clenching complained of jaw muscle fatigue and temporomandibular joint (TMJ) disorder.[35,36]

Evidence supporting the use of plastic night guards is anecdotal, as is support for behavioral methods, such as relaxation training.[37] However, at least one scoping review reported reduced bruxism associated with occlusal splints.[38] Elimination of gum chewing has been shown to be effective in helping to manage facial muscle pain and headache.

Dental Erosion

Dental erosion is a chemical process that leads to irreversible acid demineralization of tooth structure. Acids that cause dental

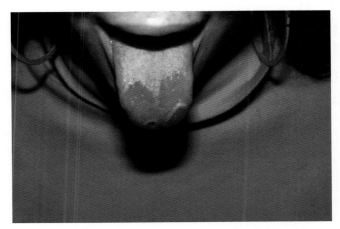

• **Fig. 20.8** Benign Migratory Glossitis, or Geographic Tongue. (From Kliegman RM, St. Geme JW, Blum NJ, et al, eds. *Nelson Textbook of Pediatrics.* 21st ed. Elsevier; 2020.)

erosion can be classified as intrinsic or extrinsic. Intrinsic acids include stomach acid introduced into the oral cavity by gastroesophageal reflux disorder (GERD), and/or vomiting. Extrinsic acids include acidic beverages, methamphetamines, citrus fruits (e.g., sucking on lemons), and medications (e.g., chewable vitamin C tablets). Factors that can aggravate dental erosion include xerostomia (dry mouth) secondary to decreased salivary flow, medications that interfere with saliva composition or production (e.g., clonidine), dental attrition, and dental abrasion. Children and adolescents with bulimia nervosa frequently present with dental erosion. Children with asthma also have greater amounts of dental erosion, which may be due to increased gastroesophageal reflux, medications, or an increased consumption of erosive beverages taken to counteract the drying effect of inhalers.

Clinical manifestations of dental erosion include smooth, cupped-out teeth on chewing surfaces, fillings that are raised above the normal level of the tooth, overly shiny silver fillings, enamel cuffing along the gums, and tooth hypersensitivity. Mild to moderate dental erosion may be associated with complaints of tooth hypersensitivity. The differential diagnosis includes abrasion caused by gritty substances (coarse toothpaste or toothbrushes with hard bristles) and attrition caused by mechanical forces (tooth grinding [bruxism] or brushing too hard). Tooth decay should also be in the differential.

Early detection, diagnosis, and treatment of dental erosion are critical. Hot and cold sensitivity can be managed by using "sensitive teeth" fluoridated toothpastes, topical fluoride treatments, or silver diamine fluoride applied by the dentist. Unless the erosion is deep, fillings are not required. Typically, the problem can be managed by identifying and eliminating the etiologic agent. Over-the-counter products, such as soft toothbrushes, low-abrasive fluoridated toothpaste, and fluoride rinses, are helpful. Severe dental erosion can lead to dental nerve (pulp) exposures, which can necessitate root canal treatment.

Fluorosis

Fluorosis is a complication of too much systemic fluoride exposure during the years of enamel development. With the increased availability of fluoride toothpaste, surveys showed there has been an increase in all levels of fluorosis.[39] In mild cases, the fluorosis appears as lacey white streaks that are largely unnoticeable. Moderate fluorosis is similar in appearance but covers more of the tooth. In rare cases, severe fluorosis (Fig. 20.9) appears as pitting and brown spots in the enamel. When the risk for caries is high, the benefit of fluoride outweighs the risk of mild or moderate fluorosis.[17]

Diastema

A space between any two neighboring teeth is referred to as a *diastema*. During the mixed dentition stage, when both primary and permanent teeth are present, a midline space between the upper front teeth is normal. There may also be diastemas present between other teeth. If the teeth are not otherwise crowded or misaligned, these spaces usually close by the time the permanent maxillary canines fully erupt, and referral is not needed. Diastemas caused by missing incisors or midline supernumerary teeth will persist in the permanent dentition stage and require early referral.

Another cause of a diastema is a prominent labial frenulum, which is the tissue connecting the upper lip to the area of the gums between the front upper teeth (Fig. 20.10). Sometimes the

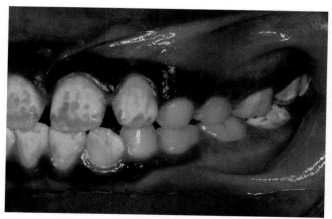

• **Fig. 20.9** Severe Fluorosis. (From Neville BW, Damm DD, Allen CM, et al, eds. *Oral and Maxillofacial Pathology.* 4th ed. Elsevier; 2016.)

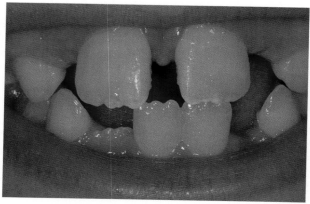

• **Fig. 20.10** Diastema: Labial Frenum. (Courtesy Donald L. Chi, DDS, PhD, Associate Professor, Department of Oral Health Sciences, University of Washington School of Dentistry.)

frenulum is large and appears to be causing the space between the front teeth. In general, the space closes as the jaws grow, and referral is not needed. Unnecessary or premature excision can result in scarring.

Gingival Hyperplasia

Gingival hyperplasia is a fibrous enlargement of gingival tissue around the teeth. The enlargement is typically caused by drugs (e.g., phenytoin, cyclosporine, nifedipine), hormones, chronic inflammation, or leukemia. It can also be idiopathic. The gingival tissue varies, appearing either normal, red-blue, or lighter than the surrounding tissue. It may be spongy or firm. In general, individuals are asymptomatic. Treatment consists of improved oral hygiene and 0.12% chlorhexidine gluconate mouth rinse. In cases in which the overgrowth interferes with chewing, gingivectomy is required.

Halitosis (Bad Breath)

Halitosis is primarily associated with poor oral hygiene and/or tooth decay; however, its presence may signal systemic disease, sinusitis, sleep apnea, and/or airway-related conditions. Halitosis is more common in individuals who are mouth breathers, who have postnasal drip or dry mouth, or who use tobacco products.

Recent research found that the microbiome composition and abundance of the tongue coatings shifted before the onset of halitosis in preschool children.[40] PCPs should encourage a healthy balanced diet, proper oral hygiene including regular brushing (including the tongue), flossing, and dental visits, as well as avoiding sugar-containing breath mints and other candies that might cause tooth decay or erosion. Artificially sweetened gum or mints may be helpful. Children and their parents/caregivers who have not had their teeth cleaned or an oral examination within the past 6 months should be referred to a dentist. For those with oral dryness, bioactive enzyme mouthwashes and lozenges are available over the counter.

Malocclusion

Malocclusions have their basis in hereditary and environmental factors. Environmental factors include the premature loss of teeth due to trauma, caries, ectopic eruptions, and/or persistent use of a pacifier and/or thumbsucking beyond infancy. Southeast Asian populations have the greatest degree of severe malocclusion. Malocclusions include anterior and posterior crossbites, as well as open bites. An *anterior* crossbite is due to crowding where one or more teeth are either behind or in front of the teeth in the opposing jaw while the others are in good alignment. With a *posterior* crossbite, one or more of the upper teeth is inside the opposing lower tooth. With an anterior *open* bite, the front teeth do not touch together when the back teeth are biting; these children may have a habit of passing their tongues through the space. They can also have problems speaking or chewing and swallowing.

Malocclusion may have serious esthetic implications, affecting the self-esteem of the child or adolescent. Orthodontic treatment is not always available or affordable for many; however, whenever possible, PCPs should engage these dental health specialists for early preventive treatment if possible.

Mucocele

A mucocele is a salivary gland lesion caused by a blockage of a salivary gland duct. It is most common on the lower lip and has the appearance of a fluid-filled vesicle or a fluctuant nodule normal in color with the overlying mucosa. The most probable cause is trauma or a habit of lip biting. The individual should be referred to an oral surgeon for surgical excision (Fig. 20.11).

Pericoronitis

Pericoronitis is due to a partially erupted lower wisdom tooth with a tissue flap covering part of the crown. A foreign body, such as a piece of food, is forced under the flap, causing a localized infection. In some cases, upper wisdom teeth will erupt with the crown rubbing against the buccal mucosa and cause pain. Partially erupted wisdom teeth can create an environment in which the distal surface of the second molar becomes decayed because it cannot be cleaned. The gum tissue partially covering the tooth is inflamed and painful, and fever may be present. The tissue flap may show trauma from biting.

Not all wisdom teeth need to be removed. Most teeth that are fully covered in bone do not need to be removed and carry no significant risk. Similarly, if there is space for the erupting teeth, there is no reason to remove them. It is appropriate to wait for the teeth to fully erupt as much as they can because this maximizes the chance that they will not need to be removed and minimizes

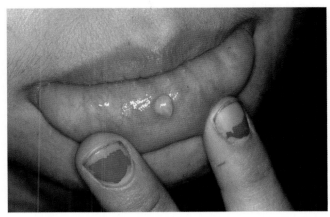

• **Fig. 20.11** Mucocele. (From Kliegman RM, St. Geme JW, Blum JN, et al, eds. *Nelson Textbook of Pediatrics.* 21st ed. Elsevier; 2020.)

injuries associated with the surgery. Impacted teeth, unerupted teeth with cysts, and upper teeth that have erupted toward the buccal mucosa should be examined and assessed for surgical removal.

Removal of wisdom teeth always requires a risk-benefit calculation because there is significant morbidity associated with the surgery. Temporary or permanent nerve damage is possible, as is TMJ disorder.[41] A common complication of wisdom tooth surgery is alveolar osteitis or dry socket. This painful condition is associated with the loss of the normal clot in the healing socket that exposes bone. Smoking and the use of oral contraceptives are risk factors. Pretreatment rinsing with 0.12% chlorhexidine gluconate mouth rinse reduces the risk of complications. Treatment at the time of surgery with a nonsteroidal antiinflammatory may reduce the extent of swelling postoperatively. Pain and foul taste in the mouth are the main symptoms, beginning 4 to 5 days after surgery. Referral to the dentist is imperative.

Ranula

A ranula is a cyst filled with mucin from a ruptured salivary gland. It most often appears as a large, soft, mucous-containing swelling in the floor of the mouth. The cyst should be excised by an oral surgeon (Fig. 20.12).

Temporomandibular Joint Disorder

TMJ disorder includes chronic facial pain and mandibular dysfunction and is multifactorial in origin. Studies suggest that the onset of most TMJ disorders increases with age and with greater occurrence during adolescence. Prevalence rates range from 4.2% to 25% in those 5 to 19 years old. Females have significantly higher rates (correlated to onset of puberty) than males.[42] Third molar (i.e., wisdom teeth) removal can result in TMJ disorder.[41]

Clinical symptoms may include self-reported facial (e.g., face, neck, temples, or jaw) pain once or more times per week associated with limitation in normal ability to open the mouth wide or with chewing; jaw locking; painful clicking, popping, or grating in jaw joint; and/or change in occlusion. On examination, the facial muscles are tender to palpation, often unilaterally, but there is usually no swelling or skin bruising. The individual will be afebrile. Tooth pain, if present, is nonspecific. There may be a deviation to the painful side when the mouth is opened. Pain,

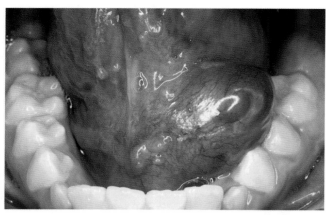

• **Fig. 20.12** Ranula of the Floor of the Mouth. (From Neville BW, Damm DD, Allen CM, et al, eds. *Oral and Maxillofacial Pathology*. 4th ed. Elsevier; 2016.)

particularly in the chewing muscles and/or jaw joint, is the most common symptom.

The differential diagnoses include infection of the face, ear, or a possible abscessed tooth; traumatic injury (e.g., fracture/dislocation of the jaw); myositis; sinusitis; headaches; neoplasm; arthritis; collagen diseases (e.g., SLE); congenital and developmental anomalies of the joint (rare); and capsulitis.

Conservative treatment should always be the first course of treatment because invasive, irreversible approaches have not proven effective (surgery, bite appliances, orthodontics, jaw implants, adjusting the bite).[43] Recommendations include avoiding extreme jaw movements, soft diet, muscle relaxation and gentle stretching exercises, application of ice packs, analgesics, and antiinflammatory medication. A short-term, removable plastic splint over the upper or lower teeth may be fitted by a dentist to see if pain relief is achieved.

Evidence does not support the supposition that chewing gum, bad bite, or orthodontic care causes TMJ disorder, but chewing gum may exacerbate it. Botox is currently being studied in adults to see if it might be a useful treatment for chronic TMJ disorder.[44] Botox use in children and young teenagers should be avoided. As the bone mass of the TMJs has not fully matured at these young ages, reducing muscle pull around the TMJs as a result of Botox injections is contraindicated. Individuals who do not respond to the basic recommendations need referral to specialized centers with expanded oral health teams that include dentists and psychologists, because adaptive behaviors to the discomfort or pain include being anxious or depressed, avoiding social interaction, developing other physical symptoms (e.g., migraines, tension headaches, back pain, ulcers, colitis), or seeking pharmacologic relief.

Traumatic Injuries to Oral Structures

Injuries to the face usually result in trauma to the soft tissues of the mouth, teeth, or jaws. Such trauma is one of the most common presentations of young children to dentists. Dental injuries occur secondary to falls, motor vehicle accidents, violence, abuse, contact with hard objects, and sporting activities. Although fewer traumas are seen from supervised, organized sports where children now wear mouth guards, a disproportionate amount of trauma results from unsupervised activities, such as skateboarding. Upper incisors are particularly vulnerable to dental injuries.

Age is a significant consideration in trauma to teeth. Most injuries cluster in three age groups: 1 to 3 years old (falls, physical abuse), 7 to 10 years old (bicycle and playground accidents), and 16 to 18 years old (sports injuries, fights, vehicular accidents). It is important to rule out physical abuse because the orofacial region is commonly traumatized during such episodes. The PCP should be alert to the possibility of a closed head or neck injury if severe trauma is reported. If child abuse is suspected, call the child abuse hotline.

Clinical Findings

Because a dental injury may become the subject of litigation, a thorough history and examination is mandatory. When possible, an injury should be photographed.

History

- Circumstance—When and how did the trauma occur?
- Presence and/or history of other injuries?
- Safety—Is there any concern for the safety of the child and/or family?
- Family history—Is there a history of physical abuse or drug or alcohol use in the family?
- Impact—Are any problems or limitations occurring because of the trauma?
- Immunizations—Tetanus within the last 5 years? (This question is especially important with soil-contaminated wounds or with complete displacement of a tooth from its socket.)
- Recent dental work—For children presenting with trauma to the inside of the cheek, tongue, or lip, did the child recently receive local anesthetic for dental treatment?

Physical Examination

Blunt trauma tends to cause greater damage to soft tissues and supporting structures, whereas high-velocity or sharp injuries cause luxation (i.e., dislocation) and fractures of the teeth. Children with sports-related injuries can have teeth that are avulsed, fractured loosened, or displaced from their normal position.

The examination should include:
- Soft tissue: palpate jaws and facial skeleton for potential fracture.
- Skin: assess for extraoral lacerations and facial wounds.
- Intraoral mucosa: assess for wounds, swelling, and bruising of the oral mucosa, gingiva, tongue, cheeks, and palate.
- Assess teeth for:
  - Displaced, loose, missing, fractured teeth
  - Root fracture: caused by injury to the tooth root
  - Bite problems: check for abnormalities in occlusion
  - Pulp exposure: bleeding from the broken stump of the tooth itself
  - Color change: intact tooth turning dark from internal bleeding and trauma
  - Jaw movement: deviation to one side, pain on opening, decreased range of motion

Management

Most minor injuries to the oral soft tissues do not require suturing unless bleeding is a problem. Wound care should consist of irrigating the area with sterile saline and prescribing water-based 0.12% chlorhexidine gluconate mouth rinse 2 to 3 minutes twice daily. Avoid alcohol-based rinses, as use of these rinses may be painful. Children with avulsed and fractured teeth, those unable to bite normally, and those with jaw injuries should be referred to a dentist promptly to avoid tooth abscesses, dental pain, and problems with the eruption of permanent teeth.

Complications

Tooth Avulsion

Avulsed primary teeth should not be replanted. If permanent teeth are knocked out, timing is important, and the following instructions can be provided over the phone. The child should be referred to a dentist at the same time.

Replant an avulsed permanent, clean tooth immediately. If the tooth is dirty, rinse it gently under cold running water (for <10 seconds), and then replant it.[35] Do not rub the root surface. If the tooth can be replanted, have the child bite gently on a handkerchief or clean cloth to keep the tooth in place. The dentist will be able to ensure that the tooth is in the right position and stabilized. If unable to immediately replant the tooth, store the tooth in cold milk, physiologic saline, or saliva to prevent dehydration. The prognosis for successful replantation decreases with time. A tooth that is allowed to dehydrate will not be viable after 1 hour; however, it is still important to have a dentist evaluate as soon as possible because there are some interventions that can be taken for a tooth that has been out of its socket for longer than 60 minutes.

Tooth Fracture

If possible, have the child keep the pieces of permanent incisors and place them in saline or water to prevent drying. Sometimes the dentist can temporarily repair the tooth if the fragment is large enough. Tooth fractures with bleeding from the stump are emergencies. Simple fractures not involving the pulp or nerve tissue are not emergencies but still need attention/repair.

Patient/Family Education

Trauma compromises a previously healthy dentition and affects self-esteem and quality of life. In some cases, the traumatized tooth may be asymptomatic and appear to be clinically normal. This tooth can subsequently become darker or can become spontaneously symptomatic, with the child reporting cold sensitivity, pain on chewing, or unprovoked pain.

It is important to identify and educate children who are at high risk for dental trauma–related injuries. Children and teenagers who participate in sports should be encouraged to wear mouth guards and helmets. Parents and coaches should also encourage youths to remove all intraoral piercings (e.g., tongue and lip rings or studs) while participating in sports. Parents, coaches, and physical education teachers should be alerted to the importance of including ViaSpan or Hanks' Balanced Salt Solution in first-aid kits to manage tooth avulsions.

Lifestyle Choices That Affect Dental Health

Oral and Intraoral Piercings and Tattoos

Adolescents may have piercings in the tongue and lower lip or tattoos on the buccal mucosa of the lips. Tissue around tongue studs may be infected, as evidenced by inflammation, swelling, and pain. The inflammation and pain may be an allergic response to the metals in the studs or piercings, particularly nickel. There also may be gum recession or fractures of the lower anterior teeth from metal studs, which can habitually click against the teeth. Tongues, especially after stud insertion, can become swollen.

Of note is that the mouth heals quickly, and the inflammatory response should be resolved within 8 to 10 days without treatment. Swelling beyond this time period suggests infection or allergic response. Infection should be treated with 0.12% chlorhexidine gluconate mouthwash twice per day for at least 1 week and a broad-spectrum systemic antibiotic, such as penicillin or clindamycin. If mouth tissue is infected, the ornament should be removed, at least temporarily. If an allergic reaction to nickel is suspected, changing to gold or silver is advised. The PCP should ensure vaccinations are current, especially tetanus and hepatitis B. Deep neck infection, airway obstruction, bleeding, nerve damage, tooth fracture, systemic infections, and hepatitis have been noted. Adolescents contemplating or who have oral piercings should be counseled about:

- Potential for acquiring an infectious disease
- Using regulated practitioners for piercing
- Ensuring sterile equipment and noble metals are used
- Completing a hepatitis B vaccination series *before* seeking piercing
- Potential damage to the teeth and gums
- Need to remove studs and piercings during sports

Smokeless Tobacco Use and Vaping

Smokeless tobacco is a highly addictive substance. Because it is held in the oral cavity, it not only allows nicotine to enter the bloodstream, but it is also detrimental to oral health. Popular cultural events (e.g., baseball) and heroes/role models (e.g., rodeo riders, baseball players) can make the habit look "cool." Its popularity has also been attributed to intensive promotion and flavors, being viewed as a way to lose weight, and a way to get nicotine without having to frequent restricted smoking areas.

Vaping and electronic cigarettes (e-cigarettes) have also become increasingly popular among youth. In 2022, 3.3% of middle school students and 14.1% of high school students reported vaping in the past 30 days.[36] Studies have reported a significant positive association between vaping and caries risk as well as associations between vaping and untreated tooth decay.[45] Vaping also appears to lead to changes in the oral microbiome, which may be one explanation for changes in caries risk.[40] Most youth appear to be unaware of the potential oral health effects of vaping.[46]

Betel nut (areca) may be crushed and chewed alone or combined with tobacco and held in the cheek like smokeless tobacco. It is the fourth most commonly used drug in the world, is carcinogenic, and legal in the United States. Nearly 70% of adolescents in the Federated States of Micronesia use betel nut at least once per month, which is a growing concern for the mainland United States because of high rates of migration from the Pacific Islands.[47]

PCPs should examine the posterior buccal vestibule of the lower jaw and the anterior buccal vestibule of the upper jaw. These are the areas where smokeless tobacco and betel nut are commonly held in the mouth. The intraoral findings include leukoplakia (matted white plaques on the soft tissues of the oral cavity), erythroplakia (matted red plaques), gingivitis and gum recession (particularly in the lower jaw), periodontitis, stained teeth, halitosis, and tooth decay (associated with tobacco products that have added sweeteners).

Individuals who use tobacco products and vape should be assessed for willingness to undergo tobacco cessation treatments. Active family involvement in the lives of children can help to prevent the start of vaping and smokeless tobacco use. If children have relatives who smoke, use smokeless tobacco products or are vaping, PCPs may need to focus family tobacco cessation efforts to encourage healthy adolescent behaviors. Complications include lip and oral cancer, gingivitis, gum recession, periodontitis, and stained teeth. Further studies on the oral effects of e-cigarettes are emerging.

Tooth Whitening (Bleaching)

Tooth whitening and bleaching are popular with youth as adolescents can be particularly self-conscious of discoloration of the teeth. Tooth whitening may be indicated for permanent teeth discolored or stained by trauma, fluorosis, tetracycline use during tooth development, or foods and caffeinated beverages. A pretreatment evaluation by a dentist is recommended prior to bleaching to determine the etiology of the discoloration and any contraindications to the bleaching. The AAPD recommends judicious use of these products, particularly in a child with mixed primary and permanent teeth.

Tooth whitening can involve the use of over-the-counter kits, in-office treatment, or take-home bleaching trays that are customized by a dentist. The in-office tooth whitening process involves repeated short-term exposure of teeth to carbamide peroxide (typically in the range of 10%–38%) until desired results are achieved. Over-the-counter kits include lower concentration carbamide peroxide in trays or hydrogen peroxide in strips. Most products are used for 2-week periods. There are also numerous gels, rinses, gums, toothpastes, and paint-on films. Higher concentrations of hydrogen peroxide are more effective than lower concentrations. Up to 66% of those using bleaching agents can experience hypersensitive teeth and soft tissue/gum irritation, usually in the initial bleaching stages.[48] Teeth will generally return to their normal sensation, gum status, and color if treatments are not repeated.

PCPs can educate parents that permanent teeth are naturally darker than primary teeth. Unless there are major esthetic concerns that could affect a child's psychosocial development, tooth whitening should not be undertaken until all permanent teeth have fully erupted. This measure will also prevent shade mismatching that can occur when teeth are whitened during the mixed dentition stage.

Eating Disorders

PCPs and dentists may be the first provider to recognize an adolescent with an eating disorder. Purging by vomiting can result in halitosis, dry mouth, tooth erosion, translucency, and sensitivity. Stomach acid damages the teeth, notably inside the upper front teeth.

Dental Care for Children With Special Health Care Needs

Children with special health care needs including congenital heart disease, facial clefts, esophageal defects, generalized hypotonia, muscular dysfunction, or intellectual and developmental disability often require additional preventive strategies and individualized dental appointments based upon their particular needs and conditions. At-risk children also include those with neuropsychological conditions (e.g., intellectual and developmental disability, autism spectrum disorder); sensory challenges (e.g., blindness, visual impairment, deafness, and hearing impairments); musculoskeletal or other structural difficulties (e.g., osteogenesis imperfecta, cerebral palsy, spina bifida, cleft lip/palate, paralysis); and chronic diseases (e.g., asthma, cardiovascular disorders, cystic fibrosis, chronic renal failure, diabetes mellitus, bleeding disorders, malignant disease, and epilepsy).

Preterm infants born with special health care needs may be more vulnerable to structural tooth defects, which can lead to increased risk for tooth decay. Some individuals have a higher incidence of oral disease either because of a systemic problem or because of the secondary effects on tooth development, diet, medications, or the inability of caretakers to clean or maintain the teeth.

Risks include:
- *Diet.* Children with special healthcare needs often have feeding problems, nutritional alterations/needs, and challenges. In addition, food is often retained in the mouth for a long time before it is swallowed. For children with reduced salivary secretion or impaired self-cleaning mechanisms of the oral cavity, restrictions in cavity-causing foods are necessary to prevent tooth decay.
- *Medications.* Ideally, medications should be taken at mealtime if possible. Rinsing the mouth and teeth with water after a meal may help if brushing is not feasible. Water or non-sweetened beverages should be recommended for drinks between meals. Phenytoin commonly causes gingival hyperplasia. Box 20.1 lists classes of drugs that may reduce salivation and thereby increase susceptibility to caries.
- *Muscular function.* Hypotonia may influence mouth breathing and salivation and cause drooling or chewing problems. Impaired manual dexterity may make it difficult for children to perform preventive oral hygiene routines. Hypertonia may result in extensive tooth wear as a result of grinding of teeth. Children with feeding tubes face additional challenges because oral health may be challenging.

PCPs are advised to ask about the status of dental visits and whether routine oral hygiene is being maintained. In addition, the following topics should be covered:
- *Topical fluorides.* A child with reduced salivary secretion, impaired muscular function, or with a cavity-causing diet may need an intense fluoride program in addition to careful oral hygiene. PCPs can apply 5% sodium fluoride topical varnish every 3 months or prescribe a fluoride rinse, gel, or high-fluoride (1.1% sodium fluoride) toothpaste for home use. Carefully monitor the teeth of these patients and make prompt referrals when problems are noted.
- *Topical iodine.* The teeth and gums can be painted with topical PVP-iodine once every 4 to 6 months. As previously discussed, there is evidence that topical 10% povidone-iodine suppresses tooth decay–causing flora without major changes in the overall

---

• BOX 20.1 Classes and Examples of Drugs Associated With Decreased Salivation and Xerostomia

- Analgesics: nonsteroidal anti-inflammatory drugs, narcotic analgesics
- Antidepressants: fluoxetine, amitriptyline
- Antiemetics: promethazine, metoclopramide
- Antihistamines: diphenhydramine, promethazine
- Antihypertensives: β-blockers, diuretics, angiotensin-converting enzyme inhibitors
- Antipsychotics: clozapine, chlorpromazine, risperidone

flora.[23] Children who have had major dental treatment because of extensive dental caries are obvious candidates for repeated iodine treatments. Iodine can be painted on the teeth at the same visit in which fluoride varnish is applied with the iodine wiped off with gauze before applying the varnish. PCPs can do this treatment if there is limited access to pediatric dental services.

References

1. Centers for Medicaid and Medicare Services (CMS). Dental Coverage in the Market Place. https://www.healthcare.gov/coverage/dental-coverage/.
2. American Academy of Pediatrics. Oral Health. https://www.aap.org/en/patient-care/oral-health/.
3. US Department of Health and Human Services. *Oral Health Strategic Framework*; 2014-2017. https://www.ncbi.nlm.nih.gov/pubmed/26957659.
4. Institute of Medicine (IOM) and National Research Council (NRC). *Improving Access to Oral Health for Vulnerable and Underserved Populations*. http://www.nationalacademies.org/hmd/~/media/Files/Report%20Files/2011.
5. American Academy on Pediatric Dentistry Council on Clinical Affairs. Policy on the dental home. *Pediatr Dent*. 2018;40(6):29–30.
6. Afeiche MC, Koyratty BNS, Wang D, Jacquier EF, Lê KA. Intakes and sources of total and added sugars among 4 to 13-year-old children in China, Mexico and the United States. *Pediatr Obes*. 2018;13(4):204–212.
7. American Academy of Pediatric Dentistry (AAPD). Policy on Social Determinants of Children's Oral Health and Health Disparities. *Oral Health Policies & Recommendations*; 2022. https://www.aapd.org/research/oral-health-policies--recommendations/social_determinants/.
8. Lewis CW. Teeth: small but mighty and mighty important. A comprehensive review of children's dental health for primary care clinicians. *Curr Pediatr Rev*. 2020;16(3):215–231.
9. US Food and Drug Administration (FDA). Dental Amalgam Fillings. https://www.fda.gov/medical-devices/dental-devices/dental-amalgam-fillings.
10. Noor Mohamed R, Basha S, Virupaxi SG, Idawara Eregowda N, Parameshwarappa P. Hypomineralized primary teeth in preterm low birth weight children and its association with molar incisor hypomineralization-a 3-year-prospective study. *Children*. 2021;8(12).
11. DeSeta M, Holden E, Siddik D, Bhujel N. Natal and neonatal teeth: a review and case series. *Br Dent J*. 2022;232(7):449–453.
12. McNeil DW, Randall CL, Cohen LL, et al. Transmission of dental fear from parent to adolescent in an Appalachian sample in the USA. *Int J Paediatr Dent*. 2019;29(6):720–727.
13. Gupta N, Sandhu M, Sachdev V, Jhingan P. Comparison of visual examination and magnification with DIAGNOdent for detection of smooth surface initial carious lesion-dry and wet conditions. *Int J Clin Pediatr Dent*. 2019;12(1):37–41.
14. Chi DL, Momany ET, Jones MP, et al. An explanatory model of factors related to well baby visits by age three years for Medicaid-enrolled infants: a retrospective cohort study. *BMC Pediatr*. 2013;13:158.
15. Beil HA, Rozier RG. Primary health care providers' advice for a dental checkup and dental use in children. *Pediatrics*. 2010;126(2):e435–e441.
16. Anil S, Anand PS. Early childhood caries: prevalence, risk factors, and prevention. *Front Pediatr*. 2017;5:157.
17. American Academy on pediatric dentistry liaison with other groups committee; American Academy on pediatric dentistry council on clinical affairs. Policy on use of fluoride. *Pediatr Dent*. 2017;39(6):49–50.
18. Mickenautsch S, Yengopal V. Caries-preventive effect of high-viscosity glass ionomer and resin-based fissure sealants on permanent teeth: a systematic review of clinical trials. *PLoS One*. 2016;11(1):e0146512.
19. Chi DL. Parent refusal of topical fluoride for their children: clinical strategies and future research priorities to improve evidence-based pediatric dental practice. *Dent Clin North Am*. 2017;61(3):607–617.
20. U.S. Preventive Services Task Force. Screening and interventions to prevent dental caries in children younger than 5 years. *JAMA*. 2021;32621:2172–2178.
21. Centers for Disease Control and Prevention (CDC). My water's fluoride: water with fluoride protects teeth from tooth decay. https://nccd.cdc.gov/doh_mwf/default/AboutMWF.aspx.
22. Tut OK, Milgrom PM. Topical iodine and fluoride varnish combined is more effective than fluoride varnish alone for protecting erupting first permanent molars: a retrospective cohort study. *J Public Health Dent*. 2010;70(3):249–252.
23. Milgrom P, Tut O, Rothen M, Mancl L, Gallen M, Tanzer JM. Addition of povidone-iodine to fluoride varnish for dental caries: a randomized clinical trial. *JDR Clin Trans Res*. 2021;6(2):195–204.
24. Frencken JE. Atraumatic restorative treatment and minimal intervention dentistry. *Br Dent J*. 2017;223(3):183–189.
25. Innes NP, Evans DJ, Bonifacio CC, et al. The hall technique 10 years on: questions and answers. *Br Dent J*. 2017;222(6):478–483.
26. Vasudavan S, Grunes B, Mcgeachie J, Sonis AL. Antibiotic prescribing patterns among dental professionals in Massachusetts. *Pediatr Dent*. 2019;41(1):25–30.
27. Periodontal diseases of children and adolescents. *Pediatr Dent*. 2017;39(6):431–439.
28. Lim GXD, Yang J. Effect of silver diamine fluoride on hyperplastic gingivitis in an adult with intellectual disability-A case report. *Spec Care Dentist*. 2022;42(1):73–79.
29. Goldman RD. Acyclovir for herpetic gingivostomatitis in children. *Can Fam Physician*. 2016;62(5):403–404.
30. Bruney TL, Scime NV, Madubueze A, Chaput KH. Systematic review of the evidence for resolution of common breastfeeding problems-Ankyloglossia (tongue tie). *Acta Paediatr*. 2022;111(5):940–947.
31. O'Shea JE, Foster JP, O'Donnell CP, et al. Frenotomy for tongue-tie in newborn infants. *Cochrane Database Syst Rev*. 2017;3(3):CD011065.
32. Santa Maria C, Aby J, Truong MT, Thakur Y, Rea S, Messner A. The superior labial frenulum in newborns: what is normal?. *Glob Pediatr Health*. 2017;4. 2333794X17718896.
33. Lin LZ, Xu SL, Wu QZ, et al. Exposure to second-hand smoke during early life and subsequent sleep problems in children: a population-based cross-sectional study. *Environ Health*. 2021;20(1):127.
34. Martins IM, Alonso LS, Vale MP, Abreu LG, Serra-Negra JM. Association between the severity of possible sleep bruxism and possible awake bruxism and attrition tooth wear facets in children and adolescents. *Cranio*. 2022:1–7.
35. Andersson L, Andreasen JO, Day P, et al. International Association of Dental Traumatology guidelines for the management of traumatic dental injuries: 2. Avulsion of permanent teeth. *Dent Traumatol*. 2012;28(2):88–96.
36. Park-Lee E, Ren C, Cooper M, Cornelius M, Jamal A, Cullen KA. Tobacco product use among middle and high school students—United States, 2022. *MMWR Morb Mortal Wkly Rep*. 2022;71(45):1429–1435.
37. L RG. Treating bruxism in children. *Decis Dent*. 2018;4(2):53–56.
38. Chisini LA, San Martin AS, Cademartori MG, Boscato N, Correa MB, Goettems ML. Interventions to reduce bruxism in children and adolescents: a systematic scoping review and critical reflection. *Eur J Pediatr*. 2020;179(2):177–189.
39. Neurath C, Limeback H, Osmunson B, Connett M, Kanter V, Wells CR. Dental fluorosis trends in US oral health surveys: 1986 to 2012. *JDR Clin Trans Res*. 2019;4(4):298–308.
40. Yang I, Rodriguez J, Young Wright C, Hu YJ. Oral microbiome of electronic cigarette users: a cross-sectional exploration. *Oral Dis*. 2022.

41. Huang GJ, Cunha-Cruz J, Rothen M, et al. A prospective study of clinical outcomes related to third molar removal or retention. *Am J Public Health*. 2014;104(4):728–734.

42. American Academy of Pediatric Dentistry (AAPD). *Acquired Temporomandibular Disorders in Infants, Children, and Adolescents. The Reference Manual of Pediatric Dentistry*. Chicago, Ill: American Academy of Pediatric Dentistry; 2021:426–434. 2021.

43. National Institutes of Dental and Craniofacial Research (NIDCR) and National Institutes of Health (NIH). TMJ Disorders. https://www.nidcr.nih.gov/sites/default/files/2017-12/tmj-disorders.pdf.

44. De la Torre Canales G, Poluha RL, Pinzón NA, et al. Efficacy of botulinum toxin type-a i in the improvement of mandibular motion and muscle sensibility in myofascial pain TMD subjects: a randomized controlled trial. *Toxins*. 2022;14(7).

45. Irusa KF, Finkelman M, Magnuson B, Donovan T, Eisen SE. A comparison of the caries risk between patients who use vapes or electronic cigarettes and those who do not: a cross-sectional study. *J Am Dent Assoc*. 2022;153(12):1179–1183.

46. Martell KM, Boyd LD, Giblin-Scanlon LJ, Vineyard J. Knowledge, attitudes, and practices of young adults regarding the impact of electronic cigarette use on oral health. *J Am Dent Assoc*. 2020;151(12):903–911.

47. Milgrom P, Tut OK, Gilmatam J, Gallen M, Chi DL. Areca use among adolescents in Yap and Pohnpei, the Federated States OF Micronesia. *Harm Reduct J*. 2013;10:26.

48. Policy on the use of dental bleaching for child and adolescent patients. *Pediatr Dent*. 2018;40(6):92–94.

21
Pediatric Injury Prevention

JAIME PANTON AND DAWN LEE GARZON

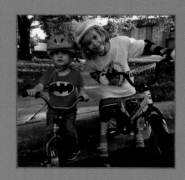

Injuries are the leading cause of pediatric deaths among those older than 1 year of age, causing more death and disability than the other top causes combined.[1] They are classified as unintentional or intentional. *Unintentional* injuries (UIs) are injuries that are unplanned and without intent to harm the child. These injuries include motor vehicle crashes (MVC), drowning, falls, fires, poisonings, and other causes (Table 21.1). Conversely, *intentional* injuries result from purposeful inflicted harm, either to oneself or another and include suicide, homicide, or child maltreatment (physical abuse, sexual abuse, emotional abuse, or neglect). See Chapter 22 for a discussion about intentional injuries and child maltreatment.

Unintentional Injuries

Globally, much progress has been made to decrease rates of childhood mortality related to preventable causes. Yet UIs are still a leading cause of death around the world. UIs are not simply accidents caused by chance but are predictable and preventable occurrences, hence the change in terminology from *accidental* to *unintentional*. The most common fatal UI in early childhood is drowning.[2] In older children and adolescents, MVC have historically caused more injury deaths; however, gun violence is currently the leading cause of death in this population in the United States.[3] Known UI risks include individual factors, such as male gender, age (younger children have the highest rates of UI, adolescents have the highest fatality rates), inattention, oppositionality, temperament, and risk-taking behaviors. Environmental risk factors include the presence of neighborhood hazards, multiple children in the home, single parents, as well as lower family socioeconomic status and education level. Young children depend on adults to prevent injury; those under 6 years of age may be able to recite safety rules, but do not always follow them and/or lack the ability to detect risk in different contexts. Therefore it is critical that parents have a realistic understanding of their child's developmental ability. Parents who overestimate their child's abilities (e.g., the 6-year-old who always knows to check for cars before he crosses the street) or underestimate their child's abilities (e.g., the parent who thinks their 15-month-old will not climb up stairs without a parent being there) may place their children at risk for injury because of inadequate supervision.

Principles of Injury Control

The most effective injury prevention education focuses on specific, useable information that decreases injury risk, rather than broad, nonspecific recommendations. Decreasing injury risk is based on an injury control framework, such as the Haddon Matrix, which identifies factors that contribute to injury (Table 21.2). Originally drawn from infection control theory, this theory isolates individual and environmental factors in the preinjury, injury, and post event timeframes that affect whether injury occurs and determines the severities of those injuries.

Passive injury prevention strategies, which involve the implementation of safety measures that do not require parents to change their behavior to make the environment safer for their children, are the most effective approach to reducing injury. These strategies include everyday modification of items in the child's environment, such as the use of child-resistant caps on medicines and cleaning products, and safety design in toys.

Another approach includes environmental modification, such as the use of smoke and carbon monoxide detectors, safe roadway design to reduce traffic volume and speed in residential neighborhoods, window locks, and firearm safety locks. Pediatric primary care providers (PCPs) should advocate for local and national injury prevention strategies and support programs such as the Safe Kids USA campaign (www.safekids.org). They should also support injury prevention legislation, promote initiatives to ensure consumer product safety, and implement public health strategies to decrease injury. Public and consumer awareness is crucial for successful prevention programs and PCPs are trusted sources of information about safe, developmentally appropriate toys and products.

Emergency preparedness is important for all PCPs and families. Although most individuals with serious injuries go to emergency departments or urgent care clinics, it is important for PCPs to remain current in basic cardiac life support (BCLS) and injury management as a severely injured child may present in primary care settings. Likewise, all parents and caregivers should be encouraged to enroll in a basic BCLS program that includes pediatric life support training and choking prevention, as well as reviewing basic first aid measures.

Injury Control

UI control (previously referred to as *injury prevention*) involves the use of both passive and active strategies that impact individual, social, physical, environmental, and vector/vehicle contributory factors. As noted earlier, the most effective strategies are *passive*, such as instituting graduated driving laws, requiring booster seats for older children, using safe road design, requiring minimal safety features for consumer products, and improving access to emergency services if injuries occur. In contrast, *active* strategies are when an individual takes part in the injury prevention plan, such

TABLE
21.1

TABLE 21.1 Common Causes of Unintentional Injury-Related Death by Age

Age	Mechanism of Injury Death	Anticipatory Guidance[a]
Newborn/neonate (0–1 month) Infant (1 month–1 year)	1. Accidental suffocation 2. MVC 3. Drowning	• Back to sleep in parent's room but not in parent's bed • Review car seat safety guidelines, instruct parent/caregiver not to drive under the influence
Early childhood: toddler (1–2 years) and preschool (3–5 years)	1. Drowning 2. Falls 3. MVC	• Constant supervision around water (pools, bathtubs, lakes, etc.) • Personal flotation devices (life jackets, not floaties) • Swim lessons beginning by age 4 years • Adequate fencing around pools • Do not leave child unattended near or inside of a vehicle
Middle childhood (6–10 years)	1. MVC 2. Drowning 3. Fires/burns	• Review car seat safety guidelines at every well visit • Consistent use of seatbelts • Swim lessons • Adult supervision around water • If on a boat or watercraft, wear Coast Guard–approved life jacket • Functioning smoke alarms in the home
Early adolescence (11–14 years) Middle adolescence (15–17 years) Late adolescence (18–24 years)	1. MVC 2. Poisoning 3. Drowning	• Prevent distracted driving • Consistent seatbelt use • Homes free of firearms • If a firearm is in the home, it must be stored unloaded and locked with ammunition stored separately

[a]Modified from Hagan JF, Shaw JS, Duncan PM. *Bright Futures: Guidelines for Health Supervision of Infants, Children, and Adolescents.* 4th ed. American Academy of Pediatrics; 2017.

MVC, Motor vehicle crash.

TABLE
21.2

TABLE 21.2 Haddon Phase Factor Matrix for Understanding a Bicycle Injury in a 5-Year-Old Child

Injury Phase	INJURY FACTORS			
	Individual	Agent	Physical Environment	Social Environment
(Pre)event Fall precursors	Inattention, bike riding skills, ability to respond to balance changes, sensory deficits	Speed, bald tires, worn brakes	Busy street, road hazards, steep grade on hill, visibility	Does not own bicycle helmet, parental supervision, residential street speed limits, beliefs about injury control
Event What forces cause injury	Ability to control bicycle, distractions, clothing that protects skin from friction forces (road rash)	Head hits the road without a helmet, gravitational forces, child skids across the road, road surface type	Wet road, surface hardness, high curb on roadside, presence of vehicle on the road	Adult witnessing injury, understanding of injury severity, child injured in a location where they can be easily reached, bicycle helmet laws
(Post)event Injury treatment and recovery	Child's health, ability of wrist fracture and skin to heal, extent of concussion	Did bicycle land on child?	Distance to emergent care, difficulty transporting child to care, quality of care	Ability to afford health care, ability to access follow-up care, family's ability to care for the injuries, social support

as a childproofing cabinets and/or drawers containing medications and/or toxic substances.

There are three levels of injury control: primary, secondary, and tertiary. *Primary* interventions focus on how injuries can be prevented (e.g., anticipatory guidance). *Secondary* levels of prevention focus on decreasing injury severity and include strategies like seat belt and home smoke detector use. *Tertiary* prevention focuses on reducing morbidity and mortality once the injury occurs (e.g., on-scene management of injury).

Injury control requires a multidimensional approach that includes education about how to provide a safe environment and developmentally appropriate supervision, advocating for public health policies that influence injury outcomes, and advocating for safe design and consumer awareness. Effective injury control strategies are developmentally grounded and focus on modifiable risk factors. Anticipatory guidance provided by PCPs at well-child visits should be developmentally appropriate. This includes assessing injury control techniques used within the home, reinforcing positive behaviors, and counseling about additional safety risks.[4] Written materials, audiovisual presentations, peer counseling, and one-to-one interaction with a health professional are all effective teaching and learning strategies, as well as online resources like www.safekids.org and www.healthchildren.org to help parents find safety information at home. PCPs should provide safety information in moderate doses, with reinforcement or repetition at subsequent visits. Research suggests parents only retain a certain amount of information; therefore only about four or five of the most developmentally appropriate teaching points should be discussed. Injury control education should be tailored to the individual/family context and risk. For example, if firearm deaths are a leading cause of death in the area, anticipatory guidance should focus on safe storage of firearms or removing firearms from the home. Counseling should also be specific. For example, teaching parents how to purchase the appropriately sized bicycle helmet is more effective than general statements such as "always wear a helmet."

Common Injury Mechanisms

Motor Vehicle–Related Injuries

MVCs are a leading cause of pediatric injury, death, and disability. In 2019 nearly 3000 infants, children, and adolescents under 21 years of age died in MVCs, and over 10,000 were involved in nonfatal crashes.[5] The greatest way to modify pediatric MVC outcomes is through the use of restraint systems appropriate for the individual's size and developmental stage. Known adolescent risk factors are driver distraction, substance use, risk-taking behaviors, and relative driving inexperience. All-terrain vehicles (ATVs), snowmobiles, motorcycles, and other motorized vehicles also contribute to adolescent risk factors.

Passenger restraint systems, including use/placement of infant, child, and booster seats and seatbelts effectively prevent significant injury. It is important to select and install child car seats according to the manufacturer's recommendations (Fig. 21.1).

Current child restraint guidelines call for the following[6]:

- Infants and toddlers should be kept rear-facing as long as possible, at least until they outgrow the maximum height and weight for their car seat.
- Young children who have outgrown rear-facing seats should transition to a forward-facing restraint that includes a harness until they outgrow the height and weight maximums for their car seat.

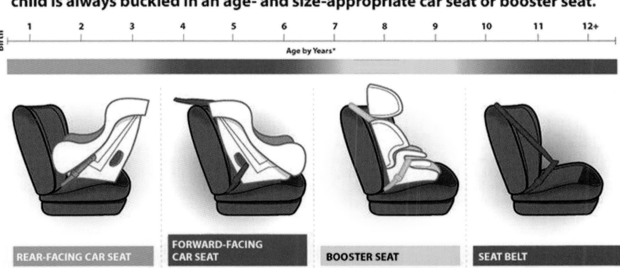

Using the correct car seat or booster seat can be a lifesafer: make sure your child is always buckled in an age- and size-appropriate car seat or booster seat.

Age by Years*

REAR-FACING CAR SEAT

Birth until age 2-4

Buckle children in a rear-facing car seat until they reach the maximum weight or height limit of their car seat. Keep children rear-facing as long as possible.

FORWARD-FACING CAR SEAT

After outgrowing rear-facing seat until at least age 5

When children outgrow their rear-facing car seat, they should be buckled in a forward-facing car seat until they reach the maximum weight or height limit of their car seat.

BOOSTER SEAT

After outgrowing forward-facing seat and until seat belts fit properly

Once children outgrow their forward-facing seat, they should be buckled in a booster seat until seat belts fit properly. Proper seat belt fit usually occurs when children are 4 feet 9 inches tall and age 9-12.

SEAT BELT

Once seat belts fit properly without a booster seat

Children no longer need to use a booster seat once seat belts fit them properly. Seat belts fit properly when the lap belt lays across the upper thighs (not the stomach) and the shoulder belt lays across the chest (not the neck).

Keep children ages 12 and under properly buckled in the back seat. Never place a rear-facing car seat in front of an active air bag.

Recommended age ranges for each seat type vary to account for differences in child growth and height/weight limits of car seats and booster seats. Use the car seat or booster seat owner's manual to check installation and the seat height and weight limits, and proper seat use.

Child safety seat recommendations: American Academy of Pediatrics.
Graphic design: adapted from National Highway Traffic Safety Administration.
www.cdc.gov/motorvehiclesafety/cps

• **Fig. 21.1** How to Select the Correct Car Seat. (From Centers for Disease Control and Prevention: Child Passenger Safety Infographics. https://www.cdc.gov/vitalsigns/childpassengersafety/infographic.html.)

- Once a harnessed car seat is outgrown, children should remain in booster seats until they are 4 feet 9 inches tall and are between 8 and 12 years old.
- Seat belts should not be used without a booster until the *shoulder belt* fits across the child's mid-chest, not the face or neck, and the *lap belt* fits across the pelvis, not the lower abdomen. The child needs to be able to sit in the car with legs bent and without slouching. Both shoulder/chest and lap restraints should always be used.
- Children should not sit in the front seat until they are 13 years old.

Adolescent drivers require additional injury control strategies, including[4]:

- Comprehensive graduated driving laws that help decrease deaths and injuries caused by inexperience, controlling movement from the learner's permit to the independent license, limiting nighttime driving, limiting passengers for teen drivers, and setting a minimum age for full licensure. These laws vary from state to state, so PCPs should be aware of rules in their area.
- Parents adding their own safety rules/driving agreement that cover restrictions, rules, and consequences for violations (see https://www.healthychildren.org/English/ages-stages/teen/safety/Pages/Teen-Driving-Agreement.aspx).
- Distraction is a leading reason for MVC. Technology, including phones and other electronic devices, should always be placed in "driving mode" so the devices are unable to be used when moving. There are also apps that prevent texting while driving (see www.distraction.gov).
- Adults should model safe driving behaviors, including seatbelt use, never driving when under the influence, avoiding aggressive driving, and never using technology while driving.

Falls

Falls are the leading cause of nonfatal injuries for all children over 1 year old. They occur with simple slips and falls, falls from a height (e.g., stairs, windows, balconies, playground equipment), during sports, and secondary to infant walker/equipment use or playsets, in homes, schools, neighborhoods, community playgrounds, childcare, and other settings.

Important components of fall control education include:

- Always watch children on playground equipment. Ensure that there is sufficient padding from either wood chips or sand. Grass does not absorb fall energy well.
- Place skid pads underneath carpets and rugs. Remove rugs that still slide even with skid pads.
- Place gates at the top and bottom of staircases. Consider using guard rails to prevent young children from getting access through spindles.
- Be cautious about leaving furniture and items that can be easily moved to allow a young child to reach areas by climbing.
- Use window guards on open windows above ground level.
- Always use helmets when using wheeled toys, skates, scooters, skateboards, and bicycles. Recommend wrist guards and knee/elbow pads when skating and skateboarding.

Drowning

Drowning is the leading cause of death in children ages 1 to 4 years old. It is also a leading cause of death in adolescence, when males have almost 10 times higher drowning death rates compared to females.[7] Supervision and environmental modification to decrease water access are leading protective factors for drowning.

Drownings occur in bodies of water (e.g., lakes, rivers, oceans), swimming pools, bathtubs, and from falling headfirst into buckets, toilets, or other containers with liquids.

Injury control to prevent drowning occurs by teaching families to:

- Never leave young children unattended when they are around water, including bathtubs, small/portable pools, hot tubs/spas, above- and below-ground pools, and natural water features like creeks and ponds. Do not assume that drowning children make noise.
- Be attentive and avoid being distracted when watching children around water. This includes avoiding technology, conversations with others, and alcohol or other substances.
- Everyone should learn basic water skills (e.g., how to float, basic swimming). Lessons can begin as early as age 1 year old, but the evidence for lessons before that age is lacking.[8]
- Fence off pools with a latched gate.
- Use personal flotation devices whenever near or in bodies of water.
- Never leave unattended buckets of water or other liquids around. A young child can drown in as little as one inch of standing water left in a bucket or container.

Fires and Burns

Burns are usually caused by scalding liquids in infancy and early childhood, while flames cause most burns in older children. Young children's burns commonly occur when they splash themselves by pulling objects filled with hot liquids (e.g., grabbing pot handles from the stove, pulling tablecloths/table runners and causing hot food or liquids spill, bathing in water that is too hot) or playing with lit candles and/or matches. Older children may mistakenly start fires or be burned with intentional fires. Residential fires can also occur from space heaters, smoking in bed, cooking, and electrical shorts.

Key points for anticipatory guidance regarding home and environmental safety issues related to burn prevention include:

- Install and maintain smoke detectors and carbon dioxide alarms in the home, on every floor, and near rooms where people sleep.
- Set the hot water heater thermostat at 120°F or lower.
- Turn pot handles away from the stove edge and use back burners if possible.
- Never leave cooking food on the stove unattended.
- Create and practice a family fire escape plan for the home.
- Be careful about leaving hot mugs and bowls within reach of infants and young children.
- Use table runners and tablecloths with caution as they can be used to pull hot items down on young children.
- Place barriers in front of open fireplaces or heating stoves to limit access to young children.
- Never leave space heaters within reach of young children, and never leave them unattended.
- Ensure cords from hot appliances (e.g., irons, hair straighteners, curling irons) are not left in reach of young children.
- Make sure ground-fault circuit interrupters (GFCIs) are functional and socket protectors and/or child-proof electrical outlets are in use in homes with young children.
- Review and reinforce injury prevention (e.g., scald prevention, safekeeping of matches and cigarette lighters, safe use of electric cords and outlets), especially after a burn injury occurs.
- Teach burn first-aid measures (e.g., submerge minor burned area in tepid water; do not use butter, margarine, and oil-based

creams and lotions; rinse chemical burns in cold water; and flush skin thoroughly for at least 20 minutes).

Poisoning

Poisoning is a major cause of pediatric injury. In the United States (US), more than 2.1 million poison exposure calls were made to the National Poison Control Center in 2020, with peak incidence of poisonings occurring in 1- to 2-year-olds. In younger children, 99% of poison exposures are unintentional, but in adolescence, 64% are intentional. In children 6 years of age and younger, the top causes of fatality from poisoning include fumes, gases, and vapors; analgesics; unknown drugs; and batteries.[9] Disk, coin, and button batteries and magnets in any body cavity require urgent attention and care because both can cause serious complications (e.g., corrosion of tissues, gastrointestinal perforation) and risk of death.

The American Association of Poison Control Centers (AAPCC) recommends the following to prevent childhood poisoning:

- Store the following away (out of the child's sight), in their original containers, and in cabinets with child-resistant locks:
  - All medications and pharmaceuticals, including over-the-counter (OTC) medications, vitamins, and supplements
  - Tobacco, e-cigarette products, cannabis products, and alcohol
  - Laundry and cleaning supplies
  - Pesticides and insect repellents
  - Disk, coin, button batteries
  - Any type of oil, lubricant, or other chemical
  - Personal care products, including cosmetics, contact lens cleaner, and hand sanitizer

  Other important strategies include:
- Never mix cleaning chemicals. Read and follow cleaning product label instructions.
- Apply insect repellent according to label instructions, not on hands, and wash off after returning indoors.
- Detect invisible threats (see Chapter 3) such as carbon monoxide, asbestos, radon.
- Do not share medicines with anyone else. Be cautious not to use more than one medication with the same active ingredient.
- Ensure proper medication disposal: visit http://dispose-mymeds.org, ask a pharmacist, or call the Poison Control Center (800-222-1222). Some communities host medicine take-back programs.
- Encourage smoking cessation for caregivers who use tobacco, nicotine, or cannabis products.
- Avoid poisonous plants and mushrooms (varies by region).
- Store and prepare food safely. Visit https://www.goodsafety.gov for more information.
- Remind parents that cosmetics and personal care products, cleaning substances, and analgesics are the top overall causes of pediatric exposures in children younger than 6 years old.
- Address poisoning from laundry detergent packets and pods, analgesics (especially opioids), and cannabis products at opportune healthcare visits. The broad category of analgesics includes acetaminophen, ibuprofen, and aspirin in addition to opioids and other analgesics. The regional Poison Control Center should be consulted in the case of any child ingestion or supratherapeutic doses (suspected or known; intentional or unintentional).
- Adolescents are more likely to intentionally abuse OTC medications, prescribed medications, and/or chemicals and illicit drugs. They are also at higher risk of attempting or completing suicide using poisons, OTC medications, or prescription medications.

Violence

Violence is the outcome of aggressive behavior that becomes destructive and results in physical injury to people or damage to property. Characteristic features of violence are listed in Box 21.1. Although there are major differences in rates of violence-related injuries and death by racial/ethnic groups, the majority of homicides involve people who know each other and are of the same race.[10] Shockingly, 14 youths die each day from homicide and about 1300 youths are treated daily for violence-related injuries.[11] Males are more likely to perpetrate and be victims of physical violence, whereas females are more frequently victims of bullying.[12] Gun-related deaths have now surpassed MVC as the leading overall cause of death of those under age 20 years of age,[3] with homicide being the leading cause of death in Black adolescents and young adult males.[2]

Children from all socioeconomic backgrounds, genders, races, and communities experience violence either directly or indirectly. Effective management depends on understanding the major influences and key risk factors that contribute to or sustain violence, especially seeking out those factors that are modifiable through individual and/or collective actions. Exposure to violence can significantly affect short- and long-term physical and mental health. The direct and indirect costs of violence are also immense, not only in the public health costs, but also in loss of productivity and decreased quality of life.

Clinical Findings

The assessment of youth who are victims of, witnesses to, or perpetrators of violence should focus on key pieces of historical information and the presence of risk factors to help determine the child or adolescent's current safety and potential for future violence. It is important to document findings carefully as medical records can be used as legal evidence in criminal proceedings.

Youth who experience violence need a trauma-informed approach to determine the circumstances of their violent events. They should be treated as minors first with the goal of not further victimizing them. The Substance Abuse and Mental Health Services Administration (SAHMSA) lists six principles of trauma-informed care, including safety; trustworthiness and transparency; peer support, collaboration, and mutuality; empowerment, voice, and choice; and cultural, historical, and gender issues. They also

---

• BOX 21.1 Characteristics of Violence

Continuity: Once it is used as a coping mechanism, violence becomes a habit that is hard to break.

Reciprocity: Violence generates violent behavior in others, increasing tension and eliciting negative responses.

Sameness: One form of violence becomes as acceptable as another. As its use becomes more common, violence permeates all of one's life.

Addiction: Violence gives a sense of power and control that, although temporary, is addictive.

Limitations of options or alternative actions: Reasoning is difficult in violent situations, and problem-solving abilities are not used.

Escalation: Violence begets more frequent and more intense violence, with potential for serious sequelae.

have additional PCP resources at https://www.thenationalcouncil.org/program/center-of-excellence/.

Management

The best way to approach violence is through targeted, evidence-based prevention strategies. The PCP also often gets involved with the care of minor trauma resulting from assault, counseling after an incident of violence or threat of violence, and the prevention of youth violence. The following are the key points in the management of minor trauma:

- Treat minor trauma and/or refer as indicated for further treatment.
- Screen for alcohol and drugs.
- Report the incident to law enforcement.
- Refer to a social worker or pediatric mental health professional and community programs, as appropriate.
- Work with children, adolescents, and parents or caregivers to identify ways to prevent violence (e.g., discuss how they can incorporate protective factors into their family life [see Chapter 6]).

Gun Violence Prevention

Prevention of gun violence includes the following[13]:

- The safest home is a firearm-free home; but if firearms are in the home, emphasize safe storage by keeping the weapon unloaded with ammunition locked away separately.
- Use trigger locks and gun safes to store guns away from children.
- Ask parents about guns in the home and encourage families to ask about guns in homes their children and adolescents visit.
- Stress the removal of guns in the homes of children and adolescents with mental health disorders, substance abuse, and/or history of suicide attempt.
- Make every attempt to limit exposure to violent media.
- Advocate for effective gun violence policies (see https://www.napnap.org/napnap-urges-government-to-address-gun-violence/).

Intimate Partner Violence

Intimate partner violence (IPV) is violence that occurs between individuals in a close relationship. One out of six children in the United States are exposed to IPV.[14] It occurs across the pediatric lifespan, and those who witness this type of violence are often victimized themselves. IPV includes physical violence, sexual violence, and/or emotional abuse and threats. It occurs in all socioeconomic, racial, genders, religious, cultural, and community groups. However, individuals experiencing poverty and those who identify as gender minorities have higher prevalence rates, often as a result of structural oppression related to racism, classism, xenophobia, and other causes.[14] IPV not only leaves physical and emotional injuries, but children and adolescents can also be physically injured during intimate partner disputes, either by getting "caught in the crossfire" or in attempts to intervene. Children and adolescents who witness violence are often emotionally traumatized, and exposure to relational violence can also lead to poor academic and social outcomes. As with other adverse childhood experiences (ACEs), there appears to be a dose-response relationship between IPV and poor outcomes—the more severe or chronic the exposure, the poorer the child/adolescent outcomes.

Clinical Findings

Although most professional organizations recommend screening for IPV, the effectiveness of screening is unclear, and it is difficult to identify families where IPV occurs. IPV occurs in all strata of society and, even when identified on screening questionnaires, victims are often reluctant to disclose their victimization due to fear of consequences. For adolescents who present with physical findings of trauma (e.g., bruising, edema, musculoskeletal injury), assess for history that is inconsistent with physical examination findings or for the presence of a partner whose behaviors raise suspicion for abuse or human trafficking (see Chapter 22).

Management

Care of families experiencing IPV requires a multidisciplinary, well-coordinated approach and referral and consultation with specialty treatment centers, social workers, and community health agencies. The PCP plays an important central role in ensuring the needs of the children in homes with IPV are treated and have close follow up. In most states, PCPs are mandated to report a minor's exposure to IPV to child protective services (CPS) because it is considered a form of emotional child abuse. State agencies can further assess the family functioning and offer resources to help the perpetrator, the adult victim, and the children who are also being victimized.

Patient Education and Prevention

The goal is to prevent IPV before it starts. Educating children and adolescents about healthy behaviors and relationships that can assist them in avoiding dating relationships that include violence. PCPs should assess and monitor for negative effects of children witnessing conflict between adults, specifically parents. More community resources are needed for prevention of IPV in adults, and further research on prevention and treatment of IPV is needed. One training resource for PCPs is the Sexual Behaviors Traffic Light Tool, available at https://www.brook.org.uk/training/wider-professional-training/sexual-behaviours-traffic-light-tool/ which has training modules for providers to assist in recognizing trauma related to IPV.

References

1. O'Donnel EP, Canares TL. Accidents waiting to happen: a review of unintentional household injuries in children. *Pediatr Rev.* 2021;42(3):109–122.
2. Centers for Disease Control and Prevention. *Child Health*; 2022. https://www.cdc.gov/nchs/fastats/child-health.htm.
3. Lee LK, Douglas K, Hemenway D. Crossing lines: a change in the leading cause of death among U.S. children. *N Engl J Med.* 2022;386(16):1485–1487.
4. Hagan JF, Shawn JS, Duncan PM. *Bright Futures: Guidelines for Health Supervision of Infants, Children, and Adolescents.* 4th ed. American Academy of Pediatrics; 2017.
5. National Highway Transportation and Safety Administration. Traffic safety facts 2019 data. https://crashstats.nhtsa.dot.gov/Api/Public/ViewPublication/813122.
6. Durbin D, Hoffman BD. Council on injury. Violence and poison prevention: child passenger safety. *Pediatrics.* 2018;127(4):1–18.
7. West BA, Rudd RA, Sauber-Schatz EK, Ballesteros MF. Unintentional injury deaths in children and youth, 2019-2019. *J Safety Res.* 2021;78:322–330.
8. Denny SA, Quan L, Gilchrist J, et al. Technical report: prevention of drowning. *Pediatrics.* 2021;148(2):1–23.

9. National Poison Control Center. *Poison Statistics National Data*; 2020. https://www.poison.org/poison-statistics-national.

10. Beck AJ. *Race and Ethnicity of Violent Crime Offenders and Arrestees, 2018*. US Department of Justice Statistical Brief; 2021.

11. Centers for Disease Control and Prevention. *National Centers for Excellence in Youth Violence Prevention*; 2019. https://www.cdc.gov/violenceprevention/youthviolence/yvpc/index.html.

12. Youth.gov. Federal data. https://youth.gov/youth-topics/violence-prevention/federal-data.

13. American Academy of Pediatrics. Firearm-related injuries affecting the pediatric population. *Pediatrics*. 2011;130(5):e1416–e1423.

14. Randell KA, Ragavan MI. Intimate partner violence: identification and response in pediatric health care settings. *Clin Pediatr*. 2020;59(2):109–115.

22

Child Maltreatment

GAIL A. HORNOR

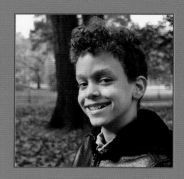

Child maltreatment is a pediatric health care problem of epidemic proportions, a problem that all pediatric healthcare providers (PCPs) must be able to recognize and address. According to the US Department of Health & Human Services (DHHS),[1] 618,000 American children suffered child maltreatment in 2020, resulting in death for 1750 children. Overall, three-fourths of those children (76.1%) experienced neglect, 16.5% experienced physical abuse, 9.4% experienced sexual abuse, and 0.2% were sex trafficked.[1] The majority of abused children (90.6%) were victimized by a biological parent. The true number of child maltreatment victims is difficult to quantify. These official numbers represent child maltreatment cases reported to child protective services (CPS) and investigated and substantiated by CPS, typically requiring collaborating evidence. These numbers are truly only the tip of the iceberg regarding the epidemiology of child maltreatment. Considering sexual abuse alone, retrospective studies of adults indicate that one in five victims never disclose their victimization.[2]

Child maltreatment is defined by the federal Child Abuse Prevention and Treatment Act (CAPTA) as "any recent act or failure to act on the part of a parent or caretaker which results in death, serious physical or emotional harm, sexual abuse or exploitation; or an act or failure to act, which presents an imminent risk of serious harm."[3] These are considered minimal standards and serve as guidelines for states to define and manage child maltreatment. Healthcare workers, including nurses and advanced practice nurses, are mandated by law to report any suspicion of child maltreatment to CPS and law enforcement (LE) to ensure the child's safety.[3] Despite this legal mandate, only 11.6% of reports of suspected child maltreatment in 2020 were made by healthcare personnel.[2]

There are a number of known risk factors for child maltreatment (Box 22.1). Young children are at increased vulnerability for fatal child maltreatment with 67.8% of fatalities involving children less than 3 years of age and nearly half (46.9%) occurring in children less than 1 year of age.[2] Nearly three-fourths (73.7%) of children who die as a result of child maltreatment die from neglect and 42.6% from physical abuse. Child maltreatment occurs in all ethnic, religious, and sex groups; however, females are more likely to suffer sexual abuse and sex trafficking than are males.[2] Children with special behavioral, developmental, or healthcare needs are at greater risk for child maltreatment than their typically developing peers. Certain familial factors increase child maltreatment risk including domestic violence, parental/caregiver mental health concerns or mental disability, parental/caregiver substance abuse, poverty, parental/caregiver history of being abused or neglected, and parental/caregiver use of corporal punishment.[4]

The landmark Adverse Childhood Experiences (ACE) Study[5] solidified our knowledge that psychosocial traumas in childhood, including child maltreatment and its risk factors, can result in negative adult mental and physical health outcomes in a dose-related gradient. Child maltreatment is a significant contributor to a variety of poor health outcomes including depression, anxiety, suicide, substance abuse, cancer, heart disease, lung disease, and early death.[6] Child maltreatment is indeed a significant public health problem.

There are different types of child maltreatment: physical abuse, sexual abuse, emotional abuse, medical child abuse, and neglect. It is not unusual for a child to experience more than one type of maltreatment. According to the US DHHS,[7] 15.5% of child maltreatment victims suffered more than one type of child abuse or neglect in 2019. It is crucial that all pediatric PCPs be able to recognize all types of child maltreatment and provide prompt, evidence-based intervention.

General Child Maltreatment Assessment

Pediatric PCPs must be alert to the possibility of child maltreatment. The overriding goals of assessment are (1) promptly identifying child maltreatment, (2) reporting maltreatment concerns to the appropriate governmental agencies to prevent further abuse, and (3) linking patients with appropriate evidence-based interventions to lessen the negative consequences of abuse. Each form of child maltreatment has specific diagnostic studies used in identification and assessment. However, general assessment and intervention guidelines exist to assist clinicians when evaluating for all forms of child maltreatment. Child abuse specialists and local child advocacy centers (CACs) are valuable resources, when available, to assist the PCP in assessing and managing youth with maltreatment concerns. PCPs should be knowledgeable regarding child abuse resources available in their own community.

A thorough psychosocial assessment should be completed to identify both risk factors and protective factors. Several evidence-based screening tools are available (Box 22.2). A suspected child maltreatment report should never be based solely upon the presence of familial risk factors. Even if concern for child maltreatment is not present, PCPs can address child maltreatment risk factors as part of secondary prevention by linking the parent or family with evidence-based interventions to address risks.

All states have mandatory reporting laws requiring healthcare professionals to report suspicion of child maltreatment to CPS and LE. Once made, the CPS (also known by various other names, such as *Social Services*, *Department of Human Services*, or

BOX 22.1 Child Maltreatment: Child and Familial Risk and Protective Factors

Child Risk Factors

- Prematurity
- Irritable baby, colic, crying
- Developmental delay
- Chronic health concerns
- Behavioral difficulties
- Physical disability
- Multiple gestation

Familial Risk Factors

- Caregiver mental health concern
- Caregiver substance abuse concern
- Household domestic violence
- Caregiver history of being maltreated in childhood or adolescence
  - Sexual abuse
  - Physical abuse
  - Emotional abuse
  - Neglect
  - Medical child abuse
  - Child protective services involvement
- Previous or current familial involvement with child protective services
- Previous or current familial involvement with LE
- Financial stressors: food or housing insecurity
- Teen parent

Protective Factors

- Social supports
- Parent self-efficacy
- Sense of competency in child rearing
- Higher parental education

Modified from Centers for Disease Control & Prevention. *Preventing Child Sexual Abuse*; 2021. https://www.cdc.gov/violenceprevention/childsexualabuse/fastfact.html; and Lane W. Prevention of child maltreatment. *Pediatr Clin North Am.* 2014;61:873–888.

BOX 22.2 Psychosocial Screening Tools

- Safe Environment for Every Kid: https://seekwellbeing.org/
- Bright Futures Pediatric Intake/Family Psychosocial Screen: https://www.brightfutures.org/mentalhealth/pdf/professionals/ped_intake_form.pdf
- American Academy of Family Physicians Social Needs Screening Tool: https://www.aafp.org/dam/AAFP/documents/patient_care/everyone_project/hops19-physician-form-sdoh.pdf
- Centers for Medicare & Medicaid Services Accountable Health Communities Screening Tool: https://innovation.cms.gov/files/worksheets/ahcm-screeningtool.pdf
- IHELP: https://pubmed.ncbi.nlm.nih.gov/26183003/
- We Care: https://www.ncbi.nlm.nih.gov/pubmed/17766528

to trauma-informed mental health treatment to prevent trauma symptoms from developing or worsening.[10]

Child Maltreatment Intervention Guidelines and Management Strategies

PCPs should have a basic understanding of the most common evidence-based mental health interventions used to treat trauma-exposed children and adolescents (see Chapter 29). The treatment model with the highest degree of empirical support for the treatment of traumatized children is trauma-focused cognitive behavioral therapy (TF-CBT). Eye movement desensitization and reprocessing (EMDR) is effective in controlling trauma symptoms in pediatric patients with post-traumatic stress disorder especially when used in conjunction with TF-CBT.[13] Adolescents who experience trauma may also exhibit emotional dysregulation and present with histories of self-injurious behaviors, suicidal ideation/attempts, and poor relationships with others.[10] Dialectical behavior therapy (DBT) has proven efficacy in addressing emotional dysregulation in trauma-exposed adolescents.[14] Pediatric PCPs must be knowledgeable about local trauma-informed mental health services available to victims of child maltreatment.

Parent and Family Education and Prevention

Pediatric PCPs play an integral role in the prevention of child maltreatment. Key to building resilience in families while preventing child maltreatment is to devise interventions that strengthen protective factors while reducing risk factors.[15] Practice interventions to prevent child maltreatment are best understood by using the public health framework.[16] This framework includes primary prevention programs that target all pediatric patients and families regardless of known child maltreatment risk factors, secondary prevention programs that target families with known child maltreatment risk, and tertiary prevention programs that prevent adverse outcomes in survivors and prevent recurrence of child maltreatment.[17] Evidence-based interventions with proven efficacy in the prevention of child maltreatment include primary, secondary, and tertiary prevention.[8]

Primary prevention includes:

1. Anticipatory guidance for parents/caregivers:
   - Encouraging and modeling positive parenting
   - Having realistic behavioral expectations of their children
   - Using effective discipline—discouraging corporal punishment
   - Creating "no hit zones" (see https://nohitzone.com/)

Department of Family and Youth Services) referral typically is forwarded to the CPS agency in the county where the youth resides (some states have a state-wide referral line). CPS investigates and takes action to ensure the youth's safety.[8] If indicated, a LE referral is made to the jurisdiction where the abuse occurred. Law enforcement (LE) conducts a separate investigation to determine if criminal charges are merited. Both civil and criminal liability protection are guaranteed to mandated reporters acting within their professional role when making a report. Reporting laws and procedures differ among states; PCPs should contact their state agency charged with child protection for guidelines regarding reporting laws and procedural polices related to child maltreatment. If doubt exists regarding reporting child maltreatment, consult with a child abuse specialist.

Children who have experienced one form of psychosocial trauma are at increased risk to experience multiple traumatic events.[10] When concerns for child maltreatment arise, the PCP must screen for trauma symptoms including anxiety, depression, irritability, anger, and other internalizing and externalizing behavioral symptoms (see Chapter 29).[11] Children exposed to trauma manifest many of the disruptive behaviors, impulsivity, and executive dysfunction commonly associated with attention-deficit/hyperactivity disorder.[12] However, not all individuals exposed to trauma or traumatic events develop trauma-related psychopathology. To prevent the damaging and lifelong effects that trauma can have on a young person's life, it is imperative to refer survivors

• BOX 22.3 **Child and Caregiver Sexual Abuse Education**

Child
- Explain to the child that everyone has private parts—parts of their body that no one should touch, kiss, tickle, hurt, or put anything in.
  - What are your private parts?
- Have the child verbally tell you or point to their private parts.
  - What should you do if anyone bothers or tries to bother your private parts?
  - Do you tell or keep it a secret?
  - Who could you tell if anyone bothered your private parts?
  - Has anyone ever touched, tickled, kissed, or hurt your private parts?
- Make sure the child can name at least two adults.

Caregiver
- Most children who are sexually abused are not abused by a stranger.
- Children was most at risk of being sexually abused by someone they know, trust, and love.
- Never leave your child with someone you do not know well.
- Never leave your child with anyone who has a history of sexually abusing a child.
- People who sexually abuse children are at high risk for abusing again.
- Teach your child the correct anatomical name for their genitals.
- Pedophiles often present as normal, healthy individuals. They may be married and have children, even grandchildren.
- Pay attention if an adult likes to spend a lot of alone time with your child.
- Most children who are sexually abused will have no physical sign, even when examined by a doctor or nurse.
- If you have concerns about sexual abuse, share them with your child's health care provider, teacher, counselor, or child protective services.
- If your child discloses sexual abuse, always report to CPS.

2. Anticipatory guidance for parents/caregivers regarding challenging developmental stages: crying (discuss abusive head trauma, shaking baby syndrome (see Chapter 10); tantrums (see Chapters 6 and 11); toileting (see Chapter 17), and adolescence (see Chapter 13)
3. Perform an anogenital examination at every episodic wellness visit and use it as an opportunity to educate patients and parents/caregivers regarding genitalia (see Box 22.3).
4. Screening for psychosocial risk factors:
   - Universal for all patients and families/caregivers
   - Screen for psychosocial risk factors and be familiar with all available community resources
   - Telehealth may offer more opportunities for psychosocial screening for adolescents
   - Offer interventions to address identified challenges
5. Early childhood educational opportunities in Head Start and Community Child Care Centers

Secondary prevention includes:
1. Child maltreatment risk factors identified on screening:
   - Link with appropriate community resources
   - Monitor to ensure linkage is completed and maintained
   - Instances when families fail to link to or maintain links to resources may raise concerns for child safety; report to CPS and LE as indicated
2. Home visitation programs
   - Nurse Family Partnership (https://www.nursefamilypartnership.org/)
   - Families First Home Visiting Program (https://www.gov.mb.ca/healthychild/familiesfirst/)

- Healthy Families America (https://www.healthyfamiliesamerica.org/)
- Parents as Teachers (https://parentsasteachers.org/)
3. Parenting training programs such as Triple-P Positive Parenting Program and ACT—Parents Raising Safe Kids Program (see Chapter 6)

Tertiary prevention includes:
1. Prompt identification of child maltreatment victims
2. Report to CPS and LE
3. Screen victims for trauma symptoms
   - Provide trauma-informed primary mental healthcare
   - Refer to mental health specialists when indicated
4. Familial risk factors for Child Maltreatment
   - Refer for intensive or specialized mental health services like Parent-Child Interaction Therapy (PCIT) and Multisystemic Therapy for Child Abuse & Neglect (MST-CAN)

Physical Abuse

Physical abuse is the intentional use of physical force by a parent or caretaker that results in physical injury.[4] The injury can be the result of a parent or caregiver striking, shaking, biting, throwing, burning, or committing another violent act towards an infant, child, or adolescent that usually occurs in a moment of anger or frustration. Physical abuse can also result from excessive corporal punishment, deliberate assault, or torture. Physical abuse causes a variety of injuries including bruises, burns, and other cutaneous findings; intraoral injuries; subconjunctival hemorrhages; skeletal injuries (fractures); abdominal trauma; and head trauma among others.

Physical injuries that appear relatively minor to the examining clinician can result in significant consequences for the child if they remain unreported. Approximately 20% to 25% of children who are diagnosed with physical abuse have suffered previous sentinel injuries that went unidentified or unreported.[18] The landmark sentinel injury study[19] revealed that 27.8% of infants less than 1 year of age with definite physical abuse injuries had a previous unreported injury. The most common sentinel injuries were bruising (80%) and intraoral injuries (11%). Unreported sentinel injuries allow children to return to unsafe environments, placing them at risk to experience additional, often escalating physical abuse.[20]

Clinical Findings

Physically abused infants and children present in a variety of ways including:
- A child or a parent/caregiver discloses an intentional injury.
- Another individual (whether or not they are a mandated reporter) reports an intentional injury.
- A parent/caregiver seeks care for an illness or injury and may or may not be aware that their child was abused.
- A PCP notes an undisclosed injury during a routine physical examination.

Regardless of how an individual with suspected child abuse presents, a detailed history of the injury must be obtained. The purpose of obtaining a detailed history of injury is not to identify the perpetrator of the abuse but rather to identify or eliminate physical abuse suspicion. The history should be obtained from both the parent/caregiver and the patient, when developmentally and medically possible. The patient and the parent/caregiver should be separated during history taking. Open-ended questions should be used to elicit a free injury narrative. If clarification is

• BOX 22.4   Detailed Injury History

Timeline of Injury
- Begin with when the child last appeared healthy
- Child's behavior before, during, and after the injury
- Narrative of the day's activities
- Events leading up to the injury
- Feeding times and quality
- Level of responsiveness
- Identify caregivers at the time of injury
- Individuals present at the time of injury
- Developmental level of child

From Lane W. Prevention of child maltreatment. *Pediatr Clin North Am.* 2014;61:873–888.

needed, the clinician can then ask more direct questions (Box 22.4). Certain historical indicators should raise concerns for possible physical abuse[21]:
- No history is given for the injury.
- Conflicting or inconsistent histories are given to explain the injury.
- The history is inconsistent with the injury.
- The history given is inconsistent with the child's developmental level.
- There is a significant delay in seeking medical care.
- The parents/caregivers seek medical care from a variety of care sites so that a pattern of repeated injuries cannot be detected by clinicians.

Whenever a child presents with an injury, whether intentional or unintentional, a thorough head-to-toe physical examination is indicated. Clinical examination findings without a clear injury history should raise concerns for physical abuse.[21] Other symptoms concerning for physical abuse include bruising, other cutaneous injuries, or fractures in an infant or non-ambulatory child or on protected areas of the body such as chest and back; cutaneous injuries that are extensive, have distinct patterns, or occur on locations suspicious for abuse including the ears, abdomen, genitals, chest, and neck; rib, scapula, sternum, classic metaphyseal, and spinal process fractures; extensive bruising or other cutaneous injuries; bruising or other skin injuries with distinct patterns; and intracranial and abdominal trauma.

Child and Family Medical History

Whenever there is a concern for physical abuse, obtain:
- Child history:
  - Newborn screening results
  - Prenatal and birth history and developmental history noting any delay of developmental milestones
  - Abnormal umbilical cord bleeding and/or umbilical cord present beyond 5 to 6 weeks
  - Bleeding from circumcision/surgeries
  - Abnormal bruising
  - Bleeding disorder
  - Skeletal disorder
  - Metabolic disorder (renal or liver disease).
  - Presence of blue sclera (osteogenesis imperfecta)
- Family history
  - Abnormal bruising or hemorrhage during delivery/surgeries
  - Easy fractures
  - Bleeding disorder

- Metabolic disorder (renal or liver disease)
- Skeletal disorder
- Dental abnormalities
- Short stature
- Multiple miscarriages
- Childhood deaths
- Blue sclera

Differential Diagnosis

Underlying medical conditions can result in findings that mimic physical abuse. The differential diagnosis depends upon the type of injury present. Obtaining a thorough medical history of both child victim and family/caregiver is crucial.
- *Bruising:* Trauma—unintentional versus inflicted/abuse; coagulopathy; congenital dermal melanocytosis (pigmented birthmarks), urticaria pigmentosa, Henoch-Schönlein purpura, cultural practices, coining, or spoon rubbing
- *Intraoral injury:* Trauma—unintentional versus inflicted/abuse
- *Subconjunctival hemorrhage:* Trauma—unintentional versus inflicted/abuse; injury following persistent vomiting or coughing
- *Burns:* Trauma—unintentional versus inflicted/abuse; bullous impetigo, phytophotodermatitis, perianal streptococcus, diaper dermatitis resulting from use of laxative with senna
- *Skeletal injuries and fractures:* Trauma—unintentional versus inflicted/abuse; metabolic bone disorder—osteogenesis imperfecta, rickets, scurvy; congenital syphilis
- *Abdominal trauma:* Trauma—unintentional versus inflicted/abuse; coagulopathy (hematoma injuries)
- *Abusive head trauma (AHT):* There is an extensive differential diagnosis, but the clinical history and a thorough physical examination can distinguish between AHT and other medical conditions.[22] Trauma—unintentional versus inflicted/abuse; birth trauma (typically resolves by 4–6 weeks of age); coagulopathy; infection-meningitis, encephalitis; metabolic/genetic disorders—glutaric aciduria type 1, pyruvate carboxylase deficiency
- *Intracranial pathology:* Tumors, benign enlargement of the subarachnoid space

Bruising

Youth presenting with bruising or petechiae concerning for physical abuse need assessment to rule out an underlying bleeding disorder that predisposes them to bruising or petechia. A hematology consult is indicated if lab results are abnormal. Laboratory assessment is indicated when the only injury noted is a clearly patterned injury for which the child gives a clear history of abuse (Fig. 22.1). For example, a child gives history of being struck with a switch and has thick linear marks that are the only bruises or injuries noted on the child's body. See Chapter 25 for the assessment, management, and follow-up of ecchymoses.

Skeletal Injuries and Fractures

The physical abuse evaluation of skeletal injuries and fractures includes any injury or fracture that is inconsistent with the parental or caregiver history, particularly when the developmental stage of the child is inconsistent with the injury history. Obtaining a radiographic skeletal survey with any suspicious skeletal fracture. Refer to Chapter 40 for the assessment and management of fractures.

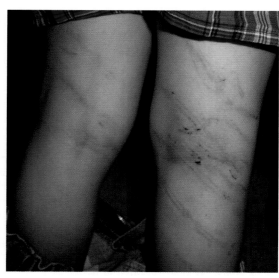

• **Fig. 22.1** Patterned Skin Injury.

Abdominal Trauma

Abdominal injuries are the second leading cause of death by physical abuse.[23] Significant force is required to inflict an abdominal injury. Symptoms of abdominal trauma are often delayed and nonspecific and include abdominal pain, emesis, abdominal rigidity, and tenderness. Abdominal bruising may or may not be present. Abdominal injuries from child maltreatment can affect any of the abdominal structures and include lacerations, hematomas, and other diffuse visceral injuries. Patients who present with suspicious abdominal injuries or concern for bleeding such as a liver or duodenal hematoma, should have coagulation studies assessed including aspartate aminotransferase (AST)/alanine aminotransferase (ALT) levels and lipase levels. Elevated levels could indicate abdominal trauma. Consultation with a child maltreatment specialist should be obtained before ordering an abdominal computed tomography (CT) scan.

Abusive Head Trauma

Abusive head trauma (AHT), previously known as *shaken baby syndrome*, is the leading cause of death and long-term disability in infants resulting from physical abuse.[24] Infants and young children are at particular risk for AHT. The Centers for Disease Control and Prevention define AHT as an injury to the skull or intracranial contents of an infant or child less than 5 years old that is caused by inflicted shaking, blunt impact, or both.[25] Crying in infants less than 12 months old is thought to be the primary trigger for AHT. Clinical signs and symptoms of AHT range from mild or asymptomatic to a more severe presentation with complete cardiopulmonary arrest.[22] AHT signs and symptoms are often nonspecific including altered mental status, loss of consciousness, limpness, vomiting, seizure, poor feeding, or cardiopulmonary compromise.[24]

The cardinal AHT injury is a subdural hematoma, which is present in about 80% to 90% of AHT cases among infants and toddlers.[26,27] Other AHT injuries include subarachnoid hemorrhage, axonal injury, gliding contusions, cortical tears, intracerebral edema, and cerebral ischemia.[22] Retinal hemorrhages are present in approximately 85% of children with AHT.[24] The mechanism of retinal hemorrhage injury is traction on the retina by the vitreous humor as the eye moves back and forth within the

orbit during the quick lateral forces that occur when the child is being shaken. Retinal hemorrhages result from conditions other than physical abuse, such as leukemia, meningitis, and hypertension. However, extensive retinal hemorrhage involving all layers of the retina, extending to the ora serrata, and involving retinal tears or schisis are pathognomonic for AHT.[24] Rib fractures, especially posteriorly located, occur in victims of AHT due to forceful chest squeezing and resulting thoracic compression.

Leg metaphyseal fractures may occur due to the legs jerking back and forth during the shaking episode.[28] Skull fractures, when present, result from blunt force trauma from the child being struck in the head or colliding with an object. Spinal cord injury may be noted in cases with severe AHT[22]; the most common spinal cord injury noted is ligamentous or soft tissue injury in the cervical spine region caused by hyperflexion.[29] Cutaneous AHT comorbidities include bruises, abrasions, and scalp edema. See Chapter 41 for the assessment, management, and follow-up for the individual with a traumatic brain injury.

Diagnostic Studies

Diagnostic testing is based upon the injury type and the patient's age. Consulting with a child abuse specialist can help determine appropriate testing to order. There are circumstances when the most appropriate option is to refer a child with more extensive injuries to the emergency department for a physical abuse workup. Whenever a concern for physical abuse arises, the following workup is indicated regardless of injury type. Physical abuse workup (for any identified injury concerning for physical abuse) includes:

- Skeletal survey should be obtained in all cases involving children younger than 2 years old. Repeat in 2 weeks to ensure that any acute fracture missed on the initial skeletal survey is ultimately diagnosed once healing or callus formation is present.
- Aspartate aminotransferase (AST), alanine aminotransferase (ALT), and lipase level in children younger than 6 years of age.
- Abdominal computed tomography (CT) is indicated in individuals with an AST/ALT elevated above 80 or grossly elevated lipase if abdominal bruising is present.
- Head CT without contrast for all infants less than 7 months of age presenting with any injury concerning for physical abuse. Consider a head CT without contrast for children between 7 months old and 5 years old who present with concern for head trauma (e.g., neurologic symptoms, head or ear bruising, intraoral trauma, or subconjunctival hemorrhage)

Management Strategies

If physical abuse is suspected, these management strategies should be followed in addition to the primary, secondary, and tertiary strategies. The provider must:

- Report any suspicion of physical abuse to CPS and LE.
- Thoroughly and precisely document statements made by parent/caregiver and child.
- Photo-document all cutaneous injuries.
- Refer for appropriate medical treatment depending on type and severity of injury.
- The American Academy of Pediatrics (AAP) recommends providers disclose to parents/caregivers that a referral to CPS and LE has been made. This may be difficult, but transparency is crucial in maintaining the patient/provider relationship.[30]

- Consult with child abuse specialist and/or local Child Advocacy Center as needed for assessment and diagnosis.
- Refer for trauma-informed mental health services (dependent upon the age of the child). Need for ongoing services is dependent upon the length and severity of the abuse, as well as other trauma exposures.

Sexual Abuse

Sexual abuse is a problem of epidemic proportions. The CDC (2021)[4] states that approximately one in four girls and one in 13 boys experience sexual abuse at some point in childhood or adolescence. Sexual abuse is defined as the involvement of an individual less than 18 years of age in sexual activity that violates the societal laws or social taboos, and that the child/adolescent does not fully comprehend, is not developmentally prepared for, and does not or is unable to consent to.[4] Youth sexual abuse involves both touching and nontouching behaviors. Nontouching sexual abuse acts include exposure to pornography, taking or posting sexual photos or images of the youth, or forcing the youth to watch adults engaged in sexual activity. Touching sexual abuse acts range from fondling of the breasts, genitalia, or buttocks to oral, anal, or vaginal penetration. These acts can be a one-time incident or can occur multiple times, sometimes over a span of many years.

Nearly all (91%) of youth sexual abuse is perpetrated by an individual known to the minor and/or their family.[4] The perpetrator is often someone they know, trust, and even love. The majority of sexual abuse perpetrators are male; however, females are also sexual abusers.[31] Adolescents are responsible for perpetrating approximately 20% to 28% of youth sexual abuse.[32] Victims are often reluctant to disclose their abuse for a variety of reasons including fear, guilt, embarrassment, threats, family loyalty, and concerns regarding consequences of disclosure.[33]

Prepubertal children normally engage in sexual behaviors, which is developmentally appropriate. However, there are circumstances when these behaviors become concerning. Sexual behaviors in prepubertal children that are considered normal and age-appropriate sexual behaviors versus problem sexualized behaviors are listed in Box 22.5 (also see Chapter 7). Although problem sexualized behaviors can result from sexual abuse victimization, studies indicate that exposure to pornography is more predictive of engagement in problem sexualized behaviors.[34] The expanded access to pornography places children and adolescents at risk for online sexual solicitation. Online sexual solicitation occurs when children and adolescents are asked to engage in sexual activities, sexual talk, or give personal sexual information. Online sexual solicitation of a minor by an adult or an age-inappropriate adolescent is sexual abuse, whether or not offline sexual contact occurs.[35]

Commercial sexual exploitation of children (CSEC), also known as *child sex trafficking*, is a form of sexual abuse. CSEC is defined as a range of crimes and activities involving the sexual abuse or exploitation of a minor for the financial benefit of any person, or in exchange for anything of value given or received by any person.[36] CSEC involves engaging a child under the age of 18 years in prostitution, pornography, stripping, escort services, or other sexual services. A strong correlation exists between experiencing sexual abuse and entry into CSEC.[37] Other CSEC risk factors include substance misuse, preexisting mental health problems, involvement with CPS, placement in foster care, runaways/homelessness, multiple sexual partners, and sexually transmitted infections (STIs).[38] PCPs should be knowledgeable regarding CSEC indicators to be better equipped to recognize potential

---

• BOX 22.5   Age-Appropriate Sexual Behaviors vs. Problem Sexualized Behaviors

Normal Age-Appropriate Behaviors
- Masturbation
- Touching own genitals
- Sex play involving
  - Age mates (age difference of ≤4 years)
  - Touching and looking at genitals

Problem Sexualized Behaviors
- Object insertion into another child's vagina or anus
- Sex play involving one or more of the following
  - 4 years age difference between children
  - Oral-genital contact
  - Oral-anal contact
  - Anal-genital contact
  - Genital-genital contact
  - Digital penetration of vagina or anus
  - Involvement of force, threat, or bribes

---

victims, and they must understand that CSEC is a form of sexual abuse and therefore concerns must be reported to CPS and LE. Knowledge of available local resources is critical when identifying CSEC victims. The National Human Trafficking Hotline (888-3737-888) and the National Human Trafficking Resource Center (https://humantraffickinghotline.org/) are equipped with call specialists who are experts in human trafficking and available to provide guidance with screening questions for patients to assist providers, identify local available resources, and speak directly to the patient.[10]

Clinical Findings

Sexual abuse is typically revealed by patient disclosure to a non-healthcare professional. However, there are occasions when a youth may reveal sexual abuse symptoms during a healthcare visit. This occurs when the youth makes a sexual abuse disclosure to the PCP, the parent/caregiver shares concerns of sexual abuse based upon statements made by the youth or other circumstances, a concerning anogenital finding is noted on examination, or a PCP notes positive laboratory result such as an STI or pregnancy. Victims of sexual abuse rarely present with abnormal anogenital examination findings. On average, less than 10% of victims have an abnormal anogenital examination and less than 5% have an STI.[37]

An anogenital examination is an essential element of every well child visit and provides the youth with an opportunity to disclose victimization. When talking with a patient about possible sexual victimization, the PCP should follow a few basic principles: separate the youth from parent/caregiver, ask open-ended questions, and avoid leading them into disclosure. Reassure the patient that the health care provider is a safe person to talk about anything that happened to their body. Obtain just enough information to elicit or eliminate a suspicion of sexual abuse: who perpetrated the sexual abuse; what happened (brief statement of what body part touched what body part of their body); where it occurred (to determine law enforcement jurisdiction); and when it happened (to determine need for an acute examination including forensic evidence collection by a health care provider with specialized training). Documentation of any disclosure must be thorough and include accurate recording of the language used by the patient and parent/caregiver.

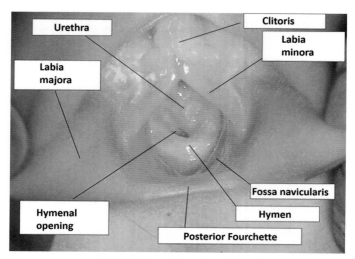

• **Fig. 22.2** Normal Prepubertal Female.

A basic knowledge of normal anogenital anatomy and a good light source are necessary tools for conducting a thorough anogenital examination (Fig. 22.2). Use the face of a clock to describe examination findings related to all structures within the vulvar vestibule including the hymen.[39] Hymenal opening visualization is an essential element of a thorough anogenital examination. Variations in normal hymen morphology exist; these have been present since birth and are not indicative of trauma or sexual abuse. There may be mounds, tags, or shallow clefts anywhere along the anterior or posterior hymenal rim, which may be normal vaginal variations. Typical findings include an uninterrupted hymenal tissue from 3 o'clock to 9 o'clock. A healed hymenal transection extending entirely through the hymen between 3 o'clock and 9 o'clock, scar of the posterior fourchette, or perianal scar are diagnostic of trauma and without a clear history of accidental injury are concerning for sexual abuse even without a disclosure of abuse. These are rare and subtle findings and should be confirmed by a health care provider with expertise in sexual abuse examinations. Acute ano-genital injury including bruising, petechiae, abrasions, bleeding, transections, or lacerations of anogenital structures identified on examination are also diagnostic of trauma and concerning for sexual abuse if a clear and consistent history of accidental trauma is not provided.

Children or adolescents disclosing sexual abuse or assault (or those with acute anogenital injury that raises concerns for abuse) that occurred acutely need an immediate sexual abuse examination. The acute sexual abuse case is defined by local jurisdictional policy but is typically 72 hours since abuse or assault in prepubertal children and 96 to 120 hours for adolescents 13 years and older.[40,41] These examinations are typically completed in an emergency department or a child advocacy center (CAC) by a nurse or doctor with specialized training in sexual abuse examination (medical forensic examination). This type of assessment involves taking an abuse history (forensic interview), performing the examination, collecting forensic evidence, obtaining STI and pregnancy testing as appropriate, and providing STI and pregnancy prophylaxis as indicated. Children and adolescents presenting for care beyond the acute window do not require forensic evidence collection or STI/pregnancy prophylaxis but require the gathering of the abuse/assault history, anogenital examination, and STI testing.

It is best practice that an expert in the medical examination of children with concerns for sexual abuse conduct the evaluation, and referral is essential. Pediatric PCPs must be knowledgeable regarding local resources. A child advocacy center (CAC) provides a multidisciplinary team assessment for sexual abuse. The child or adolescent receives a forensic interview that is video recorded and conducted by a social worker or other professional trained to interview in a forensically sound, child friendly manner. A physical examination is conducted by an Advanced Practice Registered Nurse (APRN) or physician with specialized sexual abuse examination training. CPS and LE are present to observe and provide input to the forensic interview and meet with the child and parent/caregiver. Also, a victim witness advocate from the local prosecutor's office is available to assist the child and family with the court process. The patient and family are also linked with appropriate community resources such as trauma-informed mental health services.

CSEC victims often do not view themselves as victims and most often do not self-disclose victimization.[10] CSEC victims may present with certain red flags including reluctance to answer questions, tattooing or branding that is not easily explained, or be accompanied by a controlling, often older boyfriend or other friend who is unwilling to leave the bedside and insists upon answering questions.[42] The AAP[43] recommends asking the following three questions when the PCP is concerned about possible CSEC victimization:

- Has anyone ever asked you to have sex in exchange for something you wanted or needed (money, food, shelter, or other items)?
- Has anyone ever asked you to have sex with another person?
- Has anyone ever taken sexual pictures of you or posted such photos?

The pediatric PCP must report any suspicion or sexual abuse, including CSEC, to the appropriate CPS and LE agencies even if referring for care by a child abuse specialist. The pediatric PCP must assure the child and family of continued support and ensure that they are linked with appropriate intervention, such as trauma-informed mental health services.

Diagnostic Studies

Although STIs are uncommon in the sexually abused population, testing for STIs is indicated under certain circumstances (Table 22.1). Children with positive STI results from any orifice should be tested for other STIs to ensure that, at minimum, testing for chlamydia, gonorrhea, trichomonas, syphilis, HIV, hepatitis B, and hepatitis C have been completed. Before treating a prepubertal child for an STI, a confirmatory specimen should be collected for testing. A test of cure specimen should also be collected 3 to 4 weeks after treatment. A dirty urine rapid nucleic acid amplification test (NAAT) is the preferred method of testing for chlamydia, gonorrhea, and trichomonas in males of all ages and prepubertal females. Vaginal NAAT may provide more sensitive testing for chlamydia, gonorrhea, and trichomonas in the pubertal female. Serology testing for HIV, syphilis, and hepatitis should be repeated 6 weeks, 3 months, and 6 months following the latest incident of sexual abuse. When serology testing has been completed 6 months or greater from the latest incident of sexual abuse, no further testing is indicated. Prepubertal siblings or a prepubertal child testing positive for an STI should also be evaluated for child sexual abuse.

TABLE 22.1	Indications for Sexually Transmitted Infection Testing
Sexual Transmission	**Screening Test**
Genital contact Unexplained genital injury Genital discharge	Urine or vaginal NAAT for chlamydia, gonorrhea, trichomonas HIV, RPR, Hep B surface antigen, Hep C antibody
Anal-genital contact Unexplained genital injury Anal discharge	Anal NAAT for chlamydia, gonorrhea, trichomonas HIV, RPR, Hep B surface antigen, Hep C antibody
Oral-genital contact (victim's mouth to perpetrator's genitals or anus)	Oral NAAT for chlamydia, gonorrhea
Oral-genital contact (perpetrator's mouth to victim's genitals)	Urine or vaginal NAAT for chlamydia, gonorrhea, trichomonas
Oral-genital contact (perpetrator's mouth to child's anus)	Anal NAAT for chlamydia, gonorrhea, trichomonas

HIV, Human immunodeficiency virus; *NAAT*, Nucleic acid amplification test; *RPR*, rapid plasma reagin.

TABLE 22.2	Significance of Positive Result for Sexually Transmitted Infection Screening
Sexually Transmitted Infection	**Mode of Transmission**
Gonorrhea (oral, genital, anal) Chlamydia (genital, anal) Trichomonas (genital)	Transmitted by sexual contact (report), unless there is evidence of perinatal transmission, or clearly documented but rare nonsexual transmission
Syphilis	Transmitted by sexual contact (report), unless there is evidence of perinatal transmission or clearly documented but rare nonsexual transmission
HIV	Transmitted by sexual contact (report) if perinatal or blood transfusion transmission has been ruled out
Anogenital warts	May be sexually transmitted and nonsexually via perinatal transmission, autoinoculation (child with wart on hand touches their genitals), and inoculation
Anogenital herpes	May be sexually transmitted and nonsexually via perinatal transmission, autoinoculation (child with oral herpes touches hand to mouth to genitals), or inoculation
Molluscum contagiosum	Most likely not sexually transmitted

A positive STI laboratory result can have strong forensic value in the prepubertal patient and non–sexually active adolescent. See Table 22.2 for interpretation of the relationship between a positive STI result and sexual abuse or assault. Perinatal transmission of gonorrhea does not present beyond the neonatal period, but perinatal chlamydia transmission can present up to 3 years after exposure.[44] The perinatal transmission of trichomonas is rare and thought to not persist beyond 3 years of age.[44] Anogenital warts (HPV) and anogenital herpes can be sexually and nonsexually transmitted. Children with anogenital warts or anogenital herpes need further assessment for possible sexual abuse. They need a forensic interview, anogenital examination by a professional with specialized training in sexual abuse examination, and STI testing including chlamydia, gonorrhea, trichomonas, HIV, syphilis, and hepatitis B and C. Anogenital warts in young children are most likely perinatally acquired. The incubation for HPV is unknown. Adams et al.[44] states that anogenital warts first presenting at age 5 years or older increase concern for sexual transmission, and a report to CPS and LE may be indicated with the caveat that nonsexual transmission is also possible. Anogenital herpes is most often transmitted by autoinoculation: a child with oral herpes touching their mouth and then touching their genitals. If there is no history of oral herpes in a child with genital herpes, including a parental or caregiver history of oral herpes, a report to CPS and LE should be considered, again with the caveat that nonsexual transmission is also possible. If a child with anogenital warts or herpes gives a history of sexual abuse, has an anogenital examination with findings concerning for sexual abuse, or is positive for another STI, a report to CPS and LE is indicated.

Differential Diagnosis

The differential diagnosis for sexual abuse is limited. The differential diagnosis for youth with acute or nonacute anogenital injury is unintentional versus inflicted injury (sexual abuse). Unintentional injuries, such as straddle injuries, result from blunt force trauma.[45] Typically, the child falls and straddles an object such as a chair edge or playground equipment, with the impact of the fall involving the genitalia. The site of impact is often to the anterior genitalia, usually external to the hymen, and injury is most often unilateral. However, occasionally penetrating trauma to the hymen and other genital structures occurs.[46]

There are conditions that mimic anogenital injury and raise concerns for possible sexual abuse including urethral prolapse, lichen sclerosis, venous congestion, perianal strep infection, molluscum contagiosum, failure of midline fusion, or anal fissures.

Management Strategies

If sexual abuse is suspected, the provider must:
- Report any suspicion of sexual abuse to CPS and LE.
- Document thoroughly and precisely statements made by parent/caregiver and child.
- Photo-document all cutaneous injuries and anogenital injuries.
- Refer for assessment and examination by a pediatric PCP with expertise in sexual abuse care.
- Consult with child abuse specialist and/or local Child Advocacy Center (CAC) as needed for assessment and diagnosis.
- Refer for trauma-informed mental health services (dependent upon the age of the child). Need for ongoing services is dependent upon the length and severity of the abuse, as well as other trauma exposures.

Children and adolescents presenting with concerns of acute sexual abuse or assault need STI prophylaxis. See Chapter 35 for treatment, management, and follow-up of HIV prophylaxis in children and adolescents.

Medical Child Abuse

Medical child abuse (MCA), formerly known as *Munchausen syndrome by proxy,* is a rare but potentially deadly variant of child maltreatment that involves the parent/caregiver using the pediatric HCP and system as the instrument of abuse. The parent/caregiver exaggerates or falsifies illness symptoms that cannot be verified, or they purposely induce physical or psychological symptoms in a minor.[46] The true incidence of MCA is difficult to quantify as this form of child maltreatment often goes unrecognized and unreported even when recognized.[47] Approximately 0.5 to 2.0 per 100,000 children under the age of 16 years are victims of MCA.[48] The true number of MCA victims may be even higher. Studies suggest that pediatric HCPs require a higher degree of certainty before reporting MCA to CPS than other forms of child maltreatment.[49] Pediatric PCPs are educated to trust a child's parent/caregiver to provide an accurate history of their child's illness. This innate trust of the parent/caregiver history provides an opportunity for parent/caregiver to insist on more invasive testing and procedures, despite provider reservations,[49] thus providing opportunity for MCA. Further confounding the issue of making an accurate MCA diagnosis, approximately 30% of victims have a true underlying medical disorder with a parent/caregiver who, at some point in the medical treatment, begins the exaggeration, fabrication, or induction of illness symptoms.

The median age at MCA diagnosis is between 14 months and 2.7 years; younger children are more vulnerable, but 25% of victims are older than 6 years of age. In cases of long-standing MCA, the child may take on the sick role themselves.[48] It is not unusual for siblings to also suffer MCA,[47] many with symptoms or illnesses similar to the identified MCA victim.

MCA focuses on what (abuse) and how (medically) a child experienced harm,[48] and perpetrator motivation is not relevant to this basic truth. However, it is important the pediatric PCPs possess a basic understanding of MCA perpetrators to be better able to identify victims. MCA perpetrators are almost exclusively female (97.6%) and the mother of the child (95.6%).[50] Most perpetrators are married and employed in a healthcare occupation or, if not, appear medically savvy and knowledgeable.[47] Nonoffending fathers may be completely unaware of what is happening with their child's medical care and believe the mother's statements regarding the child's health—believing the child is ill, or they have concerns and challenge the mother without success.

MCA can result in serious physical and mental health consequences, even death.[51] See Box 22.6 for a listing of the potential consequences of MCA.

Clinical Findings

The possible presentations of MCA are endless as any illness symptom can be exaggerated or fabricated, and many can be induced.[51] See Box 22.7 for possible MCA presentations. The presence of certain clinical findings should trigger the pediatric HCP to be concerned about MCA:
- A child's diagnosis does not match objective findings
- Inconsistent illness histories given by one parent/caregiver

> **• BOX 22.6 Possible Consequences of Medical Child Abuse**
>
> **Physical Health**
> - Repeated unnecessary medical tests, procedures, and treatment
>   - Pain
>   - Anxiety
>   - Psychological distress
>   - Potential complications resulting in physical health consequences including death
>   - Hospital admissions
>   - Illness/complications
>   - Death
>
> **Developmental Functioning**
> - Developmental or social delays
>   - Frequent hospitalizations
>   - Physical limitations secondary to testing, treatment, or diagnosis
>   - Low or interrupted school attendance and education
>   - Few normal school activities
> - Assumption of sick role with use of a wheelchair or feeding tubes
>
> **Psychological Health**
> - Social isolation
> - Distorted view of their health
> - Anxiety regarding their health
> - Collude with the illness presentation
> - Develop a factitious or somatoform disorder
> - Emotional and/or behavioral problems
>
> Modified from Bass C, Glaser D. Early recognition and management of fabricated or induced illness in children. *Lancet.* 2014;383(9926):1412–1421; and Jenny C, Metz J. Medical child abuse and medical neglect. *Pediatr Rev.* 2020;41:49–60.

- Signs and symptoms of illness present only in the presence of one parent/caregiver
- Illness does not respond to normal treatments
- Parent/caregiver insistence of invasive procedures
- Lack of parent/caregiver relief when told their child is improving or does not have an illness
- History of unusual or unexplained illness in parent/caregiver or siblings
- Doctor shopping[48]

Diagnostic Studies

There are no diagnostic studies used to confirm MCA, and minimizing testing is important in evaluating suspected MCA.

Differential Diagnosis

The differential diagnosis in cases of MCA is fundamentally true illness versus MCA.

Management Strategies

Consult a child abuse specialist to assist in making the MCA diagnosis. Report suspicion of MCA to CPS and LE. Thorough and precise documentation of statements made by parent/caregiver and child. Refer for trauma-informed mental health services (dependent upon the age of the child). Need for ongoing services is dependent upon the length and severity of the abuse, as well as other trauma exposures.

• BOX 22.7 Possible Presentations of Medical Child Abuse

Neurological
- Apparent life-threatening event, seizures, ataxia
- Gait abnormality, muscle weakness
- Paralysis, chronic headaches, nystagmus, blindness

Gastrointestinal
- Diarrhea
- Vomiting
- Bleeding, including hematemesis and blood in stool
- Anorexia
- Unexplained weight loss
- Refusal or inability to eat by mouth
- Disorders leading for need for parental nutrition

Urological
- Hematuria
- Proteinuria
- Urolithiasis
- Urinary tract infections
- Nocturia

Renal
- Hypertension
- Hypernatremia
- Hypokalemia
- Renal failure

Rheumatologic
- Arthritis
- Arthralgia
- Systemic autoinflammatory disease

Ear Injuries and Trauma
- Chronic otitis media
- Hearing loss
- Otorrhea
- Swallowing disorder

Allergies
- Food
- Environmental
- Rash

Dermatologic
- Erythema
- Vesicles
- Scratches
- Lacerations
- Burns
- Rashes

Developmental
- Developmental delay
- Attention-deficit/hyperactivity disorder
- Psychosis

Endocrine
- Polydipsia, polyuria
- Diabetes
- Hypoglycemia
- Glycosuria

Infection
- Fever
- Sepsis
- Unusual bacteria at site of infection
- Multiple unusual organisms at the same time of low pathogenicity

Respiratory
- Respiratory arrest
- Apnea
- Cystic fibrosis
- Bleeding from respiratory tract
- Intractable asthma

Modified from Bertuill C, Cochat P. Munchausen syndrome by proxy and pediatric nephrology. *Nephrol Ther.* 2017;13:482–484; and Doughty K, Rood C, Patel A, Thackeray J, Brink F. Neurological manifestations of medical child abuse. *Pediatr Neurol.* 2016;54:22–28.

Emotional Maltreatment

Emotional or psychological maltreatment is a repeated pattern of damaging interactions between a child or adolescent and one or more parent/caregiver that becomes typical of the relationship and harms the youth's self-worth or emotional wellbeing.[5] These behaviors convey messages to youth that they are unvalued, worthless, unwanted, or unloved. This harmful interaction pattern often becomes chronic and pervasive within the parent-child relationship.[52] Emotional maltreatment is differentiated into two broad categories: emotional abuse and emotional neglect. Emotional abuse involves acts of commission such as verbal hostility, taunting, belittling, and rejection. Emotional neglect involves acts of omission: failure to meet the emotional needs of the child. An emotionally neglectful parent is emotionally unavailable, detached, avoidant, and unresponsive to their child's needs or desires.

According to the DHHS,[53] nearly 40,000 American children suffered emotional maltreatment in 2019. The reported number of emotional maltreatment victims represents the tip of the iceberg. Based on retrospective studies of adults who were asked if they experienced emotional maltreatment as a child, the number becomes significantly higher. In a community sample of adults, 14% of females and 10% of males reported childhood emotional abuse. In addition, the landmark ACEs study[54] described not only the prevalence of emotional maltreatment, but also its interrelatedness with other forms of child maltreatment and psychosocial trauma. One-fourth (25%) of ACE study participants reported childhood emotional maltreatment (10% reported emotional abuse and 15% emotional neglect). Among participants reporting emotional abuse, 80% also reported experiencing physical abuse, 42% sexual abuse, and 58% neglect. ACE participants reporting emotional neglect also reported experiencing physical abuse (40%), sexual abuse (36%), and neglect (37%). Emotional maltreatment was also strongly associated with parental substance abuse (49%), parental mental illness (44%), parental separation/divorce (44%), and domestic violence (38%). Children experiencing emotional maltreatment often suffer multiple trauma exposures.

The following parent/caregiver behaviors are emotionally abusive, especially if severe or repetitive[55]:

1. *Spurning:* Belittling, degrading, shaming, or ridiculing a child; criticizing or punishing a child in a way that singles them out; humiliating a child.
2. *Frightening or terrorizing:* Committing or threatening to perpetrate violence or life-threatening acts against a child, a child's loved ones, or a child's treasured objects.
3. *Corruption:* Encouraging the development of inappropriate or antisocial behaviors by modeling, encouraging, or permitting developmentally inappropriate or antisocial behaviors such as criminal activity, substance use, sexual activity or pornography, or inappropriate language; and encouraging or forcing the abandonment of developmentally appropriate autonomy or interfering with cognitive development.
4. *Absence of emotional responsiveness:* Ignoring a child or never expressing affection, caring, and love for a child.
5. *Rejection:* Avoiding a child or pushing him or her away; withholding love.
6. *Isolation:* Placing unreasonable limitations upon freedom of movement or social interaction.
7. *Inconsistent parenting:* Placing conflicting demands and expectations on a child.
8. *Neglect:* Failing to provide for a child's mental health, medical, and emotional needs.
9. *Domestic violence:* Allowing a child to witness domestic violence.

Children who experience emotional maltreatment suffer a unique form of trauma. The weapons used against them are not visible such as hands, belts, cords, or sexual acts, but rather ugly, hurting words or cold, uncaring silence.[52] Although no physical pain or sexual contact is ever endured, the consequences can be just as severe and long-lasting. Experiencing emotional maltreatment has been linked to a variety of short- and long-term consequences including posttraumatic stress disorder (PTSD), depression, suicide, substance abuse, and obesity. Emotional maltreatment occurring very early in life, before 5 years of age, can result in significant consequences including failure to thrive and attachment disorders. Emotional maltreatment is associated with a number of behavioral concerns extending into adulthood including anger, aggression, relationship difficulties, borderline tendencies, anxiety, and somatic complaints.

Clinical Findings

Prompt identification of emotional maltreatment and appropriate intervention are crucial to decrease long-term sequelae for victims. However, accurately diagnosing emotional maltreatment can be difficult. Most often, it is the child's behavioral or mental health difficulties or some form of other family problems that first raises the concern of possible maltreatment. On occasion, the pediatric PCP may observe parent-child interactions in the clinical setting that raise concern for possible emotional maltreatment. Most often, the pediatric PCP will need the input of other professionals including mental health therapists, school officials and teachers, and childcare workers involved with the child and family to make the diagnosis of suspected emotional maltreatment.

When suspicions of possible emotional maltreatment arise, the pediatric PCP should talk with the child and parent/caregiver separately. Screening questions to ask parents/caregivers to elicit information regarding their feelings about parenting their child include:

1. What kind of child is _____?
2. Are they easy to care for?
3. Tell me something good/positive about _____?
4. What is hard/difficult about _____?

Children age 3 years and older can also be asked a few screening questions:

1. How are things at home? At dad's?
2. How do you get along with mom/dad/step-dad/step-mom?
3. Tell me something you like to do with mom/dad/step-dad/step-mom?
4. Tell me something you like about mom/dad/step-dad/step-mom?
5. Tell me something you don't like about mom/dad/step-dad/step-mom?
6. Does anyone make you feel scared, sad, or dumb?

A thorough physical examination must be completed. The pediatric PCP understands that emotional maltreatment coexists with other forms of child maltreatment; therefore an injury assessment for physical or sexual abuse is important. The child's growth chart may yield valuable information: weight loss or gain may be one of the few physical symptoms of emotional maltreatment.

Pediatric PCPs should gather and process information garnered from observations of child, parent/caregiver interactions, familial psychosocial history, emotional maltreatment screening questions, and reports from other involved professionals to assist determining the possibility of emotional maltreatment.[52] Collaboration with a child abuse specialist is helpful in confirming concerns of emotional maltreatment. If suspicions for emotional maltreatment are raised, a referral to CPS and LE is indicated.

Diagnostic Studies

There are no diagnostic studies to aid in making the diagnosis of emotional maltreatment.

Differential Diagnosis

The differential diagnosis for emotional maltreatment is limited to behavioral or mental health concerns versus emotional maltreatment. The pediatric PCP must recognize that the three are often intertwined and can occur simultaneously. Also, behavioral and mental health concerns can develop as the result of emotional maltreatment. Children with behavioral and mental health concerns are also at heightened risk of experiencing emotional maltreatment.

Management Strategies

For children presenting to the pediatric PCP with behavioral or mental health concerns, emotional maltreatment should always be included in the differential diagnosis and must be appropriately assessed. Referral to a pediatric mental health professional skilled at trauma-informed mental health is crucial to further explore the possibility of emotional maltreatment. The pediatric PCP must also recognize that adults perpetrating emotional maltreatment need mental health intervention so that they can understand, recognize, and change their own behavior.[52] Management strategies include:

- Consult a child abuse specialist to assist in making the emotional maltreatment diagnosis.
- Report any suspicion of sexual abuse to CPS and LE.

- Thorough and precise documentation of statements made by parent/caregiver and child.
- Refer for trauma-informed mental health services (dependent upon the age of the child). Need for ongoing services is dependent upon the length and severity of the abuse, as well as other trauma exposures.
- Referral for mental health services for offending caregiver/parent.

Child Neglect

Neglect is the most common and deadliest form of child maltreatment[57] According to the DHHS,[53] over 40,000 American children experienced neglect in 2019. Of the 1840 children who died as a result of child maltreatment in 2019, 55.6% of their deaths were attributed to neglect. Neglect is associated with a variety of additional negative immediate and long-term consequences including behavioral problems, developmental delay, physical injury, and mental and physical health concerns. Neglect is indeed a significant pediatric health care problem, and it is imperative that pediatric PCPs identify neglect in their patient populations and intervene appropriately. Neglect is defined as the failure of a parent/caregiver to provide a minor with basic necessities, such as clothing, food, housing, health care, emotional nurturance, or supervision with the potential of harming them.[57] Neglect results in actual harm or the risk of harm.[58] Neglect involves acts of omission, whereas other forms of child maltreatment involve acts of commission. Despite the significant numbers of youth affected by neglect and its potential for serious consequences, neglect is often an underrecognized form of child maltreatment.[59]

Clinical Findings

There are different neglect subtypes (Table 22.3). When the pediatric PCP assesses for possible neglect, it is critical to assess for potential barriers limiting parent/caregiver ability to provide adequate care for the child. A major factor negatively impacting parent/caregiver ability to provide adequate care is poverty.[58] Poverty affects nearly every neglect subtype including medical, dental, supervision, and physical. Parent/caregiver cognitive, mental health, physical health, or substance abuse concerns may affect their ability to understand the importance of providing adequate care, from health care to love and nurturance. Caregivers with these concerns may not know how to meet even the most basic needs of their child. Cultural and/or religious beliefs may also impact parent/caregiver ability to meet their child's needs at a level deemed adequate by the larger society.[56] Parents/caregivers of the Jehovah Witness or Christian Scientist faith may have religious beliefs that contradict clinical practice guidelines and further consultation with a child maltreatment specialist is required. Certain cultures also engage in folk practices to heal illness, which may affect caregiver decisions to seek health care when their child is ill.

Differential Diagnosis

The differential diagnosis when concerns for neglect arise includes willful neglect versus neglect arising from parental/caregiver barriers to providing adequate care. Willful neglect involves a parent/caregiver who knows how to seek necessary resources for their children but refuses to do so.

TABLE 22.3 **Child Neglect Subtypes**

Subtype	Definition	Presentation
Medical	Needed medical care offering net benefit that was recommended, understood, and accessible was not provided or care was not sought for an obviously ill child	Exacerbation of an acute or chronic condition Significant delay in seeking care
Dental	Failure of parent/caregiver to seek and follow through with treatment necessary to ensure a level or oral health essential for adequate function and freedom from pain and infection	Dental caries Dental infection Dental pain
Physical	Failure to provide basic needs such as nutrition, hygiene, shelter, or clothing	Failure to thrive Obesity Noncompliance to prescribed diet Homelessness Unsafe and/or unclean living conditions
Supervision	Failure to provide adequate supervision for a child's age and developmental level resulting in harm or risk of harm	Injury (preventable) Ingestions Car seats, seat belts Guns, other weapons Physical abuse or sexual abuse (when left with an inappropriate caregiver)
Emotional	Failure to provide adequate nurturance, affection and/or psychologic support	Behavior concerns Depression or anxiety Aggression Suicide attempts

From Fortin K. When child neglect is an emergency. *Clin Pediatr Emerg Med.* 2020;21(3):1–8.

Management Strategies

As with all forms of child maltreatment, early recognition of neglect and linkage with appropriate intervention is critical in lessening negative sequelae. Because of their relationships with patients and families, pediatric PCPs are in a unique position to identify child neglect. The pediatric PCP must make one essential decision: did parent/caregiver action or lack or action result in serious or potentially serious physical, emotional, or developmental harm to the patient? If the answer is "yes," then a referral to CPS and LE is indicated. Important information to garner, not only to assist in the reporting decision but also, if reported, to share with CPS and LE, includes an assessment of possible barriers affecting the parent/caregiver's ability to provide adequate care for the youth.

If the pediatric PCP determines that the care of the youth does not warrant a neglect referral to CPS and LE, then the PCP must work closely with the parent/caregiver to develop a care plan to ensure that the child's needs continue to be met, optimally at a higher level.[57] The plan of care should include:

- Report any suspicion of physical abuse to CPS and LE.
- Thorough and precise documentation of statements made by parent/caregiver and child.
- The AAP recommends providers disclose to parents/caregivers that a referral to CPS and LE has been made. This may be difficult, but transparency is crucial in maintaining the patient/provider relationship.[30]
- Consult with child abuse specialist and/or local Child Advocacy Center as needed for assessment and diagnosis.
- Referral for parent-training program.
- Referral for early childhood education.
- Refer for trauma-informed mental health services (dependent upon the age of the child). Need for ongoing services is dependent upon the length and severity of the abuse, as well as other trauma exposures.

The PCP must discuss the care plan with the parents/caregivers and ensure their understanding of, and agreement with, the plan. The plan must be fully documented in the medical record. Referral to appropriate community agencies is indicated, such as parent-training programs, early childhood education, or substance abuse treatment programs. Close follow-up with the patient and family is indicated to ensure that the child's needs continue to be adequately addressed.

References

1. US Department of Health & Human Services. *Child Maltreatment 2020*; 2022. https://www.acf.hhs.gov/cb/report/child-maltreatment-2020.
2. Tener D, Murphy S. Adult disclosure of child sexual abuse: a literature review. *Trauma Violence Abuse*. 2015;16(4):391–400.
3. Child Welfare Information Gateway. *About CAPTA: A Legislative History*; 2019. https://www.childwelfare.gov/pubpdfs/about.pdf.
4. Centers for Disease Control & Prevention. *Preventing Child Sexual Abuse*; 2021. https://www.cdc.gov/violenceprevention/childsexualabuse/fastfact.html.
5. Felitti V, Anda R, Nordenberg M, Williamson M, Edwards B. Relationship of childhood abuse and household dysfunction to many of the leading causes of death in adults: the adverse childhood experiences study. *Am J Prevent Med*. 1996;14:245–258.
6. Hornor G, Bretl D, Chapman E, et al. Child maltreatment screening and anticipatory guidance: a description of pediatric nurse practitioner practice behaviors. *J Pediatr Health Care*. 2017;31(6):1–12.
7. US Department of Health & Human Services. *Child Maltreatment 2019*; 2021. https://www.acf.hhs.gov/cb/report/child-maltreatment-2019.
8. Hornor G. Child maltreatment prevention: essentials for the pediatric nurse practitioner. *J Pediatr Health Care*. 2022;36(2):193–201.
9. McMahon-Howard J, Reimers B. An evaluation of a child welfare training program on the commercial sexual exploitation of children (CSEC). *Evaluation and Program Planning*. 2013;40:1–9.
10. Hornor G, Davis C, Sherfield J, Wilkinson K. Trauma-informed care: essential elements for pediatric health care. *J Pediatr Health Care*. 2019;33(2):214–221.
11. Sege R, Amaya-Jackson L, American Academy of Pediatrics Committee on Child Abuse and Neglect. Clinical considerations related to the behavioral manifestation of child maltreatment. *Pediatrics*. 2017;139(4):e1–e13.
12. Schilpzand E, Sciberras E, Aliaix E, et al. Trauma exposure in children with and without ADHD: prevalence and functional impairment in a community-based study of 6-8-year-old Australian children. *Eur Child Adolesc Psychiatry*. 2018;27(69):811–819.
13. Karadag M, Gokcen C, Sarp A. EMDR therapy in children and adolescents who have post-traumatic stress disorder: a six-week follow up study. *Int J Psychiatry Clin Pract*. 2020;24(1):77–82.
14. Perry-Parish C, Copeland-Linder N, Webb L, Sibinga E. Mindfulness-based approaches for children and youth. *Curr Prob Pediatr Adolesc Health Care*. 2016;46:172–178.
15. Vanderbilt-Adriance E, haw D. Protective factors and the development of resilience in the context of neighborhood disadvantage. *J Abnormal Child Psychol*. 2008;36:887–901.
16. US Department of Health & Human Services. *Framework for Prevention of Child Maltreatment*; 2017. https://www.childwelfare.gov/topics/preventing/overview/framework/.
17. Ashraf I, Pekarsky A, Race J, Botash A. Making the most of clinical encounters: prevention of child maltreatment. *Pediatr Clin North Am*. 2020;67:481–498.
18. Rangel E, Cook B, Bennett B, Shebesta K, Ying J, Palcone R. Eliminating disparity in evaluation for abuse in infants with head injury: use of a screening guide. *J Pediatr Surg*. 2009;44(6):1229–1234.
19. Sheets L, Leach M, Koszewski T, Lessmeier A, Nugent M, Simpson P. Sentinel injuries in infants evaluated for child physical abuse. *Pediatrics*. 2013;131(4):701–707.
20. Berger R, Lindberg D. Early recognition of physical abuse; Bridging the gap between knowledge and practice. *J Pediatr*. 2018;204:16–23.
21. Henry M, Wood J. What's in a name: sentinel injuries in abused infants. *Pediatr Radiol*. 2021;51:861–865.
22. Kazmir S, Rosado N. Abusive head trauma: a review of current knowledge. *Clin Pediatr Emerg Med*. 2020;21(3):1–11.
23. Hoehn E, Wilson P, Riney L, Ngo V, Bennett B, Duma E. Identification and evaluation of physical abuse in children. *Pediatr Ann*. 2018;47(3):e97–e101.
24. Berkowitz C. Physical abuse of children. *N Engl J Med*. 2017;376(17):1659–1666.
25. Parks S, Amnest J, Hill H, Karch D. *Pediatric Abusive Head Trauma: Recommended Definitions for Public Health Surveillance and Research*. Atlanta, GA: Centers for Disease Control and Prevention; 2020. https://www.cdc.gov/violenceprevention/pdf/pedheadtrauma-a.pdf.
26. Kemp A. Abusive head trauma: recognition and the essential investigation. *Arch Dis Child Educ Pract Ed*. 2011;96(6):202–208.
27. Rambaud C. Bridging veins and autopsy findings in abusive head trauma. *Pediatr Radiol*. 2015;45:1126–1131.
28. Leaman L, Hennrikus W, Bresnahan J. Erratum to: identifying non-accidental fractures in children aged <2 years. *J Child Orthoped*. 2016;10:467.
29. Orman G, Kralik S, Meoded A, Desai N, Risen S, Huisman T. MRI findings in pediatric abusive head trauma: a review. *J Neuroimag*. 2016;30:15–27.
30. Christian C, Committee on Child Abuse and Neglect. The evaluation of suspected child physical abuse. *Pediatrics*. 2015;135(5):e1337–e1354.

TABLE 23.1	Factors That Influence Adherence to Taking Prescribed Pediatric Medications

Factors That Influence Adherence	Interventions That Improve Adherence
Length of treatment: Longer treatment contributes to poorer adherence.	*Shorten length of treatment if possible* (e.g., if multiple antibiotic regimens are equally as effective, select the one with the fewest therapy days).
Medical condition: Adherence rates vary with chronic illnesses, frequency of medication changes, lack of physical symptoms, need to master medication administration techniques, lack of immediate medication benefits.	*Develop creative solutions to encourage adherence* (e.g., sticker charts; pill boxes; calendars; link dose to a personal daily habit, such as teeth brushing). Determine how drug regimen fits into patient's lifestyle and try to modify it to increase adherence; repeat short educational instructions at every visit (include verbal and written instructions); assess for depression. Discuss barriers (e.g., does child have other priorities? Does treatment create a negative identity?) and their underlying assumptions. Engage a family member or caregiver who will assist the pediatric patient with their medications at home. Provide continuity of care.
Doses per day: The more medication doses that need to be administered per day, the poorer the adherence rate. This is particularly true with working parents and pediatric patients in school who often miss mid-day doses.	*Simplify dosing regimen.* Minimize the number of doses per day and the medication volume to promote adherence. If possible, consider dispensing two bottles of a prescription medication so that some may be stored at home and some at school or day care. (This may be limited by insurance coverage and the ability to obtain two bottles.)
Palatability and ease of ingestion: Unpalatable medications are resisted, and some pediatric patients have preferences for certain formulations (i.e., prefers suspension due to difficulty swallowing pills)	*Prescribe medications in a higher concentration, when possible, to reduce the volume required.* For example, when prescribing 250 mg of penicillin VK, select the suspension that includes 250 mg/5 mL rather than 125 mg/5 mL to reduce the medication amount the patient needs to swallow *Choose the best-tasting medication, prescribe chewables or oral disintegrating tabs, or mask the taste.* If a medication has the same efficacy profile, the best-tasting (though that may not mean it tastes good) medication is easier to administer during infancy and early to middle childhood. Pharmacies may be able to flavor medications to match preferences and promote adherence (see Additional Resources). Use flavoring syrups or crush tablets and mix with palatable semi-solid foods, such as chocolate syrup, jam, applesauce, or pudding. Before crushing any tablet or mixing a medication, check to determine if the medication can be safely crushed and confirm food is compatible with the medication. *Facilitate the swallowing of pills and capsules.* Encourage the patient to sit up straight with their head centered and tilted back slightly. After taking a few "practice" swallows of water or another liquid that the medication can be administered with, place the pill on their tongue and encourage them to swallow more liquid. Collaboration with colleagues in child life and other support services may also help
Expense: Out-of-pocket costs may be difficult for some families to meet. Insurance coverage may not include medications.	*Choose the medication that has the lowest out-of-pocket expense for the family.* Prescribe generics when appropriate and offer information about insurance coverage and resources (e.g., discount cards, mail-order pharmacies, and medication assistance programs).
Belief systems: Religious and spiritual beliefs concerning medication containing ingredients of animal origin; concern with the safety profile and long-term effects of medications; seeing medication as a "crutch"; or if children/teens view themselves as "addicts" are all beliefs that affect adherence.	*Explore beliefs that interfere with medication adherence with open-ended questions. Counsel medication use issues with ethical and cultural sensitivity.* Specifically address safety and side effects of drug regimen and elicit concerns. Use motivational interviewing techniques (see Chapter 6).
Social determinants of health: Issues such as access to health care, insurance coverage, access to transportation, poverty, and limited literacy all impact adherence to a treatment regimen.	*Assess the family for challenges that affect successful outcomes.* Assess literacy and health literacy levels.

Modified from CDC. Social determinants of health: know what affects health. https://www.cdc.gov/socialdeterminants/about.html; 2021; and Teaching your child how to swallow pills. https://kidshealth.org/en/parents/swallowing-pills.html; 2019.

influences, of health including healthcare access and quality, neighborhood and built environment, and economic stability of the family.[15]

The term *adherence* is currently used to describe whether a patient is taking the recommended pharmaceutical or following a recommended treatment regimen. Providers need to assess the patient and/or parent's barriers to medication adherence.

Nonadherence needs to be proactively managed to improve clinical outcomes and cost-effectiveness. Table 23.1 discusses general factors that contribute to lower adherence rates and suggests strategies to increase those rates. A myriad of research studies about adherence have led to the following conclusions:

- Adherence is not a steady state; therefore, adherence needs to be assessed as part of each office visit.

- Open-ended questions that allow the patient/parent an opportunity to describe their adherence may provide more accurate information.
- There are several strategies for the assessment of medication adherence. Self-report questionnaires, validated tools developed for caregivers and children, and structured interviews are effective strategies for measuring adherence.[16]
- Use objective measurements to determine the adherence level, including strategies such as therapeutic drug monitoring, pickup and refill rates, and medication counting during visits.[16]
- Adolescents are less likely to be adherent to medication regimens in some settings. Adherence rates in this age group can be increased with interventions including mobile gaming interventions, mindfulness training, praise text messaging, and web-based education.[17–21]
- Patients/families benefit from ongoing, interprofessional education and psychosocial support throughout the treatment continuum, with emphasis on strategies to promote adherence.[22,23]
- Age-appropriate incentivization is especially effective when used in combination with other promotion strategies, such as motivational intervention, education, and technology use.[22]
- A provider is more effective when practicing active listening, providing emotional support, using plain language, giving brief but complete instructions, and having the pediatric patient and/or parent repeat instructions or "teach back," allowing adequate time for visits, using a wide range of teaching tools, and involving office staff in teaching activities.
- Language barriers and health literacy impact medication adherence and errors.[24–26] Strategies to overcome limited health literacy include providing verbal instructions, using pictures and other visuals, and utilizing language that can be completely understood by patients.
- Incorporate all modes of teaching styles. The use of tools and emerging technologies can be effective in improving adherence rates. These tools include pictogram-based instruction sheets; telephone counseling; video or mobile games to improve knowledge, disease management adherence, and clinical outcomes; mobile phone apps; short, weekly text messages; pill boxes and organizers; hands-on demonstrations; and electronic monitoring devices that record inhaler use (see Additional Resources).[27–31]
- Written instructions increase adherence rates. Consumer medication information (CMI) leaflets dispensed through retail pharmacies are intended to be short and comprehensive. They are written by third-party drug information companies and are not FDA approved or regulated. Patient package inserts (PPIs) are developed by the pharmaceutical manufacturer and discuss risk information; they are lengthy, detailed, and intended for the use of medical providers.
- Establishing a provider/pharmacist collaborative management program may improve adherence rates.[23]
- Providers should self-critique treatment biases they have toward ethnically and socially diverse populations and overcome any cultural barriers.[26]

Disposal of Pharmaceuticals

The preferred method of medication disposal is through a drug take-back program, which is available in communities across the nation (See additional resources). If families are not able to access a take-back program, there are safe ways to dispose of some medications at home. The FDA developed a "flush list" of medications that can be flushed down the toilet. Although there is concern about the environmental and human health risks associated with flushing medications down the toilet, the FDA determined that the risk of accidental exposure to such medications outweighs the potential risks. For medications that are not on the flush list, disposal in home trash requires a process described by the FDA. Medicine should be mixed with coffee grounds, cat litter, or another undesirable substance before being sealed in a container that is thrown in the trash. Advise families to remove all personal information from medication packaging.[32] In addition, the Drug Enforcement Agency has information regarding prescription take-back days and authorized collectors on their website (see Additional Resources).

Overprescribing Antibiotics: A Continuing Problem

Approximately 2.8 million illnesses and 35,000 deaths in the United States are attributed to antimicrobial-resistant infections each year.[33] In response to this serious public health threat, a National Action Plan for Combating Antibiotic-Resistant Bacteria was developed in 2015. The current plan describes a coordinated, strategic plan to reduce infections and antibiotic use from 2020 to 2025. Five goals were identified, with several objectives for each, including improved outpatient antibiotic use, support for healthcare providers to promote recommended antibiotic use practices, and support for policies to improve antibiotic use across healthcare settings.[34]

The most prescribed class of medications in pediatrics are antibiotics, and the majority of these are prescribed in the outpatient setting (e.g., clinics, emergency departments, urgent care centers, telehealth appointments, and other venues).[35] An estimated 30% of prescribed antibiotics are unnecessary. The most common antibiotic misuse indication is acute upper respiratory infections, including acute otitis media and pharyngitis.[36] There is also evidence that patients who receive an antibiotic during their first episode of bronchitis are more likely to have a second episode of bronchitis and to receive another antibiotic than those who did not get an antibiotic prescription during their initial episode.[37] These data support the need for antimicrobial stewardship programs. The goals of pediatric antimicrobial stewardship programs include using antibiotics appropriately, at correct doses and duration, and limiting the spectrum of the antibiotic to the infection being treated.[35] Strategies to achieve these goals include clinician education, standardized protocols, improved family communication, clinical decision support, and systematic approaches to situations such as negative culture results.[35] Antibiograms support PCP decision-making and promote the selection of an antibiotic with known effectiveness in the geographic area of the prescriber. Diagnostic stewardship further supports antimicrobial stewardship by requiring characteristic findings of various infections before prescribing antibiotics.[35] Antimicrobial stewardship programs are proven to be effective, and the collaboration between the government, providers, healthcare facilities, and the community outlined in the National Action Plan has the potential to decrease the threat of antimicrobial resistance.

Guidelines for Writing a Prescription

Before prescribing a medication, the PCP must take several critical steps to ensure the prescription is appropriate and rational. Make a specific diagnosis, consider pathophysiologic implications, and identify a therapeutic objective. Once those steps are complete, identify the appropriate drug, consider the appropriate dosing regimen, plan for monitoring, identify an endpoint, and share that information with the patient and caregivers. Write prescriptions in a manner that conveys accurate information to the pharmacist, the patient, the parent, and other clinicians accessing the patient's chart.[38]

Prescriptions include information regarding the prescriber (including name, license, and contact information) and the patient (including name, address, and often the date of birth). The body of the prescription includes information regarding the medication prescribed. The specific medication (brand name or generic) prescribed is the first element; this includes the medication name and strength in metric units. The quantity to be dispensed should reflect the anticipated therapy duration. This may be enough for a 7-day treatment course, such as in the case of an antibiotic for a bacterial infection, or a 1-month or 90-day supply for ongoing treatment of a chronic condition. The PCP must also consider if there is a risk of an overdose or toxicity associated with dispensing larger amounts or prolonged courses of the medication. Next, provide complete directions for use, including the medication amount, administration route, dosing frequency, and duration of therapy. The number of refills provided is guided by the anticipated therapy duration and consideration of whether or not effectiveness is established (i.e., initiating a new medication for a chronic illness that requires reassessment before refilling the medication).[38]

Prescription errors are a common threat to patient safety across the continuum of care. Among the most common errors in prescriptions are dose or timing errors related to poor writing, omitted information, and inappropriate medication choice for specific situations. Online resources are available to help reduce or document prescribing errors, including the Institute for Safe Medication Practices and National Coordinating Council for Medication Error Reporting and Prevention Program (see Additional Resources). Electronic prescribing led to several changes in prescribing practices, and an estimated 70% of prescriptions are now e-prescribed in the United States.[38] While this presents an opportunity for the PCP to gain information from the health plan regarding formulary, decision support regarding potential interactions, and more efficient transactions between prescribers and pharmacies, it does present new challenges. Prescription errors due to pull-down drug lists contribute and other unique factors to electronic prescribing are common.[38] Enhance prescribing accuracy by following the guidelines listed in Box 23.1.

Complementary and Integrative Therapies

Families of pediatric patients are increasingly interested in complementary and integrative therapies, requiring PCPs to be knowledgeable and aware of reliable resources to support the safe and effective application of desired therapies. Common indications for complementary therapies include back or neck pain, head or chest colds, musculoskeletal conditions, anxiety or stress, and attentional-deficit/hyperactivity disorder. Increased utilization with children and youth living with chronic illnesses has been reported.[39] The National Center for Complementary and Integrative Health (NCCIH) defines complementary health as the use of a nonmainstream approach used together with conventional medicine. Integrative health is a coordinated combination of conventional and complementary approaches with an emphasis on

---

• BOX 23.1 Guidelines for Accurate Prescribing

- Eliminate drug abbreviations.[a]
- Use computer-generated prescriptions whenever possible.
- Provide concise dosage information[a]:
  - Use metric measures, such as milligrams or milliliters, rather than designating tablet, vial, teaspoon, tablespoon, or dropper. Most parents, including those who are non-English speakers or who have low literacy, can follow instructions on the use of metric measures.
  - Select "unit" rather than a "U," which can be mistaken for a zero or a number.
  - Select "international unit" rather than IU, which can be mistaken for IV or the number 10.
  - Avoid a trailing or terminal zero (e.g., 9.0 mg) because the decimal point may be missed. Type or write 9 mg instead.
  - Lead with a zero before a decimal point (e.g., 0.15 mg) so that the decimal point is not missed.
  - Avoid using decimal points whenever possible (e.g., write 300 mg instead of 0.3 g).
- Do not use abbreviations for body parts[a] (e.g., o.d. [oculus dextra] for right eye).
- Avoid vague instructions that might cause confusion when patient is taking several drugs (e.g., avoid "take as directed" or "prn" without stipulating indications for which drug should be taken).
- Specify number of pills to be dispensed rather than stating a time duration.
- Adding refills for an acute treatment confuses duration of therapy and may preclude patient returning for a necessary recheck appointment.
- State indication or purpose of drug (alerts pharmacist and other physicians to appropriateness of medication and aids in counseling). For example, state the medication is for a respiratory or skin condition (preprint the body system directly on the prescription for easy check-off).
- Add supplemental information (e.g., avoid sun exposure; do not take with grapefruit juice; take with food).
- Remain alert to lethal doses and compromising pathologic conditions (e.g., compromised renal or hepatic functions) that might affect drug levels. Prescriptions of controlled substances should adhere to current regulations.

Specific Considerations for Written Prescriptions
- Limit each prescription to one medication.
- Ensure the prescriber's name, license classification, and contact information (address and telephone number) are printed on the prescription so the pharmacist can contact the prescriber with any questions.
- If a handwritten prescription is needed, print name of medication in block letters rather than write the name in cursive. Write "daily" rather than qd, which can be mistaken for qid.
- Write "every other day" rather than qod, which can be mistaken for qid and qd.
- Use generic, official, or trademarked name; avoid chemical names or coined names.

[a]A complete list of abbreviations to avoid when writing prescriptions is available from https://www.ismp.org/recommendations/error-prone-abbreviations-list.

IV, Intravenous; *qd,* quaque die (every day); *qid,* quarter in die (four times a day); *qod,* quaque altera die (every other day).
Modified from Lofholm PW, Katzung BG. Rational prescribing and prescription writing. In: Katzung BG, Vanderah TW, ed. *Basic and Clinical Pharmacology.* 15th ed. McGraw-Hill; 2021; and National Coordinating Council for Medication Error Reporting and Prevention. Recommendations to enhance accuracy of prescription/medication order writing; 2014. https://www.nccmerp.org/recommendations-enhance-accuracy-prescription-writing

---

the care of the whole person. It is important to differentiate these models from alternative healthcare, which is the application of a nonmainstream approach in the place of conventional medicine or the use of therapies that are not evidence-based in the place of conventional care.[39,40]

The NCCIH is a center of the National Institutes of Health (NIH) with the mission of defining the usefulness and safety of complementary and integrative interventions through rigorous scientific investigation. Objectives of the NCCIH include the advancement of fundamental science and methods, improved care for hard-to-manage symptoms, health promotion and disease prevention, enhanced research regarding complementary and integrative health, and dissemination of evidence-based information.[40] Subgroups of complementary health are described by their primary therapeutic input, including nutritional (e.g., vitamins, minerals, herbs, probiotics), psychological (e.g., mindfulness, meditation), physical (e.g., massage, spinal manipulation), and combinations (e.g., yoga, acupuncture, mindful eating).[41]

Patient-Provider Communication Regarding the Use of Complementary Medicine

The topic of complementary medicine use must be broached nonjudgmentally to encourage disclosure, help the family clarify safety issues, and explore how complementary therapies might fit into a patient's management plan. Nondisclosure may be related to fear of PCP disapproval, inadequate time, failure of the PCP to ask about such therapies, and belief that complementary medicine was safe.[42] On the contrary, reasons for disclosure include concerns about safety, desire for additional information, and belief that the PCP would be supportive of the use of complementary medicine.[42] Some questions that may support the PCP to inquire about the use of complementary medicine include:

- What complementary medicine products is the patient taking, including herbal, natural, or nutritional supplements?
- What complementary medicine *therapies* are being used (e.g., acupuncture, chiropractic, massage)?
- What other practitioners is the child seeing?
- What other kinds of activities are being used to address a particular problem?
- Has the complementary treatment helped the problem?

Consistently incorporating questions about complementary medicine helps facilitate an open, honest dialogue between the PCP and the patient/family. Conveying respect for the families' values and beliefs supports their disclosure. When a PCP identifies that a patient is receiving complementary or integrative therapies, they can share evidence-based information and effectively monitor treatment response.[39]

Safety Considerations of Complementary and Integrative Medicine

It is particularly important to ascertain the safety of certain treatment modalities by learning about complementary products that the patient may be using, including side effects, possible interactions with other medications, and mechanisms of action. Unlike conventional pharmaceuticals, the FDA does not approve dietary supplements before they are marketed. Rather than providing evidence to the FDA to substantiate safety, the manufacturer submits a notification to the FDA with information that supports their belief that the supplement is expected to be safe.[43] To evaluate for interactions between natural health products and medications, PCPs may refer to the Natural Medicines database, NCCIH herb-drug interactions clinical digest for clinicians, or other trusted pharmacology resources (see additional resources). It is critical to refer to an interaction checker each time a PCP learns that a patient utilizes a complementary therapy, as information in this

• BOX 23.2 Key Guidelines for Use of Herbal and Dietary Supplements

- Use only single-herb supplements instead of combinations to prevent side effect confusion.
- Emphasize that "natural" does not mean "safe."
- Stop some herbal supplements at least 1 week before any scheduled surgical procedure to prevent any alterations in coagulation, blood pressure, or interactions with anesthesia; communicate cessation to the surgeon.
- Exercise caution when purchasing herbal products over the internet.
- Avoid the use of herbs starting with the letter "G"—ginkgo, ginseng, garlic, ginger, or green tea if the patient is taking warfarin or a drug that is metabolized using the hepatic cytochrome P450 enzyme system. Some "G" herbs can either potentiate or inhibit the drug, therefore altering the therapeutic effect or causing adverse effects.
- Research the natural health products (NHPs) as thoroughly as possible and look for these labels:
  - US Pharmacopeia (USP) Dietary Supplement Verified seal: Product meets certain standards for contamination, adulteration, manufacturing processes, and pharmacologic properties.
  - National Sanitation Foundation (NSF) International: Sets standards, tests, and certifies products and systems, including Good Manufacturing Processes (GMP) for cleanliness, maintenance, and documented quality checks.
  - Natural Products Association (NPA; formerly National Nutritional Food Association TruLabel program): Includes a GMP process and a Natural Seal certification process that ensures ingredient quality and purity.
  - Consumer Lab (CL): Tests dietary supplements for composition, potency, purity, bioavailability, consistency of products.
  - Generally Recognized as Safe (GRAS) in the United States: Recognized as generally safe for its intended purpose as part of the Federal Food, Drug, and Cosmetic Act.
- Herbal and NHPs manufactured and imported from Europe are generally regarded as safe because they have to comply with standards set by Commission E (Europe's equivalent of the FDA).
- In England, an herbal product is licensed and meets standards of safety and quality if it has a Marketing Authorization (MA) or Traditional Herbal Registration (THR) scheme number on the label.
- Use websites, such as the American Botanical Council HerbClip Database, to determine if the product has been tested or reviewed. The Natural Medicines Comprehensive Database offers evidence-based information on safety, efficacy, interactions, and side effects for brand-name conventional and NHPs. The National Center for Complementary and Integrative Health (NCCIH) provides a list of herbal products that have been studied for specific conditions by that organization. The American Herbal Products Association (AHPA) evaluates herbal safety for all botanical ingredients sold in North America. Each herb is placed in one of three safety and interactions classes.

field continues to evolve. Guidelines to support the PCP's advice about herbal and dietary supplements are described in Box 23.2.

Additional Resources

Clinical Pharmacogenetics Implementation Consortium Guidelines: https://cpicpgx.org/guidelines/

Drug Enforcement Agency (DEA): Disposal of Pharmaceuticals: www.deadiversion.usdoj.gov/drug_disposal/index.html

European Medicines Agency: https://www.ema.europa.eu/en/human-regulatory/overview/paediatric-medicines-overview

Food and Drug Administration: Current and Resolved Drug Shortages: https://www.accessdata.fda.gov/scripts/drugshortages/

Food and Drug Administration (FDA): Disposal of Pharmaceuticals: https://www.fda.gov/consumers/consumer-updates/where-and-how-dispose-unused-medicines

Food and Drug Administration (FDA): MedWatch: The FDA Safety Information and Adverse Event Reporting Program: www.fda.gov/Safety/MedWatch/default.htm

Food and Drug Administration (FDA): Pediatric Labeling Changes: www.accessdata.fda.gov/scripts/sda/sdNavigation.cfm?sd=labelingdatabase

Institute for Safe Medication Practices: www.ismp.org

The Joint Commission National Patient Safety Goals: https://www.jointcommission.org/standards/national-patient-safety-goals/

National Association of Boards of Pharmacy: https://nabp.pharmacy/

National Coordinating Council for Medication Error Reporting and Prevention: www.nccmerp.org/about-medication-errors

National Center for Complementary and Integrative Health: https://www.nccih.nih.gov/

Natural Medicines: https://naturalmedicines.therapeuticresearch.com/

National Center for Complementary and Integrative Health Herb-Drug Interactions: https://www.nccih.nih.gov/health/providers/digest/herb-drug-interactions

References

1. *2022 National Patient Safety Goals.* 2021. https://www.jointcommission.org/standards/national-patient-safety-goals/.
2. Pediatric committee advises FDA on medical product research, labeling, and adverse events. aap.org. https://publications.aap.org/aapnews/news/20248/Pediatric-committee-advises-FDA-on-medical-product?searchresult=1.
3. Paediatric medicines: Overview. https://www.ema.europa.eu/en/human-regulatory/overview/paediatric-medicines-overview.
4. Edwards E. The U.S. needs to reimagine its pharma supply chain. https://hbr.org/2021/08/the-u-s-needs-to-reimagine-its-pharma-supply-chain.
5. Hibma JE, Giacomini KM. Pharmacogenomics. In: Katzung BG, Vanderah W, eds. *Basic and Clinical Pharmacology.* 15th ed. McGraw-Hill; 2021.
6. Koren G. Special aspects of perinatal and pediatric pharmacology. In: Katzung BG, Vanderah W, eds. *Basic and Clinical Pharmacology.* 15th ed. McGraw-Hill; 2021.
7. Van den Anker J, Reed MD, Allegaert K, Kearns GL. Developmental changes in pharmacokinetics and pharmacodynamics. *J Clin Pharmacol.* 2018;58(S10):S10–S25.
8. Law RM, Ngo MA, Maibach HI. Twenty clinically pertinent factors/observations for percutaneous absorption in humans. *Am J Clin Dermatol.* 2020;21:85–95.
9. Neville KA, Frattarelli DAC, Galinkin JL, et al. Committee on Drugs. Policy statement: off-label use of drugs in children. *Pediatrics.* 2014;133(3):563–567.
10. Allen HC, Garbe MC, Lees J, et al. Off-label medication use in children, more common than we think: a systematic review of the literature. *J Okla State Med Assoc.* 2018;111(8):776–783.
11. Pediatric research equity act. https://www.fda.gov/drugs/development-resources/pediatric-research-equity-act-prea.
12. Pediatric labeling changes. https://www.fda.gov/science-research/pediatrics/pediatric-labeling-changes.
13. Pediatrics fact sheet from the National Ambulatory Medical Care Survey. https://www.cdc.gov/nchs/data/namcs/factsheets/NAMCS_2014_15_Pediatrics-508.pdf.
14. Carmody JK, Gutierrez-Colina AM, Hommel KA. Fact sheet: adherence to pediatric medical regimens for chronic disease. Pedspsych.org. https://pedpsych.org/fact_sheets/medical_regimens/.
15. CDC: Social determinants of health: know what affects health. https://www.cdc.gov/socialdeterminants/about.html.
16. Al-Hassany L, Skoosterboer SM, Dierckx B, et al. Assessing methods of measuring adherence in chronically ill children: narrative review. *Patient Prefer Adherence.* 2019;13:1175–1189.
17. Radovic A, Badawy SM. Technology use for adolescent health and wellness. *Pediatrics.* 2020;145(suppl 2):S186–S194.
18. Sayegh C, Im D, Moss IK, et al. Randomized pilot trial of praise text messages to improve medication adherence among adolescents and young adults with liver transplants. *Pediatr Transplant.* 2022:e14361.
19. Scalzi LV, Hollenbeak CS, Maschuilli E, et al. Improvement of medication adherence in adolescents and young adults with SLE using web-based education with and without a social media intervention, a pilot study. *Pediatr Rheumatol Online J.* 2018;16(1):18.
20. Sibinga EMS, Webb L, Perin J, et al. Mindfulness instruction for medication adherence among adolescents and young adults living with HIV: a randomized control trial. *AIDS Care.* 2022;34(12):176.
21. Whiteley L, Brown L, Lally M, et al. A mobile gaming intervention to increase adherence to antiretroviral treatment for youth living with HIV: development guided by the information, motivation, and behavioral skills model. *JMIR Mhealth Uhealth.* 2018;6(4):e96.
22. Coyne KD, Trimble KA, Lloyd A, et al. Interventions to promote oral medication adherence in the pediatric chronic illness population: a systematic review from the Children's Oncology Group. *J Pediatr Oncol Nurs.* 2019;36(3):219–235.
23. Kini V, Ho M. Interventions to improve medication adherence. *JAMA.* 2018;320(23):2461–2473.
24. Glick AF, Farkas JS, Mendelsohn AL, et al. Discharge instruction comprehension and adherence errors interrelationship between plan complexity and parent health literacy. *J Pediatr.* 2019;214:193–200.
25. Licari A, Castagnoli R, Ciprandi R, et al. Inadequate literacy is associated with uncontrolled asthma in adolescents. *Ann Allergy Asthma Immunol.* 2021;127(5):598–600.
26. McQuaid EL, Landier W. Cultural issues in medication adherence: disparities and directions. *J Gen Intern Med.* 2018;33:200–206.
27. Alberts NM, Badawy SM, Hodger J, et al. Development of the InCharge health mobile all to improve adherence to hydroxyurea in patients with sickle cell disease: user-centered design approach. *JMIR Mhealth Uhealth.* 2020;8(5):e14884.
28. Badawy SM, Cronin RM, Hankins J, et al. Patient-centered eHealth interventions for children, adolescents and adults with sickle cell disease: systematic review. *J Med Internet Res.* 2018;20(7):e10940.
29. Ramsey RR, Plevinsky JM, Kollin SR, et al. Systematic review of digital interventions for pediatric asthma management. *J Allergy Clin Immunol Pract.* 2020;8(4):1284–1293.
30. Schandevyl GV, Casimir G, Hanssens L. A medication-adherence enhancing simulation intervention in pediatric cystic fibrosis. *J Child Health Care.* 2022;26(2):275–289.
31. Wu YP, Linder LA, Kanokvimankul P, et al. Use of a smartphone application for prompting oral medication adherence among adolescents and young adults with cancer. *Oncol Nurs Forum.* 2018;45(1):69–76.
32. Disposal of unused medicines: What you should know. https://www.fda.gov/drugs/safe-disposal-medicines/disposal-unused-medicines-what-you-should-know.
33. About antimicrobial resistance. https://www.cdc.gov/drugresistance/about.html.
34. National action plan for combating antibiotic-resistant bacteria. https://www.hhs.gov/sites/default/files/carb-national-action-plan-2020-2025.pdf.
35. Gerber JS, Jackson MA, Tamma PD, et al. Committee on Infectious Diseases. Policy statement: antibiotic stewardship in pediatrics. *Pediatrics.* 2021;147(1):e2020040295.
36. Poole NM, Frost H. Targets and methods to improve outpatient antibiotic prescribing for pediatric patients. *Infect Dis Clin North Am.* 2022;36(1):187–202.
37. Morgan JR, Carey KM, Barlam T, et al. Inappropriate antibiotic prescribing for acute bronchitis in children and impact on subsequent episodes of care and treatment. *Pediatr Infect Dis J.* 2019;38(3):271–274.

38. Lofholm PW, Katzung BG. Rational prescribing and prescription writing. In: Katzung BG, Vanderah W, eds. *Basic and Clinical Pharmacology*. 15th ed. McGraw-Hill; 2021.

39. McClafferty J, Vohra S, Bailey M, et al. Pediatric integrative medicine. *Pediatrics*. 2017;140(3):e20171961.

40. National Center for Complementary and Integrative Health. https://www.nih.gov/about-nih/what-we-do/nih-almanac/national-center-complementary-integrative-health-nccih.

41. The NIH almanac: National Center for Complementary and Integrative Health. https://www.nih.gov/about-nih/what-we-do/nih-almanac/national-center-complementary-integrative-health-nccih.

42. Foley H, Steel A, Cramer H, Wardle J, Adams J. Disclosure of complementary medicine use to medical providers: a systematic review and meta-analysis. *Sci Rep*. 2019;9(1):1573.

43. FDA. Questions and answers on dietary supplements. https://www.fda.gov/food/information-consumers-using-dietary-supplements/questions-and-answers-dietary-supplements.

24

Pediatric Pain and Fever Management

HELEN N. TURNER AND JAIME PANTON

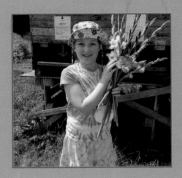

This chapter focuses on two common yet potentially challenging pediatric signs and symptoms—fever and pain. Each can occur alone or together. The chapter begins with a discussion of pain, followed by fever, and calls attention to pediatric considerations and overlapping pharmacologic management.

Pediatric Pain

Overview

Before the mid-1980s, it was thought infants did not feel or remember pain so treating it was not necessary. In addition, there were concerns pain medications were not safe for pediatric patients; however, our understanding of pain in pediatric patients and its management has evolved. Providers are now obliged to minimize pain associated with disease and medical care and have the necessary resources to do so safely and effectively.

Early painful experiences are significant events and can produce long-term consequences for the child. Preterm infants are particularly vulnerable and undergo numerous painful procedures. Studies document that early and undertreated pain has long-term negative physiologic and psychological consequences, such as increased pain sensitivity, decreased effectiveness of analgesia during subsequent procedures, persistent pain, increased stress responses, and behavior and learning difficulties.[1]

Standards for pediatric care necessitate incorporating pain management and prevention in every treatment plan, from minor painful procedures to more serious illnesses or injuries and persistent pain. Understanding nociception, types, mechanisms, and sources of pain is critical to developing a successful treatment regimen. Nociception is the neural process of encoding noxious stimuli, which results in pain perception. It is a four-part process (transduction, transmission, perception, modulation) as sensory nerve endings (nociceptors) are activated by chemical, mechanical, thermal, or mixed stimuli and are processed (Fig. 24.1). Pain assessment, diagnosis, and treatment are determined by the type of pain (Box 24.1) and the mechanism or etiology of the pain (Box 24.2). The neural foundations and pathways necessary for nociception develop early in fetal life. Myelinization of the brainstem and the thalamic tract is complete at approximately 32 weeks of gestation and the beginning of the neuronal pain-inhibiting mechanism appears. These mechanisms continue developing well past the newborn period. Because of neural plasticity, newborns

subjected to repetitive acute pain may develop central neural changes that predispose them to pain vulnerability, negative cognitive effects, and opioid tolerance.[2]

Pain is defined as an "unpleasant sensory and emotional experience associated with or resembling that associated with, actual or potential tissue damage."[3] Pain lasting 3 to 6 months, or longer than the expected healing time for an injury, is labeled persistent pain. Up to 30% of children experience persistent pain, with the most commonly reported being headaches, abdominal pain, and musculoskeletal pain. Those with persistent pain are also at greater risk for anxiety, depression, and sleep disturbances, and they may experience more emotional and functional problems than their peers. Persistent pain negatively affects children's school attendance, participation in hobbies, appetite, and quality of life, and results in increased healthcare service utilization. Because it is not always feasible to eliminate pain, effective management with minimal side effects and return of function are the primary goals of treatment.

Factors Influencing Pediatric Pain Management

Physiologic

- Pain has an evolutionary purpose—the brief painless interval postinjury allows the fight or flight response to occur and then incites injury awareness that provokes withdrawal from the painful stimuli.
- Genetics and age influence levels of neurotransmitters or medication responses.
- Established pain is more difficult to control, making pain prevention and timely pain management critical goals.
- Persistent pain is rarely associated with sympathetic nervous system arousal. Children with persistent pain may not appear to be in pain, and this lack of outward expression of symptoms may impede pain evaluation and treatment.

Social-Emotional

- Individual physiologic and social-emotional states influence pain perception and response.
- Developmental stages (e.g., cognitive, emotional, physical), age, and temperament significantly affect pain interpretation,

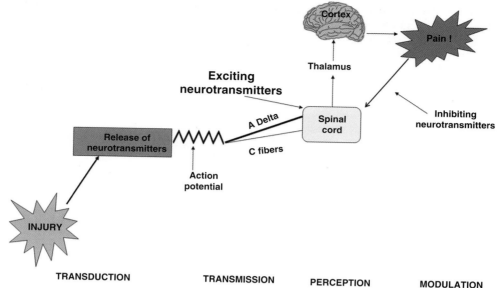

• **Fig. 24.1** Nociception. *Transduction:* Painful or noxious stimuli are translated into electrical signals at sensory nerve endings and forwarded to the spinal cord via A-delta fibers and C fibers. A-delta fibers are large, myelinated, fast, and when activated result in sharp, stinging sensations. In contrast, C fibers are small, unmyelinated, slow, and their activation results in dull, aching, burning, and diffuse sensations. *Transmission:* Electrical impulses are forwarded through the sensory nervous system through both the peripheral and central nervous systems. *Perception:* The emotional and physical experience of pain. *Modulation:* Alteration of information by endogenous mechanisms results in lessening or amplification of the pain signal. (From Czarnecki ML, Turner HN, eds. *Core Curriculum for Pain Management Nursing.* 3rd ed. Elsevier; 2018.)

• BOX 24.1 Types of Pain

- *Procedural (incidental):* Short-term acute pain caused by medical investigations and treatment.
- *Acute:* Sudden onset, usually associated with trauma, injury, or medical case and resolves in a predictable and expected timeframe.
- *Persistent:* Pain that continues beyond the expected healing time. Persistent pain no longer has a purpose. Factors not necessarily related to the initial cause of the pain may perpetuate it.
- *Recurrent:* Returning or occurring again following a pain-free period.
- *Mixed:* Acute pain in the setting of persistent pain.

• BOX 24.2 Mechanisms of Pain

- Nociceptive pain: occurs when nociceptors (mechanical, chemical, thermal) are stimulated
  - *Somatic:* From bones, joints, muscles, and skin; may be superficial or deep
  - *Visceral:* From viscera or pleura
- Neuropathic pain
  - *Central:* Disease or injury of the central nervous system (CNS)
  - *Peripheral:* Disease or injury of the peripheral nervous system (PNS)
  - *Mixed:* Combined dysfunction of CNS and PNS
- Inflammatory pain
  - Inflammatory process itself alters nociceptors such that threshold to response is lowered
  - Nerve recruitment occurs
  - Wind-up (dysregulation of amplification and modulation) occurs
- Psychogenic pain
  - Not a diagnostic term
  - Psychological factors play a significant role
  - Report of pain may not match symptoms
  - Pain is real!

---

expression, and control. Therefore pain management must be tailored.

- Cognitive factors include the child's memory, level of understanding, sense of control, attachment of meaning to a painful situation, and expectations regarding pain.
- Emotional factors include anxiety, fear, frustration, anger, and depression.
- Consider the biophysical, social, emotional, and spiritual impact of persistent pain.
- Involve patients and families in the pain management plan, including assessment, management, and education. Educate parents about their role in engaging and providing distraction and comfort to their child during and after painful procedures (e.g., vaccinations, ear examinations, incision, and drainage procedures). Educate the parents of children with persistent pain to manage pain and support the child in developing strategies to effectively cope with pain.
- Consider culture, family learning patterns, and language barriers (e.g., pain beliefs, folk remedies, and how pain is expressed).
- Others' reactions to a child's pain influence the treatment plan and should be included in the plan. Family harmony and conflict are both pediatric pain influencers.
- Socioeconomic status and other social determinants of health impact access to medications, treatments, and pediatric pain specialists.
- Work to resolve disparities in access to specialized pain care and treatment related to race, ethnicity, culture, and geographic location.

Barriers to Effective Pain Management

Barriers to effective pain management can occur in three areas: the patient and family, the primary care provider (PCP), and the healthcare system. Each of these barriers, alone or in combination, results in inadequate pain control. PCPs must be cognizant of any barriers and the negative effect they have on the effectiveness of pain management strategies.

Patient and Family

- Fear of the possible treatment (e.g., getting an injection, addiction) or not acknowledging they have pain.
- Difficulty conceptualizing, quantifying, and/or communicating their pain experience.
- Avoidance and fear of worsening or progression of the disease.
- Cultural differences in the significance of pain, and pain expression and treatment.

Primary Care Provider

- Outdated knowledge (e.g., the persistent belief that infants and children do not feel pain, or if they do, there is no consequence).
- Not up to date regarding current assessment, treatment options, and pain physiology.
- Inaccurate assumption that pediatric pain management takes too much time and effort.
- Fear of adverse side effects of analgesic medications (e.g., respiratory depression, addiction).
- Personal values and beliefs about the meaning and value of pain.

Healthcare System

- Restrictions on certain analgesic medications related to diagnosis, age, or off-label use.
- Limited insurance coverage for nonpharmacologic modalities.
- Legislative barriers to PCP ability to prescribe opioids.
- Failure to hold providers accountable for pain care.
- Lack of developmentally appropriate pain assessment tools.

Pain Assessment

A systematic approach to pediatric pain assessment begins by obtaining a pain history from the child and parent, beginning with what words they use for pain (e.g., "owie," "boo-boo," "ouchie," "hurt") and using these words. Pain evaluation in children must be multidimensional, including behavioral observations and physiologic findings, which requires collecting data about how the child describes the pain and related symptoms, assessing for physiologic and emotional manifestations of pain, and investigating other potential contributors to the child's pain. Developmental and cultural considerations must also be considered, including whether distress behaviors manifested by verbal/nonverbal children indicate pain or another cause (e.g., anxiety, fear, stress, fatigue, hunger).

Self-report is the gold standard for assessment, but it is dependent on the child's cognitive ability to understand pain severity on a continuum.[4] Children as young as 3 years old may be capable of quantifying their pain and translating it to a visual representation; however, it is important to remember that young children have limited life experience and when asked if this is the worst pain they ever felt, are truthful when they say yes. Factors influencing self-report of pain include:

- Situational influences (e.g., setting, the person asking, what the child expects to happen as a result of their answer).
- Some children may *underreport* pain if they fear their pain may upset their parents, or if they are concerned the treatment (e.g., injection) may be worse than the pain.
- Some children *overstate* their pain to receive increased attention, which is often a previously learned behavior.
- Various factors and perceptions affect a child's report of pain, including nausea, anxiety, fear of talking to a healthcare provider, disappointing or bothering others, receiving an unpleasant medication, or the need to be rehospitalized. Young children may confuse fear of pain with actual pain, while adolescents may purposefully underreport their pain or deny being in pain because they do not want to miss an athletic event or disappoint their teammates.
- Children with developmental delays may have difficulty, be less precise in their reports, or be unable to communicate their pain; however, self-report is always preferred over observational tools if possible. Extra effort is needed here, as these children are no less sensitive to painful stimuli than children with typical development.

Developmental factors must be considered in pain assessment. Infant and toddler assessment relies on pain-related behaviors, typically nonverbal responses (e.g., facial expression, limb movements, crying). Many toddlers use their own words to indicate pain and report its general location but cannot describe pain severity. Most preschoolers do best with three choices (e.g., "none," "a little," or "a lot") while some may be able to use pain scales with visual cues. During middle childhood, they are able to describe the location, intensity, and quality of their pain, adding further descriptive and contextual details as they enter adolescence.

Reliable, valid, sensitive, and easily understood tools, specific to acute or persistent pain, should be used; however, they should not be the sole determinant for evaluation or treatment. Self-report tools, pain journals, and other objective measures are helpful to quantify pain before treatment and evaluate the treatment effectiveness and multiple web-based tools are available. For children not yet able or refusing to self-report, observational pain scales are available. Commonly used pediatric pain scales are summarized in Table 24.1, but again, pain assessment is not complete until the PCP considers self-report data as well as individual and contextual factors related to the child's clinical history, child and family preferences, and responses to previous treatments.

Pain History

A systematic interval history and physical examination are needed when pain does not abate as expected or there is a change in its quality, intensity, duration, or location (see Box 24.3 for helpful mnemonics). The following information should be obtained:

- Intensity (mild, moderate, severe, overwhelming)
- Location (including areas of radiation and referral)
- Quality—how pain is described by the child or parent (e.g., stinging, burning, throbbing, squeezing feeling, "big ouchie") and any pain behaviors noted
- Aggravating or alleviating factors
- Timing and duration (e.g., when it started, any identifiable cause, present all the time or comes and goes, worse in the morning or evening, wakes the child from sleep)
- Any associated symptoms, such as nausea, anxiety, tingling, tachycardia, or diaphoresis

TABLE 24.1　Commonly Used Pediatric Pain Scales

Scale	Population	Comments
Observational		
Premature Infant Pain Profile (PIPP)	Premature infants	
Neonatal Pain, Agitation, and Sedation Scale (N-PASS)	Premature infants and neonates	Some evidence for use with older infants; quantifies both pain and sedation
Neonatal Infant Pain Scale (NIPS)	Premature and term infants	
COMFORT Behavior Scale	Noncommunicating children with cognitive impairment	
Crying, Requires oxygen, Increased vital signs, Expression, Sleeplessness (CRIES)	Infants ≤6 months	
Faces, Legs, Activity, Cry, Consolability (FLACC)	2 months–4 years Noncommunicating children with cognitive impairment	
Revised FLACC (rFLACC)	Noncommunicating children with cognitive impairment	Allows for addition of child-specific behaviors
Individualized Numeric Rating Scale (INRS)	Noncommunicating children with cognitive impairment	Pain cues based on parent/caregiver input
Self-Report		
Wong-Baker Faces	≥4 years	End anchors may lead to underreporting of pain
Faces Pain Scale Revised (FPS-R)	≥4 years	
Visual Analog Scale (VAS)	≥4 years	
Oucher	≥4 years	Multiple ethnic versions available
Poker Chip	≥4 years	
Eland Color Tool	≥4 years	
Numeric	≥8 years	Child must be able to understand seriation or rank and order

---

• BOX 24.3　Pain History Mnemonics

QUESTT is a classic strategy for *how* to evaluate a child's pain:
- **Q**uestion
- **U**se pain rating scales
- **E**valuate behavior
- **S**ecure parents' involvement
- **T**ake cause of pain into account
- **T**ake action and evaluate

PAINED identifies the specific elements *(what)* of an assessment:
- **P**lace: Location(s) of pain; keep in mind the possibility of radiating or referred pain; using a body diagram can be helpful
- **A**mount of pain: Pain intensity score, duration of pain, the pattern of onset (e.g., continuous or intermittent)
- **I**ntensifiers: What makes the pain worse (e.g., position, movement, or time of day)?
- **N**ullifiers: What makes the pain better (e.g., position, heat or cold, or medications)?
- **E**ffects: Consequences of pain medication (e.g., relief or side effects) and effects of pain on activities of daily living and quality of life
- **D**escription: Quality of pain (e.g., dull, sharp, aching, stabbing, or cramping)

- Past pain experience(s), including the child's memory of a painful experience and the treatment
- Cultural or family beliefs about pain and treatment

Physical Examination

Note the child's appearance, posture, and gait. Carefully inspect for any signs of trauma and palpate for areas of hypersensitivity and tenderness in muscles or tendon insertion sites. *Behavioral* indicators or nonverbal cues are also important indicators of pain (Box 24.4) and may be the only indicator of pain, especially in preverbal or nonverbal children. Infants in pain tend to sleep less, are irritable and agitated, feed poorly or refuse to feed, and have increased muscle tone. Older children may sleep to cope with pain, meaning sleep is not necessarily an indication the child is comfortable. It is important to remember behaviors in cognitively impaired children are particularly individualized and may differ from those more typically associated with pain. *Physiologic* indicators and parameters (e.g., heart rate, oxygen saturation, respiratory rate/pattern, blood pressure), diaphoresis, palmar sweating, and pallor can be seen but they are neither sensitive nor specific indicators of pain, particularly in children

BOX 24.4 Examples of Behavioral Indicators of Pain

- Vocalizations
  - Crying
  - Whimpering
  - Whining
- Facial expressions
  - Grimacing
  - Tightly closed eyelids
  - Grinding or clenching teeth
- Breath holding
- Body positioning
- Changes in sleep patterns (more or less)
- Actions
  - Rubbing or touching the painful site
  - Avoiding the painful site
  - Guarding the affected area
  - Withdrawal from touch
  - Protecting an injured limb
- Social withdrawal
- Vigilance
- Anger

with persistent pain. Pulse oximetry readings may decrease due to increased oxygen consumption or breath-holding. Other physiologic responses to pain include changes in metabolic functioning (e.g., hypermetabolism, hyperglycemia, lipolysis), decreased gut motility, sodium and water retention, and cytokine production.

Laboratory and Imaging Studies

Diagnostic testing is not usually indicated. Consider checking a vitamin D level as there is some evidence to suggest low levels may contribute to pain and may increase inflammatory cytokines.[5]

Management of Pediatric Pain

The goal of pediatric pain management is to reduce pain safely and effectively, limit side effects, and minimize medication use. Positive outcomes of effective pain management include improved function (ability to perform daily activities), increased life satisfaction for the child/family, an enhanced recovery process, and a positive script related to pain and its management for future use as the child matures. In some situations (e.g., after surgical procedures, severe burns, persistent pain), complete "freedom" from pain may not be possible. The PCP has a number of options to alleviate pain, including multimodal, developmentally appropriate, nonpharmacologic, and pharmacologic interventions. Multimodal therapy is more effective than high-dose single medications and reduces the risk of toxicity and adverse side effects.[6] Table 24.2 provides examples and strategies for common painful acute conditions.

Pharmacologic Considerations

There may be interactions between nutraceutical or natural preparations and medications used to manage pain, so it is imperative to know all the substances a child/family is using for the PCP to provide appropriate counseling regarding potentially undesirable or dangerous interactions. It is also important to anticipate known side effects of medications such as opioids (Table 24.3) and proactively work to prevent or mitigate them.

TABLE 24.2 Common Acute Painful Pediatric Conditions and Pain Relief Strategies

Condition	Pain Relief Strategies
Otalgia	Acetaminophen or NSAIDs Warmed compresses pressed against the ear
Pharyngitis	Acetaminophen or NSAIDs Antibiotics if GABHS Saltwater gargles Anesthetic lozenges for an older child
Stomatitis	NSAIDs Bland diet Saline mouth rinses for older children Diphenhydramine-calcium carbonate (in a 1:1 preparation) to coat the mucous membranes Sucralfate
Musculoskeletal injury	**RICE**: **R**est, **I**ce, **C**ompression, and **E**levation Immobilization of affected area Cold for the initial 48–72 hours NSAIDs
Fractures and sprains	NSAIDs Opioid analgesics if severe fracture or sprain Topical NSAIDs give relief in soft tissue trauma, strains, and sprains
Laceration	LET procedure: Use on open wounds that are simple lacerations of head, neck, extremities, or trunk that are <5 cm in length; use 3 mL max; place LET mixed with cellulose on open wound and cover with occlusive dressing, or place two cotton balls soaked with LET in the wound Contraindications: Allergy to amide anesthetics, gross contamination of wound; do not use on mucous membranes, digits, genitalia, ear, or nose

GABHS, Group A β-hemolytic streptococcal infection; *LET*, lidocaine (4%), epinephrine (0.1%), and tetracaine (0.5%); *NSAIDs*, nonsteroidal antiinflammatory drugs.

One consideration in administering analgesics is whether there is a need to maintain serum concentration levels. While medicating around the clock (i.e., regardless of pain intensity at the time of administration) is a long-held practice in some situations, there is limited evidence to recommend around-the-clock administration over "prn" or as-needed therapy.[7] Another consideration is the child's response to previous pain medications and doses. Box 24.5 highlights age-related differences in analgesia responses.

Procedural Pain Management

Box 24.6 provides examples of common pediatric painful procedures. Proper planning and preparation for any procedure will make it easier for the PCP, less distressing for the family, and provide the opportunity for a child to demonstrate mastery of appropriate coping techniques. The PCP should:

TABLE 24.3	Management of Common Opioid Side Effects	
Side Effect	Considerations	Medications
Nausea	Exclude other processes, such as bowel obstruction Consider switching to a different opioid Use antiemetics	Metoclopramide Ondansetron
Pruritus	Exclude other causes, such as drug allergy Consider switching to a different opioid Use antipruritics	Diphenhydramine Hydroxyzine
Constipation	Encourage water, fruit, vegetables, and a high-fiber diet if appropriate Regular use of stimulant and stool softener laxatives	Docusate Bisacodyl Polyethylene glycol

- Employ a multimodal (physical, psychological, pharmacologic) approach to pain management before, during, and after those procedures that may cause pain or anxiety for the child. Note: Emergent procedures do not negate the use of combination relief and many interventions can be implemented without time delay.
- Engage supportive family members as they are critical in the alleviation of a child's pain and anxiety.
- Administer intramuscular injections using a rapid injection technique without aspiration.
- Avoid placing the child supine or in a vulnerable position during painful procedures. Holding an infant/young child in a bear hug and/or placing an older child in a sitting position is preferable.

Before the Procedure
- Educate about the procedure and comfort management options; tailor information to meet the patient and family needs.
- Consider preprocedural dosing with acetaminophen and/or an appropriate nonsteroidal antiinflammatory drug (NSAID) to mitigate postprocedural pain.
- Establish a mutually agreed upon developmentally appropriate comfort plan for use during the procedure (Table 24.4).

During the Procedure
- Use a procedure room, if available.
- If pain or anxiety are not well controlled during the procedure, stop the procedure and provide additional comfort measures.
- One person should provide calm, verbal coaching and leadership and ensure the environment remains safe and relaxed for the patient and family.

After the Procedure
- Discuss and evaluate the procedure with the patient and family.

- Document procedure, patient's experience, and recommendations for future procedures.
- Develop and implement a comfort plan for postprocedure pain as needed.

One example of a common pediatric procedure is male circumcision (Box 24.7).

Acute Pain Management

Refer to a current pediatric dosing reference for specific dosing and time intervals. For *mild pain*, combining acetaminophen and an NSAID is effective and safe; however, NSAIDs should be used with caution in infants less than 6 months old. For *moderate to severe pain*, the use of an oral opioid (e.g., oxycodone, hydrocodone, morphine) may be considered, and coadministration of acetaminophen and/or NSAIDs reduces opioid consumption significantly. Because of concerns about respiratory depression, the US Food and Drug Administration has published contraindications for the use of codeine and tramadol in children[8];

- Tramadol and codeine should not be used in children under 12 years old.
- Tramadol should not be used in children under 18 years old for tonsillectomy and adenoidectomy pain.
- Tramadol and codeine should not be used in children between 12 and 18 years who are obese or have conditions such as obstructive sleep apnea or severe lung disease.

Persistent Pain Management

Persistent pain is most successfully treated by a coordinated, planned, interprofessional approach, including disciplines such as medicine, psychology, physical therapy, occupational therapy, and nursing. It is essential that all team members communicate a consistent message as an integrated team. The use of psychological interventions (e.g., relaxation, parent interventions, cognitive strategies) are key management components to reduce persistent pediatric pain, as they help reduce pain symptoms and disability posttreatment.

The PCP must also be diligent in assessing for the presence or development of other issues, including sleep disturbances, adverse childhood experiences, depression, anxiety disorders (e.g., situational, separation, social), posttraumatic stress disorder, panic disorder, and/or obsessive-compulsive disorders, as these comorbidities impact pain experience and coping. Because PCPs serve in the central position or "hub" of coordination (see Chapter 1), they provide continuity, as well as integrate subsequent care, regardless of where the care is delivered and who provides it. This is especially important in the management of persistent pain, which requires a comprehensive multimodal treatment plan focused on improving quality of life and daily functioning.

Pharmacologic Measures

NSAIDs and acetaminophen are commonly used to treat persistent pain. Gabapentin is frequently used to treat neuropathic pain and due to few adverse side effects is considered first-line therapy. As noted earlier, having the child or parent use a pain intensity rating scale and keep a diary of the child's activities and pain help evaluate treatment effectiveness, specifically focusing on whether

---

- Infants (until approximately 6 months of age) have delayed hepatic enzyme maturation resulting in altered drug metabolic inactivation. Analgesics metabolized in the liver, such as opioids, have a prolonged elimination half-life in newborns and young infants.
- Glomerular filtration is reduced in the first few weeks of life, which results in slower elimination of opioids and their active metabolites.
- Toddlers' and preschool children's renal clearance of analgesics is greater than adults.
- Neonates and young infants have decreased plasma protein binding for many drugs, resulting in greater concentrations of pharmacologically active unbound medication.

- Circumcision
- Heel stick, capillary sampling
- Tape removal
- Intramuscular or subcutaneous injection
- Urinary catheterization
- Dressing change
- Wound care
- Suture placement/removal
- Occupational or physical therapy consultations
- Cast application
- Nasopharyngeal swabs or scraping
- Lumbar puncture
- Venous or arterial sampling or catheterization.

---

symptoms/functioning have improved and if any side effects are present.

If a child's pain is not able to be controlled, referral to pain management specialists is indicated. The following therapies may be considered:

- Antidepressants (e.g., selective serotonin reuptake inhibitors [SSRIs], serotonin-norepinephrine reuptake inhibitors [SNRIs], tricyclics [TCAs], atypicals), opioids, anticonvulsants, muscle relaxants, and other selected medications.
  - These patients require close monitoring for worsening of depression, suicidality, and unusual behavior, especially during the first few weeks of therapy.
  - Educate family members to closely observe the patient and communicate changes in the patient's condition.
- Botulinum products may be used for certain pain conditions in children such as seventh cranial nerve disorders, dynamic muscle contractures associated with cerebral palsy, and migraine headaches.
  - Pain specialists work with children and their families during the administration of this drug, but the PCP should be familiar with adverse and life-threatening reactions associated with this drug.
- Invasive techniques, such as neuroablative procedures and spinal cord stimulation, are occasionally used, but as a last resort.

Nonpharmacologic Measures

Nonpharmacologic measures include physical therapy, relaxation, massage, guided imagery, biofeedback, hypnosis, heat and cold, and distraction. In addition, transcutaneous electrical nerve stimulation (TENS), art and music therapy, craniosacral therapy, acupuncture, and psychological therapy are often integrated as part of the multimodal management of persistent pain.

Parental strategies that encourage optimal coping with persistent pain include:

- Not giving excessive attention, special privileges, or rewards when child reports pain, but encouraging normal activities, within reason, during pain episodes (e.g., going to school, doing chores).
- Encouraging quiet, low-key activities, especially when the child cannot go to school or participate in other events, as playing games and/or excessive screen time may reinforce the child not wanting to participate in "well" activities.
- Lessening the focus on pain by not repeatedly asking the child about the presence of pain.
- Engaging the child in self-management. When the child reports pain, ask, "What do you think you can do to help lessen your pain?" and encouragement of nonpharmacologic strategies.

Specific Disease-Related Pain Protocols

The PCP should be aware of clinical practice guidelines addressing pain management related to common pediatric disorders. Two examples are: sickle cell anemia (https://www.nhlbi.nih.gov/health/sickle-cell-disease) and arthritis (https://www.arthritis.org/juvenile-arthritis).

Partnership in Care

Several critical elements related to pain management and administration of pain medications must be emphasized to parents and children, including:

- Take pain medication only as prescribed.
- Store pain medications under lock and key and properly dispose of them when no longer needed.
- Anticipate and correct misinformation/myths related to addiction and the use of opioids, if applicable.
- Use multimodal pain management. Medication alone is not sufficient to manage persistent pain, and cognitive-behavioral therapies are helpful in acute pain situations.
- Counsel about the dangers of mixing alcohol with opioids, using opioids for conditions other than for which they were prescribed, and the importance of not sharing medications.
- Stay informed about current and emerging prescribed, over-the-counter (OTC), and natural therapies being used in pain management.
- Remember that pain medication used for more than 10 to 14 days may need to be tapered, rather than abruptly stopped.
- Remember that pain medication works most effectively when taken before the onset of severe pain.
- Be prepared for common side effects of pain medicine, including constipation, dizziness, nausea, drowsiness, sweating, and flushing.
- Assess for improvement in daily function and decrease of pain and related symptoms.

TABLE 24.4 **Procedural Pain Management Techniques, by Age**

Age	Physical/Psychological Interventions Recommended for Use Before Pharmacologic Measures	Pharmacologic Interventions	Onset of Pharmacologic Action
Preterm neonate	• Developmental positioning • Swaddling • Breastfeeding (before, during, after the procedure) • Skin-to-skin contact • Nonnutritive sucking • Oral sucrose • Music (as appropriate)	• Acetaminophen if appropriate • Topical anesthetic cream	• 30 min • 30 min
Neonate (≥37 weeks' gestation)–3 months	• Procedure room[a] • Swaddling • Breastfeeding (before, during, after the procedure) • Skin-to-skin contact • Nonnutritive sucking • Oral sucrose • Music	• Topical anesthetic cream (maximum application duration 1 h)[b,c] • Acetaminophen if appropriate • Urojet (sterile) lidocaine jelly for urinary catheterization • For patients >6 weeks old: atomized/intranasal midazolam for sedation during procedures	• 30 min • 30 min • 1–2 min • 5 min; max effect, 10 min
3–6 months	• Procedure room[a] • Swaddling • Nonnutritive sucking • Oral sucrose • Breastfeeding (before, during, after the procedure) • Skin-to-skin contact • Nonnutritive sucking • Music • Approved pet therapy	• Topical anesthetic cream[b,c] • LET procedure[d] • Acetaminophen if appropriate • Urojet (sterile) lidocaine jelly for urinary catheterization • Viscous lidocaine for nasogastric tube insertion • Atomized/intranasal midazolam for sedation during procedures	• 30–60 min • 1–2 min • 30 min • 1–2 min • Use to lubricate tip of tube • 5 min; Max effect: 10 min
7–12 months	• Procedure room[a] • Nonnutritive sucking • Oral sucrose to encourage sucking • Breastfeeding (before, during, after the procedure) • Singing/music • Distraction • Positioning for comfort[b] • Approved pet therapy • Ice/cold pack application	• Topical anesthetic cream[b,c] or • 1% lidocaine via J-tip device or • 1% lidocaine intradermal injection • LET procedure[d] • Acetaminophen or NSAID if appropriate • Urojet (sterile) lidocaine jelly for urinary catheterization • Viscous lidocaine for NGT insertion • Atomized/intranasal midazolam for anxiety	• 30–60 min • 30–60 s • 30–60 s • 1–2 min • 30 min • 1–2 min • Use to lubricate tip of tube • 5 min; max effect, 10 min
1–2 years	• Procedure room[a] • Nonnutritive sucking • Singing/music • Distraction • Positioning for comfort[b] • Hand holding • Reading/telling stories • Medical play • Television/games • Approved pet therapy • Ice/cold pack application	• Topical anesthetic cream[b,c] or • 1% lidocaine via J-tip device or • 1% lidocaine intradermal injection or • Vapocoolant (ethyl chloride) or • Bacteriostatic saline injection • LET procedure[d] • Nitrous oxide gas for anxiolysis • Acetaminophen or NSAID if appropriate • Urojet (sterile) lidocaine jelly for urinary catheterization • Atomized/intranasal lidocaine for NGT insertion • Intranasal midazolam for anxiety	• 30–60 min • 30–60 s • 30–60 s • Immediate • 30–60 s • 1–2 min • 2–3 min • 30 min • 1–2 min • Immediate • 5 min; max effect, 10 min

TABLE 24.4	Procedural Pain Management Techniques, by Age—Cont'd		
Age	**Physical/Psychological Interventions Recommended for Use Before Pharmacologic Measures**	**Pharmacologic Interventions**	**Onset of Pharmacologic Action**
2–5 years	• Procedure room[a] • Singing/music • Distraction • Positioning for comfort[b] • Hand holding • Reading/telling stories • Medical play • Television/games • Guided imagery (≥3 years) • Blowing bubbles/deep breathing techniques (≥3 years) • Tactile stimulation before injection (≥4 years) • BuzzyBee • Approved pet therapy • Ice/cold pack application	• Topical anesthetic cream[b,c] *or* • 1% lidocaine via J-tip device *or* • 1% lidocaine intradermal injection *or* • Vapocoolant (ethyl chloride) *or* • Bacteriostatic saline injection • LET procedure[d] • Nitrous oxide gas for anxiolysis • Acetaminophen or NSAID if appropriate • Urojet (sterile) lidocaine jelly for urinary catheterization • Cetacaine spray for NGT placement • Viscous lidocaine for NGT insertion • Atomized/intranasal lidocaine for NGT insertion • Atomized/intranasal midazolam for anxiety	• 30–60 min • 30–60 s • 30–60 s • Immediate • 30–60 s • 1–2 min • 2–3 min • 30 min • 1–2 min • Immediate • Immediate • Immediate • 5 min; max effect, 10 min
6 years and older	• Procedure room[a] • Positioning for comfort[b] • Reading/telling stories • Blowing bubbles/deep breathing techniques • Medical play • Hand holding • Television/games • Guided imagery • Music • Tactile stimulation before injection • BuzzyBee • Approved pet therapy • Ice/cold pack application	• Topical anesthetic cream[b,c] *or* • 1% lidocaine via J-tip device *or* • 1% lidocaine intradermal injection *or* • Vapocoolant (ethyl chloride) *or* • Bacteriostatic saline injection • LET procedure[d] • Nitrous oxide gas for anxiolysis • Acetaminophen or NSAID if appropriate • Urojet (sterile) lidocaine jelly for urinary catheterization • Cetacaine spray for NGT placement • Viscous lidocaine for NGT insertion • Atomized/intranasal lidocaine for NGT insertion • Atomized/intranasal midazolam for anxiety	• 30–60 min • 30–60 s • 30–60 s • Immediate • 30–60 s • 1–2 min • 1–2 min • 30 min • 1–2 min • Immediate • Immediate • Immediate • 5 min; max effect, 10 min

[a]L.M.X.4 contraindicated with an allergy to amide anesthetics.

[b]EMLA is contraindicated in patients with congenital or idiopathic methemoglobinemia or in infants less than 12 months old who are being treated with sulfas, acetaminophen, benzocaine, chloroquine, dapsone, nitrofurantoin, phenobarbital, phenytoin, or quinine.

[c]Topical anesthetic cream refers to EMLA and L.M.X.4.

[d]LET procedure: use on simple lacerations of head, neck, extremities, or trunk that are <5 cm in length; use 3 mL max; place LET mixed with cellulose on the open wound and cover with an occlusive dressing, or place two cotton balls soaked with LET in the wound. Contraindicated with allergy to amide anesthetics, gross contamination of wound; do not use on mucous membranes, digits, genitalia, ear, or nose.

EMLA, Eutectic mixture of local anesthetics; *LET*, lidocaine 4%, epinephrine 0.1%, and tetracaine 0.5%; *L.M.X.4*, liposomal 4% lidocaine cream; *NGT*, nasogastric tube; *NSAID*; nonsteroidal antiinflammatory drug.

• Follow-up assessments determine whether optimal pain control is being achieved, evaluate whether pharmacologic side effects are minimized or effectively managed, and ensure the causative factor of the pain was correctly identified.

Pediatric Fever

Overview

Fever is an abnormal elevation of body temperature that occurs as part of a specific biologic response mediated and controlled by the central nervous system (CNS). It is one of the most common reasons that parents seek healthcare advice. It results from an alteration in the thermoregulatory center of the preoptic nuclei of the anterior hypothalamus in response to exogenous pyrogens (e.g., bacteria). More specifically, endotoxins generate the release of endogenous pyrogens (e.g., cytokines), regulate inflammatory cell production (e.g., C-reactive protein [CRP], haptoglobin ceruloplasmin, amyloid A, fibrinogen), release prostaglandin E, and raise the thermoregulatory set point.[9] The production of heat is the result of increased cellular metabolism, involuntary shivering, autonomic responses such as vasoconstriction, and behavioral responses such as covering oneself.

Before Procedure

- Acetaminophen 15 mg/kg 1 h before the procedure
- Topical anesthetic cream
- Hold and comfort infant (breastfeed if possible) while supplies are gathered
- Position infant in a semi-recumbent position on a padded surface with arms swaddled
- Maintain thermoregulation of the environment to prevent cold stress

During Procedure

- Analgesic/comfort techniques: in addition to at least one anesthetic
- Administer 24% sucrose or breast milk orally 2 min before penile manipulation
- Injectable anesthetic options (injection techniques should use slow injection speed, small-gauge needle, warmed solution)[a]:
  - Subcutaneous block (circumferential at midshaft or at the level of the corona at 10- and 2-o'clock positions) or
  - Dorsal penile nerve block
- Pacifier for nonnutritive sucking, if sucrose or breast milk contraindicated

Following Procedure

- Remove infant from restraint immediately, soothe, and return to parent
- Continue oral acetaminophen (15 mg/kg) around the clock every 4–6 h for at least 24 h
- Instruct family on the administration of acetaminophen and circumcision care

[a]AAP Committee on Fetus and Newborn and Section on Anesthesiology and Pain Medicine. Prevention and Management of Procedural Pain in the Neonate: An Update. *Pediatrics.* 2016;137(2):e20154271.

Fever, or pyrexia, is typically defined as 38°C (100.4°F) or higher; hyperpyrexia in children is an elevated temperature above 40°C (104°F). Fever can be infectious or noninfectious. Although viral infections are responsible for most children's fevers, the differential for fever includes bacterial infection, reaction to immunizations, autoimmune and inflammatory disease, cancer (e.g., leukemia, lymphoma), medication (antibiotics, antiseizure), tissue damage, and/or other disease states. Fever in neonates is usually the result of congenital infections or infections acquired at delivery (e.g., Group B streptococci), in the newborn nursery or neonatal intensive care unit, at home (e.g., pneumococcal or meningococcal infection), and those acquired as a result of anatomic or physiologic dysfunction (e.g., renal). Temperatures higher than 105.8°F (41°C) are rarely of infectious origin, but due to CNS dysfunction (e.g., malignant hyperthermia, drug fever, heat stroke).

Parents are often concerned about fever, what it means, and its possible harmful effect on their child. Some fear all fevers are dangerous and believe any fever over a certain point is "too high" or serious and associated with brain damage or seizures. There is no evidence that a fever leads to long-term complications or brain damage, with the exception of when it occurs as a result of heat stroke, febrile status epilepticus, or malignant hyperthermia.[10] Many others believe a fever should be treated or it will continue to rise. Further, most parents think once a medication is given, the fever should resolve completely.

Fever Assessment

The most accurate, yet invasive, measurement of fever is rectal thermometry. In general, rectal temperatures are used if a precise measurement is required and no other route is easily accessible.[11] Rectal temperatures are contraindicated in cases of neutropenia, bleeding disorders, or necrotizing enterocolitis.[10] Oral thermometry is a more comfortable method commonly used in children old enough to cooperate, which is generally around 4 to 5 years of age. It is less accurate than a rectal measurement, but more accurate than axillary measurement; however, results can be impacted by mouth breathing, tachypnea, exercise, recent intake of hot or cold drinks, and thermometer position. Axillary thermometry is used in cases of neutropenia, though the result is typically lower than with rectal thermometry. Infrared thermometry is measured using the tympanic membrane or forehead/temporal artery. A tympanic membrane temperature measurement can be affected by poor positioning, the presence of cerumen, and/or otitis media. Positioning is paramount, as the tip should be inserted into the canal and create a seal, after manipulating the ear to open the canal, in the same manner as a proper otoscopic examination. Otherwise, the reading measures the temperature of the air, ear canal, skin, or cerumen. Proper positioning can be challenging for parents. Infrared contact and no contact forehead thermometers measure the amount of heat produced by temporal arteries at the surface of the skin on the forehead; however, they can be affected by recent sun or cold exposure, sweating, and vascular changes. Placement in the middle of the forehead or temple varies with equipment being used. Both tympanic and temporal thermometers are well tolerated and easy to use; however, the rectal temperature remains the gold standard, especially for neonates and infants, unless it is contraindicated for a medical reason.

History and Physical Examination

Overall appearance of the child is often more important than the actual temperature. A careful history and physical examination are critical and include:

- Type of thermometer used to record temperature
- Duration and degree of fever
- Associated symptoms: vomiting, diarrhea, respiratory symptoms, rash (particularly petechiae or purpura), feeding pattern, irritability, inconsolability, change in play activities, lethargy, decreased level of consciousness, poor/absent eye contact, failure to recognize parents, lack of interaction with persons or objects in the environment
- Review of known exposures (family illness, contacts with other ill children, daycare); recent travel history
- Past medical history of chronic illness, malignancy, splenectomy, shunt, indwelling catheter, immunologic disorders, recurrent or serious bacterial infection (SBI)
- Neonatal history of complications, prior antibiotics, prior surgeries, or hyperbilirubinemia
- Current medications, including antipyretics, antibiotics, herbs, and dietary supplements
- Immunization history, particularly with Hib conjugate and pneumococcal conjugate vaccines

All patients should be fully undressed to undergo a complete physical examination. When febrile, the overall clinical appearance of the child should be considered first. A toxic, or ill-appearing child is considered at risk of serious bacterial infection until proven otherwise and needs a thoughtful workup. Those with a high fever due to a more benign illness usually do not appear ill, but may be subdued by parent report. Important considerations that indicate serious illness include:

- Is the child lethargic, fussy, irritable, inconsolable?
- Is there airway, breathing, and circulation (ABCs) compromise?
- Are there symptoms suggestive of serious bacterial illness (e.g., fever, bulging fontanel, respiratory system changes, lethargy, and other CNS symptoms, evidence of skin infection or rashes, skin perfusion, and turgor)?

Management of Pediatric Fever

Fever as a Friend?

Fever can have positive benefits, including decreased pathogen replication.[12] It can also be curative and maximize antimicrobial treatment. Further, it is often self-limited. Fever phobia is common among parents who have little knowledge about the beneficial role it may play, therefore educating parents can be helpful in lowering their anxiety. Teaching points include fever is a symptom or normal response to fighting an infection; fever itself is not dangerous; brain damage does not occur at temperatures under 107.8°F.[10,12] In healthy children, fever less than 39°C (102°F) can be managed without pharmacological treatment, unless the child has other symptoms. Fever may exacerbate underlying disorders; therefore antipyretics may be appropriate.[12]

Nonpharmacologic Measures

Strategies for fever control include:
- Adequate hydration
- Reassurance to parents and advice that not all fevers need to be treated
- Appropriate clothing; do not bundle in additional clothing or coverings
- Ambient environment temperatures of around 72°F (22°C)

Pharmacologic Measures

- Antipyretic agents (e.g., acetaminophen, ibuprofen) work by inhibiting prostaglandin synthesis without affecting the baseline body temperature.[13] If parents choose to alternate antipyretics (e.g., alternate acetaminophen with ibuprofen), the PCP should assist the parent with creating a dosing schedule as to not overmedicate. Table 24.5 provides antipyretic dosages.

- Naproxen sodium is marketed as a "fever reducer"; however, it has not been well studied as an antipyretic in children and should not be used for this purpose.
- Acetylsalicylic acid (aspirin) should never be used in pediatric patients as it may trigger Reyes syndrome or lead to bleeding, except as prescribed by a specialist for other significant benefits that outweighs the risk.

Fever Without Focus or Source

Fever without focus (or source) is an acute febrile illness in a child under 36 months of age in which the etiology of the fever is not apparent after a careful history and physical examination. Approximately one-third of children in this age range (0–36 months) do not have localizing signs of infection. Further, the younger the child, the greater the concern about the possibility of an SBI or invasive bacterial illness, especially because of their decreased immunologic competence. Although the cause of the majority of fevers is a viral infection (e.g., enterovirus, influenza, respiratory syncytial virus [RSV], rotavirus, adenovirus, parainfluenza), an evaluation for a bacterial disease is still necessary.[14] In the past, all neonates and infants under 90 days of age received a complete sepsis workup; however, due to the advent of the *Haemophilus influenza* type b and *Streptococcus pneumonia* vaccines, the incidence of SBI is greatly reduced. Currently, the most common SBIs that cause fever in infants are urinary tract infection (UTI), meningitis, and bacteremia.[14] Children from birth to 24 months of age are at the greatest risk for unsuspected occult bacteremia, with *Escherichia coli* as the most common cause. It is also the leading cause of UTI and meningitis in this age group, with group B *Streptococci* the next most common.

The American Academy of Pediatrics (AAP) endorses the use of an age-based algorithm for clinical decision-making in febrile infants. The updated AAP guideline on the management of well-appearing febrile infants ages 8 to 60 days stratifies the algorithm by ages 8 to 21 days, 22 to 28 days, and 29 to 60 days[15] (Figs. 24.2–24.4). Most experts still agree any ill-appearing neonate and infant older than29 days requires a full workup for SBI, hospital admission, and antibiotics.[14]

Clinical Findings

For the neonate with a temperature of 38°C (100.4°F) or higher, focus should be on the presenting illness, prenatal history and

TABLE 24.5	Antipyretics: Infants and Children Up to 12 Years of Age	
Drug	**Dosage**	**Comments**
Acetaminophen	10–15 mg/kg every 4–6 h PO (not to exceed five doses/24 hours) *or* 10–20 mg/kg every 4–6 h per rectal suppository as needed (not to exceed five doses in 24 hours)	Drug of choice. Temperature reduced by 1.8–3.6°F (1–2°C) within 2 hours; 15 mg/kg/dose as effective as ibuprofen at 10 mg/kg/dose
Ibuprofen	For temperatures <102.5°F (39°C): 5 mg/kg/dose every 6–8 hours as needed
For temperatures ≥102.5°F (39°C): 10 mg/kg/dose every 6–8 hours as needed	Use in children 6 months–12 years old; a maximum daily dose of 40 mg/kg; temperature stays lower for a longer period of time with ibuprofen vs. acetaminophen
Use with caution if decreased liver function, asthma, or coagulation disorder

PO, Orally.

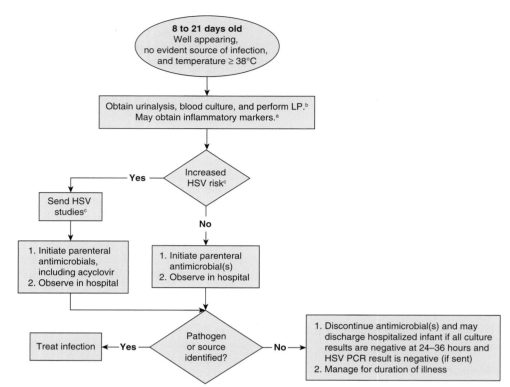

8 to 21 days old
Well appearing,
no evident source of infection,
and temperature ≥ 38°C

Obtain urinalysis, blood culture, and perform LP.[b]
May obtain inflammatory markers.[a]

Increased
HSV risk[c]

Send HSV
studies[c]

1. Initiate parenteral
   antimicrobials,
   including acyclovir
2. Observe in hospital

1. Initiate parenteral
   antimicrobial(s)
2. Observe in hospital

Treat infection

Pathogen
or source
identified?

1. Discontinue antimicrobial(s) and may
   discharge hospitalized infant if all culture
   results are negative at 24–36 hours and
   HSV PCR result is negative (if sent)
2. Manage for duration of illness

• **Fig. 24.2** Algorithm for 8- to 21-Day-Old Infants. [a]Laboratory values of inflammation are considered elevated at the following levels: (1) procalcitonin >0.5 ng/mL, (2) CRP >20 mg/L, and (3) ANC >4000, >5200 per mm³. Although we recommend all infants in this age group have a complete sepsis workup, receive parenteral antimicrobial agents, and be monitored in a hospital, knowing IM results can potentially guide ongoing clinical decisions. [b]Send CSF for cell count, Gram stain, glucose, protein, bacterial culture, and enterovirus PCR (if available) if pleocytosis is present and during periods of increased local enterovirus prevalence. [c]HSV should be considered if the mother has genital HSV lesions or fever from 48 hours before to 48 hours after delivery and in infants with vesicles, seizures, hypothermia, mucous membrane ulcers, CSF pleocytosis in the absence of a positive Gram stain result, leukopenia, thrombocytopenia, or elevated alanine aminotransferase levels. For further discussion, see the current *Red Book*. Recommended HSV studies are CSF PCR; HSV surface swabs of the mouth, nasopharynx, conjunctivae, and anus for an HSV culture (if available) or PCR assay; alanine aminotransferase; and blood PCR. *ANC,* Absolute neutrophil count; *CRP,* C-reactive protein; *CSF,* cerebrospinal fluid; *HSV,* herpes simplex virus; *IM,* intramuscular; *PCR,* polymerase chain reaction. (From Pantell RH, Roberts KB, Adams WG, et al. Clinical practice guideline: evaluation and management of well-appearing febrile infants 8 to 60 days old. *Pediatrics.* 2021;148 [2]:e2021052228.)

care, birth history, including intrapartum fever and maternal group B *Streptococcus* status, and postnatal care. In a young infant who has begun to develop a more complex immune system, consideration of vaccine status, and recent immunizations are also pertinent.

Clinical assessment of appearance is key and can give a fairly accurate impression of the child's status, as well as the severity of illness. Taking the time to pause to note general appearance, work of breathing, and circulation (Pediatric Assessment Triangle) provides this key initial assessment, along with the parent's/PCP's feeling that something is not right. Evaluation for red flags (Box 24.8) is also critical.

Diagnostic Studies. Diagnostic studies, which are ordered based on age and symptoms, include:
- Urinalysis/culture obtained by catheterization or suprapubic needle aspiration
- Complete blood count (CBC) with differential, absolute neutrophil count (ANC), and blood culture. Note: With *E. coli* being the most common bacterial organism in neonates and infants under 60 days of age, white blood cell (WBC), ANC, and bands are less helpful. Procalcitonin (PCT) is now the most accurate marker for bacterial infections.[15]
- CRP

- Alanine aminotransferase and aspartate aminotransferase, if herpes suspected
- Cerebrospinal fluid (CSF)/culture (bacterial and viral); consider herpes simplex virus (HSV) polymerase chain reaction (PCR)
- Chest radiograph if respiratory symptoms not indicative of bronchiolitis (cough, tachypnea, grunting)
- Stool culture if diarrhea with blood or mucus in stool
- RSV or influenza PCR if in season
- Consider SARS-CoV-2 PCR, especially with history of exposure

Management

Management decisions are based on age, presentation, and clinical and diagnostic findings. All neonates under 22 days of age with fever should be hospitalized and receive a full septic workup including, but not limited to, a CBC with differential, blood cultures, catheterized urinalysis with urine culture, a lumbar puncture to examine the CSF for infection and HSV. A chest radiograph and stool cultures may be done as indicated. After evaluation, antibiotics (Table 24.6) and possibly acyclovir are started empirically until the results of all cultures are known and a clearer picture of the illness is identified. Infants in the fourth week of life have

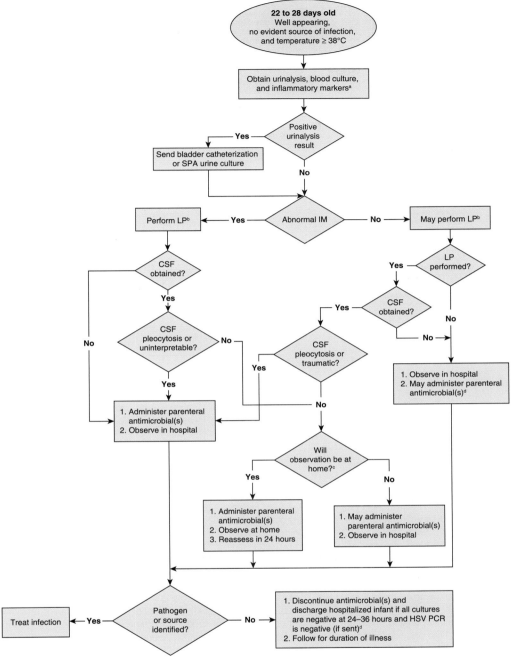

• **Fig. 24.3** Algorithm for 22- to 28-Day-Old Infants. [a]If available, procalcitonin (PCT) should be obtained along with ANC. If PCT is unavailable, ANC and CRP should be obtained, and a temperature >38.5°C is considered abnormal. PCT is considered abnormal at >0.5 mg/mL; CRP is considered abnormal at >20 mg/L; ANC is considered abnormal at >4000 when used in conjunction with PCT or >5200 when PCT is unavailable. [b]LP is recommended before administration of antimicrobial agents because interpreting CSF after the administration of antimicrobial agents is difficult. However, the risk of meningitis in 22- to 28-day-old infants is lower than that in infants <22 days old in several studies. Therefore in some circumstances, clinicians may elect to defer an LP and initiate antimicrobial agents, recognizing the potential risk of partially treated meningitis. Send CSF for cell count, Gram stain, glucose, protein, bacterial culture, and enterovirus PCR (if available) if pleocytosis is present and during periods of increased enterovirus prevalence. HSV can occur in this age group. HSV should be considered in infants with vesicles, seizures, hypothermia, mucous membrane ulcers, CSF pleocytosis in the absence of a positive Gram stain result, leukopenia, thrombocytopenia, or elevated alanine aminotransferase levels. For further discussion, see the current *Red Book*. Recommended HSV studies: CSF PCR; HSV surface swabs of mouth, nasopharynx, conjunctivae, and anus for HSV culture (if available) or PCR assay; alanine aminotransferase; and blood PCR. [c]Infant may be managed at home if parent and clinician agree that the following are present: reliable phone and transportation, parent willingness to observe and communicate changes in condition, and agreement to the infant being reevaluated in 24 hours. [d]If CSF is positive for enterovirus, clinicians may withhold or discontinue antimicrobial agents and discharge at 24 hours, provided they meet other criteria for observation at home. *ANC*, Absolute neutrophil count; *CRP*, C-reactive protein; *CSF*, cerebrospinal fluid; *HSV*, herpes simplex virus; *IMs,* inflammatory markers; *LP*, lumbar puncture; *PCR*, polymerase chain reaction; *SPA,* suprapubic aspiration. [From Pantell RH, Roberts KB, Adams WG, et al. Clinical practice guideline: evaluation and management of well-appearing febrile infants 8 to 60 days old. *Pediatrics* 2021;148 (2):e2021052228.]

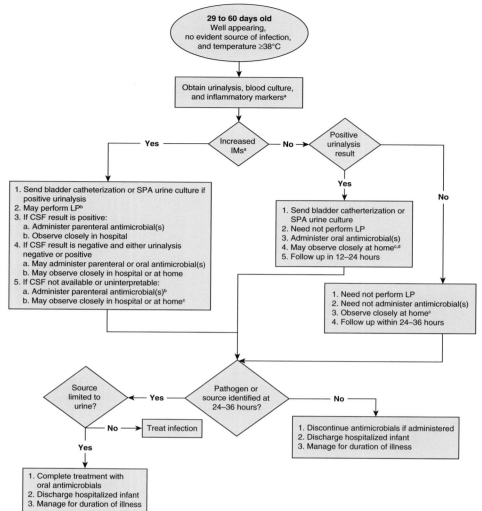

• **Fig. 24.4** Algorithm for 29- to 60-Day-Old Infants. [a]If available, procalcitonin (PCT) should be obtained along with ANC. If PCT is unavailable, ANC and CRP should be obtained, and a temperature >38.5°C is considered abnormal. PCT is considered abnormal at >0.5 mg/mL; CRP is considered abnormal at >20 mg/L; ANC is considered abnormal at >4000 when used in conjunction with PCT or >5200 when PCT is unavailable. [b]Send CSF for cell count, Gram stain, glucose, protein, bacterial culture, and enterovirus PCR (if available) if CSF pleocytosis is present and during periods of increased local enterovirus prevalence. Although uncommon in this age group, HSV should be considered when there is a maternal history of genital HSV lesions and in infants with vesicles, seizures, hypothermia, mucous membrane ulcers, CSF pleocytosis in the absence of a positive Gram stain result, leukopenia, thrombocytopenia, or elevated alanine aminotransferase levels. For further discussion, see the current *Red Book*. Recommended HSV studies are CSF PCR; HSV surface swabs of mouth, nasopharynx, conjunctivae, and anus for HSV culture (if available) or PCR assay; alanine aminotransferase; and blood PCR. If CSF is unobtainable or uninterpretable, there are insufficient data to make a specific recommendation. Options include the following: observe without treatment for a period of time and, depending on infant clinical condition, repeat LP and/or laboratory markers; begin empirical antimicrobial agents and reassess in 24 hours on the basis of infant response and results of blood culture; if CSF is bloody or antimicrobial agents have previously been started, analysis by multiplex PCR can add additional information; consult with local a pediatric infectious disease specialist. [c]Infant may be managed at home if parent and clinician agree that the following are present: reliable phone and transportation, parent willingness to observe and communicate changes in condition, and agreement to the infant being reevaluated in 24 hours. [d]Most 29- to 60-day-old infants with negative IM and urinalysis results may be observed at home. However, hospital observation is an option for infants when there are barriers to follow-up. *ANC,* Absolute neutrophil count; *CRP,* C-reactive protein; *CSF,* cerebrospinal fluid; *HSV,* herpes simplex virus; *IM,* intramuscular; *LP,* lumbar puncture; *PCR,* polymerase chain reaction. (From Pantell RH, Roberts KB, Adams WG, et al. Clinical practice guideline: evaluation and management of well-appearing febrile infants 8 to 60 days old. *Pediatrics* 2021;148 [2]:e2021052228.)

lower rates of bacteremia compared with infants 2 to 3 weeks of age. Therefore well-appearing infants 22 to 28 days of age, with no clear source of infection, may or may not be observed in the hospital, depending on CSF results. Those not admitted require antibiotic administration, reliable means of contact, transport, and follow-up within 24 hours.[15]

The young infant (29–60 days), if ill appearing, should be admitted with complete diagnostic evaluation and followed clinically as described above. If the infant appears to be healthy with no chronic problems and was full term with an uncomplicated nursery course, a full septic workup may not be indicated, and management is based on the examination and data collected. After

• BOX 24.8 Red Flags for Serious Bacterial Infection in Infants and Children With Fever

- Age <1 month old
- Toxic or ill appearing neonate, infant, or child regardless of age, risk factors, or degree of fever
- Pallor, mottled, ashen blue color
- Decreased activity (poor feeding, no smile, decreased response to stimuli, lethargy, weak, high-pitched cry)
- Tachypnea or tachycardia
- Capillary refill >3 seconds
- Decreased urine output
- Chronic illness or underlying condition (including prematurity)
- Unreliable caretakers
- Bulging fontanel
- Nonblanching skin rash

TABLE 24.6 Empiric Antimicrobial Regimens for Well-Appearing, Febrile Infants Between 8 and 60 Days of Age

Age	Antibiotic Regimen[a]
8–21 Days of Age	
UTI	Ampicillin *and* ceftazidime *or* gentamicin
Bacterial meningitis	Ampicillin *and* ceftazidime
No source identified	Ampicillin *and* ceftazidime *or* gentamicin
22–28 Days of Age	
UTI	Ceftriaxone
Bacterial meningitis	Ampicillin *and* ceftazidime
No source identified	Ceftriaxone
29–60 Days of Age	
UTI	Ceftriaxone (parental) *or* cephalexin (enteral)
Bacterial Meningitis	Ceftriaxone *or* ceftazidime *and* vancomycin
No source identified	Ceftriaxone

[a]All cultures should be obtained before antibiotic administration.

[b]Ill appearing, hypothermia, abnormal neurologic status or seizures, vesicular rash, exposure to HSV, hepatosplenomegaly.

HSV, Herpes simplex virus; *UTI*, urinary tract infection.

Modified from Pantell RH, Roberts KB, Adams WG, et al. Evaluation and management of well-appearing febrile infants 8 to 60 days old. *Pediatrics.* 2021;148(2):e2021052228. Erratum *Pediatrics.* 2021;148(5).

an initial evaluation, the infant who meets low-risk criteria (Box 24.9) can be sent home with strict follow-up, including reevaluation in 12 to 24 hours, ensuring access to emergency care if the condition worsens (see Box 24.8), and daily follow-up of culture results, with an immediate return if cultures become positive. If there is any uncertainty about the family's ability to follow up or provide care, the infant should be admitted.[15] If low-risk criteria are not met, admission and further evaluation are necessary.

The evaluation of the well-appearing infant 60 to 90 days of age should include urinalysis and urine culture, and possibly a CBC with differential, blood culture, PCT, and a respiratory viral panel. An exception could be the infant who received immunizations within the past 24 hours and has a temperature that is below 38.6°C (101.5°F). Otherwise, management proceeds for the 28- to the 60-day-old infant.

Any child under 3 years of age with fever without focus warrants a urinalysis and urine culture. Any of the following findings can constitute a preliminary diagnosis of UTI: positive urine leukocyte esterase, nitrite, leukocyte count, or Gram stain (see Chapter 42).

Fever of Unknown Origin

The definition of *fever of unknown origin* (FUO) in children is a temperature of 38°C (101°F) or higher on several occasions, for more than 3 weeks' duration, and with failure to reach a diagnosis despite at least 8 days of investigation.[16] The PCP must continue to review, rethink, and reevaluate historical, clinical, and laboratory data, with an infectious disease consultation often recommended. Many FUOs are atypical presentations of common disorders, most notably infections (accounting for more than one-third of cases) or rheumatologic and connective tissue diseases (e.g., juvenile idiopathic arthritis, systemic lupus erythematosus). In school-aged children, the most common causes of FUO are UTI/pyelonephritis, respiratory illness, localized infection (abscess, osteomyelitis), juvenile arthritis, and, rarely, leukemia. In adolescents, the more common causes include tuberculosis, inflammatory bowel disease, autoimmune disorders, abscesses, chlamydia, and lymphoma, as well as the causes listed for school-aged children. In the United States, infectious diseases associated with most diagnoses of FUO include Epstein-Barr virus, cat-scratch disease *(Bartonella henselae),* Lyme disease, and osteomyelitis.[16] Neoplastic conditions and AIDS generally have symptoms other than just fever (see Chapters 35 and 38).

• BOX 24.9 Low Risk Criteria for Young Infant With Fever of Unknown Origin

- Well appearing, easily consolable
- Previously healthy infant with uncomplicated nursery stay, no chronic problems
- Full term (>37 weeks)
- No focal bacterial infection
- No systemic antibiotics within 72 hours
- Negative urinalysis (WBC <5–10/hpf; neg leukocyte esterase and nitrate, negative Gram stain)
- WBC >5000 and <15,000 mm^3
- ANC ≤1500 bands/mL
- Procalcitonin <0.3 ng/mL
- No discrete infiltrates on CXR, if done
- Stool smear negative, if done

ANC, Absolute neutrophil count, *CXR*, chest radiograph; *WBC*, white blood cell count.

Clinical Findings

History. A carefully detailed history helps distinguish between recurrent fever episodes and those that need further evaluation. Recurrent fevers that resolve with well periods between suggest an etiology of multiple self-limiting infections. The history should include:

- A careful analysis of symptoms or signs, a meticulous review of systems, history of the fever pattern, and patient's age

- Note of past medical history of recurrent infections, surgery, transfusions, and contact with ill individuals
- Medication use, including over-the-counter and herbal/natural/dietary supplements
- Family medical history, including autoimmune disease or inflammatory bowel disorder; genetic background (inherited periodic fever syndromes [e.g., familial Mediterranean fever, hyperimmunoglobulinemia D with periodic fever syndrome], tumor receptor-associated periodic syndrome)
- Family pets, including reptiles, pet immunization history, or exposure to wild or other domestic animals
- Unusual dietary habits (eating squirrel, rabbit, unusual animal meat)
- History of pica; history of travel (location; travel immunizations; water/food ingested; if returned home with travel souvenirs containing dirt, rocks, earth-contaminated artifacts)

Physical Examination. The physical examination should begin with a general assessment of the patient's appearance, activity, vital signs, and growth parameters. Special attention needs to be paid to:

- Skin rashes, lesions, nail-fold capillary abnormalities; sweating
- Mouth: smooth tongue with the absence of fungiform papillae; the presence of candidiasis, ulcers, dental abscess, or abnormal dentition
- Throat: exudate, erythema
- Local or generalized lymphadenopathy or hepatosplenomegaly
- Palpation/percussion of sinus and mastoid areas for tenderness; tap upper teeth
- Eye examination noting exudate, erythema, palpebral/bulbar conjunctivitis, conjunctival hemorrhages, and papillary reaction. A complete ophthalmologic examination is indicated to fully evaluate for uveitis, chorioretinitis, or proptosis.
- Deep tendon reflexes and joint examination; palpation of bones for tenderness or swelling
- Pelvic examination may be indicated in adolescent females and testicular examination in males; genital ulcers may be noted in females or males.
- Rectal examination and guaiac test. If rectal examination is warranted, the PCP should discuss the invasiveness of the examination and prepare the child and family.

Diagnostic Studies. Laboratory and diagnostic studies are dependent on the child's history and physical examination. Studies may include:

- CBC with differential and smear, erythrocyte sedimentation rate, CRP, PCT, and liver chemistries
- Serologic tests for specific diseases
- Aerobic blood cultures (may require serial specimens to rule out endocarditis, osteomyelitis, or deep abscesses)
- Urinalysis/culture
- Mantoux skin test or interferon-gamma release assay
- Chest, sinus, mastoid, and/or gastrointestinal tract radiographs
- Heterophil antibody and antinuclear antibody titer (older children)
- Echocardiogram, if subacute endocarditis is suspected; radionuclide scans, total body computer tomography scan, magnetic resonance imaging, ultrasound
- Biopsy

- If bone marrow biopsy, cultures for bacteria, acid-fast bacillus, and fungus

Management

Infectious disease consultation may be advised with consideration of hospitalizing the child if there is evidence of systemic illness or failure to thrive, the child is very young, parental anxiety is extreme, or an extensive workup is planned. Otherwise, the child should be followed with frequent visits, documented fever patterns, and other specialized tests if screening tests indicate the need, or if other physical findings develop. Treatment is based on the evolving clinical picture and empirical use of antibiotics should be avoided.

References

1. Wrona S, Czarnecki M. Pediatric pain management. *Am Nur Jour.* 2021;16(3):6–12.
2. Committee on Fetus and Newborn and Section on Anesthesiology and Pain Medicine. Prevention and management of procedural pain in the neonate: an update. *Pediatrics.* 2016;137(2):e20154271.
3. International Association for the Study of Pain (IASP). *IASP Terminology*; 2020. https://www.iasp-pain.org/resources/terminology/#pain.
4. Hauer J, Jones BL. *Evaluation and Management of Pain in Children*; 2021. Retrieved from https://www.uptodate.com/contents/evaluation-and-management-of-pain-in-children?search=pediatric%20pain&source=search_result&selectedTitle=1~150&usage_type=default&display_rank=1.
5. de Oliveira DL, Hirotsu C, Tufik S, et al. The interfaces between vitamin D, sleep and pain. *J Endocrinol.* 2017;234:R23–R36.
6. Nicholas 4th, TA, Robinson R. Multimodal analgesia in the era of the opioid epidemic. *Surg Clin North Am.* 2022;102(1):105–115.
7. Hobson A, Wiffen PJ, Conlon JA. As required versus fixed schedule analgesic administration for postoperative pain in children. *Cochrane Database Syst Rev.* 2015 Feb 26;2015(2):CD011404.
8. US Food and Drug Administration. *FDA Restricts Use of Prescription Codeine Pain and Cough Medicines and Tramadol Pain Medicines in Children.* Recommends Against Use in Breastfeeding Women; 2017. https://www.fda.gov/drugs/drug-safety-and-availability/fda-drug-safety-communication-fda-restricts-use-prescription-codeine-pain-and-cough-medicines-and.
9. Lye PS, Densmore EM. Fever. In: Kliegman RM, Lye PS, Bordini BJ, Toth H, Basel D, eds. *Nelson Pediatric Symptom-Based Diagnosis.* Elsevier; 2018:701.
10. Rose E. Pediatric fever. *Emerg Med Clin North Am.* 2021;39(3):627–639.
11. Chiocca EM. *Advanced Pediatric Assessment.* 3rd ed. Springer; 2020.
12. Nield LS, Kamat D. Fever. In: Kliegman RM, S. Geme J, eds. *Nelson Textbook of Pediatrics.* 21st ed. Elsevier; 2020:1386–1388.
13. Paul IM, Walson PD. Acetaminophen and ibuprofen in the treatment of pediatric fever: a narrative review. *Curr Med Res Opin.* 2021;37(8):1363–1375.
14. Brower L, Shah SS. Fever without a focus in the neonate and young infant. In: Kliegman RM, S. Geme J, eds. *Nelson Textbook of Pediatrics.* 21st ed. Elsevier; 2020:1389–1392.
15. Pantell RH, Roberts KB, Adams WG, et al. Evaluation and management of well-appearing febrile infants 8 to 60 days old. *Pediatrics.* 2021;(2):148:e2021052228. Erratum Pediatrics. 2021;148(5).
16. Steenhoff AP. Fever of unknown origin. In: Kliegman RM, S. Geme J, eds. *Nelson Textbook of Pediatrics.* 21st ed. Elsevier; 2020:1397–1402.

25

Pediatric Injuries and Toxic Exposures

SARA D. DEGOLIER

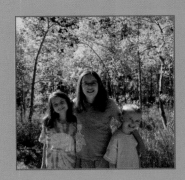

According to the Centers for Disease Control and Prevention (CDC), more than 4.4 million children ages 0 to 19 years were treated for nonfatal injuries in the emergency department (ED) setting in 2020.[1] Mechanical energy transfer (e.g., rough or hard surfaced objects lacerate or scrape the skin) is the most common type of pediatric injury. Physical injury to the body occurs in many ways, ranging from burns to toxic ingestions including environmental toxins and heavy metals, all of which can lead to cellular damage of organ systems. The abnormal transfer of energy is recognized as the underlying etiology of most pediatric injuries, whether it be by mechanical, thermal electric, chemical, or radiation between a moving and stationary object.

Three main components are essential to the management of an injured child: obtaining an appropriate history, identifying the mechanism of the injury, and performing a thorough physical examination. The assessment should occur within the first 5 minutes of initial contact and include:

- Respiratory status, airway, circulation, and vital signs
- Brief history (allergies, medications, past medical history)
- Events surrounding the injury (including mechanism)
- Rapid assessment of essential organ status and cardiopulmonary resuscitation, if indicated
- Stabilization of the injuries and preparation for transport to the ED if indicated

If the injury is life-threatening or there is deterioration in the child's condition, a trauma severity assessment must also be performed immediately. Once the patient is stabilized, a secondary assessment can be completed, including a complete physical examination with vital signs and laboratory and radiographic studies, as indicated.

Injuries can be either intentional or unintentional. The pediatric primary care provider (PCP) should always consider nonaccidental trauma (NAT) or child maltreatment (i.e., child abuse) when a child presents with an injury and the parent/caregiver's explanation for the injury is not consistent with the injury itself or if there are discrepancies in the history, an absent or partial history, a history that changes each time the parent gives the history, or a history with improbable or illogical explanations of the injury.[2] (see Chapter 22).

Trauma to the Skin and Soft Tissue

Abrasions

Abrasions are superficial skin injuries, often the result of falls or friction that involve epidermal trauma. However, the depth of skin tissue involvement varies depending on the amount of force and friction. The most serious form of abrasion is an avulsion, which results in the loss of epidermal, dermal, and subcutaneous layers.

Clinical Findings

History and Physical Examination. Determine the extent of the abrasion and the presence of dirt, grime, and/or foreign objects or material (e.g., tar) or if the skin appears scraped off with or without oozing of serous fluid and/or blood. Increasing pain, swelling, warmth, erythema, and/or red streaking away from the injured area suggest ongoing injury, deep injury (e.g., avulsion) or secondary infection. Assess the surrounding tissue for circulation, sensation, motion, and function.

Management

Most abrasions can be managed at home unless the abrasion is deep, involves a large area, is associated with severe pain, or has a significant amount of dirt, grime, tar, or a foreign object in the wound. Because the primary focus is prevention of infection, any immunocompromised pediatric patient should be further assessed by their PCP either by phone and/or office visit.

The preferred method for cleansing abrasions is gentle irrigation with copious amounts of water or normal saline (300–1000 mL depending on the surface area of the wound) although scrubbing with soap or an antibacterial cleanser using a wet gauze or soft surgical nail brush is sometimes warranted. Povidone-iodine, alcohol, and hydrogen peroxide should not be used on open wounds. Dirt or debris should be adequately removed as a secondary infection may occur. Pieces of loose skin can be removed with sterile scissors. Some foreign objects are easily removed with tweezers.

Small abrasions can be left open to the air but often require a small bandage for protection. Because larger abrasions heal quicker if kept moist, cover larger abrasions and abrasions of the hands, feet, and areas overlying joints with a sterile nonadherent dressing and antibiotic ointment (e.g., Bacitracin). Elbows or knees are vulnerable to cracking or reopening of the wound because of constant movement and stretching of the joints. Instruct the parent to wash the abrasion at least every 24 hours and reapply the dressing and antibiotic ointment until a protective dry scab forms. Provide families with instructions regarding the signs and symptoms of infection and follow up.

Puncture Wounds

Puncture wounds are typically classified as superficial or deep. Glass, wood splinters, toothpicks, needles, nails, metal, staples, thumbtacks, and bites are common sources of injury. Although most puncture wounds heal without problems, some are complicated by infection that can then lead to cellulitis, fasciitis, septic arthritis, or soft tissue abscesses.

Staphylococcus aureus and *β-hemolytic streptococci* are normal flora of the skin and common causes of secondary infections in puncture wounds. *Pseudomonas aeruginosa,* which colonizes on rubber soles of shoes, is a common pathogen for plantar puncture wounds when the puncture occurs through the sole of a shoe. Osteomyelitis can occur if the puncture wound also penetrates a bone or joint, with common bacteria including *P. aeruginosa* in nondiabetic patients and *S. aureus* in diabetic patients.[3] Cat and dog bites can cause *Pasteurella multocida* and *Capnocytophaga* wound infections.

Infection risk varies with the wound location and depth as well as the ongoing presence of a foreign object. Deep penetrating injuries to the forefoot with a dirty object, especially those involving the plantar fascia, have a higher infection risk than wounds to the arch or heel area. The forefoot has less overlying soft tissue than other plantar surfaces and is the major weight-bearing area of the foot; therefore cartilage and bone can be involved. The metatarsophalangeal joint region is also at high risk for the same reasons.

Clinical Findings

History. The assessment of a minor puncture wound begins by excluding more serious and occult injuries. Important information includes:

- Date/time of injury and history of wound care provided at time of injury and thereafter
- Identification of the penetrating object and estimated depth of penetration
- Location and condition (rusty, jagged, smooth) of the penetrating object and whether all or part of the foreign object was removed
- Type and condition of footwear worn or if the child was barefoot
- Tetanus immunization status
- Presence of any medical condition that increases the risk for infectious complications

Physical Examination. Plantar wounds are best examined while the patient is prone. With use of a good light source, note circulation, movement, and sensation of the surrounding area. Determine involvement of underlying tissue or bone structures. Evaluate neurologic status, as well as vascular and tendon injury.[3] A tourniquet and or blood pressure cuff can be briefly applied if the wound is bleeding and causing visualization to be difficult.[4] Assess the wound for length and depth, presence of debris or penetrating object, and signs of infection.

Examination findings consistent with *cellulitis* include:

- Localized pain or tenderness, swelling, and erythema at the puncture site (may be more obvious at dorsum of the foot for plantar puncture wounds)
- Fever
- Pain with flexion or extension of the involved extremity (e.g., for plantar puncture wounds, pain along the plantar aspect of the foot during extension or flexion of the toes may indicate deep tissue injury with a higher infection risk)

- Decreased ability to bear weight

Examination findings consistent with *osteomyelitis-osteochondritis* include:

- Extension of pain and swelling around the puncture wound and the adjacent bony structures
- Point tenderness over the bone
- Fever and/or increasing erythema
- Decreased use of the affected extremity

Examination findings consistent with *pyarthrosis* (septic arthritis) include:

- Pain, swelling, warmth, and erythema over the affected joint
- Decreased range of motion and weight bearing of the affected joint
- Fever

Diagnostic Studies. Obtain plain film radiographs if there is suspicion of a retained foreign object if the wound is caused by a piece of glass, a nail, or something breakable, small, or thin, or if there was penetration of a joint space, bone, growth cartilage, or the plantar fascia. Radiographs are also helpful if there is a concern for deep infection (e.g., fever, pain with passive movement, progressive pain over time, joint swelling, crepitus, disproportionate pain at the wound site).[3] Most metal, glass, and foreign objects are *radiopaque* and visible on a plain radiograph. Ultrasound is best for evaluation of *radiolucent* foreign objects, including wood and plastic. Computed tomography (CT) and magnetic resonance imaging (MRI) can also be used for penetrating foreign body evaluation. For example, MRI can be helpful in identification of nonmetallic objects and should be considered when other diagnostic identification attempts of the suspected penetrating foreign body have been unsuccessful.[3] Bone scans are sensitive but not specific for osteomyelitis, however, they do not reveal early osteomyelitis. In contrast, MRI identifies subperiosteal abscess and early edema before radiographic changes occur.

Obtain laboratory studies and imaging if osteomyelitis is suspected.[5]

- A complete blood count (CBC). White blood cell elevation often indicates infection.
- Erythrocyte sedimentation rate (ESR) and C-reactive protein (CRP) are nonspecific inflammatory markers that help diagnose bony inflammation and infection.
- A wound or blood culture is typically indicated before starting antibiotics, especially if the wound appears infected.

Management

The circumstances surrounding the penetrating injury and the presenting symptoms are the best indicators of whether the injury is superficial and will heal uneventfully.

- Ensure the patient has adequate pain control before cleaning the wound.
- Cleanse the skin surface surrounding the wound with iodine-containing or antiseptic solution such as chlorhexidine.[3] After cleansing, irrigate the wound with sterile normal saline.[6]
- Use scissors or a scalpel to remove devitalized tissue or accumulated debris.[7] Ensure that there are no foreign objects present.
- Obtain imaging studies as indicated. Refer to orthopedic surgery immediately if imaging studies demonstrate that the foreign object invaded bone, growth cartilage, or a joint space. Always suspect a retained foreign object if the puncture wound is infected, the infection is not responding to antibiotic therapy, or if pain is still present weeks after the injury. Surgical debridement should be used when there is suspicion of a deep space

infection, infection secondary to a retained foreign object, or a rapidly progressing infection.[3]

- Following cleansing, cover the wound with a simple bandage and let heal by secondary intention. Deeper wounds that require exploration should have a small, sterile, dampened saline gauze placed to keep the edges open to prevent superficial skin closure and promote healing. Remove the gauze 2 to 3 days after placement. Consultation with a surgical subspecialist (e.g., plastic surgery) is recommended for repair and treatment of complex facial animal or human bite wounds.[8]
- Simple, uncomplicated puncture wounds do not need antibiotics except with signs of infection or with cat bites, hand, foot, or genitalia wounds, a puncture near a joint or bone, or the wound is deep or contains debris (Table 25.1). Tetanus prophylaxis should be given, if indicated. A recheck appointment should be scheduled 48 hours from the start of antibiotics for the patient receiving outpatient therapy.
- Consider surgical debridement for removal of a foreign object or abscess drainage with infected puncture wounds.
- Treatment for severe infections, such as septic arthritis and osteomyelitis, includes surgical debridement and parenteral antibiotics.

Patient and Parent Education

Home care management for a puncture wound includes:
- Cleanse the wound twice daily and when wound soiling occurs. Use warm water and soap.
- Apply Bacitracin or triple antibiotic and cover the wound with a dressing.
- Observe closely for signs and symptoms of infection. If infection is suspected, notify the PCP immediately; rapid reevaluation is necessary. Further evaluation is required if a puncture wound continues to cause localized or spreading pain or discomfort.

Lacerations

Lacerations are associated with occult injuries to the deeper tissues and require careful exploration. The most common lacerations result from shear, tension, or compression injuries.

Shear injuries are caused by sharp objects and tend to cause minimal damage to the tissues surrounding the injury. They heal quickly and have a low risk of wound infection. The danger of shear injuries is the potential for damage to nerve, tendon, and vascular structures. These injuries often require a more comprehensive assessment and/or complicated repair and should be referred to the ED.

Tension injuries are caused from stresses on the skin, usually secondary to blunt force of an object at less than a 90-degree angle. Skin tears due to the stress often cause irregularly shaped injury edges accompanied by damage to surrounding tissues. A classic example of a skin tear is when a falling child hits their head against the dull edge of a piece of furniture.

Compression injuries are crush injuries, usually involving blunt force of an object at a 90-degree angle. This type of laceration usually has irregular, often stellate wound edges. Compression injuries can cause significant injury to adjacent tissues and have a high incidence of wound infections.

Clinical Findings

History. Patient history when assessing a laceration includes:
- Details and mechanism of injury.
- How long ago did the injury occur? (NOTE: Length of time since injury can influence the treatment plan for the patient).
- Does the child have allergies to antibiotics or anesthetics?
- What is the child's tetanus immunization status? Is there a need for further immunization?

Physical Examination. Key points in the examination of a laceration include:
- A neurovascular examination, including evaluation of pulses, motor function, and sensation distal to the laceration.
- Assessing range of motion, especially with the distal forearm, wrist, and hand due to the high potential for tendon injury.
- Determining whether the wound edges approximate and the degree of tension at the wound site.

Management

Providers may repair the wound using sutures, staples, surgical glue, or Steri-Strips or tape. Minor lacerations to the scalp, arms, and legs are commonly managed by PCPs. Wounds to

TABLE 25.1 Oral Antibiotic Prophylaxis After Puncture Wounds

Type	First Line	Alternative
Human bites Cover for *Staphylococcus aureus, Streptococcus viridans, Eikenella corrodes*	Amoxicillin clavulanate 3–5 days	Cefuroxime, penicillin V, doxycycline, ciprofloxacin, levofloxacin, or trimethoprim-sulfamethoxazole (TMP-SMX) plus clindamycin or metronidazole
Animal bites Cover for *Pasteurella multocida, Pasteurella canis, Staphylococcus aureus* (dog and cat bites)	Amoxicillin clavulanate 3–5 days	Cefuroxime, penicillin V, doxycycline, ciprofloxacin, levofloxacin, or trimethoprim-sulfamethoxazole (TMP-SMX) plus clindamycin or metronidazole
Plantar wounds Cover for *Pseudomonas aeruginosa*	Levofloxacin 3–5 days	Consult with infectious disease as may require IV therapy

Modified from Baddour LM, Harper M. Animal bites (dogs, cats, and other animals): evaluation and management. In: Post T, ed. UpToDate; 2021. https://www.uptodate.com/contents/animal-bites-dogs-cats-and-other-animals-evaluation-and-management?search=human%20bites&source=search_result&selectedTitle=5~90&usage_type=default&display_rank=6; Baddour LM, Harper M. Human bites: evaluation and management. In: Post T, ed. UpToDate; 2021. https://www.uptodate.com/contents/human-bites-evaluation-and-management?search=human%20bite&source=search_result&selectedTitle=1~91&usage_type=default&display_rank=1; and Baddour LM, Brown AM. Infectious complications of puncture wounds; In: Post T, ed. UpToDate; 2020. https://www.uptodate.com/contents/infectious-complications-of-puncture-wounds?search=infectious%20complications%20of%20puncture%20wounds&source=search_result&selectedTitle=1~88&usage_type=default&display_rank=1.

the face, hands, or genital areas should generally be referred to the ED for further evaluation by specialists (e.g., hand surgeon, plastic/reconstructive surgeon). Others points for consideration include:

1. *Decision to close the wound.* Most wounds are closed using a primary closure as soon as possible after the injury. This approach speeds healing, prevents infection, and improves the cosmetic result. Delayed closure can increase the risk of infection. Some researchers suggest a "golden period" for wound closure of 6 hours; however, wounds considered low risk for infection can be closed up to 12 to 24 hours after the injury.[9] In pediatrics, wound infection rates are generally between 2% and 10%.[9] The likelihood of scarring increases with wound infection. Other guidelines to consider in wound closure include the following:
   - Most facial wounds should be closed within 24 hours after initial injury to provide the child with the optimal cosmetic outcomes. Depending on the severity of the laceration or potential for infection, repair, and management may require referral to the ED.
   - Infection risk is inversely related to blood flow. The lower the blood flow, the higher is the infection risk (e.g., hand or foot laceration is more likely to become infected than a scalp laceration because the extremities have lower blood perfusion).
   - Contaminated wounds, crush wounds, and lacerations in immunocompromised children are at high risk for infection and should be closed within 6 hours of injury.
   - Animal and human bites should be left open for healing by granulation and reepithelialization (e.g., secondary intention). Scarring increases with this method, but the benefits of improved healing and decreased infection outweigh this.
   - Delayed primary closure involves closing a wound 3 to 5 days after initial injury. This approach is recommended for heavily contaminated wounds and those associated with extensive damage, crush injuries, and explosion injuries. Initial management of such injuries includes wound cleansing, debridement, and sterile dressing. Close follow-up is recommended to check for infection and for wound closure.
2. *Hair.* Hair near the wound usually creates minimal difficulty during repair. Do not shave hair because it increases the risk of infection. Instead, clip the hair with scissors, if needed, to visualize the wound during closure. Eyebrow hair should not be removed because this may lead to abnormal or slow regrowth.
3. *Wound cleansing.* Irrigation is the preferred method of wound cleansing, as it reduces bacterial contamination and prevents subsequent infection. Tap water and sterile normal saline are equally safe to use. A general rule for the saline irrigation volume is to use 100 mL of normal saline per centimeter of the wound. More solution may be needed if the wound is unusually large or contaminated. Use a large irrigating syringe (20–50 mL) to provide enough force to cleanse the wound. A splash guard attached to the syringe is recommended to reduce splatter during irrigation. It is important to remove all foreign debris to decrease infection risk. Chlorhexidine or povidone-iodine surgical scrub preparations may be used to clean the skin *surrounding* the wound but are not recommended for use in the wound itself. Hydrogen peroxide and alcohol are not recommended.

4. *Wound exploration.* Explore wounds for the presence of foreign objects, deep tissue layer damage, injury to nerve or blood vessel, or joint involvement. It is imperative to determine the wound depth. Probe the wound with a cotton-tipped swab, a hemostat, or a needle holder. Deep lacerations should be closed in an ED by layered closure. If tendon injury is suspected or if bone is exposed, consult, and refer to an orthopedist.
5. *Wound debridement.* Unattached loose tissue may be gently removed with sterile instruments. Debridement is advantageous because it removes wound contaminants and approximates wound edges. This allows for easier wound repair and cosmetic acceptability after the wound heals. Although it is helpful to excise necrotic skin, excessive trimming of irregular lacerations should not be attempted as it can create a defect that is subsequently difficult to close or increase tension at the wound margin, making scarring more likely.
6. *Wound closure.* Several methods are available for wound closure:
   - *Traditional sutures* involve "sewing" the skin together with a surgical needle and suture. This procedure usually requires an injection and/or topical use of an anesthetic. Simple, uncomplicated lacerations to the scalp, trunk, arms, or legs may be closed with sutures (i.e., primary closure). In general, an *absorbable* suture material is used for closure of structures deeper than the epidermis as well as simple facial lacerations, and *nonabsorbable* sutures are used to close the outermost layer of a laceration. See Table 25.2 for recommended suture material type, size, and removal guidelines.
   - *Staples* can be used for the scalp, trunk, and extremities (excluding hands and feet) to provide a more rapid closure time. Laceration repair with staples is associated with a lower infection rate than with sutures but can be more painful to remove and may not be as cosmetically appealing when healed. Staples should not be used if MRI or CT is necessary.
   - *Surgical tape* (e.g., Steri-Strips) is used for small superficial wounds. Surgical tape cannot be used on wounds in moist areas or in areas of tension, such as flexor or extensor surfaces. Surgical tape should also be avoided in small children, who will most likely remove the tape prematurely.
   - *Topical skin adhesive* (i.e., skin glue) is used for simple lacerations with clean edges. The adhesive is applied on top of the skin while the edges of the wound are held together. Adhesive in the wound or between wound margins should be avoided. Skin glue takes less time to apply than stitches and forms a strong, flexible bond over the top of the wound. Topical skin adhesive should not be used on areas of skin where there is tension, such as over a joint, because of the high probability of the wound reopening and thus requiring healing by secondary closure, causing increased risk of scarring. A bandage is not required for cover after tissue repair with skin glue. The topical skin adhesive sloughs off the wound as it heals, usually in 7 to 10 days, and does not require a return visit for removal. Infection risk is minimal due to antimicrobial properties of the adhesive. Minimal scarring is associated with this method of laceration repair; however, it is not recommended for lacerations with irregular borders or puncture wounds.
7. *Dressing.* The purpose of dressings is primarily to protect, compress, absorb, and/or immobilize, as well as improve

TABLE 25.2   Suture Material, Size, and Removal Guidelines

Body Region	Nonabsorbable[a]	Absorbable[b]	Duration (Days)
Scalp	5-0 or 4-0	4-0	5–7
Face	6-0	5-0	3–5
Eyelid	7-0 or 6-0	—	3–5
Eyebrow	6-0 or 5-0	5-0	3–5
Trunk	5-0 or 4-0	3-0	5–7
Extremities	5-0 or 4-0	4-0	7–10
Joint surface	4-0	—	10–14
Hand	5-0	5-0	7
Foot sole	4-0 or 3-0	4-0	7–10

[a]Examples of nonabsorbable sutures. Nylon is good for skin closure; polypropylene specifically is good for scalp and eyebrows.

[b]Examples of absorbable sutures. Vicryl, surgical gut plain, and surgical gut chromic are good for subcutaneous closure. Monocryl is good for subcuticular closure. Vicryl rapine is good for mucosa and dermis closure.

From The Johns Hopkins Hospital. *Harriet Lane Handbook.* 22nd ed. Philadelphia: Elsevier; 2021.

healing and cosmetic outcomes. A simple repaired laceration may be covered with an adhesive bandage. For more complex repairs, dress the wound with nonadherent gauze for the first layer followed by a second layer of plain gauze (if needed), and secured in place with adhesive tape or elasticized gauze (e.g., tubular net bandage).

8. *Immunization.* Give tetanus booster or tetanus immunoglobulin as indicated.

9. *Antibiotics.* Antibiotic prophylaxis of clean wounds is not indicated. Its use in contaminated wounds may be helpful, but careful wound cleaning with extensive irrigation followed by prompt wound closure (when indicated) are the most effective safeguards in preventing infection in most wounds.

10. *Suture and staple removal.* The timing for removal of staples and sutures depends on the wound and location (see Table 25.2).

Patient and Parent Education

Instructions for wound care at home are best given in writing and should include:

- Signs and symptoms of infection that warrant an early recheck (redness, swelling, discharge, increased pain).
- Instructions about cleansing and bandaging the wound. For surgical tape and topical skin adhesive, do not use topical antibiotic ointment or lotions because they will remove the adhesive.
- Limiting vigorous physical activity. Patient should return for reevaluation for any bleeding or dehiscing of the wound.
- Return appointment for staple removal or with nonabsorbable suture use.

Burns

In 2020 just over 74,000 ED visits for nonfatal fire or burn injuries and 278 fatalities occurred in children ages 0 to 19 years.[1] Intentional burns are a common form of NAT (e.g., child abuse) and every burn injury should be evaluated carefully.

Common causes of burn injuries include grills, hot soups or water, curling irons, house fires, and appliances (e.g., stove, coffee pot). Younger children tend to sustain more scald injuries, while older children tend to incur burns from flame and direct fire contact. Scald burns can cause deeper injuries, depending on the length of time the skin remains in contact with the substance (i.e., the longer contact, the deeper the burn). Thermal burns are more likely to be deeper, involving more skin layers in infants and children than in adolescents and adults because they have thinner skin. Residential fires typically lead to serious injury or death.

Burns are classified by depth of injury, percentage of body surface area (BSA) involved, location of the burn, and association with other injuries. The classification system for burns includes superficial (first degree), partial thickness (superficial or deep; second degree), and full thickness (third degree). The term *fourth-degree burn* identifies burns that extend into the muscle, fascia, and/or bone and are potentially life-threatening.[10]

- *Superficial burns* involve only the epidermis. The skin is erythematous, blanching, inflamed, dry, and painful, but there are no blisters. Superficial burns typically heal in 3 to 6 days, have little risk of scarring, and require only symptomatic treatment. Sunburn is a common example of a superficial burn.
- *Partial-thickness burns* involve the epidermis and the dermis to a variable degree.
- *Superficial* partial-thickness burns are erythematous, blanching, very painful, mottled, moist, and blistered. These burns can initially appear to be superficial and within 12 to 24 hours develop blisters, classifying the burn as partial thickness instead. They usually heal in 7 to 21 days; scarring may occur.
- *Deep* partial-thickness burns appear pale and yellow and are less painful and weepy than superficial partial-thickness burns. Deep partial-thickness burns take longer to heal (2–9 weeks) and are more likely to scar.
- *Full-thickness burns* destroy the epidermis and dermis completely. The skin appears whitish (a waxy white appearance)

or leathery. The surface is dry and nontender. Fluid losses can be profound with this burn. These usually require skin grafting, cause permanent scarring, potential contractures, and take several weeks to heal.

- *Full-thickness burns with extension into deep tissue* involve destruction and/or extensive injury of muscle, fascia, nerves, tendons, vessels, and bone. They typically require surgical intervention and skin grafting.

Burns involving large body surfaces generally vary in depth across the wound. Burn wounds are dynamic, and the effect of dermal ischemia (affected by infection, exposure, and dehydration) is not often apparent at the initial assessment. Their depth can change from day to day. The percentage of BSA and the part(s) of the body affected are also key factors to determine treatment, disposition, and prognosis (Table 25.3). Multiple methods estimate the burn BSA (e.g., Lund Browder Chart, Rule of Nines, Palm Method). For example, the palm (excluding the fingers) is approximately 0.5% of total BSA (TBSA) and the entire palmar surface including fingers is 1% of BSA in children and adults.[11] Software for calculating BSA in pediatric burn victims is available at www.sagediagram.com/. It is also often embedded in electronic health records.

Clinical Findings

History. The following information should be obtained:

- Description of how the burn occurred, including agent and length of time agent was in contact with the skin, circumstances surrounding the injury, when it occurred, and likelihood of other injuries, such as trauma or smoke inhalation
- Initial and subsequent treatment of the burn
- Previous history of burn and other injuries
- Other current medical problems, medications, allergies, and tetanus status
- Suspicion of NAT if the injury does not match the history and mechanism described

Physical Examination. The examination should begin with an airway assessment, as the most common cause of death during the first hour after a burn injury is respiratory impairment. Any sign of airway compromise should warrant administration of 100% oxygen via a nonrebreather mask and hospital transport via ambulance for further management. Airway complications should be suspected if there is history of exposure to flame, smoke, or chemicals, if the exposure was in an enclosed place, or there was loss of consciousness.[12] Concern for respiratory complications should also be considered if there are facial burns, singed nasal hairs or

TABLE 25.3 Estimation of Surface Area Burned Based on Age

Area	AGE (YEARS) Birth to 1	1–4	5–9	10–14	15+	Adult
Head	19	17	13	11	9	7
Neck	2	2	2	2	2	2
Anterior trunk	13	13	13	13	13	13
Posterior trunk	13	13	13	13	13	13
Right buttock	2.5	2.5	2.5	2.5	2.5	2.5
Left buttock	2.5	2.5	2.5	2.5	2.5	2.5
Genitalia	1	1	1	1	1	1
Right upper arm	4	4	4	4	4	4
Left upper arm	4	4	4	4	4	4
Right lower arm	3	3	3	3	3	3
Left lower arm	3	3	3	3	3	3
Right hand	2.5	2.5	2.5	2.5	2.5	2.5
Left hand	2.5	2.5	2.5	2.5	2.5	2.5
Right thigh	5.5	6.5	8	8.5	9	9.5
Left thigh	5.5	6.5	8	8.5	9	9.5
Right leg	5	5	5.5	6	6.5	7
Left leg	5	5	5.5	6	6.5	7
Right foot	3.5	3.5	3.5	3.5	3.5	3.5
Left foot	3.5	3.5	3.5	3.5	3.5	3.5

This modification by O'Neill of the Brooke Army Burn Center Diagram shows the change in surface area of the head from 19% in an infant to 7% in an adult. Proper use of this chart provides an accurate basis for subsequent management of the burned child.

From Joffe MD. Burns. In: Fleisher GR, Ludwig S, Henretig FM, et al. eds. *Textbook of Pediatric Emergency Medicine.* 8th ed. Lippincott Williams & Wilkins; 2021.

soot over the nares or oral cavity, hoarseness, stridor, retractions, tachypnea, cough, wheezes, rales, or rhonchi.[12] Once the airway is stable, the physical examination requires determination of:

- Percentage of BSA affected (see Table 25.3)
- Mechanism of burn and associated injuries
- Burn distribution and pattern with particular concern for circumferential burns to the thorax that may cause poor chest expansion and declining oxygen saturation
- Burn depth: superficial, partial thickness, or full thickness
- Assessment of the extremity vascular status
- Presence of any complicating medical condition(s)
  Diagnostic Studies.
- CBC: an elevated hematocrit secondary to fluid loss. Initial white blood cell elevation is always secondary to an acute phase reaction but may later indicate infection.
- A basic metabolic panel may reveal elevated potassium due to cell breakdown. Blood urea nitrogen (BUN) and creatine kinase assess renal function, rhabdomyolysis, and tissue perfusion.
- A urinalysis and specific gravity help determine hydration status, and the presence of myoglobin may suggest acute tubular necrosis secondary to muscle tissue destruction and breakdown.

Differential Diagnosis

Chapter 22 discusses intentional burn injuries resulting from NAT. Scalded skin syndrome caused by staphylococcal infection can cause skin exfoliation, but the clinical presentation clearly differentiates it from an acute burn injury.

Management

Determining the need for admission to a hospital or burn center involves many factors, including burn depth, percentage of BSA affected, and mechanism of the burn injury. Other considerations include the risk of infection, pain control, functional and cosmetic outcomes, and family/home situation. Pediatric burn patients who meet the following criteria should be admitted to the hospital or burn center for further management[13,14]:

- Burns involving more than 20% TBSA
- Partial-thickness burns involving more than 10% TBSA
- Full-thickness burns involving more than 5% TBSA
- Circumferential burns
- Burns overlying joints and/or involving critical areas, such as the hands and feet, genitalia, and perineum
- Chemical burns, electrical burns (including lightning injury)
- Respiratory involvement, inhalation injury
- Suspicion of NAT or unsafe home environment
- Presence of an underlying chronic illness
- Pain control
- Burn debridement is needed
- Major trauma

The outpatient treatment of minor burns is an option for superficial and partial thickness burns of less than 10% of BSA. Further referral and consultation with a burn specialist depends on the severity and location of the burn. Box 25.1 outlines the primary care management of superficial and partial-thickness burns.

BOX 25.1 Management of Superficial and Partial-Thickness Burns in the Primary Care Setting

Management of Superficial Burns[a]

- Cleanse the burn and surrounding skin with water and mild soap.
- Burns with an intact epidermis, such as superficial or superficial partial-thickness wounds, do not require a topical antimicrobial agent.
- Superficial burns usually do not require a dressing.
- Aloe vera has antibacterial properties and may be used to help with skin healing and soothing. Lanolin may cause itching and is not recommended.
- Administer analgesics, such as acetaminophen or ibuprofen, as indicated.

Management of Superficial Partial-Thickness Burns[a]

- Administer adequate analgesic medication. Sedatives may be needed before performing wound care and for breakthrough pain. Switch to over-the-counter acetaminophen or ibuprofen as the pain subsides.
- Cleanse the wound with mild soap and tap water.
- Leave small blisters intact as they provide a biological dressing and will rupture spontaneously and heal. Consider rupturing and unroofing the blister if large blisters are noted.[b]
- Gently debride open blisters to remove devitalized tissue and residue from prior dressing changes.[b]
- Superficial partial thickness burns with an intact epidermis do not require a topical antimicrobial agent.
- To prevent infection in any nonsuperficial burn, apply bacitracin or 1% silver sulfadiazine cream to the clean debrided area followed by the

application of a nonadherent dressing such as Xeroform, Mepitel, or Adaptic. Next apply a dry fluffy elastic gauze outer dressing such as kerlix.

- One percent silver sulfadiazine cream (1% SSD) is an antimicrobial and soothing agent but should not be used if the patient has a sulfa allergy or the patient is younger than 2 months of age. Also, 1% SSD is oculotoxic and should not be used near the eyes.
- Biologic and or synthetic dressings may be more beneficial depending on the burn. Consult with a burn specialist if considering use.
- An option for partial-thickness burn management is the use of nano crystalline silver dressings such as Aquacel Ag and Acticoat. This dressing is impregnated with silver ion, which helps prevent infection and a potential antiinflammatory action. These dressings are typically applied after complete burn cleansing and debridement. The burned area is then covered with sterile gauze and managed with close wound monitoring and weekly dressing changes.[c]
- Assess the burn the day after injury and then weekly (or more frequently if needed) to ensure proper healing and absence of infection. Dressing changes, debridement, and wound cleansing frequency vary from twice a day to weekly depending on the type dressing, and as needed for soaked or soiled dressings until the burn has healed.
- Itching occurs commonly during the healing process, often triggered by activity, heat, and stress. Use mittens for young children to prevent scratching if itching occurs. If needed, administer an antihistamine, such as diphenhydramine.
- Individuals with circumferential extremity burns may need to be admitted to the hospital for observation to monitor for compartment syndrome.

[a]Wiktor A, Richards D. Treatment of minor thermal burns. In: Post T, ed. UpToDate; 2021.https://www.uptodate.com/contents/treatment-of-minor-thermal-burns?search=Treatment of minor thermal burns.&source=search_result&selectedTitle=1~150&usage_type=default&display_rank=1
[b]Germann GK, Reichenberger M. The burned hand. In: Wolfe SW, Pedersen WC, Kozin SH, Cohen MS. eds. *Green's Operative Hand Surgery*. 8th ed. Elsevier, 2023:2121–2152.
[c]Tenenhaus M, Rennekampff HO. Topical agents and dressings for local burn wound care. In: Post T, ed. UpToDate; 2021.https://www.uptodate.com/contents/topical-agents-and-dressings-for-local-burn-wound-care?search=Topical agents and dressings for local burn wound care&source=search_result&selectedTitle=1~150&usage_type=default&display_rank=1

Patient and Parent Education

The following points are important components of patient and parent education:

- Injury prevention strategies (see Chapter 21).
- The serious or long-term consequences of burns. For example, frequent and significant sunburns during early childhood can predispose to skin cancers in later life. Electric burns cause thermal injury to skin (contact burn). If an arc is created and there is passage of electrical current through the body, there is a potential for cardiac dysrhythmias and neurologic impairment.
- The extent of scarring is difficult to predict with certainty. Scarring depends on depth of the burn, length of time needed for healing, whether grafting was done, and the child's age and skin color. Burn scars remain immature for the first 12 to 18 months and their color and texture will change over time. Most minor scald injuries from hot liquids heal quickly with little or no scarring.

Contusions and Hematomas

A *contusion,* or bruise, is an injury in which the skin is not broken but the trauma causes effusion into muscle and subcutaneous tissue with injury to the vessels and possibly the nerves. In children, contusions can occur anywhere on the body but are most often seen on the extremities. Contusions are common in pediatrics. They are caused by blunt trauma, most often because of falling or bumping into objects during play. Participation in contact sports puts children and adolescents at increased risk for contusions. Bruises to the trunk, face, or head are red flags for possible NAT and a careful history must be taken to determine whether the explanation is consistent with the injury.

Hematomas are localized collections of extravasated blood that are confined within a space or potential space. Hematomas can be associated with most types of minor and major wounds; they must be observed closely for signs of infection and, in some instances, drained.

Clinical Findings

History and Physical Examination. The following should be determined:

- History of excessive bleeding or easy bruising, or slow healing
- Circulatory status and discoloration, involvement of underlying structures
- Motor and sensory function: sensation, mobility, and range of motion

    Referral is needed if there is any evidence of circulatory compromise.

Differential Diagnosis

Type A or B Hemophilia, von Willebrand disease, and conditions that cause purpura should be considered. Myositis ossificans (i.e., bone forms inside muscle or soft tissue), a complication of trauma, is rarely seen in children.

Management and Complications

The following is a phased treatment plan for contusions involving extremities[15]:

- *Phase 1.* Prescribe protection, rest, ice, compression, and elevation (mnemonic: PRICE). Protect and rest the affected joint or limb during the acute phase. Consider use of slings, elastic wraps, or crutches depending on severity and location of the contusion. Apply ice to the injury for 20 minutes 3 to 4 times a day until the swelling improves or resolves. Apply a pressure bandage (e.g., Ace wrap) to help prevent further edema or bleeding but ensure it is not too tight and affecting circulation. Elevate the affected body part (ideally, above the level of the heart) to help with venous blood return and decrease edema. Acetaminophen and a nonsteroidal antiinflammatory drug (NSAID), such as ibuprofen, are good analgesia choices.
- *Phase 2.* While healing, improve strength and range of motion of the injured extremity. Start range-of-motion and strengthening exercises as soon as possible to help the recovery process and not delay a return to normal activity. When the limb is pain-free, gradually remove supportive/protective devices, and start to return to normal daily living activity. Consider low impact sport (e.g., swimming) for exercise.
- *Phase 3.* Continue to progress towards baseline sports and activities. Near normal strength and flexibility of the injured extremity is achieved.
- *Phase 4.* Full function of extremity with range of motion and strength back to baseline for sports, fun, and activities of daily living. If after returning to full function and activities the pain returns, limit sports activities for 1 to 2 days, return to the use of ice as stated earlier and then gradually return to sports/play.
- Reserve radiographs for suspected foreign object or fracture. Refer severe injuries or persistent pain despite the above management treatment for orthopedic management.
- Most contusions heal quickly without sequelae. However, severe trauma to the extremities can lead to myositis ossificans or compartment syndrome.

Patient and Parent Education

Highlight the expected progression in color changes of ecchymosis (e.g., purple to green) and the potential for ecchymosis to migrate to surrounding tissues. Arrange for follow-up if discomfort persists or increases. Review injury prevention efforts. The degree of injury and resolution of symptoms determine return to activities. Physical therapy or an athletic trainer may facilitate return to activities of daily living and/or sports.

Bites and Stings

Animal and Human Bites

Pets, stray animals, or humans (e.g., other children) are sources of pediatric bite injuries. For infants and young children, animal bites involve the head and neck, while older children commonly have upper extremity bites. In contrast, human bites mostly occur on the upper extremities.

Each year an estimated 4.5 million dog bites, 400,000 cat bites, and 250,000 human bites occur, with children sustaining more animal bites than adults.[16] In pediatrics, males are attacked more often than females. Dog and cat bites are most often from animals known to the child. The rate of infection from a dog or human bite is between 5% and 20%, and as high as 50% from a cat bite,[17] as cat bites cause puncture wounds that tend to be deep. Dog bites cause abrasions, puncture wounds, and lacerations, with or without associated tissue avulsion. Other animal bites that have been known to occur include rodents, rabbits, ferrets, reptiles, monkeys, and farm animals (e.g., pigs, horses, cattle).[18] All human bite wounds, regardless of mechanism of injury, are at high risk for infection and joint compromise. Closed or clenched-fist bites are serious indirect human bites that are typically the result of fighting. They occur when a fist hits another's teeth resulting in a puncture or laceration, as well as surrounding tissue/joint injury.

Clinical Findings

History and Physical Examination. Ask about the circumstances surrounding the bite including the type of animal, domesticated or feral/wild animal, provoked or unprovoked attack, and location of the attack. The wound should be assessed for the presence of foreign material and the status of underlying structures, along with the type, size, and depth of injury. For example, if the bite is on an extremity, assess its range of motion and sensory intactness, while with deep facial bite injuries, assess functioning of the facial nerve. A diagram of the injury should be recorded in the chart. It is best to photograph the injury. Drug allergies and immunization status should also be ascertained.

Diagnostic Studies. Obtain aerobic and anaerobic cultures if wound infection is suspected.[17] A radiograph of the affected part should be obtained if it is likely that a bone or joint could have been penetrated or fractured or if retained foreign material may be present.

Differential Diagnosis and Management

The differential diagnosis includes lacerations or puncture wounds from other causes.

Management involves both physical and psychologic care of the child and includes[14]:

- Appropriate analgesia or anesthesia.
- Debridement of avulsed or devitalized tissue and removal of foreign matter.
- For some bites, irrigation with normal saline using high pressure (>5 pounds per square inch) and high volume (>1 L). Puncture wounds from cat bites should not be irrigated to limit spread of infection; instead, soak the wound in a diluted solution of tap water and povidone-iodine for 15 minutes.
- Tetanus booster if indicated.
- Rabies prophylaxis if indicated (consult with local animal control or public health department on post-exposure prophylaxis). For dog bites, rabies risk is low in developed countries and is rarely indicated. The CDC also provides guidelines on rabies prophylaxis (see Additional Resources).
- A 3- to 5-day course of prophylactic antibiotics for immunosuppressed children and for all human and cat bites, and for the following bite types or wound characteristics: hand, puncture, overlying bone fracture, substantial crushing tissue injuries, those that require debridement, or those involving tendons, muscles, or joint spaces. Prophylactic antibiotics for low-risk dog bite wounds do not decrease incidence of infection and is not recommended. Prescribe a broad-spectrum antibiotic, such as amoxicillin clavulanate (first choice). Treat penicillin-allergic individuals with an extended spectrum cephalosporin or trimethoprim-sulfamethoxazole plus clindamycin.[19]
- Deciding whether bite wounds should be closed primarily with delayed closure (3–5 days after injury) or allowed to heal by secondary intention (leaving the wound open). Factors to consider are the type, size, and depth of the wound; the anatomic location; presence of infection; the time interval since the injury; and the potential for cosmetic disfigurement. Surgical consultation should be obtained for all deep or extensive wounds and those involving the bones, joints, or hands. Because of the excellent blood supply to the face, facial lacerations are at less risk for infection. Many plastic surgeons advocate primary closure of thoroughly irrigated and debrided facial bite wounds within 5 to 6 hours of injury. PCPs may refer patients with concerns about scarring or facial wounds for plastic surgery repair.
- Bites involving the hand or foot should not be sutured but allowed to drain. Hand and foot bites less than 1.5 cm are best healed by secondary intention; bites greater than 1.5 cm should have delayed primary closure.
- Bite wounds more than 8–12 hours old should not be sutured; facial wounds may be sutured up to 24 hours.
- A single layer of nonabsorbable sutures is best (avoid multiple closure layers and allow for gaps in between sutures).
- Obtain a surgical consult if there is evidence of or concern about nerve, tendon, and/or ligament injury or if a joint space was involved. Hospitalization, reconstructive surgery, and long-term follow-up may be indicated.
- Discuss the child's fears and management of any behavioral problems that may result (see Chapter 6).
- Deciding whether to report animal bites to animal control requires PCP knowledge of local Animal Laws and Policies and contacting the local Health Department's Office of Animal Control.

Complications

Secondary infection is the most common complication of mammalian bites and can lead to cellulitis and osteomyelitis, thus requiring hospitalization. *Streptococcus viridans* and *S. aureus* are common aerobic organisms associated with infected human bites; anaerobic infection is also possible. The most common gram-positive bacteria from dog and cat bites is *S. aureus*. Species of gram-negative bacteria (e.g., *P. multocida* and *P. canis* from dog and cat bites and *Eikenella corrodens* from human bites) can also cause infections.[19] The potential for rabies, human immunodeficiency virus (HIV), and hepatitis B and C exposure must also be considered.

Patient and Parent Education

Preventive education and actions should include[16]:

- All children, especially those younger than 5 years of age, should always be supervised when interacting or playing with animals.
- Nontraditional pets carry an increased risk of infection and injury, especially for kids who are immunocompromised.
- Avoid adopting or bringing wild animals into the home.
- Instruct children to never handle or play with wild animals or domestic animals that are not known by the child.

Hymenoptera (e.g., Bees, Wasps, Ants)

Bees, hornets, yellow jackets, fire and harvester ants, and wasps belong to the Hymenoptera order of insects and have common venom antigens. Among the Hymenoptera order, the Vespidae (e.g., hornets, wasps, yellow jackets), Apidae (e.g., honeybees, bumblebees), and Formicidae (e.g., fire ants) families can cause allergic reactions from their sting. Cross-reactivity of the allergens present within the Vespidae family venoms, but not within/across Formicidae and Apidae families.[20] Immunoglobulin E–dependent hypersensitivity is the underlying cause of local or systemic symptoms.

Bees and wasps ordinarily do not sting unless frightened, bothered, or hurt. In contrast, yellow jackets are aggressive. Fire ants may cause multiple, painful stings. Reactions to stings can vary from mild, local responses to life-threatening anaphylaxis with wheezing and urticaria. Most individuals experience only a local reaction, but some suffer severe systemic reactions, which can progress to medical emergencies unless prompt intervention is initiated.

Clinical Findings

History and Physical Examination. The PCP should ask about a past history of a local or systemic reaction following an insect bite. The physical examination findings include:

- Mild reactions consist of local redness, pruritus, pain, edema, and possibly generalized urticaria.
- Severe reactions, including anaphylaxis, include local signs and urticaria, plus any of the following: watery eyes, difficulty breathing, swallowing, or wheezing hoarseness, thickened speech, gastrointestinal disturbances, abdominal pain, dizziness, weakness, confusion, collapse, unconsciousness, even death.
- Fire ant bites can cause vesicles that develop into sterile pustules.

Diagnostic Studies. For systemic reactions, refer to an allergist for venom-specific immunoglobulin E testing and identification after resolution of the reaction.

Differential Diagnosis and Management

The differential diagnosis includes other insect bites, folliculitis, or urticaria. The following management steps are taken:

- For *mild local* reactions:
  - Remove visible stingers with the edge of a sharp object gently scraped over the bite, taking care to not squeeze the attached venom sac.
  - Apply cool compresses or use cool baths.
  - Administer an antihistamine, such as diphenhydramine dosed every 4 to 6 hours at 6.25 mg (maximum 37.5 mg/day) for children 2–5 years old; 12.5–25 mg (maximum 150 mg/day) for 6–11 years old; and 25–50 mg (maximum 300 mg/day) for 12 years and older or hydroxyzine 2 mg/kg/day, in divided doses every 6–8 hours daily (50 mg/day maximum under 6 years old; 50–100 mg/day maximum over 6 years old). For pruritus, refer to a pediatric drug formulary for further dosing information.
  - Topical glucocorticoid creams or ointments may help reduce itching.
- For *moderate to severe* reactions:
  - Moderate reactions may need to be treated with oral antihistamines, corticosteroids, and inhaled bronchodilators (if wheezing).
  - Institute emergency measures for treatment of anaphylactic reactions and transport to the ED via emergency medical services (EMS) as quickly as possible.
  - Hospitalize for anaphylactic shock.
  - Epinephrine: 0.01 mg/kg (0.01 mL/kg/dose of 1 mg/mL solution) intramuscularly, not to exceed 0.3 mg to 0.5 mg, every 5–15 minutes. Usually, the patient will respond after one or two doses.
  - Give antihistamines immediately following epinephrine (and repeated every 6 hours for up to 3 days) but not as a substitute for epinephrine. Give both histamine type 1 (H_1) and type 2 (H_2) blockers to reduce hives; this is more effective than giving an H_1 blocker alone.
  - Glucocorticoids have been used to prevent biphasic reactions and in patients with asthma in the management of anaphylaxis. The practice of treating patients in anaphylactic shock with glucocorticoids is becoming controversial

because of increasing evidence that it may not be helpful in the acute phase of management.[21]
- Nebulized albuterol (2.5 mg for <30 kg; 5 mg for >30 kg/per dose repeated every 15 minutes as needed for bronchospasm or wheezing).
- Administer high-flow oxygen (warm humidified) by nonrebreather mask.

Referral to an allergist is indicated for any child who has life-threatening respiratory symptoms (e.g., stridor, wheezing) or hypotension. Venom immunotherapy desensitization is highly effective in preventing further systemic reactions. Children younger than 16 years old who have only urticaria or angioedema do not require venom immunotherapy, because few will have systemic reactions with subsequent stings.

Patient and Parent Education

Key issues to discuss with moderate to severe reactions include:
- Importance of wearing a medical alert tag or bracelet.
- Proper use of an insect sting kit that includes two self-injectable epinephrine pens and the need to have a kit always readily available for emergency use
- Prevention of stings by avoiding areas likely to be infested with these insects, not wearing bright-colored clothing, and not using perfumed products.

Mosquitoes, Fleas, and Chiggers

Mosquito bites are the most common insect bites for infants and children. Mosquitoes are vectors of many diseases, and their bites cause irritating local skin reactions. Flea and chigger (i.e., *red bug, harvest mite*) bites produce local skin eruptions. Fleas that commonly attack humans in the United States include the human, cat, and dog flea. Chigger mites live on grain stems, shrubs, grass, and vines and attach to human or animals that pass by. The larvae of mites secrete an irritating substance that causes the skin eruption characteristic of chigger bites. There is a seasonal pattern to mosquito, flea, and chigger bites, which varies depending on region.

Clinical Findings

History. The following may be reported:
- Mosquito and flea bites: known bite or presence of cat, dog, or furry animal in child's environment; complaints of a brief stinging sensation followed by itching.
- Chigger bites: complaints of itching followed by dermatitis; history of playing or walking in grassy areas, parks, or other mite habitat near woods and water.

Physical Examination.
Mosquito bites are characterized by:
- Local irritation in unsensitized children; in sensitized children pruritic/urticarial wheals that last several hours to days or persistent firm papules or nodules.
- Central punctum (sometimes noted).
- Secondary impetigo from scratching of skin lesions.
- *Skeeter syndrome* (large, local areas of edema, erythema, and warmth) is a significant allergic reaction to the mosquito saliva that is difficult to distinguish from secondary infection, except that it occurs within hours of the bite.

Flea bites are characterized by:
- Urticarial wheal or papule surrounded by redness in a sensitized person; may progress into bullae, especially in young children.

- Central hemorrhagic puncta (often noted).
- Grouping of multiple lesions, commonly found on arms, ankles, legs, feet, thighs, waist, buttocks, and lower abdomen; classic linear configuration referred to as the "breakfast, lunch, and dinner" sign.

Chigger bites are characterized by the following:
- Discrete, bright-red papules 1–2 mm in diameter that often have hemorrhagic puncta.
- Lesions mainly seen on legs (sock area) and belt line but can be widespread.
- Wheals, papules, or papulovesicles in sensitized individuals.
- Bullae or purpuric lesions with secondary hypersensitivity reaction.
- Intense pruritus, peaks on the second day, decreases over the next 5–6 days, but can persist for months.
- Possible secondary impetigo from scratching lesions.
- May see the embedded chiggers. The presence of fleas or harvest mites is diagnostic; otherwise, no diagnostic studies exist.

Differential Diagnosis and Management

The diagnosis is often obvious, but the differential diagnosis can include insect bites that produce similar papular, vesicular lesions, or other skin conditions.

Management consists of controlling pruritus, include:
- Cool compresses
- Topical corticosteroids (e.g., 1% hydrocortisone cream)
- Topical antipruritic agents, such as calamine lotion; avoid topical diphenhydramine
- Oral antihistamines (e.g., diphenhydramine) if topical corticosteroids do not provide relief
- Removal of embedded chiggers (can be withdrawn by covering the insect with alcohol, mineral oil, nail polish, or ointment)
- Colloidal oatmeal baths (clean tub thoroughly after bath to avoid fall risk from oil residue).
- Treatment of secondary skin lesions, as indicated
- Elimination of fleas by treating animals and cleaning carpets, bedding, upholstered furniture; avoid areas that are potentially infested with mosquitoes, fleas, or chiggers
- Insecticides should be used with caution

Patient and Parent Education

Prevention includes eliminating mosquitoes, fleas, and chiggers from the environment, or preventing their contact with the skin.
- Use insect repellents (generally effective against mosquitoes and harvest mites).
- Wear protective clothing to cover the body and tuck pants into shoes or socks.
- Wear neutral-colored clothes (white, green, tan, and khaki do not attract mosquitoes).
- Avoid scented hair sprays, powders, soaps, lotions, creams, and perfumes because they can attract all forms of stinging insects.
- Mosquitoes are attracted to bright clothing and sweaty skin; drawn to humans by scent.
- Treat suspected animal carrier for fleas, and spray carpets and other infested areas; spray yards and grassy places for fleas in those environments that the child frequents.
- Vacuum carpets daily if fleas are seen on household pets.
- Avoid playing in areas of harvest mite habitat.
- Remove areas of standing water to decrease mosquito breeding.

Spiders and Scorpions

Spiders

Most spider bites are innocuous and do not cause reactions. If reactions occur, they are generally a minor, localized response that can be mistaken for a flea, bedbug, or other insect bite. Most spiders cannot bite humans because of their short and fragile fangs. Almost all spiders avoid humans unless provoked. The two main spiders common in the North American continent that can cause serious complications are the black widow (*Latrodectus mactans*) and the brown recluse (*Loxosceles reclusa*).

The *black widow* spider has a globular body about 1 cm across that is shiny black with a red or orange hourglass marking on its underside. It is found throughout the United States. It prefers to live in cool, dark, dry places in buildings and little-used or less frequented structures and outbuildings (e.g., wood piles, garages, basements, tool sheds). This spider often spins its web on outdoor furniture, which explains why many black widow spider bites occur around the genitals and buttocks. The black widow has neurotoxic venom.

The *brown recluse,* one of the most dangerous spiders in the United States, has an oval light fawn to dark chocolate-brown body; it is approximately 1-cm long (adults range from 1–5 cm in total length) with a dark brown violin-shaped band extending from its eyes partially down its back. It is endemic in the Midwest and Southeast but has been reported in larger cities outside their typical geographic pattern.[22] The brown recluse spider typically lives in dark, dry places (e.g., attics, basements, boxes) and storage closets among clothes. When living outdoors it resides in grasses, rocky bluffs, and barns. It is not aggressive and typically bites only in self-defense. Brown recluse spider venom is cytotoxic and hemolytic causing soft tissue destruction due to a combination of enzymes and spreading factors.

Scorpions

At least 30 of the 1400 reported scorpion species in the world can produce fatal stings.[23] Scorpions have a stinging apparatus in their tail. They are nocturnal and found in the Southwestern and Southern United States. Scorpions commonly live in cool, dark places during the day and are known to crawl into sleeping bags, shoes, and discarded clothing. They prefer to avoid stinging unless they are provoked or attacked.[24] Human stings by scorpions are usually accidental and most commonly occur when a person unintentionally steps on a scorpion or reaches under wood or rocks.[23]

Clinical Findings

History and Physical Examination. Assess for known history of a spider or scorpion bite or exposure to an environment where they live. Spider description can help in identification.

The characteristic bite features are:
- *Black widow spider* bites[25]:
  - Are initially asymptomatic or include mild site pain.
  - The bite wound most often has a center punctum with a blanched circular patch and a surrounding erythema.
  - Symptoms start 30–120 minutes after the bite and may include tremors, weakness, shaking of the affected extremity, local paresthesias, diaphoresis, headaches, nausea, and vomiting.
  - Muscle pain is the most common symptom and usually occurs in the back, extremity muscles, or abdomen. Severe abdominal pain is characteristic, with abdominal wall rigidity that can be confused with acute surgical conditions such

as appendicitis or cholecystitis. Muscle pain is self-limited and resolves within 24–72 hours without treatment.

- Muscle rigidity and tenderness may also be noted adjacent to the bite site and include myoclonus of the affected limb.
- Facial swelling and generalized erythema are common pediatric occurrences. Young infants and children are often distressed, inconsolable, and refuse to eat. There may be a history of using a crib that was just taken from storage.
- Vital signs are normal in 70% of patients, but tachycardia, tachypnea, and hypertension have been noted secondary to anxiety, venom effects, or pain.
- Rare findings include pulmonary edema, cardiovascular collapse, cardiomyopathy, priapism, rhabdomyolysis, hematuria, Horner syndrome, compartment syndrome, toxic epidermal necrolysis, latrodectus facies (i.e., lacrimation, blepharospasm, master trismus, periorbital edema, grimacing), and death.
- *Brown recluse spider* bites[26]:
  - Brown recluse bites typically occur on the inner thigh, upper arm, or thorax and look like two small punctum marks with surrounding erythema contained within a red plaque or papule. Central pallor eventually is noted around the punctum marks but is not usually seen immediately after the bite. The bite site can also become vesicular.
  - Initial bite is typically painless, but some report a burning sensation or pain. Pain may develop 2–8 hours following the initial bite and increase in severity with resolution within 1 week of onset.
  - The wound may develop a dark, depressed center over 24–48 hours, resulting in a dry, ulcerative eschar. The ulcerative wound may evolve into a necrotic region several days following the bite. The necrotic and ulcerative regions are more common with bites over fatty areas like the buttocks and thighs. Necrotic lesions may expand for up to 10 days before healing, usually over several weeks, usually without needing surgical repair, and without permanent scarring.
  - Some patients develop itching or a morbilliform rash.
  - Systemically, malaise, nausea, vomiting, fever, pallor, jaundice, or myalgias may occur.
  - Rarely, complications of acute hemolytic anemia, disseminated intravascular coagulopathy, myonecrosis, angioedema, coma, renal failure, myonecrosis, rhabdomyolysis, and/or death occur.
- *Scorpion* bites[23]:
  - In the United States and Mexico, most scorpion bites cause local symptoms or are painless with minimal swelling. Most puncture sites are difficult to see.
- Bites from *Centruroides exilicauda*, *C. noxious*, and *C. suffusus* are the most dangerous scorpion bites, as they can cause:
  - Paresthesias, remote pain, and unexplained agitation with uncontrollable crying
  - Systemic reactions including abnormal eye movements, blurred vision, restlessness, fasciculations, shaking, limb and body jerking movements, stridor, wheezing, respiratory failure, hyperthermia, hypersalivation, rhabdomyolysis, multiple organ failure, pancreatitis, sterile cerebrospinal fluid pleocytosis, metabolic acidosis, and death.
  - Children have a higher risk than adults of severe symptoms and death secondary to a scorpion bite.

Differential Diagnosis and Management. Differential diagnoses include other spider bites and conditions that result in similar cutaneous manifestations, systemic findings, or both. When venomous spider bites are suspected or confirmed, refer to the appropriate medical specialist or toxicologist.

Treatment includes:

- *Black widow spider bites*: Cleansing the wound with soap and water, and administering pain medication, antiemetics, tetanus prophylaxis, and muscle relaxants (e.g., benzodiazepines) as needed.[27] For severe symptoms, consult with a medical toxicologist or a provider with experience in black widow bites.
- *Brown recluse bites*: Tend to heal without incident; however, bites with necrotic centers generally require tetanus prophylaxis, pain medication, cold compress application, extremity elevation, and surgical excision and skin grafts if extensive necrosis occurs.
- *Scorpion stings*: May be managed immediately with cold compress application, elevation of the affected area, staying calm, and administering acetaminophen or ibuprofen for pain control. In the hospital setting, antivenin is administered, when available. Intensive care is needed for sedation and management of cardiorespiratory and neurologic complications.

Patient and Parent Education. The focus of patient and parent education is prevention. Careful monitoring of environments where spiders live and prompt treatment, if bitten, are important. Use caution when near woodpiles and attics, and always shake out shoes and sleeping bags before using them.

Snakebites

Worldwide, there are 600 different species of venomous snakes causing somewhere between 81,000 to 138,000 deaths per year.[28] Approximately 5000 snake bites are reported to the American Association of Poison Control Centers annually and most occur on the lower extremities.[29] Venomous snakes include *Crotalinae* snakes, from the Viperidae family or pit vipers (e.g., rattlesnakes, cottonmouths, water moccasins, copperheads), and the *Elapid* (coral snake). Southern, Southeastern, and Western states, including Texas, Florida, California, Arizona, Louisiana, Georgia, and North Carolina, account for the highest venomous snakebite rates due to the warmer climate).[30] The snake injects venom that contains a variety of toxins into the soft tissue that may be carried throughout the body via the blood and lymph systems. Snake venom can be cytotoxic, hemotoxic, cardiotoxic, and neurotoxic. *Cytotoxic* venom presents with localized pain, swelling, and ecchymosis; compartment syndrome and necrosis may develop in severe cases. *Hematotoxic* effects include hemolysis, fibrinogen activation, and thrombocytopenia. *Cardiotoxic* effects include hypotension, increased capillary permeability, and myocardial depression have also been observed secondary to venomous snake bites. *Neurotoxic* effects include taste abnormalities, local paresthesias, seizures, altered mental status, and fasciculations. Venomous snake bites may cause rhabdomyolysis, vomiting, nausea, diaphoresis, increased salivation, respiratory distress, and shock. Rattlesnake bites typically produce more severe signs and symptoms than cottonmouths. Copperheads cause local cutaneous symptoms such as soft tissue swelling and pain, not systemic symptoms.[30]

Clinical Findings

History. Ask about the type of snake (e.g., description, characteristics) and the appearance and progression of findings following the bite. Pit vipers have a large triangular head and vertically oriented elliptical pupils, unlike the round pupils of nonvenomous snakes. Copperheads and rattlesnakes have diamond-shaped patterns of varying colors. Coral snakes have blackheads, followed by yellow and red bands that are followed by black bands.

Physical Examination. Characteristic features of envenomation include the following:

- Severe local reaction soon after the bite with intense pain, burning, discoloration, edema, and hemorrhagic effects.
- Proximal extension of ecchymosis and swelling during the first few hours after the bite with later fluid-filled or hemorrhagic bullae and necrosis.
- Peripheral and central neurologic symptoms, including worsening weakness, numbness or tingling of the face and/or extremities, diplopia, and lethargy.
- Increased salivation, metallic taste in the mouth, sweating, nausea, and vomiting.
- Evidence of hematologic coagulopathy, such as hematemesis, melena, and hemoptysis.
- Respiratory distress and shock that can lead to death.

Diagnostic Studies. Coagulation studies, other laboratory tests, and an electrocardiogram, as indicated.

Management

For nonvenomous bites, clean the wound, give tetanus prophylaxis if necessary, and administer appropriate pain medication. Antibiotics are not recommended unless there are signs of infection noted. Manage pain as indicated. If there is uncertainty about the identity of the snake, contact poison control and observe for venomous symptoms for at least 3–4 hours.

If a venomous snakebite is suspected, the effects depend on the size of the child, site of the bite, type of snake, and degree of envenomation, and the treatment effectiveness. Snakebite treatment for individuals with more than local symptoms or those with suspected envenomation includes rapid transportation to a medical center, referral to appropriate medical specialists, antivenin therapy, and treatment for shock and respiratory difficulties. Up to a quarter of venomous snake bites are asymptomatic "dry" bites. Antivenom (polyvalent crotaline antivenom IV) is indicated for pit viper bites that cause systemic symptoms, coagulopathy, or progressing local injury, ideally within 6 hours of envenomation but later administration has been proven to also be therapeutic.[31]

Patient and Parent Education

Prevention of snakebites is important. Families who live or vacation in areas where pit vipers are found should be familiar with emergency snakebite first-aid, which includes[29]:

- Remove the victim from the area where the snakebite occurred staying safe as the rescuer.
- Remove jewelry, watches, or constrictive clothing from the affected extremity.
- Immobilize the affected extremity at the level of the heart initially and minimize the individual's movements.
- Consider the best position for the affected extremity to decrease systemic venom absorption and also decrease local injury. Position the victim supine.
- Do not give drugs, such as narcotics that could impair clinical evaluation.
- Cleanse the wound with soap and water.
- Do not use a tourniquet, compression dressing, or ice packs, as it may increase damage.
- Do not cut the bite area and attempt to suction out the venom.
- Transport immediately for medical evaluation ideally in a supine position.

Heat and Cold Injuries

Frostbite

Frostbite occurs when ice crystals form within the soft tissues due to cold exposure. The frozen tissue impairs circulation to the affected area and results in vasoconstriction and vaso-occlusion. This causes microvascular changes, cellular destruction, and the release of damaging inflammatory mediators. Frostbite most commonly involves distal, relatively poorly perfused regions of the body, such as fingertips, toes, earlobes, and the nose. In children, areas with poor heat-generating ability and insulation, including the cheeks and chin, are at high risk for frostbite. Any skin areas exposed to prolonged cold can be affected.

Exposure to temperatures ranging from 28.4°F to 14°F (–2°C to –10°C) can cause frostbite. The effects of cold are potentiated by factors such as exposure duration, increased wind velocity, dependency of the extremity (limb in a dependent, not elevated position), emollient application, fatigue, injury, high altitude, immobility, and general health. Exposure to very cold chemicals (e.g., liquid nitrogen or oxygen) produces instant frostbite.

Clinical Findings

History. The provider should assess the following:

- Exposure to cold temperatures
- Sensory changes (e.g., initial pain, then numbness if deeply frostbitten)
- Complaints of throbbing pain after thawing

Physical Examination. Typical initial findings include the following:

- Affected area is cold.
- Skin is red or hyperpigmented at first, then appears pale or waxy white or in individuals with darker skin becomes hypopigmented or slightly yellow or may have a bluish tint or dark pigmented tint if deeply frostbitten.
- In early stages, tissue blanches; in later stages, it feels doughy or rock hard.

The extent of tissue damage becomes apparent after rewarming. Deep frostbite occurs when tissues are icy hard and without deep tissue resilience. Deep frostbite causes the following signs and symptoms with rewarming:

- Cyanosis or mottling
- Erythema and swelling
- Numbness that evolves into complaints of burning pain
- Vesicles and bullae that appear within 24–48 hours
- Gangrene in severe frostbite.

Table 25.4 describes a four-level system to classify frostbite. This classification system is now used less frequently because it is difficult to predict the extent of tissue damage at initial presentation of injury. A simplified classification that is more common places frostbite into two categories including: superficial or mild (no loss of tissue) and deep or severe (loss of tissue).

Differential Diagnosis and Management

The differential diagnosis includes other conditions that produce similar cutaneous manifestations and injury. A history of exposure to extreme temperatures is the key to the diagnosis.

Treatment of mild frostbite includes the following:

- Cover affected area with other body surfaces and warm clothing
- Elevate the affected area if possible

TABLE 25.4	Frostbite Categories	
Category by Degree	Description	Complication
Frostnip	Redness, central pallor, edema, transient discomfort (numbness and tingling)	No tissue destruction; reversible within a few hours
Second	Notable erythema and swelling; numbness becomes burning pain in 12–24 h; bullae and vesicles form	Sensory neuropathy and cold sensitivity are residuals after healing, some soft tissue loss
Third	Hemorrhagic bullae or waxy mummified skin	Extensive tissue loss, unlikely amputation
Fourth	Involvement of full-thickness skin, muscle, tendon, bone	Amputation is likely

- Avoid pressure or any rubbing of the affected area
- Pain control as needed, preferably with NSAIDs
- *Do not apply topical dry heat*; this practice is dangerous and can cause tissue damage.

Treatment of severe frostbite requires specialist management and includes:

- Rapid rewarming procedures, pain management, medical and surgical management of tissue necrosis, infection prevention, and possible amputation
- Tetanus prophylaxis is recommended for all individuals with severe frostbite, as it is a known complication.

Patient and Parent Education

Child and parent education about frostbite prevention and initial management is important. Essential points include the following:

- Use of appropriate clothing when exposed to extreme cold temperatures
- Survival skills for travelers, hikers, or winter sports participants exposed to cold temperatures or who become lost
- Immediate rewarming of whitened or hypopigmented skin by covering with warm clothing or another body surface
- Danger of rubbing affected area with snow or ice or massaging; these practices are contraindicated because they lead to mechanical trauma.

Hypothermia

Hypothermia occurs when the body's core temperature falls below 95°F (35°C), a point where it loses its ability to generate sufficient heat to maintain bodily functions. Body heat is lost by heat radiation to nearby objects, moisture evaporation from the skin and respiratory system, heat convection from the skin's surface into cooler air, or heat conduction to objects with direct body contact. Wind, moisture, and lack of appropriate clothing or shelter exacerbate cool ambient temperatures. Although most cases are seen in winter, hypothermia can occur in other seasons during wet, windy weather. It can also occur quickly with cold-water immersion.

Children are at increased risk of hypothermia because of their relatively larger BSA, proportionately larger head, smaller body fluid volume, less developed temperature-regulating mechanisms, and decreased body fat. Children are also less able to independently leave a cold environment and are more likely to wander off from adult supervision. Those at high risk include newborns, particularly low-birth-weight or premature infants, very young children, and children who are ill, fatigued, poorly nourished, or have also experienced trauma.

Hypothermia results in cutaneous vasoconstriction and increased heat production by shivering and thyroxine releases. Hypothermia not associated with environmental exposure may be a sign of other life-threatening illnesses or injuries (e.g., malnutrition, anorexia nervosa, illness, adrenal insufficiency, hypothyroidism, hyponatremia, sepsis, central nervous system (CNS) injury or anomalies, hypoglycemia, major trauma, burns, drug overdose, medications, and NAT).[32] Secondary hypothermia is beyond the scope of this discussion.

Clinical Findings

History, Physical Examination, and Diagnostic Studies. Assess exposure to low ambient temperatures and risk factors (e.g., age, physical condition).

Signs of early- to late-stage hypothermia include:

- Decreasing body temperature
- Shivering stops in moderate hypothermia
- Pallor or blue lips and skin
- Disorientation, listlessness, sleepiness
- Decreased pulse and respiration
- Decreasing neurologic status and eventually coma and death. There are no diagnostic studies for hypothermia.

Differential Diagnosis and Management

Shock is the primary differential. For mild hypothermia [core body temperature 90°F–95°F (32°C–35°C)] remove the child from the cold environment, replace wet clothing, and provide warm liquids. Warm water baths can be effective. When the body cools and can no longer generate adequate heat, external heat sources must be provided. Use warm blankets, heat lamps, hot-water bottles, or, if none of these are available, place the child skin-to-skin in a sleeping bag or under a blanket with a person of normal body temperature. Heated humidified oxygen should be provided for all hypothermic children. Administration of warmed IV normal saline should be considered for treatment of mild hypothermia and is a necessity for treatment of moderate to severe hypothermia. Immediately refer hypothermic patients to emergency care for stabilization and treatment due to risk of cardiovascular instability and shock.

Patient and Parent Education

Instruct children, teens, and parents about the risks of hypothermia. Emphasize the need to monitor children's activities in cold weather and to provide adequate supervision and protection from exposure. The higher metabolic rate of normal, healthy children keeps them warm, and they may not feel the effects of short-term cold exposure. Thus, they may not want a jacket, sweater, hat, or mittens when their parents believe they need them. Families or teens on camping trips or traveling in uninhabited areas should have a survival kit.

Hyperthermia

Hyperthermia is a life-threatening increase in body core temperature. Heat cramps, heat exhaustion, and heatstroke are types of hyperthermia discussed in Chapter 18.

Acute Pediatric Poisoning

Poisoning occurs when a substance that interferes with normal body function is taken in by ingestion, inhalation, absorption, or injection. Poisoning generally refers to exposure and symptoms that are acute in nature. Toxic environmental exposures are more often chronic or insidious in nature (see also Chapter 3) and will be discussed later in this chapter.

Clinical Findings

History. The history often provides clues to an acute poisoning exposure. It can be as straightforward as a reported exposure, a witnessed exposure, or a parent suspecting an exposure. Some parents may be unwilling/unable to provide details or the exposure went unrecognized. The history should include:

- Circumstances surrounding the possible exposure (e.g., location, activity just before onset of symptoms, timing).
- Cosmetics, personal care products, cleaning products, analgesics, cough and cold preparations, other medications (obtain a list), topical agents, plants, herbs, pesticides, and vitamins that the child has access to. Unknown pills or chemicals may be identifiable by consultation with a regional poison control center.
- Illicit or recreational drug use in the home.

Physical Examination. Common clinical manifestations seen on physical examination of a poisoning (Box 25.2) include symptoms associated with an acute exposure. Physical examination should be tailored to exposure and condition and include neurologic examination and assessing for signs of hypoxemia.

Management and Patient/Family Education

If the history or physical examination is suspicious of either an acute or suspected chronic exposure, the PCP should call the Poison Control Center 800-222-1222 for advice while simultaneously attending to basic life support and consideration for transfer. If the individual demonstrates organ instability or failure, call 911 for rapid transfer to a tertiary care center via ambulance for further management and care.

Basic life support focuses on airway, breathing, and circulation. For the poisoned (or suspected poisoned) child, additional considerations include neurologic examination, the need for empiric treatment (if poison identified), and emergent decontamination. Administer supplemental oxygen if the patient exhibits respiratory impairment, altered mental status, and/or requires antidote therapy (e.g., naloxone for opioid poisoning). Altered mental status could be a sign that the child is unable to maintain their airway or respiratory drive on their own and needs additional respiratory support. Those with depressed mental status, diminished respirations, miotic pupils, or other concerning evidence of opioid intoxication should receive naloxone via intravenous, intramuscular, subcutaneous, or intranasal route—not oral.

Decontamination strategies vary depending on the poison and are guided by poison control centers or a toxicology team. Inducing

> ### • BOX 25.2 Clinical Manifestations of Poisoning in Children
>
> - Heart Rate: bradycardia, tachycardia
> - Respirations: bradypnea, tachypnea
> - Blood pressure: hypotension, hypertension
> - Temperature: hypothermia, hyperpyrexia (differing from hyperthermia)
> - Neurologic:
>   - Central nervous system depression, including coma
>   - Agitation
>   - Delirium/psychosis
>   - Seizures
>   - Ataxia
>   - Weakness/paralysis
>   - Tremors/myoclonus
>   - Choreoathetosis
>   - Rigidity
> - Ophthalmologic:
>   - Miosis
>   - Mydriasis
>   - Nystagmus
> - Dermatologic:
>   - Jaundice
>   - Cyanosis
>   - Pink or red
> - Odors from patient:
>   - Acetone (fruity)
>   - Bitter almond
>   - Garlic
>   - Oil of wintergreen
>   - Gasoline, turpentine, kerosene
>   - Rotten eggs

vomiting should not occur unless under the direction of poison control. General decontamination includes the following options:

- Ocular: copious saline lavage
- Skin: copious water rinse or gentle soap and water
- Gastrointestinal: dilution; gastric emptying; activated charcoal administration; catharsis; whole bowel irrigation (after consulting poison control).

Excretion of absorbed toxins can be enhanced by multidose activated charcoal, diuresis/urinary alkalization, dialysis, and hemoperfusion (similar to hemodialysis). Many antidotes and decontamination therapies require hospitalization. Referral to a mental health specialist is needed for the child or adolescent with intentional self-poisoning. Any child with concern for intentional poisoning by proxy (i.e., medical child abuse, formerly known as Munchausen syndrome by proxy) should be promptly reported to Child Protective Services.

All families should have the phone number of their local Poison Control Center posted in a prominent location (e.g., refrigerator) in their homes. Stickers with this number should be given out by PCPs as part of routine well-child care.

Common Environmental Toxins: Heavy Metals and Pesticides

Common environmental toxins including lead, mercury, arsenic, and pesticides are discussed in this section. See Chapter 3 for a general review of toxicology and known toxic and toxicant environmental hazards.

Lead

Clinical Findings

History. Every infant and child seen by a PCP should have a history taken to determine risk for lead exposure. Boxes 3.1 and 3.2 in Chapter 3 contain information regarding environmental history screening. Noteworthy risk factors include:

- The child exhibits pica.
- The child lives near a lead smelter, battery recycling plant, or industry likely to release lead.
- A family member or caregiver works with lead-based materials (e.g., welding, art materials, cosmetics, construction, boatyards).
- Household members engage in hobbies that might include ceramics, stained glass, making own fishing tackle.
- Painted or unusual materials are burned in wood stoves or fireplaces.
- Use of complementary, herbal, or folk remedies.
- Food is prepared or stored in imported pottery, metal containers, or washed in water obtained from contaminated pipes.

Physical Examination. Clinical signs of lead toxicity may not be noted during the physical examination as lead retained by the body is stored in the bones (and teeth) over time and is not measured by blood lead levels (BLLs), which more often reflect recent exposure. One child can have high BLLs (e.g., 45 mcg/dL) with no obvious clinical signs on physical examination while another may complain of severe GI problems with a lower lead level (e.g., 15–20 mcg/dL). Many children have subclinical effects or have symptoms attributed to other conditions such as anemia, constipation, abdominal pain, impaired hearing, learning disabilities, delayed growth, and/or hyperactivity. At higher levels, lead affects vitamin D metabolism, nerve conduction velocities, and hemoglobin synthesis that can lead to myocardial excitability, increased intracranial pressure, seizures, coma, and death. Many children do not demonstrate signs of acute toxicity until they have high lead levels.

Diagnostic Studies. All children at risk should be screened at 1 and 2 years of age for lead. Immigrant children or children from 3–6 years of age who have not been previously tested should also be screened. Children who have any sign of lead toxicity should be screened. If an elevated lead level is present, an assessment of free erythrocyte protoporphyrin and zinc protoporphyrin, and iron deficiency screening, including serum ferritin, are helpful in determining diagnosis and management.

Differential Diagnosis

GI infections, other causes of anemia, growth retardation, behavior disorders, attention-deficit/hyperactivity disorder (ADHD), and CNS infections should be considered in the differential diagnosis.

Management

Management involves preventing lead exposure, monitoring BLLs, correcting dietary deficiencies (if present), investigating, and removing lead (i.e., lead abatement) from the child's daily environment, and treating the child for toxicity (Table 25.5). Other children in the same household or environment where exposure could have occurred should be tested and treated as indicated.

In cases of lead toxicity (≥2 mcg/dL):
- Inform caregiver of level of toxicity.
- Provide caregiver dietary and environmental education.
- Remove child from source of lead if known.
- Report to public health department.

- Initiate environmental investigation (some health departments may do this).
- Initiate lead hazard control/abatement.
- Follow up BLL every 3 months until BLL declines.
- Refer to social services as indicated.

Chelation therapy is recommended for levels higher than 45 mcg/dL[33] to treat acute, severe, and life-threatening poisoning. It is also critical that providers do follow-up testing for children with positive lead screens until levels return to normal. Further guidance on lead poisoning treatment is available from the CDC.[33]

Patient and Parent Education

Inform parents that chelation therapy leads to a rapid fall in BLL, but most children have a rebound increase within days or weeks of treatment and repeated treatment may be necessary.

Prevention of lead poisoning is a public health responsibility, and public health officials use geographic information systems to identify high-risk areas. Population-based screening programs in Head Start classrooms can also identify prevalence of lead toxicity in children and promote early intervention programs. PCPs play a critical role in the process of preventing lead toxicity in children and should take a lead exposure history on all children and families and identify all children who need to be screened, retested, and require appropriate intervention and treatment.

Parents need to be informed that it is critical to have professional assessment of the level of home contamination and professional abatement may be necessary. Public health officials can work with parents to identify ways to control lead dust and paint chips in older homes and can work with landlords on lead abatement of properties.

Other strategies parents can use include:
- Damp-mop and damp-dust with household cleaners or lead-specific cleaning products (e.g., Ledizolv) twice weekly to decrease lead dust in the air; do not dry mop or sweep.
- Pick up and dispose of paint chips with a disposable rag or paper towel soaked in phosphate cleaner.
- Run water until temperature changes to flush pipes of lead sediment.
- Do not store or cook food in lead crystal or pottery.
- Remove work clothes/shoes and wash hands before entering home if job is lead related.

Mercury

Clinical Findings

History. The signs and symptoms of mercury poisoning are easily attributed to other processes. A careful history is essential to identify any possible exposures. Questions should focus on potential exposure (e.g., industrial exposure, mercury spills, consumer goods, and diet) and whether others in the household are experiencing similar symptoms (see Chapter 3, Boxes 3.1 and 3.2).

Physical Examination. In the case of a known or suspected mercury exposure, complete a full examination with special attention to the following systems:

- *Respiratory:* Elemental mercury vapors can cause chemical pneumonitis or necrotizing bronchitis, potentially progressing to acute respiratory distress syndrome and respiratory failure.
- *Neurologic:* Subacute exposures may cause insomnia, photophobia, decreased deep tendon reflexes, forgetfulness, loss of appetite, tremors, peripheral neuropathy, visual impairments, or behavioral changes (e.g., mood swings, nervousness, excessive shyness).

- *Skin/musculoskeletal:* Acrodynia is an idiosyncratic hypersensitivity reaction and usually occurs secondary to dermal or mucosal exposure to elemental/inorganic mercury. It is characterized by a hyperkeratotic erythematous papular often desquamating rash commonly found on the palms, soles, and face.[34] Other symptoms of acrodynia include irritability, weakness, swelling, and paresthesias.
- *GI:* Gingivostomatitis may result from chronic exposure. Acute exposure such as the ingestion of button batteries may cause corrosive gastroenteritis, hematemesis, and pain with cardiovascular collapse or renal failure.
- *Renal:* Renal tubular dysfunction and hypertension may develop.

Diagnostic Studies. Blood mercury levels can determine acute mercury exposure; however, due to mercury's half-life of 60–70 days, the result may not accurately reflect the toxicity level. A blood level of less than 10 mcg/L is considered normal, but a normal level may not exclude mercury poisoning. A 24-hour urine sample can also be collected (<20 mcg/L is considered nontoxic). Urine samples are considered more accurate in monitoring of treatment and exposure. Radiographs have also been used to aid in diagnosis. The specific type of suspected or known exposure (elemental, inorganic, or organic mercury; acute or chronic) will determine the best test, and its timing, in a specific circumstance. Poison control center personnel can assist with these determinations.

Differential Diagnosis

The differential diagnosis includes other poisonings, CNS, psychiatric conditions, or Kawasaki disease. A high level of suspicion about environmental exposures is important when evaluating any rash. A patient with neurologic symptoms, along with rash, should always be evaluated for mercury and other poisonings.

Management

The initial management is mercury source removal from the child's environment. Public health officials should investigate and determine any sources of mercury and require a hazardous materials team or Environmental Protection Agency (EPA)-certified contractor for abatement. Other children in the environment should be evaluated for possible mercury poisoning. Consult with a pediatric toxicologist and the regional poison control center or pediatric environmental health specialty unit (PEHSU) regarding patient management.

Patient and Parent Education

Education should focus on increasing awareness of sources of mercury and ways to prevent or limit exposure. Review common household items that contain mercury, such as older thermometers, healthcare supplies, antiques, and/or fluorescent light bulbs (including compact fluorescents lights). These should be recycled in accordance with local recommendations for hazardous materials. The EPA has specific instructions on how to clean up small mercury spills available at https://www.epa.gov/mercury/what-do-if-mercury-thermometer-breaks.

As with all environmental toxicants, PCPs and community activists should maintain awareness of local environmental issues (e.g., mercury emissions from industrial plants) and actively participate in legislation and regulatory efforts to decrease pollution and thus improve the health of children. The EPA and US Food and Drug Administration (FDA) have advice on fish consumption in children and women of childbearing age by promoting varieties of fish low in mercury (Box 25.3). Further information on regional varieties of fish lower in mercury can be accessed at https://www.fda.gov/media/102331/download.

Arsenic

Clinical Findings

History and Physical Examination. An exposure history is essential to determine the arsenic poisoning source and to form the differential diagnoses. Physical signs and symptoms depend on the exposure dose, route, and duration (see Box 3.1). The following symptoms and conditions can occur with arsenic poisoning:

- *Cardiovascular:* Hypotension, shock, arrhythmias, edema
- *Respiratory:* Respiratory tract irritation, pulmonary edema, bronchitis, pneumonia
- *Neurologic:* Sensorimotor peripheral axonal neuropathy, neuritis, muscle cramps, headache, weakness, lethargy, delirium, encephalopathy, hyperpyrexia, tremor, seizure, coma
- *GI and hepatic:* Garlic odor of breath, abdominal pain, nausea, vomiting, thirst, anorexia, gastroesophageal reflux, diarrhea, dysphagia, transaminitis, liver necrosis, cholangitis
- *Renal:* Hematuria, oliguria, proteinuria, uremia, tubular necrosis
- *Hematologic:* Hemolysis, anemia, leukopenia, thrombocytopenia, disseminated intravascular coagulation
- *Dermal:* Mees' lines (transverse white lines in nail beds developing weeks to months after exposure), dermatitis, melanosis or pigment changes, hyperkeratosis
- *Other:* Rhabdomyolysis, conjunctivitis

Diagnostic Studies. A 24-hour urine sample is the most accurate measurement of arsenic levels. Any random arsenic urine concentration levels greater than 50 mcg/L should be further tested with a 24-hour arsenic urine concentration level.[34] If the arsenic concentration level remains elevated, consult with a pediatric toxicologist to determine if exposure warrants laboratory evaluation and treatment. Serum levels can also be measured but are less accurate because the half-life is very short.

Management

Minimizing exposure by identifying and removing the arsenic source is of utmost importance. For severe exposures, acute stabilization with gut decontamination (e.g., activated charcoal, gastric lavage) or chelation may be necessary. Monitor renal and hematologic function acutely and on follow-up. Treatment should be in consultation with a pediatric toxicologist.

Patient and Parent Education

Parents and PCPs can work with schools and communities to assess for and manage arsenic contamination of play structures. Test water supplies that are suspected to be contaminated. Bottled water, distilled water, or home treatment units that remove arsenic should be used if drinking water is contaminated. Healthcare providers should support regulatory standards for the production and use of arsenic-containing products to ensure protection of children's health.

Pesticides

Clinical Findings

Adverse effects of pesticide exposure can be acute or chronic and can affect all body systems, depending on the nature of the toxin and the extent of exposure. In acute exposure, assessment is the same

TABLE 25.5	Management Recommendations for Lead Poisoning[a]

Screening Sample: Blood Lead Levels	Action to Be Taken	Follow-up Blood Lead Levels Monitoring
<3.5 mcg/dL	Not considered lead poisoning: • Provide caregiver/parent dietary and environmental education regarding lead • Assess development, and dietary intake especially iron and calcium • Iron deficiency increases ingested lead absorption • Conduct a history of the family and child's environment (include parent occupation due to potential to bring lead exposure into the home) to determine if child is exposed to a lead source (e.g., pre-1978 housing) • Provide appropriate resources such as Social Services, Women, Infants and Children (WIC), Department of Housing and Urban Development (HUD), or Pediatric Environmental Heath Specialty Units (PEHSU)	• Medicaid/Medicare patient retest guidelines: 12 and 24 months of age; 24–72 months without a history of previous screening • Non-Medicare/Medicaid patient retest guidelines: ongoing monitoring for changes in environment and intervention/testing as needed

≤3.5–19 mcg/dL	• Obtain confirmatory venous level only if screening level was not venous (BLL 3.5–9 mg/dL; within 3 months), BLL 10–19 mcg/dL; within 1 month)
	• Report results to Health Department
	• Help arrange a home environmental investigation through the Department of Housing and Urban Development (HUD)
	• Follow actions listed for BLL <3.5 mcg/dL
	• Evaluate for iron deficiency
		• Early follow-up (two to four tests):
		  • For BLL 3.5–9 mcg/dL; 3 months
		  • For BLL 10–19 mcg/dL; 1–3 months
		• Later follow-up (after BLLs decline):
		  • For BLL 3.5–9 mcg/dL; 6–9 months
		  • For BLL 10–19 mcg/dL; 3–6 months

20–44 mcg/dL	• Confirmatory venous blood test if screening level was not venous within 2 weeks • Follow recommendations for BLL <3.5–19 mcg/dL • Consider obtaining abdominal radiograph to evaluate for chips of lead-based paint or radiopaque foreign bodies • Obtain complete history and physical with emphasis on etiology of lead exposure • Consult with PEHSU and or Poison Control Center for further management (bowel decontamination may be needed	• Early follow-up (two to four tests): 2 weeks–1 month • Later follow-up (after BLLs decline); 1–3 months
≥45 mcg/dL	• Confirmatory venous blood test if screening level was not venous within 48 hours • Follow recommendations for BLL <3.5–44 mcg/dL • Perform complete history and physical with thorough neurologic exam • Obtain abdominal radiograph, if needed • Initiate bowel decontamination • Obtain prechelation laboratory studies including: complete blood count, electrolytes, BUN, creatinine, liver transaminase enzyme levels, and a urinalysis • Consider admission to hospital if unable to find a lead safe living environment for the child, if the lead exposure is still possible, or if the source of lead exposure is not known • Hospitalize immediately for signs of lead toxicity: abdominal pain, nausea, confusion, weakness, coma and or seizures • Consult a medical toxicologist for further management, which usually includes gastrointestinal decontamination and or chelation therapy • Contact Poison Control Center (1-800-222-1222) or PEHSU	• Follow-up BLLs are recommended as soon as possible

BLL, Blood lead level.

[a]Child has risk factors from screening criteria and/or there are no local or state guidelines on when to screen for lead levels.

Data from Centers for Disease Control and Prevention. Recommended actions based on blood lead level: summary of recommendations for follow-up and case management for children. https://www.cdc.gov/nceh/lead/advisory/acclpp/actions-blls.htm?CDC_AA_refVal=https%3A%2F%2Fwww.cdc.gov%2Fnceh%2Flead%2Facclpp%2Factions_blls.html; and Pediatric Environmental Health Specialty Units. Recommendations on Management of Childhood Lead Exposure: A Resource for Clinicians; 2021. https://www.pehsu.net/_Library/facts/PEHSU_Fact_Sheet_Lead_Management_Health_Professionals_9_2021.pdf.

as with general poisoning. Acute poisoning with organophosphates or carbamates results in clinical signs of cholinergic excess (e.g., tearing, salivation, bronchospasm, urination/incontinence, emesis, diarrhea, diaphoresis). Neurologic disorders may become apparent 24–96 hours after exposure and delayed neurotoxicity may occur weeks after exposure. Nephrotoxicity has also been reported.

Management

Specifics of exposure management depend on the type of pesticide, the amount, patient symptoms, and route of exposure. Information on ingredients and immediate treatment is generally available on product labels. Patients/parents may be able to provide the clinician with the pesticide label. When treating an individual who may have been exposed to pesticides, information about the implicated pesticides is available from the National Pesticide Information Center (http://npic.orst.edu/). The EPA's Worker Protection Standard (WPS) requires workers access to information on all pesticides currently in use. Under the WPS, this information can be obtained from employers or manufacturers usually in the form of a safety data sheet.[35] Treatment focuses on basic life support (as necessary) and the following:

- Antidote therapy (depends on the specific pesticide)
- Decontamination (e.g., remove patient's clothes; wash skin; gastric decontamination as indicated). Note that pesticides may penetrate standard healthcare personnel gloves; special protective gear may be required.
- Consultation with a poison control center (acute) and/or PEHSU (acute or chronic)
- Seizure control
- Report pesticide exposure to the local and state health department

Patient and Parent Education

The risks pesticides present to children are significant in short- and long-term health outcomes, and acute or chronic exposure to pesticides may occur in unanticipated ways. Because exposures are additive, patterns of multiple contaminations must be recognized and a plan to regulate overall exposure developed. Families can choose foods that are local, in season, and organically grown as much as possible (see Chapter 3). Not all foods labeled as organic are the same; check US Department of Agriculture labels, which include "100% organic," "organic" (i.e., at least 95% organic content), "made with organic" (i.e., 70% organic content for up to three ingredients), and "organic components" (i.e., products with <70% organic content). Organic foods are often more expensive than conventional foods, thus income disparities and environmental justice issues are important considerations. Regulation of pesticide use on foods should be considered to provide all children with safe foods and produce. Families should be advised to buy organic foods or pesticide-free foods whenever possible, until improved agricultural regulations are in place to decrease pesticide content.

Education and awareness are key to preventing pesticide poisoning in children. Steps can be taken to reduce or eliminate pesticide use, which in turn reduces exposure. Integrated pest management (IPM) combines physical, cultural, biologic, and other means of pest control without use of or with minimal use of pesticides timed to limit exposures. IPM is a coordinated use of pest and environmental information to prevent unacceptable levels of pest damage by the most economical means with the least possible hazard to people, property, and the environment.[36] This involves pest prevention and nonchemical management methods as first-line measures. Some examples of IPM include using cats by farmers to catch mice rather than using rodenticides, using bait traps for cockroaches rather than chemical sprays (in schools and homes), using boiling water to kill weeds, and caulking cracks in walls to prevent pest entry.

Additional Resources

Advice about Eating Fish: For Those Who Might Become or Are Pregnant or Breastfeeding and Children Ages 1-11 Years: https://www.fda.gov/food/consumers/advice-about-eating-fish

American Association of Poison Control Centers (Poison Control Center): www.aapcc.org/; (800-222-1222 for 24/7 hotline)

American Burn Association: www.ameriburn.org

Asbestos: OSHA Standards. https://www.osha.gov/SLTC/asbestos/standards.html

Pediatric Environmental Health Specialty Units (PEHSU) Recommendations on Management of Childhood Lead Exposure: A Resource for Clinicians: https://www.pehsu.net/_Library/facts/PEHSU_Fact_Sheet_Lead_Management_Health_Professionals_9_2021.pdf

Sage II Burn Diagramming: www.SageDiagram.com (free calculator to estimate BSA and fluid resuscitation requirements)

References

1. Centers for Disease Control and Prevention. *Injury Prevention & Control: WISQARS Injury Data*; 2021. https://www.cdc.gov/injury/wisqars/.

2. Chiesa A, Sirotnak AP. Child abuse & neglect. In: Hay WW, Levin MJ, Abzug MJ, Bunik M, eds. *Current Diagnosis & Treatment: Pediatrics*. 25th ed. McGraw-Hill; 2020:208–216.

3. Baddour LM, Brown AM. In: Post T, ed. *Infectious Complications of Puncture Wounds*. UpToDate; 2020. https://www.uptodate.com/contents/infectious-complications-of-puncture-wounds?search=infectious%20complications%20of%20puncture%20wounds&source=search_result&selectedTitle=1~88&usage_type=default&display_rank=1.

4. Chorley J. In: Post T, ed. *Forefoot and Midfoot Pain in the Active Child or Skeletally Immature Adolescent: Overview of Causes*. UpToDate; 2020. https://www.uptodate.com/contents/forefoot-and-midfoot-pain-in-the-active-child-or-skeletally-immature-adolescent-overview-of-causes?search=forefoot%20and%20midfoot%20pain%20in%20the%20active&source=search_result&selectedTitle=1. ~. 150&usage_type=default&display_rank=1.

5. Rhodes JT, Tagawa A, Niswander C, Comer W, Erickson MA, De S. Orthopedics. In: Hay WW, Levin MJ, Abzug MH, Bunik M, eds. *Current Diagnosis & Treatment: Pediatrics*. 25th ed. McGraw-Hill; 2020:811–836.

6. Baddour LM, Harper M a. In: Post T, ed. *Animal Bites (Dogs, Cats, and Other Animals): Evaluation and Management*. UpToDate; 2021a. https://www.uptodate.com/contents/animal-bites-dogs-cats-and-other-animals-evaluation-and-management?search=human%20bites&source=search_result&selectedTitle=5~90&usage_type=default&display_rank=6.

7. Armstrong DG, Meyr AJ. In: Post T, ed. *Basic Principles of Wound Management*. UpToDate; 2021. https://www.uptodate.com/contents/basic-principles-of-wound-management?search=clinical%20manifestations%20and%20initial%20management%20of%20animal%20and%20human%20bites&topicRef=7674&source=see_link#H55268712.

8. Hollander JE. In: Post T, ed. *Assessment and Management of Facial Lacerations*. UpToDate; 2021. https://www.uptodate.com/contents/assessment-and-management-of-facial-lacerations?search=animal%20bies&topicRef=7671&source=see_link.

9. Cho CS. Minor trauma. In: Shaw KN, Bachur RG, Chamberlain JM, Lavelle J, Nagler J, Shook JE, eds. *Fleisher and Ludwig's Textbook of Pediatric Emergency Medicine.* 8th ed. Wolters Kluwer; 2021:1153–1169.

10. Rice PL, Orgill DP. In: Post T, ed. *Assessment and Classification of Burn Injury.* UpToDate; 2020. https://www.uptodate.com/contents/classification-of-burn-injury?search=classification%20of%20burns&source=search_result&selectedTitle=1~24&usage_type=default&display_rank=1.

11. Antoon AY, Donovan MK. Burn injuries. In: Kliegman RM, St. Geme J, Blum NJ, et al., eds. *Nelson's Textbook of Pediatrics.* 21st ed. Elsevier; 2020:614–623.e1.

12. Micak RP. In: Post T, ed. *Inhalation Injury from Heat, Smoke or Chemical Irritants.* UpToDate; 2022. https://www.uptodate.com/contents/inhalation-injury-from-heat-smoke-or-chemical-irritants?search=inhalation%20injury%20from%20heat&source=search_result&selectedTitle=1~150&usage_type=default&display_rank=1.

13. Chilukuri N. Traumatic injuries. In: Kleiman K, Mcdaniel L, Molloy M, eds. *The Harriet Lane Handbook.* 22nd ed. Elsevier; 2021:33–51.e3.

14. Orsborn J, Braund C. Emergencies and injuries. In: Hay WW, Levin MJ, Abzug MJ, Bunik M, eds. *Current Diagnosis & Treatment: Pediatrics.* 25th ed. McGraw-Hill; 2020:305–327.

15. Karlin AM, Goyeneche NP, Murphy KP. Management of musculoskeletal injury. In: Kliegman RM, St. Geme J, Blum NJ, et al., eds. *Nelson's Textbook of Pediatrics.* 21st ed. Elsevier; 2020:3685–3700.e1.

16. Bula-Rudas FJ, Olcott JL. Human and animal bites. *Pediatr Rev.* 2018;39(10):490–500.

17. American Academy of Pediatrics (AAP). Bite wounds. In: Kimberlin DW, Barnett ED, Lynfield R, Sawyer MH, eds. *Red Book: 2021 Report of the Committee on Infectious Diseases.* AAP; 2021:169–175.

18. Hunstad DA. Animal and human bites. In: Kliegman RM, St. Geme J, Blum NJ, et al., eds. *Nelson's Textbook of Pediatrics.* 21st ed. Elsevier; 2020:3816–3819.e1.

19. Koutroulis I, Argawal D. Environmental emergencies, radiological emergencies, bites and stings. In: Shaw KN, Bachur RG, Chamberlain JM, Lavelle J, Nagler J, Shook JE, eds. *Fleisher and Ludwig's Textbook of Pediatric Emergency Medicine.* 8th ed. Wolters Kluwer; 2021:680–723.

20. Golden DBK. Insect allergy. In: Burks AW, Holgate ST, O'Hehir RE, et al., eds. *Middleton's Allergy Principles and Practice.* 9th ed. Elsevier; 2020:1247–1260.e1.

21. Cardana V, Ansotegui IJ, Ebisawa M, El-Gamal Y, et al. World allergy organization anaphylaxis guidance 2020. *World Allergy Organ J.* 2020;13(10).

22. Otten EJ. Venomous animal injuries. In: Walls RM, Hockberger RS, Gausche-Hill M, eds. *Rosen's Emergency Medicine Concepts and Clinical Practice.* 9th ed. Elsevier; 2017:698–714.

23. LoVecchio F. In: Post T, ed. *Scorpion Envenomation Causing Neuromuscular Toxicity (United States, Mexico, Central America, and Southern Africa).* UpToDate; 2022. https://www.uptodate.com/contents/scorpion-envenomation-causing-neuromuscular-toxicity-united-states-mexico-central-america-and-southern-africa?search=scorpion%20envenomation&source=search_result&selectedTitle=1~9&usage_type=default&display_rank=1.

24. Mayo Clinci. Scorpion sting. www.mayoclinic.org/diseases-conditions/scorpion-stings/basics/causes/con-20033894?p=1

25. Swanson DL, Vetter RS, White J. In: Post T, ed. *Clinical Manifestations and Diagnosis of Widow Spider Bites.* UpToDate; 2021. https://www.uptodate.com/contents/clinical-manifestations-and-diagnosis-of-widow-spider-bites?search=clinical%20manifestations%20and%20diagnosis%20of%20widow%20spider%20bites&source=search_result&selectedTitle=1~150&usage_type=default&display_rank=1.

26. Vetter RS, Swanson DL. In: Post T, ed. *Bites of Recluse Spiders.* UpToDate; 2020. https://www.uptodate.com/contents/bites-of-recluse-spiders?search=bites%20of%20recluse%20spiders&source=search_result&selectedTitle=1~150&usage_type=default&display_rank=1.

27. Vetter RS, Swanson DL, White J. In: Post T, ed. *Management of Widow Spider Bites.* UpToDate; 2021. https://www.uptodate.com/contents/management-of-widow-spider-bites?search=management%20of%20widow%20spider%20bites&source=search_result&selectedTitle=1~150&usage_type=default&display_rank=1.

28. White J. In: Post T, ed. *Snakebites Worldwide. Clinical Manifestations and Diagnosis.* UpToDate; 2020. https://www.uptodate.com/contents/snakebites-worldwide-clinical-manifestations-and-diagnosis?search=snakebites%20worldwide:%20clinical%20manife&source=search_result&selectedTitle=1~150&usage_type=default&display_rank=1.

29. Seifert SA. In: Post T, ed. *Bites by Crotalinae Snakes (Rattlesnake, Water Moccasins [cottonmouths], or Copperheads) in the United States: Clinical Manifestations, Evaluation, and Diagnosis.* UpToDate; 2020. https://www.uptodate.com/contents/bites-by-crotalinae-snakes-rattlesnakes-water-moccasins-cottonmouths-or-copperheads-in-the-united-states-clinical-manifestations-evaluation-and-diagnosis?search=bites%20by%20crotalinae&topicRef=121865&source=see_link#H3.

30. Seifert SA. In: Post T, ed. *Bites by Crotalinae Snakes (Rattlesnakes, Water Moccasins [cottonmouths], or Copperheads) in the United States: Management.* UpToDate; 2021. https://www.uptodate.com/contents/bites-by-crotalinae-snakes-rattlesnakes-water-moccasins-cottonmouths-or-copperheads-in-the-united-states-management?search=bites%20by%20crotalinae&topicRef=6595&source=see_link#H377516135.

31. Wang GS, Rumack BH, Dart RC. Poisoning. In: Hay WW, Levin MJ, Abzug MJ, et al., eds. *Current Diagnosis & Treatment: Pediatrics.* 25th ed. New York: McGraw-Hill; 2020:328–356.

32. Corneli HM, Kadish H. In: Post T, ed. *Hypothermia in Children: Clinical Manifestations and Diagnosis.* UpToDate; 2021. https://www.uptodate.com/contents/hypothermia-in-children-clinical-manifestations-and-diagnosis?search=hypothermia%20in%20chidlren:%20clinical%20manifestations%20and%20diagnosis&source=search_result&selectedTitle=1~150&usage_type=default&display_rank=1.

33. Centers for Disease Control and Prevention. Recommended actions based on blood lead level: summary of recommendations for follow-up and case management for children. https://www.cdc.gov/nceh/lead/advisory/acclpp/actions-blls.htm?CDC_AA_refVal=https%3A%2F%2Fwww.cdc.gov%2Fnceh%2Flead%2Faccloppp%2Factions_blls.html

34. Kao LW. Chronic poisoning: trace metals and others. In: Goldman L, Schafer A, eds. *Goldman-Cecil Medicine.* 26th ed. Elsevier; 2020:87–93.e2.

35. Environmental Protection Agency. *Pesticides; Agricultural Worker protection Standard Revisions*; 2015. https://www.federalregister.gov/documents/2015/11/02/2015-25970/pesticides-agricultural-worker-protection-standard-revisions.

36. Environmental Protection Agency. *About Pesticide Registration.* https://www.epa.gov/pesticide-registration/about-pesticide-registration.

26

Pediatric Palliative Care

DEANNA SCHNEIDER

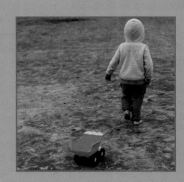

The word *palliate* comes from the Latin *pallium,* the cloak garment worn by ancient Romans. Palliative care is, at its simplest, an approach to care that cloaks the many objective and subjective symptoms of illness. The World Health Organization (WHO) defines palliative care as "an approach that improves the quality of life of patients (adults and children) and their families who are facing problems associated with life-threatening illness. It prevents and relieves suffering through the early identification, correct assessment, and treatment of pain and other problems whether physical, psychosocial, or spiritual."[1] The WHO first defined pediatric palliative care (PPC) in 1998 as "the active total care of the child's mind, body and spirit, which also involves giving support to the family."[2] The defining principles of palliative care are found in Box 26.1.[3]

PPC is a comprehensive approach that is a vital component of patient- and family-centered care. Quality palliative care can be delivered from the time of diagnosis with a serious illness, during the illness course, at the end of life, and through family bereavement. While it is typically provided to those with a serious illness, the principles of care can be applied to any patient. PPC can be provided at any age, including prenatally,[4] and in any setting—hospital, outpatient clinic, hospice center, long-term care facility, private residence, and homeless shelter, among others. All members of the care team can provide PPC, regardless of site or field of practice.[4] Fig. 26.1 describes the components of palliative services care that providers can deliver across the care continuum.

The American Academy of Pediatrics (AAP) has long noted the importance of the medical home in patient- and family-centered care[5] and the role for pediatric providers in the provision of palliative care. In 2003 the Institute of Medicine (now known as the National Academy of Medicine) issued a seminal report, *When Children Die: Improving Palliative and End-of-Life Care for Children and their Families*, noting the important role the medical home and all pediatric healthcare providers play in ensuring children receive comprehensive care and relief from all forms of suffering throughout their illness course.[6] Furthermore, the National Academy of Medicine, in their 2015 report *Dying in America,* noted that many of the palliative care needs of patients can and must be addressed by front-line providers.[7] Pediatric primary care providers (PCPs) are in a unique position to combine the strength of their medical home relationship and front-line provider role with the tenets of palliative care to provide high-quality, compassionate, comprehensive care to all patients and families.

Levels of Palliative Care

Not every patient needs the full scope of intensive, expert-level palliative care. Palliative care can be defined along two tiers: primary and specialty.[8] Primary PPC is delivered by all clinicians, regardless of diagnosis, including basic symptom management; effective communication; psychosocial, emotional, and spiritual support; and engaging in shared decision-making. Specialty PPC involves care delivered by clinicians trained in the specialty of hospice and palliative care. They collaborate with the primary team to assist in treatment of complex physical, psychological, social, and spiritual symptoms. Specialty PPC providers are experts in managing refractory symptoms, complex family situations, and circumstances that are unclear or where conflict exists. Hospice care is often confused with specialty PPC; however, hospice care is provided at the end-of-life with a focus on treating the symptoms the patient may be experiencing, not curing the underlying illness. End-of-life care is a component of the expertise of specialty PPC providers, but primary PPC providers may also be involved in providing end-of-life hospice care.[9] Palliative care can be part of the care plan at any time alongside illness-directed therapies.[10]

Interdisciplinary Team

Fundamentally, the practice of palliative care is interdisciplinary; caring for mind, body, spirit, and family requires a team of people. Interdisciplinary care of the patient and family requires the collaboration over time by healthcare professionals with a variety of backgrounds. Box 26.2 lists some of the common members of the interdisciplinary team. Teams vary depending on available resources; however, the role of this group is to collectively accompany and support the patient and family throughout illness, death, and bereavement. The National Coalition of Hospice and Palliative Care Guidelines for Quality Care specify the essentials for provision of quality palliative care; this includes the team meeting regularly to discuss patient care and the functioning of the team.[4] PCPs are essential members of the interdisciplinary team. Both the AAP[11] and National Association of Pediatric Nurse Practitioners (NAPNAP)[12] have endorsed the use of these guidelines for the care of children and families.

The tenets of palliative care are founded in nursing practice. The modern hospice movement began with the founding of St. Christopher's Hospice in the United Kington in 1967 by Dame Cicely Saunders, who was trained as a registered nurse, social worker, and physician.[13] Nurse practitioners are uniquely positioned to not

• BOX 26.1 Principles of Palliative Care

Palliative care is care that:
- Considers the child/patient and family as the center of the unit of care
- Provides relief from pain and other distressing symptoms
- Affirms life and regards dying as a normal process
- Intends neither to hasten or postpone death
- Integrates the psychological and spiritual aspects of patient care
- Offers a support system to help patients live as actively as possible until death
- Offers a support system to help the family cope during the patient's illness and in their own bereavement
- Uses a team approach to address the needs of patients and their families, including bereavement counseling, if indicated
- Aims to enhance quality of life and may also positively influence the course of illness; is applicable early in the course of illness, in conjunction with other therapies that are intended to prolong life, and includes those investigations needed to better understand and manage distressing clinical complications

The WHO's definition of palliative care for children is care that:
- Involves active total care of the child's body, mind, and spirit and also involves giving support to the family
- Begins when illness is diagnosed and continues regardless of whether or not a child receives treatment directed at the disease
- Requires healthcare providers to evaluate and alleviate a child's physical, psychological, and social distress
- Requires a broad interdisciplinary approach, one that includes the family and makes use of available community resources; it can be successfully implemented even if resources are limited
- Can be provided in tertiary care facilities, in community health and hospice centers, and in children's homes
- Should be developmentally appropriate and in accordance with family values

Modified from Wolfe J, Hinds PS, Sourkes BM. The language of pediatric palliative care. In: Wolfe J, Hinds PS, Sourkes BM, eds. *Interdisciplinary Pediatric Palliative Care.* ed 2. Oxford University Press; 2022; and World Health Organization. I*ntegrating Palliative Care and Symptom Relief into Paediatrics: A Who Guide for Health Care Planners, Implementers and Managers.* WHO; 2018.

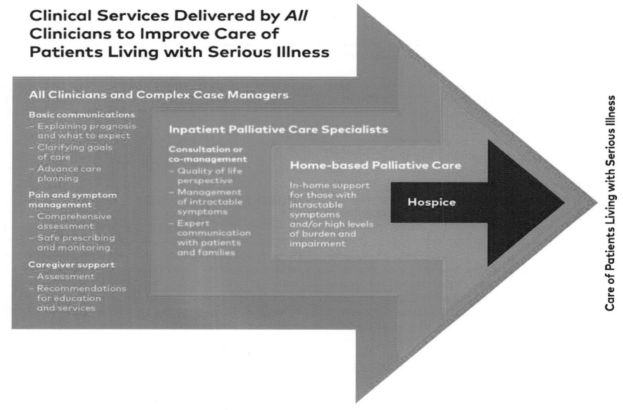

• **Fig. 26.1** Palliative Care Components Delivered Across the Care Continuum. (From Center to Advance Palliative Care: Improving value in a large health system by transforming the care of people living with serious illness: a case study from Trinity Health System. https://www.capc.org/documents/download/655/.)

only be active contributors to the interdisciplinary team, but leaders who are able to combine their foundation in nursing with their skills of advanced practice to ensure excellence in pediatric palliative clinical care, education, administration, policy, research, and social justice advocacy for patients, families, and the profession.[14]

Epidemiology of Pediatric Palliative Care

Each year, approximately 45,000 infants, children, and adolescents die in the United States. They represent an important population when it comes to evaluating how palliative care services

BOX 26.2 Common Interdisciplinary Team Members

- Nurses, both primary and specialty
- Nurse practitioners, both primary and specialty
- Physicians, both primary and specialty
- Nurse coordinators, case managers
- Social workers
- Chaplains
- Pharmacists
- Child life specialists
- Nutritionists
- Therapists: physical, occupational, speech, respiratory, massage
- Expressive art therapists: art, music, dance, animal/pet
- Integrative medicine practitioners: reiki, acupuncture, aromatherapy
- Community health workers: emergency medical technicians, paramedics
- Bereavement coordinators
- Psychologists
- Teachers
- Community members: coaches, volunteers, school communities

Modified from National Consensus Project for Quality Palliative Care. *Clinical Practice Guidelines for Quality Palliative Care.* 4th ed. National Coalition for Hospice and Palliative Care; 2018; and Battista V, LaRagione G. Pediatric hospice and palliative care. In: Ferrell BR, Paice JA, eds. *Oxford Textbook of Palliative Nursing.* Oxford University Press; 2019.

can be used to improve healthcare and quality of life for children and families. The majority of pediatric deaths occur within the first year of life, and many of those are within the first hours of life.[7] Beyond the first year, children between the ages of 1 and 19 years are most likely to die from unintentional injury, followed by malignancy, and congenital/chromosomal conditions. A distinction can be made between the children whose deaths arose from sudden injuries or were unforeseeable from those children with chronic conditions and whose deaths were expected. While there is still a role for PPC in situation of unforeseeable deaths, particularly in bereavement services, those with anticipated deaths provide an opportunity for PPC services to be of significant benefit.[7]

Finding reliable statistics for the number children in the United States with conditions warranting palliative care is difficult. Foremost, there is no uniform definition of which conditions warrant palliative care because conditions can vary related to the patient's subjective experience of suffering.[7] In addition, it is difficult to parse out the many conditions with anticipated death due to the diversity of illnesses, challenges of prognostication, the use of variable definitions and terminology, and complex datasets.[15] This has made reliable statistical analysis challenging.

The most thorough epidemiologic study of pediatric palliative and end-of-life care was reported in *Dying in America* and revealed that[7]:

- Children with complex chronic conditions (i.e., conditions that are likely to last longer than 6 months unless death occurs, require care by pediatric subspecialists and often time in the hospital) are most likely to have neonatal diagnoses, followed by cardiovascular and neurologic conditions, and then malignancies.
- Children with multiple complex chronic conditions (i.e., one complex chronic condition as defined earlier) have a heightened risk of readmission, extensive healthcare use, and death.
- Most children, including those with unforeseeable deaths, die in the hospital.

- Compared to previous years, there was an increase in proportion of children with complex, chronic conditions dying at home, underscoring the importance of community resources, including hospice.

The 2019 Center to Advance Palliative Care's report of pediatric hospice and palliative care patients found approximately 41% of patients were aged 1 year or younger, 25.6% were between 2 and 17 years of age, and 13.4% were over 18 years of age. The top diagnosis seen was cancer followed by prematurity, neurologic conditions, congenital disorders, and children with complex chronic conditions.[16]

Role of the Primary Care Provider in Holistic Care

Referral

While the tenets of palliative care can be applied to any patient interaction, certain populations may benefit most from a comprehensive, palliative approach (Table 26.1). Illness trajectories in children are varied and often unpredictable (Fig. 26.2). Children with complex, chronic conditions in particular benefit from integration of palliative care early in their course of care. PCPs play an essential role in identifying these children, integrating primary PPC practices into their care plans, and referring to specialty PPC providers as appropriate.

TABLE 26.1 Conditions That Benefit From Pediatric Palliative Care

Condition	Examples
Cure is possible, but may not succeed	• Cancer, especially with poor prognosis • Irreversible organ failure • Complex or severe congenital or acquired heart disease
Intensive treatment is available to prolong and maintain quality of life, but premature death is still possible	• Cystic fibrosis • Severe immunodeficiency • High-risk solid-organ transplant • Chronic or severe respiratory failure • Muscular dystrophy, severe and progressive neuromuscular diseases • Complex congenital syndromes • Severe chromosomal disorders
Progressive conditions with no curative options where treatment after diagnosis is almost exclusively palliative	• Progressive metabolic disorders (e.g., Tay-Sachs disease) • Batten disease • Severe forms of osteogenesis imperfecta
Conditions involving severe, nonprogressive disability resulting in extreme vulnerability to health complications	• Severe cerebral palsy with recurrent infection or difficult-to-control symptoms • Severe neurologic sequelae of infectious disease • Hypoxic or anoxic brain injury • Brain malformations (e.g., holoprosencephaly, lissencephaly)

Modified from The Together for Short Lives (formerly the Association for Children's Palliative Care [ACT]) Life-limiting/Life-threatening Condition Categories: http://www.togetherforshortlives.org.uk/professionals/childrens_palliative_care_essentials/approach; and Harrop E, Edwards C. How and when to refer a child for specialist paediatric palliative care. *Arch Dis Child Educ Pract Ed.* 2013;98(6):202–208.

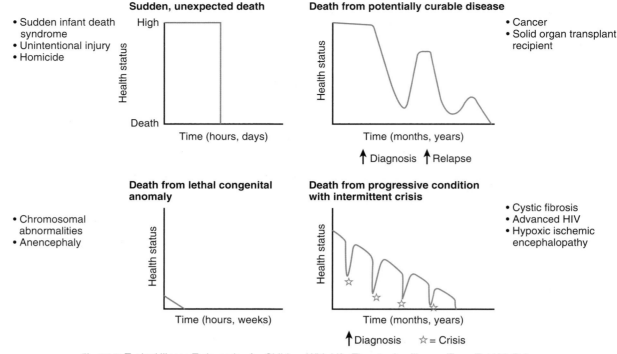

Sudden, unexpected death

- Sudden infant death syndrome
- Unintentional injury
- Homicide

Time (hours, days)

Death from potentially curable disease

- Cancer
- Solid organ transplant recipient

Time (months, years)

↑ Diagnosis ↑ Relapse

Death from lethal congenital anomaly

- Chromosomal abnormalities
- Anencephaly

Time (hours, weeks)

Death from progressive condition with intermittent crisis

- Cystic fibrosis
- Advanced HIV
- Hypoxic ischemic encephalopathy

Time (months, years)

↑ Diagnosis ☆ = Crisis

• **Fig. 26.2** Typical Illness Trajectories for Children With Life-Threatening Illness. (From Field M, Behrman R, editors. *When Children Die: Improving Palliative and End-of-Life Care for Children and Their Families.* National Academies Press; 2003:74.)

• BOX 26.3 Situations When Referral to Pediatric Palliative Care Specialists May Be Warranted

- Symptoms of distress (physical, emotional, social, spiritual) are complex and/or difficult to control
- Life-sustaining therapies are required
- Care is being transitioned to a focus on comfort and/or in the home
- Discontinuation of nonbeneficial life-sustaining therapies is being discussed
- End-of-life care is warranted
- Family situation is complex
- There is conflict within the family or medical team
- Healthcare team in need of support

Modified from Sreedhar SS, Kraft C, Friebert S. Primary palliative care: skills for all clinicians. *Curr Prob Pediatr Adolesc Health Care.* 2020;50(6):100814; Moore D, Sheetz J. Pediatric palliative care consultation. *Pediatr Clin North Am.* 2014;61(4):735-747; and Feudtner C, Kang TI, Hexem KR, et al. Pediatric palliative care patients: a prospective multicenter cohort study. *Pediatrics.* 2011;127(6):1094-1101.

Timely referral for PPC services is critical. Referral can occur at any point in the disease process, as early as diagnosis, and should be used throughout illness course to support the patient and family. PPC services should not be restricted to those with a terminal prognosis and can be implemented when goals of care and treatments are focused on cure.[17,18] Box 26.3 denotes situations where referral to PPC specialists may be warranted. In addition, facilitating communication and/or providing decision-making support is a frequent reason for consultation with a PPC specialist.[10] Screening tools are available to assist clinicians in evaluating the palliative care needs of pediatric patients and their families. These help PCPs in identifying and referring patients and families for PPC services.

Communication

Effective communication is essential to forming trusting relationships, facilitating decision-making, and enhancing quality of life. The true heart of palliative care is effective, collaborative, and compassionate communication within a trusting relationship between the patient, family, and care team. This lays the foundation for managing symptoms, assisting with decision-making, supporting care logistics, and providing truly holistic supportive care (Fig. 26.3).[19] PCPs, pediatric providers in particular, possess many of the communication skills necessary for providing effective palliative care. They can build trusting, long-term, collaborative relationships with patients and families, engage in shared decision-making, and provide individualized care to patients and families across a variety of settings. These skills are not only the foundations of family-centered pediatric practice and the medical home model, but also the foundations of palliative care.

The AAP defines the Pediatric Medical Home as being "accessible, family-centered, continuous, comprehensive, coordinated, compassionate, and culturally effective."[20] As the "hub" of the medical home, the PCP has an established relationship with the patient and family. The PCP's understanding of the patient and family's communication preferences, cultural practices, social background, education, spiritual practices, community involvement, and available sources of support lays the foundation for the provision of PPC. Sensitivity about these factors is critical for pediatric providers engaging in shared decision-making and discussions surrounding goals of care.[21] The partnership of the medical home and PPC is especially integral to the care of children with complex or chronic illness. In addition, in the face of a new diagnosis, patients and families rely on strong connections with their PCPs who can act as a trusted resource, source of support, and guide in a new and unfamiliar world of chronic illness.[10]

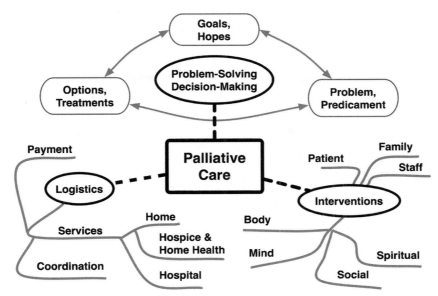

• **Fig. 26.3** Collaborative Communication in Pediatric Palliative Care. (From Feudtner C. Collaborative communication in pediatric palliative care: a foundation for problem-solving and decision-making. *Pediatr Clin North Am.* 2007;54[5]:583-607.)

PCPs should be comfortable ensuring patients and families understand the child's illness, its trajectory, and prognosis. They should be able to provide anticipatory guidance and acknowledge uncertainty when prognosis is unclear.[8,22]

Trusting relationships with medical providers are key, particularly when it comes to making decisions around goals of care. PCPs are ideally suited to ascertain patient's and family's goals and use that information to provide treatment options, discuss risks and benefits of those options, and help patients and families make decisions regarding care.[22] A variety of circumstances should prompt the clinician to consider discussing goals of care (Table 26.2). This discussion should not be considered a "one-and-done," but instead an ongoing conversation with points for "regoaling" to adjust the plans as clinical situations change.[23] Families should be given proper anticipatory guidance regarding the typical trajectory of illness and time to weigh the risks and benefits of certain interventions with relation to the child's quality of life and family values.[24] While these discussions can involve decisions surrounding end-of-life care, those decisions are not necessarily the ultimate goal. The aim of these conversations should be aligning the family's hopes and goals for their child in the context of their family with the medical care decisions.[10]

When discussions surrounding goals of care involve formalized end-of-life care decisions, this is considered advance care planning (ACP). For children with life-limiting illness it is best to have these conversations outside of crisis situations to allow the patient and caregivers time to think, reflect, and not make decisions under stress. While any member of the team can engage in the discussion, the clinician who has knowledge of the family and is able to consistently provide anticipatory guidance should develop and manage the ACP.[10] In many cases, this is the PCP. A variety of

TABLE 26.2	Triggers for Goals of Care Discussions	
Trigger	**Example**
New diagnosis of chronic or life-threatening condition	Cancer, muscular dystrophy, complex congenital heart disease, extreme prematurity with significant complications, end-stage renal disease
Exacerbations of chronic conditions	Worsening pain, dyspnea, fatigue, constipation, consideration of starting new technology, decreased activities of daily living, perceived decrease in quality of life
Transitions of care	Preprocedural medical clearance, hospital discharge, referral to new specialist team or location of care

Modified from Sreedhar SS, Kraft C, Friebert S. Primary palliative care: skills for all clinicians. *Curr Prob Pediatr Adolesc Health Care.* 2020;50(6):100814; and Ahia CL, Blais CM. Primary palliative care for the general internist: integrating goals of care discussions into the outpatient setting. *Ochsner J.* 2014;14(4):704–711.

resources exist to facilitate these conversations with options based upon the age and development of the patient and family. One such tool is the Five Wishes program, which provides ACP guidance for organizations, healthcare providers, patients, and families. Their Five Wishes document is commonly used in those 18 years and up, and in some states is a legal ACP document when completed. Voicing My Choices is designed for adolescents and young adults, while My Wishes is tailored to younger children. All of these are available at https://fivewishes.org. Incorporating members of the interdisciplinary team to facilitate expression of the child's goals and wishes can be helpful. When these conversations (and documents, if used) are completed, it is important to share the information with other care providers so they can act as a roadmap for care based upon the core values of the child and family. Completion of a Do Not Resuscitate/Do Not Intubate document, or similar order in accordance with state regulations, may be required to ensure this information is available both inside and outside of the child's home.[10] The PCP plays an important role in disseminating this information into the community, particularly the school setting where school nurses can incorporate the ACP documents into the student's individualized healthcare plan.

Clinicians may not feel comfortable having these conversations alone. When conducted by a PPC specialist, the PCP can be an important participant, enriching the discussion with their long-standing relationship with the child and family. Although preparing providers to comfortably have these conversations independently is beyond the scope of this chapter, there are many resources available to support clinicians in receiving education to gain these essential skills (see resources at the end of this chapter). Reaching out to local PPC specialists for additional training, and to practice and fine tune skills, can also be helpful.

Symptom Management

Symptom management is a cornerstone of palliative care. It requires scrupulous assessment and treatment of not only physical symptoms, but also emotional, social, spiritual, and cultural suffering that affects the quality of life for children and families. Children with illness, especially when complex or chronic in nature, face extraordinary challenges on many fronts. The experience of a distressing symptom is a highly personal experience, and understanding the experience of the child and family, and the reverberations that result, is essential to the practice of PPC.[25] Assessment requires obtaining an appropriate history and the use of developmentally appropriate assessment tools, when available. Treatment requires a broad approach incorporating many members of the interdisciplinary team to minimize distress and optimize comfort and quality of life for the patient and family.

Physical

Children with chronic illness suffer from a variety of symptoms that greatly affect their quality of life, including pain, fatigue, nausea, constipation, pruritis, dyspnea, depression, anxiety, sleep disturbances, anorexia, muscle spasms, seizures, increased respiratory secretions, and neuroirritability, among others. Children may experience one, a few, or all of these symptoms over the course of their illness with an increase in symptom burden typically seen towards end of life.[26] PPC specialists receive extensive training in the treatment of these conditions; however, all clinicians should have some familiarity with the basic treatment for these conditions to alleviate suffering and distress. Two of the most common symptoms are pain and fatigue.

Pain. Pain is among the most distressing and prevalent symptoms experienced in children and is frequently encountered in palliative care. As with many diagnoses, obtaining a thorough history is essential and can often provide clues as to the cause. Clinicians should attempt to illicit the pain history from the child as much as possible, with parents offering observations regarding changes in pain behavior and factors that may alleviate or exacerbate pain, among others. A thorough pain history includes provoking factors,

quality of the pain, radiation, severity, and timing factors. Use of age and developmentally appropriate scales, such as the Neonatal Infant Pain Scale (NIPS), Pediatric FACES, and Face, Legs, Activity, Cry, Consolability (FLACC) scale may be appropriate. Parents are essential partners in interpreting behaviors and assessing pain in children with considerable medical complexity who cannot report pain (e.g., severe cerebral palsy or severe neurologic injury). For children with significant impairments, use of pain scales such as the revised FLACC or Individualized Numeric Rating Scale should be considered. A component of the pain assessment also involves assessing the associated psychosocial components. What does pain mean to the child and the family? How is the child and family able to tolerate pain and discomfort? What is the patient and family's previous experience with pain and the various management modalities? Answers to these questions help further guide management. Refer to Chapter 24 for additional discussion of pain in the pediatric patient.

Management of pain requires both pharmacologic and nonpharmacologic approaches. Children with serious illness often experience pain involving multiple pathophysiologies; therefore a multimodal approach is warranted. Treating the underlying cause is always best, when feasible. Complementary approaches such as Reiki, yoga, hypnosis, music, massage, guided imagery, and acupuncture can be effective. Other members of the interdisciplinary team including social work, psychology, chaplaincy, child life, and other therapists can also be helpful in crafting interventions. Pharmacologic therapies can be employed when warranted. Dosage and administration recommendations for these medications can be found in a variety of readily available resources. PCPs should have some level of comfort in managing pain, particularly in patients where PPC is warranted.

Fatigue. Fatigue is a symptom frequently experienced by children with life-threatening illness. It rarely occurs in isolation, typically presenting with pain and sleep disturbances. Distinct from the usual fatigue experienced by healthy individuals, fatigue in children with serious illness is persistent and can be unrelated to the amount of rest a patient receives. It interferes with function, is distressing in nature, and can affect physical, social, and psychological wellbeing. Fatigue is frequently experienced by children undergoing cancer treatment, but can also be seen in rheumatologic conditions, epilepsy, cystic fibrosis, and advanced heart disease.[27]

The first step in managing fatigue is its recognition. PPC providers should routinely inquire about fatigue, which helps to validate patient experience and can provide significant benefit.[27] The National Comprehensive Cancer Network recommends routine screening for fatigue using a simple numeric rating scales of various ranges, depending on age, to screen for fatigue beginning as young as 5 to 6 years.[28] In addition, a variety of tools exist to assess fatigue in more detail including the Childhood Fatigue Scale,[29] the Patient-Reported Outcomes Measurement Information System (PROMIS) Pediatric Fatigue measure,[30] and PedsQL Multidimensional Fatigue Scale.[31] Treatment of fatigue typically requires education, counseling, and nonpharmacologic approaches; pharmacologic approaches are infrequently warranted. Patients and families should be given anticipatory guidance regarding the likelihood of children experiencing fatigue as caregivers can associate fatigue with disease progression. Patients and families should be educated on the important role of structured sleep as able and maintaining routine. Exercise interventions in some patients have shown promise, as have mind-body interventions such as massage, acupressure, and relaxation techniques. Also, clinicians should evaluate and treat underlying causes such as anemia, the use of sedating medications, and inadequately treated pain and other symptoms.[27]

Emotional, Social, Spiritual, and Cultural Care

PPC is best delivered by an interdisciplinary team adept at addressing all aspects of suffering. In addition to assisting with symptom management, care from allied specialties provides immeasurable benefit to comprehensive care for PPC patients and families. Children and families experiencing serious, chronic, or complex illness experience distress in many aspects of their lives. Integrating psychosocial care into PPC requires a careful and thorough assessment of the following for the patient and family[32]:

- Developmental level and ability to complete appropriate developmental tasks
- The experience of emotional symptoms by the child and family members
- Practical factors affecting the family, such as financial status, living situation, and social supports
- Religious or spiritual/existential background, practices, related beliefs, rituals, and practices of the patient and family

Pediatric PCPs are already experts in completing developmental and cognitive assessments in children and families, although these assessments may be more challenging in children with serious illness. These children are often limited in their abilities to engage in age-appropriate activities, which can delay attainment of psychosocial developmental milestones. Symptoms associated with serious illness can also cause developmental regression and result in changed parenting behaviors, such as parents feeding and bathing children who were previously independent in these tasks. These alterations in caregiving behaviors are not surprising given the diagnosis of a serious illness in a child significantly alters the developmental paths of families. This can cause significant distress in any member of the family; however, just because children are diagnosed with a serious condition does not mean that they cannot continue to progress through normal stages of development. Achieving normal developmental milestones in the face of a serious illness can be a means of coping and a real source of joy for children and families. Assessing patient and family goals, encouraging activities in alignment with these goals, and designing interventions to best support children and families to reach them are important care considerations. Child life specialists can be invaluable in assessing and crafting interventions in these situations.

Providers should conduct a thorough assessment of the child and family psychosocial needs and involve other allied specialists as needed. For example, colleagues in psychology or psychiatry can assess emotional and psychological distress; social work can evaluate social supports and needs; and chaplains can evaluate spiritual distress, beliefs, and practices. Not only can consultations with various members of the interdisciplinary team assist with assessment, but they can facilitate open discussions, build relationships, engage in therapeutic interventions, and create a supportive network prepared to care for the many facets of life affected by the diagnosis of illness in a child. Not all of these consultations need to happen at once. The needs of PPC families change as children and families develop, illness states change, and treatment plans are adjusted. The involvement of interdisciplinary team members may vary to best meet patient and family needs at any time.

Emotional Needs. Emotional distress is a common finding in children and families dealing with significant illness in a child; anxiety and depression are seen frequently. It is important to note that physical and emotional symptoms are interrelated, and both

must be addressed to relieve distress. Approximately 20% to 35% of children with a chronic illness have an anxiety disorder[33] and children with chronic illness have a 22% higher prevalence of depression compared to their peers who are not physically ill.[34] Both anxiety and depression occur on a spectrum of severity, from least to most: normal, developmental variation, problematic, and clinical disorder. Increasing frequency, symptoms lasting longer than 2 weeks, or significant impairment in functioning and/or quality of life should prompt a more thorough evaluation. Anxiety and/or depression may emerge at points throughout the various stages of illness, and at some points, these responses are to be expected. Nonpharmacologic approaches are the mainstay of treatment for many of these conditions, although for extreme symptoms pharmacologic management may be warranted. Supportive counseling and cognitive-behavioral techniques such as relaxation exercises, medication, and hypnotherapy can be helpful. Creative arts therapies and complimentary techniques such as yoga and aromatherapy can also provide great benefit.[33]

Social Needs. Caring for a child with a significant illness places a great deal of stress on the patient and family. Attending to the social needs of a child with chronic illness requires an understanding of their developmental stage, their personal social goals, talents, and preferences. Many pediatric PCPs choose to use a standardized assessment tool such as the Home & Environment, Education & Employment, Activities, Drugs, Sexuality, Suicide/Depression (HEADSS) to obtain a social history,[35] which would be appropriate. In the case of children with medical complexity, a modification of the HEADSS tool that includes assessment of Ancillary service use and Transition or goals of care plans, the HEADS AT, can also be helpful.[36] Regardless of tool use, an assessment should include asking about friends, school, activities enjoyed, favorite television shows or video games, and so forth. Chronic illness can significantly affect the ability of the child to participate in those activities and therefore cause distress. Finding ways for children to continue to participate in activities that bring them joy is essential to the holistic provision of PPC. The PCP plays an important role as a liaison with the community to ensure that the social needs of PPC patients and families are met to the greatest extent possible.

The practical challenges for families caring for an ill child cannot be underestimated. They have frequent contact with the medical system, which can impact children and caregivers alike. Caregiver stress can affect their employment status, health insurance coverage, transportation needs, childcare, basic cost of living expenses, and the many other needs for everyday life of a family. Social workers are indispensable members of the interdisciplinary team who can assist families with these needs. They are skilled clinicians who can provide emotional support and guidance for families, assess for caregiver and family challenges, and connect families with the appropriate resources.

Spiritual and Cultural Needs. Understanding the spiritual and cultural beliefs and practices of PPC patients and families plays an important role in understanding their values, guiding principles, and sources of support. Spiritual practices frequently involve the formal practice of a religion, which can be closely intertwined with cultural practices. Because every family is different, providers should conduct a broad assessment of cultural and spiritual practices. Spiritual beliefs, practices, and values play an important role in coping[37] and decision-making[38] for patients and families. Chaplains have an important role in supporting patients and families in this manner, although any member of the interdisciplinary team can provide spiritual support. Regardless of their affiliation status with an organized religion, spiritual support should be offered to all PPC patients and families. Assessing for cultural practices is also important as they may or may not be connected to religious or spiritual beliefs. There is great variation in practices, particularly surrounding illness and death. Understanding the individual beliefs and practices of the family helps the care team align care with those beliefs and provide individualized, holistic care to the child and family.

Supporting Families Through the Impact of Illness

The diagnosis of a life-threatening illness in a child has a significant impact on the family that requires support from the entire community. Such a diagnosis signals a significant shift in dynamics and the loss of "normal" for the entire family.[39] Many children and families report the experience of "riding the rollercoaster" of "good days and bad days."[39] Affected children can lose interpersonal relationships, control over their bodies, personal identity, and the ability to make many choices, among many other things. The impacts of this distress extend to caregivers, siblings, and other extended family members.

Caregivers of children with complex, chronic, life-limiting illnesses face significant stressors balancing caring for their sick child with other family responsibilities, their own physical health, social life, finances, education, and careers. This stress can be further compounded when the child nears the end of their life. These caregivers are more likely to struggle with both physical and mental health issues.[40] A recent survey of parents of children with medical complexity found that approximately 20% report poor or fair mental health and 36% did not know where to go for help in their community when they encounter difficulties.[41] PCPs caring for these children should be proactive in identifying coping strategies and providing resources of support in the community, which can involve palliative care services (see Additional Resources at the end of this chapter).

Siblings of children with complex, life-threatening conditions can go through several challenges related to having a severely ill child in their family. They can experience complex emotions including rivalry, jealousy, and anger towards their sibling and resent the perceived loss of parental attention while still being fearful for their sibling's health.[42] They can lose a sense of self and be known as the sibling of the child with the disease. They may also take on caretaking duties for their ill sibling or assume roles previously carried out by their parents, further challenging their self-concept.[39] Notably, assuming caring responsibilities is not necessarily harmful; in fact, they may be beneficial in empowering siblings to be involved in the family act of caring for the ill child.[43] Still, siblings of children with life-limited illness have increased levels of stress, depression, anxiety, behavioral problems, and lower quality of life.[40] PCPs are in a prime position to support siblings through these myriad challenges (e.g., academic and peer-related difficulties at school)[44] and must be aware of the potential for developing these complications and provide careful assessment, diagnosis, and management. Identifying support systems is essential, including those at school and elsewhere in the community (see chapter resources for sibling support).

Children and families are often an active part of a larger community that includes schools, faith organizations, arts, and sports activities, among many others. A diagnosis of a significant illness ripples into the community. PCPs should reach out to key community members—teachers, coaches, faith leaders—and form collaborative relationships to ensure the child and family continue to receive appropriate care in those settings. PCPS often work with school nurses and teachers to ensure students have appropriate accommodation plans and facilitating connections with in-hospital education services for when children are admitted to the hospital or return to their school setting. School communities must be knowledgeable about illness conditions and the plan of care for these patients. PCPs should work closely with health providers in the school to ensure they remain updated regarding the child's plan of care to receive needed symptom management during school hours. Regular collaboration with school and other key community members is essential to the provision of holistic PPC.[45]

Care Delivery

Care Coordination

Care coordination, an essential component of providing comprehensive PPC, is founded on effective communication between all members of the care team. Children with serious illness and medically complex care needs have complex networks of care crossing numerous settings and institutions. They are frequently cared for by caregivers at home, especially towards the end of their lives[26] with PPC and hospice services for additional support. Caregivers, regardless of whether PPC services are offered in the hospital or at home, value coordinated care and management of this complex network. Effective care coordination is associated with improved care quality and outcomes for the child and family including improved quality of life, symptom management, and death in preferred location. This makes the provision of high-quality care coordination of particular interest to PPC providers.

Despite the broad interest in care coordination by many parties including families, caregivers, care networks, and payers, many different activities are often performed under this umbrella although no uniform definition exists.[46] The AAP defines care coordination as care that centers on the family; is planned, proactive, and comprehensive in focus; promotes self-care skills and independence; and emphasizes cross-organizational relationships.[47] Care coordination can occur in several settings including primary care practices, tertiary care centers, or community agencies outside of the practice setting. Regardless of setting, a key first step is assessment of needs in the primary care setting,[46] making PCPs ideally positioned to provide care coordination for children requiring PPC services. Nurse practitioners, with advanced training in assessment, diagnosis, treatment, and holistic care skills, are well suited to performing the necessary skills of communication, collaboration, and systems knowledge required for high quality care coordination. Unfortunately, despite the clear benefits to care coordination for PPC patients and families, it remains a resource-heavy and time-consuming endeavor that is poorly reimbursed.[48] Much work remains to be done to overcome these barriers to ensure that all children, particularly those in need of PPC services, can receive coordinated care to achieve optimal outcomes.

Funding/Insurance Coverage for Palliative and Hospice Care

When not provided by hospital-based specialty teams, palliative care services are provided in the community by hospice providers who frequently offer both palliative care and hospice services. Palliative care services in the home are essentially treated like visiting nurse services, although the nurses are trained in principles of palliative care, and payment goes through regular insurance. Typically, for adults near the end of their life on Medicare or Medicaid benefits, receiving hospice services requires a person to elect their hospice benefit. In this case, there is a certification that someone has a life expectancy of 6 months or less and that they will forgo curative treatments. When that benefit is elected, Medicare and Medicaid will pay the hospice provider a set rate for services rendered and the hospice is responsible for making sure the patient and family are supplied with all of the medications, supplies, and services required. This process works well for adults; however, it has presented challenges for children.

Children with chronic, complex health conditions comprise a significant portion of children appropriate for PPC services. Medicaid is an important source of funding for health insurance coverage for this population. According to the latest statistics from the Kaiser Family Foundation, approximately 51% of children with these needs have health coverage through private insurance, 8% have private insurance supplemented with Medicaid or Children's Health Insurance Program (CHIP) coverage, and approximately 36% receive coverage through Medicaid/CHIP only.[49] Historically, the requirement that patients on Medicaid and/or CHIP forgo curative therapies was a significant barrier to the utilization of hospice services because these children frequently require long-standing therapies to maintain their quality of life. Acknowledging this barrier, PPC advocates lobbied for change. In 2010, with the enactment of the Patient Protection and Affordable Care Act, Section 2302 named Concurrent Care of Children, that barrier was removed. The concurrent care model now allows children to receive hospice services in conjunction with curative therapies; Medicaid and/or CHIP will continue to pay for both services. While the life expectancy guidelines of less than 6 months still apply, this change has allowed more children to receive needed services. A number of states, through waiver programs, have also enacted special programs for children to receive palliative care services earlier.[50]

While this closed a gap in coverage to hospice care for children, there remain challenges when it comes to receiving payment for some palliative care services. Reimbursement in many areas is inadequate for some supportive care services (e.g., psychology, social work, bereavement) that are characteristic of PPC, which can make it challenging to sustain comprehensive services.[51] For the PCP in the community, partnering with a PPC specialist service adept at navigating these many nuances of financing palliative care services for children can be helpful.

Barriers to Pediatric Palliative Care

Despite significant improvements in the provision of PPC services, barriers to care still exist and services are still underutilized. Common challenges include patients and families, healthcare professionals, and systems/organizational barriers. Many patients and families still hold the misconceptions that palliative care is limited to care at the end-of-life and can only be implemented when there are no further curative options; however, through education and shared patient experiences, these attitudes may be changing. A recent study of pediatric cancer patients and families demonstrated that families had very few negative attitudes towards early initiation of palliative care.[52] Framing PPC as a way to provide care for the whole person as a member of the team may be a reasonable approach when faced with this barrier.[53]

Despite the introduction of palliative care concepts early in training programs, and educational outreach directed towards practicing providers, many may still be reluctant to utilize palliative care services for their patients. This may be due to misconceptions similar to those of patients and families. In addition, some providers may not fully understand the depth and breadth of what palliative care offers and therefore think that there would be significant overlap in services.[51] Continued advocacy for the integral role of PPC services in high-quality patient care is warranted.

While the provision of high-quality PPC for children with serious illnesses is now an expected standard of care, there are a number of barriers at the systems/organizational level that make the implementation and provision of PPC difficult. There is currently a shortage of providers certified to provide specialty PPC[10,51] and variable access to pediatric hospice and palliative care services across the country, particularly in the home setting. As technology improves, and more children with complex healthcare needs are surviving longer, the needs for PPC are expected to grow. Other providers will need to step in to bridge these gaps. In addition, the reimbursement challenges previously noted are a barrier to creating sustainable programs. Programs are further faced with challenges in providing coordinated palliative care for children across increasingly complex and fragmented healthcare organizations where care is delivered in multiple settings, clinics, and by a variety of providers.[51] Training PCPs and other providers in the provision of PPC, and advocating for improved reimbursement for services, will help to ensure the needs of these children and families are met.

After the Death of a Child

Even when expected, the death of a child is always tragic and grieving the loss of a child is never easy. Families frequently develop strong connections to the child's medical team and can feel abandoned once their child dies. They also fear that their children may be forgotten by those who knew them. PCPs play an important role by maintaining their longitudinal relationships with families and continuing to support them in their bereavement. In the period immediately following the child's death, clinicians can express condolences by sending cards, making a phone call, or attending remembrance services.

If the family has additional children, the PCP might continue to see the family for sibling healthcare needs. Surviving siblings can have a variety of responses to the death of a sibling. Their grief can be complicated and affect their psychosocial health lifelong. Fifty percent or more of bereaved siblings have behavior problems including difficulty with anger, aggression, guilt, nightmares, separation anxiety, fear of being alone, hopelessness, trouble concentrating, poor school performance, and suicidal thoughts and attempts. They can suffer from depression, posttraumatic stress disorder, and may even require psychiatric hospitalization.

Siblings may present to the PCP with increased frequency in the first 13 months following their sibling's death peaking in the first 6 months, and then again at 12 to 13 months. They often have complaints of gastrointestinal problems, allergies, gynecologic problems, headaches, infections, eye problems, and anxiety. Illicit substance use can increase in the year following the sibling's death.[54] These frequent visits in the initial period following the sibling's death, possibly a reflection of parental hypervigilance, provide an opportunity for the PCP to continue to support the family.[55] The PCP needs to carefully assess these children, provide appropriate and compassionate anticipatory guidance to parents, and be vigilant in evaluating for psychosocial complications in the bereaved family.

Additional Resources

Center to Advance Palliative Care: https://www.capc.org/

Center to Advance Palliative Care, Clinical Training Recommendations for All Clinicians Caring for Pediatric Patients with Serious Illness: https://www.capc.org/training-recommendations-pediatrics/

Complex Child Magazine: https://complexchild.org

Courageous Parents Network: https://courageousparentsnetwork.org/

Education in Palliative and End-of-Life Care (EPEC): https://www.bioethics.northwestern.edu/programs/epec/

End-of-Life Nursing Education Consortium (ELNEC)–Pediatric: https://www.aacnnursing.org/ELNEC

International Children's Palliative Care Network eLearning: https://www.icpcn.org/icpcns-elearning-programme/

FastFacts For Physicians: https://www.mypcnow.org/#!fast-facts/c6xb

- Delivering Bad News Part 1: https://www.mypcnow.org/fast-fact/delivering-bad-news-part-1/
- Delivering Bad News Part 2: https://www.mypcnow.org/fast-fact/delivering-bad-news-part-2/
- Discussing DNR: https://www.mypcnow.org/fast-fact/discussing-dnr-orders-part-1/
- Advance Care Planning in Chronic Illness: https://www.mypcnow.org/fast-fact/advance-care-planning-in-chronic-illness/
- Sibling Grief: https://www.mypcnow.org/fast-fact/sibling-grief/

Describing Pediatric Palliative Care Concepts to Patients and Families: https://www.mypcnow.org/fast-fact/describing-pediatric-palliative-care-concepts-to-patients-and-families/Getpalliativecare.org: https://getpalliativecare.org/

National Hospice and Palliative Care Organization: https://www.nhpco.org/resources

National Organization for Rare Diseases: www.rarediseases.org. Palliative Care: Conversations Matter: https://www.ninr.nih.gov/newsandinformation/conversationsmatter/palliative-care-for-children

Pediatric Palliative Care Coalition: https://www.ppcc-pa.org/

The Conversation Project: https://theconversationproject.org/

VitalTalk: www.vitaltalk.org

References

1. World Health Organization. *Fact Sheet: Palliative Care*. https://www.who.int/news-room/fact-sheets/detail/palliative-care.
2. World Health Organization. *Cancer Pain Relief and Palliative Care in Children*. https://apps.who.int/iris/handle/10665/42001.
3. Wolfe J, Hinds PS, Sourkes BM. The Language of pediatric palliative care. In: Wolfe J, Hinds PS, Sourkes BM, eds. *Interdisciplinary Pediatric Palliative Care*. 2nd ed. Oxford University Press; 2022.
4. National Consensus Project for Quality Palliative Care. *Clinical Practice Guidelines for Quality Palliative Care*. 4th ed. National Coalition for Hospice and Palliative Care; 2018.
5. The medical home. *Pediatrics*. 2002;110(1 Pt 1):184–186.
6. Institute of medicine committee on palliative and end-of-life care for children and their families. In: Field MJ, Behrman RE, eds. *When Children Die: Improving Palliative and End-of-Life Care for Children and their Families*. National Academies Press; 2003.
7. *Dying in America: Improving Quality and Honoring Individual Preferences Near the End of Life*. National Academies Press; 2015.
8. Quill TE, Abernethy AP. Generalist plus specialist palliative care: creating a more sustainable model. *N Engl J Med*. 2013;368(13):1173–1175.
9. Lindley LC, Nageswaran S. Pediatric primary care involvement in end-of-life care for children. *Am J Hosp Palliat Care*. 2017;34(2):135–141.
10. Sreedhar SS, Kraft C, Friebert S. Primary palliative care: skills for all clinicians. *Curr Prob Pediatr Adolesc Health Care*. 2020;50(6):100814.
11. American Academy of Pediatrics. Clinical practice guidelines for quality palliative care. *Pediatrics*. 2019;143(1).
12. National Association of Pediatric Nurse Practitioners. Supported Position Statements and Other Documents. https://www.napnap.org/supported-position-statements-and-other-documents/.
13. Battista V, LaRagione G. Pediatric hospice and palliative care. In: Ferrell BR, Paice JA, eds. *Oxford Textbook of Palliative Nursing*. Oxford University Press; 2019.
14. Cormack CL, Dahlin C. The pediatric palliative APRN: leading the future. *J Pediatr Health Care*. 2022;34(4):381–387.
15. van der Lee JH, Mokkink LB, Grootenhuis MA, et al. Definitions and measurement of chronic health conditions in childhood: a systematic review. *JAMA*. 2007;297(24):2741–2751.
16. Rogers M, Kirch R. Spotlight on Pediatric Palliative Care: National Landscape of Hospital-Based Programs, 2015-16. https://www.capc.org/blog/palliative-pulse-palliative-pulse-july-2017-spotlight-pediatric-palliative-care-national-landscape-hospital-based-programs-2015-2016/#:~:text=Palliative%20care%20service%20penetration%20is,the%20way%20up%20to%2015%25.
17. Section on Hospice and Palliative Medicine and Committee on Hospital Care. Pediatric palliative care and hospice care commitments, guidelines, and recommendations. *Pediatrics*. 2013;132(5):966–972.
18. Linebarger JS, Johnson V, Boss RD, et al. Guidance for pediatric end-of-life care. *Pediatrics*. 2022;149(5).
19. Feudtner C. Collaborative communication in pediatric palliative care: a foundation for problem-solving and decision-making. *Pediatr Clin North Am*. 2007;54(5):583–607, ix.
20. American Academy of Pediatrics NRCfPF-CMH. What Is Medical Home? https://medicalhomeinfo.aap.org/overview/Pages/Whatisthemedicalhome.aspx.
21. Knapp C, Baker K, Cunningham C, et al. Pediatric palliative care and the medical home. *J Palliat Med*. 2012;15(6):643–645.
22. Yu JA, Schenker Y, Maurer SH, et al. Pediatric palliative care in the medical neighborhood for children with medical complexity. *Fam Syst Health*. 2019;37(2):107–119.
23. Hill DL, Miller V, Walter JK, et al. Regoaling: a conceptual model of how parents of children with serious illness change medical care goals. *BMC Palliat Care*. 2014;13(1):9.
24. Heckford E, Beringer AJ. Advance care planning: challenges and approaches for pediatricians. *J Palliat Med*. 2014;17(9):1049–1053.
25. Sourkes BM. Children's experience of symptoms: narratives through words and images. *Children (Basel)*. 2018;5(4).
26. Feudtner C, Kang TI, Hexem KR, et al. Pediatric palliative care patients: a prospective multicenter cohort study. *Pediatrics*. 2011;127(6):1094–1101.
27. Ullrich C, Jacobs S, Hinds PS. Fatigue. In: Wolfe J, Hinds PS, Sourkes B, eds. *Interdisciplinary Pediatric Palliative Care*. Oxford University Press; 2022.
28. Jankowski C, Berger AM, Aranha O, et al. *Cancer-Related Fatigue*; 2022. https://www.nccn.org/guidelines/guidelines-detail?category=3&id=1424.
29. Hockenberry MJ, Hinds PS, Barrera P, et al. Three instruments to assess fatigue in children with cancer: the child, parent and staff perspectives. *J Pain Symptom Manag*. 2003;25(4):319–328.
30. HealthMeasures. List of Pediatric Measures; 2022. https://www.healthmeasures.net/explore-measurement-systems/promis/intro-to-promis/list-of-pediatric-measures.

31. Varni JW, Burwinkle TM, Katz ER, et al. The Pedsql in pediatric cancer: reliability and validity of the pediatric quality of life inventory generic core scales, multidimensional fatigue scale, and cancer module. *Cancer*. 2002;94(7):2090–2106.

32. McSherry M, Kehoe K, Carroll JM, et al. Psychosocial and spiritual needs of children living with a life-limiting illness. *Pediatr Clin North Am*. 2007;54(5):609–629, ix-x.

33. Samsel C, Perko K, Wiener L, et al. Psychological symptoms. In: Wolfe J, Hinds PS, Sourkes B, eds. *Interdisciplinary Pediatric Palliative Care*. 2nd ed. Oxford University Press; 2022.

34. Pinquart M, Shen Y. Depressive symptoms in children and adolescents with chronic physical illness: an updated meta-analysis. *J Pediatr Psychol*. 2010;36(4):375–384.

35. Goldenring JM, Rosen DS. Getting into adolescent heads: an essential update. *Cont Pediatr*. 2004;64+.

36. Sadof M, Gortakowski M, Stechenberg B, et al. The "HEADS AT" training tool for residents: a roadmap for caring for children with medical complexity. *Clin Pediatr (Phila)*. 2015;54(12):1210–1214.

37. Reynolds N, Mrug S, Wolfe K, et al. Spiritual coping, psychosocial adjustment, and physical health in youth with chronic illness: a meta-analytic review. *Health Psychol Rev*. 2016;10(2):226–243.

38. Malcolm HV, Desjardins CM, Ferrara B, et al. Parental use of religion and spirituality in medical decision-making. *J Health Care Chaplain*. 2021;27(3):146–158.

39. Havill N, Fleming LK, Knafl K. Well siblings of children with chronic illness: a synthesis research study. *Res Nurs Health*. 2019;42(5):334–348.

40. Feudtner C, Nye RT, Boyden JY, et al. Association between children with life-threatening conditions and their parents' and siblings' mental and physical health. *JAMA Netw Open*. 2021;4(12):e2137250.

41. Bayer ND, Wang H, Yu JA, et al. A national mental health profile of parents of children with medical complexity. *Pediatrics*. 2021;148(2).

42. Tregidgo C, Elander J. The invisible child: sibling experiences of growing up with a brother with severe haemophilia-an interpretative phenomenological analysis. *Haemophilia*. 2019;25(1):84–91.

43. Kelada L, Wakefield CE, Drew D, et al. Siblings of young people with chronic illness: caring responsibilities and psychosocial functioning. *J Child Health Care*. 2021:13674935211033466.

44. Gan LL, Lum A, Wakefield CE, et al. School experiences of siblings of children with chronic illness: a systematic literature review. *J Pediatr Nurs*. 2017;33:23–32.

45. Davis KG. Integrating pediatric palliative care into the school and community. *Pediatr Clin North Am*. 2016;63(5):899–911.

46. Kuo DZ, McAllister JW, Rossignol L, et al. Care coordination for children with medical complexity: whose care is it, anyway? *Pediatrics*. 2018;141(suppl 3):S224–S232.

47. Council on Children with Disabilities and Medical Home Implementation Project Advisory Committee. Patient- and family-centered care coordination: a framework for integrating care for children and youth across multiple systems. *Pediatrics*. 2014;133(5):e1451–e1460.

48. Ronis SD, Grossberg R, Allen R, et al. Estimated nonreimbursed costs for care coordination for children with medical complexity. *Pediatrics*. 2019;143(1).

49. Williams E, Musumeci M. Children with special health care needs: coverage, affordability, and HCBS access. https://www.kff.org/medicaid/issue-brief/children-with-special-health-care-needs-coverage-affordability-and-hcbs-access/.

50. Lotstein DS, Lindley LC. Improving home hospice and palliative care policies. *Pediatrics*. 2019;144(2).

51. Haines ER, Frost AC, Kane HL, et al. Barriers to accessing palliative care for pediatric patients with cancer: a review of the literature. *Cancer*. 2018;124(11):2278–2288.

52. Levine DR, Mandrell BN, Sykes A, et al. Patients' and parents' needs, attitudes, and perceptions about early palliative care integration in pediatric oncology. *JAMA Oncol*. 2017;3(9):1214–1220.

53. Kaye EC, Friebert S, Baker JN. Early integration of palliative care for children with high-risk cancer and their families. *Pediatr Blood Cancer*. 2016;63(4):593–597.

54. Rosenberg AR, Postier A, Osenga K, et al. Long-term psychosocial outcomes among bereaved siblings of children with cancer. *J Pain Symptom Manage*. 2015;49(1):55–65.

55. Brooten DA, Youngblut JM, Roche RM, et al. Surviving siblings' illnesses, treatments/health services over 13 months after a sibling's death. *J Child Fam Stud*. 2018;27(6):2049–2056.

27

Congenital and Inherited Disorders

MARTHA DRIESSNACK AND SANDRA DAACK-HIRSCH

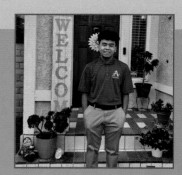

This chapter focuses on children with congenital and inherited disorders. The chapter begins with a brief review of genetic contributions to disorders, patterns of inheritance, and insights into obtaining a family health history and conducting a pediatric assessment using a genetic/genomic lens. The concept of epigenetics, types of genomic testing, and some of the ethical challenges are introduced. The chapter concludes with an overview of common congenital and inherited disorders, emphasizing clinical findings and the role of the primary care provider (PCP) as a member of a larger team of experts, including genetic healthcare professionals and counselors.

Genetic Contribution to Disorders and Patterns of Inheritance

The term genetic disorder is in some ways an antiquated term, as nearly all diseases and disorders are now thought to have a genetic component (i.e., caused in whole, or in part, by changes in DNA sequence or gene expression). The genotype associated with a particular disease can be inherited, arise spontaneously, or be acquired over a lifetime. For example, some diseases are caused by inherited mutations, others are caused by spontaneous mutations that occur during the development of the gametes or in early human development (de novo), and most forms of cancers are the result of acquired mutations in a gene or group of genes that occur during a person's life. Mutations that are acquired during a person's life happen at the somatic level and occur either randomly as a result of a random event or environmental exposure.

Genetic contributions traditionally fall into one of four categories: (1) single-gene disorders, (2) chromosome disorders, (3) multifactorial disorders, or (4) mitochondrial disorders. Each is discussed, along with an overview of both mendelian and non-mendelian inheritance patterns.

Single-Gene Disorders

Single-gene disorders occur when the mutation affects one gene. Some examples of single-gene disorders that should be familiar to PCPs are sickle cell disease, thalassemia, neurofibromatosis, hemophilia, Duchene muscular dystrophy, cystic fibrosis, fragile X syndrome, polycystic kidney disease, Marfan syndrome, and Tay-Sachs disease.

Patterns of Inheritance

Mendelian Inheritance Patterns. Disorders caused by mutations in a single gene are typically inherited in one of several patterns, commonly referred to as *mendelian* patterns of inheritance. They include *autosomal dominant* (AD), *autosomal recessive* (AR), and *X-linked* dominant or recessive.

Autosomal Dominant. This type of single-gene disorder is characterized by the inheritance of a single copy of a mutated gene located on one of the autosomal chromosomes (chromosomes 1–22). The gene mutation is passed on from one parent; the paired gene from the other parent is normal (Fig. 27.1). The parent passing on the gene mutation typically has the disorder, although there may be variable expression. The risk of each offspring inheriting the mutation from an affected parent is 50%, regardless of sex and independent of having an affected sibling. Children without the abnormal gene will neither develop the disorder nor pass a disease-causing mutation on to their offspring.

The PCP reviewing a child's family history should consider AD inheritance when a specific phenotype (1) appears in a family generation after generation (vertical transmission), (2) both sexes appear equally affected, and (3) male-to-male transmission occurs. However, penetrance, expressivity, pleiotropy, variable age of onset, and anticipation can interfere with one's ability to recognize AD inheritance (Table 27.1). Further, some AD disorders, such as achondroplasia, have a high rate of de novo (new) mutations, making it highly likely that the family history will be negative for additional affected relatives.

Examples of disorders with an AD inheritance pattern include Huntington disease, Marfan syndrome, hereditary nonpolyposis colorectal cancer, hereditary breast/ovarian cancer syndrome, Noonan syndrome, achondroplasia, familial hypercholesterolemia, hypertrophic cardiomyopathy, and neurofibromatosis type 1.

Autosomal Recessive. This type of single-gene disorder requires the inheritance of two copies of a mutated gene (one from each parent) located on one of the autosomal chromosomes (chromosomes 1–22). Offspring who inherit only one abnormal gene in the pair are considered carriers and typically do not manifest the disease; they can pass the affected allele to their children who are

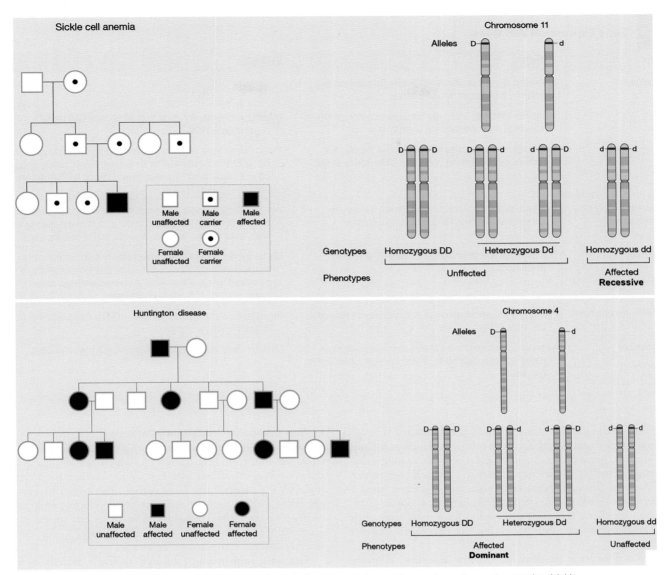

• **Fig 27.1** Patterns of Inheritance. Sample three-generation pedigrees for autosomal recessive (sickle cell anemia) and autosomal dominant (Huntington disease). (From National Human Genome Research Institute. https://www.genome.gov/genetics-glossary/Autosomal-Recessive-Disorder/.)

also typically unaffected. For offspring whose parents both carry an AR mutation, there is a 25% chance of inheriting the mutation from both parents and developing the associated disorder, a 50% chance of inheriting one copy and becoming a carrier, and a 25% chance of not inheriting either mutation (see Fig. 27.1).

The PCP reviewing a child's family health history should consider AR inheritance when (1) a specific phenotype affects multiple siblings (horizontal transmission), and (2) both sexes are affected. The phenotype is not typically seen in every generation; however, a family's geographic ancestry or ethnic background, as well as consanguinity (genetic relatedness), increases the likelihood of AR disorders, making it more likely that the family will have affected family members in several generations. Examples of AR disorders include Tay-Sachs disease, cystic fibrosis, albinism, phenylketonuria (PKU), galactosemia, thalassemia, sickle cell anemia, and Canavan disease. Examples of geographic ancestry or ethnic background increasing risk for AR disorders include (1) gene mutations associated with cystic fibrosis, which occur most frequently in populations of European descent, and (2) gene mutations associated with sickle cell anemia, which occur more

frequently throughout sub-Saharan Africa, the Middle East, and the Indian subcontinent.

X-Linked. Although X-linked inheritance patterns have traditionally been separated into subcategories of X-linked dominant or recessive, there is a move toward collapsing these categories, considering X-linked inheritance patterns across a spectrum. However, for the purposes of this chapter, they are presented separately.

When a disorder is classified as *X-linked recessive*, it usually occurs in males (see Fig. 27.1). This pattern is seen because males have only one X chromosome, so a single, abnormal, recessive allele on that X chromosome is enough to cause the disease. When the father is affected, none of his sons will be affected and all of his daughters will be *carriers*. If the mother is a carrier (one abnormal gene on one of her X chromosomes), there is a 50% chance that each son will be affected. Daughters have a 50% chance of being a carrier (like their mothers). Although females can have an X-linked recessive disorder, it is rare and is often less severe compared to males.

When reviewing a child's family history, the PCP should consider X-linked recessive inheritance when a specific phenotype

TABLE 27.1	Gene Expression Variables	
Term	**Definition**	**Examples**
Penetrance	Proportion (%) of individuals with a specific genotype that exhibit the corresponding phenotype	
	Complete: Everyone with a specific disease genotype (100%) manifests the corresponding phenotype	Huntington disease. For those with 40 or more CAG repeats, penetrance is 100%.
	Incomplete: Some (varying percentages) of the affected individuals manifest the phenotype while others do not.	Breast cancer from *BRCA1* or *BRCA2* mutation. For example, the cumulative risk estimates for developing breast cancer by age 80 years have been estimated to be 72% for *BRCA1* carriers and 69% for *BRCA2* carriers.
Expressivity (variable expressivity)	Degree to which a phenotype is expressed can vary by compilation and/or severity, even within families.	Van der Woude syndrome. Affected family members can have one or more of the following traits: cleft lip, cleft palate, cleft lip and plate, lower lip pits, lower lip mounds, and or missing teeth.
Pleiotropy	One genotype results in multiple, seemingly unrelated phenotypes.	Marfan syndrome. From joint hypermobility and limb elongation to aortic and heart disease and vision problems caused by a dislocated lens in either one or both eyes; varies in severity, timing of onset, and rate of progression.
Variable age of onset	Phenotypic expression emerges at varying ages even within the same family.	Hypertrophic cardiomyopathy (HCM). HCM can manifest from birth to age 80 years and beyond.
Anticipation	A phenotype becomes more severe and/or appears at an earlier age as a disorder is passed from one generation to the next.	Myotonic dystrophy, Fragile X syndrome, Huntington disease

is noted in males almost exclusively and is transmitted through maternal lines. Examples of X-linked recessive disorders include Fabry disease, hemophilia A and B, glucose-6-phosphate dehydrogenase (G6PD) deficiency, Wiskott Aldrich syndrome, protan/deutan forms of color blindness, and Duchene muscular dystrophy. However, as with AD inheritance, some disorders (e.g., Duchene muscular dystrophy) have high rates of de novo (new) mutations, thus rendering the past family history negative.

When a disorder is classified as *X-linked dominant*, it means that a single abnormal gene on the X chromosome gives rise to the disease. If the father is affected (abnormal gene on his X chromosome) and the mother is not, 100% of his female offspring will inherit the disease-causing allele, but none of his male offspring will. This is because daughters inherit their father's X chromosome, whereas sons inherit their father's Y chromosome. In contrast, if the mother is affected (abnormal gene on an X chromosome) and the father is not, each offspring (daughter/son) has a 50% chance of inheriting the disease-causing allele and manifesting the disorder, as mothers have two X chromosomes to pass on. In aggregate, more females are affected with X-linked dominant disorders compared to males, and they often appear to have a less severe phenotype. In contrast, males have a more severe phenotype, and the phenotype is often lethal in males, accounting for fewer living males with the disorder.

The PCP reviewing a child's family history should consider X-linked dominant inheritance when (1) a specific phenotype affects both sexes in each generation, (2) the phenotype is less severe in females, (3) there is a history of early death in male infants and fetuses, and (4) there is a lack of male-to-male transmission. Examples of disorders with X-linked dominant inheritance include Rett syndrome and vitamin D–resistant rickets.

Non-mendelian Inheritance Patterns

Mitochondrial Inheritance. Another inheritance pattern arises from the mitochondrial (mt)DNA, which accordingly is called *mitochondrial inheritance* (see Fig. 27.1). Mothers alone pass on mtDNA (i.e., matrilinear or maternal inheritance) because only egg cells contribute mitochondria to the developing embryo. Disorders that arise from mutations in mtDNA can appear in every generation and affect both sexes. On average, males are more severely affected compared to females.

Genomic Imprinting. Children typically inherit two copies of genes, one from their mother and one from their father, and both copies are active (i.e., turned on) in the cells together. However, in some cases, only one copy needs to be expressed and the other copy is "turned off" or silenced during embryogenesis. The decision as to which gene remains working and which is silenced depends on the parent of origin. Only a small number of genes go through genomic imprinting, which occurs when the origin of the gene (maternal vs. paternal) is marked (imprinted) on the gene during the formation of egg or sperm cells through methylation. Imprinted genes tend to cluster together in the same regions of certain chromosomes.[1] Improper imprinting results in a child having two active copies or two inactive copies. Two major clusters of imprinted genes have been identified in humans, on chromosomes 11 and 15. Prader-Willi syndrome occurs when the paternally derived genes located in a specific chromosome 15 region are either improperly imprinted or deleted, whereas Angelman syndrome occurs when the maternally derived genes in the same area are either improperly imprinted or deleted. Thus, the developing embryo does not detect a paternal or maternal copy of chromosome 15, producing one syndrome or the other. Beckwith-Wiedemann and Russell-Silver syndromes are other examples of disorders influenced by genomic imprinting.

Uniparental Disomy. When an individual receives two copies of one chromosome, or a part of a chromosome, from one parent and none from the other parent, uniparental disomy (UPD) is the result. This individual will be homozygous for every gene located on that chromosome, which increases the possibility of inheriting an AR disorder. UPD can occur as a random event during the formation of egg or sperm cells or may happen in early fetal development.

In many cases, UPD has no effect on a child's health or development because most genes are not imprinted. Thus, it does not matter if a child inherits both copies from one parent or one copy from each parent. However, in some cases, maternal or paternal inheritance of a specific gene is important. Examples of disorders that arise from UPD include Prader-Willi and Angelman syndromes, which are also discussed under genomic imprinting. Prader-Willi syndrome (caused by UPD) happens when the fetus inherits two maternal chromosome 15 (and no paternally derived chromosome 15). Angelman syndrome (caused by UPD) happens when the fetus inherits two paternal chromosome 15 (and no maternally derived chromosome 15).

Chromosome Disorders

Chromosome disorders occur with changes in the number or structure of an entire chromosome or large chromosomal segments. For example, Down syndrome (trisomy 21) is caused by an extra copy of chromosome 21, and chronic myeloid leukemia (CML) results from a translocation in which portions of chromosomes 9 and 22 are exchanged, resulting in an abnormal allele.[1] Other examples of chromosomal disorders that should be familiar to providers in primary care are cri-du-chat syndrome (5p–), Williams syndrome, and 22q11 deletion syndrome, also referred to as *DiGeorge syndrome* and *velocardiofacial syndrome*.

There are also chromosomal disorders of the sex chromosomes, such as Klinefelter syndrome (XXY), which is caused by an extra X chromosome, and Turner syndrome (XO), which is caused by the absence of an X chromosome. Another type of chromosomal disorder is called *mosaicism*, which occurs when an altered chromosomal arrangement occurs in some cells but not in others within the same individual. The clinical symptoms are usually milder, and the prognosis improves with fewer numbers of cells involved.

When taking a family history, PCPs should remember there is a high frequency of chromosomal disorders in spontaneous abortions and stillbirths. Further, the prevalence of chromosomal disorders because of nondisjunction increases with advancing maternal age.

Multifactorial Disorders

Multifactorial disorders result from a combination of genetic and environmental factors. Recurrence risks are based on empirical statistics—observations based on data collected from thousands of family histories transformed into probabilities. These disorders cluster in families; the exact recurrence risk is difficult to predict because the individuals' or couples' precise genetic and environmental risks are usually not known. Therefore a population-based recurrence risk rather than a personal recurrence risk is given. One example of a multifactorial disorder includes neural tube defects (NTDs), such as spina bifida or anencephaly. NTDs appear in females more often than in males, and once a child is born with an NTD, the chance for those parents to have another child with an NTD increases (see Online Mendelian Inheritance in

Man [OMIM] in the Additional Resources). The rate of NTDs decreases with sufficient maternal folic acid supplementation. Therefore the CDC recommends that all females of childbearing age consume 0.4 mg (400 mcg) of folic acid daily. In contrast, the rate of NTDs increases when mothers have uncontrolled diabetes or take certain medications (e.g., valproic acid). The specific combination of genetic factors and how they interact with each other or other environmental factors is unknown. Other examples of multifactorial disorders that should be familiar to PCPs are congenital heart defect, club foot, cleft lip/palate, pyloric stenosis, Hirschsprung disease, hip dysplasia, and asthma.

Teratogenic Disorders

A teratogen is any agent that results in or increases the incidence of, a congenital malformation. Although teratogens have traditionally been considered environmental toxins that alter critical embryonic and fetal development, it appears that genomic factors have significant modifying effects on the teratogen. The same teratogenic exposure can induce a severe malformation in one embryo but not in another, even though the timing and dose of the exposure are similar.[2] A teratogen may also affect the embryo at one developmental point but not at a different one. The Organization of Teratology Information Specialists (OTIS) provides healthcare providers and the public with evidence-based information about exposures during pregnancy and while breastfeeding (see Mother-ToBaby in the Additional Resources). One of the most notorious teratogens is thalidomide. However, clinicians today are probably more familiar with fetal alcohol spectrum disorder, which results from prenatal exposure to alcohol. Teratogenic exposures also include viruses such as rubella, cytomegalovirus, and toxoplasmosis; medications such as warfarin, lithium, tetracycline, and phenytoin; and maternal conditions such as type 2 diabetes and PKU.

Mitochondrial Disorders

Mitochondrial disorders are caused by mutations in mtDNA (i.e., nonchromosomal DNA) and are typically progressive disorders affecting the brain and muscles. Mitochondrial disorders are characterized by exclusively maternal (matrilinear) transmission (see Non-mendelian Inheritance). When many normal mitochondria are present, the effects of the aberrant mtDNA may be minimal. Examples of disorders with mitochondrial inheritance include Leber hereditary optic neuropathy (LHON), myoclonic epilepsy with ragged red fibers (MERRF), and mitochondrial encephalomyopathy, lactic acidosis, and stroke-like episodes (MELAS).

Epigenetics

Epigenetics is the study of gene expression changes that occur without a change in DNA sequence.[1] Epigenetics regulates which genes get turned on and off. Understanding the epigenome is increasingly important in the identification and treatment of pediatric diseases and developmental disorders. Unlike the genome, the epigenome is modifiable. The epigenome consists of molecular compounds that "mark" the genome and modify genetic expression by telling a gene or several genes what to do, when to do it, and where to do it. DNA methylation, histone modification, and/or micro-RNA (miRNA) are examples of three types of epigenetic modifications. *DNA methylation* involves the addition of a methyl (CH_3) group to the DNA, which modifies gene expression by turning the gene(s) off. *Histone modification* involves adding or subtracting molecules that in turn change how tightly coiled a segment of DNA is around its corresponding histone. DNA that is tightly coiled is closed to transcription, and therefore genes cannot be expressed, whereas loosely coiled DNA is open to transcription and subsequent expression. *miRNA* regulates the expression of target genes through posttranscriptional gene silencing. Different experiences or exposures may influence the epigenetic profile, including chemical exposures, diet, endocrine disruptive compounds, hypoxia, maternal physical state and age, placenta size, smoking, stress, and trauma. Epigenetic changes that occurred during an individual's embryonic development or in early childhood may contribute to common disorders, such as asthma, obesity, heart disease, hypertension, diabetes, and obesity.[3]

Care for Children With Congenital or Inherited Disorders

The pediatric PCP is ideally situated to evaluate and comanage children with a wide array of congenital or inherited disorders. With the support of existing health supervision guidelines, PCPs provide primary care, anticipate areas of medical vulnerability, and advocate for the prevention of secondary disability. In addition to providing ongoing primary care for infants, children, and adolescents with congenital or inherited disorders, the American Academy of Pediatrics (AAP) also states that pediatric PCPs should consider the genetic implications of common pediatric conditions, as disease causation of many common pediatric conditions, including asthma, allergy, autism, cancer, cardiac conditions, developmental delay, mental health disorders, and obesity, is being reconceptualized, recognizing that all diseases are located on the spectrum of genetic influence.

This section covers assessment, with an emphasis on the family health history, physical findings and cues, diagnostic studies, and clinical guidelines. It also introduces the genetics referral and how the PCP can assist families in creating an emergency plan for their children. Family and professional resources are highlighted.

Assessment

Family health history and the recognition of genetic red flags provide the foundation from which care evolves. Emphasis is on understanding genetic screening, working with children and families to understand the implications of a genetic workup and diagnosis, and coordinating care with genetic specialists. A complete head-to-toe physical and developmental assessment, combined with a comprehensive family health history, are important in identifying inherited and congenital disorders.

Family Health History and Pedigree

For the PCP, taking the time to collect a family health history in the form of a pedigree can be just as important as obtaining information from a laboratory test, yet this effort is often underused or absent in today's increasingly time-constrained visits. Most disorders have some genetic component, and the pattern of inheritance may become apparent based on the number and pattern of affected individuals in a family.

Three-Generation Pedigree. The family health history in the form of a pedigree is a valuable visual record of genetic links and health-related information. It should include at least three generations and is much more helpful in visual form, rather than in commonly used lists or narrative formats. Specific questions to use

when conducting a comprehensive family health history are listed in Table 27.2. Insights about family health are gained, not only because families share genes, but also because they share environments, behaviors, and culture—all of which contribute to common health problems. See Fig. 27.1 for the exemplars of pedigrees highlighting different patterns of inheritance.

All PCPs should be able to obtain, record, and interpret a three-generation pedigree, which includes the health status of an individual's first-, second-, and third-degree relatives (three generations). Sometimes asking about only two generations, or in some cases asking about four generations, may be more appropriate, depending on the trait or disorder and family size (see Table 27.3 for the proportion of genetic material shared according to family relationships).

TABLE 27.2	Family Health History: Questions for Inherited Conditions
Question	**Rationale/Comments**
Was anyone in the family born with a birth defect?	To identify conditions that affect others in the family. If answer is yes, try to get more information about the nature of the congenital anomaly.
Has anyone in the family had a stillborn baby? A baby who died early? A baby who died unexpectedly?	To identify unrecognized syndrome. Babies who died very early may have inheritable metabolic disorders. Distinguish sudden unexplained infant death from sudden infant death syndrome.
Is there any chance that you and your partner are blood-related? Is there any history of consanguinity/incest in your extended family? Is this pregnancy a product of incest?	Consanguinity of partners closer than first cousins is a risk factor for autosomal recessive disorders. If yes, recommend genetics consultation.
Is there anyone in your family who routinely sees a healthcare provider for a specific condition?	Significant if early onset or two or more close relatives are affected. Ask about hearing/vision, growth disorders. Genetic heart disease and genetic cancer risks are important. If yes, recommend genetic consultation and monitoring.
Have you/your partner, or any of your/your partners' parents/siblings, had three or more miscarriages? Any infertility issues?	May indicate a chromosome translocation. If yes, order a karyotype of the mother or father (or both). Difficulties becoming/maintaining a pregnancy may indicate a genetic syndrome
Does anyone in the family have learning problems, intellectual disabilities, behavioral disorders, or developmental delays?	Look for multiple family members affected or associated with dysmorphic features. If yes, recommend genetic consultation.
What is your/your partner's ethnic background and geographic heritage?	Discovering where an individual's ancestors come from can help identify certain ethnic and/or population risk factors.

TABLE 27.3	**Relationships and Shared Genetic Material**	
Degree of Relationship	Relative Designation	Percentage of Shared Genes
First degree	Parents, children, full siblings	50% for parents and children; on average 50% for siblings
Second degree	Grandparents, grandchildren, aunts, uncles, nieces, nephews, half siblings	On average 25%
Third degree	First cousins	On average 12.5%

There is a set of standardized, internationally adopted pedigree symbols.[4] In 2020 Sheehan et al. proposed nomenclature to represent transgender and gender-nonconforming patients.[5] Standard pedigree symbols are found in Fig. 27.2. Symbols for phenotypic gender include a square for males; a circle for females; and a diamond for persons with gender not specified, a congenital disorder of sex development, transgendered individuals, or when it is not clinically relevant to assign a gender.[4] For transgender and gender-nonconforming people whose gender identity may differ from their biological sex, depict their gender identity and denote their biological sex.[5] For example, use a diamond symbol to depict someone who identifies as gender neutral and denote their biological sex (e.g., XY) under their symbol. Both gender identity and biological sex have health implications. For instance, when tracking a family history of cancer of reproductive organs, knowing the biological sex is important to ensure correct screening guidelines are offered. An overview of the symbols, as well as how to connect them to illustrate various family relationships, is provided in Figs. 27.2 and 27.3. Multiple internet resources are also available to assist children, families, and providers in obtaining and documenting family health histories, including Pedigree by the National Human Genome Research Institute (https://www.genome.gov/genetics-glossary/Pedigree) and Genetic Alliance's "Does It Run in the Family?" Toolkit (https://doesitruninthefamily.org/).

The process of constructing a family pedigree should begin with the nuclear family, followed by adding aunts and uncles, cousins, and grandparents. For all persons included in the pedigree, it is important to record their date of birth or age, relevant symptoms, traits, and disorders, as well as the ages of diagnosis and the ages at and causes of death. It is also important to record miscarriages, stillbirths, infertility, and any children relinquished for adoption. An additional query should be made about the presence or possibility of consanguinity or incest. When pieces of family history are missing, note the information as missing because the absence of information does not mean the individual has not acquired genetic risk.

Genetic Red Flags. Genetic red flags indicate the potential for genetic risk. For some providers, it is easiest to remember simple rules (e.g., rule of too/two) or mnemonics (e.g., SCREEN, F-GENES) to remember the important components to look for or ask about when obtaining a family health history (Table 27.4).

In general, providers should pay attention if one or more of these genetic red flags emerge when taking a family health history: (1) multiple affected members with the same related disorder; (2)

earlier age at onset than expected for the disorder; (3) a condition or disorder seen in the less-often affected sex; (4) the appearance of a disease in the absence of any known risk factors; (5) at-risk ethnicity or ancestral background; (6) unusual close biological relationships, such as consanguinity; (7) multifocal or bilateral occurrence in paired organs; (8) intellectual impairment with or without major or minor malformations; (9) females experiencing three or more miscarriages; and (10) individuals with two or more major malformations.

Physical Findings Indicating Inherited or Congenital Disorders

It is important to identify red flags in the history and physical findings that suggest the presence of an inherited or congenital condition. Findings that are particularly notable include physical abnormalities (e.g., multiple café-au-lait spots, growth problems, and congenital anomalies) and neurologic abnormalities (including hearing loss, vision loss, developmental delay, intellectual disability, hypotonia, progressive muscle weakness, and hard-to-control seizure disorders). PCPs can hone their abilities by familiarizing themselves with advanced anthropomorphic measurement skills and by reviewing detailed descriptions and photographs of children and adults with various inherited and congenital disorders (see Positive Exposure in the Additional Resources).

Minor and Major Anomalies

The classification of features can appear somewhat arbitrary. A congenital anomaly or birth defect is an abnormality of structure or function that is present at birth. A physical finding is referred to as a *major* anomaly if it impairs normal body function (e.g., congenital heart disease, cleft palate), whereas a *minor* anomaly is more of a cosmetic variation, without impairing function (e.g., clinodactyly, small ear). This distinction is made because a genetic etiology is often considered when an individual has one major or more than two minor anomalies. Minor anomalies in the head, neck, and hand account for the majority of all minor anomalies (Table 27.5).

Malformations are birth defects that result from an intrinsic process, such as altered genetic or developmental processes. They typically result in a basic alteration in structure and occur early in embryologic or fetal development (e.g., cleft palate, anencephaly, limb agenesis). Deformities and disruptions are defects that result from an external process, resulting in an abnormal shape or positioning of a body part or organ. A *deformity* results from a distortion by a physical force, such as oligohydramnios on an otherwise normal structure (e.g., club foot), whereas a *disruption* is a destruction of a tissue or structure that was previously normal (e.g., amniotic bands). In contrast, *dysplasia* is used to reflect abnormal cellular organization within tissues that results in a structural change (e.g., achondroplasia). When there is a set, recurrent pattern of features or malformations that has a known genetic component, it is called a *syndrome*. An *association*, on the other hand, is a group of anomalies that occurs more frequently than would be expected by chance alone. Associations do not have a predictable pattern or a unified etiology (e.g., VACTERL). PCPs need to think in terms of phenotypic analysis and description, which begins with a complete physical and developmental assessment.

Genetic Testing

No single genetic test can identify all disorders. Equally important is the understanding that findings from genetic testing completed

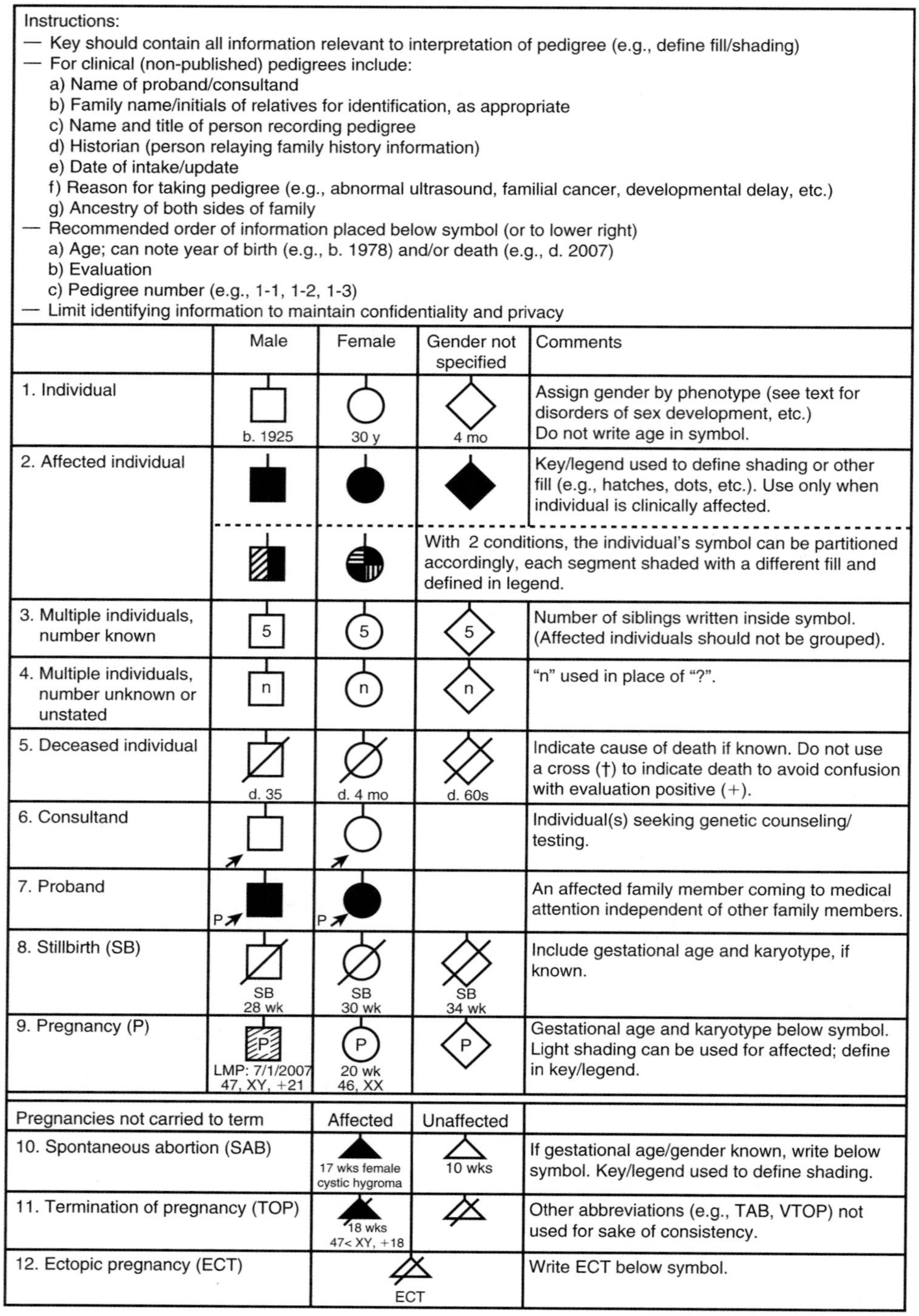

Instructions:
— Key should contain all information relevant to interpretation of pedigree (e.g., define fill/shading)
— For clinical (non-published) pedigrees include:
  a) Name of proband/consultand
  b) Family name/initials of relatives for identification, as appropriate
  c) Name and title of person recording pedigree
  d) Historian (person relaying family history information)
  e) Date of intake/update
  f) Reason for taking pedigree (e.g., abnormal ultrasound, familial cancer, developmental delay, etc.)
  g) Ancestry of both sides of family
— Recommended order of information placed below symbol (or to lower right)
  a) Age; can note year of birth (e.g., b. 1978) and/or death (e.g., d. 2007)
  b) Evaluation
  c) Pedigree number (e.g., 1-1, 1-2, 1-3)
— Limit identifying information to maintain confidentiality and privacy

	Male	Female	Gender not specified	Comments
1. Individual	b. 1925	30 y	4 mo	Assign gender by phenotype (see text for disorders of sex development, etc.) Do not write age in symbol.
2. Affected individual	■	●	◆	Key/legend used to define shading or other fill (e.g., hatches, dots, etc.). Use only when individual is clinically affected.
				With 2 conditions, the individual's symbol can be partitioned accordingly, each segment shaded with a different fill and defined in legend.
3. Multiple individuals, number known	5	5	5	Number of siblings written inside symbol. (Affected individuals should not be grouped).
4. Multiple individuals, number unknown or unstated	n	n	n	"n" used in place of "?".
5. Deceased individual	d. 35	d. 4 mo	d. 60s	Indicate cause of death if known. Do not use a cross (†) to indicate death to avoid confusion with evaluation positive (+).
6. Consultand				Individual(s) seeking genetic counseling/testing.
7. Proband	P	P		An affected family member coming to medical attention independent of other family members.
8. Stillbirth (SB)	SB 28 wk	SB 30 wk	SB 34 wk	Include gestational age and karyotype, if known.
9. Pregnancy (P)	P LMP: 7/1/2007 47, XY, +21	P 20 wk 46, XX	P	Gestational age and karyotype below symbol. Light shading can be used for affected; define in key/legend.

Pregnancies not carried to term	Affected	Unaffected	
10. Spontaneous abortion (SAB)	17 wks female cystic hygroma	10 wks	If gestational age/gender known, write below symbol. Key/legend used to define shading.
11. Termination of pregnancy (TOP)	18 wks 47< XY, +18		Other abbreviations (e.g., TAB, VTOP) not used for sake of consistency.
12. Ectopic pregnancy (ECT)	ECT		Write ECT below symbol.

• **Fig 27.2** Pedigree Model. Common pedigree symbols, definitions, and abbreviations. (Modified from Bennett RL, French KS, Resta RG, et al. Standardized human pedigree nomenclature: update and assessment of the recommendations of the National Society of Genetic Counselors. *J Genet Couns.* 2008;17[5]:424–433.)

for one individual can impact other family members. While there is increasing availability and use of genetic screening and testing in pediatrics, when presymptomatic and carrier testing or whole genome sequencing is under consideration, the ethical stance is shifting to specify that the best interest of the child should be the driving force, rather than parental discretion. The current AAP policy statement on genetic screening and testing in infants, children, and adolescents also emphasizes this, stating that any decision about whether to offer genetic screening and/or testing should be informed by the "best interest of the child."[6] The Genetic Testing Registry (GTR) is a robust resource for healthcare providers that provides current information about available genetic tests and where they can be done [see Genetic Testing Registry under Additional Resources).

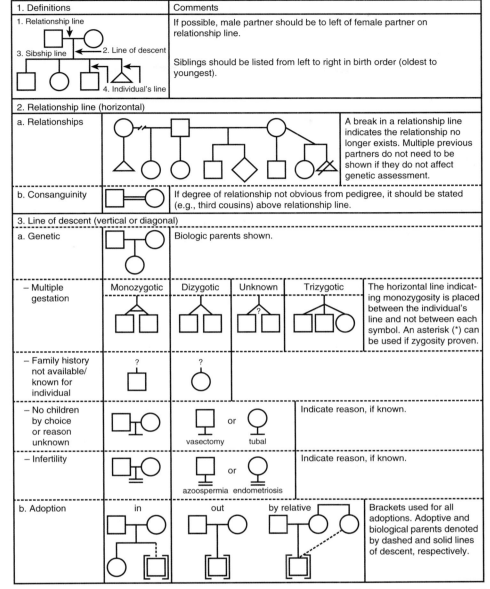

• **Fig 27.3** Pedigrees Line Definitions. (Modified from Bennett RL, French KS, Resta RG, et al. Standardized human pedigree nomenclature: update and assessment of the recommendations of the National Society of Genetic Counselors. *J Genet Couns.* 2008;17[5]:424–433.)

Screening

Screening is used in asymptomatic populations to identify individuals who need further evaluation or testing. Pediatric PCPs need to be familiar with newborn and prenatal screening. The family health history and specific tests that screen for disorders increasingly thought to have a genetic basis, such as autism, are also important. Similarly, a family health history can reveal certain forms of cancer (e.g., familial adenomatous polyposis) and cardiovascular diseases (e.g., hypertrophic cardiomyopathy and familial hypercholesterolemia) with variable age of onset, which subsequently have genetic testing and disease screening implications for pediatric patients.

Newborn Screening. Newborn screening is used to identify inherited and congenital disorders that benefit from early diagnosis and treatment. Today, effective newborn screening involves a sophisticated network of coordinated efforts among public health agencies, PCPs, and specialists. It involves individual and family education, mass screening for a select subset of congenital or inherited conditions, and short- and long-term follow-up plans for newborns whose results are positive. Each state determines the conditions included on its newborn screening panel; however, there is a national Recommended Universal Screening Panel (RUSP) that currently lists 35 core conditions and 26 secondary conditions for which every baby should be screened. The RUSP serves only as a guide for states; it is not a law. Clinicians should check the Advisory Committee on Heritable Disorders in Newborns and Children and Baby's First Test (see Additional Resources), where the latest information on the conditions included in each state's newborn screening is continually updated.

Following up on a positive newborn screen can be stressful for both the clinician and the family. Being well prepared makes

TABLE 27.4 Red Flags: Mnemonics

Mnemonic	Meaning
Rule of Too/Two	*Too* many of something: e.g., *too* tall, *too* short, *too* early, *too* young, *too* different, *or* *Two* birth defects, *two* cancers, *two* in a family, or *two* generations involved
SCREEN	**S**ome **C**oncerns about traits or diseases that run in the family **R**eproductive problems History of **E**arly disease, death, or disability **E**thnicity of the patient **N**ongenetic risk factors or conditions that run in the family
F-GENES	**F**amily history: multiple affected siblings in the same or individuals in multiple generations **G**roups (two or more) of congenital anomalies or anatomic variations **E**xtreme or exceptional presentation of a common condition(s), including early onset, recurrent miscarriage, bilateral disease **N**eurodevelopmental delay or degeneration (regression) **E**xtreme or exceptional pathology **S**urprising laboratory values

TABLE 27.5 Physical Assessment: Minor Malformations/Variations

General	Short or tall stature Body/limb disproportion Failure to thrive or obesity
Craniofacial features	Unusual head shape, circumference, fontanels Synophrys (fused eyebrows) Long eyelashes Hyper- or hypotelorism Epicanthal folds Up/down slanting and/or short palpebral fissures Heterochromia, ptosis, cataract, glaucoma Low nasal bridge Abnormal ear position, shape, tags, pits Short, long, or flattened philtrum Malar flattening Prominent metopic ridge Bifid uvula, high arched or cleft palate Natal teeth, central incisor Micrognathia
Hands and feet	Abnormal creases Short or long digit(s) Prominent digital pads Clinodactyly (incurved fingers) Syndactyly (fused digits) Polydactyly Camptodactyly (bent or flexed) Dysplastic nails
Hair and skin	Abnormal hair line or color Increased numbers or anterior location of hair whorl Hirsutism Hypo- or hyperpigmented patches Pigmented nevi
Neck	Short, webbing
Chest	Widely spaced or supernumerary nipples Abnormal chest shape
Abdomen, genitalia	Redundant umbilicus Shawl scrotum

the initial contact with the family more effective. The American College of Medical Genetics and Genomics (ACMG) developed ACTion (ACT) sheets that provide clinicians with the steps to be taken after an initial positive screening result with an accompanying algorithm. Their website contains the latest versions of the ACT sheets, which are regularly revised based on new tests and information (see Additional Resources).

Prenatal Screening. Screening and diagnostic tests to detect inherited and congenital disorders are standard prenatal care. Prenatal screening and testing are typically offered to all females to screen for common syndromes (e.g., Down syndrome) and congenital anomalies (e.g., NTDs), or to select females who might be at higher risk based on age, ancestral, or ethnic background or who have a specific family history of the disorder. All forms of genetic testing for the specific purpose of diagnosing a fetus can be performed directly on the fetus by collecting fetal cells through chorionic villus sample (CVS), amniocentesis, or cell-free DNA screening (examines fetal DNA found in the maternal bloodstream). In contrast, preimplantation testing is used to detect genetic changes in embryos before they are implanted to initiate pregnancy in the female.

Diagnostic Genetic Testing

Diagnostic testing is used to confirm a diagnosis and is used in a symptomatic individual or in response to a positive screening test. Specific practice guidelines help providers choose tests to order. For example, a chromosomal test would be used to confirm Down syndrome (trisomy 21) in a newborn, while a molecular genetic test designed to identify missing or duplicated sections in the dystrophin gene [Xp21.2] would be used to confirm Duchenne muscular dystrophy in a preschool male with delayed gross motor development and elevated creatine kinase (CK)/creatine phosphokinase (CPK) levels.

The main types of diagnostic genetic testing include karyotype, fluorescence in situ hybridization (FISH), biochemical testing, chromosomal microarray, molecular testing, and next-generation sequencing (Table 27.6). *Karyotyping* identifies and evaluates the size, shape, and number of chromosomes. *FISH* locates and detects a specific area of a particular chromosome, including subtle missing, additional, or rearranged chromosomal material by labeling a known chromosome sequence with fluorescent tags to see the location of genetic material. Unlike karyotyping, FISH does not have to be performed on cells that are actively dividing, making it more versatile. *Biochemical testing* studies the amount, activity level, or structure of proteins and enzymes that result from gene mutations. Many metabolic syndromes are screened for and diagnosed using biochemical testing. *Chromosomal microarray* (CMA) detects microdeletions or duplications of small DNA segments in any of the chromosomes but does not detect specific gene mutations. CMA is now the recommended first-line genomic test for children with neurodevelopmental disorders, including atrial septal defect, unexplained developmental delays, and intellectual disability, irrespective of having concomitant congenital anomalies.[7]

Molecular testing detects specific single-gene mutations (e.g., deletions, insertions, and single base pair changes) known to cause single-gene disorders. Molecular techniques directly detect aberrant sequence changes in a targeted gene or a short length of DNA, and indirectly detect aberrant changes in DNA structure by identifying size variations in fragments of DNA from the targeted locus or gene. *Next-generation sequencing* detects sequence changes among many genes as well as several sequence changes with one test.

Carrier Testing

Carrier testing is used to identify individuals who have one copy of a gene mutation that causes a known disorder in their offspring when two copies are present (AR disorders) or in X-linked disorders. In recessive disorders, individuals with one copy are often referred to as having the trait or being a carrier, rather than having the disease. Carrier testing is typically offered to individuals who are planning a family, focusing on information about the couple's risk of having a child with an AR or X-linked disorder. For example, parents can be tested to see if they are carriers of one of the mutations causing cystic fibrosis or to determine if they have sickle cell or thalassemia traits. Carrier testing identifies nonmanifesting female carriers of X-linked diseases such as Duchenne muscular dystrophy and hemophilia. Carrier testing in pediatrics is controversial. The AAP and ACMG do not recommend routine carrier testing in children and youth, except when the carrier status has medical implications in childhood or for pregnant adolescents.

Other Testing

Predictive or *presymptomatic* tests are used when asymptomatic individuals are interested in learning if they have a gene mutation associated with a disorder and are typically offered when there is a family history of a single-gene disorder. This type of testing identifies mutations that increase an individual's *risk* of developing an inherited disorder (such as breast or colon cancer, Huntington disease, and hypertrophic cardiomyopathy) before they actually manifest signs or symptoms of the disease. The results help individuals and their providers make decisions about the need for increased screening, preventative measures, life planning, and reproductive planning. In general, these tests are not done in pediatric patients because they are often associated with an adult symptom onset. It is considered more ethical for individuals to make the decision about receiving this information for themselves when they are adults. However, there are single-gene disorders that can and do manifest in children and adolescents, such as certain forms of hypertrophic cardiomyopathy and colon cancer. The use of predictive or presymptomatic testing should be guided by the best interests of the child with parental input.[8,9]

Pharmacologic testing (PGx testing) examines a person's genes to identify how drugs would move through the body, be broken down, or affect the body.[10] The primary purpose of PGx testing is to help clinicians identify the best drug or best drug dose for a person given their genotype. The Clinical Pharmacogenomics Implementation Consortium (CPIC) is an international consortium of professional volunteers and staff who promote the use of pharmacogenomic tests for patient care. One of the biggest barriers to the implementation of pharmacogenomic testing in primary care is the difficulty in translating genetic laboratory test results into actionable prescribing decisions. CPIC's goal is to offset the translation barrier. To facilitate the clinical implementation of pharmacogenomic tests, CPIC created, curated, and published peer-reviewed, evidence-based, updatable, and detailed gene/drug clinical practice guidelines.

Forensic testing is most often used in pediatric practice to establish biological relationships between individuals, such as establishing paternity. Forensic testing can also be used to identify victims of a catastrophe and crime victims or suspects.

General Guidelines

PCPs may lack adequate information about every rare, congenital, or inherited disorder, but they are experts in the primary care of infants, children, and adolescents and also care for their families. Being diagnosed and living with a rare, congenital, or inherited disorder can be overwhelming and isolating for the individual and their families. All involved experience a variety of challenges, including having limited information, financial or economic burden, abrupt changes to daily activities and roles, as well as new and/or unanticipated caregiving responsibilities. It is important to create an environment in which patients and families can talk about their needs and reach out for the support they need.

There are many resources for the PCP who cares for an individual with a congenital or inherited disorder. PCPs should be aware of current regional, national, and global resources for different disorders, as well as for the child/family just diagnosed or

TABLE 27.6	Genetic Testing			
	Karyotype	Fluorescence In Situ Hybridization (FISH)	Chromosomal Microarray (CMA)	Molecular Testing
Detects *large* deletions or duplications	X	X	X	
Detects deletions or duplication in *part* of a chromosome		X	X	
Detects *small* deletions or duplications			X	
Detects translocations	X			
Detects sequence changes in DNA or RNA for markers or mutations of potential or actual disease				X

growing up with the disorder.[11] For example, the Genetic Alliance is an especially useful PCP and family resource, especially its search tool (https://geneticalliance.org/disease-infosearch). This database contains information on thousands of congenital and inherited disorders manifested in infants, children, and adolescents (or affecting them in the future) along with links to educational materials as well as general and disorder-specific advocacy and support organizations.

Each affected patient/family needs an individualized plan of care. Table 27.7 highlights common clinical findings and primary care needs for a cross-section of the more familiar congenital and inherited disorders. In addition, the AAP developed disease-specific health supervision guidelines and periodicity schedules for many inherited disorders, including achondroplasia, Down

syndrome, Fragile X syndrome, Marfan syndrome, neurofibromatosis type I, Noonan syndrome, Prader-Willi syndrome, sickle cell disease, Turner syndrome, and Williams syndrome. Each guideline provides assessment needs by age, clinical cautions, vaccine considerations, and current and emerging research findings (see Additional Resources). For example, there are recommendations for pediatric PCPs and families affected by the diagnosis of Down syndrome that outlines primary care guidelines for the entire pediatric lifespan, beginning with prenatal identification and continuing with age-specific health supervision guidance. In addition, there are many syndrome-specific growth charts for children with conditions that affect growth, including cerebral palsy and Cornelia deLange, Down, Marfan, Prader-Willi, Turner, and Williams syndromes (Figs. 27.4 and 27.5).

TABLE 27.7 Selected Congenital and Inherited Disorders: Clinical Findings and Primary Care Issues

Disorder	Common Findings	Primary Care Issues
22q11.2 deletion syndrome (see Fig. 27.4) • Also known as DiGeorge or velocardiofacial syndrome • In most cases, syndrome occurs for first time in the affected person; about 10% are inherited (autosomal dominant) • Caused by variants in *TBX1* gene (22q11.2)	• Unusual facies; long tubular nose, low-set/crumpled ears, epicanthus, hypertelorism, malar hypoplasia • Palate abnormalities • Congenital heart defect(s) • Polydactyly, vertebral anomalies • Hypotonia • Early feeding problems • Constipation • Chronic otitis media, sinusitis	• Monitor growth using syndrome-specific growth chart (https://22q.org/symptoms-care/growth-charts/) • Monitor vision/hearing; strabismus and conductive hearing loss are common • Communication disorders, including delayed speech, hypernasality • Immunodeficiency; more likely to develop autoimmune disorders • Developmental delay, learning disabilities • More likely to develop personality and psychiatric disorders
Achondroplasia • Most common disorder associated with disproportionate short stature • Variants in *FGFR3* gene (4p16.3) known to cause this disease • Autosomal dominant inheritance	• Disproportionate short stature, short limbs • Infantile hypotonia • Macrocephaly • Dysmorphic midface, frontal bossing, depressed nasal bridge, anteverted nares, crowded teeth • Cervical spinal canal stenosis • Thoracolumbar kyphosis, lumbar hyperlordosis • Trident hands, brachydactyly, limited elbow extension • Knee joint hypermobility • Bowlegs	• Monitor growth using achondroplasia-specific growth chart (https://www.achondroplasia-growthcharts.com/) • Monitor OFC as hydrocephalus is a lifelong risk but is most likely to develop during first 2 years • Ensure medication doses are appropriate for age *and* size • Use achondroplasia-specific early development charts; most children have delayed motor milestones but not cognitive • Persistent or recurrent middle-ear dysfunction common; annual hearing evaluations recommended • Craniocervical junction compression risk; rear-facing car seat provides the best protection and positioning angle for any child with macrocephaly or skeletal dysplasia • Anesthesia risk; use care when manipulating the neck; avoid spinal anesthesia • Spinal cord compression, stenosis (manifests in older children with numbness, weakness, and altered deep tendon reflexes) • Avoid devices that cause curved "C" sitting, such as umbrella-style strollers, infant carriers, and soft canvas seats during first year of life • Avoid walkers, jumpers, and backpack carriers until child can bear weight (which should occur no later than 2–2.5 years) • GER, snoring are common; monitor for obstructive sleep apnea • Restrictive pulmonary disease; avoid living at high elevation • Higher risk for hyperhidrosis as child ages Health supervision guidelines available at (https://publications.aap.org/pediatrics/article/145/6/e20201010/76908/Health-Supervision-for-People-With-Achondroplasia?searchresult=1)

TABLE 27.7 Selected Congenital and Inherited Disorders: Clinical Findings and Primary Care Issues—Cont'd

Disorder	Common Findings	Primary Care Issues
Angelman syndrome • Complex genetic disorder that primarily affects the nervous system • Most cases caused by a deletion in maternal chromosome 15	• Pale hair, skin, eyes • Unusual facies: periorbital edema; small, widely spaced teeth; wide mouth (ear-to-ear smile); prominent lower lip • Global developmental delays, intellectual disability, severe speech impairment but adequate receptive language • Acquired microcephaly, seizures • Hypotonic trunk with hypertonic limbs (commando crawl) • Abnormal gait, arms held high/flexed elbows; problems with movement and balance (ataxia) • Feeding and growth problems • Abnormal sleep patterns including decreased need for sleep, delayed sleep onset, and overall poor sleep • Unusual behavior (happy and excitable), sticking out tongue, hand flapping, loves water, spontaneous (persistent) smile, fits of laughter	• Monitor severe developmental delays, learning disabilities, and speech, as there is often absence or near absence of speech • May not develop expressive language but usually understands simple commands; older children and teens may learn to communicate through gesturing and communication boards • Easily excited (distinctive behavioral cluster), hypermotoric and hyperactive, active explorers, often may appear to be constantly in motion, increased safety concerns • Sleep disorders, reduced need for sleep • Increased feeding difficulties, GER risk • Increased seizure risk beginning at age 2 years • Ataxia; some children never walk • Normal pubertal progression • Increased scoliosis risk
Beckwith Wiedemann syndrome • Overgrowth syndrome • Most common cause is abnormality of genes on chromosome 11 that undergo genomic imprinting	• Large placenta, long umbilical cord • Omphalocele or umbilical hernia, visceromegaly • Hypoglycemia (newborn) • LGA, with increased growth after birth (macrosomia) • Abnormal enlargement of one side of the body or structure (hemi-hyperplasia); becomes less apparent over time • Macroglossia; malocclusion, maxillary underdevelopment • Unusual facies: ear creases, pits	• Suspect syndrome in all LGA newborns, anticipate neonatal hypoglycemia • Monitor for feeding problems secondary to macroglossia; can also cause difficulties in speaking (articulation) and breathing • Monitor growth, limb length discrepancies, hemi- or hypertrophy/hyperplasia • Growth begins to slow by about age 8 years; adults with this condition are not unusually tall • Monitor alpha-fetoprotein levels regularly until age 4 years, abdominal ultrasounds every 3 months until age 8 years • Increased Wilms tumor (nephroblastoma) and hepatoblastoma risk, which is greatest before age 8 years • Increased incidence of renal anomalies
Down syndrome (Trisomy 21) (see Fig. 27.4) • Chromosomal disorder (extra chromosome); one of three types: complete, mosaic, translocation	• Hypotonia (infant) • Critical congenital heart defects (CCHD) common • Brachycephaly, short neck, excess nape of neck skin • Midface hypoplasia, flattened nasal bridge, small mouth, protruding tongue, small ears, narrow canals • Eyes: Brushfield spots, epicanthal folds with upslanting palpebral fissures, higher incidence of myopia and cataracts • Hands: short and wide with short fingers, single palmar crease, clinodactyly • Feet: exaggerated space/plantar groove between great and second toes • Short stature • Global developmental delay; mild to moderate cognitive impairment • Behavioral: short attention span, impulsive behavior, poor judgment	• Monitor growth using syndrome-specific growth chart (https://www.cdc.gov/ncbddd/birthdefects/downsyndrome/growth-charts.html) • Review newborn hypothyroidism screening; obtain annual and/or systematic hypothyroidism screening • Examination for CCHD, ongoing cardiac evaluations • Use syndrome-specific health maintenance guidelines • Ongoing ophthalmologic exam for cataracts • Newborn hearing screening, followed by ongoing otologic/hearing evaluation • Monitor for obstructive sleep apnea • Monitor for atlantoaxial instability; if any signs of cervical myelopathy, obtain radiograph, refer to neurosurgery • Monitor for neurologic conditions (e.g., infantile spasms, seizures, TIAs/stroke (Moyamoya malformation)) • Monitor for secondary disorders • Higher risk of developing duodenal atresia, celiac disease, hypothyroidism, diabetes (especially type 1), leukemia, Alzheimer disease (as adult) Health supervision guidelines available at (https://publications.aap.org/pediatrics/article/149/5/e2022057010/186778/Health-Supervision-for-Children-and-Adolescents?_ga=2.258752778.1062493642.1657330211-292422022.1653702194)

Continued

TABLE 27.7	Selected Congenital and Inherited Disorders: Clinical Findings and Primary Care Issues—Cont'd

Disorder	Common Findings	Primary Care Issues
Fragile X syndrome (see Fig. 27.4) • Most common form of inherited developmental disability • Caused by variance in *FMR1* gene • Individuals with only a small change in the gene may not have any signs or symptoms; those with bigger changes have more severe signs and symptoms	• Premature ovarian failure (menopause) in females is common • Unusual facies: prominent forehead, long narrow face, prominent jaw, high-arched palate, dental crowding, protuberant ears (develop late childhood/early adolescence) • Hypotonia, irritability, feeding problems, GER • Strabismus, refractive errors, nystagmus, ptosis • Recurrent or chronic OM and sinusitis • Connective tissue dysplasia (e.g., velvet-like skin, joint hypermobility, especially fingers), pes planus, congenital hip dysplasia, clubfoot, scoliosis • Short stature • Obstructive sleep apnea • Cognitive disabilities ranging from learning disabilities to severe intellectual disabilities • Speech and language problems, especially in boys • Social and behavioral/emotional issues; hypersensitivity to sensory stimuli, stereopathies, aggression (males) and shyness (females)	• Genetic testing is indicated for any male child with developmental delay or borderline intellectual disability • Anticipate delayed toilet training, enuresis • Moderate to severe cognitive deficits • Language delay is common, especially in conversational speech • Avoid excessive stimulation (e.g., large crowds, loud noises); provide earphones to decrease hypersensitivity • Monitor for behavior problems, including ADHD, emotional lability, irritability, and temper tantrums • Annual audiologic evaluation for conductive hearing loss • Orthopedic referral for connective tissue dysplasia issues • Ophthalmologic evaluation annually for strabismus, refractive errors • Monitor for inguinal hernia and macro-orchidism (begins ~9 years of age) • Increased incidence of autism, seizures (decreases by adolescence), hypertension, mitral valve prolapse risk Health supervision guidelines available (https://publications.aap.org/pediatrics/article/127/5/994/64903/Health-Supervision-for-Children-With-Fragile-X?autologincheck=redirected)
Klinefelter syndrome • Sex chromosome disorder in males • Extra X chromosome (47,XXY)	• Early: weak muscles, slow motor development (e.g., taking longer than average to sit, crawl, walk), and delayed speech • Cryptorchidism or hypospadias • Often have learning disabilities, mild speech/language delays, reading disorders; tend to have better receptive than expressive language skills • Shy, withdrawn, often immature • Absent, delayed, or incomplete puberty; small penis, small testes, reduced testosterone production (primary testicular insufficiency) • Reduced amount of facial/body hair • Gynecomastia, decreased muscle mass and bone density • Tall, with long arm span, longer legs, broader hips; scoliosis is common • Dental decay	• Monitor growth and development • Suspect any male with delayed pubertal progression, gynecomastia, low testosterone • Evaluate for testosterone replacement therapy • Annual thyroid screen • Monitor for scoliosis • Attend to dental care • Speech therapy • Monitor for anxiety, depression, impaired social skills, emotional immaturity or impulsivity, ADHD, limited problem-solving skills (executive functioning) • As they age, at risk for developing metabolic syndrome, involuntary trembling (tremors), breast cancer (for those with gynecomastia), osteoporosis, and autoimmune disorders
Marfan syndrome (see Fig. 27.5)	• Variable facial features, including long, narrow face, deep-set, downward-slanting eyes, malar hypoplasia, and micrognathia resulting in dental crowding • Myopia, ectopia lentis (hallmark), retinal detachment, glaucoma, and early cataract formation • Often tall for age, extremities disproportionately long in comparison with trunk; altered arm span to height ratio; arachnodactyly • Paucity of muscle mass and fat stores • Hypertension • Postural hypotension, low pressure headaches due to dural ectasia • Aortic root dilation, aortic tear/rupture, aortic valve prolapse/regurgitation, tricuspid valve prolapse, mitral valve prolapse/regurgitation • Spontaneous pneumothorax, reduced pulmonary reserve, and obstructive sleep apnea • Skeletal issues, including pectus deformities, scoliosis, thoracic kyphosis, protrusion acetabuli, pes planus, reduced elbow mobility, and increased laxity of other joints (see Fig. 27.5) • Stretch marks (lower back, inguinal, axillary regions) commonly across lower back, inguinal, and axillary regions (perpendicular to axes of growth) • Hernias (recurrent, incisional) common	• Monitor growth using Marfan-specific growth chart • Peak growth velocity occurs up to 2 years early • Excessive linear growth of long (tubular) bones; taller than predicted for family; altered arm span to height ratio; bones of hands and fingers are elongated but palm is normal, giving rise to positive thumb and wrist signs • Monitor for orthopedic conditions, including joint laxity, protrusion acetabuli, scoliosis, thoracic kyphosis, pes planus; pectus abnormalities are common • Many clinical features are age dependent (e.g., ectopia lentis, aortic dilation, dural ectasia, protrusion acetabuli) • Annual ophthalmology screen; myopia is common and progresses rapidly; ectopia lentis is a hallmark feature; increased risk of retinal detachment, glaucoma, and early cataract formation • Cardiac screening with echocardiogram throughout life; age of onset and rate of progression of aortic dilation are highly variable; β-blockers are often prescribed; decongestants and psychostimulants should be used with caution • Ongoing BP monitoring • Restricted participation in contact and competitive sports, as well as isometric exercise; aerobic activities in moderation • Increased spontaneous pneumothorax, reduced pulmonary reserve, and sleep apnea risk Health supervision guidelines and growth charts available https://publications.aap.org/pediatrics/article/132/4/e1059/64837/Health-Supervision-for-Children-With-Marfan?autologincheck=redirected

TABLE 27.7   Selected Congenital and Inherited Disorders: Clinical Findings and Primary Care Issues—Cont'd

Disorder	Common Findings	Primary Care Issues
Neurofibromatosis type 1 (NF1; von Recklinghausen disease) • Progressive, multisystem disorder primarily involving skin and nervous system caused by mutation in the *NF1* gene (chromosome 17) • Autosomal dominant inheritance	Two or more signs are required: • ≥6 café-au-lait spots 5 mm diameter (prepubertal)/15 mm (postpubertal) diameter • ≥2 neurofibromas or 1 plexiform neurofibroma • Axillary and inguinal freckling • Optic glioma • ≥2 Lisch nodules (iris hamartomas) • Associated osseous lesion (e.g., sphenoid wing dysplasia, cortical thickening of cortex in long bones) • First-degree relative with NF1 Clinical features are age dependent: • Café-au-lait spots are usually the initial manifestation (birth-infancy) • Plexiform neurofibromas are usually congenital (on face, trunk extremities) • Axillary and inguinal skinfold freckling typically develops between 3 and 5 years • Dermal neurofibromas typically develop prepubertally (increasing in size and number in puberty) Other clinical features: • Macrocephaly • Short stature • Seizures, learning disabilities, speech problems, hyperactivity	• Monitor growth using syndrome-specific growth chart; macrocephaly and short stature are common; puberty growth spurt is reduced • Annual ophthalmology screen; optic glioma present with visual loss, severe proptosis, and/or hydrocephalus in young children; Lisch nodules typically develop in early adolescence (slit-lamp exam) • Monitor for learning disabilities, with deficits in visual-spatial perceptual skills and poor fine-motor coordination leading to reading, spelling, and handwriting issues • Monitor BP (hypertension) as a screen for renal artery stenosis, aortic stenosis, and pheochromocytoma (adult) • Advise use of sunscreen • Precocious puberty may occur but need to rule out optic glioma as etiology • The number of neurofibromas increases over time; some get large or become cancerous • Caution with sports and activities if neurologic changes or hypotonia is present Health supervision guidelines available (https://publications.aap.org/pediatrics/article/143/5/e20190660/37168/Health-Supervision-for-Children-With?searchresult=1)

Prader Willi syndrome (PWS) (see Fig. 27.4)
• Associated with lack of expression of several genes on the paternally inherited chromosome 15
• Multiple mechanisms:
  • Microdeletion
  • Maternal uniparental disomy imprinting
  • Balanced translocation
  • NOTE: Absence of the same genes on the maternal chromosome 15 causes Angelman syndrome (see earlier)
	First phase (infant):
	• Significant hypotonia and early feeding problems; need for assisted feeding is nearly universal from birth to 6 months (e.g., tube feedings; feeding adaptations, such as Haberman nipple)
	Second phase (children):
	• Involves hyperphagia, behavioral problems, and obesity-related health concerns
	Other findings:
	• Hypothalamic insufficiency
	• Central obesity, short stature, scoliosis
	• Strabismus, myopia/hyperopia
	• Reduced salivation, enamel hypoplasia
	• Global developmental delay, mild to moderate intellectual disability, increased seizure risk (associated with fever)
	• Motor delays, poor coordination
	• Behavioral phenotype: tantrums, stubbornness, rigidity, compulsivity, skin picking, high pain tolerance, ADHD
	• Premature (isolated) adrenarche is common; hypogonadism (undescended testes, scrotal hypoplasia, small phallus/clitoris)
		• Monitor growth using Prader Willi-specific growth charts (https://www.pwsausa.org/resources/medical-issues-a-z/)
		• Anticipate and help family plan for behavioral issues: temper tantrums, obsessive behaviors, perseverant speech, skin picking (perianal, intertriginous folds), elopement (running away)
		• Challenges for PCP: high pain threshold complicates timely assessment of illness or injury; children with PWS rarely vomit
		• Generalized hypothalamic insufficiency is characteristic, including growth hormone
		• Reduced salivation leads to increased caries risk as early as 1 year of age; involve pediatric dentistry early; increased dental cleanings needed
		• Hypogonadism: trial of hCG is recommended for males, as anesthesia during infancy is high risk secondary to hypotonia
		• Annual vision and hearing screens
		Health supervision guidelines available (https://publications.aap.org/pediatrics/article/127/1/195/30016/Health-Supervision-for-Children-With-Prader-Willi_

Continued

TABLE 27.7 Selected Congenital and Inherited Disorders: Clinical Findings and Primary Care Issues—Cont'd

Disorder	Common Findings	Primary Care Issues

Turner syndrome (see Fig. 27.4)
• Female sex chromosome disorder (XO)
	• Short neck with webbing and low posterior hairline
	• Facies: ptosis; posteriorly rotated ears, narrow canals
	• Short stature; hip dysplasia, scoliosis, kyphosis
	• Extremities: short legs, short 4th/5th metacarpals, hyperconvex nails
	• Increased risk for:
	  • Cardiac defects (e.g., aortic root dilation, bicuspid aortic valve, coarctation of aorta)
	  • Kidney anomalies (e.g., horseshoe kidney, double collecting system, increased urinary tract infection
	  • Autoimmune disorders: celiac, thyroid, JRA
	• Vision: strabismus
	• Hearing: chronic OM with conductive hearing loss
	• Delayed puberty, infertility
	• Nonverbal (e.g., math) learning disabilities are common
		• Monitor growth using syndrome-specific growth chart (http://jspe.umin.jp/medical/files_chart/TSGC_eng.pdf)
		• Short stature is expected; GH treatment typically begun early (~4–5 years of age); monitor for kyphosis, scoliosis, lordosis
		• Annual hearing exam, recurrent otitis media, progressive midfrequency sensorineural hearing loss
		• Ongoing vision assessment, strabismus
		• Careful monitoring for cardiac issues, including cardiac defects, hypertension, hyperlipidemia
		• Annual thyroid screen (hypo- or hyperthyroidism); monitor for celiac disease
		• Ongoing assessment for celiac disease (tissue transglutaminase immunoglobulin A)
		• Supplemental estrogen therapy for sexual development and preservation of bone mineral density (late childhood, early adolescence)
		• Early-onset osteopenia/osteoporosis, vitamin D supplementation, appropriate estrogen therapy, exercise
		• Tendency to form keloids
		Health supervision guidelines available (https://publications.aap.org/pediatrics/article-abstract/111/3/692/79886/Health-Supervision-for-Children-With-Turner?redirectedFrom=fulltext)

VACTERL association
• Nonrandom association of birth defects that affect multiple body systems
	• No clearly established set or validated diagnostic criteria; no laboratory test can diagnose or rule out VACTERL association
	• Children typically have *at least three* characteristic features: (V) vertebral abnormalities; (A) anal atresia; (T) tracheoesophageal (TE) fistula; (E) esophageal atresia; (R) renal and radial, and (L) other limb
	• Less frequent:
	  • Single umbilical artery
	  • Growth deficiencies; FTT
	  • Facial asymmetry (hemifacial microsomia)
	  • External ear malformation
	  • Intestinal malrotation
	  • Genital anomalies
	• Intelligence is usually typical
		• Management is complex; directed toward the specific malformations and related symptoms that occur in each individual, which often vary greatly
		• Two-stage approach to treatment:
		  • Correct conditions that are incompatible with life (e.g., severe cardiac malformations, imperforate anus, and TEF)
		  • Close monitoring for other features and long-term sequelae (e.g., scoliosis, incontinence)

Williams syndrome (see Fig. 27.4) • Chromosomal microdeletion (chromosome 7)	• Infantile hypercalcemia • Low birth weight; reduced muscle tone • Infants are often irritable and colicky, with feeding problems that impede weight gain • Aversion to physical contact; sensitivity to loud noise • Can be missed in infancy, as dysmorphic facies are subtle but tend to become more distinctive with advancing age • Facies: puffy eyes, short/upturned nose with broad nasal tip, wide mouth, widely spaced teeth, full lips, micrognathia • Long neck, sloping shoulders • Clinodactyly, pectus excavatum, short stature • Personality: overfriendly • Mild to moderate delays in cognitive development, learning difficulties, delayed speech • Cardiovascular disease (narrowed arteries)	• Monitor growth using syndrome-specific growth chart (https://www.williamssyndrome.ca/williams-syndrome-growth-charts/) • Often presents to PCP with difficulty feeding, GER, colic, and FTT • Infantile hypercalcemia (early hallmark) contributes to irritability, vomiting, constipation, and muscle cramping; resolves in late childhood but abnormalities (e.g., hypercalciuria, nephrocalcinosis) in calcium and vitamin D metabolism are lifelong • Vitamin D issues: do not suggest multivitamin preparations containing vitamin D; recommend diligent sunscreen to minimize production of vitamin D • Annual or close monitoring of urine (urinalysis), urinary calcium/creatinine ratio, total calcium, and serum creatinine; consider UTI in children with fever • Ongoing cardiac evaluations; supravalvular aortic stenosis, coarctation of the aorta, renal artery stenosis, hypertension • Children can be overfriendly resulting in personal safety issues • Close monitoring of hearing; recurrent otitis media is common (sensorineural hearing loss) • Chronic abdominal pain is common in adolescents Health supervision guidelines available (https://publications.aap.org/pediatrics/article/145/2/e20193761/68224/Health-Care-Supervision-for-Children-With-Williams?searchresult=1)

ADHD, Attention-deficit/hyperactivity disorder; *ASD*, atrial septal defect; *BP*, blood pressure; *FTT*, failure to thrive; *GER*, gastroesophageal reflux; *GH*, growth hormone; *hCG*, human chorionic gonadotropin; *JRA*, juvenile rheumatoid arthritis; *LGA*, large for gestational age; *OFC*, occipital frontal circumference; *OM*, otitis media; *PCP*, primary care provider; *TEF*, tracheoesophageal fistula; *TIA*, transient ischemic attack; *UTI*, urinary tract infection.

Data from MedlinePlus, National Library of Medicine: http://medlineplus.gov.

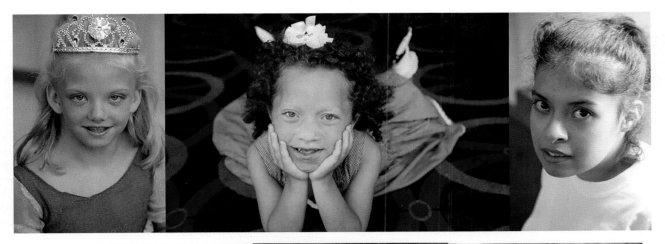
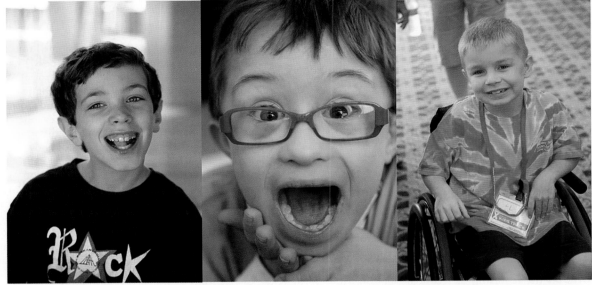
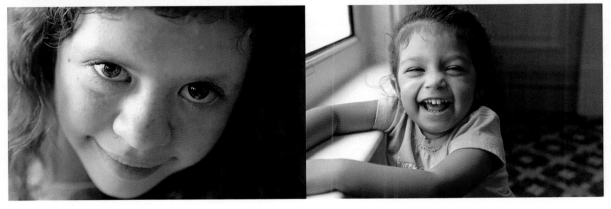

• **Fig 27.4** Children With Congenital and/or Inherited Disorders. *Top to bottom, left to right:* Children with Turner syndrome, Noonan syndrome, Prader-Willi syndrome, Fragile X syndrome, Down syndrome, Duchenne muscular dystrophy, Williams syndrome, and chromosome 22q11.2deletion. (Courtesy PositiveExposure.org.)

Genetics Referral

The PCP is the first-line point of entry; that is, the one who decides which children warrant attention and further testing, retesting, monitoring, and referral. The PCP's role is to help the family find a genetic specialist or counselor; initiate referrals with screening pedigrees, medical records, and other information; and evaluate the family's understanding of the need for a referral to genetic professionals. It is important to prepare the patient and family for the consultation and referral so that they understand the role of the specialist in the patient's overall care. The PCP should anticipate the need for the family to

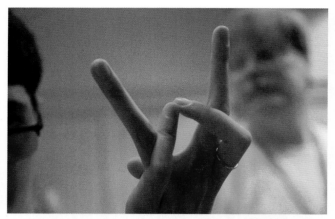

• **Fig 27.5** Marfan syndrome Hyperelasticity. (Courtesy PositiveExposure. org.)

obtain additional family health history and records, specialized neurodevelopmental testing, imaging and diagnostic studies, and child/family photographs. For those who live beyond the pediatric lifespan, genetic specialists also provide continuity of care as adolescents transition from pediatric to adult PCPs and specialists.

Genetic consultation and/or *referral* should be considered in the following circumstances: (1) a positive history for an inherited disorder, (2) physical findings and dysmorphic features on physical exam consistent with a known syndrome, (3) known inborn errors of metabolism, or (4) noted developmental, growth, or structural anomalies. Genetic specialists not only provide guidance in terms of ordering appropriate tests, but they navigate this evolving field with expertise in diagnosis, understanding inheritance patterns and recurrence risk, genetic testing, nuanced mechanisms of congenital and/or inherited disorders, and evolution of clinical manifestations across the lifespan. They also follow emerging ethical concerns and evolving perspectives on the reporting of secondary findings in clinical exome and genome sequencing.[12]

Comanagement with a genetic specialist offers many benefits, especially in terms of access to emerging evidence and high-value child/family support resources.

Genetic counseling is one specific aspect of the genetic specialist referral. Families often need ongoing support as they consider genetic information when making health-related decisions that affect their own personal physical and reproductive health, as well as the lives of their child, other children, and extended family. Genetic counselors facilitate families' understanding of the diagnosis of concern, its life course, and its management. In addition, they facilitate an understanding of how genetics/genomics influence disease (risk of recurrence, carrier status, etc.), identify strategies to address recurrence risk and assist individuals and families to choose a plan of action. Genetic counselors help individuals and families cope with a diagnosis, its prognosis, and the risk of recurrence, all of which are complex issues. They can also be engaged to support the family and the PCP when needed for difficult end-of-life conversations (e.g., postmortem investigations). Once the family has genetic counseling, the child's PCPs should reinforce genetic counseling information, assess the family's need for return genetic counseling, refer to local specialists and support services when appropriate, and advocate for the child/family within the community and the healthcare system.

Creating an Emergency Plan

Genetic specialists, in collaboration with PCPs, can help families create an emergency plan, which is a set of instructions that outlines when, where, who, and how to contact emergency personnel should their child need emergent care. The plan can be in letter form for the family to use when needed (e.g., Emergency letter for families [MSUD, Division of Metabolic Genetics, UUHSC]). While emergency plans should identify the child's diagnosis (or diagnoses), clinical findings, health status, current medications, allergies, and immunizations, they also need to highlight common presenting problems and findings with specific management strategies and professional pediatric and subspecialty contact information, especially for emergency care providers who may have limited knowledge regarding congenital and inherited disorders. With many genetic conditions (e.g., inborn errors of metabolism), an illness or surgical procedure may become life-threatening if certain precautions are not followed.

Ethical Issues

From the inception of the Human Genome Project, the National Human Genome Research Institute (NHGRI) had the foresight to anticipate the string of ethical, legal, and social issues that would arise as part of advancing the science of genomic research. Housed within NHGRI is the Ethical, Legal, and Social Implications (ELSI) program. A few of the ethical issues inherent to the identification of inherited disorders include the right to privacy and confidentiality, the right to know and not know, the duty to warn, disclosure of secondary findings, and genetic discrimination.

The Genetic Information Nondiscrimination Act (GINA) protects individuals from the misuse of genetic information in health insurance and employment and removes barriers to the use of genetic services. GINA does not affect health care. However, under GINA, *health insurers* cannot use an individual's genetic information to set eligibility requirements, establish insurance premiums, or request certain genetic tests. Further, *employers* cannot request, require, or purchase genetic information about an employee or family member, and they cannot use an individual's genetic information in decisions about job hiring, firing, assignments, or promotions. Unfortunately, GINA does not provide protection when a condition is already diagnosed or manifest, even if that condition is genetic. Further, GINA does not apply to life, disability, or long-term insurers. The types of genetic information protected under GINA include family health history, carrier testing, prenatal genetic testing, predictive testing, and other assessment of genes, mutations, gene products (biochemical products such as enzymes and proteins), and chromosomal changes. A few groups are exempt from GINA, including members of the military, veterans receiving care through the Veterans Administration, those using the Indian Health Service, and federal employees enrolled in the Federal Employees Health Benefits program. However, military, veterans, and federal employees have other protections that mirror GINA.

Additional Resources

Family Resources

Autism Speaks: https://www.autismspeaks.org/science/initiatives/autism-genome-project
Baby's First Test: http://www.babysfirsttest.org/
Centers for Disease Control and Prevention (CDC):
• Folic acid: https://www.cdc.gov/ncbddd/folicacid/index.html

- Family history: https://www.cdc.gov/genomics/famhistory/index.htm

Genes in Life: http://www.genesinlife.org/

Genetic Alliance Disease InfoSearch: http://www.geneticalliance.org/

MotherToBaby: https://mothertobaby.org/

National Organization for Rare Disorders (NORD): https://rarediseases.org/

Professional Resources

Honing Physical Assessment Skills

- *Diagnostic Dysmorphology* (1990), by Jon M. Aase, is one of the classic, most comprehensive, and detailed textbooks on dysmorphology.
- *Genetics and Genomics in Nursing and Health Care*, 2e (2018), by Theresa A. Beery, M. Linda Workman, and Julia A. Eggert, includes a detailed chapter on congenital anomalies, basic dysmorphology, and genetic assessment, including measurements, drawings, and photographs.
- *Medical Genetics in Pediatric Practice* (2013), by Robert A. Saul (Editor) and the American Academy of Pediatrics (AAP) Committee on Genetics, provides focused information for clinicians on the clinical features (including pictures), laboratory diagnosis, and management needs for specific genetic conditions from achondroplasia to Williams syndrome.
- *Positive Exposure* (http://positiveexposure.org/): Rick Guidotti, an award-winning fashion photographer, extends his talent to help transform public perceptions of children and adults living with genetic, physical, and behavioral differences. His refreshing yet realistic images provide a different lens for PCPs.

Genetics and Genetic Disorders

- American College of Medical Genetics and Genomics (http://acmg.net) ACT Sheets and algorithms describe short-term actions the PCP should follow when communicating with the family and determining the appropriate steps in the follow-up of the infant with a positive screen, including an algorithm that presents an overview of the basic steps involved in determining the final diagnosis in the infant.
- American Academy of Pediatrics (AAP) examples of disorder-specific health supervision guidelines:
  - Health Supervision for People With Achondroplasia: https://publications.aap.org/pediatrics/article/145/6/e20201010/76908/Health-Supervision-for-People-With-Achondroplasia?searchresult=1?autologincheck=redirected
  - Health Supervision for Children and Adolescents With Down Syndrome: https://publications.aap.org/pediatrics/article/149/5/e2022057010/186778/Health-Supervision-for-Children-and-Adolescents?_ga=2.258752778.1062493642.1657330211-292422022.1653702194
  - Health Supervision for Children With Fragile X Syndrome: https://publications.aap.org/pediatrics/article/127/5/994/64903/Health-Supervision-for-Children-With-Fragile-X
  - Health Supervision for Children With Neurofibromatosis Type 1: https://publications.aap.org/pediatrics/article/143/5/e20190660/37168/Health-Supervision-for-Children-With?searchresult=1
  - Health Care Supervision for Children With Williams Syndrome: https://publications.aap.org/pediatrics/article/145/2/e20193761/68224/Health-Care-Supervision-for-Children-With-Williams?searchresult=1
- MedlinePlus: Genetics: https://medlineplus.gov/genetics/. Information for the general public about the main features/inheritance of genetic conditions, the normal function of related genes and chromosomes, and how genetic variations contribute to conditions. Includes the educational handbook "Help Me Understand Genetics," which explores topics in genetics ranging from the basics of DNA to precision medicine.
- National Center for Advancing Translational Sciences Genetic and Rare Diseases Information Center: https://rarediseases.info.nih.gov/
- Gene Reviews: https://www.ncbi.nlm.nih.gov/books/NBK1116/. Point-of-care resource for busy PCPs that provides clinically relevant and medically actionable information for inherited conditions in a standardized journal-style format, covering diagnosis, management, and genetic counseling for patients and their families.
- Genetic Alliance webinars: https://geneticalliance.org/events/webinars. A nonprofit organization that offers webinars about newborn screening, genetic testing regulation, and family health history.
- Genetic Testing Registry: https://www.ncbi.nlm.nih.gov/gtr/. Central location for genetic test information, including the test's purpose, methodology, validity, evidence of the test's usefulness, and laboratory contacts and credentials.
- National Human Genome Research Institute (NHGRI):
  - Pedigree: https://www.genome.gov/genetics-glossary/Pedigree
  - Integrating genomics into clinical practice toolkit: https://www.genome.gov/minc
- OMIM: http://omim.org. A comprehensive, authoritative compendium of human genes and genetic phenotypes that is freely available and updated daily.

References

1. National Library of Medicine. *Help me understand genetics.* https://medlineplus.gov/genetics/understanding/.
2. Kaleelullah RA, Garugula N. Teratogenic genesis in fetal malformations. *Cureus.* 2021;13(2):e13149.
3. Puumala SE, Hoyme HE. Epigenetics in pediatrics. *Pediatr Rev.* 2015;36(1):14–21.
4. Bennett RL, French KS, Resta RG, et al. Standardized human pedigree nomenclature: update and assessment of the recommendations of the National Society of Genetic Counselors. *J Genet Couns.* 2008;17(5):424–433.
5. Sheehan E, Bennett RL, Harris M, Chan-Smutko G. Assessing transgender and gender non-conforming pedigree nomenclature in current genetic counselors' practice: the case for geometric inclusivity. *J Genet Couns.* 2020;29:1114–1125.
6. American Academy of Pediatrics Committee on Bioethics, Committee on Genetics, and American College of Medical Genetics and Genomics Social, Ethical, and Legal Issues Committee. Ethical and policy issues in genetic testing and screening of children. *Pediatrics.* 2013;131:620–622.
7. Martin CL, Ledbetter DH. Chromosomal microarray testing for children with unexplained neurodevelopmental disorders. *JAMA.* 2017;317(24):2545–2546.
8. Hamid R. New guidelines on genetic testing and screening in children. *AP Grand Rounds.* 2013;30:36.
9. Driessnack M, Daack-Hirsch S, Downing N, et al. The disclosure of incidental genomic findings: an "ethically important moment" in pediatric research and practice. *J Comm Genet.* 2013;4(4):435–444.

10. Cheek DJ, Bashore L, Brazeau DA. Pharmacogenomics and implications for nursing practice. *J Nurs Scholarsh*. 2015;47:496–504.

11. Carroll JC, Morrison S, Miller FA, et al. Anticipating the primary care role in genomic medicine: expectations of genetics health professionals. *J Community Genet*. 2021;12:559–568.

12. Miller DT, Lee K, Abul-Husn NS, et al. ACMG SF v3.1 list for reporting of secondary findings in clinical exome and genome sequencing: a policy statement of the American College of Medical Genetics and Genomics (ACMG). *Genet Med*. 2022;24(7):1407–1414.

28

Neonatal Disorders

KATHERINE NEWNAM AND NAN M. GAYLORD

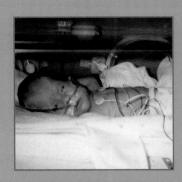

Neonatal survival depends on the successful systematic transition during the process of birth. The neonatal period is remarkable for the vast array of biophysiologic changes that must occur as the neonate transitions from intrauterine to extrauterine life, including cardiopulmonary, thermometabolic regulation, nutrition, elimination, and acquired immunity. Infant death (birth–28 days) declined by 2.9% from 558.3 per 100,000 live births in 2019 to 541.9 per 100,000 in 2020 in the United States with congenital malformations and low birth weight remaining the greatest risk factors.[1] Two-thirds of deaths within the first year of life continue to occur primarily in infancy with the highest risk in the first hour of life, followed by the first 24 hours of life.[2]

The most common challenges are referred to as the *neonatal energy triangle*, which includes hypoxia, hypothermia, and hypoglycemia. Although interlinked, each element can independently alter normal metabolic adaptation at birth.[3] Recognition and treatment of these conditions are the cornerstone of "golden hour" protocols to initiate care in a systematic, organized manner to rapidly stabilize the neonate to reduce the progression of illness and/or injury. Effective resuscitation and postresuscitation care are critical to reducing the incidence of asphyxia, a major cause of neonatal mortality and morbidity.[4]

An understanding of fetal development, needs, risks, and pertinent psychosocial and biophysical findings is necessary for primary care providers (PCPs), to assist the neonate's transition to extrauterine life. This knowledge coupled with careful and systematic assessment will provide the PCP with critical information to guide routine and specialized care. A holistic approach will focus on aspects of psychosocial transitions and strategies to best provide family support, education, and guidance to aid with successful adaptation. This chapter focuses on common perinatal and neonatal issues, diseases, injuries, and conditions, building on the global newborn care content described in Chapter 9.

Pathophysiology

High-Risk Pregnancy

Many newborn problems are due to poor and/or incomplete transition to extrauterine life, which can be secondary to premature birth, congenital anomalies, and/or adverse effects of delivery (e.g., birth asphyxia) (see Chapter 9; Fig. 9.1). High-risk pregnancies are those with factors that increase the chances of spontaneous abortion, fetal demise, premature rupture of membranes and/or delivery, intrauterine growth restriction (IUGR), and multiple fetal and maternal diseases, infections, or disorders. Identification of high-risk pregnancies is a key step toward anticipating

or preventing neonatal problems (Box 28.1) through specialized obstetric care.[5] Obtaining a three-generation pedigree can also be helpful in highlighting genetic risk factors (see Chapter 27).

Acquired Health Problems

In utero exposure to poor nutrition, alcohol, drugs, infection, and maternal conditions (e.g., hypertension and diabetes) can result in an increased risk for preterm birth and/or fetal abnormalities. The risk for neonatal problems correlates with certain maternal demographics (age, race) and socioeconomic factors (see Box 28.1). During the COVID-19 pandemic, pregnant females were at increased risk of severe illness due to the immune-compromised state of pregnancy. The risk of preterm delivery, and poor maternal and/or fetal outcomes were associated with COVID pneumonia.[6]

Perinatal Complications and Injuries

The term *birth injury* includes mechanical and anoxic trauma incurred by the newborn during labor and delivery. Predisposing risk factors for birth injury include macrosomia, prematurity, cephalopelvic disproportion, dystocia, prolonged labor, and breech presentation. Birth injuries include caput succedaneum, cephalohematoma, subgaleal hemorrhage, skull fractures, subconjunctival and retinal hemorrhages, intracranial hemorrhage, nerve palsies (brachial, phrenic, facial), fractured clavicle or humerus, ruptured liver or spleen, and hypoxic-ischemic insults.[5] Infants who sustain birth injuries need observation and/or treatment immediately following birth. PCPs who attend deliveries or care for newborns should be familiar with perinatal conditions that correlate with a higher risk of primary or secondary injury and be prepared to intervene quickly using the most up-to-date Newborn Resuscitation Program (NRP) guidelines.[7]

Immediately After Birth

The first minute of life is referred to as the *golden minute*. This critical time requires careful assessment and appropriate intervention to support infant survival. Improved neonatal outcomes have been correlated with delayed umbilical cord clamping for at least 30 to 60 seconds following delivery.[8] NRP guidelines (2021) include an initial rapid assessment that includes three key questions: (1) appears to be term gestation, (2) adequate breathing and crying, and (3) good muscle tone and movement.[7] When these are present, routine care is initiated, providing warmth and positioning the infant skin to skin on the mother's chest. Continued assessments are standard care to identify physiologic change and rapidly intervene as required. Resuscitation efforts may be necessary if the newborn does not meet adequate thresholds for heart rate,

• BOX 28.1   Factors Associated With High-Risk Pregnancies

Demographic and/or Social Factors
- Maternal age <20 years or >40 years
- African American race
- Developmentally delayed mother or low educational status
- Illicit drug, alcohol, cigarette use
- Poverty, unemployed, homelessness
- Unmarried or lack of social support
- Emotional or physical stress, including depression and other mental health problems
- Poor access to or use of prenatal care, underinsured, or uninsured

Medical History
- Diabetes mellitus
- Hypertension, maternal hypercoagulable state, sickle cell disease, congenital heart disease
- Autoimmune disease, including rheumatologic illness (SLE)
- Chronic medication
- Sexually transmitted infections (colonization: herpes simplex, GBS, syphilis, HIV)

Prior Pregnancy
- Intrauterine fetal demise or neonatal death
- Previous infertility
- Prematurity or low birthweight infant
- Intrauterine growth retardation
- Congenital malformation
- Incompetent cervix
- Blood group sensitization, neonatal jaundice
- Neonatal thrombocytopenia
- Hydrops
- Inborn errors of metabolism

Current Pregnancy
- Uterine bleeding (abruptio placentae, placenta previa)
- Infection
- Inception by reproductive technology
- Poor weight gain or abnormal fetal growth
- Multiple gestations, parity of more than 5
- Preeclampsia or eclampsia
- Premature rupture of membranes
- Short interpregnancy time
- Polyhydramnios or oligohydramnios
- High or low maternal serum alpha-fetoprotein

Labor and Delivery
- Premature labor (<37 weeks) or prolonged labor
- Postdates (>42 weeks) or prolonged gestation
- Fetal distress
- Immature L/S ratio: absent phosphatidylglycerol
- Breech presentation
- Meconium-stained fluid
- Nuchal cord
- Forceps or cesarean delivery
- Apgar score <4 at 1 min

Neonate
- Birth weight <2500 g or >4000 g
- Birth before 37 or after 42 weeks of gestation
- Male sex
- SGA or LGA
- Hypoglycemia
- Tachypnea, cyanosis
- Congenital malformation
- Pallor, plethora, petechiae

GBS, Group B streptococcus; *HIV,* human immunodeficiency virus; *LGA,* large for gestational age; *L/S,* lecithin-sphingomyelin ratio; *SGA,* small for gestational age; *SLE,* systemic lupus erythematosus.
From Kilpatrick SJ, Papile LA, Macones GA, eds. *Guidelines for Perinatal Care.* 8th ed. American Academy of Pediatrics and American College of Obstetricians and Gynecologists; 2017.

respiratory rate, and/or color. Apgar scoring is universally recognized as a newborn assessment of wellbeing.[9] It does not guide or determine the need for resuscitation based on a standardized algorithm of assessment and decision points provided by NRP guidelines (Fig. 28.1).[7] The 1-minute Apgar score assesses how well the newborn tolerated the birthing process, and the 5-minute Apgar score assesses how well the newborn is adapting to her/his new environment (see Chapter 9, Table 9.1).[10,11]

Premature and Special Needs Newborns

Premature and special needs newborns (e.g., congenital anomalies, disease states, social situations) require early and ongoing assessment, newborn and family intervention, and referral to primary care or specialist providers (Box 28.2). Before discharge, neonatal providers ensure that adequate family support, education, and specialized newborn developmental follow-up are in place.[12]

Common Neonatal Conditions

Skin

Amniotic Band/Constriction Syndrome

In utero fibrous strands that encircle fetal parts can cause permanent depression, deformity, and/or amputation of the entrapped tissue. Found in otherwise normal infants, these bands are thought to result from intrauterine rupture of amnion-producing fibrous strands that attach to the affected tissue. Although uncommon, amniotic band/constriction syndrome has been associated with abnormalities that include craniofacial anomalies, and thoracic or abdominal wall defects. The defect may be detected by prenatal ultrasound, and treatment depends on the severity of the deformities.[13] Constriction bands on the limbs are often managed in consultation with plastic surgery. Prognosis is widely variable and depends on the severity, extent, and location of findings.[14]

Branchial Cleft and Thyroglossal Cysts and Sinuses

Branchial cleft cysts and sinuses in the neck region can be unilateral or bilateral, open onto the cutaneous surface, or drain into the pharynx. They are located along the anterior border of the sternocleidomastoid muscle and form because of improper closure during embryonic life. Defects formed at the second branchial cleft cyst are most common, and these anomalies may be inherited as autosomal dominant traits. Up to 50% of children with branchial cleft cysts will develop a midline neck mass with or without secondary infection requiring treatment. Thyroglossal duct cysts are defects located in or near the midline of the neck with an extension up to the base of the tongue. Thyroglossal cysts occasionally contain aberrant thyroid tissue and mucinous material and may present as an upper respiratory infection.[15] Once these anomalies are discovered, surgical consultation is required.

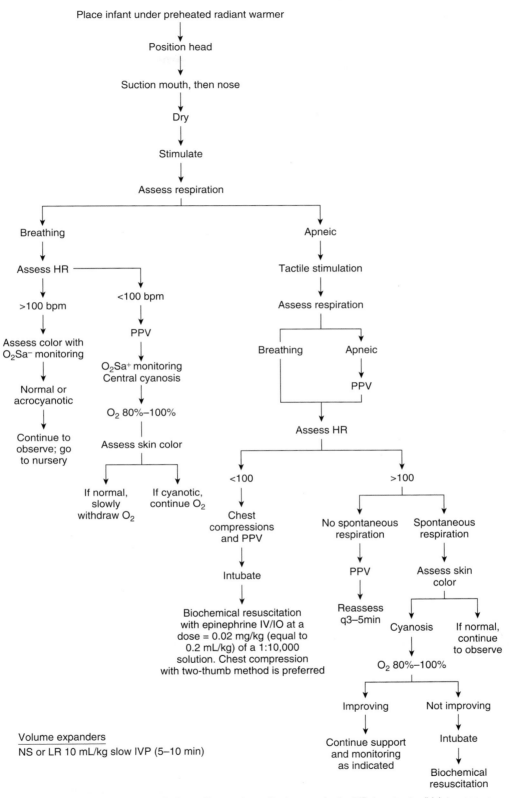

Place infant under preheated radiant warmer
↓
Position head
↓
Suction mouth, then nose
↓
Dry
↓
Stimulate
↓
Assess respiration

Breathing
↓
Assess HR
↓
>100 bpm
↓
Assess color with O$_2$Sa$^-$ monitoring
↓
Normal or acrocyanotic
↓
Continue to observe; go to nursery

<100 bpm
↓
PPV
↓
O$_2$Sa$^+$ monitoring
Central cyanosis
↓
O$_2$ 80%–100%
↓
Assess skin color
→ If normal, slowly withdraw O$_2$
→ If cyanotic, continue O$_2$

Apneic
↓
Tactile stimulation
↓
Assess respiration
→ Breathing
→ Apneic
↓
PPV
↓
Assess HR

<100
↓
Chest compressions and PPV
↓
Intubate
↓
Biochemical resuscitation with epinephrine IV/IO at a dose = 0.02 mg/kg (equal to 0.2 mL/kg) of a 1:10,000 solution. Chest compression with two-thumb method is preferred

>100
→ No spontaneous respiration
↓
PPV
↓
Reassess q3–5min

→ Spontaneous respiration
↓
Assess skin color
→ Cyanosis
↓
O$_2$ 80%–100%
→ Improving
↓
Continue support and monitoring as indicated
→ Not improving
↓
Intubate
↓
Biochemical resuscitation

→ If normal, continue to observe

Volume expanders
NS or LR 10 mL/kg slow IVP (5–10 min)

• **Fig. 28.1** Resuscitation in the Delivery Room. *bpm,* Beats per minute; *HR,* heart rate; *IV,* intravenous; *IVP,* intravenous pressure; *LR,* lactated Ringer solution; *NS,* normal saline; *O$_2$,* oxygen; *PPV,* positive pressure ventilation. (From AWHONN, Baker B, Janke J, eds. *Core Curriculum for Maternal-Newborn Nursing.* 6th ed. Elsevier; 2024.)

• BOX 28.2 Guidelines for Discharge and Follow-up of the High-Risk Neonate

Discharge Planning

- Demonstrate adequate weight gain, temperature control in open crib for 24 h, competent feeding without cardiorespiratory compromise, and mature and stable cardiorespiratory function for 5 to 7 days without caffeine.
- Ensure adequacy of immunizations based on infant's chronologic age and appropriate metabolic screenings are completed.
- Screen for anemia and nutritional risks; begin therapy, if indicated.
- Conduct fundoscopic evaluation if necessary.
- Ensure appropriate hearing screen has been completed.
- Identify all active medical or social problems through a review of the medical record and physical examination of infant; ensure home readiness has been evaluated, especially for the technologically dependent child.
- Complete car seat evaluation. Limit long car rides for 6 months and have another adult in the back when possible.
- Review with a family member the medications, feeding schedules, well-child care, signs of illness, change in health status, safety instruction, and appropriate response and follow-up for infants with active medical conditions.
- Identify family and community resources if infant is to be discharged on home oxygen therapy.
- Ensure adequate training of at least two appropriate family members in cardiopulmonary resuscitation (CPR) and, if applicable, home apnea monitor or other equipment use.
- Consider the need for: a home visit to assess environment, a visiting nurse, social services, respite care, support groups, early intervention services, referral to the Women, Infants, and Children (WIC) program, and/or a lactation consultant if breastfeeding.
- Ensure that follow-up care is arranged to include a primary care provider, neurodevelopmental follow-up, and surgical or other subspecialty providers, if indicated.

Follow-up Planning

- Schedule follow-up hearing screen (if necessary) for infants with craniofacial abnormalities, in utero infections, birthweight less than 1500 g, meningitis, exchange transfusion for hyperbilirubinemia, ototoxic medications exposure, Apgar score of ≤4 at 1 min or ≤6 at 5 min, ≥5 days of mechanical ventilation, diagnosis of a syndrome associated with hearing loss, failed initial screening, or family history of deafness.
- Ensure that by about 4 to 6 weeks of chronologic age a dilated binocular indirect ophthalmoscopic examination has occurred for neonates with a birthweight of 1500 g or less or with a gestational age of <32 weeks, a birthweight between 1500 and 2000 g, or gestational age of more than 32 weeks with an unstable clinical course. Additional examinations may be recommended based on the results of this first evaluation.
- Primary care follow-up visits every 1 to 2 weeks, especially if infant is on oxygen therapy and/or a cardiorespiratory monitor.
- Of prime interest at each routine primary care outpatient visit should be growth and development, preventative care, guidance, parental education with referral for additional evaluations if any concerns are identified. Ensure that the referral to Early Intervention program is complete.

From Interdisciplinary Guidelines and Recommendations for NICU discharge preparation and transition planning. *J Perinatol.* 2022;42:suppl 1.

Head, Eyes, Ears, Nose, and Throat

Cleft Lip and Palate

Clefts of the lip and/or palate (CLP) can be occult, involving only the soft palate or merely a small notch in the vermilion border to a complete separation of skin, muscle, mucosa, gum, tooth, and boney structures. Most CLP are immediately recognizable disruptions of normal facial structure. They represent embryonic failures in development that can occur in isolation or as part of a broad range of chromosomal, mendelian, or teratogenic syndromes, therefore a genetics consultation is recommended. When they occur together, they are known as *orofacial clefts.*[16] Collectively, CLP has a major clinical impact requiring surgical, dental, orthodontic, speech, hearing, and psychological treatments or therapies throughout childhood. They are among the most common birth defects worldwide, occurring more often in males than in females.[17]

Clinical Findings
- Varying degrees of cleft
- Interruption or cleft of the gum (alveolus)
- Unilateral or bilateral
- Involvement of the soft and/or hard palate
- A bifid uvula may indicate a submucosal cleft palate

Management and Complications. Referral to a craniofacial or an ear, nose, and throat (ENT) specialist is required as the staged surgical repair and timing are individualized based on the location and severity of the defect. Special feeding techniques are used until surgery can be performed. Breastfeeding and bottle feeding may be successful depending on the severity of the cleft, and an occupational or speech therapist can provide additional resources. Interprofessional team management is now standard, both in the short and long term, as specialized feeding equipment, speech therapy, hearing, dental/orthodontic, and ENT care will be ongoing, along with patient/family psychosocial education and support. Acute and chronic challenges such as middle ear, nasopharyngeal, and sinus infections, as well as associated hearing loss, can occur. Malposition of the maxillary arches and/or teeth may require orthodontic correction.[16]

Congenital Cataracts, Glaucoma, and Retinopathy of Prematurity

See Chapter 30 for descriptions of the most frequent congenital eye disorders.

Cardiovascular Disorders

See Chapter 33 for a discussion of the most commonly occurring cardiovascular conditions.

Respiratory Conditions

Transient Tachypnea of the Newborn

Transient tachypnea of the newborn (TTN) results from the incomplete evacuation of fetal lung fluid in near/full-term infants, leading to decreased pulmonary compliance and tidal volume, and increased dead space. Clearance of the fetal lung fluid occurs through active epithelial sodium channels (ENaC) that encourage reabsorption of the fluid, impeding gas exchange. This condition occurs most commonly in cesarean delivery without labor, precipitous delivery, breech position, second twin, history of maternal asthma, and macrosomia.[18] The primary differential diagnoses are respiratory distress syndrome (RDS) and pneumonia (Table 28.1). TTN is self-limited tachypnea with a respiratory rate >60 breaths/min, and retractions with/without grunting. Diagnosis is by exclusion with supportive care the hallmark of treatment.[19]

History and Clinical Findings
- Tachypnea, expiratory grunting, intercostal retractions
- No adventitious auscultation findings

TABLE 28.1	Clinical Comparison of Transient Tachypnea of the Newborn and Respiratory Distress Syndrome	
Transient Tachypnea of the Newborn	**Respiratory Distress Syndrome**	
Seen in infants delivered at or near term, often in infants born by cesarean section	Found almost always in premature infants, with the greatest incidence in infants weighing <1500 g	
Increased respiratory rate is present; grunting and intercostal retractions are not always present	Usually, respiratory rate is increased, infants grunt at expiration, nasal flaring is noted, and sternal and intercostal retractions are common	
Cyanosis is not a prominent feature	Cyanosis in room air is a prominent feature	
Air exchange is good; rales and rhonchi are usually absent	Auscultation reveals diminished air entry	
Begins at birth, usually resolving in the first 24–48 h of life	Progressive respiratory distress in the first hours of life	
Chest radiograph shows central perihilar streaking with slightly enlarged heart and fluid in the fissure	Chest radiograph demonstrates reticulogranular, ground-glass appearance, and air bronchograms	
Typical course involves gradual decrease in respiratory rate with resolution in about 72 h	Course variable depending on infant's gestational weight and age; usually, respiratory distress syndrome improves after 5 days of life	
No specific therapy other than maintaining oxygenation is usually necessary	Artificial surfactant and antenatal administration of steroids to the mother can reduce the severity of this disease; mechanical ventilation is common	

- Occasionally requires minimal oxygen
- Usually resolves within 24 to 48 hours

Diagnostic Studies. A chest radiograph shows prominent pulmonary vascular markings, fluid lines along fissures, over aeration, flat diaphragms, and occasionally pleural fluid.

Management and Prognosis. If the infant is not in significant respiratory distress, close observation, and transcutaneous oxygen saturation monitoring (oximetry) is sufficient until the absorption of fetal lung fluid is complete and tachypnea resolves. The need for supplemental oxygen therapy should be based on close oxygen monitoring. Intravenous (IV) fluid management and/or gavage feeding may be indicated based on the degree of tachypnea. The use of mechanical ventilation in TTN is rare. Infants usually recover rapidly within 24 to 48 hours without intervention.[19]

Neonatal Respiratory Distress Syndrome

Neonatal respiratory distress syndrome (NRDS), formerly known as *hyaline membrane disease*, results from surfactant deficiency disorder (SDD) that results in alveolar atelectasis (see Table 28.1). Most cases of NRDS occur in newborns born before 37 weeks' gestation with the incidence of NRDS inversely related to the degree of prematurity. NRDS can also be due to genetic problems

resulting in pulmonary hypoplasia or poor lung development. A rare autosomal recessive condition, surfactant protein B or C deficiency can be fatal even in term infants.[20] Antenatal steroids, postnatal surfactants, and newer ventilation techniques have reduced mortality from RDS to approximately 10%.[21]

History and Clinical Findings
- Sibling who had RDS
- Maternal diabetes
- Cesarean delivery or induction of labor before the baby is 39 weeks' gestation
- Problems with the delivery that reduces blood flow to fetus/newborn (e.g., asphyxia, cold stress, infection)
- Multiples (twins or more)
- Preterm, precipitous, or cesarean delivery

Physical Examination
- Dyspnea with rapid and progressive respiratory distress and/or apnea
- Tachypnea, grunting, intercostal retractions, nasal flaring, duskiness, and/or cyanosis
- Breath sounds may be normal but often are diminished with harsh tubular quality
- Fine rales on deep inspiration

Diagnostic Studies. A radiograph of the chest shows a fine reticular granularity of the parenchyma and air bronchograms. Blood gas results indicate hypoxemia, hypercarbia, and mixed metabolic/respiratory acidosis.

Management, Prognosis, and Prevention. Supportive care includes thermoregulation, fluid management, and respiratory support to establish functional residual capacity (FRC). Nasal continuous positive airway pressure (CPAP), and noninvasive and invasive mechanical ventilation are used as indicated to support the inadequate pulmonary gas exchange. The administration of synthetic corticosteroids to females expected to deliver prematurely is indicated to reduce the severity and mortality due to RDS as well as the incidence of severe intraventricular hemorrhage (IVH), necrotizing enterocolitis (NEC), and neurodevelopmental impairment. After delivery, the immediate introduction of exogenous surfactant to the newborn has been found to reduce mortality rates and improve short-term respiratory status in preterm infants. The overall prognosis depends on the severity of the disease and the gestational age and birthweight of the infant. The only fully effective preventive measure is the elimination of prematurity.[21]

Meconium Aspiration Syndrome

Meconium aspiration syndrome (MAS) occurs most commonly in term or postterm infants. This syndrome is a serious pulmonary disorder characterized by small airway obstruction, chemical pneumonitis, and secondary respiratory distress. In utero fetal distress and anoxia increase intestinal peristalsis and relax the anal sphincter, resulting in the release of meconium into the amniotic fluid. Thick meconium is aspirated either in utero or with the first breath. Approximately 10% to 15% pass meconium before delivery but only 5% of these infants develop respiratory problems.[22]

Clinical Findings
- Meconium in the amniotic fluid and below the vocal cords on resuscitation
- Tachypnea, intercostal retractions, grunting, and cyanosis within hours of delivery

Diagnostic Studies. A chest radiograph shows patchy infiltrates, coarse streaking of both lung fields, and flattening of the diaphragm.

Management, Prognosis, and Prevention. An infant born with thick meconium in the amniotic fluid but who is vigorous (strong respiratory effort, good muscle tone, and a heart rate of higher than 100 beats per minute [bpm]) does not require intubation and suctioning as had been previously recommended.[7] Continue to provide supportive care and standard management of respiratory distress. Resuscitation of the depressed infant with MAS follows the same recommendations as for an infant with clear fluid,[23] including standard management of respiratory distress.[7] MAS has an increased risk for spontaneous pneumothorax. Severe meconium aspiration cases may require treatment for pulmonary hypertension (PPHN) including inhaled nitrous oxide (iNO) and in severe cases, extracorporeal membrane oxygenation (ECMO). The mortality rate is increased in infants born with meconium staining. MAS accounts for a significant proportion of neonatal deaths. Residual lung problems are possible, and central nervous system (CNS) injury from asphyxia can occur.[22]

Gastrointestinal and Abdominal Conditions

Esophageal Atresia and Tracheoesophageal Fistula

Esophageal atresia (EA), a blind pouch that occurs in the esophagus with or without an associated fistula, termed *tracheoesophageal fistula (TEF)* is the most common congenital defect of the esophagus. EA with or without TEF occurs in 1 in 3500 to 4000 births.[24] This defect is classified into five types; most infants (87%) have type C, consisting of a proximal blind pouch with the associated fistula connecting the distal esophagus and the trachea (Fig. 28.2). Affected infants born prematurely and those that have associated cardiac anomalies have the highest risk for mortality. About 50% of infants with EA have an associated defect. A cluster of associated defects termed *VACTERL syndrome* is highly correlated with EA. This syndrome consists of *v*ertebral dysgenesis, *a*nal atresia [imperforate anus], *c*ardiac anomalies, *t*racheo*e*sophageal fistula, *r*enal anomalies, and *l*imb anomalies. An evaluation for associated findings, especially cardiac, renal, and vertebral, is warranted following the diagnosis of EA or TEF.[25]

History and Clinical Findings. The history includes maternal polyhydramnios and the inability to pass a nasogastric tube into the stomach during resuscitation at birth or afterward in the nursery, especially in a child with respiratory distress, vomiting, or excessive oral secretions. Feedings typically increase these early symptoms. The diagnosis may be suspected prenatally with maternal polyhydramnios and when a small or absent stomach sac or blind pouch is found on prenatal ultrasonography but is difficult to diagnose prenatally and may need additional evaluation.[26]

Physical Examination
- Respiratory distress
- Excessive or frothy oral secretions that require frequent suctioning
- Choking, coughing, and cyanosis, particularly during feedings
- Spitting or vomiting

Diagnostic Studies. Chest and abdominal radiographs show the nasogastric tube coiled in the pouch in the thoracic region confirms EA, and air in the stomach suggests an associated TEF. Carefully performed water-soluble radiographic evaluation of the upper esophagus demonstrates the anatomy of the atresia and the presence of an associated TEF.

Differential Diagnosis. RDS, MAS, diaphragmic hernia, and congenital heart disease should be considered.

Management, Complications, and Prognosis. This is a surgical emergency requiring immediate intervention. A nasogastric tube with suction is inserted into the blind pouch to prevent aspiration until surgical repair can be accomplished. Preoperatively, the infant should be placed in a prone position and orally suctioned frequently.[27] Pneumonia, atelectasis, aspiration, postoperative strictures, and repeated surgery are possible complications. The survival rate postoperatively approaches 100% unless other congenital anomalies are present. Approximately 50% of affected infants have other congenital anomalies.[25]

Duodenal Atresia

Duodenal atresia (DA) is a complete obstruction of the duodenum, ending blindly just distal to the ampulla of Vater. DA occurs in about 1 in 10,000 births and accounts for 25% to 40% of all types of intestinal atresia. It is associated with prematurity in 50% of cases, and other congenital anomalies commonly occur with DA. Associated anomalies include congenital heart disease, malrotation, renal anomalies, EA with or without TEF, and annular pancreas. Complex congenital heart disease has the highest associated mortality. About half of the patients with DA have chromosome abnormalities with the highest incidence (30%) in those children with trisomy 21.[28]

History and Clinical Findings. The history includes maternal polyhydramnios and is more common in prematurity and in infants with chromosomal abnormalities, especially trisomy 21. The infant presents with bilious vomitus, absence of abdominal distention, and jaundice.

Diagnostic Studies. Abdominal radiographs show a "double-bubble" pattern in the upright position secondary to air in the stomach and a distended duodenum.

Differential Diagnosis. Malrotation, volvulus, and duodenal obstruction are secondary to other reasons.

Management, Complications, and Prognosis. Surgical intervention is indicated once the diagnosis of DA has been made. Feedings should be discontinued, IV fluid management, and gastric decompression through low continuous suction as aspiration of gastric contents can occur as a complication of this condition. The long-term prognosis is excellent but greatly depends on early identification and treatment. Associated anomalies may also play a role in mortality and morbidity. Evaluation for associated anomalies, such as heart disease, skeletal anomalies, and renal abnormalities, is warranted.[28]

Malrotation With Volvulus

Malrotation occurs when there is an incomplete rotation of the intestine during development. This abnormal position of the intestine increases the incidence of volvulus, a loop of the bowel that becomes twisted around the superior mesenteric artery leading to vascular compromise and tissue necrosis. This condition in the newborn period presents with intermittent or acute pain, and intestinal obstruction with vomiting. It occurs in 1 in 500 live births, half of whom present with symptoms in the first month of life.[29]

Clinical Findings. Physical findings include abdominal distension and bilious vomiting.

Diagnostic Studies. Intestinal obstruction is demonstrated on the plain abdominal radiograph. Contrast studies demonstrate a "bird's-beak" obstruction in the proximal duodenum and a spiral (corkscrew) configuration of the duodenum.

Differential Diagnosis. Duodenal obstruction or atresia and annular pancreas are in the differential diagnosis.

Management, Complications, and Prognosis. In the symptomatic infant, fluid replacement and surgical repair are indicated.

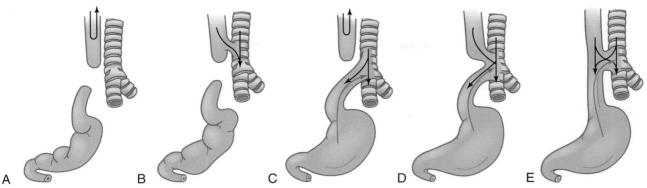

• **Fig. 28.2** Five Types of Esophageal Atresia and Tracheoesophageal Fistulae. (A) Simple esophageal atresia. The proximal esophagus and distal esophagus end in blind pouches, and there is no tracheal communication. Nothing enters the stomach; regurgitated food and fluid may enter the lungs. (B) Proximal and distal esophageal segments end in blind pouches, and a fistula connects the proximal esophagus to the trachea. Nothing enters the stomach; food and fluid enter the lungs from the mouth. (C) Proximal esophagus ends in a blind pouch, and a fistula connects the trachea to the distal esophagus. Air enters the stomach; regurgitated gastric secretions enter the lungs through the fistula. (D) A fistula connects both proximal and distal esophageal segments to the trachea. Air, food, and fluid enter the stomach and the lungs from the mouth; regurgitated gastric secretions enter the lungs through the fistula. (E) A simple tracheoesophageal fistula is present between an otherwise normal esophagus and trachea. Air, food, and fluid enter the stomach and the lungs from the mouth through the fistula; regurgitated gastric secretions enter the lungs through the fistula. Of esophageal anomalies, 85% to 90% are the type shown in part C; 6% to 8% are the type shown in part A; 3% to 5% are the type shown in part E; and fewer than 1% are the types shown in parts B and D. (From Rogers J. *McCance & Huether's Pathophysiology*. 9th ed. Elsevier; 2024.)

The prognosis depends on early identification of the volvulus and rapid surgical repair. Perforation, necrosis of the bowel, sepsis, and peritonitis are possible complications.[29]

Pyloric Stenosis

Pyloric stenosis is caused by a hypertrophic pyloric muscle, resulting in a narrowing of the pyloric sphincter. Pyloric stenosis occurs in 1 to 3 per 1000 live births, with a four- to sixfold increase in males compared with females.[30] It tends to be familial and is seen more commonly in White first-born males.

History and Clinical Findings
- Regurgitation and nonprojectile vomiting typically after the first week of life that progresses to nonbilious, progressive projectile vomiting around 2 to 3 weeks old.
- Insatiable appetite with weight loss, dehydration, and constipation.
- A distinct "olive" mass might be palpated in the epigastrium to the right of the midline.
- Reverse peristalsis visualized across the abdomen is frequently reported in the literature but is rarely seen in practice.
- There is an association of pyloric stenosis with the administration of oral erythromycin in the first 2 weeks of life.

Diagnostic Studies. The most common test is ultrasound with measurement of the pyloric muscle thickness. If ultrasound is unavailable or inconclusive, an upper gastrointestinal series demonstrates a "string sign," indicating a fine, elongated pyloric canal.

Management and Prognosis. Surgical intervention (pyloromyotomy) is corrective. Vomiting and fluid and electrolyte imbalance should be analyzed and corrected before surgery. Feedings should be introduced gradually. The prognosis is excellent.[30]

Hirschsprung Disease (Congenital Aganglionic Megacolon)

Hirschsprung disease is an absence of ganglion cells in the bowel wall, most often from the anus to the rectosigmoid region in 80%

of cases, resulting in a portion of the colon having no motility.[31] This disorder occurs in 1 in 5000 births. It is the most common cause of neonatal colon obstruction and accounts for approximately 33% of all neonatal obstructions. The disease is familial, affects males four times more commonly than females, is associated with various syndromes, and is common in children with trisomy 21. A thorough physical examination should be performed to identify additional anomalies that are sometimes present.[32]

History and Clinical Findings
- Failure to pass meconium within the first 48 hours of life
- Dilation of the proximal bowel
- Distended abdomen with bilious vomiting
- Failure to thrive, poor feeding
- Chronic constipation, vomiting, abdominal obstruction
- Diarrhea, explosive bowel movements, or flatus
- Down syndrome

Diagnostic Studies. Radiographs (plain or with contrast) indicate dilated bowel loops (Fig. 28.3). A rectal section biopsy to identify the absence of ganglion cells and identify a transition zone is the gold standard for diagnosis and treatment plan.

Differential Diagnosis. The differential diagnosis includes ileal atresia with microcolon, small left colon syndrome, and meconium plug/ileus syndrome (often associated with cystic fibrosis [CF]). In the older child, the differential diagnosis includes acquired functional megacolon, colonic inertia, chronic idiopathic constipation, lower spine malformations, and constipation.

Management. Surgical resection of the affected bowel is indicated, with or without a colostomy.[32]

Imperforate Anus

Imperforate anus is the lack of a rectal opening and occurs in about 1 in 3000 births. This defect is grouped according to the endpoint, either high or low lesions. The low lesion is where the rectum descends into the sphincter complex. Most infants with imperforate anus have an associated fistula. Infants with a

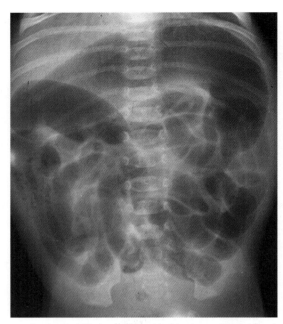

• **Fig. 28.3** Dramatic Dilation of Bowel Consistent With Hirschsprung Disease. (Courtesy Lawrence H. Robinson, Professor of Radiology and Pediatrics, University of Texas Medical School, Houston.)

diagnosis of imperforate anus have an association with another anomaly, often VACTERL syndrome. Congenital heart disease, EA, intestinal atresia, annular pancreas, intestinal malrotation or duplication, bilateral absence of the musculus rectus abdominis, trisomy 21, finger and hand anomalies, omphalocele, bladder exstrophy, and exstrophy of the ileocecal area are among the associated conditions.[33]

History and Clinical Findings. The history includes failure to pass meconium or the passage of meconium from an unexpected location. Findings may include no obvious anal orifice or lack of opening in the rectal area. In girls, stool passage may occur through a rectovaginal fistula, and in boys a fistula in the median raphe or to the bladder can be identified. The diagnostic studies to evaluate this condition vary depending on clinical findings including plain films, ultrasound, and urinalysis.

Management. Immediate surgical consultation and repair based on high/low lesion with or without patent fistula. Performing a colostomy may be indicated. Long-term management related to bowel functioning is often needed as some children will have challenges with bowel emptying or incontinence.[33]

Omphalocele and Gastroschisis

An omphalocele is a protrusion of the sac of the intestines into the base of the umbilical cord where the intestines are covered by the peritoneum without overlying skin. The occurrence is 1 in 5000 to 10,000 births.[30] Gastroschisis is similar in the appearance of intestinal contents with or without abdominal organs that protrude through the abdominal wall with no protective peritoneal covering. Gastroschisis occurs in about 1 in 10,000 to 20,000 live births. With omphalocele, serious associated conditions occur in 50% to 70% of newborns including congenital diaphragmatic hernia (CDH), and a variety of cardiac problems. Approximately 30% of infants with omphalocele have chromosomal abnormalities (trisomy 13 and 18). Concomitant hypoglycemia and macroglossia suggest Beckwith-Wiedemann syndrome. Associated congenital anomalies are rare with gastroschisis.[34]

Clinical Findings. Examination reveals a saclike protrusion covered by the peritoneum without overlying skin at the mid-abdomen.

Management and Complications. At delivery, maintain body temperature. The infant with gastroschisis typically has exposed organs placed into a sterile bowel bag with the application of warmed saline-soaked gauze to reduce fluid loss across exposed intestines. Decompress the bowel with the placement of a suction catheter and place the infant side lying to reduce vascular compromise of the tissue. A surgical silo of gastric contents may be necessary with large defects. When the infant is stable, surgical closure repair is indicated. Ileus is a common postoperative complication with a reduced incidence in those infants fed their mother's own milk.[35]

Necrotizing Enterocolitis

NEC is an intestinal infection characterized by varying degrees of mucosal or transmural intestinal necrosis. NEC is the most common life-threatening emergency of the gastrointestinal tract during infancy.[36] Radiologic evidence of pneumatosis intestinalis confirms the diagnosis. Classified as medical or surgical NEC based on evidence of intestinal perforation that requires immediate surgical intervention. The usual onset is within the first 2 weeks of life, but it can be later in very low birth weight infants. The cause is likely multifactorial with increased risk based on the degree of prematurity, immature intestinal immunity, and presence of microbial dysbiosis. The condition is less common in infants who receive breast milk feedings, strict antibiotic stewardship, and systematic feeding protocols in place.[37] Infants that have immature colons that have become necrosed from trauma or injury are at an increased risk of developing this condition. NEC occurs in 1% to 5% of neonates in the neonatal intensive care unit (ICU), with the highest risk to those infants born preterm, especially the extremely or very low birthweight premature infants. While NEC is most common in preterm infants, the condition is also seen in full-term infants; particularly those with a history of birth asphyxia, congenital heart disease, and after rotavirus infections.[36]

History and Clinical Findings
- Prematurity, small for gestation (SGA), asphyxia, polycythemia
- Maternal hemorrhage, preeclampsia, cocaine exposure in utero
- Exchange transfusions, umbilical catheters
- Congenital heart disease
- Abdominal distention, vomiting, bloody stools (25%)
- Apnea, lethargy, hypotension
- Evidence of disseminated intravascular coagulation (DIC), rapid progression of shock

Diagnostic Studies
- Sepsis evaluation should be completed.
- An abdominal radiograph (anteroposterior/left lateral view) shows pneumatosis intestinalis, a specific air pattern. Examination for evidence of portal venous gas and/or free air that indicates intestinal perforation.

Differential Diagnosis. The differential diagnosis includes sepsis, intestinal obstruction, volvulus, Hirschsprung disease, anal fissures, and neonatal appendicitis.

Management, Complications, and Prognosis
- Prescribe systemic antibiotics following sepsis workup.
- Stop feedings, initiate gastric suctioning, maintain electrolyte balance, and provide respiratory support including supplemental oxygen as needed.
- Initiate surgical consultation.
- Obtain serial abdominal radiographs to follow the course of the disease.

The mortality rate is 10% to 30%. Ileus and perforation are early complications. Sequelae to NEC include feeding intolerance, stricture formation, and short-bowel syndrome, especially after intestinal resection.[36]

Meconium Ileus

Meconium ileus is intestinal obstruction caused by meconium bowel impaction. Meconium ileus is associated with CF and maternal polyhydramnios. About 80% to 90% of patients with meconium ileus have CF and 10% to 15% of patients with CF have meconium ileus. In simple cases, the distal 20 to 30 cm of ileum can be disimpacted through water-soluble enemas in radiology.[29]

History and Clinical Findings
- Failure to pass meconium within 48 hours of life
- Progressive abdominal distention (rarely present at birth) and persistent bilious vomiting

Diagnostic Studies. A radiograph shows bowel loops of varying width, often with a grainy appearance due to trapped gas bubbles at the points of the impacted viscid meconium.

Management and Prognosis. Treatment is individualized including high enemas (with water-soluble contrast material) with about a 50% success rate. Laparotomy with a surgical plan based on the degree of pathology. The survival rate is excellent. Underlying disorder identification should be considered including CF testing. Referral to a gastrointestinal specialist may be necessary, and to a CF team if confirmed.

Diaphragmatic Hernia

In diaphragmatic hernia, abdominal contents herniate into the thoracic cavity. A diaphragmatic hernia is rarely caused by trauma. It is typically a failure of the pleuroperitoneal canal to close completely during embryologic development with size ranging from a small opening to complete agenesis of the diaphragm. It occurs on the left side 80% to 90% of the time with a frequency of 1 in 2000 to 5000 live births and is twice as likely to occur in females. While most cases of CDH are sporadic, up to 30% have associated anomalies including CNS lesions, EA, omphalocele, and cardiac defects and have been linked to trisomy 21, 18, and 13.[38]

History and Clinical Findings. These lesions are often diagnosed on prenatal ultrasound. After birth, immediate respiratory failure occurs secondary to pulmonary hypoplasia coupled with pulmonary hypertension. The degree of respiratory distress is related to the amount of functional lung capacity. Any newborn with respiratory distress should be evaluated for diaphragmatic hernia.
- Respiratory distress with tachypnea, cyanosis, absence of breath sounds
- Scaphoid abdomen, bowel sounds heard in the chest (rare)
- Heart tones best heard in the contralateral chest

Diagnostic Studies. A chest radiograph shows fluid and air-filled loops of the intestine in the chest. The mediastinum is displaced toward the unaffected side, usually to the right.

Management and Prognosis
- As soon as the diagnosis is suspected, the infant should be positioned with the head and chest higher than the abdomen.
- Rapid intubation and intensive respiratory support, including mechanical ventilation, high-frequency ventilation, iNO, and may include ECMO.
- Surgery, with intensive respiratory and metabolic support.

The survival rate is about 70%, depending on the size of the defect, degree of lung hypoplasia, and birth location. Centers of excellence have reported survival rates to 85% and fetal surgical interventions show promise.[38]

Umbilical Hernia

An umbilical hernia is a weakness or imperfect closure of the umbilical ring. Low birth weight and Black race are predisposing factors for the presence of an umbilical hernia.

Clinical Findings. Findings include a reducible soft swelling in the umbilical area often associated with diastasis recti.

Management, Prognosis, and Education. Surgery is not required unless the hernia persists beyond about 5 years of age, strangulates, becomes nonreducible, or dramatically enlarges in size. Incarceration is extremely rare. Most umbilical hernias resolve spontaneously by 1 year old, but some can take up to 4 to 5 years to resolve. Lesions with fascial defects greater than 2 cm in diameter have a lower rate of spontaneous closure.[34] Counsel parents to avoid taping coins or placing bellybands over the umbilicus. These efforts do not help, can contribute to an infection, and are a choking risk if swallowed.

Genitourinary and Renal Conditions

Hydrocele and Inguinal Hernia

See Chapter 42 for a discussion of hydrocele and inguinal hernia.

Acute Kidney Injury (Previously Known as Acute Renal Failure)

Acute kidney injury (AKI) refers to the discrete loss of kidney function and marked decline in the glomerular filtration rate (GFR) stemming from prerenal, intrinsic renal, or postrenal etiology. Newborns normally produce 1 to 3 mL/kg/h of urine and urinate within the first 48 hours of life, most within the first 24 hours of life. A stressed or sick neonate may develop decreased kidney function with urine output less than 0.5 mL/kg/h, a marker of AKI. Careful holistic assessment is necessary to establish possible causes that include stress during the prenatal period, dehydration, sepsis, anoxia, shock, administration of nephrotoxic drugs, kidney dysgenesis, obstructive uropathy, congenital heart disease, hemorrhage, and renal vein thrombosis.[39]

History and Clinical Findings
- Decreased or no urinary output; maternal oligohydramnios
- Pallor, edema, lethargy, vomiting, seizures, coma
- High or low blood pressure
- Pulmonary edema, congestive heart failure, or arrhythmias
- Abdominal mass or abdominal wall defect, myelomeningocele, or prune-belly syndrome

Diagnostic Studies (Based on Comprehensive Physical Examination and History)
- Catheterization or bladder tap to confirm the adequacy of urinary output
- Urinalysis to identify hematuria or pyuria
- Urine osmolarity, sodium, and potassium values to measure kidney filtration
- Serum blood urea nitrogen, creatinine, sodium, and potassium values to measure kidney filtration (although in the first days of life, these may reflect maternal kidney function)
- Complete blood count (CBC) including differential and platelets for evidence of thrombocytopenia, sepsis, or renal vein thrombosis
- Consider additional diagnostic testing based on symptoms, including a cardiac ECHO, and kidney ultrasound

Management and Prognosis
- Replace fluid loss (approximately 30 mL/kg every 24 hours), then restrict fluid and diet

- Maintain strict intake, output, and fluid and electrolyte balance
- Monitor blood pressure
- Dialysis is sometimes indicated
- The prognosis depends on the cause and the degree of kidney failure

Hydronephrosis

Hydronephrosis is a significant dilation of one or both kidneys caused by an obstruction of the ureteropelvic junction, posterior urethral valves, ectopic ureterocele, prune-belly syndrome, or ureteral or ureterovesical obstructions. Prenatal diagnosis is made by ultrasound and hydronephrosis may be accompanied by a distended bladder. Obstructive uropathy is slightly more common in males.[40]

History and Clinical Findings
- Findings on prenatal ultrasonogram
- Asymptomatic in early stages
- Decreased urinary output or abdominal mass

Management and Prognosis. Surgical repair may be necessary depending on the cause of the hydronephrosis. The longer the obstruction lasts, the less likely kidney function will return to normal, therefore urology follow-up is indicated by 6 to 12 months of age.[41]

Polycystic Kidney Disease

The presence of multiple kidney cysts of various sizes and shapes is the most common hereditary kidney disease. The autosomal dominant form usually appears in the fourth or fifth decade of life and is associated with hepatic cysts or cerebral aneurysms. The adult form (autosomal dominant) occurs in one in 400 to 1000 individuals; the juvenile form (autosomal recessive) is typically diagnosed during the prenatal or neonatal periods due to abdominal masses. This condition occurs in one in 10,000 to 40,000 live births.[35]

History and Clinical Findings
- Maternal oligohydramnios due to decreased fetal kidney function and results in varying degrees of pulmonary hypoplasia
- Evidence of Potter syndrome (low-set ears, micrognathia, flat nose, arthrogryposis, and IUGR)
- Abdominal lobular mass
- Hematuria
- Hypertension

Differential Diagnosis. A renal ultrasound is completed to confirm the diagnosis. Multicystic dysplastic kidney, hydronephrosis, von Hippel-Lindau disease, Wilms tumor, and renal vein thrombosis are included in the differential diagnosis.

Management and Prognosis. The infant presenting with the juvenile form of the disease typically is born with significant pulmonary hypoplasia leading to respiratory failure and requires aggressive ventilator support. These infants are at high risk for pneumothorax secondary to hypoplasia. Both forms require careful monitoring of kidney function, renal ultrasound for the enlargement of cysts, and observation for signs and symptoms of infection. Hypertension may be difficult to control. Nephrectomy may be necessary if cysts do not regress in size or complications develop. Dialysis or transplantation is sometimes considered for those infants with profound kidney failure. With severe involvement of the juvenile form, the neonate is at risk for death from pulmonary or renal insufficiency.

Renal Artery or Vein Thrombosis

A vascular clot typically forms in the intrarenal venous circulation and then extends to the main renal vein and may extend to the inferior vena cava. Injury to the kidney occurs when there is decreased blood flow to the kidney due to thrombus formation.[42]

History and Clinical Findings. This condition is associated with asphyxia, dehydration, shock, sepsis, hypercoagulable states, and maternal diabetes. Sudden onset of gross hematuria may be noted. Findings include a firm flank mass. Ultrasonography shows a marked enlargement of the kidney. Doppler flow studies show reduced flow to affected kidney(s), typically unilateral. The hematocrit is low, and the urine contains protein and often blood.[42]

Differential Diagnosis. Other causes of hematuria (e.g., hydronephrosis, cystic disease, Wilms tumor, hemolytic-uremic syndrome, and renal abscess) are included in the differential diagnosis.

Management
- Maintain fluid and electrolyte balance and treat renal insufficiency
- Monitor blood pressure
- Anticoagulation therapy used with caution
- Nephrectomy is not necessary unless chronic infection or uncontrollable hypertension occurs

Neuroblastoma

A neuroblastoma is a solid tumor of unknown cause that originates from neural crest tissue along the craniospinal axis. Typically, the tumor develops in the abdomen, most commonly in the adrenal gland but can develop at any site along the sympathetic nervous system. These tumors resemble other small round "blue cell tumors" such as rhabdomyosarcoma, Ewing sarcoma or non-Hodgkin lymphoma. About 600 new cases of neuroblastoma are diagnosed each year; it is the most diagnosed neoplasm in neonates. Genetic mutations of the *BARD1* gene are more likely to be associated with neuroblastoma.[43]

Clinical Findings
- An unexplained fever, mass, and symptoms related to the site of the tumor
- Ascites and/or firm, irregular, nontender mass in the abdomen
- Pallor, hypotension, irritability
- Possible external tumors in newborns, such as skin lesions similar to those present during congenital rubella syndrome
- Signs and symptoms reflect the tumor site and may be varied resulting in delayed diagnosis

Diagnostic Studies. The following help to assess and stage the disease:
- CBC, basic chemistry panel
- Renal radiographs to detect calcifications
- Ultrasound, computed tomography (CT) or magnetic resonance imaging (MRI) of the abdomen
- Radiograph or CT scan of the chest
- Skeletal survey or bone scan
- Urine catecholamines, homovanillic acid, and vanillylmandelic acid
- Bone marrow aspirate and biopsy
- Lymph node survey for metastatic spread

Differential Diagnosis. Wilms tumor, hydronephrosis, renal vein thrombosis, and lymphoma are included in the differential diagnosis.

Management and Prognosis. Although some neuroblastomas regress without therapy (usually only those in children younger than 1 year old), treatment generally involves surgical removal followed by radiation therapy or chemotherapy. The prognosis depends on the age of the patient, the level of metastasis, and the stage of the tumor.[44]

Renal Agenesis

Renal agenesis is the failure of the kidney to form. Unilateral agenesis occurs in one in 450 to 1000 births. Bilateral agenesis is incompatible with life and occurs in one in 3000 births with male predominance. Bilateral renal agenesis is termed *Potter syndrome* with a characteristic facial appearance.[45]

History and Clinical Findings. Maternal oligohydramnios is noted in bilateral agenesis. Unilateral renal agenesis usually is detected on prenatal ultrasound or when the child is evaluated for other congenital anomalies or for urinary tract infection (UTI).
- Single umbilical artery associated with unilateral agenesis
- Associated anomalies involving the gastrointestinal or urinary tract and skeleton, especially with Potter syndrome (bilateral agenesis)
- Low-set ears, senile appearance, broad nose, and receding chin consistent with Potter syndrome

Management and Prognosis. Infants with bilateral disease often die shortly after birth due to pulmonary insufficiency. Unilateral renal agenesis is typically discovered when evaluation for other congenital defects (VACTERL).[25]

Endocrine Conditions

Congenital Hypothyroidism

Congenital hypothyroidism (CH) is included in newborn screening (NBS) of every state as the detection of the defect leads to immediate treatment with levothyroxine at 10 to 15 mcg/kg daily. Untreated CH leads to intellectual disabilities; if detected on the NBS, treatment should be initiated before 2 weeks of age to prevent adverse neurodevelopmental outcomes. The goal of treatment is to maintain consistent euthyroidism with normal thyroid-stimulating hormone (TSH) and free thyroxine (T4) in the upper half of the age-specific reference range during the first 3 years of life. Follow-up is required every 2 weeks, in consultation with the pediatric endocrinologist, until the FSH and T4 are stable then every month or two in the first 6 months of life. Even if NBS thyroid test results are normal when clinical signs and symptoms of hypothyroidism are present (such as large posterior fontanelle, large tongue, umbilical hernia, prolonged jaundice, constipation, lethargy, and/or hypothermia), measurement of serum TSH and free T4 is indicated. Despite early initiation of appropriate treatment, children with CH are at higher risk for neurocognitive and socioemotional dysfunction and, therefore require close evaluation and follow-up[46] (see Chapter 39).

Congenital Adrenal Hyperplasia

Congenital adrenal hyperplasia is described in Chapter 39.

Metabolic Conditions

Hypoglycemia

Glucose is critical for energy metabolism in the brain; a ready fuel responsible for vital functions including cerebral oxygen metabolism. In the term infant, serum glucose levels rarely fall below 35 mg/dL in the first 3 hours of life, below 40 mg/dL between 3 and 24 hours of life, or below 45 mg/dL thereafter, although there is no strong correlation between suboptimal serum glucose levels and overt symptoms.[47] Infants at higher risk of developing hypoglycemia include late preterm infants exposed to maternal steroids, SGA infants, large for gestational age (LGA) and those born to diabetic mothers, asphyxia at birth, sepsis, erythroblastosis fetalis, glycogen storage disease, or galactosemia (Table 28.2).

Management and Prognosis. Infants with symptomatic hypoglycemia, particularly low birth weight infants, LGA, and infants of diabetic mothers should receive rapid corrective treatment to reduce risk for poor intellectual development. Standard serum glucose monitoring for at risk infants is required. Therapeutic glucose gel can be used to support oral feedings in infants at risk for transient hypoglycemia.[48] Prognosis for normal intellectual function is guarded in infants with prolonged and severe hypoglycemia.[47]

Infant of a Diabetic Mother

Gestational diabetes affects approximately 2% of pregnancies and insulin-dependent diabetes occurs in 1 in 1000 adults females. An infant of a diabetic mother (IDM) is born to a mother whose pregnancy is complicated by poorly controlled gestational or chronic (type I or type II) diabetes mellitus. Maternal hyperglycemia causes fetal hyperglycemia and hyperinsulinemia, leading to increased hepatic glucose uptake and glycogen synthesis, accelerated lipogenesis, and augmented protein synthesis (see Table 28.2).[49]

Management, Complications, and Prevention. Cardiomegaly is common (30%), and heart failure occurs in 5% to 10% of infants. Congenital anomalies are increased threefold; there is a 15 times greater incidence of cardiac malformations, and lumbosacral agenesis is more common.[49] Maternal glucose supply is abruptly discontinued with the severing of the umbilical cord. The elevated maternal blood glucose level generates increased insulin production in the infant. This transiently elevated insulin level without adequate glucose stores places the IDM at increased risk for hypoglycemia. Symptomatic neonatal hypoglycemia increases the risk of impaired intellectual development. Strict management of blood glucose levels in mothers with diabetes decreases the risk of severe complications in the infant. Additional complications include surfactant deficiency leading to RDS, hyperbilirubinemia, small left colon, polycythemia, and hypertrophy of the septum with secondary heart failure.[47]

Hematologic Conditions

Polycythemia

Polycythemia is characterized by a central hematocrit of 65% or higher. The hematocrit value peaks approximately 2 to 3 hours of life and peripheral values can vary as much as 15%. Polycythemia or hyperviscosity of the blood occurs with a variety of conditions, including twin-to-twin transfusion, maternal-fetal transfusion, and delayed cord clamping. Other conditions stem from chronic fetal hypoxia resulting in stimulated erythropoietin production and increased red blood cell (RBC) production. These are IDM, cyanotic congenital heart disease, trisomy, and infants that are born growth restricted or LGA. Polycythemia occurs in 1% to 2% of term appropriate-for-gestational-age births, depending on the etiology (see Table 28.2).[50]

History and Clinical Findings
- Dehydration should be considered as a cause.
- Cyanosis (persistent fetal circulation), tachypnea, respiratory distress irritability, lethargy, feeding disturbances, early jaundice.
- Increased risk for NEC. In severe cases, stroke, seizures, and renal vein thrombosis.

Management and Prognosis. Confirmation of laboratory values should be completed before treatment. Most asymptomatic infants are normal and can tolerate hematocrit values to 70%, but

	Identification and Management of Hypoglycemia, Infant of Diabetic Mother and Polycythemia in the Newborn

TABLE 28.2

Condition	Clinical Finding	Workup	Management
Hypoglycemia	Blood glucose <30 mg/dL; infant with history of SGA; mother with poorly controlled diabetes (IDM); at risk for sepsis, asphyxia, erythroblastosis fetalis, lethargy, poor feeding, regurgitation, apnea, jitteriness, pallor, sweating, cool extremities and seizures	Serum glucose—measure within 1 h of birth, every 2 h until 6–8 h of life, then every 4–6 h until 24 h of life	Give normoglycemic high-risk infants oral or gavage feedings with breast milk or formula at 1–3 h of life and continue every 2–3 h for 24–48 h; IV glucose at 8 mg/kg/min if serum glucose less than 30 to 35 mg/dL and oral feedings poorly tolerated
Infant of diabetic mother (IDM)	IDM: Large, plump infant; puffy facies; plethora; hyperactivity first 3 days; ± hypotonicity, lethargy, poor suck; ± cardiomegaly and murmur	Intensive observation and care Serum glucose—measure within 1 h of birth, then frequently for the next 6–8 h, especially for macrosomia or growth restriction	If clinically well and normoglycemic, start oral or gavage feedings with infant formula or breast milk within 2–3 h old and continue at 3-h intervals; If infant is unable to tolerate oral feeding, discontinue feeding and give 10% glucose by peripheral IV infusion at a rate of 4–8 mg/kg/min; Treat hypoglycemia, even in asymptomatic infants, with IV infusions of glucose
Polycythemia	Cyanosis, tachypnea, respiratory distress; hyperbilirubinemia; infant with history of diabetic mother; IUGR, postmaturity, SGA exposed to chronic hypoxia; recipient of twin–twin transfusion; delayed clamping of umbilical cord; plethora; and feeding disturbance	Hematocrit ≥65%	Phlebotomy and replacement with saline or albumin or partial exchange transfusion to reduce hematocrit to 50%

IUGR, Intrauterine growth restriction; *IV,* intravenous; *SGA,* small for gestational age.
From Kleinman K, McDaniel L, Molloy M. *The Harriet Lane Handbook.* 22nd ed. Elsevier; 2021.

close observation and serial monitoring including bilirubin levels are recommended. Adequate hydration including IV fluids or partial exchange transfusion with normal saline for extreme levels may be indicated. Long-term problems may include speech deficits, abnormal fine motor control, reduced intelligence quotient (IQ), and other neurologic abnormalities may develop. Neurodevelopmental follow-up is indicated for these infants.[51]

Vitamin K Deficiency Bleeding in the Newborn

Previously termed *hemorrhagic disease of the newborn,* this transient but severe form of hemorrhage can lead from mild to significant bleeding risk. Transient vitamin K-dependent clotting factor deficiencies lead to Vitamin K–dependent bleeding (VKDB). Vitamin K deficiency is caused by a lack of free vitamin K in the mother and the absence of bacterial intestinal flora normally responsible for the synthesis of vitamin K in the infant. Vitamin K–dependent clotting factors (II, VII, IX, and X) are normal at birth, but decrease within 2 to 3 days, increasing the incidence of early-onset bleeding in all newborns. Breast milk is a poor source of vitamin K; late-onset bleeding (occurring 1–3 months after birth) is rare but may be seen in exclusively breastfed infants. A particularly severe form of the deficiency of vitamin K–dependent coagulation factors occur in the first day of life in infants whose mothers received the anticoagulant warfarin, antiseizure medications (phenytoin, phenobarbital), and some cholesterol-lowering medications.[52]

History and Clinical Findings
- Antiseizure medication (phenytoin or phenobarbital), warfarin used by the mother

- Prematurity
- Exclusive breastfeeding without vitamin K supplementation
- Failure to administer parenteral vitamin K at birth
- Neonatal hepatitis or biliary atresia
- Gastrointestinal, nasal, subgaleal, or intracranial bleeding or bleeding at the site of an injection or circumcision

Diagnostic Studies. Prothrombin time, blood coagulation time, and partial thromboplastin time are prolonged.

Differential Diagnosis. Neonatal hemorrhage may result from DIC or congenital bleeding disorders unrelated to vitamin K deficiency.

Management, Prognosis, and Prevention
- In the child with evidence of hemorrhagic disease, an IV infusion of 1 to 5 mg of vitamin K is needed. Improvement of coagulation defects and cessation of bleeding should occur within a few hours.
- If a newborn is delivered at home, confirm that vitamin K was given.
- Prevention of early- and late-onset bleeding is achieved by routinely giving 1 mg of natural oil-soluble vitamin K intramuscularly within 1 hour of birth.
- Prognosis of a child sustaining a hemorrhagic event depends on the site and extent of bleeding.
- Some parents object to parenteral vitamin K. Oral formulations are available but are unlicensed and ineffective against the early onset of disease as the peak efficacy of oral vitamin K is 24 hours with continued dosages required over the first 3 to 4 months of life. Full efficacy of parental vitamin K is obtained 4 to 6 hours after injection and the infant is fully protected against VKDB.[53]

Anemia

Anemia is characterized by less than the normal range of hemoglobin for birthweight and postnatal age. Anemia may be chronic or acute and caused by multiple factors before, during, or immediately after birth. Clinical implications range from asymptomatic to life-threatening symptoms. Prenatal and delivery courses should be examined for possible etiology of anemia.[54]

History and Clinical Findings

- Congenital aplastic or hypoplastic anemia
- Twin–twin transfusion
- Unexpected tearing or separation of the umbilical cord resulting in neonatal blood loss
- Internal hemorrhage (fracture, cephalhematoma, internal organ trauma, gastrointestinal, pulmonary, or another injured organ)
- Umbilical stump or circumcision bleeding
- Hemolysis
- Pallor, congestive heart failure, and shock are possible

Management and Prognosis. A complete examination of medical history with the determination of classification of anemia: blood loss, erythrocyte destruction, or underproduction of RBCs. Treatment depends on the cause and symptoms. An asymptomatic full-term infant with a hemoglobin level of 10 g/dL might be observed, whereas a symptomatic neonate born after abruptio placentae or with severe hemolytic disease of the newborn requires transfusion. Treatment with blood should be balanced by concern about transfusion-acquired infection with cytomegalovirus (CMV), HIV, and hepatitis B and C viruses. The prognosis depends on the cause and severity of the anemia.[54]

Blood in Vomitus or Stool

Evidence of bright red or dark red blood in the vomitus or stool without clinical evidence of blood loss. This newborn problem is often caused by maternal blood ingestion during delivery.

Clinical Findings. Visible bright red or dark red blood in vomitus or stool.

Diagnostic Studies. Baseline hematocrit may be indicated. Blood of maternal origin can be differentiated from infant blood by testing for fetal hemoglobin using the alkali denaturation test.[55]

Differential Diagnosis. The differential diagnosis includes infant gastrointestinal bleeding caused by trauma, bowel duplication, intussusception, volvulus, bowel hemangioma or telangiectasia, rectal prolapse, vitamin K deficiency, or anal fissure.

Management. No treatment is necessary if blood is of maternal origin, although the breakdown of maternal blood may exaggerate neonatal jaundice.

Hyperbilirubinemia

Hyperbilirubinemia, a relatively common neonatal condition, is often termed *neonatal jaundice.* The yellow discoloration of the infant's skin and/or sclera is correlated with the bilirubin accumulation in the skin and subcutaneous tissue that occurs when the serum bilirubin is above approximately 6 mg/dL.[56] The appearance of neonatal jaundice is apparent in a cephalocaudal progression, starting on the head and face, at a serum level of approximately 5 mg/dL with progression toward the chest, abdomen, and finally the entire body including the lower extremities when serum levels approach 20 mg/dL.[57]

Distinction between physiologic and pathologic hyperbilirubinemia is determined by factors that include the onset of jaundice, the rate of rise, clinical history, and risk factors. Nonpathologic or physiologic hyperbilirubinemia typically appears during the first week of life and reflects an imbalance between bilirubin production and excretion[58] (see Chapter 9). Breastfed infants have bilirubin levels that are typically higher than formula fed infants with levels that peak around 3 to 5 days of life and can be complicated by decreased fluid and caloric intake, dehydration, or the delayed passage of meconium. Although this condition can be serious if left untreated, most infants recover with close observation, monitoring, and adequate nutrition and fluid intake.

Pathologic hyperbilirubinemia is a serious condition associated with an underlying problem that causes a significant and rapid rise in the bilirubin level, often within the first day of life.[59] Conditions leading to pathologic hyperbilirubinemia include impaired hepatic function, increased hemolysis from viral or bacterial infection, isoimmune hemolytic disease (ABO or Rh incompatibility), metabolic disease, abnormal shape of the RBCs (glucose-6-phoshate dehydrogenase deficiency, pyruvate kinase deficiency), or perinatal complications such as asphyxia, hypothermia, and hypoglycemia. Elevated bilirubin levels in the newborn infant typically come from the destruction of hemoglobin or abnormal excretion or absorption that can occur under conditions that include polycythemia, isoimmune hemolytic disease, hemolysis, drug toxicity, or structural defects of the RBCs. Each of these clinical conditions associated with pathologic hyperbilirubinemia requires specialized treatment with serum bilirubin levels typically exceeding 13 mg/dL by 48 hours of age (Fig. 28.4).[60]

Bilirubin has two forms: unconjugated (indirect) and conjugated (direct). Unconjugated fat is soluble and can be toxic to tissues. The conjugated bilirubin is water soluble and not toxic to tissues. Kernicterus, also called *bilirubin encephalopathy,* is the most serious complication of hyperbilirubinemia. It occurs when circulating bilirubin that is not bound to albumin crosses the blood-brain barrier, leading to bilirubin-induced neurologic dysfunction. Although rare, this condition can cause hypertonicity, irritability, apnea, seizures, and neurologic devastation.[56]

Clinical Findings

- Anemia
- Hemolytic disease
- Inborn errors of metabolism
- Early severe bilirubin levels
- Hemolytic anemia associated with ethnic or geographic origin
- Hepatobiliary disease
- Sibling who required phototherapy
- ABO or Rh incompatibilities
- Sepsis risk
- Polycythemia (increased with delayed cord clamping)
- Macrosomia, idiopathic diabetes mellitus
- Maternal drug use

Physical examination includes jaundice within the first 24 hours of life or rapid escalation of jaundice, petechiae, cephalohematoma, occult bleeding, bruising, hepatosplenomegaly, or signs of sepsis. Clinical examination and transcutaneous monitoring can provide estimates only, and serum measurement is the gold standard of care for infants at risk for hemolysis or pathologic jaundice.[61]

Diagnostic Studies

- Transcutaneous bilirubin level
- Total and direct serum bilirubin level
- ABO, Rh, blood type, isoimmune antibodies of mother, Coombs test on infant
- Hemoglobin, hematocrit, reticulocyte count
- CBC with differential
- Serologic assays to rule out congenital syphilis
- Maternal serologies

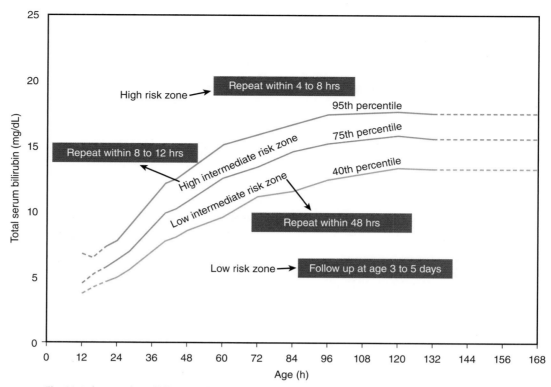

• **Fig. 28.4** Approach to Follow-up Time for Repeat Jaundice and Bilirubin Evaluation Based on Predischarge Bilirubin Testing. (Modified from Bhutani VK, Johnson L. A proposal to prevent severe neonatal hyperbilirubinemia and kernicterus. *J Perinatol.* 2009;29:S61–S67.)

Differential Diagnosis. Common differential diagnosis related to jaundice seen in the first 3 to 7 days of life include physiologic conditions (e.g., breastfeeding jaundice), polycythemia, or excessive bruising. Pathologic differentials include bacterial sepsis, urinary tract infection, syphilis, or TORCH infections. Polycythemia may also contribute to rapid hemolysis with elevated bilirubin levels.[57]

Management, Complications, and Prevention. Prevention of neurotoxicity related to hyperbilirubinemia is the goal of therapy. Typically, phototherapy is considered first-line treatment, coupled with adequate hydration through oral intake. Maintain thermal homeostasis during phototherapy treatment, which is thought to reduce bilirubin levels through excretion of unconjugated bilirubin through urine and stool passage. Delivery of phototherapy includes fluorescent light bank, halogen spotlight, fiberoptic or light-emitting diode (LED) systems, and a bilirubin blanket or bassinet system that supports phototherapy above and below the infant's resting position. The infant is unclothed with eyes shielded for protection. Turning every 2 to 4 hours is supported during phototherapy with close observation for skin integrity. The bilirubin blanket allows holding of the infant with possible home therapy.[62]

Orthopedic Conditions

Fractured Clavicle and Brachial Palsy

See Chapter 40 for information about fractured clavicles and branchial palsy in the neonate.

Polydactyly and Syndactyly

Early in gestation, around 41 to 43 days, rudimentary formation of fingers and toes begins. This is the most common time for syndactyly and/or polydactyly to occur. Syndactyly, the webbing or fusing of digits may include tissue and/or boney structures. The finding may be complete fusion that is to the nailbed, or incomplete. Polydactyly, the more common variant, varies from a skin tag to a fully formed finger or toe with a nail; they most commonly extend from the postaxial side. Postaxial polydactyly is an inherited condition in the African American population. In the Asian and White population, preaxial duplication is more common. Syndactyly and polydactyly occur in isolation or as part of a variety of syndromes.[63,64]

History and Clinical Findings. A positive family history is found in 30% of cases.[63,64] In polydactyly, a floppy digit is seen on the foot or hand. It varies in degree of formation. Syndactyly is the webbing of two digits, partially or to the tip of the digit.

Management. For polydactyly, surgical removal of the floppy extra digit is indicated. If the digit is stabilized by bone, surgical removal is deferred until the patient is older, when the function can be assessed. Surgical separation of syndactyly is recommended by at least 2 to 3 years of age.[65] Close physical examination for other congenital anomalies is recommended.

Central Nervous System Conditions

Congenital Hydrocephalus

Congenital hydrocephalus is the result of various conditions that impair the circulation of/absorption of cerebrospinal fluid (CSF) or an overaccumulation of CSF by the choroid plexus in the brain. This increase in the CSF causes the increased size of the ventricles at birth, placing pressure on adjacent structures or reducing the growth of the cerebral structures. Obstructive or noncommunicating hydrocephalus is most common in children. Malformations, infections, IVH, and disorders in brain development can lead to congenital hydrocephalus. The incidence and clinical presentation vary depending on etiology. Cranial ultrasonography shows dilated ventricles. Often an MRI is obtained to further define the anatomy.[66]

History and Clinical Findings
- Head circumference >99% at delivery, enlarging or rapidly increasing in size
- Cranial sutures separated by large, tense fontanelles
- Signs of increased intracranial pressure (ICP; prominent scalp veins, sun-setting eyes, apnea, bradycardia)

Management. There should be close monitoring of clinical changes that may indicate increasing ICP. Medications that decrease CSF production (e.g., acetazolamide), a ventriculoperitoneal shunt, or both are used. Referral to a pediatric neurosurgeon should be prompt. Refer to Chapter 41 for ongoing management of hydrocephalus.

Intraventricular Hemorrhage

IVH occurs when the fragile capillaries rupture typically in the periventricular white matter or choroid plexus structures. The bleeding is deposited within the lateral ventricles of the brain and may result in secondary obstructive hydrocephalus. IVH usually occurs within the first 72 hours of life and is staged I–IV based on ventricular size and hemorrhagic extension into the white matter. The incidence of IVH decreases with increasing gestational age. Infants weighing <1000 g are particularly prone to severe IVH.[67]

History and Clinical Findings
- Risk factors (prematurity, RDS, hypoxic-ischemic or hypotensive injury, increased or decreased cerebral blood flow, hypertension, hypervolemia, and reduced vascular integrity)
- Majority of cases are asymptomatic
- Diminished or absent Moro reflex, apnea
- Poor muscle tone, lethargy, somnolence
- Periods of pallor or cyanosis
- Inadequate suck
- High-pitched, shrill cry; seizures
- Bulging fontanel or rapid increase in head circumference

Diagnostic Studies. Ultrasonography is used to identify and classify IVH into grades I to IV. Screening cranial ultrasounds are routinely performed on all premature infants. The initial screening typically is done between 7 and 14 postnatal days, and follow-up studies are done based on the infant's clinical course and initial findings.[68]

Management, Prognosis, and Prevention. Prevention and treatment may include the following:
- Prevention
  - Glucocorticoid is given antenatally for pregnancies 24 to 34 weeks gestational that are at risk for preterm delivery to reduce the severity of RDS and associated complications.
  - Supportive care including meticulous fluid and electrolyte management and avoidance of wide swings in blood pressure.
  - Careful respiratory care to avoid hypocarbia and hypoxia.
  - Minimal stimulation and midline position initially to support neuroprotection.
  - Delayed cord clamping has shown an early reduction in preterm infants.
- Treatment
  - Acetazolamide decreases CSF production.
  - Repeated lumbar punctures.
  - Ventriculoperitoneal shunt or external ventriculostomy.

The outcome is related to white matter involvement and the presence of periventricular leukomalacia (PVL). IVH with grade III or IV lesions is associated with the most adverse functional delay.[69]

Hypoxic-Ischemic Encephalopathy

There are three stages of newborn hypoxic-ischemic encephalopathy (HIE) (stages I, II, and III, or mild, moderate, and severe based on Sarnet scoring)[70] (Table 28.3). Brain damage results from fetal hypoxia or ischemia over an extended period followed by metabolic and/or respiratory acidosis. Compensatory mechanisms, such as shunting blood through the ductus to maintain brain, heart, adrenal, kidney, liver, and intestine perfusion ultimately fail if the insult is severe. Depending on the organ(s) most damaged, a variety of signs and symptoms can be seen; 20% to 30% of infants with HIE die in the neonatal period, and up to 30% to 50% develop permanent neurodevelopmental disabilities. Causes of the initial hypoxic or ischemic insult include abruptio placentae, hemorrhage, cord compression, mechanical injury, severe maternal hypertension or diabetes, and inadequate resuscitation of the infant.[71]

Clinical Findings. Infants can have apnea, pallor, cyanosis, and bradycardia unresponsive to stimulation. Seizure activity can be a consequence of a hypoxic-ischemic event.

Management and Prognosis. Term infant management includes a whole body or selective cerebral hypothermia for 72 hours with gradual rewarming.[72] Imaging including MRI is indicated in these patients following normothermia. For preterm and term infants, symptom management includes seizure control and end-organ damage management. The prognosis depends on the effectiveness of managing the underlying symptoms. Severe complications (hypoxia, hypoglycemia, shock) and encephalopathy characterized by flaccid coma, apnea, and seizures are associated with a poorer prognosis. An infant who remains neurologically abnormal after the initial recovery phase (2 weeks) is more likely to have sustained permanent neurologic impairment. A low Apgar score at 20 minutes, absence of spontaneous respirations, and persistence of abnormal neurologic signs at 2 weeks of age predict death or severe cognitive and motor deficits; Apgar scores assessed at 1 and 5 minutes are far less predictive of outcome.[10] Neurology consultation is indicated for initial and ongoing care recommendations (see Chapter 41).

Myelomeningocele

A myelomeningocele is the result of failure to close the posterior neural tube and the vertebral column. This is the most severe form of a classification of neural tube defects (NTD) that include spina bifida occulta, meningocele, encephalocele, caudal regression, tethered cord, and others. Myelomeningocele occurs in 1 in 4000 live births.[73] Genetic and environmental factors play a causative role (see Chapter 41 for more information).

History and Clinical Findings
- Decreased prenatal intake of folic acid and/or exposure to hyperthermia or valproic acid
- Sac-like cyst containing meninges and spinal fluid covered by a thin layer of partially epithelialized skin; 75% found in the lumbosacral area
- Flaccid paralysis of lower extremities
- Absence of deep tendon reflexes
- Lack of response in lower extremities to touch and pain
- Lack of urinary continence with frequent urinary dribbling

Management, Prognosis, and Prevention. Surgical repair, sometimes in utero in advanced centers, and multidisciplinary

TABLE 28.3	Hypoxic-Ischemic Encephalopathy in Term Infants		
Signs	**Stage 1**	**Stage 2**	**Stage 3**
Level of consciousness	Hyper alert	Lethargic	Stuporous, coma
Muscle tone	Normal	Hypotonic	Flaccid
Posture	Normal	Flexion	Decerebrate
Tendon reflexes/clonus	Hyperactive	Hyperactive	Absent
Myoclonus	Present	Present	Absent
Moro reflex	Strong	Weak	Absent
Pupils	Mydriasis	Miosis	Unequal, poor light reflex
Seizures	None	Common	Decerebration
Electroencephalogram findings	Normal	Low voltage changing to seizure activity	Burst suppression to isoelectric
Duration	<24 h if progresses, otherwise; may remain normal	24 h–14 days	Days to weeks
Outcome	Good	Variable	Death, severe deficits

Modified from Sarnat H, Sarnat M. Neonatal encephalopathy following fetal distress: a clinical and electroencephalographic study. *Arch Neurol.* 1976;33:696; and Kliegman RM, Stanton BF, St Geme JW, et al, eds. *Nelson Textbook of Pediatrics.* 21st ed. Elsevier; 2020.

supportive management are indicated. The mortality rate is 10% to 15% in aggressively treated children with most deaths occurring before 4 years old. At least 70% have normal intelligence, but seizure disorders, hydrocephalus, learning disabilities, and neurogenic bowel and bladder are more common than in the general population.[73] Prenatal folic acid supplementation (400 mcg/day) with a daily multivitamin helps prevent neural tube defects and should be taken by all females of childbearing age.[74] Prenatal vitamins have at least 400 mcg of folic acid/vitamin; however, additional folic acid supplementation (4000 mcg) is recommended for females who have had a previous child with a neural tube defect.[75]

Infections of the Newborn

Four mechanisms for acquiring neonatal infections exist:
- Transplacental, when the mother acquires an organism that invades her bloodstream and passes through the placenta
- Vertical, when organisms in the vagina invade the uterine amniotic fluid
- Exposure during the birth process
- Horizontal, when the newborn is exposed to environmental agents after birth

Syphilis is transplacentally acquired; herpes, gonorrhea, group B streptococcus (GBS), *Listeria, Escherichia coli,* and *Chlamydia trachomatis* are typically vertically acquired.[76] Staphylococcal infection, a common skin flora in humans, is the most prevenient horizontal infection with transmission typically by unwashed hands.[77]

Risk factors for newborn sepsis include early rupture of amniotic membranes, preterm labor, prolonged rupture of membranes, maternal fever, maternal diagnosis of chorioamnionitis, maternal tachycardia, fetal tachycardia, and malodorous amniotic fluid. The neonate with sepsis can be asymptomatic or, due to delayed immune response to local infection, display nonspecific infection symptoms, such as poor feeding or temperature instability.[76]

Organisms quickly invade the systemic circulation, and significant deterioration occurs before it can be clinically recognized. Because of the serious nature of neonatal sepsis, a newborn with significant risk factors or a clinically unstable neonate without perinatal risk factors warrants investigation, sepsis evaluation, and initiation of appropriate antibiotics (Box 28.3).[78]

Toxoplasmosis

Toxoplasmosis is caused by *Toxoplasma gondii,* an obligate intracellular protozoan. *T. gondii* infects most species of warm-blooded animals, particularly cats. Cats excrete oocysts in their stools; intermediate hosts include cattle, pigs, and sheep. Humans become infected by the consumption of poorly cooked meat or by accidental ingestion of oocysts from soil or in contaminated food. The incidence in the United States is 1 in 1000 to 8000 births. Depending on the timing of the infection, 17% to 65% of untreated females who acquire toxoplasmosis during gestation transmit the parasite to their fetuses.[79]

History and Clinical Findings
- Prematurity and low Apgar scores
- Infants with congenital infection may be asymptomatic at birth[64]
- Jaundice, anemia, hepatosplenomegaly
- Chorioretinitis, microcephaly

Diagnostic Studies. CT of the brain shows calcifications or hydrocephalus. The CSF shows high protein, low glucose, and evidence of *T. gondii.* Serum-specific immunoglobulin G (IgG), IgM, and IgA antibodies against toxoplasmosis are elevated.

Differential Diagnosis. Sepsis, syphilis, and hemolytic disease are considered in the differential diagnosis.

Management, Prognosis, and Prevention. Pyrimethamine plus sulfadiazine (with folic acid supplementation) for up to 1 year is often recommended. Treatment usually eliminates the manifestations of toxoplasmosis, such as active chorioretinitis, meningitis, encephalitis, hepatitis, splenomegaly, and thrombocytopenia. However,

BOX 28.3 Neonatal Sepsis

History
- "Not doing well"
- Temperature instability (often hypothermia)
- Jitteriness
- Poor feeding, vomiting
- Irritability or lethargy
- Apnea or respiratory distress
- Seizures

Physical Examination
- Jaundice
- Pallor
- Petechiae or purpura
- Rash
- Hepatosplenomegaly
- Poor tone and perfusion
- Tachycardia or bradycardia
- Tachypnea
- Cyanosis, grunting, flaring, retractions

Laboratory Evaluation
- Blood for CBC with differential, platelet count, and culture (evaluating for anemia; increase or decrease in WBC count with left shift; thrombocytopenia); serum ammonia for urea cycle defects
- Urine for analysis and culture typically not done in the first 72 h of life because of low yield
- CSF often obtained for protein, glucose, cell count, and culture (sample evaluated for elevated protein and WBC; decreased glucose level)

Management
- Combination of broad-spectrum antibiotic coverage for gram-positive cocci, gram-negative bacilli, and *Listeria* are recommended. Consider adding coverage for herpes infection when suspected. *Listeria* is treated with ampicillin; *GBS* can be treated with the penicillins and the cephalosporins; gram-negative organisms are well covered by aminoglycosides and some cephalosporins.

CBC, Complete blood count; *CSF*, cerebrospinal fluid; *GBS*, group B streptococcus; *WBC*, white blood cell.

infants with extensive involvement at birth often have mild to severe impairment of vision, hearing, cognitive function, and other neurologic functions. No protective vaccine is available. Pregnant females should be informed not to handle raw meat or contaminated cat litter, to wash fruits and vegetables before consumption, to cook meat and eggs well, and to drink pasteurized milk.[79]

Congenital Rubella

Rubella is a ribonucleic acid (RNA) virus. It is transmitted by person-to-person contact; the virus infects the placenta and is transmitted to the fetus. It occurs more frequently in the winter and spring.

History and Clinical Findings
- Maternal infection before 16 weeks of gestation results in the highest rate of congenital defects
- Negative maternal rubella titers at beginning of pregnancy
- As many as 50% of infected females are asymptomatic[80]
- May be asymptomatic in the newborn period
- Unilateral or bilateral cataracts, glaucoma, microphthalmia, and hearing loss
- Growth restriction

- Cardiac abnormalities in half of the affected children, patent ductus arteriosus has the highest incidence
- "Blueberry muffin" skin lesions, congenital heart disease
- Intellectual disability

Diagnostic Studies. The diagnosis of rubella typically is made through the measurement of serum immunoglobulins. Alternatively, the rubella virus can be isolated from nasopharyngeal secretions, conjunctiva, urine, stool, and CSF.[80]

Management and Prevention. No specific drug therapy is available. Monitoring and intervention for developmental, auditory, visual, and medical needs improve the quality of life for these children. Congenital rubella has been significantly reduced because of the widespread administration of an effective vaccine with caution in those communities with high vaccine resistance.[81] All females of childbearing age should have rubella serology titers as part of routine prenatal care, and the vaccine should be given to IgG-seronegative, nonpregnant females.

Cytomegalovirus

CMV, a member of the herpesvirus family, is transmitted via intimate and household contact with virus-containing secretions and blood products. When CMV is introduced into a household, it is common that all members will acquire the infection. CMV transmission to the infant occurs via the placenta, passage through an infected maternal genital tract, or postnatally by ingestion of CMV-positive human milk. Infections occur worldwide and most humans are infected by the time they reach adulthood. About 0.5% to 1% of all live-born infants are infected in utero and excrete CMV at birth. As many as 90% of infected newborns are asymptomatic. Fetal damage is worse following an infection in the first half of the pregnancy. Infection can be primary (new exposure in a previously CMV-negative mother) or nonprimary (acquisition of a different strain or reactivation of an existing strain).[80,82]

History and Clinical Findings
- Maternal infection (although many females are asymptomatic)
- SGA and/or IUGR
- Jaundice, hepatosplenomegaly
- Petechial rash, chorioretinitis
- Cerebral calcifications, microcephaly, hearing loss

Diagnostic Studies. CMV is isolated in urine, saliva, or other body fluid cultures; recovery of the virus from a target organ is strong evidence of its pathology. Detection of viral deoxyribonucleic acid (DNA) by immunofluorescence antibody (IFA) is available. Proof of congenital infection requires obtaining specimens within 2 to 4 weeks of birth. Viral isolation or a strongly positive test for serum IgM anti-CMV antibody, especially with a fourfold rise in titers, is considered diagnostic.

Management, Prognosis, and Prevention. Treatment of symptomatic infants with oral ganciclovir for 6 months has shown promise in improved audiologic and neurodevelopmental outcomes at 2 years of age.[83] The prognosis of symptomatic congenital CMV infection is poor; a 3% to 10% mortality rate is seen, and up to 50% of children have isolated sensorineural hearing loss. Between these two extremes, psychomotor retardation, microcephaly, seizures, chorioretinitis, optic atrophy, intellectual disability, and learning disabilities are seen. Susceptible pregnant females exposed to the urine and saliva of CMV-infected children who attend daycare centers are at high risk for acquiring the infection.[83] Reinforce hand washing and simple hygienic measures in this population.

Group B Streptococcus

GBS, a gram-positive diplococcus, is a leading cause of sepsis in infants from birth to 3 months old, resulting in significant perinatal morbidity and mortality rates. The early-onset disease usually occurs within the first 24 hours of life but can occur in the first 6 days of life and is often related to maternal obstetric complications. The late-onset disease occurs after 6 days of life and can be seen as late as age 3 months, usually presenting with bacteremia or meningitis.[83,84]

The organism colonizes the maternal genitourinary and gastrointestinal tracts. Pregnant females are usually asymptomatic, but they can manifest chorioamnionitis, endometritis, or UTI. Infants born of females who are highly colonized are more likely to become infected. GBS is acquired by newborns following vertical transmission (e.g., ascending infection through ruptured amniotic membranes or contamination following passage through the colonized birth canal). As many as 50% of infants with the early-onset disease are symptomatic at birth. The highest attack rate of early-onset GBS is in high-risk deliveries, premature SGA infants, very low birth weight infants, or those with prolonged ruptured membranes. Full-term infants account for 50% of cases. Colonization of pregnant females and newborns ranges from 15% to 35%. The incidence of early-onset GBS disease declined from one to four cases per 1000 live births to 0.24 cases per 1000 live births due to widespread chemoprophylaxis.[84,85]

History and Clinical Findings
- Infants born before 37 weeks of gestation
- Rupture of membranes ≥18 hours
- Maternal fever during labor >100.4°F (40°C) oral
- Previous delivery of a sibling with invasive GBS disease
- Maternal chorioamnionitis including rupture of membranes and maternal fever with at least two of the following symptoms:
  - Maternal tachycardia (heart rate >90 bpm)
  - Fetal tachycardia (heart rate >170 bpm)
  - Maternal leukocytosis (white blood cell count >15,000/mm^3)
  - Uterine tenderness
  - Foul-smelling amniotic fluid
  Infant symptoms include:
- Poor feeding, temperature instability
- Cyanosis, apnea, tachypnea, grunting, flaring, and retracting
- Seizures, lethargy, bulging fontanelle
- Rapid onset and deterioration

Diagnostic Studies. Cultures of blood, CSF, or both are definitive; Gram stain of body fluids typically sterile is presumptive evidence of infection. Focal infections are rare (joint, soft tissue, UTI) but should be considered.

Differential Diagnosis. RDS, amniotic fluid aspiration syndrome, persistent fetal circulation, infection or sepsis from other organisms, and metabolic problems are included in the differential diagnosis.

Management, Prognosis, and Prevention. Initiate antibiotic therapy with a penicillin (usually ampicillin) and an aminoglycoside, often gentamicin, until GBS has been differentiated from *E. coli* or *Listeria* sepsis or other organisms.[84] Duration of therapy is 10 (bacteremia without focus) to 14 days (uncomplicated meningitis) minimum. Consultation with pediatric infectious disease specialists is recommended.

Screening of all pregnant females for GBS at 35 to 37 weeks of gestation is recommended. Antepartum treatment of asymptomatic mothers carrying GBS is not recommended. The mortality rate of early-onset disease is as high as 20%; the mortality rate is highest in very low birth weight infants and in those with low neutrophil count (<1500/mm^3), low Apgar scores, hypotension, apnea, and a delay in antimicrobial therapy initiation. Chemoprophylaxis of high-risk, colonized, pregnant females is effective for preventing early-onset GBS infection. The American Academy of Pediatrics (AAP) developed consensus guidelines that outline screening and risk-based GBS prevention.[84] Treatment consists of IV penicillin or ampicillin given to high-risk females at the onset of labor, repeated every 4 hours until the infant is born.

Listeriosis

Listeria monocytogenes is a small gram-positive rod isolated from soil, streams, sewage, certain foods, silage, dust, and slaughterhouses. This organism is widespread in nature. Foodborne disease transmission is generally related to soft-ripened cheese, whole and 2% milk, uncooked hot dogs, undercooked chicken, raw vegetables, and shellfish. The newborn infant acquires the organism transplacentally, by aspiration or ingestion at the time of delivery. Late-onset disease (typically at 8–30 days) is also possible, usually presenting with meningitis and a fatality rate of approximately 25%.[86]

History and Clinical Findings
- Brown-stained amniotic fluid
- Generalized symptoms of sepsis
- Whitish posterior pharyngeal and cutaneous granulomas
- Disseminated erythematous papules on skin

Diagnostic Studies. Culture blood, CSF, meconium, and urine. The CSF shows elevated protein, depressed glucose, and a high leukocyte count. Cultures of the placenta and amniotic fluid also may be helpful.

Management and Prognosis
- Administer IV ampicillin and an aminoglycoside (gentamicin) as initial therapy for severe infections. Be mindful of the emergence of multiantibiotic resistance.
- The duration of therapy is 14 days for infections without meningitis and at least 21 days for infections with meningitis.[86]

Transplacentally acquired listeriosis often results in spontaneous abortion. The death rate of premature infants with *Listeria* pneumonia noted within 12 hours of birth approaches 100%. The mortality rate varies from 14% to 56% if the disease develops within the first week of life, and it is especially high in premature infants. Intellectual disability, paralysis, and hydrocephalus occur in survivors of *Listeria* meningitis.[86]

Congenital Varicella

Varicella-zoster virus (VZV) is a herpesvirus. Humans are the only infection source for this highly contagious virus. The infectivity rate for congenital varicella syndrome is 2% when exposure occurs between 7 and 20 weeks of gestation.[87]

History and Clinical Findings
- History of maternal chickenpox infection
- Limb atrophy
- Scarring of the skin in a dermatomal distribution
- Microcephaly
- Eye manifestations

Diagnostic Studies. Diagnosis of congenital VZV is made by a history of maternal infection, and viral DNA identification by a polymerase chain reaction in tissue samples.

Management, Prognosis, and Prevention. Experts recommend acyclovir for pregnant females with varicella, especially in the second or third trimester.[80] Varicella-zoster immune globulin (VariZIG) is recommended for the term newborn infant whose mother had chickenpox onset within 5 days before delivery or within 48 hours after delivery. All exposed premature infants younger than 28 weeks of gestation or 1000 g or less birthweight should receive VariZIG; exposed premature infants 28 weeks of gestation and older whose mothers lack serologic evidence of disease, or a reliable history of the disease also require VariZIG.[81] Despite having received VariZIG, about 50% of infants may still develop a mild varicella infection. If VariZIG is not available, then immunoglobulin intravenous is recommended. VariZIG is not indicated if the mother has varicella-zoster (shingles) only. Airborne and contact precautions are recommended for neonates born to mothers with varicella for 21 days from the last exposure or 28 days if they received VariZIG.

Target prevention efforts to potential mothers. Varicella vaccination is recommended for nonpregnant females of childbearing age who have no history of varicella infection (see Chapter 19).[87]

Sexually Transmitted Infections

Gonorrhea

Neisseria gonorrhoeae is a gram-negative diplococcus that occurs only in humans. The organism lives in exudate and secretions of infected mucous membranes and is transmitted primarily through sexual contact and birth. Gonococcal infections in the newborn are acquired primarily during delivery.[88]

History and Clinical Findings. There is a history of maternal gonococcal infection. Findings include conjunctivitis, and rarely septicemia, pneumonia, or joint infection.

Diagnostic Studies. Cultures of eye and body fluids (blood, joint fluid, abscess) are positive for *N. gonorrhoeae*.

Management and Prevention. Administer a single dose of intramuscular ceftriaxone 25 to 50 mg/kg (not to exceed 125 mg) for the prophylaxis of infants born to mothers with active gonorrhea. Because gonorrheal conjunctivitis can rapidly lead to blindness, all infants are given eye prophylaxis at birth with erythromycin 0.5% ophthalmic ointment.[80]

Chlamydia

Chlamydial infection is caused by an obligate intracellular parasite, *Chlamydia trachomatis*, and is the most common sexually transmitted infection in the United States. Acquisition occurs in approximately 50% of infants born vaginally to infected mothers and in some infants delivered by cesarean section with intact membranes. The risk of developing conjunctivitis is 25% to 50% in infants who have acquired *C. trachomatis*; the risk of pneumonia is 5% to 30%.[89]

History and Clinical Findings
- History of maternal chlamydial infection
- Conjunctivitis a few days to several weeks after birth
- Infant commonly afebrile with normal activity level
- Symptoms of pneumonia at 2 to 19 weeks after birth

Diagnostic Studies
- Although not approved by the US Food and Drug Administration, nucleic acid amplification tests (NAATs) have published sensitives and specificities as high as those for culture.
- Routine bacterial cultures are not helpful.
- When NAATs are not available, Gram stain and culture of discharge from the eye must include epithelial cells from the palpebral conjunctival sac because chlamydia is an obligate parasite and cells are necessary for diagnosis.

Management and Prevention. Oral erythromycin or azithromycin will be given for both conjunctivitis and pneumonia.[80,89] Appropriate treatment of the pregnant female before delivery prevents disease in the newborn. Prophylaxis with oral erythromycin of the asymptomatic infant born to an untreated but *Chlamydia*-positive female is generally contraindicated because of the increased risk of developing hypertrophic pyloric stenosis.

Syphilis

Congenital syphilis is caused by the spirochete *Treponema pallidum*, transferred vertically from an infected mother to an infant. The national rate of congenital syphilis was 57.3 per 100,000 live births in 2020, a 254% increase since 2016.[72] Routine maternal serologic testing is legally required during prenatal care in all states. Following treatment, evidence of serologic response to therapy is required.[90,91]

History and Clinical Findings
- Maternal primary or secondary infection and positive serologic testing
- Most neonates are asymptomatic at birth
- Failure to thrive, restlessness, fever, persistent rhinorrhea
- Maculopapular or bullous dermal lesions, hepatosplenomegaly

Diagnostic Studies. Individualize evaluation depending on the adequacy of maternal syphilis treatment and follow-up. Consultation with an infectious disease specialist may be indicated. CSF evaluation shows high protein, low glucose, high white blood cell count, and positivity on Venereal Disease Research Laboratory (VDRL) test. Serum liver enzymes are elevated with liver involvement and the serum rapid plasma reagin test is positive.[91]

Management and Prognosis. For proven or highly probable congenital syphilis, the Centers for Disease Control and Prevention (CDC) recommends 10 consecutive days of crystalline penicillin G 100,000 to 150,000 units/kg/day. Infants with abnormal CSF evaluations should have a serologic test for treponemal titers at age 6 to 12 months.[80] For infants with less certain evidence of syphilis, alternative regimens are available; reference to the latest CDC guidelines or the AAP Red Book is recommended. Untreated congenital syphilis can lead to severe multiorgan involvement including boney deformities, blindness, hearing loss, anemia, and jaundice.[72] Infants who are appropriately treated have a good prognosis.

Herpes Simplex Virus

Three clinically distinguishable categories of herpes simplex virus (HSV) (Fig. 28.5) infection exist: (1) disseminated disease; (2) CNS disease; and (3) disease restricted to the skin, eyes, and mouth.[64] HSV is transmitted by direct contact with infected maternal genitalia during the birth process. Transplacental transmission occurs but has been reported in only a few cases. The risk of neonatal infection is highest with primary genital infection (see Chapter 35).

History and Clinical Findings. The mother may have active lesions and deliver vaginally. Vesicles in the skin, eye, and mouth are found. Signs or symptoms of encephalitis, pneumonia, or sepsis also can be present.

Diagnostic Studies. The virus is isolated in tissue cultures obtained from vesicles, nasopharyngeal or conjunctival swabs, urine, stool, and tracheal secretions; alternatively, vesicle scrapings can be evaluated for antigens with rapid diagnostic tests.

Management, Prognosis, and Prevention. Acyclovir is given for 14 days (skin, eyes, and mouth infection), and up to 21 days (disseminated or involving the CNS) for HSV.[80] In addition,

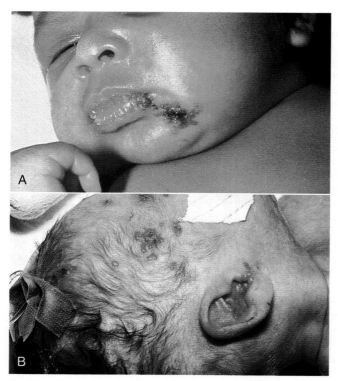

• **Fig. 28.5** Herpes Simplex Virus. (From Cohen BA. *Pediatric Dermatology*. 5th ed. Elsevier; 2022.)

treatment with ophthalmic drugs (1% trifluridine, 0.1% iododeoxyuridine, or 0.15% ganciclovir) is used for infants with ocular involvement.[80] Despite effective antiviral therapy, disseminated neonatal HSV infections and localized encephalitis are associated with considerable morbidity and mortality. Some healthcare providers provide antiviral therapy in the final weeks of pregnancy for females with a history of HSV. The risk of acquiring this serious infection is lowered by performing cesarean delivery before rupturing of membranes in any pregnancy in which signs or symptoms of HSV infection occur.

Human Immunodeficiency Virus

The human immunodeficiency virus (HIV), a retrovirus, is transmitted to the newborn via the placenta or at birth secondary to exposure to maternal blood[92] (see Chapter 35).

Drug Exposure

Neonatal Opioid Withdrawal Syndrome/Neonatal Abstinence Syndrome

Although the incidence varies by location, ethnicity, and socioeconomic status, there has been a significant increase in opioid use disorder (OUD) during pregnancy, now estimated to affect 8.8 in 1000 births.[93] Other substances are often used in combination with opioids including tobacco, alcohol, marijuana, and benzodiazepines complicating the symptoms and timing of neonatal withdrawal. Complications of maternal drug abuse include a higher risk of infection including syphilis, gonorrhea, hepatitis, and HIV; psychiatric, nervous, and emotional disorders; and abruptio placentae. Elimination of in utero drug exposure can occur only if high-risk mothers are identified and referred to a substance abuse prevention program with medication-assisted therapy (MAT) available.[94]

The use of nonprescription substances and/or prescription medications place the infant at risk for poor neurologic outcomes and withdrawal symptoms at birth. Drugs of abuse generally can be divided into opioids, CNS stimulants, CNS depressants, and hallucinogens. The onset of neonatal symptoms ranges from birth to 14 days, although most infants demonstrate symptoms of withdrawal by day 5. Symptomatic neonates need both pharmacologic and nonpharmacologic intervention for withdrawal symptoms; asymptomatic neonates need nonpharmacologic interventions using family engagement and Eat, Sleep, and Console therapy as described below[95] (Fig. 28.6). When opioid taper therapy is required, infants are typically admitted to the ICU for close monitoring. The use of an objective scoring tool such as the Neonatal Drug-Withdrawal Scoring System helps guide therapy.[96] Table 28.4 is a relatively simple numeric system using a value of 4 as an indication of significant withdrawal signs. A more comprehensive scoring system (21 symptoms and a different assigned score for each) is the Modified Finnegan's Neonatal Abstinence Scoring Tool.[97] Pharmacologic treatment guided by this scoring system can be used in conjunction with nonpharmacologic management including Eat, Sleep, and Console therapy.[98] This specialized care includes rooming with the mother/family member, low stimulation environment (dimmed lights, muted television/low noise), staff engaged with family to support and guide care, and immediate response to crying with feeding on demand. This therapy has been shown to reduce the need for pharmacologic intervention, ICU admissions, and hospital length of stay.[94,98]

Cocaine (Crack) and Methamphetamine Exposure

Cocaine is a local anesthetic and CNS stimulant that some believe to be a teratogen that crosses the placenta. Methamphetamine is a highly addictive CNS stimulant and its known impact on pregnancy is limited.

History and Clinical Findings
- Maternal exposure to drug, and a positive maternal and/or infant urine drug screen
- Premature labor
- Abruptio placentae
- IUGR
- Fetal asphyxia with meconium staining is possible
- Some infants may be small, irritable and hyperactive. Many infants show no adverse effects from maternal use and no clinically documented neonatal withdrawal syndrome has been identified.[99]

Management, Complications, and Prevention
- Do not breastfeed because both drugs are detectable in breast milk and impact a mother's judgement.
- Close neurodevelopmental follow-up and testing are necessary through the first several years of age.
- Involve the Department of Child and Family Services.

Heroin and Methadone Exposure

Heroin and methadone are narcotics that cross the placenta.
History and Clinical Findings
- Maternal exposure to heroin or methadone
- Urine drug screen positive for opiates in mother and/or infant
- Increased incidence of stillbirths and SGA infants, but not congenital anomalies
- Tremors and hyperirritability are often coarser than those with hypoglycemia
- Limbs rigid and hyperreflexia, fist sucking
- Skin abrasions secondary to hyperactivity

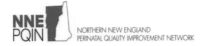 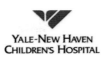 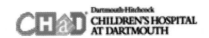

EATING, SLEEPING, CONSOLING (ESC) CARE TOOL

- Assess infant **after feedings**, preferably while **skin-to-skin or held swaddled** by mother/caregiver.
- Review baby's **ESC** behaviors **since last assessment 3–4 hours ago** using **Newborn Care Diary** with parents.
- If infant with **"Yes"** for any **ESC** item or receiving **"3s"** for **"Soothing Support Used to Console Infant"**, perform **team huddle** with mother/parent & RN to **determine non-pharm interventions that can be optimized** further.
- If infant **continues with "Yes"** for any **ESC** item or **"3s"** for **"Soothing Support"** despite **optimal non-pharm care** and **symptoms felt likely due to NAS**, perform **full team huddle** with mother/parent, RN, and Infant Provider to determine if medication treatment is needed.

See back of sheet for definition of items.

TIME					
EATING					
Poor eating due to NAS? Yes / No					
SLEEPING					
Sleep < 1 hr due to NAS? Yes / No					
CONSOLING					
Unable to console within 10 min due to NAS? Yes / No					
Soothing support used to console infant: Soothes with little support: 1 Soothes with some support: 2 Soothes with much support or does not soothe in 10 min: 3					
PARENTAL / CAREGIVER PRESENCE					
Parental / caregiver presence since last assessment: No parent present: 0 1 - 59 minutes: 1 1 hr – 1 hr 59 min: 2 2 hr – 2 hr 59 min: 3 3 hr+: 4					
MANAGEMENT DECISION					
Recommend a team huddle? Yes / No					
Management decision: Optimize non-pharm care: 1 Initiate medication treatment: 2 Other (please describe):					
NON-PHARM INTERVENTIONS					
Rooming-in: Increased / Reinforced					
Parental presence: Increased / Reinforced					
Skin-to-skin contact: Increased / Reinforced					
Holding by caregiver/cuddler: Increased / Reinforced					
Swaddling: Increased / Reinforced					
Optimal feeding: Increased / Reinforced					
Non-nutritive sucking: Increased / Reinforced					
Quiet environment: Increased / Reinforced					
Limit visitors: Increased / Reinforced					
Clustering care: Increased / Reinforced					

• **Fig. 28.6** Eating, Sleeping, Consoling (ESC) Care Tool Grading Scale. (Courtesy Boston Medical Center Corporation, Dr. Matthew Grossman and Children's Hospital at Dartmouth-Hitchcock, 2017. https://www.cffutures.org/files/QIC_Resources/Learning_with_the_Expert/Eat_Sleep_console_manual_with_tools_Yale_Boston_NNEPQIN.pdf.)

TABLE 28.4 Neonatal Drug-Withdrawal Scoring System

Signs	SCORE			
	0	1	2	3
Tremors (muscle activity of limbs)	Normal	Minimally increased when hungry or disturbed	Moderate or marked increase when undisturbed; subside when fed or held snugly	Marked increase or continuous even when undisturbed, going on to seizure-like movements
Irritability (excessive crying)	None	Slightly increased	Moderate to severe when disturbed or hungry	Marked even when undisturbed
Reflexes	Normal	Increased	Markedly increased	
Stools	Normal	Explosive, but normal frequency	Explosive, more than 8 days	
Muscle tone	Normal	Increased	Rigidity	
Skin abrasions	No	Redness of knees and elbows	Breaking of the skin	
Respiratory rate/minute	<55	55–75	76–95	
Repetitive sneezing	No	Yes		
Repetitive yawning	No	Yes		
Vomiting	No	Yes		
Fever	No	Yes		

From Lipsitz PJ. A proposed narcotic withdrawal score for use with newborn infants: a pragmatic evaluation of its efficacy. *Clin Pediatr.* 1975;14(6):592–594.

- Tachypnea, poor feeding, high-pitched cry
- Vomiting, diarrhea
- Low birth weight or SGA

Heroin withdrawal symptoms occur in the first 48 hours of life in 75% of affected newborns, depending on the daily maternal dose, duration of addiction, and most recent maternal dose. Symptoms of methadone withdrawal occur in up to 90% of affected newborns. A higher incidence of symptomatology is seen if the last dose was taken within 24 hours of birth. Overall, the withdrawal syndrome is more severe and more prolonged with methadone than with heroin.[100]

Differential Diagnosis. The differential diagnosis includes hypoglycemia and hypocalcemia.

Management and Prevention. Supportive management, such as swaddling, frequent feedings, and protection from external stimuli is needed. Education regarding sudden infant death syndrome is imperative because these infants are at increased risk. Child protective services must be involved before discharge. Medications (e.g., morphine, clonidine, buprenorphine, phenobarbital, and methadone) can be used if symptoms—such as severe irritability, vomiting and diarrhea, seizures, temperature instability, or severe tachypnea—are noted. Pregnant females who are addicted to heroin should be encouraged to enter a treatment program for MAT.

Additional Resources

American Academy of Pediatrics: www.aap.org
Birth Defect Research for Children: www.birthdefects.org
Centers for Disease Control and Prevention (CDC), birth defects: www.cdc.gov/ncbddd/birthdefects/index.html
Centers for Disease Control and Prevention (CDC), infectious disease information: www.cdc.gov/DiseasesConditions/
American Cleft Palate-Craniofacial Association (ACPA): www.cleftline.org
Group B Strep Association: https://gbss.org.uk
Compassionate Friends: www.compassionatefriends.org
Infant Loss Resources: http://infantlossresources.org/ (limited to State of Missouri)
March of Dimes: www.marchofdimes.com (local chapters available)
National Association of Pediatric Nurse Practitioners: www.napnap.org
National Center on Substance Abuse and Child Welfare: https://ncsacw.acf.hhs.gov/topics/infants/
National Perinatal Association: www.nationalperinatal.org

References

1. Driscoll AK, Ely DM. *NCHS Data Brief: Trends in Infant Mortality in the United States, 1995-2018*; 2021. www.cdc.gov/nchs/data/nvsr/nvsr70/nvsr70-06-508.pdf.
2. US Department of Health and Human Services, Centers for Disease Control and Prevention, National Center for Health Statistics. *NCHS Data Brief, No. 427*; 2021. https://www.cdc.gov/nchs/data/databriefs/db427.pdf.
3. Aylott M. The neonatal energy triangle. Part 1: metabolic adaptation. *Paediatr Nurs.* 2006;18(6):38–42.
4. Sharma D. Golden hour of neonatal life: need of the hour. *Matern Health Neonatol Perinatol.* 2017;3:16.
5. Kilpatrick SJ, Papile LA, Macones GA, eds. *Guidelines for Perinatal Care.* 8th ed. American Academy of Pediatrics and American College of Obstetricians and Gynecologists; 2017.
6. Centers for Disease Control and Prevention (CDC). *COVID-19 during Pregnancy.* https://www.cdc.gov/coronavirus/2019-ncov/vaccines/recommendations/pregnancy.html

7. American Academy of Pediatrics (AAP) and American Heart Association. Eds. Weiner GM, Zaichkin J, Kattwinkel J. *Textbook of Neonatal Resuscitation*. 8th ed. American Academy of Pediatrics.

8. American College of Obstetricians and Gynecologists. Delayed umbilical cord clamping after birth. ACOG Committee Opinion No. 814. *Obstet Gynecol*. 2020;136:e100–e106.

9. American Academy of Pediatrics (AAP) Committee on Fetus and Newborn. The Apgar score. *Pediatrics*. 2015;136(4):819–822.

10. Apgar V. A proposal for a new method of evaluation of the newborn infant. *Curr Res Anesth Analg*. 1953;32:260–267.

11. Simon LV, Hashmi MF, Bragg BN. APGAR Score. In StatPearls, May 23, 2022. https://www.ncbi.nlm.nih.gov/books/NBK470569/#_NBK470569_pubdet_.

12. Smith V. NICU discharge preparation and transition planning. *J Perinatol*. 2022;42:4–5.

13. Singh AP, Gorla SR. Amniotic Band Syndrome. In: StatPearls, January 2022.

14. McKinney JM, Rac MW, Gandhi M. SMFM fetal anomalies consult series #2: extremities. *Am J Obstet Gynecol*. 2019;221(6):B2–B18.

15. Abidi NY, Martin KL. Cutaneous defects. In: Kliegman RM, St Geme JW, eds. *Nelson Textbook of Pediatrics*. 21st ed. Elsevier; 2020:3456–3458.

16. Dhar V. Cleft lip and palate. In: Kliegman RM, St Geme JW, eds. *Nelson Textbook of Pediatrics*. 21st ed. ; 2020:1915–1917.

17. Mai CT, Isenburg JL, Canfield MA, et al. National population–based estimates for major birth defects, 2010–2014. *Birth Defects Res*. 2019;111(18):1420–1435.

18. Ahlfeld SK. Transient tachypnea of the newborn. In: Kliegman RM, St Geme JW, eds. *Nelson Textbook of Pediatrics*. 21st ed. Elsevier; 2020:941.

19. Lubbers L., Eckland W. Respiratory system. In: Kenner C., Boykova, eds. Neonatal Nursing Care Handbook, 3rd ed. NewYork: Springer Publishing Company:3-44.

20. Litao MK, Hayes D, Chiwane S, et al. A novel surfactant protein C gene mutation associated with progressive respiratory failure in infancy. *Pediatr Pulmonol*. 2017;52(1):57–68.

21. Ahlfeld SK. Respiratory distress syndrome. In: Kliegman RM, St Geme JW, eds. *Nelson Textbook of Pediatrics*. 21st ed. Elsevier; 2020:932–936.

22. Ahlfeld SK. Meconium aspiration. In: Kliegman RM, St Geme JW, eds. *Nelson Textbook of Pediatrics*. 21st ed. Elsevier; 2020:941–942.

23. American College of Obstetricians and Gynecologists (ACOG) Committee Opinion no. 689. Delivery of a newborn with meconium-stained amniotic fluid. *Obstet Gynecol*. 2017;129:e33–e34 (Reaffirmed 2021).

24. Cassina M, Ruol M, Pertile R, et al. Prevalence, characteristics, and survival of children with esophageal atresia: a 32-year population-based study including 1,417,724 consecutive newborns. *Birth Defects Res A Clin Mol Teratol*. 2016;106:542.

25. Khan S, Matta SK. Esophageal atresia and tracheoesophageal fistula. In: Kliegman RM, St Geme JW, eds. *Nelson Textbook of Pediatrics*. 21st ed. Elsevier; 2020:1929–1931.

26. Garabedian C, Verpillat P, Czerkiewicz I, et al. Does a combination of ultrasound, MRI, and biochemical amniotic fluid analysis improve prenatal diagnosis of esophageal atresia? *Prenat Diagn*. 2014;34(9):839–842.

27. van der Zee DC, Tytgat SHA, van Herwaarden MYA. Esophageal atresia and tracheo- esophageal fistula. *Semin Pediatr Surg*. 2017;26(2):67–71.

28. Maqbool A, Bales C, Liacouras CA. Intestinal atresia, stenosis, and malrotation. In: Kliegman RM, St Geme JW, eds. *Nelson Textbook of Pediatrics*. 21st ed. Elsevier; 2020:1950–1953.

29. Maqbool A, Liacourus CA. Malrotation. In: Kliegman RM, St Geme JW, eds. *Nelson Textbook of Pediatrics*. 21st ed. Elsevier; 2020:1952–1953.

30. Maqbool A, Liacouras CA. Pyloric stenosis. In: Kliegman RM, St Geme JW, eds. *Nelson Textbook of Pediatrics*. 21st ed. Elsevier; 2020:1946–1948.

31. Maqbool A, Fiorino KN, Liacouras CA. Motility disorders in Hirschsprung disease. In: Kliegman RM, St Geme JW, eds. *Nelson Textbook of Pediatrics*. 21st ed. Philadelphia: Elsevier; 2020:1955–1958.

32. Maqbool A, Liacouras CA. Congenital aganglionic megacolon (Hirschsprung disease). In: Kliegman RM, St Geme JW, eds. *Nelson Textbook of Pediatrics*. 21st ed. Elsevier; 2020:1961–1964.

33. Shanti CM. Surgical conditions of the anus and rectum. In: Kliegman RM, Stanton BF, St Geme JW, et al., eds. *Nelson Textbook of Pediatrics*. 21st ed. Elsevier; 2020:2055–2061.

34. Nathan AT. The umbilicus. In: Kliegman RM, St Geme JW, eds. *Nelson Textbook of Pediatrics*. 21st ed. Elsevier; 2020:975–976.

35. Storm AP, Bowker RM, Klonoski SC, et al. Mother's own milk dose is associated with decreased time from initiation of feedings to discharge and length of stay in infants with gastroschisis. *J Perinatol*. 2020;40:1222.

36. Brown R. Necrotizing enterocolitis. In: Kliegman RM, St Geme JW, eds. *Nelson Textbook of Pediatrics*. 21st ed. Elsevier; 2020:951–953.

37. Gephart SM, Newnam K, Wyles C, et al. Development of the NEC-Zero toolkit: supporting reliable implementation of necrotizing enterocolitis prevention and recognition. *Neonatal Netw*. 2020;39(1):6–15.

38. Ahlfeld SK. Diaphragmatic hernia. In: Kliegman RM, St Geme JW, eds. *Nelson Textbook of Pediatrics*. 21st ed. Elsevier; 2020:944–946.

39. Devarajan P. Renal failure. In: Kliegman RM, St Geme JW, eds. *Nelson Textbook of Pediatrics*. 21st ed. Elsevier; 2020:2769–2774.

40. Elder J. Congenital anomalies and dysgenesis of the kidneys. In: Kliegman RM, St Geme JW, eds. *Nelson Textbook of Pediatrics*. 21st ed. Elsevier; 2020:2786–2788.

41. Pennesi M, Amoroso S, Bassanese G, et al. Frequency of urinary tract infection in children with antenatal diagnosis of urinary tract dilatation. *Arch Dis Child*. 2020;105(3):260.

42. Devarajan P. Anatomic and Vascular abnormalities associated with hematuria. In: Kliegman RM, St Geme JW, eds. *Nelson Textbook of Pediatrics*. 21st ed. Elsevier; 2020:2742–2748.

43. Harrison A. Neuroblastoma. In: Kliegman RM, Stanton BF, St Geme JW, et al., eds. *Nelson Textbook of Pediatrics*. 21st ed. Elsevier; 2020.

44. Sharma R, Mer J, Lion A, et al. Clinical presentation, evaluation and management of neuroblastoma. *Pediatr Rev*. 2018;39(4):194–203.

45. Elder J. Obstruction of the urinary tract. In: Kliegman RM, St Geme JW, eds. *Nelson Textbook of Pediatrics*. 21st ed. Elsevier; 2020:2800–2810.

46. Rose SR, Wassner AJ, Kupper A, Wintergest NH, et al. Section on endocrinology executive committee, council on genetics executive committee; congenital hypothyroidism: screening and management. *Pediatrics*. 2023;151(1): e2022060419.

47. Spearling MA. Hypoglycemia. In: Kliegman RM, Stanton BF, St Geme JW, et al., eds. *Nelson Textbook of Pediatrics*. 21st ed. Elsevier; 2020:848–849.

48. Newnam KM, Bunch M. Glucose gel as a treatment strategy for transient neonatal hypoglycemia. *Adv Neonatal Care*. 2017;17(6):470–477.

49. Sheanon NM, Muglia LJ. The endocrine system. In: Kliegman RM, Stanton BF, St Geme JW, et al., eds. *Nelson Textbook of Pediatrics*. 21st ed. Elsevier; 2020:982–985.

50. Kleinman K, McDaniel L, Molloy M. *The Harriet Lane Handbook*. 22nd ed. Philadelphia: Elsevier; 2021.

51. Niss O, Ware RE. Neonatal polycythemia. In: Kliegman RM, Stanton BF, St Geme JW, et al., eds. *Nelson Textbook of Pediatrics*. 21st ed. Elsevier; 2020:971–972.

52. Tarango C, Ware RE. Hemorrhage in the newborn infant. In: Kliegman RM, Stanton BF, St Geme JW, et al., eds. *Nelson Textbook of Pediatrics*. 21st ed. Elsevier; 2020:972–973.

53. Centers for Disease Control and Prevention (CDC). *Facts about Vitamin K Deficiency Bleeding*; 2017. cdc.gov/ncbddd/vitamink/facts.html.

54. McGann PT, Ware RE. Anemia in the newborn infant. In: Kliegman RM, St Geme JW, eds. *Nelson Textbook of Pediatrics*. 21st ed. Elsevier; 2020:961–967.

55. AAP Committee on Fetus and Newborn and ACOG Committee on Obstetric Practice, Kilpatrick SJ, Papile LA. In: Macones GA, Watterberg KL, eds. *Guidelines for Perinatal Care*. 8th ed. AAP and ACOG; 2017.

56. Pace EJ, Brown CM, DeGeorge KC. Neonatal hyperbilirubinemia: an evidence-based approach. *J Fam Pract*. 2019;68(1):E4–E11.

57. Shaughnessy EE, Goyal NK. Digestive system disorders. In: Kliegman RM, St Geme JW, eds. *Nelson Textbook of Pediatrics*. 21st ed. Philadelphia: Elsevier; 2020:954–959.

58. Maisels JJ, Watchko JF. Neonatal hyperbilirubinemia. In: Fanaroff AA, Fararoff JM, eds. *Klaus & Fanaroff's Care of the High-Risk Neonate*. 7th ed. Elsevier; 2020:310–345.

59. Kemper AR, Newman TB, Slaughter JL, et al. Clinical practice guideline revision: management of hyperbilirubinemia in the newborn infant 35 or more weeks of gestation. *Pediatrics*. 2022;150(3): e2022058859.

60. Bhutani V, Johnson L. A proposal to prevent severe neonatal hyperbilirubinemia and kernicterus. *J Perinatol*. 2009;29(suppl 1):S61–S67.

61. Stark, AR, Bhutani, VK. Neonatal hyperbilirubinemia. In E. C. Eichenwald, AR Hansen, FC Martin & AR Stark (Eds.), Cloherty and Stark's Manual of Neonatal Care 8th ed. (pp 482-490). Wolters Kluwer.

62. Reyna, BA The infant at risk. In Core Curriculum for Maternal-Newborn Nursing. Eds: B. Baker, J. Janke. 6th ed.. Elsevier.

63. AAP Committee on Fetus and Newborn and ACOG Committee on Obstetric Practice. In: Kilpatrick SJ, Papile LA, Macones GA, Watterberg KL, eds. *Guidelines for Perinatal Care*. 8th ed. AAP and ACOG Publishers; 2017.

64. Carrigan RB. The upper limb. In: Kliegman RM, St Geme JW, eds. *Nelson Textbook of Pediatrics*. 21st ed. Elsevier; 2020:3651–3656.

65. Winell D. Polydactyly. In: Kliegman RM, St Geme JW, eds. *Nelson Textbook of Pediatrics*. 21st ed. Elsevier; 2020.

66. Little KJ, Cornwall R. Congenital anomalies of the hand: principles of management. *Orthop Clin North Am*. 2016;47(1):153–168.

67. Kinsman S, Johnston MV. Congenital anomalies of the central nervous system. In: Kliegman RM, St Geme JW, eds. *Nelson Textbook of Pediatrics*. 21st ed. Elsevier; 2020:3063–3082.

68. Greenberg JM. Overview of morbidity and mortality, intraventricular hemorrhage. In: Kliegman RM, St Geme JW, eds. *Nelson Textbook of Pediatrics*. 21st ed. Elsevier; 2020:863–866.

69. Watterberg KL. Brain injury: hemorrhagic and periventricular white matter brain injury. In: *Guidelines for Perinatal Care*. 8th ed. AAP and ACOG Publishers; 2017:411–412.

70. Sarnat H, Sarnat M. Neonatal encephalopathy following fetal distress: a clinical and electroencephalographic study. *Arch Neurol*. 1976;33:696. cited in Kliegman RM, Stanton BF, St Geme JW, et al., eds. Nelson Textbook of Pediatrics. 21st ed. Elsevier; 2020.

71. Novak CM, Ozen M, Burd I. Perinatal brain injury: mechanisms, prevention, and outcomes. *Clin Perinatol*. 2018;45(2):357–375.

72. Cho KH, Davidson JO, Dean JM, Bennet L, Gunn AJ. Cooling and immunomodulation for treating hypoxic-ischemic brain injury. *Pediatr Int*. 2020;62(7):770–778.

73. Thomas CW, Merhar SL. Nervous system disorders. In: Kliegman RM, Stanton BF, St Geme JW, et al., eds. *Nelson Textbook of Pediatrics*. 21st ed. Elsevier; 2020:3053–3063.

74. American Academy of Pediatrics (AAP). Folic acid for the prevention of neural tube defects. *Pediatrics*. 1999;104(2):325–327.

75. Viswanathan M, Treiman KA, Kish-Doto J, et al. Folic acid supplementation for the prevention of neural tube defects: an updated evidence report and systematic review for the US Preventive Services Task Force. *JAMA*. 2017;317(2):190–203.

76. Martin RJ, Fanaroff AA, Walsh MC. *Fanaroff & Martin's Neonatal-Perinatal Medicine: Diseases of the Fetus and Infant*. 11th ed. Elsevier; 2019.

77. Böhne C, Knegendorf L, Schwab F, et al. Epidemiology and infection control of Methicillin-resistant Staphylococcus aureus in a German tertiary neonatal intensive and intermediate care unit: a retrospective study (2013–2020). *PLoS One*. 2022;17(9):e0275087.

78. Weiss AK, Balamuth FB. Triage of the acutely ill child. In: Kliegman RM, Stanton BF, St Geme JW, et al., eds. *Nelson Textbook of Pediatrics*. 21st ed. Elsevier; 2020:526–529.

79. McLeod R, Boyer KM. Toxoplasmosis (*Toxoplasma gondii*). In: Kliegman RM, St Geme JW, eds. *Nelson Textbook of Pediatrics*. 21st ed. Elsevier; 2020:1865–1876.

80. American Academy of Pediatrics (AAP). In: Kimberlin DW, Barnett ED, Lynfield R, Sawyer MH, eds. *Red Book: 2021 Report of the Committee on Infectious Diseases*. 32nd ed. American Academy of Pediatrics; 2021.

81. Cherry J, Baker A. Rubella virus. In: Cherry JD, Harrison GJ, Kaplan SL, eds. *Feigin and Cherry's Textbook of Pediatric Infectious Diseases*. 8th ed. Elsevier; 2019:1601.

82. Britt WJ. Cytomegalovirus. In: Kliegman RM, St Geme JW, eds. *Nelson Textbook of Pediatrics*. 21st ed. Elsevier; 2020:1718–1723.

83. Lachenauer CS, Wessels MR. Group B Streptococcus. In: Kliegman RM, St Geme JW, eds. *Nelson Textbook of Pediatrics*. 21st ed. Philadelphia: Elsevier; 2020:1450–1455.

84. Centers for Disease Control and Prevention (CDC). Prevention of perinatal group B streptococcal disease—revised guidelines from CDC, 2010. *MMWR Recombs Rep*. 2010;59(RR–10):1–36.

85. Puopolo KM, Lynfield R, Cummings JJ. American Academy of pediatrics, committee on fetus and newborn, committee on infectious diseases. Management of infants at risk for group B streptococcal disease. *Pediatrics*. 2019;144(2):e20191881.

86. Murray TS, Baltimore RS. Listeria monocytogenes. In: Kliegman RM, St Geme JW, eds. *Nelson Textbook of Pediatrics*. 21st ed. Elsevier; 2020:1463–1465.

87. LaRussa MG. Varicella-zoster virus. In: Kliegman RM, St Geme JW, eds. *Nelson Textbook of Pediatrics*. 21st ed. Elsevier; 2020:1708–1715.

88. Centers for Disease Control and Prevention (CDC). Sexually Transmitted Diseases (STDs). https://www.cdc.gov/std/dstdp/.

89. Kohlhoff SA, Hammerschlag MR. Chlamydia pneumonia/Chlamydia trachomatis. In: Kliegman RM, St Geme JW, eds. *Nelson Textbook of Pediatrics*. 21st ed. Philadelphia: Elsevier; 2020:1614–1618.

90. Centers for Disease Control and Prevention (CDC). Syphilis. https://www.cdc.gov/std/statistics/2020/overview.htm#Syphilis/.

91. Patterson MJ, Davies HD. Syphilis (Treponema pallidum). In: Kliegman RM, Stanton BF, St Geme JW, et al., eds. *Nelson Textbook of Pediatrics*. 21st ed. Philadelphia: Elsevier; 2020:1582–1599.

92. Workowski KA, Bolan GA, Centers for Disease Control and Prevention (CDC). Sexually transmitted diseases treatment guidelines, 2015. *MMWR Recomm Rep (Morb Mortal Wkly Rep)*. 2015;64(3):1–140.

93. Patrick SW, Barfield WD, Poindexter BB. Committee on fetus and newborn, committee on substance use and prevention; neonatal opioid withdrawal syndrome. *Pediatrics*. 2020;146(5):e2020029074.

94. Hudak ML, Tan RC. American Academy of pediatrics (AAP) committee on drugs and committee on fetus and newborn. Neonatal drug withdrawal. *Pediatrics*. 2012;129(2):540–560.

95. Grossman MR, Berkwitt AD, Osborn RR, et al. An initiative to improve the quality of care of infants with neonatal abstinence syndrome. *Pediatrics*. 2017;139(6):e20163360.

96. Lipsitz PJ. A proposed narcotic withdrawal score for use with newborn infants: a pragmatic evaluation of its efficacy. *Clin Pediatr*. 1975;14(6):592–594.

97. Finnegan LP. Neonatal abstinence syndrome: assessment and pharmacotherapy. In: Nelson N, ed. *Current Therapy in Neonatal-Perinatal Medicine*. 2nd ed. BC Decker; 1990.

98. Grisham LM, Stephen MM, Coykendall MR, Kane MF, Maurer JA, Bader MY. Eat, Sleep, Console approach: a family-centered model for the treatment of neonatal abstinence syndrome. *Adv Neonatal Care*. 2019;19(2):138–144.

99. Fill MM, Miller AM, Wilkinson RH, et al. Educational disabilities among children born with neonatal abstinence syndrome. *Pediatrics*. 2018;142(3):e20180562.

29

Neurodivergence and Behavioral and Mental Health Disorders

DAWN LEE GARZON AND NANCY BARBER STARR

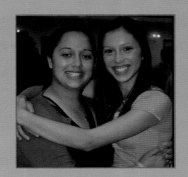

The term *mental health disorder* describes conditions that affect behavioral, emotional, and neurologic development and include disorders related to toxic stress and adverse childhood experiences (ACEs). *Neurodevelopmental disorders* are conditions that affect development and are characterized by delays, deficits, or impairments in personal, social, academic, or occupational functioning. More specifically, both types of challenges affect emotions, behaviors, attention, memory, learning ability, socialization, self-regulation, and self-control. Neurodevelopmental disorders as defined in the DSM-5TR include autism spectrum disorder (ASD), attention–deficit/hyperactivity disorder (ADHD), specific learning disorder, intellectual disorders, communication disorders, tic disorders, and motor disorders.[1] The term *behavioral health* includes emotional health issues, substance use and abuse, and neurodevelopmental and mental health disorders. It is a broader and preferred term to mental health and is used commonly in clinical practice. There are many reasons for pediatric behavioral health issues, including exposure to environmental toxins, such as lead and mercury, genetic inheritance, chronic toxic stress, insufficient opportunities to develop coping and resiliency, and ACEs, among others.

Epigenetics, or the role of nongenetic influences of gene expression, is a significant contributor to behavioral health disorders. Known epigenetic influences of behavioral health include trauma, ACEs, and toxic stress, including child maltreatment, harsh caregiving, caregiver psychopathology, poor nutrition, hormones, environmental toxins, low social support, substance abuse, unsafe environmental conditions, chronic financial disadvantage, and dysfunctional family interactions.[2] A number of suspected epigenetic influences remain the subject of ongoing scientific investigation. These include global environmental changes that affect the maternal-fetal environment, alterations in the microbiome of the urogenital and gastrointestinal tracts, and mutigenerational ribonucleic acid changes and their effects on neuronal development when disease burden increases in subsequent generations.[3] Common childhood stressors that negatively impact pediatric behavioral health include parental divorce or separation, domestic violence, child abuse or neglect, death of a parent or sibling, natural disasters, familial mental illness, exposure to media reports of traumatic events, school problems, interpersonal conflict, and/or prolonged separation (e.g., incarceration or military deployment) from a loved one.

The COVID-19 pandemic and the subsequent public health response resulted in dramatic changes in the lives of children, adolescents, and adults. Children and adolescents were particularly vulnerable during the pandemic; 1% of youth experienced significant school disruptions and the resulting social isolation and lost peer interaction.[4] Multiple studies demonstrate increasing rates of pediatric depression and anxiety, especially in vulnerable populations including neurodivergent individuals and those from racial, gender, and sexually marginalized groups.[4,5]

The 2019 America's Children: Key National Indicators of Well-Being report showed that 6% of responding parents identified their 4- to 17-year-old children as having severe emotional difficulties, impaired concentration, challenging behavior, or inability to get along well with others.[6] Significant problems were identified for 7% of males and 4% of females. In 2019 approximately 16% of the adolescents between 12 and 17 years old experienced a major depression episode in the previous year, an increase from the previous reported years of 2014 (11%) and 2004 (9%). Children living in families with incomes below the federal poverty level were significantly more likely to have serious behavioral issues than those whose family incomes were at least twice the federal poverty level (8.6% vs. 5.0%). Children living with a relative or guardian (9%) or only with their mother (8%) were more likely to have significant problems compared with children living in two-parent families (5%) or only with their fathers (4%).[6]

Children and adolescents in the United States are not receiving the behavioral health care they need. National estimates indicate that annually 20% of US children are diagnosed with a mental health or substance use disorder (SUD), and almost 40% of adolescents meet criteria for a mental health disorder before age 18 years.[7] Those with a psychiatric diagnosis represent the most severely impaired; those with mild symptoms often go unrecognized. Less than half of the children and adolescents with behavioral health issues obtain any treatment for their condition, and of those that do, even fewer receive evidence-based care.[8] There is a particular shortage of pediatric behavioral health providers and child psychiatrists, especially in rural areas and for children and teens from lower socioeconomic backgrounds. This was the rationale for the development of the pediatric primary care mental health specialist certification, thus allowing for recognition of advanced expertise of pediatric nurse practitioners with demonstrated expertise in primary care mental health. Primary care providers (PCPs) must take active roles in the identification of and early intervention for children and adolescents with mental health disorders. Bright Futures calls for assessment of family psychosocial functioning at all routine health supervision visits and routine screening for mental health issues using validated instruments for older school-age children and adolescents.[9]

Early behavioral health influences include the child's genetic composition and intrauterine exposures and the effects of maternal health status on the developing fetus. Known maternal factors that influence child behavioral health include maternal nutrition, especially vitamin B_{12}, folate and folic acid intake, and maternal stress including behavioral health, experiencing a natural disaster or chronic toxic stress, and maternal sustained psychosocial stress (see Chapter 6 for additional information). There are known genetic links for conduct disorder (CD), bipolar disorder, depression, schizophrenia, ADHD, substance abuse, antisocial behavior, generalized anxiety disorder (GAD), and obsessive-compulsive disorder (OCD), among others.

From infancy through early adulthood, changes in the limbic system, specifically the amygdala and hippocampus, influence emotional development and the emergence of affective disorders, substance abuse, and high-risk behaviors. However, none of these brain differences alone are necessary or sufficient for psychopathology to develop. Rather, environmental strengths and vulnerabilities, and cumulative life experiences strongly influence the number and severity of symptoms and the adaptive competencies that individuals display at any age. Activation of the hypothalamic-pituitary-adrenal (HPA) axis triggers release of cortisol, and elevated serum cortisol levels are toxic to central nervous system (CNS) neurons, inhibiting the growth of dendrites and neurons, and causing neuronal apoptosis. There are profound effects of chronic stress during the final phase of brain growth when the brain prunes away unused neurons and dendritic connections. This results in actual changes to brain structures. For example, research demonstrates that adults who experienced child maltreatment have changes to the cortical structure including thickening of the frontotemporal and occipital regions.[10]

Neurodiversity is a concept that explains neurodevelopmental issues as differences or variations in brain structure or wiring rather than abnormalities. This framework allows patients and families to approach challenges as differences rather than deficits, and it offers the perspective that the goal is to support those who are neurodiverse to enable them to participate and reach their maximum potential. This perspective is especially useful in removing barriers and advocating for a variety of teaching strategies with learning and attention issues. However, to receive support and services, a disability must be identified.

Neurodevelopmental disorders are disorders of brain function in three main areas: motor, cognition, and social behavior. Each area has an associated *spectrum* and *continuum*: the spectrum ranges from mild to severe, and the continuum represents the associated deficits or comorbidities and how they affect the other areas of function. The motor stream consists of gross motor, fine motor, and oral motor (speech, chewing, and swallowing) skills. On the mild end, this may look like a clumsy child or dysgraphia. The cognitive stream includes intellectual ability, language and communication, and nonverbal skills. On the mild end, this may look like a slower learner or letter identity and position difficulties. The social-behavior stream includes social abilities, attention, and impulse/hyperactive dimensions. On the mild end, this may look like a shy, inattentive, or hyperactive child.

Assessment and Management of Behavioral Health Disorders

A behavioral health disorder is a sustained behavior change resulting in functional impairment. Nonimpairing behaviors do not reach the threshold of becoming a behavioral health disorder. Because these problems cover a broad range of behavioral, emotional, and psychological disorders, many of which include genetic influences, the accurate identification of emotional, social, behavioral, and mental health status requires a thorough history and a physical examination. A targeted history should focus on child behavior and functional impairment (see Chapter 6). The physical examination detects underlying physical conditions that can cause behavioral or emotional changes. PCPs must recognize that common illness symptoms, such as fever, can change a child's behavior because of malaise, arthralgias, pain, or other physical symptoms.

Making Mental Health and Behavioral Diagnoses

Making behavioral health diagnoses is often difficult. PCPs must decide whether behaviors are within normal limits for age, temperament, family, health, and other factors. Comorbidities are common. In practice, several things may need to be addressed: the behavior, the family effects, nutrition, sleep, and other interrelated issues. In many cases, a behavioral health specialist such as a clinical psychologist or psychiatrist may be required to assist in diagnostic decision-making. In general, always address the most troublesome symptoms and behaviors first. For example, if an adolescent has significant symptoms of depression with suicidal ideation and inattention with hyperactivity, it is important to address the depression first given the risk of not treating it and the comorbid inattention caused by both depression and ADHD.

Management Strategies

After the diagnosis, the PCP must decide how to manage or comanage problems with other pediatric specialists, where appropriate. Pediatric PCPs manage more behavioral health problems than ever before, largely because of the scarcity of behavioral health services or inadequate insurance coverage that makes behavioral health care out of reach for many families. However, many PCPs lack adequate education to manage complex problems. In addition, it is financially difficult for many busy primary care practices to offer the extended appointments needed for high-quality behavioral health care, and reimbursement for these services is different than that provided for medical care.

Evidence demonstrates the best outcomes occur when behavioral health and primary care are integrated; however, this model is not standard, and PCPs must plan for how to manage children and youth with behavioral health issues. This includes, but is not limited to, determining referral sources to therapists and other behavioral health providers, identifying appropriate screening tools, and educating themselves about behavioral health. There are very good education programs available through organizations like The Reach Institute (www.thereachinstitute.org), Project Teach (www.projectteachny.org), and the National Association of Pediatric Nurse Practitioners (NAPNAP) (www.napnap.org). Almost half of the states in the United States have free phone consultation with a psychiatrist or other behavioral health provider to help PCPs identify and manage affected youth. A list of participating states and contact information is available at http://web.jhu.edu/pedmentalhealth/nncpap_members.html.

As a rule, if the cause of the problem is a life event with acute, short-term consequences (such as the death of a pet or a friend moving away) or a common developmentally normal but troublesome behavior (e.g., temper tantrums or sibling rivalry), it can be managed in the primary care setting. More enduring problems, such as loss of a parent or major depression, may require collaboration or consultation with or referral to a pediatric behavioral health specialist.

Appropriate care of pediatric behavioral disorders always requires an interprofessional approach. Pharmacotherapy alone is never appropriate, nor should it be used without a thorough evaluation. Clinical practice guidelines further emphasize the need for treatments to be evidence-based and inclusive of short- and long-term follow-up plans. All ethical issues regarding consent and assent are especially important in mental health care. Caregivers and patients should be aware of treatment risks, benefits, and alternative options.

PCPs can find information from the Developmental Behavioral and Mental Health special interest group of the NAPNAP, which has a comprehensive website for providers at www.dbmhresource. org/. In addition, the American Academy of Pediatrics (AAP) provides information about evidence-based psychosocial interventions at https://downloads.aap.org/AAP/PDF/crpsychosocialinterventions.pdf. This resource is updated multiple times a year and includes a wealth of information about evidence-based diagnosis and management of pediatric behavioral health disorders, training resources, and links to practice guidelines and screening resources.

Common Behavioral Health Disorders

Anxieties: Anxiety

Anxiety causes apprehension and differentiates from fear in that the stimuli is unknown or nonspecific. It is a normal developmental phenomenon that is experienced by every person at some point and may serve to heighten the senses and help in stressful situations. Anxiety is an evolutionary protective mechanism that allows an individual to identify and protect oneself from dangerous or threatening circumstances. In excessive and inappropriate amounts, anxieties have profound effects on social interactions and daily functioning. Anxious responses include somatic symptoms mediated by the autonomic system and include tachycardia, tachypnea, hypertension, gastrointestinal distress, tremor, diaphoresis, and enhanced vigilance and reactivity. Anxiety that persists at high levels and causes maladaptive behavior warrants diagnosis and treatment. Anxiety disorders include conditions associated with childhood such as separation anxiety disorder (SAD), GAD, social anxiety disorder, panic disorder, and agoraphobia. SAD, GAD, and social anxiety are often referred to as the *pediatric anxiety disorder triad,* as they often happen in the same individual and have similar life courses and treatments. Anxiety disorders are some of the most common child and adolescent psychiatric conditions, affecting 7% of youth worldwide and 20% to 30% of people in the United States over a lifetime.[8] Prevalence for social anxiety in 13- to 17-year-olds is 7%. Anxiety disorders are often comorbid with other psychiatric conditions, cause social functioning impairments, and are significantly more likely to occur if the caregivers has an anxiety or mood disorder.[8] Different anxiety disorders emerge at different developmental stages, but the median age of onset is age 11 years.[8] Separation anxiety occurs mostly in early childhood, social anxiety in middle childhood and early adolescence, and panic disorders, GAD, and agoraphobia in late adolescence. Children with early onset anxiety generally have greater impairment of social and

personal development, and thus a much greater likelihood of poor subjective views of their personal mental and physical health, social relationships, career satisfaction, and home and family relationships in adolescence and adulthood.

Risk factors include (1) genetics (familial heritance and specific gene loci), (2) temperamental disposition for behavioral inhibition and/or shyness, and (3) social environment or life circumstances (e.g., parental distress, dysfunction, or trauma). Youth with anxiety disorders are at high risk for comorbid mood disorders, ADHD, learning and language disorders, eating disorders, OCDs, and substance abuse.

Anxieties: Separation Disorder

The essential feature of SAD is an abnormal reaction to real, impending, or imagined separation from major attachment figures, home, or familiar surroundings. Separation anxiety is a normal developmental phenomenon from about 7 months old through early childhood. Some infants and toddlers experience excessive levels of distress with separation from their major caregiver and they cry, cannot be comforted, or refuse to be cared for and comforted by a competent, substitute caregiver. Alternatively, older infants, toddlers, and preschoolers may act aggressively toward the substitute caregiver or intentionally injure themselves.

SAD is the most common pediatric anxiety disorder, causing difficulty with separation and interfering with daily activities and developmental tasks. It is one of the leading reasons for referral to mental health professionals and is estimated to affect 1% to 4% of the population with a mean age of onset between 6 and 7 years; however, clinical presentation frequently is delayed by months to years following symptom onset.[11] SAD is a risk factor for the future development of panic disorder and depression in adolescence or adulthood and evolves from the interaction among physiologic, cognitive, and overt behavioral factors in response to life events that threaten safety, primary relationships, or both. Among infants and young children, only about 10% of those affected by separation anxiety are referred for care despite the concerns of most parents. Often, older children are brought to the PCP when the disorder results in school refusal or somatic symptoms. A significant number of children with school refusal have SAD, and many of these have comorbid depression. Sleep problems and impaired social interactions are also common.

Clinical Findings

The following are symptoms and behaviors seen in individuals with SAD:

- Excessive or developmentally inappropriate anxiety about separations
- Unrealistic worry about harm to self or loved ones, or fears about abandonment during periods of separation
- Reluctance to sleep alone or sleep away from home
- Persistent avoidance of being alone
- Nightmares about separation
- Physical complaints and signs of distress in anticipation of a separation
- Social withdrawal during separations
- Environmental stress, parental dysfunction, and maternal anxiety and depression are risk factors especially when accompanied with symptoms of panic disorder or agoraphobia, the fear of being outside the home, in crowds, or places they will not be able to easily leave.

The Spielberger State-Trait Anxiety Inventory for Children (STAIC) is a 20-item, self-report scale useful with children 9 to 12 years old; it can also be used with high reading–skill younger children and low reading–skill adolescents. The Generalized Anxiety Disorder-7 (GAD-7) is a 7-item scale normed for 12 years old and older. The Screen for Child Anxiety Related Disorders (SCARED) is a 41-item self-report scale with both parent and child versions available in the public domain for use in 8- to 18-year-olds.

Differential Diagnosis

Differential diagnoses include other anxiety disorders not associated with separation. It is essential to identify past traumatic experience or situations (e.g., sexual or physical abuse) as anxiety is a typical response to trauma or posttraumatic stress. Depression, social phobia/anxiety, and ADHD are common comorbidities. Problems at home can cause or exacerbate school refusal. For instance, a child may want to stay at home if the child worries about the caregiver's safety when they are alone.

Management

SAD is best treated as a family system or relationship-based problem. Symptom relief is the priority in school-age children. Identifying and treating the source of the problem is the first line of treatment for infants and young children and a secondary focus of treatment for school-age children and adolescents. Note the role of attachment figures and refer the child to a therapist for psychoeducational, behavioral, and cognitive-behavioral interventions. Eighty percent to 90% of youth respond to a combination of psychoeducation and parental education/training. PCPs can help patients identify their anxious feelings and physical responses to their anxiety. Caregivers benefit from learning how to help their children identify feelings of anxiety and by supporting them during exacerbations. Pharmacotherapy is not particularly helpful in reducing symptoms and should only be used if the patient fails to respond to nonpharmacologic intervention and has considerable impairment in function, and thus merits referral to a pediatric behavioral health provider.

Anxieties: Generalized Anxiety Disorder

GAD is both cognitive and obsessive in nature and causes excessive anxiety, worry, and apprehension generalized to several events or activities. These anxieties do not focus on a specific person, object, or situation, nor are they the result of a recent stressor. Individuals with GAD might be characterized as "worriers," or they might see themselves as being "overwhelmed" or "stressed out." The diagnosis is usually made in late middle childhood and adolescents aged 9 to 18 years old and affects approximately 2% of the general population with 1% showing signs of significant impairment.[12] There are clear genetic influences of GAD, especially in females.

Clinical Findings

Major symptoms of GAD are:
- Worry about future events and/or preoccupation with past behavior
- Feelings of being overwhelmed
- Poor-quality sleep
- Fatigue not explainable by other conditions
- Muscle tension
- Irritability and tantrums in young children
- Overconcern about competence and marked preoccupation with performance
- Significant self-consciousness and unusual need for reassurance
- Restlessness, difficulty concentrating

- Somatic complaints without a physical basis
- Comorbidity with other anxiety disorders, ADHD, or mood disorder

Differential Diagnosis

Differential diagnoses include anxiety due to a medical condition, substance or medication-induced anxiety disorder, panic disorder, separation anxiety, and adjustment disorder associated with a specific stressor. It is important to pay attention to cues that point to traumatic experiences or conditions as the source of anxiety symptoms and to symptoms suggestive of the presence of pediatric acute onset neuropsychiatric syndrome (PANS; see OCD).

Management

The treatment of preschool children and toddlers generally focuses on behavioral and family interventions with the best response coming with interventions that incorporate cognitive behavior therapy (CBT) with a caregiver component (Fig. 29.1). Preschoolers may benefit from play therapy. Refer the older child or adolescent to a pediatric mental health therapist for symptom treatment using mindfulness, psychodynamic therapy, or CBT. Individual and/or family counseling helps identify the source of anxiety and to assist with family discord. Treatment outcomes are more positive when caregivers are involved in interventions that target familial contextual processes. Younger children in middle childhood benefit from a combination of cognitive-behavioral strategies and family intervention. Individual and group treatments or child- and family-focused treatments are equally effective, and follow-up data demonstrate that treatment gains are maintained up to several years after treatment.

Pharmacologic intervention in combination with psychotherapy is advisable for older children and adolescents (see Fig. 29.1). Evidence points to the safety and efficacy of the selective serotonin reuptake inhibitors (SSRIs), especially sertraline and fluoxetine; two serotonin and norepinephrine reuptake inhibitors (SNRIs), venlafaxine and duloxetine; and other medications like buspirone and hydroxyzine (Table 29.1). Benzodiazepines are not recommended because of cognitive impairment and concerns about tolerance and dependency.

Obsessive-Compulsive Disorder

Obsessions are recurrent thoughts, images, or impulses that are disturbing to the child or adolescent and difficult to dislodge. They often involve a sense of risk or fear of harm to the child or family members; concerns about contamination are common. Compulsions are repetitive behaviors or mental acts that the child feels driven to perform with the aim of reducing the anxiety associated with obsessions and include behaviors such as washing (e.g., hands, objects, or body), counting, or arranging objects. Recurrent worries, rituals, and superstitious games are common in children at various stages of development; these behaviors result in mild anxiety but do not cause distress. OCD differs from normal child behavior in that it results in marked distress; is time consuming (individuals often spend a minimum of 1 hour a day engaged in the behavior); and interferes with the child's social, familial, or academic function. Abnormal compulsive behavior is distinguished by a sense of urgency or a profound discomfort until the ritual is completed. Children and adolescents often deny the fear and lack recognition of the "senselessness" of the ritual and try to hide their illness often out of embarrassment. Obsessive thoughts are intrusive, recurrent, and disturbing, and unlike anxious worries, are generally unrelated to events or situations.

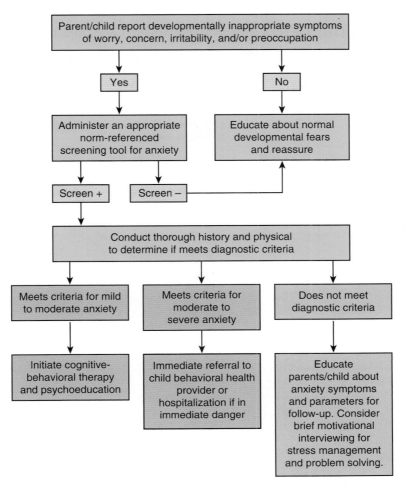

• **Fig. 29.1** Primary Care Management of Pediatric Anxiety Disorders.

OCD has environmental and genetic influences and has prevalence rates of 1% to 4% worldwide.[13] OCD is more common in males (3:2) before adolescence, but sex-based differences disappear after puberty. Most adults with OCD report experiencing initial symptoms in late childhood or adolescence. Like most psychiatric conditions, OCD is a chronic disease, and if untreated can result in lifelong disease and significant loss of quality of life.

There are strong familial patterns of transmission, and the link between genetics and OCD is strong. A subgroup of pediatric patients with OCD and Tourette syndrome is diagnosed with PANS, also known as *pediatric autoimmune neuropsychiatric disorder, associated with streptococcal infection* (PANDAS), a condition believed to be the result of autoimmune responses following group A β-hemolytic streptococci (GABHS) infection. PANDAS diagnostic criteria include dramatic onset of OCD or tic disorder in children between 3 years old and puberty shortly following GABHS infection and symptom exacerbation. However, it is important to note that this diagnosis remains controversial and has been since it was first established in the mid-1990s, with ongoing conflicting evidence as to the validity of the diagnosis. OCD is a chronic condition, and about half of all affected individuals have comorbid psychiatric conditions, typically other anxiety disorders, major depression, ADHD, or substance abuse disorder. Disruptive behavior disorders and learning disorders are also common comorbidities.

Clinical Findings

OCD is characterized by obsessions and compulsions, as previously defined. Children may not recognize that their obsessions or compulsions are excessive or unreasonable, so insight into the behaviors is important. The most common obsession is fear of contamination that results in compulsive washing and avoidance of "contaminated" objects. Other common obsessive worries include fears about safety (their own or their parents), exactness or symmetry, and religious sinfulness (scrupulosity). Common compulsions include repetitive counting, arranging, or touching patterns, and compulsive rechecking (doors, homework, and exam items). High anxiety levels are common if they are unable to perform their obsession "until I get it right." Other core symptoms include impulsivity, sexual obsessions, aggression, emotional lability, anger, and food rituals and/or obsessions.[13] Children with PANS/PANDAS often have additional symptoms like enuresis, irritability, behaviors consistent with behavioral regression (e.g., "baby talk"), impaired memory, separation anxiety, and nightmares.

Differential Diagnosis

To assess context and severity of symptoms, PCPs should obtain information from the child, parents, family members, and teachers. A diagnosis of OCD is warranted if the content of the obsessions and compulsions is unrelated to another mental health disorder (e.g., social phobia, trichotillomania [pulling out hair],

TABLE 29.1 Evidence-Supported Drug Therapy for Common Mental Health Conditions in Childhood

Drug Class and Examples	Conditions Treated	Primary Care Drug Interactions	Common Side Effects
Selective Serotonin Reuptake Inhibitor			
Fluoxetine (FDA approved 8+ for MDD, 7+ for OCD)	Anxiety; MDD, OCD, selective mutism, PTSD	Multiple drug interactions Contraindicated drugs: MAOIs, tryptophan, St. John's wort, thioridazine, and TCAs	Headache, nervousness, insomnia or sedation, fatigue, nausea, diarrhea, dyspepsia, appetite loss
Escitalopram (FDA approved 12+ for MDD)	MDD, anxiety, OCD, PTSD	Same as above but better drug interaction profile	Same as above
Fluvoxamine (FDA approved 8+ for OCD)	MDD, anxiety, OCD	Increased risk of bleeding: NSAIDs, aspirin, warfarin	Same as above
Sertraline (FDA approved 6+ for OCD)	MDD, OCD, anxiety, PTSD	Same as above Diet: may interact with grapefruit juice	Same as above
Serotonin Norepinephrine Reuptake Inhibitor			
Duloxetine (FDA approved 7+ for GAD)	MDD, GAD, PTSD	Multiple drug interactions Risk for toxic levels: SSRIs, amphetamines, guanfacine-potentiates BP effects	Nausea, headache, dizziness, diaphoresis, behavior activation
Venlafaxine	MDD, GAD, PTSD	Same as above Discontinuation syndrome common	Same as above
Mood Stabilizer			
Lithium	Bipolar disorder, CD	Multiple drug interactions Risk for toxic drug levels: NSAIDs, metronidazole, and a wide range of antihypertensives	Weight gain, acne, sedation, tremors, GI upset, hair loss Diet: limit caffeine, alcohol; ensure maintain fluid intake; maintain salt intake
Second-Generation Antipsychotics			
Risperidone (FDA approved 5+ ASD with aggression, 11+ BPD, 13+ schizophrenia)	Aggression CD ODD Schizophrenia Tourette syndrome	Multiple drug interactions Avoid: St. John's wort Potentiates: antihypertensives	Orthostatic hypotension, sedation, syncope, tachycardia, insomnia, agitation, headache, dizziness, seizures, rash, weight gain, nausea, vomiting, diarrhea, polyuria, weight gain, elevated lipids, hyperglycemia, rhinitis, suicidal ideation Can cause increased prolactin levels
Aripiprazole (FDA approved 6+ ASD, 10+ BPD, 13+ schizophrenia)	BPD Schizophrenia Aggression with ASD	Same as above	Same as above
Olanzapine (FDA approved 13+ for schizophrenia and BPD)	BPD Schizophrenia	Same as above	Same as above
Quetiapine (FDA approved 10+ BPD, 13+ schizophrenia)	BPD Schizophrenia	Same as above	Same as above Hypertension

ASD, Autism spectrum disorder; *BPD,* bipolar disorder; *CD,* conduct disorder; *FDA,* US Food and Drug Administration; *GAD,* generalized anxiety disorder; *GI,* gastrointestinal; *MAOI,* monoamine oxidase inhibitor; *MDD,* major depressive disorder; *NSAID,* nonsteroidal antiinflammatory drug; *OCD,* obsessive-compulsive disorder; *ODD,* oppositional defiant disorder; *SSRI,* selective serotonin reuptake inhibitor; *TCA,* tricyclic antidepressant.

ASD, eating disorder, and body dysmorphic disorder). Medical conditions that mimic OCD include autism, carbon monoxide poisoning, tumors, encephalitis, traumatic brain injury, Prader-Willi (compulsive eating), drug side effects (stimulants), and rheumatic fever. Providers should assess developmental history to determine delays and/or difficulties. School performance may be impaired, and OCD may mimic learning disorders when children have compulsions to reread or rewrite or have pathologic perfectionism. Caregivers of children with secretive rituals may bring their child to primary care with complaints of skin rashes (dermatitis, chapped hands), temper tantrums, declining school performance, or sudden food or activity aversions. Individuals with self-injurious behavior (see Chapter 13) physically harm themselves to decrease mental anguish; however, this disorder is distinct from the rituals of OCD.

Assessment should include symptom description and context, frequency, and effect on daily functioning. It is important to note how these behaviors contribute to difficulties in home, school, and other domains. Six screening questions can be used to determine OCD pathology (Box 29.1). Children with suspected PANS/PANDAS and unclear history of recent upper respiratory tract infection should have confirmation of streptococcal infection either by throat culture or ASO titer. Screening with a norm referenced instrument like the Children's Yale-Brown Obsessive-Compulsive Scale (CY-BOCS) are preferred.

Management

OCD treatment decisions should center on the degree of child impairment. If the child's symptoms do not interfere with the child's life and do not cause undue distress, medications, and intensive therapy can be deferred (see Chapter 6 for alternative strategies to promote mental health). Optimal treatment involves an individualized and developmentally appropriate approach that centers on child and family therapy to help the child learn to manage his or her anxiety and distress. CBT provides the best long-term effectiveness for OCD and is considered first-line therapy for all children and adolescents with mild to moderate OCD.[13] Individuals with moderate to severe disease (e.g., causes excessive distress, leads to significant social isolation or inability to perform developmentally normal tasks, or occurs with significant comorbid psychopathology) should receive pharmacologic management. SSRIs are first-line pharmacologic agents and have the greatest efficacy of all drug classes; however, overall drug response rates are 40% to 60%.[13] Individuals who do not respond to CBT, who experience increasing symptom severity during treatment, who show signs of psychosis and/or suicidality, and who do not respond to SSRIs should be emergently referred to a child behavioral health provider.

Children with suspected PANS/PANDAS are best managed by referring to a PANS/PANDAS specialist. The current clinical practice guideline for the management of PANS/PANDAS indicates that the cornerstone for the pharmacologic treatment is immunotherapies, but these are reserved for individuals with neuroinflammation or who show signs of autoimmune sequelae. Immunotherapies include immunomodulators and antiinflammatory medications including corticosteroids.[14] All individuals with suspected PANS/PANDAS should be treated with appropriate antibiotics at the time of initial diagnosis, but prophylactic antibiotics are not universally recommended.[15]

Tic Disorders

Tic disorders are characterized by sudden, repetitive, fast, unconscious motor movements or vocalizations. A combination of multiple motor and at least one verbal tic that begin before age 18 years, persists for more than 1 year, and is not caused by another medical condition or substance is called *Tourette syndrome*.[1] All children have some repetitive habits (such as finger sucking or hair twirling), and many of these are adaptive behaviors that help decrease stress or help them calm or emotionally regulate. Habits

are pathologic when they have no clear purpose and result in physical or social impairment. Tic disorders cause significant anxiety for affected children and often result in impaired self-esteem, bullying, and emotional or academic problems.

Chronic tic disorders affect 1% to 2% of the population, and transient tic disorders affect 5% of the population. There is an estimated 70% to 85% heritability of tic disorders in first-degree relatives with a greater prevalence in males than females (2–4:1).[1] Most motor tics start in early childhood, between 4 and 6 years old, with peak intensity occurring in preadolescence between 10 and 12 years old.[1–16] Eye blinking is the most common initial tic, and most individuals with tics endorse an intense sensation that precedes the tic and an intense impulse to engage in the motor activity that is only relieved by performing the action in a specific way. Children with neurodevelopmental disorders, including ASD and ADHD, have greater risk of developing tics than their nonaffected peers.

Clinical Findings and Diagnostic Studies

Motor tics can be simple (involving a single muscle group) or complex (complicated movements like jumping or a series of simple tics). Common simple tics include blinking, twitching of hands or limbs, shoulder shrugging, tongue thrusting, or squinting. Other common tic behaviors include trichotillomania, bruxism (tooth grinding), skin pulling, and nail biting. Verbal tics include vocalizations or pushing air through the nose. Grunting sounds and/or clearing the throat are common. Obscene gestures and swearing are rare. Symptoms generally worsen during periods of stress, fatigue, or anxiety. Most individuals with tic disorders can unconsciously or consciously suppress tics when they intensely concentrate on other things like homework or games, when they become aware of others actively evaluating their tics, and when social pressure against tics is high. It is not uncommon for tics to improve during clinical evaluation, so videos of tic expression at home and in nonclinical settings may help clinicians understand actual tic intensity and impairment. The Yale Global Tic Severity Scale is the gold standard and most common used assessment tool in clinical practice. This semistructured interview is valid for use with 6- to 17-year-olds and assesses both tic type and the resulting impairment.

There are several potential organic causes of new onset tic disorders, many of which are the result of autoimmune processes that affect the CNS and are triggered by acute infections, such as GABHS.[16] Those affected with tics secondary to an underlying neurologic disorder will present with changes in their neurologic examination, most commonly changes in mental status and/or loss of fine motor skills (e.g., loses ability to draw figures or penmanship becomes impaired).

Management

Mild tics do not require treatment. Children with moderate to severe tics that disrupt self-esteem or impair socialization best respond to psychotherapy, specifically comprehensive behavioral intervention for tics (CBIT). The focus of treatment is to extinguish the tic, to increase children's awareness of the behaviors, and to teach another behavior to engage in when they feel they are about to have a tic behavior. Best responses are often obtained with older children and adolescents. Common reminder strategies include using an elastic bandage over a digit to discourage thumb sucking, using an elastic hair band to make it difficult to grasp hair, or placing a rubber band that can be gently pulled when a child is aware of engaging in a tic behavior. Positive reinforcement is another effective extinguishing strategy. It is important to note that tics cannot be extinguished when the child is not interested in stopping the habit. Because of their lower side effect profiles and their effects on comorbid ADHD, alpha-2 adrenergic agonists (e.g., clonidine and guanfacine) are first-line therapies for the management of mild to moderate tics. For moderate to severe symptoms, common psychopharmaceuticals include SSRIs and atypical antipsychotics (e.g., risperidone).

Posttraumatic Stress Disorder

Posttraumatic stress disorder (PTSD) describes a characteristic set of symptoms that develops following actual or threatened exposure to a severe stressor or trauma. The trauma may result from a single event ("one sudden blow" trauma) or variable, multiple long-standing events, such as ongoing maltreatment. According to the *Diagnostic and Statistical Manual of Mental Disorders,* 5th edition text revision (DSM-5TR), the criteria for PTSD for children and adolescents older than 6 years include[1]:

1. Witnessing or experiencing a traumatic event(s) that resulted in risk of death or serious injury to oneself or a loved one.
2. Experiencing event(s) that resulted in fear, helplessness, recurrent distress, flashbacks, or a sense of numbness and loss of awareness, avoidance of distressing memories, or nightmares.
3. Symptoms that cause increased arousal, excessive startle, altered mood and emotional response, intrusive thoughts, nightmares, and continued avoidance of reminders of the trauma.
4. Symptoms that last at least 1 month and cause significant impairment in social, cognitive, or school functioning.
5. Acute symptoms that last less than 3 months and chronic symptoms that last more than 3 months.

Trauma exposure is a key feature of the diagnosis of PTSD. Unfortunately, there are those who are skeptical about whether children suffer from PTSD. Parents and teachers frequently minimize traumatic effects, perhaps to relieve themselves of vicarious distress or to reassure themselves that their children have not suffered harm. Children experience trauma with a cognitive understanding of their age at the time of the trauma, and even as they age, their memories are the memories of the child they were then.

Substantial PTSD rates are documented for children who experience maltreatment. Children experience PTSD following exposure to any traumatizing experience including natural disasters and witnessed violence. Three factors consistently influence the severity of the response: (1) severity of the trauma exposure, (2) parental/caregiver distress related to the trauma, and (3) temporal proximity to the event. Evidence demonstrates that between 15% to 43% of females and 14% to 43% of males experience at least one trauma during childhood and adolescence and 3% to 15% of females and 1% to 6% of males develop PTSD.[17] The rate of PTSD is high among those who have been physically and sexually abused. The closer the perpetrator is in relation to the victim, the greater the trauma (e.g., PTSD is more likely when the perpetrator is a member of the immediate family as opposed to an extended family member, family friend, or stranger).

Clinical Findings

A diagnosis of PTSD requires that the child demonstrate specific behaviors following trauma[1]:

1. The child repeatedly reexperiences a set of symptoms from each of the three following categories:
   - Recurrent and intrusive memories of the trauma
   - Nightmares of monsters or threats to self or others, or nightmares about a specific event

- Distress caused by cues that symbolize or resemble an aspect of the trauma, including physiologic reactivity.
2. The child demonstrates three of the following symptoms, reflecting avoidance of stimuli associated with the traumatic event(s) and numbing of general responsiveness. These symptoms must not have been present before the trauma:
   - Avoidance of reminders of the trauma
   - Efforts to avoid thoughts, feelings, or conversations linked to the trauma
   - Amnesia for an important aspect of the trauma
   - Detachment or estrangement from others
   - Emotional constriction (restricted range of affect)
   - Diminished interest in or participation in usual activities
   - A sense of a foreshortened future
3. Two persistent symptoms of increased arousal must be new to the child, present for at least 1 month, and cause clinically important distress or negatively affect functioning, including the following:
   - Sleep disturbances
   - Hypervigilance
   - Difficulty concentrating
   - Exaggerated startle response
   - Agitated or disorganized behavior
   - Irritability or angry outbursts, extreme fussiness, or tantrums

Among infants, toddlers, and preschoolers, symptoms must be understood within the context of the trauma itself, the child's temperament and personality, and the caregiver's ability to support the child and provide a sense of safety and protection. Table 29.2 includes a listing of PTSD symptoms by age group.

Pediatric PTSD assessment requires careful and direct clinical interviews with the patient and caregivers. If the identified traumatic event involves a caregiver as the perpetrator of child maltreatment or domestic violence, the nonoffending caregiver or other caretaker should be interviewed. During assessment, do not use prompting or leading questions. Instead ask questions about whether someone has invaded the patient's privacy, how it happened, and how the injuries occurred. Assessment includes

TABLE 29.2	Posttraumatic Stress Disorder Symptoms by Age Group
Age Group	**Common Symptoms**
Infancy	Feeding problems, failure to thrive, sleep problems, irritability
Early childhood	Sleep problems, nightmares, developmental regression, aggression, extreme temper tantrums, anxiety symptoms, sudden worsening of fears, irritability, avoidance symptoms
Middle childhood	Sleep problems, nightmares, developmental regression, repetitive play themes, social withdrawal, may have partial amnesia of events, new onset anxiety or fears, panic attacks, impaired concentration, impaired school performance, avoidance symptoms or hypervigilance, somatic complaints
Adolescence	"Acting out," nightmares, insomnia, extreme startling, social withdrawal, fears, anxiety, panic attacks, depression, anger or rage, internalizing, suicidal ideation, impaired concentration, impaired school performance, hypervigilance

the nature of the trauma and the consequent symptom pattern. Screen by identifying TRAUMA symptoms:

- **T**rauma—known traumatic experience
- **R**eexperience—includes flashbacks and nightmares
- **A**voidance—avoids stimuli associated with the event
- **U**nable to function
- **M**onth or longer
- **A**rousal—is hypervigilant, has sleep disturbances, concentration difficulties, or an exaggerated startle response.

Differential Diagnosis

PTSD is the most severe and prolonged stress response to trauma. Adjustment disorders result in anxiety, depression or mixed symptoms and occur commonly with stressful transitions (e.g., moving, starting a new school, birth of a sibling, divorce), but they do not involve the avoidance, dissociation and hypervigilance seen with PTSD. Anxiety disorders, the most common differential diagnosis, are distinguished by not being precipitated by a traumatic event. Acute stress disorder is distinguished by the symptom pattern occurring and resolving within a 4-week period after the traumatic event. Recurrent intrusive thoughts occur in OCD but are experienced as inappropriate and are not related to an experienced trauma as they are in PTSD. Flashbacks also connect to the event and involve a feeling of reliving the event in PTSD, whereas hallucinations and other perceptual disturbances are unrelated to exposure to trauma. Comorbid conditions in preschoolers differ from those of adults and older children. Oppositional defiant disorder (ODD) is most common, followed by SAD and ADHD. Major depressive disorder (MDD) is very unlikely.

Management

Referral to a pediatric behavioral health specialist is crucial and a report to social service agencies is essential for children younger than 18 years who have witnessed or experienced violence. Many child abuse intervention centers are prepared to accept referrals, assess, and direct management of children who have witnessed violence. Psychotherapy is the first-line treatment for PTSD, and the best evidence coming from trauma-focused CBT.[18] Eye movement desensitization and reprocessing therapy (EMDR) is not as well studied in children as adults but shows promise as an effective therapy strategy.

Medications should be reserved for moderate to severe and unresponsive cases and children who fail therapy should be referred to behavioral health specialists before starting medications for symptom management. Adrenergic receptor blockers like propranolol, clonidine, and guanfacine may be effective at decreasing somatic symptoms (e.g., racing heart rate and hyperpnea) associated with posttraumatic stress responses. Anxiety and depressive symptoms respond well to SSRIs. Prazosin is used to help decrease nightmares.

Crisis intervention is often necessary for the child as well as the parents. PCPs should educate themselves about trauma and PTSD so they can provide high quality psychoeducation to parents and pediatric patients. The National Child Traumatic Stress Network has lots of evidence-based information about childhood trauma (www.nctsn.org).

Mood Disorders: Depression

There are three categories of depression that occur during childhood and adolescence: (1) MDD, (2) persistent depressive disorder, and (3) adjustment disorder with depressed mood. MDD is defined as either a depressed or irritable mood or a markedly decreased interest and pleasure in almost all the usual activities, or both, for a period of at least 2 weeks.[1] A persistent depressive disorder is characterized by depressed or irritable mood for most days for at least 2 years that is less intense but more chronic than major depressive episodes. Adjustment disorder with depressed mood typically occurs within 3 months after a major life stressor, involves less-severe symptoms, and is relatively mild and brief.

There are multiple subtypes of MDD. Children and adolescents with psychotic depression (e.g., affected individuals hallucinate or have delusions) have a greater incidence of adverse long-term outcomes, resistance to psychopharmacotherapy, and a much higher risk of developing bipolar depression. Seasonal affective disorder is most common during the fall and winter months when there is less daylight. Premenstrual dysphoric disorder occurs within a week of menstruation and lasts until a few days after menstruation.

Depression is uncommon in the preadolescent years with only 2% of 6- to 11-year-olds diagnosed with depression, a rate that increases to 8% of 12- to 17-year-olds with approximately 20% of adolescents experiencing symptoms of depression within the previous year.[7,19] Of those with depression who are diagnosed, as many as two-thirds of youths with depression are identified by their PCPs.[20] Adolescent depression has biological (e.g., sexual maturation and the influence of the sex hormones), social environment (e.g., greater social and academic expectations, greater exposure to negative events), and developmental (e.g., increased autonomy and abstract thinking) factors. Vulnerability to depression is created by an interplay of genetic, biological, biochemical, and psychosocial forces. Genetic factors underlie the risk for major depression, especially for earlier disease onset. Children of depressed parents are 3 to 4 times more likely to be diagnosed with depression than their peers.

Three biological theories of depression are used to understand the psychopharmacology of depression: (1) impaired neurotransmission, (2) endocrine dysfunction, and (3) biological rhythm dysfunction. Given a biological predisposition, certain life events may trigger the onset of depression. These include loss of a parent or significant other, losses that accompany a disability or injury, family dysfunction, chronic adversity, exposure to traumatic events, and physical or sexual abuse. There is a high risk of recurrent depression persisting into young adulthood.

An important feature of early-onset depression is the potential for the condition to be the initial symptoms of bipolar depression (see later). As many as one-third of preadolescent children who meet criteria for major depression develop bipolar depression. Psychiatric comorbidity with depression is common. The most common comorbidity with depression is anxiety (up to 70%). Other comorbid conditions include disruptive behavior disorders, eating disorders, substance abuse and/or dependence, learning disorders, stress disorders, and ADHD. Depression is also comorbid with chronic medical conditions, especially those with a neurologic component, such as brain injury, learning disorder, migraine headaches, and epilepsy.

Clinical Findings

Older children and adolescents with depression usually present with symptoms like those of adults. School-aged children rarely spontaneously admit to depression symptoms. Parents and teachers may report decreased mood, impaired concentration, inattention, irritability, fluctuating mood, temper tantrums, social withdrawal, somatic complaints, agitation, separation anxiety, or behavioral problems. Males are more likely to have externalizing symptoms (e.g., aggression, acting-out, anger), and females are more likely to have internalizing symptoms (e.g., somatic complaints, feelings of sadness, feelings of worthlessness). Females have two times higher depression rates than males after puberty, but prepubertal sex rates are roughly equal. Major depressive symptoms represent a persistent change that occurs across settings, activities, and relationships and causes the child distress, impaired functioning, or developmental alteration. Infants and young children may present with failure to thrive, speech and motor delays, repetitive self-soothing behaviors, withdrawal from social interaction, poor attachment, and loss of developmental skills. Infants may not respond to extra efforts to soothe or engage them.

Children in early childhood may lack energy, be too eager to please others, be excessively or unusually clingy or whiney, and have developmentally inappropriate problems with separation. Preschoolers with MDD may present with sad or grouchy mood, lack of pleasure in play or activity, poor appetite and weight loss, sleep problems, low energy and activity levels, low self-esteem, or increased death or suicide play or talk.

During middle childhood, youth with depression may be irritable, angry, or hostile or have externalizing behaviors, such as hyperactivity, aggression, irritability, or reckless behavior. Frequent school absences, perhaps because of school phobia, poor academic performance secondary to impaired concentration and fatigue, and other school problems are common. On the other hand, school-age children may have internalizing symptoms, such as boredom, lack of interest in playing with friends, social withdrawal, somatic complaints (e.g., stomachaches, headaches, muscle aches, or tiredness), eating or sleeping disturbances, enuresis, or encopresis. Some children with depression describe themselves in negative terms, whereas others, to compensate for feelings of poor self-worth, become preoccupied with attempting to please others.

Depression symptoms in adolescents include impulsivity, fatigue, hopelessness, antisocial behavior, substance use, restlessness, grouchiness, aggression, hypersexuality, and problems with family members or at school. Social withdrawal, manifested as shyness, boredom, or a lack of motivation, is common. Substance abuse is a significant comorbidity, and some substances (alcohol, cannabis, MDMA ["ecstasy"] and stimulant withdrawal) exacerbate or cause depressive symptoms.

It is essential to speak directly with the child or adolescent because it is thought that half of depression cases are missed when only parents are interviewed. Parents often mistake withdrawal, fatigue, and irritability as being "normal" adolescent moodiness. The following symptoms are common:
- Depressed mood: Sad, "blue," down, angry, bored
- Loss of interest and pleasure in usual activities, feeling numb or "meh"
- Change in appetite or weight (loss or increase)
- Insomnia or hypersomnia
- Low energy and fatigue
- Difficulty concentrating; indecision
- Feelings of worthlessness or inappropriate or excessive guilt
- Recurrent thoughts of death or suicidal ideation

A diagnosis of MDD is made if there have been at least 2 weeks of depressed mood or loss of interest and at least four additional symptoms of depression. The symptoms cause considerable distress and impairment in social and academic functioning and cannot be caused by bereavement.[1] Therefore it is important to assess the following:
- Recent life events and losses
- Family history of depression or other psychiatric disorders
- Family dysfunction
- Changes in school performance

- Risk-taking behavior, including sexual activity and substance use
- Deteriorating relationships with family
- Changes in peer relations, especially social withdrawal

Mild depression impacts daily life but affected individuals still function and complete normal tasks although doing so requires a lot of energy because of lack of motivation. Mild MDD causes lower scores on standardized assessments, shorter symptoms duration, and results in five to six MDD symptoms with mild functional impairment. In moderate depression, what began as a decreased interest in engaging in activities becomes a complete lack of interest and affected individuals often express concern about their inability to function and complete tasks. Its severity lies between mild and severe disease. Severe depression is demonstrated by increased agitation, psychosis, and suicidality and will often demonstrate all the depression symptoms. Current clinical practice guidelines state all adolescents with a minimum of five symptoms who have clear suicidality and a plan or recent attempt, who are psychotic, have a first-degree relative with bipolar disorder, or who have significant impairment including being unable to leave the home, have severe depression.[20] Undiagnosed and untreated/undertreated depression can be fatal. In 2020 suicide was the third leading cause of death for 14- to 24-year-olds.[21] Possible warning signs for suicide are listed in Table 29.3.

Both patient self-report and clinician-completed rating scales are available. Table 29.4 contains a listing of these scales.

Differential Diagnosis

Some medications and certain chronic illnesses (hypothyroidism, adrenal insufficiency, epilepsy, metabolic disease, sleep disorders, hepatitis, multiple sclerosis, inflammatory bowel disease, and type 1 diabetes) predispose children and adolescents to depression. If a substance (e.g., medication, toxin, or drug of abuse) is related to the mood disturbance, a substance-induced mood disorder is diagnosed. Medications that commonly cause depressive symptoms include β-blockers, benzodiazepines, nonsteroidal antiinflammatory drugs (NSAIDs), stimulants, clonidine, corticosteroids, oral contraceptives, and isotretinoin. Infections, lead intoxication, anemia, eating disorders, mitral valve prolapse, premenstrual syndrome, and neurologic disorders mimic depression in children and adolescents. In general, a physical examination and screening laboratory tests are necessary to rule out organic causes. Suggested diagnostic testing for an individual with new symptoms of depression include complete blood count (CBC), vitamin D, pregnancy testing, Epstein-Barr titers, thyroid panel, liver function testing, urinalysis, and drug screening.

Depressive symptoms in response to a psychosocial stressor are diagnosed as adjustment disorder, which has a good short-term prognosis and does not predict later dysfunction. With SAD, depressive symptoms usually arise only in the context of separation and resolve quickly with reunion; however, concomitant depressive disorder is not uncommon. A depressive episode with irritable mood can be difficult to distinguish from a manic episode with irritable mood; careful evaluation of the presence of manic symptoms (e.g., excessive activity, inflated self-esteem, little need for sleep, talkativeness) is required. Irritability alone is not sufficient to diagnose mania or hypomania. Many adolescents and adults who develop mania had preponderantly depressive symptoms in childhood. Family history of bipolar depression is an important risk factor. Depression can be differentiated from the irritability and inattention of ADHD in that children with MDD are not usually impulsive. In addition, they typically have a normal attention span before the onset of symptoms.

TABLE 29.3 Suicide Warning Signs

Area of Functioning	Signs[a]
Behavior changes	Accident prone or risk taking Drug and alcohol abuse Physical violence toward self, others, or animals Appetite loss Sudden alienation from family, friends, coworkers Worsening performance at work or school Putting personal affairs in order Loss of interest in personal appearance Disposal of possessions Writing letters, notes, or poems with suicidal content; talking about suicide Buying a gun or other weapon Isolation and withdrawal
Changes in mood	Expressions of hopelessness or impending doom Explosive rage Dramatic affect swings Crying spells Sleep disorders—insomnia, hypersomnia, or sleep interruption Talking about suicide
Changes in thinking	Preoccupation with death Difficulty concentrating Irrational speech Hearing voices, seeing visions Sudden interest (or loss of interest) in religion
Major life changes	Death of a family member or friend (especially by suicide) Separation or divorce Public humiliation or failure Serious illness or trauma Loss of financial security Recent relationship loss (e.g., first love)

[a]These signs must be interpreted in context. Many of them are common outside the realm of presuicidal behavior.

TABLE 29.4 Diagnostic Rating Scales for Depression Diagnosis

Scale	Appropriate Ages
Child Behavior Checklist (CBCL)	1.5–5 and 6–18 years
Children's Depression Rating Scale-Revised (CDRS-R)	6–12 years
Children's Depression Inventory (CDI)	6–18 years
Center for Epidemiologic Studies-Depression Scale (CES-D)	Adolescents
Depression Self-Rating Scale	Adolescents
Pediatric Symptom Checklist (PSC)	4 years to adolescent
Patient Health Questionnaire-9 (PHQ-9) and PHQ-9 Modified for Teens	6–10 years and 11 years to adolescent

Management

The first goals of management are to determine suicidal risk and intervene to prevent suicide. Suicidal risk is greatest during the first 4 weeks of a depressive episode. Patients with acute suicidal intent that includes a plan, psychosis, risk of abuse, and unstable behavior require immediate psychiatric evaluation. Cumulative suicidal risks—prior suicidal behavior or attempts, depression, and alcohol, tobacco, or drug abuse/dependence—require behavioral health intervention and immediate referral must be made. Attention must also be paid to establish a safe environment (e.g., removal or placing firearms in a gun safe with ammunition locked in a separate location, knives, and medications including over-the-counter medications, acetaminophen containing medications, and those containing iron). Families of adolescents with depression may be noncompliant with recommendations to secure firearms in the home despite compliance with other aspects of treatment. Vigilant follow-up in this regard is crucial. Other PCP management strategies include referral to community resources, such as hotlines and community mental health centers, and to identify an emergency plan for the family should the patient become actively suicidal, psychotic, or a danger to others. It is important to note that suicidal ideation often increases during the treatment phase known as *emergence*. Emergence occurs in the first week to month of treatment when the patient's energy levels increase, but feelings of hopelessness and helplessness have not yet receded. Complete a safety plan to help the patient and family members identify resources, coping strategies, and individual patient warning signs. A Stanford Brown suicide safety plan template can be found online at the https://suicidesafetyplan.com/forms/. The US national suicide hotline can be reached by dialing 988 from any cellular or landline.

A major depressive episode requires intervention by a behavioral health specialist. Unfortunately, only about half of all individuals with depression achieve full remission of their symptoms. Therapies typically include CBT in a group or individual psychotherapy format. Group CBT may help adolescents. Often, family therapy or psychoeducation is indicated. See Fig. 29.2 for primary care management of pediatric depression.

Available studies do not support the efficacy of tricyclic antidepressants and older medications for depression in young children, and they may be harmful.[19] Although the 2004 "black box" warning for SSRIs occurred because of concerns of increased suicidality with use of these medications, randomized controlled trials of pediatric depression consistently demonstrate that best treatment responses come from combinations of CBT and SSRIs and suicide rates are higher when patients are not treated with medications than when psychopharmacologic therapies are used. CBT has a protective effect against suicide. Currently, there are only a few antidepressants the US Food and Drug Administration (FDA) approved for use in children and adolescents (see Table 29.1). The FDA specifically recommends against the use of paroxetine in children and adolescents because of the 3.5-fold increased risk for suicide. A general rule of antidepressant dosing is to start low and slowly increase. It takes 4 to 6 weeks for maximum response, but medication doses can be adjusted to improve response every 2 to 4 weeks if significant side effects are absent. Activation (e.g., elevated energy without mood change) and mania can occur in patients secondary to treatment with antidepressants. Therefore it is critical to teach caregivers about symptoms that merit immediate evaluation, including decreased impulse control, marked elevated mood, acting out, fearlessness, and risk taking. For patients with psychosis, child behavioral health specialists often add antipsychotics like risperidone or olanzapine to the therapeutic drug plan.

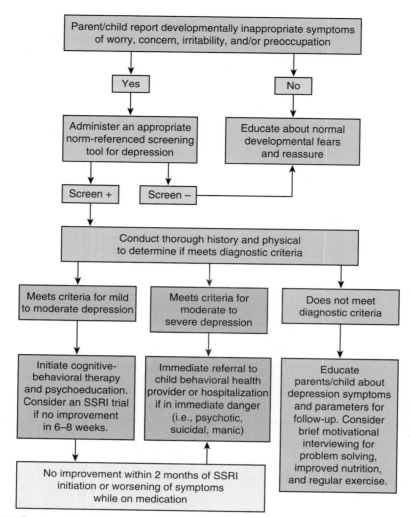

Parent/child report developmentally inappropriate symptoms
of worry, concern, irritability, and/or preoccupation

Yes → Administer an appropriate norm-referenced screening tool for depression

No → Educate about normal developmental fears and reassure

Screen + / Screen −

Conduct thorough history and physical to determine if meets diagnostic criteria

Meets criteria for mild to moderate depression

Meets criteria for moderate to severe depression

Does not meet diagnostic criteria

Initiate cognitive-behavioral therapy and psychoeducation. Consider an SSRI trial if no improvement in 6–8 weeks.

Immediate referral to child behavioral health provider or hospitalization if in immediate danger (i.e., psychotic, suicidal, manic)

Educate parents/child about depression symptoms and parameters for follow-up. Consider brief motivational interviewing for problem solving, improved nutrition, and regular exercise.

No improvement within 2 months of SSRI initiation or worsening of symptoms while on medication

• **Fig. 29.2** Primary Care Management of Pediatric Depression. *SSRI,* Selective serotonin reuptake inhibitor.

Close follow-up is recommended for all children and adolescents with depression, especially when symptoms are significant enough to merit pharmacotherapy. Providers should make phone contact with the patient and/or family within 3 days and see the patient every 1 to 2 weeks until stable or with any future medication changes. The first 4 weeks of treatment are critical. Once stable, maintenance visits can occur at 3-month intervals. Consider decreasing medication doses if patients are stable and asymptomatic for 6 to 12 months.

Prognosis

MDD is a chronic condition with a high rate of recurrence. Although most children and adolescents recover from an MDD episode, the probability of recurrence is 60% within 2 years and 75% by 5 years. Poor long-term outcomes are associated with severe or frequent disease, and patients with significant family dysfunction, low socioeconomic status, and history of abuse or family strife.

Mood Disorders: Bipolar Disorder

Bipolar disorder, formerly known as *manic depression,* is characterized by unusual shifts in mood, energy, and functioning and may begin with manic, depressive, or a mixed set of manic and depressive symptoms. Most adults with bipolar disorder report their initial symptom was depression, and those who develop symptoms in childhood are significantly more likely to develop severe disease, to be hospitalized frequently, and have a less favorable life course. It is a recurrent disorder, and nearly all of those (90%) who have a single manic episode will have future episodes. Approximately 0.6% to 2% of children younger than 18 years meet the diagnostic criteria for bipolar disorder.[22] The risk of suicide in bipolar depression is the highest of all the psychiatric disorders.

A characteristic pattern usually evolves, with manic episodes following major depressive episodes 60% of the time.[1] Most individuals with bipolar disorder return to a full level of functioning between episodes; 30% experience persistent mood lability, work impairment, and interpersonal difficulties.[1] Sometimes psychotic symptoms develop after several days or weeks of manic symptoms. Such features tend to predict that the individual with subsequent manic episodes will again experience psychotic symptoms.

Multiple theories explain the cause of bipolar disorder, but no definitive cause is known. Biological influences include structural changes in the third ventricle, the white matter, the prefrontal cortex, the amygdala, and the basal ganglia. There is evidence of a genetic influence for bipolar disorder from twin studies and adoption studies;

bipolar disorder tends to cluster in families. Parents who are bipolar are at greater risk for having bipolar children. The most common onset of symptoms occurs between 15 and 19 years old. There is no differential incidence based on race, ethnicity, or sex. Children with ADHD seem to be vulnerable to bipolar illness, or it may be that ADHD is a misdiagnosed early sign of the mania to come. If children are also bipolar, treatment of ADHD with psychostimulants or antidepressants may precipitate a manic episode. Antidepressants also precipitate mania and the onset of bipolar illness.

Clinical Findings

Bipolar disorder in childhood or early adolescence appears to be a different, more severe form of the illness than that which occurs with late adolescence or in adulthood. The early-onset form is characterized by irritability and continuous, rapid-cycling, and mixed-symptom state that may also co-occur with disruptive behavior disorders (e.g., ADHD or CD); features of ADHD or behavior disorder are often early symptoms. Prepubertal and early adolescent bipolar disorder is consistent with no differences according to gender, puberty, or comorbid ADHD. In the late adolescent or adult form, the hallmark features include classic manic episodes, episodic patterns of mania and depression, and relative stability between episodes. Symptoms include the following:[1]

- Severe mood changes—extreme irritability or overly elated and silly
- Inflated self-esteem or grandiosity—"I am the GOAT (greatest of all time)!" "I am the best football player in the world."
- Increased energy and physical agitation
- Decreased need for sleep (sleeps few hours or no sleep for days without fatigue the following day)
- Talkativeness or compulsion to talk; frequent topic changes or cannot be interrupted
- Racing thoughts
- Distractibility, with attention moving constantly from one thing to another
- Increase in goal-directed activity (socially or at school)—get "stuck" on activities and cannot stop doing them, suddenly cleans or reorganizes their room and redecorates after weeks of having little energy
- Risk-taking behaviors or activities; taking "more dares"
- Hypersexuality in talk, thoughts, feelings, or behaviors
- Psychosis—visual or auditory hallucinations
- Suicidal thoughts and behaviors.

Most adolescents experience depression as their initial symptom. The most common symptoms of mania include irritable mood and grandiosity, elevated mood, decreased sleep, racing thoughts, poor judgment, flight of ideas, and hypersexuality. With mania, children appear to be the happiest of people, but the happiness and laughter do not match the situation or context. Grandiosity may manifest in efforts to correct teachers or critique their efforts, seeing themselves as above rules and laws; seeing themselves as possessing incredible physical skills (e.g., believing they can jump down a flight of stairs without difficulty); or devoting time to an activity for which they have no talent, but they see themselves as being a master. Children's sleep difficulties (a hallmark sign) are reflected in high activity levels before bed (e.g., rearranging the furniture), whereas adolescents need little sleep at all. Risk-taking behavior ranges from children climbing excessively high trees or hopping between rooftops to adolescents driving recklessly and speeding. In adolescents, manic episodes are more likely to include psychotic features and may be associated with school truancy, school failure, substance use, or antisocial

behavior. The child or adolescent who has depression but also manifests symptoms of ADHD that seem severe (e.g., extreme temper outbursts and mood changes) should be evaluated by a child behavioral health specialist with experience in bipolar disorder. Symptoms are manifested in relatively age-specific ways.

Assessment for comorbid conditions is important. Anxiety disorders, including panic disorder, affect about half of patients with bipolar disorder. Other common comorbidities include ADHD, disruptive behavior disorders, and substance abuse disorders.

Differential Diagnosis

A manic episode must be distinguished from a mood disorder caused by a medical condition (e.g., brain tumor) and a substance-induced mood disorder (e.g., laughing fits with marijuana, amphetamine highs followed by withdrawal "crashes," perceptual distortions or hallucinations of hallucinogens). Distinguishing bipolar disorder from ADHD can be a challenge. ADHD, like mania, is characterized by excessive activity, poor impulse control, and impulsive judgment. However, ADHD lacks a clear onset or episodes, mood disturbances, and psychotic features. Recent evidence suggests that children with ADHD are vulnerable to bipolar disorder and that pharmacological treatments may precipitate manic episodes, so providers should carefully evaluate and refer any child treated for ADHD who does not respond to therapy or who experiences a sudden worsening of agitation while using ADHD medications.

Management

Referral to a child behavioral health provider is critical if bipolar disease is suspected. Current recommendations for pharmacologic treatment include the use of mood stabilizers, such as lithium, alone or in combination with antiseizure medications (e.g., valproic acid) and atypical antipsychotics (e.g., risperidone). Neither antidepressants nor stimulants have proven efficacy. Antidepressant use may potentiate manic responses. Lithium use must be carefully monitored. The best clinical responses occur when pharmacotherapy is combined with individual and family psychotherapy. Therapy should focus on minimizing comorbidities, enhancing problem-solving and communication skills, and reducing negative self-thoughts. Other nonpharmacologic interventions with proven effectiveness include stress reduction, healthy diet, routine exercise, and developing good sleep hygiene.

Attention-Deficit/Hyperactivity Disorder

Definition and Diagnostic Criteria

ADHD is one of the most diagnosed disorders in childhood. It is a neurodevelopmental disorder because it has a clear neurologic base with symptoms that profoundly affect the behavior of individuals across many settings in their lives. It is a chronic condition that persists for many into adolescence and adulthood. ADHD symptoms affect cognitive, educational, behavioral, emotional, and social functioning. Its core symptoms include developmentally inappropriate inattention, hyperactivity, and/or impulsivity observed in at least two settings (home, school, or work) that impair social, academic, and/or occupational functioning. Symptoms severity ranges from one individual to the next (mild, moderate, and severe), and the scope and severity of behaviors may change as an individual matures. ADHD criteria are listed in Table 29.5.

ADHD affects executive functions and self-regulation and has significant impact on social relationships. Children may present with struggles in the classroom, difficulties with peers, or trouble regulating their behavior or emotions. Because ADHD symptoms

TABLE 29.5	DSM-5TR Criteria for Attention-Deficit/Hyperactivity Disorder

A persistent pattern of inattention and/or hyperactivity-impulsivity that interferes with functioning or development, as characterized by (1) and/or (2):

Symptom	Criteria
(1) Inattention	Six (or more) of the following symptoms have persisted at least 6 months to a degree that is inconsistent with developmental level and that negatively impacts directly on social and/or academic/occupational activities: **Note:** The symptoms are not solely a manifestation of oppositional behavior, defiance, hostility, or a failure to understand tasks or instructions. For adolescents (age 17 years and older), at least five symptoms are required. • Often fails to give close attention to details or makes careless mistakes in schoolwork, at work, or during other activities (e.g., overlooks or misses details, work is inaccurate) • Often has difficulty sustaining attention in tasks or play activities (e.g., has trouble remaining focused during lectures, conversations, or lengthy reading) • Often does not seem to listen when spoken to directly (e.g., mind seems elsewhere, even in the absence of any obvious distraction) • Often does not follow through on instructions and fails to finish schoolwork, chores, or duties in the workplace (e.g., starts tasks but quickly loses focus and is easily sidetracked) • Often has difficulty organizing tasks and activities (e.g., difficulty managing sequential tasks; difficulty keeping materials and belongings in order; messy, disorganized work; has poor time management; fails to meet deadlines) • Often avoids, dislikes, or is reluctant to engage in tasks that require sustained mental effort (e.g., schoolwork or homework; for older adolescents and adults, preparing reports, completing forms, reviewing lengthy papers) • Often loses things necessary for tasks or activities (e.g., school materials, pencils, books, tools, wallets, keys, paperwork, eyeglasses, mobile telephones) • Is often easily distracted by extraneous stimuli (for older adolescents and adults, may include unrelated thoughts) • Is often forgetful in daily activities (e.g., doing chores, running errands; for older adolescents and adults, returning calls, paying bills, keeping appointments)
(2) Hyperactivity/impulsivity	Six (or more) of the following symptoms have persisted for at least 6 months to a degree that is inconsistent with developmental level and negatively impacts directly on social and academic/occupational activities: **Note:** The symptoms are not solely a manifestation of oppositional behavior, defiance, hostility, or a failure to understand tasks or instructions. For older adolescents and adults (age 17 and older), at least five symptoms are required. • Often fidgets with or taps hands or feet or squirms in seat • Often leaves seat in situations when remaining seated is expected (e.g., leaves his or her place in the classroom, in the office or other workplace, or in other situations that require remaining in place) • Often runs about or climbs in situations where it is inappropriate. (Note: In adolescents or adults, may be limited to feeling restless • Often unable to play or engage in leisure activities quietly • Is often "on the go" acting as if "driven by a motor" (e.g., is unable to be or uncomfortable with being still for extended time, as in restaurants, meetings; may be experienced by others as being restless or difficult to keep up with) • Often talks excessively • Often blurts out an answer before a question has been completed (e.g., completes people's sentences; cannot wait turn in conversation) • Often has difficulty waiting his or her turn (e.g., while waiting in line) • Often interrupts or intrudes on others (e.g., butts into conversations, games, or activities; may start using other people's things without asking or receiving permission; for adolescents and adults, may intrude into or take over what others are doing)

- Several inattentive or hyperactive-impulsive symptoms were present prior to age 12 years.
- Several inattentive or hyperactive-impulsive symptoms are present in two or more settings (e.g., at home, school, or work; with friends or relatives: in other activities).
- There is clear evidence that the symptoms interfere with, or reduce the quality of, social, academic, or occupational functioning.
- The symptoms do not occur exclusively during schizophrenia or another psychotic disorder and are not better explained by another mental disorder (e.g., mood disorder, anxiety disorder, personality disorder, substance intoxication or withdrawal).
- Specify whether:
  - **Combined presentation:** If both inattentive and hyperactivity-impulsivity criteria are met in the past 6 months
  - **Predominantly inattentive presentation:** If inattention criteria are met but hyperactivity-impulsivity criteria are not met for the last 6 months
  - **Predominantly hyperactive/impulsive presentation:** If hyperactivity-impulsivity criteria are met and inattention criteria are not met for the last 6 months

From American Psychiatric Association (APA). *Diagnostic and Statistical Manual of Mental Disorders, Text Revision DSM-5-TR.* APA; 2022.

cross over so many settings and often persist into adulthood, this condition has a major effect on the individual, family, and community (Table 29.6). Families report significantly higher levels of stress when they include children with ADHD; individuals with ADHD have difficulties with peer relationships, increased non-fatal injuries, and issues with driving (traffic violations and accidents). There are significant direct and indirect costs to individuals and families, including parental days of missed work due to the child's school and medical appointments, patient evaluation and treatment expenses that are not covered by health insurance (e.g., psychological or educational testing beyond that done at the school), and medication and mental healthcare costs.

ADHD prevalence rates vary depending on the source, criteria used to make the diagnosis, and the ages sampled. It is more common in males than females, and females tend to have more problems with inattention. ADHD affects approximately 10% of all children between 3 and 10 years of age in the United States.[7] There is evidence that children living in urban settings, white children, and children from with public insurance and who are more than 200% below the federal poverty line are more likely to have a formal ADHD diagnosis than their peers.[7]

It is important to ascertain if the symptoms are caused by ADHD with comorbidity or if the comorbid disorder is masquerading as ADHD as the approach to treatment may be very different. In addition, some coexisting conditions manifest over time, so monitoring for these conditions after assessment is critical.

Genetics, Neurobiological Pathophysiology, and Environmental Factors

Attention is a complex and multilayered neurologic activity requiring the function and interconnection of several different brain areas. Structural and functional imaging demonstrate smaller

brain volume in the accumbens, amygdala, and hippocampus in addition to the caudate and putamen regions.[23] Anomalous brain development (reductions in gray matter) in preschoolers 4 and 5 years of age (youngest studied) correlated with behavioral symptoms.[24]

There is no single cause for ADHD; research indicates that it is primarily a genetic disorder with environmental factors that modulate the biochemical predisposition. Genetic variations include deletions and duplications of DNA segments (copy number variants) involved with the manufacture and regulation of noradrenaline and dopamine. Individuals with ADHD have less neurotransmitters in certain brain regions. Dopamine and noradrenaline help alert, maintain attention and appropriate internal arousal, and inhibit external distraction.

Identified risk factors include alcohol and tobacco use during pregnancy, premature and low birth weight, exposure to environmental toxins (lead) in pregnancy or in early childhood, brain injury, and ACEs. Maternal inflammation during pregnancy is theorized to cause reduced infant brain circuitry thus affecting key pathways connecting the executive hub and deeper emotional processing regions and affecting working memory.[24]

The faster pace and demands of society also impact the child with ADHD. Schools have longer school days, increasingly complex tasks, a higher pupil to teacher ratio, more lecture versus active learning, increased homework, emphasis on timed tasks and tests, and reduced art, music, and physical education classes. Untreated, children with ADHD can struggle with learning, social relationships, self-management and self-esteem, employment (lower socioeconomic status, higher unemployment rates), more traffic violations and higher motor vehicle accident rates, difficult family interactions including marital discord and divorce, and increased risk of substance abuse, depression, and anxiety.

Clinical Findings and Assessment

Often, the child presents after being referred by a childcare provider, the school, or the parent/guardian. Concerns may include the inability to sustain attention, curb activity level, or inhibit impulsivity (core symptoms). However, concerns may be related to memory, emotional control, organization, planning or inhibiting thoughts or actions (executive functions or cognitive control), and/or difficulty with peers, following classroom rules, or regulating behavior. ADHD symptoms affect the domains where children and adolescents work on developmental mastery—school, peers, family life, sports, and recreational activities. It is important for the provider to inquire about all these areas.

The components of the ADHD assessment include interviewing the parent and youth, physical examination, standardized ADHD assessment scales from several different sources (parents, caregivers, teachers, childcare programs, and/or sports coaches) to assess for impairment in multiple domains, and other pertinent evaluations, such as school testing and psychological or other mental health evaluations. A comprehensive history for ADHD assessment is outlined in Table 29.7.

Perform a complete physical with a focus on the following:
- Vital signs—weight, height, body mass index, blood pressure, pulse, and head circumference in young children
- Vision and hearing screening
- General observation of the child's behavior (may or may not present with ADHD symptoms in the clinical setting); observe the parent-child interaction

TABLE 29.6	Attention-Deficit/Hyperactivity Disorder Impairments Across the Life Span
Life Stage	**Impairment**
Middle childhood	Academic difficulties including: • Needs for special education (high comorbidity with learning disabilities) • Grade retention • Classroom behavior management issues • Difficulties with friendships and peer relationships • Behavioral difficulties at home and other settings (childcare, sports, after-school programs) • High comorbidity with other childhood psychiatric problems • Associated difficulties (at higher rates than non-ADHD children) with sleep disorders, enuresis, encopresis
Adolescence	Academic difficulties including: • Need for special education (high comorbidity with learning and emotional disabilities) • School failure and dropout • Social difficulties with peer relationships • Substance abuse (in untreated ADHD) • High comorbidity with other psychiatric disorders (depression, anxiety, conduct disorder) • High-risk behaviors leading to greater accident rates • Involvement in juvenile criminal activities
Adulthood	Difficulties include: • Fewer employment possibilities and higher rates of unemployment • Higher risk of tobacco, drug, and alcohol abuse • Higher risk of motor vehicle accidents • Marital discord and higher divorce rates • Increased incidence of criminal involvement

ADHD, Attention-deficit/hyperactivity disorder.

TABLE 29.7	Attention-Deficit/Hyperactivity Disorder History
Assessment Area	**Suggested Topics to Explore**
Chief complaint and history of present problem	Major areas of concern and beliefs about root cause of problem First awareness of problem and previous evaluations and results Medication history for behavioral, emotional, or learning problems
Birth history	Prenatal history: maternal illnesses; medications, recreational drugs, alcohol, and tobacco use during pregnancy Birth and postpartum complications, prematurity, low birth weight or intrauterine growth retardation, anoxia, difficult delivery, birth defects Neonatal behavior: feeding, sleep, temperament problems
Family and environmental history	ADHD, neurologic problems, learning difficulties Mental health history of first- and second-degree family members, behavior problems in other family members Genetic disorders: cognitive disorders, growth disorders, neurofibromatosis Drug or alcohol abuse (current and/or past), involvement with law enforcement, weapons in the home
Medical history	Chronic diseases, current medication use, environmental allergies Hospitalizations, prolonged illness Trauma history (head injury, frequent injuries) Poisoning, lead, or environmental exposures Neurologic status, seizures, tics, uncontrolled twitches Cardiovascular history including personal and family history of cardiovascular disease, sudden cardiac death, and arrythmia
Developmental history	Milestones: motor, personal/social, language, cognitive Strengths (e.g., personality, activities, friendliness) and weaknesses
Behavioral history	Frequency with which child complies when told to do something Methods used at home to improve behavior and effectiveness Parenting skills and style, cultural beliefs, and agreement about child management Counseling history for child or family (or both)
ADHD history	Attention: paying attention, sustaining attention, listening, following through, organization, reluctant to engage in activities that need sustained attention, hyperfocusing on activities of interest, loses things, forgetful, ability to follow three or four step commands Activity: fidgets, leaves seat, runs or climbs when inappropriate, has difficulty with quiet games, talks excessively, has problems waiting turn, interrupts, "on the go"
Academic history	Child's progress at each grade level (strengths seen) Adjustment problems at school, child's history with peers, friendships Difficulties with specific skills: reading, writing, spelling, math, concepts Performance problems: attention, grades, participation, excessive talking, disturbing others, fighting, bullying, teasing, abusive language, not completing work School assistance: tutoring, counseling, special help
Activities of Daily Living	
Feeding	Ability to sit through a complete meal, messy and clumsy with utensils, dishes, and glasses Inadequate caloric intake can be result of symptoms
Elimination	Enuresis, encopresis
Sleeping	Difficulty falling asleep, night waking, needs less sleep than other family members Complains about fatigue interfering with completion of tasks
Activity	Amount and activity or exercise Amount and details of screen time
Family relationships	General family relationships (child and parents/siblings) Home, day care, and school environments Births, deaths, marriage, and family transitions, recent moves; parental deployment, separation, divorce, remarriage Violence: domestic, current, or past abuse of parent or child; problems with the law; weapons in the home Inadequate social and relational skills: lies, steals, plays with fire, hurts animals, is aggressive with other children, talks back to adults
Mental health, coping, and stress tolerance	Difficulty maintaining routines Struggles with self-concept and low self-esteem Family stress (e.g., parent job loss or change, financial problems) and coping patterns Outbursts of temper, low tolerance for frustration Moody, worried, sad, quiet, destructive, fearful, or fearless, self-deprecating Somatic complaints
School & teacher history	Level of performance (below potential for achievement) Tends to miss the point of conversations and activities Often does things the hard way in absence of established routines Information from school about child's strengths, weaknesses, difficulties, academic management of issues

ADHD, Attention-deficit/hyperactivity disorder.

- General—dysmorphic stigmata suggestive of genetic syndrome or prenatal exposure to drugs or alcohol
- Skin—café-au-lait spots; signs of abuse
- Ear, nose, and throat (ENT)—signs of past recurring otitis media (scarring of tympanic membranes), signs of respiratory allergies, enlarged tonsils, sleep apnea
- Cardiovascular—heart sounds and rhythm, murmur, pulses
- Neurologic—general screening examination—mental status, speech and language, motor skills, and general cognition and mental process as appropriate for age
- Screening for iron deficiency, lead, and thyroid dysfunction, if indicated
- Obtain individual and family history of cardiovascular disease including conduction disorders like Wolff-Parkinson-White syndrome and long QT syndrome

Scales and Diagnostic Tools, Differential Diagnosis, and Comorbidities

Use of ADHD-specific behavior rating scales provides the most objective data to assess the scope and severity of the symptoms and is useful to monitor change once treatment begins. Several different behavioral scales evaluate ADHD symptoms, and some also screen for executive function and comorbidities. Common screeners include the Vanderbilt ADHD Scales, the ADHD Rating Scale IV, Conner Parent and Teacher Rating Scales, and the Child Attention Profile. All can be found online, some at no charge. Consistent use of one scale is recommended to become familiar with the scoring and interpretation. Scales should be completed independently by individuals who know the youth; obtain assessments from at least two different domains (e.g., home, school, and daycare). As children get older, obtain information from teachers who work with the student; this information provides valuable insight into symptom variation at different hours of the day and clues about learning difficulties.

Management

Diagnosis and Initial Meeting With Families. Once the PCP collects all data from the history and physical examination, behavioral rating scales from various domains, and any other evaluations (school reports, psychoeducational testing, mental health assessment), it is important to assess the onset, duration, the settings where impairment is present, and the nature and degree of symptoms and functional impairment. Use clinical judgment to determine the effect of symptoms on academic achievement and classroom performance; family, peer, and authority relationships; sports and recreation participation; and behavioral and emotional regulation with thoughtful consideration of the possibility of coexisting conditions. Compare these data to the diagnostic criteria to identify if ADHD is present and which subtype best describes the symptoms.

It is imperative to set aside sufficient time to discuss the findings in detail with the family. This discussion should be comprehensive and strengths-based to help the parents understand their child's attentional difficulties as part of an inclusive picture of their functioning. Families may need education about developmental concerns, academic performance issues, learning disabilities, medical diagnoses, social concerns, family issues and stressors, and associated coexisting mental health diagnoses. For children not meeting the criteria for ADHD who do not have another condition identified, it is equally important to meet with their families to review findings and establish a plan that

includes close monitoring and further evaluation of learning or behavior problems.

It is imperative for PCPs to identify the child's and family's strengths and to build on those during the entire diagnostic and treatment process. It is worthwhile to share the perspective that, although some of these traits are a problem in childhood, the high energy, creativity, humor, and flexibility in ideation can actually lead to a successful career—note some of the very famous and successful people with ADHD (e.g., Albert Einstein, Bill Gates, Michael Phelps, and Walt Disney). The hyperfocus that comes with ADHD can actually be a "superpower" of sorts, and once tapped into can help the individual be highly successful in their field of choice.

PCPs are care coordinators to help facilitate strong family-school partnerships. Care plans should focus on the areas of the youth's functional impairment: academic achievement; relationships—parent, peer, sibling, and adult authority; social skills—sports and recreational participation; and behavior and emotional regulation. A key element is having three specific, measurable short-term target goals at a time from the areas that are most impaired, incorporating the child's strengths and resiliency (Box 29.2).

Family Education and Support. Education focuses on parent-child management techniques. The chronic nature of ADHD affects family functioning and treatment compliance. Parents often must educate others: family, other parents, teachers, coaches and caregivers about their child's special needs. Likewise, education of the child or adolescent is critical. Providers should have several resources available that they are familiar with and feel comfortable about recommending to families.

It is necessary to help parents understand the diagnosis complexity, to deal with feelings of shock, confusion, or guilt, if present. The diagnosis of a child is often the first clue to the eventual diagnosis of a sibling or parent who has similar difficulties. ADHD symptoms impact the already complex relationships within a family, so ongoing support is important. As a culture, we value attention and impulse control with educational standards centered on these values. Perceptions about parenting and childrearing, beliefs about medication and the healthcare system in general, family, and social networking roles in managing child behavior problems, and parents' own experiences with school are all factors that shape the approach to seeking care, diagnosis, and treatment. Families may have differing understanding of what constitutes a behavior problem. Providers should be open and honest in the discussion of diagnoses and all treatment options and include key family members in collaborative decision-making, striving to become more aware of the community and the patient's cultural values.

Children with ADHD often struggle with self-esteem as they attempt to meet expectations placed on them. It is crucial to identify their areas of strength and promote mental health to develop those areas rather than constantly focusing on remediating areas of weakness (see Chapter 6). Help parents focus on the many positive attributes, sometimes called "superpowers," of ADHD: being innovators, dreamers, creative thinkers and problems solvers, highly sensitive, humorous, doers, risk takers, and persistent.

Behavior Management, Parent Skills Training, and Counseling. Behavior management modifies behavior and physical and social environments and is effective in decreasing core ADHD symptoms. Behavior management alone should be used if the child is younger than 6 years, symptoms are mild, or if the patient has ADHD symptoms but does not meet full DSM criteria. Medication paired with behavior management is used

---

• BOX 29.2 **Potential Goals for Family Support for Youth With ADHD**

Family Support

- *Routines, rules, and family relationships* are key. Home should be a safe place where one feels valued. Life with ADHD is stressful for the youth and family, and keeping family ties strong helps ease the stress.
- *Family meetings* provide opportunity to discuss structure, rewards, and consequences, and plan and problem solve to keep communication lines open.
- *Support and advocacy groups* help manage daily problems that come from living with ADHD.
- *Family therapy or counseling* is used short term to aid with specific family situational goals. It is especially helpful if there is aggressive behavior or problems related to anxiety, self-esteem, and depression or if other family members (especially siblings) need psychological assessment or support.
- *"Coaching"* helps a youth develop difficult skills. It helps with problem solving, time management, organizational skills, and learning strategies (how to be an active learner, learning to learn, and learning how to organize learning).

Home Management

- *Environmental management:* A calm, predictable home with clear, consistent morning and evening routines is extremely helpful for the child with ADHD. Providing an organized place for everyday things to go is another way to provide structure.
- *Homework support* is essential (see Box 29.4). Monitor for mental fatigue.
- *Exercise:* Aerobic exercise improves clinical, cognitive, and scholastic performance because it increases dopamine, serotonin, and norepinephrine levels. Scheduling daily time to be active and expend energy, especially before school, helps children with ADHD stay regulated. Martial arts and other sports that demand discipline and self-control are useful.
- *Downtime or senseless fun:* Children with ADHD need more time for typical childhood activities, including downtime and time to daydream.

Time in less-structured activities improves self-directed executive function.

- *Technology:* Many children with ADHD love computers, smartphones, and tablets; they produce neat results, never criticize, offer second and third chances, help with spelling and organization, and provide novel stimulation and opportunities for relaxation. Keep an open mind to their use but ensure they are not used to the point of social isolation.
- *Nutrition:* Regular mealtimes with healthy portion sizes provides necessary energy. Small meals with the morning dose of stimulant medication can decrease stomachaches. Instant breakfast drinks and other high-calorie foods supplement calories when the child has low caloric intake because of difficulty sitting through meals or side effects of medications.
- *Sleep:* Many youth with ADHD have trouble falling or staying asleep and do not require as much sleep as other people. It is important to ask if the child is sleeping well and staying in bed the entire night. Ritualized bedtime routines are important including massage, deep breathing, and relaxation techniques. Melatonin (1–6 mg/day) or an antihistamine may be helpful; however, long-term use of these agents is not recommended.
- *Patience, unconditional love, and support* are especially important for individuals with ADHD because they face challenges throughout their day. Plan a daily "time in" for 15 to 20 minutes with undivided parent attention focused on a child-selected activity.
- Complementary treatments may have some benefit.

Friends and Activities

- *Areas of strength* should be developed (music, sports, computer) rather than always focusing on areas of weakness. Camps, clubs, and appropriate work provide avenues for development of skills and new friendships.
- *Activities* of the child's choosing in areas of strength or developmentally appropriate work help build peer relationships and self-esteem.
- *Friendships* may come easier with provided structure (going to a movie or a sporting event) within a time frame the child can handle.
- *Musical training* develops and maintains certain executive functioning skills helpful to children with ADHD.

ADHD, Attention-deficit/hyperactivity disorder.

---

when there is a poor response to medication alone, there are psychosocial stressors or coexisting conditions, or when the parents desire it. Children and adolescents who receive both medication and behavior management show greater parent and teacher satisfaction and lower medication dosages than those receiving monotherapy.

Calm parenting is very successful with an ADHD child; it is a combination of positive parenting with the addition of the essential component of deepening the bond between parent and child. Strategies are: staying cool, "Do you realize…?" instead of reacting and becoming frustrated; looking for the parent role in the issue; knowing how the child is hardwired and differentiating between what is a core ADHD symptom and what is truly rebellion; and remembering to play and connect. Parenting programs can help caregivers set up rewards and reinforcers for positive behavior, give clear and effective commands and structure, and establish safe and consistent discipline strategies. The goal of parent skills training is for parents to learn ways to optimize their child's success by giving the child direction, setting goals and limits to improve compliance, increasing self-esteem, enhancing the parent-child relationship, and reducing struggles in the home. Three essential components include: (1) increasing positive parent-child interactions, (2) practicing different scenarios with the child, and (3)

learning time-out/disciplinary consistency. If parents disagree about management or do not get along, this approach is not likely to work.

Therapy can help parents learn to parent effectively, foster improved communication, and help children learn self-regulation skills. As a child with ADHD approaches middle school, high school, and college age and the child assumes more responsibility for their school and schedule, new approaches are needed. These may be times of strain for the family, and counseling may be needed.

Educational and Adaptive Supports. It is essential for the PCP to work with the family and the school to set reasonable expectations and help develop a plan for the child to be successful in school. The PCP can provide information on the common features of ADHD and how they relate to the child's previous and current school problems, give expectations for the patient's clinical course, and suggestions for intervention strategies. For the child, a developmentally appropriate explanation and demystification of ADHD are essential knowing how attention works and identifying their own strengths and attributes, as well as the areas of weakness that need support. It is particularly important to have a good match between teacher and student. Communication with the school personnel is imperative to provide specific teacher-focused information about diagnosis and difficulties in all identified areas and to address appropriate intervention strategies and modifications. Many teachers are familiar with ADHD and many schools have behavior management programs or interventions to enhance academic and social functioning. Most children benefit from either a 504 plan with accommodations or an Individualized Education Program (IEP) for academic learning or behavior (see Chapter 6 and Box 29.3).

Classroom behavior management helps improve attention in the classroom, increases productivity, and decreases disruptive behavior. Common techniques include increased structure and behavior contracts with goals and positive reinforcement; using a token economy (earning or losing points that can be exchanged for privileges or items); creating a periodic behavior report card (e.g., daily or weekly progress notes); and/or study or organizational skills training. Other considerations are brain/energy breaks (a set time to stretch, get up, and walk around), secret signals to indicate need for a break, and allowing them opportunities to move (fidget toys, standing, or pacing while working). Peer intervention strategies, either in groups or in pairs, help reduce inappropriate or disruptive behaviors.

Adaptive technology (AT) assists individuals with ADHD and should be included in any 504 or IEP. Examples of AT that are readily available include: voice-activated and word prediction software to help with writing papers, note-taking pens that download into a computer, visual thinking tools, electronic organizers, cell phones or tablets with timers and reminders, and a multitude of apps.

Homework is often a challenge for parents who want their children to do well and children who have trouble focusing after a long day at school. Helping parents plan a home routine is essential (Box 29.4). Children with ADHD often work best in nontraditional study areas—sitting in places other than a table and chair or while moving (see Chapter 6 for sensory techniques). Parents should monitor assigned homework and how the child manages it, communicating with teachers if modifications are needed. The PCP should recognize homework struggles may also be symptoms of a learning disability and may need further evaluation. While important to give time off during summer and other breaks, it is essential to structure plans to provide stress-free activities and hands-on learning.

Pharmacologic Management. Medications effectively reduce core symptoms and are recommended for children who meet the

---

• BOX 29.3 Classroom Accommodation Suggestions for Children With Attention-Deficit/Hyperactivity Disorder

Memory and Attention
- Seat the child close to the teacher away from heavy traffic areas (e.g., doorways).
- Keep oral instructions brief and provide repetitions; avoid multiple commands.
- Provide written directions—broken down or simplified, if needed.
- "Walk" the child through assignments to ensure they are understood.
- Break tasks and homework into small tasks.
- Use visual aids, hands-on, and experiential teaching methods rather than strict lecture style.
- Teach active reading with underlining and active listening with note taking.
- Provide remedial help in small sessions.
- Teach subvocalization (saying words in your head while reading) to aid memorizing.
- Establish a signal that reminds the child to focus and return to task.
- Allow nondistracting motor activity during tasks requiring concentration (e.g., squeezing a ball, using popping toys, or fingering Velcro to replace pencil tapping).
- Allow earplugs if they have auditory processing sensitivities.

Impulse Control
- Allow for freedom of movement as much as possible (e.g., classroom helper).
- Never punish the child by taking away physical education, recess, or other physical activity outlets.
- Teach the child to review quality of work before turning it in.

Classroom Atmosphere
- Provide a structured classroom with clear expectations.
- Use moderate, consistent discipline.
- Rely on positive reinforcement for good behavior.
- Provide a quiet place to work in the classroom (headsets with select music may block out distractions).

Organizational Skills
- Establish a daily checklist of tasks.
- Use a daily planner. List homework assignments with due dates and needed resources.
- Divide notebook into three sections: work to be completed, work completed, and work to save.
- Color code class material to help organize.
- Follow up on homework not turned in.
- Allow extra time to gather necessary items, pack backpack, etc.
- Consider using an e-book that can be accessed at multiple locations or obtain an extra set of textbooks for use at home.
- Teach strategies for time management and basic study skills.
- Develop planning skills.

Productivity Problems
- Divide tasks into manageable sections that allow for breaks.
- Reduce the amount of homework and written classwork.
- Modify the number of math problems to be completed.
- Request test modifications—quiet location and extra time.
- Use assistive technology—dictation software, calculator, audio books, and note-taker pen.

Written Expression
- Give extra time to complete written tests and assignments.
- Provide help with handwriting.
- Allow child to dictate reports and take tests orally.
- Reduce the quantity of written work required.
- Grade papers on content rather than untidy work, spelling errors, or poor handwriting.

Self-Esteem
- Celebrate progress.
- Encourage performance in areas of child's strength.
- Use positive reinforcement and avoid public behavior correction.
- Give hand signals only the child can see as private reminders of appropriate behavior.

Social Relationships
- Provide feedback about behavior involving other children.
- Make sure other children do not believe that the child is doing less or is allowed unacceptable behavior; change the rules for all children if necessary.

• BOX 29.4 **Tips for Home-Based Homework Support**

- Provide a quiet location to work with minimal distractions. Consider using white noise of soft instrumental music in the background. Set up a workstation equipped with necessary materials.
- Establish a homework time as early as possible to prevent the child from being too tired but allow a break after school.
- Establish a homework plan: review assignments and make a schedule for completion, breaking tasks into small, manageable pieces.
- Help the child get started. Monitor without taking over. Praise effort; do not insist on perfection.
- Use a timer to help with time management. Structure time for breaks as often as every 15 minutes, if needed. Encourage movement during breaks.
- Permit time for editing so the child does not lose points due to simple errors. Help to study for tests.
- Provide incentives to help motivation.
- Identify another student to contact for clarification.

ADHD diagnostic criteria. Medication alone is usually not as effective as medication combined with behavior therapy. Stimulants are the most effective medications and are considered the cornerstone for ADHD management, but nonstimulants (selective norepinephrine-reuptake inhibitors and α_2-adrenergic agonists) are also efficacious. Medication selection depends on the patient's age, how long and when symptoms occur, comorbid conditions, and insurance coverage. Clinicians can readily find information about medications from online sources and prescribing guides; however, one of the most up-to-date sources is the ADHD Medication Guide available at http://adhdmedicationguide.com. This source includes information about all medications currently available in the United States including dosing, medication formulations, and color photos of all brand name preparations. The PCP should focus on finding the medication and dosage that best fits the patients' needs.

Stimulants. The first-line medications for uncomplicated ADHD treatment are the stimulants, methylphenidate and amphetamine compounds.[25] Both are equally effective but the most common side effects of insomnia and anorexia are more common with amphetamines. Stimulants work by increasing the availability of dopamine and norepinephrine at the neuron synapses by blocking their reuptake in key areas of the brain. This action is theorized to allow the child to exhibit more purposeful, goal-oriented behavior by focusing attention, lessening impulsiveness, and decreasing motor activity. Between 70% and 90% of children respond positively to stimulant medications (approximately 40% respond to methylphenidate and 40% respond to amphetamines) although there is no predictor for which one will work best.[25] If a patient is a nonresponder to the highest tolerated dose of one stimulant group, then it is appropriate to try another stimulant in the same class or try one from the different class. Start stimulants at low doses and watch for common and rare side effects, titrating up to minimize core ADHD symptoms with minimal adverse effects. Individuals with inattentive symptoms often respond well to lower doses, whereas children with hyperactive symptoms often require moderate to high doses. In general, the long-acting forms are preferred because no midday school dosing is required, thus providing smoother coverage, greater convenience, improved compliance, and less stigma. Short-acting medications are often selected for initial dosing, for third (afternoon) doses, for dosage

titration, or if patients have significant withdrawal symptoms from long-acting formulations.

When working with the adolescent, it is important to assess for substance abuse and, if identified, refer for treatment before prescribing stimulants. If no risk is detected but there are concerns about stimulant diversion (e.g., selling the drug to other students) and abuse, methylphenidate is the preferred stimulant but lisdexamfetamine and dermal preparations should be considered as they are less likely to result in diversion.[26] Alternatively, many clinicians elect to use a nonstimulant drug in these circumstances. It is important to focus on the patient's substance abuse first, and then focus on the ADHD. Failure to treat ADHD symptoms can result in anxiety, academic failure, and social difficulties, each of which can be triggers for substance abuse.

Preschoolers, those 4 to 5 years old, need special consideration and care when symptoms and behaviors of ADHD are present. It is important to remember that inattention, hyperactivity, and impulsivity are developmentally typical in this age group; therefore ADHD represents a *developmentally excessive* presentation. As a result, diagnosis must include evaluation of information from at least two teachers or community sources.[25] PCPs must always be aware that ADHD symptoms in preschoolers are often related to other conditions such as language disorders, hearing loss, intellectual disorders, genetic disorders, ASD, or another psychopathology. Behavioral therapy, especially classroom interventions and parent training, is the recommended first line of treatment. However, medication can be considered for a child with moderate to severe dysfunction, who has at least 9 months of symptoms, with dysfunction in more than one domain (e.g., home, daycare, preschool), and/or who has an inadequate response to behavioral therapy. Adderall is the only FDA-approved stimulant for children as young as 3 years old; however, the current clinical practice guidelines state this medication should be avoided in children under 6 years old.[25] Methylphenidate is the first-line medication to be considered if behavioral interventions are not sufficient to help the 4- to 5-year-old; atomoxetine and clonidine may also be considered. Use caution to start at the lowest doses possible and although there are multiple liquid and chewable formulations commercially produced, they are often difficult to find in local pharmacies and not covered by insurance.

When dosing stimulants, it is important to remember that:
- Dose response is unique to each individual and should be adjusted for age, body weight, degree of impairment, and specific symptoms
- Begin dosing at the low end and titrate up every 1 to 3 weeks while monitoring for symptom improvement and side effects
- Approximately one-third of individuals achieve best clinical response at the low dose, one-third at mid-dose range, and one-third require the higher doses
- The dosing goal is maximum reduction of ADHD core symptoms with minimal side effects
- Change to a different medication, the other stimulant group, or a nonstimulant medication if the child is at the maximum dose without adequate response or is having significant side effects
- Instruct families to monitor for benefit and adverse effects
When a change in medication is needed, consider the following:
- An amphetamine is approximately 1.5 times as potent as methylphenidate
- Stimulant medications increase heart rates by an average 1 to 2 beats per minute and increase blood pressure an average of

4 mm Hg systolic and diastolic, they may also worsen underlying arrythmias[25]

- Simulants are associated with decreased growth velocity, especially in the first 3 years of treatment. Average height difference at end of puberty is 3 to 4 cm.[25]

Common adverse effects of the stimulants include decreased appetite, weight loss, insomnia, stomachache, and headache. Adjustments to the medication administration time and the relationship to food intake sometimes alleviate side effects. With time, these symptoms often resolve but must be monitored. If they persist, decreasing the dose or switching the medication may help. Emotional lability and irritability, especially if persistent and not just the result of the medication wearing off, can indicate the need to adjust the dose, change the medication, or revisit the diagnosis. Contraindications to stimulants include psychosis, unstable cardiovascular disease, underlying arrythmia, or any previous untoward reactions to stimulant medication. Transdermal patches may cause skin irritation where the patch is applied; this may improve by alternating sites, using good skin care, and liberal skin moisturization. Topical steroid may help irritation or itching, although caution should be used if applying under the patch as it may cause increased skin absorption.

The FDA issued a black box warning linking stimulant use with an increased risk, although extremely rare risk, of sudden cardiac death in adolescents. Subsequent research demonstrates that pediatric patients on stimulants have the same sudden cardiac death rates as their peers who do not use stimulants.[25] Any patient with an individual or family history of sudden cardiac death, specific cardiac symptoms, Wolff-Parkinson-White syndrome, long QT syndrome, or any signs of active cardiovascular disease should have additional evaluation to determine the risk of using atomoxetine or stimulants to treat their ADHD.[25] Cardiovascular screening includes (1) assessing for a cardiac history of shortness of breath with exercise, exercise intolerance, fainting or seizures with exercise, palpitations, elevated blood pressure, previously detected cardiac abnormalities, rheumatic fever, cardiomyopathy, and/or dysrhythmia; (2) a family cardiac history of sudden unexplained or cardiac death before age 50 years, or any familial rate, rhythm, or structural cardiac problems; and (3) performing a complete physical examination paying special attention to the cardiovascular system. If the cardiac history and examination are negative, no further tests are recommended before starting ADHD medication. If there are any positive findings in the history or examination, a consultation with a pediatric cardiologist is necessary before initiating medication.[25]

Approximately 20% of all children develop tics, although often these are mild and simple in complexity and typically resolve within a year. Up to 20% of children with ADHD develop a chronic tic disorder, and over half of children with Tourette syndrome or chronic tic disorder have coexisting ADHD (see earlier discussion of tics). Typically, ADHD symptoms emerge before tic onset. The FDA issued a contraindication for methylphenidate and a warning for amphetamine in patients with preexisting tic disorders or those with a family history of Tourette syndrome; however, stimulants are unlikely to evoke or exacerbate tics and may improve tic symptoms and reduce oppositional behaviors. Stimulants may exacerbate anxiety disorders. Options for children with tics include low-dose, short- or long-acting stimulants, α-agonists, or nonstimulants. If tics emerge on ADHD medication, are not severe or disturbing to the child or adolescent, and the medication is beneficial, it is acceptable to continue stimulant treatment.

Nonstimulant Medications. There are two nonstimulants with specific FDA approval for use in ADHD treatment: viloxazine and atomoxetine. Atomoxetine is a noncontrolled, norepinephrine reuptake inhibitor, nonstimulant medication approved for ADHD for children older than age 6 years. Unlike the stimulants, it may take up to 6 weeks of regular use before effects are noted. It should be given with food and is usually dosed once a day, but it can be given twice daily. Although it is not as effective as the stimulants, atomoxetine may be a preferable first choice if the family prefers a nonstimulant medication, a substance abuse concern exists in the family, or the child has significant side effects with the stimulants including tics, anxiety, or sleep initiation difficulties. It provides 24-hour coverage, but it must not be discontinued abruptly. Common adverse effects of atomoxetine include decreased appetite, gastrointestinal complaints (nausea, anorexia), somnolence and dizziness, and mild hypertension or tachycardia. Most side effects resolve with time—headaches are the most likely to persist—and can be managed with dose reduction or medication change. There are a few reports of liver toxicity in patients taking atomoxetine. Viloxazine (Qelbree) is a selective norepinephrine reuptake inhibitor, nonstimulant medication approved for use in children age 6 years and older. It has a side effect profile like atomoxetine and also takes up to 6 weeks for a therapeutic effect. Common side effects include increased heart rate, increased blood pressure, somnolence, headache, dizziness, nausea, and anorexia. There is no need to do liver studies before treatment with either medication; however, if evidence of jaundice or elevated liver function is found, stop the medication. Caution patients to report dark urine, flu-like illness, fatigue, abdominal pain, or nausea. Increased risk of suicidal ideation or attempts may occur in children and adolescents being treated with atomoxetine or viloxazine. Although the risk is small, parents and patients should be advised that if there is any change in mood—depression, mood lability, agitation, suicidal thoughts, or gestures—they must get care immediately. Preexisting and development of suicidal thoughts, hallucinations, psychosis, or mania are absolute contraindications, and these children need referral to a qualified behavioral health clinician. Finally, because of the possibility of clinically significant increased blood pressure or heart rate (e.g., a 15–20 mm Hg blood pressure rise or 20 beats/min pulse increase), neither medication should be used in those individuals with tachyarrhythmias or hypertension.

Extended-release guanfacine (Intuniv) and extended-release clonidine (Kapvay) are α-agonists approved for ADHD treatment in children age 6 years and older, although their efficacy is not as strong as with the other medications. They are traditionally used as adjunctive therapy not as monotherapy. Guanfacine improves oppositional symptoms in addition to ADHD core symptoms, especially impulsivity. Clonidine helps children with sleep and decreases impulsivity and aggression. These medications do not worsen tics, are typically not abused, and may help children with trouble sleeping or CD symptoms. It takes 1 to 2 weeks to appreciate any effect. Both are FDA approved as adjunctive therapy to stimulant medications and provide additional symptom reduction. A cardiovascular history and full physical examination are recommended before initiating these medications. The most common adverse effects include sedation, bradycardia, and abdominal pain. With guanfacine, these effects tend to resolve over time. Monitoring blood pressure and heart rate is important, but medications should not be discontinued unless the child becomes symptomatic (e.g., hypotensive or bradycardic). Instruct the family not to abruptly discontinue the medication because of the possibility of rebound hypertension.

Complementary Therapies. Outdoor exercise, aerobic exercise, adequate sleep, and good nutrition are key. Ensure a healthy diet with high-quality macronutrients—protein, fats, and carbohydrates. A clean, uncluttered environment and learning to manage stress are helpful. Mindfulness and yoga can help teach youth to tune out distractions and hone focus. Only prescribe zinc and iron in patients with a proven deficiency. Omega-3 fatty acids are used widely but there are limited data to support their use. A recent systematic review of herbal preparation effectiveness in ADHD treatment was consistent with prior reviews and showed no evidence for the effectiveness of Gingko biloba, St. John's wort, pine bark extract, *Valeriana officinalis,* and *Melissa officinalis.*[27] In early 2019 the FDA approved a trigeminal nerve stimulator to treat nonmedicated children with ADHD. Evidence for this approach is limited to a small study of 62 children.[28]

Follow-up and Referral

Regular child and family follow-up includes reassessment of core symptoms, functioning, and target goals; medication regimen review; education; care coordination and advocacy; and assessment of family functioning and need for family support or other resources (Box 29.5). Refer to behavioral health specialists as needed if there is a poor medication response, more than two failed medication trials, or emergent comorbidities. At times, transitions are overwhelming and referral to behavioral health for coping skills training may be helpful.

As the child matures, so does the brain, and symptomatology and coexisting conditions may change. PCPs must be attuned to these changes and provide anticipatory guidance and modify treatment plans as needed. Empowering children/adolescents to understand and comanage their condition and impairments is essential. Include management strategies, clarifying that ADHD is not a lack of intelligence, and help them build on strengths. Equip parents with proactive strategies for the home and for dealing with transitions to middle school, high school, and college or vocational studies. Families are often under stress because of the ongoing challenges and helping them learn how to cope with the stress or access behavioral health services is important. As the child nears the end of adolescence, plan for transition to adult care. Got Transition (www.gottransition.org) is a model developed to guide this practice.

When initiating medication treatment and any time there is a dose or medication change, the PCP should meet with the family to assess the effectiveness within 2 to 3 weeks of the change and monthly until the patient and the regimen are stable. It is important to note that sometimes a medication change from brand name to generic may result in symptom changes. Regular reassessment of the child's core symptoms and functioning should occur every 3 to 6 months if stable. In addition to assessing medication effectiveness, it is important to comprehensively look at the child's functioning in school, at home, at work, with peers, and in activities. Assess family functioning, including the reasonableness of parental expectations with a focus on areas where additional resources or support is needed. The Vanderbilt Scale has a follow-up version for parents and teachers that collects information about the core ADHD symptoms, level of impairment, potential side effects, and comorbid symptoms. Often families think things are going well when they may actually benefit from modifications or other support. Monitor height, weight, blood pressure, sleep,

> ## • BOX 29.5 Questions to Consider When Developing the Plan of Care for a Child/Adolescent With Attention-Deficit Hyperactivity Disorder
>
> - Does the family understand ADHD symptoms and the specific symptoms being targeted and the presence of coexisting conditions?
> - What support does the family need to set, measure, and monitor treatment goals?
> - Does the care plan address the family's care goals?
> - Does the family understand how to use behavior management techniques to respond to tantrums, oppositional behavior, or when their child does not respond to requests and commands?
> - Do they need help normalizing peer and family relationships?
> - Does the child/adolescent need help in academic areas? If so, obtain a formal evaluation and review it to distinguish work production problems secondary to ADHD from those caused by coexisting learning or language disabilities.
> - Does the child/adolescent need help becoming independent with self-care or schoolwork?
> - Does the child/adolescent or family need help with organizing, planning, or managing schoolwork?
> - Does the family need help recognizing, understanding, or managing coexisting conditions?
> - Is there a plan in place to educate the child/adolescent about ADHD and its treatment, and help the patient to understand their own strengths and weaknesses?
> - Is there an education plan in place to assist the child/adolescent to increase his or her adherence to treatments? Was the plan initiated as early as possible and is it attuned to the child's/adolescent's developmental level?
> - Does the family have a copy of the care plan? Can it be updated and used in school and other settings to allow for seamless implementation of the treatment plan?
> - Is the treatment plan family-centered and culturally grounded?
> - Are there any additional referrals or support needed?
> - How does the care plan take into consideration the complex care needs that are part of the transition of care from pediatric to adult health care? How is the patient included in this care transition?
>
> *ADHD,* Attention-deficit hyperactivity disorder.
> Modified from American Academy of Pediatrics (AAP). Supplemental Information: Implementing the Key Action Statements of the AAP ADHD Clinical Practice Guidelines: An Algorithm and Explanation for Process of Care For the Evaluation, Diagnosis, Treatment, and Monitoring of ADHD in Children and Adolescents. https://publications.aap.org/pediatrics/article/144/4/e20192528/81590/Clinical-Practice-Guideline-for-the-Diagnosis?autologincheck=redirected.

appetite, and significant symptom development such as aggression or tics. Perform an abbreviated physical examination with a focus on the cardiac system. Medication modification may include dose adjustment, a change in the dosage timing, or adding an adjunctive medication.

Many of the medication side effects can be minimized by having children and adolescents eat a healthy meal before taking their medication, ensuring medications are taken by 9 AM, taking the medication with food, or eating soon after the dose. Assess and advise about sleep hygiene. Some children taking stimulants experience "rebound" moodiness as the medication wears off, often in the afternoon after school. These symptoms can be treated by giving the child a low dose of the same stimulant in immediate release formulation in the afternoon, usually at one-third to one-half the morning dose. A trial without medications may be considered if the child is stable and doing well. It is best done at a time when there will be few transitions (i.e., not the first year of middle or high school), and not at the beginning of the school year, or during the junior or senior year of high school. If there is a decision to discontinue medication, there should be close follow-up during the first 4 weeks.

Specific Learning Disorders

Definition and Diagnostic Criteria

The DSM-5TR defines specific learning disorder (SLD) as a biological neurodevelopmental disorder that causes significant and persistent learning and academic skills acquisition difficulties that present in the early years of formal education, lasting for at least 6 months, are not attributed to an intellectual developmental disorder, external factors such as economic or environmental disadvantage, vision or hearing problems, neurological condition, or motor disorders.[1] SLD is classified as mild, moderate, or severe and results in reading, written expression, or math involvement. Key skills impacted include reading single words, reading comprehension, writing, spelling, math calculation, and math problem solving. Reading difficulties include reading rate or fluency, reading accuracy and comprehension, and foreign language. *Dyslexia* refers to difficulties with word recognition, decoding, and spelling. Difficulties in writing include spelling, punctuation, grammar, organization, and clarity of written expression. *Dysgraphia* describes difficulty with handwriting (forming letters, writing within a defined space). Math difficulties include number sense, memorizing math facts, math calculations or math reasoning, and problem solving. *Dyscalculia* describes difficulties with learning math facts and performing calculations, including making change in cash transactions. In addition to the educational difficulties, children and adolescents with learning disorders often have social and language deficits that may be present before their educational problems are evident.

It is not clear what causes learning disorders, but problems are often present from birth, and known risk factors include genetics, toxin or substance exposure, and ACEs.[29] Dyslexia, the most common SLD, includes structural brain differences in the language area. SLD affects 5% to 15% of school-aged children and is more common in males.[1] Issues with learning and attention affect one in every five children in the United States; about one-third have both disorders. SLDs affect children from all socioeconomic, racial, and ethnic groups, but are less common in upper-income children and children who are not of color. One in 16 public school students have an IEP for SLD (ADHD or dyspraxia, a motor disorder that results in poor coordination); one in 50 have accommodations through a 504 plan.[29] It is important to remember that SLDs can occur in individuals with high intelligence or "gifted" youth. This may complicate diagnosis as these youth compensate for their difficulties learning in one domain with their abilities in other areas and this may delay recognition of their condition until later in their education when more complex skills and timed learning environments exceed their capacity to overcome the SLD.[1]

Coexisting neurodevelopmental (e.g., ADHD) issues are not uncommon, and social, emotional, and behavioral challenges may result in lower academic achievement, school distress (avoidance, disengagement, or alienation), school failure (retention, expulsion, and dropping out), lower self-esteem, conduct issues, aggression, oppositionality, anxiety, and depression.[30]

Other comorbidities include chronic health problems such as fetal alcohol syndrome disorder, lead or other toxic exposure, and fragile X syndrome.

Clinical Findings and Assessment

Diagnosis with SLD cannot occur until the elementary school years but symptoms may be present during early childhood. Children with SLD have test scores and grades significantly below what is expected given cognitive ability. In early childhood, delays in attention, language, or motor skills may emerge. Preschoolers may demonstrate difficulty with repetition games, trouble learning common rhyming stories, have delayed speech acquisition, show difficulty learning their letters or numbers, or learning to recognize their own spelled name.[1] Early school-aged children may not be able to write letters, have trouble breaking words into syllables, or recognizing rhyming words. Later elementary school aged children may have difficulty connecting letters with sounds, read slowly and inaccurately, and have trouble with spelling or math facts. Adolescents may have delayed reading, poor language comprehension, difficulty solving complex math problems, or challenges with tasks involving spatial relations. As children age, they may become aware of their learning differences and demonstrate behaviors including reluctance to engage in learning (e.g., "it's boring") or oppositional behavior.

Screening and Specialty Referral for Diagnosis

Screening for SLD starts with routine developmental surveillance that includes monitoring for school performance and attendance. It helps to ask children and adolescents about what is going well and what is challenging. The Level I school performance prescreening questionnaire (Box 29.6) is a five-item instrument that can be administered at every well-child check. If school problems are suspected, a Level II school performance screener (see Box 29.6) provides a more comprehensive assessment of the child's academic performance, along with samples of schoolwork, report cards, and previously administered tests. The National Center for Learning Disabilities has a free Learning Disabilities Checklist (www.ncld.org/), organized by skill set and age group. If delays are suspected, it is extremely important to get the child evaluated and into early intervention services quickly. The family may need support and direction through the assessment process, which is often lengthy and emotional and involves interprofessional collaboration with colleagues in healthcare and educational fields.

As PCPs identify symptoms and behaviors that indicate SLD, these findings may help with understanding other causes of learning problems. Important items in the family history include dyslexia or other learning disability, decreased academic achievement, attention deficits, and grade retention or school dropout. Assess for prematurity or low birth weight, early developmental concerns or delays (especially speech/language issues), hesitancy to participate in early reading and learning activities, history of head injury or hypoxia, seizure disorder, and chronic health conditions. Assess for child connectedness to school (feels accepted, valued, respected, and included), parent's and youth's perception of the patient's efforts compared to classmates (does learning come easier, harder, the same?), perception of the root cause, and experiences with teachers, peers, and homework. It is also important to assess the patient's social competence, temperament, and coping skills. Evaluate teacher reports of academic performance, absences,

Level I School Performance Prescreening Questionnaire

- Do you have any concerns about:
  - Your child's learning or school performance?
  - Your child's attention, concentration, impulsivity, and/or hyperactivity?
  - How your child is doing in certain subjects at school? If yes, in what subjects? Reading? Writing? Math? Other?
  - How much your child enjoys school compared with friends or classmates?
- Does your child have any problems completing homework?

Level II School Performance Screener

- In what area(s) does your child have problems in school performance? Learning/achievement? Attention/concentration/memory? Behavior?
- Subjects/activities of difficulty: Reading? Math? Spelling? Writing? Speaking? Listening? Remembering? Science? Social studies? Language/grammar? Following directions? Inconsistency? Transferring knowledge from one situation to another? Organizing?
- Current grade? What grade did problems become evident? Did child repeat a grade? Was the child ever in danger of repeating a grade?
- Grades on report card? Performance on standardized testing? Is excessive amount of help needed to do homework? Is excessive amount of homework due to child not completing in school? Would grades be lower without a great amount of extra work being done at home with parents? Is homework a battle each night?
- Stressors? None? Current? At time of onset of school problems? With family? Peers? At school?
- Medical concerns? Frequent ear infections? Hearing problem? Vision problem? Prenatal/perinatal problems? Allergies? Loss of consciousness? Sleep problem? Describe.
- Strengths? Reading? Math? Spelling? Writing? Speaking? Listening? Remembering? Science? Social studies? Language/grammar? Other? Learns better by seeing versus hearing or vice versa?
- How does the child get along with peers? Involved in extracurricular activities? Type? If so, how does he or she do?
- Emotional issues: Lack of motivation? School avoidance? Homework avoidance? Seems lazy? Irritable? Anxious? Volatile? Down on self? Aggressive? Gives up easily? Refuses to work in class? Doesn't turn work in? Oppositional? Angry?
- Tested by school system? If yes, eligible for services? Receives services (types)? Found ineligible? Has received services, but they have been discontinued?

engagement, behavioral information, and educational testing results. Investigate home versus school functioning, behavioral and stress responses to problems, ability to attend to and complete tasks, and child strengths and weaknesses.

The physical examination is typically normal and includes behavioral observations, hearing and vision evaluation, sensory processing screening, neurologic changes, dysmorphic features, and assessment for minor congenital anomalies. Psychoeducational evaluation is performed by a specialist in the school system or privately and includes identification of strengths and weaknesses, assessment of cognitive ability, perceptual abilities, communicative ability, and social and emotional adaptation. Unfortunately, this process is costly and often not covered by insurance.

Management

Most children with academic struggles have more than one dysfunction. Although the educational system focuses primarily on linguistic and logical-mathematical intelligence, and many cultures esteem highly articulate or logical people, there are other types of intelligence. The theory of multiple intelligences (Table 29.8) offers that perspective. Unfortunately, many children with nonlinguistic and nonlogical-mathematical intelligence do not receive much reinforcement in school and end up being labeled learning disabled or underachievers when their unique ways of thinking and learning are not addressed by the typical classroom.

Family Education and Support. Although it is not the purview of the PCP to develop educational plans, the PCP plays a critical role in the care of children with SLD. The PCP can help identify child and family strengths, affinities, and interests to develop passions and areas of expertise. Assisting the family with interpretation of evaluations, describing lagging skills, treatment, and accommodations, and monitoring for co-occurring conditions are part of the PCP role. Encouraging parents to do research and become experts on their child's needs proves helpful, especially in planning for school. This includes helping parents and children understand the implications of a particular learning disability and its effects on peer interactions; exploring ideas and acting as a conduit to find reliable resources and others who solved similar problems; and helping devise an organized approach to respond to their child's struggles (Box 29.7). PCPs may also coach parents about demystifying the diagnosis, reminding children of their intelligence and special way of learning.

Behavior Management and Counseling. School challenges and having to work harder and longer to achieve in school may affect the child's self-esteem, ability to cope, and mental health. Participation in activities outside of school, especially those in which the child can excel, is beneficial. Remind parents that

TABLE 29.8	**Multiple Intelligences**
Intelligence	**Description**
Linguistic	Language sensitivity; language-based function (word smart)
Logical/ mathematical	Abstract reasoning, symbol manipulation, pattern detection, logical reasoning (number/reasoning smart)
Musical	Musical structure and pattern detection and production; appreciation of pitch, rhythm, musical expressiveness (music smart)
Spatial	Visual memory, visual-spatial skills, visualization (picture smart)
Body/kinesthetic	Idea representation, feeling in movement; body use, coordination, goal-directed activities (body smart)
Naturalistic	Animal and plant classification and recognition (nature smart)
Social/ interpersonal	Sensitivity and responsiveness to moods, motives, intentions, and feelings of others (people smart)
Personal/ intrapersonal	Sensitivity to self, feelings, strengths, desires, weaknesses, and understanding of intention and motivation of others (self-smart)

their relationship with the child, their attitude, and emotional support influence the child more than anything else. Providing social-emotional skills training and being alert to issues with self-esteem, self-regulation, and emerging emotional problems allows for early intervention and referral to counseling to help deal with the demands and stresses before they become overwhelming.

Educational System and Adaptive Supports. Children with neurodevelopmental problems are entitled to special education opportunities to maximize their learning potential. These are detailed in an IEP or a 504 plan with appropriate plans and accommodations. Specific, individualized, intensive instruction helps the child improve or find strategies to compensate. Assistive technologies should be included in any home and school plans. Examples of AT that are readily available include: text-to-speech software, audio books, annotation tools, voice-activated and word prediction software to help with writing papers, note-taking pens that download into a computer, graphic organizers and visual thinking tools, and a multitude of apps.

Acknowledge a child's aptitude, initiative, spirit, industry, and self-efficacy to provide tangible strengths support. The PCP may be involved in the discussion about a child's school placement (mainstream classroom, special classroom, or combination of settings); may be asked to provide relevant information related to the child's development; may advocate for the child's rights and needs; or may serve as mediator, consultant, or resource to the school.

Follow-up and Referral

Routine well care includes ongoing evaluation of the school setting, performance, and accommodations. Maintain a heightened awareness of the possibility of mental health issues and screen for comorbidities. Additional visits and referrals may be recommended to ensure the child achieves maximal potential.

Intellectual Developmental Disorder and Global Developmental Delay

Intellectual functioning, the general mental capacity to learn or understand and deal with new situations, is often measured by intellectual quotient (IQ) tests that evaluate problem-solving, language, attention, memory, and information processing. Adaptive functioning defines how well a person can care for themselves (conceptual, social, and practical skills) and how independent they are compared with others the same age.

Definition and Diagnostic Criteria

The DSM-5TR defines an intellectual developmental disorder (IDD; previously known as intellectual disability/ID) as a neurodevelopmental disorder that results in deficits in intellectual and adaptive functioning.[1] Adaptive functioning encompasses multiple domains: (1) conceptual: language, reading, writing, math, reasoning, knowledge, memory; (2) social: empathy, social judgment, communication skills, the ability to follow rules, and the ability to make and keep friends; and (3) practical: independence in personal care, job responsibilities, managing money, recreation, and organizing school and work. IDD severity is defined as mild, moderate, severe, or profound based on adaptive functioning. IQ scores are not reliable in children under 5 years old and are no longer part of the diagnostic criteria[31] (Box 29.8). The term *global developmental delays* (GDD) is used to describe children younger 5 years who have significant delays in two or more areas of development. The DSM does not have age-related diagnostic exclusions, but IDD is not typically diagnosed until after age 5 years. Two-thirds of all children with GDD will go on to be diagnosed with IDD. IDD is also often classified as unspecified ID, especially early in diagnostic evaluation.

There is no one factor that predicts the development of IDD, but there are several identified genetic, prenatal, perinatal, and postnatal risks for ID. Genetic influences of IDD include Fragile X syndrome (the most common cause), Prader-Willi syndrome, Down syndrome, Angelman syndrome, and Williams syndrome.[31] Single gene and chromosomal variants that cause changes in brain structure and function like tuberous sclerosis and Rhett syndrome also increase ID risk. In addition, there are several known environmental risk factors including prenatal factors like poor nutrition, placental insufficiency, and in utero exposures to known teratogens, alcohol, illicit substances, and maternal infections.[31] Herpes, cytomegalovirus, toxoplasmosis, rubella, parvovirus B19, syphilis, and varicella-zoster infections during pregnancy and during the perinatal period are also

---

• BOX 29.7 A Parent's Response to a Learning Disability

- Organize information about your child's learning disability—including evaluations and other material, school files, samples of work that demonstrate difficulties as well as strengths; a history of contacts with school establishing services; any services or adaptive techniques used.
- Know your child's strengths and make sure they are utilized.
- Have your child evaluated as needed and monitor your child's progress.
- Establish realistic expectations and provide opportunities for your child to assume responsibility.
- Provide your child opportunities to improve social skills and interact successfully with other children and adults.
- Work as an advocate for your child and find reasonable accommodations that work.
- Talk to your child about learning disabilities.
- Know your legal rights.

• BOX 29.8 Severity Score for Intellectual Disability

Mild (85% of individuals)
Presents during early school years; difficulties in academic settings; more socially immature than peers; concrete thinking and communication; function adaptively but need support for complex daily living

Moderate (10% of individuals)
Presents earlier than mild; learning and language difficulties in preschool; deficits in social and communication requiring support; may be able to function adaptively with training and support; may be able to be employed in jobs with minimal communication and cognitive skills needed.

Severe (3%–4% of individuals)
Limited ability to understand written language, numbers, and time; needs significant support throughout life; understanding of verbal and gestural communication and spoken language limited; requires extensive support and supervision for all daily living activities.

Profound (1%–2% of individuals)
Use of objects in a goal-directed manner for self-care or recreation; communication very limited with limited understanding and nonverbal expression; requires pervasive support and dependent in all levels of care and living.

known to have effect on the developing CNS. Lastly, perinatal risk factors include asphyxia (leading cause), prematurity, intracranial hemorrhage, low birth weight, perinatal infection, and neonatal hypoglycemia. Postnatal causes include intentional and unintentional trauma (i.e., drowning, traumatic brain injury, lead poisoning), CNS infection, chemotherapy and radiation, severe neglect and abuse, and any condition that results in significant hypoxemia.

The global incidence of IDD is estimated to be approximately 1% of the population.[31] This disorder is more common in males and 85% of those are mildly affected.[31] Co-occurring conditions are common, including sensory processing difficulties, sleep difficulties, significant hearing loss or deafness, cerebral palsy, and respiratory and gastrointestinal issues. Individuals with IDD have significantly higher risk of having a seizure disorder than their nonaffected peers. Other neurodevelopmental disorders occur in about one-third of children with IDD (ASD, ODD, ADHD, anxiety, depression, neurodevelopmental disorder associated with prenatal alcohol exposure, aggression, and self-injury).[31] Issues needing extra attention include nutrition, the potential for obesity, exercise and activity, safety, dental issues and care, sexuality and abuse, and pain management. Individuals with IDD who present with acute behavioral changes might have an underlying medical condition that causes physical discomfort or pain such as infection that is often overlooked.

Clinical Findings and Assessment

Presentation varies depending on impairment severity, with the more severe IDD recognized earlier, and milder IDD in middle childhood. Delays in receptive and expressive language, adaptive skills, fine motor deficits, problem-solving difficulties, social immaturity, and behavioral difficulties may be presenting concerns. Gross motor delays are the least likely to occur.

Screening and Specialty Referral for Diagnosis

Diagnosis begins with a thorough developmental, educational, medical, and family history (including a three-generation family history focused on neurodevelopmental issues, genetic conditions, and consanguinity). Screening for motor, language, and social skills helps to identify early signs of intellectual function and is part of the standard well child assessment conducted at the 9-, 12-, 18-, 24-, and 30-month episodic visits and is discussed in Chapters 10 and 11.[9] A complete physical and neurologic examination including vision and hearing testing is needed with a focus on head circumference, skin evaluation, and dysmorphic features. If a syndromic form is suspected, laboratory, chromosomal studies, and neuroimaging may be indicated, and referral to a genetics specialist initiated. If patient presentation is not syndromic, chromosomal microarray, fragile X testing, and karyotyping may be indicated as first-line tests, but referral to genetics is recommended as further evaluation may be needed. Many children are identified in early childhood, but others may not show symptoms until middle childhood when academic tasks and social expectations exceed their capacity. The clinical practice guidelines for the management of intellectual disorder published by the American Academy of Child and Adolescent Psychiatry (AACAP) emphasize the importance of referring children to child psychiatry when initial screening is suspicious for IDD and when diagnostic evaluation is needed and includes an algorithm for the use of genetic testing in the evaluation of an individual with suspected IDD.[31]

Neurocognitive diagnostic evaluation includes intelligence testing and adaptive testing with standardized measures and interviews typically done by a psychologist or other certified clinician. Intelligence testing is most reliable after 5 years of age using standardized tests such as the Child Wechsler Intelligence Scale, the Mullen Scale of Early Learning, the Leiter Intentional Performance Scale, or the Stanford-Binet Intelligence Scales. Assessment of adaptive functioning is done with standardized tests such as Vineland Adaptive Behavior Scales or Adaptive Behavior Assessment System. Impairment in one of the three domains (conceptual, social, or practical) requiring ongoing support is needed to qualify as impairment.

Management

Early identification and intervention support functioning in cognition, language, academics, and behavior, enabling maximum potential and minimizing functional decline. Timely identification and management of other conditions are key.

Family and Social Support. Family and social support starts with knowing the child's strengths, learning to appreciate their uniqueness, offering hope, and encouraging patience. Parents need resources to learn about the disability and connect with other parents. Assisting the family with home environmental management helps maintain a smoother, more controlled family life. Most individuals with IDD do best in environments that are predictable with consistent routines. Helping families to identify ways to implement routines and behavioral economies can benefit all family members by minimizing distress and decreasing likelihood of emotional dysregulation. Community services and educational resources are available for social, recreational, and sports opportunities (Special Olympics, Best Buddies). Though schools often manage transitional support plans, the PCP should be actively involved in assisting the family with advocacy and issues related to medical care.

Medication Management. IDD, like other neurodivergent conditions, does not resolve with medication therapy. The aim of medication use in IDD management is to help minimize problematic symptoms and behaviors and to decrease comorbidities that worsen overall functioning. Behavioral health specialists may elect to target symptoms like impulsivity with methylphenidate or aggression with risperidone using evidence-based guidelines, many of which are summarized in the AACAP guidelines.[31] However, there are currently no FDA approved medications specifically for use in this population.

Behavioral Management and Counseling. Individuals with IDD are not different than neurotypical individuals and benefit from secure emotional attachment, warm parental interaction, and developing social-emotional skills that allow enhanced peer interactions. Youth with depression, anxiety, ADHD, and other psychiatric disorders may benefit from psychosocial interventions including CBT.[31] Parents and other family members may need counseling or case management services as they deal with the diagnosis (guilt) and manage the extra burdens (financial, fatigue, isolation) required to care for a child with IDD. Siblings may need support as they are relied upon to help or are overlooked in the complexity of the family situation. Parental classes and education provide the family with behavioral management strategies (see Chapter 6).

Educational and Adaptive Support. Early intervention and support as provided through an Individualized Family Service Plan or IEP are essential. Mainstreaming with special education support teachers or aides is common for children with milder severity. Self-contained classrooms with small student-teacher ratios are helpful for those with moderate to profound severity. Additional supports may include occupational therapy, physical therapy, and speech/language therapy; accommodations may include special instruction, personnel, equipment, or strategies. By age 16 years, every adolescent should have a transitional plan in place looking toward employment, adult living skills, and recreation.

Follow-up and Referral

Management of the child with ID includes routine well-child care with special attention, follow-up, and referral as needed for co-occurring or comorbid issues. Diagnostic reevaluation is needed every 3 years as treatment of comorbidities may resolve symptoms initially diagnosed as ID.[31] As children grow and mature, needs change and lags appear more significant so staying attuned to child and family needs is important.

Aggression and Disruptive Behavior Disorders: Aggression

Aggression is a leading cause of clinic psychiatric visits and emergency department visits. It is not a DSM diagnosis but rather a symptom that occurs in many conditions and is most often associated with ASD, intellectual developmental disorder, oppositional defiant disorder, and attention deficit disorder. It usually occurs due to a combination of irritability, emotional dysregulation that exceeds coping skills, and impulsivity. Onset may occur as early as toddlerhood. It can be overt (e.g., hitting or pushing) or covert (e.g., threatening or socially ostracizing). Disruptive behavior disorders include CD, oppositional defiant disorder, disruptive mood dysregulation disorder, and intermittent explosive disorder among others.

Typical developmental aggression occurs in early childhood (age 1 to 2 years) and manifests as hitting, biting, and throwing objects. Maladaptive aggression affects males more often than females and neurodivergent individuals more than neurotypical individuals, and peaks during adolescence. Females are more likely to be socially or covertly aggressive, whereas males are more likely to be physically aggressive. Acute, stressful life events or transitions can precipitate a brief period of social aggression. There is strong genetic influence for aggressive behavior, especially in males, with twin studies demonstrating that genetics explain as much as 65% of the variance in generalized aggression. Significant risk factors include a history of maltreatment or trauma with or without PTSD; inconsistent or harsh discipline; poor parental responsiveness, especially in infancy and early childhood; weak social ties; bullying; peer influences (especially for older children and adolescents); and parental figure changes or parental rejection. Any individuals with disorders that affect the prefrontal cortex, amygdala, or hypothalamus have higher risk of demonstrating aggression.[32]

Clinical Findings

During early childhood, aggression manifests as oppositional or defiant behavior and is considered clinically significant if it interferes with normal developmental functioning. The pervasiveness, intensity, and persistence of irritable, argumentative, defiant, and easily annoyed behaviors identify a pathologic condition and may be precursors to ODD. Preschool-aged children have a basic understanding of the effect of their behavior on others and can control their behavior based on internalized norms and developing self-regulation. When social aggression becomes a pattern, peer rejection is common. Aggressive behavior at all ages involves the following: property destruction; name-calling; physically pestering and deliberately annoying others; hitting, biting, kicking, fighting; frequent peer conflict; temper tantrums; misinterpreting social cues and responding aggressively; lack of problem-solving in social situations; swearing, obscene language and gestures; excessive arguing; and/or inappropriate or aggressive sexual behaviors.

Screening should include suicidal ideation, homicidal ideation, child and family behavioral health disorders, abuse by a caregiver or peer, and substance abuse history. Table 29.9 includes screening tools for youth aggression.

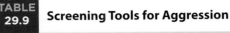

TABLE 29.9	Screening Tools for Aggression	
Scale	**Appropriate Ages**
Child Aggression Scale	5–18 years
Modified Overt Aggression Scale	Not defined but validated for use in middle childhood
Buss-Perry Aggression Questionnaire	9 years to adulthood

Modified from Austerman J. Violence and aggressive behavior. *Pediatr Rev.* 2017;38(2):69–78.

Differential Diagnosis

ODD is a pattern of problems with rules and authority figures. ODD symptoms emerge during the preschool years and persist for a minimum of 6 months. CD is a clear pattern of behavior established over a 6-month period, typically diagnosed at school age. CD differs from ODD in that it involves serious aggression toward people or animals, willful destruction of property, or theft. Typical and atypical problems can be differentiated, and children with these problems can be identified with a developmentally based DSM-5TR framework.[1] Children with externalizing ADHD symptoms may demonstrate aggression due to poor impulse control and hyperactivity.

Management

It is important to ascertain whether a difficult temperament underlies the behavioral issues, especially in conjunction with a parental temperament lack of fit. A difficult temperament may account for a child's being hard to discipline, having social behavior problems in school (e.g., poor fit with the teacher), or having poor academic achievement. In these situations, the use of positive parenting strategies does not have to change, but supportive counseling for the parents should be provided regarding temperament, its manifestations, and strategies for managing transitions and other difficult times or behaviors. A teacher conference may provide similar information and explore strategies to facilitate the child's learning and positive behavior.

When aggression is a response to acute stress, the problem usually resolves if parents and caregivers use positive caregiving strategies and facilitate developmentally appropriate coping efforts. If peer relationship development is hampered, close monitoring of and intervention with peer interactions by day care, preschool, and school personnel, especially with the parents present for observation, enhances appropriate social behavior and competence. Changing schools to lessen problems is not advised because children carry their social difficulties with them and assume the same roles in new groups. It is helpful to work with teachers to ensure that they are supportive and facilitative.

When aggression becomes a social behavior pattern, referral for intervention to a behavioral health specialist is critical. Early intervention is essential, and a focus on psychotherapy and skill building is paramount. Parental education should focus on reestablishing positive parent-child interactions, use of consistent limit setting, and teaching parents to use effective discipline. Social skills development training can help youth learn to communicate, to manage emotions, and to develop healthy coping skills. Strategies employed to manage inappropriate aggression include individual and family therapy, and school- and community-based programs. Medication therapy for underlying causes (i.e., seizure disorder, ADHD) is appropriate. If the aforementioned is not successful, behavioral health specialists may initiate a trial with an antipsychotic like risperidone or aripiprazole or they may trial an alpha-adrenergic agent like clonidine or guanfacine to decrease impulsivity and help the patient interact with psychotherapeutic approaches.[32]

Aggression and Disruptive Behavior Disorders: Conduct Disorder

CD is a repetitive and persistent pattern of behavior in which the basic rights of others or major age-appropriate societal norms and rules are violated.[1] The onset of aggressive behavior is observed in toddlerhood. Early-onset conduct problems are diagnosed from age 4 to 6 years, and a formal diagnosis is typically made when the child is age 7 years or older. The cause of the disorder rests in chronic negative circumstances, as in social aggression. CD is frequently associated with a history of harsh discipline, abuse, or neglect. Prevalence rates are approximately 2% to 4% in the general population.[1] CD is more common in males than females (3:1). However, it is thought that the prevalence data do not accurately reflect the occurrence of CD for females, because the diagnostic criteria emphasize physical aggression.

Behavioral dysregulation usually becomes problematic during the transition from early to middle childhood in large part due to the changing school structure and increasing social and peer behavioral expectations. There is a high rate of comorbidity with major depression, and the joint presence of CD and depression increases the risk for substance abuse and suicide. ADHD negatively influences the development, course, and severity of CD.

Clinical Findings

Clinical features fall into four main subgroups: (1) aggressive behavior that threatens or results in physical harm to other people or animals, (2) nonaggressive behavior that causes property damage, (3) lying or stealing, and (4) serious violation of rules or laws. Several factors are relevant to practitioners for their prognostic importance:

- How atypical the behaviors are for age or sex
- How overt versus covert are the behaviors
- The nature of any aggression
- The presence of early antisocial or psychopathic-related symptoms
  Most referrals for clinical treatment are for aggressive behaviors. Physical aggression toward others includes the following: hitting, kicking, fighting; physical cruelty to animals or people; property destruction (including fire setting); frequent temper tantrums; high rates of annoying behavior, such as yelling, whining, or threatening; disobedience to adults; lying, cheating, covert stealing; truancy and running away from home; blaming others for mistakes; using or selling illegal drugs; engaging in inappropriate or violent sexual behaviors (e.g., sexual assault); and/or academic problems.

There is growing evidence that preadolescent and adolescent females manifest CD more indirectly through verbal and relational aggression, including alienation, ostracism, and character defamation directed at the relationships between friends. With CD, social role functioning tends to be impaired with poor academic performance, poor family and peer relationships, and poor self-management. Childhood CD may predict antisocial personality disorder in adulthood. Poorer prognoses are associated with increased symptom severity.

Differential Diagnosis

ODD behaviors are typically less serious and are characterized by more disobedience than aggressiveness. ADHD is characterized by inattention, impulsiveness, and hyperactivity, but willful

destruction is uncommon. CD is distinguished from isolated acts of aggressive behavior by degree of aggression exhibited, the presence of willful defiance, and by the persistence of symptoms for a minimum of 6 months.[1] A thorough physical examination is essential to rule out organic causes of behavior and to identify evidence of abuse, neglect, and substance abuse disorders.

Management

If aggressive behavior is identified before a CD develops, preventive efforts can be implemented. Successful programs are multifaceted, including a parent-directed component (e.g., parent education and support for positive parenting strategies and healthy, consistent approaches to discipline), social-cognitive skills training, proactive classroom management and teacher training, and group therapy.[32] Effective education includes conflict resolution strategies and development of coping and resiliency skills. Once a CD is evident, referral for child and family intervention is crucial.

Safety is a priority in caring for children with aggressive and oppositional disorders. Because of the strong association of child abuse and neglect with CD, it is critical to determine the safety of the child and family members. If there is evidence of abuse or neglect, prompt referral to child protective agencies is mandatory. Potential interventions when family safety is at risk include referral for inpatient psychiatric evaluation, police notification of criminal activity, supporting the family to petition the juvenile court for services, and referral to community health services.

Family therapy can be helpful for adolescents with CD. Collaboration between the family and the school is of critical importance, and the PCP can refer the family to a community mental health center for case management services. Isolated individual treatment is not superior to parent intervention programs. Education about problem-solving skills may also be effective.

Psychopharmacologic intervention is reserved for explosive aggression and includes mood stabilizers, atypical antipsychotics, alpha-adrenergic agents, and stimulants. However, PCPs should refer patients to a behavioral health specialist for drug therapy given the high risk for substance abuse in those with CD.

Aggression and Disruptive Behavior Disorders: Oppositional Defiant Disorder

ODD is a pattern of negative, hostile, and defiant behavior that is excessive compared with other children of the same age.[1] Symptoms often occur in early childhood, from age 3 to 7 years, with the disorder typically beginning by age 8 years.

Etiologic factors include many of the parenting and family dysfunctions identified for aggression. Precursors to the disorder are common in early childhood, especially defiance and negativism. ODD is more common in males before puberty, but the gender distribution is approximately equal after puberty.

Clinical Findings

The essential feature of ODD is a recurrent pattern of behavior that is negative, defiant, disobedient, and hostile toward authority figures. Behavior is typically directed at family members, teachers, or peers that the child knows well. The child manifests the following behaviors to an extent that leads to impairment[1]:

- Actively defies or refuses adult requests or rules
- Is argumentative, angry, resentful, touchy, or easily annoyed
- Easily loses temper; is vindictive
- Blames others for own mistakes or difficulties

- Deliberately does things to annoy others
- Often sees their own behavior as justifiable, not oppositional or defiant

Differential Diagnosis

CD involves more serious violations of the rights of others and a more willful disregard of authority. Bipolar disorder often causes irritability but is also associated with depression. ADHD is associated with forgetfulness and impulsivity but individuals with ADHD always have symptoms, not only in situations that require them to be still or to apply sustained effort.[1]

Management

Attend to the early signs of defiant and oppositional behavior or aggression, or both, and educate parents about positive parenting strategies and exercising consistent, healthy discipline, which is like the management of CDs. Because these children typically do not perceive themselves as having a problem and cause distress within the family system, referral for intervention is indicated. As described for CD, parent training programs are more successful if they include information about child behavior in multiple environments (e.g., school and home) and target dysfunctional family processes. Child training groups provide added benefit if combined with parent training groups. Again, collaboration with the school is important. These multiple approaches, conducted simultaneously, are most effective. Medication therapy is reserved for moderate to severe cases that do not respond to therapy. Medications target core symptoms and include stimulants, alpha-adrenergic agents, nonstimulants like atomoxetine and viloxazine, and atypical antipsychotics.[32]

Aggression and Disruptive Behavior Disorders: Disruptive Mood Dysregulation Disorder

Disruptive mood dysregulation disorder (DMDD) is a diagnosis with core symptoms of severe irritability with resultant verbal and/or physical outbursts. It was added to the DSM-IV due to concerns for the overdiagnosis of bipolar disorder in youth. Classified in the DSM-5TR as a depressive disorder, it is characterized by consistent irritability, negative mood, and emotional outbursts that are out of proportion to the situation.[1] Diagnostic criteria require symptom onset to occur before age 10 years (it cannot be diagnosed in children younger than 6 years), symptoms to be present in at least two settings and to occur at least 3 times a week for at least a year. The prevalence of the disorder is unclear, but it is estimated to affect approximately 2% of the population and is more commonly diagnosed in males.[1] The risk factors for DMDD are like the risk factors noted for other psychiatric diagnoses resulting in aggression.[33] There is significant comorbidity with ADHD and ODD, and children with DMDD often present with depression, anxiety, and ASD.[1]

Clinical Findings

The main reason why parents and caregivers seek help for patients with DMDD is their significant irritability. This may present as temper tantrums outside the age when these are developmentally expected, significant anger in situations where such a response is unwarranted, marked impatience, or verbal and/or physical aggression towards others, most commonly parents and family members.[1,33] Other common symptoms include difficulty concentrating in situations that require mental effort and poor

psychosocial relations primarily with parents and siblings that commonly result in dysfunction. School suspensions are common, affecting a third of children with this diagnosis.[33]

Differential Diagnosis

Bipolar disorder occurs episodically while DMDD causes a persistent irritable mood. ODD is characterized by defiance and intentional disregard for authority, MDD results in similar behaviors but also includes altered mood between outbursts. Children with ASD have social and emotional challenges in interpreting cues or difficulty processing sensory input that may result in outbursts, but these occur episodically.

Management

Primary care management of children with suspected DMDD involves referral to behavioral health specialists for evaluation, diagnosis, and management. Psychotherapeutic approaches target parental skills training and patient socioemotional skills training, CBT, and dialectical behavioral therapy. The evidence for dialectical behavioral therapy is greatest with as many as 90% of patients showing significant improvement in randomized control trials.[33] Medications, when selected, target core symptoms, specifically impulsivity and irritability. The strongest evidence supports the use of antidepressants including SSRIs and some atypical antipsychotic antidepressants; stimulants especially methylphenidate; and nonstimulants including atomoxetine, clonidine, and guanfacine.[33]

Autism Spectrum Disorder

Definition and Diagnostic Criteria

ASD is a complex neurodevelopmental disorder that affects communication and behavior beginning in the first 2 years of life. According to the DSM-5TR, ASD causes social interaction impairment with additional communication impairment and restrictive, repetitive, and stereotyped behavior, interest, and activity patterns. ASD occurs on a spectrum, and there is a wide variability in symptoms ranging from mild symptoms to those with profound symptoms impacting almost all areas of daily functioning. ASD diagnostic criteria require that affected individuals show symptoms from early childhood even if they are not recognized until later in life. DSM-5TR criteria for ASD and severity levels (Box 29.9) guide diagnosis. ASD is a lifelong disorder, but symptoms can improve with early and appropriate services.

The etiology of ASD is unclear, but evidence demonstrates strong genetic etiology with familial inheritance patterns (the 4:1 male dominance, increased prevalence in siblings and concordance in twins [ranging from 37–90% in twin studies[1]], and increased risk in relatives) and association with genetic disorders (fragile X syndrome [most common single gene cause of ASD], neurofibromatosis, tuberous sclerosis, Angelman syndrome, and Rett syndrome). There are several identified genes associated with ASD; however, these are not sufficient to cause disease; that is, not all individuals with these genes show symptoms and behaviors of ASD.[1] Inherited genetic variations are important, as are de novo, or spontaneous, mutations. Interaction between multiple genes and environmental modifiers contributes to variable expression. Environmental factors are considered a "second hit" in that they modulate existing genetic factors increasing ASD predisposition: these include extreme prematurity, meconium aspiration, breech delivery, and low 5-minute Apgar scores, maternal medications that are

• BOX 29.9   DSM 5-TR Diagnostic Criteria for Autistic Disorder

- Persistent deficits in social communication and social interaction across multiple contexts, demonstrated by the following, currently or by history (examples are illustrative, not exhaustive):
  - Deficits in social-emotional reciprocity, ranging, for example, from abnormal social approach and failure to have normal back-and-forth conversation; to reduced sharing of interests, emotions, or affect; to failure to initiate or respond to social interactions.
  - Deficits in nonverbal communication used for social interaction, ranging, for example, from poorly integrated verbal and nonverbal communication; to abnormalities in eye contact and body language or deficits in understanding and use of gestures; to a total lack of facial expressions and nonverbal communication.
  - Deficits in developing, maintaining, and understanding relationships ranging, for example, from difficulty adjusting social behavior to suit various social contexts; to difficulties in sharing imaginative play or making friends; to absence of interest in peers.
  - Severity is based on social communication impairments and restricted, repetitive behavior patterns.
- Restricted, repetitive patterns of behavior, interests, or activities, as manifested by at least two of the following, currently or by history (examples are illustrative, not exhaustive):
  - Stereotyped or repetitive motor movements, use of objects, or speech (e.g., simple motor stereotypes, lining up toys or flipping objects, echolalia, idiosyncratic phrases).
  - Insistence on sameness, inflexible adherence to routines, or ritualized patterns of verbal or nonverbal behavior (e.g., extreme distress at small changes, difficulties with transitions, rigid thinking patterns, greeting rituals, need to take same route or eat same food every day).
  - Highly restricted, fixated interests that are abnormal in intensity or focus (e.g., strong attachment to or preoccupation with unusual objects, excessively circumscribed or perseverative interests).
  - Hyper- or hyporeactivity to sensory input or unusual interest in sensory aspects of the environment (e.g., apparent indifference to pain/temperature, adverse response to specific sounds or textures, excessive smelling or touching of objects, visual fascination with lights or movement).
- Symptoms must be present in infancy and early childhood (but may not become fully manifest until social demands exceed limited capacities or may be masked by learned strategies in later life).
- Symptoms cause clinically significant functional impairment in social, occupational, or other important areas.
- These disturbances cannot be better explained by intellectual disability (intellectual developmental disorder) or global developmental delay.
- **Note:** Individuals with a well-established DSM-IV diagnosis of autistic disorder, Asperger disorder, or pervasive developmental disorder not otherwise specified should be given the diagnosis of autism spectrum disorder.

Severity Level	Social Communication	Restrictive Repetitive Behaviors
Level 3: Requiring very substantial support	Severe deficits in verbal and nonverbal social communication skills cause severe impairments in functioning, very limited initiation of social interactions, and minimal response to social overtures from others. For example, a person with few words of intelligible speech, who rarely initiates interaction, and, when he or she does, makes unusual approaches to meet needs only responds to only very direct social approaches.	Inflexibility of behavior, extreme difficulty coping with change, or other restricted/repetitive behaviors markedly interfere with functioning in all spheres. Great distress/difficulty changing focus or action.
Level 2: Requiring substantial support	Marked deficits and verbal and nonverbal social communication skills; social impairments apparent even with supports in place; limited initiation of social interactions; and reduced or abnormal responses to social overtures from others. For example, a person who speaks in simple sentences, whose interaction is limited to narrow special interests, and who has markedly odd nonverbal communication.	Inflexibility of behavior, difficulty coping with change, or other restricted/repetitive behaviors appear frequently enough to be obvious to the casual observer and interfere with functioning in a variety of contacts. Distress and/or difficulty changing focus or action.
Level 1: Requiring support	Without supports in place, deficits in social communication causes noticeable impairments. Difficulty initiating social interactions, and clear examples of atypical or unsuccessful responses to social overtures of others. May appear to have decreased interest in social interactions. For example, a person who is able to speak in full sentences and engages in communication, but whose to –and– fro conversation with others fails, and whose attempts to make friends are odd and typically unsuccessful.	Inflexibility of behavior causes significant interference with functioning in one or more contexts. Difficulty switching between activities. Problems of organization and planning hamper independence.

From American Psychiatric Association (APA). *Diagnostic and Statistical Manual of Mental Disorders, Text Revision DSM-5-TR.* APA; 2022.

neurotoxic, advanced parental age, autoimmune conditions, and toxin exposure. Neuroimaging provides insights into biological differences between individuals with ASD and their nonaffected peers. These differences include increased extra-axial cerebrospinal fluid volume, enlarged amygdala volumes, and altered cerebral growth trajectory.[34]

The Centers for Disease Control and Prevention report ASD prevalence as 1.7% to 2.3%, as of 2021, with males being diagnosed at a 4:1 ratio compared to females.[35] White children are diagnosed with ASD at higher rates than Latino and Black children, and children from areas with higher mean household incomes are more likely to receive an ASD diagnosis than children from areas with lower mean household incomes.[35] ASD occurs more frequently in individuals with certain genetic or chromosomal conditions (e.g., Down syndrome, fragile X syndrome).

Clinical Findings and Assessment

Children with ASD demonstrate consistent problems with social interactions, communication, and language skills; challenges relating to people, objects, and events; abnormal responses to sensory stimuli, usually sound and tactile stimuli; and restricted, repetitive, or stereotypical behaviors and echolalia (meaningless repetition of others' speech). *Infants* may be passive, nonengaging, quiet, floppy, "difficult," colicky, or stiff and have poor eye contact or fail to respond to name or gestures. During *early childhood,* parents often become convinced that something is wrong with their child as language delays (especially expressive), lack of social relatedness, and severe behavior problems are common. If speaking, echolalia is present or the child primarily talks about specific interests and has trouble modulating their voice volume. Language delays include lack of meaningful speech, decreased gestures, and altered gaze. Approximately one-quarter of children with ASD regress in social and/or language skills between age 18 and 24 months.[36] Socially, the child exhibits detachment, decreased eye contact, a lack of reciprocity or initiating conversation, lack of fear, poor creative play, invasion of others' space, preference to be alone, and lack of social awareness. Persistent and insistent behaviors, excessive temper tantrums, repetitive movements, and a preference to line, stack, or spin toys occur. The child may have precocious or average development of rote memory skills but often without concept comprehension. By *middle childhood,* children with ASD often lack reciprocal friendships, have ritualistic behaviors, and have language, social, and behavioral problems. Transitions between places and activities are often challenging. *Adolescents* have similar behaviors. Children with level 1 autism do well in regular classrooms, and mildly affected persons can be academically successful but have social relationship problems.

Development is uneven, with occasional talent in a limited area, such as music or mathematics, coupled with severe deficits in other areas. Many children with ASD have medical comorbidities such as sleep problems, seizures, gastrointestinal problems (diarrhea, constipation, and abdominal pain), and dental disorders. About 70% of individuals with ASD have a comorbid psychiatric condition. Forty percent have two or more of the following: IDD, ADHD, anxiety, depression, and avoidant/restrictive food intake disorders.[36]

Screening and Specialty Referral for Diagnosis

Routine developmental surveillance in early childhood helps identify red flags for ASD (Box 29.10), and PCPs should be sensitive to parental concerns. The AAP recommends screening for autism at all periodic wellness visits and with autism-specific screening at both 18 and 24 months, as a negative screen at 18 months may be abnormal at 24 months.[36] The Modified Checklist for Autism in Toddlers revised with follow-up (M-CHAT-R/F) is the most used tool. Readily available online in multiple languages (http://mchatscreen.com; https://m-chat.org), it screens children 16 to 30 months of age and identifies those who need further evaluation. Other available tools include Screening Tool for Autism in Two-Year-olds (STAT, 24–35 months) and Social Communication Questionnaire (SCQ, 4+ years old). The gold standard diagnostic tools are the second edition of the Autism Diagnostic Observation Schedule (ADOS-2) and the Autism Diagnostic Interview (ADI-R), which are costly and require specialized training and therefore may require lengthy waiting lists when scheduling. The ADOS takes 45 to 60 minutes to administer, the ADI 90 to 150 minutes. Some settings use the ADOS without the ADI.

Children who fail routine developmental screening should begin an early identification process including analysis of family and provider concerns and descriptions of behavior. Family history may reveal other members with ASD, speech delay or language deficits, mood disorders, or IDs. It is important to identify individual and family medical history of seizures, hearing loss, head injury, and meningitis. Perform a complete physical examination with a focus on evaluating growth, identifying findings suggestive of genetic syndromes (e.g., skin findings, dysmorphic features) or neurologic abnormalities (e.g., macrocephaly, hypotonia), and test for iron levels and lead exposure. Comprehensive

diagnostic assessment should be done by a multidisciplinary team, ideally at a specialty center, and address core symptoms, cognition, language, and adaptive, sensory, and motor skills. Specialty assessment includes developmental, behavioral, and IQ testing; audiologic evaluation; and genetic testing with microarray. Neuroimaging, electroencephalogram, and metabolic testing may be done if indicated by examination and history. The differential diagnosis includes intellectual disorder, pragmatic social disorder, language disorder, Rett syndrome, neurodevelopmental disorders, and significant psychosocial trauma (PTSD, reactive attachment disorder, and abuse/neglect).

Management

ASD is a disorder of neurodivergence, so treatment focuses on helping youth reach their maximum potential and decreasing core symptoms. ASD diagnosis and severity determination is just the beginning of the management journey. The PCP must assist the family with ongoing routine care, developmental changes, and day-to-day behavior management as well as problems with sleep and feeding, gastrointestinal issues, and irritability. Classified as children with special healthcare needs, these children need a comprehensive plan and appropriate interventions to maximize their health outcomes during childhood and adolescence and to assist with their transitions to adult health care.

Diagnostic and Initial Meeting With Families. It is important to take time to meet with the family after a child is diagnosed with autism to ensure they understand the diagnosis and have

---

• BOX 29.10 **Red Flags for Autism Spectrum Disorder**

Social

- Lack of social smile and eye contact at 2–3 months of age
- Lack of shared spontaneous enjoyment around 9 months
- Does not respond to his or her name by 12 months
- Does not follow a point to a picture or object and look back at pointer by 12 months
- Does not point at objects to show interest (pointing at an airplane flying over) by 14 months
- Does not pretend (feed a doll) by 18 months
- Avoids eye contact and wants to be alone
- Trouble understanding other people's feelings or talking about their own feelings
- Gives unrelated answers to questions
- Loss of social abilities at any age

Language

- Delayed speech and language skills (no babbling or gesturing by 12 months; no single words by 16 months; no two-word [not echolalic] phrases by 24 months)
- Repeats words or phrases over and over (echolalia)
- Monotone intonation; speech rhythm, rate, pitch, volume, and quality of sound issues
- Speech that sounds scripted
- Difficulty with conversation where each person adds information
- Parental concern about hearing due to lack of response
- Loss of language at any age

Patterns of Behavior or Interests

- Gets upset by minor changes
- Has obsessive interests
- Flaps hands ("flapping"), rocks body, or spins in circles (these are described as self-stimulating ["stimming"] behaviors)
- Unusual reactions to the way things sound, smell, taste, look, or feel
- Self-injurious behaviors (head-banging, biting, pinching)

resources. Developing a management plan for the child with ASD is tailored based on disease severity and can be complex, requiring a multidisciplinary approach including a behavioral-developmental pediatrician or psychiatrist, an applied behavior analysis (ABA) therapist, a gastroenterologist, an allergist, a dietician, and/or speech and occupational therapists. Individuals with autism manifest different behaviors at different developmental stages, and behavioral improvements with therapy can dramatically improve quality of life, so it is important to have ongoing evaluation of the management plan to ensure its adequacy for the youth's needs.

When establishing the initial plan of care, detail essential therapies and plans for diet, gastrointestinal issues, exercise, sleep, and safety. The following therapies are recommended but may be difficult to find in many communities: ABA therapy supervised by a Board-Certified Behavior Analyst (BCBA), speech therapy, occupational therapy with a sensory processing focus (modulation for self-regulating and soothing) and assistance with play and self-help skills, and physical therapy if needed. Refer the child for dental care with a provider who is familiar with ASD issues.

Children with ASD are often picky eaters with limited diets due to atypical food preferences, food selectivity, and disruptive mealtime behaviors that may result in overweight, underweight, or development of pica. The PCP can suggest different foods and techniques as well as behavioral tips, but referral to a nutritionist and/or an occupational therapist with an emphasis in feeding (often combined in a feeding clinic) is worthwhile. Gastrointestinal issues such as abdominal pain, constipation, and diarrhea are common. The PCP should acknowledge these difficulties and work with families to monitor and find strategies to minimize issues. Exercise decreases self-stimulating behaviors and improves academic performance in children with neurodevelopmental disorders. Physical therapy and/or shoe inserts help with weak ankles or flat feet. Fifty percent to 80% of children with ASD have problems falling and staying asleep,[36] so work with parents to develop good child sleep hygiene and promptly referral for suspicion of obstructive sleep apnea (see Chapter 16). If difficulties persist, 1 to 6 mg of melatonin can be used. Safety concerns must be considered especially for nonverbal children or children with low IQ. They should always have identification with them, and local authorities should be aware of where they live if elopement is a concern. Consideration of risks related to water and fire, and safety around the house, needs to be addressed. The Autism Speaks website has a Safety Tool Kit available at https://www.autismspeaks.org/tool-kit/autism-safety-kit.

Family Education and Support. Families need support and education to manage children with autism, and siblings need help dealing with the time and attention focused on the child with ASD. Groups and mentors provide support and concrete management ideas. Helping the family find ways to enjoy the child, promote positive routine, create a calm environment, and coordinate with specialists to improve quality of life for everyone are helpful strategies. Although the prognosis for children with autism is highly variable, long-term care needs to be addressed to help those who can be fully independent, employed adults. The 100 Day Kit is a helpful, free resource created for families with children aged 4 years and under available from Autism Speaks. There is a version for young children and one for school-aged children. This kit provides families with information about diagnosis, services, and treatment, and a week-by-week plan for the first 100 days following diagnosis.

Behavior Management, Parent Skills Training, and Counseling. Behavioral management is the most important aspect of ASD management. These therapies focus on social skills development,

distress tolerance, improved communication, and developing a positive behavioral economy. Behavior plans target behaviors according to age, developmental level, and disruptiveness. PCPs can utilize the ABA approach, considering gaps in the child's skills (see Chapter 6), to help parents work through behaviors. Utilizing the child's "rigidity" to establish routine is another strategy to help the child regulate while learning flexibility with the normal variations in family life. Social stories, short descriptions of an activity, event, or situation (e.g., getting dressed, what to do in a thunderstorm), and simple visual representation of social interactions are learning tools that assist children to learn skills and behaviors.[37]

ABA therapy is the gold standard therapeutic approach for ASD treatment. It focuses on developing socially appropriate behaviors while decreasing challenging behaviors. ABA requires extensive parental education, is very time intensive and expensive, and is often not covered by insurance, thereby limiting its use by many families. Social skills training (one-on-one or in small groups), early and intense developmental work, and parenting skills training are also helpful. Parents are important collaborators at all stages—from assessment through goal development and treatment delivery. Following the family regularly allows for the identification of stressful times when referral for counseling might be helpful. Because comorbidity is common, the PCP needs to maintain ongoing surveillance for new symptoms or concerns.

Educational and Adaptive Supports. Early intense intervention is necessary to maximize educational abilities and enhance learning for children with autism. Early intervention programs, school-based special education, and information and assistance for school personnel are essential components of care. Educational needs may range from classroom modifications, the presence of additional classroom personnel, to part- or full-time special education. Care planning requires cognitive testing, and social, behavioral, and language assessment to identify the child's strengths and weaknesses. Every child with ASD needs an IEP or 504 plan. When special abilities are discovered in children with autism, attempts should be made to encourage opportunities for success in those areas. Parents should be skilled advocates for the child and protect them from unrealistic expectations of social competence when necessary. The long-term goal is to help the child to function as effectively and comfortably as possible in the least restrictive environment.

Pharmacologic Management. Although there is no medication to treat the core symptoms of autism, medications are moderately successful at treating ASD-associated behaviors. The current AAP clinical practice guidelines emphasize the use of pharmacotherapy to target irritability, anxiety, sleep disturbances, ADHD symptoms, depression, and aggression but emphasize that medication should be used in a balanced approach that minimizes side effects while maximizes child functioning.[36] Autistic children do not benefit from stimulant medications unless they also have ADHD; they are more sensitive to stimulants so the "start low, go slow" approach should be followed. Alpha-agonist (guanfacine or clonidine) or norepinephrine-reuptake inhibitors (atomoxetine, viloxazine) may prove more effective. Atypical antipsychotics, risperidone, and aripiprazole are FDA approved for irritability and explosive behaviors but are not routinely recommended. SSRIs may be used for anxiety, phobias, and compulsions but require monitoring for agitation, increased energy, and poor sleep. About one-quarter of autistic children also need antiseizure medications for seizures.

Nutrition, Complementary and Alternative Therapies. PCPs should be familiar with complementary or alternative therapies and ask families what they are using or considering. While maintaining a nonjudgmental approach, encourage the family to thoroughly research the approach they are considering, know what specific behavior they hope to affect, and attempt only one treatment at a time.

There are many studies evaluating nutrition and its effects on ASD, although to date none provide evidence-based guidelines for clinical practice. Nonetheless, it is useful for the PCP to be familiar with some of the information that families may hear or ask about. *Nutritional strategies* are either additive (supplementing with vitamins, minerals, folic acid, amino acids, omega-3 fatty acids) or they are subtractive (eliminating based on food intolerance, allergy, yeast-free, gluten-free, casein-free, ketogenic, or specific carbohydrate). There is lack of evidence-based research to support the effectiveness of these diets, and they are costly, take time to prepare, and have an effect on other family members. A few studies show amino acid depletion and bone loss. Special diets also complicate school participation. Mind-body therapies (biofeedback and neurofeedback, music therapy, yoga) and body-based practices (acupuncture, auditory integrative training, transcranial magnetic stimulation, hippotherapy, massage, Qigong) are other options.

Follow-up and Referral

In addition to ensuring the child with ASD receives regular well-child care, additional visits may be required to monitor medication, assess for common medical comorbidities, address behavioral concerns, or assist the family with establishing or modifying school plans. Monitoring family and child coping and need for additional referrals are critical care components. Beginning transitional care planning is also recommended in the teen years.

Eating Disorders

Eating disorders cause abnormal eating behaviors that are secondary to altered body image (dysmorphism). Anorexia nervosa (commonly called *anorexia*) and bulimia nervosa (commonly called *bulimia*) are the primary eating disorders of concern; however, there are other conditions in this diagnostic cluster, including eating disorders not otherwise specified, rumination disorders, pica, avoidant/restrictive food intake disorder (ARFID), and feeding disorders of infancy. Some believe obesity should be classified as an eating disorder because of the correlation between self-soothing and eating, because many obese individuals have feelings of loss of control over their eating, and symptoms of body dysmorphism. Eating disorders are complex conditions that are very difficult to treat and are associated with significant medical and mental health comorbidities. Anorexia has the highest mortality rate of all the mental health conditions. The 5-year mortality rate for anorexia is 15% to 20%, and most of these deaths are caused by electrolyte imbalance, malnutrition, and suicide. Due to the complexity of these disorders, specialty care is needed; however, PCPs play a critical role through detection and early intervention, case coordination, and monitoring for complications.

Lifetime prevalence rates for anorexia and bulimia are 0.5% and 1%, respectively. Both disorders affect females at much greater rates than males (8:1). Symptom onset usually occurs during mid to late adolescence, but preadolescent cases do occur and are associated with significantly higher morbidity and mortality. Athletes are more likely to develop eating disorders, especially those who compete in sports that are based on weight divisions (e.g., wrestling), long-distance running, and those with emphases on aesthetic lines and flexibility (e.g., dancers, gymnasts, and ice skaters). Other individual risk factors include middle to high socioeconomic status, divorced families, chronic disease (e.g., diabetes mellitus, cystic fibrosis, depression, obesity, and substance abuse), recent weight loss in a previously obese person, personality disorders (e.g., borderline, narcissistic, and antisocial), strong will, and history of child abuse. Children and adolescents with eating disorders are more likely to have parents who have a weight or fitness focus, are substance abusers, have high achievement expectations, who comment on their child's physical appearance, have difficulty expressing emotions, or who are overprotective or enmeshed with their children. Like most mental illness, there is an increasing body of evidence suggesting a strong genetic component to anorexia and bulimia that results in altered serotonin and dopamine receptors.

Clinical Findings

Diagnosing anorexia or bulimia can be difficult. Some clinical findings characteristic of these disorders occur in the healthy adolescent. For example, it is not uncommon for a 14-year-old adolescent who is neither anorexic nor bulimic to express concern about their body appearance, stating that they are too fat or unattractive. In addition, anorexic or bulimic adolescents and their families commonly hide their condition and actions, deny problems, or present a mature, self-sufficient, and successful facade. Early in the disease process, the family system may appear to be coherent, making it difficult to collect accurate data about family relations and behavior patterns that contribute to eating disorders.

Many consider anorexia and bulimia to be part of a disease continuum with categories that are more arbitrary than actual. Clinical presentations vary depending on the disease severity. Both anorexia and bulimia are associated with disordered eating and body dysmorphism with or without purging (e.g., laxative abuse, enemas, diuretics, and induced vomiting). In general, there is no loss of appetite or sense of hunger. Affected individuals often link feelings of self-worth with weight or the ability to restrict food intake despite being hungry.

Diagnostic criteria for anorexia are[1]:
- Food restriction leading to significant low body weight based on sex, age, height, and expected developmental growth pattern
- Intense fear of weight gain and "being fat"
- Body dysmorphism
- Binge eating/purging subtype, which is associated with frequent purging although bingeing episodes are rare

Diagnostic criteria for bulimia are[1]:
- Consuming large quantities of food in a short period of time (within 2 hours)
- Loss of control during binge episodes (e.g., cannot control the amount of food they eat or are shocked at amount consumed)
- Engaging in repeated behaviors to lose weight, including purging, excessive exercise, or fasting
- Binging or purging behaviors that occur at least once a week for at least 3 months

Individuals with anorexia are underweight, but children and adolescents with bulimia are often average weight to overweight. In addition to the regular primary care monitoring of weight and growth, it is important to include routine screening to detect the red flags (Table 29.10). Also helpful is the SCOFF questionnaire. This five-item screen asks the following questions:
- Do you make yourself **S**ick because you feel uncomfortably full?
- Do you worry that you have lost **C**ontrol over what you eat?
- Have you lost **O**ver 10 pounds in the last 3 months?
- Do you believe you are **F**at when others say you are thin?

TABLE 29.10	Red Flags and Signs That Indicate Need for Eating Disorder Treatment

Red Flags	Needs Treatment Signs
Reads diet books or clips dieting articles	Regularly fasts or skips meals
Visits pro-anorexia or bulimia websites (pro Anna or pro Mia)	Stops eating with family or friends
Intense focus on diet or regular dieting	Misses two or more periods during weight loss
Sudden desire to be a vegetarian	Reports binge eating
Sudden picky eating	Reports purging
Visits bathroom regularly during or after meals	Parents find laxatives or diet pills
Showers multiple times a day	Excessive exercise
Skips meals because "I ate at school" or other place away from home	Refuses to eat nondiet foods
Large amounts of missing food	Refuses to eat meals prepared by others Extreme calorie counting or portion controls

- Would you say **F**ood dominates your life?

Patients with suspected eating disorders need a thorough history and physical examination and evaluation for comorbid depression, anxiety, suicidality, and risk of physical harm. Common history findings include:

- Menstrual irregularity
- Body dysmorphism
- Preoccupation with food; often fixes elaborate meals but does not eat; rituals associated with food
- Desire to lose weight and history of dieting
- Weight fluctuation or loss
- Guilt about eating
- Hides eating or lies about having eaten or amount eaten
- Social isolation, mood changes, suicidal ideation
- Fixed, highly structured schedule; inflexible to change
- Cold intolerance, fatigue, myalgias
- Constipation, diarrhea, abdominal bloating, gastrointestinal distress
- Sore throat
- Dizziness, syncope
- Substance abuse, self-harm
- Family history of chaos, abuse, sexual abuse

Common physical findings that may indicate an eating disorder are:

- Altered growth
- Parotid gland enlargement
- Fluid retention, facial edema
- Thin body type, low body temperature
- Hypotension, bradycardia, orthostatic hypotension, shallow respirations
- Dental enamel erosion, dental caries
- Russell sign (e.g., knuckle cuts, calluses, or abrasions from inducing vomiting)
- Thinning hair, alopecia, decreased deep tendon reflexes
- Abdominal distention, altered bowel sounds
- Lanugo, dry skin

- Muscle atrophy
- Mental torpor

Differential Diagnosis

Inflammatory bowel disease and peptic ulcer disease result in chronic pain and microscopic or gross bleeding. CNS lesions cause focal neurologic signs. Hormonal and metabolic diseases cause symptoms like polyphagia, polydipsia, polyuria, abnormal hair growth, and goiter. Immune disorders are associated with frequent, rare, and opportunistic infections. Other mental health differential diagnoses include OCD, SUD, and major depression.

Diagnostic Studies

Laboratory testing is done to ascertain the degree of electrolyte imbalance and malnutrition and to rule out other causes of weight loss and amenorrhea. Suggested diagnostic testing for an individual with a suspected or newly diagnosed eating disorder includes: CBC (anemia), serum electrolytes (potassium, sodium, phosphorous, magnesium, and acid-base imbalance), fasting glucose (diabetes), thyroid studies (hyperthyroidism), liver function testing, follicle-stimulating hormone (FSH), luteinizing hormone (LH), urinalysis, electrocardiogram (for premature ventricular contractions and QT prolongation), and bone density (if amenorrheic to assess for osteopenia).

Management

Management of children and adolescents with anorexia or bulimia is difficult, in part because the child, family, and even the healthcare provider often deny the significance of the problem. Therefore referral to behavioral health specialists, especially those with a subspecialization in treating eating disorders is needed. Even though early detection and treatment are helpful to reduce physical complications, diagnosis can be complicated, and treatment may be inadequate. Because the issue is not food, but rather sociopsychological dynamics of control in the child's life, effective treatment is complex and long term. Eating disorders are managed with a multifaceted approach with emphasis on nutritional rehabilitation, pharmacotherapeutics (e.g., antidepressants, atypical antipsychotics), and individual, family, and group therapy. Intensive, inpatient management is warranted for medical instability, psychosis or self-destructive behavior, and failure to improve with outpatient therapy.

Many children and adolescents with eating disorders require inpatient management, especially if there are fluid and electrolyte imbalances, cardiovascular instability, or significant mental illness. Individual and family therapy is critical. Pharmacologic approaches include antidepressants and atypical antipsychotics, but their use is controversial in many cases. The role of the PCP in the management of eating disorders is primarily that of screening and early identification. Weight gain during refeeding is expected to occur at 1.1 pounds (0.5 kg) per week.[38] Close monitoring for refeeding syndrome is warranted. This is a rare, potentially life-threatening condition that occurs in the first days of enteral or parenteral feeding and results in severe fluid and electrolyte imbalance. Symptoms include confusion, severe irritability, organ dysfunction, and seizures.

Complications

Anorexia has the highest mortality rate of all mental health disorders. The complications of anorexia or bulimia include death, usually secondary to cardiac arrhythmia, hypokalemia, congestive heart failure, or suicide; altered metabolism (chronic); alcohol and drug addictions; osteoporosis; gastrointestinal disturbance: ulcers; motility disorders; fertility problems; gynecologic problems related to prolonged amenorrhea; growth retardation; and dehydration.

Substance Use Disorder

Substance use is a precursor to abuse or dependence, and regular use clearly increases the risk for developing an SUD. However, the use of substances per se is not sufficient for a diagnosis of SUD. Substance abuse is a maladaptive pattern of the use of alcohol or drugs manifested in significant impairment or distress. The criteria for SUD in the DSM-5TR is divided into specific categories (alcohol, caffeine, cannabis, tobacco, and so on), and in adults, it includes tolerance, withdrawal, and compulsive substance use.[1] For children and adolescents, tolerance and loss of control are not good indicators for a diagnosis. Instead, substance-related blackouts, craving, and impulsive sexual or risk-taking behavior are more important criteria.

The cause of SUD is multifaceted. Many contributing factors exist, including:

- Genetic vulnerability (family history)
- Parental substance use
- Dysfunctional family relationships (i.e., rigidity, distant relationships, neglect) and negative life events
- Psychiatric conditions (e.g., CD, ADHD, depression), low self-esteem, poor body image, ineffective coping (poor emotional regulation, poor problem-solving skills)
- Poor sleep hygiene
- School failure
- Low religiosity
- Competitive athleticism
- Adverse life events and trauma response.

Precipitating life events tend to center around loss of relationships (e.g., parental separation, divorce, or death; death of a close friend) and chronic negative circumstances (e.g., parental substance abuse, maltreatment).

Data from the Youth Risk Behavior Survey indicate that 29% of teens reported drinking alcohol and 21% reported using marijuana within the previous month.[39] Approximately 14% of high school students binge drink and 7% report opioid misuse. Nearly half of problem drinkers are thought to try alcohol by age 10 years and two-thirds by age 13 years. Most adolescents who use drugs do not progress to abuse or dependence. Peer influence is not as important in substance abuse as previously thought; it remains important in substance use. Males use both alcohol and drugs of all kinds at higher rates than females. For both males and females, abuse of alcohol and other drugs is negligible from 10 to 13 years old, but doubles between adolescence (12–16 years old) and late adolescence (17–20 years old), peaks between 18 and 25 years old, and declines thereafter. The percentage of students reporting lifetime use of alcohol, marijuana, cocaine, synthetic marijuana, methamphetamine, and heroin use has decreased in the past decade.[39]

Clinical Findings

Identifying an adolescent's problem with substance abuse requires a careful assessment, conducted with an accepting, nonjudgmental, nonthreatening, matter-of-fact attitude. The covert nature of substance abuse and the dynamic of denial make it crucial to avoid a critical tone (see Chapter 13 for discussion of adolescent risk behaviors).

Interviewing the adolescent and obtaining collateral from the parents/caregiver is a key strategy for obtaining information about etiologic factors and behavioral, cognitive, emotional, and physical changes that they have observed in the adolescent. However, it is essential that the adolescent is interviewed alone at every visit to assess mental health and family issues. When talking about substance use with an adolescent, it is important to begin with general questions that are not overly personal. Begin by asking the adolescent about acquaintances or friends who smoke, drink, or use drugs; whether anyone in the family has had problems with these; and what the adolescent does with friends when they get together. It is helpful to ask about experimentation, under what circumstances it occurs, and the adolescent's feelings about it. To obtain a chronologic history of tobacco, alcohol, or drug use, it may be helpful to approach the subject by inquiring about prescription drugs and moving to illicit substances. The key is to remain nonjudgmental to elicit information that will indicate whether the adolescent is experimenting, a regular user, or dependent on substances. Ask about the adolescent's source of drugs or alcohol; the adolescent who uses substances provided by a friend, family member, or acquaintance is less advanced than one who purchases them directly. The practitioner should ask, "What? How much? How often? When? How? Where? With whom? Does the patient use substances at parties, home, school, alone, or with friends?"

Adolescents who screen positive should receive Screening, Brief Intervention, and Referral to Treatment (SBIRT). Information and training can be found at https://www.samhsa.gov/sbirt.

The CRAFFT questionnaire (https://crafft.org/) is an age-appropriate screening instrument for substance abuse in the primary care setting. Positive responses to two or more items indicate a high likelihood for substance abuse and merits further evaluation and treatment.

Significant behavioral changes that may reflect drug use or exposure include the following:

- Infancy and early childhood: Excessive crying; poor feeding or failure to thrive; irritability, jitteriness, or excessive lethargy; poor eye contact; sleep disorders
- Middle childhood and adolescence: Decreased school performance; lethargy, hyperactivity or agitation, hypervigilance, decreased attention; disinhibition; risk-taking behavior; repeated absences or suspensions from school; marked oppositionality; loss of interest in previously enjoyed activities; withdrawal from family and usual friends, or change in friends to those involved in drugs and alcohol; irritability, fighting, or acting out; hypersexuality; exaggerated mood swings; sleep pattern changes or nightmares; altered menstruation; and change in appetite (from anorexia to unusual hunger)

Mood changes include swings from depression to euphoria, nervousness, unreasonable anger, and frequent expressions of hopelessness or failure. Low self-esteem typically characterizes those who abuse substances.

Physical signs that indicate a substance use problem include the following:

- Weight loss
- Red eyes with inhaled or smoked substances
- Hoarseness, chronic cough, wheezing, frequent "colds" or "allergy" symptoms, epistaxis, and perforations of nasal septum with cocaine and inhalant use
- Accidents, trauma, injuries
- Intoxication
- Complete or partial amnesia for events during intoxication with alcohol and date rape drug use
- Dilated or constricted pupils
- Gynecomastia, irregular periods, small testes with marijuana
- Needle tracks occur with intramuscular steroids or intravenous use
- Generalized pruritus with opiate use

- Reflux, diarrhea, gastritis, and constipation with opiate and alcohol use
- Perioral sores or pyodermas from huffing and bagging

Differential Diagnosis

Substance abuse is distinguished from social drinking or non-pathologic substance use by the presence of compulsive use, craving, or substance-related problems. SUDs are comorbid most often with CD, depression, and anxiety.

Diagnostic Studies

Urine toxicology can be helpful to verify adolescent truthfulness, although a positive drug screen result does not indicate substance abuse or dependence; it only indicates substance use. A negative drug screen result does not rule out an SUD. The approximate duration that drugs can be detected in the urine is as follows[40]:
- Alcohol—10 to 12 hours
- Amphetamines—2 to 4 days
- Cocaine and its major metabolite—1 to 3 days
- Benzodiazepines—1 day to 1 week
- Barbiturates—1 day to 1 week
- Opiates—2 to 5 days
- Marijuana—up to 30 days

Duration of detection from last substance use varies according to the laboratory and type of test used. All urine tests should be validated by measuring specific gravity to ensure sample is not very dilute urine (creatinine between 2 and 20 mg/dL).[40]

Management

Exposure to tobacco, alcohol, and illicit substances begins in early childhood as young children observe those around them. The pediatric PCP should discuss parental modeling for the use of alcohol, tobacco, and other substances in early childhood during routine well-child visits. It is important to educate school-age children and their parents about substance use and its consequences. Parents must be educated that "just say no" education is not evidence based. For adolescents, a direct assessment and an interview about substance use are essential. Parents should be advised not to involve their child in their own substance use. Something as seemingly innocuous as "getting dad a beer from the refrigerator" gives the child practice in alcohol use.

Substance abuse must be treated, and prompt referral to substance abuse treatment is crucial. The initial goal is to help adolescents take positive steps toward changing their substance use and abuse behavior. If the adolescent denies a problem, efforts should focus on helping the adolescent modify their willingness to change. Providers should ask open-ended questions and acknowledge positive steps. Providing information about substance use, clarifying reported negative consequences, creating doubts about substance use, and raising awareness of the risks related to current use including the risks of not changing are helpful strategies. It is important to remain empathic and yet emphasize the adolescent's responsibility to make healthy choices. If the adolescent does not have chronic use, harm prevention is the goal of the intervention. Guide the adolescent to examine his or her substance use responsibly and identify ways to prevent harmful consequences.

If the adolescent progresses to chronic substance use, several options exist. Outpatient or day treatment programs are effective for those who can live and be managed at home. For adolescents with more serious addiction, comorbid psychiatric conditions, or suicidal ideation, residential treatment or hospitalization may be necessary. Given the prominence of family dysfunction and family life events as contributors to SUD, family-based treatment programs are essential. Family treatment, rather than family psychoeducation or family support groups, is superior to other modalities. Follow-up assessments should include substance use issues and other predictors of use: stress or negative life events, depression or negative affect regulation, and the presence of positive support within or outside of the family. Self-help or 12-step groups are an essential element in the recovery process for many but do not work for everyone.

References

1. American Psychiatric Association (APA). *Diagnostic and Statistical Manual of Mental Disorders, Text Revision Dsm-5-TR*. APA; 2022.
2. Barker ED, et al. Annual research review: DNA methylation as a mediator in the association between risk exposure and child and adolescent psychopathology. *J Child Psychol Psychiatry*. 2017;59(4):303–322.
3. Monaco AP. An epigenetic, transgenerational model of increased mental health disorders in children, adolescents and young adults. *Eur J Human Genet*. 2020;29:10.
4. Bartek N, et al. Addressing the clinical impact of COVID-19 on pediatric mental health. *J Pediatr Health Care*. 2021;35(4):10.
5. Samji H, et al. Review: mental health impacts of the COVID–19 pandemic on children and youth—a systematic review. *Child Adolesc Ment Health*. 2021;27(2):10.
6. Federal Interagency Forum on Child and Family Statistics. *America's Children: Key National Indicators of Well-Being, 2021*. US Government Printing Office; 2021.
7. Bitsko RH, et al. Mental health surveillance among children—United States, 2013–2019. *MMWR Suppl*. 2022;71(2):1–42.
8. Walter HJ, et al. Clinical practice guideline for the assessment and treatment of children and adolescents with anxiety disorders. *J Am Acad Child Adolesc Psych*. 2020;59(10):1107–1124.
9. Hagan J, Shaw JS, Duncan PM. *Bright Futures: Guidelines for Health Supervision of Infants, Children, and Adolescents*. Bright Futures/American Academy of Pediatrics; 2017.
10. Price M, et al. Examination of the association between exposure to childhood maltreatment and brain structure in young adults: a machine learning analysis. *Neuropsychopharmacology*. 2021;46(11):1888–1894.
11. Feriante J, Bernstein B, Separation Anxiety. *StatPearls*; 2022. https://www.ncbi.nlm.nih.gov/books/NBK560793/.
12. National Institute of Mental Health. Generalized Anxiety Disorder. www.nimh.nih.gov/health/statistics/generalized-anxiety-disorder.
13. Nazeer A, Latif F, Mondal A, et al. Obsessive-compulsive disorder in children and adolescents: epidemiology, diagnosis and management. *Translat Pediatr*. 2020;9(suppl 1):S76–S93.
14. Frankovich J, et al. Clinical management of pediatric acute-onset neuropsychiatric syndrome: part ii—use of immunomodulatory therapies. *J Child Adolesc Psychopharmacol*. 2017;27(7):574–593.
15. Cooperstock MS, et al. Clinical management of pediatric acute-onset neuropsychiatric syndrome: part iii—treatment and prevention of infections. *J Child Adolesc Psychopharmacol*. 2017;27(7):594–606.
16. Ueda K, Black KJ. A comprehensive review of tic disorders in children. *J Clin Med*. 2021;10(11):2479.
17. National Center for PTSD. *How Common Is PTSD in Children and Teens?* 2014. www.ptsd.va.gov/understand/common/common_children_teens.asp.
18. Smith P, et al. Practitioner review: posttraumatic stress disorder and its treatment in children and adolescents. *J Child Psychol Psych*. 2018;60(5).

19. Cheung AH, et al. Guidelines for adolescent depression in primary care (GLAD-PC): II. treatment and ongoing management. *Pediatrics*. 2007;120(5):e1313–e1326.

20. Zuckerbrot RA, et al. Guidelines for adolescent depression in primary care (GLAD-PC): part I. Practice preparation, identification, assessment, and initial management. *Pediatrics*. 2018;141(3):e20174081.

21. Centers for Disease Control and Prevention. *Ten Leading Causes of Death and Injury*; 2019. www.cdc.gov/injury/wisqars/Leading-Causes.html.

22. Van Meter A, et al. Updated meta-analysis of epidemiologic studies of pediatric bipolar disorder. *J Clin Psychiatry*. 2019;80(3).

23. Hoogman M, et al. Subcortical brain volume differences in participants with attention deficit hyperactivity disorder in children and adults: a cross-sectional mega-analysis. *Lancet Psychiatr*. 2017;4(4):310–319.

24. Jacobson LA, et al. Anomalous brain development is evident in preschoolers with attention-deficit/hyperactivity disorder. *J Int Neuropsychol Soc*. 2018;24(6):531–539.

25. Wolraich ML, et al. Clinical practice guideline for the diagnosis, evaluation, and treatment of attention-deficit/hyperactivity disorder in children and adolescents. *Pediatrics*. 2019;144(4):e20192528.

26. Barbaresi WJ, et al. Society for developmental and behavioral pediatrics clinical practice guideline for the assessment and treatment of children and adolescents with complex attention-deficit/hyperactivity disorder. *J Dev Behav Pediatr*. 2020;41:S35.

27. Anheyer D, et al. Herbal medicines in children with attention deficit hyperactivity disorder (ADHD): a systematic review. *Compl Ther Med*. 2017;30:14–23.

28. US Food and Drug Administration. US FDA permits marketing of first medical device for treatment of ADHD. https://www.fda.gov/news-events/press-announcements/fda-permits-marketing-first-medical-device-treatment-adhd.

29. Horowitz SH, et al. *The State of Learning Disabilities: Understanding the 1 in 5*. National Center for Learning Disabilities; 2017. www.ncld.org/research/state-of-learning-disabilities/executive-summary.

30. Donolato E, et al. Research review: language and specific learning disorders in children and their co–occurrence with internalizing and externalizing problems: a systematic review and meta–analysis. *J Child Psychol Psychiatry*. 2021;63(5):507–518.

31. Siegel M, et al. Practice parameter for the assessment and treatment of psychiatric disorders in children and adolescents with intellectual disability (intellectual developmental disorder). *J Am Acad Child Adolesc Psychiatry*. 2020;59(4):468–496.

32. Connor DF, et al. Maladaptive aggression: with a focus on impulsive aggression in children and adolescents. *J Child Adolesc Psychopharmacol*. 2019;29(8):576–591.

33. Bruno A, et al. Focus on disruptive mood dysregulation disorder: a review of the literature. *Psychiatry Res*. 2019;279:323–330.

34. Hiremath CS, et al. Emerging behavioral and neuroimaging biomarkers for early and accurate characterization of autism spectrum disorders: a systematic review. *Transl Psychiatry*. 2021;11(1).

35. Maenner MJ, et al. Prevalence and characteristics of autism spectrum disorder among children aged 8 years — autism and Developmental Disabilities Monitoring Network, 11 Sites, United States, 2018. *MMWR Surveill Summ*. 2021;70(11):1–16.

36. Hyman SL, et al. Identification, evaluation, and management of children with autism spectrum disorder. *Pediatrics*. 2020;145(1):2019–3447.

37. National Autistic Society. Social Stories and Comic Strip Conversations. www.autism.org.uk/advice-and-guidance/topics/communication/communication-tools/social-stories-and-comic-strip-coversations.

38. Mehler P, Andersen A. *Eating Disorders: A Comprehensive Guide to Medical Care and Complications*. 4th ed. Johns Hopkins University Press; 2022.

39. Jones CM, et al. Prescription opioid misuse and use of alcohol and other substances among high school students — youth risk behavior survey, United States, 2019. *MMWR Suppl*. 2020;69(1):38–46.

40. Hadland SE, Levy S. Objective testing. *Child Adolesc Psychiatr Clin North Am*. 2016;25(3):549–565.

30

Eye and Vision Disorders

TERI MOSER WOO

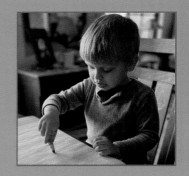

Eye disorders occur most often in the very young or elderly, except for eye trauma, refractive errors, and other select disorders (e.g., retinoblastoma). Infants and children are particularly susceptible to permanent central visual loss (amblyopia), opacities (congenital cataracts), refractive errors not associated with amblyopia, strabismus (ocular misalignment), and other conditions that interfere with visual acuity (ptosis, anisometropia). With early detection and correction, these conditions do not lead to permanent loss in the mature central visual system of the older child or adult.[1] When caring for children with eye disorders, priorities include promoting optimal growth and development of the ocular structures and maximizing visual acuity. To this end, primary care providers (PCPs) seek to promote good vision and eye health, detect abnormalities, treat those conditions that fall within their scope of practice, refer patients with conditions requiring an ophthalmologist's expertise, and provide education and reassurance to parents and children.

Standards for Visual Screening and Care

Pediatric-focused vision objectives in *Healthy People 2030*[2] include:
- Increase the proportion of preschool children (5 years old and younger) who receive vision screening.
- Reduce vision loss in children and adolescents (17 years old and younger).
- Increase state surveillance of tracking eye health and access to eye care.
- Reduce vision loss due to refractive errors.
- Increase access to vision services in community health centers.
- Understand factors that impact use of protective eyewear in occupational and recreational settings.
- Understand the impacts of screen time on eye development and vision loss.

The US Preventive Services Task Force (USPSTF) guidelines for vision screening for children 6 months to 5 years old recommend that screening tests have reasonable accuracy in identifying strabismus, amblyopia, and refractive errors in children 3 to 5 years old.[3] Providers should be alert for signs of ocular misalignment when examining infants and children. Treating strabismus and amblyopia early greatly reduces long-term amblyopia and improves visual acuity.

The American Academy of Pediatrics (AAP), American Association of Certified Orthoptists, American Association for Pediatric Ophthalmology and Strabismus (AAPOS), and the American Academy of Ophthalmology (AAO) jointly recommend that well-child examinations should include ocular history, vision assessment, external inspection of the eyes (e.g., pupils, red reflex), lids, and ocular mobility. This also includes an evaluation of fixation and following (binocularly and monocularly) starting at birth, with patched visual acuity screening starting at 3 years old (Tables 30.1–30.3). Instrument-based vision screening for amblyopia, high refractive error, and strabismus can start in the pediatric office at age 18 months and continue until age 5 years, when traditional vision screening can be performed. If the child is uncooperative, retesting should occur 6 months later. Inability to fix and follow after age 3 months warrants a referral to a pediatric ophthalmologist or an eye specialist trained to treat pediatric patients. Subsequent visual testing should occur at 4 and 5 years of age and every 1 to 2 years until age 18 years.[4] A subjective historical assessment should occur during visits at all other ages. Children who are difficult to screen after two attempts or who demonstrate any other eye abnormalities should undergo photoscreening to detect amblyopia, media opacities, and treatable ocular disease processes with referral to an ophthalmologist as indicated.[4]

For high-risk children, the AAO[4] recommends that asymptomatic children have a comprehensive examination by an ophthalmologist if they have any of the following:
- Vision screening failure or inability to be screened in primary care.
- A vison complaint or observed abnormal visual behavior.
- Health or developmental problems that place the child at risk for developing eye problems (e.g., prematurity, Down syndrome, juvenile idiopathic arthritis, neurofibromatosis, or diagnostic evaluation of a complex disease with ophthalmologic manifestations).
- A family history of conditions that cause or are associated with eye or vision problems (e.g., retinoblastoma, significant hyperopia, strabismus (particularly accommodative esotropia), amblyopia, congenital cataract, or glaucoma.

Development, Physiology, and Pathophysiology of the Eye

Development of the Ocular Structures

At 21 days of gestation, ocular tissue is visible on each side of the head. By the end of the eighth week of pregnancy, the eyelids are completely formed, and the upper and lower lids fuse to seal the eye while it develops. At 16 weeks of gestation, the eyes are fully anterior. By the seventh month of pregnancy, the fetus can open its eyes. Development of the eye as a visual organ is not complete at birth, yet newborns have the ability to fix their gaze, follow an object to midline, and react to a change in the intensity of light.

TABLE 30.1	Normal Visual Developmental Milestones
Age	**Milestone**
Birth–2 weeks	Infant sees and responds to change in illumination; refuses to reopen eyes after exposure to bright light; increasing alertness to objects; fixes on contrasts (e.g., black and white); jerky movements; pupillary reaction present
By 2–4 weeks	Infant fixes and follows on an object, though sporadically
By 3–4 months	Infant recognizes parent's smile; looks from near to far and focuses close again; beginning development of depth perception; follows 180-degree arc; reaches toward toy; few exodeviations; esotropia abnormal
By 4 months	Color vision near that of an adult; tears are present
By 6–10 months	Infant fixes on and follows toy in all directions; movements smooth
By 12 months	Vision is close to fully developed

TABLE 30.2	Visual Acuity Norms (Snellen Equivalents)	
Age	**Forced-Choice Preferential Looking (FPL)**	**Age Visual-Evoked Potential (VEP)**
Birth	20/400	20/800
2 months	20/400	
4 months	20/200	20/600
6 months	20/150	20/400
12 months	20/50	20/20
18–24 months	20/25 or 20/20	
5 years	20/25 or 20/20	

Over the first 2 to 3 months of extrauterine life, the ability to focus develops as the eyes become coordinated horizontally and vertically. By 3 months old, infants can follow moving objects; by 4 months old, they can indicate visual recognition of familiar objects. The shape and contour of the eyeball change, and visual acuity and binocularity gradually increase with age. The volume of the orbit doubles by the time the child is 1 year old and almost doubles again by age 6 to 8 years. Eye growth is completed at age 10 to 13 years. The corneal dimension, however, changes minimally from the full-term newborn to adulthood.

During early childhood, the visual pathways that ensure central vision are developing. The brain must receive equally clear, bilaterally focused images at the same time for this development to occur. The adult visual field is obtained by age 10 years. The visual pathways are amenable to the greatest corrective influences (e.g., adequate treatment of amblyopia) until age 7 to 8 years. Research has demonstrated that the visual system of teens and adults with amblyopia might still retain substantial plasticity into adulthood.[5]

Anatomy and Physiology of the Eye

The eyeball consists of three layers of tissue: the fibrous tunic, the vascular tunic, and the inner tunic or retina. The fibrous tunic consists of the sclera and the cornea. The vascular tunic, the middle layer, is composed of the choroid, the ciliary body, and the iris (Fig. 30.1). All the structures of the eye are dedicated to accurate and efficient functioning of the innermost layer of the eyeball, the retina. The optic disc consists only of nerve fibers (no rods or cones), so no visual images are formed here. Thus, it is referred to as the *blind spot*.

The inside of the eyeball consists of the anterior and posterior cavities (see Fig. 30.1). The anterior cavity is divided into anterior and posterior chambers. The anterior chamber lies between the cornea and the iris. The posterior chamber lies between the iris and the suspensory ligament. Aqueous humor circulates throughout these chambers to maintain intraocular pressure (IOP) and link the circulatory system with the avascular lens and cornea. The other cavity within the eyeball, the posterior cavity, lies between the lens and the retina. The gelatinous vitreous humor found in this cavity contributes to the maintenance of IOP and holds the retina in place. The lens, which separates the cavities, hangs by the suspensory ligament. Six muscles guide movement of the globe. Four rectus muscles (superior, inferior, lateral, and medial) move the eyeball up, down, in, and out, respectively. Two oblique muscles (superior and inferior) rotate the eyeball on its axis. Cranial nerve (CN) III (oculomotor), CN IV (trochlear), and CN VI (abducens) innervate these muscles.

The focusing of light rays involves four basic processes: (1) refraction of light rays, (2) accommodation of the lens, (3) constriction of the pupil, and (4) convergence of the eyes. *Refraction* is the bending of light rays as they pass from one transparent medium (air) to another (cornea or lens). The lens modifies the degree of refraction to create the sharpest image on the retina. *Accommodation* is the ability of the lens to focus on close objects by increasing its curvature. The normal eye refracts light rays from an object 20 feet away to focus a clear image onto the retina; hence the fraction 20/20 is used to denote the accepted standard of normal vision. The circular muscle fibers of the iris, which contract in response to light, cause constriction of the pupil. Regulating the light entering the eye can also facilitate production of a precise image. To maintain single binocular vision, close objects require the eyes to rotate medially so that the light rays from the object hit the same points on both retinas. This rotation is called *convergence*. A normal neonate demonstrates disconjugate eye movements, but convergence and accommodation normally develop by 3 to 4 months old, with parallel alignment by 5 to 6 months old without nystagmus or strabismus. Jerky eye movements can be seen until 2 months old, after which time smooth tracking movements are expected.

After an image is formed on the retina, light impulses are converted into nerve impulses and transmitted to the visual centers located in the occipital lobes of the cerebral cortex. Lesions in various places along the neural tracts from the eye to the cortex cause different types of loss of visual fields (Fig. 30.2).

Pathophysiology of the Eyes

Potential problems with the eyes or visual system can take the form of specific disorders, infections, or injuries. The most common eye disorders interfering with vision are refractive errors (myopia, hyperopia, astigmatism, and anisometropia). Less common disorders include strabismus, amblyopia, ptosis, nystagmus, cataracts, glaucoma, retinopathy of prematurity (ROP), and retinoblastoma.

| TABLE 30.3 | Recommended Ages and Methods for Pediatric Eye Evaluation Screening |

Recommended Age	Method	Indications for Referral to an Ophthalmologist
Newborn–3 months	Ocular history	
	Red reflex	Abnormal or asymmetric
	Inspection	Structural abnormality
3–6 months (approximately)	Ocular history	
	Fix and follow	Failure to fix and follow in a cooperative infant
	Red reflex	Abnormal or asymmetric
	Inspection	Structural abnormality
6–12 months and until child is able to cooperate for verbal visual acuity	Ocular history	
	Fix and follow with each eye	Failure to fix and follow
	Alternate occlusion	Failure to object equally to covering each eye
	Corneal light reflex	Asymmetric
	Red reflex	Abnormal or asymmetric
	Inspection	Structural abnormality
	Photoscreening	Abnormal finding
3 years and older and every 1–2 years after 5 years	Ocular history	
	Visual acuity[a] (monocular)	36–47 months: 20/50 or worse 48–59 months: 20/40 or worse >5 years: 20/30 or worse, or two lines of difference between the eyes 36–47 months: must correctly identify the majority of the optotypes on the 20/50 line to pass 48–59 months: must correctly identify the majority of the optotypes on the 20/40 line to pass
	Corneal light reflex/cover-uncover reflex	Asymmetric/ocular refixation movements
	Red reflex	Abnormal or asymmetric
	Inspection	Structural abnormality
	Photoscreening or autorefraction	Abnormal findings
	Attempt ophthalmoscopy	

[a]Pictures (Lea Hyvärinen [LH/LEA] symbols or Allen cards for age 2 to 4 years); "tumbling E" or HOTV for ≥age 4 years; or vision testing machines.

Data from American Academy of Pediatrics (AAP) Committee on Practice and Ambulatory Medicine and Section on Ophthalmology, American Association of Certified Orthoptists, American Association of Pediatric Ophthalmology and Strabismus, American Academy of Ophthalmology (AAO). Eye examination in infants, children, and young adults by pediatricians: policy statement, *Pediatrics.* 2003;111(4):902–907; and American Association of Pediatric Ophthalmology and Strabismus (2014) Vision screening recommendations.

Infections and injuries may be relatively minor and superficial or critical and involve deep tissues of the eye. Certain systemic diseases (e.g., juvenile rheumatoid arthritis) and medications (e.g., steroids) can also affect the eyes and warrant extra assessment measures.

Assessment

Assessment of the eye, as with all body systems, requires a thoughtful history, careful physical examination, and certain specialized screening tests.

History

- General medical history, including birth weight; pertinent prenatal, perinatal, postnatal factors (e.g., prematurity, infections); past hospitalizations and surgery; general health and development
- Family medical history of ocular problems including eye surgeries: glaucoma, blindness, poor vision, difficulty walking in dim light, photophobia, use of lenses or contact lenses, lazy eye, strabismus, nystagmus, leukokoria, retinoblastoma, congenital cataracts
- History of chronic systemic disease in patient or family: e.g., inflammatory bowel disease; connective tissue disorders; cardiac defects of Marfan syndrome; midfacial hypoplasia; abnormalities of teeth, or urinary tract; neurologic or skin anomalies; developmental delay; intellectual disability; diabetes; sickle cell hemoglobinopathies; Tay-Sachs disease; tuberculosis
- Presence of allergies and specific allergens

- Current medications (e.g., steroids); past or present substance abuse
- Child's ocular history, including:
  - Date (and results) of the last vision screening and prior eye problems or diseases, including diagnoses and treatments
  - If history of eye injury: Unilateral or bilateral injury? Were there visual changes or photophobia? What treatment was received?

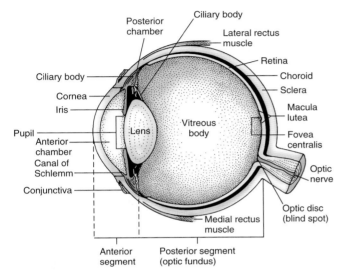

• **Fig. 30.1** Anatomy of the Eye. (From Ignatavicius DD, Workman LM, Rebar CR, et al. *Medical-Surgical Nursing: Concepts for Interprofessional Collaborative Care*, ed 10. Elsevier; 2021.)

- Prescription and use of eyeglasses or contact lenses: Does the child have glasses that were prescribed? Are they used? If not, why?
- Use of sunglasses with ultraviolet (UV) protection and protective eyewear for sports activities
- History of double vision or concussion.
- Symptoms or indications of eye dysfunction or disease:
  - Older children may report visual loss or change in vision, such as blurring, diplopia, spots, and halos. Younger children may be observed to have problems with fixing or focusing (holding objects up close to see), tracking, squinting, head tilt, eye-hand coordination, grasp, gait, balance, behavior, and changes in the ability to maintain eye contact, eyelid droop.
  - Photophobia may present as irritability, shielding, or rubbing of the eyes.
  - Swollen eyelids, pruritus, excessive tearing or discharge, erythema, burning, eye fatigue, strabismus
  - Constant blinking, chronic bulbar conjunctival injection

Physical Examination

The physical examination can be challenging depending on the child's age. The components need to be performed quickly to accommodate the child's short attention span and tolerance. Knowledge of visual developmental milestones is essential in assessing a child's visual capabilities (see Table 30.1):

- Gross inspection should be made of the external structures with a penlight (lids, bulbar and palpebral conjunctiva, cornea, lacrimal structures, and the size, symmetry, and reactivity of the pupils), orbits, eye muscle balance, and mobility.

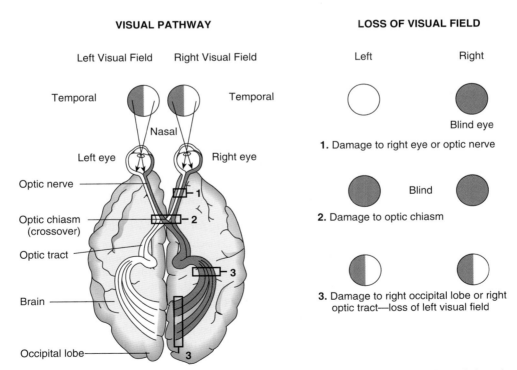

• **Fig. 30.2** Visual Pathway. On the right are diagrams of the visual fields with areas of blindness darkened to show the effects of injuries in various locations. (From VanMeter KC, Hubert RJ. *Gould's Pathophysiology for the Health Professions*, ed 7. Elsevier; 2023.)

- The red reflex is tested in all ages. It needs to be assessed for color, intensity, and clarity (opacities or white spots). A rule of thumb is that if the examiner cannot see into the eye (e.g., absent red light reflex), the patient cannot see out.
- In children older than 5 years, funduscopic examination allows for visualization of the retina, choroid, fovea, macula, optic disc and cup, and entry and exit of the vessels and nerves.
- Examination of the eye for possible foreign body is sometimes facilitated by using a cotton-tipped applicator to evert the eyelid. Eyelid eversion is accomplished by having the patient look down while the examiner grasps the lashes with the thumb and index finger, places the applicator in the middle of the lid, pulls the eyelid down and out, and everts it over the applicator.
- Growth parameters (especially head growth and shape) and the head and neck or other structures should be examined if a systemic condition is suspected.

Screening Tests

Conducting Screening Tests

Fatigue, hunger, anxiety, and environmental distractions can interfere with vision testing in children and adolescents. Testing should always precede the administration of immunizations or any procedure that might cause discomfort. While testing, observe children for behavior indicating that they are having difficulty, such as straining, squinting, excessive blinking, head tilting or shaking, or thrusting the trunk or head forward. The tendency to peek out from behind the eye shield may or may not reflect difficulty; the child may do so out of a desire to be successful and please the tester. The examiner should resist the tendency to correct a mistake or give the child nonverbal clues that can influence the results. Three-year-old children who have difficulty performing any of the vision tests in the PCP's office should be tested again within 6 months; those unable to perform when older than 4 years should be retested in 1 month. A child who is uncooperative on the second attempt should be referred for a formal examination.[4]

Red Reflex

The red reflex should be tested at every well examination, including the initial newborn examination. Performing the red reflex (Bruckner) test allows the clinician to detect the presence of asymmetric refractive errors, strabismic deviations, and abnormalities in the ocular media (e.g., cataracts, corneal abnormalities, retinoblastoma). Disease processes involving the cornea, lens, vitreous, or retina block the light from entering or exiting the pupil and result in an abnormal red reflex. The recommended technique follows:

- Darken the examination room, it is easier to detect more subtle asymmetries between the red reflexes.
- Stand an arm's length away from the infant or child and use the ophthalmoscope light set at 0 or +1 to illuminate the face.
- Look at both pupils simultaneously and separately. In children with fair skin pigmentation, the red reflex is bright red orange; in those with darker pigmentation, the red reflex is often pale appearing or dark red-brown.
- The red reflexes should be symmetric; any asymmetry, dark or white spots, opacities, or leukocoria (white pupillary reflex) requires prompt referral to an ophthalmologist.

Visual Acuity Testing

Visual acuity screening (see Tables 30.2 and 30.3) for both near and distance vision, should be performed on all children during routine health maintenance visits, when problems with visual acuity are suspected, and/or when eye trauma occurs. Children who are not reading at grade level after age 5 years should also have formal visual acuity screening.[4] If vision is normal, the child may require further cognitive or learning evaluations. If the child wears eyeglasses or contact lenses, visual acuity measurement should be obtained using corrective devices.

Color Vision Testing

The human retina contains 6 million red and green cones and approximately 1 million blue cones. Alterations in color vision occur when the normal photopigments in the photoreceptor cones are replaced with different ones. Color ranges are then interpreted or perceived differently.

Red-green color deficiency can be due to an X-linked inherited disorder or may indicate optic nerve disease. Inherited color deficiencies are more common in males than in females. In a study examining ethnicity and color blindness, the prevalence of color blindness was highest in non-Hispanic White males at 5.6%, 3.1% among Asian males, 2.6% among Hispanic males, and 1.4% among Black males. Color vision deficiency may also be acquired. A patient with acquired deficiency may have had normal color vision and then experienced color changes and losses. Diabetes, infections, optic neuritis, and toxins are systemic conditions that can lead to such losses. Blue-yellow deficiency is the most common type of acquired color deficiency.

Significant color blindness can affect school performance, have safety implications if the child is unable to distinguish traffic or vehicle brake lights, and affect career choices. Color vision is tested by using the Richmond pseudoisochromatic plates (formerly Hardy-Rand-Rittler plates) or Ishihara plates.[4] Children 3 to 4 years old are usually able to comply with testing directions, but the test does not routinely need to be administered (parents may request testing when their child is young and makes errors when asked to identify colors). In a child who is truly color deficient, the colors are not misnamed.

Peripheral Vision Testing

Examination of peripheral visual fields provides information about retinal function, the neuronal visual pathway to the brain, and the function of CN II (optic nerve). In an infant, assessment is limited to a rough estimate of peripheral visual fields by watching the child's response to a familiar object (e.g., bottle, toy) as it is brought into each of the four quadrants.[4] In children mature enough to cooperate, peripheral visual fields can be measured by confrontation or by finger counting. Peripheral visual fields should be approximately 50 degrees upward, 70 degrees downward, 60 degrees medially (toward the nose), and 90 degrees laterally.

Testing for Ocular Mobility and Alignment

The Hirschberg test (i.e., corneal light reflex) evaluates extraocular muscle function by projecting a small light source onto the cornea of the eye with the child looking straight ahead. A normal test reveals the reflected light as a small white dot symmetrically located in the same position of each eye (often slightly nasal of center).[4] The cover-uncover test and the alternating cover test should be performed with the child fixating straight ahead, first on a near point object and then on a far point object about 20 feet away (Fig. 30.3). The process is sometimes aided by asking the child questions about the object (e.g., "How many cows do you see?" in a picture that has been placed for this purpose on the wall). During the alternating cover test, the examiner rapidly

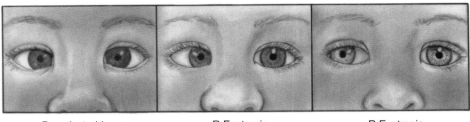

Pseudostrabismus   R Esotropia   R Exotropia

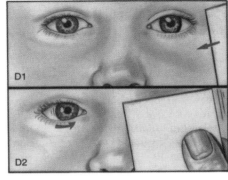

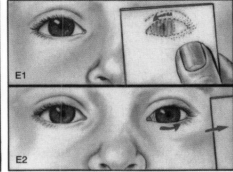

Right, uncovered eye is weaker   Left, covered eye is weaker

• **Fig. 30.3** Extraocular Muscle Function Testing (Corneal Light Reflex and Cover Test). (From Jarvis C. *Physical Examination and Health Assessment*, ed 2. Saunders; 1996.)

covers and uncovers the eye while shifting between the two eyes. Any orbital movement is an indication of misalignment, and the child referred immediately to an ophthalmologist.

Assessment of Visual Loss

If significant visual disturbance is suspected after functional vision assessments have been performed, the child should be referred immediately to an ophthalmologist.

Diagnostic Studies

Photo Screening and Autorefractors

Photoscreeners and autorefractors may be used to screen for optical and physical abnormalities of the eyes and can be used to screen children at preventive visits in the pediatric office.[1] Photoscreeners can assess the red-light reflex and high refractive error, and screen for amblyopia and strabismus. Photoscreening of preschoolers for amblyopia is more accurate than using an eye chart.[6] Autorefractors may be used to determine the refractive error of each eye. Medial opacities and refractive errors can be discerned using instrument-based screening in preverbal or developmentally delayed children. Instrument-based vision screening has had extensive validation and is a reliable, alternative method for visual screening in children under 5 years of age or who are not able to use vision charts.

Laboratory and Imaging Studies

Cultures and Gram stain of eye discharge are done if identification of infection or organisms would be helpful in guiding management. Ultrasound (not to be used in cases of a suspected ruptured globe), computed tomography (CT), or magnetic resonance imaging (MRI) is sometimes useful in determining a diagnosis of orbital cellulitis, trauma, or tumor, or in substantiating a concern about the central nervous system (CNS). An MRI should not be used in the case of a suspected intraocular metal foreign body.

Fluorescein Staining

Fluorescein staining may be used to determine the extent of damage to the corneal or conjunctival epithelium due to trauma, infection, or exposure to a foreign body. After applying fluorescein, examine the cornea with a cobalt blue filter light; any injury will take up the fluorescein stain and appear as a greenish area. Too much of the stain will cloud the entire cornea.

Management Strategies

Referral for Ophthalmologic and Specialty Management

Although any child with pathologic conditions of the eye should be referred to an ophthalmologist, optometrists can be a valuable resource in caring for children with refractive errors or certain common eye conditions (e.g., corneal abrasions, foreign bodies). Pediatric providers should acquaint themselves with the statutory guidelines for scope of practice and prescription privileges as designated by the state boards of optometry within their state to optimize referral possibilities. See Table 30.4 for guidance on when to refer for a more comprehensive examination.

Ophthalmologic or optometric management of potential or present central vision deficiencies may include the following strategies:

Occlusion

Patching, occlusive contact lens, and optical penalization or pharmacologic penalization with 0.5% or 1% atropine may be used in young children to treat strabismus and improve or prevent amblyopia by blocking vision in the sound eye.

TABLE 30.4	Indications for a Comprehensive Pediatric Medical Eye Evaluation	
Indication	**Specific Examples**	
Risk factors (general health problems, systemic disease, or use of medications that are known to be associated with eye disease and visual abnormalities)	• Prematurity (birth weight less than 1500 g or gestational age 30 weeks or less) • Retinopathy of prematurity • Intrauterine growth retardation • Perinatal complications (evaluation at birth and at 6 months) • Neurologic disorders or neurodevelopmental delay (at diagnosis) • Juvenile idiopathic arthritis (at diagnosis) • Thyroid disease • Cleft palate or other craniofacial abnormalities • Diabetes mellitus (5 years old after onset) • Systemic syndromes with known ocular manifestations (at 6 months or at diagnosis) • Chronic systemic corticosteroid therapy or other medications known to cause eye disease • Suspected child abuse	
Family history of conditions that cause or are associated with eye or vision problems	• Retinoblastoma • Childhood cataract • Childhood glaucoma • Retinal dystrophy/degeneration • Strabismus • Amblyopia • Eyeglasses in early childhood • Sickle cell anemia • Systemic syndromes with known ocular manifestations • Any history of childhood blindness not due to trauma in a parent or sibling	
Signs or symptoms of eye problems by history or observations by family members[a]	• Defective ocular fixation or visual interactions • Abnormal light reflex (including both the corneal light reflections and the red fundus reflection) • Abnormal or irregular pupils • Large and/or cloudy eyes • Drooping eyelid • Lumps or swelling around the eyes • Ocular alignment or movement abnormality • Nystagmus • Persistent tearing, ocular discharge • Persistent or recurrent redness • Persistent light sensitivity • Squinting/eye closure • Persistent head tilt • Learning disabilities or dyslexia	

[a]Headache is not included because it is rarely caused by eye problems in children. This symptom should first be evaluated by the primary care physician.

From American Academy of Ophthalmology (AAO): Pediatric eye evaluations PPP—2017. https://www.aao.org/preferred-practice-pattern/pediatric-eye-evaluations-ppp-2017.

Corrective Lenses

In children, eyeglasses or contact lenses are used to correct refractive errors. Gas-permeable or soft contact lenses can be successfully worn by children as young as 8 years with no higher incidence of corneal problems than adults.[7] Silsoft silicon polymer lenses may be used in aphakic infants and can be worn 24 hours a day for as long as 1 week.[8] Contact lenses (including daily wear [hard lenses] and soft, extended, or disposable wear lenses), in addition to the cosmetic benefit, can provide better refractive error correction than eyeglasses, thereby enhancing visual acuity and the total corrected field of vision. Studies have also shown that their use improves how children feel about their appearance, their athletic abilities, and peer acceptance.[7] The Centers for Disease Control and Prevention (CDC) have recommendations for parents considering contact lenses for their children.[9]

"Plano" lenses (noncorrective, decorative, or theatrical contact lenses used for cosmetic purposes) are available for purchase from nonvision care resources. Severe eye injuries (including blindness) result when people bypass the usual regulatory safeguards (proper fit, adequate instruction on use, and hygiene). Such cases prompted the AAO to sponsor legislation that required the US Food and Drug Administration (FDA) to regulate these lenses as medical devices. The law requires that these types of lenses be properly fitted and dispensed by prescription only from a qualified eye care professional. Another type of plano lens includes those with light-filtering tints. These block or enhance certain colors and are designed for sports use by tennis players, golfers, baseball players, spectators, trap shooters, and skiers. Regardless of federal regulations, over-the-counter decorative contact lenses are still illegally sold on the market.[10] Risks of nonprescription contacts, including corneal abrasions and ulcers, infection, and scarring may lead to blindness.[11]

Keratorefractive (laser-assisted in situ keratomileusis [LASIK]) surgery is undergoing worldwide research for its applicability in children with low to moderate myopia, severe anisometropia, bilateral high ametropia, and refractive amblyopia. However, its use remains controversial. In the United States, LASIK surgery is FDA approved for age 18 years and older.[12] The AAO discourages LASIK surgery in individuals younger than 18 old and provides guidelines regarding suitable candidates for the procedure.[13] General guidelines for glasses and contact lenses can be found in Box 30.1.

Ophthalmic Medications

Caution and precision must be exercised when administering ocular medications to children, because their smaller body mass and faster metabolism may potentiate the action of the drugs and result in adverse ocular and systemic side effects. Topical ophthalmic medications, such as antibiotics, mydriatics, and corticosteroids, are frequently found in ointment or solution vehicles. These topical agents are primarily used for treating disorders affecting the anterior segment of the eye. Solubility is one of several factors that influence the absorption of topical ophthalmic medications. Those that are water soluble (e.g., anesthetics, steroids, and alkaloids) penetrate the corneal epithelium easily. Fat-soluble preparations (e.g., most antibiotics) do not penetrate the epithelium of the cornea unless it is inflamed.

Topical Antibiotics

Prescription of topical antibiotics is ideally based on empirical evidence of infection. Topical ophthalmologic preparations, such

BOX 30.1 Recommendations for Use of Corrective Lenses

Eyeglasses

- Glasses must be changed frequently in children because of head growth.
- Parents should assess the fit of the eyeglasses monthly and watch for behavior that indicates discomfort in a preverbal child (e.g., constantly removing glasses, rubbing at the frames or face).
- Polycarbonate lenses are lightweight, strong, and shatterproof; scratch-resistant coating is recommended.
- Silicone nose pads with nonskid surfaces prevent glasses from slipping.
- Comfort cables secure frames by wrapping around the child's ears and are available for children 1–4 years old. Straps are recommended for infants younger than 1 year old and allow them to roll and lie down.
- Flexible hinges allow outward bending for easy removal by the child.
- Match the frame to the child's facial shape and features to encourage compliance; if old enough, allow the child to choose the frames.
- To encourage compliance with infants and children, do not fight them when they remove glasses; be persistent, replace the glasses, and provide distraction. Parents may need to set the glasses aside for a few hours before trying again. Seek counsel from the prescribing provider for further help.
- Tinted lenses can be used for photosensitivity; ultraviolet (UV) light filters are helpful with aphakia (absence of lens), congenital absence of iris, and albinism.
- Do not place the glasses down with lenses in contact with hard surfaces.
- Clean glasses daily with liquid soap and a soft cloth. (Do not use paper products.)

Contact Lenses

- Contact lenses are appropriate for children 8 years and older; children need to be able to demonstrate ability to manage lens hygiene, including insertion and removal.
- Daily disposable soft lenses are convenient and eliminate the need for cleaning and storage, making their use appealing for children and adolescents.
- Contact lenses are helpful for an aphakic child who would otherwise need very thick glasses that distort images.
- Wear protective outer eyewear for sports.
- Do not wear contact lenses if one or both eyes are inflamed or when using topical ophthalmic medications.
- Children with recurrent conjunctival or corneal infections, inadequate tears, severe allergies, or excessive exposure to dust or smoke should not wear contact lenses.
- Omit wearing extended-wear contact lenses (usually worn overnight) for 1 night a week to perform lens hygiene procedures.
- Educate regarding proper care of contact lens.

as fluoroquinolones, sulfacetamide, bacitracin, and bacitracin/polymyxin B, are effective and rarely produce a hypersensitivity reaction. Topical penicillins, on the other hand, are to be avoided. The pros and cons of these antibiotics are addressed in later sections of this chapter. Ophthalmic ointments may be preferred over solutions for use in children, especially infants, because they last longer, do not sting, do not need to be given as often, and are less likely to be absorbed into the lacrimal passage.

Ophthalmic Corticosteroids

Although ophthalmic corticosteroids are effective in the treatment of ocular inflammation and traumatic iritis (excluding ocular allergy), a patient with a condition severe enough to warrant consideration of corticosteroid use should be referred to an ophthalmologist. Steroids are associated with numerous complications, such as an increased incidence of herpes simplex keratitis and corneal ulcers, fungal keratitis, corneal perforation and intraocular sepsis, glaucoma, slowed healing of corneal abrasions and wounds, increased IOP, cataract formation, and permanent loss of sight. A child receiving long-term ophthalmologic steroids should be assessed frequently for signs of adrenal suppression or other side effects. Encourage parents to keep scheduled tonometry appointments at 2- to 3-month intervals.

Other Topical Preparations

Topical decongestants or antihistamines or a combination of mast cell stabilizers and nonsteroidal antiinflammatory drugs (NSAIDs) are used in treating various ophthalmologic conditions. Over-the-counter vasoconstrictors or vasoconstrictor-antihistamine preparations can be tried first for mild allergic conjunctivitis. Cycloplegic agents are used for iritis.

Systemic Medications

In ocular infections involving the posterior segment and the orbit, systemic antibiotic preparations are necessary. A combination of topical and systemic antibiotics can also be used. In general, these conditions warrant referral to an ophthalmologist. Systemic drugs may also cause damage to the eyes (Table 30.5).

Eye Injury Prevention

Ocular trauma is the leading cause of monocular blindness in children, with males at higher risk of eye trauma than females.[14] Ninety percent of the injuries could be prevented by using protective eyewear.[15] Most injuries are the result of sports (50% of all eye injuries), toy darts, sticks, stones, fireworks, paintball sports, other projectiles, and alpine skiing.[15] Other causes include battered child syndrome (40% have ocular findings); birth trauma; fingers, fists, or other body parts in the eye; fireworks (firecrackers, sparklers, rockets); and auto airbags. The areas most affected by superficial trauma include the cornea, conjunctiva, and sclera; the most serious eye injuries involve the cornea, iris, lens, and optic nerve and may result from anterior chamber hyphema, vitreous hemorrhage, or retinal tear or detachment.

Prevent Blindness recommends parental supervision and child education regarding eye injury prevention as essential to minimize eye injuries. Prevention includes fundamental concepts, such as understanding the dangers to sight, finding and removing hazards, and watching children closely.[16] Specific prevention steps include:

- In the home, use safety gates and cushion or pad sharp corners, store sharp utensils and tools out of reach of children, and store chemicals securely.
- Toys should be age appropriate and without sharp or rigid points.
- Wear safety glasses or goggles to protect against flying particles when working outside or mowing.
- Restrain children in cars with age- and weight-appropriate restraints and car seats, and do not allow children younger than 12 years to sit in the front seat of an automobile. Limit and supervise the use of laser pointers, BB guns, air rifles, paintball devices, darts, and fireworks.

Sunglasses

Ultraviolet A (UVA) and ultraviolet B (UVB) radiation from the sun can damage the lens and retina of the eye and cause cataracts and other conditions harmful to vision later in life (e.g., macular

TABLE 30.5	Systemic Drugs, Herbs, and Nutritional Supplements That Can Cause Ocular Side Effects	

Drug	Ocular Side Effects	Intervention
Aminoglycoside Antibiotics (high doses)	Retinal hemorrhages, retinal edema	Monitor peak levels of aminoglycosides to stay in therapeutic range
Corticosteroids (prednisone at dosage of 15 mg/day for ≥1 year)	Cataracts, increased IOP	Monitor with ophthalmologic examinations
Digoxin at moderately toxic ranges	Snowy, flickering, yellow vision	Resolves when drug is administered in correct range
Isoniazid in greater than recommended dosages	Loss in color vision, decreased visual acuity, and visual field changes	Effects are reversible only if discovered early Ophthalmologic examination is indicated before treatment and every 6 months; any changes warrant stopping isoniazid and referring to an ophthalmologist
Isotretinoin	Pseudotumor cerebri (after initiating treatment) with resultant blurred vision, visual field loss, and varying visual acuity changes, including optic neuritis, dry eye, decreased night vision, and transitory myopia	Monitor for symptoms. Annual eye examination recommended while on isotretinoin
Minocycline hydrochloride	Pseudotumor cerebri and orthostatic blackouts, evidenced by blurred vision, visual field loss, varying visual acuity changes, diplopia; scleral pigmentation	Monitor for symptoms; scleral pigmentation may not resolve
Amiodarone	Amiodarone-induced kera–topathy, halos around lights and/or a decrease in vision, blurred vision	If possible, stop amiodarone
Phenytoin and carbamazepine	Blood levels in moderately toxic ranges can produce diplopia, blurred vision, nystagmus; sensitivity to glare	Resolve when therapeutic doses are within normal ranges
Topiramate	Acute angle closure glaucoma; mydriasis; ocular pain; decreased visual acuity (myopia)	Onset of symptoms within 3–14 days after medication started; Stop medication Treatment may include cycloplegics, hyperosmotic therapy, and topical antiglaucoma medications
Quetiapine	Cataracts	Monitor with ophthalmologic examinations
Oral contraceptives (estrogen and/or progesterone)	Optic neuritis, pseudotumor cerebri, dry eyes	Monitor
Fluoxetine/SSRIs	Dry eye, blurred vision, mydriasis, photophobia, diplopia, conjunctivitis, and ptosis, potential for angle closure glaucoma in first month of SSRI use if high doses (>20 mg/day) used	Monitor
Chloroquine and hydroxychloroquine	Retinopathy, blurred vision, macular degeneration with long term use	Baseline fundus exam and at 5 years. After 5 years fundus exam every 1–3 years. Males should have baseline color vision test to rule out congenital color deficiency vs toxicity
Herbs		
Canthaxanthin (taken to produce artificial suntan; food coloring)	Decreased visual acuity; retinopathy	
Cassava (with prolonged usage)	Decreased visual acuity; retinopathy	Contains natural cyanide, so it is important that this plant is processed correctly
Datura (may be used by those with asthma, influenza, coughs)	Mydriasis	
Ginkgo biloba	Retrobulbar and retinal hemorrhage; hyphema	
Licorice	Decreased visual acuity	
Vitamin A	Intracranial hypertension	

IOP, Intraocular pressure; *SSRI,* selective serotonin reuptake inhibitor.

Data from Constable PA, Al-Dasooqi D, Bruce R, et al. A review of ocular complications associated with medications used for anxiety, depression, and stress. *Clin Optom (Auckl).* 2022;14:13–25; Prakash B, Kumar HM, Palaniswami S, Lakshman BH. Ocular side effects of systemic drugs used in dermatology. *Indian J Dermatol.* 2019;64(6):423–430; and Stone A. Systemic Rx, ocular side effects: an update. *EyeNet Magazine.* 2021.

degeneration). Sunlight has more UVA than UVB, but UVB is more damaging. Sunglasses should be used to minimize such damage by absorbing these light wavelengths, even if wearing UV-treated contact lenses. It is never too early to start wearing sunglasses. Wearing a hat with a wide (3-inch) brim with sunglasses reduces the UV rays that reach the eyes by half.[17]

Sunglasses should fit well and have large-framed wraparound lenses with side shields to provide the best protection. They should provide 99% to 100% protection from the UVA and UVB short waves.[17] The lens and frame should be constructed of nonbreakable plastic or polycarbonate and be large enough to shield eye from all angles. Darker colors or polarized lenses alone do not offer the protection that is needed unless they specifically state otherwise. Sunglasses that are for fashion purposes or that do not list the UV protective wave spectrum should be avoided, including inexpensive novelty store glasses. In addition to the requisite UVA and UVB protection, the American Optometric Association recommends purchasing only lenses that state that they screen out 75% to 90% of visible light, are gray (for best color perception), and cause no distortion in vision.[18]

Sports Protection

Sports-related eye injuries result in 30,000 emergency department visits a year, yet 90% of serious eye injuries can be avoided by wearing proper eye protection.[19] Eye protection is recommended for any child or adolescent participating in sports that have a high eye injury rate, specifically hockey, fencing, boxing, full-contact martial arts, racquetball, lacrosse, squash, basketball, baseball, tennis, badminton, soccer, volleyball, water polo, fishing, golf, field hockey, paintball games, pool activities, and football. Specific protective eyewear that is labeled ASTM F803 approved should be used for playing sports.[17] Polycarbonate or wire mesh hockey face masks should be approved by the Hockey Equipment Certification Council or the Canadian Standards Association.[19]

Protective eyewear should be properly fitted and selected specifically for the sport. A complete list of recommended eyewear for each sport is available at the AAO website (www.aao.org). The list serves as a useful handout for parents. A headband or wraparound earpieces should be used to secure the glasses. Sports eye guards should have protective lenses designed to stay in place or pop outward in case of a blow to the eye.[16] Athletes who need prescription eyewear can either choose polycarbonate lenses in a sports frame that is rated for the specific sport, wear polycarbonate contact lenses plus the appropriate protective eyewear, or wear an attached over-the-glasses eye guard that also meets sport specifications. Younger children who do not fit into manufactured protective eyewear may be fitted with 3-mm polycarbonate lenses, although adequate protection cannot be guaranteed and perhaps another choice of sport should be discussed.

Protective eyewear is mandatory for all functionally one-eyed individuals (with best corrected vision worse than 20/40 in the poorer-seeing eye) or for any athlete who has had eye surgery or trauma or whose ophthalmologist recommends eye protection.[16,20] In addition, these children or adolescents should not participate in boxing or full-contact martial arts. Caution is also recommended for these individuals if they choose to wrestle, even though there is a low rate of reported injury.

Laser Pointers

Lasers are rated on a scale of I to IV, with class I lasers used in laser printers and class IV used in research lasers. The FDA strengthened its message to manufacturers regarding the labeling and safety of laser pointers, stating class IIIa lasers may be used as pointers, but class IIIb (laser light shows, industrial lasers) and class IV lasers should not be used.[21] Although harmless when used as intended by lecturers, potential injury from direct, intentional, or prolonged exposure to the retina is of concern if the pointers are used as toys. Permanent retinal damage has been recorded from children playing with laser pointers who initially presented asymptomatically.[22] Therefore any suspicion of laser eye injury should be referred to an eye specialist for evaluation.

Computer and Technology Use

Computer vision syndrome is well documented and can lead to eyestrain, headaches, blurred vision, dry eyes, and neck and shoulder pain.[23] Eye strain is seen with computer, tablet, and smart phone use in children and young adults.[24] During the COVID-19 pandemic shutdown, increased computer use in children and adolescents increased myopia significantly over a 6-month period, with worsening associated with less time outside and increased time spent online.[25] AAPOS[26] recommends following the SCREENS mnemonic to keep developing eyes healthy while using technology:

Screen limits: Older children who use digital screens for school work should have limited use of screens for recreation. Children under 2 years should have no screen time outside of video phone time, and 2 to 5 years of age children should limit screen time to 1 hour a day.

Comfort: Screens should be at eye level and at least 25 inches from the eyes. Ideally, any television watching is from a greater distance to relax the eyes.

Rest: Children should take frequent breaks from screens to decrease eye strain. The 20/20/20 rule recommends that children take a 20 second break every 20 minutes and focus on something 20 feet away to allow their eyes to relax.

Eye drops. If screen use leads to dry eyes not relieved by blinking, over-the-counter eye lubricants should be used.

Exit outside: Children need exposure to sunlight and physical activity and should be encouraged to play outdoors for 1 to 2 hours a day, as exposure to natural light can decrease the development of myopia.

No nighttime screens: It is recommended to stop screen time at least 1 hour before bedtime to minimize effects on sleep.

Screen settings: Screen settings should be set with decreased brightness and increased contrast to decrease eye strain.

Vision Therapy, Lenses, and Prisms

Vision therapy, lenses, and prisms are controversial methods of treatment claimed by some to be effective therapy for those with learning disabilities and dyslexia. These interventions consist of (1) visual training, including muscle exercises, ocular pursuit, tracking exercises, or "training" glasses (with or without bifocals or prisms); (2) neurologic organizational training (laterality training, crawling, balance board, perceptual training); and (3) wearing of colored lenses.

In a joint statement, the AAP, AAPOS, American Association of Corporate Optometrists (AACO), and AAO state that vision problems can interfere with learning; however, there is insufficient evidence to support the contention that vision abnormalities cause disabilities, including dyslexia.[27] The joint statement further notes that the literature supporting vision therapy is "poorly validated," anecdotal, and consists of poorly controlled studies. Recommendations regarding vision care for children with learning disabilities include the following[27]:

- PCPs should perform periodic eye and vision screening for all children according to national standards and refer those who do not pass screening to ophthalmologists.
- Children with a suspected or diagnosed learning disability in which vision is believed to play a role by parents, educators, or physicians should be referred to a pediatric ophthalmologist.
- Ophthalmologists should identify and treat any significant ocular or visual disorder.
- PCPs should recommend an evaluation for learning differences and dyslexia, use of only evidence-based treatments, and educational accommodations in school districts.
- Diagnostic and treatment approaches for dyslexia that lack scientific evidence of efficacy (e.g., behavioral vision therapy, eye muscle exercises, colored filters, and lenses) are not endorsed or recommended.

Managing a child with academic difficulties requires a multidisciplinary approach involving educational, psychological, and other medical specialists. Screening for ocular defects early is a routine part of primary care practice, and eye defects should be referred to the appropriate eye specialist.

Visual Disorders

Refractive Errors and Amblyopia

Alterations in the refractive power of the eye include myopia, hyperopia, astigmatism, accommodation, and anisometropia. In a healthy eye, light from a distant object focuses directly on the retina. When variations in axial length of the eyeball or curvature of the cornea or lens exist, light focuses in front of or behind the retina. This abnormal focusing produces an alteration in the refractive power of the eye that results in a visual acuity deficit. Box 30.2 provides more complete definitions.

Refractive errors are the most common visual disorders seen in children. Approximately 9% of children 5 to 17 years of age have significant refractive errors (0.75 diopters or more).[13] Myopia may be present at birth, but it is more likely to develop between 6 and 9 years old with increased prevalence after the adolescent growth spurt.[13] Mild hyperopia is normal in a young child but should decrease rapidly between age 7 and 14 years. There appears to be genetic and environmental impacts on the development of myopia, with the prevalence of myopia up to 80% in East Asian

---

• BOX 30.2 Descriptive Terms for Refractive Errors

Myopia, or nearsightedness, exists when the axial length of the eye is increased in relation to the eye's optical power. As a result, light from a distant object is focused in front of the retina rather than directly on it and child sees close objects clearly, but distant objects are blurry.

Hyperopia, or farsightedness, exists when the visual image is focused behind the retina. As a result, distant objects are seen clearly, but close objects are blurry.

Astigmatism exists when the curvature of the cornea or the lens is uneven; thus, the retina cannot appropriately focus light from an object regardless of the distance, making vision blurry close up and far away. Rarely, can be caused by an alteration in the corneal sphere caused by a soft tissue mass on the inner aspect of the eyelid, such as a chalazion or hemangioma.

Anisometropia is a different refractive error in each eye consisting of any combination of refractive errors discussed earlier, or occurring with aphakia.

---

countries.[13] In a large study of preschool children in Los Angeles, Latino children had worse visual acuity than other races/ethnicities.[28] AAO practice guidelines recommend children spend increased time outdoors to protect against myopia, based on studies indicating increased myopia with more time spent indoors.

Amblyopia affects 3% to 5% of children and is usually a unilateral deficit in which there is defective development of the visual pathways needed to attain central vision.[29] Clear focused images fail to reach the brain and result in reduced or permanent loss of vision. The condition is varies according to the structural or refractive problem that is causing the poor visual image to reach the brain: *deprivational,* or obstruction of vision (e.g., caused by ptosis, cataract, nystagmus), *strabismic* (caused by strabismus or lazy eye), or *refractive* (myopia, hyperopia, astigmatism, anisometropia).

Definitions of varying degrees of visual impairment include:
- Legal blindness: Best corrected distance acuity in the better eye is less than 20/200, a visual field restriction in the better eye of less than 20 degrees, or both.
- Low vision: Corrected acuity is in the 20/70 to 20/200 range; these individuals generally meet requirements for special education.

Clinical Findings
- Squinting
- Fatigue
- Headaches (rare)
- Pain in or around eyes
- Dizziness
- Mild nausea
- Developmental delay
- Tendency to cover or close one eye when concentrating
- Family history of refractive errors, strabismus, or amblyopia

Management
- Refer to an ophthalmologist or optometrist for prescription corrective lenses.
- Once a refractive error has been determined or if a child is wearing glasses, an annual refraction and evaluation is recommended.
- Moderate amblyopia usually responds to 2 hours of daily patching or weekend atropine (produces cycloplegia of nonamblyopic eye, blurring the vision).
- Support and reassurance according to the child's developmental level are needed during the period of adjustment to contact lenses or eyeglasses. Infants and toddlers need distraction with consistent replacement of glasses once removed. Verbal children may be aided by positive reinforcement, such as sticker charts.
- Untreated or inadequately treated amblyopia in young childhood results in irreversible and lifelong visual loss.[13]

Strabismus

Strabismus is a defect in ocular alignment, or the position of the eyes in relation to each other; it is commonly called *lazy eye.* In strabismus, the visual axes are not parallel because the muscles of the eyes are not coordinated; when one eye is directed straight ahead, the other deviates. As a result, one or both eyes appear crossed. In children, strabismus may be manifested as a phoria or a tropia (Box 30.3). Pseudostrabismus is present when the sclera between the cornea and the inner canthus is obscured by closely placed eyes, a flat nasal bridge, or prominent epicanthal folds

Phoria is an intermittent deviation in ocular alignment that is held latent by sensory fusion. The child can maintain alignment on an object. Deviation occurs when binocular fusion is disrupted (i.e., cover/uncover test).
Tropia is a consistent or intermittent deviation in ocular alignment. A child with a tropia is unable to maintain alignment on an object of fixation. Intermittent tropia may occur when a child is tired.
Phorias and tropias are classified according to the pattern of deviation seen:
- *Hyper-* (up) and *hypo-* (down) are used to classify vertical strabismus.
- *Exo-* (away from the nose) and *eso-* (toward the nose) describe horizontal deviations.
- *Cyclo-* describes a rotational or torsional deviation.

(Fig. 30.3). In children older than 7 to 9 years who have acquired tropia, double vision occurs. In those younger than 6 to 7 years, cortical suppression of vision in the deviated eye results, which stops the diplopia but leads to amblyopia. Exodeviations may be constant or intermittent—the intermittent type occurs more often. Both types of strabismus may be hereditary or the result of various eye diseases (e.g., neuroblastoma), trauma, systemic or neurologic dysfunction that paralyzes the extra ocular muscles, uncorrected hyperopia, craniofacial abnormalities, accommodation, and accommodative convergence. Esotropia, where the eye deviates inward, is associated with a history of prematurity, low birth weight, cerebral palsy, and hydrocephalus.[31] Risk factors for exotropia, where the eye deviates outward, include prematurity, genetic disorders, maternal substance abuse during pregnancy, and decreased vision.[30]

The incidence of ocular misalignments is approximately 1% to 6%, and each type varies by population (e.g., there are more exodeviations in Japan and more esodeviations in Ireland). Accommodative esotropia is most visible when the child is looking at a near object, occurs between 1 and 8 years old (average between 2 and 3 years old), and may occur intermittently. Children with esotropia generally have hyperopia of +3.00 diopters.[31]

Variable alignment with transient esotropia is common in the newborn and is normal in the first three months. However, infants ≤4 months old who have constant esotropia and infants >4 months old who have persistent esodeviation or esotropia (even if intermittent) should be referred to an ophthalmologist.[32] Congenital esotropia is ascribed to an infant with an onset younger than 6 months who did not have a deviation as a newborn. Accommodative esotropia is an inward deviation caused by high hyperopia.[31]

Clinical Findings

- Intermittent exotropia in normal children 6 months to 4 years who are ill or tired or when they are exposed to bright light or with sudden changes from close to distant vision. It is more often seen when the child is looking with distant fixation.
- When only one eye is affected, the child always fixates with the unaffected eye.
- When both eyes are affected, the eye that looks straight at any given time is the fixating eye.
- The angle of deviation may be inconsistent in all fields of gaze, often changing with some forms of strabismus.
- Persistent squinting, head tilting, face turning, over-pointing, awkwardness, marked decreased visual acuity in one eye, or nystagmus may be seen.

- Cataracts, retinoblastoma, anisometropia, and severe refractive errors are found infrequently.
  Diagnostic Techniques. The corneal light reflection technique and the cover-uncover and alternating cover tests are used to screen for strabismus. Asymmetry of light reflection on the cornea is indicative of a deviation in ocular alignment. The cover-uncover test is used to detect tropias, whereas the alternating cover test detects phorias (Fig. 30.3). The photoscreener can also be used to detect strabismus.

Management

- Any ocular misalignment seen after 4 months old is considered suspicious, and the infant should be referred. Hypertropia or hypotropia, exotropia, acquired esotropia or exotropia, cyclovertical deviation, or any fixed deviation is an indication for referral to ophthalmology as soon as it is first observed.
- The unaffected ("good") eye is occluded (using an adhesive bandage eyepatch, an occlusive contact lens, or an overplussed lens), which forces the child to use the deviating eye. Surgical alignment of the eyes may be necessary, but this does not preclude additional amblyopia therapy.
- Corrective lenses alone improve amblyopia.[29] Assessment for amblyopia should be done at every visit, even after straightening the eyes, because changes in alignment can occur through the fifth year.
- Botulinum toxin (Botox) may be used as an alternative to surgery in patients with mild esotropia.[31]

Although response to treatment is more rapid in younger children, age should not be used as the deciding factor for referring a child with amblyopia. Typically, change is minimal in children over 12 years, but there have been reports of improvement with treatment even into adulthood.

Blepharoptosis

Blepharoptosis or ptosis is drooping of the upper eyelids affecting one or both eyes. It can be congenital or acquired, secondary to trauma or inflammation. Congenital ptosis is caused by striated muscle fibers of the levator palpebral superioris muscle being replaced by fibrous tissue. It can be inherited in an autosomal dominant fashion with incomplete penetrance (see Chapter 27). Other possible etiologies include trauma to CN III during the birthing process, trauma to the eyelid or neck, chronic inflammation (particularly of the anterior segment of the eye), or a neuromuscular disorder (myasthenia gravis, botulism, muscular dystrophy).[32] Parents may remark that one eye appears smaller. In severe cases, children may assume a "chin-up" head position and/or adapt by raising their brow.

Management

- Refer to an ophthalmologist. If vision is compromised, surgery is performed to prevent amblyopia and developmental delays. Surgical correction depends on the degree of muscle compromise.[33]
- Correct any underlying systemic disease.
- Evaluate for anisometropia (unequal refractive errors in each eye), anisocoria, and decrease in pupillary light reflex.

Nystagmus

Nystagmus is the presence of involuntary, rhythmic movements that may be pendular oscillations or jerky drifts of one or both eyes. Movement is horizontal, vertical, rotary, or mixed, and is classified as congenital or acquired. Congenital nystagmus is present in the first 6 months of life; acquired nystagmus occurs at a later age. Nystagmus can occur in association with genetic mutations, including albinism or trisomy 21, with up to 30% of children with Down syndrome developing nystagmus.[34] CNS abnormalities (e.g., intracranial mass, congenital optic nerve abnormalities) can also contribute to nystagmus, as well as trauma, medications, and radiation. The child may have a history of prematurity, intraventricular hemorrhage, intrauterine psychogenic drug exposure, developmental delays, hydrocephaly, or be an infant of a mother with gestational diabetes. Nystagmus can be inherited, sometimes with a strong family history.

Clinical Findings

The clinician should observe the nystagmus and note as much as possible about the type of movement (up, down, sideways), frequency (number of oscillations per a time unit), distance of movement, field(s) of gaze within which the nystagmus is evident (e.g., field of gaze straight ahead, left, or up), and any compensatory head or neck postures of the child. The movements may be constant or varied, depending on the direction of gaze and head position. Latent nystagmus only manifests when one eye is covered.[35] Infantile idiopathic nystagmus (oscillation of newborn's eyes) is common and exists for a short time during the neonatal period, while opsoclonus (involuntary oscillation) that persists or occurs beyond the initial weeks of life indicates a pathologic condition and requires referral to ophthalmology.

Management and Prognosis

Management consists of treating any underlying systemic disorder and referring the patient to an ophthalmologist. Any acquired nystagmus is most worrisome and requires prompt evaluation. Prognosis is varied, with sometimes only a slightly decreased acuity (20/50 or better) and other times with severe disability (20/200).[34]

Cataracts

Cataract, a partial or complete opacity of the lens affecting one or both eyes, is the most common cause of an abnormal pupillary reflex (Fig. 30.4). The incidence of cataracts is approximately 3 to 4 out of 10,000 live births in the United States, with a variable incidence worldwide.[36] Cataracts may occur spontaneously or be genetic. More than 15 genes are associated with cataract formation. If there is a positive family history of cataracts, a referral to a geneticist is indicated. Cataracts can be the result of infection (e.g., congenital rubella, cytomegalovirus, toxoplasmosis), trauma to the eye (including physical abuse, airbag deployment), metabolic disease (e.g., galactosemia, hypocalcemia), long-term use of systemic corticosteroids or ocular corticosteroid drops, prematurity, CNS anomalies (e.g., craniosynostosis, cranial defects), and demyelinating sclerosis and ataxia-telangiectasia.[36] They may also be seen in children who have other ocular abnormalities, such as strabismus or pendular nystagmus, and in children with type 1 diabetes mellitus, atopic dermatitis, or Marfan syndrome.

Clinical Findings

- A history of maternal prenatal infection, drug exposure, or hypocalcemia may be elicited.
- Cataract appears as an opacity on the lens, either unilateral or bilateral.

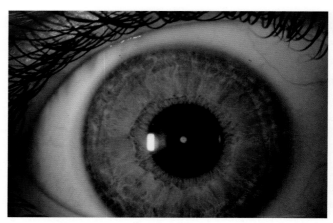

• **Fig. 30.4** Anterior Polar Cataract. A small anterior polar cataract generally results in minimal visual deprivation but is commonly associated with anisometropic amblyopia. (From Lyons CJ, Lambert SR. *Taylor and Hoyt's Pediatric Ophthalmology and Strabismus*, ed 6. Elsevier; 2023.)

- Visual acuity deficits vary.
- A pale red reflex in darker skinned individuals should not be confused with a cataract.

Management

Management depends on the size, density, and location of the cataract. Recommended laboratory workup of a child with bilateral congenital cataracts includes toxoplasmosis, rubella, cytomegalovirus, herpes simplex, and HIV (TORCH) titers, the Venereal Disease Research Laboratory (VDRL) test, serum calcium and phosphorus levels, and urine testing for reducing substances.[36] Genetic testing is recommended if the child has dysmorphic features. A small, partial congenital, or infantile cataract can be monitored over several years for a progression that could produce amblyopia; some types of cataracts do not progress. Patients should be monitored by an ophthalmologist, as amblyopia may develop. Surgical removal of the lens optically clears the visual axis. The resultant aphakic refractive error can be corrected with a permanent intraocular implant, the use of a contact lens, or glasses, although lenses are often very thick causing magnification and limitation of visual fields. Ophthalmic surgeons may insert an intraocular lens into the posterior chamber to partially correct aphakia (absent lens), with residual refractive error corrected with corrective lenses.

Complications

Complications include amblyopia, residual anisometropia, aniseikonia (unequal ocular image between eyes), or intraocular competition. Complications of surgery include infection, retinal detachment, glaucoma, displacement of the intraocular lens, or development of vitreous cloudiness.[36]

Prognosis and Prevention

The ultimate degree of visual function depends on the cataract type, age at time of surgery, underlying disease(s), age of onset and duration, and presence of amblyopia or other ocular abnormalities. If the cataract is dense and present at birth, outcomes are better if removed within the first few weeks of life or before 2 months of age, because amblyopia may occur due to visual deprivation.[36] Visual outcomes are variable, with poorer results seen with congenital unilateral cataracts than with congenital incomplete bilateral cataracts.

Children with a history of cataract surgery may exhibit later inflammatory sequelae, glaucoma, retinal detachment, secondary membranes, and orbital architectural distortions. Use of UV protectant sunglasses is essential in the prevention of cataract formation.

Glaucoma

Glaucoma is a disturbance in the circulation of aqueous fluid that results in an increase in IOP and subsequent damage to the optic nerve. It can be classified according to age at the time of its appearance and type of structural abnormality or other associated conditions. Primary congenital glaucoma is present at birth; infantile glaucoma develops in the first 1 to 2 years of life; juvenile glaucoma occurs after age 3 years. Most glaucoma has no identifiable cause and is considered primary. Secondary glaucoma is associated with another condition. Primary glaucoma occurs because of a congenital abnormality of the structures that drain the aqueous humor. Fortunately, it is rare and generally caught early. The incidence is approximately one in 10,000 live births in the United States, and more common in males at a 3:2 ratio of males to females.[37]

Ten percent of cases are present at birth, and 80% are diagnosed by 12 months of age. About 10% to 40% of primary cases are hereditary, and those with high carrier rate of *CYP1B1* gene (2p21) have a higher prevalence of glaucoma.[37] It is also seen in association with dominantly inherited conditions, such as neurofibromatosis or aniridia; diffuse facial nevus flammeus (port-wine stain); Sturge-Weber, Marfan, Hurler, or Pierre Robin syndromes; intraocular hemorrhage; or intraocular tumor. There is a higher incidence in children with a history of cataract removal.[38]

Secondary or juvenile glaucoma occurs when the drainage network for aqueous humor becomes obstructed after ocular infection, trauma, systemic disease, or long-term corticosteroid use.

Clinical Findings

Parents may report that something is unusual about their child's eyes, such as cloudiness or a blue tint to the eyes. This occurs more often in unilateral glaucoma when the orbital size discrepancy is more noticeable. The clinician should then note the following symptoms of infantile glaucoma:
- Classic triad of tearing, photophobia, and excessive blinking or blepharospasm caused by irritation (manifests only 30% of patients)
- Infants may turn away from light
- Hazy corneas
- Corneal edema
  Corneal and ocular enlargements are common in infants and young children. Bulbar conjunctival erythema and visual impairment may occur. If the condition is bilateral, parents may not notice any difference in the size of the corneas.
  Symptoms of secondary glaucoma include the following:
- Extreme pain, vomiting
- Blurred or lost vision
- Tunnel vision
- Pupillary dilation
- Erythema (often in only one eye)
- Change in configuration of optic nerve cupping with asymmetry between the eyes and loss of vision over time

Management

Early diagnosis is important. The goal is normalization of IOP and prevention of optic nerve damage along with correction of associated refractive errors and prevention of amblyopia.

- Prompt recognition and referral to an ophthalmologist. Examination under anesthesia may be required to get an accurate IOP reading.[37]
- Primary treatment is surgery as early as possible (often multiple surgeries are required). Medications may be used as part of the medical management:
  - Systemic (azetazolamide or methazolamide) or topical (dorzolamide or brinzolamide drops) carbonic anhydrase inhibitors will reduce IOP.
  - Beta-blockers (timolol and betaxolol) or combined beta-blocker/carbonic anhydrase inhibitor drops may be used.[37]
  - Drug therapy may be difficult because of its prolonged nature, drug side effects, and adverse system effects.
- Parent and patient education must emphasize the importance of medication compliance and discourage excessive physical or emotional stress and straining during defecation.
- A medical identification tag should be worn at all times.
- Follow-up is for life, often every 3 to 6 months.
- Ophthalmoscopic examination (including tonometry) is needed for every member of the family.

Complications and Prognosis

Myopia, amblyopia, and strabismus are not uncommon in children with glaucoma. In addition, permanent vision loss secondary to stretching of the cornea and sclera with resultant scarring and glaucomatous optic nerve damage can also occur. Eighty percent to 90% of infants who receive prompt surgery and long-term monitoring will do well, but blindness occurs in 2% to 15% of childhood patients.[37]

Retinopathy of Prematurity

ROP is a multifactorial retinal vascular pathologic disease primarily caused by early gestational age with low birth weight. It involves the abnormal growth of the retinal vessels in incompletely vascularized retinas of premature infants. Previously ROP was called *retrolental fibroplasia*. An international classification system provides guidance for understanding this disease and for predicting outcome. ROP is classified according to the distance to which the vascularization has progressed away from the optic nerve (zone I, II, or III), severity of inflammatory changes (stage 1 through 5), duration (clock hours), and extent of disease (recorded as hours of the clock).[36]

Developing retinal vessels grow outward from the optic nerve. The immature and incompletely vascularized retina is in a state of hypoxia, which stimulates the production of vascular endothelial growth factor (VEGF). Requisite levels of VEGF are needed to maintain the integrity of and stimulate retinal vessel growth. Exposure to supplemental oxygen presents an additional risk factor. Higher oxygen concentrations produce lower VEGF levels and result in slowed vessel growth. Over several weeks, an avascular retina becomes ischemic, and, in turn, stimulates renewed VEGF production. The increase in VEGF stimulates vessel growth but not necessarily in an ordered manner. ROP occurs primarily in premature infants born at or less than 28 weeks of gestation or weighing less than 1500 g. The overall incidence of ROP in all newborns is 0.12%, with the risk in high risk very premature infants under 1250 g up to 68%.[39] Other risk factors for ROP in premature infants include intraventricular hemorrhage, sepsis, respiratory distress syndrome, and mechanical ventilation.[36]

Clinical Findings

ROP is initially diagnosed by a pediatric ophthalmologist while the infant is in the neonatal intensive care unit(NICU) or nursery, with first examination based on gestation at birth (at 31–34 weeks postconception) and chronologic age.[40] All infants born at gestational age 30 weeks or earlier require an ophthalmologic examination. An infant (especially if full/near term) not previously diagnosed with ROP with detached retinas or leukocoria needs an ophthalmologic evaluation to rule out genetic disorders (e.g., Norrie syndrome, familial exudative vitreoretinopathy [X-linked recessive]).

Management

ROP progresses at variable rates. Initial ophthalmologic examinations should be done on all infants born at less than 30 weeks' gestation or weighing 1500 g or less or those born at more than 1500 g or 29 to 34 weeks with an unstable course during hospitalization.[40] The PCP's role in managing ROP is to ensure that all infants fitting these criteria (even in those whose ROP resolved or who did not have ROP) receive the initial and follow-up ophthalmologic examinations (within 2 weeks or less after discharge) by a specialist experienced in examining preterm infants. The PCP further needs to:

- Discuss with parents the implications of their child's disease.
- Monitor for late sequelae or ROP progression (e.g., strabismus, pseudostrabismus, amblyopia, myopia, anisometropia, leukocoria, and cataracts).
- Assist children who have sequelae to maximize their potential by referring to early intervention services for low-vision children, to low-vision community support services, and to family support groups.
- Refer all children for yearly ophthalmologic follow-up if ROP required any treatment (even if ROP has resolved completely); less frequent follow-up is needed if no treatment was needed.

Cryosurgery or laser photocoagulation is used to arrest the progression of abnormally growing blood vessels; argon and diode laser is treatment of choice.[40] Off-label use of intravitreal anti-VEGF monoclonal antibodies bevacizumab (Avastin), ranibizumab (Lucentis) and aflibercept (Eylea) have been used successfully in treatment of ROP and may be used in conjunction with laser treatment.[36]

Complications

Complications can arise secondary to ROP or the treatment. Retinal detachment, strabismus, amblyopia, cataracts, serious myopia, nystagmus, astigmatism, anisometropia, uveitis, hyphema, macular burns, occlusion of the central retinal artery, glaucoma, and cicatrix (residual retinal scars) leading to later vision loss are possible.[40]

Prevention

Minimizing or preventing ROP can be accomplished by decreasing the occurrence of premature births and closely monitoring the oxygen needed to keep oxygen saturation at 90% to 95%.

Retinoblastoma

Retinoblastoma is an intraocular tumor that develops in the retina. Although it is rare, this malignant tumor of the retina is the most common tumor in childhood (4% of cancers in children younger than 15 years old).[41] Age-adjusted incidence is one in 15,000 to 18,000 live births with two-thirds diagnosed before age 2 years, and 95% diagnosed before age 5 years.[42] Single or multiple tumors may be found in one or both eyes. Most children have unilateral tumors (60%), but 40% will have bilateral tumors.[43]

Hereditary and nonhereditary forms occur, and carrier and prenatal diagnosis is possible. Mutation of the *RB1* gene (13q14.2) occurs in hereditary retinoblastoma (40%) and is known as *germinal retinoblastoma*. All bilateral disease is considered hereditary, and 15% of unilateral disease involves germline mutation.[43] It is critical to determine whether the initial mutation is germline, as the ongoing management of the patient and family members will be determined by whether there is a gene mutation or 13q deletion. These patients are at risk for additional retinoblastoma tumors and second primary malignancies throughout life.[42] There is some evidence that human papillomavirus (HPV) is associated with retinoblastoma development in children in developing countries, with HPV 16 and HPV 18 both contributing to the development of retinoblastoma in children in India with no family history.[44,45]

The diagnosis of retinoblastoma in developing countries can be delayed and the care suboptimal due to poor education, lower socioeconomic conditions, and inadequate access to health care. The extraocular spread of retinoblastoma due to delayed diagnosis makes the possibility of death a real concern in developing countries.

Screening Guidelines

The AAP, AACO, AAPOS, and AAO[46] recommend all infants and children should have a red reflex examination before discharge from the newborn nursery, and at every health maintenance visit. The American Association of Ophthalmic Oncologists and Pathologists with support of the AAPOS and the AAP have developed screening guidelines for children at risk of retinoblastoma[42]:

- Screen at-risk children from birth to age 7 years. If children are known *RB1* mutation carriers, they should be screened every 1 to 2 years after age 7 years.
- All children at *high* risk require serial dilated fundus examinations by an ophthalmologist familiar with retinoblastoma monthly for the first 12 months of life, every 2 months between 12 and 24 months, every 3 months between 24 and 36 months, every 4 months between 36 and 48 months, and every 6 months from 48 months to 7 years.
- Children at *intermediate* risk should be screened monthly for the first 3 months of life, every 2 months from age 3 to 12 months, every 3 months from 12 to 36 months, every 4 to 6 months from 36 to 60 months, and every 6 months from 5 to 7 years.
- Genetic testing for the patient with retinoblastoma, parents, and siblings.

Clinical Findings

- Positive family history of strabismus is the most common finding.
- Unilateral or bilateral leukocoria (white pupil), described often as an intermittent glow, glint, gleam, or glare by parents, usually in low-light settings or noted in photographs taken with a flash; also called *cat's eye reflex*.
- Decreased visual acuity.
- Abnormal red reflex, nystagmus, glaucoma, orbital cellulitis, and photophobia (causes pain), hyphema, hypopyon (pus in anterior chamber of eye), or signs of global rupture are possible.

Diagnosis is made via ophthalmic examination under anesthesia, ultrasound, or MRI. CT scans are no longer recommended in children due to high radiation exposure and the risk of radiation-induced second cancers.

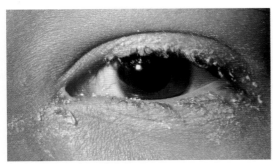

• **Fig. 30.5** Bacterial Conjunctivitis. (From Palay DA, Krachmer JH. *Primary Care Ophthalmology*, ed 2. Mosby; 2005.)

Management

Refer a patient with any abnormal findings suspicious of retinoblastoma to an ophthalmologist for diagnosis and management by a multidisciplinary team. An international classification system for intraocular retinoblastoma lists the criteria of tumors based on their size, location, number, and degree of invasiveness or seeding. Depending on the diagnosis, treatment may involve cryotherapy, laser photocoagulation, episcleral plaque brachytherapy, intravitreous chemotherapy, or enucleation.[47] Early detection and advances in treatment, such as ophthalmic artery chemosurgery and intravitreous chemotherapy, have led to less enucleation, preserving sight. In those with advanced tumors requiring enucleation, a hydroxyapatite implant or porous polyethylene is placed at the time of enucleation. Siblings and parents should receive a referral for examination of the fundi and genetic testing and counseling.

Frequent follow-up (every 2–4 months for at least 28 months or until 5 years old if heritable form) to assess treatment and monitor for recurrence is important. Close to half of children will develop new or recurrent ocular tumors that require further treatment.

Complications and Prognosis

Retinoblastoma has a high cure rate (95%) in the United States, children with unilateral retinoblastoma having the best prognosis.[43] In countries with poor resources, the survival rate may be less than 30%. Children with germinal retinoblastoma have increased risk of other cancers outside the eye and require lifelong follow-up. These subsequent neoplasms are the most common cause of death, contributing to more than 50% of deaths for children with bilateral disease. Most commonly these are pinealoma, osteosarcoma, cancers of the soft tissues, and melanoma.[43] Those who survive are at high risk for cataracts, vitreous hemorrhage, neovascular glaucoma, lacrimal duct or gland injury, impaired orbit bone growth, radiation retinopathy, optic neuropathy, or bone marrow suppression. Late effects of retinoblastoma therapy include diminished orbital growth, visual-field deficits, and hearing loss.

Infections

Conjunctivitis

An estimated 6 million cases of bacterial conjunctivitis occur in the United States annually, at an estimated cost of $800 million each year.[48] Conjunctivitis is an inflammation of the palpebral and occasionally the bulbar conjunctiva (Fig. 30.5). It is the most frequently seen ocular disorder in pediatric practice. In pediatric patients, bacteria are the most common cause of infection

(50%–75%) and there is a seasonal occurrence, most commonly from December to April. Pathogens include *Haemophilus influenzae, Streptococcus pneumoniae,* and *Moraxella* species with both gram-negative and gram-positive organisms implicated.[49]

Conjunctivitis also occurs as a viral or fungal infection or as a response to allergens or chemical irritants. Bacterial conjunctivitis is often unilateral, whereas viral conjunctivitis is most often bilateral. Unilateral disease can also suggest a toxic, chemical, mechanical, or lacrimal cause. Blockage of the tear drainage system (e.g., from meibomianitis or blepharitis), injury, foreign body, abrasion or ulcers, keratitis, iritis, herpes simplex virus (HSV), and infantile glaucoma are other known causes. Patient age is a major indicator of etiology (Table 30.6).

Conjunctivitis in the Newborn (Ophthalmia Neonatorum)

Ophthalmia neonatorum or *neonatal blennorrhea* is a form of conjunctivitis that occurs in the first month of life. In most states, newborn conjunctivitis is a reportable infectious disease. It occurs in 0.3% to 11% of newborns. *Chlamydia trachomatis* is the most common cause of ophthalmia neonatorum, and 25% to 50% of newborns with a mother positive for *C. trachomatis* at the time of delivery will contract the disease.[50] Various bacteria account for 30% to 50% of cases (*Staphylococcus, Streptococcus, Pseudomonas, H. influenzae, Escherichia coli, Corynebacterium* species, *Moraxella catarrhalis, Klebsiella pneumoniae, Pseudomonas aeruginosa*). *Neisseria gonorrhoeae* and HSV are also seen.[50] Gonococcal conjunctivitis accounts for less than 1% of cases but is the most serious cause of ophthalmia neonatorum due to concerns of the bacteria causing blindness.[50]

Clinical Findings
History and Physical Examination
- Septic conjunctivitis caused by:
  - Bacterial infection usually occurs from 5 to 14 days of life.
  - *C. trachomatis* usually begins between 5 to 14 days of life; it can also occur in newborns born via cesarean section with intact membranes.
  - *N. gonorrhoeae* usually appears in the first 3 to 5 days of life (up to 29 days).
  - HSV presents at birth or in the first 4 weeks of life.
  Symptoms most commonly seen include the following:
- Chemical-induced conjunctivitis frequently manifests as nonpurulent discharge and edematous bulbar and palpebral conjunctiva.
- *C. trachomatis* causes moderate eyelid swelling and palpebral or bulbar conjunctival injection and moderate thick, purulent discharge.
- *N. gonorrhoeae* causes acute conjunctival inflammation, lid edema, erythema, and excessive, purulent discharge.
- Bacteria present with conjunctival erythema, purulent discharge.
- HSV causes mild conjunctivitis, erythema, corneal opacity, serosanguineous discharge, and vesicular rash on eyelids and is often unilateral.

There may be a maternal history of vaginal infection during pregnancy or current sexually transmitted infection (STI).

Diagnostic Studies. Swabs and scrapings must be done. Gram and Giemsa staining, direct immunofluorescent monoclonal antibody staining, cultures, enzyme-linked immunosorbent assay (ELISA), or polymerase chain reaction (PCR) testing can be used. Any infant younger than 2 weeks with ophthalmia neonatorum should be tested for gonorrhea. A culture for gonorrhea (on chocolate agar or Thayer-Martin medium) or aggressive scraping for a

TABLE 30.6 Types of Conjunctivitis

Type	Incidence/Etiology	Clinical Findings	Diagnosis	Management[a]
Ophthalmia neonatorum	Neonates: *Chlamydia trachomatis, Staphylococcus aureus, Neisseria gonorrhoeae,* HSV	Erythema, chemosis, purulent exudate with *N. gonorrhoeae*; clear to mucoid exudate with chlamydia	Culture (ELISA, PCR), Gram stain, rule out *N. gonorrhoeae,* chlamydia	Saline irrigation to eyes until exudate gone; follow with erythromycin ointment For *N. gonorrhoeae*: ceftriaxone or IM or IV For chlamydia: erythromycin or possibly azithromycin PO For HSV: antivirals IV or PO
Bacterial conjunctivitis	In neonates 5–14 days, preschoolers, and sexually active teens: *Haemophilus influenzae* (nontypeable), *Streptococcus pneumoniae, S. aureus, N. gonorrhoeae*	Erythema, chemosis, itching, burning, mucopurulent exudate, matter in eyelashes; incidence increases in winter	Cultures (required in neonate); Gram stain (optional); chocolate agar (for *N. gonorrhoeae*); rule out pharyngitis, *N. gonorrhoeae,* AOM, URI, seborrhea	Neonates: Erythromycin 0.5% ophthalmic ointment ≥1 year: Fourth-generation fluoroquinolone For concurrent AOM: Treat accordingly Warm soaks to eyes 3 times a day until clear No sharing towels, pillows No school until treatment begins
Chronic bacterial conjunctivitis (unresponsive conjunctivitis previously treated as bacterial in etiology)	School-age children and teens: bacteria, viruses, *C. trachomatis*	Same as above; foreign body sensation	Cultures, Gram stain; rule out dacryostenosis, blepharitis, corneal ulcers, trachoma	Depends on prior treatment, laboratory results, and differential diagnoses Review compliance and prior drug choices of conjunctivitis treatment Consult with ophthalmologist
Inclusion conjunctivitis	Neonates 5–14 days and sexually active teens: *C. trachomatis*	Erythema, chemosis, clear or mucoid exudate, palpebral follicles	Cultures (ELISA, PCR), rule out sexual activity	Neonates: erythromycin or azithromycin PO Adolescents: doxycycline, azithromycin, EES, erythromycin base, levofloxacin PO
Viral conjunctivitis	Adenovirus 3, 4, 7; HSV, herpes zoster, varicella	Erythema, chemosis, tearing (bilateral); HSV and herpes zoster: unilateral with photophobia, fever; zoster: nose lesion; spring and fall	Cultures, rule out corneal infiltration	Refer to ophthalmologist if HSV or photophobia present Cool compresses 3 or 4 times a day
Allergic and vernal conjunctivitis	Atopy sufferers, seasonal	Stringy, mucoid exudate, swollen eyelids and conjunctivae, itching (key finding), tearing, palpebral follicles, headache, rhinitis	Eosinophils in conjunctival scrapings	Naphazoline/pheniramine, naphazoline/antazoline ophthalmic solution (see text) Mast cell stabilizer (see text) Refer to allergist if needed

[a]See text for dosages.

AOM, Acute otitis media; *EES,* erythromycin ethylsuccinate; *ELISA,* enzyme-linked immunosorbent assay; *HSV,* herpes simplex virus; *IM,* intramuscular; *IV,* intravenous; *PCR,* polymerase chain reaction; *PO,* (by mouth, orally); *URI,* upper respiratory infection.

Gram stain is used for diagnosis. (Do not just sample the purulent discharge.) If gonorrhea is suspected, also check for *C. trachomatis*.
Management
- Irrigate the eyes with sterile normal saline until clear of exudate.
- Gonococcal conjunctivitis: In the newborn, gonococcal conjunctivitis requires intramuscular (IM) ceftriaxone (25–50 mg/kg, not to exceed 125 mg) given once.[51] If there are extraocular manifestations, such as scalp lesions, a 7-day course of IM or intravenous (IV) ceftriaxone is warranted. Ceftriaxone is not given to neonates with hyperbilirubinemia; cefotaxime 100 mg/kg IV or IM is an alternative.[51] Ocular morbidity (corneal infection with possible scarring or perforation) can result if infection is missed.
- Nongonococcal conjunctivitis: A topical ophthalmic antibiotic preparation, such as erythromycin 0.5% ointment, trimethoprim-polymyxin B, or fluoroquinolone drops, is indicated.[49] The eyes should be cleansed with water or saline applied to cotton balls before instilling the ointment into the lower conjunctival sac.

- Herpes simplex conjunctivitis: Immediate referral for hospitalization and topical and systemic antivirals are needed. Spread of virus to the CNS, mouth, and skin is of concern.
- *Chlamydia:* Assess for systemic infection (pharyngitis, ear infection, pneumonia). Chlamydial conjunctivitis is treated with systemic erythromycin (50 mg/kg/day in four divided doses for 14 days) or azithromycin (20 mg/kg for 3 days).[52] Topical treatment is not indicated because it does not lower the risk for a subsequent pneumonia caused by *Chlamydia* (see Inclusion Conjunctivitis in the next section).
- Mothers and their sexual partners should receive treatment if gonococcal and/or chlamydial infections occur in their newborns.

Prevention. To prevent ophthalmia neonatorum, prophylactic administration of antibiotic eye medication within 1 hour of vaginal delivery or delivery via cesarean is indicated.[51] The recommended antibiotic is erythromycin ointment 0.5% (0.25–0.5-inch strip to each eye). Prophylaxis may be delayed for up to an hour to facilitate parent-infant bonding.[51] Prophylaxis is required by law in most states and territories to prevent gonococcal conjunctivitis in the newborn. However, prophylaxis does not prevent neonatal chlamydial conjunctivitis or extraocular infection. It should be determined at the time of the first visit whether infants born at home have received this prophylaxis.

Inclusion Conjunctivitis (Chlamydia)

Inclusion conjunctivitis is usually caused by one of eight known strains of *C. trachomatis* and is most often seen in a neonate or sexually active adolescent. Neonates usually demonstrate symptoms within the first 5 to 14 days of life (up to 6 weeks), whereas *N. gonorrhoeae* symptoms are usually detected earlier. Nasopharyngeal infection with *C. trachomatis* is found in 50% of infants with inclusion conjunctivitis.[53] *C. trachomatis* conjunctivitis in sexually active persons is usually through direct contact with infected genital secretions and presents with nonpurulent erythematous injection of the conjunctiva.

Clinical Findings
History and Physical Examination
- Maternal history of an STI or a history of a sexual partner with an STI.
- Conjunctival erythema and mild to severe mucopurulent to bloody discharge, usually bilateral.
- Follicular reaction (large, round elevations) in the conjunctiva of the lower eyelids; conjunctiva may bleed if stroked.
- Associated cervicitis, urethritis, or rectal infection.

Infants may have symptoms suggestive of chlamydial pneumonia at 1 to 3 months old.

Diagnostic Studies. To achieve a definitive diagnosis of *Chlamydia* conjunctival cells, not just eye discharge, must be collected.[53] Direct fluorescence antibody [DFA] tests are the only FDA-approved test for conjunctival swabs; nucleic acid amplification tests (NAAT) are not approved for conjunctival testing.[53] Specimens are obtained by everting the eyelid and using a Dacron-tipped swab or the swab in the test kit. Scrapings must contain epithelial cells because *Chlamydia* is an obligate intracellular organism. A specimen should also be gathered appropriately to test for gonorrhea because of the comorbidity of these two organisms. Ocular morbidity can result if gonorrhea is missed (see Chapter 32 for guidance on pneumonia caused by *C. trachomatis*).

Management. Systemic therapy is required for treatment of conjunctivitis caused by *C. trachomatis* due to high incidence of concurrent nasopharynx, lung, and genital tract infections in infants and genital infections in adolescents.[53] Treatment options have expanded from the traditional use of oral erythromycin ethylsuccinate (EES) to azithromycin. There is an increased incidence of idiopathic hypertrophic pyloric stenosis (IHPS) in infants younger than 6 weeks following systemic EES. However, this has not altered the recommendation of EES as the preferred treatment. Newborns treated with EES should be monitored for signs of developing IHPS.

Treatment recommendations include:
- A 14-day course of oral EES. A second 14-day course may be required because the failure rate with EES is 10% to 20%. EES may be repeated; oral azithromycin is also effective.[53] Providers are encouraged to use systemic EES with caution; if no other alternatives are viable, they need to have a high index of suspicion for the development of IHPS.
- Azithromycin 20 mg/kg daily for 3 days for infants.
- Doxycycline, azithromycin, ofloxacin, or levofloxacin can be used in young adults.
- Topical ointment (erythromycin, moxifloxacin) is sometimes recommended despite systemic drug treatment; the AAP notes that such concurrent treatment is unnecessary and ineffective.[53]
- Mothers of infants with *C. trachomatis* conjunctivitis, partners of such mothers, and partners of sexually active adolescents also need examinations and treatment for 2 weeks with tetracycline or erythromycin.

Complications. Complications include chlamydial pneumonia (5%–20% of infants will develop pneumonia if their mother has a chlamydial infection at delivery), nasopharyngeal colonization (in up to 50% of infants treated for inclusion conjunctivitis), or gastroenteritis in infants.[53] Complications may occur 6 to 8 weeks following the conjunctivitis.

Bacterial Conjunctivitis

Acute bacterial conjunctivitis (commonly called *pinkeye*) is a contagious and easily spread disease. *H. influenzae* is the most common organism isolated in children who are younger than 7 years old.[49] *S. pneumoniae, M. catarrhalis,* and adenovirus are also common pathogens. It is most common in the winter and in early childhood (see Fig. 30.5).

Clinical Findings
- Key findings:
  - Erythema of one or both eyes, usually starting unilaterally and becoming bilateral
  - Yellow-green purulent discharge
  - Encrusted and matted eyelids on awakening
- Burning, stinging, or itching of the eyes and a feeling of a foreign body
- Photophobia
- Petechiae on bulbar conjunctiva
- Symptoms of upper respiratory infection, otitis media, or acute pharyngitis

Vision screen should be normal and documented in the patient's record

Diagnostic Studies. Routine culture testing is *not necessary.* Gram stain and culture can be done if the conjunctivitis is chronic, recurrent, or difficult to treat. An in-office rapid antigen test with high sensitivity and specificity for adenovirus is available and may be warranted to decrease inappropriate prescribing of antibiotics for viral conjunctivitis.

Differential Diagnosis. Bacterial conjunctivitis requires consideration of nasolacrimal duct obstruction in infants, ear infection,

Kawasaki syndrome, foreign body, corneal abrasion, uveitis, herpetic conjunctivitis, poor compliance, or wrong choice of drug. Cultures or scrapings are appropriate for unresolved infection.

Management. Bacterial conjunctivitis is considered a self-limited disease (unless caused by gonorrhea or *Chlamydia*) that usually resolves within 8 to 10 days. However, because both gram-negative and gram-positive organisms have been implicated, children who receive topical antibiotics demonstrate faster clinical improvement, can return to day care or school faster, and cause less parental work loss.[49] The common practice of prescribing antibiotics for conjunctivitis, however, has led to an increasing rate of drug resistance. It is imperative that providers make their diagnosis judiciously and then treat with an effective drug that is more likely to be tolerated and taken as directed. For this reason, older children and teens may be treated conservatively without using antibiotics. This prevents the overuse of antibiotics and takes into consideration the self-limited nature of this disease.

Choose broad-spectrum coverage that has the lowest resistance rate, greatest compliance, and best penetration of tissues. The cost of ophthalmic antibiotics varies significantly. If patients have a large copayment for brand-name drugs or if they lack paid drug coverage, cost should be factored in when prescribing for this self-limited disease.

Parents can be instructed to put pressure over the lacrimal duct when instilling the medication to prevent drainage into the nasolacrimal system. If improvement is not seen in 3 days after treatment is initiated, refer to or consult with an ophthalmologist. Contacts should not be worn during conjunctivitis treatment, disposable lenses should be discarded, and permanent contacts sterilized before reinserting.

For uncomplicated bacterial conjunctivitis, treatment includes[49]:
- Trimethoprim sulfate plus polymyxin B sulfate ophthalmic solution for 5 to 7 days.
- Erythromycin 0.5% ophthalmic ointment is recommended for patients with sulfa allergy and for infants for 7 days.
- Fluoroquinolone ophthalmic drops including ciprofloxacin, gatifloxacin, levofloxacin, moxifloxacin, or ofloxacin may be prescribed for children older than 12 months for 5 to 7 days (regimens vary by medication).

The aminoglycosides (neomycin, tobramycin, gentamicin) are to be avoided because of possible hypersensitization, severe allergic reactions, and increasing resistance.

Conjunctivitis-Otitis Syndrome. This syndrome is usually caused by *H. influenzae*. Treat for the otitis media (see Chapter 31). Concurrent use of a topical antibiotic is not necessary.

Patient Education. If only one eye is involved, it is likely that the infection will spread within 1 to 2 days to both eyes. The patient (or parent) is instructed to do the following:
- Cleanse the eyelashes several times a day with a weak solution of no-tears shampoo and warm water. The importance of wiping from the inner canthus outward and using a different cloth or cotton ball for each eye should be emphasized.
- Use warm soaks 3 or 4 times a day to relieve itching and burning.
- Instill the prescribed ophthalmic solution or ointment into the lower conjunctival sac. A moistened cotton swab may be used to facilitate instillation of ointments. Dosing while the child is sleeping greatly increases compliance and effectiveness.
- Wash hands frequently and avoid shared linens to limit spread of the infection.

Treat seborrheic dermatitis on the scalp and face if present (see Chapter 37 for treatment recommendations). Daycare center exclusion policies vary, with some allowing return once the treatment is started, while others allow return only after completing 1 to 2 days of treatment. Improvement should be seen within 48 hours. If medication compliance is not in question and improvement is not seen within 72 hours of administration, the PCP should consider referral to an optometrist or ophthalmologist.

Complications. If the infection proves recalcitrant to treatment, eye pain is present, vision is blurred, or ophthalmoscopic examination reveals a bulging iris and a contracted, fixed pupil, suspect more serious inflammation of the uveal tract (iritis, cyclitis, or choroiditis). Refer immediately to an ophthalmologist to avoid ocular morbidity.

Trachoma

Trachoma is a chronic infectious disease of the eye caused by one of the two *C. trachomatis biovars* that exist in the world characterized by follicular keratoconjunctivitis with neovascularization of the cornea. It is contagious, often spreads by direct contact with eye, nose, or throat secretions of infected persons, contact with towels or washcloths contaminated by secretions, or spreads by flies attracted to the eyes. Although rare in the United States, it is the second leading cause of blindness in the world, with 21 million people living with active trachoma worldwide. It is endemic in Africa and found in the Middle East, Southeast Asia, and Northwest India.[54] The peak incidence of active infection is in children 4 to 6 years of age, with scarring and blindness occurring in adults. The World Health Organization recommends community or mass antibiotic treatment within a region when the prevalence of trachoma in children is greater than 10%. Trachoma may be treated with azithromycin with the number of doses dependent on the overall prevalence of trachoma in the local community.[54]

Viral Conjunctivitis

Viral conjunctivitis is usually caused by an adenovirus but can also be caused by herpes simplex, herpes zoster, enterovirus, molluscum contagiosum, or varicella virus. It is more common in children older than 6 years and in the spring and fall (see Table 30.6). Adenovirus causes 65% to 90% of viral conjunctivitis.[49]

Clinical Findings
- Key findings:
  - Tearing and profuse clear, watery discharge
- Fever, headache, anorexia, malaise, upper respiratory symptoms (pharyngitis-conjunctivitis-fever triad) with adenovirus
- Pharyngitis with enlarged preauricular nodes
- Itchy, red, and swollen conjunctiva
- Hyperemia and swollen eyelids
- Photophobia with measles or varicella rashes.
- Herpetic vesicles on the eyelid margins and eyelashes (marginal blepharitis) or on the conjunctiva and cornea (keratoconjunctivitis)

Management
- Good hygiene is essential. Viral conjunctivitis is self-limited and should resolve in 7 to 14 days. Conjunctivitis is often difficult to distinguish from keratitis. If there is any question about diagnosis, refer for ophthalmologic assessment.
- Warm or cold compresses and artificial tears can be used.
- Prophylaxis with antibiotics is not recommended.
- Antihistamine or vasoconstrictive ophthalmic solutions may be used for symptomatic relief.

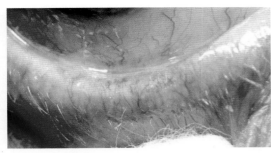

• **Fig. 30.6** Allergic Conjunctivitis. (From Palay DA, Krachmer JH. *Primary Care Ophthalmology*, ed 2. Mosby; 2005.)

- If HSV infection is suspected, immediate referral to an ophthalmologist is indicated. Topical corticosteroids should be avoided because they may worsen the course.
- Molluscum on the eyelid margins requires referral for excision.

Conjunctivitis-Pharyngitis Syndrome. This syndrome is more likely to be caused by adenovirus than by a bacterium and the PCP should treat accordingly.

Complications. Involvement of deeper layers of the cornea (keratitis) can occur and must be differentiated from conjunctivitis. Scarring of the cornea resulting in blindness is a significant complication of HSV infection. If in any doubt, refer to an ophthalmologist for a slit-lamp examination.

Allergic Conjunctivitis

Allergic conjunctivitis usually occurs in childhood but can occur after adolescence (Fig. 30.6). In a patient with allergic conjunctivitis, there is inflammation of the ocular surface in response to an allergen. The onset of symptoms may be chronic or sudden (within 30 minutes) after exposure to an environmental allergen such as animal dander, with itching, tearing, chemosis, and eyelid edema that resolves within 24 hours once exposure to the allergen ends. Seasonal allergies affect 15% to 40% of the population.[49]

- *Perennial conjunctivitis* is chronic conjunctivitis that is related to year-round exposure to allergens such as dust mites, animal dander, and molds. Perennial conjunctivitis is usually mild and waxes and wanes throughout the year.
- *Seasonal* allergic conjunctivitis ("hay fever") is characterized by mild injection and swelling and is associated with exposing the eyes to outdoor pollens and may be associated with generalized allergic reaction including nasal congestion (allergic rhinoconjunctivitis). *Atopic keratoconjunctivitis* occurs in those with atopic dermatitis and/or asthma, affecting the lower tarsal conjunctiva, usually occurring in late adolescence, and is notable for significant (beyond that seen in allergic conjunctivitis) itching, burning, and tearing that is often chronic.
- *Giant papillary conjunctivitis* occurs most often in contact lens wearers, occurring 10 times more frequently in those wearing soft contacts than hard contacts.

Clinical Findings
- Key finding: severe itching and tearing
- Family history of atopy or seasonal allergies
- Rhinitis, eczema, asthma
- Acute attacks precipitated by allergens (e.g., pollen, animals, molds, dust, dust mites, occasionally food)
- Redness and swelling of the conjunctiva or eyelid (or both)
- Follicular reaction of the conjunctiva
- Stringy, mucoid discharge
- Bilateral involvement most common

- Cobblestone papillary hypertrophy in the tarsal conjunctiva

Vision screening should be normal and documented in patient's record.

Diagnostic Studies. Conjunctival or nasal smears (using Wright stain) reveal numerous eosinophils.

Management
- Prevention is best; avoid allergens.
- For mild cases, saline solution or artificial tears are administered along with cool compresses. Refrigerated eye drops are more soothing. Pharmacologic treatment includes topical decongestants, oral or topical antihistamines, topical mast cell stabilizers, or topical NSAIDs.[49] Topical decongestants like naphazoline hydrochloride ophthalmic solution do not decrease the allergic response, but do relieve erythema, injection, and lid edema.
- A combination antihistamine-decongestant is more effective than either agent alone; naphazoline hydrochloride plus antazoline ophthalmic solution can be used sparingly to reduce ocular congestion, irritation, and itching.
- Topical mast cell stabilizers may be helpful for maintenance therapy, chronic allergies, or vernal conjunctivitis and are available over the counter:
  - Cromolyn sodium 4% on a regular basis
  - Nedocromil sodium 2% or lodoxamide tromethamine 0.1%
- Topical olopatadine hydrochloride 0.1% is a mast cell stabilizer combined with an antihistamine for children older than 3 years old. Topical NSAIDs, like ketorolac tromethamine 0.5%, provide relief of itching and burning though it often stings when applied.
- The ophthalmic histamine 1 (H_1) blockers ketotifen or levocabastine can be prescribed for allergic conjunctivitis and ocular pruritus.
- Topical steroids should not be used because of possible side effects (increased IOP, potential for viral infection, contraindication with herpes, potential to cause cataracts, and poor corneal healing). An ophthalmologist should be consulted if a patient's condition warrants considering topical corticosteroids.

Patients may be treated with systemic antihistamines (fexofenadine, loratadine, or cetirizine) if systemic symptoms are present (see Chapter 36 for management of allergies):
- Refer to an allergist for allergen immunotherapy when rhinitis is present because therapy can lead to better control without need for medication.
- Refer to an ophthalmologist if unresponsive to treatment or if the following is present: corneal abrasions, impaired vision, need for corticosteroids, severe keratoconjunctivitis, or atypical manifestations.
- Maintain a high threshold of suspicion for herpes-induced blepharitis or atopic keratoconjunctivitis if pain is present.

Complications. Some forms of allergic conjunctivitis (e.g., vernal conjunctivitis) can lead to corneal ulceration, scarring and vision loss, corneal degeneration, and changes in the corneal curvature.

Blepharitis

Blepharitis is an acute or chronic inflammation of the eyelash follicles or meibomian sebaceous glands of the eyelids (or both). It is usually bilateral. The two types of blepharitis are anterior and posterior. *Posterior* blepharitis occurs when there is inflammation at the inner portion of the eyelid at the Meibomian glands. Diseases with chronic inflammation such as rosacea or seborrheic dermatitis may be source of posterior blepharitis. *Anterior* blepharitis may be caused by seborrhea or staphylococcal bacteria, which colonize the eyelid.[55] *Demodrex folliculorum* is a parasite that may cause chronic anterior blepharitis, presenting with cylindrical sleeves of dandruff around the eyelashes. Blepharitis may also be caused by allergic contact dermatitis, eczema, or psoriasis.[55]

Clinical Findings

- Swelling and erythema of the eyelid margins and palpebral conjunctiva
- Flaky, scaly debris over eyelid margins on awakening
- Gritty, burning feeling in eyes
- Mild bulbar conjunctival injection
- Ulcerative form: hard scales at the base of the lashes (if the crust is removed, ulceration is seen at the hair follicles, the lashes fall out, and an associated conjunctivitis is present)
  Differential Diagnosis. Pediculosis of the eyelashes.

Management

Explain to the patient that this may be chronic or relapsing. Instructions for the patient include:

- Scrub the eyelashes and eyelids with a cotton-tipped applicator or clean washcloth containing a weak (50%) solution of no-tears shampoo to maintain proper hygiene and debride the scales. Rinse well after washing.
- Use warm compresses for 5 to 10 minutes at a time 2 to 4 times a day and wipe away lid debris.
- Lid massage 2 to 4 times a day to express Meibomian secretions.
- At times antistaphylococcal antibiotic (e.g., bacitracin or erythromycin 0.5% ophthalmic ointment) is used once daily at bedtime until symptoms subside and for at least 1 week thereafter. Ointment is preferable to eye drops because of increased duration of contact with the ocular tissue. Azithromycin 1% ophthalmic solution for 4 weeks may also be used for posterior blepharitis.[55]
- Treat associated seborrhea, psoriasis, eczema, or allergies as indicated.
- Remove contact lenses and wear eyeglasses for the duration of the treatment period. Sterilize or clean lenses before reinserting.
- Purchase new eye makeup; minimize use of mascara and eyeliner.
- Use artificial tears for patients with inadequate tear pools.
  Chronic staphylococcal blepharitis and meibomian keratoconjunctivitis respond to oral antibiotics. Doxycycline, minocycline, or tetracycline can be used chronically in children older than 8 years. Azithromycin for 5 days may be used in younger children who do not respond to topical treatments.

Hordeolum

Commonly called a *stye,* hordeolum is an infection of either the sebaceous glands (Zeis or Molls glands), the eyelids (external hordeolum), or the meibomian glands of the eyelid (internal hordeolum). The most common causative organism is *S. aureus* or, rarely, *P. aeruginosa.*[56]

Clinical Findings

A tender, swollen red furuncle is seen. In an *external* hordeolum, the swelling is generally smaller, superficial, and located along

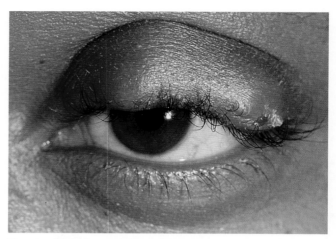

- **Fig. 30.7** Chalazion and External Hordeolum. (From Yanoff M, Duker JS. *Ophthalmology,* ed 6. Elsevier; 2023.)

the lid margin. An *internal* hordeolum is larger and may point through the skin or conjunctival surface. The patient complains of a foreign body sensation. An internal hordeolum on the palpebral conjunctiva can be inspected by rolling back the eyelid (Fig. 30.7).

Differential Diagnosis. If the hordeolum does not resolve, consider cellulitis of the lid or orbit, sebaceous cell cancer, or pyogenic granuloma.

Management

- Rupture often occurs spontaneously when the furuncle becomes large, and a point develops. Removal of an eyelash near the furuncle frequently promotes rupture.
- Warm, moist compresses 3 to 4 times/day, for 10 to 15 minutes, facilitate the process of rupturing.
- Hygiene for the eye can be maintained by scrubbing the eyelashes and eyelids with a cotton-tipped applicator or clean washcloth containing a weak (50%) solution of no-tears shampoo once or twice a day.
- At times, antistaphylococcal ointment (e.g., 0.5% erythromycin) is effective.
- Steroids are not indicated.
- Refer to an ophthalmologist for incision and drainage if the hordeolum does not rupture on its own after coming to a point or for multiple or recurrent hordeolum.

Chalazion

Chalazion is a chronic sterile inflammation of the eyelid resulting from a lipogranuloma or blockage of the meibomian glands that line the posterior margins of the eyelids (see Fig. 30.7). It is deeper in the eyelid tissue than a hordeolum and may result from an internal hordeolum or retained lipid granular secretions.

Clinical Findings

Initially, mild erythema and slight swelling of the involved eyelid are seen. After a few days the inflammation resolves, and a slow growing, round, nonpigmented, painless (key finding) mass remains. It may persist for a long time and is a commonly acquired lid lesion seen in children (see Fig. 30.7).

Management

- Acute lesions are treated with hot compresses.

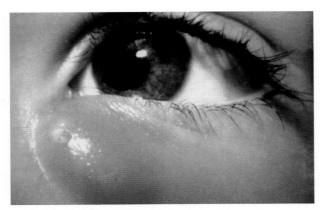

• **Fig. 30.8** Dacryocystitis. (From Walls RM, Hockberger RS, Gausche-Hill M, et al. *Rosen's Emergency Medicine: Concepts and Clinical Practice*, ed 10. Elsevier; 2023.)

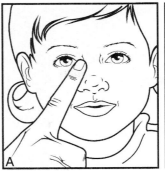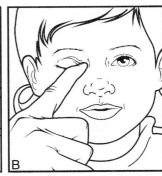

• **Fig. 30.9** Technique to Clear Nasolacrimal Duct Obstruction. (A) Incorrect technique. (B) Correct technique. The finger is pushing behind the bone, "in and up." Note that the fingertip is not visible in the proper technique.

• Refer to an ophthalmologist for surgical incision or topical intralesional corticosteroid injections if the condition is unresolved or if the lesion causes cosmetic concerns. A chalazion can distort vision by causing astigmatism because of pressure on the orbit.

Complications

Recurrence is common. Fragile, vascular granulation tissue called *pyogenic granuloma* that enlarges and bleeds rapidly can occur if a chalazion breaks through the conjunctival surface.

Nasolacrimal Duct Conditions: Dacryostenosis and Dacryocystitis

Nasolacrimal duct obstruction, or dacryostenosis, is an abnormal obstruction of the nasolacrimal duct (imperforate valve of Hasner) that prevents tears from flowing into an opening in the nasal mucosa. Nasolacrimal duct obstruction is fairly common in neonates (up to 6% of live births),[33] thought to be due to a membrane at birth that covers the nasolacrimal duct, which then fails to break down quickly. It may also occur at any age secondary to trauma to the duct or to a chronic duct obstruction complicated by an upper respiratory infection. The condition is also found more frequently in those with craniofacial disorders and trisomy 21 (Down syndrome). Congenital failure of the duct to canalize may be unilateral or bilateral, and clinical signs appear 2 to 6 weeks after birth when tear production develops. Duct blockage usually resolves spontaneously in 90% of infants by 12 months of age. Bacterial overgrowth may occur resulting in excessive mucus production. Dacryocystitis is an inflammation of the involved nasolacrimal duct, and infection in the lower eyelid can result (Fig. 30.8).

Clinical Findings

• Continuous or intermittent tearing, stickiness, and mucoid discharge at the inner canthus that can become purulent with possible expression of purulent material
• Blepharitis in lids and lashes
• Occasional nasal obstruction and drainage
• Expression of thin mucopurulent exudate from the punctum lacrimale
• Tenderness and swelling over the lacrimal duct (can be exquisite) (see Fig. 30.8)
• Eyelids stuck shut on awakening

• Edema and erythema of the tear sac (most prominent in the triangular area just below the medial canthus)
• Excoriation and thickening of the periorbital skin
• Conjunctival injection is not common.
• Mucocele of inner canthal tendon (unusual; presents as a bluish mass)
  Diagnostic Studies
• Fluorescein dye, instilled bilaterally in the inferior conjunctival sac and checked at 2 and 5 minutes with a cobalt blue light source, will disappear if duct is patent.
• A white blood cell (WBC) count (elevated) and cultures are obtained from the expressed exudate if the inflammation is severe.
  Differential Diagnosis. Punctual or canalicular atresia, ophthalmia neonatorum, infected sebaceous cysts, conjunctivitis, foreign body, congenital glaucoma, dacryocele, intraocular inflammation, and nasal mucosal edema are differential diagnoses.[33]

Management

The treatment goals are to minimize stagnation in the tear duct and prevent infection.
• Daily (Crigler) massage of the lacrimal sac may be performed to facilitate canalization of the duct. The technique involves placing a clean finger over the medial canthus and pressing in a posterior direction until the fingertip enters the space behind the inferior bony orbital ridge. Gentle pressure applied in a downward and medial direction transmits hydrostatic force through the nasolacrimal duct to the obstruction (Fig. 30.9). This technique should be performed about 10 times, 2 or 3 times a day. The eyelid should be cleaned with plain water after massage.[33]
• Bacterial conjunctivitis or excessive mucopurulent exudate is most commonly *S. pneumoniae* (35%) or *H. influenzae* (20%) and may be treated with erythromycin ophthalmic ointment, or the fluoroquinolones (moxifloxacin, ciprofloxacin, ofloxacin, norfloxacin) for 1 to 3 weeks with massage and frequent cleansing of secretions. The duct may open spontaneously with resolution of the bacterial infection.
• Saline drops into the nose, followed by aspiration before feeding and at bedtime, help relieve any concurrent nasal congestion.

If the mucopurulent exudate persists for 1 to 2 weeks despite the recommended interventions, the infant or child needs a referral to an ophthalmologist regardless of age. Some ophthalmologists may probe the duct in an infant as early as age 6 months,

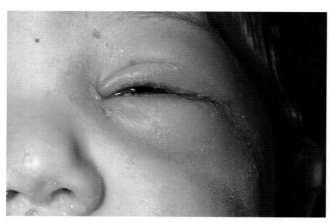

• **Fig. 30.10** Preseptal Cellulitis due to *Haemophilus influenzae* in a 6-Month-Old Infant. (From Lyons CJ, Lambert SR. *Taylor and Hoyt's Pediatric Ophthalmology and Strabismus*, ed 6. Elsevier; 2023.)

whereas others wait until 9 to 12 months of age. Early in-office probing is less expensive and does not require anesthesia, but it does require a skilled ophthalmologist. If probing fails to alleviate the problem, which is unusual, surgery may be required for placement of a tube stent or for a dacryocystorhinostomy.

Dacryocystitis may be acute or chronic and is evidenced by erythematous swelling below the medial canthal area. Treatment of dacryocystitis is warm compresses and oral or parenteral antibiotics with gram-positive coverage. When fever, marked erythema, swelling, tenderness, and toxic appearance occur, hospitalization is indicated for parenteral antibiotics. Periorbital or orbital cellulitis is a complication of chronic dacryocystitis.

Preseptal Cellulitis

Preseptal cellulitis, previously known as *periorbital cellulitis*, or inflammation of the tissues surrounding the involved eye, is often associated with trauma or focal infection near the eye, eyelid abscess, or sinusitis.[57] In preseptal cellulitis, the infection is anterior to the orbit septum and does not involve the orbit or other eye structures (Fig. 30.10). Orbital cellulitis is a more serious infection involving tissues posterior to the orbit septum.

It is most commonly seen in children up to 6 years old. It can also occur with infected lacerations, abrasions, insect stings or bites, impetigo, or a foreign body where the infection is spread via venous or lymphatic channels. It may also be secondary to paranasal sinusitis. The etiology is often unknown, but the bacteria most commonly responsible for periorbital cellulitis are gram-positive streptococcal organisms and *S. aureus*. Until the introduction of the *H. influenzae* type B vaccine, *H. influenzae* was a common organism.[57]

Clinical Findings
- Usually afebrile; if fever present, consider orbital cellulitis
- Swelling and erythema of tissues surrounding the eye; upper lid affected more often than the lower lid
- Deep red eyelid (Note: color is purple-blue with *H. influenzae* infection)
- History of sinusitis, insect bite, or eye trauma
- Symptoms of bacteremia may indicate orbital cellulitis
- Orbital discomfort or pain, proptosis, or paralysis of extraocular muscles occurs with orbital cellulitis.

Diagnostic Studies. Diagnostic studies are not usually required for preseptal cellulitis. Depending on the severity and speed of progression of the cellulitis, the following are useful in evaluating for orbital cellulitis[57]:
- Visual acuity, extraocular movement, and pupillary reaction testing
- Complete blood count with differential; WBC count usually greater than 15,000, if bacteremic
- Culture any eyelid wound and/or blood cultures, if febrile
- CT scan to rule out sinusitis, orbital cellulitis, or subperiosteal abscess

Differential Diagnosis. Conjunctivitis (bilateral conjunctival inflammation), cavernous sinus thrombosis, and orbital cellulitis (proptosis, limited extraocular movement, and reduced visual acuity) are the differential diagnoses in children; in neonates, consider conjunctivitis, dacryocystitis, and ruptured dacryocystocele.

Management
Management must be made on a case-by-case basis. Referral to an ophthalmologist is needed when proptosis, ophthalmoplegia, or changes in visual acuity occur; these conditions are suggestive of orbital cellulitis. Moderate to severe cases of cellulitis, a child younger than 1 year old, a poor response to outpatient management, or a purulent wound near the eyelid require hospitalization and IV administration of antibiotics followed by a 10-day course of oral antibiotics.[57]

The child may be managed as an outpatient if older than 1 year, the cellulitis is mild, the orbit is not involved (full eye movements are present, no pain with eye movement, visual changes, or ptosis), and the child exhibits no symptoms of systemic bacterial sepsis.

Outpatient management consists of:
- Oral antibiotics to complete 7- to 14-day course. Amoxicillin with clavulanic acid, cefdinir, and cefpodoxime are first-line choices for treatment.
- Warm soaks to the periorbital area every 2 to 4 hours for 15 minutes may provide comfort and speed healing.
- If a rapid clinical response is not seen, further evaluation and treatment should be done. The parent/caregiver is advised to call immediately if there is any change in condition.
- Reexamine the patient in 24 hours. Failure to improve in 24 hours indicates a need for hospitalization and parenteral antibiotics, usually ceftriaxone or other third-generation cephalosporin. The child is monitored daily until blood cultures are negative for 48 hours or clinical improvement is seen.

Complications
Complications include orbital cellulitis or extension of the infection into the orbit, subperiosteal or orbital abscess, optic neuritis, retinal vein thrombosis, panophthalmitis, meningitis, epidural and subdural abscesses, and cavernous sinus thrombosis.

Keratitis and Corneal Ulcers

Inflammation of the cornea (keratitis) can cause a dramatic alteration in visual acuity and can progress to corneal ulceration and blindness. It is a medical emergency and requires prompt referral to an ophthalmologist. A corneal ulcer begins as a well-defined infiltration at the center or edge of the cornea and subsequently suppurates and forms an ulcer that may penetrate deep into the corneal tissue or spread to involve the width of the cornea. Involvement is usually unilateral. The causative agents include viruses (HSV-1, varicella-zoster, hepatitis C), bacteria (*H. influenzae, Moraxella, S. aureus, S. pneumoniae, Pseudomonas, N. gonorrhoeae*, Enterobacteriaceae [including *Klebsiella, Enterobacter, Serratia*, and *Proteus*]), fungi (rare), and protozoa. Less common causes include an allergic reaction, conjunctivitis, systemic infections, toxic chemicals, and the use of corticosteroids. Contact lens wearers are at higher risk of keratitis, particularly if the wearer does not care for their contact lenses.[9]

The most common risk factor for keratitis is trauma, which can result from wearing extended-wear contact lenses or having poor contact lens hygiene. Other high-risk factors include age (younger than 30 and older than 50 years), sex (males more than females [secondary to increased ocular trauma]), smoking, low socioeconomic status, and vitamin A deficiency.

Clinical Findings

Symptoms vary in intensity according to the depth and extent of ulceration. The following are reported or seen:
- Exposure to an infected individual
- History of illness, eye trauma, extended contact lens wear, foreign body, or history of recent antibiotic treatment for conjunctivitis that was unresponsive
- White lesions on cornea
- Vesicles on the skin or eyelids and herpes lesions elsewhere on the body
- Severe pain, sensation of a foreign body ("gritty"), and photophobia
- Tearing, erythema, and spasms of the eyelid
- Inflamed eye
- Blurred vision
- Occasional corneal opacification
- Area staining green with a fluorescein strip (Note: If herpes, a dendritic ulcer is seen)

Management

When a corneal ulcer is suspected, the child should be referred immediately for a slit-lamp examination. Delay can result in loss of vision in the eye. Do not attempt to treat. Visual acuity outcome is good when these ulcers are treated aggressively with the appropriate agent.
- Steroids should never be used.
- Treatment with antivirals, such as trifluridine or vidarabine, may be used to speed healing in herpes simplex infections.
- Complications include corneal opacification, scarring, and loss of vision if treatment is delayed.

Inflammation of the Uveal Tract

Inflammation of the uveal tract (iris, ciliary body, choroids) and other ocular structures is often called *uveitis* (Fig. 30.11). The inflammation may be anterior (affecting the iris, ciliary body, or both) or posterior (affecting the choroid). Adjacent ocular structures can also be involved, including the retina, vitreous, sclera, lens, and optic nerve. The inflammation may be acute or chronic. In the United States, 5% to 10% of patients with uveitis are children; prevalence in children with juvenile idiopathic arthritis (JIA) is 4% to 38%.[58] Many causes have been implicated with idiopathic cause the most common. Known etiologies include infections, and systemic diseases such as JIA and Kawasaki disease.[59]

Clinical Findings
- Key findings:

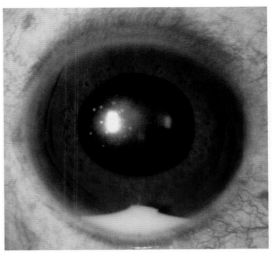

- **Fig. 30.11** Uveitis. (From Palay DA, Krachmer JH. *Primary Care Ophthalmology*, ed 2. Mosby; 2005.)

  - Acute onset of pain
  - Red eye
  - Photophobia
  - Blurred or decreased vision
- Excessive tearing and eyelid edema.
- Conjunctival erythema.
- Circumcorneal injection.
- Hypopyon (pus layer in the bottom of the anterior chamber) (see Fig. 30.11).
- Cloudy appearance of the eye with a bulging iris and a contracted, irregular, or fixed pupil (see Fig. 30.11).
- If chronic, there may be no ocular pain, photophobia, redness, or tearing.
- May be a history of prior viral infection, joint pain, trauma, gastrointestinal problems

Management

Evaluate and treat any underlying systemic disease. Refer the patient to an ophthalmologist; definitive diagnosis is made by slit-lamp examination. The prognosis is improved with early treatment. Cycloplegics and topical or systemic corticosteroids (depending on the cause of the inflammation) are often used in treatment. Cycloplegic-mydriatics are used regularly to prevent posterior synechiae (adhesions of iris to lens and cornea); NSAIDs may be used as adjunct treatment.

Complications

Anterior and posterior synechiae, changes in IOP, corneal edema, various degrees of visual impairment, papillary scarring, retinal detachment, glaucoma, enucleation, and cataracts are possible complications.

The Injured Eye

Subconjunctival Hemorrhage

Subconjunctival hemorrhage is splotchy bulbar conjunctival redness that spontaneously occurs or is secondary to increased intrathoracic pressure (from coughing, sneezing, straining, or trauma) that results in the bursting of conjunctival vessels. It is commonly found in neonates as a benign occurrence to a vaginal delivery. The hemorrhages are painless and usually spontaneously resolve within 2 to 3 weeks. No treatment is indicated unless there is pain, vision loss, or photophobia, which indicate a referral to an ophthalmologist. Spontaneous hemorrhages can (rarely) occur with hypertension, diabetes mellitus, and blood dyscrasias, or can be a sign of a ruptured globe if there is a history of trauma.[60]

Eyelid Contusion ("Black Eye")

An eyelid contusion is usually a result of blunt injury to the eye and surrounding tissues. The result is bruising, swelling, and often an impressive appearance ("black eye"). If the child complains of increased pain or swelling, decrease in visual acuity, double vision, flashing lights or "floaters," or develops a bilateral "raccoon eyes" appearance, an ophthalmologic evaluation is needed to rule out a more serious eye injury (e.g., ruptured globe, basilar skull fracture, detached retina, hyphema). It also should alert the PCP to the possibility of child maltreatment. Examine all eye structures before excessive swelling sets in. Treatment consists of elevating the head and intermittent ice compresses for 48 hours.

Corneal Abrasion

Damage to or loss of the epithelial cells of the cornea in the form of a corneal abrasion or tear is relatively common. Scratches from forceps delivery, paper, brushes, fingernails, contact lens overuse, improperly fitted cosmetic contact lenses, airbag deployment, plants, or foreign body in the conjunctival sac are often responsible.

Clinical Findings

- Evidence and sensation of a foreign body
- Severe pain and photophobia
- Tearing and blepharospasm
- Decreased vision
- Conjunctival erythema

On examination, disrupted tear film over the corneal epithelium is seen with a penlight.

Fluorescein staining with superficial uptake is indicative of a minor corneal abrasion. If the fluorescein staining goes deeply into the cornea, subepithelial corneal damage (e.g., corneal ulceration or corneal tear) is possible. Vertical striations on the cornea suggest a foreign body embedded under the eyelid.

Management

- Refer severe corneal injuries or possible subepithelial damage to an ophthalmologist. Refer those who wear contact lenses with an abrasion to an ophthalmologist to rule out bacterial corneal infection. A prophylactic topical antibiotic (e.g., ciprofloxacin or ofloxacin) may be prescribed in these circumstances to cover *Pseudomonas.*
- If no symptoms of corneal infection, use topical antibiotics (0.5% erythromycin ointment [preferred as more lubricating] or polymyxin/trimethoprim, ciprofloxacin, or ofloxacin drops) 4 times daily for 3 to 5 days.[61]

The use of a patch does not improve healing or decrease pain and a poorly applied patch may cause a corneal abrasion. If a patch is used, it should be used for no longer than 24 hours. An abrasion generally heals in 24 to 48 hours. If responding, continue the ointment for 2 to 3 days.

Abrasions in young children should be followed daily until healed. If pain continues past 48 hours, they should be referred

for slit-lamp examination within 24 to 36 hours. If no improvement is seen after 24 to 48 hours or if symptoms worsen, refer to an ophthalmologist. Use elbow restraints for the infant to ensure that the eye is not rubbed or further irritated.

- Oral analgesics or ophthalmologic NSAIDs (e.g., ketorolac 0.5%) may be used to ease the discomfort. Do not use topical anesthetics, because they are toxic to the epithelium.
- Do not use topical steroids.[61]

Foreign Body

A superficial foreign body in the eye is usually lodged on the surface of the eye or superficially in the cornea. It rarely results in serious trauma but may penetrate the globe (intraocular) with more serious consequences. Foreign bodies commonly occur in younger children during play and in older children during sports; they can include dirt, dust, metallic particles, or alkaline products from the deployment of an airbag.

Clinical Findings

Be sure to include in the history if the individual was working on a metal-on-metal activity. The following may be noted:
- Pain and foreign body sensation
- Foreign body visible in the conjunctival sac
- Tearing, inflammation, photophobia
- Irregular or peaked pupil
- Opaque lens
- Perforating wound to the cornea or iris

Fluorescein staining may be useful if no foreign body is visualized.

Diagnostic Studies. Ultrasonography or CT scan may be needed, depending on the foreign body and its location. An MRI is contraindicated.

Management

- Never remove an intraocular foreign body (including a metal object or fragment) and never remove a foreign body if the history indicates that a projectile object was possibly involved in the injury or patient has had LASIK procedure. Refer immediately to an ophthalmologist.
- View the upper bulbar conjunctiva by having the patient look down while the upper lid is pulled away from the globe and the upper recess illuminated. Evert the eyelid to visualize the superior tarsal conjunctiva.
- Use of a topical anesthetic facilitates patient cooperation.
- If not visualized but suspected, remove an extraocular foreign body via irrigation with sterile saline or eye irrigant.
- If the object is visualized, either irrigate or gently lift object away with a moistened cotton-tipped swab (after instillation of topical anesthetic). The latter technique should be used only for cooperative individuals and for small foreign bodies to avoid further trauma to the epithelial surface.
- If any difficulty is encountered, stop all efforts, and refer the patient immediately to an ophthalmologist. Treat with antibiotic ointment (erythromycin 4 times/day) until seen by ophthalmologist.[61]
- After removing any extraocular object, instill fluorescein stain and inspect the cornea with cobalt-blue light to look for green staining or lines; check visual acuity. Follow guidelines for managing a corneal abrasion.
- Reschedule the patient in 24 hours or refer to an ophthalmologist for follow-up.

- In the case of an airbag deployment (talc, cornstarch, and/or baking soda are released), irrigate the eyes with sterile saline or eye irrigant and carefully examine the eye(s) for further evidence of trauma.

Complications

Sympathetic ophthalmia, chronic siderosis, or uveitis of the injured eye can occur any time from 10 days to many years after a penetrating injury of the globe.

Burns

Burns to the eyes and surrounding tissues can be *thermal* (caused by exposure to steam, flame, intense heat [e.g., touching cornea with a curling iron], cinders, or cigarettes), *chemical* (e.g., cleaning agents, fertilizers, pesticides, battery fluid, laboratory products), or induced by *UV li*ght (e.g., bright snow, laser pointers, sunlamp). The amount of damage to the eye is directly related to the length of exposure and the nature of the source of the burn.[62] Chemical burns are true emergencies because of the progressive damage that can occur and require immediate referral to ophthalmology. Alkaline solutions are especially damaging. Burns on the eyelids are classified and treated the same as burns elsewhere on the body.

Clinical Findings

- Pale or necrosed appearance of the surrounding skin and eyelids
- Opacity of corneal tissue
- Visual impairment (decreased acuity)
- Initial exquisite pain or delayed complaints of pain (e.g., in UV burns, pain emerges about 6 hours after exposure)
- Photophobia
- Tearing within 12 hours of exposure
- Swollen corneas
- Fluorescein stain revealing pinpoint uptake

Management

- Instill a topical anesthetic if available.
- Chemical burns require immediate, ongoing, copious irrigation.[62] With the eyelids held apart, instill a steady, gentle solution of tepid water, saline, or Ringer irrigation for 20 to 30 minutes or until the pH of the tear film is 7.3 to 7.7. The pH should be rechecked after 30 minutes to ensure it maintains this level. Refer to an ophthalmologist after irrigation to determine the extent of the damage. Do not patch the eye; allow tearing to continue to cleanse the eye. Cool compresses applied to the surrounding skin may be comforting. Hospitalization may be needed for sedation and analgesia.
- Thermal burns may be treated the same way as corneal abrasions.
- UV burns are treated by using topical antibiotic prophylaxis, patches, and analgesics. Healing should occur in 1 to 2 days.

Lacerations of the Orbit

Lacerations from injuries cause perforation of the cornea and lead to uveal prolapse. They are described as to whether they are of the anterior segment (cornea, anterior chamber, iris, lens) or posterior segment (sclera, retina, vitreous).

Clinical Findings

The clinical findings (only a few of the more obvious are mentioned here) depend on which segment is involved.

- Anterior segment: irregular pupil (retracted or peaked), iris prolapse
- Posterior segment: poor red-light reflex, decreased vision, black tissue, or fluid seen under the conjunctiva

Management

Apply an eye shield (can be made from a cup) to protect the eye. Refer the patient immediately to an ophthalmologist to rule out damage to the globe and surrounding structures.

Traumatic Hyphema

A hyphema is an accumulation of visible blood or blood products in the anterior chamber of the eye and is the result of blunt trauma to the globe without penetration or perforation. Hyphemas may also occur after intraocular surgery.[63] This condition is most often caused by balls, fists or fingers, elbows, rocks, exploding airbags, and sticks. High-risk sports associated with hyphema include baseball, hockey, racquetball, and squash, with the stick or racket often responsible for the injury. It may also occur in infants with birth trauma or in patients with retinoblastoma, abnormal iris vessels (rubeosis), leukemia, juvenile xanthogranuloma of the iris, or abnormal hematologic profiles, such as sickle cell trait or disease, or secondary to child abuse.

Clinical Findings

Vision, pupil motility, the lids and adnexa, the cornea and anterior segment, and the red-light reflex should be assessed. An open globe must be excluded before any examination that would increase IOP.[63] The following may be noted:

- History of traumatic eye injury
- Somnolence (often associated with intracranial trauma)
- Blood appearing as a dark red fluid level between the cornea and iris on gross examination or as a hazy-appearing iris
- Inability to detect a bilateral red-light reflex
- Pain, photophobia, and tearing
- Visual acuity changes and impaired vision (light perception and hand motion perception)
- Abnormal pupillary reflex

Management

The goals of treatment include resolving the hyphema, making the patient comfortable, and preventing complications. There is a risk of recurrent bleeding. The following steps should be taken:

- Refer the patient immediately to an ophthalmologist. A slit-lamp examination is indicated.
- Restrict oral intake until the child has been seen by an ophthalmologist.
- Place a perforated eye shield (not a patch) over the eye; avoid pressure to prevent reinjury.
- If a hematologic disorder is detected, ensure quick intervention and close follow-up.
  The following steps are commonly recognized for treatment of a traumatic hyphema:
- Outpatient management is acceptable for those with a small hyphema (grade I). Elevate the head of the bed to 45 degrees. The child should wear a Fox eye shield; maintain bed rest with bathroom privileges for 5 days, participate in no strenuous activities for 10 days, and have daily eye examinations to check for blood staining and IOP. Cycloplegic agents may be used.[63]
- Children should be hospitalized with a hyphema of grade II or III, those with sickle cell, if there is an increase in IOP, or if there is a question about compliance with outpatient treatment.

- Acetaminophen is the analgesic of choice; avoid aspirin and NSAIDs because they may add to the risk of a rebleed. Sedatives may be necessary in pediatric patients.
- Treat nausea and prevent vomiting.
- Surgery may be necessary to remove the trapped blood from the chamber for the following reasons: (1) if it is causing an increase in IOP; (2) in sickle cell patients, to prevent corneal blood staining; (3) if the hyphema remains without some clearing in the first 4 days; or (4) if a clot is pressing against the corneal epithelium.
- After hospital discharge, the child should be followed closely by an ophthalmologist because long-term monitoring is necessary to detect possible traumatic cataract, retinal detachment, or glaucoma.

Complications

A second hemorrhage can occur within 3 to 5 days of the first, increasing the risk of glaucoma, amblyopia, or corneal blood staining that can result in permanent visual loss. The larger the hyphema, the more likely the child is to rebleed. Patients with abnormal hematologic profiles (e.g., sickle cell hemoglobinopathies) are more likely to have visual loss because of optic atrophy.[63]

Success in treatment is determined by the recovery of visual acuity. A small grade I hyphema will lead to permanent visual loss (worse than 20/50) in less than 10% of cases. When less than a third of the anterior chamber is filled with blood, approximately 80% regain acuity of 20/40 or better. When more than half (but less than total) of the chamber is filled, this same visual acuity is regained in about 60%. However, only 35% of those with total hyphema will have this return in acuity. Patients should be followed by an ophthalmologist due to elevated risk of developing glaucoma.[63]

Retinal Detachment

Retinal detachment is detachment of the neurosensory retina from its retinal pigment epithelium base within the globe. It is rare in children, so suspicion should be high for traumatic causes (e.g., child abuse), a congenital abnormality or syndrome (aphakia, cataracts or Ehlers-Danlos, Stickler, Marfan, or Norrie syndromes), or specific disease (ROP, viral retinitis, retinoblastoma, or various retinopathies).[63] Children who have had cataract surgery are at increased risk of retinal detachment, with an overall 10-year risk of 5.5%.[64] There may be concurrent ocular disease or a family history of retinal detachment.

Clinical Findings

- Blurry vision that becomes progressively worse
- Dark cloud in one visual field, flashing lights, or a "shower of floaters"
- Darkening of retinal vessels on funduscopic examination
- Gray elevation at the site of detachment

Management

Instruct the patient not to eat and refer to an ophthalmologist for evaluation emergently.

Orbital Hematoma and Contusion of the Globe

This condition is usually the result of a blow to the globe. The degree of damage depends on the energy of the object hitting the globe. Such injuries commonly occur because of sports activities, motor vehicle accidents, assault, BB gun accidents, or airbag deployment.

Clinical Findings

- Milky white appearance of the retina
- Visual acuity changes
- Severe bruising of the eyelids and periorbital tissues
- Lens dislocation, retinal detachment, or edema
- Vitreous, retinal, or choroid hemorrhage
- Rupture of the eyeball

Management

Refer the patient immediately to an ophthalmologist. A closed head injury, damage to the skull, and facial bone fractures need to be ruled out via CT scan, MRI, or ultrasound radiography. Occasionally, cryopexy or laser photocoagulation surgery is needed for contusions of the globe.

Complications

Possible complications include permanent visual loss, retinal necrosis, subretinal hemorrhage, and retinal or macular holes.

Orbital Fractures

An orbital fracture is a fracture of the walls of the orbit secondary to blunt trauma to the orbital rim or eye(s). Orbital fractures are most common among adolescent and young adult males.[65] The orbital floor is thin and subject to fracture. The inferior rectus muscle may become caught in the fracture site. The usual cause of an orbital fracture is a blow or blunt trauma to the orbit (e.g., ball, fist, motor vehicle accident [hitting the dashboard], or fall).

Clinical Findings

- Pain, diplopia
- Numbness below orbit
- Ecchymosis of the lids, nosebleed, trouble chewing
- Limited ocular movement (especially upward) and weakness in downward movement
- Globe displacement with a sunken-eye appearance or a protruding eye
- Bony discontinuity or "step-off"
- Subcutaneous emphysema in surrounding tissues and edema
- Enophthalmos (recession of the eyeball within the orbit)
- Corneal laceration
- Irregular pupil
- Hyphema or absent red reflex

Diagnostic Studies. CT scan is the best imaging modality and is preformed if the patient has evidence of fracture upon examination, limited extraocular motility, decreased visual acuity, pain or inability to perform an accurate examination.[65]

Management

- An orbital fracture is an ophthalmologic emergency requiring immediate intervention and referral. Diagnostic studies are performed to rule out injury to the skull and cranial contents. Open reduction may be necessary if any of the orbital bones are displaced or to rule out displacement of the globe or enophthalmos.
- Ice the injury intermittently for 48 hours and have the patient sleep with the head of bed elevated.[65] Antibiotic prophylaxis to cover sinus pathogens is recommended if the patient has an orbital fracture into the sinus.[65]
- Nasal decongestants may also be used to reduce nose blowing and sniffling.

Deformities of the Eyelids

Entropion

Entropion is a condition in which the eyelids invert so that the cilia or epithelium rubs against the corneal surface, causing abrasion or irritation. The upper and lower eyelids may be involved. There is a rare congenital form. Examination reveals evidence of lid laxity. Pain or irritation and photophobia are typical symptoms. Complications include corneal scarring and corneal infections. Management involves surgical intervention, and the patient should be referred to an ophthalmologist.[66]

Ectropion

Ectropion is a rare condition in which the eyelid margins evert. The condition may be congenital, seen after infection, or secondary to scarring after trauma, radiation, or prior surgery. It can be confused with euryblepharon (a congenital eyelid anomaly). Management involves lubrication for mild cases; surgery is indicated for chronic or symptomatic cases. The patient should be referred to an ophthalmologist for management.[67]

Euryblepharon

Euryblepharon is a congenital eyelid anomaly that appears as a wide palpebral fissure with the appearance of a sagging half of the lower eyelid (temporal side) or a pulling away of the lid from the orbit. It can have a genetic etiology (e.g., Down syndrome), be associated with other ocular anomalies (e.g., congenital cleft lip, strabismus, congenital ptosis), or be seen in association with nonocular anomalies (e.g., hypospadias, inguinal hernias, dental anomalies). It is often confused with ectropion. It is usually a mild cosmetic condition that the child may outgrow. No treatment is indicated unless chronic tearing or exposure keratitis occurs; in such cases, reconstruction can be considered.

Additional Resources

American Academy of Ophthalmology: www.aao.org
American Association for Pediatric Ophthalmology and Strabismus: www.aapos.org
Grajewski Lyra (GL) Foundation for Children with Glaucoma: www.gl-foundation.org
InfantSEE: www.infantsee.org
National Center for Children's Vision and Eye Health: http://nationalcenter.preventblindness.org/
National Eye Institute: www.nei.nih.gov
Prevent Blindness: www.preventblindness.org

References

1. AAP, AAPOS, AACO and AAO Hoskins Center for Quality Eye Care. *Procedures for the Evaluation of the Visual System by Pediatricians: Clinical Report*; 2016. https://www.aao.org/clinical-statement/procedures-evaluation-of-visual-system-by-pediatri.
2. Office of Disease Prevention and Health Promotion Vision Workgroup *Healthy People 2030: Vision Workgroup*. U.S. Department of Health and Human Services (HHS). https://health.gov/healthypeople/about/workgroups/vision-workgroup.
3. U.S. Preventive Services Task Force. Vision screening in children aged 6 months to 5 years: US preventive services Task force recommendation statement. *JAMA*. 2017;318(9):836–844.
4. American Academy of Ophthalmology (AAO). *Pediatric Eye Evaluations Preferred Practice Pattern*; 2017a. https://www.aao.org/preferred-practice-pattern/pediatric-eye-evaluations-ppp-2017.
5. Xie JZ, Tarczy-Hornoch K, Lin J, Cotter SA, Torres M, Varma R. Multi-ethnic pediatric eye disease study group. *Ophthalmology*. 2014;121(7):1469.
6. Huang X, Xia H, Zhang Q, et al. New treatment for amblyopia based on rules of synaptic plasticity: a randomized clinical trial. *Sci China Life Sci*. 2022;65:451–465.
7. Vaughan J, Dale T, Herrera D. Comparison of photoscreening to chart methodology for vision screening. *J Sch Nurs*. 2022;38(3):306–310.
8. Stewart A. *Infant Aphakia: Putting Study Results into Practice*. AAO. *EyeNet Magazine*; 2017. https://www.aao.org/eyenet/article/infant-aphakia-putting-study-results-into-practice.
9. Centers for Disease Control and Prevention (CDC). *Children and Contact Lenses*; 2021. https://www.cdc.gov/contactlenses/children-and-contact-lenses.html.
10. Centers for Disease Control and Prevention (CDC). *Healthy Contact Lens Wear and Care: Decorative Contact Lenses*; 2019. www.cdc.gov/contactlenses/decorative-contacts.html.
11. Dang S. *Avoid These Four Dangers of Non-prescription Contact Lenses*; 2021. https://www.aao.org/eye-health/tips-prevention/avoid-these-four-dangers-of-non-prescription-conta.
12. US Food and Drug Administration (FDA). *When Is LASIK Not for Me?*; 2018. https://www.fda.gov/medical-devices/lasik/when-lasik-not-me.
13. American Academy of Ophthalmology (AAO). *Amblyopia Preferred Practice Pattern*; 2017. https://www.aao.org/preferred-practice-pattern/amblyopia-ppp-2017.
14. Matsa E, Shi J, Wheeler KK, et al. Trends in US emergency department visits for pediatric acute ocular injury. *JAMA Ophthalmol*. 2018;136(8):895–903. Erratum JAMA Ophthalmol. 2018;136(8):959.
15. Justin GA. *Eye Injury Prevention*; 2022. https://eyewiki.org/Eye_Injury_Prevention#Eye_injury_prevention.
16. Prevent Blindness. Your child's sight: Protect your child from eye injuries. www.preventblindness.org/protect-your-child-eye-injuries.
17. Prevent Blindness. Choosing UV protection. www.preventblindness.org/choosing-uv-protection.
18. American Optometric Association (AOA). Ultraviolet (UV) protection. https://www.aoa.org/healthy-eyes/caring-for-your-eyes/uv-protection?sso=y.
19. Turbert D, Shelton B. *Sports Eye Safety*; 2021. https://www.aao.org/eye-health/tips-prevention/injuries-sports.
20. American Academy of Pediatrics (AAP) and American Academy of Ophthalmology (AAO). *Communications Advisory Board. Protective Eyewear for Young Athletes*. American Academy of Ophthalmology Policy Statement; 2013. https://www.aao.org/education/clinical-statement/protective-eyewear-young-athletes.
21. US Food and Drug Administration (FDA). Important information for laser pointer manufactures. https://www.fda.gov/Radiation-EmittingProducts/RadiationEmittingProductsandProcedures/HomeBusinessandEntertainment/LaserProductsandInstruments/ucm116373.htm.
22. Chen Y, Cunningham A, Kotagiri A. The danger of laser pointer-induced retinal damage in children: a large United Kingdom case series and survey of public awareness. *J Pediatr Ophthalmol Strabismus*. 2022:1–8.
23. American Optometric Association (AOA). *Computer Vision Syndrome*; 2022. www.aoa.org/patients-and-public/caring-for-your-vision/protecting-your-vision/computer-vision-syndrome?sso=y.
24. Wang J, Li M, Zhu D, et al. Smartphone overuse and visual impairment in children and young adults: systematic review and meta-analysis. *J Med Internet Res*. 2020;22(12):e21923.
25. Chang P, Zhang B, Lin L, et al. Comparison of myopic progression before, during, and after COVID-19 lockdown. *Ophthalmology*. 2021;128(11):1655–1657.

26. American Association for Pediatric Ophthalmology and Strabismus (AAPOS). Screen time and online learning. https://aapos.org/glossary/screen-time-and-online-learning.

27. AAP, AAPOS, AACO and AAO Hoskins Center for Quality Eye Care. *Joint Statement: Learning Disabilities, Dyslexia, and Vision—Reaffirmed*; 2014. https://www.aao.org/clinical-statement/joint-statement-learning-disabilities-dyslexia-vis.

28. Margines JB, Haung C, Young A, et al. Refractive errors and amblyopia among children screened by the UCLA preschool vision program in los angeles county. *Am J Ophthalmol.* 2020;210:P78–P85.

29. Bascal DA, Ribot FM, Feldman BH, et al. Amblyopia. https://eyewiki.org/Amblyopia.

30. Bacal DA, Koretz Z, Prakalapakorn SG, et al. Exotropia. https://eyewiki.org/Exotropia.

31. Suh DW, Grigorian AP. Esotropia. https://eyewiki.org/Esotropia.

32. Coats DK, Paysse EA. *Causes of Horizontal Strabismus in Children*; 2023. Available at: https://www.uptodate.com/contents/causes-of-horizontal-strabismus-in-children?search=infants%20and%20esotropia%20&source=search_result&selectedTitle=1~26&usage_type=default&display_rank=1.

33. Alsuhaibani A, Al-Zubidi N, Plemel D, et al. Blepharoptosis. http://eyewiki.org/Blepharoptosis.

34. American Academy of Ophthalmology (AAO). *Clinical Guidelines: Childhood Nystagmus Workup*; 2020. https://www.aao.org/disease-review/clinical-guidelines-childhood-nystagmus-workup.

35. Kim J, Konda S. Nystagmus. http://eyewiki.org/Nystagmus.

36. Heidar K. *Cataracts in Children, Congenital and Acquired*; 2021. http://eyewiki.org/Cataracts_in_Children,_Congenital_and_Acquired.

37. Clark RA. *Glaucoma, Congenital or Infantile*; 2021. http://eyewiki.org/Glaucoma,_Congenital_Or_Infantile.

38. American Association for Pediatric Ophthalmology and Strabismus (AAPOS). *Glaucoma for Children*; 2021. https://aapos.org/glossary/glaucoma-for-children.

39. Dougherty M, Wittenborn J, Phillips E. *Published Examination-Based Prevalence of Major Eye Disorders*; 2018. EyeConditionExamLiteratureReviewVEHSS.pdf.

40. Heidar K, Miller AM, Stevenson E, et al. *Retinopathy of Prematurity*; 2022. http://eyewiki.org/Retinopathy_of_Prematurity.

41. U.S. National Library of Medicine (NLM). *Retinoblastoma*; 2018. http://ghr.nlm.nih.gov/condition/retinoblastoma.

42. Skalet AH, Gombos DS, Gallie BL, et al. Screening children at risk for retinoblastoma. *Ophthalmology.* 2018;125(3):453–458.

43. Choe C & O'Brien. Retinoblastoma. https://eyewiki.org/Retinoblastoma.

44. Naru J, Aggarwal R, Singh U, et al. HPV-16 detected in one-fourth eyes with retinoblastoma: a prospective case-control study from North India. *J Pediatr Hematol Oncol.* 2016;38(5):367–371.

45. Soltani S, Tabibzadeh A, Yousefi P, et al. HPV infections in retinoblastoma: a systematic review. *J Clin Lab Anal.* 2021;35(10):e23981.

46. American Academy of Pediatrics (AAP). American association of certified orthoptists (AACO), American association for pediatric ophthalmology and strabismus (AAPOS), American academy of ophthalmology (AAO). Visual system assessment in infants, children and young adults by pediatricians. *Pediatrics.* 2016;137(1):28–30.

47. Schaiquevich P, Francis JH, Cancela MB, et al. Treatment of retinoblastoma: what is the latest and what is the future. *Front Oncol.* 2022;12. 822330.

48. Pepose JS, Sarda SP, Cheng WY, et al. Direct and indirect costs of infectious conjunctivitis in a commercially insured population in the United States. *Clin Ophthalmol.* 2020;14:377–387.

49. Lopez Montero, MC. Conjunctivitis. https://eyewiki.org/Conjunctivitis.

50. American Academy of Pediatrics Committee on Infectious Diseases. Chlamydia trachomatis. In: Kimberlin DW, Barnett ED, Lynfield R, Sawyer MH, eds. *Red Book: 2021-2024 Report of the Committee on Infectious Diseases*. American Academy of Pediatrics; 2021a:1023–1024.

51. American Academy of Pediatrics Committee on Infectious Diseases. Gonococcal infections. In: Kimberlin DW, Barnett ED, Lynfield R, Sawyer MH, eds. *Red Book: 2021-2024 Report of the Committee on Infectious Diseases*. American Academy of Pediatrics; 2021b:342.

52. American Academy of Pediatrics Committee on Infectious Diseases. Nongonococcal, nonchlamydia ophthalmia. In: Kimberlin DW, Barnett ED, Lynfield R, Sawyer MH, eds. *Red Book: 2021-2024 Report of the Committee on Infectious Diseases*. American Academy of Pediatrics; 2021c:974.

53. American Academy of Pediatrics Committee on Infectious Diseases. Chlamydia trachomatis. In: Kimberlin DW, Barnett ED, Lynfield R, Sawyer MH, eds. *Red Book: 2021-2024 Report of the Committee on Infectious Diseases*. American Academy of Pediatrics; 2021c:263.

54. International Trachoma Initiative. *Zithromax Management Guide*; 2020. https://www.trachoma.org/zithromax-management-guide.

55. Tonk RS. Blepharitis. American Academy of Ophthalmalogy EyeWiki. Retrieved from https://eyewiki.org/Blepharitis.

56. Baharestani S, Stye. https://eyewiki.org/Stye.

57. Monsivais-Rodriguez FV. Preceptal cellulitis. https://eyewiki.org/Preseptal_Cellulitis.

58. Maleki A, Anesi SD, Look-Why S, et al. Pediatric uveitis: a comprehensive review. *Surv Ophthalmol.* 2022;67(2):510–529.

59. Shin Y, Kang JM, Lee J, et al. Epidemiology of pediatric uveitis and associated systemic diseases. *Pediatr Rheumatol.* 2021;19:48.

60. Gardiner MF. *Conjunctival Injury*; 2022. UpToDate www.uptodate.com/contents/conjunctival-injury.

61. Jacobs DS. Corneal abrasions and corneal foreign bodies: Management.https://www.uptodate.com/contents/corneal-abrasions-and-corneal-foreign-bodies-management.

62. Soleimani M, Naderan M. Management strategies of ocular chemical burns: current perspectives. *Clin Ophthalmol.* 2020;14:2687–2699.

63. Oldham GW. *Hyphema*; 2022. https://eyewiki.org/Hyphema.

64. Agarkar S, Gokhale VV, Raman R, et al. Incidence, risk factors, and outcomes of retinal detachment after pediatric cataract surgery. *Ophthalmology.* 2018;125(1):36–42.

65. Neuman MI, Bachur RG. *Orbital Fractures*; 2022. UpToDate www.uptodate.com/contents/orbital-fractures.

66. Weber AC, Chundury RV. Entropion. http://eyewiki.org/Entropion.

67. Belliveau MJ. *Ectropion*; 2022. http://eyewiki.org/Ectropion.

31

Ear and Hearing Disorders

ADEBOLA M. OLAREWAJU

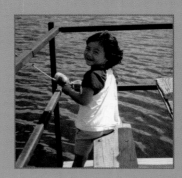

The ear serves two functions—hearing and equilibrium. Any dysfunction of the external or internal ear structures or surrounding tissues can cause global developmental delays with lifelong effects as adequate hearing is important for speech and language acquisition, academic performance, and socialization. Pediatric primary care providers (PCPs) must understand ear anatomy and physiology and be able to identify, assess, and diagnose ear disorders in children. The management of acute and chronic ear disorders is also discussed in this chapter.

Embryonic Development

Ear development begins during the third week of gestation and is complete by the third month of fetal life. An insult to the fetus during this time can cause irreparable damage to the ear and negatively affect hearing. The ear and kidney develop at a slightly different gestational periods, but a developmental malformation of the renal system or ear should alert the PCP to potential malformation or dysfunction in the other system.

Anatomy and Physiology

The ear has three main structures: the external, middle, and inner ear.

The *external* ear consists of the pinna (or auricle), the auditory canal (or meatus), and the tympanic membrane (TM). The external ear collects and transmits sound waves from outside the ear to the middle ear and requires patency of the external auditory canal (EAC). The canal contains glands that secrete sweat, sebum, and cerumen that help lubricate the hair follicles as well as trap and remove dust, pollen, pollution, and small foreign bodies to aid in debris removal. The auditory canal starts at the outer ear and ends at the TM. The canal moves sound waves from the pinna to the TM at the proximal end of the EAC. The TM separates the external ear from the middle ear.

The *middle* ear consists of the structures between the TM and the oval window and includes the ossicles, oval window, round window, and eustachian tube. The ossicles—the malleus, incus, and stapes—conduct sound waves from the EAC to the inner ear. The malleus lies against the TM, the incus lies between the malleus and stapes, and the stapes rests against the oval window. Vibrations across the TM, ossicles, and oval window cause the fluids of the inner ear to stimulate the cochlea resulting in sound perception.

The eustachian tube serves as the ventilation system to the middle ear, linking the middle ear with the posterior aspect of the palate. The function of the eustachian tube is to: (1) ventilate the middle ear to equalize middle ear pressure with atmospheric pressure, and (2) drain secretions from the middle ear into the nasopharynx. The muscles surrounding the eustachian tubes contract during yawning and swallowing and impact the opening and closing of the eustachian tubes in the posterior palate.

The *inner* ear consists of the cochlea (hearing) and the semicircular canals (equilibrium/balance). The sound waves that reach the cochlea are transmitted by the organ of Corti to the auditory (acoustic) nerve (cranial nerve [CN] VIII) and then to the auditory cortex of the brain's temporal lobe. The equilibrium receptors in the semicircular canals and vestibule of the inner ear respond to changes in movement direction and help maintain equilibrium. The vestibular nerve transmits information related to motion and position to the ocular and postural muscles, brainstem, and cerebral cortex.

Pathophysiology

Defense Mechanisms

The pathological processes that affect the ear are usually localized; however, they can also be related to systemic dysfunction or disorders. Common localized pathologic conditions include viral, bacterial, or fungal infections; foreign bodies; and trauma. Systemically, neurologic dysfunction, poor immunologic competence, and congenital anomalies can affect the ear and its function. Debris produced by keratinizing cells in the EAC form *cerumen* (i.e., "ear wax"), which is lubricated and extruded by the cilia. The acidic pH in the ear canal prevents the growth of pathogenic bacteria, and the surface lining of the external ear is water resistant as well as having ample blood and lymph supplies. These characteristics and the antibacterial properties of cerumen help protect against invading microorganisms. The proximal end of the EAC has more nerve fibers, which cause discomfort when touched. This discomfort serves as a protective function by deterring the insertion of foreign bodies into the ear, thus preventing damage to the middle ear. The structures for both hearing and equilibrium are deep within the skull, which provides additional protection to the inner ear. External influences, such as excessive environmental noise, can cause irreparable damage to the hearing structures.

Assessment of the Ear

Clinical Findings

History

The health history should include:
- Pain: onset, location, quality, duration, alleviating, or aggravating factors

Newborn/Infancy
- Does not startle at loud noises.
- Does not turn to the source of a sound after 6 months of age.
- Does not say single words, such as "dada" or "mama" by 1 year of age.
- Does not turn head to voice.
- Seems to hear some sounds but not others.
- Suspected or confirmed congenital or inherited condition associated with hearing loss, such as:
  - Usher, Waardenburg, Pendred, CHARGE, Alport, Stickler, Treacher Collins, or branchio-oto-renal syndromes or osteogenesis imperfecta.

Early/Middle Childhood
- Delayed or unclear speech
- Difficulty following instructions
- Teacher concerns about paying attention
- Often saying "Huh?" or "What?"
- Turning the volume on television or radio up very high

- Associated symptoms (e.g., fever, upper respiratory infection, cough symptoms)
- Itching and/or discharge
- Exposure to risk factors (e.g., tobacco smoke, bottle propping, pacifier use, childcare attendance, swimming)
- Known ear conditions (e.g., effusion in middle ear, otitis media, trauma)
- Prior history of meningitis (because of associated hearing loss)
- Tinnitus or hearing loss (Box 31.1)
- Craniofacial abnormalities (e.g., cleft palate) or syndromes associated with craniofacial anomalies affecting ear/hearing (e.g., Turner syndrome, Down syndrome, 22q11.2 deletion syndrome)
- Family history of ear dysfunction, hearing loss, or history of kidney malformation
- Prematurity (e.g., very low birth weight, low Apgar score, mechanical ventilation)
- Developmental milestones for speech and hearing-impaired children (Table 31.1)

Physical Examination

The physical examination should include:
- A visual inspection of the external ear structures for symmetry, ear shape (presence of helix, antihelix, fully formed pinna), ear/skin abnormalities (e.g., Darwinian tubercle, preauricular tags, pits, sinus), any discharge.
- The inner and outer canthi of the eye should align or form a straight line with the superior portion of the pinna. If the pinna inserts below this line, the ear is considered low-set, which can be associated with inherited syndromes.
- Assess for preauricular skin tag, pits, and/or sinus, which can be an isolated finding or associated with hearing loss, renal disorders, and genetic syndromes (e.g., branchio-oto-renal syndrome).
- Palpate the external ear and the mastoid process for tenderness and inflammation.
- Examine surrounding lymph nodes: preauricular/parotid, postauricular/mastoid.
- Otoscopic examination is often best accomplished using a soft-tipped speculum (see Chapter 5, Fig. 5.1) or at the end of the

TABLE 31.1   Developmental Milestones for Hearing-Impaired Children

Age Range	Developmental Milestones
Newborn/infant (0–1 year)	Language development: Deaf children exposed early to sign language develop language similarly to hearing children exposed to spoken language. Deaf children exposed to both spoken and sign language learn both and progress as hearing children. Deaf children exposed only to spoken language have language delays. Language output is decreased around 6–9 months old
Early childhood	
1–2 years	Language output decreased
3–5 years	May have early processing delays. Symbolic play may be delayed if language skills are decreased
Middle childhood (6–10 years)	May have concrete processing delays. Decreased self-concept
Adolescence (11–18 years)	Increased adjustment problems and decreased social maturity. Decreased self-concept. May have formal processing delays

physical examination as it can be painful if an ear speculum contacts the sensitive external canal wall.
- Examine younger child seated or secured on the parent's lap. For infants and small children, pull the helix down, out, and back to enhance visualization of the EAC and TM before inserting the speculum. In older children and adolescents, lift the ear up and back, slightly away from the head, as with adults.
- Examine the EAC for redness, edema, or discharge. Assess the surface of the TM, the bony (malleolus) processes, and cone of light (Fig. 31.1).
- Note air-fluid level or bubbles behind the TM or any retraction, bulging, perforation, fibrosis, redness, or color alteration.
- Assess TM mobility using pneumatic otoscopy. Use of a soft-tipped otoscopic speculum (see Fig. 5.1) can improve occlusion by creating a good seal.

Cerumen Removal

The removal of cerumen is essential when it impedes the examination or alters hearing. This can be accomplished by mechanical removal or by cerumenolytics with or without irrigation. Proper restraint is essential during the procedure. Infants or young children may be swaddled, as movement during manual extraction can cause injury to the external canal. The best results occur with the instillation of a cerumenolytic agent followed by water ear irrigation.

Common *cerumenolytics* include hydrogen peroxide and docusate sodium (Colace), both of which are water-based, or mineral oil. Irrigation is accomplished by using a bulb syringe, ear

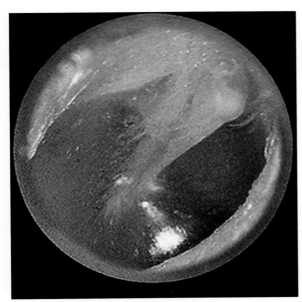

• **Fig. 31.1** Normal Tympanic Membrane. (From Ball JW, Dains JE, Flynn FA, et al. *Seidel's Guide to Physical Examination*. 10th ed. Elsevier; 2023.)

irrigation bottle, or water jet on low setting. Water-based cerumenolytics disintegrate the wax, whereas oil-based products soften the wax. Irrigation should not be attempted if there is a suspected TM perforation or if the child has tympanostomy tubes.

Mechanical removal requires skill and special instrumentation (e.g., plastic or metal curettes, microsuction, curettage, ear forceps). The PCP should carefully explain the procedure to parents and inform them that the ear canal is extremely sensitive and fragile and bleeds easily when touched. Use of a lighted instrument (e.g., curette) with magnification is helpful. PCPs and parents typically prefer the irrigation technique over mechanical removal of cerumen.[1] For children with chronic cerumen impactions that affect hearing, routine otic drops containing carbamide peroxide may be needed to keep the EACs clear of cerumen.

Hearing Screening

The American Academy of Pediatrics' Early Hearing Detection and Intervention (EHDI) 1-3-6 guidelines include: hearing screening completion by *1 month* of age, diagnosis of any hearing loss by *3 months* of age, with hearing aid selection and fitting within 1 month of confirmation of hearing loss if parents choose that option, and entry into early intervention services by *6 months* of age. The newborn hearing evaluation is administered with the Automated Auditory Brainstem Response (AABR), Otoacoustic Emissions (OAE), or both. Both approaches have high sensitivity and specificity, and relatively low cost, and can be done while the newborn is asleep. Newborns identified with potential hearing loss through newborn screening have earlier referral, diagnosis, and management than those identified later in infancy or early childhood.[2]

In addition to newborn screening, the Joint Committee on Infant Hearing (JCIH) recommends assessing hearing and speech development regularly reevaluated at appropriate intervals across the pediatric lifespan.[3] Infants who pass newborn screening but have other risk factors for hearing loss should have at least one diagnostic audiology assessment by 9 months of age.[4] The American Academy of Pediatrics (AAP) Bright Futures guidelines recommend pure-tone audiometry at 4, 5, 6, 8, 10, 13, 16, and 20 years of age, with subjective assessment at other ages.[3] More frequent hearing, speech-language, and communication screenings are indicated for children at high risk for hearing loss, including those with craniofacial anomalies, persistent or recurrent acute otitis media (AOM), middle ear effusion (MEE), and those with chronic exposure to loud noise.

Diagnostic Studies

- **Evoked otoacoustic emission** (EOAE) testing is the method of hearing screening used for universal newborn screening. The normal-hearing ear emits detectable sounds called *spontaneous otoacoustic emissions* when stimulated. EOAE shows the cochlea's outer hair cells are functioning appropriately and hearing is likely intact. EOAE is efficient, highly sensitive, and easy to perform in a quiet room with a cooperative, quiet, or sleeping infant, which makes it conducive for newborns. EOAE does not quantify hearing deficit and may not identify auditory nerve dysfunction.

- **Auditory brainstem response** (ABR) measures sound-induced electrical signals in the cochlea and the functioning of the peripheral auditory system and neurologic pathways related to hearing. Although it is not a direct measure of hearing, ABR indicates hearing thresholds. The ABR is useful in identifying hearing loss in newborns, as well as infants or children unable to cooperate with EOAE or pure-tone audiometry. Occasionally, sedation is required for infants and children who are unable to successfully cooperate to complete the test. Neurologic abnormalities may affect the interpretation of ABR results.

- **Pure tone audiometry** assesses hearing loss in older children through adulthood. It measures hearing in decibels (dBs) at varying frequencies (Tables 31.2 and 31.3). Twenty dB is about as loud as a whisper, 40 dB is normal speaking loudness, and 90 dB produces pain. The frequencies of normal speaking range from 250 to 4000 Hz. Hearing loss, especially in the higher frequencies (2000–6000 Hz), can cause significant problems in understanding speech. Screening audiograms test hearing at 20 dB and frequencies of 500, 1000, 2000, and 4000 Hz and are useful in office and school settings. If a more detailed audiogram is needed, the PCP should refer the child/teen to an audiologist.

- **Conditioned play audiometry** (CPA) can be used for children with a developmental age of at least 2.5 years. The child is taught to perform a simple task, such as placing a block in a bucket, when they are presented with a sound, rather than raising a hand.

- **Pneumatic otoscopy** assesses TM mobility in response to pressure changes. A good seal with the ophthalmoscope speculum is required. Brisk movement of the membrane should be seen; altered mobility may be due to fluid in the middle ear or tympanosclerosis. Detecting MEE is key to establishing the diagnosis of otitis media with effusion (OME).

- **Tympanometry** evaluates the function of the middle ear by assessing the movement of the TM. TM movement is translated into a graph called a *tympanogram* (Fig. 31.2). Type A tympanogram has a compliance peak between ±100 mm H_2O and reflects a healthy TM; type B tympanogram has no peak or a flattened wave and suggests effusion, perforation, or the presence of a pressure-equalizing tube (Fig. 31.3); type C tympanogram has a sharp peak between –100 and –200 mm H_2O and reflects negative ear pressure.

TABLE 31.2   Audiologic Tests for Infants and Young Children

Test	Characteristics	Age Range	Advantages	Disadvantages
Behavioral observation audiometry (BOA)	Behavioral test: Responses to noisemakers or calibrated sounds are observed	0–5 months	Low cost	Insensitive to unilateral or less than severe hearing loss; highly subject to observer bias; child tires rapidly when subjected to repeated stimuli
Visual reinforced audiometry (VRA)	Behavioral test: Child is given an animated toy for turning to sounds	5–24 months	Low cost; child responds at softer levels and for longer periods compared with BOA	Insensitive to unilateral loss (unless earphones used); need two examiners to reduce bias
Play audiometry	Behavioral test: Child is trained to respond to tones by playing a game	2–5 years	Low cost; can detect unilateral and mild hearing loss	Requires cooperation of child
Screening audiometry	Behavioral test: Child raises hand or responds verbally to tones at fixed levels (20–25 dB)	4 years and older	Can be performed by trained paraprofessional in most children 4 years and older; can detect unilateral and mild hearing loss	Further tests required if failed
Otoacoustic emission (OAE)	Physiologic test: Response of inner ear to brief clicks or tones is measured with specialized instrument	All ages	Child's response not needed; takes less than 2 minutes if child is quiet; can be performed by a trained paraprofessional; low cost; can detect unilateral and mild hearing loss	Cannot tell type or degree of loss; further tests required if failed
Auditory brainstem response (ABR) audiometry	Physiologic test: Averaged number of responses of brainstem to brief tones or clicks	All ages	Child's response not needed; can detect unilateral and mild loss; can determine degree and slope of loss (with tone bursts and bone conduction testing)	Requires audiologist and equipment to administer and interpret; expensive; requires sedation beyond about 6 months old

TABLE 31.3   Evaluation of Audiometric Results

Average Threshold at 500–2000 Hz (Decibels)	Description	Significance
–10 to +15	Normal	
16–25	Slight loss (minimal)	Difficulty hearing faint speech, slight verbal deficit
26–40	Mild loss	Auditory learning dysfunction, language, or speech problems
41–55	Moderate loss	Trouble hearing conversational speech; may miss 50% of class discussion
56–70	Moderately severe loss	
71–90	Severe loss	Educational retardation, learning disability, limited vocabulary
90+	Profound loss	

Laboratory tests are rarely indicated, unless questions remain regarding perinatal infection, systemic illness, or concomitant kidney dysfunction. Exudate from AOM with perforation may be cultured.

Hearing Impairment: Sensorineural, Conductive, and Mixed Hearing Loss

Normal hearing thresholds are between 0 to 20 dB. Hearing loss is defined as pure-tone hearing loss greater than 20 dB at any frequency and ranges from mild to profound loss (deaf), affects one or both ears, and low to high frequencies. The overall prevalence of hearing loss is estimated to be 1.7 per 1000 infants screened and 5 per 1000 in children 3 to 17 years old.[4] Approximately 50% to 60% of hearing loss in infants is related to a genetic syndrome.[5,6] More than 400 genetic conditions involve hearing loss,[5] and almost half of congenital hearing loss is attributed to a mutation in the connexin gene family, with most mutations occurring on the *GJB2* (13q12.11) gene.[7] A referral for genetic testing is key if genetic hearing loss is suspected. Thirty percent of hearing loss in newborns is due to environmental causes, such as maternal infection during pregnancy (e.g., Rubella, cytomegalovirus) or complications at the time of delivery.[4]

There are three types of hearing loss or impairment: sensorineural (inner ear issue), conductive (outer or middle ear issue), and mixed.

A normal tympanogram is depicted below. Four features of the tympanogram can be used to evaluate the ear under test:

❶ **Static admittance (Peak Y_a)** is a measure of the height of the tympanometric peak. Given appropriate norms, static admittance is a useful indicator of middle ear disease.

❷ **Equivalent ear canal volume (+200 Vea)** is the admittance value determined with an ear canal air pressure of +200 d_aP_a (dekapascals). An abnormally high equivalent ear canal volume suggests the presence of a tympanic membrane perforation, or a patent tympanostomy tube.

❸ **Tympanometric peak pressure (TPP)** is the position of the tympanometric peak on the pressure axis. TPP is an imprecise measure of the middle ear pressure. By itself, TPP is not an accurate indicator of middle ear disease.

❹ **Tympanometric gradient (GR)** or **tympanometric width** is a measure of the width of the tympanometric peak. Defined as the pressure interval required for a 50% reduction of peak eardrum admittance, tympanometric width is a good indicator of the presence of **middle ear effusion**.

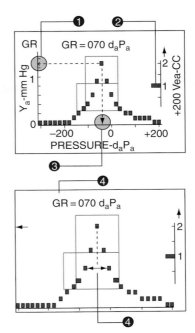

• **Fig. 31.2** Normal Tympanogram.

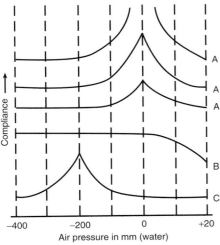

• **Fig. 31.3** Five Types of Tympanogram Curves. In general, an A curve indicates a normal tympanic membrane, a B curve is abnormal, a C curve may be abnormal, and a D curve (not shown) indicates hypermobility. A D curve (not shown) indicates hypermobility, which may be normal in infants.

Sensorineural hearing loss (SNHL) is most commonly associated with dysfunction or damage to the inner ear (e.g., the cochlea) or the auditory nerve (CN VIII). It can be congenital or acquired, mild or severe, and is almost always permanent. Environmental causes include exposure to excessive noise over time. Prenatal and perinatal causes include intrauterine infections (e.g., cytomegalovirus), toxic chemicals, and erythroblastosis fetalis.

Conductive hearing loss (CHL), either congenital or acquired, is caused by a problem in the outer ear or middle ear. It results from blocked sound wave transmission from the EAC to the inner ear and the causes include AOM, OME, foreign body, aural canal stenosis or atresia, ossicular malformations, cerumen impaction, TM perforation, cholesteatoma, and otosclerosis. In CHL, the cochlea and auditory nerve function normally, but the hearing loss is usually in the range of 20 to 60 dB.

Mixed hearing loss involves a combination of SNHL and CHL. Abnormalities occur in the outer, middle, and/or inner ears. CHL occurs when the nerves or nuclei of the central nervous system are impaired either in the pathways to the brain or in the brain.

Clinical Findings

History. Hearing loss is often a "silent disease." The PCP needs to be alerted to SNHL risk factors, especially in newborns, which include:

- Birth weight less than 1500 g
- Severe respiratory depression at birth (e.g., Apgar score of 0–3 at 5 minutes, failure to initiate a response by 10 minutes, or hypotonia at up to 2 hours old), also referred to as *birth asphyxia* or *hypoxic ischemic encephalopathy*
- Neonatal Extracorporeal membrane oxygenation (ECMO
- Neonatal intensive care unit admission for 5 days or longer
- Prolonged mechanical ventilation for more than 10 days
- Persistent pulmonary hypertension
- Long QT syndrome (usually profound hearing loss)
- Congenital infections (e.g., toxoplasmosis, bacterial meningitis, syphilis, rubella, cytomegalovirus, herpes)
- Metabolic disorders (e.g., phenylketonuria, galactosemia)
- Endocrine disorders (e.g., adrenal hyperplasia, hypothyroidism)
- Craniofacial anomalies, including morphologic abnormalities of the pinna and ear canal.
- Genetic syndromes associated with hearing loss (e.g., Usher, Alport syndrome, branchio-oto-renal syndrome, Down syndrome, Neurofibromatosis [NF1, NF2], osteopetrosis, sickle cell disease, Treacher Collins syndrome, Waardenburg syndrome).
- Hyperbilirubinemia requiring exchange transfusion or causing kernicterus
- Family history of hereditary childhood SNHL
- Ototoxic drug exposure (e.g., gentamicin, furosemide)

In addition, risk factors for hearing loss in infants and early childhood include:

- Parental concern regarding hearing, speech, language, or developmental delay
- Kidney malformation or malfunction
- Neurodegenerative disorders (e.g., Hunter syndrome) or sensorimotor neuropathies (e.g., Friedreich ataxia, Charcot-Marie-Tooth disease)
- Head trauma with loss of consciousness or skull fracture (especially basal skull or temporal bone fractures)
- Bacterial meningitis

Other risk factors or indicators of hearing loss in older children and adolescents include:

- Failure to respond to auditory stimuli, delayed speech development, speech that is monotone and difficult to understand, speaking avoidance
- Failed school screening audiogram; decreased note taking; seeming to misunderstand, ignore, confuse, or miss what is being said
- Aggressive behavior, increased physical complaints, difficulty in school and social situations
- Environmental exposure to loud noises like firecrackers, pistols, firearms, loud music, and machines (e.g., snowmobiles, farm equipment, lawn mowers)
- History of head or neck irradiation

Physical Examination

- Ears: Preauricular tags, pits, or sinus, auricular malformation, abnormal TM, or impaired mobility with pneumatic otoscopy
- Eyes: Cataracts, corneal opacities, coloboma, blindness, nystagmus, exophthalmos, night blindness, heterochromia iridis, or blue sclerae (associated with genetic disorders such as osteogenesis imperfecta and Ehlers-Danlos syndrome that can cause SNHL)
- Note craniofacial abnormalities, low-set ears or abnormalities of the pinna and ear canal associated with SNHL, or note a white forelock on hairline as seen in Waardenburg syndrome

Diagnostic Studies. Hearing screening and evaluation as presented above.

Differential Diagnosis

Differential diagnoses for:

- *Conductive loss* includes cerumen impaction, OME, AOM, or AOM with TM perforation.
- *Congenital SNHL* includes infection, malformation, perilymph fistula, inherited disorders, prematurity, hyperbilirubinemia, infection, ototoxic drug exposure, noise exposure, trauma, tumor (rare in children without NF2), or heavy metals.

With any significant hearing loss, comorbidities may exist, including developmental and speech and language delays, family disruptions, depression, and associated genetic disorders.

Management

For *suspected* hearing loss, the PCP should:

- Evaluate and treat AOM and OME if present.
- Screen for hearing loss if bilateral MEE is present for 3 months or longer and refer to otolaryngology as indicated.
- If the child fails screening, refer to an audiologist for full evaluation. If hearing impairment or hearing loss is identified, then referral to otolaryngology is indicated.
- Refer families for genetic counseling if heritable causes are suspected.
- Encourage the use of amplification devices early as appropriate to improve school readiness and engagement.

Cochlear implants with an external speech processor are used for profound SNHL. Cochlear implants provide direct electrical stimulation to the auditory nerve. They are usually used in children with bilateral, severe SNHL and require a dedicated family and educational support system. Note: Children with cochlear implants may not be able to undergo standard magnetic resonance imaging (MRI) so consult with an otolaryngologist before ordering one.

Bone-anchored hearing implants may be used when auricular or postauricular aids cannot be used. They increase audibility in noisy situations, improve speech understanding, and help with sound localization through temporal bone sound conduction.

- Ensure a family-centered approach in making decisions regarding interventions for the child.
- Refer to/work with the public school district for evaluation for special education and classroom support for hearing impairment and preferential classroom seating.

Optimizing the care of a child with hearing loss or hearing impairment requires a multidisciplinary approach and interprofessional team, including the PCP, otolaryngologist, audiologist, speech–language pathologist, and, if indicated, a sign language specialist, a developmental linguist, and teacher(s) trained to work with the deaf and hearing impaired. From an information-processing perspective, early management goals are directed at providing stimuli that the infant and child can use to understand and interact with the environment.

Complications

Significant hearing loss impedes speech, language, cognitive development, and social interaction skills.

Developmental and Behavioral Effects

Most hearing-impaired children have some functional hearing. Developmental milestones for hearing-impaired children can be found in Table 31.1. Factors affecting their behavioral and developmental outcomes include the type and degree of hearing loss, the etiology of the loss (with comorbidities), the age of hearing loss onset and identification, the timing and appropriateness of educational interventions, and the family environment. The four main areas affected by hearing loss are (1) delay in the development of receptive and expressive communication skills, (2) reduced academic achievement due to language deficit causing learning problems, (3) communication difficulties causing social isolation and poor self-concept, and (4) impact on vocational choices. Children who experience difficulty with language development due to hearing deficits may also exhibit a decreased ability to communicate their needs and thoughts. They generally do well on nonverbal and performance measures of intelligence but score below average in abstract concepts and language abilities. In early childhood, schooling focuses on communication development, which may cause less focus on instruction in other areas, and lower scores in reading comprehension and math (Box 31.2).

Hearing-impaired children may manifest more behavioral and emotional problems than normal-hearing children, with impulsivity and aggression most common. Unless parents/families focus on communication, children with hearing loss may not receive the same nurturing and social support as their hearing counterparts. For example, if a child learns American Sign Language (ASL) but parents/siblings do not, communication opportunities are lost. Teens with hearing loss often face identity confusion because they compare themselves to their hearing peers, have academic challenges because they miss information or have a difficult time

• BOX 31.2 Effects of Hearing Loss on Development

Vocabulary
- Vocabulary develops more slowly.
- Learns concrete words more easily (e.g., "cat," "jump," "five," and "red") than abstract words (e.g., "before," "after," "equal to," and "jealous").
- Difficulty with function words (e.g., "the," "an," "are," and "a").
- The gap in vocabulary between children with normal hearing and those with hearing loss widens with age; there is no "catch up" without intervention.
- Has difficulty understanding words with multiple meanings (e.g., "bank" can mean the edge of a stream or a place for saving money).

Sentence Structure
- Comprehends and produces shorter and simpler sentences.
- Has difficulty understanding/writing complex sentences (e.g., relative clauses ["The teacher whom I have for math was sick today"] or passive voice ["The ball was thrown by Mary"]).
- Often cannot hear word endings, such as "-s" or "-ed," leading to misunderstandings and misuse of verb tense, pluralization, nonagreement of subject and verb, and possessives.

Speaking
- Often cannot hear quiet speech sounds, such as "s," "sh," "f," "t," and "k," and may not include them in speech, making the child difficult to understand.
- May not hear their own voices when they speak, thus speaking too loudly or not loud enough, use too high a pitch or sound like they are mumbling because of poor stress, poor inflection, or poor rate of speaking.

Academic Achievement
- Difficulty with all areas, especially reading and mathematical concepts.
- Children with mild to moderate hearing losses, on average, achieve one to four grade levels lower than their peers with normal hearing, unless appropriate management occurs.
- Those with severe to profound hearing loss usually achieve skills no higher than the third- or fourth-grade level unless appropriate educational intervention occurs early.
- The gap in academic achievement between children with normal hearing and those with hearing loss widens as they progress in school.
- Level of achievement is related to parental involvement and the quantity, quality, and timing of the support services children receive.

Social Functioning
- Severe to profound hearing loss children often report feeling isolated, without friends, and unhappy in school, particularly when their socialization is limited with other children whose hearing loss is limited.
- Social problems appear more frequently in children with a mild or moderate hearing loss than severe to profound loss.

Data from the American Speech-Language-Hearing Association. Effects of Hearing Loss on Development. http://www.asha.org/public/hearing/disorders/effects.htm.

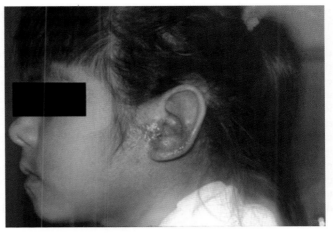

• **Fig. 31.4** Acute Otitis Externa With Purulent Drainage From Ear Canal. (From Cherry JD, et al. *Feigin and Cherry's Pediatric Infectious Diseases*, 8th ed. Elsevier; 2019.)

in class discussion, and experience depression or low self-esteem from feelings of being different.

Habilitation and Assistive Devices and Amplification Devices. Many technologic advances are available, including alert and warning devices, such as strobe lights and vibrating wake-up alarms, text messaging and email, closed-captioned television, videos, and phones, service animals, and social network sites. If children or teens use sign language, they should be provided with an interpreter during healthcare visits to ensure communication.

Amplification from a very early age is crucial in improving speech, language, and cognitive abilities of hearing-impaired children. Different types of hearing amplification have different purposes, and wireless and Bluetooth technologies have vastly improved the flexibility and use of these devices. Hearing assistive technology systems, including teacher microphone systems, frequency modulation systems, infrared systems, induction loop systems, and one-to-one communicators, may be used with or without amplifiers. Sound field systems amplify sound throughout a room, not just to an individual. Body-worn hearing aids with a lead to earphones are not common but may be used for children younger than 3 years, and those in need of more powerful or durable amplification. Postauricular devices may be used as early as 4 weeks of age, and postauricular external canal devices are frequently used in early childhood and as children grow. For external ear devices, ear molds are used and must fit well. Ear molds must be revised initially every 3 to 6 months, then annually after 4 to 6 years of age. Ear molds for external ear devices should be washed with soap and water each night and cleaned carefully to avoid clogging. Continuous high-pitched sounds from the hearing aid may be a sign that the ear molds do not fit properly. Avoidance of infection in the external ear canal includes ear-adjusting molds to reduce irritation and using petroleum jelly to decrease friction. If an otitis externa infection occurs, ear molds should be removed, cleaned, and not replaced for 1 to 2 days in bacterial infection and 3 to 5 days for fungal infections (Fig. 31.4).

Noise-Induced Hearing Loss

Noise is usually considered loud, harsh, unpleasant, or unwanted sound. *Noise pollution* is the presence of irritating, distracting, or physically dangerous noise. Sound has qualities of frequency or pitch (measured in cycles per minute and stated in hertz [Hz]), intensity or loudness (measured in dB sound pressure levels [SPLs]), periodicity, and duration (either continuous, short-term, or episodic). The human voice is approximately 50 to 60 dB SPL, blow dryers or food processors are 80 to 90 dB SPL, and jackhammers are 130 dB SPL. The National Institute for Occupational Safety and Health (NIOSH) defines hazardous noise as 85 dB for an average of 8 hours of sound exposure.[8] Hazardous noise is a common cause of SNHL in children, and the pattern of damage depends on the frequency, intensity, and duration of the noise.

Any structure in the ear can be permanently damaged by noise at a 140-dB SPL or greater.

Humans are subject to noise-induced hearing loss (NIHL) and tinnitus from exposure to continuous noise or to sudden acoustic trauma that causes damage to the hair cells of the cochlea due to excessive vibration. Extreme noise can rupture the TM. Noise of more than 85 dB but less than 140 dB leads to temporary hearing loss—most often in the 4000 Hz range. Permanent hearing loss can result from one exposure to a sudden, extreme noise (greater than 120 dB in children) of short duration, or from ongoing lower levels of noise. Permanent loss is often in the 3000 to 6000 Hz range. Music listened to with headphones, ear buds, and at concerts; firecrackers; electrical tools; and airport noise can contribute to hearing loss. Chronic, everyday noise causes sleep disturbance, distraction, impairment of cognitive function (e.g., poor reading comprehension, decreased memory), and an increased stress response (e.g., increased heart rate, blood pressure, adrenaline, cortisol production), which, in turn, result in irritability, poor coping, and lower achievement in children. Newborns are particularly vulnerable, and it is important to recognize that excessive noise in hospital nurseries and intensive care units may have short- and long-term effects on growth and development.

Clinical Findings

History. A careful history includes the following:
- Type(s) of noise in the environment
- Exposure to chronic noise
- Episodic acoustic trauma
- History of ear disease
- History of prematurity or exposure to ototoxic drugs

Physical Examination. Visual examination of the TM with insufflation or pneumatic otoscopy should be done at every well-child visit. Tympanography can help rule out chronic MEE.

Management

NIHL is 100% preventable. The goals are to:
- Increase awareness of hazardous noise in the home environment.
- Well-child visits should include a targeted history related to the child's noise environment. All families should be given information on excessive noise, its relationship to the auditory system, and how to avoid exposure to hazardous noise.
- Parents and children should be encouraged to minimize noise, including efforts to:
  - Reduce excessive noise from television and car radios.
  - Use ear buds and headphones cautiously; volume should allow the child/adolescent to hear normal conversation.
  - Avoid hazardous sounds (e.g., loud music, firecrackers) and other sources of episodic, extreme noise (e.g., crowd noise at concerts, sports events).
  - Create a "quiet" zone in the home setting. Mitigate exposure to noise.
- Wear earplugs to protect against "unavoidable" occupational noise (e.g., when electrical ss or other loud tools are used).
- Reduce hazardous noise in the environment and increase awareness of hazardous noise among children, teens, and families.

Foreign Body in the Ear Canal

Foreign bodies in the ear canal are seen by PCPs, in emergency departments, and by otolaryngologists. The foreign bodies include food, toy pieces, beads, disk batteries, paper, cotton swab, and/or insects, to name a few. They are usually placed into the ear canal by the child; however, it is important to remember that plant materials can be intentionally inserted into the EAC as a form of native remedy.

Clinical Findings

History. The history often reveals:
- Child report of putting something into their ear or having something thrown at them
- Complaints of itching, buzzing, fullness, or an object in the ear
- Persistent cough or hiccups
- Unilateral otalgia and otorrhea (bloody or purulent)

Some children may be asymptomatic despite the presence of a foreign body in the canal.

Physical Examination. A foreign body is visible with the naked eye or by otoscopic examination.

Management

Adequate visualization in a cooperative child is key to successful removal of the foreign body in the EAC. Foreign bodies in the lateral one-third of the ear canal are the easiest to remove. Those trapped in the medial two-thirds of the ear canal are more difficult to remove because the canal narrows and is increasingly vascular and sensitive.
- Soft, irregularly shaped objects are generally graspable with a bayonet forceps, alligator forceps, or curved hook.
- Round or breakable objects can be removed using a wire loop, a curette, or right-angle hook slowly advanced beyond the object and withdrawn carefully. If available, a lighted curette can illuminate the ear canal and assist in foreign body removal.
- Irrigation can only be done if the TM is intact. Use body temperature fluid and a commercial irrigator or 60-mL syringe with an angiocatheter on the end.
  - Irrigation can push the object farther into the ear canal, so care should be taken when attempting to flush out a foreign body.
  - Do not irrigate if the object is a disk battery, the TM is not intact, or if it is made of organic material (corn, peas, and so on), because moisture may cause the object to expand and become more difficult to remove.
- Disk, coin-shaped, or button batteries must be removed emergently as disk batteries exposed to moisture leak corrosive material causing severe tissue damage and possible hearing loss.
- Spherical objects are the most difficult to remove and often require referral to an otolaryngologist.
- If the object is made of iron, nickel, or cobalt, a tiny, but powerful magnet may be used for retrieval.
- Insects in the ear canal should be suffocated with mineral oil, then the ear can be irrigated, or the child can be referred for otolaryngology for removal.
- Refer to otolaryngologist when:
  - The foreign body cannot be extracted on the first few attempts or cannot be removed without risking damage to the external canal or TM.
  - There is worsening pain.
  - Child is uncooperative.
  - The object is lying on the TM or has been in the canal over 24 hours.
- Post removal, topical antibiotic drops with steroid are recommended for drainage/infection, to prevent infection if the canal is damaged during the removal, and to decrease inflammation.

Complications

Infection, perforation of the TM, and damage to the ossicles are possible if the object is not removed.

Ear Conditions in Children

Otitis Externa

Otitis externa (OE) ("swimmer's ear") is a diffuse inflammation of the EAC but can also involve the pinna or TM. Inflammation is evidenced by (1) simple infection with edema, discharge, and erythema; (2) furuncles or small abscesses that form in hair follicles; or (3) infection of the superficial layers of the epidermis. It can also be classified as mycotic OE, caused by fungus, or as chronic external otitis, a diffuse low-grade infection of the EAC. Severe infection or systemic infection can occur in children who have type 1 diabetes mellitus, are immunocompromised, or who received head and neck irradiation.

OE results when the protective barriers in the EAC are damaged by mechanical or chemical mechanisms. OE is usually caused by retained moisture in the EAC that changes the usually acidic environment to a neutral or basic environment, thereby promoting bacterial or fungal growth. The chlorine in swimming pools kills the normal ear flora, allowing the growth of pathogens, which is why it is seen most often in swimmers. Further, regular cleaning of the EAC removes cerumen, which is an important water and infection barrier. Soapy deposits, alkaline topical medications, debris from skin conditions, local trauma, sweating, allergy, stress, and hearing aids can also cause OE.[9]

OE is most often caused by *Pseudomonas aeruginosa* and *Staphylococcus aureus,* but it is not uncommon for the infection to be polymicrobial. Furunculosis of the external canal is generally caused by *S. aureus* and *Streptococcus pyogenes*. Otomycosis is caused by *Aspergillus* or *Candida* and can result from systemic or topical antibiotics or steroids. Otomycosis is more common in children with type 1 diabetes mellitus or immune dysfunction, and in these cases is most commonly caused by *Aspergillus niger, Escherichia coli,* or *Klebsiella pneumonia. Group B streptococci* are a more common cause in neonates.

Long-standing ear drainage may suggest a foreign body, chronic middle ear pathology (e.g., cholesteatoma), or granulomatous tissue. Bloody drainage may indicate trauma, severe otitis media, or granulation tissue. Chronic or recurrent OE may result from eczema, seborrhea, or psoriasis. Eczematous dermatitis, moist vesicles, and pustules are seen in acute infection, whereas crusting is more consistent with chronic infection.

Clinical Findings

History
- Itching and irritation
- Pain that is disproportionate to what is seen on examination
- Pressure and fullness in ear
- Conductive or SNHL, or otorrhea
- EAC or periauricular edema, and preauricular and postauricular lymphadenopathy with more severe disease
- Extension to the surrounding soft tissue results in the obstruction of the canal with or without cellulitis

Physical Examination. Findings on physical examination include the following:
- Pain, often quite severe, with pushing the tragus or pulling the pinna during otoscopic examination
- Swollen EAC with debris, making visualization of the TM difficult or impossible
- Occasional regional lymphadenopathy (pre-/post-auricular)
- Tragal tenderness with a red, raised area of induration that can be deep and diffuse or superficial and pointing, which is characteristic of furunculosis
- Red, crusty, or pustular spreading lesions
- Pruritus associated with thick otorrhea (can be black, gray, blue-green, yellow, or white) and black spots over the TM are indicative of mycotic infection
- Dry-appearing canal with atrophy or thinning of the canal and no cerumen visible with chronic OE
- Presence of tympanostomy or pressure-equalizing (PE) tubes or TM perforation

Diagnostic Studies. Culturing the ear discharge is not routine but may be indicated if clinical improvement is not seen during or after treatment, severe pain persists, in neonates and immunocompromised children, or chronic or recurrent OE is suspected. Culturing requires a swab premoistened with sterile nonbacteriostatic saline or sterile water.

Differential Diagnosis

Differential diagnoses include AOM with perforation, tympanostomy tube otorrhea (TTO), chronic suppurative otitis media (CSOM), necrotizing OE, cholesteatoma, mastoiditis, posterior auricular lymphadenopathy, dental infection, and eczema.

Management

The management of OE includes:
- Eardrops are the mainstay of OE therapy (Table 31.4). Symptoms should markedly improve within 7 days, but resolution of the infection may take up to 2 weeks. Treat with eardrops until all symptoms resolve.
  - Eardrops containing acetic acid or antibiotic with and without corticosteroid drops are the treatment of choice. Neomycin-containing drops should not be used if the TM is not intact, because these drugs are known to cause damage to the cochlea and hypersensitivity.
  - Quinolone medications are effective against *Pseudomonas, S. aureus,* and *Streptococcus pneumoniae,* if the OE is a complication of AOM.
- Systemic antibiotics should not be used unless there is extension of infection beyond the ear or host factors that require more systemic treatment (severe OE, systemic illness, fever, lymphadenitis, failed topical treatment).
- Drops should be administered with the child lying down with the affected ear upward and instilled until the canal is filled, pumping the tragus to ensure filling. The child should remain lying down for 3 to 5 minutes, leaving the ear open to the air.
- If the infection is severe and not improving in the first 2 to 3 days, reexamine patient and consider a change in diagnosis and/or treatment. Consider referral to the otolaryngologist for debridement and suction.[11]
- Avoid cleaning, manipulating, and getting water into the ear. Swimming is prohibited during acute infection.
- Administer analgesics for pain.
- Debridement with calcium alginate swabs is indicated once the inflammatory process subsides and enhances the effectiveness of the ototopical antibiotic drops. Lance a furuncle that is superficial and pointed with a 14-gauge needle. If it is deep and diffuse, a heating pad or warm oil-based drops can speed resolution.

TABLE 31.4	Commonly Used Topical Preparations for Otitis Externa and Analgesia				
Product Name (Manufacturer)	Antibiotic	Steroid	Acid	Comments	
Antibiotics (Not Ototoxic)					
Ciprodex (Alcon)	Ciprofloxacin	Dexamethasone		Use ≥6 months old Contains steroid	
Floxin Otic (Daiichi Pharmaceutical)	Ofloxacin	None	Acetic and boric	Does not contain steroid	
Vasocidin ophthalmic (Ciba Vision Ophthalmics)	Sulfacetamide sodium	Prednisolone sodium phosphate		No documented ototoxicity with either agent Excellent broad-spectrum coverage Contains steroid	
Antibiotics (Only Use With Intact TM)[a]					
Cortisporin Otic Susp Pediotic (King Pharmaceutical)	Polymyxin B and neomycin	Hydrocortisone	Hydrochloric acid	May be painful on instillation Neomycin may cause cutaneous irritation Not to be used if TM integrity unknown	
Cipro HC Otic (Alcon Labs)	Ciprofloxacin	Hydrocortisone	Glacial acetic acid	Use ≥1 year old Contraindicated with TM perforation	
Cleansing and Antipruritic Agent (Only Use With Intact TM)[a]					
Domeboro Otic (Bayer Pharmaceutical Division)	None	None	Acetic acid	Excellent choice for cleansing of the EAC Aluminum acetate helps to prevent itching Not to be used if TM integrity is unknown	

EAC, External auditory canal; *TM*, tympanic membrane.

[a]Ototoxic if TM perforation present.

- If infection is present, clear the canal by using water or an antiseptic solution followed by a warm-water rinse. Apply an antibiotic ointment (mupirocin) twice a day for 5 to 7 days, or retapamulin in children over 9 months of age if resistant to mupirocin. The child should avoid touching the ear.
- Fungal OE is uncommon and more likely related to chronic OE or follows treatment with topical and/or systemic antibiotics. *Aspergillus* and *Candida* species are the most common pathogens in OE.[11] Treatment consists of antifungal solutions, such as clotrimazole-miconazole or nystatin.

If the child has not improved (relief of otalgia and itching) within 72 hours, recheck to confirm diagnosis.[11] Lack of improvement may be due to an obstructed ear canal, foreign body, poor adherence, or contact sensitivity among other things. Routine follow-up is not needed unless symptoms worsen after treatment or there is no improvement in a week. A referral to an otolaryngologist is indicated.

Complications

Infection of surrounding tissues, irritated furunculosis, and malignant OE with progression and necrosis caused by *Pseudomonas* are possible complications. Involvement of the parotid gland, mastoid bone, and infratemporal fossa is rare.

Prevention

The patient should be instructed to do the following:
- Avoid water in the ear canals.
- Use ear plugs during water sports.

- Use a blow dryer on warm setting to dry the EAC.
- Avoid persistent scratching or cleaning of the external canal.
- Avoid prolonged use of cerumenolytic agents.
- If the child uses hearing aids, they should be removed nightly and cleaned.

Acute Otitis Media

AOM is an acute infection of the middle ear (Fig. 31.5). It is important that clinicians accurately diagnose otitis media to reduce overtreatment and antibiotic resistance.[12] The following three components are needed to diagnose AOM[13]:
- Recent, abrupt onset of middle ear inflammation and effusion (ear pain, irritability, otorrhea, and/or fever)
- Moderate to severe bulging TM (mild bulging if onset <48 hours), limited or absent mobility by pneumatic otoscopy, air-fluid level behind TM, and/or otorrhea
- Signs and symptoms of middle ear inflammation confirmed by distinct TM erythema or ear pain (holding, tugging, rubbing the ear)

Characteristics of different types of AOM are defined in Table 31.5. AOM often follows eustachian tube dysfunction (ETD). Infants and young children are prone to ETD because of the proximity to the adenoids, the horizontal orientation of the eustachian tube (takes an adult orientation in middle childhood), and narrow diameter of the tube, but it also occurs in older children. Common causes of ETD include upper respiratory infections, craniofacial anomalies (e.g., cleft palate), allergies, adenoid hypertrophy, and tobacco smoke exposure. ETD leads to functional eustachian tube obstruction and inflammation that decreases the protective

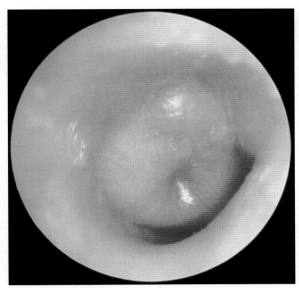

• **Fig. 31.5** Acute Otitis Media. (From Slater T, Waduud MA, Ahmed N. *Pocketbook of Differential Diagnosis.* 5th ed. Elsevier; 2021.)

TABLE 31.5　Types of Acute Otitis Media

Type	Characteristics
Acute otitis media (AOM)	Suppurative effusion of the middle ear
Bullous myringitis	AOM in which bullae form between the inner and middle layers of the TM and bulge outward
Persistent AOM	AOM that has not resolved when antibiotic therapy has been completed or AOM recurs within days of treatment
Recurrent AOM	Three separate bouts of AOM within a 6-month period or four within a 12-month period; often a positive family history of otitis media and other ENT disorders

ENT, Ear, nose, and throat; *TM,* tympanic membrane.

virtually disappeared from the middle ear fluid of children with AOM.[15] With the introduction of the 13-valent *S. pneumoniae* vaccine, the bacteriology of the middle ear is likely to continue to evolve. Bullous myringitis is almost always caused by *S. pneumonia.* Nontypeable *H. influenza* remains a common cause of AOM. It is the most common cause of bilateral otitis media, severe TM inflammation, and otitis-conjunctivitis syndrome. *M. catarrhalis* obtained from the nasopharynx is increasingly more beta-lactamase positive, but the high rate of clinical resolution in children with AOM from *M. catarrhalis* makes amoxicillin a good choice for initial therapy.[14] *M. catarrhalis* rarely causes invasive disease. *S. pyogenes* (group A B-hemolytic streptococcus) occurs in less than 5% of cases.[16] Acute mastoiditis is a complication of AOM with the most common pathogens being *S. pneumoniae* and *S. pyogenes.*[17] Although a virus is usually the initial causative factor in AOM, strict diagnostic criteria, careful specimen handling, and sensitive microbiologic techniques have shown that the majority of AOM is caused by bacteria or bacteria and virus together.[18]

Clinical Findings

History
Rapid onset of:
- Ear pain that may interfere with activity and/or sleep, especially when lying flat
- Irritability and ear pulling in an infant or young child
- Otorrhea
- Fever

Other key risk factors or symptoms include prematurity, craniofacial anomalies, or congenital syndromes associated with craniofacial anomalies, sustained pacifier use, childcare attendance, disrupted sleep or inability to sleep, lethargy, dizziness, tinnitus, unsteady gait, diarrhea and vomiting, sudden hearing loss, stuffy nose, rhinorrhea, and sneezing.

Physical Examination
- Presence of MEE, confirmed by pneumatic otoscopy, tympanometry, or acoustic reflectometry, as evidenced by:
  - Bulging TM (see Fig. 31.5)
  - Decreased TM translucency

ciliary action in the eustachian tube. Eustachian tube obstruction causes negative pressure as air absorbs in the middle ear (see Fig 31.5). The negative pressure pulls fluid from the mucosal lining and causes fluid accumulation that may be colonized by bacteria and result in purulent fluid. Infants and young children have shorter, more horizontal, and more flaccid eustachian tubes that are easily disrupted by viruses, which predisposes them to AOM. Adult morphology is not reached until early adolescence; however, significant differences are noted by 8 years of age.

Respiratory syncytial virus and influenza are two of the viruses most responsible for the increase in the incidence of AOM seen from January to April. Other risk factors associated with AOM are listed in Box 31.3. *S. pneumoniae,* nontypeable *Haemophilus influenzae,* and *Moraxella catarrhalis* are the most common infecting organisms in AOM.[14]

S. pneumoniae continues to be the most common bacteria responsible for AOM, although the strains of *S. pneumoniae* in the heptavalent pneumococcal conjugate vaccine (PCV7) have

- Absent or decreased TM mobility
- Air-fluid level behind the TM
- Otorrhea

Signs and symptoms of middle ear inflammation include amber color TM, which is usually seen in OME and white or yellow TM, which may be seen in either AOM or OME.[11] In addition, the following TM findings may be present:

- Increased vascularity with obscured or absent landmarks (see Fig. 31.5).
- Red, yellow, or purple TM. (Redness alone should not be used to diagnose AOM, especially in a crying child.)
- Thin-walled, sagging bullae filled with straw-colored fluid seen with bullous myringitis.

Diagnostic Studies. Pneumatic otoscopy is the simplest and most efficient way to diagnose AOM. Type B tympanometry reflects effusion. Tympanocentesis identifies the infecting organism and is helpful in the treatment of infants younger than 2 months. In older infants and children, tympanocentesis is rare and useful only if the patient is toxic or immunocompromised, or in the presence of resistant infection or acute pain from bullous myringitis. If a tympanocentesis is warranted, the PCP can refer the patient to an otolaryngologist for the procedure.

Differential Diagnosis

Differential diagnoses include OME, mastoiditis, dental abscess, sinusitis, lymphadenitis, parotitis, peritonsillar abscess, trauma, ETD, impacted teeth, temporomandibular joint dysfunction, and immune deficiency. Any newborn or young infant (2 months or younger) with AOM should be evaluated for fever of unknown etiology.

Management

Many changes have been made in the treatment of AOM because of the increasing rate of antibiotic-resistant bacteria related to the injudicious use of antibiotics. Ample evidence demonstrates that symptom management may be all that is required in children with MEE without other symptoms of AOM.[11] Treatment is based on the child's age, illness severity, and the certainty of diagnosis. Table 31.6 outlines the recommendation for the diagnosis and subsequent treatment of AOM.

1. Pain management is the first principle of treatment with weight-appropriate doses of children's ibuprofen or acetaminophen to decrease discomfort as well as fever. Distraction or external use of heat or cold may be of some use.
2. Antibiotics are effective, if indicated (Table 31.7).
3. Amoxicillin remains the first-line antibiotic for AOM if there has not been a previous treated AOM in the previous 30 days, there is no conjunctivitis, and no penicillin allergy.[11] β-lactam coverage (amoxicillin/clavulanate, third-generation cephalosporin) is recommended when there is a history of recurrent otitis that has not responded to amoxicillin or a history of amoxicillin in the previous 30 days, an allergy to penicillin, or the child has concurrent conjunctivitis.
4. If the child is younger than 2 years, treatment with amoxicillin or amoxicillin/clavulanate for 10 days; for children older than 2 years, treatment for 5 to 7 days.
5. Ceftriaxone may be effective for the vomiting child, the child unable to tolerate oral medications, or the child who has failed amoxicillin/clavulanate.
   - Clindamycin may be considered for ceftriaxone failure but *only* used if susceptibilities are known.

TABLE 31.6	Treatment Guidelines for Acute Otitis Media (AOM)
Diagnosis	**Treat**
Any child with moderate/severe bulging TM with otorrhea not associated with AOM	Yes
Any child with mild bulging of the TM with recent (<48 h) onset pain (holding, tugging, and so on) or intensely erythematous TM	Yes
Infants ≥6 months of age with severe signs of AOM (fever >102.2°F [39°C], otalgia for ≥48 h)	Yes
Any child 6–23 months old with acute bilateral otitis media without severe symptoms, without fever, and sick less than 48 h	Yes
Children ≥24 months old with unilateral AOM without severe symptoms and fever <102.2°F (39°C)	Provide prescription and/or wait Close follow-up
Children ≥24 months old without severe symptoms	Provide prescription and/or wait Close follow-up
Children not treated and no improvement in 48–72 h	See the patient again Clinician discretion whether or not to treat

TM, Tympanic membrane.

From Lieberthal AS, Carroll AE, Chonmaitree T, et al. The diagnosis and management of acute otitis media. *Pediatrics.* 2013;131(3):e964–e999.

- Prophylactic antibiotics for chronic or recurrent AOM are *not* recommended.
6. Observation or "watchful waiting" for 48 to 72 hours (see Table 31.6) allows the patient to improve without antibiotic treatment. Pain relief should be provided, and a means of follow-up must be in place. Recommendations for follow-up include parent-initiated visit/phone call for worsening or no improvement; scheduled follow-up appointment; routine follow-up phone call; or a prescription sent to pharmacy to be started if the child's symptoms do not improve or if they worsen in 48 to 72 hours.
7. Routine follow-up is not needed if the child improves within 48 hours. If the child has not shown improvement in ear symptomatology after 48 to 72 hours, the child should be seen to confirm or exclude the presence of AOM. If the initial management option was an antibacterial agent, the agent should be changed.

Management of Persistent and Recurrent Acute Otitis Media

- *Persistent* AOM occurs when antibiotic therapy is completed and AOM is still present or AOM recurs within days of treatment.
  - Retreatment with a broader-spectrum antibiotic is suggested.
  - Persistent MEE is common after resolution of acute symptoms and should not be seen as a need for continuing antibiotics (see Otitis Media with Effusion section).

TABLE 31.7 Medications Used to Treat Acute Otitis Media

Drug	Dosage	Comments
Amoxicillin	80–90 mg/kg/day divided twice a day (maximum dose 2–3 g daily)	First choice unless allergy 10 days for children <2 y and all children with severe symptoms 7 days for children 2–5 years with mild to moderate symptoms 5–7 days for children >6 y with mild to moderate symptoms Consider watchful waiting in patients 6–23 months with unilateral nonsevere symptoms
Amoxicillin-clavulanate	80–90 mg/kg/day divided twice a day (maximum dose depends on formulation of drug)	Clavulanate <10 mg/kg/day Good beta-lactamase coverage Costly and more likely to cause diarrhea
Azithromycin	10 mg/kg/day on day 1 (maximum dose 500 mg/day) then 5 mg/kg/day on days 2–5 given daily (maximum dose 250 mg/day)	Children older than 6 months need 5-day treatment course Macrolide primarily used because of penicillin allergy Should not be used as first-line treatment due to high resistance
Cefdinir	14 mg/kg/day daily or divided twice a day (maximum dose 600 mg/day)	Broad-spectrum Third-generation cephalosporin Causes red stool Alternative if penicillin allergy
Cefixime	8 mg/kg daily or divided twice a day (maximum dose 400 mg/day)	Broad-spectrum Third-generation cephalosporin Reduced efficacy against *Streptococcus pneumoniae*
Cefpodoxime	10 mg/kg/day daily divided twice a day (maximum dose 400 mg/day)	Broad spectrum of coverage Third-generation cephalosporin Alternative if penicillin allergy
Ceftriaxone	50 mg/kg/day IM (maximum dose 1 g/day) for 1 or 3 days	Costly Third-generation cephalosporin Alternative if penicillin allergy
Cefuroxime	15–30 mg/kg/day divided twice a day (maximum dose 500 mg/day) 250 mg every 12 h for 2–12 years old 250–500 mg every 12 h for 12 years or older	Broad spectrum of coverage Costly Most potent second-generation cephalosporin Poor taste
Clindamycin	30–40 mg/kg/day given divided 3 times a day (maximum dose 1.8 g/day)	Should not be used unless culture and sensitivities are done

IM, Intramuscular.

Data from Taketomo CK, Hodding JH, Kraus DM. *Pediatric Dosage Handbook.* 28th ed. Lexi-Comp; 2021.

- *Recurrent* AOM is defined as more than three distinct and well-documented bouts of AOM in 6 months or four or more episodes in 12 months.

An otolaryngology referral is indicated when appropriate therapy for otitis media fails. Placement of tympanostomy or PE tubes can help relieve discomfort, reduce time with OME, improve hearing, and decrease the likelihood of further infection.[19] Indications for tympanostomy and the insertion of PE tubes is discussed below.

Other Treatment Issues

- The PCP is encouraged to maintain understanding of current recommendations for AOM management because of rapid changes in resistance patterns and newly developed treatments.
- Decongestants and antihistamines are not indicated.
- Antimicrobial ototopical drops (ofloxacin or ciprofloxacin) or ophthalmic drops (tobramycin or gentamicin) are indicated if the TM is perforated, the child has otorrhea, or the child has patent, draining PE tubes.
- Xylitol, a sugar found in fruits and birch bark, has bacteriostatic effects against *S. pneumoniae* and interferes with bacterial adhesion to mucous membranes. It appears to have some suppressive effects in preventing ear infections. Xylitol is available in an oral solution, lozenges, and chewing gum. The lozenges and chewing gum are more effective than the oral solution. Children younger than 2 years cannot have chewing gum or lozenges. Xylitol must be given 3 to 5 times a day on a regular basis to be effective.
- There is no safe or effective herbal treatment for AOM or OME.

Complications

Persistent AOM, persistent OME, TM perforation, OE, mastoiditis, cholesteatoma, tympanosclerosis (Fig. 31.6), hearing loss of

25 to 30 dB for several months, ossicle necrosis, pseudotumor cerebri, cerebral thrombophlebitis, and facial paralysis are possible complications.

Prevention and Education

The following interventions, shown to be helpful in preventing AOM, should be encouraged:
- Exclusive breastfeeding until at least 6 months of age[20]
- Avoid bottle propping, feeding infants lying down, and passive smoke exposure
- Pneumococcal 20 vaccine
- Annual influenza vaccine

- Xylitol liquid or chewing gum, as tolerated
- Choose licensed daycare facilities with fewer children, if possible
- Educate regarding the problem of drug-resistant bacteria and the need to avoid antibiotic use unless absolutely necessary.
- If antibiotics are used, the child needs to complete the entire course of the prescription and follow up if symptoms do not resolve.

Otitis Media With Effusion

The diagnosis of OME is made in the presence of MEE without signs or symptoms of acute ear infection (Fig. 31.7). MEE decreases the mobility of the TM and interferes with sound conduction. OME can occur spontaneously with ETD caused by an inflammatory process after AOM, viral illness, anatomic abnormalities, barotrauma, allergies, or a combination of these conditions (see Figs. 31.7 and 31.8). ETD changes the middle ear mucosa in the following sequence: (1) increased mucus production, (2) the mucus absorbs water as the mucosa becomes viscous, and (3) fluid becomes stuck behind the TM. Bacterial biofilms may explain the persistence of OME. Biofilms are mixed microorganisms enclosed in a polymeric matrix that adhere to surfaces, such as the middle ear mucosa. Risk factors for chronic OME are listed in Box 31.4.

Clinical Findings

History. Children with OME are often afebrile and asymptomatic. Some children may present with intermittent complaints of mild ear pain, fullness in the ear ("popping" or feeling of "talking in a barrel"), as well as dizziness or impaired balance. The older child may complain of hearing loss, while the young child may request that you speak louder or require a higher volume than usual for the radio or television.

Physical Examination. Pneumatic otoscopy reveals decreased TM mobility. An abnormal-appearing TM, often described as dull, varying from bulging and opaque with no visible landmarks

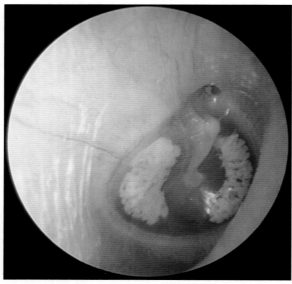

• **Fig. 31.6** Tympanosclerosis. (From Swartz MH. *Textbook of Physical Diagnosis: History and Examination.* 8th ed. Elsevier; 2021.)

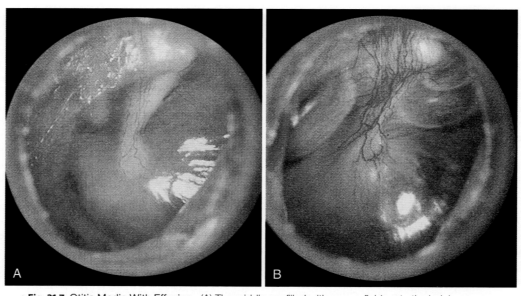

• **Fig. 31.7** Otitis Media With Effusion. (A) The middle ear filled with serous fluid; note the bulging appearance and distorted light reflex. (B) Air-fluid levels in upper middle ear. (Courtesy of Richard A. Buckingham MD, Abraham Lincoln School of Medicine, University of Illinois, Chicago. In Seidel HM, Ball JW, Dains JE, et al. *Mosby's Guide to Physical Examination.* 8th ed. Elsevier; 2015.)

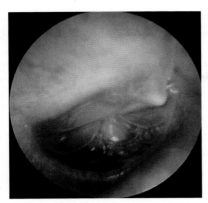

• **Fig. 31.8** Middle Ear Effusion With Air Bubbles. (From Dhingra PL, Bluestone CD, Klein JO. *Otitis Media in Infants and Children.* 2nd ed. Elsevier; 1995.)

<table>
<tr><td>• BOX 31.4</td><td>Risk Factors for Hearing Loss Caused by Otitis Media With Effusion</td></tr>
</table>

If two or more present:
- OME present for ≥2 months
- Speech development slower than peers
- Speech less clear than previously
- Decrease talking
- Less responsive to name and other familiar sounds
- Says "Huh?" or "What?" frequently
- Sits close to TV or wants volume louder
- Has difficulty learning (reading, spelling)
- Hyperactive or overly inattentive

OME, Otitis media with effusion.

---

to retracted and translucent with visible landmarks and an air-fluid level or bubble (see Figs. 31.7 and 31.9). Examine head and neck structures for abnormalities.

Diagnostic Studies. The tympanogram is flat-type B. The audiogram can show hearing loss ranging from mild to moderate (25–60 dB).

Differential Diagnosis

Differential diagnoses include AOM, all causes of hearing loss and anatomic abnormalities, and persistent unilateral OME can indicate a nasopharyngeal lesion or mass.

Management

Recommendations for management of OME in children 2 months to 12 years include[21]:
1. Pneumatic otoscopy to document OME, particularly in children with ear pain and/or hearing loss. Tympanometry may be indicated in children to confirm OME diagnosis.
2. Watchful waiting for 3 months from date of diagnosis. An age-appropriate hearing test should be performed if OME persists for 3 months or longer.
3. Intranasal steroids or systemic steroids, system antibiotics, antihistamines, and decongestants are not recommended.
4. Children at risk for speech, language, and learning problems should be identified and promptly referred for hearing, speech, and language evaluation.
   - At-risk children are defined as having developmental delays because of sensory, physical, cognitive, or

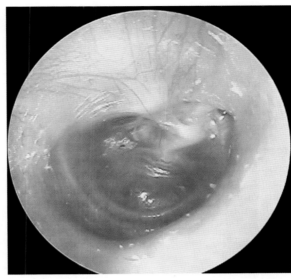

• **Fig. 31.9** Tympanic Membrane Retraction. (From Emmett SD, Kokesh J, Kaylie D. Chronic ear disease. *Med Clin North Am.* 2018;6:1063–1079.)

behavioral factors (e.g., hearing loss independent of OME, speech or language delays, pervasive or other developmental disorders, syndromes or craniofacial disorders, blindness, and/or cleft palate).
5. Reevaluate a child with OME every 3 months until the effusion resolves, or every 3 to 6 months for children with chronic OME. The PCP should document resolution of OME in the medical record.
6. Communication is key to families understanding the duration and course of OME, the need for follow-up, and the associated sequelae including potential hearing impairment and impact on speech and language development.
7. Referral to an otolaryngologist is recommended when otoscopy suggests possible or impending structural damage of the TM, significant hearing loss is identified, and/or for chronic or persistent OME for more than 6 months.
8. In a child younger than 4 years, insertion of PE tubes is performed for persistent or chronic OME with associated sequelae; adenoidectomy is not recommended unless an indication exists other than OME. In a child 4 years old or older, insertion of PE tubes by otolaryngology and/or adenoidectomy is recommended for OME.

Complications

Complications include recurrent AOM and hearing loss that may be transient CHL, or with persistent OME, permanent high-frequency SNHL.

Tympanostomy or Pressure-Equalizing Tubes

Insertion of tympanostomy tubes is one of the most common ambulatory surgeries performed in pediatrics in the United States.[19] Tympanostomy or PE tubes are most often inserted because of persistent middle ear fluid, frequent ear infections, or ear infections that persist after antibiotic therapy (see the previous discussion on referral for OME). Criteria for referral to otolaryngology when managing children 6 months to 12 years of age include:
- Bilateral OME for 3 months or more, unilateral OME for 6 months or more, or recurrent episodes of OME with

cumulative duration of OME for more than 6 of the previous 12 months
- CHL associated with MEE
- Recurrent or recurrent AOM
- Prevention of acquired cholesteatoma due to a retraction pocket of the TM

It is important to clearly communicate to families the importance of referral and possible long-term sequelae of hearing loss from persistent MEE.

Management

Viral myringitis or early AOM without otorrhea in a child with tympanostomy or PE tubes usually resolves spontaneously. TTO can occur within the first few weeks of ear tube placement and should self-resolve.[19] Approximately 7% of children experience recurrent otorrhea while the PE tubes remain in place.[19] It usually occurs when a child with tubes has an upper respiratory infection. TTO usually involves the same bacterial pathogens seen in AOM. Combination antibiotic and corticosteroid otic drops are the preferred treatment for TTO.[19] Otic medications are listed in Table 31.4.

A child with PE tubes does not need to take precautions during bathing, showering, or surface swimming, unless recurrent TTO or instructed otherwise by their otolaryngologist.[19] Swimming in lake water should be avoided due to the inherent bacteria level of stagnant water. Most tympanostomy or PE tubes come out spontaneously. If the tube is extruded and there are persistent ear complaints, or if it remains in the TM for more than 2 or 3 years, the child should see an otolaryngologist.[19]

Complications

Complications of tympanostomy or PE tubes include otorrhea, OE, granuloma, cholesteatoma, tube obstruction, persistent TM perforation, retraction pocket, and tympanosclerosis. Bacterial biofilms can form on implanted prostheses and tend to be antibiotic resistant. If the biofilm is antibiotic resistant, the PE tubes will likely have to be replaced by the otolaryngologist if the child has persistent symptoms.

Perforated Tympanic Membrane

Spontaneous perforated or ruptured TMs are associated with AOM, occurring in up to approximately 30% of younger children with a middle ear infection.[22] Children with a perforation are more likely to have had AOM in the past. The pain associated with the AOM generally improves significantly once the rupture occurs and there is usually profuse otorrhea. The fluid that drains from the ruptured TM usually contains the same virus and bacteria that is associated with TTO. Nontypeable *H. influenza* and *S. pneumonia* are the most common pathogens in AOM with tympanic membrane perforation.[22] *S. aureus* has been detected mostly in children with previous episodes of AOM with tympanic membrane perforation.[22] Most ruptures heal without intervention in 1 to 3 months.

Traumatic TM perforations are caused by blows to the ear, blasts (fireworks), improper ear cleaning, and insertion of foreign bodies. Perforating the TM is not necessarily painful, and most children will present with acute onset of bleeding from the ear. Traumatic perforations are less likely to heal spontaneously and can be prone to infection and hearing loss.

Clinical Findings

History, Physical Examination, and Diagnostic Studies
- The child may be asymptomatic. After perforation, the child may feel immediately better. Children may present with whistling sounds during sneezing or nose blowing or hearing loss.
- TM perforation is evident on otoscopic examination. Profuse otorrhea from the perforation may decrease TM visibility.
- Tympanogram will be flat (type B).
- Follow-up hearing test once the acute infection clears or the traumatic perforation heals.

Differential Diagnosis

Include AOM, TTO, or nonaccidental trauma (e.g., boxed ears).

Management

The goal of therapy is to control the otorrhea and watchful waiting to ensure healing of the perforation. If the perforation was caused by an AOM, treat the ear with otic drops (see Table 31.4), analgesics if needed, and oral antibiotics (see Table 31.7). Other treatment considerations include:
- Perforation makes the ear more susceptible to infection if water enters the EAC. The perforation of the TM is a contraindication to swimming, getting water into the ears when shampooing, and irrigation for cerumen removal.[23] It is important to keep the ears dry.
- Small perforations are not usually repaired unless there is a quality-of-life issue. Perforations caused by acute infection tend to heal spontaneously. Primary care follow-up is important to assure there are no sequelae from the perforation.
- Hearing loss is the most common sequelae of a TM perforation. The degree of hearing loss can range from mild to severe depending on the size and location of the perforation.
- Referral to the otolaryngologist is indicated if there is significant hearing loss or structure damage noted on otoscopy.

Auricular Hematoma

Auricular hematoma (i.e., "wrestler's ear" or cauliflower ear) occurs from blunt trauma to the ear from activities such as wrestling, martial arts, or boxing results in a tear in the perichondrial blood vessels causing hematoma formation. The hematoma in the subperichondrial space stimulates asymmetrical cartilage formation resulting in ear deformity. Prompt drainage of the blood and ear bolstering to prevent reaccumulation of blood is needed.

Clinical Findings

History and Physical Examination. The history should include mechanism of the blunt trauma as well as safety of home and school environment for the child or adolescent. Note: Children on anticoagulants may develop a hematoma after minor trauma. Other symptoms include:
- Auricular swelling and/or tenderness
- Blood on the outside of the ear
- Erythema or ecchymosis to the overlying skin

Differential Diagnosis

Infections of the middle ear cartilage or inflammation from the autoimmune condition relapsing polychondritis may look similar on physical examination.

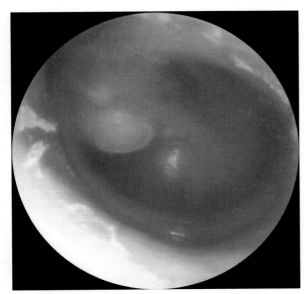

• Fig. 31.10 Cholesteatoma Behind Intact Tympanic Membrane. (From Flint PW, Haughey BH, Lund VJ, et al. *Cummings Otolaryngology: Head and Neck Surgery.* 7th ed. Elsevier; 2021.)

Management and Complications

Patients with an auricular hematoma should be referred to otolaryngology as soon as possible and within 7 days of the trauma to prevent the formulation of granulation tissue and asymmetrical cartilage growth in the ear. Reaccumulation of the hematoma or an untreated hematoma can result in permanent deformity, scar formation, perichondritis, infection, and/or necrosis.

Cholesteatoma

Cholesteatoma is an epidermal inclusion cyst derived from abnormal growth of keratinizing squamous epithelium in the temporal bone (Fig. 31.10). As the cholesteatoma grows and increases in size, it can destroy the surrounding structures. Chronic otorrhea, ossicular erosion, and hearing loss follow. Any child with ongoing otorrhea that does not resolve with appropriate antibiotic treatment should be referred to an otolaryngologist to rule out cholesteatoma. Permanent hearing loss, facial nerve paralysis, meningitis, and brain abscess are rare but potential complications of untreated cholesteatoma.

Cholesteatomas can be congenital or acquired. *Congenital* cholesteatomas are rare, small, and self-contained at birth, initially appearing as a pearly white mass behind the TM. *Acquired* cholesteatomas are localized exclusively in the middle ear, and further divided into primary acquired and secondary forms. *Primary* acquired cholesteatomas arise from negative middle ear pressure that causes TM retraction and subsequent accumulation of an erosive keratin-filled cyst in an intact TM, usually in the region of the pars flaccida. *Secondary* acquired cholesteatomas are the result of epithelial migration into the middle ear through a perforated TM caused by infection or trauma.

Clinical Findings

History and Physical Examination. The history may be negative with congenital cholesteatomas, while the history for acquired cholesteatoma might include:

- Chronic otitis media with ongoing, malodorous purulent otorrhea

- Vertigo and hearing loss
- History or presence of tympanostomy or placement of PE tubes

On physical examination, a pearly white lesion is seen on or behind the TM. Congenital cholesteatomas are often in the most anteroinferior position behind the TM (see Fig. 31.10).

Differential Diagnosis

Differential diagnoses include tympanosclerosis (see Fig. 31.6), debris from chronic OME, malignant rhabdomyosarcoma, and aural polyps. Aural polyps are considered cholesteatomas unless proven otherwise.

Management and Complications

Cholesteatoma is managed surgically. Accurate diagnosis and immediate referral to an otolaryngologist for surgical excision are needed. Complications include irreversible structural damage, permanent bone damage, facial nerve palsy, hearing loss, and intracranial infection, especially in untreated cases.

Mastoiditis

Mastoiditis is a suppurative infection of the mastoid cells that may occur with AOM or follow an AOM. The mucoperiosteal lining of the mastoid air cells becomes inflamed, with subsequent progressive swelling and obstruction caused by drainage from the mastoid. It is now rare in children since the introduction of the *H. influenzae* (HIB) and the *S. pneumoniae* or pneumococcal (Prevnar 13 [PCV13] or Pneumovax 23 [PPSV23]) vaccine. Other causative invasive organisms identified include *M. catarrhalis, S. aureus, S. pyogenes,* and *Mycobacterium tuberculosis* (rare). Gram-negative *E. coli, Proteus,* and *Pseudomonas* are more common in chronic mastoiditis, more virulent infections, and young infants. Intracranial complications of mastoiditis are common and may develop despite treatment.

Clinical Findings

History, Physical Examination, and Diagnostic Studies
- Concurrent, recurrent, or persistent otitis media unresponsive to antibiotic therapy
- Fever and otalgia.
- Postauricular swelling:
  - Infants may have edema above the ear, displacing the pinna inferiorly or laterally.
  - Older children have edema that pushes the earlobe superiorly and laterally.
- Computed tomography (CT) or MRI provide definitive anatomical information and should be ordered with/by otolaryngology either before or after hospitalization.
- Tympanocentesis with culture and Gram stain help identify the offending organism.

Differential Diagnosis

Postauricular inflammation or swelling such as lymphadenopathy, periauricular cellulitis, perichondritis of auricle, mumps, or mastoid tumors.

Management

Urgent ear, nose, and throat referral is imperative. Hospitalization, intravenous antibiotics, and often surgical intervention with myringotomy, PE tube placement, and mastoidectomy are required.

Telehealth

Over the last decade, telehealth has been a growing field that has allowed remote clinical visits between providers and patients. Within the last few years, telehealth has become important in maintaining continuity of care and ensuring access to healthcare during pandemics. Although telehealth visits are beneficial, they come with challenges. It is important to obtain a thorough history because the examination is often limited to the external ear, unless families have access to specialized devices paired with their smartphone that allow for inspection of the ear canal and middle ear. There are also several applications for basic audiometry that can be paired with smart devices if needed. However currently, tele-audiometry is not the gold standard for hearing examinations. Determine if it is appropriate for the child to be seen remotely based on the complaint. For new ear complaints that may require intervention, a face-to-face appointment should be scheduled. For recurrent ear complaints (e.g., otorrhea) that often respond well to standard treatment or watchful waiting, a telehealth visit can be utilized.

Additional Resources

American Cleft Palate-Craniofacial Association (ACPA): www.cleftline.org

American Society for Deaf Children (ASDC): www.deafchildren.org

Beginnings for Parents of Children with Hearing Loss and Their Families: http://ncbegin.org/

Cochlear Implant Awareness Foundation: www.ciafonline.org/

Family Voices: www.familyvoices.org

Imagery Language and Visual Communication: www.handspeak.com

My Baby's Hearing: www.babyhearing.org

National Association of the Deaf (NAD): https://www.nad.org/

National Family Association for Deaf-Blind (NFADB): www.nfadb.org

National Institute on Deafness and Other Communication Disorders (NIDCD): www.nidcd.nih.gov

References

1. Horton GA, Simpson MTW, Beyea MM, et al. Cerumen management: an updated clinical review and evidence-based approach for primary care physicians. *J Prim Care Community Health*. 2020;11:1–5.
2. Yoshinago-Itano C, Manchaiah V, Hunnicutt C. Outcomes of universal newborn screening programs: systematic review. *J Clin Med*. 2021;10(13):2784–2807.
3. The Joint Committee on Infant Hearing (JCIH). Year 2019 position statement: Principles and guidelines for early hearing detection and intervention programs. *J Early Hear Detect Interv*. 2019;4(2):1–44.
4. American Academy of Pediatrics. *Preventive Care/Periodicity Schedule*; 2021. https://www.aap.org/en/practice-management/care-delivery-approaches/periodicity-schedule/.
5. Centers for Disease Control and Prevention (CDC). *Hearing Loss in Children*; 2021. www.cdc.gov/ncbddd/hearingloss/data.html.
6. Gettelfinger JD, Dahl JP. Syndromic hearing loss: a brief review of common presentations and genetics. *J Pediatr Genet*. 2018;7:1–8.
7. Beach R, Abitbol JM, Allman BL, et al. GJB2 mutations linked to hearing loss exhibit differential trafficking and functional defects as revealed in cochlear-relevant cells. *Front Cell Dev Biol*. 2020;8:15.
8. Centers for Disease Control and Prevention (CDC). *Loud Noise Can Cause Hearing Loss*; 2019. https://www.cdc.gov/nceh/hearing_loss/what_noises_cause_hearing_loss.html.
9. Smith ME, Hardman JC, Mehta N, et al. Acute otitis externa: consensus definition, diagnostic criteria and core outcome set development. *PLoS One*. 2021;16(5):e0251395.
10. Rosenfeld RM, Schwartz SR, Cannon CR, et al. Clinical practice guideline: acute otitis externa. *Otolaryngol Head Neck Surg*. 2014;150(suppl 1):S1–S24.
11. Wiegand S, Berner R, Schneider A, et al. Otitis externa. *Dtsch Arztebl Int*. 2019;116(13):224–234.
12. Schilder AGM, Marom T, Bhutta MF, et al. Panel 7: otitis media: treatment and complications. *Otolaryngol Head Neck Surg*. 2017;156(suppl 4):S88–S105.
13. Schilder AGM, Rosenfeld RM, Venekamp RP. Acute otitis media and otitis media with effusion. In: Lesperance MM, ed. *Cummings Pediatric Otolaryngology*. 2nd ed. Elsevier; 2021.
14. Venekamp RP, Sanders SL, Glasziou PP, et al. Antibiotics for acute otitis media in children. *Cochrane Database of Sys Rev*. 2015;6:CD000219.
15. Palmu AA, Lahdenkari M. Early vaccine-type pneumococcal acute otitis media does not predispose to subsequent otitis when compared with early acute otitis media due to other bacterial etiology. *Pediatr Infec Dis J*. 2018;37(6):592.
16. Lieberthal AS, Carroll AE, Chonmaitree T, et al. The diagnosis and management of acute otitis media. *Pediatrics*. 2013;131(3):e964–e999.
17. Cassano P, Ciprandi G, Passali D. Acute mastoiditis in children. *Acta Biomed*. 2020;91(1-S):54–59.
18. Van Dyke MK, Pircon JY, Cohen R, et al. Etiology of acute otitis media in children less than 5 years of age: a pooled analysis of 10 similarly designed observational studies. *Pediatr Infec Dis J*. 2017;36(3):274–281.
19. Rosenfeld RM, Tunkel DE, Schwartz SR, et al. Clinical practice guideline: tympanostomy tube in children (update). *Otolaryngol Head Neck Surg*. 2022;166(1):S1–S55.
20. Køvel-Hanquist A, Djurhuus B, Homøe P. The effect of breastfeeding on childhood otitis media. *Curr Allergy Asthma Rep*. 2017;17(7):45.
21. Rosenfeld RM, Shin JJ, Schwartz SR, et al. Clinical practice guideline: otitis media with effusion (update). *Otolaryngol Head Neck Surg*. 2016;154(IS):S1–S41.
22. Principi N, Marchisio P, Rosazza C, et al. Acute otitis media with spontaneous tympanic membrane perforation. *Eur J Clin Microbiol Infect Dis*. 2017;36:11–18.
23. Hardman J, Muzaffar J, Nankivell P, et al. Tympanoplasty for chronic tympanic membrane perforation in children: systematic review and meta-analysis. *Otol Neurotol*. 2015;36(5):796–804.

32

Respiratory Disorders

JENNIFER SONNEY AND JESSICA PECK

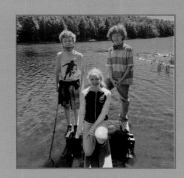

Respiratory conditions are a frequent cause of illness in children and represent a common reason for seeking pediatric care. A thorough understanding of pulmonary anatomy, physiology, and pathophysiology is essential to determining appropriate care of a child with a respiratory condition. Providers need to conduct a comprehensive respiratory history, perform a systematic and complete pulmonary examination, and, if indicated, order laboratory testing and radiographic examinations. A systematic approach to the care of a child with a respiratory condition is important to determine an accurate diagnosis and facilitate the development of a successful treatment plan.

Respiratory System

Pulmonary Anatomy

The lungs are situated within the thoracic cavity, with the right and left lung separated by the heart and the left lung with a characteristic cardiac notch. The right lung is comprised of three lobes: right superior (upper) lobe, right middle lobe, and right inferior (lower) lobe. The right superior and middle lobes are divided by the horizontal fissure, whereas the right middle and inferior lobes are divided by the oblique fissure. The left lung is comprised of two lobes, the left superior (upper) lobe and left inferior (lower) lobe, divided by the oblique fissure. The visceral pleura covers the lungs, whereas the parietal pleura lines the inner thoracic cavity.

The upper respiratory tract includes the nostrils, nasopharynx, larynx, eustachian tubes, sinuses, and extrathoracic trachea. The lower respiratory tract includes the intrathoracic trachea, bronchi, and bronchioles. Gas exchange occurs within the alveoli and depends on a rich alveolar-capillary network. This gas exchange portion of the lung is referred to as the *parenchyma*. The chest wall is comprised of bony structures, the ribs, sternum, and vertebra as well as muscles of respiration, including the diaphragm and the internal and external intercostals.

Airway Generations and Structure

The intrathoracic trachea branches into the right and left mainstem bronchi. The airways progressively branch from bronchi to bronchioles. The airway diameter diminishes with each airway branching, or generation; at each division point, the airway branches into two smaller airways. There are anywhere from 10 to 23 airway generations to reach the alveoli.[1] Terminal bronchioles branch to respiratory bronchioles, with each feeding one acinus, or cluster of alveoli. The conducting zone includes the trachea through the terminal bronchioles and constitutes anatomic dead

space, as there is no gas exchange that occurs within this zone. The respiratory bronchioles and their corresponding alveoli constitute the respiratory zone, where gas exchange occurs.

Airway structure varies throughout the tracheobronchial tree. The trachea is lined with ciliated pseudostratified columnar epithelium with dense mucous glands. C-shaped cartilaginous rings provide rigid structure and support to the trachea to prevent collapse. The open portion of the C-shaped ring, comprised of smooth muscle, is where the esophagus is located.[1] The mainstem bronchi have similar epithelial lining and C-shaped rings. The right mainstem bronchus is more vertically situated than the left, which makes foreign body (FB) aspiration more common in the right mainstem bronchus. Bronchial generations get their airway structure from cartilaginous plates, rather than C-shaped rings, that progressively diminish in size and density with each generation. Bronchioles have no cartilage, making them more prone to collapse. Bronchial airways are lined in ciliated columnar epithelium, whereas bronchioles are lined in ciliated cuboidal epithelium. The alveolus is comprised primarily of thin squamous epithelial cells, called *type 1 cells*, which creates a large, thin-walled surface area for gas exchange to occur. Scattered among the type 1 cells are type 2 cells, which secrete alveolar fluid and surfactant, which prevent alveolar collapse.[1]

Mechanics of Breathing

The elasticity of the lungs causes a natural tendency to recoil at rest, similar to a deflating balloon. In contrast, the chest wall at rest naturally pulls outward. Together, these forces are at equilibrium during rest to maintain lung inflation. Inhalation and exhalation occur due to atmospheric and intrapulmonary pressure differences; gas (air) flows from high to low pressure. During inhalation, intrapulmonary pressure drops compared to atmospheric pressure and air flows in. Conversely, exhalation occurs when intrapulmonary pressure exceeds atmospheric pressure, causing air to flow out.

Inhalation is considered an active process with the diaphragm constituting the primary muscle of respiration. Upon contraction, the domed diaphragm flattens, placing downward traction on the lungs and creating negative intrapulmonary pressure.[1] At the same time, the external intercostal muscles contract to cause anteroposterior and lateral movement of the rib cage, increasing the thoracic cavity further contributing to negative intrapulmonary pressure. The sternocleidomastoid is considered an accessory muscle of inspiration and may be recruited to further support inhalation, such as during exercise, coughing, sneezing, or with certain conditions, such as asthma. Exhalation is typically a passive process whereby the diaphragm and external intercostals relax, causing the thoracic cavity to reduce. The resulting positive intrapulmonary pressure exceeds atmospheric pressure and air flows out. Active exhalation may occur during exercise, sneezing, coughing, or certain conditions such as asthma. Abdominal and internal intercostal muscle contraction forces the diaphragm upward, and internal intercostal contraction returns the ribs to neutral position.[1] The medulla controls automatic breathing, though this may be overridden by higher brain centers.

Gas exchange depends on alveolar ventilation and perfusion. Ventilation refers to air flowing in and out of the alveoli, whereas perfusion refers to blood flow to the alveolar-capillary network. Ventilation entails inhaled air, with a high proportion of oxygen and low proportion of carbon dioxide (CO_2), traveling at a relatively high velocity through the conducting airways to the terminal bronchioles. Air flow continues through the terminal bronchioles, to the respiratory bronchioles, and into the alveolus via diffusion. Deoxygenated blood with high CO_2 content flows from the right ventricle to the pulmonary arteries, which then perfuse the pulmonary capillaries. Red blood cells within the pulmonary capillary release CO_2, which diffuses across the alveolar-capillary membrane into the alveolus. Within the alveolus, inhaled oxygen diffuses across the alveolar-capillary membrane and binds with the red blood cell, which then travels to the pulmonary veins to the left atrium, left ventricle, and systemic circulation. Following this gas exchange, air that is exhaled from the alveolus has a higher proportion of CO_2 compared to oxygen.

Pulmonary Defense

The pulmonary system has numerous ways in which it protects itself, including mechanical and biologic processes. Mechanical defenses include warming and humidifying inspired air, filtration and impaction, mucociliary clearance, and airway reflexes. Inhaled air is warmed and humidified as it passes through the nose, nasopharynx, and oropharynx. This warming and humidification protect the lower airways and alveoli from drying. The nose has a large surface area on which particles larger than 10 μm are filtered, essentially functioning as a trap, to prevent them from entering the lower airways.[1] Smaller particles that bypass nasal filtration may become impacted when inhaled air changes direction in the nasopharynx. Particles that bypass these defenses and enter the conducting airways encounter the mucociliary defenses. The ciliated epithelium of the conducting airways is lined in mucus produced by goblet cells. The mucus traps particles and the cilia sweep the particles up toward the pharynx, a process referred to as the *mucociliary escalator*. Trapped particles may then be swallowed or expelled by coughing, sneezing, or expectorating. Other protective mechanisms are the airway reflexes, including coughing, sneezing, and bronchoconstriction, which prevent particle penetration of the airways and/or expel the particle from the airway.

Biologic processes that protect the respiratory system include phagocytosis, lymphatic absorption, enzymatic destruction, and immunologic reactions. Macrophages within the alveoli or interstitium phagocytize foreign material to then be removed via the mucociliary escalator or lymphatic system. Various enzymatic defenses, part of the innate immune system, also are active in defending the lung. Finally, adaptive or acquired immune-mediated mechanisms constitute another pulmonary defense mechanism.[1]

Pediatric Respiratory System

Pulmonary Development

Pediatric pulmonary development begins prenatally and continues through childhood. Pulmonary development includes the embryonic, pseudoglandular, canalicular, saccular, and alveolarization stages; the estimated gestational weeks and postnatal ages associated with stages may overlap. During the embryonic stage, at approximately 4 to 7 weeks' gestation, primitive lung buds and major airways form. The pseudoglandular stage ranges from weeks 5 to 17 and is the critical stage for the development of conducting airways as well as the diaphragm, larynx, rudimentary cilia, and lymphatics. The canalicular stage, at 16 to 26 weeks' gestation, is characterized by the formation of rudimentary alveolar sacs and pulmonary capillary proliferation and the onset of surfactant production. The saccular stage, at approximately 24 to 38 weeks' gestation, is characterized by the expansion of air spaces that will form alveoli, increase air-blood surface membrane area, and produce surfactant for release.[2] Alveolarization, or the formation of alveoli, occurs from approximately 36 weeks' gestation through childhood. Approximately 50 million primitive alveoli are present at birth, whereas adults are estimated to have 300 million or more alveoli. The majority of alveolarization occurs by 3 years of age but may continue well into childhood or adolescence.

Sinus development also occurs prenatally and postnatally. The maxillary and ethmoid sinuses are both present at birth but not yet mature. The maxillary sinuses begin developing around 10 weeks' gestation and undergo two stages of postnatal growth, from birth to age 3 years and again from 7 to 12 years, at which point they reach maturity. The ethmoid sinuses follow a similar pattern with gestational development during weeks 13 to 17 and two postnatal growth cycles, between 1 and 4 years and again at 4 and 8 years. Sphenoid sinuses are not present at birth and undergo rapid development during early childhood, reaching maturity by 14 years. The frontal sinuses begin developing around age 6 years and reach maturity during mid-adolescence.[3] A mnemonic to remember the order of sinus development is "*m*axillaries *e*arly, *s*phenoids *f*ollow," which translates to the following order: (1) *m*axillary (2) *e*thmoids, (3) *s*phenoids, and (4) *f*rontal. The sinuses become clinically significant sites of infection around the following ages: maxillary and ethmoid sinuses, 1 to 2 years old; sphenoid sinuses, 3 to 4 years old; and frontal sinuses, 7 to 10 years old.

Anatomic Differences Compared to Adults

Numerous anatomical differences exist between the pediatric and adult respiratory system, many of which make children more prone to obstruction. Compared to adults, the pediatric head is larger in proportion to their body. This is especially prominent in infants, whose large occiput causes a natural neck flexion while supine, which compresses the upper airway. Infants are obligate nasal breathers until approximately 5 months. The tongue is large and flaccid, and the mandible is short. The epiglottis is vertically positioned, omega-shaped and flaccid. Collectively, these factors contribute to an increased potential for upper airway obstruction.

Compared to adults, pediatric airways are shorter, smaller in diameter, and have higher mucous gland density. Marginal decreases in the pediatric airway diameter from inflammation or mucus can cause airway obstruction and dramatically increase airway resistance. Pediatric airways are also more compliant than those of an adult. Changes in intrapleural pressure lead to greater changes in an infant's or young child's airway compared to the effect that it exerts on adult airways, thereby causing an increased risk of airway collapse. The pediatric chest wall and muscles of respiration also have important variations compared to adults. In infancy and early childhood, the chest is cylindrically shaped with relatively horizontal ribs, which limits capacity for thoracic expansion. Similarly, increased chest wall compliance and immature muscles of respiration make infants and young children less capable of handling a sustained increase in respiratory workload that occurs during severe pulmonary illnesses. Chest wall shape grows laterally and vertically as the child ages, leading to more vertical positioning of the ribs and increased thoracic capacity. Alveolarization during infancy and childhood highlights the dramatic changes in physiologic capacity for gas exchange compared to adulthood.

Pathophysiology

Lung conditions are often classified as obstructive or restrictive processes. Obstructive processes increase airflow resistance, usually the result of one or more of the following: intraluminal material (e.g., secretions, tumors, or foreign matter); mural thickening (e.g., edema or hypertrophy of the glands or mucosa); contraction of smooth muscle (e.g., spasm); and extrinsic compression. These factors rarely occur in isolation. Conversely, restrictive processes are characterized by restricted expansion of the lung, which may be caused by conditions impairing the parenchyma, pleura, chest wall, or neuromuscular function.[4] Restrictive conditions are less common in pediatric patients and are characterized by reduced lung capacity and resting lung volume, though airway resistance is not affected. Although uncommon, mixed obstructive, and restrictive conditions also may occur.

Obstructive Processes

Airway obstruction is the underlying etiology for the most common pediatric pulmonary conditions and can be partial or complete. In partial airway obstruction, airflow and secretion drainage are impaired, thus compromising ventilation. Partial obstruction may be caused by a narrowing of the airway lumen, such as occurs with inflammation, which produces turbulent airflow and adventitious lung sounds. Partial obstruction may also be caused by check-valve or ball-valve obstruction from foreign material partially occluding an airway. With ball-valve obstruction, inhalation is not typically impaired. However, during exhalation, the foreign material will lodge within the airway, causing a partial or complete obstruction of the airway lumen. In complete obstruction, neither airflow nor drainage of secretions occurs. Complete occlusion compromises alveolar emptying, impairs gas exchange, and may lead to atelectasis.

Upper Airway Obstruction

Airway obstruction that occurs at or above the extrathoracic trachea generally disrupts inhalation more than exhalation. Complete obstruction is a medical emergency that results in death if left untreated. Depending on the severity of a partial obstruction, dyspnea, stridor, and retractions may occur. Cough may remove nonfixed upper airway obstructions, though compromised inspiratory airflow limits coughing effectiveness. The sound produced by coughing may indicate the level of airway obstruction and assists in making a diagnosis. Laryngeal obstructions produce a cough that sounds croupy or barking, whereas obstruction in the trachea or major bronchi produces a brassy sound.

Lower Airway Obstruction

Lower airway obstruction generally disrupts exhalation more than inhalation. Lower airway obstruction may occur anywhere within the lower airway, though bronchioles are the most significantly affected given their small diameter. Complete obstruction prevents airflow to the affected airway, impairs gas exchange, and may lead to atelectasis. A large portion of the lower airway needs to be involved before symptoms become apparent; a small area of atelectasis does not produce obvious clinical manifestations. The usual obstructive mechanisms involve spasm, accumulation of secretions, edema of the mucous membrane, extrinsic compression, or any combination of these factors. Increased airway resistance leads to a prolonged exhalatory phase and may require active exhalation, or the use of accessory muscles to overcome airway resistance. An increased anteroposterior diameter of the chest may occur due to insufficient chest excursion, which is sometimes referred to as a "barrel chest." Percussion of a hyperinflated chest elicits hyperresonance. Symptoms worsen as the obstruction increases. Mild obstruction is marked by reduced respiratory rate and increased tidal volume; severe obstruction is characterized by increased respiratory rate, the use of accessory muscles, anxiety, and cyanosis.

On auscultation, wheezing may be appreciated as air passes through the narrowed lumen. Fine crackles (formerly called *rales*) are intermittent, nonmusical, short, explosive, clicking, or rattling sounds best heard on mid to late inspiration and occasionally, on exhalation. These sounds are gravity dependent, not transmitted to the mouth, and are unaffected by cough. They are heard in pneumonia and interstitial lung disease and are caused by airways suddenly opening after having been previously closed. Coarse crackles are nonmusical, short, and explosive sounds that are heard on early inspiration and throughout expiration. They are intermittent bubbling or brief popping sounds that are longer in duration than fine crackles. Course crackles may be affected by cough and are more common during inspiration. They may indicate intermittent airway opening and may be related to excessive airway secretions.

Restrictive Processes

Airway restriction is less common in pediatric patients and is characterized by airflow limitation and decreased total lung capacity. The etiology is diverse and includes interstitial inflammation and fibrosis; respiratory muscle weakness as seen in spinal muscular atrophy; decrease in outward recoil of the chest wall as seen in scoliosis; alveolar destruction such as pneumonia or acute lung injury; and space occupying problems such as a lung tumor, pneumothorax, effusion, or cyst. Key characteristics of restrictive lung conditions are the limited ability to expand the lung, resulting in decreased lung capacity, a low resting lung volume, and a higher respiratory rate.[4]

Alterations in Pulmonary Defense

The respiratory defense system is at risk for compromise from numerous environmental factors. Inhalation of cold air is irritating to the lower airways. Similarly, inhalation of dry air, such as during mouth breathing, inhalation of inadequately humidified supplemental oxygen, or tracheostomy placement, may cause drying of the mucous membrane and impaired ciliary motility. Hypothermia, hyperthermia, morphine, codeine, and hypothyroidism can also adversely impact mucociliary defenses. Damage to airway epithelial cells may be caused by a variety of substances and gases, such as sulfur, nitrogen dioxide, ozone, chlorine, ammonia, and smoke. Phagocytic activity may be impaired by numerous substances or conditions, including ethanol ingestion, cigarette smoke, hypoxemia, malnutrition, hypothermia, corticosteroids, narcotics, and some anesthetic gases.

Recent acute viral infections may temporarily impair immunodefenses. Recurrent respiratory infections in children, though, merit investigation for immunodeficiency or other underlying diseases, such as primary ciliary dyskinesia or cystic fibrosis (CF). The mnemonic SPUR helps clarify which children may require an immunodeficiency workup: *s*evere infection, *p*ersistent infection and poor recovery, *u*nusual organisms, and *r*ecurrent infection.[5] While children may have six to 10 colds per year, three or more annual episodes of bronchitis, bronchiolitis, or pneumonia or other conditions should trigger further evaluation for possible immunodeficiency workup (see Chapter 36).

Respiratory Failure

Respiratory failure occurs when the pulmonary system is unable to achieve adequate oxygenation and/or ventilation to support bodily functions. Many conditions may lead to respiratory failure, generally falling within one of two categories: hypoxemic respiratory failure, or low arterial oxygen, and hypercarbic respiratory failure, or high arterial CO_2.[6] Common signs of impending respiratory failure include tachypnea, tachycardia, increased work of breathing, and altered mental status. A rapid history and physical examination are needed to identify the type and cause of respiratory failure to appropriately intervene.

Assessment of the Respiratory System

History

The history provides valuable information about the causes, progression, and potential complications of a child's respiratory condition. The physical examination and diagnostic testing allow the provider to determine the extent of respiratory distress.

- Onset: When did the condition start? Describe the onset of symptoms? Is this a new or recurrent onset? Was there any recent travel within the past 6 months? Is there any preexisting condition? Because the potential long-term impacts of COVID-19 in children are still uncertain, a history of prior COVID-19 infection should be elicited with a report on course of illness if applicable.
- Promoting, preventing, precipitating, palliating factors:
  - *Contacts:* Are any family members or close contacts (e.g., daycare, school) ill with similar signs and symptoms?
  - *Prevention:* Which over-the-counter (OTC) medications or supplements (e.g., herbs, botanicals, or vitamins) does your child routinely take? Tell me about your handwashing practices. Do you encourage extra water intake? Are all routinely recommended pediatric immunizations up to date, including seasonal vaccination for both influenza and COVID-19?
  - *Progression:* Are the respiratory signs or symptoms increasing in severity, lessening, or about the same? Is your child easily fatigued or less active, having trouble sleeping, or working harder to breathe?
  - *Treatment:* What OTC or prescription medications, herbs, supplements, or natural remedies have been used? What

other treatment modalities have been used, including cultural practices or home remedies? Have you been prescribed any antibiotics in the last 4 to 6 weeks?
- Quality or quantity: How severe are the symptoms? Is the illness interfering with school attendance or play? Are breathing problems affecting your child's ability to sleep?
- Region or radiation: Does your child complain of chest, stomach, or back pain?
- Severity, setting, simultaneous symptoms, or similar illnesses in the past:
  - *Key signs and symptoms:* Has your child had symptoms or signs of a daytime or nighttime cough, fever, vomiting, malaise, runny nose, sore throat, mouth sores, increased respiratory work of breathing, discoloration in nasal drainage or sputum, or blue skin color around the mouth? Table 32.1 lists key characteristics and causes of cough.
  - *Associated symptoms:* Has there been a change in appetite or eating? Any rashes, headaches, or stomach pain?
  - *Similar illnesses in the past:* Does your child have a history of chronic illness including respiratory tract infections, allergies, or asthma? How many similar infections has your child had in the last year (e.g., croup, pneumonia, sinusitis, strep throat, or frequent colds)?
- Temporal factors: Was the onset rapid or slow? How long has it lasted? How has it changed over time? Are there any other factors that seem to impact their symptoms (e.g., outside or environmental exposure, activity or exertion)?
- Family history:
  - Do others in the family have a history of allergies or asthma?
  - Is there any family history of immunodeficiency, ear-nose-throat, or respiratory problems?
  - Does anyone in the family have a genetic disorder, such as CF?
- Review of systems: Note any infections, constitutional symptoms, or congenital problems that might have a respiratory component.
- Environment: Does anyone in the family or in other care settings smoke? Does the child live or attend school in an urban or industrial area subject to air pollution (e.g., near a major highway, industrial plant, or bus terminal)?

Physical Examination

When assessing respiratory conditions or level of respiratory distress, examine the total presentation and not just individual isolated findings. Consider anxiety level, respiratory rate and rhythm, use of accessory muscles, color, breath sounds, grunting, and pulse oximetry results. Information pertinent to the physical examination of a child with suspected respiratory disease includes the following:
- Accurate measurement of vital signs and observation of general appearance:
  - Normal respiratory rate is age dependent and, if elevated, is a key indicator of lower respiratory tract involvement (Table 32.2).
  - Anxiety level, nasal flaring, and "prefers to stay upright" are useful indicators of significant respiratory distress. Grunting is associated with small airway disease. Changes in skin color may be subtle or obvious, depending on the level of deoxygenation and dermatologic differences in diverse populations with variations in skin color. Care should be taken by pediatric providers to evaluate for implicit bias when examining patients with racial and ethnic backgrounds

TABLE 32.1	Key Characteristics of Cough, Common Causes, and Questions to Ask in a Pediatric History	
Key Characteristics to Consider	Description and Questions to Ask
Age	Infants less than 1 mo with pneumonia may not have a cough
Quality	Staccato-like (*Chlamydia trachomatis* in infants); barking or brassy (croup, tracheomalacia, habit cough); paroxysmal or inspiratory whoop (pertussis); honking (psychogenic) Is the cough wet or dry?
Duration	*Acute* (most causes are infectious and last less than 2 wk), *subacute* (cough lasts from 2–4 wk); *recurrent* (associated with allergies and asthma), or *chronic* (lasting greater than 3 mo [e.g., CF, asthma]) Is cough continuous or intermittent?
Productivity	Mucous-producing or nonproductive? Younger children do not expectorate
Timing	During the day, night (associated with asthma), or both? Associated with exercise?
Family history	Is there a history of CF in the family? What genetic diseases run in the family?
Effect on caregiver and child	What are caregiver's responses to cough? Is it causing loss of sleep and work time? Are there concerns the child may have something seriously wrong?
Associated symptoms	High fever in acutely ill child: can be bacterial or viral infection (pneumonia). Rhinorrhea, sneezing, wheezing, atopic dermatitis, pale boggy mucosa: associated with asthma and allergic rhinitis. Malaise, sneezing, watery nasal discharge, mild sore throat, no or low fever, not ill appearing: typical of URI. Tachypnea: pneumonia or bronchiolitis in infants (infants may not have a cough)
Exposure to infection or travel	Travel history (areas of tuberculosis or novel coronaviral infection)? Is there a household member being treated for a cough illness?
Causes	
Congenital anomalies	Tracheoesophageal fistula, vascular ring, laryngeal cleft, vocal cord paralysis, pulmonary malformations, tracheobronchomalacia, congenital heart disease
Infectious agent	Viral (RSV, adenovirus, parainfluenza, HIV, metapneumovirus, human bocavirus), bacterial (tuberculosis, *Bordetella pertussis*, *Streptococcus pneumoniae*, *Haemophilus influenza*, *Moraxella catarrhalis*), fungal, and atypical bacteria (*Chlamydophila* and *Mycoplasma pneumoniae*)
Allergic condition	Allergic rhinitis, asthma
Other	FB aspiration, gastroesophageal reflux, psychogenic cough, environmental triggers (air pollution, tobacco smoke, wood smoke, glue sniffing, volatile chemicals), CF, drug induced, tumor, congestive heart failure

CF, Cystic fibrosis; *FB*, foreign body; *HIV*, human immunodeficiency virus; *RSV*, respiratory syncytial virus; *URI*, upper respiratory infection.

TABLE 32.2	Normal Respiratory Rates in Children	
Age (Years)	Respiratory Rate (Breaths/Min)
0–1	24–38
1–3	22–30
4–6	20–24
7–9	18–24
10–14	16–22
15–18	14–20

different from their own. Some studies suggest overestimation of arterial oxygen saturation with pulse oximetry for patients with darker skin tones. While more research is needed, care should be taken to eliminate racial bias associated with medical technologies in care delivery.[7,8]

- Inspection:
  - Nose: Inspect for rhinorrhea—clear, mucoid, mucopurulent; foreign bodies, erosion, polyps, lesions, bleeding, septal position, and mucous membrane color.
  - Throat, pharynx, and tonsils: Inspect for lesions, vesicles, exudate, enlargement of any structure, or other abnormalities. It is important to examine the entire tonsil to make sure there are no abscesses in a child with a severe sore throat; however, if epiglottitis is a consideration, never inspect the mouth or attempt to elicit a gag reflex unless clearly indicated and adequately prepared to do so in an emergency department setting.
  - Chest: Observe respiration depth, symmetry, and rhythm. Atypical findings in any of these assessment parameters should raise clinician index of suspicion for lower respiratory tract involvement. Note the use of accessory muscles and presence of retractions. In infants, early retractions are best observed on the chest along the posterior axillary line. A prolonged expiratory phase is associated with lower airway respiratory obstruction.

- Palpation or percussion of the chest: Percuss for signs of dullness or hyperresonance caused by consolidation, fluid, or air trapping.
- Auscultation of the chest:
  - Upper tract: Pathology frequently causes noisy breathing, snoring, stridor, and musical or wheezing tracheal breath sounds and can be a source of referred breath sounds. Have the child take a deep breath by having them blow out the light on the otoscope or blow paper off your hand.
  - Lower tract: Pathology is suggested with the presence of fine crackles, coarse crackles, rhonchi, pleural friction rub, wheezing, and bronchial breath sounds.

Diagnostic Studies

Diagnostic procedures used to evaluate and manage respiratory illness in children include the following:

- Monitoring oxygenation. Pulse oximetry can be used to spot check or continuously measure pulse rate and is a noninvasive method of monitoring arterial oxygen saturation. The oxyhemoglobin saturation percentage (SpO_2) is digitally displayed. Results generally correlate well with simultaneous arterial oxygen saturation (SaO_2). Continuous outpatient measurement of oxygen saturation in diseases like bronchiolitis is no longer recommended and may be responsible for the increasing admission rate for bronchiolitis.[9] With anoxia, there is a rise in organic phosphate content within the red blood cells (RBCs) resulting in more oxygen (O_2) available to tissues. People living at higher elevations suffer from chronic hypoxia. When first arriving at a high elevation, many individuals experience a transient mountain sickness with symptoms that include headache, insomnia, irritability, breathlessness, nausea, and vomiting. This phenomenon lasts approximately 1 week before acclimatization begins. The affected person begins to experience increased production of RBCs. Functional nonpathologic right ventricular hypertrophy may occur if the condition persists. These effects last as long as the person remains at high elevation. Severe altitude sickness can lead to cerebral and pulmonary edema and can be life-threatening.
- Monitoring CO_2 in acute care settings. Monitoring CO_2 can be done by a transcutaneous measurement (TCOM) or nasal cannula/endotracheal end tidal CO_2 monitoring. TCOM involves a small patch placed on the abdomen or chest measuring CO_2 diffusing to the surfaces. It can be affected by extreme obesity or poor peripheral perfusion. Nasal cannula provides a noninvasive way of monitoring for hypoventilation or apnea but may underestimate accurate CO_2 levels, meaning elevated readings need further investigation.[10]
- Blood gas studies. These studies are used in acute care settings to assess possible respiratory compromise. A rising partial arterial pressure of carbon dioxide ($PaCO_2$) is an ominous sign.
- Rapid diagnostic testing. Testing for bacteria, viruses, and fungal infections performed by CLIA-waived tests now include more accurate second-generation antigen assays, newer molecular testing with real-time polymerase chain reaction (PCR), and increased antigen detection sensitivity at the point of care.[11] The US Food and Drug Administration (FDA) approved molecular tests for the pediatric population include testing for group A beta--hemolytic *Streptococcus* (GABHS), respiratory virus panels including respiratory syncytial virus (RSV), influenza, *Bordetella pertussis, Chlamydophila pneumoniae, Mycoplasma pneumonia,* and *Bordetella parapertussis*

and *holmesii*. The rapid digital immunoassays and molecular testing for influenza A and B have a higher sensitivity and can improve management for selected populations,[11] but can be expensive with inequitable access. Newer GABHS molecular point of care tests have specificity and sensitivity over 95%; therefore back-up cultures are not indicated if these tests are negative. This testing should be done only if doing so contributes to the child's treatment decision.[12]

- Radiographic imaging to assess respiratory disease should be obtained in accordance with clinical guidance and best-practice principles of imaging with consideration of risks of radiation exposure. Imaging can include radiographs, ultrasonography, magnetic resonance imaging (MRI), and computed tomography (CT) of the sinuses, soft tissues of the neck, and chest. Abnormalities of the nasal mucosa may reflect inflammation. Imaging in acute rhinosinusitis (ARS) is not indicated as CT demonstrates abnormality in 80% of patients with uncomplicated upper respiratory infection (URI). Chest radiographs should be ordered with both posteroanterior and lateral positions, as lesions may be obscured by a singular view.
- Pulmonary function tests (spirometry) are discussed in Chapter 36 in the section on asthma.
- Other specialized tests, including sweat testing, cultures, and blood work, are addressed under the specific condition. Children with unusual signs and symptoms, chronic or recurrent respiratory conditions should be referred to a pulmonary specialist for further evaluation. Fluoroscopy is useful in the evaluation of stridor and abnormal movement of the diaphragm. Endoscopy (bronchoscopy and laryngoscopy), bronchoalveolar lavage, percutaneous tap, lung biopsy, and microbiology studies can be helpful if used appropriately. Contrast studies (e.g., barium esophagogram) are useful for patients with recurrent pneumonia, persistent cough, tracheal ring, or suspected fistulas. Other imaging studies that might be needed to assess these children include bronchograms (useful in delineating the smaller airways), pulmonary arteriograms (evaluation of the pulmonary vasculature), and radionuclide studies (evaluation of the pulmonary capillary bed).

Basic Respiratory Management Strategies

General Measures

There are several essential and basic measures related to the prevention of respiratory illnesses, including avoidance of smoke and exposure to secondhand smoking or vaping, effective hand-washing practices, and recommended childhood immunization. Children who are significantly ill or have unusual manifestations need referral to or consultation with a pediatric subspecialist or acute care provider. For those with mild or moderate respiratory illnesses, the following general management measures are applicable:

- *Fluid:* Hydration is important to keep mucous membranes and secretions moist. Intake of fluids should be encouraged, and caregivers should be given guidelines regarding the type, amount, and frequency of fluids and feedings.
- *Oxygen administration:* The use of supplemental oxygen is important to help relieve hypoxemia in most children who have acute respiratory distress. Depression of the respiratory drive is possible with supplemental oxygen administration if central nervous system (CNS) chemoreceptors are blunted by hypercapnia. Children at risk for blunted ventilation are those with issues related to chronic hypercapnia and are generally easily

recognized because they tend to have chronic severe respiratory diseases such as CF and bronchopulmonary dysplasia (BPD; also called *neonatal chronic lung disease*). In acute situations, administer oxygen using an appropriately sized mask or a high-flow oxygen source held near the child's face if a mask frightens the child. While ideally a child's oxygen should range between 95% and 100%, new guidelines for bronchiolitis allow an infant to go home when the oxygen ranges between 90% and 95%.[13] Children with oxygen saturation less than 85% and those with significant distress initially evaluated in an outpatient setting should be transported via emergency medical services to an acute care setting for management. Some children with preexisting medical conditions such as cardiac congenital anomalies may have low oxygen saturations as a baseline of their condition and oxygen administration can sometimes be harmful.

- *Humidification:* A cool-mist humidifier provides moisture to the nares and oropharynx in a dry environment during a common cold. The tank and parts exposed to water should be cleaned frequently (Box 32.1). Vaporizers are no longer recommended.
- *Normal saline (NS) nasal drops, rinses, or spray:* Use before feedings, sleep, and when mucus is thick or crusted. Follow by suctioning the nares gently with a bulb syringe. Saline nasal rinses are widely available commercially and are helpful for older children and adolescents (see Box 32.1).
- *Bulb syringe:* Infants are preferential nose breathers; therefore caregivers should be instructed in gentle and intermittent use of the nasal bulb syringe to relieve obstruction of the infant's nares. Improper use can cause irritation, inflammation, and respiratory obstruction from tissue damage. Providers should give written instructions and in-person demonstration (see resources for guidelines).

Medications

There is lack of evidence to recommend any OTC cold and cough medications for children. Prescriptive recommendations should be carefully considered based on symptom presentation and evidence for safe administration.[14] The following pharmacologic agents may be considered to treat symptoms of respiratory illnesses:

- *Analgesics and antipyretics:* Acetaminophen (for ages newborn and up with provider recommendation or starting at age 12 weeks for OTC administration) and ibuprofen (for infants ages 6 months and older) may be recommended for short-term relief of pain or fever. Dosing should be based on a current and accurate weight with clear caregiver instruction.
- *Decongestants:* The use of decongestants does not shorten the course of a disease. Due to the risk of overdose, unsupervised ingestions, potential for harm, and little evidence of efficacy, use of decongestants and/or OTC cough medication is no longer recommended for children younger than 6 years. The FDA issued warnings not to prescribe any cold medications containing codeine or hydrocodone to pediatric patients under 18 years of age due to serious side effects, deaths, and addiction potential.[15]
- *Expectorants:* Water is one of the most effective expectorants. OTC agents provide some symptomatic relief but do not shorten the course of respiratory illnesses. Although expectorants like guaifenesin are approved for use in children over 2 years of age, they are not recommended for use in children less than 6 years old.[15] While guaifenesin has a safety profile with

over 50 years of use in the United States, common side effects include gastrointestinal (GI) upset, dizziness, and headache.[16]
- *Antihistamines:* Although antihistamines are commonly prescribed for persistent cough, they are not recommended.[17] The FDA recommended in 2008 that children less than 2 years of age not use cough and cold medicines. Although prescribing patterns of opioid-containing cough medication decreased, use of antihistamines rose, especially for children younger than 12 years of age, making antihistamines one of the most prescribed pediatric medications despite guidelines to the contrary.[18]
- *Zinc and vitamin C:* Interest in the use of zinc and vitamin C to treat or prevent respiratory illness was revived in the emergence of the COVID-19 pandemic. Research on their efficacy and safety is inconclusive, making confident recommendation difficult.[19]
- *Probiotics:* The use of probiotics in the pediatric population has demonstrated best efficacy in cases of acute gastroenteritis and prevention of antibiotic-associated diarrhea but has limited demonstrated efficacy for respiratory infections. Scientific research to support broader recommendations for routine use is lacking in standardized study design, standard application

---

• BOX 32.1 Education for at-Home Care of the Child With a Respiratory Tract Infection

General Management Issues to Discuss

Fluids: Provide guidance on type, amount, and frequency of fluids.

Humidification: For croup, consider advising caregiver to take the child out into the cold night air or open a freezer door. In dry climates, cool-mist humidifiers may help in common colds; provide clear guidance on the importance of cleaning of nebulizers and humidifiers (see bullet about care of nebulizers and humidifiers).

Saline nose drops or spray: Use before feedings and when mucus is thick or crusted. Follow with bulb syringe suctioning.

Bulb syringe: Educate caregivers on safe use of intermittent suctioning with the bulb syringe.

Encourage frequent hand washing and avoidance of exposure to smoke or secondhand smoke.

Other Educational Topics to Cover
- Indications for immediate reevaluation of child:
  - Signs and symptoms of respiratory distress
  - Other indicators of worsening of illness (e.g., toxic appearance [mild or moderately ill looking], malaise, feeding difficulty)
- Provide guidance on expected improvement in child's symptoms and what to do if symptoms do not improve as expected.
- Provide clear instructions about medications: provide instructions regarding how much medication to give, when to give it, what side effects to watch for, how long to give medication, and necessity of completing any course of antibiotics.
- Infection control information if needed: provide information regarding handwashing and disposal of infected secretions; CDC has excellent written and video education materials available on handwashing at www.cdc.gov/Features/HandWashing.
- Care of nebulizers and humidifiers: to prevent growth of organisms, nebulizers and humidifiers should be cleaned daily with soapy water, rinsed thoroughly, soaked for one half hour in a solution of one part vinegar to two or three parts distilled water, and then air-dried. Control III disinfectant is a commercial product that can be substituted for vinegar; however, this approach may be cost-prohibitive.
- Provide instructions regarding next return visit.

CDC, Centers for Disease Control and Prevention.

of rigor, and indications for dose, strains, and treatment regimens. Probiotic supplements are associated with a low risk of adverse events and are generally well tolerated, although efficacy is questionable.[20]

Antibiotic Stewardship

The efforts by the Centers for Disease Control and Prevention (CDC) and the American Academy of Pediatrics (AAP)[21] for antibiotic stewardship encourages providers to avoid the use of antibiotics for viral infections.[22] While there has been progress in antibiotic stewardship,[23] data suggest that 30% of antibiotics used in an outpatient setting are unnecessary.[22] There are geographic differences in the United States with lower rates of antibiotic prescriptions in the Pacific regions and the highest rate in the East South-Central regions.[24]

Patient and Family Education

Frequent hand washing and avoiding touching the eyes and nose prevent the spread of infection. Always educate about the dangers related to exposure to smoking or vaping and secondhand smoking or vaping exposure and the need to avoid this respiratory trigger. Teach the child and other family members how to cough/sneeze into sleeve, dispose of tissues, and use hand sanitizers because these measures decrease the spread of infections. Caregivers should be educated about assessment and management of changes in the child's condition. Significant educational issues are identified in Box 32.1.

Upper Airway Conditions: Infectious

Upper Respiratory Infection

A URI or the common cold is a frequent problem seen in pediatric practice, and caregivers often seek information from their child's primary healthcare provider as to whether their child's symptoms represent a typical URI or indicate the beginning or advancing signs of a more serious illness. Children have on average 2 to 10 colds per year with daycare attendance increasing the occurrence up to 14 URIs per year.[25] The typical course of these illnesses is an initial low-grade fever with a sore throat that progresses to rhinorrhea, cough, and congestion. The average duration is 7 to 9 days; the peak is generally on the third day when purulent discharge may be noted. There is a slow resolution with clear nasal discharge by day 10.

Viruses cause most URIs, with 50% caused by more than 100 serotypes of rhinoviruses, peaking in the spring and fall. URIs are generally most contagious in the first 3 days of illness and can shed for up to 2 weeks.[26] Parainfluenza viruses, RSV, adenoviruses, coronavirus, human bocavirus, and human metapneumovirus are also common agents.[25] Daycare and preschool attendance are associated with an increased number of URIs in young children that spread to school-age children in the family. Acquisition of viruses occurs by hand contact of the infected surface to the nose or conjunctiva, inhalation of small airborne particles, or by deposition of large particles that land directly on the conjunctiva or nasal mucosa. Transmission by direct contact is the most efficient pathway for infection with rhinovirus and RSV.[27]

Viral infection of the nasopharyngeal mucosa initiates a host response that produces symptoms of a URI. Once the virus is deposited on the nasal mucosa, it attaches to cell receptors and achieves cell entry. Potent cytokines including interleukin (IL)-8 attract large number of neutrophil cells by 6 hours after infection. As a result, vascular permeability increases, causing the leak of plasma proteins into nasal secretions. Bradykinins cause pharyngitis and rhinitis. The presence of polymorphonuclear leukocyte (PMN) enzymatic activity changes the color of nasal mucus (i.e., yellow to green mucus); however, this change in color does not necessarily indicate the presence of bacterial infection.

Clinical Findings

Symptoms of a viral URI include nasal congestion, cough, sneezing, rhinorrhea, fever, hoarseness, and pharyngitis. The symptoms typically worsen over the first 1 to 3 days of illness, with a plateau effect and should decrease or resolve by the end of 10 days.

History. The following may be reported:
- Gradual onset and low-grade fever, especially in younger children
- Prominent nasal symptoms of rhinorrhea (key finding)
- Sore throat and dysphagia; mild cough and poor sleep
- After a variable period of 1 to 3 days, nasal secretions are thicker and more purulent, leading to nasal excoriation

Physical Examination. Virus-specific findings include:
- Mild conjunctival injection; red nasal mucosa with secretions of varying colors depending on the degree of nasal mucosa destruction and PMN activity; mild erythema of the pharynx
- Anterior cervical lymphadenopathy with freely movable, soft nodes less than 2 cm
- Chest clear to auscultation and without increased work of breathing

Diagnostic Studies. A throat culture is not recommended if there are nasal symptoms with complaints of throat pain. If the presenting symptom is a sore throat rather than rhinitis, a rapid antigen detection test (RADT), or a rapid strep test, should be considered.

Differential Diagnosis

The most common differentials are allergic rhinitis, rhinosinusitis, and adenoiditis (Table 32.3).

Management

Only supportive care is needed for a viral URI. See the Respiratory Management Strategies section and Box 32.1. Antibiotics are not appropriate treatment. The child should receive symptomatic relief for fever, pain, and nasal congestion using an antipyretic and NS irrigation. Fluid intake should be encouraged.

Complications

Common colds are self-limiting but secondary bacterial infections including otitis media, pneumonia, and sinusitis can occur. Children with worsening symptoms after 3 days, severe symptoms at any point in time, or symptoms lingering beyond 10 days should be carefully evaluated.

Rhinosinusitis

Rhinosinusitis is an inflammatory condition that may or may not be infectious. Bacteria form biofilms, which are a matrix of polysaccharides, proteins, and nucleic acids. These films allow bacteria to aggregate in a protective environment, such as the sinuses, and are responsible for antimicrobial resistance.[28] The maxillary and anterior ethmoid sinuses are most frequently involved in children because they are present at birth, but only the ethmoidal sinuses are pneumatized.

TABLE 32.3	**Differentiations of Common Upper Respiratory Infections in Children**					
Site of Infection	Symptoms	Duration of Symptoms	Etiologic Agent	Management	Duration of Treatment	Comments
The common cold (viral URI)	Malaise, sneezing, watery nasal discharge, mild sore throat, may have a fever, not ill appearing	0–10 days	Parainfluenza, RSV, adenovirus, coronavirus,	No antibiotics; symptomatic treatment (e.g., saline nose drops, increased fluids); for infants, bulb-syringe suctioning of the nose before meals and sleep; for older children, consider a cool-mist humidifier	As long as symptoms last	If lasts longer than 10–14 days, consider other diagnosis (e.g., rhinosinusitis)
Acute rhinosinusitis	Persistent nasal symptoms for more than 10 days with URI, nasal drainage (purulent or discolored), cough Acute presentation with or without low-grade fever, purulent rhinitis	10–30 days		Amoxicillin, or amoxicillin-clavulanic acid	10 days	By 7 days, should be asymptomatic; change antibiotics 48–72 h after start of treatment if no response
Subacute rhinosinusitis	Same as above but persistent for at least 30 days	30–84 days	Same as above; may be β-lactamase producing	Amoxicillin-clavulanic acid		If initial acute infection did not clear, need to switch antibiotics
Chronic/recurrent rhinosinusitis	Malaise, easy fatigability, unilateral or bilateral nasal discharge, postnasal discharge, nasal obstruction if middle turbinate significantly obstructed	Recurrent >10 to <28 days but symptom free for at least 10 days in between bouts Chronic >84 days	Same as above plus α-hemolytic streptococci and *Staphylococcus aureus*	Amoxicillin-clavulanic, azithromycin, staph coverage	3–6 wk	May need endoscopic sinus surgery if no response to prolonged medical management; investigate differential diagnoses or underlying issues (e.g., allergic rhinitis)

CRS, Chronic rhinosinusitis; *RSV*, respiratory syncytial virus; *URI*, upper respiratory infection.

Rhinosinusitis can be divided into acute or chronic designations. ARS involves inflammation of the mucosal lining of the nasal passages and paranasal sinuses. Acute bacterial sinusitis is a complication of a viral URI.[29] Sinusitis results because of several anatomic factors including inflammation of the sinus mucosa obstructing the sinus ostia, nasal polyps, allergic rhinitis, and underlying conditions such as ciliary dyskinesia, CF, and immunodeficiency. It presents in three ways: (1) onset of severe upper respiratory symptoms, (2) onset of upper respiratory symptoms with persistent symptoms, and (3) a "double sickening" with initial improvement followed by onset of severe disease.[28] Chronic rhinosinusitis (CRS) is diagnosed when symptoms persist for 12 weeks or longer.[29]

The most common bacterial pathogens that cause ARS include *Streptococcus pneumoniae, nontypeable, Haemophilus influenza, Moraxella catarrhalis,* and less often, *Staphylococcus aureus.*[29]

Although there is no consensus about the bacteriology of CRS, it is believed that CRS is a multifactorial inflammatory disease instead of a persistent bacterial infection. Predisposing factors for CRS include a preceding viral, bacterial, and/or fungal infection; environmental irritants; allergies; anatomic problems, including septal deviation, nasal polyps, trauma, FB, or abnormality of the ostiomeatal complex; gastroesophageal reflux; cigarette smoking; CF; primary ciliary dyskinesia; and immunodeficiencies.[30] Persistent swelling of the sinonasal mucosa impairs sinus drainage, which is associated with sinusitis.

The adenoids are believed to be a reservoir for bacterial infections that lead to nose and nasal sinus infections. That is why adenoidectomy may be indicated.[31]

The presence of antibiotic-resistant organisms is associated with the production of cephalosporinase and β-lactamase and is more common in patients in day care or with recent exposure to antibiotics.[31] The role of viruses in rhinosinusitis is not clear. Children with immunodeficiency disorders need to be treated with antibiotics that cover *Pseudomonas;* children with CF are predisposed to sinus infections with *Aspergillus* and *Zygomycetes.*

Clinical Findings

The duration of symptoms determines the classification of rhinosinusitis. The history of acute sinusitis differs from an uncomplicated URI. A child with an uncomplicated URI presents with a thick, yellow discharge on the third or fourth day without fever or with low-grade fever followed by improvement. Headache, malodorous breath, fatigue, and decreased appetite are nonspecific symptoms and therefore not helpful in the diagnosis. Box 32.2 shows major and minor criteria for sinusitis. ARS is a clinical diagnosis and should not be confirmed by any diagnostic testing including imaging.

Diagnostic Studies. Imaging studies should only be obtained if a complication is suspected. If the child is suspected of having an orbital or CNS extension of sinusitis, then contrast-enhanced CT of the brain sinuses and orbits is generally obtained due to speed and ease. An MRI with contrast is an excellent option if readily available.[31]

Differential Diagnosis

The differential diagnosis of sinusitis includes a viral URI, allergic rhinitis, nasal polyps, nasal tumors, and tension, migraine, or cluster headache. Remember that sinusitis may exacerbate asthma. Ethmoiditis can occur after a child is 6 months old, in contrast to frontal rhinosinusitis, which is first seen around 10 years of age.

Management

The healthcare provider must be cautious to not overdiagnose rhinosinusitis and overprescribe antibiotics. Chronic or recurrent rhinosinusitis may result in referral to an otolaryngologist and/or allergist.

To aid in decision-making about when to treat, the AAP developed clinical guidelines for the treatment of ARS based upon three different clinical presentations in children[32]:

- A URI with persistent nasal discharge or daytime cough lasting for more than 10 days without clinical improvement

---

- A URI that worsens or there is a new onset of fever, nasal discharge, or daytime cough after initial improvement
- A fever higher than 102.2°F (39°C) with purulent nasal discharge for at least 3 days in a child who also has sinusitis

Severe onset or a worsening course requires oral antibiotics. If the child has a persistent illness suggestive of rhinosinusitis, antibiotics can be given, or watchful waiting for 3 days can be offered. Symptomatic pain relief with acetaminophen or ibuprofen has been shown to be helpful. The sinusitis guidelines suggest treatment with amoxicillin with or without clavulanate as a first-line treatment.[31,32] Treatment length varies from 10 to 28 days. An alternative to this is to continue treatment for 7 days after the child is completely free of any signs or symptoms.

Treatment considerations include the following:
- Amoxicillin at a standard dose of 45 mg/kg/day divided in two doses is the first-line treatment in communities with low incidence of nonsusceptible *S. pneumoniae.* In communities with an incidence of more than 10% resistance to *S. pneumonia*, amoxicillin should be used at 80 to 90 mg/kg/day divided every 12 hours (maximum dose: 1000 mg/dose).
- In patients younger than 2 years, daycare attendees, recent antimicrobial use, or in patients with moderate to severe illness, amoxicillin-clavulanate at 80 to 90 mg/day of amoxicillin component divided every 12 hours and only use the 600 mg/5 mL formulation.
- In children with vomiting, a single dose of 50 mg/kg of ceftriaxone can be given either intravenously (IV) or intramuscularly (IM).
- In patients with allergy to amoxicillin, the type of allergic reaction determines the antibiotic. If the child has a serious type 1 immediate or accelerated reaction, the cephalosporins cannot be used. However, if they have a non–type 1 hypersensitivity reaction, they can safely be treated with one of the third-generation, cephalosporin antibiotics—cefdinir, cefpodoxime, or cefuroxime.

The management of CRS is more complicated because bacteria are generally only one of other contributing factors. Referral to an otolaryngologist is often needed as an adenoidectomy is an effective first-line procedure for children under 12 years. Surgical drainage by an otolaryngologist, treatment of allergies and control of allergic rhinitis by an allergist, or both may be necessary.

Additional management considerations include the following:
- Decongestants and antihistamines: There is evidence to support the use of topical decongestants.[29] There are no data to support the use of either topical or oral antihistamines as an adjuvant therapy.
- Intranasal corticosteroids: There is insufficient evidence to support the use of intranasal steroids in ARS or CRS, though inflammation is often a factor in CRS.
- Saline irrigation: NS is used to mechanically clean the nasal passages of mucus, biofilms, antigens, cytokines, inflammatory mediators, and thin secretions, and moisturize the nasal passages. While the 2013 clinical guidelines do not support or negate the use of saline,[32] there is evidence to support the use of NS in adults, though evidence is lacking in children.[29]
- Analgesics: Comfort measures include the use of acetaminophen and ibuprofen for severe pain.
- Ensure adequate hydration.

Complications

Orbital complications are common and usually occur following ethmoid sinusitis.[33] Complications of eye involvement include

---

> ### • BOX 32.2 Criteria for Bacterial Sinusitis
>
> **Major Criteria**
> - Facial pain or pressure (second major criteria is needed)
> - Facial congestion or fullness
> - Nasal congestion/obstruction
> - Nasal discharge, purulence, or discolored postnasal discharge
> - Hyposmia or anosmia
> - Fever (acute sinusitis requires a second major criteria)
> - Purulence on intranasal examination
>
> **Minor Criteria**
> - Headache
> - Fever
> - Halitosis
> - Fatigue
> - Dental pain
> - Cough
> - Ear pain, pressure, or fullness

presptal cellulitis, orbital cellulitis, and subperiosteal and orbital abscess. While orbital cellulitis is manifested by swelling and erythema of the eyelids, proptosis, decreased extraocular movements, and altered vision, an orbital abscess can lead to proptosis, ophthalmoplegia, and ultimately vision loss. Children with findings concerning for orbital involvement should be admitted for evaluation and IV antibiotics. Pediatric presentation of subperiosteal orbital abscess may need immediate surgical evaluation. Early identification and intervention can preserve eye function and decrease morbidity and mortality. Further extension can lead to a cavernous sinus thrombosis (CST). A CST starts with periorbital edema with chemosis and headaches and can advance to cranial nerve palsies as the infection invades the cavernous sinus.[33]

Intracranial complications are more likely from frontal sinusitis and include Pott's puffy tumor, epidural abscess, subperiosteal abscess, brain abscess, venous thrombosis, and meningitis. The child with Pott's puffy tumor or osteomyelitis of the frontal bone presents with frontal bone tenderness and swelling on the forehead. A neurosurgical consult should be obtained. An infectious disease and otolaryngology consult is important with these complications.

Prevention

Prevention of sinusitis includes allergy and gastroesophageal reflux management, influenza vaccine, and relief of nasal airway obstruction.

Pharyngitis, Tonsillitis, and Tonsillopharyngitis

Pharyngitis is an inflammation of the mucosa lining the structures of the throat, including the tonsils, pharynx, uvula, soft palate, and nasopharynx. It can be due to infectious agents or noninfectious causes such as environmental exposures, allergic responses, referred pain, or oncological causes. Most children with pharyngitis have an acute illness involving an inflammatory response such as erythema, exudate, or ulceration.

If there are nasal symptoms with pharyngitis, it is called *nasopharyngitis,* but if there are no nasal symptoms, the illness is called *pharyngitis* or *tonsillopharyngitis.* Most cases of pharyngitis are viral in nature.[34] and typically include adenovirus, Epstein-Barr virus (EBV), parainfluenza, influenza, herpes simplex virus (HSV), cytomegalovirus (CMV), enterovirus, and human immunodeficiency virus (HIV). While adenoviruses are more likely to cause pharyngitis as a prominent symptom, other viruses (e.g., rhinovirus) cause rhinorrhea or cough as predominant features. Adenoviruses are generally self-limiting illnesses in children under 5 years old. By the age of 10 years, most children have had at least one episode of adenovirus infection.[35] Enterovirus (coxsackievirus, echovirus), herpesvirus, and EBV are also common. Viral infections occur year-round, but adenovirus presenting as pharyngoconjunctival fever occurs in outbreaks during the summer due to contaminated swimming pools and school exposure, particularly in kindergarten.[36] Hoarseness, cough, coryza, conjunctivitis, and diarrhea are classic features of a viral infection.[34]

GABHS is the most common bacterial cause of pharyngitis and tonsillitis in all pediatric patients, but most commonly between 5 and 11 years of age. It accounts for 15% to 35% of infections in children with acute sore throat and fever.[37] Other less common causes of bacterial pharyngitis in children include group C and group G streptococci, which can cause pharyngitis and other more severe infection. *M. pneumoniae* and *C. pneumoniae* are associated with cough. *M. pneumonia* can cause a significant sore throat

and most commonly is accompanied with lower tract symptoms. *Neisseria gonorrhoeae* can cause pharyngitis if the patient engages in oral to genital sex with an individual who has *N. gonorrhoeae* of the genital region. *Corynebacterium diphtheria* is an extremely rare cause of pharyngitis and is primarily limited to incidence in developing countries.[38]

Clinical Findings

History. A history of pain, myalgia and arthralgia, fever, sore throat, and dysphagia may be reported in viral or bacterial presentations.

In viral illnesses, the following is commonly reported:
- Rhinitis, cough, hoarseness, stomatitis, stridor and conjunctivitis, nonspecific rash, or diarrhea
  The following characterize GABHS infection[39]
- Most commonly found in 5- to 15-year-old children; infrequent in children younger than 3 years old
- Abrupt and acute onset without nasal symptoms
- Tender lymph nodes, may or may not be enlarged
- Constitutional symptoms, such as arthralgia, myalgia, headache
- Moderate to high fever, malaise, prominent sore throat, dysphagia
- Nausea, abdominal discomfort, vomiting, headache
- Absence of rhinorrhea or cough
- Petechiae on soft palate and pharynx, swollen beefy-red uvula, red enlarged tonsillopharyngeal tissue
- Scarlet fever may be seen: scarlatiniform rash, strawberry tongue, circumoral pallor

Physical Examination

When a patient presents with only a sore throat, it is difficult to differentiate viral from bacterial causes and RADT can be positive in both acute illness and carriage states, the latter of which requires no treatment.[38]

Diagnostic Studies

The Centor criteria may be used to aid in judicious ordering of diagnostic testing to assess for GABHS and to guide index of suspicion. It consists of fever >38.5°C; swollen, tender anterior cervical lymph nodes, tonsillar exudate, and absence of cough; presence of two or more indicate a higher likelihood of GABHS and testing is indicated.[40]

It is important to reserve RADT for patients with clinical features consistent with GABHS to diagnose acute illness and avoid false-positive tests on patients who are carriers of streptococcus and do not need treatment. Testing for GABHS in children younger than 3 years and in asymptomatic household contact is not recommended.[34] Following a negative RADT with back-up culture is recommended for first and second generation testing but is generally unnecessary following newer, more accurate molecular test methods. Judicious use of RADT is needed to avoid overuse of antibiotics and maintain antimicrobial stewardship.[41]

Serological tests, such as anti–streptolysin O (ASO) and anti–deoxyribonuclease B tests (anti-DNase B) are not useful in the diagnosis of acute pharyngitis because antibody response takes 1 to 3 weeks after infection and titers remain elevated for months after an acute infection. While ASO is the most common test used to document past GABHS infection, it is also positive in the presence of group C and G infections.[42] ASO and anti-DNase B testing involves identifying antibody titers in response to streptolysin O or deoxyribonuclease B, respectively; these tests are often performed simultaneously. The ASO titer rises 1 week postinfection and peaks 3 to 5 weeks after infection. Measurement of antistreptococcal antibody titers is useful in the diagnosis of nonsuppurative complications of GABHS, such as rheumatic fever or acute glomerulonephritis. The anti-DNase B test rises 2 weeks after infection, peaks 6 to 8 weeks following infection (later than ASO) and remains elevated for months and longer than ASO.

Rare bacterial causes of pharyngitis requiring antibiotics include *C. diphtheria* and *N. gonorrhoeae*. Adolescents who have oral to genital sex and present with symptoms suggestive of GABHS should have a throat culture specific to these organisms.

If infectious mononucleosis is suspected, a complete blood count (CBC) identifies lymphocytosis with atypical lymphocytes. This is a nonspecific test, because reactive (atypical) lymphocytes can occur with EBV and acquired CMV infections, as well as viral hepatitis, rubella, roseola, and mumps. Heterophile antibody testing (Mono Spot) for infectious mononucleosis can be helpful in school-age children and adolescents after the first week of infection but commonly yields false negatives.

Management

Supportive care alone is generally recommended for pharyngitis with viral etiology, including management with antipyretics and adequate fluid intake. Antibiotics should only be used in symptomatic GABHS when the RADT or throat culture is positive. Antibiotic stewardship is critical to decrease the rise of antibiotic resistance associated with overuse.[43] The goal of antibiotic therapy is to shorten the course and severity of bacterial illness, prevent spread to others, and prevent development of suppurative and nonsuppurative complications. Treatment must be initiated within 9 days of symptom onset to prevent nonsuppurative complications of rheumatic fever. The use of β-lactam antibiotics during an acute CMV or EBV infection is not needed and can cause a diffuse, morbilliform skin eruption.[43]

The management plan of GABHS includes the following:
- Antimicrobial therapy shortens the length of the fever, decreases infectivity, lowers toxicity, and is based on positive bacterial testing results in a symptomatic patient. Penicillin (therapy of choice due to low cost, efficacy, lack of documented antibiotic resistance, and infrequent adverse reactions):
  - Penicillin V potassium: Children (<27 kg): 250 mg twice daily or 3 times daily for 10 days; children (greater than 27 kg) and adolescents: 500 mg twice daily or 3 times daily for 10 days; can do 250 mg 4 times a day with teens.
  - Amoxicillin suspension is more palatable (efficacy seems equal to penicillin): 50 mg/kg once daily (maximum dose = 1000 mg); alternate: 25 mg/kg (maximum dose = 500 mg) twice daily for 10 days.
  - Benzathine penicillin G IM: 600,000 units as a single dose if less than 27 kg; 1.2 million units as a single dose for larger children and adults.
- If allergic to penicillin:
  - Cephalexin: 20 mg/kg/dose twice daily (maximum dose = 500 mg/dose) for 10 days but should be avoided in patients with moderate hypersensitivity reaction to penicillin
  - Cefadroxil: 30 mg/kg/day divided twice daily (maximum daily dose = 1 g/day) for 10 days but should be avoided with moderate hypersensitivity reaction to penicillin
  - Clindamycin: 20 mg/kg/day in 3 divided doses (maximum dose = 900 mg/day) for 10 days
  - Azithromycin: 12 mg/kg on day 1, then 6 mg/kg once daily for 4 days. It should be noted that macrolide resistance is variable in the United States.[44]

- Clarithromycin: 7.5 mg/kg/dose to a maximum of 250 mg twice per day for 10 days.
- Supportive care: antipyretics, fluids, and rest.
- Use of corticosteroids is not indicated.
- Repeat culture is not needed except in situations where it is necessary to ensure eradication of the organism.
- Fomites on items such as bathroom cups, toothbrushes, or orthodontic devices, may harbor GABHS and should be sterilized or discarded.
- Children can return to school when they are afebrile and have been taking antibiotics for at least 12 to 24 hours.

Continued symptoms of streptococcal pharyngitis and a positive culture for streptococcus may represent treatment failure or a new infection with a different serologic type of streptococcus.[43] Nonadherence to pharmacologic therapy can explain treatment failure, and in these instances an injection of benzathine penicillin is recommended.

The mean carriage rate of GABHS is around 16%. To avoid overusing antibiotics, it is not recommended to do a follow-up culture in asymptomatic children nor to do a RADT on a patient with primarily nasal symptoms. The degree of communicability is less in carriage state due to difference in the M protein surrounding GABHS. Published guidelines do not recommend routine treatment of the carriage state except in special circumstances: (1) an outbreak in a closed community, (2) family or personal history of rheumatic fever, (3) "ping pong" spread in family members over several weeks, (4) if a tonsillectomy is being considered because of persistent symptoms related to continued carriage, or (5) a local outbreak of rheumatic fever or invasive group A strep disease.[45]

Treatment of chronic symptomatic carriage of GABHS[39]:
- Clindamycin: 20 to 30 mg/kg/day in three doses (maximum dose = 300 mg/dose) for 10 days
- Amoxicillin-clavulanic acid: 40 mg/kg/day in three doses (maximum daily dose = 2000 mg/day) for 10 days
- Penicillin V for 10 days (maximum dose = 2000 mg/day) with the use of rifampin: 20 mg/kg/day divided in two doses (maximum dose = 600 mg/day) during the last 4 days of penicillin therapy[39,44]
- Benzathine penicillin G: 600,000 units for <27 kg and 1.2 million units for 27 kg or greater, with rifampin: 20 mg/kg/day in two doses (maximum dose = 600 mg/day) for 4 days

If clinical relapse occurs, a second course of antibiotic is indicated, as discussed earlier. If recurrent infection is a problem, culturing of the family for chronic carrier state is advised.

Complications

Nonsuppurative complications of streptococcal infections include rheumatic fever, poststreptococcal reactive arthritis, and acute glomerulonephritis. Suppurative complications include cervical adenitis, rhinosinusitis, otitis media, pneumonia, mastoiditis, and retropharyngeal or peritonsillar abscess. Retropharyngeal abscess is more common in children younger than 6 years old, whereas peritonsillar abscess peaks in adolescence with an average age of 13.6 years.[34] Most peritonsillar abscesses are caused by streptococcus and Fusobacterium and are polymicrobial.

Other poststreptococcal sequela include poststreptococcal arthritis and pediatric autoimmune neuropsychiatric disorder syndrome (PANDAS). Pediatric acute-onset neuropsychiatric syndrome (or PANS) is a condition in which there is a sudden onset of obsessive-compulsive symptoms and/or severe restriction of eating, and with at least two neuropsychiatric symptoms including separation anxiety, motor abnormalities, behavior regression, poor academic performance, mood changes, urinary symptoms, and somatic symptoms.[46] PANS can result from different disease mechanisms ranging from psychological trauma to underlying neurological autoimmune, neuroinflammatory, endocrine, and postinfectious etiology. When a recent streptococcal infection is the cause, it is called *PANDAS*. The treatment of PANS and PANDAS is similar. Guidelines have a threefold approach: (1) cognitive behavioral or family therapy and/or psychotropic medications to treat the psychiatric symptoms, (2) antimicrobial therapy to treat the underlying cause of inflammation if the source can be identified, and (3) use of immunomodulatory or antiinflammatory medications to treat the immune system disturbance.[46]

Indications for Tonsillectomy and Adenoidectomy

Clinical guidelines for tonsillectomy include having more than seven episodes of throat infections in the past year or more than five episodes of throat infection in the past 2 years or at least three episodes per year for the past 3 years.[47] The definition of throat infections includes a temperature of higher than 100.9°F (38.3°C), cervical lymphadenopathy with tonsillar exudate, or a positive GABHS culture or if antibiotics had been administered in suspected or confirmed cases of GABHS. Benefits of tonsillectomy do not persist over time and quality of life was not different in either group.[47] Sleep apnea is the most common noninfectious indication for tonsillectomy and adenoidectomy. Other indications include recurrent tonsillitis, peritonsillar abscesses, periodic fever with aphthous ulcers, and adenopathy.

The chief indication for an adenoidectomy is severe nasal obstruction for more than 1 year and unresponsiveness to medical therapy including antibiotics and nasal steroids. Severe nasal obstruction presents with hyponasal speech, olfaction difficulties, and chronic mouth breathing. Refractory otitis media, chronic otitis media with effusion, and recurrent otitis media in children who had tympanostomy tubes placed are relative contraindications.[34]

Croup (Laryngotracheobronchitis)

Croup (laryngotracheobronchitis) is a common URI in children and caused by inflammation of the larynx, upper subglottic airway, and sometimes bronchi, leading to upper airway obstruction. Croup is characterized by a barky cough and is associated with varying degrees of inspiratory stridor, hoarseness, and respiratory distress. There is often a URI prodrome, including congestion, rhinitis and coryza for 1 to 2 days. Symptoms progress to include fever, hoarseness, barking cough, and stridor. Severe cases may include tachypnea and significant respiratory distress. Croup is usually a self-limited illness, though severe cases do occur and may cause severe respiratory distress or respiratory failure.

Human parainfluenza types 1 and 2 causes most cases of croup.[48] Other viral causes include influenza A and B, adenovirus, and RSV. Viral croup is most common between the ages of 5 months and 5 years, with a peak at age 2 years. Croup occurs most often in late fall and winter but can occur throughout the year. Family history of croup is common, and croup frequently recurs. Risk factors for recurrent croup include asthma, allergies, and gastroesophageal reflux.[48]

Clinical Findings

Clinical manifestations depend on the infectious agent responsible for the croup and the extent of the upper airway involvement.
History. The history typically includes the following:
- URI prodromal symptoms (congestion, rhinitis, coryza)

- Acute onset of a hoarse, barking cough (usually day 2–3 of illness
- Mild to severe inspiratory stridor
- Sleep disturbance caused by nighttime coughing (symptoms often worse at night).
- May or may not have sore throat
- May or may not have a fever
- May or may not have tachypnea and/or retractions
- Less common: mild hypoxia or cyanosis
  Physical Examination. Findings include the following:
- Fussiness, irritability is common; lethargy or inconsolability are ominous signs
- Upper respiratory findings of congestion, rhinitis, coryza
- Lower respiratory findings of:
  - Inspiratory stridor (often audible, sometimes biphasic)
  - Brassy or barking cough (harsh sounding)
  - Substernal and/or intercostal retractions
  - Prolonged inspiration
  - Varying signs of respiratory distress and pulmonary involvement (e.g., nasal flaring, grunting, retractions, cyanosis, prolonged exhalation)
  Diagnostic Studies. Croup is considered a clinical diagnosis as it is based upon history and physical examination. Chest radiographs are not routinely indicated unless there is concern for airway complication. If obtained, radiography of the neck and chest display a classic pattern of subglottic narrowing (the "steeple sign") on posteroanterior views. Routine virologic testing is not routinely obtained as it does not change the management of most children.

Differential Diagnosis

Differential diagnoses include acute epiglottitis; bacterial tracheitis, FB aspiration; retropharyngeal or parapharyngeal abscess; extrinsic compression from tumors, trauma, or congenital malformations; angioedema (anaphylaxis), infectious mononucleosis; and psychogenic stridor.[48] Epiglottitis is discussed below. Bacterial tracheitis is a rare bacterial infection of the trachea that causes epithelial sloughing and airway obstruction. It is a rapidly progressive disease accompanied by high fever. FB aspiration usually has a sudden onset without URI prodrome. Retropharyngeal abscess occurs when a suppurative lymph node ruptures into the retropharyngeal area; a penetrating FB enters the area; or diskitis, osteomyelitis, or a mediastinal infection spreads to the area. CT scan is the standard study for diagnosis; it is important that part of the mediastinum is imaged to pick up spread from this area.

Table 32.4 differentiates acute laryngotracheitis from other common causes of stridor.

Management

Overall, the management of croup aims to promote adequate respiration and is largely dependent upon the severity of disease. The Westley croup severity score is frequently used to determine severity.[49] Mild croup is characterized by a barking cough, hoarseness, no stridor at rest, and absent or mild retractions. Children with moderate croup have a frequent barking cough, stridor at rest, retractions, but no significant irritability or lethargy. In addition to a frequent barking cough and stridor at rest, severe croup is characterized by marked retractions and notable distress or agitation. Table 32.5 shows a comparison of the degrees of croup severity and associated management.

The mainstay of croup management is supportive care, including antipyretics and encouragement of fluid intake. Frequently caregivers are counseled to expose the child to cold night air or

TABLE 32.4   Differentiating Common Respiratory Diseases That Can Cause Stridor or Similar Signs

Characteristic	Epiglottitis	Laryngotracheobronchitis	Diphtheria	Foreign Body
Peak age	1–5 years old	2 years old	Any age/unimmunized	Toddlers
Onset	Rapid	Acute	Gradual onset over 1–2 days	Acute symptoms or gradual onset
Common findings	Severe sore throat, fever, irritability, muffled voice, dysphagia, dyspnea, possible drooling, progressive respiratory distress; toxic appearing, tripod position or "sniffing posture"	Hoarseness with barking cough, inspiratory stridor, and possible toxic presentation; often with URI symptoms (congestion, rhinitis, coryza), possible pharyngitis, possible fever)	Membranous nasopharyngitis, obstructive laryngotracheitis with local infection presenting as pharyngitis, bloody nasal discharge, neck swelling, cervical adenitis	Coughing and/or choking episode, dyspnea, wheezing, cyanosis, signs and symptoms of secondary infection
Respiratory efforts	Marked distress	Variable distress from mild to severe	Minor to significant signs and symptoms of obstruction	Minor to significant distress
Fever	High [ranges from 101.8–104°F (38.8–40°C)]	Variable, may be low grade or high	Low grade	Normal to low grade
CBC	High, left shift	High, left shift	Normal to slight leukocytosis, decreased thrombocyte count	Normal unless secondary infection
Organism(s)	Varies, usually group A Streptococcus	Usually parainfluenza	*Corynebacterium diphtheria*	
Specific laboratory tests	None	None	Positive culture for *C. diphtheria*	None
Radiographic view with findings	Lateral of neck/thumb sign	Lateral of neck/subglottic narrowing ("Steeple sign")	Signs of obstruction in severe cases	May see radiopaque FB, localized hyperinflation, atelectasis, opacification
Treatment	Hospitalization, respiratory support cephalosporin, corticosteroids	Varies by severity; supportive care, dexamethasone, possible racemic epinephrine, supplemental oxygen	Hospitalization, erythromycin/penicillin, antitoxin	FB removal, treatment of secondary infection or bronchospasm
Intubation	Usually necessary	May be necessary	May be necessary	Endoscopy to remove FB
Prevention	Immunization—HIB	None	Immunization—DTaP	Education on child-proofing home and monitoring child

AP, Anteroposterior; *CBC*, complete blood count; *DTaP*, diphtheria-tetanus-acellular pertussis; *FB*, foreign body; *HIB*, *Haemophilus influenzae* type B; *RSV*, respiratory syncytial virus; *URI*, upper respiratory infection.

TABLE 32.5   Croup Severity and Treatment

Symptoms and Treatment	Mild	Moderate	Severe	Impending Respiratory Failure
Symptoms	Barking cough, no stridor at rest, mild or absent retractions, no agitation	Frequent barking cough, stridor at rest, tachypnea, retractions, no significant irritability or lethargy	Frequent barking cough, stridor at rest, tachypnea, marked retractions, notable distress or agitation	Audible stridor at rest Sternal retractions Lethargy Decreased level of consciousness with dusky color
Treatment				
Education of caregiver	✓	✓	✓	✓
Corticosteroid	✓	✓	✓	✓
Nebulized epinephrine		Possible	✓	✓
Supplemental oxygen		Possible	✓	Until intubation
Intubation				✓

sitting in a steamy bathroom. Though there is no evidence to support this practice,[50] it also does not cause harm and may provide a distraction for the child and provide the caregiver a sense of doing something. Antipyretics may be administered to treat fever or discomfort with advice on proper safe dosing.

Pharmacologic management of croup varies depending on severity. Bronchodilators are not indicated as they do not treat upper airway obstruction. Cough and cold medications are not recommended.

- Mild croup
  - May administer single dose of oral dexamethasone (0.15–0.6 mg/kg, maximum of 16 mg). Oral corticosteroids have been shown to reduce symptoms within 2 hours and decrease return visits to the provider or emergency department.[50]
- Children with moderate croup (stridor at rest)
  - Single dose of oral dexamethasone (0.15–0.6 mg/kg, maximum of 16 mg)
  - May be administered nebulized racemic epinephrine to reduce airway edema by vasoconstriction of subglottic mucosa. While onset is swift, children who receive racemic epinephrine need to be monitored for several hours following the treatment due to possible worsening (rebound) symptoms.
  - Ongoing monitoring with infrequent hospitalization
- Children with severe croup
  - Single dose of oral dexamethasone (0.15–0.6 mg/kg, maximum of 16 mg)
  - May be administered nebulized racemic epinephrine to reduce airway edema by vasoconstriction of subglottic mucosa
  - Emergency department care and likely admission for ongoing respiratory monitoring and intervention

Indications for Hospitalization

Children with severe respiratory distress, severe retractions, exhibiting stridor at rest, hypoxemia, or not improving with the standard treatment should be hospitalized. Increasing obstruction of the airways causes continuous stridor, nasal flaring, and suprasternal, infrasternal, and intercostal retractions. With further obstruction, air hunger and restlessness occur and are quickly followed by hypoxia, weakness, decreased air exchange, decreased stridor, increased pulse rate, and eventual death from hypoventilation. Hospitalized children may require IV hydration if they are unable to tolerate feedings.

Complications

Bacterial superinfection is the main complication of viral croup. Viral pneumonia will occasionally complicate croup cases.

Epiglottitis

Epiglottitis is an emergent, life-threatening illness characterized by rapidly progressing inflammation of the epiglottis. Sore throat and fever may precede the rapid onset of respiratory distress and toxicity. The causative organisms have changed from *H. influenza* to group A *Streptococcus, S. pneumonia, Klebsiella spp.,* and *S. aureus.*[48] Since the introduction of routine *H. Influenzae* B (HIB) vaccination, fewer cases of epiglottitis are seen in both children and adults.

Clinical Findings

History. There is an abrupt onset of fever, irritability, muffled voice, severe sore throat, dyspnea, dysphagia leading to drooling,

and increasing respiratory distress.[48] The child looks acutely ill and toxic.

Physical Examination. If epiglottitis is suspected, the examiner must take extreme care not to upset the patient, as doing so may lead to a loss of the airway. Examiners may forego a physical examination entirely to preserve the airway while arranging for emergency transport to tertiary care.

Findings include the following:
- Toxic-appearing and anxious
- Inspiratory and sometimes expiratory stridor
- Drooling, aphonia (muffled voice), and high fever
- Rapidly progressive respiratory obstruction and prostration
- Retraction of the supraclavicular, intercostal, and subcostal spaces
- Child assumes a position of hyperextension of the neck ("sniffing posture")

In older children, one may find:
- Stridor, irritability, restlessness, and brassy cough (uncommon)
- Positions self with arms back, trunk forward, neck hyperextended, and chin thrust forward (tripod position)
- A rare, unusual finding is that of just a hoarse cough and a cherry-red epiglottis

Diagnostic Studies. Diagnostic workup must occur in a tertiary care setting with emergency airway management supplies nearby. If the possibility of epiglottitis is thought to be remote in a patient with croup, a lateral neck radiograph may be obtained before the physical examination is undertaken. Absence of the "thumb" sign on the radiograph rules out the condition. A healthcare professional capable of supporting the airway and skilled in intubation must accompany the child to the radiology department and back.

Management

Airway management is essential as the time from the onset of symptoms until respiratory arrest may only be a matter of hours. Due to the risk of sudden airway obstruction, early consultation with a pediatric otolaryngologist and anesthesiologist is key. The goal of therapy is to establish an airway and start appropriate antimicrobials. Do not place the child in the supine position and immediately transport the child to the hospital via emergency medical services. The child should be examined in the operating room by a skilled provider who can perform an emergency tracheostomy. An airway must be established, either a nasotracheal airway or a tracheostomy. The diagnosis is confirmed in the operating room by depressing the tongue to view the swollen cherry-red epiglottis. An expert in establishing an airway needs to be present because there is a risk of reflex laryngospasm, with acute and complete airway obstruction.

Treatment includes the following:
- Establish an airway, preferably by nasotracheal intubation.
- Administer IV broad-spectrum antibiotics, which can include ampicillin/sulbactam, cefotaxime, ceftriaxone, or clindamycin if penicillin allergic with the addition of vancomycin if methicillin-resistant *S. aureus* is suspected.
- Administer oxygen and respiratory support.

Epiglottitis usually resolves swiftly following parenteral antibiotics and intubation. Once stabilized and extubated, antibiotic therapy usually continues for at least 10 days. If *H. influenzae* is identified as the causative agent, rifampin prophylaxis (20 mg/kg in a single dose [maximum, 600 mg] for 4 days for infants and children and 600 mg once a day for adults for 4 days) should be given to all household contacts of the patient whose household has:

- At least one child younger than 4 years who is unimmunized or incompletely immunized.
- Children less than 12 months who have not received the primary series of HIB vaccine.
- Immunocompromised children.[44]

Complications

Complications from epiglottis involve systemic spread of the causative organism and include cervical lymphadenitis, pneumonia, otitis media, or less commonly septic arthritis or meningitis.[48]

Prevention

Routine immunization is the primary means of prevention. Hand washing is also an effective method of preventing spread of infection. See prior discussion regarding rifampin prophylaxis.

Diphtheria

Diphtheria is a rare infection of the respiratory tract caused by toxigenic strains of gram-positive *C. diphtheria* or, less commonly, *Corynebacterium ulcerans*. The toxigenic strains produce two exotoxins—enzymatically active A domain and binding B domain. The binding B domain promotes entry of A into the cell. The bacterium has four biotypes (mitis, intermedius, belfanti, and gravis) that can be toxigenic or nontoxigenic. The ability of a strain of *C. diphtheria* to produce toxin is related to bacteriophage infection of the bacterium, not to colony type.

Only six cases of respiratory diphtheria were reported in the United States from 2000 to 2018 and four toxigenic cases from 2015 to 2018.[44] The bacteria can be shed for 2 to 6 weeks in an untreated patient. Disease may be mild or asymptomatic in partially or fully immunized individuals and severe if unimmunized. With toxin production, the primary infection can become lethal.

The disease is transmitted through respiratory droplets, touching the open sores of someone with diphtheria (rare) or via fomites.[44] Asymptomatic carriers can transmit the organism. The incubation period averages from 2 to 5 days with a range of 1 to 10 days.[44] The incidence of respiratory diphtheria is greater in the fall and the winter; skin infections are more common in the summer.

Clinical Findings

History. Infection is associated with a history of low-grade fever and gradual onset of symptoms over 1 to 2 days with bacterial shedding for 2 to 6 weeks if untreated. Fully immunized individuals can carry the bacteria asymptomatically and may present with a mild sore throat.

Physical Examination. Signs of primary infection include:

- A thick, grayish, adherent pseudomembrane found in either the nasopharynx, pharynx, or trachea that bleeds on removal is the hallmark of diphtheria[38]
- Bloody nasal discharge (with membranous pharyngitis) is highly suggestive of diphtheria[44]
- Sore throat, serosanguineous or seropurulent nasal discharge, hoarseness, cough
- Extensive neck swelling with cervical adenitis (bull neck) characterizes severe disease[44] and causes airway obstruction (because of membranous obstruction of the upper airway)

- Cutaneous lesions (nonhealing ulcers with dirty gray membrane or colonization of preexisting dermatoses) infected with diphtheria (seen less often)
- Possible otic and/or conjunctival infection findings

Clinical indications of toxin production include the following: myocarditis and electrocardiographic changes, respiratory compromise, cranial nerve and local neuropathies, and peripheral neuritis.

Diagnostic Studies. A confirmatory diagnosis is based on a positive culture of *C. diphtheria*. Specimens should be obtained from the nose, throat, any skin lesions, and either beneath the membrane or from a portion of the membrane. Because a special culture medium is needed, notify the lab if *C. diphtheria* is suspected. Toxigenicity tests are performed if *C. diphtheriae* is confirmed. Culture results take 8 to 48 hours; however, treatment begins when diphtheria is suspected and should not be delayed waiting for laboratory confirmation.[44] CBC results may be normal or show a slight leukocytosis and thrombocytopenia.

Differential Diagnosis

Acute streptococcal pharyngitis and infectious mononucleosis are included in the differential diagnosis of pharyngeal diphtheria. A nasal FB or purulent rhinosinusitis can resemble nasal diphtheria; epiglottitis, laryngeal diphtheria, and viral croup can also cause obstruction.

Management

Children with diphtheria require hospitalization with early tracheostomy for airway stabilization. Treatment consists of the following:

- *Antitoxin administration (hyperimmune equine antiserum):* A single dose needs to be administered if there is a high index of suspicion before a positive culture result. Allergic reaction to the serum occurs in 5% to 20%, so a scratch test should be performed before administration. IV immunoglobulin is not FDA approved for use.[44]
- *Antimicrobial therapy:* Erythromycin given orally or parenterally for 14 days, penicillin G for 14 days either IM or IV, or penicillin G procaine IM for 14 days. This is not a substitute for antitoxin administration.
- Supportive care for respiratory, cardiac, and neurologic complications as appropriate.
- Standard and droplet precautions until two cultures are negative.[44]
- Immunization after recovery because disease does not necessarily confer immunity.
- Monitoring and antimicrobial prophylaxis of contacts regardless of immunization status.
- Care for respiratory, cardiac, and neurologic complications.

Complications and Prevention

Cranial and peripheral neuropathy, myocarditis with heart block, and upper airway obstruction occur with severe disease. Universal immunization against diphtheria with regular booster injections is the only effective method of control. Infection can occur in immunized or partially immunized children; however, the disease severity is greatly diminished in these individuals. Disease generally occurs in nonimmunized children; severe life-threatening complications in this group are high. Care of a child exposed to diphtheria includes an age-appropriate booster dose of a diphtheria toxoid containing vaccine and close surveillance.

If the contact cannot be followed, penicillin G benzathine is recommended.[44]

Pertussis

Pertussis is caused by a gram-negative bacillus, *B. pertussis*, and can be a primary infection or a reinfection. The three most common types of Bordetella species causing respiratory disease are *B. parapertussis*, *Bordetella holmesii*, and *Bordetella bronchiseptica*.[43] *B. bronchiseptica* infrequently causes respiratory infection; *B. holmesii* causes bacteremia. The infection caused by *B. pertussis* is also known as whooping cough because of the high-pitched inspiratory whoop following spasms of coughing. The cough is an attempt to dislodge plugs of necrotic bronchial epithelial tissue and thick mucus followed by a whoop to draw in oxygen.

B. pertussis produces a variety of components that are highly antigenic as well as biologically active. These include pertussis toxin (PT), adenylate cyclase toxin, dermonecrotic toxin, fimbriae, filamentous hemagglutinin, pertactin, and autotransporters. Pertactin, filamentous hemagglutinin, and fimbriae allow for bacterial adhesion, whereas PT causes lymphocytosis that irritates and inflames the ciliated epithelium lining, leading to epithelial cell damage.

B. pertussis is highly contagious, and transmission occurs by respiratory aerosols and airborne droplets; patients with a cough are more likely to be vectors. Contaminated droplets are inhaled and adhere to the ciliated epithelium of the nasopharynx. The incubation period is usually 7 to 10 days but can last up to 28 days.[51] Children are most contagious during the catarrhal stage, the first stage of illness that lasts 2 weeks.[52] The usual and most common source of transmission of *B. pertussis* infection to an infant is a mother with the disease.[53] The highest incidence of mortality occurs in infants less than 6 months old.[51]

While the acellular vaccines are safer and more efficacious than older whole cell diphtheria, tetanus, and pertussis vaccine, there has been a steady increase in pertussis rates with outbreaks occurring across the United States and the globe. Before vaccination, there were an estimated 270,000 annual cases with 10,000 deaths in the United States. In 2002 a sharp increase began with intermittent spikes in rates not seen since prevaccination.[54] Factors attributed to the increase include a shift in pertussis epidemiology, lower immunization rates, waning immunity of the acellular vaccine, lack of healthcare providers' knowledge of the clinical presentation of the disease, and changes in *B. pertussis* bacteria along with spread of other species of *Bordetella*.[55]

Clinical Findings

The clinical presentation of the disease depends on the length of time from the last vaccination (if vaccinated), age and sex of the child, the infectious species of pertussis (*B. pertussis* is more severe than *B. parapertussis*), and the amount of infectious load. The range of symptoms in children varies from an asymptomatic infection to upper respiratory tract disease to severe, progressive coughing that can last for months. There are three consecutive stages of pertussis—catarrhal, paroxysmal, and convalescent—each lasting 1 to 3 weeks without complete recovery for 2 to 3 months. Table 32.6 shows the stages of pertussis with accompanying symptoms.

In infants, particularly neonates, the clinical presentation is generally severe, and includes:
- Apnea (common) often with seizures caused by hypoxemia; tachypnea
- Cough without an inspiratory whoop; poor feeding
- Leukocytosis with a marked lymphocytosis (in the presence of illness marked by persistent cough points to *B. pertussis*)

Reinfections are common as disease immunity does not provide long-lasting protection. Coinfection with other respiratory pathogens including RSV, parainfluenza virus, *M. pneumoniae*, adenovirus, and influenza occurs.[51]

Diagnostic Studies. PCR is the primary diagnostic test used in most commercial and state laboratories for confirmation. Starting in the mid-1990s, pertussis diagnostic test options included culture, serology, direct fluorescent antibody testing, and PCR. Previously, culture was considered the gold standard, but the use of PCR has increased. Nasopharyngeal collection is done with a Dacron or calcium alginate fiber-tipped swab inserted into the nasal passage and advanced to the nasopharynx then immediately placed into a special transport medium. Culture can be negative

TABLE 32.6	Stages of Pertussis	
Stage of Pertussis	Length of Time	Manifestation
Catarrhal	2–3 wk	**Infant and child** Upper respiratory infection symptoms with mild progressive dry cough Low-grade fever (to 101°F [38.3°C]) Cough worsens as child progresses to paroxysmal stage
Paroxysmal	2–4 wk	Intense and violent coughing with 5–10 coughs with an inspiratory whoop. Cough can lead to eye proptosis and tearing, thick mucus production, and salivation Cyanosis, sweating, prostration, and exhaustion after coughing Sleep disturbed but fever absent or minimal **Adolescents** Classic paroxysm of coughing missing in up to one-third of patients Clinicians should consider pertussis if a persistent cough beyond 3 weeks
Convalescent	3 wk–6 mo	Symptoms wane over a variable period that can last months Waning of paroxysmal coughing episodes but nonparoxysmal cough can last up to 6 weeks with coughing paroxysm occurring when child gets another viral infection

Data from Kilore P, Salim A, Zervos M, et al. Pertussis: microbiology, disease, treatment and prevention. *Clin Microbiology Rev.* 2016;29(3):449–481.

if the person had been ill for 2 weeks or more, was previously vaccinated, or if antibiotics were started.[44] Bacteria are found in high number in the airways early in infection but decrease markedly in the paroxysmal stage.

PCR testing provides faster results and earlier treatment, allowing public health officials to identify pertussis cluster cases and encourage faster response to outbreaks. The test incorporates a parapertussis-specific molecular target, decreasing the false positive rate. They require a nasopharyngeal culture and must be done within 3 weeks of the cough onset. PCR testing is increasingly popular due to its improved sensitivity (70–99%) and specificity (86–100%).

The CDC and the FDA developed serologic tests that can be done up to 12 weeks after the onset of symptoms; however, the optimal time for testing is from 2 weeks to 8 weeks. This testing has utility in identifying outbreaks.

A CBC is nonspecific with leukocytosis and lymphocytosis common findings in infants and young children but rare in adolescents. A chest radiograph may be normal or have nonspecific findings such as atelectasis, peribronchial cuffing, or perihilar infiltrates.

Differential Diagnosis

Numerous infectious diseases can present with a cough including RSV, *B. parapertussis*, adenoviruses, bocaviruses, human metapneumovirus, influenza A and B, parainfluenza, and rhinovirus. Noninfectious disease triggers of coughs include gastroesophageal reflux, CF, sinusitis, aspiration pneumonia, and asthma. FBs should be included in the differential diagnosis.

Management

Treatment:
- Antibiotic treatment should be started within 6 weeks of disease onset in infants and in children and adults within 21 days. The macrolide class of drugs including azithromycin, clarithromycin, and erythromycin is recommended for all ages. However, there is an association between the development of pyloric stenosis and erythromycin in infants younger than 1 month.[44]
  - Azithromycin: The drug of choice for infants less than 1 month at 10 mg/kg in a single dose for 5 days. This same dose is used from 1 to 5 months.
  - Azithromycin: For infants 6 months and older, children, and adolescents, a 5-day treatment course is also recommended but the first day only, a single dose of 10 mg/kg/day (maximum dose of 500 mg) is given, then a single dose of 5 mg/kg/day (maximum dose of 250 mg) on days 2 to 5.
  - Clarithromycin: For infants over 1 month, children, and adolescents, 15 mg/kg/day divided every 12 hours for 7 days with a maximum dose of 1 g/day.
  - Erythromycin: For infants over 1 month to 5 months, 10 mg/kg/dose, 4 times a day for 14 days; >6 months and children, 10 mg/kg/dose, 4 times a day for 7 to 14 days, maximum daily dose 2 g/day; adolescents 500 mg 4 times a day for 7 to 14 days.
  - Sulfamethoxazole (SMX) and trimethoprim (TMP): Can be used as an alternative in infants older than 2 months who cannot tolerate macrolides; dose at TMP 8 mg/kg/day and SMX 40 mg/kg/day in divided doses every 12 hours for 14 days (maximum single dose 160 mg TMP).

- The use of corticosteroids or albuterol and other β2-adrenergic medications are not supported by controlled, prospective studies.[56]

Care of Exposed Children

Postexposure prophylaxis with a macrolide is recommended for household and close contacts irrespective of immunization status. Close contact includes household members, caretakers, healthcare workers, and any person who was within 3 to 4 feet of a symptomatic person, shared a closed space for 1 hour or more, or had direct contact with secretions of the nasal, oral, or respiratory tract. Early prophylaxis limits secondary transmission as untreated infants can have a positive nasopharyngeal culture 6 weeks after the start of illness; other persons can shed the bacteria for 3 to 4 weeks. The value of chemoprophylaxis is limited after 21 days but should be considered in high-risk household contacts (young infant, pregnant woman, or person who is in contact with infants)[44]:
- Immunization coverage with diphtheria-tetanus-acellular pertussis (DTaP) or Tdap depending on age group needs to be reviewed and appropriate acellular pertussis vaccine given.
- Students and staff in schools need to be monitored for any respiratory symptoms with exclusion and evaluation for anyone with a cough illness.
- Close monitoring of respiratory symptoms for 21 days after last contact with an infected individual.

Complications

Infants younger than 4 months have the highest rates of fatal pertussis, and infants younger than 2 months have the highest rates of hospitalizations.[39] Other complications include apnea, secondary pneumonia, convulsions, insomnia, sinusitis, otitis media, syncope, rib fracture, and weight loss.[43]

Prevention

The concept of "cocooning" around the infant is designed to protect infants from dangerous or unwanted environmental hazards.[57] Cocooning recommendations include targeted immunization strategies to immunize adults around the infant, including caretakers, grandparents over 65 years old, fathers, and mothers who were not immunized in the last trimester. In addition, all adolescents 11 to 18 years old should receive the Tdap vaccine.

In addition, the recommended guidelines for the initial series of DTaP vaccines and booster doses should be followed. Just one DTaP immunization can reduce the severity of symptoms in an infant infected with pertussis. The clinician needs to be mindful of valid contraindications to receiving pertussis vaccine. Immunity following either natural pertussis infection or illness or vaccination is not long lasting. Due to the wide range of clinical presentations in children, adolescents, and adults, persons who are either asymptomatic or think it is "just a cold" can transmit the infection to an unimmunized infant resulting in life-threatening illness. Universal immunization of children and adolescents is crucial to pertussis control.

Upper Airway: Noninfectious Conditions

Nasal Foreign Body

Young children tend to insert all types of FBs into body orifices. Objects can be noted immediately by the caregiver or lie undetected until classic symptoms appear. Jewelry beads are the most common reported FB in North America.[58]

Clinical Findings

History. A persistent or recurrent unilateral purulent nasal discharge is reported. Foul odor, epistaxis, nasal obstruction, and mouth breathing are less commonly reported symptoms. Young children often deny inserting an FB.

Physical Examination. The classic symptom of a nasal FB is unilateral, purulent, foul-smelling nasal discharge. If the FB is embedded in granulation tissue or mucosa, it may take on the appearance of a nasal mass. Other symptoms include mouth breathing, epistaxis, and nasal obstruction.

Differential Diagnosis

Nasal polyps, purulent rhinitis, adenoiditis, rhinosinusitis, and nasal tumors are conditions that cause bilateral or unilateral discharge. Two rare conditions to consider are juvenile nasopharyngeal adenofibroma and hereditary hemorrhagic telangiectasia.[59]

Management

Management involves the following:

- Properly restrain the child to avoid movement during examination. Use a head light or overhead light when possible to free provider's hands for examination.
- Elevate the child's head and suction out blood and secretions.
- Detection of an FB in the nasal cavity establishes the diagnosis.
- Removal of the nasal FB depends on its location, its composition, and the skill of the practitioner. A curette, alligator forceps, suction with narrow tips, and cotton-tipped applicators with collodion with or without topical vasoconstrictor drugs (to reduce swelling) can be used. If the object is small and 5-French catheter with a balloon can be advanced past the FB, the balloon can be inflated and gently withdrawn with the object. A Katz Extractor can be used to remove otorhino FBs.
- Otolaryngology referral is merited for young children who cannot cooperate or when the FB is extremely difficult or dangerous to remove, such as paper clips or staples. On a cautionary note, an FB can be forced deeper into the nose if the practitioner is inexperienced at nasal FB removal.

Foreign Body Aspiration

The symptoms and physical findings associated with aspiration of an FB depend on the nature of the material aspirated, plus the location and degree of the obstruction. The cough reflex protects the lower airways, and most aspirated material is immediately expelled with coughing. Onset of a sudden episode of coughing without a prodrome or signs of respiratory infection should make the provider suspicious of FB aspiration.

Objects that are either too large to be eliminated by the mucociliary system or cannot be expelled by coughing eventually lead to some form of respiratory symptomatology. An especially large FB occluding the upper airway can cause suffocation. A small object in the lower respiratory tree may not produce symptoms for days to weeks. Obstruction results from either the FB itself or secondary edema. Hot dogs are one of the most common causes of fatal aspiration. Other foods associated with choking are meats, sausages, fish with bones, popcorn, pretzel nuggets, candy (hard or sticky), whole grapes, raw vegetables (peas, carrots, celery), fruits with skins, nuts, seeds, cheese cubes, ice cubes, and peanut butter (spoonful or with soft bread). Examples of household items and toys that pose a choking risk to young children include latex balloons, coins, marbles, toys with small parts, small balls, pen or marker caps, button-type batteries, screws, rings, earrings, crayons, erasers, safety pins, small stones, and tiny figures. Although toddlers commonly aspirate FBs, aspiration occurs in children of all ages.

Most FB aspirations occur under the age 4 years with a peak incidence in toddlers between 1 and 2 years of age. In 50% of cases, there is no history of choking. In laryngeal FB aspiration, there is a rapid onset of hoarseness and the development of a chronic croupy cough with aphonia. Suspect an FB aspiration in children with sudden episode of cough, unilateral wheezing, and/or recurrent pneumonia. The child with an FB lodged in the trachea presents with a history of a brassy cough, hoarseness, dyspnea, and possibly cyanosis. The most characteristic signs of tracheal FB aspiration are the homophonic wheeze and the audible slap and palpable thud sound produced by the momentary expiratory effect of the FB at the subglottic level.

Occasionally, the FB is lodged in the bronchus or lung. Most objects are aspirated into the right lung. A careful health history may reveal a forgotten episode of choking.

Clinical Findings

History. There may or may not be a history of an initial episode of coughing, gagging, and choking. Blood-streaked sputum may be expectorated, but hemoptysis rarely occurs as an early symptom. On rare occasions, hemoptysis does occur as an initial symptom months or years after the aspiration event took place.

Physical Examination. Children with an upper airway FB present with cough, stridor, or in respiratory or cardiorespiratory arrest. If the FB goes into the lower airway they develop cough, wheezing, retractions, and have decreased breath sounds.[60] Initial clinical findings are similar in either tracheal or laryngeal FB aspiration. If the object is nonobstructive and nonirritating, few or no initial symptoms may be seen. The child may have limited chest expansion, decreased vocal fremitus, atelectasis, or emphysema-like changes with resulting hyporesonance or hyperresonance. Diminished breath sounds are often found. A small object can act as a bypass valve, and homophonic wheezes can be heard. Crackles, rhonchi, and wheezes can be present if air movement is adequate. If the acute episode is missed or not appreciated, a latent period of mild "wheezing" or cough may be evident.

Diagnostic Studies. Neck and chest radiographs in posteroanterior and lateral views should be ordered. Only radiopaque FBs are seen, but secondary signs include hyperinflation, atelectasis, or opacification of the distal lung (Fig. 32.1). Virtual bronchoscopy (CT), as well as flexible bronchoscopy, can provide a noninvasive way to diagnose an FB. If the FB cannot be removed, then a flexible bronchoscopy is done, sometimes it may be possible to remove with a foley catheter or magnet tube.[61]

Management

As noted, the history may not be positive. Therefore if a child has symptoms of an FB, a referral to a pulmonary specialist is needed. If the object is removed via bronchoscopy before permanent damage occurs, recovery is usually complete. Secondary lung infections and bronchospasms should be treated as suggested in the section on management of pneumonia in this chapter and asthma in Chapter 36.

Complications

If the FB is vegetable matter, vegetal or arachidic, bronchitis can occur. Characteristics of this severe condition can include sepsis-like fever, dyspnea, and cough. If the material has been present

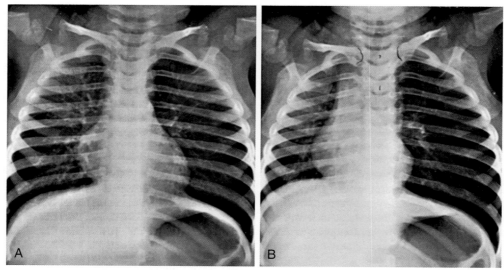

• **Fig 32.1** Foreign Body Aspiration. (A) Normal inspiratory chest radiograph in a toddler with a peanut fragment in the left main bronchus. (B) Expiratory radiograph of the same child showing the classic obstructive emphysema (air trapping) on the involved *(left)* side. Air leaves the normal right side, allowing the lung to deflate. The medium shifts toward the unobstructed side. (From Hammer AR, Schroeder JW. Foreign bodies of the airway. In: Kliegman RM, St. Geme JW, Blum NJ, et al., eds. *Nelson Textbook of Pediatrics.* 21st ed. Elsevier; 2020.)

for a long time, suppuration can occur. Lobar pneumonia, intractable wheezing, and status asthmaticus can develop. Atelectasis or emphysema, a rare occurrence, can also occur as the result of a large obstruction caused by a bronchial FB.

Prevention

Anticipatory education regarding prevention of FB aspiration should be part of well-child supervision guidance. Caregivers should be cautioned about high-risk foods (e.g., whole carrots, nuts, popcorn, and hot dogs). Young children need to be supervised closely as they put small objects into their mouths as well as when they cry, shout, run, and play with food or other objects in their mouths.

Recurrent Epistaxis

Recurrent epistaxis is common in children, with an incidence of 30% in children from birth to 5 years old and over 50% in children by age 10 years and accounts for 1 in 260 emergency department visits each year.[62,63] While it is classified into anterior and posterior epistaxis, anterior bleeding is far more common in children. Only 10% of epistaxis episodes originate in the posterior area, which are more likely to be arterial bleeds. Primary epistaxis represents about 85% of the cases.[62] Recurrent epistaxis is defined as five or more episodes per year and occurs in approximately 9% of children. Although up to 90% of these cases are self-limiting and spontaneously resolve, epistaxis can cause significant psychologic distress and negatively impact quality of life for families.[63]

Etiologies include medication and local, systemic, environmental, and idiopathic factors. A recent study found that pediatric epistaxis incidence was highest in the spring and summer months.[64] Local factors that can cause mucosal irritation resulting in bleeding include nasal trauma, allergies, septal abnormalities, neoplasia, juvenile nasopharyngeal angiofibroma in an adolescent, and inflammation. However, in children, local trauma is commonly due to digital trauma or irritation. Systemic causes include

coagulopathies, allergies, polyps, hemangiomas, FB, and viral or bacterial infections of nasal tissue. Known environmental risk factors are living in dry climates or dryness from artificial heat during winter months. Use of medications such as nonsteroidal antiinflammatory drugs (NSAIDs), anticoagulants, chronic use of topical nasal sprays containing corticosteroids or antihistamine decongestants, and topical cocaine abuse can all lead to epistaxis.

The bleeding originates from the anterior portion of the nasal septum called Little's area where Kiesselbach plexus meets under the thin nasal mucosa. The blood supply of the Kiesselbach area comes from branches of the internal carotid, which break up into the facial and internal maxillary arteries, which supply most of the face. Two of the six branches of the internal maxillary artery, the palatine, and sphenopalatine arteries, provide 80% of the blood supply with an additional 20% coming from the facial artery.[63] A coagulopathy, generally von Willebrand disease or platelet aggregation disorders, can manifest as recurrent epistaxis; a careful history will reveal hallmark clinical signs of mucocutaneous bleeding beyond epistaxis that includes easy bruising, menorrhagia, and GI bleeding.[64]

Clinical Findings

History. The following may be reported:
- Recent nasal trauma, including nose-picking
- Allergies; frequent rhinosinusitis, or a recent URI
- Unexpected bruising or bleeding from other sites; frequent nosebleeds (unilateral or bilateral).
- Tarry stools (the result of swallowed blood)

The provider should always ask about a family history of excessive bleeding episodes or bleeding disorders. Oral anticoagulants and topical nasal medication use, including topical steroid spray, nasal decongestants, or in the case of the teen, cocaine or other inhaled recreational drugs should be explored.

Physical Examination. Nares visualization using the otoscope without a tip may reveal fresh or old clots, nasal masses, FB, polyps, and/or raw, red Little's area. The nasal mucosa on the medial surface of the anterior septum may be dry, cracked, excoriated, or scabbed. It is important to evaluate Little's area in children. Signs of nasal allergy including allergic shiners, Dennie-Morgan lines, adenoidal facies, and pale boggy mucosa should be assessed.

Diagnostic Studies. A baseline hematocrit may be indicated in severe or chronic epistaxis. It can reveal anemia secondary to the bleeding. Unless the history points to a coagulopathy or the nosebleeds are recurrent and refractory to treatment, coagulation studies are not indicated.[63] If coagulopathy is suspected, order a CBC, platelet count, prothrombin time, and activated partial thromboplastin time (aPTT). If the labs are normal but the diagnosis is strongly suspected, further workup for von Willebrand disease is needed.

Differential Diagnosis

Differential diagnoses as to causes of epistaxis include tumors, juvenile nasopharyngeal angiofibroma, long-standing nasal FB, congenital bleeding disorders, idiopathic thrombocytopenia purpura (ITP), vasculitis, nasal hemangioma, hereditary hemorrhagic telangiectasia, and allergic rhinitis. A bleeding disorder is characterized by epistaxis that is severe, prolonged, and recurrent. Nonaccidental injury or coagulopathy should be considered in children younger than 2 years with spontaneous epistaxis. If epistaxis is associated with a traumatic injury, evaluate for the presence of a nasal fracture or septal hematoma. A nasal neoplasm may present with facial swelling, pain, nasal obstruction, Eustachian tube dysfunction with effusion, and cranial neuropathies with severe epistaxis. Granulomatosis with polyangiitis, a small vessel vasculitis, can present in adolescents with nasal bleeding.[63]

Management

Studies are lacking regarding the optimal management for epistaxis; however, nasal mucosal hydration techniques were found to be effective in the management of pediatric patients. Nasal cautery is a useful adjuvant for those who do not respond to the following recommended measures[63]:

- Have the child sit upright and lean forward to prevent swallowing the blood.
- Apply direct, sustained pressure at the nasal ala (pinch the nares together at the bony structure) for 5 minutes (watch the time, because perceptions of time are subjective).
- Packing and topical vasoconstrictor drugs are occasionally needed.
- Use a bedside cool-mist humidifier to moisten the air in dry climates or in winter with forced-air heating. NS nose sprays can add moisture to dry nasal mucosa.
- Apply topical antibiotic to the site of the septal scab for 2 weeks to reduce nasal colonization with *S. aureus* crusting and inflammation.
- Topical agents such as BleedCease, WoundSeal, or NasalCease are hydrophilic polymers that form an artificial scab when in contact with blood. These can be applied via a swab to the Kiesselbach's plexus area. Local applications of a solution of oxymetazoline or Neo-Synephrine (0.25% to 1%) can also be used.
- Silver nitrate sticks can be used to cauterize exposed vessels if bleeding persists; however, the site must be easily accessible, visible, and not bleeding briskly. Silver nitrate has a high failure rate and is associated with nasal septum atrophy.
- Nasal packing with absorbable oxycellulose material can be used if bleeding continues or the site cannot be localized; the

child should be referred to an ear, nose, and throat specialist for further evaluation and management.
- Treat the underlying cause of the problem (e.g., trauma from nose-picking, dry air, and/or topical nasal sprays).
- Teach caregivers to leave blood scabs alone because removal may precipitate further bleeding.

Prevention

Preventive measures include instructions on an effective nasal regimen (humidifier use and NS nose drops or sprays) to keep the nasal mucosa moist. Emollient application (saline gel, petroleum jelly, or antibiotic ointment) can be comforting but are not statistically associated with improved outcomes to decrease recurrence. If nasal corticosteroids are used, make sure that the child directs the spray laterally rather than toward the septum. This reduces epistaxis associated with nasal spray.[63]

Lower Airway and Parenchymal Conditions: Acute Conditions

Bronchitis

Bronchiolitis is the most common respiratory infection in children under 2 years and a leading cause of hospitalizations.[65] Bronchiolitis is characterized by a URI prodrome, including congestion, rhinitis, cough, and coryza. Following 1 to 3 days of URI symptoms, coughing worsens, respiratory distress and wheezing develop, sometimes with feeding disruption and/or fever. In severe cases, cyanosis, air hunger, severe respiratory distress and apnea may occur. For most children, bronchiolitis is a self-limited condition, though complete resolution may take 2 to 3 weeks. Risk factors for severe bronchiolitis include prematurity, low birth weight, under 12 weeks of age, chronic pulmonary disease, anatomic airway defects, hemodynamically significant congenital heart disease, immunodeficiency, and neurologic disease.

Approximately 80% of bronchiolitis cases are caused by RSV.[67] Other causes include rhinovirus, parainfluenza, human metapneumovirus, influenza, adenovirus, coronavirus, parainfluenza, and others. Seasonality tends to follow other respiratory illnesses, primarily occurring within autumn and winter months, though bronchiolitis occurs year-round. The most frequent mode of transmission is large droplet or self-inoculation.[66]

The pathophysiology in bronchiolitis begins with infection of the epithelial cells lining the respiratory mucosa. This infection causes bronchiolar inflammation and copious mucus production, which narrow the bronchioles and obstruct airflow. In addition, in RSV, the virus binds to bronchiolar epithelial cells and replicates, causing necrosis and ciliary dysfunction. Necrotic cellular tissue is sloughed during inhalation, with airflow carrying it into the alveolus. Exhalation lodges the debris within the alveolus, trapping air and leading to hyperinflation, ventilation/perfusion mismatch, and atelectasis.

Clinical Findings

History. The following are reported:
- Initial presentation: 1 to 3 days of URI symptoms including congestion, rhinitis, cough, coryza, and rhinorrhea
- Gradual development of worsening cough, wheezing, respiratory distress, accessory muscle use, and possible grunting, flaring, and retracting
- Low-grade to moderate fever ≤101°F (38.3°C)
- Feeding disruption

- No prodrome in some infants; rather they have apnea as the initial symptom
- Symptoms tend to peak around 3 to 5 days of illness
- Consider a secondary bacterial infection for persistent or high fever

Physical Examination. Findings include the following:
- Fussiness, irritability is common; lethargy or inconsolability are ominous signs
- Upper respiratory findings of congestion, rhinitis, coryza
- Lower respiratory findings of:
  - Tachypnea (approximately 40–80 breaths/min)
  - Substernal and/or intercostal retractions
  - Diffuse expiratory wheezing
  - Fine or coarse crackles may be heard throughout the breathing cycle
  - Varying signs of respiratory distress and pulmonary involvement (e.g., nasal flaring, grunting, retractions, cyanosis, prolonged exhalation)

Diagnostic Studies. Bronchiolitis is considered a clinical diagnosis as it is based upon history and physical examination. Chest radiographs are not routinely indicated unless there is concern for airway complication or need for admission to the intensive care unit. Hematologic testing is not recommended.[68] If a CBC is done for another reason, a mild leukocytosis may be seen with 12,000 to 16,000/mm^3. Likewise, routine virologic testing is not indicated as it does not change the management of most children with bronchiolitis. Exceptions to laboratory testing may include during hospitalization if a child will be cohorted or if quarantining will be recommended, such as with the recent COVID-19 pandemic.

Differential Diagnosis

The differential diagnosis includes asthma, pneumonia, FB aspiration, congestive heart failure among others. The best distinction between bronchiolitis and asthma is history, particularly any previous wheezing illnesses. Bacterial pneumonia presents with asymmetric breath sounds whereas bronchiolitis does not. Viral pneumonia and bronchiolitis are very difficult to distinguish, though largely are managed the same. FB aspiration is usually found in a toddler with a history of choking who then develops focal areas of wheezing. Although children with congestive heart failure can wheeze, they also show symptoms of sweating and signs of failure to thrive with a murmur and an S4 gallop rhythm.

Management

Management of bronchiolitis is largely dependent upon severity of the disease. Children with mild bronchiolitis generally are without tachypnea, have mild or no retractions, do not require supplemental oxygen, and are nontoxic. Moderate bronchiolitis is characterized by tachypnea, intercostal retractions, a need for supplemental oxygen, and a fussy or anxious disposition. Severe bronchiolitis is characterized by marked tachypnea, significant respiratory distress (i.e., nasal flaring, head bobbing, substernal or subcostal retractions), lethargy or inconsolability, and the need for supplemental oxygen, and lethargy. Children with mild bronchiolitis and no risk factors may be managed outpatient with supportive care. Children with moderate bronchiolitis, risk factors or dehydration should be managed in an urgent care or emergency department where repeated assessment is available. Those with severe bronchiolitis, O$_2$ requirement, apnea, dehydration, are under 12 weeks, or have a family unable to care for them require hospitalization.

The mainstay of outpatient bronchiolitis management is supportive care, including monitoring hydration status, nasal aspiration, and fever management. There is no evidence showing benefit from bronchodilators, racemic epinephrine, or systemic corticosteroids; for this reason, the AAP guidelines recommend against their use.[69,70] In addition, antibiotics are not indicated given the viral etiology of bronchiolitis unless a secondary bacterial infection is present, such as acute otitis media or urinary tract infection.

Recommended education for caregivers of infants and children at home:
- The management of rhinitis (use of saline drops and suctioning of nares)
- Indications for the use of antipyretics
- Signs of increasing respiratory distress or dehydration (seek immediate care)
- Guidelines for feeding an infant with signs of mild respiratory distress (amount of fluid needed per 24 hours; smaller, more frequent feedings; monitoring of the respiratory rate; and guarding against vomiting)
- Monitoring for wet diapers as an indicator of hydration
- Education that infants and children with bronchiolitis may cough for 2 to 3 weeks

Inpatient management of bronchiolitis includes supportive care. In addition, humidified supplemental oxygen and intravenous or nasogastric hydration, as clinically indicated. Hypertonic saline may be trialed, but chest physiotherapy is contraindicated.

Complications

Complications of bronchiolitis include apnea, respiratory failure, aspiration, and secondary bacterial infections. Prolonged apnea, uncompensated respiratory acidosis, and profound dehydration secondary to loss of water from tachypnea and an inability to drink are the factors leading to death in young infants with bronchiolitis. Early life bronchiolitis is considered a risk factor for subsequent wheezing and asthma by age 5 years.[71] The relationship between bronchiolitis and asthma is not well understood, though there is an association.

Prevention

Universal prevention includes hand hygiene, covering coughs and sneezes, cleaning surfaces, and avoiding close contact with others that are ill. Educate caregivers about decreasing exposure to and transmission of RSV, especially those with high-risk infants. Advice may include limiting exposure to childcare centers whenever possible; use of alcohol-based hand sanitizers or hand washing, if hand sanitizer is not available; avoiding tobacco smoke exposure; and scheduling RSV prophylaxis, if eligible. RSV prophylaxis, palivizumab (Synagis), is an RSV-specific monoclonal antibody that disrupts the replication of RSV, thus providing immunoprophylaxis for high-risk infants. Palivizumab is administered IM monthly for 5 months during respiratory season. Given the high cost, there are strict eligibility criteria that align with some of the risk factors for severe disease (refer to most recent guidelines to determine eligibility). While prophylaxis may not prevent RSV infection, it has been shown to decrease rates of hospitalization (see Chapter 35). In 2022, the FDA recommended the RSV vaccine for pregnant women to protect newborns through active immunization. Such a vaccine represents a promising approach to RSV prevention for infants.[72]

Pneumonia

Pneumonia is a lower respiratory tract infection within the parenchyma. Pneumonia acquired outside of the hospital setting is referred to as community-acquired pneumonia (CAP) whereas pneumonia acquired within the hospital may be referred to as hospital-acquired or nosocomial pneumonia. CAP is one of the leading causes of pediatric hospitalization, particularly among children under 2 years.[73] Risk factors for pneumonia include cardiopulmonary dysfunction (i.e., congenital heart disease, BPD, asthma, cystic fibrosis); disorders that may impact respiration, such as neuromuscular disorders and some GI conditions (i.e., tracheoesophageal fistula, gastroesophageal reflux); immunocompromised status; history of recurrent or severe pneumonia; and exposure to environmental smoke.

The pathophysiology of pneumonia typically begins with a viral upper respiratory tract infection that causes impairments in pulmonary defenses by altering normal secretions, inhibiting phagocytosis, modifying the normal bacterial flora, and disrupting mucociliary clearance. These impairments in host defenses create opportunity for viral or bacterial lower respiratory tract infections to develop. The subsequent immune response to the infection causes inflammation and accumulation of fluid, and white blood cells and cellular debris within the airways. In turn, small airways obstruct, alveoli collapse or fill with fluid, disrupting ventilation and perfusion. Most CAP cases in childhood are caused by infection, though pneumonia may also be caused by aspiration, hypersensitivity reactions, or other adverse reactions.[74] Historically, childhood pneumonia was primarily caused by bacterial infections. After introduction of routine childhood pneumococcal and HIB vaccines, viruses emerged as the cause of over 70% of the cases of childhood pneumonia.[73]

Pneumonia is typically classified as viral, typical bacterial, or atypical bacterial. Clinical onset and presentation may give clues to the type of pneumonia, though there is overlap in presentations and the actual cause of a pneumonia may go unknown.[73] Age influences clinical manifestations of pneumonia and differing infectious agents cause varied presentations and symptoms. Table 32.7 differentiates the various forms of pneumonia commonly found in infants, children, and adolescents. Table 32.8 shows the most common infecting organisms associated with CAP by age. Treatment is often empirical and varies with age.

Clinical Findings

The classic presentation of pneumonia includes tachypnea, cough, fever, and respiratory distress,[75] though presentations often vary. For example, neonates and young infants may have an absent cough. Clinical presentation may vary by type of pneumonia as well. Viral pneumonia tends to have an insidious onset with a URI prodrome and gradual worsening of cough. Associated symptoms often include low-grade fever and diffuse crackles and wheezing.[74] In contrast, typical bacterial pneumonia may also have a URI prodrome, but then an abrupt onset of high fever, chest pain, and possible toxicity. Typical bacterial pneumonia often has focal auscultatory findings including decreased breath sounds and crackles. Children may also experience referred symptoms, such as abdominal or shoulder pain. Atypical bacterial pneumonia usually has an abrupt onset with fever, malaise, and worsening nonproductive cough that can last weeks.[76] Auscultatory findings may include diffuse crackles or wheezes.

History. The following may be reported[73]:
In infants:
- Slower onset of respiratory symptoms, cough, wheezing, or stridor with low-grade fever suggests viral pneumonia.
- Determine mother's HIV status or infant's exposure to tuberculosis.

In children and adolescents:
- Obtain immunization history and travel history of the family.
- Assess for tuberculosis exposure, risk, history; history of vaccination against tuberculosis.
- Evaluate for sick contacts at home and possible FB aspiration.
- Initial history of a mild URI for a few days—similar for both bacterial and viral.
- Abrupt high fever with temperatures greater than 103.3°F (39.6°C), chest pain, lethargy, and dyspnea suggest bacterial pneumonia.

TABLE 32.7 Differentiating Various Forms of Pneumonia in Infants, Young Children, and Adolescents

Characteristic	Viral	Typical Bacterial	Atypical Bacterial
Common age	All ages	All ages	>5 years
Onset	Acute; gradual	Acute; abrupt	Abrupt
Clinical findings	Depends on age; URI prodrome, gradual worsening of cough, generalized crackles, wheezing	Depends on age; URI prodrome, cough, tachypnea, crackles, focal decreased breath sounds, retractions, chest pain; potential toxicity, progression to severe respiratory distress	Malaise, worsening nonproductive cough, diffuse crackles or wheezes
Fever	Present (usually low-grade)	Acute onset of fever (≥102.2°F [≥39°C])	>102.2°F (>39°C)
CBC	Normal or slight elevation of WBC	WBCs often elevated >15,000/μL	Normal
Most common organism	RSV, parainfluenza, influenza	*Streptococcus pneumoniae*	*Mycoplasma pneumonia*
Radiographic findings	Transient lobar infiltrates	Lobar consolidation	Varies, interstitial infiltrates
Treatment	Supportive care	Depends on bacteria and child's age; amoxicillin is first line	Azithromycin is first-line therapy; erythromycin; clarithromycin

CBC, Complete blood count; *RSV*, respiratory syncytial virus; *URI*, upper respiratory infection; *WBC*, white blood cell.

TABLE 32.8	Age Variants in Community-Acquired Pneumonia Microorganisms		
Age	**Viral Organisms**	**Typical Bacterial Organisms**	**Atypical Bacterial Organisms**
Infants	Respiratory syncytial virus (RSV) Parainfluenza Influenza Adenoviruses Metapneumovirus	*Streptococcus pneumoniae* *Staphylococcus aureus* *Haemophilus influenzae* *Mycoplasma pneumonia* *Mycobacterium tuberculosis* *Bordetella pertussis* *Pneumocystis jirovecii*	*Chlamydia trachomatis*
Preschool children	RSV Parainfluenza Influenza Adenoviruses Enterovirus Rhinovirus Coronavirus Metapneumovirus	*S. pneumoniae* *H. influenzae* *Streptococcus pyogenes* *S. aureus*	*M. tuberculosis* *Chlamydophila pneumoniae*
School-age children	Respiratory viruses as earlier	*S. pneumoniae* *S. aureus* *S. pyogenes*	*M. pneumoniae* *C. pneumoniae*
Adolescents	Respiratory viruses as earlier	*S. pneumoniae* *M. tuberculosis*	*M. pneumonia* *C. pneumonia*

Modified from Waseem M. Pediatric pneumonia. Medscape. https://emedicine.medscape.com/article/967822-overview#a4

- Other manifestations include restlessness, chills, apprehension, shortness of breath, malaise, and pleuritic chest pain.

Physical Examination. Closely observe the child's general appearance, noting their work of breathing, assessing for hypoxia, and evaluating tachypnea, which is the most valuable sign for ruling out pneumonia. To incentivize younger children to breathe deeply, ask them to blow a pinwheel or crumpled examination paper off your hands.

Common findings seen in all types of pneumonia include:
- Tachypnea (may be the only symptom), generally more than 60 breaths/min in infants younger than 2 months, more than 50 breaths/min in children 2 to 11 months, or more than 40 breaths/min at rest in children 1 to 5 years.
- Respiratory distress: retractions, with more severe distress (nasal flaring, grunting) less often
- Tachycardia, air hunger, and cyanosis are ominous findings
- Fine crackles, dullness, diminished breath sounds
Additional findings associated with typical bacterial pneumonia:
- Fever and hypoxia
- Splinting the affected side to minimize pleuritic pain or lying on the side in a fetal position helps compensate for decreased air exchange and improves ventilation.
- Circumoral cyanosis
- Signs of pleural effusion and signs of congestive heart failure
- Abdominal distention, downward displacement of the liver or spleen
- Progression to delirium and posturing
In viral pneumonia:
- Wheezing
- Low-grade fever
- Downward displacement of the liver or spleen
In atypical bacterial pneumonia:
- Fever

- Nonproductive cough
- Diffuse crackles or wheezes
- Repetitive, staccato cough with tachypnea, cervical adenopathy, crackles, and rarely wheezing (*C. trachomatis*)

Diagnostic Studies. A chest radiograph should not be routinely performed in children with pneumonia. If the primary care provider (PCP) has difficulty distinguishing pneumonia from other respiratory conditions, a chest radiograph may be considered, though radiologic findings for pneumonia, bronchiolitis, and asthma are quite similar. A chest radiograph should be ordered for children with hypoxemia (oxygen saturation <90%), significant respiratory distress, or if not improving after 48 to 72 hours of antimicrobial therapy.[76] Follow-up chest radiographs are not needed in patients who have an uneventful recovery. Additional diagnostic testing, such as chest ultrasound, CBC, acute-phase reactants, and blood and sputum cultures, are not indicated in the outpatient setting. PCPs may consider viral respiratory testing, such as for COVID-19 or influenza, if such infections are occurring within the community.[74,76]

Differential Diagnosis

The child's age and characteristic signs and symptoms as discussed previously can help distinguish between viral and bacterial pneumonia. Differential diagnoses to consider include bronchiolitis, congestive heart failure, acute bronchiectasis, FB aspiration, pulmonary abscess, parasitic pneumonia, and endotracheal tuberculosis. Right lower lobe pneumonia can present with abdominal pain and be confused with appendicitis. Right upper lobe pneumonia can often closely resemble meningitis as it may present with a stiff neck.

Management

All children with pneumonia require supportive care with antipyretics, hydration, rest, and suctioning, if indicated. Antibiotics

---

• BOX 32.3 Criteria for Hospital Admission for Pneumonia

Neonate to 3 Months Old
- Fever
- Poor oral intake with evidence of dehydration
- Pulmonary complications noted on radiographs: abscess, empyema, pneumatocele

Infants and Children Older Than 3 Months
- Hypoxemia with oxygen less than 90%
- Tachypnea: >60 breaths/min in infants younger than 2 months; >50 breaths/min in children 2–11 months old; or >40 breaths/min at rest in children 1–5 years old
- Respiratory rate >70 breaths/min in infants or older children >50 breaths/min indicates more severe community-acquired pneumonia
- Grunting, dyspnea, or apnea
- Poor feeding with tachycardia and signs of dehydration (slow capillary refill of >2 s) in infants
- Severe respiratory distress
- Oxygen saturation <90% with the need for supplemental oxygen (pulse oximetry reading or arterial blood gas)
- Toxic appearance
- Failure to respond to appropriate oral antibiotic

All Age Groups
- Social factors that interfere with caregiver's ability to monitor and/or care for the child at home

---

should be reserved for those with suspected bacterial infection only. Serious infections may require hospitalization for respiratory monitoring or support, including humidified oxygen, pulmonary therapy, and/or intubation. Most otherwise healthy children can be managed as outpatients, though management varies by age. Guidelines for admission are identified in Box 32.3. Guidelines for outpatient treatment of bacterial pneumonia by age and certain specific pathogens follow.[74,76] Local resistance rates may need to be taken into consideration.

- *Neonates:* Admission regardless of pathogen
- *Infants 3 Months to 5 Years:*
  - Young infants (3–6 months) may also need hospitalization.
  - If *C. trachomatis* is suspected, treat with oral azithromycin for 5 days or clarithromycin (15 mg/kg/day in 2 doses) or oral erythromycin (40 mg/kg/day in 4 doses).
  - Use caution in prescribing antimicrobials as viral causes of pneumonia predominate during early childhood.
  - Amoxicillin 90 mg/kg/day divided every 12 hours is first-line therapy. Duration of therapy is under debate, but typically ranges from 5 to 10 days.
  - Alternative antimicrobial options:
    - History of nonallergic reaction to penicillin, treat with amoxicillin
    - History of mild reaction (non–type I reaction): amoxicillin 90 mg/kg/day or third-generation cephalosporin, such as cefdinir (14 mg/kg/day in 2 doses)
    - History of type I reaction (serious allergic reaction) to penicillin, consider clindamycin (30–40 mg/kg/day in 3 doses) or levofloxacin, if susceptible (16–20 mg/kg/day in 2 doses)
  - *C. pneumonia* and *M. pneumonia* (community-acquired) are less common in this age group. Consider if a child with suspected bacterial pneumonia fails to improve after

48 to 72 hours of antimicrobials. Treat with azithromycin 10 mg/kg/day once on day 1 (maximum dose = 500 mg) and then 5 mg/kg daily for the next 4 days (maximum dose = 250 mg). Note, routine prescribing of azithromycin for CAP is contributing to resistance to macrolides.[77] Only use macrolides for CAP when there is a high index of suspicion for atypical bacterial pneumonia, otherwise follow first-line recommendations for typical bacterial pneumonia.

- *Children >5 years:*
  - Amoxicillin, 90 mg/kg/day, divided every 12 hours is first-line therapy. Duration of therapy is under debate, but typically ranges from 5 to 10 days.
  - Alternative antimicrobial options:
    - History of nonallergic reaction to penicillin, treat with amoxicillin
    - History of mild reaction (non–type I reaction): amoxicillin 90 mg/kg/day or third-generation cephalosporin, such as cefdinir (14 mg/kg/day in 2 doses)
    - History of type I reaction (serious allergic reaction) to penicillin, consider clindamycin (30–40 mg/kg/day in 3 doses) or levofloxacin, if susceptible (16–20 mg/kg/day in 2 doses)
  - If *C. pneumonia* or *M. pneumonia* (community-acquired) is suspected, azithromycin is an appropriate choice. Azithromycin 10 mg/kg/day once on day 1 (maximum dose = 500 mg) and then 5 mg/kg daily for the next 4 days (maximum dose = 250 mg). Note, routine prescribing of azithromycin for CAP is contributing to resistance to macrolides.[77] Only use macrolides for CAP when there is a high index of suspicion for atypical bacterial pneumonia, otherwise follow first-line recommendations for typical bacterial pneumonia.

Education about medication administration, hydration, fever control, and worrisome signs and symptoms is important. In the child receiving antimicrobial therapy, advise families that the child should experience improvement in clinical symptoms within 48 to 72 hours of starting antibiotics.[74] The child should be seen for reevaluation if there is no improvement or if symptoms worsen, at which time a chest radiograph and change in antibiotic is likely. Children with recurrent pneumonia diagnoses should be referred to a pulmonary specialist for further evaluation.

Prognosis

Most children with pneumonia experience an uneventful recovery, though it is important to inform caregivers that the cough may last for several weeks. Routine rechecks with chest x-rays are not recommended. If pneumonia recurs or persists for longer than 1 month, further evaluation for underlying immunodeficiency disease is indicated.

Complications

Complications associated with CAP may result from spreading of the infection, including pleural effusion, empyema, pericarditis, bacteremia, or hematologic impacts. Additional rare complications include meningitis, osteomyelitis, and/or septic arthritis.[73]

Prevention

Prevention of pneumonia begins prenatally, such as the identification and treatment of pregnant individuals. During childhood, universal vaccination against influenza, HIB, and pneumococcal infection is essential. Current guidelines limit the use of palivizumab (Synagis) prophylaxis (see Chapter 35).

Lower Airway and Parenchymal Conditions: Chronic Conditions

There are numerous chronic respiratory conditions that are encountered during childhood. Asthma is the most common chronic condition of childhood, affecting an estimated 6 million children in the United States.[78] See the Chapter 36 section on asthma for additional detail. A full review of every chronic respiratory condition is beyond the scope of this chapter, but BPD and cystic fibrosis are discussed.

Bronchopulmonary Dysplasia

BPD, also known as *chronic lung disease of prematurity*, is the most common cause of chronic lung disease in pediatrics. Premature infants born during the canalicular or saccular stages of lung development have severely diminished pulmonary development and capacity for gas exchange, often with just rudimentary alveolar sacs, reduced pulmonary capillary proliferation, and an inability to produce surfactant.[79] The definition and classification of BPD has evolved over recent decades, which has led to inconsistency in the literature. Early classification was based upon oxygen requirements at 28 days postnatal age. Presently, a BPD diagnosis is often made based on such oxygen requirements at 28 days postnatal age, but also includes grading the severity of BPD based upon the mode of oxygen delivery, with more invasive delivery associated with more severe disease.[80] It is estimated that 40% of infants born less than 28 weeks' gestation develop BPD. Risk factors for developing BPD include genetics, in utero growth failure, chorioamnionitis, preeclampsia, and exposure to tobacco or drugs.[79]

The pathophysiology of BPD has evolved as medical therapeutics became more widely accessible. Before exogenous surfactant and antenatal steroids, premature infants—typically those less than 32 weeks' gestation—would often initially develop respiratory distress syndrome, presenting with tachypnea, accessory muscle use, and progressive respiratory compromise. Intervention included oxygen supplementation and invasive ventilation, which caused a high incidence of interstitial inflammation and fibrosis. The subsequent oxidative stress and barotrauma frequently led to a diagnosis of BPD, characterized by atelectasis, hyperinflation, remodeling of the pulmonary arteries and diminished alveolarization, which is now referred to as "old BPD." Presently, antenatal surfactant and steroids are routinely administered, which has improved survival in premature infants, particularly those at much lower gestational ages. Similarly, gentler approaches to ventilation as well as revised oxygen supplementation standards have resulted in lowering oxidative stress and ventilator-associated barotrauma and an overall reduced incidence of pulmonary fibrosis. This "new BPD" is characterized by an arrest of distal lung development, with decreased lung capillaries and alveolar simplification, largely due to the earlier gestational age of premature infants.[79]

Infants with new BPD require interdisciplinary care throughout their initial hospitalization and following discharge. Most new BPD survivors experience persistent respiratory disease with recurrent wheezing that may or may not respond to bronchodilators, and numerous other acquired airway conditions. There is a high incidence of pulmonary hypertension, secondary to chronic hypoxemia, with some experiencing right ventricular hypertrophy. Gastroesophageal reflux is common due to intraabdominal pressure. Similarly, immature swallowing coordination may lead to dysphagia and aspiration. Growth concerns and nutritional challenges are very common due to high metabolic demand coupled with possible gastroesophageal reflux and/or dysphagia. In addition, there is a high incidence of neurodevelopmental delays.[79]

Clinical Findings

History. The history for a child with BPD will be comprehensive, to include respiratory, cardiac, nutrition, growth surveillance and neurodevelopmental surveillance, and assessment where indicated. In addition, the history will include care plans from various subspecialists involved in the child's care.

Management

Primary care management of infants with BPD entails serving as the medical home and ensuring ongoing surveillance and routine pediatric care are provided. Often, subspecialists are involved and include pulmonary, nutrition, respiratory therapy, speech, physical and occupational therapy, audiology, and neurodevelopment. PCP surveillance of growth and formalized developmental screening are recommended, given the high incidence of developmental delays. Children with BPD should receive routine childhood immunizations as well as evaluation for RSV prophylaxis eligibility. For children who experience recurrent wheezing, an asthma diagnosis may be appropriate, with careful monitoring for responsiveness to bronchodilator and possible inhaled corticosteroid. Further, optimal nutrition and growth will support alveolarization, which has important implications for later childhood and adulthood. Additional diagnostic testing and imaging may be indicated, such as repeat echocardiograms, depending on comorbidities and subspecialist recommendations. Readmission to the hospital is common, particularly with respiratory illnesses.

Cystic Fibrosis

CF is the most common autosomal-recessive disease, occurring in one of 15,000 to 17,000 live births, manifested by chronic obstructive pulmonary disease, GI disturbances, and exocrine dysfunction. The epidemiology and management of CF have dramatically increased life expectancy through survival rates. Beginning in the 1930s, children usually died in their first year of life while today the expected survival rate is nearly 50 years. Newer therapies that target the genetic defect are likely to further increase the life span of patients with CF, however, pulmonary manifestations will need active preventive treatments. CF occurs in approximately one in 2500 White births, one in 15,000 to 20,000 Black Americans, and one in 4000 to 10,000 Latin Americans.[81,82] Prenatal population carrier screening is correlated with decreased numbers of reported patient with CF.[82]

CF involves mutation of the CF transmembrane conductance regulator (CFTR) protein, which is expressed in epithelial and blood cells. This genetic discovery nearly 30 years ago transformed understanding and care delivery for patients. The gene is on chromosome 7 with more than 2000 CFTR mutations identified.[82] Mutations are categorized into six distinct classes, although the functional importance of only a few mutations is known. CFTR functions in sodium transport through the epithelial sodium channel, regulates the adenosine triphosphate channels, and is involved in bicarbonate chloride exchange. The *CFTR* gene defect causes defective ion transport, airway surface liquid depletion, and defective mucociliary clearance.

The diagnosis is based on evidence of CFTR dysfunction and signs and symptoms of the disease. Infants in the United States with a positive newborn screening (NBS) with inconclusive diagnostic testing are identified as having CF related metabolic syndrome; the expression *CF screen positive, inconclusive diagnosis* (CFSPED) is used in other countries. This classification is given when there is a positive NBS and either a sweat chloride value <30 mmol/L and two *CFTR* mutations, at least one of which has unclear phenotypic consequences, or an intermediate sweat chloride value of 30 to 59 mmol/L and one or zero CF-causing mutations. The CFTR-related disorder is a monosymptomatic clinical entity associated with CFTR dysfunction that does not meet the diagnostic criteria for CF. The use of atypical and nonclassical terms is not recommended.[83]

The most common defect, which is found in 70% of cases, is a deletion of phenylalanine in position 508 (D508). Polymorphism in non-*CFTR* genes may explain the difference in the manifestations of the genetic change within different families.[84] Ultimately, the resulting mucus obstruction causes inflammation and infection. Failure to conduct ions across epithelial cell membranes leads to problems in the lungs, biliary tree, pancreas, intestines, vas deferens, and sweat glands. This results in mucus thickening and targets organ damage in the lungs and exocrine glands. There is airway surface liquid depletion with inhibited transport of bicarbonate causing decreased mucociliary transport. The deficiency in mucociliary transport causes chronic inflammation and infection and, as a result of environmental insults and host defense defects, leads to bacterial colonization in trapped mucous secretions.[84] The mucus is adhesive and stringy, leading to tenacious secretions that have poor cough clearance. Osmolar fluid depletion leads to a loss of water and increased concentration of ions. In the exocrine system, subsequent pancreas, liver, and intestinal tract adhesive secretions lead to malabsorption of fat and proteins resulting from pancreatic insufficiency.

Clinical Findings

CF is a multisystem progressive illness with varying levels of severity. Table 32.9 outlines clinical manifestations seen in children at various ages. They may include the following:

- *Pulmonary:* CF is a major cause of severe chronic lung disease in children. Lungs of children with CF are normal at birth but become inflamed with chronic airway infection shortly after birth. The respiratory epithelium exhibits marked impermeability to chloride and excessive sodium reabsorption. Mucus is adherent and stringy with a need for periciliary fluid to aid in expectoration, leading to dysfunctional mucociliary transport, airway obstruction, and chronic infections. Pulmonary system manifestations vary from chronic, dry, frequent cough and sputum production to respiratory failure. Bronchitis, bronchiolitis, bronchiectasis, and pneumonia occur frequently. Bronchospasm resembling acute or chronic asthma may be present. Airways become colonized with *S. aureus, H. influenzae,* and, finally, *Pseudomonas aeruginosa. Burkholderia cepacia* is a slower-growing organism found in children with CF. Infection can present in infancy. Pulmonary disease usually becomes progressive and leads to cor pulmonale, respiratory failure, and death by adulthood. Other respiratory problems associated with CF include recurrent ARS, nasal polyps, and allergic bronchopulmonary aspergillosis, which starts by childhood and continues into adulthood. Digital clubbing is common.
- *GI tract and nutrition:* During infancy, meconium ileus, pancreatic insufficiency, and rectal prolapse can be manifestations of CF. Meconium ileus develops in up to 15% of newborns born with CF. Meconium ileus syndrome equivalent can also

TABLE 32.9	Clinical Manifestations of Cystic Fibrosis: From Neonatal Period to Adolescence
Stage of Childhood	**Clinical Manifestations**
Fetal ultrasound	Hyperechoic bowel suggestive of meconium ileus and present in 10% of fetuses with CF
Neonatal period	Meconium ileus, delayed meconium passage, meconium plug Prolonged jaundice Intestinal atresia Edema, hypoproteinemia, and acrodermatitis enteropathica due to malabsorption Hemorrhagic disease of newborn due to vitamin K deficiency
Infancy	Cough Colonization with bacteria in mucus Bacterial pneumonia Failure to thrive Hypoproteinemia, hypochloremic dehydration Abdominal distention Cholestasis Rectal prolapse Steatorrhea DIOS Hemolytic anemia

Childhood	Respiratory manifestations:
	    Chronic recurrent infection of sinuses and respiratory tract/nasal polyposis/poorly controlled asthma
	Bronchiectasis
	Allergic bronchopulmonary aspergillosis
	Digital clubbing
	GI manifestations:
	    Poor weight gain and growth
	    Steatorrhea
	    Chronic constipation
	    Rectal prolapse
	    DIOS
	Idiopathic pancreatitis/liver disease

Adolescence	ABPA Chronic pansinusitis Nasal polyposis Bronchiectasis/hemoptysis Idiopathic pancreatitis Osteoporosis Diabetes Obstructive azoospermia

ABPA, Allergic bronchopulmonary aspergillosis; *CF,* cystic fibrosis; *DIOS,* distal intestinal obstruction syndrome; *GI,* gastrointestinal.

Modified from Rosenfield M, Sontag M, Ren C. Cystic fibrosis diagnosis and newborn screening. *Pediatr Clin N Am,* 2016;63:602; and Paranjape SM, Mogayzel PJ. Cystic fibrosis. *Pediatr Rev.* 2014; 35(5):194–205.

develop in older patients, with desiccated fecal material causing GI obstruction. Eighty-five percent of affected children have failure to thrive because of pancreatic enzyme insufficiency, which leads to bulky, malodorous stools resulting in failure to thrive. Edema with hypoproteinemia may also be present. Children have thick fat-laden stools (steatorrhea), poor muscle mass, and delayed maturation. Infants with CF who are fed soy-based formulas do very poorly, and severe hypoproteinemia and anasarca quickly result. During childhood, intussusception, hepatic steatosis, biliary fibrosis, and rectal prolapse can occur. Childhood problems continue into adulthood. Clinically apparent cirrhosis occurs in 15% of patients with subsequent risk of portal hypertension. Adenocarcinoma of the digestive tract can occur. Other GI problems associated with CF include volvulus, duodenal inflammation, gastroesophageal reflux, bile reflux, fibrosing colonopathy, and poor fat absorption that leads to vitamin A, K, E, and D deficiencies with resulting anemia, neuropathy, night blindness, osteoporosis, and bleeding disorders. Distal intestinal obstructive syndrome occurs when viscous fecal matter causes blockage in the distal intestine and presents with abdominal pain and distention with pain. This occurs due to poor fat absorption, pancreatic insufficiency, and dehydration.

- *Hepatobiliary tract:* Biliary cirrhosis occurs in 2% to 3% of children with CF and is characterized by jaundice, ascites, hematemesis from esophageal varices, portal hypertension, cirrhosis, hepatomegaly, and splenomegaly. Hepatic steatosis is also a known complication of CF. Adolescent patients may experience biliary colic and cholelithiasis.
- *Endocrine:* Recurrent acute pancreatitis is not uncommon. CF-related diabetes (CFRD) with relative insulin deficiency develops as the child ages due to autolysis of the pancreas as the pancreas body becomes fatty due to thick viscous secretions. CF patients need annual blood glucose screening with up to 30% of patients developing CFRD by adulthood.[84]
- *Musculoskeletal:* Vitamin D deficiency may result in osteoporosis when bone reabsorption exceeds bone formation.
- *Reproductive:* Affected children have delayed sexual development. The vas deferens is nonfunctional and atrophied due to CFTR dysfunction, leading to azoospermia and male sterility. The incidence of inguinal hernia, hydrocele, and undescended testes is also high. Females experience secondary amenorrhea, cervicitis, and decreased fertility. A pregnancy is usually carried to term if pulmonary function is not severely compromised.
- *Sweat glands:* Excessive salt loss can lead to hypochloremic alkalosis, especially in warm weather or after gastroenteritis. Children with CF often taste salty because of elevated amounts of sodium chloride lost in endogenous sweat. Dehydration and heat exhaustion are concerns.

Diagnostic Studies. All 50 states screen newborns for CF but methods vary across requirements. NBS enables early identification of CF and referral to CF centers. Children with access to earlier routine care due to early diagnosis do better than those with a later diagnosis. All state screenings identify immunoreactive trypsinogen or trypsin (IRT) as the initial test with an IRT/IRT protocol. IRT-IRT-DNA states test IRT levels twice before DNA analysis. IRT-DNA states test IRT levels once before DNA analysis. If the IRT is elevated after one or two tests, depending on the state, or the child has a confirmed *CFTR* mutation, the primary provider is notified, and the child is referred for sweat testing. There are false-negative screens, so if an infant has symptoms and signs of CF, a sweat test should be performed. This protocol is less sensitive than the IRT/DNA algorithms (96.2–76.1%). False positives and false negatives do occur.[83]

Sweat testing should be done even if the newborn screen was negative when a child has pulmonary symptoms such as chronic cough, recurrent pneumonia, nasal polyps, and digital clubbing or systemic signs such as failure to thrive, jaundice, rectal prolapse, intussusception, prolonged jaundice, or pancreatitis. Sweat tests should be done by a trained technician at a laboratory in a care center accredited by the Cystic Fibrosis Foundation. The test is done by using gauze, filter paper, or macroduct coils to induce iontophoresis of pilocarpine to stimulate sweat production by sweat glands. Because of transient elevations of sweat chloride 24 hours after birth, testing should be deferred until 48 hours of life at a minimum. Two samples should be collected to ensure consistency and sufficiency of sample collection.[85]

Sodium chloride concentration increases with age. A concentration of sweat chloride greater than 60 mmol/L is suggestive of CF; a range of 30 to 59 mmol/L for infants less than 6 months or 40 to 59 mmol/L for older individuals suggests the need for further genetic testing. If the sweat test is less than 30 mmol/L, CF is unlikely. It is rare for someone with two mutations to have a negative sweat test. A result of greater than 60 mEq/L of chloride on two specimens is in the diagnostic range for CF. Children with CF who have hypoproteinemia may elicit false-negative sweat test results. Results of the genetic testing should be compared to the most current knowledge found at https://www.cftr2.org/. False negatives can be attributed to conditions including improper testing technique, atopic dermatitis, hypothyroidism, pancreatitis, glycogen storage disease, and malnutrition. A normal sweat test does not definitively exclude a diagnosis of CF. Genetic testing is recommended for children presenting with clinical concern in the presence of negative testing.[85]

Other diagnostic testing is indicated depending on secondary complications of CF. Glycosylated hemoglobin levels may be elevated in older children because of impaired pancreatic functioning. Pulmonary function tests are used to follow the clinical course. Liver function tests abnormalities on three tests in a 12-month period, ultrasound, and liver tissue biopsy are used to diagnose liver disease.

Management

Children with CF have complicated treatment regimens and should be monitored by an interprofessional team at a CF-accredited center. Because lung disease is the most common cause of morbidity and mortality, it is important to educate families and develop a shared treatment plan that will optimize lung functioning, prevent disease progression, and avoid complications. Treatment of CF-related lung disease requires control of airway infections, clearance of airway secretions, and decreasing lung inflammation. Pulmonary, nutritional, physical, and pharmacologic (antibiotic and antiinflammatory) therapy and psychological counseling must be individualized for children at each stage of their illness.

- Pulmonary
  - To promote airway clearance, inhaled dornase alfa (recombinant human deoxyribonuclease) selectively cleaves the DNA and reduces mucus viscosity. Hypertonic saline works by drawing water into secretions and is used to thin secretions to allow their removal. The use of postural drainage, active cycle of breathing, autogenic drainage, percussion, positive expiratory pressure, exercise, and high-frequency chest wall oscillation are done twice a day to facilitate secretion removal.
  - CFTR modulators are approved for use in about 50% of the population. It took nearly 25 years after discovering the *CFTR* gene to market ivacaftor (Kalydeco), the first CFTR modulator, indicated for children aged 6 years and older. This therapy yielded significant clinical improvements. In 2012 ivacaftor was combined with a corrector lumacaftor (Orkambi), approved for patients 12 years and older who were p.Phe508del homozygous. Again, this yielded

significant clinical improvement. A second dual combination introduced in 2018 has continued to improve sweat chloride concentrations, reduce pulmonary exacerbations, and increase quality of life.[82]

- To reduce chronic airway inflammation, high-dose ibuprofen, and oral azithromycin, dosed three times a week, are used. Although increasing research supports the practice, to date there is a lack of standard guidelines in children. Children must be screened for atypical mycobacterial infection before starting long-term azithromycin.[86] Although high-dose ibuprofen decreases neutrophil migration in children ages 6 to 17 years, the therapy is not widely used because of risk of GI bleeding and frequent drug blood level measurements. Hemoptysis can be scant (<5 mL), moderate (5–240 mL), or massive (>240 mL) and is associated with advancing lung disease as well as vitamin K deficiency. It results from the hypertrophy and proliferation of the bronchial arteries rupturing into airways because of disease progression. Management includes antibiotic therapy, cessation of the antiinflammatory drugs, and limiting therapies for airway clearance.[86]
- Pneumothorax presents as acute onset of chest pain and dyspnea and is confirmed by chest radiograph. Smaller pneumothoraces are managed by observation and discontinuation of positive pressure. Surgical or chemical pleurodesis is used in recurrent large pneumothoraces.
- Lung transplantation is a viable therapy for selected patients with terminal lung disease and is used more in Canada than in the United States.
- GI
  - Replacement with exogenous pancreatic enzyme replacement therapy (PERT) with every meal and snack along with a fat-soluble vitamin supplement is done. PERT capsules are opened but should not be crushed. Dosing ranges from 2000 to 2500 units/kg of lipase to a maximum of 10,000 units/kg/day. Higher dosing of lipase can lead to fibrosing colonopathy in a small number of patients.
  - Fat malabsorption causes deficiency of vitamins A, D, E, and K; therefore replacement must be started along with serum monitoring of the levels annually. Vitamin D deficiency can occur, resulting in osteopenia, osteoporosis, or rickets.
  - CF liver disease is managed with optimizing nutritional intake and avoiding hepatotoxic drugs.
  - Distal intestinal obstructive syndrome is managed using IV hydration, polyethylene glycol solution, and oral laxatives to promote lower bowel clearance. Sodium meglumine diatrizoate (Gastrografin) enemas can be used by an experienced radiologist in instances of a complete obstruction.[87]
- Endocrine disorder
  - Beginning at age 10 years, an oral glucose tolerance test is done annually to screen for CFRD. Hemoglobin A1C is not recommended because it underestimates overall glycemic control. Prevention of microvascular complication of diabetes including renal disease, retinopathy, and neuropathy associated with hyperglycemia is key. Ketoacidosis is rare.
  - Insulin is used to treat CFRD.

Transition From Pediatric to Adult Care
- More than 50% of patients with CF are adults. It is important to provide reproductive health care as well as to initiate care within an interprofessional team and make sure there is a transition to an adult care clinic.

Chest Wall Conditions

Pectus deformities refer to abnormalities of the sternum and adjacent ribs. Pectus excavatum (PE) is characterized by a depression in the sternum and adjacent ribs, causing the appearance of a "sunken chest," whereas pectus carinatum (PC) causes a protrusion of the sternum and adjacent ribs, sometimes referred to as "pigeon chest." Pectus deformities are caused by costochondral cartilage growth abnormalities, though the actual mechanism remains unknown. Pectus deformities may also present as a comorbidity in children with lung hypoplasia, severe chronic negative intrathoracic pressure, or certain neuromuscular conditions, such as spinal muscular atrophy. Pectus deformities are typically identified at birth, but often worsen during rapid pubertal growth.

Pectus Excavatum/Pectus Carinatum

PE accounts for more than 95% of all thoracic abnormalities, affecting an estimated 1 in 300 to 400 live births.[88] There is a male preponderance and approximately 40% of children with PE have a family history. It is believed to be an autosomal dominant trait and is also associated with inheritable connective tissue disease such as Marfan and Ehlers-Danlos syndromes. Many children with PE have no associated impairments, though many express cosmetic concerns. Severe cases of PE may impair thoracic expansion and diaphragmatic contractility, leading to reduced lung volume, chest anteroposterior diameter, and diminished cardiac stroke volume and output. When it is severe, the heart can be compressed, or displaced to the left causing the great vessel to rotate. There is an additional risk of cardiac dysrhythmias due to lower oxygen supply to the heart. The length of the sternum abnormalities and the adjacent ribs determine the degree of pulmonary and cardiac dysfunction.[88]

PC is far less common than PE, although it too has a male predominance. Clinical manifestations of PC are rare other than cosmetic concerns. There are few clinical complications compared to PE. However, PC is less easily concealed by clothes, therefore cosmetic concerns are common.

Clinical Findings

History. The history for either pectus deformity includes exercise intolerance, easy fatigability, wheezing, chest tightness, chest pain, palpitations, or dizziness. Psychological effects may be pronounced, particularly during puberty. Careful assessment of self-image and impacts on social activities is important.[89]

Physical Examination. Evaluate the anteroposterior chest diameter and chest wall motion during inhalation and exhalation to determine impacts on thoracic expansion. Also complete a careful respiratory assessment, with particular attention to signs of restricted inhalation. There are three main types of PE. The cup-shaped or classic deformity is limited to the lower part of the sternum. The flat or saucer-shaped is a long pectus that involves most of the sternum. In the asymmetric type, there is asymmetry between the left and right hemithorax with the right side more affected. The sternum is also slightly rotated in this deformity, with more than a 30-degree rotation considered a significant torsion. There are four variants of PC: chondrogladiolar, costomanubrial, horseshoe chest, or asymmetric.

Diagnostic Studies. Pectus deformity may be diagnosed clinically; however, diagnostic testing may be indicated to determine severity. Diagnostic testing may include chest CT (or other chest imaging), pulmonary function testing, echocardiogram, and stress testing. A chest CT is used to estimate the severity of the deformity using the Pectus Severity Index (PSI, sometimes referred to as *Haller index*). In PE, a PSI of greater than 2.5 is considered abnormal, and greater than 3.5 severe.[87] In PC, a PSI of less than 2.5 is considered abnormal. Pulmonary function testing is important to determine the severity of lung restriction. Body plethysmography is preferred over spirometry due to the likelihood of increased reserve volume, which is not measured in spirometry. Echocardiogram and cardiac stress testing may be indicated, depending on the severity of the deformity. All adolescents with pectus deformity should be evaluated for psychosocial impacts and quality of life.[89]

Management

Patients with severe deformity may be referred to cardiology and pulmonary for specialized diagnostic testing described above. Children with severe deformity and/or significant physiological effects should be referred to a surgeon for evaluation. Indications for surgical evaluation are based primarily on quality of life, considering the degree of psychological and physical impairment rather than the severity of the deformity. Some patients with PC may be candidates for bracing, a noninvasive intervention, which is most successful when initiated before puberty. Invasive and minimally invasive surgical options are available for PE and PC, with the less invasive repair usually preferred.

Scoliosis

The spinal curvature and rib asymmetry associated with scoliosis contribute to decreased chest wall compliance and reduced thoracic cavity capacity, thereby reducing pulmonary capacity. Pulmonary impairment has historically been attributed to moderate scoliosis (50–60 degrees), whereas those with severe curves of 90 or more degrees at risk for respiratory failure. However, pulmonary restriction due to scoliosis is an emerging area of research. Recent evidence indicates an inverse relationship between the degree of spinal curvature and lung functioning, particularly lung capacity, indicating that more intentional monitoring for pulmonary restriction may be warranted for all children and adolescents with scoliosis.[91] See Chapter 40 for scoliosis screening, identification, and management.

Monitoring and Management

While children and adolescents with scoliosis are often asymptomatic, PCPs should routinely monitor for pulmonary symptoms, including breathing disruption, exercise intolerance, or visible deformity of the spine.[92] A referral to a pulmonary specialist is indicated should any pulmonary symptoms occur. In collaboration with an orthopedic specialist, bracing or surgery may be considered to preserve pulmonary function. Bracing is typically used to prevent worsening curvature, particularly during pubertal growth. Surgical correction is reserved for moderate or severe cases of scoliosis (50 degrees or more) to correct and/or stabilize the curvature, preserve lung function, and prevent complications.[91]

Congenital Diaphragmatic Hernia

Congenital diaphragmatic hernia (CDH) is a birth defect characterized by a failure of the diaphragm to close, which results in herniation of abdominal contents into the fetal chest cavity. CDH is considered a multifactorial condition, though risk factors include maternal age, pregestational diabetes and hypertension, tobacco use, and alcohol consumption.[93] CDH may also be associated with other structural abnormalities and/or neurodevelopmental conditions. Development of the diaphragm begins in approximately week 7 of gestation; the most common diaphragmatic defects are posterolateral (known as *Bochdalek hernia*), followed by anterior (known as *Morgagni*) or the rare central hernia.[93] See Chapter 28 for additional details.

Children with CDH experience numerous cardiopulmonary abnormalities, including pulmonary hypoplasia (diminished lung development), reduced alveolarization, and impaired pulmonary vascularization function. Previously, it was presumed that the herniation of abdominal contents compressed fetal lungs, which led to pulmonary hypoplasia on the ipsilateral (affected) side of the diaphragmatic defect. However, the contralateral lung (opposite of the affected side) has been found to be hypoplastic with abnormal pulmonary vascularization as well, suggesting mechanical compression could not fully account for the pathogenesis of CDH.[93] The dual hit hypothesis for CDH emerged, with the first "hit" triggered by genetic and environmental factors, causing pulmonary hypoplasia, pulmonary vascular defects, and possible left ventricular abnormalities. The second hit was caused by mechanical compression of the abdominal contents, interfering with fetal lung growth and maturation, causing a variable degree of hypoplasia of both ipsilateral and contralateral lungs, including reduced alveolarization.

Infants with CDH require interdisciplinary prenatal, perinatal, and postnatal care. Prenatal and postnatal care are discussed in Chapter 28. Following surgical repair of the defect, ongoing pulmonary support may still be required, depending on the infant status. There is a high incidence of chronic lung disease following the neonatal period due to impaired gas exchange, with CDH survivors frequently requiring oxygen supplementation, bronchodilators for recurrent wheeze, inhaled corticosteroids, and treatment for recurrent pneumonia. Many infants with CDH develop pulmonary hypertension because of reduced pulmonary vascular bed and remodeling, with some also developing ventricular dysfunction. Pulmonary hypertension is the major contributor to the high proportion of morbidity and mortality among infants with CDH.[93] Additional health considerations among infants with CDH include a high proportion of musculoskeletal deformities (chest asymmetry, pectus deformities, scoliosis), gastroesophageal reflux, nutritional concerns and poor weight gain, hernia recurrence, and neurodevelopmental delays (motor, speech, hearing loss).[93]

Clinical Findings

History

The history for a child with a repaired CDH will include respiratory assessment including exercise intolerance, cardiac assessment, nutrition and feeding assessment, assessment of bowel movements and evidence of obstruction, growth surveillance, neurodevelopmental surveillance, and assessment where indicated.

Management

Primary care management of children with a repaired CDH entails serving as the medical home and ensuring ongoing surveillance and routine pediatric care is provided. Surveillance of growth and development is critical, with frequent weight, length, and head circumference measurements recommended. Children with a history of CDH should receive routine childhood immunizations as well as evaluation for possible RSV prophylaxis. Careful developmental surveillance with formalized developmental and neurodevelopmental evaluation is recommended. Additional diagnostic testing and imaging may be indicated, depending on whether the child experiences any respiratory, cardiac, or GI symptoms. As the child matures, the PCP will monitor for psychosocial development and intervene if the child exhibits concern for self-image or other psychosocial concerns. In addition, the PCP must coordinate with the interdisciplinary care team to ensure the child receives comprehensive care.

Additional Resources

CDC: Children with Special Health Care Needs: https://www.cdc.gov/childrenindisasters/children-with-special-healthcare-needs.html

Cincinnati Children's Hospital Medical Center: www.cincinnatichildrens.org

Cincinnati Children's Hospital Medical Center: Suctioning the Nose with a Bulb Syringe: www.cincinnatichildrens.org/health/s/suction

Cystic Fibrosis Foundation: www.cff.org

Family Voices: https://familyvoices.org/

MSD Manual: How to Remove a Foreign Body from the Nose: https://www.msdmanuals.com/professional/ear,-nose,-and-throat-disorders/how-to-do-nose-procedures/how-to-remove-a-foreign-body-from-the-nose

National Organization of Rare Diseases: Cystic Fibrosis: https://rarediseases.org/rare-diseases/cystic-fibrosis/

Seattle Children's Hospital: Clinical Standard Work Pathways: https://www.seattlechildrens.org/healthcare-professionals/gateway/clinical-resources/pathways/

Sounds of Pertussis: https://www.youtube.com/watch?v=wuvn-vp5InE&feature=youtu.be

References

1. Levitsky MG. *Pulmonary Physiology*. 10th ed. McGraw Hill; 2022.
2. Kallapur SJ, Jobe AH. Lung development and maturation. In: Martin RJ, Fanaroff AA, Walsh MC, eds. *Neonatal-Perinatal Medicine*. 11th ed. Elsevier; 2020:1124–1142.
3. Goldman-Yassen AE, Meda K, Kadom N. Paranasal sinus development and implications for imaging. *Pediatr Radiol*. 2021;51(7):1134–1148.
4. West JB, Luks AM. *West's Pulmonary Pathophysiology: The Essentials*. 10th ed. Wolters Kluwer; 2021.
5. de Benedictis FM, Bush A. Recurrent lower respiratory tract infections in children. *BMJ*. 2018;362:k2698.
6. Friedman ML, Nitu ME. Acute respiratory failure in children. *Pediatr Ann*. 2018;47(7):e268–e273.
7. Crooks CJ, West J, Morling JR, et al. Pulse oximeter measurements vary across ethnic groups: an observational study in patients with COVID-19. *Eur Respir J*. 2022;59(4):2103246.
8. Sjoding MW, Dickson RP, Iwashyna TJ, et al. Racial bias in pulse oximetry measurement. *N Engl J Med*. 2020;383(25):2477–2478. Erratum N Engl J Med. 2021;385(26):2496.
9. Schondelmeyer AC, Bettencourt AP, Xiao R, et al. Evaluation of an educational outreach and audit and feedback program to reduce continuous pulse oximetry use in hospitalized infants with stable bronchiolitis: a nonrandomized clinical trial. *JAMA Netw Open*. 2021;4(9):e2122826.
10. Humphreys S, Schibler A, von Ungern-Sternberg BS. Carbon dioxide monitoring in children-A narrative review of physiology, value, and pitfalls in clinical practice. *Paediatr Anaesth*. 2021;31(8):839–845.
11. Hanson KE, Azar MM, Banerjee R, et al. Molecular testing for acute respiratory tract infections: clinical and diagnostic recommendations from the IDSA's Diagnostics Committee. *Clin Infect Dis*. 2020;71(10):2744–2751.
12. Stace LB. Point-of-care testing in primary care. In: John RM, ed. *Pediatric Diagnostic Labs for Primary Care: An Evidence-Based Approach*. Springer; 2022.
13. Nagakura A, Morikawa Y, Takasugi N, et al. Oxygen saturation targets in pediatric respiratory disease. *Pediatr Int*. 2022;64(1):e15129.
14. Food and Drug Administration. *Should You Give Kids Medicine for Coughs and Colds?*; 2021. https://www.fda.gov/consumers/consumer-updates/should-you-give-kids-medicine-coughs-and-colds.
15. Food and Drug Administration. *FDA Acts to Protect Kids from Serious Risks of Opioid Ingredients Contained in Some Prescription Cough and Cold Products by Revising Labeling to Limit Pediatric Use*; 2018. https://www.fda.gov/NewsEvents/Newsroom/PressAnnouncements/ucm592109.htm.
16. Albrecht HH, Dicpinigaitis PV, Guenin EP. Role of guaifenesin in the management of chronic bronchitis and upper respiratory tract infections. *Multidiscip Respir Med*. 2017;12:31.
17. Chang AB, Oppenheimer JJ, Weinberger MM, et al. Management of children with chronic wet cough and protracted bacterial bronchitis: CHEST Guideline and Expert Panel Report. *Chest*. 2017;151(4):884–890.
18. Horton DB, Gerhard T, Strom BL. Trends in cough and cold medicine recommendations for children in the United States, 2002-2015. *JAMA Pediatr*. 2019;173(9):885–887.
19. Murni IK, Prawirohartono EP, Triasih R. Potential role of vitamins and zinc on acute respiratory infections including COVID-19. *Glob Pediatr Health*. 2021;8:2333794X211021739.
20. Depoorter L, Vandenplas Y. Probiotics in Pediatrics. A review and practical guide. *Nutrients*. 2021;13(7):2176.
21. Gerber JS, Jackson MA, Tamma PD, et al. Committee on infectious diseases, pediatric infectious diseases society. Antibiotic stewardship in pediatrics. *Pediatrics*. 2021;147(1):e2020040295.
22. CDC. Antibiotic Use in the United States, 2017: Progress and Opportunities. https://www.cdc.gov/antibiotic-use/stewardship-report/pdf/stewardship-report.pdf.
23. King LM, Tsay SV, Hicks LA, et al. Changes in outpatient antibiotic prescribing for acute respiratory illnesses, 2011 to 2018. *Antimicrob Steward Healthc Epidemiol*. 2021;1(1):1–8.
24. Hersh AL, Shapiro DJ, Pavia AT, et al. Geographic variability in diagnosis and antibiotic prescribing for acute respiratory tract infections. *Infect Dis Ther*. 2018;7(1):171–174.
25. Noor A, Fiorito T, Krilov LR. Cold weather viruses. *Pediatr Rev*. 2019;40(10):497–507.
26. Buensalido JA, Valencia JCB. *Rhinovirus (RV) Infection (Common Cold)*; 2019. https://emedicine.medscape.com/article/1001332-overview#a4.
27. Leung NHL. Transmissibility and transmission of respiratory viruses. *Nat Rev Microbiol*. 2021;19(8):528–545.
28. Jaume F, Valls-Mateus M, Mullol J. Common cold and acute rhinosinusitis: up-to-date management in 2020. *Curr Allergy Asthma Rep*. 2020;20(7):28.
29. Pappas DE, Hendley JO. Sinusitis. In: Kliegman RM, St Geme JW, Blum NJ, et al., eds. *Nelson Textbook of Pediatrics*. 21st ed. Elsevier; 2020:2266–2274.
30. Brook I. The role of antibiotics in pediatric chronic rhinosinusitis. *Laryngoscope Investig Otolaryngol*. 2017;2(3):104–108.
31. Quintanilla-Dieck L, Lam DJ. Chronic rhinosinusitis in children. *Curr Treat Options Pediatr*. 2018;4(4):413–424.
32. Wald ER, Applegate KE, Bordley C, et al. Clinical practice guideline for the diagnosis and management of acute bacterial sinusitis in children aged 1 to 18 years. *Pediatrics*. 2013;132(1):e262–e280.

33. Saltagi MZ, Rabbani CC, Patel KS, et al. Orbital complications of acute sinusitis in pediatric patients: management of Chandler III patients. *Allergy Rhinol (Providence)*. 2022;13:21526575221097311.

34. Bochner RE, Gangar M, Belamarich PF. A clinical approach to tonsillitis, tonsillar hypertrophy, and peritonsillar and retropharyngeal abscesses. *Pediatr Rev*. 2017;38(2):81–92. Erratum *Pediatr Rev*. 2017;38(5):240.

35. Shieh WJ. Human adenovirus infections in pediatric population - an update on clinico-pathologic correlation. *Biomed J*. 2022;45(1):38–49.

36. Scott IU. *Pharyngoconjunctival Fever*; 2021. https://emedicine.medscape.com/article/1192323-overview.

37. Mustafa Z, Ghaffari M. Diagnostic methods, clinical guidelines, and antibiotic treatment for group a streptococcal pharyngitis: a narrative review. *Front Cell Infect Microbiol*. 2020;10:563627.

38. CDC. Group. *A Streptococcal (GAS) Disease*; 2021. https://www.cdc.gov/groupastrep/diseases-hcp/strep-throat.html.

39. Kliegman RM, St Geme JW, Blum NJ, et al. *Nelson Textbook of Pediatrics*. 21st ed. Philadelphia; 2020.

40. Patel C, Green BD, Batt JM, et al. Antibiotic prescribing for tonsillopharyngitis in a general practice setting: can the use of Modified Centor Criteria reduce antibiotic prescribing? *Aust J Gen Pract*. 2019;48(6):395–401.

41. Shapiro DJ, Lindgren CE, Neuman MI, et al. Viral features and testing for streptococcal pharyngitis. *Pediatrics*. 2017;139(5):e20163403.

42. Pagana KD, Pagana TJ, Pagana TN. *Mosby's Diagnostic & Laboratory Test Reference*. 14th ed. Elsevier; 2019.

43. CDC. *Antibiotic Prescribing and Use*. US Department of Health and Human Services; 2022. https://www.cdc.gov/antibiotic-use/stewardship-report/pdf/stewardship-report.pdf.

44. American Academy of Pediatrics (AAP) and the Committee on Infectious Diseases. Summaries of infectious diseases. In: Kimberlin DW, ed. *Red Book 2021 Report of the Committee on Infectious Diseases*. 32nd ed. American Academy of Pediatrics; 2021.

45. Wald E. *Group A Streptococcal Tonsillopharyngitis in Children and Adolescents: Clinical Features and Diagnosis*. UpToDate; 2022. https://www.uptodate.com/contents/group-a-streptococcal-tonsillopharyngitis-in-children-and-adolescents-clinical-features-and-diagnosis.

46. National Institute of Mental Health. *PANDAS- Questions and Answers*; 2019. https://www.nimh.nih.gov/sites/default/files/documents/health/publications/pandas/pandas-qa.pdf.

47. Mitchell RB, Archer SM, Ishman SL, et al. Clinical practice guideline: tonsillectomy in children (update)-executive summary. *Otolaryngol Head Neck Surg*. 2019;160(2):187–205.

48. Rodrigues KK, Roosevelt GE. Acute inflammatory upper airway obstruction (croup, epiglottitis, laryngitis, and bacterial tracheitis). In: Kliegman RM, St Geme JW, Blum NJ, et al., eds. *Nelson Textbook of Pediatrics*. 21st ed. Elsevier; 2020:2266–2274.

49. Westley CR, Cotton EK, Brooks JG. Nebulized racemic epinephrine by IPPB for the treatment of croup: a double-blind study. *Am J Dis Child*. 1978;132(5):484–487.

50. Gates A, Johnson DW, Klassen TP. Glucocorticoids for croup in children. *JAMA Pediatr*. 2019;173(6):595–596.

51. Kilgore PE, Salim AM, Zervos MJ, et al. Pertussis: microbiology, disease, treatment, and prevention. *Clin Microbiol Rev*. 2016;29(3):449–486.

52. Souder E, Long SS. Pertussis in the era of new strains of Bordetella pertussis. *Infect Dis Clin North Am*. 2015;29(4):699–713.

53. Healy CM, Rench MA, Wootton SH, et al. Evaluation of the impact of a pertussis cocooning program on infant pertussis infection. *Pediatr Infect Dis J*. 2015;34(1):22–26.

54. Decker MD, Edwards KM. Pertussis (whooping cough). *J Infect Dis*. 2021;224(12 suppl 2):S310–S320.

55. Faulkner AE, Skoff TH, Tondella ML, et al. Trends in pertussis diagnostic testing in the United States, 1990 to 2012. *Pediatr Infect Dis J*. 2016;35(1):39–44.

56. Bocka JJ. *Pertussis*. Medscape. http://emedicine.medscape.com/article/967268-overview.

57. Rodrigues CMC, Plotkin SA. Impact of vaccines; health, economic and social perspectives. *Front Microbiol*. 2020;11:1526.

58. Ayotunde O, Burkard DJ, Kolacki C, et al. Nasal foreign body removal: success rates for techniques and devices. *Am J Emerg Med*. 2022;56:384–385.

59. Yan T, Goldman RD. Recurrent epistaxis in children. *Can Fam Physician*. 2021;67(6):427–429.

60. Richards AM. Pediatric respiratory emergencies. *Emerg Med Clin North Am*. 2016;34(1):77–96.

61. Choe JY, Choe BH. Foreign body removal in children using foley catheter or magnet tube from gastrointestinal tract. *Pediatr Gastroenterol Hepatol Nutr*. 2019;22(2):132–141.

62. Yan T, Goldman RD. Recurrent epistaxis in children. *Can Fam Physician*. 2021;67(6):427–429.

63. Shay S, Shapiro NL, Bhattacharyya N. Epidemiological characteristics of pediatric epistaxis presenting to the emergency department [published correction appears in Int J Pediatr Otorhinolaryngol. 2018 Dec;115:193]. *Int J Pediatr Otorhinolaryngol*. 2017;103:121–124.

64. Schinco P, Castaman G, Coppola A, et al. Current challenges in the diagnosis and management of patients with inherited von Willebrand's disease in Italy: an Expert Meeting Report on the diagnosis and surgical and secondary long-term prophylaxis. *Blood Transfus*. 2018;16(4):371–381.

65. Kirolos A, Manti S, Blacow R, et al. A systematic review of clinical practice guidelines for the diagnosis and management of bronchiolitis. *J Infect Dis*. 2020;222(suppl 7):S672–S679. Erratum *J Infect Dis*. 2020;221(7):1204].

66. Milani GP, Bollati V, Ruggiero L, et al. Bronchiolitis and SARS-CoV-2. *Arch Dis Child*. 2021;106(10):999–1001.

67. Kyler KE, McCulloh RJ. Current concepts in the evaluation and management of bronchiolitis. *Infect Dis Clin North Am*. 2018;32(1):35–45.

68. Shanahan KH, Monuteaux MC, Nagler J, et al. Early use of bronchodilators and outcomes in bronchiolitis. *Pediatrics*. 2021;148(2):e2020040394.

69. Ralston SL, Lieberthal AS, Meissner HC, et al. Clinical practice guideline: the diagnosis, management, and prevention of bronchiolitis. *Pediatrics*. 2014;134(5):e1474–e1502. Erratum *Pediatrics*. 2015;136(4):782.

70. Wang G, Han D, Jiang Z, et al. Association between early bronchiolitis and the development of childhood asthma: a meta-analysis. *BMJ Open*. 2021;11(5):e043956.

71. Pfizer. Pfizer granted FDA breakthrough therapy designation for Respiratory Syncytial Virus (RSV) Vaccine Candidate for the Prevention of RSV in Infants from Birth up to Six Months of Age by Active Immunization of Pregnant Women. March 2, 2022. https://www.pfizer.com/news/press-release/press-release-detail/pfizer-granted-fda-breakthrough-therapy-designation.

72. Katz SE, Williams DJ. Pediatric community-acquired pneumonia in the United States: changing epidemiology, diagnostic and therapeutic challenges, and areas for future research. *Infect Dis Clin North Am*. 2018;32(1):47–63.

73. Kelly MS, Sandora TJ. Community-acquired pneumonia. In: Kliegman RM, St Geme JW, Blum NJ, et al., eds. *Nelson Textbook of Pediatrics*. 21st ed. Elsevier; 2020:2266–2274.

74. Smith DK, Kuckel DP, Recidoro AM. Community-acquired pneumonia in children: rapid evidence review. *Am Fam Physician*. 2021;104(6):618–625.

75. Krafft C, Christy C. *Mycoplasma* pneumonia in children and adolescents. *Pediatr Rev*. 2020;41(1):12–19.

76. Lipsett SC, Hall M, Ambroggio L, et al. Antibiotic choice and clinical outcomes in ambulatory children with community-acquired pneumonia. *J Pediatr*. 2021;229:207–215.e1.

77. CDC. *Most Recent National Asthma Data*; 2019. https://www.cdc.gov/asthma/most_recent_national_asthma_data.htm.

78. Tracy MK, Berkelhamer SK. Bronchopulmonary dysplasia and pulmonary outcomes of prematurity. *Pediatr Ann*. 2019;48(4):e148–e153.

79. Jensen EA, Dysart K, Gantz MG, et al. The diagnosis of broncho-pulmonary dysplasia in very preterm infants. An evidence-based approach. *Am J Respir Crit Care Med*. 2019;200(6):751–759.

80. Farrell PM, White TB, Ren CL, et al. Diagnosis of cystic fibrosis: consensus guidelines from the cystic fibrosis foundation. *J Pediatr*. 2017;181S:S4–S15.e1. Erratum J *Pediatr*. 2017;184:243.

81. Scotet V, L'Hostis C, Férec C. The changing epidemiology of cystic fibrosis: incidence, survival and impact of the *CFTR* gene discovery. *Genes (Basel)*. 2020;11(6):589.

82. Cystic Fibrosis Foundation. *CF Diagnosis Clinical Care Guidelines*; 2022. https://www.cff.org/medical-professionals/cf-diagnosis-clinical-care-guidelines#cf-diagnosis-clinical-care-guidelines.

83. Meng X, Clews J, Kargas V, et al. The cystic fibrosis transmembrane conductance regulator (CFTR) and its stability. *Cell Mol Life Sci*. 2017;74(1):23–38.

84. Schmidt H, Sharma G. *Sweat Testing*. National Library of Medicine; 2022. https://www.ncbi.nlm.nih.gov/books/NBK547728/.

85. Sun J, Li Y. Long-term, low-dose macrolide antibiotic treatment in pediatric chronic airway diseases. *Pediatr Res*. 2022;91(5):1036–1042.

86. Sathe MN, Freeman AJ. Gastrointestinal, pancreatic, and hepatobiliary manifestations of cystic fibrosis. *Pediatr Clin North Am*. 2016;63(4):679–698.

87. Hebra A. *Pectus Excavatum*; 2022. https://emedicine.medscape.com/article/1004953-overview#a6.

88. Koumbourlis AC. Pectus deformities and their impact on pulmonary physiology. *Paediatr Respir Rev*. 2015;16(1):18–24.

89. Alaca N, Yüksel M. Comparison of physical functions and psychosocial conditions between adolescents with pectus excavatum, pectus carinatum and healthy controls. *Pediatr Surg Int*. 2021;37(6):765–775.

90. Kempen DHR, Heemskerk JL, Kaçmaz G, et al. Pulmonary function in children and adolescents with untreated idiopathic scoliosis: a systematic review with meta-regression analysis. *Spine J*. 2022;22(7):1178–1190.

91. US Preventive Services Task Force, Grossman DC, Curry SJ, et al. Screening for adolescent idiopathic scoliosis: US preventive services task force recommendation statement. *JAMA*. 2018;319(2):165–172.

92. Zani A, Chung WK, Deprest J, et al. Congenital diaphragmatic hernia. *Nat Rev Dis Primers*. 2022;8(1):37.

93. Gupta VS, Harting MT. Congenital diaphragmatic hernia-associated pulmonary hypertension. *Semin Perinatol*. 2020;44(1):151167.

33

Cardiovascular Disorders

JENNIFER NEWCOMBE

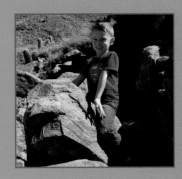

Most pediatric cardiovascular problems are due to congenital heart disease (CHD), which affects nearly 1% of all live births—or approximately 40,000 babies per year. Approximately one-quarter of these children have critical congenital heart disease (CCHD). CCHD is defined as disease requiring cardiac surgery or catheterization before 1 year of age. CHD is the leading cause of morbidity and mortality within the first year of life in children with congenital malformations.[1]

CHD survival is dependent on the defect severity and timely diagnosis.[1] CHDs may be detected by fetal ultrasound as early as 20 to 24 weeks of gestation or in the postdelivery period by pulse oximetry screening.[2] Many defects may also be detected by primary care providers (PCPs) through auscultation of a murmur during a physical examination.

This chapter presents information on both pediatric congenital and acquired heart disease. A thorough discussion of the examination and assessment of the cardiac system is included, as well as guidance for screening, identifying, and managing specific cardiovascular disorders in primary health care.

Anatomy and Physiology

Fetal Circulation

Knowledge of fetal circulation is essential for understanding the circulatory changes that occur in the newborn after delivery (Fig. 33.1). Fetal circulation has four unique features that differ from postnatal circulation:

- Blood oxygenation occurs in the placenta, not the lungs.
- Fetal pulmonary vascular resistance is high, and systemic vascular resistance is low (high pressure on the right side of the heart, low pressure on the left side).
- The foramen ovale, the opening in the septum between the two atria, permits a portion of the blood to flow from the right atrium directly to the left atrium.
- A patent ductus arteriosus (PDA) provides a connection between the pulmonary artery and the aorta, allowing blood to flow from the pulmonary artery to the aorta and bypass the fetal lungs.

Oxygen from the maternal uterine arteries diffuses into the fetal circulation via the placenta. The placenta delivers oxygenated blood through the umbilical vein to the fetus by diverting blood through the liver to the inferior vena cava (IVC) via the ductus venosus. When this well-oxygenated blood reaches the right atrium, it flows preferentially toward the atrial septum, through the foramen ovale, and into the left atrium. Oxygenated blood then flows into the left ventricle and out the aorta. Approximately two-thirds of the blood from the aorta flows toward the head and neck to ensure the fetal brain constantly receives well-oxygenated blood.[3] Venous blood returns from the head and upper extremities via the superior vena cava (SVC) to the right atrium. This blood preferentially flows toward the tricuspid valve into the right ventricle. From the right ventricle, the blood enters the pulmonary artery. Because pulmonary vascular resistance is high and systemic resistance is low, most blood in the pulmonary artery flows through the ductus arteriosus into the descending aorta to supply oxygen and nutrients to the trunk and lower extremities. Only a small amount of blood flows into the pulmonary circuit to perfuse the lungs.[3]

Fetal circulation is best described as two parallel circuits, with the left ventricle supplying blood to the upper extremities and the right ventricle serving the lower extremities and the placenta. During transition to extrauterine life, these separate blood flow circuits become a serial circuit.

Neonatal Circulation

Several complex events occur at birth that rapidly shift fetal circulation to the neonatal circulation pattern. Clamping the umbilical cord and subsequent loss of the placenta as the oxygenating organ causes an immediate circulatory change that requires the lungs to assume oxygenation. Cord clamping also causes an increase in systemic vascular resistance (systemic blood pressure [BP]). With the first breath, mechanical inflation of the lungs and an increase in oxygen saturation bring about a dramatic fall in pulmonary vascular resistance and an increase pulmonary blood flow. The increased oxygen saturation begins the process of constricting the ductus arteriosus. As the pressures within the heart become relatively higher on the left side and lower on the right, the foramen ovale closes. Functional closure of the ductus arteriosus and foramen ovale usually occurs within the first few hours to days of life, and the once-parallel pulmonary and systemic circulation now forms a closed circuit.

The obliteration of fetal structures by tissue growth or constriction is more gradual. Pulmonary vascular resistance drops gradually over the first 6 to 8 weeks of life, which protects the pulmonary circulation against volume overload in some congenital heart anomalies. If not noted earlier, shunt murmurs or symptoms of congestive heart failure (CHF) gradually become apparent as the infant approaches 8 weeks of life. At this time, pulmonary vascular resistance drops and shunting to the pulmonary bed increases.

Conditions that cause fetal shunt persistence allow unoxygenated blood to flow from the right side of the heart to the left. This may result in cyanosis or signs of congestive heart failure. Any murmur or cyanosis in a newborn merits prompt evaluation to detect and manage cardiac abnormalities.

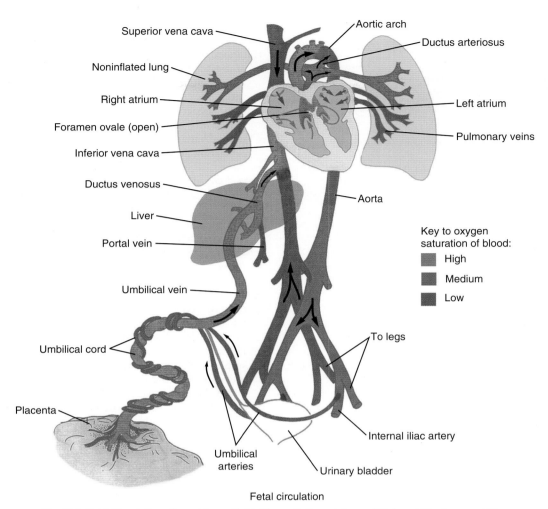

Superior vena cava
Noninflated lung
Right atrium
Foramen ovale (open)
Inferior vena cava
Ductus venosus
Liver
Portal vein
Umbilical vein
Umbilical cord
Placenta
Umbilical arteries
Aortic arch
Ductus arteriosus
Left atrium
Pulmonary veins
Aorta
Key to oxygen saturation of blood:
High
Medium
Low
To legs
Internal iliac artery
Urinary bladder

Fetal circulation

• **Fig. 33.1** Fetal Circulation. (From Murray S, McKinney E. *Foundations of Maternal-Newborn and Women's Health Nursing.* 8th ed. Elsevier; 2024.)

Normal Cardiac Structure and Function

The heart is a four-chambered muscular organ located in the mediastinum, the space in the chest between the lungs. The four chambers are divided into two larger muscular pumping chambers, the ventricles, and two smaller filling chambers, the atria. The heart has one-way valves that open and close in response to pressure changes within the heart, thus controlling blood flow from chamber to chamber. Desaturated systemic blood returns to the right atrium by way of the inferior and superior venae cavae. The blood passes from the right atrium through the tricuspid valve to the right ventricle. The tricuspid value has three cusps held in place by the chordate tendineae. The right ventricle pumps blood through the pulmonary valve into the pulmonary artery, which bifurcates into right and left arteries to allow flow into both lungs. This is where blood is oxygenated. Blood returning from the lungs enters the left atrium by way of the pulmonary veins (which contain no valves to allow easy blood flow into the atrium) and then passes through the mitral valve into the left ventricle. The high-pressured left ventricle pumps the blood through the aortic valve into the aorta to provide oxygenated blood for the systemic circulation.

Conduction System

Myocardial contraction is stimulated by electrical depolarization along the heart's conduction tract Depolarization begins at the sinoatrial (SA) node, which is high in the right atrial wall. This node acts as the heart's pacemaker by regularly beginning each heartbeat's depolarizing impulse. The depolarization wave travels from the SA node throughout the atria and produces atrial muscle contraction. The impulses move to the atrioventricular (AV) node, which is located in the lower portion of the right atrium at the junction of the atrium and ventricle. From the AV node, the depolarization wave passes through the bundle of His, with fibers extending from the AV node along the intraventricular septum. Depolarization spreads through the left and right bundle of His branches, through the Purkinje fibers, and extending into the ventricular muscle. Impulses then spread throughout the ventricles and cause contraction. The electrocardiogram (ECG) demonstrates this pattern of changing electrical impulses.

Cardiovascular System Assessment

History

Cardiac evaluation includes review of the family, maternal, fetal, neonatal, and infant medical history, in addition to growth and development. See Box 33.1 for a listing of CHD risk factors.

Physical Examination

Physical assessment of an individual with suspected CHD should be adapted to their age. Be flexible yet thorough in the evaluation and include all aspects of the physical examination in an order that best suits the patient's comfort and needs.

BOX 33.1 Risk Factors Associated With Congenital Heart Disease by Age and Family History

Perinatal
- Maternal infections and exposures (CMV, rubella, other viral syndromes)
- Maternal use of tobacco, alcohol, street drugs, retinoic acid, hydantoins, lithium, valproates, ibuprofen, naproxen, ACE inhibitors, tricyclic antidepressants, sulfonamides, sulfasalazines
- Maternal chronic disease (CHD, lupus, insulin-dependent diabetes, phenylketonuria)
- Maternal age at child's birth (increase in chromosomal abnormalities after 40 years old)
- Maternal pregnancy history (excessive weight gain, gestational diabetes)

Neonatal
- Fetal or newborn distress (aspiration, hypoxia, cyanosis)
- Prematurity (increased incidence of CHD in premature infants)
- Presence of associated anomalies (genetic or chromosomal abnormalities or syndromes)
- Neonatal infections (GBS)
- Birth weight (term infants <2500 g; SGA, less than two standard deviations from the mean for gestational age)

Infant
- Murmur at birth or early infancy
- Hypertension (at birth or beyond)
- Feeding difficulty (shortness of breath, easily fatigued, diaphoresis, poor intake)
- Cyanosis (increase with crying, feeding, exertion)
- Tachypnea (persistent, with crying, feeding)

Early/Middle Childhood, Adolescent
- Deviation from individual's normal growth and development
- Deviation from an activity level appropriate for chronologic age (unable to keep up with peers; unable to run or ride bike)
- Frequent respiratory tract infections (pneumonia, URIs that last longer than normal)
- Prior murmurs, blue spells
- Documented GABHS infection
- Hypertension (documented on a minimum of three separate visits)
- Chest pain with exertion
- Shortness of breath with exertion (beyond normal peers)
- Syncope or dizziness (especially associated with noted heart rate change)
- Tachycardia or bradycardia (fluttering in chest, racing heart)

Family History
- CHD (especially siblings, parents, first-degree relatives)
- Sudden death or premature myocardial infarction (before 50 years old; includes any deaths by drowning)
- Hypertension
- Rheumatic fever
- Genetic syndromes
- Hypercholesterolemia

ACE, Angiotensin-converting enzyme; CHD, congenital heart disease; CMV, cytomegalovirus; GABHS, group A β-hemolytic streptococci; GBS, group B streptococcus; SGA, small for gestational age; URI, upper respiratory infection.
Data from Richards A, Garg V. Genetics of congenital heart disease. Curr Cardiol Rev. 2010;6:91–97; and Sayasathid J, Sukonpan K, Somboonna N. Epidemiology and etiology of congenital heart diseases. In: Rao PS, Vidyasagar D, ed. Congenital Heart Disease: Selected Aspects. Cardiotext; 2021.

Vital Signs

Heart rate, respiratory rate, and BP vary considerably throughout childhood.

- *Heart rate* (Table 33.1): Heart rates should always be assessed by auscultation. Assessment should include rate and rhythm variations. An increased heart rate may be caused by excitement, anxiety, hyperthyroidism, heart disease, anemia, or fever. Irregularity may be caused by a normal sinus arrhythmia (the normal variation in heart rate that occurs with inhalation and exhalation and is more common in children than adults).
- *Pulses:* Palpate pulses in the upper and lower extremities and evaluate them for character (strength) and variation between the different sites. A bounding pulse may indicate a PDA or aortic insufficiency. Weak or "thready" pulses may indicate CHF or an obstructive lesion, such as severe aortic stenosis. Strong brachial pulses in conjunction with weak or absent femoral pulses may indicate coarctation of the aorta (CoA).
- *Blood pressure:* Healthy children and adolescents should have annual BP monitoring, beginning at age 3 years rather than at every health encounter. Individuals with obesity, kidney disease, diabetes, or known aortic arch disease should have BP taken at every appointment. Manual blood pressure assessment with sphygmomanometer is the preferred method. PCPs should check BPs in younger children if the index of suspicion for heart disease is high. It is important to always use a BP cuff that is appropriate for the child's size. The cuff width should be two-thirds the length of the upper arm measured from the axilla to the antecubital space. A cuff that is too narrow, too wide, or does not fit around an arm may cause an erroneous reading. Cuff sizes of 3, 5, 7, 12, and 18 cm should be on hand to accommodate the array of pediatric sizes. Initial evaluation should include pressure assessment in all four extremities: these should be equal, with pressure in the legs being slightly higher (10–20 mm Hg) in a child who walks. Measure lower extremity pressure with the stethoscope placed over the popliteal artery. If the blood pressure is higher than the 90th percentile, retake blood pressure two additional times and average the last two readings to determine the blood pressure.[4]
- *Respiratory rate:* Respiratory system evaluation includes the respiratory rate, respiratory effort, and breath sounds in all five lung lobes. It is important to evaluate the respiratory rate in a quiet infant or child. A respiratory rate greater than 40 breaths/min in a young child or 60 breaths/min in a newborn who is quiet, resting, and afebrile warrants further evaluation. An infant with CHD may be happily tachypneic and not show

TABLE 33.1 Normal Heart Rates (Beats/Min) in Infants and Children

Age	Resting (Awake)	Resting (Asleep)	Exercise/ Fever
Newborn	100–180	80–160	Up to 220
1 week–3 months	100–220	80–200	Up to 220
3 months–2 years	80–150	70–120	Up to 220
2–10 years	70–100	60–90	195–215
10–20 years	55–90	50–90	195–215

significant signs of grunting, intercostal retractions, nasal flaring, or tracheal tug (up and down movement of the trachea with each inspiration).

- *Oxygen saturation:* Oxygen saturation is an essential vital sign. Obtain oxygen saturations in newborns or children suspected of having a cardiac condition because cyanosis is not always readily perceptible. A joint statement by the American Academy of Pediatrics (AAP) and the American Heart Association (AHA) recommends that pulse oximetry screening be done on all newborns at 24 to 48 hours of life.[2]

General Appearance and Growth Parameters

The PCP should observe infants while obtaining the history and before proceeding with the complete physical examination. Observe general nutritional state, respiratory effort, color, physical abnormalities, and distress or discomfort level.

- Look for the presence of unusual facial characteristics (e.g., malformed ears, wide-spaced eyes, noticeable anomalies) or extracardiac anomalies (e.g., cleft lip or palate, polydactyly, microcephaly) that may be associated with a syndrome or chromosomal abnormality. Some children with conditions that are associated with CHD have characteristicfeatures, such as those seen with Down syndrome, Marfan syndrome (unusually tall with an arm span wider than the head-to-toe height), Turner syndrome (webbed neck, prominent ears), and fetal alcohol spectrum disorder (microcephaly and pinched facies).
- Assess overall skin color for signs of mottling or central cyanosis while the infant is at rest. Cyanosis caused by heart disease is detectable as a pale blue or ruddy red mucous membrane (lips, tongue, and nailbeds) color. The tongue is the best indicator because it lacks pigmentation and is abundantly perfused by the vascular system. Peripheral cyanosis or acrocyanosis, a blueness or pallor noted around the mouth and on the hands or feet, can be a normal variant, especially if it intensifies when the infant or young child is cold. Long-standing cyanosis may result in clubbing of the fingers and toes.
- Note any wheezing, nasal flaring, retractions, prominent neck veins, or head bobbing with respirations.
- Note peripheral or periorbital edema. Edema around the eyes may be evident in an infant with CHF even in the absence of peripheral edema of the hands or feet. True pitting edema of the feet is an unusual finding in an infant with CHF.
- Measure and plot height and weight on standardized charts including Down syndrome and Turner syndrome charts, as appropriate, at each assessment. Although many children with CHD fall within the normal height, weight, and development ranges, many individuals with heart disease experience poor weight gain, less than normal linear growth, and delays in achieving developmental milestones.

Palpation

Palpate all five areas of the chest: the aortic, pulmonic, tricuspid, and mitral areas and Erb's point (Fig. 33.2). Palpate the chest using the open palm of the hand near the base of the fingers. Gently move the hand across the chest to assess abnormal precordial activity, including pulsations, lifts, heaves, or thrills, and to determine the location of the apical impulse. The apical impulse is used to determine the heart size and is the most lateral point at which cardiac activity can be palpated. In infants and children, the impulse is normally palpated at the apex of the heart in the fourth intercostal space just to the left of the midclavicular line. At approximately 7 years old, the point shifts to the fifth intercostal

space. Cardiomegaly causes the apical impulse to shift laterally or downward.[5]

- Thrills are a palpable vibration caused by turbulent blood flow through abnormal structures or heart defects. The turbulent flow may be caused by valvular narrowing, stenosis, or defects, such as a ventricular septal defect (VSD).
- Assess peripheral pulses (radial, brachial, carotid, dorsalis pedis, and posterior tibial) for amplitude and intensity. In CoA, there may be decreased or absent femoral pulses and impulse lag with the radial pulse during simultaneous palpation. A fast pulse rate may indicate arrhythmia or CHF.
- Assess the liver and spleen for enlargement. Hepatomegaly is an important finding. Infants may normally have a palpable liver edge.
- The back should be examined for scoliosis, a finding that may be associated with CHD.

Heart Sounds Auscultation

- Auscultate the heart in the same manner for every patient by beginning at the base or apex of the heart. Ideally, assess heart sounds in a quiet environment when the patient is cooperative.
- Four individual heart sounds may be heard: S_1, S_2, S_3, and S_4. S_1 and S_2 are normal heart sounds, whereas the presence of S_3 or S_4 may indicate cardiac enlargement or volume overload.
- At each examination area, the provider should accurately identify the first (S_1) and second (S_2) heart sounds.
- S_1 has the following characteristics:
  - It is heard at the beginning of systole and indicates closure of AV valves (mitral and tricuspid). It is the "lubb" of the lubb-dupp.
  - It is often detected as a single sound. Even though the left side of the heart reacts slightly before the right side, the closure of the two values occurs so closely together that a single sound may be heard.

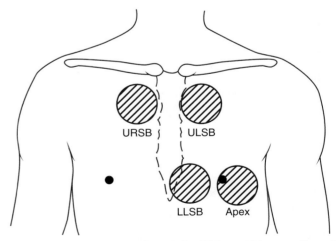

- **Fig. 33.2** Direction of Heart Sounds for Clicks and Murmurs (Auscultatory Areas Circled) With Associated Cardiac Conditions. *Upper right sternal border (URSB):* aortic valve clicks of aortic stenosis, venous hum. *Upper left sternal border (ULSB):* pulmonary valve clicks of pulmonary stenosis, pulmonary flow murmurs, atrial septal defect, patent ductus arteriosus, venous hum. *Lower left sternal border (LLSB):* ventricular septal defects, Still murmur, tricuspid valve regurgitation, hypertrophic cardiomyopathy, subaortic stenosis. *Apex:* aortic or mitral valve clicks, mitral valve regurgitation. *Erb point (left sternal border between 2nd and 3rd intercostal space):* aortic ejection click or aortic stenosis or dilated aortic root.

- It may be differentiated from early systolic clicks by the low sound frequency (clicks have a higher frequency). It is best heard with the diaphragm of the stethoscope.
  - It is usually loudest at the apex.
  - It is synchronous with the apical and carotid pulses.
- S_2 has the following characteristics:
  - It is caused of the aortic (A_2) and pulmonic (P_2) valve closure and marks the end of systole and onset of diastole. It is the "dupp" of lubb-dupp.
  - S_2 is normally split with inspiration in children because the pulmonic valve closure lags behind the aortic valve closure. S_2 becomes single with expiration. The intensity of S_2 splitting is one of the most important parts of the cardiac examination.
  - S_2 is best assessed at the upper left sternal border (ULSB) in the pulmonic area.
  - Pulmonary hypertension (HTN) causes early closure of P_2 and accentuation of S_2, which may sound like a loud, single second heart sound.
  - Absence of one of the semilunar valves (as in pulmonary atresia) causes single S_2.
  - Wide splitting of S_2, without becoming a single sound on expiration, may indicate increased pulmonary flow (typical of atrial septal defect [ASD]).
- S_3 and S_4 have the following characteristics:
  - S_3 is associated with rapid ventricular filling; it may be heard in a quiet infant or child with a rapid heart rate.
  - S_3 "gallop" is best heard at the apex with the stethoscope bell during early diastole. When combined with S_1 and S_2, S_3 sounds like the word "Kentucky." S_3 is easier to appreciate when the child is in the left lateral decubitus position.
  - S_4 is always pathologic; it is caused by increased force of atrial contraction and ventricular distention.
  - S_4 "gallop" sounds like the word "Tennessee" and is best heard in late diastole just before S_1.
  - S_4 is low-pitched and best heard at the apex with the stethoscope bell.
- Clicks: Ejection clicks are heard early in systole, immediately after S_1, and may sound like a split first heart sound. Pulmonic ejection clicks are high in frequency, vary with respiration, and disappear with inspiration. An aortic ejection click, heard best at Erb's point, is constant in intensity with a sound of a "snap" or a "click." Nonejection clicks are heard best in midsystole, or at the apex midway between S_1 and S_2 during the cardiac cycle. Clicks are best heard in the leaning forward or standing positions, can disappear with inspiration, and are due to mitral valve prolapse. Fig. 33.2 describes cardiac conditions associated with clicks.

Murmurs

All murmurs are intensified by factors that increase cardiac output (e.g., anemia, fever, exercise). It is important to remember significant heart defects may *not* cause a murmur because they may not result in turbulent blood flow (e.g., a large septal defect or nonrestrictive patent ductus). Fig. 33.2 shows auscultatory areas for different murmurs.

Criteria for Describing a Heart Murmur. Assess murmurs according to the criteria listed in Table 33.2. These are further illustrated in Fig. 33.3. Characteristics of pathologic murmurs needing referral are listed in Box 33.2. The presence of a murmur often causes great anxiety for a family. If the diagnosis is uncertain or there is a suspicion of heart disease, a referral to pediatric cardiology is warranted.

Innocent or Functional Murmurs. Up to 80% of children may have an innocent, physiologic, or "functional" murmur at some time during childhood. These are caused by normal blood flow through normal cardiac structures rather than by turbulent blood

TABLE 33.2 Describing a Heart Murmur

Heart Murmur	Description
Grade or intensity: • Does not necessarily indicate problem severity • May be altered with positional change from supine to sitting	Grade I: Barely audible; heard faintly after a period of attentive listening Grade II: Soft but easily audible Grade III: Moderately loud; no thrill Grade IV: Loud, present over widespread area; palpable thrill Grade V: Loud, audible with stethoscope barely on the chest; precordial thrill present Grade VI: Heard without stethoscope (rare)
Timing during cardiac cycle	Systolic Diastolic Continuous
Location on chest where murmur is loudest	Aortic or pulmonic listening areas, URSB, ULSB, Erb point, LLSB, apex
Radiations or transmission to other locations	To back To apex To carotids
Quality	Musical Harsh blowing
Duration	Point of onset and length of time systole and diastole murmurs last (e.g., "early systole, heard throughout cardiac cycle")
Pitch	Low Middle High

LLSB, Left lower sternal border; *ULSB,* upper left sternal border; *URSB,* upper right sternal border.

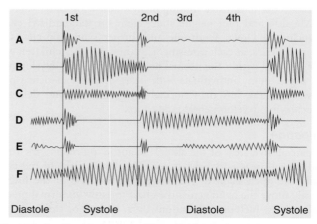

• **Fig. 33.3** Cardiac Murmurs on Phonocardiography. *A,* Normal phonocardiogram; *B,* systolic murmur (in aortic stenosis); *C,* systolic murmur (in mitral regurgitation); *D,* diastolic murmur (in aortic regurgitation); *E,* diastolic murmur (in mitral stenosis); *F,* continuous murmur (in patent ductus arteriosus). (From Khurana I, Khurana A. *Medical Physiology for Undergraduate Students.* 3rd ed. Elsevier; 2022.)

• BOX 33.2 Auscultation Findings: Innocent Versus Pathologic Murmur

Innocent Murmur

- Usually grade I to III/VI in intensity and localized
- Changes with position (sitting to lying)
- May vary in loudness or presence from visit to visit
- May increase in loudness (intensity) with fever, anemia, exercise, or anxiety
- Musical or vibratory in quality, sometimes blowing
- Systolic timing (except for venous hum, which is continuous), peaking in first half of systole
- Short duration
- Best heard in LLSB or pulmonic area (except for venous hum)
- Rarely transmitted
- May disappear with Valsalva maneuver, position, or gentle jugular pressure
- Vital signs: normal
- ECG: normal
- General health status: good

Possible Pathologic Murmur

- A murmur in a child with a syndrome associated with CHD (e.g., trisomy 21)
- Any diastolic murmur
- Any systolic murmur associated with a thrill
- Pansystolic murmurs
- Continuous murmurs that cannot be suppressed
- Systolic clicks
- Opening snaps
- Fixed splitting of the second heart sound not associated with bundle branch block
- An accentuated S_2
- S_4 gallops
- Not positional
- Grade IV/VI or higher
- Harsh quality

CHD, Congenital heart disease; *ECG,* electrocardiogram; *LLSB,* left lower sternal border.

---

flow caused by a defect or abnormal cardiac structures. Functional or innocent cardiac murmurs are common in children and may be evident in newborns. Table 33.3 describes common types of innocent murmurs; Box 33.2 describes the characteristics of an innocent murmur compared those of a pathologic murmur. Families and older children with innocent murmurs should be reassured that they are not caused by cardiac pathology. They should be informed the murmur may come and go and may be louder at times of fever, anemia, anxiety, pain, or exercise. A child's activities do not need to be limited, nor should any special precautions be taken.

Common Diagnostic Studies

If the PCP intends to refer a child for a pediatric cardiology consultation, performing routine diagnostic studies is not cost effective or necessary. The pediatric cardiology consultant can determine with greater discernment, which, if any, tests should be ordered.[5]

- Chest radiograph provides the following information: cardiac size and size of specific chambers and great vessels, cardiac contour, pulmonary blood flow status, and the lung and other surrounding tissue status (Fig. 33.4).
- ECG: The ECG monitors the electrical activity of the heart from different locations and in different planes of the body, giving information about ventricular contraction forces, heart rhythm, and the presence of hypertrophy and chamber dilation.
- Complete blood count (CBC): CBC rules out severe anemia or polycythemia as a murmur cause.
- Hyperoxia test: Supplementation of 100% oxygen results in "pinking" and increased arterial oxygen saturation when the disease is primarily pulmonary; minimal or no color improvement indicates the disease is cardiac. More commonly, simple pulse oximetry saturations are used to evaluate for cyanosis.

Other diagnostic studies usually done by cardiology may include the following:

- Echocardiogram: Echocardiography uses reflected sound waves to identify intracardiac structures and their motion. The types of recordings include two-dimensional, M-mode, contrast, Doppler, and tissue Doppler studies (Fig. 33.5). Fetal echocardiography can diagnose CHD as early as 16 to 18 weeks' gestation (high-frequency transvaginal echocardiography as early as 10 weeks' gestation), arrhythmias, and hemodynamic changes.[5]
- Cardiac catheterization: This provides information regarding the heart's anatomy, pulmonary vascular resistance, and cardiac output. This procedure can also be done to obtain a heart tissue sample, open narrow arteries or valves, or deploy devices to close holes in the heart or extra vessels.
- Magnetic resonance imaging (MRI): This is used to identify the heart structures and obtain information about chamber volumes and function.
- Exercise testing: A graded treadmill or bicycle ergometer is used to determine cardiac output (myocardial blood flow and rhythm) response to exercise and to assess endurance and capacity measurement.

Primary Healthcare Management Strategies

Due to advances in prenatal diagnosis and medical-surgical management, children with CHD are much more commonly seen in primary care than in prior decades. The goals of primary health care for a child with cardiovascular disease include the following:

- Adequate nutritional intake and optimal growth: Depending on the child's condition, diet modification to provide maximum calories or limit various types of foods may be needed. The young infant with CHF may need 24, 27, or 30 kcal per ounce formula or fortified breast milk. The child may need a nasogastric or gastric tube to obtain adequate calories because of an inadequate suck or fatigue with feeding. Children with cyanotic conditions may initially have adequate weight gain. Overweight or obese children with CHD need to be screened for associated comorbidities such as diabetes, HTN or nonalcoholic fatty liver.[6] The PCP should refer to a nutritionist, if available, for assistance with complex diets. (See Chapter 14 for further information on altered nutrition patterns.)
- Optimal psychosocial development and functioning: Discuss with the family the need to treat the child as normally as possible. Direct parents to support groups that provide informational and emotional support for all family members. Poor sibling bonding and unexpressed fears and anger in young siblings toward the child with a severe or chronic disease can affect their relationships and family dynamics for years to come. Psychological functioning and quality of life of children and adolescents with serious congenital heart defects may decrease as the number of cardiac interventions increased. PCPs should be familiar with signs of developmental delay that are common

TABLE 33.3	Common Innocent Murmurs	
Murmur	**Characteristics/Evaluation**	**Age of Occurrence**
Still's murmur	Localized between LLSB and apex Grade 1–3/6 systolic ejection (outflow murmur), decreasing with inspiration, when upright, or disappearing with Valsalva maneuver Low frequency, vibratory, musical in quality Often confused with VSD murmur	Most commonly heard at 2–7 years old
Peripheral pulmonic stenosis	Also known as *newborn pulmonary flow murmur* Heard at LUSB with radiation to back, axillae Grade 1–2/6 systolic ejection, crescendo-decrescendo	Often heard in premature infants, infants with low birth weight, and infants up to 4 months of age Need to document resolution by 4–5 months of age to rule out organic cause or valve involvement
Pulmonary ejection	Well localized to LUSB Grade 1–3/6 systolic ejection crescendo-decrescendo Heard loudest when supine and decreases or disappears with Valsalva maneuver Does not radiate Similar to ASD murmur, but S_2 is normal	Common in 8- to 14-year-olds with greatest frequency in adolescents
Venous hum	Heard best just below clavicles at either RUSB or LUSB Grade 1–3/6 low-frequency continuous murmur Loudest when sitting, diminishes or disappears when supine; can be increased by turning patient's head away from the side of the murmur, and can be obliterated by light jugular vein compression Can be mistaken for PDA	Common in 3- to 6-year-olds
Supraclavicular carotid bruit	Heard above the right or left clavicle with radiation to the neck Grade 1–3/6 holosystolic, crescendo-decrescendo Decreases or diminishes with shoulder hyperextension Can be confused with murmur of aortic stenosis	Common at any age

ASD, Atrial septal defect; *LLSB*, left lower sternal border; *LUSB*, left upper sternal border; *PDA*, patent ductus arteriosus; *RUSB*, right upper sternal border; *VSD*, ventricular septal defect.

Data from Park M. *Pediatric Cardiology for Practitioners*, 6th ed. Elsevier; 2014.

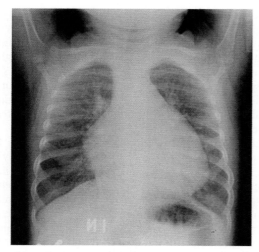

• **Fig. 33.4** Chest Radiograph of a 3-Month-Old With Ventricular Septal Defect and Congestive Heart Failure. Cardiomegaly with increased pulmonary vascular markings from pulmonary venous congestion is visible.

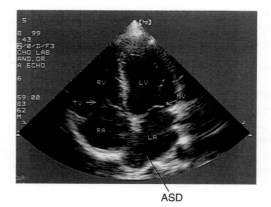

ASD

• **Fig. 33.5** Echocardiogram of a 2-Year-Old With an Atrial Septal Defect *(ASD)*. *LA*, Left atrium; *LV*, left ventricle; *MV*, mitral valve; *RA*, right atrium; *RV*, right ventricle; *TV*, tricuspid valve.

in children with congenital heart defects. Table 33.4 lists common signs that merit assessment and early intervention.

- Preventive vaccines: Live virus vaccines should be delayed until 6 months after cardiopulmonary bypass and exposure to red blood cells and plasma.[7] This most often affects 1-year-old infants who are due for varicella and measles, mumps, and rubella vaccines. Other vaccines should be given on a regular schedule. The AAP recommends providing respiratory syncytial virus (RSV) prophylaxis for infants younger than 1 year who have cyanotic or complicated CHD, especially those with CHF or pulmonary HTN. According to AAP guidelines, infants should receive a maximum of five doses (15 mg/kg intramuscularly every 30 days) during RSV season.[8] Anyone older than 19 years and spends time with infants should have the Tdap vaccine, regardless of the interval since the last Td vaccine to prevent pertussis.[9] The CDC currently recommends using a new vaccine, nirsevimab-alip (Beyfortus), as an alternative to prophylaxis.[9] Nirsevimab is a monoclonal antibody that is indicated in infants younger than 8 months born in or entering their first RSV season and again in their second season (up to 24 months) who have significant CHD. It is administered as a one-time intramuscular injection prior to the RSV season.[9]
- Prevention of avoidable complications: Emphasize preventing respiratory infections through good hand washing and avoiding contact (if possible) with others with upper respiratory infection (URI) symptoms. Vaccination against seasonal influenza is prudent for infants and family members/caregivers per Centers for Disease Control and Prevention guidelines.

TABLE 33.4	Common Signs of Developmental Delay in Children With Congenital Heart Disease
Domain	**Developmental Delay or Deficits**
Cognition	Decreased ability to process information Signs of intellectual disorder
Speech and language	Demonstrates difficulty with articulating or pronouncing language Has oral-motor delays
Motor	Demonstrates deficits in fine motor skills Has difficulties with the strength or coordination of gross motor skills as demonstrated by changes in strength, balance, endurance, manual dexterity, or visual-spatial-motor integration
Memory	Demonstrates difficulty with visual or verbal memory
Behavioral	Demonstrates symptoms of depression, anxiety, attention-deficit/hyperactivity disorder Demonstrates difficulty with emotional regulation or shows inappropriate aggression
School and social	Requires additional educational support Demonstrates difficulties communicating with peers and maintaining relationships with peers
Quality of life	Has alterations in ability to perform age-appropriate activities of daily living Has difficulties with psychosocial developmental tasks including psychosexual development

Modified from Lisanti AJ, et al. Developmental care for hospitalized infants with complex congenital heart disease: a science advisory from the American Heart Association. *J Am Heart Assoc.* 2022:e7967.

- Preventing infective endocarditis (IE): Although uncommon in children, IE (also called *subacute bacterial endocarditis* [SBE]) is associated with significant morbidity and mortality rates and warrants primary prevention when indicated. SBE prophylaxis standards for individuals undergoing dental procedures are available in Box 33.3 and Table 33.5. A high index of suspicion for IE should be maintained if any unusual clinical findings (e.g., petechiae, fever) are present after any procedure. Compared to other individuals, people affected by CHD have more severe gingival inflammatory conditions and a concomitant increase in *Haemophilus* species, *Actinobacillus actinomycetemcomitans, Cardiobacterium hominis, Eikenella corrodens,* and *Kingella* species (HACEK) and other microbes known to cause endocarditis. The reason for this is not clear. Good dental hygiene is extremely important for these individuals.
- Optimal fitness: Counsel parents and children on the importance of daily physical activity and limiting sedentary behavior. The initial goal is to develop habitual physical activity, including all types of physical movement, not just organized exercise designed to increase fitness. Certain children and adolescents, such as those with ventricular arrhythmias, need complete activity restrictions (see Chapter 18, Table 18.6 for the sports participation parameters for individuals with cardiac diseases or conditions). Children who have motor skill delays, often due to perioperative morbidity, tend to have more sedentary lifestyles and may need encouragement to become more active.
- Before discussing physical activity, physical assessment should include a detailed history of exertional symptoms, such as angina, excessive dyspnea, palpitations, dizziness, and syncope (see Chapter 18, Box 18.7 for the 14-element cardiovascular screening checklist for congenital and genetic heart disease).
- Assessment of capacity for physical activity should also include current behavior, motor skills (and expected skill development that will be required), motivation, anticipated time spent in physical activity, and type of activity. Reassure the parents that the child generally self-limits activity according to ability. If the child can comfortably talk during the activity, they will automatically limit their activity intensity. The cardiology provider should be consulted regarding exercise limitations before participation in sports or any activities that require strenuous physical exertion.
- Optimal neurodevelopmental adaptation to school and life tasks. Children who require heart surgery in the first year of

---

• BOX 33.3 Cardiac Conditions Associated With the Highest Risk of Endocarditis: Prophylaxis for Dental Procedures Recommended

- Prosthetic cardiac valve(s) or prosthetic material used for cardiac valve repair
- Previous infective endocarditis
- Congenital heart disease (CHD)
  - Unrepaired cyanotic CHD including palliative shunts and conduits
  - Completely repaired CHD with prosthetic material or device(s) by surgery or interventional catheterization, for 6 months after repair (due to the endothelialization of prosthetic material within that period)
  - Repaired CHD with residual defects (e.g., residual VSD) at the site or adjacent to the site of a prosthetic patch or device
- Cardiac transplantation recipients who have valve disease

TABLE 33.5	**Prophylactic Antibiotic Regimens for Dental Procedures**		

| Situation | Agent | REGIMEN: SINGLE DOSE 30–60 MINUTES BEFORE PROCEDURE | |
		Adults	Children
Oral	Amoxicillin	2 g	50 mg/kg
Unable to take oral medication	Ampicillin *or*	2 g IM or IV	50 mg/kg IM or IV
	Cefazolin or ceftriaxone	1 g IM or IV	50 mg/kg IM or IV
Allergic to penicillins or ampicillin—oral regimen	Cephalexin[a,b] *or*	2g	50 mg/kg
	Azithromycin or clarithromycin *or*	500 mg	15 mg/kg
	Doxycycline	100 mg	<45kg, 2.2 mg/kg >45kg, 100 mg
Allergic to penicillins or ampicillin and unable to take oral medication	Cefazolin or ceftriaxone[b]	1 g IM or IV	50 mg/kg IM or IV

[a]Or other first- or second-generation oral cephalosporin in equivalent adult or pediatric dosage.

[b]Cephalosporins should not be used in an individual with a history of anaphylaxis, angioedema or urticaria with penicillins or ampicillin.

IM, Intramuscular; *IV,* intravenous.

From Wilson WR, Gewitz M, Lockhart PB, et al. Prevention of *Viridans* group streptococcal infective endocarditis: a scientific statement from the American Heart Association. *Circulation.* 2021;143:e963–e978.

life can have significant neurodevelopmental impairment. Risk factors that predict worse neurodevelopmental outcomes include genetic syndromes, low birth weight, single ventricle physiology, low socioeconomic status, low maternal education, the need for cardiopulmonary resuscitation (CPR), duration of mechanical ventilation, duration of intensive care unit stay, gestational age at time of surgery, and preoperative intubation. Only a few of these are amenable to modification in the surgical period. However, early recognition of and intervention for developmental and cognitive delays lead to improved neurodevelopmental outcomes. Most children with neurocognitive impairment have average intelligence scores, but many have difficulties with visuospatial tasks, fine motor functions, higher-order language skills, memory, and/or attention. They may have impaired ability to coordinate lower-order skills or perform higher-order tasks. Children with delays in executive function and attention may be predisposed to mental health issues. It is important the PCP screen for psychiatric comorbidities.[6]

Referral

If a PCP suspects cardiac disease or is unsure about findings, it is best to refer the patient to a pediatric cardiologist. Findings suggestive of cardiac disease include nonstressed and presumably healthy infants with oxygen saturation less than 95%, CHF symptoms, a pathologic murmur, or a murmur that is difficult to differentiate in the presence of poor growth and development. A child with a murmur who is otherwise doing well should be referred to a pediatric cardiologist for further evaluation in a timely but not urgent manner. Newborns should be evaluated within 1 or 2 days of noticeable signs or immediately (change in breathing patterns, increased irritability, and poor feeding, and/or cyanosis) depending on their symptom severity. An older child with dizziness, chest pain with exertion, arrhythmia, dyspnea, syncope, signs of CHF, or abnormal vital signs should be referred as soon as possible.[5] Some defects, such as small VSDs or bicuspid aortic valves, escape early detection and may cause no disability. However, they should be identified as these defects pose a risk for bacterial endocarditis and thrombotic cerebrovascular accident.

Genetic Testing

Genetic testing should be performed in individuals who have, in addition to CHD, other congenital anomalies, dysmorphic features, neurocognitive deficits, growth retardation, mothers with a history of multiple miscarriages, or siblings with congenital defects.[10] Approximately 35% of CHD are attributed to genetic factors. There are several testing modalities; however, patients' clinical findings and family history determine which genetic test is appropriate. Consultation with a pediatric geneticist may be beneficial. Table 33.6 lists the most common genetic syndromes, aneuploidies, single gene defects, and microdeletions associated with heart disease.

Family Support

Families need the PCP support to help them understand the diagnosis and to cope with short- and long-term consequences. Because of the stress at time of diagnosis, many parents cannot absorb the information presented and may need multiple opportunities to ask questions.

Parents and their designated support people should clearly understand the diagnosis, have diagrams of the defect, and general information to take home for future reference. If medication is necessary, parents should understand the reason for the drug, administration regimen, and potential side effects. Parents should also understand the signs and symptoms of deterioration (e.g., CHF) and have clear information regarding how to proceed should symptoms develop. Infant and child CPR certification is critical for anyone caring for a child with a heart condition.

TABLE 33.6	Congenital Malformation Syndromes Associated With Selected Congenital Heart Disease
Syndrome	**Features**
Chromosomal Disorders	
Trisomy 21 (Down syndrome)	Endocardial cushion defect, VSD, ASD
Trisomy 21p (cat-eye syndrome)	Miscellaneous, total anomalous pulmonary venous return
Trisomy 18	VSD, ASD, PDA, TOF, coarctation of aorta, bicuspid aortic or pulmonary valve
Trisomy 13	VSD, ASD, PDA, coarctation of aorta, bicuspid aortic or pulmonary valve
Trisomy 9	Miscellaneous, VSD
XXXXY	PDA, ASD
Penta X	PDA, VSD
Triploidy	VSD, ASD, PDA
XO (Turner syndrome)	Bicuspid aortic valve, coarctation of aorta
Fragile X	Mitral valve prolapse, aortic root dilatation
Duplication 3q2	Miscellaneous
Deletion 4p	VSD, PDA, aortic stenosis
Deletion 9p	Miscellaneous
Deletion 5p (cri du chat syndrome)	VSD, PDA, ASD, TOF
Deletion 10q	VSD, TOF, conotruncal lesions[a]
Deletion 13q	VSD
Deletion 18q	VSD
Deletion 1p36	ASD, VSD, PDA, TOF, cardiomyopathy
Deletion/duplication 1q21.1	ASD, VSD, PS
Deletion 17q11 (William syndrome)	Supravalvar AS, branch PS
Deletion 11q 24-25 (Jacobsen syndrome)	VSD, left-sided lesions
Syndrome Complexes	
CHARGE association (*c*oloboma, *h*eart, *a*tresia choanae, growth *r*etardation, *g*enital, and *e*ar anomalies)	VSD, ASD, PDA, TOF, endocardial cushion defect
DiGeorge sequence, CATCH 22 (*c*ardiac defects, *a*bnormal facies, *t*hymic aplasia, *c*left palate, *h*ypocalcemia, and deletion 22q11)	Aortic arch anomalies, conotruncal anomalies
Alagille syndrome (arteriohepatic dysplasia)	Peripheral pulmonic stenosis, PS, TOF
VATER association (*v*ertebral, *a*nal, *t*racheo*e*sophageal, *r*adial, and *r*enal anomalies)	VSD, TOF, ASD, PDA
FAVS (*f*acio *a*uriculo*v*ertebral *s*pectrum)	TOF, VSD
CHILD (*c*ongenital *h*emidysplasia with *i*chthyosiform erythroderma, *l*imb *d*efects)	Miscellaneous
Mulibrey nanism (muscle, liver, brain, eye)	Pericardial thickening, constrictive pericarditis
Asplenia syndrome	Complex cyanotic heart lesions with decreased pulmonary blood flow, transposition of great arteries, anomalous pulmonary venous return, dextrocardia, single ventricle, single atrioventricular valve
Polysplenia syndrome	Acyanotic lesions with increased pulmonary blood flow, azygos continuation of inferior vena cava, partial anomalous pulmonary venous return, dextrocardia, single ventricle, common atrioventricular valve
PHACE syndrome (*p*osterior brain fossa anomalies, facial *h*emangiomas, *a*rterial anomalies, *c*ardiac anomalies and aortic coarctation, *e*ye anomalies)	VSD, PDA, coarctation of aorta, arterial aneurysms

Continued

TABLE 33.6 Congenital Malformation Syndromes Associated With Selected Congenital Heart Disease—Cont'd

Syndrome	Features
Teratogenic Agents	
Congenital rubella	PDA, peripheral pulmonic stenosis
Fetal hydantoin syndrome	VSD, ASD, coarctation of aorta, PDA
Fetal alcohol syndrome	ASD, VSD
Fetal valproate effects	Coarctation of aorta, hypoplastic left side of heart, aortic stenosis, pulmonary atresia, VSD
Maternal phenylketonuria	VSD, ASD, PDA, coarctation of aorta
Retinoic acid embryopathy	Conotruncal anomalies
Others	
Apert syndrome	VSD
Autosomal dominant polycystic kidney disease	Mitral valve prolapse
Carpenter syndrome	PDA
Conradi syndrome	VSD, PDA
Crouzon disease	PDA, coarctation of aorta
Cutis laxa	Pulmonary hypertension, pulmonic stenosis
De Lange syndrome	VSD
Ellis–van Creveld syndrome	Single atrium, VSD
Holt-Oram syndrome	ASD, VSD, first-degree heart block
Infant of diabetic mother	Hypertrophic cardiomyopathy, VSD, conotruncal anomalies
Kartagener syndrome	Dextrocardia
Meckel-Gruber syndrome	ASD, VSD
Noonan syndrome	Pulmonic stenosis, ASD, cardiomyopathy
Pallister-Hall syndrome	Endocardial cushion defect
Primary ciliary dyskinesia	Heterotaxia disorders
Rubinstein-Taybi syndrome	VSD
Scimitar syndrome	Hypoplasia of right lung, anomalous pulmonary venous return to inferior vena cava
Smith-Lemli-Opitz syndrome	VSD, PDA
TAR syndrome (thrombocytopenia and absent radius)	ASD, TOF
Treacher Collins syndrome	VSD, ASD, PDA

aConotruncal includes TOF, pulmonary atresia, truncus arteriosus, and transposition of great arteries.

ASD, Atrial septal defect; *AV*, aortic valve; *PDA*, patent ductus arteriosus; *PS*, pulmonary stenosis; *TOF*, tetralogy of Fallot; *VSD*, ventricular septal defect.

From Kliegman RM, St. Geme III GW, Blum NJ, et al. *Nelson Textbook of Pediatrics.* 21st ed. Elsevier; 2020.

Congenital Heart Disease

When an individual is diagnosed with CHD, parents may incorrectly assume they are somehow responsible for the child's defect. Healthcare professionals must be clear about what is and what is not known about CHD to help allay needless worry and guilt.

CHD is caused by a developmental alteration in, or failure of, embryonic heart development in early embryologic development. This alteration occurs in the second to eighth weeks of gestation and is caused by genetic, environmental, or multifactorial influences. Most CHD cases have no identifiable cause. The discovery of the human genome and advances in molecular techniques identified more genetic factors in CHD. This is increasingly important as more children with CHD survive into childbearing years.

A positive family history of CHD is a risk factor. The risk of reoccurrence after an affected child is about 2% to 5%. The risk is also higher if one parent has CHD. The risk of reoccurrence is higher if a mother is carrier (10%–15%) compared to a father (2%).[11]

Two percent to 4% of CHDs are caused by teratogens, maternal conditions, or environmental influences. Drugs or teratogens linked to CHD include lithium, retinoic acid, antiepileptics, ibuprofen and naproxen, angiotensin-converting enzyme (ACE) inhibitors, tricyclic antidepressants, sulfonamides, sulfasalazine, tobacco, alcohol, cocaine, and marijuana.[5] Environmental exposures to organic solvents, pesticides, and air pollution are also implicated in CHD. It is best to avoid exposure to these agents during the vulnerable period (2–8 weeks of gestation), although often women do not know they are pregnant at this stage. Maternal illnesses (e.g., diabetes mellitus, connective tissue disorders, phenylketonuria, rubella, and febrile illnesses—especially influenza) are associated with CHD[5] (see Box 33.1).

Specific Congenital Heart Diseases

Congestive Heart Failure

CHF is a progressive clinical and pathophysiologic syndrome found in many individuals with heart problems. The symptoms vary with age of the patient and the root cardiac problem (Box 33.4). Besides functional changes, CHF is marked by cardiac neurohormonal and molecular changes.

Pediatric CHF can be caused by congenital malformations leading to ventricular dysfunction, pressure, or volume overload. CHF also occurs in individuals with structurally normal hearts and is caused by cardiomyopathy, arrhythmias, ischemia, toxins, or infections (Table 33.7). The American College of Cardiology and the AHA heart failure classifications help healthcare providers categorize patients.[12]

The largest group of pediatric patients with CHF are those with excessive left-to-right shunting through unrepaired congenital defects. CHF is somewhat of a misnomer in these cases because the myocardium generally responds quite well to the challenge of excessive blood volume for a long time, and cardiac output remains adequate. However, the compensatory response to this excessive workload for the lungs and some heart chambers includes electrolyte and fluid imbalances, and neurohormonal changes. Patients with heart failure from systolic or diastolic cardiac dysfunction caused by infections, obstruction, or arrhythmias need treatment to ameliorate fluid and electrolyte imbalances, increase contractility, and decrease cardiac afterload.

Depending on the underlying pathophysiology, those with CHF have elevated neurohormonal and inflammatory mediators (aldosterone, norepinephrine, natriuretic peptides, tumor necrosis factor, and renin). Due to limited randomized controlled trials to assess the efficacy of oral therapy in CHF, understanding of the management of heart failure primarily comes from studies of adults. Large-scale studies in adult populations show the value of blocking the neurohormonal and immune mechanisms with agents such as aldosterone inhibitors, angiotensin inhibitors, and sympathetic inhibitors (β-blockers). Clinical evidence suggests pediatric patients with advanced heart failure may benefit from an aldosterone antagonist coadministered with an ACE inhibitor and a β-blocker.[12]

The traditional heart failure therapies (i.e., diuretics, inotropes, and after load reducers) are used in many heart failure cases. Patients with chronic recurrent fluid overload may benefit from fluid restriction. The degree of fluid restriction depends on diuretic refractoriness, nutritional status, and the presence of electrolyte imbalance.[12]

• BOX 33.4   Signs and Symptoms of Congestive Heart Failure

Infants
- Tachypnea
- Tachycardia
- Rales or wheezing
- Cardiomegaly and hepatomegaly
- Periorbital edema
- Poor feeding/tires easily when feeding
- Poor weight gain
- Diaphoresis

Children and Teens
- Tachypnea
- Tachycardia
- Rales or wheezing
- Cardiomegaly and hepatomegaly
- Orthopnea
- Shortness of breath or dyspnea with exertion
- Peripheral edema
- Poor growth and development

TABLE 33.7   Conditions Associated With Pediatric Congestive Heart Failure

Age	Condition
Premature infant	Patent ductus arteriosus (PDA)
Birth–1 week	Hypoplastic left heart syndrome (HLHS)
	Coarctation of the aorta (COA)
	Critical aortic stenosis
	Interrupted aortic arch
	Arteriovenous malformations
	Tachycardia
	Cardiomyopathy
1 week–3 months	Ventricular septal defect (VSD)
	Truncus arteriosus
	Atrioventricular (AV) canal (endocardial cushion defect)
	Total anomalous pulmonary venous return
	Coarctation
	Tachycardia
	PDA
	Aortic stenosis
	Tricuspid atresia
Older than 1 year	Bacterial endocarditis
	Rheumatic fever
	Myocarditis

Left-to-Right Shunting Congenital Heart Disease (Acyanotic)

Pulmonary overflow lesions result in communication between the two sides of the heart through which extra blood shunts from the high-pressure, oxygenated left side of the heart to the low-pressure, deoxygenated right side of the heart. The result is an increase in pulmonary blood flow. These lesions are acyanotic. Fig. 33.6 lists the various left-to-right versus right-to-left shunting disorders.

Atrial Septal Defect. An ASD is a defect or hole in the atrial septum and accounts for 5% to 10% of all CHD.[5] ASDs occur alone or as part of more complex heart disease. Of the four types of ASDs, the most common involves the midseptum around the

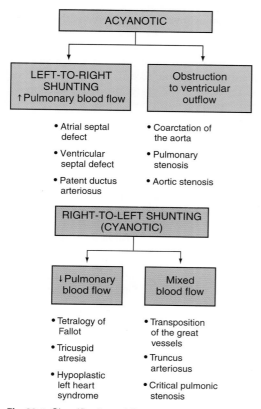

ACYANOTIC

- LEFT-TO-RIGHT SHUNTING ↑Pulmonary blood flow
  - Atrial septal defect
  - Ventricular septal defect
  - Patent ductus arteriosus

- Obstruction to ventricular outflow
  - Coarctation of the aorta
  - Pulmonary stenosis
  - Aortic stenosis

RIGHT-TO-LEFT SHUNTING (CYANOTIC)

- ↓Pulmonary blood flow
  - Tetralogy of Fallot
  - Tricuspid atresia
  - Hypoplastic left heart syndrome

- Mixed blood flow
  - Transposition of the great vessels
  - Truncus arteriosus
  - Critical pulmonic stenosis

• **Fig. 33.6** Classification of Congenital Heart Disease.

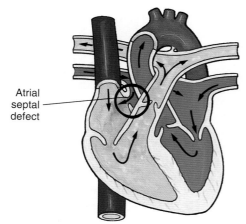

Atrial septal defect

• **Fig. 33.7** Atrial Septal Defect. (From Hockenberry MJ, Duffy EA, Gibbs K. *Wong's Nursing Care of Infants and Children.* 12th ed. Elsevier; 2024.)

foramen ovale and is called an *ostium secundum–type defect* (Fig. 33.7). Defects of the sinus venosus type occurs high in the atrial septum, near the entry of the SVC or low near the IVC and are frequently associated with anomalous pulmonary venous return. A primum ASD occurs in the lower septal portion and is most often seen in children with Down syndrome. The rarest form of ASD is an unroofed coronary sinus occurring in less than 1% of ASDs. Usually ASDs occur spontaneously; however, there are a few identified genetic mutations that cause familial ASDs such as a *ACTC1* gene mutation or *NKX2-5*.[5]

Clinical Findings

History. Most individuals with ASDs are completely asymptomatic or fatigue easily, have exertional dyspnea, are somewhat thin, and have a history of frequent upper respiratory tract infections or pneumonia. Symptoms become more common in late adolescence or early adulthood.

Physical Examination
- Typically, a murmur is not noticed until the child is 2 to 3 years old.
- Possible mild left anterior chest bulge or palpable lift at the left sternal border.
- S_1 is normal or split, with tricuspid valve closure sound accentuation.
- S_2 is often split widely and relatively fixed.
- A grade I to III/VI, widely radiating, medium-pitched, not harsh, systolic crescendo-decrescendo murmur is heard best at the pulmonic area. This murmur is not due to flow across the atrial septum but is due to increased flow across the pulmonary valve.

Diagnostic Studies
- Chest radiography may reveal cardiac enlargement, especially of the right atrium and right ventricle. The main pulmonary artery may be dilated, and pulmonary vascular markings increased.
- Obtain an ECG to assess for PR prolongation. The ECG shows right axis deviation with right atrial enlargement. Lead V_1 usually shows a right bundle branch block with an rSR pattern. P wave may be tall, showing right atrial enlargement. The PR interval may be prolonged. However, the ECG may be normal in small left-to-right defects.
- The echocardiogram identifies the specific defect location in the atrial septum and shows right-sided chamber enlargement.
- Cardiac catheterization is rarely necessary unless the diagnosis is in doubt, the site of pulmonary venous return is questionable, or when transcatheter device closure is planned.[5]

Management
- Small defects found in infancy may close spontaneously.
- Larger defects require intervention, usually after the child is 1 year old, before school entry, or when the defect is identified in an older child or adolescent. Most small to moderate ostium secundum ASDs can be closed percutaneously in the cardiac catheterization laboratory if the child weighs more than 15 kg and there are adequate margins to anchor the device. If the defect is large or unfavorable for device closure, cardiac surgery is indicated. Surgical mortality rate is less than 0.5%.[5]
- SBE prophylaxis (see Table 33.5) precautions are necessary only in the first 6 months after cardiac surgery or device closure. Low-dose aspirin is prescribed for 6 months after transcatheter device closure.[13]
- Long-term outcome is excellent after ASD repair. However, there is a small incidence of atrial arrhythmias due to the atriotomy scar.[14]

- If untreated, ASDs can result in right ventricular enlargement, fibrosis, and failure. Although rare in children, paradoxical emboli can occur (a thrombus transverses the intracardiac defect and enters the systemic circulation). Some with uncorrected ASDs develop severe irreversible pulmonary HTN that is disabling and life shortening.[5]
- Exercise restriction is unnecessary.[5]

Ventricular Septal Defect. A VSD is a hole or defect in the ventricular septum and accounts for 37% of all CHDs (Fig. 33.8).[15] There are four types of VSDs: perimembranous, supracristal (occurs in the outflow part of the right ventricle above crista supraventricularis), inlet, and muscular. The most common type is the perimembranous VSD. VSDs are associated with many congenital defects, but 95% of individuals with VSD do not have a chromosomal anomaly (see Table 33.7). Approximately 30% to 50% of these defects are small; the vast majority of these spontaneously close by 4 years of age.[5]

Clinical Findings
History
- Often, a murmur is not heard immediately after birth. When pulmonary vascular resistance falls (normally at 2–8 weeks old), more blood shunts across the VSD from left ventricle to right ventricle, and into the pulmonary circulation. This causes a classic loud murmur. Early signs and symptoms of CHF also begin at this time.
- Parents may notice the signs and symptoms of CHF (see Box 33.4).
- Small defects may be completely asymptomatic at birth and become symptomatic by 6 months old.

Physical Examination
- Small VSD
  - Harsh, high-pitched, grade II to IV/VI holosystolic murmur at lower left sternal border (LLSB).
  - All other findings within normal limits.
- Large VSD
  - Low-pitched, grade II to V/VI holosystolic murmur at LLSB.
  - VSD murmur that becomes higher pitched over time indicates the defect is becoming smaller.
  - Diastolic rumble at the apex.
  - Thrill along the left sternal border.
  - Signs of progressing CHF after the first weeks of life.
  - Presence of S_3 or S_4 gallop if patient has CHF.

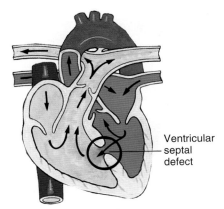

- **Fig. 33.8** Ventricular Septal Defect. (From Hockenberry MJ, Duffy EA, Gibbs K. *Wong's Nursing Care of Infants and Children.* 12th ed. Elsevier; 2024.)

Diagnostic Studies
- Chest radiography findings vary depending on the shunt's size. Children with small shunts have a normal heart size and pulmonary vascular markings that are just beyond the upper limits of normal. Those with large shunts have cardiac enlargement involving both ventricles and the left atrium, and significantly increased pulmonary vascular markings (see Fig. 33.4).
- The ECG is normal with small defects and may show left ventricular hypertrophy (LVH) or biventricular hypertrophy (BVH) with large shunts.
- Echocardiography provides defect visualization and pinpoints the exact anatomic location. In "pinhole" VSDs, a murmur may be present but a defect may not be visualized on the echocardiogram.
- Cardiac catheterization is rarely necessary except when there is a question of elevated pulmonary vascular resistance or when transcatheter closure of a muscular VSD is expected. A transcatheter device can only be used in children weighing more than 5 kg.[13]

Management
- Infants with small defects and no CHF symptoms are monitored every 6 months during the first year of life, then every 2 years thereafter to assess for VSD closure. Some defects may never close and cause no difficulty. SBE prophylaxis is not recommended.
- Larger defects that result in CHF are managed as follows:
  - Lanoxin, diuretics, ACE inhibitors, or β-blockers may be prescribed by cardiology.
  - Nutritional intake and weight gain must be monitored. It is important to teach families to fortify an infant's calories to 24, 27, or 30 kcal/oz, as needed. Arrange for enteric nutritional support via nasogastric tube for young infants struggling to meet their caloric needs.
  - Families should be taught the signs and symptoms of developing or progressing CHF.
  - Surgery or percutaneous device closure can be performed if symptomatic lesions do not improve. The long-term outcome is excellent after repair.[5] Potential complications after VSD repair include residual VSD, aortic insufficiency secondary to aortic cusp prolapse, or arrhythmias.[5]
  - SBE prophylaxis is necessary for 6 months after surgery (see Box 33.3 and Table 33.5).

Atrioventricular Septal Defect (Atrioventricular Canal Defect or Endocardial Cushion Defect). The endocardial cushion is a central cardiac structure that includes the septal portions of the mitral and tricuspid valves, the lower portion of the atrial septum, and the upper portion of the ventricular septum. Variable portions of the endocardial cushion are absent. Complete AV septal defect includes the absence of this cushion, leading to a primum ASD, a single AV valve (composed of leaflets of the intended mitral and tricuspid valves), and an inlet VSD. There may also be partial, transitional, and intermediate defects with less profound abnormalities and usually less severe CHF symptoms (Fig. 33.9). Complete or partial AV canal defects account for 4% to 5% of all CHDs.[5] Complete atrioventricular canal defect is more commonly seen in children with Down syndrome.[5]

Clinical Findings
History. Children with only a primum ASD (partial AV canal) may be asymptomatic. In infants with complete AV canal defects, parents may note signs and symptoms of CHF and failure to thrive (see Box 33.4).

Physical Examination

- Partial AV canal (primum ASD) findings are the same as those with secundum ASD. There may also be a soft blowing mitral regurgitation murmur in the apex and/or infrascapular area.
- Complete AV canal defect findings:
  - Low-pitched, grade II to V/VI holosystolic murmur at LLSB. A murmur may not be evident at birth but increases in loudness 2 to 8 weeks after pulmonary vascular resistance falls.
  - Diastolic rumble at the apex; thrill along the left sternal border.
  - Signs of progressing CHF after the first weeks of life; S_3 or S_4 gallop if CHF is present.
    - Some infants, particularly those with trisomy 21, maintain neonatal high pulmonary vascular resistance and do not show signs of CHF. Instead, they may manifest signs of pulmonary HTN including a loud single S_2, precordial heave, minimal murmur, and desaturation with agitation or effort.[5]

Diagnostic Studies

- Chest radiography findings vary depending on the size of the shunt. Children with small shunts have a normal heart size and pulmonary vascular markings just beyond the upper limits of normal. Those with large shunts (complete AV canal defect) have cardiac enlargement involving both left and right ventricles and left atrium, with increased pulmonary vascular markings (see Fig. 33.4).
- The ECG usually shows superior axis between −40 and −160 degrees. Right ventricular hypertrophy is usually present, and large shunts may cause LVH or BVH in large shunts. In 50% of children, the PR interval is prolonged.
- Echocardiography (two-dimensional, Doppler, or transesophageal) provides visualization of the ASD and VSD defect size, characteristics and size of the AV valves, and relative sizes of the ventricles.
- Cardiac catheterization may be performed if there is a question of elevated pulmonary vascular resistance or discrepancy in ventricular size.

Management

- Children with a partial AV canal defect consisting of a primum ASD and possibly a cleft mitral valve are monitored every 3 to 6 months throughout the first year of life and then twice a year until the defect is closed surgically during toddler or preschool years. They usually do not have signs of CHF but may gain weight slowly. They rarely manifest difficulty with pulmonary HTN after surgery.
- Infants with a complete AV canal defect usually need surgical correction before they reach 6 months of life. Infants who desaturate or develop CHF should see a cardiologist to determine surgical timing. Medical management before surgery may include:
  - Digoxin, diuretics, ACE inhibitors, and β-blockers.
  - Monitoring nutritional intake and weight and fortifying breast milk or infant formulas; enteric nutritional support via nasogastric tube may be needed.
  - Educating families on signs and symptoms of developing or progressing CHF.
- Surgical repair consists of defect closure and reconstruction of the common AV valve into separate tricuspid and mitral valves. Surgical mortality is between 3% and 10% for those with complete AV defects and 3% for those with partial defects.[5]
- Long-term complications include regurgitant or stenotic AV valve, arrhythmias, and pulmonary HTN.[5]
- SBE prophylaxis is indicated before surgery and 6 months after surgical repair.[5]

Patent Ductus Arteriosus. The ductus arteriosus typically closes between 12 to 72 hours after birth in term infants. However, the ductus arteriosus may remain patent in some infants, leaving a connection between the aorta and the pulmonary artery. As pulmonary vascular resistance falls, aortic blood shunts into the pulmonary artery and recirculates through the lungs (Fig. 33.10). The incidence is 5% to 10% of all CHDs, with a female to male ratio of 3:1. The frequency of a PDA increases in premature infants with decreasing gestational age; it is as high as 45% to 80% in very young infants less than 1750 g.[5] This condition occurs with many congenital malformation syndromes (see Table 33.7).

Clinical Findings

History. Individuals with a PDA may be asymptomatic if the PDA is small. Increasing signs of CHF may appear in the first

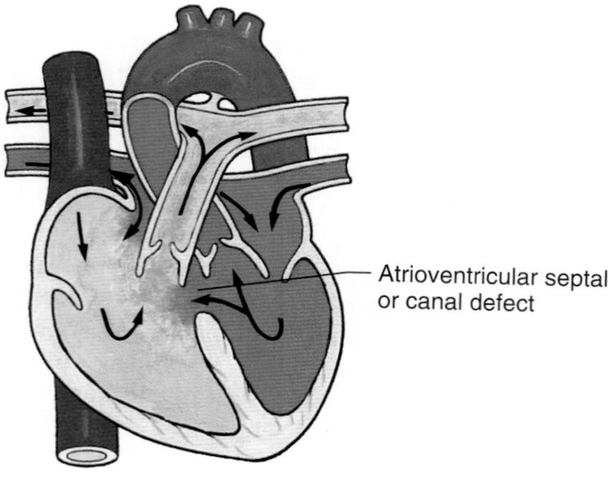

• **Fig. 33.9** Complete Atrioventricular (AV) Septal Defect. AV septal defect is also known as an AV canal defect or complete endocardial cushion defect. (From Hockenberry MJ, Duffy EA, Gibbs K. *Wong's Nursing Care of Infants and Children.* 12th ed. Elsevier; 2024.)

Atrioventricular septal or canal defect

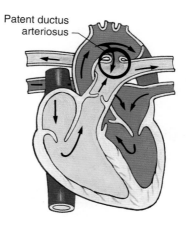

Patent ductus arteriosus

• **Fig. 33.10** Patent Ductus Arteriosus. (From Hockenberry MJ, Duffy EA, Gibbs K. *Wong's Nursing Care of Infants and Children.* 12th ed. Elsevier; 2024.)

weeks of life in infants with larger PDAs. PDAs become symptomatic by 3 months old.

Physical Examination
- In the immediate postnatal period, the murmur is soft, systolic, and heard along the left sternal border, under the left clavicle, and in the back.
- After the first weeks of life, a typical grade II to V/VI, harsh, rumbling, continuous "machinery murmur" heard in the left infraclavicular fossa and pulmonic area with a thrill at the base.
- Physical findings of CHF may be present with a large shunt.

Diagnostic Studies
- Chest radiography: The heart is not enlarged with small to moderate shunts; with larger shunts, both the left atrium and left ventricle can show enlargement. Pulmonary vascular markings may be increased.
- ECG: Large shunts may cause left ventricular hypertrophy; QRS axis is normal or rightward.
- Echocardiogram: Shows the patent ductus and usually left atrium enlargement.

Management
- Indomethacin or ibuprofen may be given to preterm infants to effect closure when there is a significant left-to-right shunt. It is contraindicated and ineffective in term or older infants.[5]
- Asymptomatic infants with a small left-to-right shunt are followed to identify spontaneous closure or to perform transcatheter device closure, preferably before 1 year old. Infants with large shunts or pulmonary HTN should have their PDA surgically closed within the first few months of life to prevent the development of progressive pulmonary vascular obstruction. Surgical ligation of the ductus is a low-risk procedure because it does not require cardiopulmonary bypass.[5]
- Interventional cardiologists close many PDAs by inserting coils or closure plugs into the shunt via cardiac catheterization. Infants must weigh more than 700 grams for this procedure.
- SBE prophylaxis precautions are recommended for the 6-month period after device closure.[16]

Right-to-Left Shunting Congenital Heart Disease (Cyanotic)

Cyanotic CHD represents 10% to 18% of all congenital heart lesions. Cardiac cyanosis is caused by obstruction of pulmonary blood flow or mixing of oxygenated and unoxygenated blood. Visible cyanosis occurs when oxygen saturation in blood reaches approximately 85%. Cyanosis is more readily apparent with polycythemia and less apparent with anemia or the presence of fetal hemoglobin. Polycythemia is a compensatory mechanism to increase the oxygen-carrying capacity in cyanotic patients; however, it increases the risk for cerebral thrombosis.[5] The most common heart conditions causing cyanosis in the immediate newborn period are listed in Fig. 33.6.

Tetralogy of Fallot. Tetralogy of Fallot (TOF; also referred to as TET) is a combination of four anatomic cardiac defects resulting in right ventricular outflow tract (RVOT) obstruction: (1) pulmonary valve stenosis, (2) right ventricular hypertrophy, (3) VSD, and (4) an aorta that overrides the ventricular septum (Fig. 33.11). It is the most common cyanotic cardiac lesion (approximately 10% of all CHDs), occurs slightly more in males, and has a spectrum of severity.[17] The most severe forms involve nonpatent pulmonary valve and artery atresia, referred to as *TOF pulmonary atresia,* and these infants are cyanotic as newborns. In the mildest form, "pink TETs," infants may not display signs of cyanosis because the valvular stenosis is mild, and their symptoms are

similar to having a large VSD. In most individuals with TOF, right-to-left shunting across the VSD and cyanosis increase over the first months of life. This results in increasing RVOT obstruction. Children with chromosome 22q11.2 deletion syndrome or Down syndrome have a higher risk of this defect.[5]

Clinical Findings
History. TOF symptom severity depends on the degree of right ventricular outflow obstruction and presence of a PDA. Symptoms include:
- Cyanosis not initially evident in cases with mild RVOT obstruction or may be present at birth (with severe obstruction). Cyanosis is usually present by 6 months of age.
- Dyspnea and cyanosis (including hypercyanotic episodes, or "TET spells") frequency increases by 2 to 4 months old, especially with crying, feeding, and/or defecation. The infant may also have a history of poor weight gain.

Physical Examination. The following findings may be evident:
- Mucous membrane cyanosis and dyspnea
- A grade III to V/VI, harsh systolic ejection murmur at the left mid- to upper sternal border (VSD murmur and symptoms of a large VSD). There may be a palpable thrill and a holosystolic murmur at the LLSB.
- Sternal lift secondary to right ventricular hypertrophy.

Diagnostic Studies
- Chest radiography may show a boot-shaped heart with decreased pulmonary vascular markings.
- ECG shows right ventricular hypertrophy, right axis deviation, and may show a conduction delay in V_1.
- An echocardiogram shows the extent of the pulmonary obstruction and demonstrates the anatomy of the overriding aorta and VSD.
- Pulse oximetry values decrease over time, with resultant increase in hemoglobin and hematocrit values.
- Cardiac catheterization may be performed to delineate location of coronary arteries before surgical correction.

Management
- In neonates with severe pulmonary obstruction, prostaglandin E_1 (PGE_1) may be used to maintain or reopen the ductus arteriosus until more definitive repair or palliation is possible.
- For hypercyanotic episodes, cradle the child in a knee-chest position, soothe the child, and give oxygen and perhaps morphine sulfate subcutaneously until the spell subsides. The

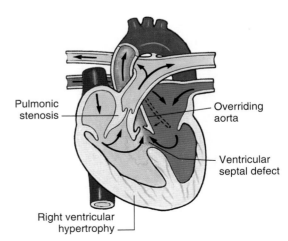

Pulmonic stenosis
Overriding aorta
Ventricular septal defect
Right ventricular hypertrophy

• **Fig. 33.11** Tetralogy of Fallot. (From Hockenberry MJ, Duffy EA, Gibbs K. *Wong's Nursing Care of Infants and Children.* 12th ed. Elsevier; 2024.)

knee-chest maneuver increases systemic resistance, decreases right-to-left shunting, and increases pulmonary blood flow, alleviating the symptoms. Immediate intervention is required for infants who are "spelling," especially if the previously mentioned maneuvers do not end the spell. Most children are surgically repaired before hypercyanotic spells begin.

- Complete repair with open-heart surgery is usually performed in infancy by closing the VSD and relieving the RVOT obstruction.
- Long-term complications after repair include pulmonary valve regurgitation and atrial and ventricular arrhythmias and require lifelong cardiology follow-up. Recent studies indicate progressive right ventricular dilation causes increasing QRS duration on ECG. QRS duration of 180 mm significantly increases the risk of ventricular tachycardia and sudden death. A cardiology consult is indicated before clearing for sports participation.[5]
- SBE prophylaxis is indicated for 6 months after repair. Patients who have pulmonary valve replacement required prophylaxis for their entire life.[16]

Transposition of the Great Arteries. Dextro transposition of the great arteries (d-TGA) results from incomplete septation and migration of the truncus arteriosus during fetal development. In d-TGA, the aorta arises from the right ventricle and the pulmonary artery arises from the left ventricle. The aorta receives the deoxygenated systemic venous blood and returns it to the systemic arteries. The pulmonary artery receives oxygenated pulmonary venous blood and returns it to the pulmonary circulation (Fig. 33.12). There may be several comorbid heart malformations with d-TGA—most commonly VSD, PDA, and coronary artery defects. The incidence is 5% to 7% of all CHDs, with a male to female ratio of 3:1.[5]

Clinical Findings
History
- Cyanosis is immediately evident within 1 hour after birth (approximately 50%) or the first day after birth. Because d-TGA allows mixing of oxygenated and unoxygenated blood, occasionally, less cyanotic infants may present as late as 3 months old.
- CHF symptoms may be present.
- Affected infants are often large for gestational age with retardation of growth and development after the neonatal period.

Physical Examination. Infants may have no murmur at birth or may have a murmur characteristic of associated lesions, such as VSD, ASD, or PDA. The S_2 is loud and single because of the anatomic placement of the great arteries.

Diagnostic Studies
- Chest radiography and ECG findings may be normal in the early newborn period, or the heart may appear egg shaped.
- ECG findings show right axis deviation and right ventricular hypertrophy.
- Echocardiography shows the pulmonary artery arising from the left ventricle and the aorta arising from the right ventricle.

Management
- Immediate referral to a pediatric cardiac center is necessary. Correction of electrolyte and acid-base imbalance may be necessary.
- Intravenous PGE_1 is administered to delay closure or reopen the ductus arteriosus.
- A balloon atrial septostomy may be performed to promote mixing of oxygenated and unoxygenated blood in the atria.
- The arterial switch (Jatene procedure) is usually performed in the first few days of life. If this is not possible, a number of other operations can be performed, such as the Nakaidoh, Damus-Kaye-Stansel, or REV procedures (réparation à l'étage ventriculaire).
- Children are monitored closely throughout life with annual echocardiogram follow-up.
- SBE prophylaxis precautions are indicated for life.[16]

Prognosis. Operative mortality is low.[18] However, long-term monitoring for the patency and growth of the coronary arteries is warranted. Neopulmonic stenosis, neoaortic regurgitation, or aortic root dilatation may occur after the arterial switch.[5] Refer any patient with a history of arterial or atrial switch to a pediatric cardiologist, especially if they have a history of palpitations, syncope, and/or shortness of breath with exertion.

Tricuspid Atresia, Hypoplastic Left Heart Syndrome, and Other Single Ventricle Defects. Tricuspid atresia, pulmonary atresia/intact ventricular septum, and hypoplastic left heart syndrome (HLHS) are the most common types of single ventricle defects. In most cases, there is functionally only one ventricle of either right or left morphology that must do the work of pumping blood to both the systemic and pulmonary circulations. Oxygenated and deoxygenated blood mix in this ventricle, and the child is cyanotic. Most of these individuals require palliative cardiac procedures to survive.

Tricuspid atresia results in a small right ventricle without access to the right atrium. Blood returning from the systemic circulation must pass over an ASD to the left atrium and then left ventricle before being pumped to either the lungs or the body (Fig. 33.13). TGA also occurs in 50% of these patients. Less than 3% of all children with CHD have tricuspid atresia; the etiology is unknown.[5]

HLHS occurs in less than 1% of congenital heart defects.[5] Intrauterine stenosis of either the mitral or aortic valves or both, results in a small left ventricle and hypoplasia of the ascending aorta and arch (Fig. 33.14). The cause is unknown, although it is linked to some genetic syndromes including Jacobsen syndrome and Turner syndrome (10% of cases). Central nervous system abnormalities are also associated with HLHS.[19]

Clinical Findings
History. Cyanosis occurs soon after birth and patients develop increased respiratory rate, fatigue with crying or feeding, and subsequent poor weight gain. This often progresses to cardiorespiratory shock as the ductus arteriosus closes.

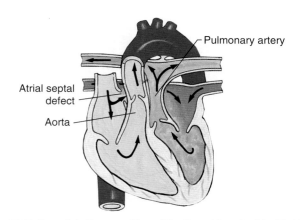

• **Fig. 33.12** Complete Transposition of the Great Vessels. (Modified from Hockenberry MJ, Duffy EA, Gibbs K. *Wong's Nursing Care of Infants and Children.* 12th ed. Elsevier; 2024.)

Pulmonary artery

Atrial septal defect

Aorta

Physical Examination
- A grade I to III/VI early systolic murmur may be present; usually a single S_2 is heard.
- Cyanosis is generally evident as soon as the ductus arteriosus closes.
- Hepatomegaly (may or may not be present).

Diagnostic Studies
- Heart size on chest radiography is generally initially normal. Cardiomegaly and decreased pulmonary blood flow occur over time.
- ECG findings depend on the type of single ventricle pathology but are always abnormal for age. Right ventricular forces are diminished in tricuspid atresia.
- Two-dimensional echocardiography is diagnostic and shows the anatomic specifics.

Management
- Intravenous PGE_1 may be indicated in newborns. Most infants receive initial palliation with aortopulmonary shunts or other procedures depending on their anatomy. At 4 to 6 months old, palliation is continued with a bidirectional anastomosis of the SVC to the pulmonary artery. The third stage of palliation (Fontan procedure) occurs at 2 to 4 years old when the IVC is connected to the pulmonary artery. Some children are considered for cardiac transplantation early in life if their anatomy is not amenable to the Fontan pathway or heart function and pulmonary vascular resistance does not allow for palliative repair.[5]
- Families require support throughout the child's life. Frequent surgeries and hospitalizations can interfere with normative social development. Early recognition and intervention for developmental delays are important.
- SBE prophylaxis is recommended while the child remains cyanotic (see Box 33.3 and Table 33.5).

Complications. Complications include development of collateral arterial and venous vessels, protein-losing enteropathy, arrhythmias, thromboembolic events including strokes, and many others. A decrease in exercise tolerance throughout life can be expected, in addition to left or right ventricular dysfunction. There may be fewer complications with surgical palliation at earlier ages. For those with severe long-term complications, heart transplantation is an option.[5]

Obstructive Cardiac Lesions

Aortic Stenosis and Insufficiency. Aortic stenosis or narrowing occurs at the aortic valvular, subvalvular, or supravalvular level. Valvular stenosis is the most common form (Fig. 33.15). The stenotic aortic valve is usually bicuspid rather than tricuspid. Stenosis causes increased pressure load on the left ventricle leading to LVH and, ultimately, ventricular failure. The imbalance between increased myocardial oxygen demand of the hypertrophied myocardium and coronary blood supply can lead to ischemia and fatal ventricular arrhythmias. The bicuspid aortic valve generally becomes more stenotic and often regurgitant (insufficient) over time. Some infants are born with critical aortic stenosis and require urgent intervention, usually a balloon valvuloplasty in the newborn period. Children with a congenital bicuspid aortic valve and without stenosis or regurgitation are at risk of developing symptoms by adolescence. Aortic stenosis occurs in 3% to 8% of all CHDs, with a male to female ratio of approximately 4:1.[5]

Clinical Findings

History
- Growth and development may be normal.
- Activity intolerance, fatigue, chest pain (angina pectoris), or syncope can develop or increase with age.

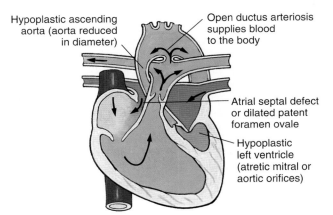

• **Fig. 33.14** Hypoplastic Left Heart Syndrome. (Modified from Hockenberry MJ, Duffy EA, Gibbs K. *Wong's Nursing Care of Infants and Children.* 12th ed. Elsevier; 2024.)

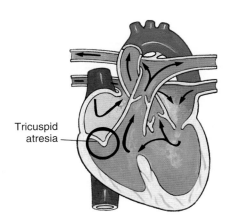

• **Fig. 33.13** Tricuspid Atresia. (From Hockenberry MJ, Duffy EA, Gibbs K. *Wong's Nursing Care of Infants and Children.* 12th ed. Elsevier; 2024.)

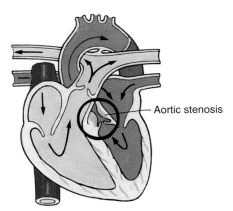

• **Fig. 33.15** Aortic Stenosis. (From Hockenberry MJ, Duffy EA, Gibbs K. *Wong's Nursing Care of Infants and Children.* 12th ed. Elsevier; 2024.)

- CHF, low cardiac output, and shock may be evident in newborns with severe aortic stenosis.
- Sudden death, presumably because of arrhythmias, can occur with exertion as stenosis severity increases.

Physical Examination

- BP may reveal a narrow pulse pressure. Moderate to severe stenosis may cause the apical impulse to be pronounced.
- A grade III to IV/VI, loud, harsh systolic crescendo-decrescendo murmur is best heard at the upper right sternal border with radiation to the neck, LLSB, and apex.
- A faint, early systolic click at the LLSB may be heard if there is a valvular lesion present.
- With aortic insufficiency, an early diastolic blowing murmur is heard at the LLSB to apex.
- In the most severe lesions, the S_2 is single or closely split; S_3 or S_4 heart sounds may also be present.
- A thrill may be present at the suprasternal notch.

Diagnostic Studies

- Chest radiographs are usually normal or may show LVH. Adults frequently develop radiographic evidence of aortic valve calcification over time.
- ECG can be normal or reveal LVH and inverted T waves.
- A 24-hour Holter monitor or 30-day event monitor demonstrates ventricular arrhythmia.
- Echocardiogram is the diagnostic examination of choice.

Management

- The treatment type and timing depend on the obstruction severity.
- Initial palliative treatment in the newborn is balloon valvuloplasty of the stenotic valve. However, the aortic valve generally needs further intervention.
- In older children, surgical division of fused valve commissures may relieve stenosis but often valve replacement is necessary for severe aortic stenosis and/or insufficiency. Unfortunately, none of the current replacement options are ideal or enduring for children. Mechanical valves are prothrombotic and require anticoagulation with warfarin. Aortic heterograph and homograft valves have limited durability and the Ross procedure requires placement of the homograft in the pulmonic position, leading to future replacements of that valve as it stenoses.[5]
- Children with subaortic stenosis require surgical resection when the gradient is greater than 35 mm Hg; patients with supravalvar aortic stenosis require resection of the narrowed area with patch material.
- Children with mild aortic stenosis can participate in all sports but should have annual cardiac examination. Those with moderate aortic stenosis should choose low-intensity sports (such as, golf, bowling, table tennis, or softball) as guided by their cardiologist. Children with severe aortic stenosis or moderate aortic stenosis with symptoms should avoid competitive or intensive sports because of the risk of sudden death from ventricular arrhythmias[5] (see Chapter 18, Table 18.6).
- Aortic root dilation (commonly seen with bicuspid or stenotic aortic valves) may require intervention to prevent aortic dissection.
- Anticoagulation is necessary with mechanical valve replacement.[5]

Pulmonic Stenosis. Normally, the pulmonary valve opens to allow the blood flow from the right ventricle into the pulmonary artery. In pulmonic stenosis, there is narrowing at the subpulmonic, valvular, or supravalvular area. Right-sided pressure increases as the ventricle pumps against the obstruction. Right ventricular hypertrophy occurs as a result of this increased load. Pulmonary stenosis can occur in the main and/or branch pulmonary arterial system. Mild pulmonic stenosis is usually identified on routine examination. Many of these children also develop poststenotic dilation of the pulmonary artery. Isolated pulmonic stenosis occurs in 8% to 12% of all CHDs[5] (see Table 33.6 for associated congenital malformation syndromes).

Clinical Findings

History

- The individual is usually asymptomatic, with a murmur noted on routine physical examination in the newborn to school-age child.
- Exertional dyspnea and fatigue are noticeable as stenosis progresses.
- Cyanosis from right-to-left shunting over the foramen ovale may be evident in the newborn with critical pulmonic stenosis.
- Growth and development are usually normal except in cases of Turner or Noonan syndrome in which short stature is common.[5]

Physical Examination

- A grade II to IV/VI, harsh, mid to late systolic ejection murmur is heard at the ULSB over the pulmonic region with transmission along the left sternal border, neck and back, and into both lung fields.
- An intermittent systolic ejection click may be evident in the pulmonic area that decreases with inspiration and increases with expiration.
- Cyanosis and symptoms of right-sided CHF can occur in the newborn with severe pulmonic stenosis.

Diagnostic Studies

- Chest radiographs may be within normal limits in infants or show prominent main pulmonary artery segments. Right-sided cardiac enlargement and decreased peripheral pulmonary vascular markings may be evident if heart failure develops.
- ECG may be normal with mild stenosis. Right axis deviation and right ventricular hypertrophy occur in moderate to severe pulmonic stenosis.
- Echocardiograms confirm the diagnosis, identify the gradient and monitor stenosis progression.
- Cardiac catheterization may be used to delineate the location of the main and branch pulmonary artery stenosis.

Management

- Balloon valvuloplasty is performed in neonates and older children with stenosis greater than 50 mm Hg. If unsuccessful, surgical valvuloplasty or replacement may be indicated. Stents and balloons are also used for branch stenosis.
- With mild stenosis, families must be encouraged to treat their children normally and not to limit their activity. Moderate stenosis can progress to severe narrowing during periods of rapid growth, such as during infancy or adolescence.[5]
- SBE prophylaxis is not necessary except in the 6-month postoperative period or if prosthetic material is used in valve repair (see Box 33.3).

Coarctation of the Aorta. CoA is a narrowing of a small or long segment of the aorta (Fig. 33.16). Coarctation may occur as a single defect resulting from a disturbance in the development of the aorta or may be secondary to constriction of the ductus arteriosus. The severity of the coarctation, its location, and the degree of obstruction determine the clinical presentation. Systolic and diastolic HTN exists in vessels proximal to the narrowing, whereas hypotension is present in vessels below the narrowing. CoA accounts for 8% to 10% of all congenital heart defects and

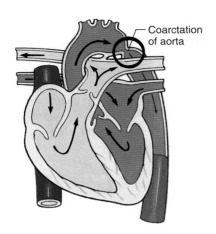

• **Fig. 33.16** Coarctation of the Aorta. (From Hockenberry MJ, Duffy EA, Gibbs K. *Wong's Nursing Care of Infants and Children.* 12th ed. Elsevier; 2024.)

occurs slightly more in males.[5] Most children with CoA have a bicuspid aortic valve. Other CHD can occur with CoA including abnormalities of the left side of the heart.

Clinical Findings

History. CoA is not always apparent in newborns until the ductus closes and blood flow decreases to the lower body. Severe coarctation in infants is apparent in the first 6 weeks; symptoms include tachypnea, poor feeding, and possibly cool lower extremities. In children 3 to 5 years old, coarctation may go unnoticed until HTN or a murmur is detected. Retrospectively, children with coarctation may have complaints of headaches or leg pain with exercise.[5]

Physical Examination

- Upper extremity HTN with lower extremity hypotension are present, although milder cases may cause only a minimal discrepancy between upper and lower extremity BPs. In severe cases, poor lower extremity perfusion may be noticed with lower body mottling or pallor.
- Delayed timing and absent or weak arterial and other distal arterial pulses may occur.
- Bounding brachial, radial, and carotid pulses may occur.
- Signs of CHF may be evident.
- A systolic ejection murmur may be detected in the left infraclavicular region with transmission to the back.
- A ventricular heave at the apex may be palpated.
- A gallop rhythm may occur in infants with CHF.

Diagnostic Studies

- Chest radiography may reveal a normal or slightly enlarged heart and normal to increased pulmonary vascular markings; rib notching may be seen.
- ECG findings depend on the severity of the lesion and the age of the child. In infants, right ventricular hypertrophy may be seen; in older children, LVH develops secondary to HTN.
- Echocardiography is helpful in confirming the diagnosis and locating the constricted aortic segment. It may also show associated cardiac abnormalities. In newborns with a PDA, diagnosis by echocardiogram can be challenging.
- MRI defines location, severity, and anatomy of the aortic arch.

Management

- In critical neonatal coarctation, PGE_1 is used to maintain or reopen the ductus.
- If possible, surgical resection of the constricted area and anastomosis of the upper and lower portions of the aorta are performed. Restenosis is more likely to occur if repair occurs before 1 year of age. Cardiologists may dilate or stent the coarcted area in recoarctation or mild coarctation. Other procedures, including bypass grafting, may be necessary with unusually long coarcted segments. Surgical mortality is rare. Some centers choose balloon valvuloplasty or stent procedures for initial coarctation management.[5]
- In older children with long-standing HTN, antihypertensive medication may be required for several months after repair.[5] Long-term prognosis is excellent unless there are associated intracardiac defects. BP should be monitored postoperatively annually to assess for recoarctation.
- Children with previous coarctation repairs may participate in competitive sports if the residual BP gradient between arm and legs is less than 20 mm Hg and peak systolic BP is normal at rest and with exercise. However, during the first year after surgery, high-intensity static exercises, such as weightlifting and wrestling, should be avoided.[5]
- Lifelong follow-up is necessary due to risk of recoarctation, residual HTN, aortic aneurysms, and problems associated with having a bicuspid aortic valve.
- SBE prophylaxis is no longer necessary except in the 6-month postoperative period or if prosthetic material is used (see Box 33.3).

Sudden Cardiac Death

The PCP has a responsibility to screen for causes of sudden cardiac death (SCD) whenever performing a sports physical examination or assessing a complaint of chest pain, syncope, or palpitations. This can be a daunting challenge because none of the common causes of SCD are easily diagnosed by history or examination. In the United States, the incidence of SCD (excludes sudden infant death syndrome) for ages 1 to 35 years is 0.8 to 2.8 per 1,000,000 person-years.[20] The most frequent cause of exercise-related SCD is cardiomyopathy, especially hypertrophic cardiomyopathy (HCM), and to a lesser extent arrhythmogenic right ventricular cardiomyopathy.[12] Both are inherited, structural abnormalities of the myocardium resulting in ventricular arrhythmias that result in death.

Other congenital structural abnormalities that cause sudden death include coronary artery anomalies, aortic dissection/rupture (usually seen in children with Marfan syndrome), mitral valve prolapse, and aortic stenosis. Congenital, electrical cardiac abnormalities also cause SCD including Wolff-Parkinson-White syndrome, congenital long QT syndromes, and Brugada syndrome.[20]

Sudden death from acquired cardiac abnormalities includes commotio cordis from blunt, nonpenetrating trauma to the midchest (e.g., blow by a baseball or other object), myocarditis, performance-enhancing drugs, and premature coronary artery disease due to familial hypercholesterolemia.[20] Commotio cordis triggers ventricular fibrillation and SCD because of the blow during the T wave timing in the cardiac cycle.

Clinical Findings

Hypertrophic and arrhythmogenic right ventricular cardiomyopathy present with a history of syncope and a family history of either of these conditions. Most individuals are asymptomatic, and arrhythmogenic right ventricular cardiomyopathy is more likely to occur in males beginning around 15 years of age. There may be reports of shortness of breath with activity, palpitations, dizziness/lightheadedness, fatigue, and chest pain/pressure with or without activity. Arrhythmias and shortness of breath with exertion occur in both conditions. Patients with HCM may have a dynamic murmur (late systolic ejection) and forceful apical beat. See Chapter 18, Box 18.7 for the 14-element cardiovascular screening checklist to use during the preparticipation physical examination for sports.

Diagnostic Studies

- HCM: Greater than 90% have an abnormal resting ECG, sustained or nonsustained ventricular tachycardia on Holter or 30-day event monitor, severe LVH on echocardiogram, and an attenuated BP response to exercise.
- Arrhythmogenic right ventricular cardiomyopathy: Changes seen with resting/ambulatory ECG, on echocardiography, and cardiac MRI studies.

Management

Cardiology referral is indicated for all children with a family history of SCD; inheritable cardiomyopathies; Marfan syndrome; chest pain of concern; syncope; acquired cardiac disease, such as Kawasaki disease; and those with known CHD, cardiac rhythm disturbances, or palpitations.

Long-Term Complications for Children and Young Adults With Congenital Heart Disease: Transitioning to Adult Care

As children grow into adulthood, they are vulnerable to a host of long-term complications depending on their disease, repair, and residual lesions. Because of the success of pediatric cardiac surgery, 90% of children born with CHD live into adulthood. As a result, there are currently more adults than children and adolescents with CHD. The adult congenital heart disease (ACHD) population exceeds 1.4 million individuals in the United States.[21]

Not all surgeries performed during childhood are corrective. Many surgeries are palliative or incompletely corrective and leave residual problems. Thus, these individuals continue to require close supervision to assess their cardiac function and need for further interventions. Despite published guidelines by the AAP and AHA concerning the need for transition of care, research indicates many adults with CHD are lost to follow-up due to lack of resources and accessibility.[21] The particular problems faced by adults with CHD are beyond the scope of this text; however, key points in the evaluation of an older child, adolescent, or young adult with CHD are detailed in Box 33.5.[22]

Acquired Heart Disease

Chest Pain

Pediatric chest pain is a common complaint but represents a serious cardiovascular problem in no more than 5% of cases.[5] Although youth of all ages can have chest pain, it is the young adolescent who most frequently presents to the emergency department or PCP with this complaint. The first goal of chest pain

evaluation is to rule out cardiac causes, which are also the main concern of most patients and their parents. Table 33.8 lists possible cardiac causes of chest pain, with corresponding history and examination findings.

The most frequent cause of chest pain is musculoskeletal, and originates in the chest wall or chest cage, is benign, and rarely

---

> **• BOX 33.5** Key Points in the Evaluation of Congenital Heart Disease in the Older Child, Adolescent, and Young Adult
>
> - *Left-sided lesions:* Those with a history of bicuspid aortic valves, subaortic stenosis, aortic valve stenosis, coarctation, or aortic aneurysm may worsen over time and present with significant stenosis or regurgitation. Symptoms include exercise intolerance, dyspnea on exertion, or atypical chest pain. Problems include arrhythmias, sudden death, endocarditis, syncope, and angina.
> - *Left-to-right shunt lesions:* Repaired or unrepaired atrial or VSDs, AV septal defect, aortopulmonary window (a hole between the aorta and the pulmonary artery), or coronary sinus fistulas may be hemodynamically significant and cause elevated pulmonary vascular resistance (resulting in right-to-left shunting through a lesion). Symptoms include arrhythmias, dyspnea on exertion, unexplained deterioration of left ventricular function, and/or left ventricular dilation. If left untreated, left-to-right shunts lead to overloading and remodeling of the pulmonary vasculature and eventually pulmonary arterial hypertension (PAH).[30] The PAH type determines the operability of shunt lesions. Patients are not surgical candidates if PAH is fixed (i.e., not reversible), also known as Eisenmenger syndrome.
> - *Chronic cyanosis:* In addition to left-to-right shunt, lesions causing Eisenmenger syndrome and chronic cyanosis also result from defects causing right ventricular outflow obstruction, baffle leaks (can occur after certain surgical procedures to correct TGA), or palliation for a single ventricle. Chronic hypoxia to vital organs, hyperviscosity, and hematologic problems (e.g., thrombocytopenia, erythrocytosis, thromboemboli, iron deficiency, and bleeding) can result.
> - *Valvar problems:* Besides aortic stenosis, other long-term valve abnormalities include mitral valve prolapse (causes mitral regurgitation) and/or pulmonary valve stenosis or regurgitation (more frequent in those with repaired TOF). Pulmonic stenosis or regurgitation can cause right ventricular remodeling, decreased exercise intolerance, arrhythmias, and sudden death.[30]
> - *Heart failure:* Can occur via many different pathways depending on the underlying disease and previous interventions. It is the leading cause of death in patients with ACHD.[30] Prolonged aortic or pulmonic valvar stenosis or regurgitation is a common mechanism for failure. In single ventricle patients, the development of systemic venous collateral vessels or arteriovenous pulmonary fistulas increases ventricular volumes. Over time, these hemodynamic problems lead to chronic cyanosis, myocardial ischemia, poor ventricular compliance, and serious ventricular arrhythmias. Management of each problem is challenging; ultimately, a heart transplant may be required.
> - *Arrhythmias and heart blocks:* The risk of sudden cardiac death (SCD) is the most significant complication facing adults with CHD. Congenital diagnoses at greatest risk for subsequent SCD include coarctation of the aorta, TOF, aortic stenosis, d-TGA with aortic stenosis, and TGA. Single ventricle patients with a Fontan procedure are also at increased risk for arrhythmias. Rhythm disturbances occur as a result of long-standing cyanosis, the aforementioned chamber dilation, increased atrial pressures, sinus node dysfunction, and extensive fibrotic suture lines.[30] Management is complex. Although episodes of palpitations or chest pain may bring those with CHD into care, they need to be referred to cardiology specialists.
>
> *ACHD,* Adult congenital heart disease; *AV,* atrioventricular; *d-TGA,* dextro-transposition of the great arteries; *SCD,* sudden cardiac death; *TOF,* tetralogy of Fallot; *VSD,* ventricular septal defect.

TABLE 33.8 Cardiac Causes of Chest Pain and Associated Findings

Condition	History	Physical Examination	Electrocardiogram	Chest Radiograph
Abnormal coronaries due to Kawasaki disease or other coronary artery disease	Previous history consistent with disease; typical exercise anginal pain	Usually normal; continuous murmur or possible fistulae	ST segment elevation ± myocardial infarction findings	Normal
Cocaine abuse	History of substance abuse	Hypertension; tachycardia	± ST elevation	Normal
Pericarditis and myocarditis	History of URI ± sharp chest pain	Friction rub; muffled heart sounds	Low QRS voltages; ST segment shift	Cardiomegaly
Postpericardiotomy syndrome	Recent heart surgery; pain positional	Muffled heart sounds; rub	ST segment elevation	Cardiomegaly
Arrhythmia	May have history of Wolff-Parkinson-White or long QT syndrome	Normal to irregular heart rate	Preexcitation, long QT, or normal QT	Normal
Aortic stenosis (severe)	History of aortic stenosis	Loud SEM at USB radiating to neck	LVH with or without strain	Prominent ascending aorta and aortic knob
Pulmonary stenosis (severe)	History of pulmonary stenosis	Loud SEM at ULSB	RVH with or without strain	Prominent PA segment
Hypertrophic cardiomyopathy (HCM)	Positive family history (in one-third of patients)	Variable murmur	LVH; deep Q/small R or QS in LPLs	Mild cardiomegaly
Mitral valve prolapse	Positive family history	Midsystolic click; thin; thoracic skeletal abnormalities	Inverted T waves in aVF	Normal except skeletal anomalies
Eisenmenger syndrome (untreated or untreatable congenital heart disease [CHD])	History of congenital heart disease	Cyanosis, clubbing, loud S_2	Right ventricular hypertrophy	Prominent PA; normal heart size

aVF, Augmented vector right; *LPL*, lateral precordial leads; *LVH*, left ventricular hypertrophy; *PA*, pulmonary artery; *RVH*, right ventricular hypertrophy; *SEM*, systolic ejection murmur; *ULSB*, upper left sternal border; *URI*, upper respiratory infection; *USB*, upper sternal border.
Modified from Park M. *Park's Pediatric Cardiology Handbook.* 5th ed. Elsevier; 2021.

requires treatment. Chest wall pain, particularly with exercise, may indicate exercise-induced bronchospasm but rarely indicates cardiac disease. Chronic chest pain that is vague and occurs over many months in a variety of circumstances, particularly around stressful events, may be psychogenic (anxiety or hyperventilation). Chest pain associated with syncope, exertional dyspnea, or irregularities in heart rhythm needs careful evaluation for a cardiac cause. Children or adolescents who have pain of cardiac origin usually describe a specific history with details that are consistent from event to event.[5]

Clinical Findings

History. A careful history and a thorough physical examination are especially important in assessing this complaint.
- Past medical history or family history of sudden death (including drownings), heart disease or condition, asthma, eczema, Marfan syndrome, and sickle cell disease.
- Sports, exercise, and activity history.
- Previous trauma or muscle strains.
- Chest pain characteristics:
  - Relationship of pain to exercise; presence of syncope, exertional dyspnea, or wheezing.
  - Presence of burning, substernal pain that worsens with reclining or with spicy foods (gastrointestinal etiology).

- Pain that is sharp or stabbing, lasting several seconds to minutes, located over the midsternum or infranipple area, and occurs with nonexertion or deep inspirations is more likely musculoskeletal in origin.
- Pain that awakens the patient is more likely organic.
- Associated symptoms, such as fever, nausea, vomiting, headaches, or choking episodes.
- Recent, major stressful events.
- Medication, tobacco, or other drug use, including oral contraceptives (embolism).

Physical Examination. A complete chest (lungs and heart) and abdominal examination should be performed. Key findings to focus on include the presence of the following:
- Cardiac murmur, rubs, or clicks.
- Point tenderness of one or more costochondral joints that exaggerates with physical activity or deep inspirations (suggests costochondritis or Tietze syndrome [if associated with warmth, swelling, or tenderness over costochondral junction]). Use the middle fingertip to palpate each costochondral and chondrosternal junction for tenderness to avoid missing this finding. Tenderness and swelling may also be present in the pectoral and shoulder carriage muscles due to overuse by excessive weightlifting or excessive electronic game playing.
- Irregular heart rhythm (cardiac disease).

- Rales, wheezing, tachypnea, and decreased breath sounds (pulmonary disease).

Diagnostic Studies. In most cases, the history and physical are sufficient to make the diagnosis; other tests are not indicated unless the following problems are suspected:

- Febrile, cardiac, or pulmonary condition: obtain a chest radiograph.
- Exercise-induced asthma: perform a pulmonary function test with exercise.
- Rhythm disturbance: order a 24-hour Holter or 30-day event monitor or stress test (or both).
- Signs of CHD, pericarditis, or myocarditis: order an ECG and consider a chest radiograph.

Differential Diagnosis

Chest pain of musculoskeletal origin includes costochondritis, Tietze syndrome, idiopathic chest pain, precordial catch syndrome, slipping rib syndrome, hypersensitive xiphoid syndrome, trauma, and muscle strain. Esophagitis, esophageal foreign body ingestion, and exercise-induced bronchospasm are additional differential diagnoses.

Management

When chest pain has no clear etiology, the child appears well, and all aspects of the evaluation are normal, reassurance is the most important treatment. Refer any child with chest pain that worsens with exercise or suggests angina, where there are positive findings on examination, abnormal ECG or chest radiograph, or a concerning personal or family history to pediatric cardiology. Musculoskeletal causes usually respond to nonsteroidal antiinflammatory drug treatment and rest.

Hypertension

Normal BP in children younger than 13 years is defined as systolic and diastolic BP less than the 90th percentile for age, sex, and height. HTN in children younger than 13 years is defined as a systolic or diastolic (or both) BP in the 95th or higher percentile for age, sex, and height on at least three separate occasions. Elevated BP is defined as average systolic or diastolic BP between the 90th and 95th percentile for age, sex, and height. For adolescents older than 13 years, systolic and/or diastolic BP ≥120/80 to 129/<80 mm Hg is considered elevated, whereas ≥130/80 mm Hg is considered hypertensive. For children younger than 13 years, stage 1 HTN is BP between the 95th and 99th percentiles for age, sex, and height. Stage 2 HTN is BP 5 mm Hg or higher or greater than the 99th percentile. For adolescents 13 years or older: stage I is systolic and/or diastolic BP ≥130/80 to 139/89 mm Hg and stage II is systolic and or diastolic BP ≥140/90 mm Hg.[4]

HTN is a significant problem affecting more males (15%–19%) than females (7%–12%).[4] HTN prevalence is higher in Hispanics and African Americans. Increasingly, children and adolescents have HTN associated with obesity, sedentary lifestyles, and stress. Secondary HTN is more common in children younger than 6 years (usually at significant or severe HTN levels). The primary cause of secondary, severe HTN is renovascular or parenchymal renal diseases. Other causes include coarctation of aorta, endocrine disorders, genetic disorders such as Williams syndrome, neurofibromatosis and tuberous sclerosis, drugs, and central nervous system tumors. Primary HTN onset is more likely to occur after 10 years of age. Neonates with HTN are generally severely ill with neurologic, cardiac, and renal symptoms.[4]

Clinical Findings

The goal of the clinical history and physical examination is to assess whether the HTN is primary or secondary to renal disease or other causes. If secondary HTN is ruled out, then the evaluation focuses on the comorbidities of primary HTN. With both types of HTN, the PCP must assess for signs of end-organ damage from prolonged HTN.[4]

History. Inquire about:

- Neonatal history of prolonged mechanical ventilation, umbilical catheterization, prematurity, or small for gestational age at birth. Poor maternal nutrition and high stress have an epigenetic effect on the embryo, making HTN more likely for the neonate.[23]
- Cause of any prior hospitalizations
- Trauma
- Diet, physical activities, and other habits (e.g., smoking, drinking, substance abuse including caffeine)
- Sleep history, particularly symptoms of sleep apnea (see Chapter 16)
- Medications taken including oral contraceptives, cold medications, steroids, and diet aids
- Chronic illness, especially renal disease, past history of urinary tract infections, diabetes, and seizures
- History of headache, chest pain, dyspnea, muscle weakness, palpitations, abdominal pain, facial palsy, decreased vision, and excessive sweating
- Family history of a first-degree relative with myocardial infarction (especially before 50 years old), stroke, HTN, diabetes, hyperlipidemia, sickle cell disease, polycystic kidney disease, neurofibromatosis, pheochromocytoma, or obesity[4]

Physical Examination. Note the following:

- Body habitus, especially overweight (body mass index [BMI]), poor growth (height, weight), or signs of metabolic syndrome
- Edema, pallor, flushing, or skin lesions suggestive of tuberous sclerosis, systemic lupus erythematosus, or neurofibromatosis
- Upper and lower extremity central pulses; absent, diminished, or pounding pulses in all extremities
- Optic fundi abnormalities, enlarged thyroid gland, abdominal mass, flank bruit, decreased visual acuity or facial palsy
- Presence of elevated BP on at least three separate occasions

Diagnostic Studies

- Laboratory evaluation of stage 1 or 2 HTN focuses on searching for the secondary HTN causes, primary HTN comorbidities, and target organ damage. The search for secondary HTN causes must be individualized based upon age, history, physical examination, and extent of BP elevation. Because many children with secondary HTN have renal or renovascular causes for BP elevation, initial laboratory studies should include tests for renal function and plasma renin levels.[4]
- Children younger than 10 years with stage 2 HTN require more aggressive laboratory evaluation compared with older children with stage 1 HTN and obesity. Screening studies for the most common secondary causes of HTN include CBC, erythrocyte sedimentation rate (ESR), C-reactive protein (CRP), urinalysis and culture, electrolytes, blood urea nitrogen, creatinine, and plasma renin levels. If renal vascular disease is suspected, the workup is best managed by a nephrologist and may include renal nuclear medicine scans, renal ultrasound, MRI, or spiral computed tomography.
- Additional organ assessments include echocardiography for LVH and CoA and a thorough ophthalmologic examination.

Management

Algorithms that categorize and illustrate management of children with high BP are found in Figs. 33.17 and 33.18.

- BP measurements should be obtained annually on all children age 3 years and older, with baseline and serial measurements documented in the child's record.
- Elevated BP: At least two follow-up BP measurements should be taken within 1 to 2 months of the initial reading to determine whether a high reading is a single, isolated event. If subsequent readings fall to less than the 95th percentile, the child should continue with routine BP checks during annual visits.
- HTN secondary to overweight can be as serious as HTN secondary to other organic disease and should be treated as such. For those with high-normal BP without any indication of organic disease, treatment should consist of nonpharmacologic intervention—diet, exercise, and weight management. Caloric restriction with exercise is more effective than caloric restriction alone.[4] Recommendations should include the following:
  - Dietary intervention to control or reduce overweight.[4] High-sodium foods and sodium supplements should be eliminated.

- Increase physical exercise and sports participation to 30 to 60 minutes a day balanced with relaxation techniques. Aerobic, not static or isometric, exercise is recommended.
- Avoid smoking, caffeine, alcoholic beverages, and illicit drug consumption.
- If the BP elevation persists, referral should be made to a nephrologist or cardiologist experienced in using antihypertensive agents in pediatric patients. Children and adolescents with confirmed BP equal to or greater than the 99th percentile should have immediate referral.[4]
- The treatment goal is to reduce systolic and diastolic BP to less than the 95th percentile. If a comorbid condition exists, the goal becomes reducing BP to the 90th percentile.
- Medication is usually provided by cardiology. Management starts with a single drug (usually an ACE inhibitor, angiotensin receptor blocker, β-blocker, long-acting calcium channel blocker, or a thiazide diuretic) at the lowest recommended dose and increased until the desired BP is reached. A second medication should be added if maximum dose is reached or if adverse side effects occur. Step-down therapy may be possible for overweight children who lose weight and achieve BP goals.[4]

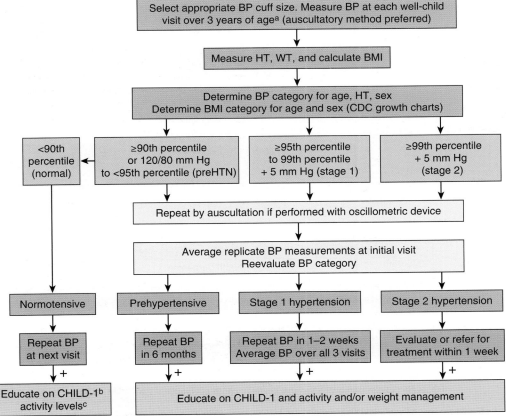

• **Fig. 33.17** Blood Pressure (BP) Measurement and Categorization Algorithm. [a]Cardiovascular health integrated lifestyle diet (CHILD-1) recommended (see Section 5, "Nutrition and Diet" in the NHLBI reference for these nutrition and diet recommendations). [b]See Section 6, "Physical Activity" in the NHLBI source for physical activity recommendations. [c]See Section 10, "Overweight and Obesity" in the NHLBI source for discussion regarding overweight and obesity. *BMI,* Body mass index; *CDC,* Centers of Disease Control and Prevention; *HT,* height; *HTN,* hypertension; *WT,* weight. (From National Heart, Lung, and Blood Institute [NHLBI]. *Expert Panel on Integrated Guidelines for Cardiovascular Health and Risk Reduction in Children and Adolescents: Full Report;* 2012. www.nhlbi.nih.gov/files/docs/guidelines/peds_guidelines_full.pdf.)

Complications

Long-term HTN leads to an increase in left ventricular mass, increased carotid intimal medial thickness, and coronary artery calcification, especially in individuals who are overweight, who have lipid and lipoprotein abnormalities, and who use tobacco. There is some evidence that HTN causes cognitive impairments in pediatric patients.[4] Yearly echocardiograms are recommended to evaluate LVH.

Patient and Family Education

Because much of HTN is related to lifestyle, prevention through optimal health promotion and maintenance is essential. Regular health maintenance including evaluation of BP and health education regarding risk factors is critical. Counseling should emphasize both behavioral modification and parental involvement. Decreasing BMI and increasing aerobic fitness reduce age-related BP elevations. Preventive measures include the following:
- Good nutrition with a moderation in dietary fat and sodium
- Prevention of overweight with diet and aerobic exercise for at least 30 minutes daily

- Stress management
- Avoiding caffeine, tobacco, and prescription or over-the-counter medications that exacerbate HTN (e.g., cold medications with ephedrine or phenylephrine, steroids)
- Monitoring BP with oral contraceptives use

Infective Endocarditis

IE (also known as SBE) is a condition in which a bacterial or fungal infection invades endocardial heart surfaces. Turbulence caused by stenotic cardiac valves, previous surgical repairs, or high-velocity jets (from blood flowing under force through a structural heart defect) traumatizes the cardiac endothelium and leads to thrombogenesis. Platelet and fibrin clumps provide a nidus for circulating bacteria or fungi (rarely). These organisms multiply, shielded from circulating white cells by the platelet-fibrin matrix, and cause further damage by destroying nearby valve tissue and extend into surrounding endothelium.[5]

Infection occurs in any age group but is rare in those without structural heart disease. The incidence of IE increased as

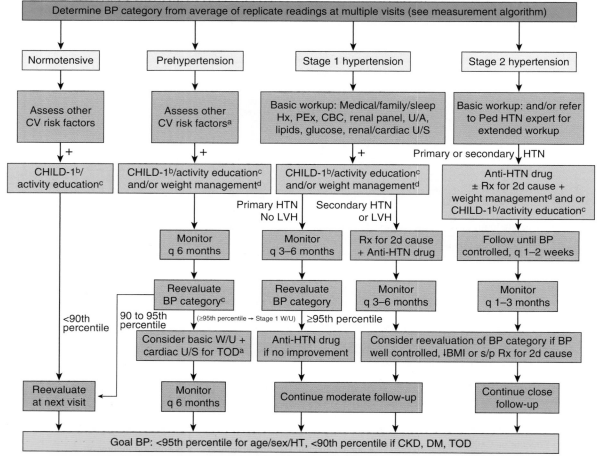

• **Fig. 33.18** Blood Pressure (BP) Management by Category Algorithm. [a]Workup (W/U) for target organ damage/left ventricular hypertrophy (TOD/LVH) if obese or (+) for other cardiovascular (CV) risk factors. [b]Cardiovascular health integrated lifestyle diet *(CHILD-1)* (see Section 5, "Nutrition and Diet" in the NHLBI source). [c]Activity education (see Section 6, "Physical Activity" in the NHLBI source). [d]Weight management for overweight and obesity (see Section 10, "Overweight and Obesity" in the NHLBI source). *2d,* Secondary; *Anti-HTN,* antihypertensive; *BMI,* body mass index; *CBC,* complete blood count; *CKD,* chronic kidney disease; *DM,* diabetes mellitus; *HT,* height; *HTN,* hypertension; *Hx,* history; *Ped,* pediatric; *PEx,* physical examination; *Q,* every; *Rx,* prescription; *s/p,* status post; *U/A,* urinalysis; *U/S,* ultrasound. (From National Heart, Lung, and Blood Institute [NHLBI]. *Expert Panel on Integrated Guidelines for Cardiovascular Health and Risk Reduction in Children and Adolescents: Full Report;* 2012. www.nhlbi.nih.gov/files/docs/guidelines/peds_guidelines_full.pdf.)

more children with CHD survive because of improved surgical interventions. In developing countries where there is a high prevalence of rheumatic heart disease, there is a concurrent increase in IE.[24] Gram-positive cocci cause 80% of cases of pediatric IE. *Staphylococcus aureus* is the most common causative organism, followed by *Streptococcus viridans*.[25] A group of gram-negative bacilli referred to as HACEK [**H**aemophilus species (*H. parainfluenzae, H. aphrophilus,* and *H. paraphrophilus), **A**. actinomycetemcomitans, **C**. hominis, **E**. corrodens,* and **K**ingella species) are less common. Children with CHD have more severe gingival inflammatory conditions, increased plaque accumulation, and more HACEK microbes, which lead to endocarditis. Fungal endocarditis is the most severe form, with increased mortality rates in immunocompromised children and neonates.[5]

Clinical Findings

History and Physical Examination
- History of underlying structural cardiac abnormality, palliative surgery for cyanotic heart disease, prosthetic aortic valve replacements, or indwelling catheters and devices (these may have been used for oncologic or neonatologic purposes).
- History of dental procedures or oral surgery that may have caused gingival or mucosal bleeding
- Intravenous drug use
- Acute manifestations: Short illness duration, prolonged low-grade fever (101°F–103°F [38.3°C–39.4°C]), myalgias, night sweats, arthralgias, headache, general malaise, decreased appetite, increased intensity of preexisting murmur, or new-onset murmur[5]
- Subacute manifestations: Low-grade or relapsing fever, progressive nonspecific symptoms (e.g., myalgias, arthralgias, headache, and general malaise)
- Neonates: Symptoms ranging from relatively few to systemic hypotension, respiratory distress, other generalized signs of sepsis, and neurologic findings
- Evidence of dental caries and/or periodontal or gingival disease
- Embolization symptoms: Hematuria, acute respiratory distress onset, splenomegaly, neurologic changes (stroke, brain abscesses, hemorrhage, meningitis), petechiae (in conjunctiva, buccal mucosa, palatal area, nailbeds, palms, and soles). The classical findings—Janeway lesions (flat, nontender lesions on palms and soles), Osler nodes (small, raised lesions on pad of fingers and toes), Roth spots (retinal hemorrhages with a central white spot), and splinter hemorrhages—occur rarely in children[5]

Diagnostic Studies
- The diagnosis is based on clinical findings and blood culture results. A persistent low-grade fever in a child with known cardiac abnormalities should be evaluated immediately with three sets of blood cultures obtained over 24 hours from different sites before the administration of empirical antibiotic therapy.[25] When three cultures are positive for the same organism, IE must be considered, and treatment instituted. Greater than 90% of those without prior antibiotic treatment will have a positive blood culture.[5]
- Some children have blood culture–negative endocarditis because of prior antibiotic administration, poor culture techniques, or fastidious organisms.[25]
- The ESR, CRP, and white blood cell count are elevated in the acute stage; anemia may be evident.
- Two-dimensional echocardiography is the main modality for detecting infection.[25]

Differential Diagnosis

The differential diagnoses include postoperative fever, collagen vascular diseases, and childhood cancers.

Management and Complications

All children with suspected IE should be hospitalized and referred to pediatric cardiology. Begin treatment as soon as IE is suspected to decrease the morbidity and mortality associated with untreated bacteremia. Give high doses of appropriate antibiotics intravenously for 4 to 6 weeks.[5]

IE can destroy the heart valves or cause disseminated sepsis. Septic and thrombotic emboli from bacterial or fungal vegetations can cause abscesses and ischemic damage to distant areas such as the brain, abdominal viscera, and extremities.[25]

Patient and Family Education

Prophylactic antibiotic therapy is given before all dental procedures involving manipulation of gingival tissue for individuals with high-risk cardiac conditions (previous endocarditis; unrepaired or palliated cyanotic CHD; prosthetic or bioprosthetic valve, shunt, or conduit; repaired CHD with residual defects adjacent to the site of the prosthetic patch or device; and heart transplant recipients) (see Box 33.3 and Table 33.5).[25]

Myocarditis

Myocarditis is a rare inflammatory illness of the muscular walls of the heart. It may go unrecognized in youth whose inflammatory process resolves spontaneously, or it may progress to fulminant disease resulting in chronic cardiomyopathy or death. Myocarditis is often caused by viral infections, most commonly adenoviruses, coxsackievirus A and B, parvovirus B19, echoviruses, and poliovirus. Influenza, cytomegalovirus, varicella, mumps, human immunodeficiency virus, RSV, rubella, COVID-19, and other viral causes. Nonviral infections (fungal, bacterial, protozoal, and rickettsial), various medications, autoimmune or inflammatory disorders (e.g., acute rheumatic fever, systemic lupus erythematosus), toxic reactions to infectious agents, or other disorders (e.g., Kawasaki disease) can also be causative factors; however, the etiology is often unknown. Myocarditis may occur in epidemics, usually in infants caused by coxsackievirus B.[26]

The myocardial inflammatory process leads to dilation of all cardiac chambers, especially the left ventricle, resulting in poor function and stretching of mitral annulus causing regurgitation. The healing process may lead to replacement of myofibers with fibroblasts and scar formation. Scarring decreases elasticity and performance and predisposes an individual to ventricular arrhythmias. Myocarditis causes approximately 8% of sudden death in young athletes.[26]

Clinical Findings

History. As the interstitial inflammation process progresses, cardiac function decreases, and CHF symptoms become evident. The following history is characteristic:
- Infants (may manifest intrauterine exposure): Fever, irritability or listlessness, pallor episodes, diaphoresis, tachypnea or respiratory distress, poor appetite, and vomiting
- Children and adolescents: Recent flu-like or gastrointestinal viral illness (10–14 days previously), lethargy, low-grade fever, pallor, decreased appetite, abdominal pain, exercise intolerance, rashes, palpitations, and respiratory distress (late finding)

Physical Examination

- Pallor, mild cyanosis, skin cool and mottled with poor perfusion (in infants)
- Rapid, labored respirations, grunting, decreased pulse oximetry reading
- Tachycardia, gallop rhythm, muffled heart sounds, apical systolic murmur, weak pulses
- Hepatomegaly, jugular venous distention (older children and adolescents)

Diagnostic Studies. Refer children with symptoms suggestive of myocarditis to a pediatric cardiologist. Diagnostic testing involves chest radiography, ECG, two-dimensional echocardiography, MRI, CBC, ESR, CRP, cardiac and liver enzymes, B-type natriuretic peptide, viral titers, blood cultures, metabolic studies (e.g., thyroid and carnitine), and viral cultures or polymerase chain reaction from the myocardial tissue.[26]

Differential Diagnosis

Differential diagnoses include sepsis, asthma, recurrent vomiting, and chronic viral illness.

Management

Treatment is supportive with bed rest and medications including diuretics, ACE inhibitors, and carvedilol. Occasionally, anticoagulation and antiarrhythmia medications may be used. Therapy modalities include the use of immunomodulators and antiviral therapy.[26] Severe cases may require mechanical ventilation, inotropic support, and mechanical circulatory assistance.[27] Recovery often takes 2 to 3 months; follow-up is lifelong.

Complications and Prognosis

Pericardial effusion and pericarditis may occur concurrently. Myocardial scarring can be a complication that causes persistent heart failure and ventricular arrhythmias. Cardiac transplantation may be necessary in some children with myocarditis. Approximately 80% of children progress to complete recovery.[26]

Pericarditis

Pericarditis is an inflammation or other abnormality of the pericardium, the sac surrounding the heart. Excess fluid accumulates in the pericardial space and causes the normally compliant pericardium to distend. As intrapericardial pressure increases, the heart compresses and limits its filling ability. Pericarditis occurs in youth without a history of cardiac disease. Viral infection (especially with coxsackievirus and adenovirus) is the most common cause of pericarditis in infants and children. Adolescents are at higher risk of pericarditis following COVID-19 vaccination.[28] Other etiologic agents include infections (tuberculosis, other bacteria), trauma, medication hypersensitivity (isoniazid, hydralazine), collagen-vascular and connective tissue diseases (acute rheumatic fever, juvenile rheumatoid arthritis, and systemic lupus erythematosus), Kawasaki disease, postsurgical complications, and systemic infection complications.[5]

Pericarditis is a serious illness that may have rapidly fatal consequences if not diagnosed and treated in a timely manner. The following findings should alert the provider to refer the patient to a pediatric cardiologist:

- History of precordial or substernal chest pain altered by respiration, coughing, or position (may not be found in small children); lethargy, loss of appetite, abdominal pain; fever, irritability; tachycardia; viral illness 10 to 14 days before onset of symptoms

- Physical examination findings: Distended neck veins; tachycardia, pericardial friction rub (an early sign heard best along the left sternal border with the patient leaning forward) or muffled heart sounds (if the effusion is large); Kussmaul sign (slow, deep respirations); pulsus paradoxus, a BP decrease of greater than 10 mm Hg during inspiration when in a supine position; hepatomegaly.
- ECG showing diffuse ST segment elevation (80%), PR depression, and T wave inversion
- Chest radiography showing enlargement of the cardiac silhouette
- Echocardiogram showing relative quantities of pericardial fluid and cavity compression if large effusion is present

Pericarditis requires inpatient management. Cardiac tamponade can occur with large or rapid effusions. There is a relapse rate of 15% if the causative agent is viral. Most youth recover fully within 3 to 4 weeks. Myocarditis is the main differential diagnosis.[5]

Multisystem Inflammatory Syndrome in Children

Patients younger than 21 years who present with fever, elevated inflammatory markers, and multisystem organ involvement (two or more systems), and a confirmed history of SARS-CoV-2 infection within the previous 4 to 8 weeks meet criteria for multisystem inflammatory syndrome in children. Clinical manifestations are similar to myocarditis and pericarditis. The most common cardiovascular complications include coronary aneurysms, myocardial ischemia, heart failure, and arrhythmias (ventricular arrhythmias, atrioventricular block, atrial tachycardia, and sinus tachycardia). These patients require close cardiac follow-up after hospital discharge and activity restriction up to 3 to 6 months depending on degree of myocardial damage.[27]

Heart Conduction Disturbances

Cardiac Arrhythmias

Arrhythmias manifest as a primary disorder or secondary to cardiac or other systemic disorders. Some of the more common arrhythmias are described in Box 33.6 (Table 33.1 lists normal heart rates.)

Clinical Findings

Slow or fast heart rate are present with a rhythm that can be regular, irregular, or regularly irregular. Arrhythmias may be accompanied by feeding difficulties in infants and exercise intolerance in older children.[5]

- Long QT syndrome: The child may be asymptomatic until experiencing syncope or sudden death from a torsades de pointes ventricular tachycardia. Family history may include syncope, sudden death, or known long QT syndrome. Congenital deafness is an additional family characteristic in one type of long QT syndrome.

Diagnostic Studies

- A 12-lead ECG is essential to document the arrhythmia.
- Supraventricular tachycardia (SVT): Wolff-Parkinson-White is one subtype of AV reentrant tachycardia in which there are markers on the resting (non-SVT) ECG that indicate an accessory pathway. These markers are delta waves, short PR interval, and prolonged QRS duration. Diagnosis is usually made when capturing SVT on an ECG, Holter monitor, or another device. A QT interval corrected for the heart rate (QTc) of greater

---

• BOX 33.6 Common Pediatric Arrhythmias

- Sinus arrhythmia: variable heart rate that increases with inspiration and decreases with expiration. This is a normal finding in children and young adolescents.
- Bradycardia or slow heart rate for age:
  - Sinus bradycardia is the most common cause of bradycardia in children and can be due to hypoxia, acidosis, increased intracranial pressure, abdominal distention, hypothermia, hypoglycemia, eating disorders, or athletic conditioning. Bradycardia can also be caused by drugs, such as β-blockers or digoxin.[5]
  - Complete AV block can either be congenital or acquired after cardiac surgery. Ninety percent of congenital cases are secondary to maternal connective tissue disorders or complex CHD (levo- or L-looped transposition of the great arteries [L-TGA]) heterotaxy.[32]
- Tachycardias:
  - Sinus tachycardia is caused by predisposing factors that increase cardiac output, including fever, anxiety, infection, drug exposure, dehydration, pain, hyperthyroidism, or anemia among many others. Treatment is directed at the underlying disorder.
  - SVTs are the most common pathologic tachycardias in children.
  - AV reentrant tachycardia is the most common SVT. In AV reentrant tachycardia, there is an additional (accessory) pathway for impulse transmission from atria to ventricles besides the normal AV node. Less commonly, this may be through a dual AV node (nodal reentrant AV tachycardia). AV reentrant tachycardias often first present in infants younger than 4 months and again in young adolescents.[5]
- Long QT syndrome–induced ventricular tachycardia: Long QT syndrome is linked to 13 different genes. The clinical manifestation is delayed repolarization (the long QT interval) visible on ECG. Genetic prolongation of the QT segment increases the susceptibility to drug-induced long QT interval. Such drugs include antiarrhythmics (e.g., amiodarone and sotalol), psychotropic drugs (e.g., haloperidol and ziprasidone), and antibiotics (e.g., ciprofloxacin, clarithromycin, and erythromycin). Lists of medications that should be avoided are available on the Internet.
- Premature atrial contraction (PAC): This arrhythmia occurs in children and adults. The PAC depolarization may or may not be conducted through the AV node. PACs in a child with an otherwise normal heart are usually benign. It is not unusual to see multiple PACs on the ECG of a newborn.
- Premature ventricular contraction (PVC): PVCs are premature QRS complexes with a prolonged duration or morphologic difference from the preceding QRS. Occasional PVCs are also seen in an otherwise healthy infants and children. PVCs that are uniform in appearance, which means they have the same QRS complex appearance every time, are usually of no consequence.

AV, Atrioventricular; *CHD,* congenital heart disease; *ECG,* electrocardiogram; *SVT,* supraventricular tachycardia.

---

than 0.44 second in males and 0.46 second in females is worthy of investigation.[5]
- Long QT syndrome: 12-lead ECG (shows a long QT interval); genetic testing
- An echocardiogram can rule out complex CHD and assesses ventricular function. A Holter monitor determines the average heart rate over a 24-hour period and helps establish rhythm-related symptoms.[5]

Management and Complications
- Bradycardia: Treat the underlying cause. Symptomatic children and those with high-grade AV block may require temporary or permanent pacing. A permanent pacemaker may be indicated if bradycardia persists after the underlying cause is treated or if there is high-grade AV block.[5]

- SVT: Vagal maneuvers, intravenous adenosine, or, if necessary, synchronized cardioversion. Long-term management involves recurrence prevention with β-blockade or, in the absence of Wolff-Parkinson-White, digoxin. Radiofrequency ablation of accessory pathway is attempted if medical therapy fails and the child is old enough for the procedure.
- Long QT syndrome: If long QT syndrome is suspected, the child should be referred to a pediatric electrophysiologist. Treatment options include β-blockers and implantable defibrillator placement. These children are at high risk of SCD.

Syncope

Syncope is a transient loss of consciousness due to a decrease in cerebral blood flow; recovery is relatively prompt. Most syncope or near syncope in children is benign, unlike older adults where cardiac causes are predominant. In assessing a syncopal episode, the provider must distinguish between a simple fainting event versus one that is a red flag for a serious cardiovascular or other medical condition.[30]

Simple or common fainting occurs in approximately 15% of children from 8 to 18 years old. The relatively syncopal high incidence contrasts with a low incidence of aborted and cardiac-related sudden death in the pediatric and young adult population.[5]

Cardiac-related syncope occurs as a result of obstruction to left ventricular filling (e.g., mitral stenosis), obstruction to left ventricular ejection (e.g., aortic stenosis), or ineffective contraction with an underlying structural, functional, or electrical heart disturbance. Syncope may be due to primary pulmonary HTN, which is often a clinically silent disease until severe symptoms are present. Syncope due to a cardiac cause often comes without prodromal symptoms or may be associated with palpitation or chest pain (angina).

In contrast, noncardiac syncope (also called *neurocardiogenic syncope* [NCS], or simply *fainting*) is neurally mediated and involves systemic vasodilation, vagally induced bradycardia, and hypotension, which result in decreased cerebral blood flow and fainting. NCS includes different overlapping subtypes, such as vasovagal syncope, vasodepressor syncope, cardioinhibitory syncope, pallid breath-holding spells (or reflex anoxic seizures), postural orthostatic tachycardia syndrome, among others. Ninety-five percent of syncope is vasodepressive or vasovagal. The incidence of simple fainting in female adolescents supersedes that of males.[5]

Additional causes of syncope include neurologic (headache, seizure, transient ischemic attack), psychiatric (depression, panic attack, functional neurologic disorder), and metabolic (drugs, carbon monoxide, electrolyte imbalance/problems). Toddlers may faint with breath-holding spells, most commonly between 6 months and 3 years old. Many of these cases resolve by 5 years old and the majority by 8 years old (after this time, they are usually classified as convulsive syncope).[5]

Clinical Findings

History
A thorough history that focuses on triggers and presyncope symptoms is the most critical test of syncopal causation (Table 33.9). Key history elements to review include:
- Triggering factor, such as exercise, pain, or an emotional event (e.g., anxiety, panic)
- Prior incident(s) of syncope or fainting (e.g., venipuncture, seeing blood, experiencing an injury)

| TABLE 33.9 | Relative Frequency of Premonitory Symptoms and Residual Findings With Common Neurally Mediated Syncope vs. More Serious Cardiac Syncope |||

	Neurally Mediated	Cardiac Syncope
Symptoms		
Premonitory symptoms	+++	±
Lightheadedness	+++	+/±
Palpitations	+	++
Occurs while upright	+++	+
Occurs while sitting	+/±	+
Emotional trigger	++	++
Exercise trigger	+	++
Residual Findings		
Pallor	+++	+/±
Incontinence	–	+
Disorientation	–	+
Fatigue	++	±
Diaphoresis	++	±
Injury	+	++

+++, Very common (>50%); ++, common (>20%); +, not rare (> ≈5%); ±, uncommon (<5%); –, rare (< ≈1%).

From Newburger JW, Alexander ME, Fulton DR. Innocent murmurs, syncope, and chest pain. In: Keane JF, Lock JE, Fyler DC, eds. *Nadas' Pediatric Cardiology.* 2nd ed. Elsevier; 2006.

- Associated injury, tonic-clonic movements, or vertigo
- Associated chest pain, palpitations, tachycardia, or bradycardia
- Family history of sudden death before age 40 years, congenital deafness, long QT syndrome, cardiomyopathy, and/or recurrent adolescent or toddler syncope that was outgrown
- Possibility of pregnancy or the use of illicit drugs; list all medications taken (including diet supplements, herbs, other botanicals, caffeine-containing and energy drinks)
- History of exercise-induced bronchospasms, respiratory distress, or other concomitant medical disorder
- Known psychological stress or stressors at home, school, or in social environments
- Standing for any length of time before the episode (indicates orthostasis); history of "head rushes" when standing up
- In a hot environment, sweating, dehydration; hunger
- Nausea, visual fields constriction ("world going dark") before episode
- Any postepisode symptoms, such as dizziness, pallor, clammy feeling, exhaustion, headache
- History of otherwise being well, active, with minimal medical issues
- Arousal after fainting within 1 to 2 minutes; recovery to full baseline state took more than 1 hour (many patients, though awake and alert, may not totally feel "like themselves" for a while)
- Stiffening, jerking motions during unconsciousness (tonic-clonic muscular contractions of face [including fixed upward deviation of eyes], trunk, and extremities mimicking epilepsy

occurs in approximately half of individuals experiencing a syncopal episode)
- Other activities before episode: hair grooming, coughing, micturition, neck stretching

Physical Examination

A detailed neurologic examination is needed if the syncopal episode suggests a seizure disorder. A cardiovascular examination is especially important. In most cases, the physical examination is completely normal.

Diagnostic Studies

Most individuals with cardiac syncope are identified either by a history of associated presyncope symptoms with exercise, abnormal ECG, family history of arrhythmia, or abnormal physical examination. The diagnosis of neurally mediated syncope can confidently be made based on history, normal examination, and normal ECG.[30] The diagnostic workup to distinguish between the two consists of:

- Orthostatic vital signs: More than a 30 mm Hg drop in BP after standing for 5 to 10 minutes, or a baseline systolic pressure of less than 80 mm Hg in an adolescent.
- Hemoglobin, if anemia is suspected: CBC, random glucose, and glucose tolerance tests have low yields and are not recommended routine tests for syncope.
- 12-lead ECG (assessing for LVH, Wolff-Parkinson-White syndrome, AV and interventricular conduction defects, electrical myopathies [e.g., long QT syndrome]): If ECG results are borderline or family history is highly suggestive of cardiac etiology, ECGs on siblings and parents may be useful. Twenty-four-hour Holter monitoring and portable 30-day event monitoring can also be beneficial.
- Echocardiography: Can be useful when history, physical, ECG, or family history suggests cardiac disease or cardiac syncope.
- Tilt table testing is not recommended for use in primary care due to poor reliability.
- Treadmill exercise testing may be used in cases of exercise-related syncope.

Differential Diagnosis/Management

If cardiac syncope is suspected, restrict the child from sports participation until referral to a pediatric cardiologist is completed. For neurally mediated syncope, education is key (cause, prevention, and how to abort a syncopal event). Prevention involves ensuring good hydration (along with decreasing caffeine and increasing sodium intake) and initiating antigravity techniques at the onset of presyncopal sensations (isometric leg or arm contractions; squatting or lying down; possibly using compression socks). The individual should rest for 5 to 10 minutes either supine or with legs up if prodromal symptoms occur before or after fainting. Concomitant cognitive-behavioral therapy is indicated for psychogenic episodes.[5]

In refractory cases, pharmacologic management by cardiology specialists may play a role, although this should not be the first-line treatment. These therapies may involve use of volume enhancement (fludrocortisone); limiting excessive catecholamine drive (using β-blockers, such as atenolol); vagolytic agents (disopyramide); and/or selective serotonin reuptake inhibitors. If drug therapy is used, the typical duration is 1 year, followed by weaning. Pacemaker implantation is used in rare cases.[30]

Differential diagnoses include migraine with confusion or stupor, seizures, hypoglycemia, hysteria, hyperventilation, vertigo, carbon monoxide poisoning, electrolyte imbalance, drugs, and cardiovascular disease, including underlying arrhythmia.

Additional Resources

American Heart Association: http://www.heart.org

Mended Hearts, Inc: http://www.mendedhearts.org

National Center for Biotechnology Information: http://www.ncbi.nlm.nih.gov.

National Institutes of Health Genetic Tests, Information About Genetic Defects or Syndromes, and Resources for Families: http://www.genetests.org

Online Mendelian Inheritance in Man: http://www.ncbi.nlm.nih.gov/omim

PediHeart: http://www.pediheart.net/ (requires a subscription)

References

1. Centers for Disease Control and Prevention. *Congenital Heart Defects (CHDs): Data & Statistics*; 2021. www.cdc.gov/ncbddd/heartdefects/data.html.
2. Martin G, Ewer A, Gaviglio A, et al. Updated strategies for pulse oximetry screening for critical congenital heart disease. *Pediatrics.* 2020;146(1):e20191650.
3. Murray S, McKinney E. *Foundations of Maternal Newborn and Women's Health Nursing.* 7th ed. Saunders/Elsevier; 2018.
4. Flynn JT, Kaelber DC, Baker-Smith CM, et al. Clinical practice guideline for screening and management of high blood pressure in children and adolescents. *Pediatrics.* 2017;140(3):1–72.
5. Park M. *Park's the Pediatric Cardiology Handbook.* 6th ed. Elsevier; 2021.
6. Park M. *Park's Pediatric Cardiology Handbook.* 6th ed. Elsevier; 2021.
7. Scott M, Neal A. Congenital heart disease. *Prim Care.* 2021;48(3):351–366.
8. Centers for Disease Control and Prevention. *General Best Practice Guidelines for Immunization: Best Practices Guidance of the Advisory Committee on Immunization Practices*; 2022. www.cdc.gov/vaccines/hcp/acip-recs/general-recs/timing.html.
9. American Academy of Pediatrics Committee on Infectious Diseases, AAP Bronchiolitis Guidelines Committee. Updated guidance for palivizumab prophylaxis among infants and young children at increased risk of hospitalization for respiratory syncytial virus infection. *Pediatrics.* 2014;134(2):415–420.
10. Centers for Disease Control and Prevention. CDC Recommends a Powerful New Tool to Protect Infants From The Leading Cause of Hospitalization. https://www.cdc.gov/media/releases/2023/p-0803-new-tool-prevent-infant-hospitalization-.html.
11. Shannon N, Chung WK. Genetic basis of human congenital heart disease. *Cold Spring Harb Perspect Biol.* 2020;12(9):a036749.
12. Meller C, Grinenco S, Aiello H, et al. *Arch Argent Pediatr.* 2020;118(2):e149–e161.
13. Price J. Congestive heart failure in children. *Pediatr Rev.* 2019;40(2):60–70.
14. Contractor T, Mandapati R. Arrhythmias in patients with atrial defects. *Card Electrophsiol Clin.* 2017;9:235–244.
15. Turner ME, Bouhout I, Petit CJ, Kalfa D. Transcatheter closure of atrial and ventricular septal defects: JACC Focus Seminar. *J Am Coll Cardiol.* 2022;79(22):2247–2258.
16. Dakkak W, Bhimji S. Ventricular septal defect. NCBI Stat Pearls. https://www.ncbi.nlm.nih.gov/books/NBK470330/.
17. Matiasz R, Rigolin VH. 2017 focused update for management of patients with valvular heart disease: summary of new recommendations. *J Am Heart Assoc.* 2018;7(1):e007596.
18. Mancini M. Tetralogy of Fallot. NORD. https://rarediseases.org/rare-diseases/tetralogy-of-fallot/.
19. Broberg CS, S, van Dissel A, Minnier J, et al. Long-term outcomes after atrial switch operation for tansposition of the great arteries. *J Am Coll Cardiol.* 2022;80(10):951–963.
20. Peyvandi S, Rollins C. Fetal brain development in congenital heart disease. *Can J Cardiol.* 2023;39(2):115–122.
21. Aro AL, Chugh SS. Prevention of sudden cardiac death in children and young adults. *Prog Pediatr Cardiol.* 2017;45:7–42.
22. John AS, Jackson JL, Moons P, et al. Advances in managing transition to adulthood for adolescents with congenital heart disease: a practical approach to transition program design: a scientific statement from the American Heart Association. *J Am Heart Assoc.* 2022;11(7):e025278.
23. Zaidi AN, Daniels CJ. The adolescent and adult with congenital heart disease. In: Allen HD, Driscoll DJ, Shaddy RE, et al., eds. *Moss and Adams' Heart Disease in Infants, Children, and Adolescents Including the Fetus and Young Adult.* 10th ed. Lippincott Williams & Wilkins; 2021.
24. Bizmark RS, Chang RKR, Tsugawa Y, et al. Impact of AHA's 2007 guideline change on incidence of infective endocarditis in infants and children. *Am Heart J.* 2017;189:110–119.
25. Dixon G, Christow G. Infective endocarditis in children: an update. *Curr Opin Infec Dis.* 2017;30(3):257–267.
26. Pomiato E, Perrone MA, Palmieri R, et al. Pediatric myocarditis: what have we learnt so far? *J Cardiovasc Dev Dis.* 2022;9(5):143.
27. Xiong H, Bingqing X, Zhu J, et al. Clinical outcomes in pediatric patients hospitalized with fulminant myocarditis requiring extracorporeal membrane oxygenation: a meta-analysis. *Pediatr Cardiol.* 2017;38(2):209–214.
28. Li M, Wang X, Feng J. Myocarditis or pericarditis following the COVID-19 vaccination in adolescents: a systematic review. *Vaccines.* 2022;10(8):1316.
29. Stasiak A, Kedziora P, Kierzkowska B, et al. Changes in the cardiovascular system in children with pediatric multisystem inflammatory syndrome temporally associated with COVID-19-A single center experience. *Int J Cardiol.* 2022:126–133.
30. Singhi P, Saini AE. Syncope in pediatric practice. *Indian J Pediatr.* 2017;85(8):636–640.
31. Thakkar AN, Chinnadurai P, Lin CH. Adult congenital heart disease: magnitude of the problem. *Curr Opin.* 2017;32(5):467–474.
32. Smith AH. Arrhythmias in cardiac critical care. *Pediatr Crit Care Med.* 2016;17(8 suppl 1):S146–S154.

34

Gastrointestinal Disorders

DANIELLE SEBBENS

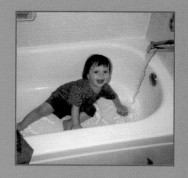

The gastrointestinal (GI) system, also known as the *digestive system,* processes the nutrients that give the body's cells the energy needed to function. Its sustained operation and maintenance are essential for the growth, development, and functioning of other organ systems. The pediatric primary care provider (PCP) is integral in caring for children with GI dysfunction. A thorough understanding of the GI system's anatomy, physiology, and common disorders is needed to assess and treat common pediatric GI problems and engage consultants as needed. This chapter focuses on common pediatric GI disorders.

Anatomy and Physiology

The GI system begins to develop during the third week of embryonic development. The primitive gut is initially formed and then divided into the fore-, mid-, and hindgut. These structures develop in an intricate and complex fashion to form the digestive tract and accessory organs. The foregut develops into the esophagus, stomach, liver, gallbladder, bile ducts, pancreas, and proximal duodenum; malformations of this part of the GI tract include esophageal atresia and biliary atresia. The midgut matures into the distal duodenum, jejunum, ileum, cecum, appendix, ascending colon and the first half to two-thirds of the transverse colon; errors in development of this section result in omphalocele, Meckel's diverticulum, and malrotation. The hindgut develops into the remaining transverse colon, descending colon, sigmoid colon, and the upper anal canal; the major pathology associated with hindgut malformation is Hirschsprung disease.

The GI tract extends from the mouth to the anus and includes the digestive organs and accessory organs including the liver, pancreas, and gallbladder. This system provides the following functions: ingestion, movement from the mouth toward the rectum, mechanical and chemical food dissolution, nutrient and water absorption, and waste product expulsion. The mouth ingests, chews, and mixes food with saliva. The tongue senses the food texture and taste, which stimulates salivation and the release of gastric juices in the stomach. The esophagus transports food from the mouth to the stomach by *peristalsis,* which is the sequential contraction and relaxation of the musculature in the esophagus. The upper esophageal sphincter prevents air from being swallowed while breathing. The lower esophageal sphincter (LES) prevents the stomach from regurgitating food, which is important because intraabdominal pressure exceeds intrathoracic and atmospheric pressures. The stomach serves as a reservoir for ingested foods. Its secretions mix with food, which is then propelled into the small intestine through the pylorus. The small intestine's primary function is absorption of nutrients (carbohydrates, fats, proteins, minerals, vitamins) into the systemic circulation.

Absorption occurs through villi, which cover the mucosal folds and serve as the functional unit of the intestine. Each villus contains an artery, a vein, and a lymph vessel that transports nutrients from the intestine into the systemic circulation. The villi are covered with enterocytes, whose major role is carbohydrate and protein digestion. Enterocytes secrete proteins and enzymes known as *brush border enzymes,* which assist in digestion. To be absorbed, carbohydrates must be converted to monosaccharides. This process begins in the mouth, where the salivary enzyme amylase breaks down complex starches into disaccharides. The brush border enzymes in the small intestine then convert disaccharides into monosaccharides (sucrose to glucose and fructose, lactose to glucose and galactose, maltose to glucose). Disaccharides remain osmotically active when this process is hindered (e.g., lactose intolerance) and can cause diarrhea. Fat absorption, which occurs mainly in the jejunum, is accomplished by adding lipases, secreted by the pancreas, and bile salts from the liver. Fats are absorbed by the lymphatic system.

Proteins are converted to amino acids by pepsin, which is secreted by the stomach and by pancreatic enzyme digestion. The resulting amino acids are further divided into smaller amino acid particles absorbed via the brush border into the systemic circulation. After appropriate absorption of nutrients, fecal liquid remains in the small intestine. This liquid is propelled by peristalsis through the large intestine, which removes the water from the fecal liquid and allows for short-term storage. The fecal mass, which consists of waste products, bacteria, intestinal secretions, and shed cells, is pushed forward into the sigmoid colon.

The entry of feces into the rectum stimulates the defecation reflex. This reflex stretches the rectal wall, relaxes the internal anal sphincter, and creates the need to defecate. If this urge is ignored, further fluid resorption occurs as the stool is retained, resulting in increased stool mass and dryness. Excessive stretching of the colon from the hard, dry stool bolus can lead to decreased peristalsis, further complicating stool retention.

Pathophysiology

The GI tract can be affected by illness, injury, or other problems that prevent it from normal function. Resulting dysfunction can be localized or systemic. Dysfunctions and include motility disorders; infection; malabsorption syndromes; impairment of digestion, absorption, and nutrition; congenital malformations and genetic syndromes; metabolic disorders; behavioral problems; injuries and trauma; and food intolerances, such as lactose and gluten intolerance due to absence of essential enzymes.

Assessment

History

Assessment of the GI system includes:

- Symptom analysis: How long has it been present? What makes it better or worse? What have you tried or attempted to treat? Has it impacted your activities of daily living?
- Associated symptoms: Any vomiting, nausea, belching, and flatulence?
- Nutritional patterns:
  - Feeding habits, nutrition history, current diet (what, when, how often, how tolerated)
  - Changes in appetite/thirst
  - Food intolerance or allergy (which foods, reaction, treatment)
- Elimination patterns: Bowel habits (frequency, consistency, associated pain, need for medications or enemas)
  - Constipation or diarrhea (definition of each, how often they occur, and treatment tried). (See Bristol Stool Chart—Chapter 17).
  - Changes in bowel pattern
- Presence/location of pain (onset, type, quality, aggravating/alleviating factors)
  - *Epigastric* pain usually indicates pain from the liver, pancreas, biliary tree, stomach, and upper part of the small bowel (duodenum).
  - *Periumbilical* pain is generated from the distal end of the small intestine, cecum, appendix, and ascending colon.
  - *Colonic* visceral pain is lower abdominal pain that can be dull, diffuse, cramping, or burning.
  - *Suprapubic* discomfort indicates distal intestine, urinary tract, and pelvic organ dysfunction.
  - *Referred* pain is a diagnostic challenge. For example, because of convergent nerve pathways, inflammation of the diaphragm can generate pain that is perceived as shoulder or lower neck pain. When visceral pain is overwhelming, referred pain occurs.
  - *Acute* continuous pain is more indicative of an acute process.
- Family history of GI disease (e.g., gallbladder disease, stomach ulcers, food allergy, inflammatory bowel disease [IBD], Hirschsprung disease).
- Past medical history related to the GI system (e.g., illnesses, surgeries, congenital disorders, such as cleft lip/palate, esophageal atresia).
- Review of systems: Apnea or asthma that may be caused by gastroesophageal reflux (GER), concerns or symptoms of cardiac insufficiency, autoimmune symptoms (e.g., rashes)

Physical Examination

When assessing a suspected GI problem, a head-to-toe physical examination is indicated.

- Plot growth parameters, including weight for length/height, noting proportionality and/or growth aberrations.
- Determine hydration status (skin turgor, mucous membranes, peripheral pulses, presence of tears, capillary filling).
- Inspect the abdomen for visible peristalsis, rashes, lesions, asymmetry, masses, organomegaly, and pulsations.
- Auscultate bowel sounds (10–30/minute for infants; 5–20/minute for children and adolescents).
- Percuss for density and to measure organs.
- Palpate both lightly and deeply.
- Assess peritoneal irritation:
  - Have the patient walk standing straight up or cough.
  - Have the patient stand on tiptoes and fall onto the heels or jump. This is the heel-jar test and is positive if it causes abdominal pain.
  - Palpate for rebound tenderness and/or positive *Rovsing sign* (palpation in the left iliac fossa produces pain in the right iliac fossa).
  - Check for the positive *obturator sign* (while supine, the patient flexes the right thigh at the hip with the knee bent and internally rotates the hip; it is positive if it induces abdominal pain).
  - Check for positive *psoas sign* (patient lies on the left side, extends and then flexes the right leg at the hip. It is positive if the maneuver induces abdominal pain.
- Perform a rectal examination. This is typically included when intraabdominal, pelvic, or perirectal disease is suspected, although it is often done in a newborn examination to assess for anal stenosis. NOTE: This examination is intrusive, and patients should be prepared.
  - Include external inspection first, followed by internal palpation for masses, stool, or irregularities. The index finger is typically used because of its increased sensitivity; however, in infants and young children, use the fifth finger. Insert a gloved, lubricated finger into the rectum. Place the other hand on the abdomen for a bimanual examination.
  - Position young patients supine with their feet held together, knees and hips flexed, and put their knees over their abdomen. Adolescent males can be lying on their side or standing with the hips flexed and the upper part of the body on the examination table. Adolescent females can lie on their side or, if a concurrent pelvic examination is to be done, in the lithotomy position.
- Perform a gynecologic examination if a pathologic pelvic condition is suspected (see Chapter 43).

Common Diagnostic Studies

Laboratory Tests

Tests may include:

- Urinalysis (UA) and urine culture
- Complete blood count (CBC) with differential
- Serum chemistry screen, liver profile, lipid profile, erythrocyte sedimentation rate (ESR), C-reactive protein (CRP), thyroid function
- Serology tests for IBD including anti-*Saccharomyces cerevisiae* antibody (ASCA) (positive predominantly in Crohn disease) and atypical perinuclear antineutrophil cytoplasmic antibody (pANCA) (positive predominantly in ulcerative colitis [UC]).
- Stool examination for ova and parasites (O&P), culture, blood, white blood cells (WBCs), pH, reducing substances
- Fecal fat collection for 72 hours to rule out fat malabsorption
- Pregnancy test
- Urine tests for gonorrhea or chlamydia, Papanicolaou (Pap) smear and vaginal cultures and smears if a pelvic or gynecologic pathologic condition is suspected

Imaging Studies

Common imaging studies used to assess the GI system include:

Radiography

- Abdominal radiographs—(Two views): supine and upright (or right side up decubitus) positions are the preliminary screening approach in children with nonspecific presentations, as it is readily available, less expensive, and utilizes lower radiation exposure than other studies.
- Upper and lower GI with fluoroscopy and barium swallow studies to demonstrate anatomy and function. An upper GI (UGI) series may be warranted to evaluate bowel obstruction (e.g., late presentation of malrotation, surgical adhesions) in patients with bilious and/or protracted vomiting. Small bowel follow-through may be added if IBD (particularly Crohn disease) is suspected. An air contrast enema can diagnose and treat intussusception.

Abdominal Ultrasonography

- No ionizing radiation, noninvasive, relatively inexpensive
- May be indicated to evaluate gallstones, appendicitis, extrahepatic bile ducts, pancreatic pseudocyst, hydronephrosis, or retroperitoneal mass
- Pelvic ultrasonography may be indicated to evaluate ovarian masses or pregnancy

Magnetic Resonance Imaging

- It may be warranted if IBD is suspected, particularly Crohn disease.

Computed Tomography

- May be warranted to evaluate retroperitoneal or intraabdominal abscesses (e.g., associated with IBD)
- Usually reserved for urgent evaluation (e.g., abscess, mass) given concerns about radiation exposure

Specialized tests may also be considered:
- Duodenal aspirate to identify existing infection
- Esophageal pH probe to establish gastroesophageal reflux disease (GERD), with a pH of less than 4 indicating a reflux episode
- Capsule endoscopy to record internal images of the gastrointestinal tract to evaluate IBD and chronic diarrhea; does not require radiation exposure
- Breath hydrogen test if lactose intolerance is suspected
- Sweat chloride test if cystic fibrosis (CF) is suspected (see Chapter 32)

Management Strategies

Medications

Multiple medications are used to treat GI disorders, including:
- Antibiotics, antifungals, or anthelmintics
- Antiemetics and antidiarrheals
- Stool softeners, laxatives, and cathartics
- Medications that promote gastric emptying and/or alter GI motility or tone (e.g., dopamine receptor antagonists, serotonin receptor agonists)
- Oral steroids, parenteral steroids, and other immunosuppressants (e.g., treatment of IBD)
- Pain medications and antispasmodics in selected acute and chronic GI conditions
- Medications that alter gastric acidity (e.g., antacids, H_2 antagonists, proton pump inhibitors [PPIs])
- Iron supplementation as supportive therapy for chronic disease
- Vitamin B_{12} injections if chronic inflammation results in malabsorption

Probiotics and Prebiotics

Prebiotics are nondigestible dietary fibers and fructo-oligosaccharides (carbohydrate molecules made up of a relatively small number of simple sugars) acquired from food and used as an energy source by the beneficial bacteria that naturally live in the intestines. Prebiotics are sometimes known as "fermentable fiber." They give the probiotic bacteria a chance to exert their influence by acting as a food source. The concept of prebiotics was first introduced in 1995 by Gibson and Roberfoid[1] as an alternative approach to modulating the gut microbiota. The role of prebiotics role in treating disease is controversial, and more studies are needed to determine their usefulness in primary care. Preliminary evidence shows that prebiotics may have a role in improving antibiotic-associated diarrhea (AAD), traveler's diarrhea, and gastroenteritis; normalizing bowel function; improving colitis; reducing irritable bowel problems; aiding calcium absorption; and boosting the immune system.[2,3] Common prebiotics include oligosaccharides and inulin. Inulin is found in more than 36,000 species of plants, including wheat, onions, bananas, garlic, asparagus, Jerusalem artichoke, and chicory.

Probiotics are beneficial bacteria. They also include live microbial food supplements or components of bacteria with demonstrated beneficial effects for the host. To be most effective, a probiotic species must survive passage through the stomach's acidic environment and thrive in and colonize the intestine, even in the presence of antibiotics. Probiotics promote healing of the intestinal mucosa by reducing gut permeability, enhancing local intestinal immune responses, and reconstituting the intestinal flora. They are often regulated as dietary supplements rather than as pharmaceuticals or biological products. There are varying requirements to demonstrate safety, purity, or potency before marketing probiotics, causing the potential for significant inconsistencies between the stated and actual contents of probiotic preparations. In the United States, dietary supplements generally do not require premarket review and approval by the Food and Drug Administration (FDA). Probiotics are used in clinical practice for a variety of purposes. Most of the identified benefits of probiotics relate to GI conditions, including irritable bowel syndrome (IBS), infectious diarrhea, AAD, and traveler's diarrhea.[4] The most widely used and researched organisms are *Lactobacillus, Bifidobacterium,* and *Saccharomyces;* however, their exact mechanism of action remains unclear. *Lactobacillus* promotes healthy bacterial flora in the digestive tract and is widely used to manage and prevent AAD, traveler's diarrhea, and infectious diarrhea. Some suggest specific strains of *Lactobacillus reuteri* may help relieve infantile colic.[2] *Bifidobacterium* is widely used to manage abdominal bloating, flatulence, and abdominal pain, all symptoms of IBS. *Saccharomyces* have some effectiveness in treating and managing AAD and infectious diarrhea.

Some of the most common uses of probiotics in the treatment of digestive disease include:
- *IBS:* Probiotics may improve symptoms of IBS, but overall conclusions are limited by inconsistency in specific probiotics studied.[3]
- *Infectious diarrhea:* Probiotics and prebiotics use is associated with duration and severity of rotavirus diarrhea, infection prevention, and reduced incidence of reinfections.[5]
- *AAD:* Probiotics may help prevent AAD through a gut barrier and restoration of gut microflora.[6]
- *Colic:* Probiotics may be used to decrease crying times and fussiness, with differences noted between infants who are exclusively breastfed and those who are not.[2]

Upper Gastrointestinal Tract Disorders

Dysphagia

Dysphagia, or difficulty swallowing, is caused by various disorders. Young children may present with the inability to swallow, while older children may relay difficulty swallowing or complain of a sensation that something is stuck in their throat (i.e., globus pharyngitis). The physiology of swallowing is complex and involves three phases: oral, pharyngeal, and esophageal. The *oral phase* involves ingestion, mastication, and the propulsion of food to the back of the mouth as a bolus. The *pharyngeal phase* includes the swallowing and transfer of food from the pharynx to the esophagus. Airway closure is critical during the *pharyngeal phase* and requires intact motor and sensory pharyngeal protective mechanisms to prevent aspiration. In the *esophageal phase*, food passes to the stomach.

Dysphagia can result from a variety of disorders or defects. *Structural defects* make swallowing solids more difficult than swallowing liquids. They include esophageal stenosis, or narrowing (e.g., stricture, web, tumor) or extrinsic obstruction (e.g., vascular ring). Nonstructural causes arise from oropharyngeal or esophageal *motility disorders* and are uncommon in pediatrics. Other causes include prematurity and neurologic impairment from disorders (e.g., cerebral palsy, muscular dystrophy). Dysphagia from *mucosal injury* most commonly occurs from GERD, eosinophilic esophagitis (EoE), or gastritis, but it can also result from caustic ingestion or medication. The number of children with swallowing difficulties has increased because medical and technological advances increased the survival of children and youth with special healthcare needs (CYSHCN) and those with sensorimotor deficits.

Clinical Findings

History
- Progressive dysfunction
- Persistent drooling or cough
- Discomfort with swallowing or a sense of food getting stuck after swallowing
- Picky eating (e.g., a child who prefers liquids to solids) or food refusal
- Halitosis
- Chest pain

Physical Examination
- Observe feeding adequacy, paying special attention to oral motor skills and swallowing safety.
- Perform a complete physical examination, paying particular attention to the mouth, throat, and neck.

Diagnostic Studies
- Lateral neck films
- Barium swallow (usually the initial procedure because it is especially effective detecting esophageal narrowing)
- Fiberoptic endoscopy swallowing evaluation
- Video fluoroscopy swallowing study
- Esophageal manometry (the gold standard for diagnosing motor disorders)
- Magnetic resonance imaging (MRI) (for structural abnormalities)
- Electromyography

Differential Diagnosis

Obstructive and compressive lesions usually cause trouble with solids only. Physiologic dysfunction is generally associated with systemic disease, and the patient has difficulty swallowing both liquids and solids. A dysfunctional feeding relationship between child and feeder can manifest as dysphagia.

Management

Dysphagia requires evaluating associated cognitive, sensory-motor, developmental, and behavioral issues. A multidisciplinary approach, involving professionals from otolaryngology, gastroenterology, nutrition, occupational therapy, psychology, and speech-language pathology, is recommended to provide a comprehensive, cost-effective evaluation and consistent care for the child and family.

Vomiting and Dehydration

Vomiting is the forceful emptying of gastric contents coordinated by the medullary vomiting center and the brain's chemoreceptor trigger zone. It is different from *regurgitation*, which is a passive reflux of gastric contents into the oral pharynx. Vomiting can be caused by GI or external disorders that can be either acute or chronic. Common descriptors include projectile (often arising from the central nervous system [CNS]) nonprojectile (often seen in GER); and bilious or nonbilious, and bloody or nonbloody. Projectile vomiting is a sudden and forceful emesis expelled up to several feet in front of the child. Bilious emesis is typically green in appearance; however, it may also be yellow-green, as both reflect bile in the stomach. Bloody emesis includes bright red-, brown-, or black-appearing vomitus. The blood volume may range from streaks or flecks to a larger volume with clots. Projectile, bilious, or bloody emesis requires urgent evaluation.

The patient's age helps to formulate an appropriate list of potential diagnoses:
- Newborn/young infant: infection, congenital GI anomaly, CNS abnormality, or inborn errors of metabolism, obstruction (e.g., pyloric stenosis)
- Older infant/early childhood: gastroenteritis, GERD, milk/soy protein allergies, pyloric stenosis or other obstructive lesion, inborn errors of metabolism, intussusception, child abuse, intracranial mass
- Middle childhood/adolescence: gastroenteritis, systemic illness, CNS (cyclic vomiting syndrome [CVS], abdominal migraine, meningitis, brain tumor), intussusception, rumination, superior mesenteric artery syndrome, pregnancy

Vomiting is one of the most common pediatric symptoms. Nonbilious vomit is generally secondary to infection, inflammation, and metabolic, neurologic, or psychological problems. An obstructive lesion generally causes bilious vomiting, while bloody vomitus usually accompanies active bleeding in the UGI tract (e.g., gastritis, peptic ulcer disease [PUD]).

Following is a list of potential causes of vomiting by site of originating disorder:
- Oropharynx: Cleft palate, laryngopharyngeal cleft
- UGI: Congenital stricture, foreign body (FB), gastritis, esophagitis, gastric web, pyloric stenosis, tracheoesophageal fistula, vascular ring, PUD
- Small intestine: Annular pancreas, choledochal cyst, intestinal atresia/stenosis, intestinal malrotation with volvulus, intestinal pseudo-obstruction
- Colon: HD, intussusception, meconium ileus, necrotizing enterocolitis, fecal impaction
- Hepatobiliary or pancreatic dysfunction
- Infections: Bacterial enteritis, otitis media, sepsis, urinary tract infection (UTI), viral gastroenteritis (VGE), hepatitis

- Neurologic: Congenital anatomic malformation, gray and white matter degenerative disorders, hydrocephalus, kernicterus, brain tumors, migraine headache, head trauma
- Other: Cow's-milk protein (CMP) allergy or intolerance, inborn errors of metabolism, intrauterine drug exposure and withdrawal, toxic ingestions, appendicitis, cyclic vomiting, pneumonia, drug or alcohol ingestion, eating disorder, pregnancy

Dehydration is the loss of water and *hypovolemia* is the loss of extracellular fluid. These terms are often used interchangeably. Dehydration is overwhelmingly caused by infectious processes, primarily viral that often cause diarrhea. Infants and children are at increased risk for dehydration due to their higher surface area-to-volume ratios, higher rate of insensible fluid loss, and inability to communicate or actively replenish losses. Depending on the cause, water and salts (e.g., sodium chloride) losses may be physiologically proportionate or disparate, producing one of three types of dehydration: *isonatremic* (isotonic), *hypernatremic* (hypertonic), or *hyponatremic* (hypotonic). When dehydration is caused by simple diarrhea, homeostatic mechanisms usually maintain sodium concentrations in the serum, resulting in isonatremic dehydration. When vomiting occurs with diarrhea and water intake is less, there is greater water loss than salt loss, leading to hypernatremic dehydration. In contrast, when there is massive stool loss of water and salt, and only water is ingested, there is a significant salt loss, potentially resulting in hyponatremia.

Clinical Findings

History. The *vomiting* history should include:
- Symptom analysis: Onset and duration of vomiting, quality/quantity, presence of blood or bile, odor; precipitating event; pain; relationship of vomiting to meals, activities, or time of day. Note: Vomiting early in the morning can indicate increased intracranial pressure.
- Recent exposures: Illness or injury, stress, travel (including camping), swimming, possibility of food poisoning or contaminated food
- Current medications (including over-the-counter [OTC], herbal, homeopathic, folk or culture-based remedies)

- Associated symptoms: Diarrhea, fever, ear pain, UTI symptoms, vision changes, cough, headache, seizures, high-pitched cry, polydipsia, polyuria, polyphagia, anorexia
- Past medical history: Illnesses, surgeries, or hospitalizations
- Family history of GI disease: Include fetal or neonatal deaths, metabolic syndrome, congenital anomaly

The *dehydration* history should include:
- Mental status and thirst
- Parental concern regarding decreased tearing or urination, or depressed fontanel newborn/infant)

Physical Examination

- Baseline: Growth parameters and vital signs, Note: Hypotension is a late manifestation of dehydration.
- Neurologic examination: Nuchal rigidity, decreased level of consciousness, and behavioral changes (e.g., irritability, lethargy). Note: Sensorium remains intact until there is greater than 6% weight loss due to dehydration.
- Abdominal examination: Distention, scars from previous surgery (may be associated with obstruction/adhesions), visible peristaltic waves.
  - Auscultate bowel sounds (i.e., increased with gastroenteritis, decreased with obstruction, absent with ileus or peritonitis)
  - Palpate for pain or rebound tenderness, organomegaly, masses
  - Rectal examination, as indicated
- Respiratory examination: Tachypnea, decreased oxygen saturation, stridor
- Dehydration assessment (Table 34.1)
  - Capillary refill time (CRT). Normal CRT is less than 2 seconds. Note: CRT, skin turgor, and tachypnea, considered together, are most helpful when determining dehydration.[7]
  - Clinical dehydration scale (CDS). The four parameters used for assessment are general appearance, eyes (sunken or not), moistness of mucous membranes, and presence of tears. (Table 34.2). Note: CDS scores predict length of stay and the need for intravenous (IV) fluids.[8]

TABLE 34.1   Pediatric Dehydration Assessment

	Mild Dehydration	Moderate Dehydration	Severe Dehydration
Weight loss (newborn/infant)	4%–5%	6%–9%	≥10% weight loss
Anterior fontanel (newborn/infant)	Normal	Mildly sunken	Very sunken
Mental status	Normal	Irritable	Lethargic/somnolent
Tears (not newborn)	Normal	Decreased	Absent
Mucous membranes	Mildly dry	Dry	Very dry
Urine output	Normal or mildly decreased	Reduced or concentrated	Anuria >8 hours
Respirations	Normal	Mildly rapid	Deep and rapid
Blood pressure	Normal	Normal to mild orthostatic hypotension (>10 mm Hg change)	Hypotension
Pulse	Normal	Rapid	Weak and rapid
Skin turgor	Normal	Decreased	Severely decreased/tenting present
Capillary refill	Normal (<2 s)	Slowed (2–4 s)	Marked delayed (>4 s)

From Zhu F. Evaluation and management of traveler's diarrhea in children. *Pediatr Clin North Am*. 2022;69(1):99–113.

TABLE 34.2 Differential Diagnosis of Vomiting

Age	Nonbilious	Bilious
Newborn and infant (0 days–1 year)	Overfeeding, physiologic reflux, milk protein sensitivity, pyloric stenosis, necrotizing enterocolitis, metabolic disorder, infection (GU, respiratory, GI), esophageal/intestinal atresia/stenosis, and Hirschsprung disease	Malrotation ± volvulus, intestinal atresia/stenosis, intussusception, pancreatitis
Early childhood (1–5 years)	Cyclic vomiting, infectious (GI, GU), toxic ingestion, diabetic ketoacidosis (DKA), CNS mass effect, eosinophilic esophagitis, posttussive, peptic disease, and appendicitis	Malrotation, intussusception, incarcerated hernia, pancreatitis, intestinal dysmotility
Middle childhood and adolescence	Eating disorders, pregnancy, CNS mass effect, eosinophilic esophagitis, DKA, peptic disease, cyclic vomiting, toxins/drugs of abuse, infectious (GI, GU), and appendicitis	Peritoneal adhesions, malrotation, incarcerated hernia, pancreatitis, and intestinal dysmotility

CNS, Central nervous system; GI, gastrointestinal; GU, genitourinary.

From Buendia M, Thoni N. Gastroenterology. In: Kleinman K, McDaniel L, Molloy M, eds. *The Harriet Lane Handbook.* 22nd ed. Elsevier; 2021:283–299.

Diagnostic Studies

- Laboratory studies:
  - CBC with differential, blood culture
  - Electrolytes, including blood urea nitrogen (BUN) and creatinine, glucose, and liver function tests
  - Serum sodium less than 130 mEq/L (hyponatremic) or greater than 150 mEq/L (hypernatremic)
  - CRP and ESR
  - Serum lactate, organic acids, and ammonia for metabolic disorders (may only be abnormal during episodes of vomiting)
  - UA and urine culture
  - Toxicology screen
  - Stool for culture and occult blood, leukocytes, parasites, fat, pH, reducing substances
  - Rapid strep test and throat culture
  - Pregnancy test
- Imaging:
  - Abdominal radiographs (suspected obstruction, FB ingestion, organomegaly, or a palpable mass)
  - Chest radiograph (suspected pneumonia)
  - Ultrasound (abscesses, masses, stenoses, cysts, appendicitis, pyloric stenosis)
  - Barium swallow or enema (malrotation, GER, masses)
  - CT or MRI (masses, inflammation, herniations, perforations, obstructions)
- Other studies:
  - Endoscopy (obstruction, hemorrhage, infection, biopsies)
  - Esophageal pH probe analysis
  - Scintiscan (e.g., MIBG neuroendocrine tumors, such as neuroblastoma, pheochromocytoma)
  - Electroencephalogram

Differential Diagnosis

See Table 34.2.

Management

Vomiting. Treatment involves initial rehydration, fluid maintenance, and ongoing loss replacement (Table 34.3):
- Identify and alleviate the cause.
- Antiemetics may be warranted. Ondansentron (Zofran), a 5-hydroxytryptamine (5-HT$_3$) receptor antagonist, combined with oral rehydration therapy, is successful for the management of vomiting in children (off-label in children under 4 years old).[9]
- Refer to a GI specialist for persistent or recurrent vomiting, or vomiting associated with a significant underlying process.

Dehydration

- Physiologically, sodium and glucose couple in transport across the intestinal brush border into the systemic circulation to maximize rehydration. Initially, administer oral fluids in frequent, small (5 mL or less) amounts. Larger amounts may be given as tolerated. Plain water, juices, soda, milk, and sports drinks should be avoided as they are hyperosmolar and do not replace glucose and electrolytes appropriately. The palatability of ORS does not affect the quantity consumed. Homemade solutions can be used when premade ORS is unavailable. Refeeding should resume as quickly as possible because the gut needs nutrition to facilitate mucosal repair following injury. Determine the degree of dehydration.
  - If *minimal, mild,* or *moderate,* oral rehydration solution (ORS) with 70 to 90 mEq/L sodium, 25 g/L glucose, 20 mEq/L potassium, 30 mEq/L base (citrate, acetate, or lactate) with a defined osmolarity of 240 to 300 mOsm/L is recommended.
  - If *severe,* immediate and aggressive intervention is needed (e.g., IV fluids).
- Pediatric subcutaneous rehydration (i.e., hypodermoclysis) using recombinant human hyaluronidase aids absorption of subcutaneous fluids reduces the risk of allergic reaction and increases absorption.[10]
- Antiemetics: A single dose of an orally disintegrating tablet of ondansetron (2 mg for children 8–15 kg, 4 mg for children 15–30 kg, and 8 mg for more than 30 kg) reduces vomiting.[11]
- Treat fever over 38.2°C.
- Monitor all output, especially urine.
- Immediately refer children with a toxic appearance, severe dehydration, projectile vomiting, abnormal physical examination, vomiting for greater than 12 hours, decreased urine output to less than 1 mL/kg/h, and/or vomiting of blood, bile, or fecal matter.

Complications

Dehydration, fluid and electrolyte imbalance, aspiration pneumonia, hemorrhage, or a tear of the esophagus are possible.

Patient and Family Education

Providing specific written information to the caregiver about the care required during oral rehydration therapy is helpful. Also include information about red flags or signs that indicate the child is not responding to treatment, including expected timeframe for improvement, or worsening.

TABLE 34.3 Treatment Based on Stages and Management of Dehydration

Degree of Dehydration	Rehydration Therapy	Maintenance	Replacement of Ongoing Losses
Minimal or none	Not applicable	0–10 kg: 100 mL/kg/24 h 10–20 kg: 1000 mL + 50 mL/kg for each kg over 10 kg >20 kg: 1500 mL +20 mL/kg for each kg over 20 kg	<10 kg body weight: 60–120 mL ORS for each diarrheal stool or vomiting episode >10 kg body weight: 120–240 mL ORS for each diarrheal stool or vomiting episode
Mild to moderate	ORS: 50–100 mL/kg body weight over 3–4 h or 10–20 mL/kg/h	Same	Same
Severe	Lactated Ringer's solution or normal saline[a] IV in boluses of 20 mL/kg body weight until perfusion and mental status improve. If after 60–80 mL/kg given, other causes of shock should be considered, then administer 100 mL/kg body weight ORS over 4 h or 5% dextrose in 1/2 normal saline IV at twice maintenance fluid rates	Same	Same: If unable to drink, administer through nasogastric tube or administer 5% dextrose in 1/4 normal saline with 20 mEq/L potassium chloride IV

Nutrition

- Continue breastfeeding.
- Lactose-containing formulas are usually well tolerated. If lactose malabsorption appears clinically substantial, lactose-free formulas can be used.
- Return to regular milk in smaller amounts more often.
- Resume age-appropriate normal diet after initial rehydration, including adequate caloric intake for maintenance.
- Complex carbohydrates, fresh fruits, lean meats, yogurt, and vegetables are all recommended.
- Avoid fatty foods and foods high in simple sugars.
- Avoid carbonated drinks or commercial juices.

[a]In severe dehydrating diarrhea, normal saline is less effective than Ringer lactate solution for treatment because it contains no bicarbonate or potassium. Use normal saline only if Ringer lactate solution is not available, and supplement with ORS as soon as the patient can drink. Plain glucose in water is ineffective and should not be used.

ORS, Oral rehydration solution.

From Burgunder L. Fluids and electrolytes. In: Kleinman K, McDaniel L, Molloy M, eds. *The Harriet Lane Handbook.* 22nd ed. Elsevier; 2021: 261–282.

Cyclic Vomiting Syndrome

CVS is an uncommon, idiopathic disorder that is characterized by recurrent, sudden-onset attacks of repeated retching and vomiting, separated by symptom-free intervals of weeks to months.[12] Accompanying symptoms include pallor, listlessness, appetite loss, nausea, diarrhea, abdominal pain, fever, dizziness, headache, and photophobia.[13]

The etiology is unclear, although it is often associated with other episodic conditions (e.g., migraine headaches, abdominal migraine). Less common is the association of CVS with mitochondrial DNA variants. Some patients report *triggers* (e.g., teething, fever, upper respiratory infection [URI]); others report *prodromes* (e.g., headache, abdominal pain, photophobia, phonophobia, vertigo).[13]

Clinical Findings

History
- Red flags (Box 34.1)
- Family history: migraine headache is common
- Phases: prodrome, vomiting, and recovery
  - Begins and ends abruptly
  - More likely to occur early in the morning (3:00–4:00 am) or upon awakening
  - Intense nausea not relieved by vomiting
  - Headache, motion sickness, photophobia, phonophobia, or vertigo may occur
- Identifiable trigger is common in children: physical stress (infection, lack of sleep, menstrual periods), psychological

• BOX 34.1 Red Flags for Cyclic Vomiting Syndrome

- Abdominal: Bilious vomiting, abdominal tenderness, and/or severe abdominal pain, hematemesis.
- Triggering events: Fasting, high-protein meal, or intercurrent illness.
- Abnormal neurologic examination: Severely altered mental status, abnormal eye movements, papilledema, motor asymmetry, and/or gait abnormality [ataxia].
- Progressive, worsening episodes or conversion to a continuous or chronic pattern.

Data from Hyams J, Di Lorenzo C, Saps M, et al. Functional disorders: children and adolescents. *Gastroenterology.* 2016;150(6):1456–1470; Dipasquale V, Falsaperla R, Bongiovanni A, et al. Clinical features and long-term outcomes in pediatric cyclic vomiting syndrome: a 9-year experience at three tertiary academic centers. *Neurogastroenterol Motil.* 2022;34(3):e14224-14230; Raucci U, Borrelli O, Nardo G, et al. Cyclic vomiting in children. *Front Neurol.* 2020;11:583425.

stress (birthdays, holidays, school), or food product (e.g., chocolate, cheese, monosodium glutamate)
- Brief prodromal period: combination of pallor, anorexia, nausea, abdominal pain
- Brief recovery period: from ill to playing again

Physical Examination. Physical examination is normal, although these children appear more ill than those with VGE. If red flags are present, further evaluation is indicated.

Diagnostic Studies. Excluding organic causes of vomiting is not required when the patient presents with clinical findings

BOX 34.2 Lifestyle Changes for Cyclic Vomiting Syndrome

1. Keep a journal of potential precipitating factors to identify triggers (75% of patients can improve with this alone):
   - Recognize the role of excitement as a trigger (e.g., downplay big events) to avoid excessive energy output.
   - Avoid trigger foods (chocolate, cheese, monosodium glutamate, hot dogs, aspartame, antigenic foods).
2. Provide supplemental carbohydrate for fasting-induced episodes or high-energy demand times (e.g., fruit juices or other sugar-containing drinks, snacks between meals, before exertion, or at bedtime).
3. Maintain healthy lifestyle:
   - Regular aerobic exercise, avoiding overexercising
   - Regular meal schedules; don't skip meals
   - Maintain good sleep hygiene
   - Maintain good hydration
   - Avoid or moderate caffeine consumption.

Data from Hyams J, Di Lorenzo C, Saps M, et al. Functional disorders: children and adolescents. *Gastroenterology.* 2016;150(6):1456–1470; Dipasquale V, Falsaperla R, Bongiovanni A, et al. Clinical features and long-term outcomes in pediatric cyclic vomiting syndrome: a 9-year experience at three tertiary academic centers. *Neurogastroenterol Motil.* 2022;34(3):e14224–14230; Raucci U, Borrelli O, Nardo G, et al. Cyclic vomiting in children. *Front Neurol.* 2020;11:583425.

BOX 34.3 Prophylactic Medication for Cyclic Vomiting Syndrome

Children ≤5 Years
- Cyproheptadine (first choice): 0.25–0.5 mg/kg/day divided bid or tid. Maximum dosage *2–6 years:* 12 mg/24 h.

Children >5 Years
- Amitriptyline (first choice): 0.1–0.25 mg/kg at bedtime, increase weekly by 0.1–0.25 until maximum dose of 2 mg/kg/24 h or 75 mg/24 h. For doses >1 mg/kg/24 h, divide daily dose bid and monitor electrocardiogram (ECG). Monitor ECG before starting and 10 days after peak dose. *Adult:* Initial 10–25 mg/dose qhs PO; reported range oSf 10–400 mg/24 h.
- Propranolol (second choice–see earlier): 0.25–1 mg/kg/day, most often 10 mg bid to tid; *<35 kg:* 10–20 mg PO tid; *≥35 kg:* 20–40 mg PO tid. Taper when discontinuing; monitor resting heart rate.

Data from Hyams J, Di Lorenzo C, Saps M, et al. Functional disorders: children and adolescents. *Gastroenterology.* 2016;150(6):1456–1470; Dipasquale V, Falsaperla R, Bongiovanni A, et al. Clinical features and long-term outcomes in pediatric cyclic vomiting syndrome: a 9-year experience at three tertiary academic centers. *Neurogastroenterol Motil.* 2022;34(3):e14224–14230; Raucci U, Borrelli O, Nardo G, et al. Cyclic vomiting in children. *Front Neurol.* 2020;11:583425.

meeting the Rome IV criteria from CVS. If red flags exist or the provider/caregiver requests further evaluation, the following are recommended:
- Electrolytes, including sodium bicarbonate (HCO_3)
- UGI radiographs (exclude malrotation)
- Abdominal ultrasound (exclude hydronephrosis)
- Hyponatremia or hypoglycemia needs further evaluation to exclude Addison disease and fatty acid oxidation

Differential Diagnosis

Symptoms experienced during the prodromal phase in patients with CVS include headache, abdominal pain, lethargy, and vertigo.[13] Migraine headaches or intraabdominal pathology are included in the differential diagnosis. Often episodes occur in the early morning and mimic symptoms of increased intracranial pressure leading to MRI to exclude cerebral abnormalities.[13]

Management

There is no definitive treatment, but some treatments (e.g., antiemetics) show benefits in a case-by-case series.[13] Management is divided into well phase and acute phase treatment.

Well Phase: Prevention and Prophylaxis. Keys to successful prevention include lifestyle modifications, trigger avoidance, stress reduction, and prophylactic medications (Box 34.2). Some examples include receiving adequate sleep to prevent exhaustion, treating allergies and sinus problems, instituting measures to reduce stress and anxiety, and avoiding foods with additives and those known to trigger episodes. Eating small carbohydrate-containing snacks between meals, before exercise, and at bedtime are also advised.[14] Additional treatments include:
- Trial of prophylactic medication (Box 34.3) if abortive therapy fails consistently or episodes are frequent and severe.
- Titrate doses every 1 to 4 weeks to achieve a therapeutic dose for at least two CVS cycles.
- Phenobarbital and supplements (L-carnitine and coenzyme Q10) have also been used.[14]

Acute Episode: Interventions
- Supportive measures: Early intervention (within 2–4 hours of onset); a dark, quiet environment; and fluid, electrolyte, and calorie replacement. If anxiety is a trigger, relaxation exercises may be helpful.
- Pharmacologic: Administer abortive therapy as early as possible.
  - Antimigraine (triptans) in children and teens older than 12 years with infrequent and mild episodes (less than one per month); sumatriptan 20 mg intranasally at onset is contraindicated if basilar artery migraine or a migraine with at least two of the following brainstem symptoms: dysarthria, vertigo, tinnitus, hypoacusis (i.e., partial or total loss of hearing), diplopia, ataxia, or decreased level of consciousness.
  - Antiemetic ondansetron (5-HT_3 receptor antagonist): orally as tablet (4 or 8 mg), disintegrating tablet (4 or 8 mg), or liquid (4 mg/5 mL). Dosage is:
    - 8 to 15 kg: 2 mg × 1
    - >15 and ≤30 kg: 4 mg × 1
    - >30 kg: 8 mg × 1
  - Sedatives for unrelenting nausea and vomiting to induce sleep: Lorazepam (with ondansetron) is most effective, but chlorpromazine with diphenhydramine can be used for acute symptom management.[14]
- Treatment of specific symptoms often include histamine 2 receptor antagonists (H_2RAs) or PPIs for epigastric or dyspeptic pain, antidiarrheals for diarrhea, short-acting angiotensin-converting enzyme inhibitors for hypertension, and anxiolytic medication for anxiety (panic) triggers.
- Complementary modalities (e.g., biofeedback, massage, imagery) have also been used.

Follow-up/Referral. Work with families to use their knowledge of their child to determine individual triggers to tailor a care plan specific to each disease stage. A referral is recommended if red flag symptoms occur or if the child does not respond to appropriate acute treatment including prophylaxis. A positive response is defined as at least a 50% reduction in episode frequency and severity of vomiting during attacks over 2 months of therapy.

Complications

Complications include dehydration, electrolyte derangement, metabolic acidosis, hematemesis, and weight loss. Ongoing esophagitis may require acid suppression. Frequent or prolonged episodes may lead to growth failure.

Abdominal Migraine

Abdominal migraine (AM) is considered on a continuum with migraine and CVS. It typically occurs in children rather than adults. The diagnosis is often difficult to determine during the first episode but becomes evident with recurrent episodes. The symptom-based diagnostic criteria for assessing functional GI disorders in pediatrics are the Rome IV criteria.[12] To make the diagnosis of AM, *all* the following criteria must have occurred at least twice and for at least 6 months before diagnosis:[12–14]

- Paroxysmal episodes: intense, acute, periumbilical, midline pain, or diffuse abdominal pain lasting 1 hour or more (should be the most severe and distressing symptom)
- Episodes separated by weeks to months
- Intervening periods of usual health lasting weeks to months
- Individual patient episodes tend to have the same pattern and symptoms each time
- Pain associated with two or more of the following: nausea, vomiting, anorexia, headache, photophobia, or pallor
- After evaluation, pain cannot be explained by another medical condition
- Present two or more times in the preceding 12 months

Several theories target the pathophysiology of AM as an alteration in gut-brain communication. Others postulate an interplay between genetic, environmental, and metabolic factors.[15] The reported incidence varies from 1% to 20% of children depending on country of origin. It tends to be more common in females (1.6:1), but rarely persists into adulthood; however, it is considered a precursor to migraine.[15] AM is considered one of the common reasons for recurrent abdominal pain in childhood.

Clinical Findings

History
- Meets Rome IV criteria for AM
- Family history of migraine or motion sickness
- Past history of motion sickness
- Most episodes last hours to days, with a 1-hour minimum
- Aura is not common but may have prodrome symptoms of fatigue and drowsiness
- Headache complaints are typically absent or uncommon

Physical Examination
- Normal physical examination, growth curves, body mass index (BMI)
- Absence of symptoms concerning for other organic GI conditions (e.g., intussusception)

Diagnostic Studies. Diagnostic studies are not indicated if the history and physical examination meet Rome IV criteria.
- UGI (if concerns for obstruction)
- Ultrasound (if concerns for a renal process/pancreatitis)

Differential Diagnosis.

The diagnosis is difficult to establish during the first episode. Disorders to exclude include obstructive GI and renal processes, biliary tract disease, recurrent pancreatitis, familial Mediterranean fever, and metabolic disorders, such as porphyria. Cyclic vomiting is a severe variant of AM.[15]

Management
- Identify and avoid triggers: Caffeine, nitrates, and amine-containing foods; excessive emotional stress; travel; prolonged fasting; altered sleep; flickering or glaring lights.
- Sleep: Often relieves symptoms.
- Medications:
  - Antiemetics may abort an attack.
  - AM should respond to migraine prophylactic therapy (cyproheptadine, amitriptyline, topiramate). A positive response helps confirm the diagnosis.

Gastroesophageal Reflux Disease

GERD refers to the reverse passage of gastric contents into the esophagus from the stomach through the LES. The etiology of GERD is unclear; however, the most likely causes include inappropriate relaxation of the LES with failure to prevent gastric acid esophageal reflux, prolonged esophageal gastric refluxate clearance, and impaired esophageal mucosal barrier function. LES function is influenced by intraabdominal pressure, hormones, neurologic control, and age. Young infants have increased intraabdominal pressure due to their inability to sit upright, which also increases the potential to regurgitate when they cough, cry, or strain. Daily regurgitation is more common in young infants than in older infants and children; its highest rates are in neonates.

Other factors that contribute to GERD are alterations in swallowing, pharyngeal coordination, esophageal motility, and delayed gastric emptying. Increased muscle tone, chronic supine positioning, and altered GI motility also exacerbate GERD.

Clinical Findings

Table 34.4 lists common signs and symptoms by age; however, there is no symptom or symptom complex that is diagnostic of GERD or predicts the individual's response to therapy. In older children and adolescents, the history and physical examination may be sufficient to diagnose GERD. The most common symptom is "heartburn"; however, many describe this discomfort as chest or sternal pain. Recurrent regurgitation, with or without vomiting, weight loss or poor weight gain, hematemesis, dysphagia, and respiratory disorders (e.g., wheezing, stridor, cough, apnea, hoarseness, recurrent pneumonia) can also be associated with GERD.

History. See Box 34.4 for history and Box 34.5 for warning signs that merit urgent investigation.

Physical Examination
- Signs of growth faltering
- Torticollis, neck arching
- Hoarseness
- Anemia
- Tooth erosion (i.e., enamel destruction from gastric acids)
- Symptoms of another primary disease with GERD as a secondary problem (e.g., facial rash, recurrent diarrhea, persistent vomiting, or early-morning vomiting)

Diagnostic Studies
- CBC with differential
- UA and urine culture
- Stool for occult blood

TABLE 34.4 Symptoms and Signs That May Be Associated With Gastroesophageal Reflux

Symptoms and Signs by Age	Symptoms and Signs for All Ages
Infancy: Regurgitation; signs of esophagitis (irritability, arching, choking, gagging, feeding aversion); growth faltering. Usually, symptoms resolve between 12 and 24 months of age. Also, obstructive apnea, stridor, lower airway disease by which reflux complicates a primary airway disease (e.g., bronchopulmonary dysplasia), otitis media, sinusitis, lymphoid hyperplasia, hoarseness, vocal cord nodules, laryngeal edema *Child and adolescent*: Regurgitation during preschool years, complaints of abdominal and chest pain, neck contortions (arching, turning of head), asthma, sinusitis, laryngitis	Recurrent regurgitation with/without vomiting Ruminative behavior Heartburn or chest pain Hematemesis Dysphagia, odynophagia Respiratory disorders, such as wheezing, stridor, cough, hoarseness, or persistent throat clearing Halitosis Esophagitis Esophageal stricture Barrett esophagus Laryngeal/pharyngeal inflammation Recurrent pneumonia Anemia Dental erosion Apnea spells BRUE (brief, resolved, unexplained event) Weight loss or poor weight gain

From Rosen R, Vandenplas Y, Singendonk M, et al. Pediatric gastroesophageal reflux clinical practice guidelines: joint recommendations of the North American Society for Pediatric Gastroenterology, Hepatology, and Nutrition and the European Society for Pediatric Gastroenterology, Hepatology, and Nutrition. *J Pediatr Gastroenterol Nutr*. 2018;66(3):516–554.

• BOX 34.4 History for the Patient With Suspected Gastroesophageal Reflux Disease

Feeding and Dietary History
- Feeding: Amount/frequency; note overfeeding
- Review preparation of infant formula (if used)
- Provider observation of the child during a feeding
- Recent changes in feeding type or technique
- Position during feeding, burping technique and frequency
- Behavior during feeding
- Choking, gagging, coughing, arching, discomfort, refusal
- Other concerning behaviors
- Torticollis
- Sandifer syndrome: torsional dystonia with arching of the back and rigid opisthotonic posturing, involving primarily the neck, back, and upper extremities
- Pattern of vomiting
- Blood or bile
- Associated fever, lethargy, diarrhea
- Medical history
- Prematurity and newborn screen results
- Growth and development, previous weight and height gain (growth charts)
- Past surgery, hospitalizations
- Recurrent illnesses, especially croup, pneumonia, asthma
- Symptoms of hoarseness, fussiness, hiccups, apnea
- Other chronic conditions
- Medications: Current, recent, prescription, nonprescription
- Family psychosocial history
- Sources of stress and/or postpartum depression
- Maternal or paternal drug use
- Family medical history
- Significant illnesses
- Family history of gastrointestinal (GI) disorders or atopy

From Rosen R, Vandenplas Y, Singendonk M, et al. Pediatric gastroesophageal reflux clinical practice guidelines: joint recommendations of the North American Society for Pediatric Gastroenterology, Hepatology, and Nutrition and the European Society for Pediatric Gastroenterology, Hepatology, and Nutrition. *J Pediatr Gastroenterol Nutr*. 2018;66(3):516–554.

Specialized tests (obtained following consultation with a pediatric gastroenterologist):
- *Esophageal pH monitoring.* Gold standard to diagnose reflux; however, the presence of reflux may not correlate with the illness severity, and some gastric contents may not be acidic. Transnasal pH placement may be uncomfortable, decrease appetite and activity, and thus underestimate the true incidence of reflux episodes. H_2 blockers are discontinued 72 hours before and PPIs 1 week before the study.
- *Multichannel intraluminal impedance* (MII) measures reflux episodes independent of the fluid's pH. pH-MII accurately detects reflux in children with respiratory events. It measures multiple indices, such as heart rate, oxygenation, sleep state, and apnea episodes. It also measures the height of refluxed material and the content and direction of the reflux (liquid, air, or both).
  - In infants and children, pH-MII optimizes the GER-symptom association yield.
  - Indications for pH-MII include (1) evaluating antireflux therapy efficacy; (2) endoscopy-negative patients with symptoms concerning for reflux despite PPI therapy in whom documentation of nonacid reflux alters clinical management; (3) evaluating tube-fed patients for reflux, because the majority of refluxate during tube feeding is nonacidic; and (4) differentiating aerophagia from GER.[16]
- *Wireless pH monitoring* is also available. A pH probe is placed transorally, temporarily attached to the esophageal mucosa, where it records events for 48 hours. The capsule typically sloughs in about 5 days. Negative aspects are failure to attach, chest pain, feeling of FB, and premature detachment.

• BOX 34.5 Red Flags Requiring Urgent Investigation in Infants With Vomiting

- Bilious vomiting
- Gastrointestinal (GI) bleeding, hematemesis, hematochezia
- Consistently forceful vomiting or onset of vomiting after 6 months old
- Growth faltering (failure to thrive)
- Recurrent respiratory infections
- Feeding problems (uncoordinated swallow, choking, or cough associated with feeding)
- Diarrhea or constipation
- Fever and/or lethargy
- Hepatosplenomegaly
- Bulging fontanelles, macrocephaly, or microcephaly
- Seizures
- Abdominal tenderness or distension
- Documented or suspected genetic/metabolic syndrome

From Rosen R, Vandenplas Y, Singendonk M, et al. Pediatric gastroesophageal reflux clinical practice guidelines: joint recommendations of the North American Society for Pediatric Gastroenterology, Hepatology, and Nutrition and the European Society for Pediatric Gastroenterology, Hepatology, and Nutrition. *J Pediatr Gastroenterol Nutr*. 2018;66(3):516–554.

- *Endoscopy* (with or without biopsy) is used to determine the severity of reflux esophagitis, exclude esophagitis and other pathologic conditions, or dilate strictures.
- *UGI series*—Only used if obstruction or a UGI anatomic abnormality is suspected.
- *Gastric emptying scan* can be used to evaluate delayed gastric motility associated with GERD.
- *Video swallow study* may be necessary to evaluate for aspiration or effective esophageal swallow if recurrent respiratory infection, persistent cough, or feeding refusal (or difficulty) is present.

Differential Diagnosis

Table 34.2 contains a list of other conditions that cause vomiting.

Management

GERD management varies depending on the age of the affected individual and is summarized in Figs. 34.1 and 34.2 and Table 34.5. A history and physical examination are typically sufficient to diagnose GERD, recognize complications, and reliably initiate treatment. It is not recommended to treat crying or to use medications to treat healthy infants with visible regurgitation.[16] A 4- to 8-week course of medication is recommended for symptomatic infants and children with typical symptoms of GERD.[16]

Pharmacologic. Acid-suppression agents (Table 34.6) are the mainstays of treatment. H$_2$RAs suppress gastric acid secretion by competitively inhibiting histamine at the parietal cell's H$_2$ receptor. Dosage varies by age, but children require a relatively higher dose than adults. H$_2$RAs are recommended, especially when PPIs are not available or are contraindicated.[16] PPIs are the most potent acid suppressants, as they block the final step in acid secretion and provide increased and faster symptom relief. They are recommended for infants and children as the first-line treatment of reflux-related erosive esophagitis.[16] Antacids, which are compounds containing different combinations (e.g., calcium carbonate, sodium bicarbonate, aluminum, magnesium hydroxide) provide rapid but short-term symptom relief by buffering gastric acid.[16] There is insufficient evidence to recommend using prokinetic agents (e.g., cisapride, metoclopramide, domperidone, bethanechol, erythromycin, baclofen) for GERD.

Nutrition. Feeding technique, volume, and frequency of feeding should follow a routine. An extensively hydrolyzed protein formula trial may be used for 2 to 4 weeks in formula-fed infants with vomiting. Thickened feedings have been a recommended treatment for GERD; however, this recommendation only decreases visible regurgitation/vomiting. Thickening feeds has no impact on other GERD-associated symptoms. When recommending thickened feeds, consider reducing feeding volume and frequency to avoid rapid weight gain.[16] An increase in caloric density may be necessary in infants with poor weight gain or weight loss. In contrast, there is no evidence to support specific dietary restrictions to decrease symptoms in older children; however, avoiding eating less than 2 hours before bedtime may be helpful. Obesity is related to an increased incidence of GERD and weight management can be a treatment component; however, the emphasis should be on healthy eating (see Chapter 14).

Lifestyle. There is evidence to support supine and left lateral positioning for infant sleep to reduce reflux episodes; however, placing an infant on their back to sleep reduces an infant's risk of sudden infant death syndrome (SIDS).[16] Based on studies in adults with GER, there may be some benefit in older children to left-side positioning during sleep or elevation of the head of the

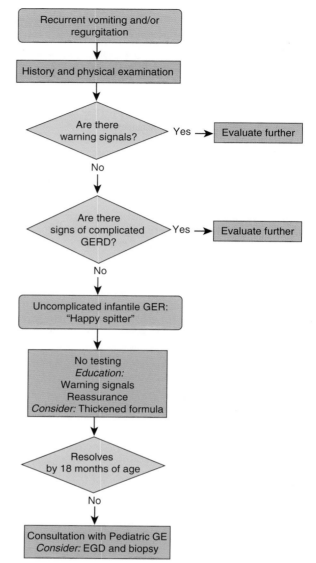

- **Fig. 34.1** Management of the Symptomatic Infant. *EGD,* Esophago-gastroduodenoscopy; *GE,* gastroenterologist; *GER,* gastroesophageal reflux; *GERD,* gastroesophageal reflux disease. (From Rosen R, Vandenplas Y, Singendonk M, et al. Pediatric gastroesophageal reflux clinical practice guidelines: joint recommendations of the North American Society for Pediatric Gastroenterology, Hepatology, and Nutrition and the European Society for Pediatric Gastroenterology, Hepatology, and Nutrition. *J Pediatr Gastroenterol Nutr.* 2018;6(3);516–554.)

bed. Note: Elevate the head of the bed by adding pillows under the mattress. Do not add pillows under the child's head because it may increase abdominal flexion and compression.

Surgical. Antireflux surgery (i.e., fundoplication) is used for infants/children who have not responded to less invasive strategies but have life-threatening complications or long-term dependence on medical therapy.

Complications

Complications include chronic cough, growth faltering, irritability, and malnutrition. Esophageal injury, secondary to GER, results in bleeding, stricture formation, and very rarely, Barrett esophagus. GERD is associated with significant asthma, recurrent

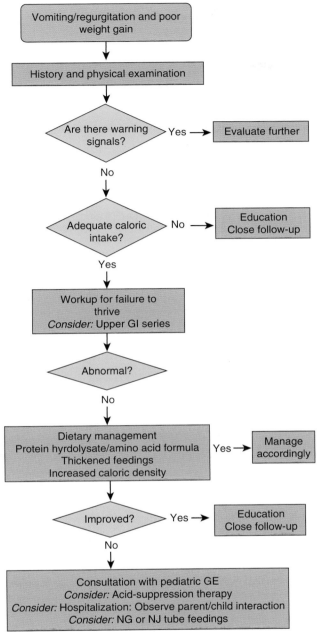

• **Fig. 34.2** Diagnostic and Therapeutic Algorithm for Typical Reflux Symptoms in the Older Child. *GE,* Gastroenterologist; *GI,* gastrointestinal; *NG,* nasogastric; *NJ,* nasojejunal; *PPI,* proton pump inhibitor. (From Rosen R, Vandenplas Y, Singendonk M, et al. Pediatric gastroesophageal reflux clinical practice guidelines: joint recommendations of the North American Society for Pediatric Gastroenterology, Hepatology, and Nutrition and the European Society for Pediatric Gastroenterology, Hepatology, and Nutrition. *J Pediatr Gastroenterol Nutr.* 2018;6(3);516–554.)

pneumonia, or laryngeal disorders. While GERD is not the cause in most infants with brief, resolved, unexplained event (BRUE), in the rare case where a relationship is suspected, pH monitoring in combination with polysomnographic recording and precise, synchronous symptom recording may aid in establishing cause and effect.

Parent and Family Education
• Regurgitation is usually self-limited, and symptoms improve as they mature.
• GERD may temporarily worsen during illness.
• Review medication information, including dosages and side effects.

Infantile Hypertrophic Pyloric Stenosis

Infantile hypertrophic pyloric stenosis (IHPS) is characterized by abnormal thickening of the pylorus muscles in the stomach, which causes narrowing of the pyloric sphincter and gastric outlet obstruction. It has a multifactorial inheritance pattern and is more common in White individuals (53%), especially those of Scandinavian ancestry, and first-born males (82.7%).[17] While relatively uncommon, pyloric stenosis repair (pylormyotomy) is still the most common abdominal surgery in the first 6 months of life.[17]

Clinical Findings
History
• Normal eating pattern or intermittent episodes of regurgitation/nonprojectile vomiting during the first few weeks of life. Nonbilious vomitus can contain blood and occur immediately after feeding
• Projectile vomiting beginning at 2 to 3 weeks old
• Hungry immediately following vomiting episode; insatiable appetite
• Constipation
Note: There is a demonstrated association of pyloric stenosis with macrolide administration in the first 2 weeks of life.[18]

Physical Examination
• Weight loss or dehydration
• A firm, nontender, hard pylorus (1–2 cm in diameter) or "olive" may be palpated in the epigastrium to the right of midline
• Reverse peristalsis visualized across the abdomen
Diagnostic Studies. Ultrasound, with measurement of the pyloric muscle thickness, is the current standard. A UGI series may be done if ultrasound is unavailable or inconclusive, or if there is a suspicion of malrotation/volvulus. In pyloric stenosis, the UGI demonstrates a "string sign," indicating a fine, elongated pyloric canal and delayed gastric emptying. Electrolyte panel may show hypokalemic, hypochloremic metabolic alkalosis.

Differential Diagnosis
It is important to rule out malrotation and volvulus, which can also present in the first month of life with bilious vomiting. Other differential diagnoses are gastroenteritis, acute renal failure, sepsis, hernia, colic, constipation, necrotizing enterocolitis, trauma, toxic megacolon, HD, testicular torsion, appendicitis, and UTI.

Management and Prognosis
Surgical intervention (pyloromyotomy) is indicated, but only after correction of fluid and electrolyte imbalance (e.g., hypokalemic, hypochloremic metabolic alkalosis). Vomiting can continue for a few days after surgery, although it is not as significant as it was preoperatively; feedings should be introduced gradually. The prognosis is excellent.

Eosinophilic Esophagitis

EoE is characterized by isolated esophageal inflammation by a specific WBC, the eosinophil. Young children may present with

TABLE 34.5	Management Strategies for Infants and Children With Gastroesophageal Reflux	
Population	**Diagnostic Tests**	**Management Strategies**
Infant with uncomplicated recurrent regurgitation (GER)	None needed	Provide parental education and reassurance. In formula-fed babies, thickened formula may reduce overregurgitation and vomiting but does not reduce reflux itself.
Infants with recurrent vomiting and poor weight gain (GERD)	Diet history, UA, CBC, serum electrolytes, BUN, serum creatinine Other tests as indicated	For breastfed infants, continue breastfeeding. For formula-fed babies, 2-week trial of extensively hydrolyzed formula or amino acid–based formula to exclude CMA. Increase caloric density. Thicken formula if needed. Educate regarding formula intake needed to sustain normal weight gain. Refer to pediatric gastroenterologist if management fails to improve symptoms and weight gain.
Infants with unexplained crying and/or distressed behavior	Evaluate for CMA, neurologic disorders, constipation, infection (especially UTIs)	Empiric trial with extensively hydrolyzed protein formula or amino acid–based formula. No evidence to support empiric use of acid suppression to treat irritable infants. If irritability persists and no condition other than GERD remains, support parents with anticipated improvement over time; evaluate to establish the relationship of reflux to feeding or to diagnose esophagitis; or trial of antisecretory therapy, although a potential risk for adverse effects. Clinical improvement following empiric therapy may result in spontaneous symptom resolution or placebo response.
Child >18 months old with chronic regurgitation or vomiting	Consider diagnosis other than GERD; testing may include upper GI endoscopy, esophageal pH/MII, and barium upper GI series	Treatment depends on diagnosis.
Heartburn in older children and adolescents	No further studies needed if problem is episodic and not severe	On-demand therapy with buffering agents, sodium alginate, or H2RA may be used for occasional symptoms. For chronic heartburn, lifestyle changes (e.g., diet change, weight loss, smoking avoidance, sleeping position, no late-night eating) and a 2-week trial with a PPI may help. Can continue PPI for up to 3 months if symptoms resolve. Persistent heartburn after that time should be referred to a pediatric gastroenterologist if needed.
Reflux esophagitis—endoscopically diagnosed	No further studies needed	PPI for 3 months is initial therapy. Trial of tapering dose and then withdrawal of PPI. Chronic relapsing esophagitis may be diagnosis if PPI cannot be withdrawn and may involve long-term therapy with PPI or antireflux surgery (i.e., fundoplication).

BUN, Blood urea nitrogen; *CBC*, complete blood count; *CMA*, cow's-milk allergy; *GER*, gastroesophageal reflux; *GERD*, gastroesophageal reflux disease; *GI*, gastrointestinal; *H2RA*, histamine 2 receptor antagonist; *MII*, multichannel intraluminal impedance; *PPI*, proton pump inhibitor; *UA*, urinalysis; *UTI*, urinary tract infection.

From Rosen R, Vandenplas Y, Singendonk M, et al. Pediatric gastroesophageal reflux clinical practice guidelines: joint recommendations of the North American Society for Pediatric Gastroenterology, Hepatology, and Nutrition and the European Society for Pediatric Gastroenterology, Hepatology, and Nutrition. *J Pediatr Gastroenterol Nutr.* 2018;66(3):516–554.

feeding refusal or growth faltering. Recurrent vomiting and abdominal pain may occur in school-age children. Older children and adolescents often present with dysphagia, chest pain, choking, and food impaction.[19]

Clinical Findings

Differentiating EoE from GERD may be difficult because both entities present with similar clinical history and physical examination findings. The only way to diagnose EoE is by upper endoscopy and biopsy; however, esophageal mucosa may appear normal in up to one-third of patients. Typical macroscopic findings include esophageal edema, longitudinal furrows, mucosal fragility, whitish exudates, transient esophageal rings (felinization), fixed esophageal rings (trachealization), diffuse esophageal narrowing, and small-caliber esophagus.[19]

Management

Objectives of EoE therapy include improvement in histology and quality of life, reduction in clinical symptoms, and prevention of complications (e.g., food impaction/stuck in the esophagus) or long-term sequelae (e.g., strictures, small-caliber esophagus).

Dietary modifications include elemental diet, empiric dietary elimination, and targeted food elimination. Elemental diet consisting of an amino acid–based formula remains the most effective and accepted dietary intervention in infants. For older children, initiating the six-food (milk, soy, egg, wheat, peanut/tree nuts, fish/shellfish) elimination diet and a referral to a pediatric allergist for identification and targeted food elimination based on allergy testing results. Although expensive and unpalatable, the elemental diet lacks all food antigens that cause eosinophil infiltration and inflammation. In affected children, an elemental diet produces

TABLE 34.6	Common Medications Used to Treat Gastroesophageal Reflux Disease	
Medication	**Pediatric Dosage**
Histamine 2 Receptor Antagonists	
Famotidine (Pepcid)	Infants: 1–3 months: 0.5 mg/kg/dose once daily for up to 8 weeks Infants >3 months –1 year: 1 mg/kg/dose twice daily for up to 8 weeks (maximum dose 40 mg/da) Children and adolescents: initially 1 mg/kg/dose every 12 h (maximum dose: 40 mg/day)
Proton Pump Inhibitors	
Lansoprazole (Prevacid)	Children 1–11 years: <30 kg: 15 mg once daily for up to 12 weeks >30 kg: 30 mg once daily for up to 12 weeks
Omeprazole (Prilosec)	Children >1 year: 5–10 kg: 5 mg once daily for up to 12 weeks 10–20 kg: 10 mg once daily for up to 12 weeks >20 kg: 20 mg once daily for up to 12 weeks
Pantoprazole (Protonix)	Infants and children <5 years: 1.2 mg/kg/day once daily for 4 weeks Children 5–11 years: <40 kg 20 mg/once/day, >40 kg = 40 mg/once/day up to 8 weeks Children and adolescents 12–16 years: 20 or 40 mg once daily for up to 8 weeks

From Buendia M, Thoni N. Gastroenterology. In: Kleinman K, McDaniel L, Molloy M, eds. *The Harriet Lane Handbook.* 22nd ed. Elsevier; 2021: p. 283–299; Rosen R, Vandenplas Y, Singendonk M, et al. Pediatric gastroesophageal reflux clinical practice guidelines: joint recommendations of the North American Society for Pediatric Gastroenterology, Hepatology, and Nutrition and the European Society for Pediatric Gastroenterology, Hepatology, and Nutrition. *J Pediatr Gastroenterol Nutr.* 2018;66(3):516-554.

nearly complete remission of EoE in 80% to 90%.[19] Medication for EoE consists of PPIs and swallowed inhaled corticosteroids (fluticasone, propionate, budesonide, ciclesonide) for 12 weeks.

Peptic Ulcer Disease

PUD consists of a group of gastric and duodenal disorders ranging from gastritis to ulceration. Peptic ulcers result from an imbalance between protective and aggressive factors. *Protective factors* include the water-insoluble mucous gel lining, local production of bicarbonate, regulation of gastric acid, and adequate mucosal blood flow. *Aggressive factors* include the acid-pepsin environment, infection with *H. pylori,* and mucosal ischemia. *H. pylori* colonization rates in the United States and Europe are less than 10%; there are much higher rates in less-developed countries.[20] Colonization likely occurs during the first years of life, but the infection often remains asymptomatic with low-grade inflammation or no mucosal changes. Zollinger-Ellison syndrome (ZES) is a rare syndrome involving refractory severe PUD caused by gastric hypersecretion due to the autonomous secretion of gastrin by a neuroendocrine tumor.

PUD results in primary or secondary ulcers. Most *primary ulcers* are duodenal, have no underlying cause, and tend to be chronic with resulting granulation tissue and fibrosis. They tend to recur and are more common in adolescents and rare in children. *Secondary ulcers* are more often gastric, generally more acute, and associated with known ulcerogenic events. Severe erosive gastropathy can result in bleeding ulcers or gastric perforations, more commonly in the stomach than duodenum. Head trauma, severe burns, use of corticosteroids, and nonsteroidal antiinflammatory drugs (NSAIDs) are associated with secondary ulcers. Aspirin or NSAIDs cause mucosal injury by direct injury or inhibiting cyclooxygenase and prostaglandin formation. Chronic therapy with these medicines causes gastric mucosal damage but is not associated with ulcer formation. Stress ulceration usually occurs within 24 hours of critical illness and may occur in 25% of critically ill children in intensive care units. Preterm and term infants in neonatal intensive care units (NICUs) can develop gastric mucosal lesions with bleeding or perforation. *Idiopathic ulcers* are found in *H. pylori*–negative children who have no history of taking NSAIDs; 20% of pediatric duodenal ulcers are of this type. A strong familial predisposition for PUD is noted, and most patients with duodenal ulcers have a positive family medical history, a key finding. There is no evidence that diet plays a role in ulcer formation.

Clinical Findings

The most common symptom of PUD is vague, dull abdominal pain; however, presenting symptoms vary by age. Neonates can present with gastric perforation. Infants usually present with feeding difficulty, vomiting, crying episodes, hematemesis, or melena. Epigastric pain and nausea are reported more often by school-age children and adolescents. The classic adult symptom of PUD is pain alleviated by food ingestion; it is present in a minority of pediatric patients.

History
- Asymptomatic or symptoms wax and wane. Remissions may last from weeks to months.
- Pain with eating, dyspepsia; can interrupt sleep.
- GI tract bleeding may be a presenting symptom; hematemesis or melena is reported in up to 50% of patients.
- Age dependent:
  - Infants: Poor feeding, GI bleeding, vomiting, intestinal perforation, slow growth; history of prematurity or NICU admission.
  - Early childhood: Poorly localized abdominal pain, vomiting, GI bleeding. May worsen after eating; irritability; anorexia.
  - Middle childhood and adolescents: Poorly localized epigastric or right lower quadrant (RLQ) pain. Pain is often described as dull, aching, and lasting from minutes to hours. Nocturnal pain is common in older children. Relief from antacids is reported by less than 40% of children. If the pain awakens the child, worsens with food, and is relieved by fasting, this may help distinguish GI pathology from psychogenic pathology, although these symptoms are infrequently described in children. Recurrent vomiting may occur.
- GI bleeding may lead to iron deficiency anemia.
- Family history of PUD.
- Predisposing factors: Alcohol, smoking, aspirin, NSAIDs, corticosteroids, emotional stress, serious systemic disease, sepsis, hypotension, respiratory failure, multiple traumatic injuries, and extensive burns.
- ZES presents with severe peptic ulceration, kidney stones, watery diarrhea, or malabsorption (fasting serum gastrin level

>200 pg/mL and baseline gastric acid hypersecretion at more than 15 mEq/h).

Physical Examination. The physical examination should include the following; however, there may be no physical findings:

- Height, weight, head circumference, BMI, and percentiles
- Vital signs
- General appearance
- Assessment of perfusion: Mental status, heart rate, pulses, capillary refill, pallor
- Assessment of hydration: Mucous membranes, skin turgor
- Abdominal examination for tenderness and hepatosplenomegaly
- Rectal examination (to assess perirectal disease)
- Females: Pelvic examination in sexually active female patients with pain
- Males: Testicular and inguinal examinations

Diagnostic Studies. Endoscopy with mucosal biopsy validates *H. pylori* infection; however, if a child has mild PUD, minimal laboratory studies are needed. Other diagnostic studies to consider include:

Laboratory Studies

- Initially (red flags for systemic disease): CBC (anemia is associated with chronic *H. pylori* infection or acute or chronic blood loss due to ulcer perforation into the abdominal cavity), albumin (low), and ESR (high). May also consider stool for guaiac and *H. pylori* (especially in children).
- If the child is unstable, severe, or has chronic, recurrent symptoms or serious complications consider:
  - Iron studies
  - *H. pylori* serology (most useful in teenagers, only helpful in children if negative due to high false-positive rate)
  - Prothrombin time and activated partial thromboplastin time (aPTT) (identify coagulopathy).
  - Electrolyte, BUN, creatinine levels (assess volume depletion)
  - Arterial blood gases (acidosis)
  - UA (hydration, infection, or stones).
  - Serum gastrin and gastrin-releasing peptide levels (in patients with refractory ulcers to exclude ZES)

Note: PPIs must be discontinued 2 weeks before gastrin level measurement. Type and crossmatch for blood may also be obtained.

Imaging Studies and Procedures

- Abdominal or chest radiograph for perforation.
- An upper GI series diagnoses about 70% of children (sensitivity higher for duodenal ulcers); however, a fibrinous clot in the ulcer may lead to false-negative findings. Barium studies have false-positive rates as high as 30% to 40%.
- Esophagogastroduodenoscopy (EGD) is the procedure of choice for detecting PUD, because it allows direct visualization of mucosa, localization of the bleeding source, and collection of biopsy specimens. It is also used therapeutically for acute bleeding.
- Angiography is sometimes done if there is a significant bleed and EGD cannot be performed.

Studies to Detect *H. Pylori*

- *Histologic examination and culture biopsies* obtained via endoscopy are the gold standard for detecting acute infection; however, it is an invasive procedure that requires anesthesia and only appropriate for persistent or recurrent infection or severe symptoms.
- *C-urea breath test* is the noninvasive diagnostic test of choice; it distinguishes between past and present infection. It is sensitive in individuals older than 2 years but requires special equipment. It should be performed off acid suppression (4 weeks) pharmacotherapy to avoid false-negative results.
- *Stool monoclonal antibody test* also distinguishes between past and present infection. It is reliable for evaluating therapy response if symptoms persist and should also be performed off acid suppression (4 weeks) pharmacotherapy to avoid false-negative results.
- *Serum immunoglobulin G (IgG) antibody titer.* A positive result (>500 units) indicates disease exposure. This test should not be the sole basis for starting therapy or used to test for eradication. It is beneficial for the initial screening to evaluate epigastric pain/dyspepsia.

Differential Diagnosis

Most youth presenting with epigastric or periumbilical pain do not have PUD, but rather functional bowel disorder, IBS, or functional dyspepsia. Differential diagnoses include all other causes of abdominal pain, especially GERD, GI bleeding, cholelithiasis, cholecystitis, pancreatitis, lactose intolerance, hyperkalemia, and hypercalcemia.

Management

The treatment goals include ulcer healing, primary cause elimination, symptom relief, and complication prevention.

- Medications:
  - H_2RAs or PPIs are first-line therapy (see Table 34.6). PPIs are most effective if taken before a meal.
  - Antacids: Liquid preparation given between 1 and 3 hours after eating and before bed.
  - *H. pylori* eradication therapy is indicated for patients with a duodenal or gastric ulcer identified by endoscopy and histopathology (Table 34.7). Compliance with the treatment regimen is the single most important determinant of eradication. Eradication rates are more than 90%. The test of cure can either be the stool antigen test or the urea breath test.
  - Empiric therapy for suspected *H. pylori* is not recommended. There is increasing antibiotic resistance to *H. pylori*. Therapy is not indicated for gastritis without PUD, recurrent abdominal pain, or for youth with asymptomatic PUD or with a family member with PUD.
- Referral to a gastroenterologist should occur if there is:
  - Lack of improvement or inability to wean off medications after eradication therapy is completed and a test of cure is negative.[20]
  - History of hematemesis, melena, occult blood in stools, anemia, and/or weight loss.
- Idiopathic ulcers: The preferred treatment is acid suppression with either H_2RAs or PPIs. Follow patients closely and, if symptoms recur, restart acid suppression treatment. PPIs are preferred for maintenance in children older than 1 year.

Complications

Obstruction can occur if inflammation and edema are extensive. Hemorrhage occurs in 15% to 20% of patients, and perforation occurs in less than 5%. Other possible complications are recurrence, gastric outlet obstruction, gastric adenocarcinoma, and gastric lymphoma. Acute hemorrhage, chronic blood loss, ulcer penetration into the abdominal cavity, or adjacent organs may produce shock, anemia, peritonitis, or pancreatitis.

TABLE 34.7	Therapies for *Helicobacter pylori* Disease in Children	
Medications	**Dosage**	
Option 1 (Three Drugs)		
Amoxicillin	500 mg (15–34 kg), 750 mg (25–34 kg), or 1 g (>35 kg) twice daily	
Clarithromycin	15 mg/kg/day up to 500 mg twice daily	
Omeprazole	20 mg BID (15–25 kg), 30 mg BID (25–34 kg), 40 mg BID (≥35 kg)	
Option 2 (Three Drugs)		
Amoxicillin	500 mg (15–34 kg), 750 mg (25–34 kg), or 1 g (>35 kg) twice daily	
Metronidazole	250 mg BID (15–34 kg), 500 mg in AM 250 mg in PM (25–34 kg), or 500 mg BID (>35 kg)	
Omeprazole	20 mg BID (15–25 kg), 30 mg BID (25–34 kg), 40 mg BID (≥35 kg)	
Option 3 (Three Drugs; 8 Years Old or Older)		
Bismuth sub salicylate	<10 years old: 262 mg QID; ≥10 years: 524 mg QID	
Amoxicillin	500 mg (15–34 kg), 750 mg (25--34 kg), or 1 g (>35 kg) twice daily	
Metronidazole	250 mg BID (15–34 kg), 500 mg in morning 250 mg at night (25–34 kg), or 500 mg BID (>35 kg)	
Option 4 (Sequential Therapy)		
	Omeprazole and amoxicillin for 5 days then omeprazole, clarithromycin, and metronidazole for 5 days at dosages above	

From Jones N, Koletzko S, Goodman K, et al. Joint ESPGHAN/NASPGHAN Guidelines for the management of *Helicobacter pylori* in children and adolescents (Update 2016). *J Pediatr Gastroenterol Nutr.* 2017;64(6):991-1003.

Patient and Family Education

Treatment success depends on the patient completing the drug regimen. This is essential for limiting antibiotic resistance and symptom improvement.[20]

Lower Gastrointestinal Tract Disorders

Foreign Body Ingestion

Most FB ingestions pass through the GI tract without consequence. Three-fourths of all FB ingestions are in patients under 5 years of age. In fact, these ingestions are so common that 20% of children have had at least one FB ingestion by their fourth birthday.[21] Most swallowed items are radiopaque, with coins and small toys and objects being the most ingested items. Older children and adolescents ingest FBs secondary to psychiatric problems or engaging in risk-taking behaviors. Small batteries and packaging challenges, including blister packs, contribute to the increased incidence of battery ingestion, despite warnings and family education.[22]

Esophageal Foreign Bodies

Esophageal FBs lodge at three spots: (1) 70% at the thoracic inlet where skeletal muscle changes to smooth muscle (between the clavicles at about C6), (2) 15% at the mid-esophagus where the aortic arch and carina overlap the esophagus, and (3) 15% at the lower esophageal sphincter. Pointed or small objects (e.g., small button batteries) can lodge anywhere along the esophageal mucosa. The initial episode involves choking, gagging, and coughing, which is sometimes followed by excessive salivation, dysphagia, food refusal, emesis/hematemesis, or discomfort/pain in the neck, throat, or sternal notch areas. Respiratory symptoms, such as stridor, wheezing, cyanosis, or dyspnea, may occur if the esophageal body impinges on the larynx or tracheal wall.[23] Drooling or pooling of secretions may be related to an esophageal FB or abrasion. Disk batteries cause a liquefactive necrosis, an electrical discharge leading to low-voltage burns, and pressure necrosis. Children who swallow lithium batteries (≥20-mm diameter) are at greatest risk of problems. Some have documented severe erosion or ulceration in as little as 2 hours after ingestion. Emergency endoscopic removal is essential.[22]

Abdominal Foreign Bodies

Most ingested objects that reach the stomach pass through the remainder of the GI tract without difficulty. Items greater than 5 cm (~2 inches) in diameter or 2 cm (~0.8 inches) thick tend to lodge in the stomach and need to be retrieved. Thin objects that are longer than 10 cm (e.g., a pen) may not make the duodenal sweep turn and need to be retrieved. In infants and 1-year-olds, FBs greater than 3 cm in length or 20 mm in diameter may not pass through the pyloric sphincter. Open safety pins or other pointed objects, such as needles or thumbtacks, also should be retrieved.

Perforation after ingestion occurs in only 1% of ingestions. Perforation occurs near physiologic sphincters, areas of angulation, gut congenital malformations, or near areas of previous bowel surgery. Coins made with nickel (i.e., all dimes, quarters, half dollars; some nickels) have been reported to interact with gastric acid to cause stomach ulceration.[22] Abdominal distention or pain, vomiting, hematochezia, and unexplained fever are symptoms related to ingestions lodging in the stomach or intestinal areas. Items that pose a greater risk include small magnets that may cling together across the bowel wall, leading to pressure necrosis; items containing lead; and batteries, if there is leakage of alkali, lithium, or mercury from battery degradation, which can result in toxicity. Nickel in coins can also lead to allergic symptoms in children with a nickel allergy.

Rectal Foreign Bodies

Children sometimes put items into their rectum. Rectal FBs may be suspicious for abuse and are of particular concern in children under 6 years of age. Small blunt objects usually will pass spontaneously, but large or sharp objects should be retrieved after sedation to relax the anal sphincter.

Clinical Findings

History, Physical Examination, and Laboratory Studies. Specific physical findings are unusual. Hypopharyngeal abrasions, streaks of blood, or edema may occasionally indicate an FB. Laboratory studies are not usually helpful, although they may be used to identify the presence of infection.

Imaging Studies. Since most FBs are radiopaque, a single anteroposterior (AP) radiograph that includes the neck, chest, and/or abdomen is usually sufficient to locate the object. Subsequent radiographs may also be useful to document movement. Esophageal objects should be precisely located with AP and lateral radiographs to make sure there are not two closely aligned objects. Note: Coins in the esophagus are usually visible in the frontal view, whereas tracheal coins are more often visible from the lateral view.[22–24] Having the patient ingest a small amount of dilute contrast material may help locate radiolucent objects. Endoscopy may be needed and allows object removal.

Management

Most patients do not require special care, except for suctioning with excessive drooling and/or pooling secretions that are overwhelming to the child. Esophageal objects should be considered impacted, and removal is mandatory, except for blunt objects that have been in place less than 24 hours. Disk batteries and sharp objects should be removed without waiting. Endoscopy is the method of choice; however, trained GI or emergency providers may use a Foley catheter to retrieve the object or bougienage (i.e., using bougie) to move the object into the stomach. Obtain a radiograph immediately before the procedure to be sure the item did not move and another radiograph following the procedure to be sure there are no retained parts or complications (e.g., pneumomediastinum).

FBs that reach the stomach usually pass through the GI tract within 2 to 3 days. Very sharp items may perforate the bowel and should be removed from the stomach (endoscopy) or surgically from the intestine. Button batteries in the stomach or intestine may be left to pass but should be removed if the family has not identified the battery in the stool after 2 to 3 days. Items may not pass through the GI tract if the child has a bowel abnormality or had bowel surgery. Laxative use and inducing vomiting are contraindicated.

Complications

When medications or toxins are ingested, a systemic reaction or toxic response can occur. Allergic reactions are also possible. The primary complication is a retained FB, which may cause erosion, abrasion, local scarring, obstruction, abscess, growth faltering, perforation, pneumomediastinum, pneumonia, or other respiratory disease. In addition, complications from ingestion or removal can occur, including traumatic epiglottitis from trauma during swallowing or a finger sweep trying to dislodge the item.

Appendicitis

Appendicitis includes inflammation, distention, and ischemia of the appendix that can result in necrosis, perforation, peritonitis, and/or abscess formation. Often following a closed-loop obstruction of the appendiceal lumen by a fecalith, lymphoid tissue, tumor, parasite, FB, or inspissated CF secretions, the appendix becomes distended, experiences increased bacterial overgrowth, and is at risk for ischemia and necrosis. Peritoneal inflammation around the infected appendix causes the characteristic symptoms. Typically, there is about a 36- to 72-hour maximum window from the onset of pain to the rupture of the gangrenous appendix. Rupture results in the release of inflammatory fluid and bacteria into the abdominal cavity, causing peritoneal infection with resultant generalized peritonitis. The infected fluid may be walled off by the omentum and loops of small bowel with resultant abscess formation and localized pain.[25]

The average age appendicitis occurs in childhood is 6 to 10 years old, with a male-to-female ratio of approximately 2:1. It is rare in infancy. The incidence is four cases per 1000 children. Perforation is most common in younger children (<5 years) and is complicated by the decreased incidence of appendicitis in this age group and the diminished ability of this age group to communicate location and type of pain.[25] Due to these factors, a timely diagnosis can be challenging to make.

Clinical Findings

Although a classic presentation is easy to discern, appendicitis mimics many other intraabdominal conditions, making diagnosis challenging.

History
- Classic presentation includes:
  - Pain: Initially poorly defined periumbilical pain (earliest sign); shifting of pain to the RLQ may occur after a few hours and becomes more intense, continuous, and localized.
  - Nausea and vomiting: Typically occur after pain; however, in retrocecal appendicitis, this may be reversed (similar to gastroenteritis, where vomiting precedes the pain).
  - Anorexia, although up to 50% of children report hunger.
  - Low-volume stool with mucus; diarrhea is atypical but occurs especially after perforation (unlike gastroenteritis, which has high-volume, watery stools).
  - Fever: Many children present as afebrile or with low-grade fever. High fever may be associated with perforation.
- Use of a standardized scoring system may be helpful (e.g., Appendicitis Inflammatory Response [AIR], Alvarado score, Raja Isteri Pengiran Anak Saleha Appendicitis [RIPASA] score specific to Asian and Middle Eastern populations, Pediatric Appendicitis Score (PAS), pediatric Appendicitis Risk Calculator [pARC]). The Alvarado score and the PAS are recommended tools for excluding acute appendicitis in children.[25]
  - A PAS of 4 or less is highly sensitive in the exclusion of appendicitis:
    - Nausea or emesis (1 point)
    - Anorexia (1 point)
    - Migration of pain to RLQ (1 point)
    - Low-grade fever (1 point)
    - RLQ tenderness on light palpation (2 points)
    - Cough, percussion, heel tapping tenderness at RLQ (2 points)
    - Leukocytosis (>10,000/mm^3) (1 point)
    - Left shift (>75% neutrophilia) (1 point)
    - Total: 10 points
- The process evolves over 12 hours, with the potential for infants and young children to become ill much more quickly.
- Following perforation, symptoms lessen, with less vomiting, fever greater than 101°F (38.3°C), and the most comfortable position being on the side with the legs flexed.
- Infants demonstrate irritability, pain with movement, and flexed hips.
- Children often become quiet or still because crying and movement hurt.

Physical Examination
- Complete physical examination. Reexamination may be needed in 4 to 6 hours.
- Presence of involuntary guarding, RLQ rebound tenderness, maximal pain over McBurney point (1.5–2 inches in from the right anterior superior iliac crest on a line toward the umbilicus) on abdominal examination (most reliable finding); percussion is best method for eliciting rebound tenderness.
- Heel-drop jarring test (on toes for 15 seconds, dropping down forcefully on heels); inability to stand straight or climb stairs;

winces when getting off examination table or riding in a car over bumps; child most comfortable with bent knees.
- Positive psoas and/or obturator sign.
- Rovsing sign (pressure deep in left lower quadrant with sudden release elicits RLQ pain) or rebound tenderness, which strongly suggests peritoneal irritation.
- Tenderness and/or mass (abscess) palpated on rectal examination.

Diagnostic Studies
- CBC with differential: Increased WBC count (>10,000) with an increased neutrophil count occurs in 70% to 90% of those with acute appendicitis; however, an elevated WBC count is not sensitive/specific to appendicitis and during the first 24 hours of symptoms, it is often within normal range.[25]
- Pancreatic (e.g., amylase, lipase) and liver enzymes to differentiate liver, gallbladder, or pancreatic issues.
- UA can show small numbers of WBCs (<20) and RBCs (<20).
- Stool may reveal blood or pus (rare finding).
- Abdominal radiographs can highlight a fecalith, especially if a rupture occurred.
- Ultrasound documents enlargement of the appendix and changes in its wall, increased field around the appendix, or an abscess. Excellent specificity, but only fair sensitivity and is operator dependent.
- CT scan with contrast has the highest accuracy, especially in adolescents. CT scan, compared with ultrasound, has higher sensitivity and specificity, is not operator dependent, and may be more cost effective in preventing an unnecessary appendectomy; however, it is a high-dose radiological procedure, which is always a consideration in children. An appendiceal diameter greater than 6 mm is considered diagnostic (in both ultrasound and CT scans).[25]
- β-Human chorionic gonadotropin test to exclude pregnancy or ectopic pregnancy.

Differential Diagnosis
The differential diagnosis includes gastroenteritis, constipation, UTI, pregnancy, pelvic inflammatory disease (PID) or organ pathologic condition, pneumonia, duodenal PUD, intestinal obstruction, peritonitis, and intussusception (child younger than 2 years with a right upper quadrant [RUQ] mass) (Fig. 34.3).

Management
- Administration of opioid narcotics to reduce acute abdominal pain does not impede the diagnostic process and does not lead to inappropriate increased CT scanning preoperatively. If perforation is suspected, give IV antibiotics.
- Surgical consultation:
  - Open appendectomy (OA) or laparoscopic appendectomy (LA) is indicated for nonperforated appendicitis. The management of perforated appendicitis remains a topic of debate, including the use of surgical intervention. An urgent appendectomy may not be indicated in cases of perforated appendicitis. Some surgeons may administer antibiotics and provide fluid resuscitation before appendectomy.
  - Nonoperative/delayed approach used if the child's clinical condition improves with antibiotic treatment. Appendectomy may be performed 8 to 12 weeks after treatment.
- Follow-up varies from 1 to 4 weeks after surgery. If appetite, bowel function, energy, and activity level are normal; no pain or fever is present; findings on physical examination are normal, and the

wound is well healed, the child can resume activity as tolerated. If the child has signs or symptoms of delayed infection, abnormal bowel function, or unexplained weight loss, refer to the surgeon.[26]

Complications
Perforation, peritonitis, pelvic abscess, ileus, obstruction, sepsis, shock, and death can occur.

Intussusception

Intussusception occurs when a section of the intestine moves into (i.e., telescopes) an adjacent part of the intestine, trapping the distal segment in the proximal bowel. It is typically ileocolic, involving the ileocecal valve, but it can be ileoileal or colocolic. Intussusception usually occurs between 5 and 10 months old and is also the most common cause of intestinal obstruction in children 3 months to 6 years old, with 80% of the cases occurring before 2 years of age. In young infants, intussusception is generally idiopathic and responds to nonoperative reduction. Some children have an identified lead point, such as polyps, Meckel diverticulum, or predisposing factor, such as Henoch-Schönlein purpura, constipation, lymphomas, lipomas, parasites, rotavirus, adenovirus, and FBs. Intussusception occurs in 1% of children with CF. Children older than 3 years are more likely to have polyps, lymphoma, Meckel diverticulum, or Henoch-Schönlein purpura at the lead point of the intussuscepted bowel; therefore a cause must be investigated. The absolute risk of intussusception is marginally increased by the rotavirus vaccination or rotavirus infection in unvaccinated individuals.[27]

Clinical Findings
History
- The classic triad, intermittent colicky (crampy) abdominal pain, vomiting, and bloody mucous stools, is present in fewer than one-quarter of cases.
  - Paroxysmal, episodic abdominal pain with vomiting every 5 to 30 minutes (occur with peristalsis). Vomiting is initially nonbilious. Some children do not have pain.
  - Screaming with the legs drawing up and periods of calm, sleeping, or lethargy between episodes.
  - Hematochezia or "currant jelly" stool (mixed with blood and mucus), possibly diarrhea.
- History of a URI is common.
- Lethargy is a common presenting symptom.
- Fever may or may not be present; can be a late sign of transmural gangrene and infarction.

Physical Examination
- Observe the infant's general appearance and behavior over time; often, the child appears glassy eyed and groggy between episodes, almost as if sedated.
- A sausage-shaped mass may be felt in the RUQ of the abdomen with emptiness in the RLQ (Dance sign); best observed the infant when quiet between spasms.
- The abdomen is often distended and tender.
- Grossly bloody or guaiac-positive stools.

Diagnostic Studies
- Abdominal flat-plate radiograph may appear normal, especially early in the course, revealing intussusceptions in only about 60% of cases (Fig. 34.4). A plain radiograph may show sparse

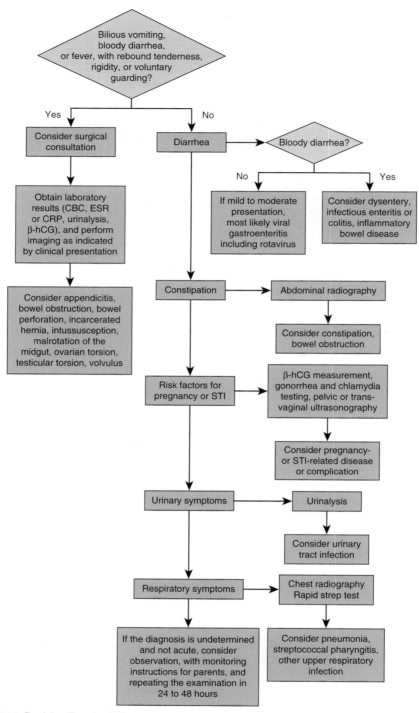

• **Fig. 34.3** Decision Tree for Differential Diagnosis of Acute Abdominal Pain. *β-hCG*, β-Human chorionic gonadotropin; *CBC*, complete blood count; *CRP*, C-reactive protein; *ESR*, erythrocyte sedimentation rate; *STI*, sexually transmitted infection. (From Schwartz MW, Curry TA, Sargent J, eds. *Pediatric Primary Care: A Problem-Oriented Approach.* 3rd ed. Mosby; 1997.)

or no intestinal gas or stool in the ascending colon with air-fluid levels and distension only in the small bowel.
• Ultrasound is the diagnostic test of choice for its high sensitivity and specificity, pathology characterization, and lack of ionizing radiation.[28] May show "target sign" (e.g., "bull's eye" or "doughnut sign") and/or a "pseudo kidney" sign.
• Air contrast enema is both diagnostic and a treatment modality.

Differential Diagnosis

The differential diagnosis includes incarcerated hernia, testicular torsion, acute gastroenteritis, appendicitis, colic, and intestinal obstruction.

Management

• Emergency management and consultation with a pediatric radiologist and surgeon are recommended.

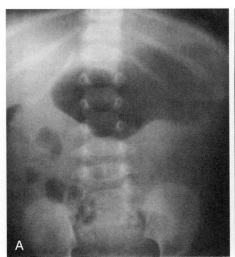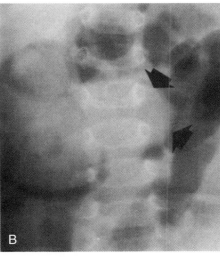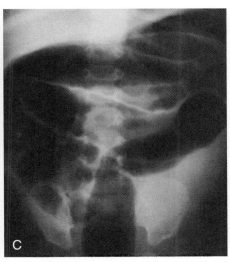

• **Fig. 34.4** Intussusception. (A) Plain abdominal radiograph demonstrating a gas-filled stomach and relatively little gas in the distal end of the bowel. This baby had typical clinical features of intussusception and a palpable upper abdominal mass. Therefore an enema with air was performed. (B) The intussusception *(arrows)* is outlined by air. (C) Reduction is proved by air refluxing into loops of small bowel. (From Burg FD, Ingelfinger JR, Wald ER, eds. *Gellis and Kagan's Current Pediatric Therapy.* 15th ed. Saunders; 1999.)

- Rehydration and stabilization of fluid status; gastric decompression.
- Radiologic reduction using a therapeutic air contrast enema under fluoroscopy is the gold standard.
- Surgery is necessary if perforation, peritonitis, or hypovolemic shock is suspected, or radiologic reduction fails.
- IV antibiotics are often administered to cover potential organisms from intestinal perforation.
- Observation following radiologic reduction is recommended (12–18 hours) as it may reoccur. Follow-up and discharge instructions include to return with any recurrence of symptoms are required, and close phone follow-up for up to 72 hours is prudent.

Complications

Complications associated with intussusception include bowel obstruction, dehydration, ischemia, and perforation. If left untreated swelling, hemorrhage, incarceration, and necrosis of the bowel requiring bowel resection may occur, along with perforation, sepsis, and shock. Recurrence of intussusception is reported in less than 10% and typically occurs within 72 hours of reduction, especially if related to an identified lead point, but can occur up to 36 months later.

Hirschsprung Disease (Congenital Aganglionic Megacolon)

HD is an absence of ganglion cells in the intestinal mesenteric and submucosal plexus, most often in the rectosigmoid region. This results in a loss of motility and functional obstruction. HD occurs in 1 in 5000 live births and accounts for approximately 40% of all neonatal bowel obstructions. The majority (80%) of individuals will have a short segment of bowel affected, while the other 20% will have long segment. Short-segment HD affects males 4 times more commonly than females, while long-segment is equally distributed. It is considered inherited, but the genetic variables are complex. Mutations in the *RET* gene are most common, with a dominant inheritance pattern; however, the inheritance is considered to have incomplete penetrance (see Chapter 27). There is an increased risk of HD in children with

trisomy 21 and several other inherited disorders (e.g., Waardenburg syndrome). Additional information is available at https://medlineplus.gov/genetics/condition/hirschsprung-disease/.

Clinical Findings

History
- Failure to pass meconium within the first 48 hours of life
- Growth faltering, poor feeding
- Chronic constipation, vomiting, abdominal obstruction
- Diarrhea, explosive bowel movements, or flatus
- Presence of other inherited disorders

Diagnostic Studies
- Abdominal radiographs show dilated bowel loops.
- Barium or other contrast dye study. No prep required.
- Anorectal manometry study: A lack of relaxation of the internal anal sphincter with balloon rectal distension suggests HD. Anorectal manometry has a reported sensitivity and specificity ranging from 88% to 94% in diagnosing HD.[29]
- HD diagnosis is established by rectal suction biopsy, which determines the absence of ganglion cells.

Differential Diagnosis

The differential diagnosis includes acquired functional megacolon, colonic inertia, chronic idiopathic constipation, obstipation, small left colon syndrome, meconium plug syndrome, and ileal atresia with microcolon.

Management

Surgical resection of the affected bowel is indicated, with or without a colostomy.

Functional Abdominal Pain Not Otherwise Specified

Children with recurrent abdominal pain with no specific organic etiology are diagnosed with functional abdominal pain-not otherwise specified (FAP-NOS), also known as *recurrent abdominal pain,* a disorder that is often a puzzling problem for providers. FAP-NOS is more common than organic reasons for abdominal pain. The Rome IV criteria are the diagnostic standards.[30] The following criteria[12] must occur at least four times per month for at least 2 months before diagnosis:

- Episodic or continuous abdominal pain that does not occur with other events (e.g., eating, menses)
- Insufficient criteria for IBS, functional dyspepsia, or abdominal migraine
- After appropriate evaluation, abdominal pain that cannot be fully explained by another medical condition

FAP-NOS is the most common pain complaint in early childhood and accounts for 2% of pediatric visits. FAP-NOS is more prevalent in females. The peak incidence of FAP-NOS occurs between 7 and 12 years old.[31] The pain is genuine, but its cause remains unclear. There is no evidence of visceral hypersensitivity in the rectum, as occurs with IBS. Affected children often have a familial predisposition for the development of physiologic pain (e.g., family history of FAP-NOS). The primary theory is FAP-NOS results from a dysregulation of the brain-gut communication axis. Feedback from a variety of sources, including genetic, physical, psychological, and environmental factors, has an impact on the CNS (brain) and GI motility (gut).[30] Approximately 25% of children worldwide meet the criteria for a functional GI disorder.

Clinical Findings

History

- Presence of Rome IV criteria for FAP-NOS
- Abdominal pain often accompanied by a dramatic reaction (e.g., clutching abdomen, doubling over, throwing self to ground)
- Symptoms may worsen in the morning, preventing the child from going to school and resulting in school avoidance
- Report that pain medications do not alleviate pain
- Obtain a review of systems, with attention to:
  - Comorbid anxiety and depression, behavioral problems
  - Illicit drug use
  - Sexual activity or abuse; possible pregnancy
- Careful psychosocial history (home, school, parents, friends, community); ACEs; secondary gains from symptoms and insufficient coping skills; endeavor to determine the degree of functional impairment
- Associated symptoms, such as headache, joint pain, anorexia, vomiting, nausea, excessive flatulence, and altered bowel pattern
- Red flags listed in Box 34.6; there is an association between these symptoms and an organic cause of the chronic pain[12]
- Family history of FAP-NOS

Physical Examination. After an initial examination, reexamination should be done during an acute episode and each subsequent visit. The physical examination is usually normal but includes:

- Plot weight, length/height, and BMI
- Vital signs
- Abdominal examination: Presence of pain, rebound tenderness, masses
- Perianal and rectal examination
- Complete neurologic examination
- Pelvic examination as indicated
- Skin and joint assessment
- Identification of red flags (see Box 34.6)

• BOX 34.6 Red Flags for Functional Abdominal Pain

Red Flags on History

- Localization of the pain away from the umbilicus, especially right or left upper quadrant
- Pain associated with a change in bowel habits, particularly chronic, severe diarrhea; constipation; or nocturnal bowel movement
- Pain associated with night wakening
- Repetitive, significant emesis, especially if bilious
- Constitutional symptoms, such as recurrent fever, loss of appetite or energy
- Recurrent abdominal pain occurring in a child younger than 4 years old
- Blood in stool or emesis
- Red flags on physical examination
- Unexplained fever
- Unintentional loss of weight or decline in height velocity
- Organomegaly
- Localized abdominal tenderness, particularly removed from the umbilicus
- Perirectal abnormalities (e.g., fissures, ulceration, or skin tags)
- Joint swelling, redness, heat, or discoloration
- Ventral hernias of the abdominal wall

Data from Hyams J, Di Lorenzo C, Saps M, et al. Functional disorders: children and adolescents. Gastroenterology. 2016;150(6):1456–1470.

Diagnostic Studies

- The Rome IV criteria states children with FAP-NOS do not require laboratory or radiology investigation. PCPs may opt for selective testing based on the history, physical examination, family history, or parental reassurance, including[12]:
  - CBC, ESR, CRP, UA, and urine culture if FAP-NOS is suspected. A biochemical profile (liver and kidney function); stool for O&P and culture; and breath hydrogen testing may be useful if indicated by the history.
  - Stool for *H. pylori* antigen.
  - Serum IgA, IgG, and tissue transglutaminase (TTG) antibody to exclude celiac disease (CD).
  - Ultrasound and esophageal pH monitoring as indicated by potential red flags.

Follow-up evaluation (e.g., CT, colonoscopy, CD serology) should be considered if positive results are noted in the initial diagnostic testing, symptoms progress, or alarm features develop.

Differential Diagnosis

The following differential diagnoses should be considered: all organic causes of abdominal pain, including urinary tract, GI tract (e.g., IBS, CD, intestinal malformations), and extraabdominal causes; malabsorption syndromes; lactose intolerance; constipation; and small intestine bacterial overgrowth (SIBO). There is no evidence that the presence of the associated symptoms, an adverse life event, or anxiety or depression helps distinguish between organic and FAP-NOS. Abdominal pain associated with depression usually includes low mood, fatigue, loss of interest, social isolation, decreased activity, impaired attention span, difficulty sleeping, and irritability while abdominal pain and school avoidance is usually associated with severe pain and anxiety only on weekday mornings.

Management

- Establish a therapeutic parent-child-practitioner relationship to improve patient satisfaction, treatment adherence, symptom reduction, and other outcomes.

- Explain the brain-gut interaction and that biopsychosocial interventions are the most effective evidence-based treatments for FAP-NOS.[30]
- Use medications judiciously. H_2 blockers should not be used unless dyspepsia is present.
- Early in the visit, discuss the possibility with the patient and parent/caregiver that the pain can be functional (inorganic). Assure them that the symptoms are real and will be addressed.
- Encourage return to school and normalization of lifestyle. Limit attention given to pain episodes.
- Consider using complementary and alternative medicine (CAM) approaches (see Chapter 23). A bland diet may be helpful if certain dietary practices seem to cause pain (e.g., a lactose-free diet with documented lactose intolerance). Avoiding sorbitol and fructose may help if malabsorption is a contributing factor. The authors of a systematic review and meta-analysis suggest that cognitive behavioral therapy (CBT) and hypnotherapy should be considered.[30]
- Explore psychological triggers and manage the pain. Discuss how stressful events and emotional issues affect pain. Suggest distraction to shift attention from the abdominal pain to other activities. School attendance is a good distraction. Biofeedback provides evidence to the patient that they can change muscle tension, skin temperature, and relaxation. Relaxation and guided imagery decrease abdominal pain.
- Identify, treat, and refer for any significant psychological issues. Psychotherapy and family therapy may be beneficial. Using a biopsychosocial approach is helpful for FAP-NOS symptoms. Refer for psychological dysfunction (maladaptive behavior, conversion reaction, depression, anxiety).
- Discuss potential alarm features (see Box 34.6) so the parents and child can identify changes in status and illness.
- Establish regular patient follow-up.

Prognosis and Complications

The prognosis is positive if FAP-NOS is managed effectively. Prompt diagnosis is important as diagnosing a functional GI disorder (e.g., FAP-NOS, IBS, functional dyspepsia, abdominal migraine) at the first visit for abdominal pain was associated with a two times greater chance of symptom control.[32] Symptoms management focuses on the acknowledgement of the abdominal pain, providing reassurance and acceptance, and modifying the environment.[33]

Irritable Bowel Syndrome

IBS is a chronic condition that occurs when altered bowel habits and bloating are not explained by structural or biochemical abnormalities.[33] There are four subgroups of IBS:
- Predominant-diarrhea (IBS-D)
- Predominant-constipation (IBS-C)
- Mixed/alternating stool forms (IBS-A)
- Unclassified (IBS-U)

Rome IV criteria for IBS must include *all* the following at least once per week for at least 2 months before diagnosis[12]:
- Change in the stool frequency
- Change in stool form (appearance)
- In individuals with constipation, the pain does not resolve with the resolution of constipation (children in whom the pain resolves have functional constipation, if it does not, they likely have IBS)
- After appropriate evaluation, the symptoms cannot be fully explained by another medical condition

IBS is the most common cause of abdominal pain in children in the Western world. It is estimated that all functional GI disorders have a pediatric prevalence of greater than 40%.[33] The pathophysiology of IBS remains poorly understood. The presumption is multifactorial and includes infection, inflammation, visceral hypersensitivity, allergy, genetic factors, psychological factors, and disordered gut motility.[33]

Clinical Findings
History
- Meets IBS Rome IV criteria
- Abnormal stool frequency (four or more stools/day and two or fewer stools/week
- Abnormal stool form (lumpy/hard or loose/watery or alternating)
- Abnormal stool passage (straining, urgency, feeling of incomplete evacuation)
- Mucus passage
- Bloating or feeling of abdominal distention
- Dyspepsia (present in 30% of pediatric patients)
- Psychosocial history, including potential triggering events and other psychosocial factors
- Family history of IBS
- Nutrition history: fiber and water intake, excessive sorbitol, fructose intake

Physical Examination
- Normal physical examination; normal growth curves and BMI
- Absence of alarm signals

Diagnostic Studies. There are no specific laboratory markers for IBS.

Differential Diagnosis
See FAP-NOS for the differential diagnoses.

Management
Treatment goals are to improve the quality of life and modify the symptoms severity by minimizing pain and normalizing stool consistency and frequency. The following therapeutic interventions are used:
- Dietary interventions
  - Fiber supplement, low fermentable oligo-di-monosaccharides and polyol (FODMAP) diet.[33]
  - Avoid trigger foods known to exacerbate pain episodes: caffeine; sorbitol; fatty food; large meals; gas-producing foods such as carbonated beverages, lactose (with lactose intolerance), and cruciferous vegetables.
- Probiotics *Lactobacillus rhamnosus* GG and *L. reuteri* are commonly used.[34,35]
- Drug therapy includes peppermint oil, tegaserod, antispasmodic agents, antidiarrheal agents, antibiotics, and amitriptyline or selective serotonin reuptake inhibitors.[34]
- Biopsychosocial therapy (e.g., hypnotherapy, CBT, yoga, acupuncture).
- Validate and explain the diagnosis to the patient and family.
- Identify and develop strategies to address triggering events and psychosocial factors.

Malabsorption Syndromes

Malabsorption syndromes are caused by congenital, inherited, and acquired conditions. They usually result in a decrease in weight, followed by height velocity deceleration. In this section, celiac disease, lactose intolerance, cow's-milk protein intolerance, and food protein immunologic enterocolitis syndrome are discussed.

Celiac Disease. *Celiac disease* (CD), also known as gluten sensitivity enteropathy, is an immune-mediated systemic disorder triggered by dietary exposure to wheat gluten and related proteins in barley and rye. It is characterized by a variable combination of gluten-dependent clinical manifestations, CD-specific antibodies, and enteropathy. A complex of genes that predispose individuals to celiac disease are members of the HLA complex located on chromosome 6. HLA-DQ2 is the most common celiac-related gene found in the general population (between 90 and 95% of people with celiac disease), followed by HLA-DQ8 (between 2.5 and 5% of celiac patients). CD frequently co-occurs with other autoimmune disorders, including diabetes mellitus type 1, Hashimoto thyroiditis, autoimmune liver disease, IgA nephropathy, and juvenile chronic arthritis.[35] CD also has a higher incidence among infants born via cesarean section. It is hypothesized that the development of enteric homeostasis in the newborn period may be altered in cesarean birth, thus increasing susceptibility. CD has a worldwide distribution, with both a global and American prevalence of 1%.[36] Increased recognition of the wide CD symptom distribution and improved screening, along with lower screening thresholds, led to diagnosing patients who would not have been diagnosed in the past. It is suggested that an increased incidence is also attributable to demographic changes, such as immigration from developing to developed countries, which increases exposure to gluten.

Clinical presentation typically occurs between 6 months and 2 years of age, with a female predominance of 2:1.[35] The classic CD clinical features include diarrhea, steatorrhea, weight loss, and growth failure. Nonclassical and symptomatic patients tend to have either mild GI symptoms, such as abdominal pain or constipation, or extraintestinal manifestations (EIM) of CD.[36] Common EIM include joint swelling, erythema nodosum, uveitis, and primary sclerosing cholangitis.

Lactose Intolerance. *Lactose intolerance* is a clinical syndrome characterized by abdominal pain, diarrhea, nausea, flatulence, and bloating that occurs after ingesting lactose-containing foods. The symptoms are caused when lactose, a disaccharide found exclusively in mammalian milk, is not absorbed secondary to a lactase enzyme deficiency. Increased lactose draws fluid and electrolytes into the intestine, resulting in osmotic diarrhea. Intestinal bacteria also metabolize excess lactose, creating methane, carbon dioxide, and hydrogen gases that lead to bloating and flatulence.[37] There are four types of lactase deficiency:

- Primary (i.e., lactase nonpersistence), is the most common cause of lactose intolerance. It typically develops after weaning but occurs at varying ages. Patients initially produce lactase but decrease lactase production as their diet becomes more varied. Its prevalence has not been established in the United States; however, it is found more often in Hispanic, Black, Ashkenazi Jewish, Asian, and American Indian populations than in White populations.
- Secondary—results from small bowel injury (e.g., gastroenteritis, chemotherapy, chronic diarrhea) and is most common in infancy.
- Congenital—extremely rare congenital absence of lactase that if left untreated, can be fatal in early infancy.
- Developmental—occurs in preterm infants (born before 34 weeks' gestation) and occurs because of the intestinal tract immaturity.

Cow's Milk Protein Intolerance/Allergy. *Cow's milk protein intolerance* (CMPI) and *cow's milk protein allergy* (CMPA) can clinically present similarly; however, CMPI is a nonallergic hypersensitivity to the proteins in cow's milk, whereas CMPA is an immunologically mediated reaction. Most CMPA is an IgE-mediated atopic disease in which atopic dermatitis, allergic rhinitis, and asthma may also be present. Some CMPA cases are cell mediated, presenting primarily with GI symptoms.[38] CMPA is the cause of approximately 2% to 7.5% of childhood food allergies globally.[38] The use of extensively hydrolyzed casein formula and *L. rhamnosus GG* supplementation may reduce inflammation, GI symptoms, and reduce disease duration.[38]

Food Protein–Induced Enterocolitis Syndrome. *Food protein–induced enterocolitis syndrome* (FPIES) is inflammation involving the small and large intestines. It is classified as a delayed hypersensitivity reaction or non-IgE–mediated GI food allergy. The acute form is more common and presents about 2 to 6 hours following ingesting a causative food, while the less common chronic form is linked to continuing exposure to the causative food. FPIES is commonly seen in infants with the introduction of infant formula and/or solids; exclusively breastfed infants present at a later age. The most common triggers are cow's milk, soy, rice, and oats, but any food can cause FPIES.[39] Typical symptoms include severe vomiting, followed by diarrhea, and then dehydration, which leads to lethargy, an unhealthy, pale appearance, growth faltering, hypotension, and nutrient deficiencies. There is often a delayed diagnosis or misdiagnosis, particularly because of the nonspecific presenting symptoms and a lack of definitive diagnostic biomarkers. It is often confused with sepsis, metabolic disease, and acute or severe gastroenteritis. Diagnosis is based on clinical history, symptoms and timing, exclusion of other causes, and ultimately symptom improvement with offending food avoidance. Definitive diagnosis may be achieved through a supervised oral food challenge. In some cases, when the clinical history includes numerous episodes of typical symptoms, a food challenge is not necessary for diagnostic confirmation. Early recognition is necessary to deter recurrent acute episodes, thus avoiding further syndrome complications, particularly nutritional deficiencies. Management is staged:

- *Initial*: Fluid replacement if profuse vomiting with dehydration is present.
  - Oral hydration is preferred and, if necessary, use IV fluids.
  - Causative food removal and continuous elimination from the diet is required.
  - Introduce new food one at a time to observe reactions.
- *Long term*: Involves dietary monitoring with a goal of allergy resolution.
  - Monitor for nutritional deficiencies, provide supplements where necessary, and develop care plans to manage the episodes.

Prognosis is usually good with a large percentage of the population achieving symptom resolution. Internationally, the age of tolerance varies based on study design, provider preference, and the food challenged.[39]

Clinical Findings

History: General for Malabsorption Syndromes. Careful medical and family medical histories are important when evaluating a malabsorption syndrome and are the key to the diagnosis. In addition, a complete nutrition and dietary intake history distinguishes between undernutrition and malabsorption. Significant historical findings include:

- Past surgical and trauma history
- Growth failure

- Delayed puberty
- A voracious appetite or particular food avoidance
- Chronic diarrhea with frequent, large, foul-smelling, pale stools
- Excessive flatus with abdominal distention
- Pallor, fatigue, hair and dermatologic abnormalities, digital clubbing, dizziness, cheilosis, glossitis, peripheral neuropathy
- Disease-specific history:
  - CD: chronic or intermittent diarrhea, persistent or unexplained GI symptoms (e.g., nausea, vomiting), sudden or unexpected weight loss, and fatigue
  - Lactose intolerance: abdominal pain, diarrhea, nausea, flatulence, and bloating
  - CMPI/CMPA: family history of allergy or atopy

Physical Examination: General
- Growth parameters and percentiles
- Skinfold thickness and lean body mass
- Examination for delayed growth and puberty (e.g., sexual maturity rating [SMR]; see Chapter 13).

Physical Examination: Disease-Specific
Celiac Disease
- Impaired growth, growth faltering, unexplained iron-deficiency anemia, abdominal distention, bloating or cramping pain.
- May have no symptoms despite evidence of small bowel changes; maintain a high suspicion for CD in children with metabolic bone disease (e.g., rickets, osteomalacia), low-trauma fractures, or those with dental enamel defects.

Lactose Intolerance
- Abdominal distention
- Increased flatus
- Symptom onset varies from 30 minutes to 2 hours after lactose ingestion

CMPI and CMPA
- Immediate[38]:
  - Anaphylaxis (rare) but can be life-threatening
  - GI: Lip or tongue edema, oral pruritus, nausea, vomiting
  - Skin: Urticaria, rash, flushing, angioedema
  - Respiratory: Nasal pruritus, sneezing, rhinitis, congestion, wheezing, dyspnea, chest tightness
- Late onset (1 hour to several days after ingestion of CMP)[38]:
  - Typically, non–IgE-mediated allergic reaction
  - Symptoms are primarily GI: Varied, including nausea, vomiting, abdominal pain, diarrhea, bloody stool, GERD-like symptoms, pyloric stenosis, malabsorption, growth faltering, IBD
  - Urticarial rash (with both IgE- and non–IgE-mediated allergy); eczema
  - Respiratory: Heiner syndrome (i.e., cow's milk–induced pulmonary disease) is rare

Diagnostic Studies: General
- Stool assessment: Occult blood, WBCs, and culture; liquid stool for pH and reducing substances; 72-hour fecal fat collection or Sudan stain for stool fat; spot stool testing for α1-antitrypsin level to establish the diagnosis of protein-losing enteropathy.
- Sweat chloride test: If steatorrhea present, evaluates for cystic fibrosis
- Stool for O&P: Giardiasis is a common intestinal infection causing malabsorption. See later discussion for symptoms suggestive of infestation.
- CBC with differential, RBC indices, iron, folic acid, and ferritin

- Serum calcium, phosphorus, magnesium, alkaline phosphatase, serum protein, liver function tests, vitamin D and its metabolites, vitamins A, B_{12}, E, and K
- Human immunodeficiency virus (HIV) testing when growth faltering and chronic diarrhea present
- Small bowel biopsy
- Plain abdominal radiographs and/or barium contrast studies, as indicated
- Abdominal ultrasound for hepatobiliary stones or masses
- Retrograde studies of the pancreas and biliary tree, if indicated
- Bone age

Disease-Specific Tests
Celiac Disease
- If there is clinical suspicion of CD, the child has an associated disorder or has a first-degree relative with CD, obtain serological testing. Patients should eat gluten in more than one meal every day for 6 weeks before testing. Recommended serologic tests including IgA tissue transglutaminase antibody (tTGA) and a total serum IgA to identify patients with IgA deficiency.[35]
- Although several commercial screening tests sold direct to consumers are available, home blood testing is not recommended.
- If serologic testing is positive, refer for endoscopy with biopsy for a definitive diagnosis. In an IgA-deficient person, obtain an intestinal biopsy even if all serologic tests are negative.[35]
- There are no published recommendations for follow-up; however, careful follow-up of growth parameters, tTGA testing after 6 months of a gluten-free diet, and then yearly is the general recommendation.[35]
- Bone density testing (skeletal changes may be the first symptom of CD).

Lactose Intolerance
- Lactose hydrogen breath test is the gold standard. Children should not take antibiotics at the time of the study because the intestinal bacteria that act on lactose may be diminished.
- A 2-week trial lactose-free diet for 2 weeks, being aware of hidden sources of lactose. Symptoms should disappear with the diet and reappear when lactose is reintroduced.
- Bone density if calcium deficiency is suspected (lactose is necessary for calcium absorption into bone, and lactose-free diets can predispose to osteoporosis).
- If a secondary cause of lactose intolerance is suspected, continue evaluation for all other causes of malabsorption.

CMPI/CMPA
- Elimination diet followed by a double-blind placebo-controlled oral food challenge.
- An allergy skin patch test may be performed.
- Serum IgE antibodies testing may be performed.
- Diagnosis of CMPI is made when there is clinical improvement on a CMP-free diet.

Differential Diagnosis
Differential diagnoses include organic and nonorganic growth faltering, colic, short stature, chronic diarrhea, CF, immunodeficiency, cholestatic liver disease, GERD, SIBO, and IBD.

Management
Celiac Disease
- A lifelong strict gluten-free diet is currently the only effective treatment. Counseling from an experienced dietitian with CD expertise is essential.[35]

- Alternative treatments are being explored, including using enzyme therapy, developing genetically engineered grains, inhibiting tTGA in the intestine, and correcting intestinal barrier defects (particularly increased permeability).

Lactose Intolerance
- Once lactose intolerance is verified, reduce lactose exposure:
  - Avoid lactose-containing milk (cow/goat) and other dairy products.
  - Use lactose-free dairy products (e.g., milk prehydrolyzed with lactase).
  - Use alternate milk sources (e.g., soy, rice).
  - Use oral lactase supplements with the first bite of lactose-containing foods. Most individuals with primary lactase deficiency can ingest small to moderate amounts of dairy products, especially if taken with other foods.
- Ensure adequate intake of calcium and vitamin D from other sources.

CMPI/CMPA[38]
- Breastfeed, if possible.
- Restrict milk and milk products from the diet of breastfeeding mothers.
- Use extensively hydrolyzed infant formula, as partially hydrolyzed formula is *not* appropriate for infants with CMPA.
- Use amino acid formula for infants who demonstrate severe allergy (e.g., prior history of anaphylaxis) or who do not respond to extensively hydrolyzed formula.
- Extensively hydrolyzed soy formula is appropriate for infants after 6 months old; before 6 months old, infants fed soy formula are at risk for nutritional deficit (e.g., decreased weight gain despite fed sufficient calories).
- Avoid the use of other mammals' milk (e.g., sheep, goat, camel) because of the risk of cross-allergic reaction.
- After 2 years old, infant formula is inappropriate but ensure daily dietary intake of 600 to 800 mg of calcium.
- Probiotics may help create tolerance.
- Patients should have injectable epinephrine (EpiPen) if anaphylaxis is a concern.
- Monitor growth and development.
- Refer to an allergist or gastroenterologist if symptoms are severe; immunotherapy is not recommended.
- Annual reevaluation of sensitivity, preferably an oral food challenge under medical supervision.

Complications and Prognosis
Celiac Disease. Growth failure is the primary complication of CD. With delayed diagnosis or inadequate treatment, there is a risk for fractures, osteomalacia, and osteoporosis, lymphoma, autoimmune diseases (e.g., type 1 diabetes, Hashimoto thyroiditis), primary biliary cirrhosis, and primary sclerosing cholangitis. Sensory peripheral neuropathy may be related to gluten sensitivity.[35] Although rare, celiac crisis, consisting of abdominal distention, explosive watery diarrhea, dehydration with hypoproteinemia, electrolyte imbalance, hypotensive shock, and lethargy can be the first indication of CD. Prognosis is improved with adherence to lifelong gluten-free diet.

Lactose Intolerance. Unabsorbed lactose does not cause clinical intestinal damage despite clinical symptoms. Bone density loss may occur with inadequate calcium and vitamin D intake.

CMPI/CMPA. CMPI usually resolves by 1 to 3 years old. When patients only have GI symptoms, CMPI typically resolves completely. CMPA cannot be reversed. There is a high likelihood of other food allergies developing in patients with CMPI. Complications include rickets, poor growth, and growth faltering.

Intestinal and Rectal Polyps

Intestinal polyps in children may be benign or present a risk for subsequent cancer or other conditions (e.g., anemia). Solitary or juvenile polyps are the most common (90%). They are most often found in early childhood (4–5 years old) in the rectosigmoid area. The incidence is about 2% in children younger than 10 years and are considered negligible or at no malignancy risk. Polyps are also associated with autosomal dominant disorders, including familial adenomatous polyposis (FAP), juvenile polyposis syndrome, phosphatase and tensin homolog hamartoma tumor syndrome, and Peutz-Jeghers syndrome.

Clinical Findings
History
- May be asymptomatic.
- Obtain careful family history/three-generation pedigree to identify individuals at risk for polyposis.
- Hematochezia (painless, bright red rectal bleeding). Blood coats/mixes with the stool. Bleeding can be daily, intermittent, or infrequent. Large volume blood loss is extremely rare.
- For FAP: Nonspecific complaints, diarrhea, constipation, or changes in bowel habits.

Physical Examination
- Anorectal examination to identify polyp or other rectal bleeding source.
- Note pallor (caused by anemia from GI hemorrhage) and edema (caused by hypoproteinemia from protein-losing enteropathy) indicate heavy polyp burden.
- For FAP, assess for ophthalmologic changes (e.g., hypertrophy of retinal pigment), dental anomalies (e.g., supernumerary/unerupted teeth), osteomas of skull, jaw, or extremities, and multiple lipomas.

Diagnostic Studies
- CBC with differential and ESR, CRP, prothrombin time, and APTT.
- Fecal occult blood test, even if blood appears to be present.
- Stool culture for bacterial pathogens and O&P.
- Diagnostic test of choice: colonoscopy to the terminal ileum with biopsy.
- Endoscopy (if concerned about gastric or duodenal polyps). Small-bowel video capsule endoscopy may be used.
- Barium contrast of upper intestine.

Management
- Refer to a pediatric gastroenterologist for management and follow-up screening.
- Resection of the polyp(s), usually with diagnostic or surveillance screening.
  - If multiple polyps are present, bowel resection (colectomy) is common.
  - For familial adenomatous polyposis, colectomy is standard therapy.
- Children with one to two juvenile colonic polyps usually need no further follow-up.

TABLE 34.8	Features of Crohn Disease and Ulcerative Colitis	
Feature	**Crohn Disease**	**Ulcerative Colitis**
Age at onset	10–20 years	10–20 years
Area of bowel affected	Can affect any part of GI system; often in terminal ileum or colon; may be small bowel only; small bowel and cecum; small bowel and colon; or colon only; occasionally isolated perianal disease	Affects colon/rectum; entire colon may be inflamed (pancolitis); may have subtotal colitis or "ileal backwash" (i.e., superficial inflammation of ileum proximal to splenic flexure); may be left-sided (distal to splenic flexure); may have proctitis (limited to rectum or distal 15 cm)
Distribution	Segmental; disease-free "skip" areas common	Continuous distal to proximal
Endoscopic, radiographic, or biopsy findings	Noncaseating granulomas located in inflamed mucosa; cobblestone appearance of bowel wall; linear/serpiginous ulcers and transverse fissures; fixation and separation of loops; small bowel strictures/stenoses; bowel or perianal fistulas; perianal abscesses or large (>5 mm) skin tags	Superficial inflammation of mucosa; friable tissue with exudates and granularity; loss of vascular pattern; small perianal skin tags (<5 mm)
Intestinal symptoms	Abdominal pain, diarrhea, anorexia, weight loss	Abdominal pain with or around time of stooling, bloody diarrhea, urgency, and tenesmus
Extraintestinal manifestations seen more often in Crohn disease than ulcerative colitis; similar types for both conditions	Ophthalmologic conditions (uveitis, iritis, conjunctivitis) more likely in Crohn disease	Primary sclerosing cholangitis more likely in ulcerative colitis

GI, Gastrointestinal.
Data from Orlanski-Meyer E, Aardoom M, Ricciuto A, et al. Predicting outcomes in pediatric ulcerative colitis for management optimization: systematic review and consensus statements from the pediatric inflammatory bowel disease -Ahead program. *Gastroenterology*. 2021;160(1):378–402; Ricciuto A, Aardoom M, Orlanski-Meyer E, et al. Predicting outcomes in pediatric Crohn's disease for management optimization: systematic review and consensus statements from the pediatric inflammatory bowel disease-Ahead program. *Gastroenterology*. 2021;160(1):403–436.

- Follow-up is required if:
  - Family history of polyps (i.e., all children are at risk for polyposis).
  - Child has three or more polyps on colonoscopy.
  - Polyps are found outside the colon.
  - Extraintestinal symptoms are present.
- Additional follow-up varies by condition and severity.
  - Testing to determine gene mutation(s) is usually done at 8 to 10 years old. Genetic counseling may be recommended.
  - Ophthalmologic evaluation may be recommended.

Complications

Children with inherited disorders/multiple polyps are at risk for adult colorectal, gastric, duodenal, pancreatic, and extraintestinal cancer (usually appearing after 40 years of age). Psychological issues related to having a hereditary condition with uncertain long-term outcomes (i.e., high risk for malignancies) can cause family problems.

Anal Fissure

Anal fissures are small tears in the anal mucosa most typically due to the passage of frequent or hard stools. Anal stenosis or other trauma can also be causative factors. Anal fissures are the most common cause of pediatric rectal bleeding.

Clinical Findings

History and Physical Examination. History typically includes crying with bowel movement, bright red (blood) streaks in the stool or diaper, and stool withholding. Physical examination reveals small tears in the anal mucosa. Tears are best visible with the child in the knee-chest position and the anus slightly everted. An otoscope with a large speculum is needed if the external fissures are not readily visible. A digital examination with the fifth finger excludes anal stenosis.

Differential Diagnosis

Differential diagnoses include other sources of lower intestinal hemorrhage, such as infection, formula intolerance, necrotizing enterocolitis, intussusception, juvenile polyps, hemolytic-uremic syndrome, Henoch-Schönlein purpura, irritable bowel disease, and vascular lesions. Sexual abuse should be considered in children with large, irregular, or multiple fissures.

Management

- Treat constipation.
- Local wound care should include sitz baths twice a day and the application of 0.5% hydrocortisone cream or lubricating jelly to the anus.

Patient/Family Education

- Preventive measures (e.g., avoiding constipation, encouraging regular toileting habits, avoiding laxatives/enemas).
- Recurrence is common. Fissures cause painful stooling, cycles of stool withholding and encopresis.

Inflammatory Bowel Disease

IBD is a chronic relapsing inflammatory disease that can involve any part of the GI tract. It includes Crohn disease, UC, and unclassified IBD (IBDU)[40] (Table 34.8). Crohn disease and UC share a similar clinical presentation; however, they affect distinct parts of the GI tract with a different extent of gut wall inflammation. IBD is a multifactorial disease stemming from the impact of both environmental and genetic components on the intestinal microbiome. Understanding of IBD genetics is evolving and the incorporation of a genetic panel covering key genes enhances the diagnosis and evaluation of IBD; however, PCPs should consult a specialist before recommending genetic testing to their patients (see Chapter 27).

Children often present with atypical features, making definitive diagnosis challenging.[41] Several indices assess and classify IBD. The Pediatric Ulcerative Colitis Activity Index (PUCAI) defines severe disease with a score of at least 65 points and provides a range of scores that monitor disease severity and treatment progress.[42,43] The Pediatric Crohn Disease Activity Index (PCDAI) is used in clinical practice and research to assess disease severity and to enhance clinical decision making.[43]

The incidence of IBD is increasing worldwide, especially Crohn disease and pediatric-onset IBD. North America has the highest incidence of IBD in the world.[40] IBD occurs at any age, with a peak onset between 15 and 30 years. Up to 25% of cases occur in children and adolescents, and 4% are found in children younger than 5 years. IBD in infants is extremely rare. In contrast to adults, children diagnosed with IBD are more likely to have Crohn disease than UC, have more severe or extensive disease (both Crohn disease and UC), vague symptoms, extraintestinal symptoms (e.g., anemia), and more relapses.[43] In the United States, the prevalence of pediatric IBD was 77 per 100,000 in 2016, which is about 16,000 children with UC and 34,000 with Crohn disease, and 7000 with IBD.[44] These numbers reflect a 133% increase in pediatric IBD prevalence since 2007.[45]

Crohn Disease

Crohn disease is a chronic disease with dysregulated inflammation and cytokine production in the intestinal tract. It can involve any part of the GI tract, although the terminal ileum and colon are most affected. Inflammation is usually transmural, affecting the entire wall of the intestine, creating fissures and fistulas. The unaffected areas of the intestine are called *skip areas*. The exact cause is unknown, although the likely etiology is an environmental exposure that triggers an abnormal immune reaction in a genetically susceptible individual. Crohn disease peaks in adolescence and early adulthood, then again in middle adulthood (50–70 years); however, rates are increasing in the 10 to 17 age subgroup. Further, 25% to 40% of cases are diagnosed in childhood and adolescence. Inflammation of the UGI tract is reported in approximately half of children at the IBD initial assessment.[41]

Clinical Findings

History
- Fever, usually low grade, of unknown etiology
- Weight loss (average of 5–7 kg)
- Delayed growth velocity, short stature, delayed bone age
- Arthralgias and arthritis in large joints, occasional joint destruction
- Obstructive symptoms associated with meals, bloating, early satiety
- Pain in the umbilical region and RLQ; may awaken at night
- Anorexia
- Malabsorption and lactose intolerance
- Diarrhea (with/without blood or mucus), pain with stooling
- Jaundice

- Oral aphthous ulcers, especially during exacerbations of the illness
- Tobacco use history
- Positive family history

Physical Examination
- Review and measure growth.
- Abdominal examination: RLQ tenderness, mass.
- Perianal skin tags, deep anal fissures, and perianal fistulas strongly suggest Crohn disease.
- Digit clubbing is due to mucosal inflammatory change and fibrosis or platelets sensitivity in the microvasculature with release of platelet-releasing growth factor.
- Erythema nodosum (i.e., panniculitis) is common.

Diagnostic Studies
- Inflammatory markers: ESR, CRP
- Nutritional status: Albumin, total protein, consider iron panel, calcium, zinc, alkaline phosphatase, folate, vitamin B_{12}
- Blood: CBC with differential, consider liver enzymes, aspartate aminotransferase (AST), alanine aminotransferase (ALT), total bilirubin, γ-glutamyltransferase (GGT); amylase; lipase
- Stool: Routine culture, O&P, *Clostridium difficile* (with recent antibiotic use), blood, WBCs, and fecal α1-antitrypsin:
  - Fecal calprotectin assay is an appropriate initial test in a child with recurrent abdominal pain or to assess for disease flare when stool changes occur.[46]
- Radiologic studies: Bone age (usually delayed by 2 years), bone density, plain abdominal films, upper GI series with small bowel follow-through, abdominal CT with contrast
- Ileocolonoscopy is a first step to assess for Crohn disease.
- Other endoscopic studies include small bowel capsule endoscopy, push enteroscopy, single- or double-balloon enteroscopy, interoperative enteroscopy, or spiral enteroscopy.
  - Upper endoscopy is recommended because up to one-half of children have upper GI involvement on initial evaluation.[41]
- Screen for tuberculosis in an at-risk child (see Chapter 35). Note: Biologic agents used in Crohn disease therapy can activate latent TB.

Differential Diagnosis

Differentials should include rheumatoid arthritis, systemic lupus erythematosus, hypopituitarism, acute appendicitis, peptic ulcer, intestinal obstruction, intestinal lymphoma, anorexia, chronic granulomatous disease, sarcoidosis, and growth failure.

Management

The goals of therapy are to (1) control the disease, (2) prevent relapses, and (3) achieve normal nutrition, growth, and lifestyle. Treatment combines pharmacologic, nutritional, surgical, and psychosocial interventions, including:
- Refer to a pediatric gastroenterologist for a colonoscopy, endoscopy, definitive diagnosis, consultation, and follow-up care.
- In the United States, pharmaceutical management is most common. In Europe, exclusive enteral nutrition (EEN) is used as first-line therapy for mild to moderate disease. EEN improves growth, healing of the mucosa, and overall nutrition status.[47,48]
- Medications:
  - Corticosteroids (e.g., prednisone, budesonide) are used orally, rectally, or intravenously for acute inflammation of mild to moderate disease. They are not intended for use in remission.

- 5-aminosalicylates (balsalazide, sulfasalazine, olsalazine, and mesalamine) are used orally or rectally for mild disease to control inflammation.
- Immunomodulator agents (azathioprine, 6-mercaptopurine, methotrexate, and cyclosporine) for severe small or large bowel disease, steroid-dependent or refractory disease, severe fistula, and growth failure.
- Biologic agents (e.g., infliximab, a chimeric, antitumor necrosis factor α [anti–TNF-α] antibody) for steroid-dependent or refractory disease, perirectal fistula, and maintenance of remission can be given alone or in combination with immunomodulators. One IV infusion of infliximab induces remission in Crohn disease. Greater mucosal healing follows treatment with immunomodulators and biologic agents than with corticosteroids; improved growth is seen with early anti–TNF-α treatment.[48]
- Antibiotics are used for acute infections (ampicillin, gentamicin, clindamycin, ciprofloxacin, or metronidazole).
- Adjunctive therapies (e.g., growth hormone) are not commonly prescribed.
  - Growth impairment, more common in males than females. This continues to be studied and is thought to be associated with underlying inflammation and sex-specific molecular pathways.[49]
- Hospitalization (severe disease) with total parenteral nutrition, nasogastric tube for decompression, or surgery.
- Surgery may still be required for patients with refractory disease or those who are intolerant of medication side effects and for pediatric patients with poor growth and unresponsiveness to medical therapy.[46]
- Ongoing monitoring of growth and pubertal changes.
- Ophthalmologic examination to exclude underlying ophthalmologic disease manifestations (e.g., uveitis, scleritis).
- Nutritional counseling, especially during remission to prevent or correct malnutrition and maintain and promote growth (see Chapter 14).
- Encourage participation in social activities, such as support groups (e.g., Team Challenge, a fund-raising running event for Crohn disease and UC) and Crohn disease camps.
- Refer for individual and family therapy, as indicated.

Complications

Intestinal obstruction with scarring and strictures is the major complication of Crohn disease. Growth failure (especially linear growth) is also common. Fistula and abscesses can occur; however, perforation and hemorrhage are rare. Primary sclerosing cholangitis, pancreatitis, pericarditis, arthritis, and peripheral neuropathy are other complications of Crohn disease.[50,51] Treatment with corticosteroids or immunosuppressive drugs increases the risk for opportunistic infections and inadequate response to immunizations.[52] As with many chronic illnesses, the patient and family are at risk for social functioning difficulties, anxiety, depression, somatization disorders, and school difficulties.

Prevention and Prognosis

It is important to follow recommended therapy to prevent sequelae. Crohn disease is progressive and without a cure, although about 55% of individuals are in remission at any one time, and only about 1% of individuals experience continuous active disease. One systematic review reported older age (>13 years) was a possible predictor for bowel surgery; however, no prognostic association was made based on sex, family history, or disease location at the time of diagnosis.[53]

Ulcerative Colitis

UC is a chronic disease characterized by diffuse inflammation of the rectal and colonic mucosa. UC involves the rectum in 95% of cases and may extend continuously and circumferentially to more proximal parts of the large intestine.[54] Pediatric patients, especially those younger than 10 years old, may appear to have no lesions in the rectum, leading to a misdiagnosis of Crohn disease. The exact cause is unknown, but there are multiple antecedents including heredity, diet, environment, immunologic alterations, and ineffective mucosal integrity. UC occurs twice as frequently in pediatrics as adults. The annual incidence, which occurs primarily in North America and Europe, is 1 to 4 per 100,000.[54]

Clinical Findings
History
- Fever
- Weight loss (average of 4 kg)
- Delayed growth and sexual maturation
- Arthritis and arthralgias of the large joints
- Anorexia
- Diarrhea
- Lower abdominal cramping and left lower quadrant pain
- Increased pain before stooling and passing flatus
- Stool with bright red blood and mucus
- Nocturnal stooling
- Oral aphthous ulcers
- Skin lesions (e.g., erythema nodosum, pyoderma gangrenosum, diffuse papulonecrotic eruptions)

Physical Examination
- Careful growth measuring/monitoring and SMR.
- Complete physical examination with particular attention to pallor, iris/uvea inflammation, oral ulcers, skin rash, abdominal pain, perianal disease, and joint inflammation/tenderness.
- Abdominal examination can reveal rebound tenderness if UC is severe.

Diagnostic Studies
- CBC with differential, iron-binding capacity, total protein, albumin, ESR, and CRP
- Stool for WBCs, blood, and culture (bloody diarrhea with negative stool culture characteristic of UC)
- Bone age (usually delayed up to 2 years)
- Colonoscopy (diffuse mucosal inflammation)
- Perinuclear neutrophil cytoplasmic antigen (positive in 60–70% of cases)
- Fecal calprotectin assay[54]

Differential Diagnosis

Differential diagnoses include Shigella, Salmonella, Yersinia, Campylobacter, E. coli, C. difficile, IBS, self-limited colitis, and Crohn disease.

Management

The goals of therapy are to (1) control the disease, (2) prevent relapses, and (3) achieve normal nutrition, growth, and lifestyle. Treatment combines pharmacologic, nutritional, surgical, and psychosocial interventions, including:
- Referral for consultation, colonoscopy, biopsy/definitive diagnosis, and close follow-up care.
- Pharmacologic options: Treatment for UC are complex and require an individualized approach. Patients with

mild-to-moderate disease can usually be managed in the out-patient setting, whereas severe UC warrants inpatient care.

- Mild to moderate UC: Topical mesalamine, oral 5-amino-salicylates, or topical steroids with topical mesalamine as a superior first-line agent.
- Moderate-to-severe UC: Systemic steroids for 1 to 2 weeks until clinical response is established followed by a slow steroid taper.
- Thiopurines: Azathioprine and 6-mercaptopurine have limited utility in the acute setting. Adverse effects include fever, rash, nausea, diarrhea, arthralgia, thrombocytopenia, leukopenia, infection, pancreatitis, hepatitis, non-Hodgkin lymphoma, and hepatosplenic T-cell lymphoma.
- Biologic agents e.g., (infliximab, adalimumab, golimumab) for induction of remission and maintenance in steroid-refractory and moderate to severe disease.
- Hydrocortisone rectal preparation for tenesmus.
- Cyclosporine monotherapy is as effective as or more effective than corticosteroids for the initial treatment of fulminating disease.
- Probiotics (e.g., VSL#3, *Saccharomyces boulardii*) may benefit when used with other therapies in mild to moderately active disease.
- Curcumin (i.e., active ingredient in turmeric) may assist in maintaining inactive disease.
- Iron supplementation to correct anemia, multivitamin.
- Nutrition:
  - Diet: Due to potential nutritional deficiencies, exclusion diets to induce remission or for remission maintenance should not be followed.[54]
  - Lactose is poorly tolerated.
  - Parenteral or enteral nutritional supplements (60–70 kcal/kg/day) may be used.
  - Refer for nutritional therapy to prevent or correct malnutrition and maintain and promote growth.
- Monitor growth.
- Surgery may be indicated; complete proctocolectomy with permanent ileostomy is curative.
- Referral to ophthalmology to rule out ophthalmologic manifestations of the disease (e.g., episcleritis, blurred/loss of vision, light sensitivity).
- Refer for psychosocial therapy as indicated. Depressive disorders are common.
- Assess immunization status and ensure the child is up to date; there is controversy regarding immunizing with live vaccines (e.g., varicella) primarily attributed to the belief that immunosuppressive therapy with steroids and biologics will impact the effectiveness of vaccination.[52] There is no evidence to support a lower immune response to vaccination in patients with IBD, but immunosuppressed patients should not receive live vaccine.[52]

Complications

Complications include growth failure, toxic megacolon, intestinal perforation, liver disease, sepsis, colon cancer (a long-term sequela 1–2% per year after 10 years of disease), arthritis, uveitis, malnutrition, as well as behavioral and emotional problems similar to those individuals with Crohn disease

Prevention and Prognosis

Follow the recommended therapy to optimize remission, maintain inactive disease state, and prevent complications. Prognosis is

good for patients with mild disease and those who respond quickly to initial therapy. Those with untreated or poorly treated disease are at increased risk for colectomy and colon cancer. Offering psychological support is highly recommended because the impact on quality of life can impact the entire family.[54]

Growth Faltering

Failure to thrive was a broadly used term referring to poor weight gain relative to age as determined by standardized growth charts. Its use has decreased in favor of the terms growth deficiency, growth delay, protein-energy malnutrition, faltering weight, and growth faltering. Growth faltering should be considered if any of the criteria in Box 34.7 are found. Growth faltering occurs secondary to (1) inadequate caloric intake, (2) inadequate caloric absorption, and/or (3) excessive caloric expenditure. In 90% of growth faltering cases there is no underlying medical condition.[55] In the United States, the prevalence ranges from less than 2% to 10%.[56] Youth living in poverty and those from developing countries with higher malnutrition rates and/or HIV infection are more likely to have growth faltering. Onset of growth faltering between 2 weeks and 4 months of age is usually associated with congenital disorders, serious somatic illness, and abnormal mother-infant interactions. Onset between 4 and 8 months of age in otherwise healthy children is usually associated with feeding problems. In chronic cases, weight for height may appear to be normal because of decreased growth velocity.

Clinical Findings and Risk Factors

Clinical findings include poor weight gain associated with poor intake, vomiting, food refusal, food fixation or intense preoccupation with food, abnormal feeding practices, anticipatory gagging, irritability, chronic physical problems in any body system, or psychosocial problems. Inborn errors of metabolism should be suspected with a history of acute, severe, and potentially life-threatening symptoms, liver dysfunction, recurrent vomiting, neurologic symptoms, cardiomyopathy, vision or hearing impairment, renal symptoms, dysmorphic features, organomegaly, and high anion gap acidosis, lactic acidosis, or hypoketotic hypoglycemia. In more severe cases, height, head circumference, and developmental progress may also be affected.

Growth faltering is rarely associated with adequate caloric intake.[55] There is no association between micronutrient deficiencies and growth faltering in those children who lack an underlying medical diagnosis.[55,57] A careful and detailed history may provide clues to aerodigestive, GI, anatomical, or developmental issues that contribute to growth faltering. Excessive consumption of an unbalanced diet should be considered, commonly excess milk and/or juice.[56] The nutritional history should include questions regarding infant formula preparation (e.g., If powder is used, how much water is mixed in? Is prepared formula being diluted with water?). These questions can provide clues to the patient's caloric intake. Low activity level, food restriction, and/or feeding rituals and poor appetite are predictive of nonorganic causes (e.g., inadequate caloric intake) while vomiting, diarrhea, irregular bowel movements, and abdominal distention are typical of organic causes (e.g., malabsorption/excessive expenditure of calories). Vomiting and abdominal distention were noted to be of particular significance. Hospitalized infants experiencing neglect, the most common cause of growth failure, usually have average or greater weight gain while hospitalized, thus helping exclude organic causes.[58] A thoughtful approach to the history (medical, developmental-behavioral, nutritional, social), thorough physical examination, and limited laboratory evaluation is needed when assessing children with growth faltering.

History. General parental concerns about the child's weight and growth must be addressed. Look for conditions that would negatively affect the patient's growth potential, increase caloric needs, decrease caloric availability or use, affect the individual's ability to feed or willingness to feed, or factors that might affect the parent's ability or interest in feeding their child.

Prenatal
- Maternal health, including chronic illness, such as diabetes mellitus, HIV, cytomegalovirus (CMV), infection; maternal habits such as nutrition, illicit substance, alcohol, nicotine use
- Obstetric complications, such as toxemia, placental insufficiency, hemorrhage, multiple pregnancies

Neonatal
- Premature birth
- Birth weight, Apgar scores, complications, length of stay in the hospital, congenital anomalies, neurologic insults, newborn screening results, weight for gestational age
- Intraventricular hemorrhage, seizures, hypoxia, extreme hyperbilirubinemia, infection

Postnatal Health
- Hospitalizations, medications, surgeries, accidents, illnesses
- Serious or recurrent infections
- Recurrent symptoms, such as vomiting, diarrhea, wheezing, snoring
- Chronic health conditions (Table 34.9)
- Collection and interpretation of growth data, percentiles, BMI, height for weight over time
- Stooling and voiding history: Diarrhea, constipation, vomiting, poor urine stream
- A careful review of systems

Developmental History
- Developmental and behavioral history
- Infant/child temperament

Family and Psychosocial History
- Family composition, caregiving environment, daycare, family support, poverty, parent-child relationship, parenting attitudes, typical day
- Family health history: Size and growth of family members, siblings or family members who have developmental disabilities, inherited diseases that may affect growth and development

Physical Examination
- Weight, length/height, and occipital frontal (head) circumference (in those younger than 2 years old) plotted on standardized growth curves and percentiles, including weight for height and BMI

TABLE 34.9	Major Causes of Growth Faltering (Failure to Thrive)
System	**Cause**
Gastrointestinal	GER, Crohn disease, pyloric stenosis, cleft palate or cleft lip, lactose intolerance, Hirschsprung disease, CMPI, hepatitis, cirrhosis, pancreatic insufficiency, biliary disease, IBD, malrotation (without volvulus), malabsorption, alkaline foods
Cardiac	Cardiac diseases leading to congestive heart failure
Renal	UTI, renal tubular acidosis, diabetes insipidus, chronic kidney disease
Pulmonary	Asthma, bronchopulmonary dysplasia, CF, anatomic abnormalities of the upper airway; obstructive sleep apnea; recurrently infected adenoids and tonsils
Endocrine and metabolic	Hypothyroidism, diabetes mellitus, adrenal insufficiency or excess, parathyroid disorders, pituitary disorders, growth hormone deficiency; inborn errors of metabolism
Neurologic	Mental retardation, cerebral hemorrhage, degenerative disorders, cerebral palsy
Infectious	Parasitic or bacterial GI tract infections, TB, HIV
Congenital	Many genetic abnormalities
Malignancy and autoimmune disorders	Many cancers of childhood, collagen-vascular disease, juvenile idiopathic rheumatoid arthritis
Nutritional	Lack of calories, lack of micronutrients including vitamin A, zinc, iron
Hematologic	Hemoglobinopathies (e.g., sickle cell disease)
Prenatal	Small for gestational age, perinatal infection
Psychosocial	Depression, anorexia nervosa, bulimia, maternal depression, child abuse or neglect, ADHD, autism, chronic pain
Environmental toxins	Heavy metal poisoning; other toxins

ADHD, Attention-deficit/hyperactivity disorder; *CF*, cystic fibrosis; *CMPI*, cow's-milk protein intolerance; *GER*, gastroesophageal reflux; *GI*, gastrointestinal; *HIV*, human immunodeficiency virus; *TB*, tuberculosis; *UTI*, urinary tract infection.

Data from Puls HT, Plencner L, Krager M, Frazier TN, Hall M, Bettenhausen JL. The diagnostic accuracy of in-hospital weight gain for differentiating neglect from other failure to thrive etiologies. *Hosp Pediatr.* 2018;8(10):620–627.

- Skinfold measurements: Subcutaneous fat loss; general wasting (more common in developing countries; seen with malignancy, HIV, cerebral palsy, inflammatory diseases)
- Vital signs
- Hydration status
- Presence of dysmorphic features
- Skin, hair, nails, and mucous membranes: Scaling skin (seen with zinc deficiency); rough or hard skin (with hypothyroidism); edema (with protein deficiency); alopecia (with hypervitaminosis, kwashiorkor, or syphilis); hair color or texture changes

TABLE 34.10	Evaluation Studies for Growth Faltering (Failure to Thrive)

General Category	Associated Conditions	Physical Findings	Diagnostic Evaluation
Inadequate intake	Poor food intake Chronic illness Inappropriate type/volume of feeding Anorexia, bulimia Food not available, parental withholding Poverty, neglect	Signs of neglect or abuse, minimal subcutaneous fat, protuberant abdomen	Complete dietary history Complete psychosocial evaluation Basic metabolic profile, vitamin D (calcidiol), lead, zinc, iron screening, albumin for protein status in severe growth faltering
Inadequate absorption	GI causes (malabsorption, chronic vomiting, pancreatic insufficiency, celiac disease, chronic reflux, IBD) Chronic renal disease, CF, inborn errors of metabolism, infestations	Dysmorphism suggestive of chronic disease, organomegaly, skin/mucosal changes	CBC/ESR, basic metabolic profile, serum electrolytes (include total CO_2 to rule out renal tubular acidosis), UA and urine culture, sweat test, stool studies for fat, reducing substances, O&P, and culture Review of newborn metabolic screening tests Extremity radiographs if indicated (e.g., rickets)
Excessive energy expenditure	Hyperthyroidism, chronic disease (cardiac, renal, endocrine, hepatic), malignancy	Dysmorphisms, skin dysmorphology, cardiac findings, abdominal mass or lymphadenopathy, hepatosplenomegaly	TSH, CBC/ESR, serum protein, albumin, alkaline phosphatase, BUN, creatinine, liver function tests Chest radiograph Renal ultrasound and voiding cystourethrography
Defective energy utilization	Genetic, familial short stature, small for gestational age, hypothyroidism	Short stature, dysmorphisms, decreasing height growth with symmetric weight to height	Thyroid studies, HIV screening Karyotype (especially in small girls for Turner syndrome) Bone age Developmental testing Growth hormone (expensive, often done later in evaluation)

BUN, Blood urea nitrogen; *CBC*, complete blood count; *CF*, cystic fibrosis; *ESR*, erythrocyte sedimentation rate; *GI*, gastrointestinal; *HIV*, human immunodeficiency virus; *IBD*, inflammatory bowel disease; *O&P*, ova and parasites; *TSH*, thyroid-stimulating hormone; *UA*, urinalysis.

Data from Tang M, Adolphe S, Rogers SR, Frank D. Failure to thrive or growth faltering: Medical, developmental/behavioral, nutritional, and social dimensions. *Pediatr Rev.* 2021;42(11):590–603.

(with zinc deficiency, Menkes kinky hair disease); spoon-shaped nails (with iron deficiency or GI diseases); cyanosis (with heart disease); and labial fissures (with vitamin deficiency)
- Evidence of abuse or neglect: Unexplained burns or skin lesions; fractures; retinal hemorrhages; unwashed skin; diaper rash; untreated impetigo; uncut or dirty fingernails; soiled clothing
- Oral findings: Dental caries, tonsillar hypertrophy, submucosal cleft palate, or tongue enlargement (may require oral-motor function studies, including lip, tongue, and swallowing assessment)
- Respiratory compromise (with CF, bronchopulmonary dysplasia)
- Cardiovascular examination for congenital heart disease
- Abdominal: Lymphadenopathy, hepatosplenomegaly, masses, distention (with malignancy, inborn errors of metabolism, and immunodeficiency)
- Endocrine: Thyroid enlargement, precocious or ambiguous sexual development
- Neuromuscular tone and strength, cranial nerves for swallowing (cerebral palsy)
- Hypertonicity or hyperreflexia for cerebral palsy

Diagnostic Studies
- Feeding assessment: Nutritional and feeding history for calorie, protein, and micronutrient intake
  - Quality of food for age and ability to suck, chew, and swallow
  - Social nature of the feeding event and family eating patterns (meals and patient feeding)

- Feeding history: Caloric intake; feeding behavior; feeding cues; hunger and satiety cues; progression to solids; feeding frequency; amount taken per feeding; formula preparation (over dilution)
- 24-hour diet recall for infants, 3-day diet history for older children eating solid foods
- Parent understanding of nutrition and feeding of infants and children
- Consider social determinants of health; food insecurity[56]
- Developmental assessment (see Chapters 9–13)
- Laboratory and imaging studies (Table 34.10)

Differential Diagnosis
See Tables 34.9 and 34.10.

Management
Management is best addressed through a collaborative, interprofessional, culturally sensitive team that includes pediatrics (with specialty consultants for specific medical conditions), nutrition (may include lactation specialist), mental health, and other community resources (e.g., Women, Infants, and Children [WIC] program, food stamps, Medicaid, housing authorities), and social work personnel. Community nurse home visits can aid in observations (mealtime behaviors, such as food refusal, spitting, food throwing, oral retention), assessment, and support.
- Manage treatable causes with prompt attention to urgent, life-threatening medical conditions.
- Restore nutritional intake and appropriate intake patterns.

- Provide nutritional rehabilitation: Vitamin supplementation with iron, zinc, and minerals; calorically enriched formula and foods (up to 150 cal/kg/day for infants <6 months old). In older infants and toddlers, solids should be offered before liquids and should not be force-fed.
- The expected normal weight gain by age should be:
  - Birth to 3 months: 25 to 30 g/day
  - 3 to 6 months: 15 to 20 g/day
  - 6 to 12 months: 10 to 15 g/day
  - 12 months and older: 5 to 10 g/day
- Provide parent education and support and improve parent-child interaction.
- Treat underlying chronic conditions.
- Make referrals as needed, including feeding clinics.
- Evaluate for normal weight gain every 1 to 3 weeks. Catch-up growth can occur rapidly but can take up to 2 weeks before growth occurs with more involved cases. Monitor for gaining too much weight resulting in being overweight.
- Hospitalize for evaluation and intervention to protect from abuse when intentional etiology is suspected, avoid further starvation and sequelae, manage extreme patient-child-parent interaction problems, provide care when outpatient management is not feasible or practical, and provide more intensive care after the failure of outpatient management.

Prognosis

Nutrition management aims to achieve symmetry of weight and height and genetic growth potential. Nutritional effects of chronic conditions may persist if not treated with the primary condition. Outcomes are variable depending on the underlying condition and severity.

Most patients achieve expected growth and development. However, because critical brain growth occurs in the first 6 months of life, nutritional insufficiency in an infant can severely affect long-term development and social and emotional health. Subtle neurodevelopmental abnormalities, the home environment, and the quality of caregiver nurturing can affect outcomes. Growth faltering may result in long-term detrimental effects—short stature, lower cognitive functioning, poor academic functioning, and increased risk for adult disease including cardiovascular disease, obesity, hypertension, and diabetes.[56]

Diarrhea

Acute and chronic diarrhea results from alterations in the normal functioning of the intestinal system. The altered intestinal mechanisms that cause diarrhea vary; briefly, diarrhea may result from:

- Nonabsorbable solutes in the GI tract occur when fluids exceed the transport capacity or when water-soluble nutrients are not absorbed (osmotic diarrhea). Such nutrient malabsorption and excessive fluid intake account for most chronic diarrhea; dumping syndrome, lactase deficiency, overfeeding, and malabsorption syndromes are causative conditions.[59]
- Invasion, inflammation, and release of toxins by bacteria or viruses (such as in traveler's diarrhea) that decrease absorption and increase secretion and transportation of electrolytes and water from mucosal crypt cells in the small intestine into the bowel lumen (secretory diarrhea). For example, viruses injure the absorptive mature mucosal surface cells, thereby altering the release of disaccharides and preventing the conversion of carbohydrates to monosaccharides necessary for normal absorption. Congenital disorders, mucosal disorders, and tumors can also lead to secretory diarrhea.
- Mutations in the ion transport proteins, such as chloride-bicarbonate exchange.

- Alterations in the anatomy of the intestinal surface or functional ability due to inflammation or surgical procedures (e.g., short bowel syndrome, Crohn disease, IBS) with a subsequent fluid, electrolyte, macronutrient, and micronutrient loss, and abnormal peristalsis.
- A change in intestinal motility either increased or decreased (e.g., irritable bowel, bacterial overgrowth due to stasis [pseudo-obstruction], toddler's diarrhea).
- Altered immune function.

Acute Diarrhea

The terms *acute gastroenteritis, acute diarrhea,* or *diarrheal disease* are based on different definitions, but all describe GI infection caused by microorganisms.[60] With acute diarrhea, there is a disruption of the normal intestinal net absorptive versus secretory fluid and electrolyte mechanisms, resulting in excessive fluid loss into the intestinal lumen. This leads to dehydration, electrolyte imbalance, and in severe cases, death in those also malnourished. In infants, diarrhea commonly causes increased stool frequency, resulting is twice as many bowel movements per day. For children older than 1 year, diarrhea is defined as four or more loose, watery stools in a 24-hour period. The duration lasts up to 14 days.

Viruses injure the absorptive surface of mature villous cells, which reduces the amount of fluid absorbed. Some release a viral enterotoxin (e.g., rotavirus). Water and electrolyte loss ensues, and there are watery diarrhea volumes, even if the child is not being fed. Bacterial and parasitic agents adhere and translocate, causing noninflammatory diarrhea. Bacteria damage the intestinal mucosa anatomy and functional ability by direct invasion. Some bacteria release endotoxins, whereas others release cytotoxins that result in the excretion of fluid, protein, and cells into the intestinal lumen and, in some cases, cause an inflammatory response. Abnormal peristalsis for any reason can result in acute diarrhea. The enteric pathogens spread through the fecal-oral route and by ingesting contaminated food or water.

Worldwide, the burden of acute diarrhea is huge, resulting in 3 to 5 billion cases and nearly 2 billion deaths (20% of total child deaths) in children younger than 5 years (particularly vulnerable). Developing countries also see their share of the disease burden (approximately 10%) attributable to poor water, sanitation, and hygiene.[60] Globally, females have higher rates of *Campylobacter* species infections and hemolytic uremic syndrome; otherwise, the case incidence shows no sex difference. Nontyphoidal *Salmonella, Shigella, Campylobacter, E. coli* organisms (bacteria); rotavirus, norovirus, enteric adenovirus (viruses); and *Giardia, Cryptosporidium,* and *Strongyloides* (parasites) cause the most disease. *Shigella, E. coli, Giardia lamblia, Cryptosporidium parvum,* and *Entamoeba histolytica* are particularly infectious in small amounts.

In the United States, those most vulnerable include American Indian and Alaska Native infants and children, where remote residential locations or living on reservations compromises sanitation and safe water supplies and where severe rotavirus diarrhea occurs. About 200,000 hospitalizations in the United States occur annually due to diarrheal illness, with 300 deaths. The most common viral pathogens are noroviruses and rotavirus, followed by adenoviruses and astroviruses. Food-borne bacterial or parasitic diarrheal diseases are most commonly due to *Salmonella* and *Campylobacter* species, followed by *Shigella, Cryptosporidium, E. coli* O157:H7, *Yersinia, Listeria, Vibrio* (*Vibrio cholerae*), and *Cyclospora* species. *C. difficile* associated with pseudomembranous colitis and diarrhea after the use of antibiotics; it is not the causative agent in most AAD in children in the United States.[61]

Tables 34.11 and 34.13 list the characteristics of diarrheal diseases caused by bacteria, viruses, and parasites that a PCP is more likely to

TABLE 34.11   Diarrhea: Common Bacterial and Viral Pathogens

Etiology	Incubation Period	Signs and Symptoms	Duration of Illness	Route of Transmission	Laboratory Testing	Treatment and Complications
Campylobacter jejuni	2–5 days, but can be longer	Diarrhea (foul smelling), cramps, fever, nausea and vomiting; diarrhea may be bloody in neonates. Occurs in warm weather months	2–10 days	Raw and undercooked poultry, unpasteurized milk, contaminated water; low inoculum dose produces infection	Routine stool culture; Campylobacter requires special media and incubation temperature; positive gross blood, leukocytes; CBC: ↑WBCs	Rehydration is mainstay. Azithromycin, erythromycin, and metronidazole shorten the duration of illness when given early, and usually eradicates the organism from stool within 2–3 days
Clostridium difficile	Unknown	Variety of symptoms and severity seen: mild to explosive diarrhea, bloody stools, abdominal pain, fever, nausea, vomiting. Mild to moderate illness characterized by watery diarrhea, low-grade fever, and mild abdominal pain	During or after several weeks of antibiotic use; can occur without being associated with such treatment	Acquired from environment or from stool of other colonized or infected people by the fecal-oral route	Stool cultures; enzyme immunoassay for toxin A, or A and B; positive gross blood, leukocytes; CBC: ↑WBCs; ESR normal	Discontinue current antibiotic (any antibiotic, but notably ampicillin, clindamycin, 2nd/3rd-generation cephalosporins). Fluids and electrolyte replacement usually sufficient. If antibiotic still needed or illness is severe, treat with oral metronidazole (drug of choice in children) or vancomycin for 7–10 days. Supplement with probiotics; *Lactobacillus* GG, *Saccharomyces boulardii* recommended. Complications include pseudomembranous colitis, toxic megacolon, colonic perforation, relapse, intractable proctitis, death in debilitated children
Enterohemorrhagic *Escherichia coli* (EHEC) including *E. coli* O157:H7 and other Shiga toxin–producing *E. coli* (STEC)	1–8 days	Severe diarrhea is often bloody, abdominal pain, and vomiting. Usually little or no fever. More common in children <4 years old	5–10 days	Undercooked beef, especially hamburger, unpasteurized milk and juice, raw fruits, vegetables (e.g., sprouts, spinach, lettuce), salami (rarely). Contaminated water; petting zoos	Stool culture; *E. coli* O157:H7 requires special media to grow. If *E. coli* O157:H7 suspected, specific testing must be requested. Shiga toxin testing may be done using commercial kits; forward positive isolates to public health laboratories for confirmation and serotyping. Stool grossly positive for blood	Supportive care: Monitor CBC, platelets, and kidney function closely. *E. coli* O157:H7 infection also associated with HUS, which can cause lifelong complications. Studies indicate antibiotics may promote development of HUS

TABLE 34.11   Diarrhea: Common Bacterial and Viral Pathogens—cont'd

Etiology	Incubation Period	Signs and Symptoms	Duration of Illness	Route of Transmission	Laboratory Testing	Treatment and Complications
Enterotoxigenic *E. coli* (ETEC) and enteroadherent *E. coli* (frequent cause of traveler's diarrhea)	1–3 days	Watery diarrhea, abdominal cramps, some vomiting; often cause of mild traveler's diarrhea	3 to >7 days	Water or food contaminated with human feces	Stool culture ETEC requires special laboratory techniques for identification. If suspected, request specific testing	Supportive care: antibiotics rarely needed except in severe cases. Recommended antibiotics include TMP-SMX, azithromycin, ciprofloxacin, and metronidazole
Listeria monocytogenes	Variable, ranging from 1 day to more than 3 weeks	Rare, but serious Fever, muscle aches, and nausea or diarrhea Pregnant women may have mild flulike illness, infection can lead to premature delivery or stillbirth Older adults or immunocompromised patients may have bacteremia or meningitis Infants infected from mother at risk for sepsis or meningitis	Variable	Thrives in salty and acidic conditions, such as fresh soft cheeses, ready-to-eat deli meats, hot dogs; also unpasteurized milk, inadequately pasteurized milk; multiplies at low temperatures, even in properly refrigerated foods	Blood or cerebrospinal fluid cultures; asymptomatic fecal carriage occurs; stool culture usually not helpful; antibody to listeriolysin O may be helpful to identify outbreak retrospectively	Initial therapy with IV ampicillin and an aminoglycoside usually gentamicin, recommended for severe infections
Adenovirus, enteric	3–10 days	Children >2 years old	Variable	Fecal-oral, throughout year; remains viable on inanimate objects	Stool specimen for adenovirus antigen via rapid commercial immunoassay techniques or per electron microscopy	Supportive care: monitor intake and hydration status Preventive care: good hand washing and diapering precaution
Norovirus	12–48 h	Abrupt-onset watery diarrhea, nausea, vomiting, abdominal cramps	24–60 h Often associated with closed venues (childcare centers, cruise ships)	Fecal-oral; contaminated food (ice, shellfish, ready-to-eat foods [e.g., salads, bakery products], or water)	No commercial assay available; CDC can support laboratory evaluation or state and local health department laboratories can perform RT-PCR assays	Supportive care: may need to treat dehydration and/or electrolyte imbalance Preventive care: hand hygiene, clean surfaces and food preparation areas; no swimming in recreational venues for 2 weeks after symptoms resolve
Rotavirus	1–3 days; prevalent during cooler months in temperate climates	Acute-onset fever, vomiting, and watery diarrhea occur 2–4 days later in children <5 years old, especially those between 3 and 24 months old	3–8 days	Fecal-oral; viable on inanimate objects; rarely contaminated water or food	Enzyme immunoassay and latex agglutination assays for group A rotavirus antigen; virus can be found by electron microscopy and specific nucleic acid amplification methods	Supportive care: may need to correct dehydration and electrolyte imbalances. Oral IG has been used in those immunocompromised Preventive care: rotavirus vaccine; hygiene and diapering precautions in day care facilities

Continued

TABLE 34.11 Diarrhea: Common Bacterial and Viral Pathogens—cont'd

Etiology	Incubation Period	Signs and Symptoms	Duration of Illness	Route of Transmission	Laboratory Testing	Treatment and Complications
Salmonella spp.	1–3 days	Diarrhea, fever, abdominal cramps, rebound tenderness, vomiting. *Salmonella typhi* and *Salmonella paratyphi* produce typhoid with insidious onset characterized by fever, headache, constipation, malaise, chills, and myalgia; diarrhea is uncommon, and vomiting is not usually severe	4–7 days	Contaminated eggs, poultry, unpasteurized milk or juice, cheese, contaminated raw fruits and vegetables (alfalfa sprouts, melons) *S. typhi* epidemics are often related to fecal contamination of water supplies or street-vended foods	Routine stool cultures; positive leukocytes and gross blood CBC: WBC can be slightly ↑ with left shift, ↓, or normal	Supportive care: *only consider antibiotics* (other than for *S. typhi* or *S. paratyphi*) for infants <3 months old, those with chronic GI disease, malignant neoplasm, hemoglobinopathies, HIV, other immunosuppressive illnesses or therapies If indicated, consider ampicillin or amoxicillin, azithromycin, or TMP-SMX; if resistance shown to any of those, use IM ceftriaxone, cefotaxime; or azithromycin or quinolones A vaccine exists for *S. typhi* in certain cases
Shigella spp.	Varies from 1–7 days, but typically is 1–3 days	Abdominal cramps, fever, and diarrhea; Stools may contain blood and mucus Seen most commonly in those 6 months to 3 years old	4–7 days	Food or water contaminated with human fecal material Usually person-to-person spread, fecal-oral transmission Ready-to-eat foods touched by infected food workers (e.g., raw vegetables, salads, sandwiches)	Routine stool cultures; gross blood, leukocytes. CBC: normal or slightly ↑ WBCs with left shift	Supportive care: if antibiotics indicated (severe disease, dysentery, immunocompromised), test first for susceptibility. Oral ampicillin (amoxicillin less so) or TMP-SMX recommended in the United States; for organism resistance, use IM ceftriaxone for 2–5 days; PO ciprofloxacin; azithromycin (oral cephalosporins not useful). If child is at risk of malnutrition, supplement with vitamin A (200,000 international units) No swimming in recreational pools/slides for 1 week after symptoms resolve
Yersinia enterocolitica and *Y. pseudotuberculosis*	Typically, 4–6 days with a range of 1–14 days	Appendicitis-like symptoms (diarrhea and vomiting, fever, and RLQ pain) occur primarily in older children and young adults May have a scarlatiniform rash or erythema nodosum with *Y. pseudotuberculosis* Seen in all ages	1–3 weeks, usually self-limiting	Undercooked pork, unpasteurized milk, tofu, contaminated water Infection has occurred in infants whose caregivers handled chitterlings	Stool, vomitus, or blood culture *Yersinia* requires special medium to grow. If suspected, must request specific testing Serology is available in research and reference laboratories.	Supportive care: if septicemia or other invasive disease occurs, antibiotic therapy with gentamicin or cefotaxime (doxycycline and ciprofloxacin also effective) after susceptibility testing is done

CBC, Complete blood count; *CDC*, Centers for Disease Control and Prevention; *ESR*, erythrocyte sedimentation rate; *GI*, gastrointestinal; *HIV*, human immunodeficiency virus; *HUS*, hemolytic uremic syndrome; *IG*, immunoglobulin; *IM*, intramuscular; *IV*, intravenous; *RLQ*, right lower quadrant; *RT-PCR*, reverse transcription-polymerase chain reaction; *TMP-SMX*, trimethoprim-sulfamethoxazole; *WBC*, white blood cell.

Data from Lo Vecchio A, Conelli ML, Guarino A. Infections and chronic diarrhea in children. *Pediatr Infect Dis J.* 2021;40(7):e255–e258; Florez ID, Niño-Serna LF, Beltrán-Arroyave CP. Acute infectious diarrhea and gastroenteritis in children. *Curr Infect Dis Rep.* 2020;22(2):4; McDonald LC, Gerding DN, Johnson S, et al. Clinical practice guidelines for Clostridium difficile infection in adults and children: 2017 update by the Infectious Diseases Society of America (IDSA) and Society for Healthcare Epidemiology of America (SHEA). *Clin Infect Dis.* 2018;66(7):e1–e48; Shane AL, Mody RK, Crump JA, et al. 2017 Infectious Diseases Society of America clinical practice guidelines for the diagnosis and management of infectious diarrhea. *Clin Infect Dis.* 2017;65(12):e45–e80.

TABLE 34.13   Common Parasitic Illnesses (Protozoa and Helminths)—cont'd

Etiology	Incubation Period	Signs and Symptoms	Duration of Illness	Route of Transmission	Laboratory Testing	Treatment[a]
Taenia (tapeworm) (*T. saginata* [beef]; *T. solium* [pork])	2–3 months after larvae ingested to feces excretion	Worm(s) may be seen in perianal region May be asymptomatic or have abdominal pain, nausea, diarrhea, excessive appetite	Several years before cysticercosis symptoms evident	Fecal-oral from ingestion of water or food contaminated with eggs or from ingested cysts or larvae in inadequately cooked pork or beef	Stool microscopy: ova seen	Praziquantel, niclosamide, nitazoxanide Complications: systemic cysticercosis from *T. solium* (viscera, brain, muscle invasion with possible seizures)
Trichuris trichiura (whipworm)	12 weeks	Asymptomatic unless infestation is heavy; abdominal pain, tenesmus, bloody diarrhea with mucus; can mimic IBD; growth retardation		Fecal-oral from contaminated soil (where eggs incubate), water, and/or food (embeds in mucosal lining of large intestines). Not spread person to person	Stool microscopy or concentration techniques	Mebendazole, albendazole, ivermectin for 3 days; can reexamine stools after 2 weeks to ensure resolution Complications: chronic colitis, rectal prolapse, compromised nutritional status, growth retardation

[a]See Table 34.14 for dosages.

CBC, Complete blood count; CT, computed tomography; IBD, inflammatory bowel disease; PCR, polymerase chain reaction; TMP-SMX, trimethoprim-sulfamethoxazole.
Data from Chitunda K, Kelly P. Parasitic infections of the gut in children. Paediatr Int Child Health. 2019;39(1):65–72; Hodges P, Kelly P. Intestinal parasites. In: Guandalini S, Dhawan A, eds. Textbook of Pediatric Gastroenterology, Hepatology and Nutrition. Springer; 2022: p. 219–229; Committee on Infectious Diseases, American Academy of Pediatrics. Kimberlin DW, Barnett ED, Lynfield R, Sawyer MH. Red Book: 2021–2024 Report of the Committee on Infectious Diseases. American Academy of Pediatrics; 2021.

- Dietary history (including the amount of fruit juices or high-carbohydrate fluids ingested per day)
- Stool consistency, blood, mucus, pus, particles of food
- Stool incontinence
- Exposure to illness (including day care; contact with pets or other animals)
- Prior treatments for diarrhea (dietary, drug, or home treatments)
- Recent travel

Physical Examination. Look for physical findings associated with the underlying pathologic condition:
- Assessment of hydration status
- Weight and height measurements; document weight loss
- Growth retardation
- Skin and hair condition, the color of skin, and conjunctivae
- Vital signs
- Palpation of the thyroid for enlargement
- Increased heart rate
- Respiratory symptoms
- Finger clubbing
- Abdominal examination
- Rectal examination (skin tags, impaction, tenderness)

Diagnostic Studies
- Stool: culture, O&P (best done on three specimens collected on separate days), pH (normal stool pH >5.5 indicates negative carbohydrate.), reducing substances, occult blood, leukocytes, fat and fecal elastase (to evaluate for pancreatic insufficiency)
- CBC with differential, electrolytes, and albumin
- UA and culture in young children

The following are ordered as indicated by the history, physical examination, and in consideration of the differential diagnoses:
- ESR, CRP
- Hormonal studies to assess for secretory tumors (vasoactive intestinal peptide, gastrin, secretin, urine assay for 5-HT)
- Breath hydrogen test for lactose or sucrose intolerance (challenging to assess in infants)
- Viral serologies, such as HIV or CMV
- Sweat chloride test
- Endoscopy, barium studies

Differential Diagnosis. See Table 34.12.

Management
- Treat the underlying cause.
- Chronic nonspecific diarrhea (toddler's diarrhea): Normalize the diet; remove offending foods and fluids; eliminate sorbitol and fructose-containing fluids; reduce fluid intake to no greater than 90 mL/kg/24 hours (give half of the fluid as milk [whole or 2%]); increase fat intake to 35% up to 40% of the diet and increase fiber to bulk up stools.
- Treat carbohydrate malabsorption by decreasing lactose or sucrose; add lactase or sacrosidase as indicated by a particular carbohydrate intolerance.
- Postgastroenteritis malabsorption syndrome (evidenced in infants with weight loss and fat globules in the stool) give a pre-digested formula (e.g., Pregestimil, Alimentum), if tolerated for 3 to 4 weeks (use elemental formula if those are not tolerated).
- Refer the following patients to a gastroenterologist: Newborns with diarrhea in the first hours of life; patients with growth delay or failure or abnormal physical findings (anorexia, abdominal pain, chronic bloating, vomiting, weakness); or those with severe illness.

Complications. Malnutrition, growth failure, and cognitive/developmental impairments (found more in developing countries) can occur.

Intestinal Parasites

Various protozoa and helminths invade the GI tract and cause disease. In developing countries, infections are more likely to be endemic and have major public health impact. Protozoa multiply within the human body, whereas helminths do not. All parasites are associated with diarrheal symptoms and spread by fecal contamination due to poor water and sewage disposal practices. Cysts of these parasites are often resistant to chlorine.

Helminths are worms: nematodes (roundworms), cestodes (tapeworms), and trematodes (flatworms) that most commonly reside in the human intestines but do not multiply there. One route of infection is fecal-oral contact with eggs or cysts excreted from the initial vector via ingestion of contaminated food or water. Some helminths (hookworms and whipworms) release larvae into the soil; humans become infected when they walk barefoot on contaminated soil and the larvae penetrate the skin. These larvae then travel to the lungs and intestines. Eggs also excrete in the stool; poor sanitary disposal of human waste into soils affords the further potential for ingestion via contamination of food and water. They are found worldwide, principally in tropical and subtropical developing countries. In industrialized countries, the infestation is found in those who travel to endemic areas, the immunocompromised, and immigrants from endemic regions. Their insidious nature causes chronic health and nutritional problems that impair the physical and mental growth of children. Enterobius vermicularis (pinworm), Ascaris lumbricoides (roundworm), and Taenia (tapeworm) are some of the more common intestinal parasites that affect the pediatric population.[63]

Clinical Findings, Management, and Differential Diagnosis

See Tables 34.13 and 34.14 for clinical findings and management. The differential diagnosis includes all other causes of infectious and noninfectious diarrhea.

Patient and Family Education

Most parasitic infestations can be prevented by good hand washing and sanitation. The following preventive measures are recommended:
- Travelers to developing countries need to eat only foods that can be peeled or have been cooked. Ice, "washed" foods, and tap water can be contaminated. Bottled or treated water is advised for drinking and brushing teeth. Shoes should be worn when walking on potentially contaminated soil.
- G. lamblia: Encourage good hand hygiene. Avoid unpasteurized milk. Prevent contamination of water sources. Treat questionable water with iodine, boil for 20 minutes, or use commercial filters to filter contaminated water. Exclude symptomatic children and staff from school and daycare until asymptomatic.
- E. vermicularis: Avoid scratching; wash sheets and clothing in hot water and detergent.
- A. lumbricoides: Appropriate food preparation is necessary to prevent infection. When human feces are used for fertilizer, thoroughly cook or soak fruits and vegetables in diluted iodine solution before consuming. Periodic, empiric treatment of children may prevent nutritional and cognitive deficits in endemic areas.
- Taenia: Avoid raw or undercooked beef or pork.

Congenital Gastrointestinal Disorders

See Chapter 28.

TABLE 34.14	Medications for Parasite Infestations	
Drug	**Dosage**
Albendazole (Albenza): Take with food. The tablet may be crushed or chewed and swallowed with a drink of water.	*Ascariasis:* 1 year old: 200 mg once- repeat in 2 weeks; >2 years old: 400 mg once- repeat in 2 weeks *Taenia solium:* 15 mg/kg/day in 2 doses × 8–30 days; can be repeated as necessary (maximum 400 mg per dose)
Mebendazole (Emverm): Tablet may be crushed, mixed with food, swallowed whole, or chewed.	*Pinworms:* 100 mg once; may need to repeat in 3 weeks Whipworms, roundworms, and hookworms: 100 mg twice daily for 3 days *Toxocariasis:* 100–200 mg twice daily for 5 days
Ivermectin (Stromectol): Take on an empty stomach.	All ages: 150–200 mcg/kg/dose once
Metronidazole (Flagyl)	30–50 mg/kg/day in 3 doses × 7–10 days (maximum 500–750 mg per dose) *Giardia lamblia:* 15 mg/kg/day in 3 doses × 5 days (maximum 250 mg per dose)
Nitazoxanide (Alinia): Administer with food, shake suspension well before use.	1–3 years old: 100 mg BID × 3 days 4–11 years old: 200 mg BID × 3 days 11 years old to adult: 500 mg BID × 3 days
Paromomycin: Administer with or without meals, protect from moisture.	25–35 mg/kg/day in 3 doses × 7 days
Praziquantel (Biltricide): Administer tablets with water during meals; do not chew due to bitter taste.	*Tapeworm:* 5–25 mg/kg once *Liver Fluke:* 25- 75 mg/kg in 3 doses in 1 day
Pyrantel pamoate (Reese's Pinworm): Over the counter. May be mixed with milk or fruit juice. Shake suspension well.	11 mg/kg daily (maximum 1 g) × 3 days Use with caution in children <2 years old
Tinidazole (Tindamax)	*Giardia lamblia:* 50 mg/kg once (maximum 2 g)

Medication choices and dosages are dependent upon child's condition at diagnosis and parasite. Consult CDC or latest recommendations for treatment regimens.

Data from Hodges P, Kelly P. Intestinal parasites. In: Guandalini S, Dhawan A, eds. *Textbook of Pediatric Gastroenterology, Hepatology and Nutrition.* Springer; 2022: p. 219–229; Committee on Infectious Diseases, American Academy of Pediatrics. Kimberlin DW, Barnett ED, Lynfield R, Sawyer MH. *Red Book: 2021–2024 Report of the Committee on Infectious Diseases.* American Academy of Pediatrics; 2021.

Additional Resources

American Gastroenterological Association: www.gastro.org
American Society for Parenteral and Enteral Nutrition (ASPEN): www.nutritioncare.org
Canadian Celiac Association: www.celiac.ca
Celiac Disease Foundation: http://celiac.org
National Celiac Association: www.nationalceliac.org
Crohn's and Colitis Foundation: www.crohnscolitisfoundation.org
Cyclic Vomiting Syndrome Association www.cvsaonline.org
Improve Care Now (IBD Resources): www.improvecarenow.org
International Foundation for Gastrointestinal Disorders (IF-FGD): www.iffgd.org
National Institute of Diabetes and Digestive and Kidney Diseases: www.niddk.nih.gov
North American Society for Pediatric Gastroenterology, Hepatology, and Nutrition (NASPGHAN): www.naspghan.org
The Oley Foundation: www.oley.org
Rehydration Project: http://rehydrate.org/solutions/homemade.htm
Rome Foundation: Functional Gastrointestinal Disorders: www.the romefoundation.org

Acknowledgment

We acknowledge Elizabeth E. Willer and Belinda James-Petersen, the chapter authors in the previous edition.

References

1. Gibson G, Roberfroid M. Dietary modulation of the human colonic microbiota: introducing the concept of prebiotics. *J Nutr.* 1995;125(6):1401–1412.
2. Zermiani A, Soares A, deMoura B, et al. Evidence of Lactobacillus reuteri to reduce colic in breastfed babies: systematic review and meta-analysis. *Complement Ther Med.* 2021;63:1–9.
3. Ford A, Harris L, Lacy B, et al. Systematic review with meta-analysis: the efficacy of prebiotics, probiotics, synbiotics and antibiotics in irritable bowel syndrome. *Aliment Pharmacol Ther.* 2018;48:1044–1060.
4. Zhu F. Evaluation and management of traveler's diarrhea in children. *Pediatr Clin North Am.* 2022;69(1):99–113.
5. Yang Y, Pei J, Qin Z, et al. Efficacy of probiotics to prevent and/or alleviate childhood rotavirus infections. *J Funct Foods.* 2019;52:90–99.
6. Guo Q, Goldenberg J, Humphrey C, et al. Probiotics for the prevention of pediatric antibiotic-associated diarrhea. *Cochrane Database Syst Rev.* 2019;4(4):CD004827.
7. Caruggi S, Rossi M, DeGiacomo C, et al. Pediatric dehydration assessment at triage: prospective study on refilling time. *Pediatr Gastroenterol Hepatol Nutr.* 2018;21(4):278–288.
8. Guarino A, Ashkenazi S, Gendrel D, et al. European society for pediatric gastroenterology, hepatology, and Nutrition/European society for pediatric infectious diseases evidence-based guidelines for the management of acute gastroenteritis in children in Europe: updated 2014. *J Pediatr Gastroenterol Nutr.* 2014;59(1):132–152.
9. Fugetto F, Filice E, Biagi C, et al. Single-dose of ondansetron for vomiting in children and adolescents with acute gastroenteritis-an updated systematic review and meta-analysis. *Eur J Pediatr.* 2020;179:1007–1016.
10. Florez I, Nino-Serno L, Beltran-Arroyave C. Acute infectious diarrhea and gastroenteritis in children. *Curr Infect Dis Rep.* 2020;22(2):1–12.

11. Burgunder L. Fluids and electrolytes. In: Kleinman K, McDaniel L, Molloy M, eds. *The Harriet Lane Handbook.* 22nd ed. Elsevier; 2021:261–282.

12. Hyams J, Di Lorenzo C, Saps M, et al. Functional disorders: children and adolescents. *Gastroenterology.* 2016;150(6):1456–1470.

13. Dipasquale V, Falsaperla R, Bongiovanni A, et al. Clinical features and long-term outcomes in pediatric cyclic vomiting syndrome: a 9-year experience at three tertiary academic centers. *Neuro Gastroenterol Motil.* 2022;34(3):e14224–e14230.

14. Raucci U, Borrelli O, Nardo G, et al. Cyclic vomiting in children. *Front Neurol.* 2020;11:583425.

15. Lenglar L, Caula C, Moulding T, et al. Brain to belly: abdominal variants of migraine and functional abdominal pain disorders associated with migraine. *J Neurogastroenterol Motil.* 2021;27(4):482–494.

16. Rosen R, Vandenplas Y, Singendonk M, et al. Pediatric gastroesophageal reflux clinical practice guidelines: joint recommendations of the North American Society for Pediatric Gastroenterology, Hepatology, and Nutrition and the European Society for Pediatric Gastroenterology, Hepatology, and Nutrition. *J Pediatr Gastroenterol Nutr.* 2018;66(3):516–554.

17. Donda K, Asare-Afriyie B, Ayensu M, et al. Pyloric stenosis: national trends in the incidence rate and resource use in the United States from 2012 to 2016. *Hosp Pediatr.* 2019;9(12):923–932.

18. Rosenthal Y, Chodick G, Grossman Z, et al. The incidence of infantile hypertrophic stenosis and its association with folic acid supplementation during pregnancy: a nested case-control study. *J Pediatr Surg.* 2019;54(4):701–706.

19. Bhesania N, Selvakumar P, Patel S. Eosinophilic esophagitis: a review of the pediatric population and consideration of upcoming therapies. *J Gastroenterol Hepatol.* 2022;37(3):420–427.

20. Jones N, Koletzko S, Goodman K, et al. Joint ESPGHAN/NASPGHAN Guidelines for the management of Helicobacter pylori in children and adolescents (Update 2016). *J Pediatr Gastroenterol Nutr.* 2017;64(6):991–1003.

21. Orsagh-Yentis D, et al. Foreign-body ingestions of young children treated in US emergency departments: 1995-2015. *Pediatrics.* 2019;143:5.

22. Mubarak A, Benninga M, Broekaert I, et al. Diagnosis, management, and prevention of button battery ingestion in childhood: a European Society for Paediatric Gastroenterology Hepatology and Nutrition position paper. *J Pediatr Gastroenterol Nutr.* 2021;73(1):129–136.

23. Oliva S, Romano C, DeAngelis P, et al. Foreign body and caustic ingestions in children: a clinical practice guideline. *Dig Liver Dis.* 2020;52(11):1266–1281.

24. Dipasquale V, Romano C, Iannelli M, et al. Managing pediatric foreign body ingestions: a 10-year experience. *Pediatr Emerg Care.* 2020;38(1):E268–E271.

25. Di Saverio S, Podda M, De Simone B, et al. Diagnosis and treatment of acute appendicitis: 2020 update of the WSES Jerusalem guidelines. *World J Emerg Surg.* 2020;15(1):27.

26. Ingram MC, Harris C, Studer A, et al. Distilling the key elements of pediatric appendicitis clinical practice guidelines. *J Surg Res.* 2021;258:105–112.

27. Vetter V, Pereira P, Benninghoff B. Rotavirus vaccination and intussusception: a paradigm shift? *Hum Vaccin Immunother.* 2020;17(1):278–282.

28. Kelley-Quon L, Arthur LG, Williams R, et al. Management of intussusception in children: a systematic review. *J Pediatr Surg.* 2021;56:587–596.

29. Ambartsumyan L, Smith C, Kapur RP. Diagnosis of Hirschsprung disease. *Pediatr Dev Pathol.* 2020;23(1):8–22.

30. Gordon M, Sinopoulou V, Tabbers M, et al. Psychosocial interventions for the treatment of functional abdominal pain disorders in children: a systematic review and meta-analysis. *JAMA Pediatr.* 2022;176(6):560–568.

31. Robin SG, Keller C, Zwiener R, et al. Prevalence of pediatric functional gastrointestinal disorders utilizing the Rome IV criteria. *J Pediatr.* 2018;195:134–139.

32. Trivić I, Hojsak I. Initial diagnosis of functional gastrointestinal disorders in children increases a chance for resolution of symptoms. *Pediatr Gastroenterol Hepatol Nutr.* 2018;21(4):264–270.

33. Rexwinkel R, Vlieger AM, Saps M, et al. A therapeutic guide on pediatric irritable bowel syndrome and functional abdominal pain-not otherwise specified. *Eur J Pediatr.* 2022;181:2603–2617.

34. Wallace C, Gordon M, Sinopoulou V, et al. Probiotics for management of functional abdominal pain disorders in children. *Cochrane Database Syst Rev.* 2021:11.

35. Hill HD, Fasano A, Guandalini S, et al. NASPGHAN Clinical report on the diagnosis and treatment of gluten-related disorders. *J Pediatr Gastroenterol Nutr.* 2016;63(1):156–165.

36. Bingham SM, Bates MD. Pediatric celiac disease: a review for non-gastroenterologists. *Curr Prob Pediatr Adolesc Health Care.* 2020;50(5).

37. Misselwitz B, Butter M, Verbeke K, et al. Update on lactose malabsorption and intolerance: pathogenesis, diagnosis, and clinical management. *Gut.* 2019;68(11):2080–2091.

38. Nocerino R, Bedogni G, Carucci L, et al. The impact of formula choice for the management of pediatric cow's milk allergy on the occurrence of other allergic manifestations: the atopic march cohort study. *J Pediatr.* 2021;232:183–191.

39. Nowak-Węgrzyn A, Chehade M, Groetch M. International consensus guidelines for the diagnosis and management of food protein-induced enterocolitis syndrome: executive summary-workgroup report of the adverse reactions to foods committee, American Academy of Allergy, Asthma & Immunology. *J Allergy Clin Immunol.* 2017;139(4):1111–1126.

40. Sýkora J, Pomahačová R, Kreslová M, et al. Current global trends in the incidence of pediatric-onset inflammatory bowel disease. *World J Gastroenterol.* 2018;24(25):2741–2763.

41. Abuquteish D, Putra J. Upper gastrointestinal tract involvement of pediatric inflammatory bowel disease: a pathological review. *World J Gastroenterol.* 2019;25(16):1928–1935.

42. Orlanski-Meyer E, Aardoom M, Ricciuto A, et al. Predicting outcomes in pediatric ulcerative colitis for management optimization: systematic review and consensus statements from the pediatric inflammatory bowel disease Ahead Program. *Gastroenterology.* 2021;160(1):378–402.

43. Shaoul R, Day A. An overview of tools to score severity in pediatric inflammatory bowel disease. *Front Pediatr.* 2021;9:615216.

44. Ye Y, Manne S, Treem WR, et al. Prevalence of inflammatory bowel disease in pediatric and adult populations: recent estimates from large national databases in the United States, 2007-2016. *Inflamm Bowel Dis.* 2020;26(4):619–625.

45. Goyal A, Zheng Y, Albenberg LG, et al. Anemia in children with inflammatory bowel disease: a position paper by the IBD committee of the North American Society of Pediatric Gastroenterology, Hepatology and Nutrition. *J Pediatr Gastroenterol Nutr.* 2020;71(4):563–582.

46. Mitchel E, Rosh J. Pediatric management of Crohn's disease. *Gastroenterol Clin N Am.* 2022;52(2):401–424.

47. Verburgt CM, Ghiboub M, Benninga MA, et al. Nutritional therapy strategies in pediatric Crohn's disease. *Nutrients.* 2021;13(1):212.

48. van Rheenen PF, Aloi M, Assa A, et al. The medical management of paediatric Crohn's disease: an ECCO-ESPGHAN guideline update. *J Crohns Colitis.* 2021;15(2):171–194.

49. Gupta N, Lustig R, Andrews H, et al. Sex-specific pathways lead to statural growth impairment in children with Crohn's disease. [published online ahead of print, 2022 May 29]. *J Pediatr.* 2022:S0022–S3476.

50. Laborda TJ, Jensen MK, Kavan M, Deneau M. Treatment of primary sclerosing cholangitis in children. *World J Hepatol.* 2019;11(1):19–36.

51. Fousekis FS, Theopistos VI, Katsanos KH, Christodoulou DK. Pancreatic involvement in inflammatory bowel disease: a review. *J Clin Med Res.* 2018;10(10):743–751.

52. Dembiński K, Dziekiewic M, Banaszkiewicz A. Immune response to vaccination in children and young people with inflammatory bowel disease: a systematic review and meta-analysis. *J Pediatr Gastroenterol Nutr.* 2020;71(4):423–432.

53. Ricciuto A, Aardoom M, Orlanski-Meyer E, et al. Predicting outcomes in pediatric Crohn's disease for management optimization: systematic review and consensus statements from the pediatric inflammatory bowel disease-Ahead program. *Gastroenterology.* 2021;160(1):403–436.

54. Turner D, Ruemmele FM, Orlanski-Meyer E, et al. Management of paediatric ulcerative colitis, part 1: ambulatory care-An evidence-based guideline from European Crohn's and Colitis Organization and European Society of Paediatric Gastroenterology, Hepatology and Nutrition [published correction appears in J Pediatr Gastroenterol Nutr. 2020;71(6):794]. *J Pediatr Gastroenterol Nutr.* 2018;67(2):257–291.

55. Hong J, Park S, Kang Y, et al. Micronutrients are not deficient in children with nonorganic failure to thrive. *Pediatr Gastroenterol Hepatol Nutr.* 2019;22(2):181–188.

56. Tang M, Adolphe S, Rogers SR, et al. Failure to thrive or growth faltering: medical, developmental/behavioral, nutritional, and social dimensions. *Pediatr Rev.* 2021;42(11):590–603.

57. Selbuz S, Kırsaçlıoğlu CT, Kuloğlu Z, et al. Diagnostic workup and micronutrient deficiencies in children with failure to thrive without underlying diseases. *Nutr Clin Pract.* 2019;34(4):581–588.

58. Puls HT, Plencner L, Krager M, et al. The diagnostic accuracy of in-hospital weight gain for differentiating neglect from other failure to thrive etiologies. *Hosp Pediatr.* 2018;8(10):620–627.

59. Lo Vecchio A, Conelli ML, Guarino A. Infections and chronic diarrhea in children. *Pediatr Infect Dis J.* 2021;40(7):e255–e258.

60. Florez ID, Niño-Serna LF, Beltrán-Arroyave CP. Acute infectious diarrhea and gastroenteritis in children. *Curr Infect Dis Rep.* 2020;22(2):4.

61. McDonald LC, Gerding DN, Johnson S, et al. Clinical practice guidelines for Clostridium difficile infection in adults and children: 2017 update by the Infectious Diseases Society of America (IDSA) and Society for Healthcare Epidemiology of America (SHEA). *Clin Infect Dis.* 2018;66(7):e1–e48.

62. Steele MK, Wikswo ME, Hall AJ, et al. Characterizing norovirus transmission from outbreak data, United States. *Emerg Infect Dis.* 2020;26(8):1818–1825.

63. Parasites. Centers for Disease Control and Prevention. https://www.cdc.gov/parasites/children.html.

64. Chu C, Rotondo-Trivette S, Michail S. Chronic diarrhea. *Curr Probl Pediatr Adolesc Health Care.* 2020;50(8):100841.

65. Shane AL, Mody RK, Crump JA, et al. Infectious Diseases Society of America clinical practice guidelines for the diagnosis and management of infectious diarrhea. *Clin Infect Dis.* 2017;65(12):e45–e80.

66. Chifunda K, Kelly P. Parasitic infections of the gut in children. *Paediatr Int Child Health.* 2019;39(1):65–72.

67. Hodges P, Kelly P. Intestinal parasites. In: Guandalini S, Dhawan A, eds. *Textbook of Pediatric Gastroenterology, Hepatology and Nutrition.* Springer; 2022:219–229.

68. Committee on Infectious Diseases, American Academy of Pediatrics, Kimberlin DW, Barnett ED, Lynfield R, Sawyer MH. In: *Red Book: 2021–2024 Report of the Committee on Infectious Diseases.* American Academy of Pediatrics; 2021.

35

Infectious Diseases

ANDREA ACHENBACH, JODI BLOXHAM, AND NAN M. GAYLORD

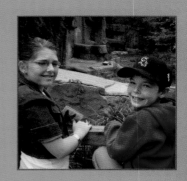

Infectious diseases are the leading causes of illness in infants and children despite advances in public and personal health, antimicrobial use, and active and passive vaccination. The ability to distinguish serious infections from those that resolve with minimal or no intervention is an important skill for primary care providers (PCPs). The ability to effectively communicate with, educate, and support frustrated and anxious parents is nearly as important as the medical care provided to the sick child. In addition, PCPs must include preventive education, including vaccinations, in the routine delivery of primary health care.

Pathogenesis of Infectious Diseases

Researchers from the National Institutes of Health Common Fund Human Microbiome Project (2020)[1] are mapping the normal microbial makeup of healthy individuals. This project found that approximately 100 trillion microorganisms (mostly bacteria, but also viruses and fungi) abound in the body (the brain, spinal fluid, blood, urine, lungs, and tissues are inherently sterile) and for the most part live in harmony with their human hosts, contributing to human survival. Bacteria outnumber human cells by 10 to 1 and can weigh 2 to 7 pounds, depending upon an individual's size.[1,2] A recent study of the virome (viruses hosted by the human body) shows the number of viruses is similar to the number of bacterial and human cells.[3]

The normal human flora, or "normal microbiota" (Table 35.1), remain throughout life unless environmental changes affect them. Studies show that humans are losing some of their microbial diversity.[4] It is believed that this loss is caused in part by antibiotic overuse, cesarean sections, and modern sanitation practices. This loss may account for the increase in asthma, allergies, diabetes, obesity, and possibly some forms of colorectal cancer.[4]

It is estimated that only 10% of pathogens attributed to causing human diseases are identified. Although viruses are the most frequent cause of childhood infectious illnesses, bacterial infections, particularly of the skin and mucosal surfaces, are also common. Bacteria are ubiquitous in the environment. They are intercellular microorganisms that carry all their requirements and mechanisms for growth and multiplication with them. Most grow on nonliving surfaces and some live at temperature extremes. They have many shapes, including curved rods, spheres, rods, and spirals. Each bacterium has its own unique mode(s) of transmission and mechanisms of colonization and pathogenesis. Humans are inoculated with important bacteria on the skin, especially in moist areas, and mucosal surfaces such as the upper respiratory, urinary, and gastrointestinal (GI) tracts during vaginal birth or shortly afterward.

Most bacteria are harmless and are the first line of defense against colonization by potentially pathogenic organisms.

Microbiotas are degraded toxins and are required for digestion and immune system maturation. Infectious disease results when the balance between harmless colonization and protective immunity is disrupted in favor of the harmful proliferation of a microorganism. Bacteria are adept at adapting, as evidenced by increasing resistance to antibiotics.

In comparison, viruses (Latin noun meaning *toxin* or *poison*) are submicroscopic particles that invade a host cell, redirect the normal cell's functions, and effectively transfer genetic information (deoxyribonucleic acid [DNA] and ribonucleic acid [RNA]) to replicate viral particles. Viruses need to have a living host to multiply. Viruses are rarely dangerous because of their inability to simultaneously meet three criteria necessary for virulence, to: (1) inflict serious harm, (2) remain unrecognized by the immune system, and (3) spread efficiently. Some viruses control bacteria; these are referred to as *bacteriophages,* or "eaters of bacteria." These phages are numerous in the environment and practically harmless to humans. Vaccines prevent the spread of some viruses, and antiviral medications help slow down their reproduction in some cases. Newer research focuses on human resident viruses (human virome), and there is an indication that viruses play a part in the human defense system.[3] The human immune system is complex and provides many layers of disease protection. Skin and mucosal surfaces are barriers to microorganism invasion, and antibodies and immune cells defend the body in general and specific ways against pathogen invasion. Microorganisms may breach the immune barrier of the skin and mucosa by binding to cell surface structures. For example, the influenza virus uses hemagglutinin protein to attach to cell membranes and invade the respiratory mucosa. Disease caused by microbial pathogens results from infected cell and tissue destruction and from normal cell function disruption. Some disease symptoms are caused by the immune system's response to infection, resulting in local or systemic inflammatory responses. Biotechnology is developing bacterial-based treatments to allow bacteria to enter cells and trigger intense immune responses, much like vaccines.

Clinical Findings

History

Most pediatric infectious illnesses are diagnosed solely based on history and physical examination. A comprehensive history generates and helps prioritize the individual's differential diagnoses based on symptomatology and history. Many symptoms are shared by different illnesses making establishing differential diagnoses challenging (e.g., fever is most commonly associated with infectious illnesses but also occurs with rheumatologic or oncologic diseases). Crucial aspects of the history that help distinguish

TABLE 35.1   Common Distribution Sites of Normal Microflora[a] Found in Humans

Bacterium	Very Commonly or Commonly Found in These Locations	Notes
Aerobic Bacteria		
Gram Positive		
Staphylococcus aureus	Skin, hair, naso-oropharynx, lower GI, cerumen, vagina	Rarely found in the anterior vagina and conjunctiva; trachea, bronchi, lungs, and sinuses; High levels of MRSA bacteria in the nose may indicate MRSA colonization in other parts of the body, specifically the axilla, groin, and perineum
Staphylococcus epidermidis	Skin, hair, naso-oropharynx, adult vagina, urethra, conjunctiva, ear (including cerumen), lower GI	Occasionally found in the vagina of prepubertal females; found in low quantities in "normal" urine, probably as a result of contamination from urethra and skin
Staphylococcus saprophyticus	Skin, mucous membranes, vagina, perineum	Most common cause of UTI in sexually active women
Streptococci • S. mitis • S. mutans • S. pneumoniae (Pneumococcus, Diplococcus) • S. pyogenes (group A)	Skin, pharynx, mouth; less commonly in adult vagina and urethra; rare lower GI Mouth, pharynx Nasopharynx, mouth; rarely found in conjunctiva, nose, vagina Mouth, pharynx; rarely skin, conjunctiva, adult vagina, lower GI	 Is potentially pathogenic Common cause respiratory tract and ear infections; pathogen of sepsis, pneumonia, meningitis Common cause of skin and pharyngeal infections
Bifidobacterium bifidum	Lower GI	
Enterococcus faecalis	Lower GI, postpubertal vagina; mouth, anterior urethra; rarely pharynx	Is potentially pathogenic
Propionibacterium acnes	Skin (rarely seen in children before age of 10 years); external ear	Commonly involved in acne vulgaris during puberty
Gram Negative		
Acinetobacter spp.	Skin; less commonly respiratory tract, mouth, GI	Has the potential of causing pathogenic outbreaks and developing antibiotic resistance
Corynebacterium	Skin, conjunctiva, naso-oropharynx, mouth, lower GI, anterior urethra, adult vagina	
Citrobacter diversus	Lower GI	Possible cause of UTI
Escherichia coli	Lower GI, vagina, mouth, anterior urethra; rarely found in conjunctiva, nose, pharynx	Has the potential of being a pathogen
Haemophilus influenzae	Nasopharynx, mouth; rarely conjunctiva, ear	Cause of upper respiratory tract, ear, and eye infections
Kingella kingae (formerly referred to as Moraxella kingae)	Pharynx	Has the potential of being a pathogen (cause of invasive infections in young children)
Klebsiella pneumoniae	Nose, colon, axillary area	Associated with neonatal sepsis; UTIs
Lactobacillus spp.	Pharynx, mouth, lower GI, adult vagina	
Moraxella catarrhalis	Nasopharynx	Implicated in otitis media
Morganella morganii	Lower GI	
Mycobacterium spp.	Skin, lower GI, anterior urethra; rarely nasopharynx	
Mycoplasma	Mouth, pharynx, lower GI, vagina; rarely anterior urethra	Implicated in upper and lower respiratory tract infections
Neisseria spp. (e.g., N. mucosa)	Nose, pharynx (100% of population), conjunctiva, mouth, anterior urethra, vagina	Nonpathogenic species
N. meningitidis	Nose, pharynx, mouth, vagina	Significant cause of meningitis and sepsis in children. Accounts for >90% of invasive meningococcal disease cases worldwide

Continued

TABLE 35.1   Common Distribution Sites of Normal Microflora[a] Found in Humans—Cont'd

Bacterium	Very Commonly or Commonly Found in These Locations	Notes
Proteus spp.	Skin, nasopharynx, mouth, lower GI, vagina, anterior urethra; rarely in conjunctiva	
Pseudomonas aeruginosa	Lower GI; rarely in pharynx, mouth, anterior urethra; colonization in lungs of patients with cystic fibrosis; small numbers can be found on the skin	Has the potential of being a pathogen
Anaerobic Bacteria		
Bacteroides spp.	Lower GI, anterior urethra; rarely adult vagina	Has the potential of being a pathogen
Clostridium spp.	Lower GI; rarely mouth	Has the potential of being a pathogen
Streptococcus spp.	Mouth, colon, adult vagina	
Spirochetes (a distinct form of bacteria)	Pharynx, mouth, lower GI	
Fungi		
Actinomycetes spp.	Pharynx, mouth	
Candida albicans	Skin, conjunctiva, mouth, lower GI, adult vagina	Can be found in voided urine but is a contaminant
Cryptococcus spp.	Skin	
Protozoa	Mouth, lower GI, adult vagina	

[a]Normal microflora in humans consists of indigenous microorganisms that colonize human tissues and live in a mutualistic state without producing disease. An individual's microflora depends on genetics, age, sex, stress, nutrition, and diet. A pathogen is a microorganism (or virus) that produces disease. Normal flora can become pathogens when a host is compromised or weakened (endogenous pathogen); other microorganisms invade a host during times of disease only (obligate pathogens) or lowered resistance (opportunistic pathogens). Skin microflora also includes yeast (Malassezia furfur), molds (Trichophyton mentagrophytes var. interdigitale), and mites (Demodex folliculorum). The normal flora found in the vagina depends on one's age, pH, and hormonal levels. Cerumen contains some antimicrobial elements to discourage growth of pathogenic P. aeruginosa and S. aureus. The cervix is normally sterile but can demonstrate flora similar to those in the upper area of the vagina. Greater than 500 species of bacteria are identified in the colon. The flow of tears and inherent antibacterial lysozymes prevent the growth of flora in the conjunctiva.

GI, Gastrointestinal; MRSA, methicillin-resistant Staphylococcus aureus; spp., species; UTI, urinary tract infection.

Data from Carroll KC, Hobden JA, Miller S, et al., eds. Jawetz, Melnick, & Adelberg's Medical Microbiology. 27th ed. New York: McGraw-Hill; 2016; Cystic Fibrosis Foundation. Pseudomonas aeruginosa; 2015. https://www.cff.org/Life-With-CF/Daily-Life/Germs-and-Staying-Healthy/What-Are-Germs/Pseudomonas/; and Todar K. The normal bacterial flora of humans. Todar's Online Textbook of Bacteriology, 2008–2012. www.textbookofbacteriology.net/normalflora.html.

infectious illnesses from other types of diseases or assist in determining the responsible pathogen include careful questioning of:

- The history of present illness with a careful analysis of the presenting symptoms: When did the symptoms start? What other symptoms were associated with the illness? Were there periods when the patient seemed improved or even back to normal?
- A comprehensive past medical history: Determine the place of birth and past acute or chronic illnesses that increase specific illness risk. A history of asthma in a teenager with fever and cough, for example, is suspicious of atypical pneumonia.
- Current and recent medications: Recent antibiotic use may negate culture results or contribute to resistant infections (e.g., methicillin-resistant Staphylococcus aureus [MRSA] infection). Include any nonprescription, herbal, or natural health usage.
- Immunizations: Adherence to recommended vaccine schedules,[22] including age and spacing of vaccines, is an important consideration if the child's symptoms suggest a vaccine-preventable disease.
- Family history, particularly noting infectious illness: History of any first- or second-degree relative with a known immune deficiency, with numerous infections or difficulty recovering from infections, or with a history of recurrent miscarriages raises suspicion of an immune deficiency. A strong history of autoimmune disease in the family may suggest possible rheumatologic diagnoses as opposed to an infectious process.

- Social history: Daycare or school attendance or living in a crowded setting increases exposure to viral infections. A sexual history (see Chapter 7 is important to accurately assess the sexually active adolescent and to identify those with high-risk sexual practices.
- Exposure history, including any known contacts with individuals with similar symptoms: A comprehensive, in-depth exposure history helps diagnose infections caused by epidemic illness (e.g., influenza) and those that might otherwise not be considered. Ask about contact with individuals with known illnesses or at high risk for certain illnesses, or contact with animals (e.g., at farms or animal markets) or animal by-products (e.g., hides, waste, blood), insects, or snakes (e.g., bites). A history of travel to tropical countries or areas with endemic illnesses is important (e.g., Lyme disease [LD], malaria, dengue, or parasitic illnesses), as well as the lodging accommodations during travel (e.g., possible exposure to parasites). Other important exposures include environmental tobacco smoke or mold, and swimming in rivers, flood waters, or other waterways.
- Complete review of symptoms: Some illness-presenting features may be discounted or forgotten by children or parents and recalled only when asked direct questions.
- Diet history: Any ingestion of raw milk or raw/undercooked meats and/or fish; history of pica.

Physical Examination

A complete physical examination is necessary; however, the differential diagnoses generated during history taking allows the examiner to focus on certain examination aspects. Physical findings that may be noted with infectious diseases include:

- Abnormal vital signs such as fever, tachypnea, or hypotension, which are concerning for dehydration and/or septic shock.
- Irritability is nonspecific in ill children but may raise concern for meningitis or Kawasaki disease. Lethargy raises concern for meningitis and sepsis, particularly in infants and younger children.
- A stiff or painful neck is suggestive of meningitis.
- A new murmur may herald the possibility of endocarditis or rheumatic fever.
- Refusal to walk can be a manifestation of deep tissue infections (e.g., pyomyositis), osteomyelitis, septic arthritis, or meningitis.
- Skin or mucous membrane changes such as exanthema or enanthema, are common with a viral illness, and characteristic rashes of specific illnesses such as chickenpox.

Laboratory and Imaging Studies

Laboratory studies measure the host-pathogen damage-response framework. Inflammation or tissue damage stimulates proinflammatory cytokines, which activate proteins referred to as *acute-phase reactants*. There is no single marker with the necessary sensitivity, specificity, or predictive values to serve as a stand-alone test upon which to initiate therapy for suspected serious infection. Likewise, testing cannot positively confirm when to stop therapy for proven infection.[6] New bloodstream infections/sepsis biomarker types are continuously under investigation.[6]

In selected circumstances, laboratory evaluation clarifies a differential diagnosis or rules out a serious illness that may be under consideration. When in doubt, it may be helpful to consult with knowledgeable laboratory personnel or an infectious disease expert. The following should be taken into consideration when ordering diagnostic studies:

- The quality of the specimen sent to the lab strongly affects the reliability of the results. For example, pus aspirated from a skin infection is generally more likely to grow the pathogen of concern than a surface swab. The collection site of the microbiologic specimen needs to be appropriately cleansed with sterile saline, 70% alcohol, and/or iodine to minimize possible skin contamination.
- Sample collection timing affects the accuracy of results. Bacterial cultures collected after the antibiotic administration may be negative even with active infection. Acute and convalescent titers or certain blood chemistries help to make a diagnosis or monitor treatment response.
- Laboratory tests require a certain volume or quantity to ensure valid and reliable results. Be prepared to prioritize test requests when a limited quantity is collected. For example, if a catheterized urine specimen only yields 7 mL, it may be more important to get a urine culture than a urinalysis.
- Microbiologic samples may require special handling and should be transported to the laboratory promptly. Contact the laboratory if there is any question regarding the sample collection and transport.

The Centers for Disease Control and Prevention (CDC) lists the notifiable infectious diseases and conditions that must be reported to local public health authorities or their agents. In many cases, this reporting is done by the laboratory, but there are some conditions the provider may treat without obtaining a laboratory specimen such as LD. Providers should be familiar with the list, known as the National Notifiable Diseases Surveillance System.[7]

Complete Blood Count. From an infectious disease standpoint, the white blood cell (WBC) count is generally the most useful piece of information obtained from the complete blood count (CBC). Leukocytosis, or elevated WBC count, occurs in bacterial infections and leukopenia, or decreased WBC count, occurs in some viral infections. A WBC differential helps to identify the infectious organism. Bacterial infections often, but not always, cause increases in the neutrophil or polymorphonuclear cell count and may elevate bands (immature neutrophils), and viral infections often cause elevated lymphocyte counts and/or atypical lymphocyte production. Long-term use of certain medications (some of which decrease counts), age, steroid use (may increase counts), and the clinical state (e.g., overwhelming sepsis) can affect WBCs. Chronic inflammatory processes, such as anemia, can decrease red blood cell (RBCs) numbers.

Platelet Count. Thrombocytosis, or elevated platelet count, occurs during the active phase of acute infection and correlates with concurrent elevations in C-reactive protein (CRP) and erythrocyte sedimentation rate (ESR).

C-Reactive Protein. CRP is one the serum acute phase reactants that increase in the presence of acute inflammation and specific pathogens. CRP is synthesized in the liver within 4 to 6 hours after tissue injury, peaking at 36 hours.[8] CRP is sometimes used as part of the workup for infants at risk of septicemia; however, its diagnostic value for influencing clinical judgment remains weak. CRP is more specific than WBC in detecting bacterial infections but cannot be utilized solely for clinical decision-making. Serial CRPs 24 to 48 hours after the onset of symptoms are recommended and help monitor the body's response to treatment in certain infections (e.g., in neonatal sepsis and osteomyelitis). Inflammatory processes other than infection may elevate CRP, including maternal and perinatal factors, trauma, rheumatologic diseases, cardiac failure, and oncologic diseases. Persistent CRP elevations may be related to treatment failure and conditions such as adiposity, birth control pill use, and pregnancy.

Procalcitonin. Serum procalcitonin (PCT) is a biomarker that differentiates certain viral infections from serious bacterial infections. PCT is a protein that has an activity similar to hormones and cytokines and is released by the liver 4 hours after tissue injury, peaks at 6 hours, and sustains the peak for 8 to 24 hours. PCT levels tend to rise and fall quicker than CRP during the onset and control of bacterial infections when compared to CRP and other biomarkers. It is important to note that PCT is not accurate in fevers less than 2 hours in duration.[8] It may prove to be a valuable tool when the ability to draw and process blood cultures is limited. Levels increase in individuals with bacteremia and reflect the severity of the illness. The evidence establishes its usefulness and it has higher sensitivity and specificity than CRP[6] for predicting pyelonephritis, pneumonia, early-onset sepsis in premature infants, bacterial infection in febrile neutropenic children with cancer, diarrhea-associated hemolytic-uremic syndrome, bacterial causes of acute hepatic disease, bacterial versus aseptic meningitis, and various diseases or conditions that involve inflammatory processes (e.g., posttraumatic sepsis, Crohn disease). At this point, it should only be used with other clinical and diagnostic data when making diagnostic and management decisions. Rapid test kits are available.

Erythrocyte Sedimentation Rate. The ESR is another measure of inflammation and reflects RBCs settling faster when acute-phase proteins (such as fibrinogen) are present in serum than when they are not. Although the ESR is not a specific test for infection, it is useful in evaluating fever of unknown origin (FUO) and, like CRP, is used to monitor therapy response. A low sedimentation rate (<10 mm/h) makes bacterial infection an unlikely cause of prolonged unexplained fever. Viral infections result in mean ESR values around 20 mm/h (90% <30 mm/h), except for adenovirus, which is associated with values higher than 30 mm/h. An ESR greater than 50 mm/h in children warrants further evaluation.[9]

During the waxing and waning period of infection, the ESR tends to increase and resolve slower than CRP. ESR is useful to evaluate the effectiveness of therapy when long-term antibiotics are needed. It is used when managing diseases in which treatment effectiveness is judged, in part, by ESR normalization such as osteomyelitis. Similar to the CRP, the ESR elevates in noninfectious conditions that cause inflammation (e.g., rheumatoid arthritis, inflammatory bowel disease, and vasculitis). Anemia also causes a nonspecific ESR increase.

Cultures, Stains, and Antimicrobial Susceptibility Testing. The usefulness of microbiologic testing depends on the quality of the sample and on the correct choice of test for the given clinical situation. Details of appropriate tests for given infections are discussed in the sections about specific infectious agents.

The presence of purulence assists in the diagnosis of some infections. Staining methods are useful in certain clinical situations, such as when fungal or other infections are suspected. Antigen detection immunofluorescence or antibody assays (e.g., complement fixation tests [CFTs], immunofluorescence techniques, and enzyme-linked immunosorbent assays [ELISAs]) are used to diagnose viral infections. There are many diagnostic staining methods available.

Fluid and tissue specimens can be sent for bacterial, viral, or fungal cultures; however, the laboratory may need to be notified for instruction on certain pathogens for the most accurate evaluation of the sample (e.g., pertussis). Antibody bacterial susceptibility can be obtained from cultured samples, especially if organism resistance is suspected because of community resistance patterns.

Other Technologies. DNA and RNA testing are common in the in-patient setting and are used more frequently in primary care practice. These tests use polymerase chain reaction (PCR) and screen for multiple organisms using one sample. Pathogens commonly detected by PCR include *Neisseria gonorrhoeae, Chlamydia trachomatis,* human immunodeficiency virus (HIV), *Bordetella pertussis,* herpesviruses, and enteroviruses. Newer technologies include molecular fingerprinting for nosocomial infection and microarrays to differentiate between viral and bacterial pathogens. Several experimental assays are under investigation that should be more accurate than the CRP and PCT. Further studies are needed to confirm if RNA biosignatures can differentiate between viral and bacterial infections.[8]

Immunoserology. In specific situations, tests that rely on antibody generation may be useful. Various methods (e.g., hemagglutination, enzyme immunoassays [EIAs], latex agglutination, complement fixation, immunofluorescence, and neutralization assays) detect the presence of antibodies to specific infectious organisms such as HIV, West Nile virus (WNV), *Bartonella henselae,* and *Mycoplasma pneumoniae.*

Imaging Techniques. Radiographs, computed tomography (CT) scans, magnetic resonance imaging (MRI), echocardiography, and ultrasounds assist in the diagnosis of bone, sinus, lung, skin, viscera, brain, and heart infections. Several nuclear imaging techniques evaluate for the presence of bone infections, tumors, fractures, urinary backflow blockage, heart conditions, GI bleeding, and thyroid disorders.

General Management Strategies

Preventing Infection Spread

Thorough and frequent hand washing is the most effective means of preventing infection spread. In addition to educating parents and children on the importance of proper hand washing, it is crucial that PCPs practice proper hand washing. Alcohol-based hand rubs may be substituted for soap and water in most cases.[9a] However, they are ineffective in controlling the spread of *Bacillus anthracis* and *Clostridium difficile.* It is recommended that gloves and washing hands with soap and water be used when in contact with children with *B. Anthracis* and *C. difficile–associated* disease and/or in outbreak settings.[9a]

Specific handwashing guidance that should be given to children and parents includes:
- Wash hands after using the bathroom, before meals, and before preparing food. The proper technique includes scrubbing with soap and water for at least 20 seconds (the time it takes to sing "Happy Birthday" twice), rinsing with warm water, and drying hands completely.
- Avoid finger-nose and finger-eye contact, particularly if exposed to someone with a cold.
- Use a tissue to cover the mouth and nose when coughing or sneezing to help prevent the spread of pathogens. If a tissue is unavailable, use the upper sleeve (not the hands).

Antibiotic Use

In the United States, more than 2.8 million people become infected, at least 35,000 people die, and others die from complications stemming from an antibiotic-resistant infection annually.[9b] The World Health Organization (WHO) estimates worldwide there are 700,000 deaths caused by multidrug resistance bacteria, of which 200,000 are newborns. The WHO also reports that multidrug-resistant bacterial infections in pediatric patients constitute approximately 30% of total cases reported.[10] Antibiotics are often prescribed for conditions that do not require their use and inappropriate prescribing patterns contribute to the emergence of resistant bacteria. This is particularly troublesome for children in group childcare settings. PCPs should educate children and parents about the role and efficacy of antibiotics and assume a more "targeted therapy" approach when prescribing.

The CDC provides brochures, posters, and information sheets that may help explain the importance of judicious antibiotic use. Knowledge about emerging resistance patterns, and susceptibility patterns of bacterial agents within their practice communities will better arm the provider to appropriately prescribe antibiotics (see Chapter 23 for a further discussion about the overuse of antibiotics).

Preventing Infection Through Vaccines

Immunizations are the mainstay of pediatric infectious disease prevention. Vaccines reduce the burden of mortality and morbidity due to infectious diseases around the world and are cost-effective. See Chapter 19 for a full discussion on immunizations.

Children in childcare settings have increased infectious disease rates, principally respiratory and GI infections. In addition, these children are more likely to receive antibiotic treatment and acquire antibiotic-resistant organisms than children not in childcare.[11] Infections typically spread in these settings are listed in Table 35.2.

Specific Viral Diseases

Enteroviruses

Nonpolio Enteroviruses

Ten to 15 serotypes account for most diseases from more than 100 nonpolio RNA enterovirus serotypes. There are four genomic classifications: human enteroviruses (HEVs) A, B, C, and D. Coxsackieviruses and echoviruses are subgroups of HEVs. Hand-foot-mouth, herpangina, pleurodynia, acute hemorrhagic conjunctivitis, myocarditis, pericarditis, pancreatitis, orchitis, and dermatomyositis-like syndrome are manifestations of infection. Enteroviruses are the most common cause of aseptic meningitis and are associated with paralysis, neonatal sepsis, encephalitis, and respiratory and GI symptoms. The specific serotype may not be unique to any given disease.[12]

As evidenced by the name, enteroviruses concentrate on the GI tract as their primary invasion, replication, and transmission site; they spread by fecal-oral contamination, especially in diapered infants and young children. They are also transmitted via the respiratory tract and vertically either prenatally, during parturition, or during breastfeeding by an infected mother who lacks antibodies to that serotype. Transplacental infection can lead to serious disseminated disease in the neonate involving multiorgan systems (liver, heart, meninges, and adrenal cortex).

Children become infected with nonpolio enteroviruses at any time of year, but there is a higher incidence of infection in summer and fall. Infants younger than 12 months old have the highest prevalence rate. Illness occurs more frequently in males; in those living in crowded, unsanitary conditions; and in those of lower socioeconomic status. Children with asthma have a higher risk for severe symptoms when infected with nonpolio enteroviruses.[12] Infection ranges from asymptomatic to undifferentiated febrile illness, to severe illness. Young children are more likely to be symptomatic. The incubation period is 3 to 6 days (less for hemorrhagic conjunctivitis). After infection, the virus sheds from the respiratory tract for 1 to 3 weeks and from the GI tract for several weeks to months; it is viable on environmental surfaces for long periods.

Nonpolio enteroviral infection is not a reportable disease, nor is it routinely tested for in the clinical setting, so the overall incidence rate is not known. The CDC administers the National Respiratory and Enteric Virus Surveillance System and the National Enterovirus Surveillance System to monitor detection patterns of respiratory and enteric adenoviruses. Recent outbreaks

TABLE 35.2 Pathogens and Modes of Transmission in Childcare Settings

Modes of Transmission	Bacteria	Viruses	Parasites, Fungi, Mites, and Lice
Respiratory	Haemophilus influenzae type B Neisseria meningitides Group A Streptococcus (GAS) Streptococcus pneumonia Bordetella pertussis Mycobacterium tuberculosis Kingella kingae (also known as Moraxella kingae)	Adenovirus Coronavirus Influenza A and B Measles Mumps Varicella-zoster Metapneumovirus Parainfluenza Parvovirus B19 Respiratory syncytial virus Rhinovirus	
Fecal-oral	Campylobacter jejuni Salmonella spp. Shigella spp. Clostridium difficile Aeromonas Plesiomonas Escherichia coli O157:H7	Enteroviruses (including genus Klebsiella) Hepatitis A virus Rotavirus Calicivirus Astrovirus Norovirus (Norwalk) Enteric adenovirus	Cryptosporidium parvum Giardia lamblia Enterobius vermicularis
Person-to-person via skin contact	Group A Streptococcus (GAS) Staphylococcus aureus	Herpes simplex Varicella-zoster Molluscum contagiosum	Pediculus capitis Sarcoptes scabiei Trichophyton spp. Microsporum spp.
Contact with blood, urine, or saliva		Cytomegalovirus (CMV) Hepatitis B and C Herpes simplex Human immunodeficiency virus (HIV)	

Data from Collins JP, Pickering LK. Infections associated with group childcare. In: Long SS, Prober CG, Fisher M, eds. *Principles and Practice of Pediatric Infectious Diseases.* 5th ed. Elsevier; 2018:25–32; and American Academy of Pediatrics (AAP) Committee on Infectious Diseases, Kimberlin DW, Barnett, ED, et al., eds. *Children in Group Child Care and Schools: Red Book: 2021 Report of the Committee on Infectious Diseases.* 32nd ed. American Academy of Pediatrics; 2021:116–121.

of acute flaccid myelitis (AFM), where there is limb paralysis similar to poliomyelitis, prompted investigations into etiology. There was an increase in the incidence of AFM in the United States in 2014, 2016, 2018, and 2021. The peaks of AFM coincided with peaks in enterovirus cases. Epidemiologic studies are ongoing. The CDC provides clinical guidance for AFM.[12]

Clinical Findings

History. General symptoms include:

- A mild upper respiratory infection (URI) is common and may include complaints of pharyngitis, fever, emesis, diarrhea, anorexia, coryza, abdominal pain, rash, and headache.
- Nonspecific febrile illness of at least 3 days: In young children, there is an undifferentiated abrupt-onset febrile illness (101–104°F [38.5–40°C]) associated with myalgias, malaise, irritability; fever may wax and wane over several days.
- Onset of viral symptoms within 1 to 2 weeks after delivery for neonates infected transplacentally.

Physical Examination. General findings include mild conjunctivitis, pharyngitis, and/or cervical adenopathy. Other findings include:

- Skin: Rash may be macular, maculopapular, urticarial, vesicular, or petechial. It may imitate the rash of meningitis, measles, or rubella.
- Herpangina: There is a sudden onset of high fever (up to 106°F [41°C]) lasting 1 to 4 days. Anorexia, pharyngitis, and dysphagia are common, with emesis and abdominal pain in 25% of cases. Small vesicles (from one to more than 15 lesions of 1–2 mm each) appear and enlarge to ulcers (3–4 mm) on the anterior pillars of the fauces, tonsils, uvula, and pharynx and the edge of the soft palate. The vesicles commonly have red areolas up to 10 mm in diameter. This self-limiting infection usually lasts 3 to 7 days.
- Acute lymphonodular pharyngitis: This manifests as acute pharyngitis lasting approximately 1 week.
- Hand-foot-mouth disease: This is a clinical entity with fever, vesicular eruptions in the oropharynx that may ulcerate, and a maculopapular rash involving the hands and feet. The rash evolves to vesicles, especially on the dorsa of the hands and the soles of the feet and lasts 1 to 2 weeks (Fig. 35.1).
- Aseptic meningitis: The usual signs are fever, stiff neck, and headache. Altered sensorium and seizures are common. Most cases appear in epidemics or as unique cases; most patients recover completely.
- Paralytic disease: A Guillain-Barré–type syndrome is described in the literature.
- Congenital or neonatal infection: The neonatal infection often manifests as a sudden onset of emesis, coughing, anorexia, fever or hypothermia, rash, jaundice, irritability, cyanosis, tachycardia, and dyspnea. It is often mistaken for pneumonia. The latter three symptoms can progress to myocarditis and congestive heart failure (CHF). Infants can have cardiac collapse, hepatic and adrenal necrosis, intracranial hemorrhage, and death. For those who survive severe disease, the recovery can be rapid.
- Acute hemorrhagic conjunctivitis: Characterized by sudden eye pain, photophobia, blurred vision, tearing, and conjunctival erythema and infection. Most patients recover in a few weeks.
- Pleurodynia (Bornholm disease or devil's grip): This condition usually occurs in epidemics, but some isolated cases occur. It is most often caused by type B disease, but echoviruses are implicated. There may be a prodrome before the onset of chest pain consisting of headache, malaise, anorexia, and myalgia.

The onset of chest or upper abdominal pain can be sudden, pleuritic in nature, and is aggravated by deep breathing, coughing, or sudden movements. The pain occurs in waves of spasms that last several minutes to several hours and is described by individuals as feeling like being stabbed with a knife or being squeezed in a vise. It can be mistaken for coronary artery disease, pneumonia, or pleural inflammation. Low to high fever occurs, and a pleural friction rub often is heard. The disease generally lasts from 3 to 6 days (up to a few weeks).

- Orchitis: This type B infection is clinically similar to mumps.
- Myocarditis or pericarditis: HEVs are the identified cause in 25% to 35% of myocarditis and pericarditis cases. Symptoms range from mild to severe (sudden death), and male adolescents and young adults are particularly vulnerable.[11]
- Respiratory symptoms are frequently reported before the onset of fatigue, dyspnea, chest pain, CHF, and dysrhythmias. Wheezing, asthma exacerbation, apnea, respiratory distress, pneumonia, otitis media, bronchiolitis, croup, parotitis, and paroxysmal thoracic pain may be seen.

Diagnostic Studies. PCR assay is highly sensitive for all enteroviruses, results can be available in hours, and the test is more sensitive than cell culture. Cultures can be obtained from a throat swab, stool, rectal swab, nasopharyngeal aspirates, cerebrospinal fluid (CSF), vesicle fluid, tissue biopsy, conjunctival swab, urine, and blood.[11] Serology for serotype-specific immunoglobulin (Ig) M antibodies or other testing is less useful than culture or PCR.

Differential Diagnosis and Management. The differential diagnosis includes other causes of the aforementioned symptoms (e.g., viral or bacterial infections [pneumonia, meningitis, sepsis], or connective tissue diseases). There is no specific therapy available. Immune globulin intravenous (IVIG) is helpful in some chronic and life-threatening infections. The use of antiviral therapy is under study or development, although none are currently

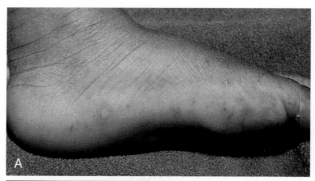

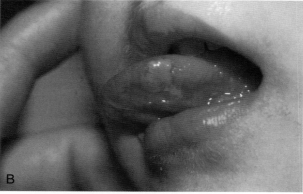

• **Fig. 35.1** Hand-Foot-Mouth Rash.

commercially available (e.g., pleconaril and pocapavir).[11] Fluoxetine has in vitro activity against group B and D enteroviruses, but studies have not shown any benefit clinically.[11] Enteric precautions and good hand washing are the only efficient control measures.

Poliovirus Infections

Poliovirus is an enterovirus with three serotypes (types 1, 2, and 3). It causes disease that ranges from an asymptomatic illness to severe central nervous system (CNS) involvement. Humans are the only documented source of infection. Transmission is through fecal-oral and respiratory routes. Almost all cases in North America occur in individuals exposed to children who received oral poliovirus vaccine in another country.[11] There have been wild-type poliovirus importations into countries previously deemed polio-free (United States, United Kingdom, Israel, Somalia, Burkina Faso, Uganda, Ethiopia, Ghana, Yemen, and Eritrea), and polio is endemic in Pakistan, Nigeria, and Afghanistan. Through the efforts of the Global Polio Eradication Initiative, the incidence of polio worldwide remains low; however, reemergence is a concern. Wild-type polioviruses are easily transmitted into previously deemed polio-free countries. Poliomyelitis should be considered in any unimmunized or underimmunized child who has a nonspecific febrile illness, aseptic meningitis, or paralytic symptoms (paralysis occurs in <1% of infections). Asymptomatic disease occurs in about 72% of those infected, symptomatic flu-like symptoms occur in 24%, and extremity weakness or paralysis occurs in approximately 1% of those infected.[7]

Viral culture is the diagnostic test of choice, obtained from stool and throat (two samples taken 24–48 hours apart) as soon as polio is suspected and at least within 14 days of the onset of symptoms. The wild-type virus must be differentiated from the vaccine-acquired type. The CSF may be normal or show changes based on the degree of CNS involvement. Antibody titers vary from the acute phase and those taken 3 to 6 weeks later. Polio is a reportable disease. In cases of paralytic polio, those infected must notify local and state health departments within 4 hours of diagnosis; nonparalytic polio requires notification at the local and state levels within 24 hours of diagnosis.[7]

Differential Diagnosis and Management. Polio is rare. Differential diagnoses include other conditions causing flaccid muscular weakness and/or paralysis: acute flaccid myelitis, Guillain-Barré syndrome, peripheral neuritis, transverse myelitis, encephalitis, vaccine-associated paralytic poliomyelitis (VAPP) (only occurs following live virus [oral] vaccination), rabies, tetanus, botulism, demyelinating encephalomyelitis, tick-bite paralysis, WNV, spinal cord tumors, familial periodic paralysis, myasthenia gravis, and hysterical paralysis. Conditions that cause decreased limb movement or pseudoweakness are also differential diagnoses and include unrecognized sciatic nerve trauma, toxic synovitis, acute osteomyelitis, acute rheumatic fever, scurvy, and congenital syphilitic osteomyelitis.

Management is supportive and directed at minimizing skeletal deformity in the disease's paralytic form. Both nonparalytic and mild paralytic cases can be managed on an outpatient basis, but otherwise, individuals should be hospitalized. During the early disease stages, advise individuals against increasing their physical activity, exercising, or becoming fatigued because these factors may increase the risk of paralytic disease.[7]

Hepatoviruses

Hepatitis A Virus

Hepatitis A virus (HAV) is an RNA-containing virus belonging to the Picornaviridae family, comprised of five genera (enteroviruses, rhinoviruses, hepatoviruses, cardioviruses, and aphthoviruses). HAV causes a primary infection in the liver. It is highly contagious and commonly spreads through person-to-person contact and fecal-oral spread via food and water contamination and rarely via contaminated blood transfusion. It accounts for most of the acute and benign viral hepatitis in the United States and worldwide. There is no seasonal or geographic variance.

Transmission occurs readily in households and childcare centers; risk factors include personal contact with an infected individual, international travel, recognized foodborne outbreak, men who have sex with men, and illicit drug use. In children younger than 6 years, about 30% are symptomatic; few of these have jaundice.[13] This high anicteric incidence allows considerable spread of disease to adult caretakers in childcare settings. Infants are protected by maternal antibodies during the first few months of life. Older children and adults tend to be more symptomatic. Incidence rates are similar across all age groups and geographic regions.

The incubation period is 15 to 50 days (average 28–30 days). The period of contagion occurs during viral shedding, usually for 1 to 3 weeks. The highest period of infectivity is up to 2 weeks before the onset of illness until 1 week after the onset of jaundice, although neonates and young children may shed the virus in their stool for longer periods.

Clinical Findings

1. Preicteric (prodromal) phase: This phase manifests as an acute febrile illness and includes malaise, nausea, anorexia, emesis, digestive complaints, fever (rarely higher than 102°F [38.9°C]), headache, and occasional abdominal complaints. This phase goes unnoticed in many children. There may be dull right upper quadrant pain; some children have only mild URI and GI symptoms along with a transient fever.
2. Icteric phase: Jaundice appears shortly after symptom onset (70% of older children and adults)[11] and lasts from a few days to almost a month; it may be subtle in children. Urine darkens, and stools become clay colored. Often, these are the only apparent signs of illness. Diarrhea is common in infants, whereas constipation is more common in older children and adults. Patients feel sick. Infants have poor weight gain during the icteric phase. Mild hepatomegaly and tenderness, posterior cervical adenopathy, and a tender spleen (10%–20% incidence) may occur.
3. Convalescent phase: Jaundice, abdominal pain and tenderness, and fatigue abate. Appetite returns. Complete clinical and laboratory recovery occurs by the ninth week in HAV.[14]

Diagnostic Studies. Serologic testing is widely available. IgM-specific antibodies indicate recent infection. These are replaced by IgG-specific antibodies 2 to 4 months later and are indicators of past infection. Aspartate aminotransferase (AST) and alanine aminotransferase (ALT) elevations usually occur, may precede symptoms by a week or more, and indicate the degree of hepatic inflammatory injury. Elevations are also seen in γ-glutamyl transpeptidase and serum bilirubin (rarely above 10 mg/dL); mild lymphocytosis may be present.

Differential Diagnosis. Includes any cause of jaundice.
- Infancy: Physiologic jaundice, hemolytic disease, galactosemia, hypothyroidism, biliary metabolic disorders, biliary atresia, α1-antitrypsin deficiency, and choledochal cysts. Hypervitaminosis A causes yellow pigmentation (carotenemia) of the skin and is often mistaken for jaundice in infants and young children. Infections, such as those referred to as TORCH (toxoplasmosis, other [syphilis, varicella-zoster, parvovirus B19], rubella, cytomegalovirus [CMV], and herpes infections) also cause hepatitis.

- Older infants, children, and adolescents: Differential diagnoses include hemolytic-uremic syndrome, Reye syndrome, malaria, leptospirosis, brucellosis, chronic hemolytic diseases with gallstone development, Wilson disease, cystic fibrosis, Banti syndrome, collagen-vascular disease (e.g., systemic lupus erythematosus [SLE]), infectious mononucleosis syndrome (IMS), CMV, coxsackievirus, toxoplasmosis, Weil disease, yellow fever, acute cholangitis, amebiasis, and hepatitis B, C, and D. Drugs and poisons such as pyrazinamide (PZA), isoniazid (INH), valproic acid, acetaminophen overdose, zoxazolamine, gold, cinchophen, phenothiazines, and methyltestosterone also cause hepatitis.

Management, Complications, and Prevention. Treatment is supportive. Good hand hygiene after diaper changes is a crucial preventive measure, especially for childcare personnel. Ig or HAV vaccine use within 2 weeks of exposure is discussed earlier in this chapter (Table 35.3). Those with acute infections who work as food handlers or in schools/childcare settings should be excluded for 1 week after symptom onset.[11] Although patients can become very ill, most individuals with HAV recover completely. Fulminant hepatitis with liver failure is rare. There is no chronic disease. Complete recovery is anticipated within 1 to 2 months with rate relapses lasting up to 6 months. Prevention includes good personal hygiene, safe drinking water, and routine HAV vaccine for those age 12 months and older.

Hepatitis B Virus

HBV is a double-stranded DNA containing the Hepadnaviridae family of viruses. It is highly contagious and causes severe liver disease. The most common method of transmission is percutaneous or from mucosal exposure to contaminated blood/serum, semen, vaginal secretions, and other bodily fluids, including but not limited to amniotic, cerebrospinal, and pleural. It is not spread by the fecal-oral route. HBV can survive in a dried state for more than 1 week, but it is highly susceptible to common household disinfectants, such as 1:10 diluted bleach. Prolonged percutaneous contact with contaminated fomites, such as toothbrushes and razors, are a source of infection.

The major reservoirs for HBV are healthy chronic carriers and patients with acute disease. Approximately 880,000 to 1.89 million people have chronic HBV in the United States, and approximately 296 million worldwide. Unimmunized children who immigrated to the United States from sub-Saharan Africa and East Asia and other high-endemic areas pose the highest infection risk. Transmission is rare within the United States because of the high pediatric HBV immunization coverage. Perinatal transmission is highly efficient during birth from female carriers (HBsAg-positive or hepatitis Be antigen [HBeAg]-positive, or both) to the newborn. In utero transmission is rare because HBV is a large molecule and rarely crosses the placenta. The infection rate is 70% to 90% if both maternal antigen markers are positive and 5% to 20% if the mother is HBsAg-positive but HBeAg-negative.[11]

Whether one eventually develops a chronic infection depends on the age at infection and the rate of HBeAg loss. More than 90% of infected infants develop a chronic infection after exposure. Twenty-five percent to 50% of children who acquire the infection between 1 and 5 years old (as compared to about 5% exposed as adults) develop chronic HBV infection. Twenty-five percent of chronically infected children die prematurely of cirrhosis or liver cancer (CDC, 2018f). Individuals who abuse intravenous (IV) drugs, engage in sexual activity with multiple partners, or men who have sex with men have the greatest HBV risk. Healthcare workers exposed to blood, blood products, or blood-contaminated body fluids, those working with the developmentally disabled, and chronic renal dialysis patients are also high-risk. Tattooing or body piercing with contaminated instruments is another route of infection.

Clinical Findings. The incubation period is 45 to 160 days (an average of 90 days). HBV illness ranges from asymptomatic seroconversion to fulminating disease and death. HBV usually has a gradual onset. Most children who acquire HBV at an early age are asymptomatic. Some have minimal nonspecific constitutional complaints, such as fever, nausea, and minimal hepatomegaly. Arthralgia and skin problems, such as urticaria or other rashes, are often the first apparent signs. Papular acrodermatitis is described in infants. Acute HBV infection is somewhat similar to the icteric phase of HAV, but it is usually more severe. Skin, mucous membranes, and sclerae are icteric. The liver is enlarged and tender.

Diagnostic Studies. Screen all pediatric patients who missed the HBV birth dose, especially if their parents were born in regions of high-HBV endemicity. Serologic tests include HBsAg, hepatitis B core antigen (HBcAg), HBeAg, and antibodies to these antigens. The results help determine the stage of infection (Table 35.4) and changes in liver enzymes indicate the degree of injury. Serum transaminases (serum glutamic-oxaloacetic transaminase (SGOT), AST, serum glutamate pyruvate transaminase (SGPT), and ALT) elevate. Prothrombin time can elevate, especially in fulminating disease. Hybridization assays, nucleic acid amplification testing (NAAT), and PCR are also available.

Differential Diagnosis and Management. Any cause of jaundice is included (see HAV).

Therapy for acute infection is supportive and prevented by active and passive vaccination (see Chapter 19). A pediatric hepatitis B specialist should be consulted for the management of suspected HBV reactivation or for chronic hepatitis B due to the risk of developing hepatocellular carcinoma. Infants who are breastfeeding are not at high risk. The US Food and Drug Administration (FDA) approved four medications chronic hepatitis B treatment: Interferon-alfa (≥12 months old); entecavir (≥2 years old); tenofovir disoproxil fumarate (≥3 years old); and tebivudine (≥16 years old). Additional information on antiviral therapies for HBV and practice guidelines is found on the American Association of the Study of Liver Diseases website (www.aasld.org). Those with chronic infection should receive a yearly liver ultrasound, testing of liver function and α-fetoprotein concentration, and vaccination for HAV.[11]

Complications and Prevention. Liver failure, cirrhosis, and hepatocellular carcinoma are complications of chronic infection. The initial infection can be prevented with hepatitis B vaccination. Transmission in utero or during labor to newborns and postexposure prophylaxis (PEP) is covered in Chapter 19.

Hepatitis C Virus

Hepatitis C virus (HCV) is a single-stranded RNA virus with seven genotypes and more than 50 subtypes. The most common genotype in the United States is genotype 1a.[1] The virus is transmitted by contact with infected blood, blood products, or unsafe drug injection practices. The estimated prevalence in the United States is 1.3% (about 4 million people) and 170 million people worldwide.[15] The prevalence in children of all ages is difficult to establish with estimates ranging from approximately 0.1% to 0.4%. Those who do not go on to develop chronic hepatitis C (15–25%) spontaneously clear the virus without treatment.

TABLE 35.3 Immunoglobulins Used in Children in the United States

Immunoglobulin	Reference Name	Indications for Use	Comments
Botulism immune globulin intravenous	BIG-IV	Botulism toxin A or B in infants <1 year old	Available as BabyBig from California Department of Health Services (510-231-7600). A HBAT may be indicated for life-threatening food-borne botulism (other than infant botulism) but risk must be weighed against side effects (fever, serum sickness, anaphylaxis); only available from CDC (770-488-7100)
Cytomegalovirus immune globulin intravenous	CMV-IGIV	For stem cell or organ transplants; studies ongoing to evaluate use for CMV transmission to newborns	Used in combination with IV ganciclovir to treat CMV pneumonia. In hematopoietic stem cell transplant recipients, CMV-IGIV and ganciclovir administered intravenously have been reported to be synergistic in treatment of CMV pneumonia
Diphtheria antitoxin (from equine sera)		Life-threatening *Corynebacterium diphtheriae* disease	Only available from CDC to treat life-threatening diphtheria; preferred route of administration is IV. Anaphylaxis and delayed serum sickness are possible adverse reactions and need to be weighed against risks of disease Tests for reaction to animal sera should be performed
Hepatitis B immune globulin	HBIG	Prophylaxis for those unvaccinated or undervaccinated; who have discrete identifiable exposure to blood; exposed to body fluids that contain blood: • Newborns whose mothers are HBsAg positive • Household contacts <12 months old who have received only one prior HBV vaccine and the second dose is not due • Sexual contact or needle-sharing with known HBsAg-positive cases, including sexual assault or abuse victims • Individuals with percutaneous or permucosal exposure to body secretions of known cases	If mother's HBsAg status is unknown before delivery, infants should receive both HBV vaccine and HBIG within 12 h of birth or 24 h of blood exposure; vaccines administered after birth should be given at different injection sites. HBIG can be given within 7 days of delivery if mother tests positive for HBsAg postpartum but it is less effective Sexual partners of known cases: give HBIG and HBV vaccine up to 14 days after last exposure; repeat vaccine at 1 and 6 months Household contacts <12 months old: HBIG and three doses of HBV vaccine. If >12 months old, follow index case's antibody profile (if a carrier, vaccinate all household members). If children and adolescents have documented Hep B series and unknown seroconversion status, a booster dose is indicated Hepatitis B vaccine can be used for postexposure prophylaxis if given within 12–24 h after exposure
Immune globulin	IG	Hepatitis A prophylaxis: • Household contacts and sexual partners of known cases • Persons accidently inoculated with a contaminated needle • Newborn infants of infected, jaundiced mothers • People with open lesions directly exposed to body secretions of known cases • Children in schools where more than one case is reported • All children and employees of childcare centers where a case is reported • Custodial care residents and staff in close contact with an active case • Persons traveling to developing countries for <3 months • Can give HAV vaccine concurrently with IG, if warranted, for those traveling internationally	Give within 2 weeks of exposure; can be used in children <2 years old; is thimerosal-free; >85% effective; dosage for those with continuous exposure to HAV differs from that given for short-term exposure HAV vaccine is used for postexposure prophylaxis if given within 14 days of exposure

Continued

TABLE
35.3 **Immunoglobulins Used in Children in the United States—Cont'd**

Immunoglobulin	Reference Name	Indications for Use	Comments
		Measles prophylaxis: • To prevent or modify infection in unvaccinated children <1 year old and others at higher risk of complications who have been exposed to measles • IGIV is recommended for pregnant women and the immunocompromised who are without immunity	Not indicated in those who have had one dose of vaccine at ≥12 months old, unless immunocompromised Given within 6 days after exposure. The dose for those immunocompromised differs according to the type and degree of immunodeficiency, whether IGIV has been given, and prior dosage amounts of IG
		Rubella prophylaxis: • Modifies or suppresses the clinical manifestations of the disease, urine shedding, and decreases the rate of viremia For use in: • Early pregnancy after confirmed exposure and only if termination of pregnancy is not an option • Infants after maternal exposure • Older children not vaccinated with known exposure or at serious risk (immunocompromised)	If pregnant woman is exposed to wild rubella or because of being accidently vaccinated within 28 days of conception, fetus has theoretic risk of 1.3% of congenital rubella; refer to OB-GYN Administration of IG and the absence of clinical manifestation of maternal rubella infection do not guarantee the infant will be born without congenital rubella syndrome. IgM antibody (not IgG) after IG can be used to determine maternal infection after exposure
Immune globulin intravenous	IGIV	FDA-approved for treating primary immunodeficiencies, chronic lymphocytic leukemia, bone marrow transplantation, HIV in children, ITP, Kawasaki disease; IGIV contains measles antibodies sufficient for measles prophylaxis (see Immune globulin)	Off-label use, including treatment for toxic shock syndrome, has created shortages
Rabies immune globulin (human)	HRIG, RIG	For postexposure prophylaxis for rabies; used in conjunction with rabies vaccine	Consult with local health authorities before use
Respiratory syncytial virus immune globulin	RSV-IGIV (RespiGam)	Reduces risk of RSV bronchiolitis or pneumonia in high-risk children Provides additional protection against other respiratory viral illnesses; may be preferred over palivizumab in children with immune deficiencies or for premature infants before discharge in the RSV season for the first month of prophylaxis	Palivizumab, a monoclonal antibody, is generally preferred over RSV-IGIV (see Chapter 32)
Tetanus immune globulin	TIG	For individuals with tetanus-prone wounds who are undervaccinated (fewer than three tetanus toxoid vaccine doses) or whose vaccination status is unknown For individuals with tetanus infection in combination with antibiotics (metronidazole or penicillin G) For immunodeficient patients, including those with HIV; they should be considered undervaccinated regardless of actual tetanus toxoid status	Tetanus-prone wounds include those contaminated with dirt (especially if around horses), feces, or saliva; puncture wounds; avulsions; wounds acquired as a consequence of missiles, burns, crushing, or frostbite In infants <6 months old without the initial three-dose series, decision to use TIG depends on mother's tetanus toxoid immunization history at the time of delivery and if the wound is tetanus prone (e.g., out-of-hospital delivery and umbilical cord cut with nonsterile implement) TIG is given IM plus a dose of tetanus toxoid vaccine If TIG not available, IGIV may be considered (not licensed for this use in the United States); equine TAT is another alternative to TIG (not available in the United States)—hypersensitivity testing required before use of TAT Smaller dose is administered for tetanus neonatorum

TABLE 35.3 Immunoglobulins Used in Children in the United States—Cont'd

Immunoglobulin	Reference Name	Indications for Use	Comments
Vaccinia immune globulin intravenous	VIG-IGIV	Being held in reserve to prevent or manage complications of smallpox; can be used in individuals receiving an experimental vaccine that involves a vaccinia carrier virus	Only available from CDC
Varicella immune globulin	VariZIG (varicella-zoster immune globulin)	Given to those exposed to varicella infection who are most susceptible to varicella and most likely to develop the disease and in whom complications of the infection would result: • Household contacts • Playmates with face-to-face contact (5 min–1 h) • Infant whose mother had varicella onset 5 days or less before delivery or within 48 h after delivery • Immunocompromised children and adolescents without history of varicella, varicella immunization, or known to be susceptible • Hospitalized preterm infants 28 weeks or more gestation whose mother lacks history of varicella or serologic evidence of protection • Hospitalized preterm infants <28 weeks' gestation or <1000 g birth weight exposed in neonatal period regardless of mother's history or VZV serologic evidence[a] • Other conditions: See CDC guidelines	Available from FFF Enterprises 24 h/day (1-800-843-7477); strict adherence to forms and protocols required Administered within 96 h of exposure; may be of benefit if given within 10 days[70] Not indicated in infants whose mothers had zoster infection In the absence of VariZIG, IGIV or acyclovir may be considered[a]

[a]Consult with an expert in infectious disease or the CDC.

CDC, Centers for Disease Control and Prevention; *CMV*, cytomegalovirus; *FDA*, US Food and Drug Administration; *HAV*, hepatitis A virus; *HBAT*, heptavalent equine antitoxin; *HBsAg*, hepatitis B surface antigen; *HBV*, hepatitis B virus; *HIV*, human immunodeficiency virus; *IG*, immune globulin; *IgG*, immunoglobulin G; *IgM*, immunoglobulin M; *IM*, intramuscular; *ITP*, idiopathic thrombocytopenia purpura; *IV*, intravenous; *IVIG*, intravenous immunoglobulin; *OB-GYN*, obstetrics and gynecology; *RSV*, respiratory syncytial virus; *TAT*, tetanus antitoxin.

Data from Goddard AF, Meissner HC. Passive immunization. In: Long SS, Prober CG, Fischer M, eds. *Principles and Practice of Pediatric Infectious Diseases.* Elsevier; 2017:37–43; and Kimberlin DW, Brady MT, Jackson MA, Long SS, eds. *Red Book: 2018 Report of the Committee on Infectious Diseases.* 31st ed. American Academy of Pediatrics; 2018.

TABLE 35.4 Interpretation of Serologic Markers for Hepatitis B Virus Infection

SEROLOGIC MARKER				
HBsAg	Anti-HBs	IgM Anti-HBc	Total Anti-HBc	Interpretation
−	−	−	−	Susceptible; never infected
+	−	−	−	Acute infection, early incubation; transient, up to 3 weeks after vaccination
+	−	+	+	Acute infection
−	−	+	+	Acute infection, resolving
−	+	−	+	Past infection, recovered, and immune
+	−	−	+	Chronic infection
−	−	−	+	False positive (i.e., susceptible) past infection, or "low level" chronic infection
−	+	−	−	Immune from vaccination

Anti-HBs, Antibody to hepatitis B surface antigen; *HBsAg*, hepatitis B surface antigen; *IgM anti-HBc*, immunoglobulin M antibody to hepatitis B core antigen; *total anti-HBc*, total antibody to hepatitis B core antigen.

From Thio CL, Hawkins C. Hepatitis B and hepatitis D viruses. In: Bennet JE, Dolin RD, Blaser MJ, eds. *Principles and Practice of Pediatric Infectious Diseases.* 9th ed. Elsevier; 2020.

However, HCV infection causes the highest rate of chronic infection and liver disease (70%–80% of adults) of all the hepatitis viruses; the incidence of chronic liver failure in children is about 5% but increases with the duration of infection.[11]

Perinatal transmission is the major pediatric infectious route: approximately six out of every 100 infants born to HCV-positive mothers become infected. Mothers who are HCV-positive have a two- to threefold increased risk of transmitting the virus to their infants. Vaginal birth and breastfeeding do not contribute to higher transmission rates and women with HCV alone should not be discouraged from experiencing either.[16] Infants who acquire HCV via vertical transmission have a high rate of spontaneous resolution, approaching 50%, usually by 24 months old but some as late as 7 years old. Older children experience spontaneous resolution at a rate of 6% to 12%.

The most common means of HCV transmission in the United States is from injection drug use, infecting an estimated one-third of injection drug users between the ages of 18 and 30 years old.[17] Men who have sex with men are also at increased infection risk. Strict blood product screening and manufacturing practices in the United States significantly reduced the risk of transmission.

Clinical Findings. HCV has an incubation period ranging from 2 weeks to 6 months (average 45 days). Symptom onset is often insidious; most children are asymptomatic. Flu-like prodromal symptoms (jaundice, nausea, anorexia, upper right quadrant abdominal pain) may occur in 20% to 30% of older children and adults.[19] Chronic hepatitis with cirrhosis is a late occurrence, often 20 to 30 years later. Fulminant infection is uncommon. Teenagers may be identified as HCV-positive when screened for other reasons (e.g., a school blood donation drive).

Diagnostic Studies. There is no serologic marker for acute infection. Screening and diagnosis of HCV include IgG antibody EIA for anti-HCV, enhanced chemiluminescence immunoassay, and HCV RNA PCR. Early in the infection, false negative results occur. Most individuals seroconvert within 15 weeks postexposure or within 5 to 6 weeks after the onset of illness. A newborn can be anti-HCV-positive from maternal transfer for up to 18 months, so testing should ideally be done after that time. Liver function tests are indicated and liver enzymes may go up and down with some near-normal levels for many years; a liver biopsy is confirmatory but not necessary in most pediatric patients as it does not affect the treatment decision).[15] A table with the interpretation of the results of tests for HCV infection is available from the CDC.[18] at

Differential Diagnosis and Management. Differential diagnoses include HAV and HBV and other causes of chronic hepatitis (see HAV).

Children with HCV infection should be referred to an infectious disease or GI specialist for monitoring and treatment consideration. The FDA approved several drug regimens for HCV treatment in children 3 years and older. It is recommended that all children 3 years or older with HCV are treated with an age-appropriate medication regimen.[19] Treatment for HCV is rapidly advancing. The American Association for the Study of Liver Disease and Infectious Disease Society of America provides a continually updated website with HCV antiviral treatment guidelines.[20] Administer HAV and HBV vaccines to prevent further liver complications. Liver damage can be exacerbated by comorbid conditions such as cancer, iron overload, thalassemia, or HIV. Drugs such as acetaminophen or antiretroviral medications need to be closely monitored; monitor serum hepatic transaminases closely. Children with HCV infection need not be excluded from childcare facilities.[11] Individuals with HCV should be discouraged from using alcohol to prevent further liver injury and from sharing razors and toothbrushes; condom use should be encouraged.

Complications and Prevention. The course of HCV is generally mild even with cirrhosis. Liver transplantation is an option in severe cases although reinfection after transplant is common and progressive. The outcome of chronic HCV disease in children is

less known. Ig is not recommended for prophylaxis after exposure. Research into developing a vaccine is ongoing.

Hepatitis D Virus

Hepatitis D virus (HDV) is caused by an RNA virus that is structurally different from HAV, HBV, and HCV. HDV infection is uncommon in children but must be considered in cases of fulminant hepatitis or hepatic failure. It cannot cause infection unless the child also is infected with HBV, which it needs to replicate. Transmission is through parenteral, percutaneous, or mucosal contact (including sexual) with infected blood and can be acquired either as a coinfection with or superinfection with chronic HBV. Incubation is 2 to 8 weeks. In the United States, it is diagnosed most commonly in drug users, individuals with hemophilia, and immigrants from Southern Italy and parts of Eastern Europe, South America, Africa, and the Middle East. Mother-to-newborn transmission is rare.[11] Infection is detected by IgM antibody to HDV. There is no vaccine against HDV. However, the HBV vaccine prevents HDV because it is comorbid with HBV. Those with chronic HBV should take precautions against being infected.

Hepatitis E Virus

Hepatitis E virus (HEV) is an RNA virus in the Hepeviridae family; certain strains have zoonotic hosts (e.g., swine, nonhuman primates). It is passed via the fecal-oral route. Contaminated water is the most common reservoir. It is an acute infection with symptoms that resemble those of other viral hepatitis infections. Symptomatic individuals are usually older adolescents and young adults; pregnant women especially in the third trimester are vulnerable to serious illness. Children are either asymptomatic or experience mild symptoms. If symptoms appear, they do so within 15 to 60 days (mean of 40 days) after exposure. Endemic areas include India, the Middle East, parts of Africa, Southeast Asia, and Mexico. Most cases in the United States occur in immigrants or visitors from these locations. Clinical symptoms include jaundice, malaise, anorexia, fever, abdominal pain, and arthralgia; these are similar to HAV symptoms but are often more severe. Laboratory studies include IgM and IgG anti-HEV, but these can be unreliable. Definitive diagnosis is determined by the detection of viral RNA in serum or stool using reverse transcriptase–PCR (RT-PCR) assay. Treatment is supportive; there is no approved vaccine in the United States. Good hand hygiene is crucial. Chronic infection is rare, and recovery is usually complete. The overall mortality rate is 4% or less; however, in pregnant women, the mortality rate can reach 25%.[21]

Herpes Family of Viruses

The herpes family of viruses is large with several features in common: all infect humans, the viruses establish latency for the life of the host, and reactivation is controlled by immune function. Most active infections are self-limited. The infection becomes serious and life-threatening when the cellular immune system is compromised or naive, such as in the newborn. This family of viruses includes herpes simplex virus (HSV) types 1 and 2; varicella-zoster virus (VZV); Epstein-Barr virus (EBV); CMV; and human herpesvirus 6, 7, and 8 (HHV-6, HHV-7, and HHV-8). HSV-1, HSV-2, and VZV are all members of the herpesvirus subfamily with neurotropic characteristics and latency in the sensory ganglia. HSV-1, HSV-2, VZV, EBV, HHV-6, and HHV-7 are discussed in the following sections. See Chapter 28 for a discussion of perinatally acquired CMV infection and other resources for a discussion about HHV-8.

Herpes Simplex Virus

HSV is among the most widely disseminated infectious agents in humans; it is a double-stranded DNA virus and there are two types. HSV-1 is traditionally associated with orolabial lesions or oral secretions and typically infects the mouth, lips, and eyes and can progress to the CNS. HSV-2 is traditionally shed from genital lesions and genital secretions and is most associated with genital and neonatal infections. Both HSV types can occur anywhere on the body due to contact with infected lesions, for example, herpetic whitlow, a finger abscess caused by HSV-1. Although HSV-2 accounts for 70% to 85% of neonatal cases, both types are equally devastating to a newborn.[11] HSV-1 virus is typically the causative agent in primary infections in children 6 months to 5 years of age and most often presents as gingivostomatitis. Distribution is worldwide, but the infection is more frequent in crowded environments. It is spread by intimate, direct contact usually by an adult with or without symptoms. There is no seasonal variation.

HSV-2 infections usually occur following sexual activity. Sexual abuse must always be ruled out when the infection is found in non neonates; for this reason, determining the type of virus and assessing the lesion location is always important. Neither HSV type is transmitted by inanimate objects, such as toilet seats. Neonatal HSV-2 infection is primarily transmitted from the mother as the infant passes through an infected birth canal with viral migration to the neonate's conjunctiva, nose, and/or mouth mucosa, or broken skin due to forceps, for example. Infection also occurs with cesarean births. The risk of infection for an infant born to a mother with a primary genital infection, who is shedding HSV at delivery, is 10 to 30 times more likely. However, approximately 75% of infants with congenital HSV infection are born to women without a history or clinical findings of an active HSV infection during pregnancy. HSV incidence is 1 in 2000 live births in the United States depending upon demographics and geographic area. HSV transmission to the infant from a mother with active HSV genital lesions during delivery is 25% to 60%. However, an infant born to a mother shedding the HSV virus from reactivation during pregnancy is 2%. Mothers can inoculate their babies from oral, breast, or skin lesions. Fathers and other caregivers can inoculate infants with nongenital lesions from the mouth or hands. There can be lateral transmission from an infected baby in the nursery due to inadequate hand hygiene by hospital personnel.[11]

The period of communicability for HSV-1 and HSV-2 (for nonneonates) is 2 days to 2 weeks. Some cases of perinatal infection occur more than 6 weeks after birth depending on when the fetus was exposed. Infection can be transmitted during either primary or recurrent infections, whether symptomatic or asymptomatic.

Clinical Findings. History and physical findings are determined by the viral port of entry, age, state of health, and immune competence. Eczema alone or in combination with other manifestations is a complicating factor. Clinical findings, diagnosis, management, and treatment of the most seen infections in children and adolescents due to HSV-1 and HSV-2 are discussed in other chapters (i.e., gingivostomatitis, neonatal herpetic infection, eczema herpeticum, herpes vulvovaginitis, herpes labialis, and herpes keratoconjunctivitis). A few general observations follow:

- Neonatal infection: The neonate is always symptomatic; infection is described by the extent and location of disease: disseminated (approximately 25% of cases); CNS (approximately 30% of cases); and skin, eye, and/or mouth (SEM) (approximately 45% of cases). The disseminated disease presents around days 10 to 12 of life with multiple organ failure; two-thirds develop concurrent encephalitis. Almost half of the infants with the disseminated disease never develop the characteristic vesicular rash. CNS disease presents around 16 to 19 days of life with neurologic manifestations of focal/generalized seizures, lethargy and/or irritability, and poor feeding. The majority of these infants develop herpetic lesions during the course of the illness. SEM manifests itself around days 10 to 12 of life[11] (see Chapter 28).

- Traumatic herpetic infection: This is a localized infection that occurs in a susceptible child because of abrasion, teething, finger sucking, laceration, or burn that is inoculated with herpesvirus by an orally infected parent who kisses the "booboo" or from autoinoculation. Vesicles appear at the site of the lesion. There may be fever, constitutional symptoms, and regional lymph node involvement. Athletic activities such as wrestling and rugby have been implicated in mucocutaneous herpetic lesions.

- Acute herpetic meningoencephalitis: After the neonatal period, infection with HSV-1 is a leading cause of intermittent, nonepidemic encephalitis in children and adults in the United States. Encephalitis can be focal, mimicking a mass lesion. Diagnosis is made by brain biopsy. In contrast, HSV meningitis is usually a relatively benign disease most often caused by HSV-2.

- Recurrent infections: The body does not eradicate the virus; the virus lies dormant, and recurrent infections are common. Recurrent infections occur either as herpes labialis or genital herpes. Some incidences of recurrent aseptic meningitis are attributed to HSV infection.

Diagnostic Studies. Intrapartum cultures from mother and infant should be obtained no later than 12 and 24 hours after birth if a neonatal infection is suspected. Tests may include viral culture, cytology-Pap smears, Tzanck stains, ELISA, fluorescent techniques, glycoprotein G assay, blood or CSF PCR in neonates, or histologic evaluation and viral culture from a brain biopsy in individuals with encephalitis. Obtain cultures in neonates from skin vesicles, mouth, nasopharynx, eyes, blood, rectum, and CSF. An ophthalmic examination and MRI to establish baseline brain anatomy are recommended for all infants with neonatal HSV, regardless of diagnosis classification. Serologic tests are not helpful in neonates. In disseminated disease, elevated transaminase and/or radiographic evidence of HSV pneumonitis may be seen.[11]

Differential Diagnosis and Management. The diagnosis is not difficult if vesicles are present. Coxsackievirus can cause vesicular stomatitis. Neonatal HSV disease should always be suspected in cases of neonatal respiratory distress or sepsis.

The management of HSV infections is discussed in other chapters (i.e., gingivostomatitis, neonatal herpetic infection, eczema herpeticum, herpes vulvovaginitis, herpes labialis, and herpes keratoconjunctivitis). Parenteral acyclovir is the treatment of choice in life-threatening illnesses, neonatal infections, or disease in immunocompromised patients. A repeat lumbar puncture is recommended at the end of parenteral treatment for infants with CNS involvement.[11]

Oral acyclovir suppressive therapy for 6 months after parenteral treatment of acute neonatal disease reduces the recurrence of mucocutaneous lesions and improves neurodevelopmental outcomes. The absolute neutrophil count should be monitored in infants at 2 weeks and 4 weeks after initiating therapy and then monthly during the treatment period.[11] If neutropenia occurs, stop acyclovir therapy until the neutrophil count recovers, then restart therapy. Any suspected new lesion(s) should be cultured.

Infants born to women with active recurrent genital infection are generally not given empiric antiviral medication, but instead are closely monitored by parents and providers over the following 6 weeks. Basic preventative measures include careful hand hygiene before and after handling newborns and refraining from kissing or nuzzling (masks can be worn until lesions crust over) by those with active herpes labialis infection.

Complications. Most HSV infections are mild. However, bacterial superinfection is always a potential problem. Any patient with evidence of HSV ocular involvement must be referred to an ophthalmologist immediately.

The morbidity and mortality associated with neonatal herpetic infection significantly improve with aggressive antiviral therapy (acyclovir). When treated appropriately, 1-year mortality is 29% for disseminated disease and 4% for CNS disease. Poor neurologic outcomes occur in 17% of neonates with disseminated disease and 69% with CNS disease. Aggressive acyclovir therapy results in SEM infections remaining limited to the mucocutaneous tissues and preventing disseminated or CNS disease.[11]

Patient and Family Education
- Toddlers and infants with primary gingivostomatitis who drool should be excluded from childcare centers if they cannot control their saliva. Children with recurrent "fever blisters" may attend school. Cover recurrent HSV lesions with a bandage in children with active nonmucosal involvement.
- Wrestlers and rugby players should be excluded from competition for 3 to 8 days (see Chapter 18).
- All pregnant women must be asked about HSV infection in themselves and their sexual partners. Signs and symptoms of HSV should be carefully monitored throughout pregnancy.
- During labor, all women must be questioned about HSV and carefully examined for signs and symptoms of infection. Cesarean delivery is indicated in women with apparent infection unless membranes are ruptured for more than 4 to 6 hours. Scalp monitoring should be avoided in infants of women with a history of HSV infection.

Infectious Mononucleosis Syndrome

More than 90% of IMS cases are caused by EBV, a member of the herpes viruses. The remaining cases are attributed to acute CMV, *Toxoplasma gondii,* adenovirus, viral hepatitis, HIV, and possibly rubella. Approximately 90% of US adults have a history of infection.[11] Almost all older children and adolescents in developing countries and poor urban settings in developed countries are seropositive for EBV. In these children, primary exposure occurs in infancy or early childhood, tends to produce only mild symptoms, and is subclinical. Infection in children younger than 4 years old occurs less frequently in affluent populations in developed countries; one-third of cases occur during adolescence or young adulthood.[11] The mode of transmission is personal contact, penetrative sexual contact, and the exchange of saliva. EBV is transmitted by blood transfusion or transplantation. The virus lives outside the body in saliva for several hours. Infection is common in early life, more so among those in lower socioeconomic groups. Endemic IMS is most common in adolescents in the school system and those enlisted in the military.[11] Because the IMS virus is found in the saliva and blood of both clinically ill and asymptomatic infected persons for many months, the period of communicability is difficult to assess. The incubation period is thought to be from 30 to 50 days. It is mildly contagious.

Clinical Findings. IMS affects the primary lymphoid tissue and peripheral blood. Lymphoid tissue—regional lymph nodes, tonsils, spleen, and liver—is enlarged. Atypical lymphocytes are seen in the peripheral blood. The disease spectrum ranges from asymptomatic to fatal infection. Almost all body organs are involved, including but not limited to the lungs, heart, kidneys, adrenals, CNS, and skin. Symptoms are variable and last up to 2 to 3 weeks. Clinical presentation typically occurs in three phases: *prodrome, acute,* and *resolution.* During the *prodrome* phase, symptoms are mild and may include malaise, fatigue, and possibly fever, and it is difficult to distinguish IMS from other viral infections. The *acute* phase follows with the classic symptoms of fever (100.4°F [38°C] to 104.9°F [40.5°C]), pharyngitis, malaise, and fatigue. Physical findings include discrete, nontender, nonerythematous lymphadenopathy, and tonsillopharyngitis (exudative in approximately half of the patients). Hepatomegaly and splenomegaly may occur and require physical contact and sports restrictions. Skin rash occurs in up to 20% of cases, usually on the trunk, arms, and palms, and is more common in those treated with antibiotic therapy, namely the penicillins. It can be maculopapular, urticarial, scarlatiniform, hemorrhagic (rarely), or nodular and usually occurs during the first few days of symptom onset and lasts 1 to 6 days. IMS associated with EBV is closely associated with several distinct disorders, including X-linked lymphoproliferative syndrome, Burkitt lymphoma, and Hodgkin disease. After several days (or up to 3–4 weeks), the *resolution* phase begins with a gradual decrease in fatigue and fever; organomegaly may take 1 to 2 months to resolve.[11]

Diagnostic Studies. The CBC classically demonstrates lymphocytosis with more than 10% atypical lymphocytes. Elevated liver enzymes are typical. Monospot and the serum heterophile tests are positive in 85% of infected patients older than 4 years old (often negative in those younger than 4 years). Children older than 4 years usually must be ill for approximately 2 weeks before seroconverting. Viral culture and Epstein-Barr-specific core and capsule antibody testing are usually used for diagnosis if the primary screening test results are negative and there is continued suspicion of IMS (e.g., in younger children). Depending on the specific EBV antigen system tested, levels are detectable for years after infection. PCR assay for the detection of EBV is available and is useful in evaluating if the child is immunocompromised or has a chronic complex medical condition.[11]

Differential Diagnosis and Management. IMS is in the differential diagnosis of almost every infectious disease. Conditions and infections typically associated with a mononucleosis-like syndrome are gram-positive alpha and beta-hemolytic streptococcal pharyngitis, leukemia, lymphoreticular malignancies, adenoviruses, toxoplasmosis, CMV, rubella, HIV, hepatitis, SLE, drug reactions, and diphtheria.

Treatment is supportive with adequate bed rest for debilitated cases, over-the-counter pain relievers, fluids, and increased calories. Corticosteroids and acyclovir are not recommended for routine, uncomplicated disease; penicillin products should not be given. Contact sports and strenuous exercise should be avoided for 21 days after the onset of symptoms and especially in those with hepatosplenomegaly (see Chapter 18 for return-to-play sports participation recommendations). Symptoms generally resolve within 2 to 4 weeks; fatigue and weakness may persist for up to 6 to 12 months after severe infection.[11]

Complications and Patient and Family Education. Healthy children and youth experience few sequelae. Rare complications include splenic rupture, neurologic complications (from aseptic meningitis, encephalitis, myelitis, optic neuritis, cranial nerve palsies, Guillain-Barré syndrome), thrombocytopenia, agranulocytosis, hemolytic anemia, orchitis, myocarditis, or chronic IMS. The virus increases the risk of Hodgkin disease. Death is rare. There is no clear evidence that supports an association between EBV infection and chronic fatigue syndrome.[11]

Persons with a recent history of IMS or an infectious mononucleosis-like disease should not donate blood or organs. Sharing food and drinks with infected individuals needs to be avoided to reduce the risk of acquiring EBV-associated IMS.[11]

Roseola Infantum (Exanthem Subitum)

HHV-6 and HHV-7 are members of the *Roseolovirus* genus in the Betaherpesvirinae subfamily of HHVs. HHV-6 is responsible for most roseola infantum cases (exanthema subitum or sixth disease) and is associated with other diseases, including encephalitis, especially in immunocompromised hosts. A small percentage of children with roseola have a primary infection with HHV-7. Humans are the only natural reservoir. The method of transmission is not completely understood, but the virus is probably spread via the oral, nasal, and conjunctival routes from close contacts. Transmission is suspected to occur prenatally (1%) or during or after birth. The disease is most common in children between 7 and 24 months old after protective maternal antibodies wane. It is rare in children younger than 3 months old or older than 4 years old. Most children are HHV-6 seropositive by 4 years old, and about 85% are seropositive for HHV-7 by adulthood. Reactivation of infection can occur in those who are immunocompromised. Visits to emergency departments by infants are common because of associated fevers, toxicity, and/or seizures. The disease occurs worldwide, year-round, and shows no gender preference. The incubation period has a mean of 9 to 10 days. The period of communicability for HHV-6 is unknown and for HHV-7 is likely greatest during the fever phase before the rash erupts.[11]

Clinical Findings. There is a sudden onset of high fever from 101°F to more than 103°F (38.3°C to more than 39.5°C) for 3 to 7 days, but the child does not seem ill. Approximately 20% of all emergency department visits for children with fevers, ages 6 to 12 months are attributed to HHV-6. However, during high fevers, irritability and malaise may be noted. There may be URI signs; cervical and posterior occipital lymphadenopathy; lethargy; infected palpebral conjunctiva; eyelid edema; GI complaints; reddened tympanic membranes; and occasionally, a febrile convulsion (10–15%). As the fever breaks, a diffuse, nonpruritic, discrete, rose-colored maculopapular rash, 2 to 3 mm in diameter,

appears (Fig. 35.2). It fades on pressure and rarely coalesces. The roseola exanthema is similar to the rash of rubella. The rash lasts from hours to 2 to 3 days, begins on the trunk, and spreads centrifugally. In the rare case of CNS involvement, the anterior fontanelle may bulge.[11]

Diagnostic Studies. The diagnosis of roseola exanthema is usually made clinically and diagnostic studies are not indicated. If serology is done (the diagnosis is unclear or symptoms are severe or unusual), the WBC count is distinctive, showing a decrease for age initially, dropping further by the third or fourth day, and then returns to normal. It tends to follow the fever pattern. Another serologic test involves isolating HHV-6 for peripheral blood mononuclear cells and documenting a significant rise in antibody titer; however, test results vary widely, so diagnosing unequivocal acute infection is problematic. Serial titers 2 to 3 weeks apart are more reliable. Fourfold increases in HHV-6 or HHV-7 IgG antibodies suggest active infection. Virus cultures are helpful. A rapid HHV-6 culture is available. An RT-PCR assay distinguishes between acute and latent infection.

Differential Diagnosis, Management, and Complications. The clinical course usually makes this illness easy to diagnose. The differential diagnoses include most viral rashes, scarlatina, and drug hypersensitivity. A roseola-like illness is also associated with parvovirus B19, echovirus 16, other enteroviruses, measles, and adenoviruses. Until the rash develops, fever without focus and bacterial sepsis are in the differential diagnoses. If a febrile seizure occurs, add meningitis to the differential diagnosis. Management is supportive. Use acetaminophen if the child is uncomfortable with the fever. There are no practical means of prevention. Complications include febrile convulsions, meningoencephalitis, encephalitis, and hemiplegia.

Varicella Zoster Virus

VZV is a common, highly contagious herpes virus. Chickenpox is the primary illness. It derives its name not from chickens but from the propensity of the lesions to resemble chickpeas. Shingles (herpes zoster) is the reactivation infection of latent VZV acquired during varicella infection (see Chapter 37).

Humans are the only infection reservoir; illness is spread by direct contact, droplets, and airborne transmission. Victims of shingles are infectious and can cause primary varicella illness. Immunity is usually lifelong; reinfection is rare and when it does occur, symptoms are usually mild. Immunocompromised patients risk developing generalized zoster. The disease peaks in those aged 10 to 14 years, although the overall incidence decreased in all age groups from prevaccine levels (after licensure in 1995, incidence declined 90% by 2005 with further reduction after the second dose was made routine in 2006).[22] Distribution is worldwide and endemic in most large cities. Epidemics occur at irregular intervals; the highest incidence is in late winter and spring in temperate climates. Mild varicella breakthrough infection occurs in approximately 10% to 20% of those previously vaccinated; however, the vaccine is 97% protective against severe disease.[23]

The incubation period is 10 to 21 days (mean of 14–16 days). The period of communicability is 1 to 2 days before the rash erupts until all lesions crust over (about 3–7 days). Communicability is prolonged in individuals who received varicella immune globulin (VZIG) or immune globulin intravenous (IGIV).[11]

Clinical Findings. The following two phases are seen in varicella:
1. *Prodrome:* Not always present. It is composed of low-grade fever, listlessness, headache, backache, anorexia, mild abdominal

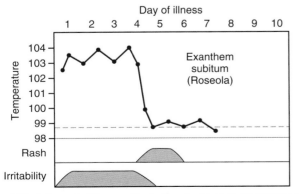

• **Fig. 35.2** Schematic Diagram Illustrating the Symptoms of Roseola.

pain, and occasionally URI symptoms. These symptoms may occur 1 to 2 days before the onset of the second phase.

2. *Rash:* Classic appearance. It is centripetal, beginning on the scalp, face, or trunk. Crops of generally highly pruritic lesions progress from spots to "teardrop vesicles" that cloud over and umbilicate in 24 to 48 hours. After a few days, all morphologic forms are seen simultaneously. The average number of lesions in unvaccinated individuals is about 300.[24] Scabs last from 5 to 20 days, depending on the depth of the lesions. There can be a fever of 105°F (40.6°C). The more severe the rash, the higher the fever. Lesions can develop on all mucosal tissues, mouth, pharynx, larynx, trachea, vagina, and anus. Breakthrough varicella disease can occur more than 42 days after vaccination and should be regarded as contagious.[24]

Diagnostic Studies. As the incidence of varicella disease has decreased, many providers may be unfamiliar with the clinical presentation of the disease, especially in individuals with mild cases and few lesions. Diagnostic studies play an important role in these instances. For both unvaccinated and vaccinated persons, the most reliable method for diagnosing VZV is the PCR (preferred) or direct fluorescent antibody done from scrapings of a vesicle base during the first 3 to 4 days posteruption. Tzanck smears of lesions demonstrate multinucleated giant cells containing intranuclear inclusion bodies but are not specific for VZV. A positive serologic test for varicella-zoster IgM antibody is confirmatory. Compare serial IgG antibody titers from acute and convalescent samples to confirm the diagnosis. Culture the virus from vesicular fluid, CSF, and biopsy of tissue, but the sensitivity of this method is less than that of the PCR. The WBC count is usually within normal limits.

Differential Diagnosis and Management. The rash is the classic symptom; therefore the diagnosis is usually clinical. Fig. 35.3 shows differences in the distribution of the maculopapular eruptions and prodromal symptoms between scarlet fever, chickenpox, and smallpox. Occasionally, impetigo, cigarette burns, and insect bites cause diagnostic confusion in children with a mild rash. Other infections that can be confused with varicella include eczema herpeticum, HSV, and Stevens-Johnson syndrome.

Chickenpox is usually a benign infection in healthy children. Treatment is supportive and includes the management of pruritis with antihistamines or oatmeal baths, acetaminophen for fever, and antistaphylococcal penicillin or cephalosporins for bacterial superinfections. Evaluate children for invasive disease who present with fever for more than several days or increasing temperatures 4 or more days after the appearance of the rash. Aspirin is contraindicated because of the risk of Reye syndrome. The use of ibuprofen for fever is questionable because of a possible causal relationship with bacterial superinfections.[25]

Intravenous acyclovir is efficacious for immunocompromised individuals and for those with severe disease. See Table 35.3 regarding the use of VZIG; it is not effective after the disease progresses. Oral acyclovir is not routinely recommended for most children. When given to otherwise healthy children within 24 hours after eruption of the rash, there is a modest decrease in the symptoms and illness duration. Indication for oral acyclovir use is available from the AAP *Red Book*.[11] It should be considered for use in pregnant women with varicella, especially in their second or third trimester. The safety of acyclovir to the fetus in the first trimester is uncertain.

Complications. The following complications can occur: pyodermas (about a 5% incidence, causing serious invasive disease with *Streptococcus* and *Staphylococcus*); idiopathic thrombocytopenic purpura (ITP) (1%–2%); pneumonia (smoking is a risk factor); CNS complications (e.g., encephalitis and Reye syndrome); and, rarely, glomerulonephritis, orchitis, hepatitis, toxic shock, osteomyelitis, necrotizing fasciitis, myositis, myocarditis, arthritis, and appendicitis. Primary varicella is rarely fatal, and since the licensure of the varicella vaccine, the highest mortality occurs in newborns and immunocompromised children.[25] Neonatal involvement is directly tied to the timing of the maternal infection with varicella. See Chapter 28 for a discussion about congenital varicella syndrome.

Patient and Family Education
- Asymptomatic children exposed to chickenpox may attend school for about 1 week before quarantining. If they show signs of illness, they must be kept home for 1 week. If they do not break out in a rash, they may return to school. Children with active disease are to be kept home until all lesions are dry.
- Exposed patients: VZIG use was discussed earlier and can cause asymptomatic infection. Individuals who receive VZIG should obtain age-appropriate varicella immunization (unless contraindicated) in 5 months. The AAP *Red Book* and the CDC website include further recommendations regarding VZIG for the immunocompromised.

Influenza Viral Infections

Influenza viruses are orthomyxoviruses with three antigenic types: A, B, and C. Types A and B cause epidemic disease; type C causes sporadic mild influenza-like illness in children. Type A is further classified into two surface proteins—hemagglutinin (HA) and neuraminidase (NA). Three HA subtypes and two NA types cause disease in humans (e.g., H1N1, HIN2, and H3N2). Variant influenza viruses also infect humans and originate from swine and domestic or wild avian sources. Influenza is a highly contagious disease and is spread from person to person by direct contact, droplet contamination, and fomites recently contaminated with infected nasopharyngeal secretions.

Typical Influenza

In temperate climates, typical influenza epidemics occur in the winter months, last approximately 4 to 8 weeks, and peak 2 weeks after the index case. Influenza illness circulates year-round in countries closest to the equator. In recent years, some epidemics lasted 3 months due to more than one strain of virus circulating within a community. Children, particularly school agers, can shed the virus longer than adults (10 days vs. 5 days) and are particularly prolific community transmitters. After a newly shifted subtype emerges, the highest incidence of the illness occurs in healthy children 5 to 18 years old. Children younger than 2 years, especially infants younger than 6 months old, individuals 65 years and older, and those with chronic diseases have high hospitalization rates. Children under 5 years old with high-risk conditions account for most pediatric deaths.[11] According to the CDC, an average of 37,643 deaths annually are associated with influenza.[26]

The incubation period is 1 to 4 days. Patients become infectious 24 hours before the onset of symptoms. Viral shedding usually peaks by day 3 and ceases 7 days after the onset of the illness.[30]

Clinical Findings. Classic clinical symptoms include a sudden onset of high fever (102–106°F [38.8–41°C]), headache, chills, coryza, vertigo, pharyngitis, pain in the back and extremities, and a dry hacking cough that resembles pertussis. Emesis, diarrhea, croup, conjunctival infection, and epistaxis occur in young children. Infants can become septic. In severe infection, there may

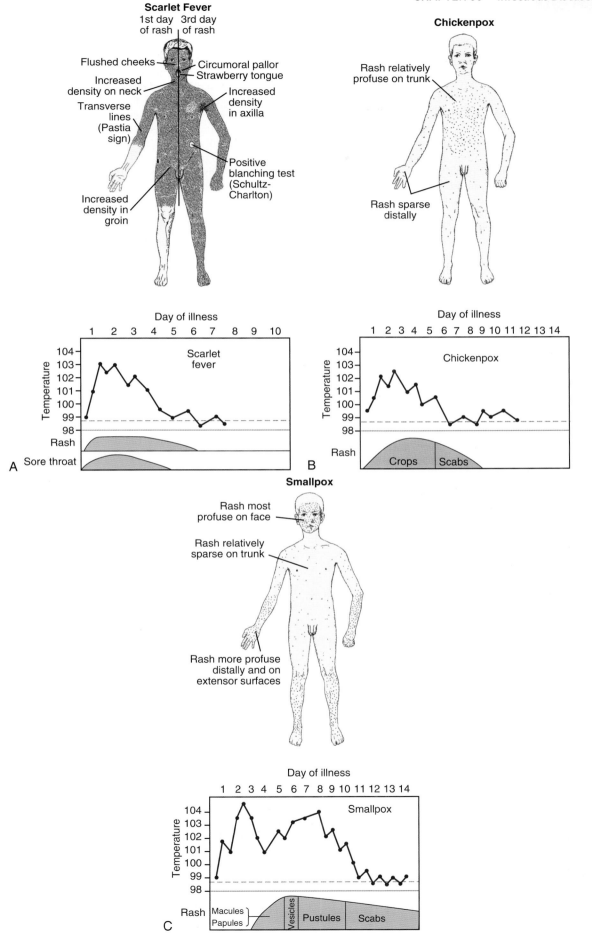

• **Fig. 35.3** Differences in Distribution of the Maculopapular Eruptions of Scarlet Fever, Chickenpox, and Smallpox.

be involvement of the lower respiratory tract with atelectasis or infiltrates. Severe influenza-associated myocarditis (evidenced by weak heart sounds and rapid, weak pulse) results in distention of the right side of the heart and CHF. Acute symptoms generally last 2 to 3 days, rarely over 5 days.

Diagnostic Studies. Rapid influenza diagnostic tests have limited sensitivities and predictive values. They are useful when determining the etiology of a respiratory disease outbreak in certain settings such as schools, camps, and hospitals, or if the child was recently exposed to pigs, poultry, or other animals, or had exposure to novel influenza A infection. A negative result should not determine the treatment course (e.g., antiviral treatment), or actions to protect others at risk for complications.[27] Special viral cultures taken from the nasopharyngeal or nasal cavity by swab, nasal wash, or aspirate (varies by test) within 72 hours of illness onset can isolate the virus in 2 to 6 days and confirm the diagnosis. Other tests for influenza virus include serology (acute and convalescent sera), PCR, immunofluorescent assay (IFA), and rapid molecular assays. A CBC may show leukopenia.

Differential Diagnosis, Management, and Complications. The differential diagnosis includes other viral respiratory infections (e.g., common cold, parainfluenza, respiratory syncytial virus [RSV], rhinovirus, avian flu), allergic croup, epiglottitis, and bacterial pulmonary infections (e.g., *M. pneumoniae*).

Treatment is supportive (bed rest, fluids, over-the-counter antipyretics). Advise children and parents of symptoms that warrant further medical consultation (e.g., dehydration, difficulty breathing, muscle weakness). Promote hand hygiene, barrier protection such as masks and gowns, and social distancing. Four antiviral medications are approved for the treatment or chemoprophylaxis of influenza A and B strains in the United States (i.e., zanamivir, oseltamivir, peramivir, or baloxavir in the United States) and are reserved for the following[28]:

- Patients with immunosuppression
- Children younger than 2 years
- Children with chronic illnesses [pulmonary (including asthma), cardiovascular (excludes hypertension alone), renal, hepatic, hematologic (including sickle cell disease), metabolic disorders (including diabetes mellitus), neurologic and neurodevelopment conditions (including seizure disorders), intellectual disability, moderate to severe developmental delay, muscular dystrophy, or spinal cord injury]
- Pregnant or postpartum females (within 2 weeks of delivery)
- Individuals younger than 19 years on long-term aspirin therapy or salicylate-containing medications
- Children residing in population-dense housing circumstances
- Children who are morbidly obese (i.e., BMI is 40 or greater)
- Children in residential care facilities

When antivirals are indicated, start treatment as soon as possible after illness onset (preferably within 48 hours of symptom onset). The FDA recommends oseltamivir to treat influenza in those 2 weeks or older and for chemoprophylaxis in those age 1 year or older. The AAP and CDC endorse its use to treat influenza in those under 2 weeks old and as chemoprophylaxis in those 3 months to 1 year old (CDC, 2022). Antiviral effectiveness varies from year to year based on the virus and strains present. PCPs can consult the CDC website "FluView Interactive" (https://www.cdc.gov/flu/weekly/fluviewinteractive.htm) for information regarding circulating strains and antiviral resistance patterns within their geographic regions during influenza season.

Complications include Reye syndrome, respiratory infections (acute otitis media ([AOM], pneumonia), acute myositis, toxic shock, myocarditis, cystic fibrosis, and asthma exacerbations caused by bacterial superinfection, usually with *H. influenzae*. Aspirin should never be given to persons with influenza.

Patient and Family Education. The influenza vaccine should be widely promoted (see Chapter 19). The CDC recommends the influenza vaccine for everyone 6 months of age and older. Although not mandated by any professional organization, the Infectious Diseases Society of America (IDSA), the Society for Healthcare Epidemiology of America (SHEA), and the Pediatric Infectious Diseases Society (PIDS) recommend that all healthcare providers receive yearly influenza vaccine to protect themselves and prevent the spread of this disease to their patients and families.

Highly Pathogenic Avian Influenza

The highly pathogenic avian influenza A (HPAI H5N1 or, simply H5N1) virus potentially acquires genes from the influenza virus that affects other species. It spreads quickly and morphed into a more pathogenic virus than when it first emerged in 1996. There is little natural immunity in humans; fortunately, the disease in humans is uncommon, and the virus has not yet mutated to be efficiently transmitted from person to person. To date, only humans who had direct contact with sick or dead poultry, wild birds, or who visited live poultry markets are at high risk for virus acquisition. The outbreak worldwide has not diminished significantly, and healthcare providers in the United States should remain on alert. Human cases are reported in Asia, Africa, the Pacific, Canada, Europe, and Near East. The highest number of cases occur in Indonesia, Egypt, and Vietnam.[29]

Humans who acquire the disease may experience a range of mild to severe symptoms. Symptoms include fever (often >100.4°F [38°C]), cough, pharyngitis, malaise, myalgia, abdominal pain, diarrhea, and respiratory symptoms progressing to pneumonia with shortness of breath, difficulty breathing, and hypoxia. Complications of severe infection include acute respiratory and multiorgan system failure leading to death. To date, the mortality rate in humans is approximately 60%.[30] A vaccine for HPAI H5N1 was recently developed. If avian influenza is suspected, the CDC provides guidance in obtaining specimens, monitoring suspected cases, and advising precautions for those traveling to endemic locales. The United States banned the import of birds (dead or alive) and bird products (including hatching eggs) from H5N1-affected countries. A list of countries is available from the CDC.

Other Viral Diseases

Human Immunodeficiency Virus

HIVs, serotypes HIV-1 and HIV-2, are retroviruses that cause human disease. Retroviruses are RNA viruses that must make a DNA copy of their RNA to replicate. HIV cells enter a target CD4+ T cell and, using the reverse transcriptase enzyme, convert their RNA into DNA that integrates with the T-cell DNA within the cell nucleus, permanently infecting the host cell. Through the processes of transcription, translation, and maturation, the HIV genes convert into messenger RNA and leave the nucleus. Eventually, new virions bud from the CD4+ T cells, infect other cells, and the cycle repeats. HIV persists in infected individuals for life; latent virus protein remains in cells of the blood, brain, bone marrow, and genital tract even when the plasma viral load cannot be detected. Both serotypes cause clinically indistinguishable diseases; most infections worldwide are attributed to HIV-1. HIV-2 is generally limited to West Africa. Three genetic groups of HIV exist: major (M), outlier (O), and new (N). Group M viruses are the most prevalent worldwide. Group M is divided into eight genetic subtypes (subtypes A thru K). Each subtype has its own geographic distribution.[11]

The worldwide burden of HIV/acquired immune deficiency syndrome (AIDS) remains high, with approximately 38 million individuals infected with HIV at the end of 2021. Africa is the most affected region and accounts for approximately 60% of all people with newly diagnosed infections.[31] There are approximately 1.7 million children living with HIV. Antiviral treatment is increasingly available in low- and middle-income countries; however, pediatric coverage with these drugs is lagging compared to adults.[30] Limited resources in some countries also make unscreened blood products a means of transmission.

In the United States in 2020, there were an estimated 30,692 new HIV infections—down from 39,640 in 2019.[32] The HIV acquisition rate among infants continued to decrease in the United States. Overall infection rates among adolescents and young adults aged 13 to 24 years also decreased. HIV infection rates among men who have sex with men aged 13 to 24 years increased. Increased infection rates occur disproportionately among adolescents of minority race or ethnicity.[32] A decreased infection rate across the United States is thought to be a result of primary prevention efforts to decrease mother-to-child transmission (MTCT) and antiretroviral therapy (ART) availability for children with HIV.

Humans are the only known reservoir for HIV-1 and HIV-2. Although there are AIDS-like syndromes in other primates and felines, the infection does not spread from pets, animals, or insects. HIV isolates blood (lymphocytes, macrophages, and plasma), CSF, pleural fluid, cervical secretions, human milk, feces, saliva, and urine. However, only blood, semen, cervical secretions, and human milk transmit infection. Transmission is through intimate sexual contact, sharing contaminated needles (inconclusive mode for HIV-2), receiving contaminated blood or blood products, perinatal exposure, and breastfeeding. HIV-2 has lower transmissibility rates than HIV-1.[33]

HIV transmission to infants occurs in several ways. In-utero transmission accounts for about 30% of infections (usually occurs by 10 weeks of gestation and is associated with early, severe newborn disease); intrapartum transmission (at least 60%; from infected blood and cervicovaginal secretions in the birth canal or microtransfusions between mother and fetus during labor); or postpartum transmission via breast milk (15%; transmission rates range from 33% to 50% globally in resource-poor countries). The risk of an untreated HIV-infected woman giving birth to an infected infant with HIV-1 is 25% to 35% (4% or less for HIV-2).[33] In vaginal twin deliveries, the firstborn twin has a greater risk of developing HIV than the second. Other risk factors for increased transmission include maternal drug use, premature rupture of membranes more than 4 hours before the onset of labor, low birth weight, and premature birth before 34 weeks.[34]

Mother-to-child transmission (MTCT) has been virtually eliminated in the United States due to rigorous, universal antenatal HIV testing, combination ART use, cesarean births, and breastfeeding abstaining.[34] Breast milk HIV transmission contributes to MTCT. The CDC and the AAP recommend that HIV-infected women in the United States do not breastfeed. In resource-limited areas, the WHO recommends mothers living with HIV exclusively breastfeed for the first 6 months of life when receiving ART.[35]

The incubation period is variable. HIV infection symptom onset in infants untreated perinatally occurs as early as 2 months.[33]

The infection has a latency period longer than 5 years. Disease progression is faster with earlier mortality in children born to mothers with advanced infection, low CD4+ T-lymphocyte count, and who have high viral loads. In sub-Saharan Africa, approximately 30% of infants untreated with antiviral medication succumb to the disease by 1 year old, and more than 50% die before they turn 2 years. Children untreated that live in the United States and Europe have a mortality rate between 10% and 20%.

Clinical Findings. HIV infection is often experienced as an influenza-like illness (fever, rash, pharyngitis, lymphadenopathy, and myalgias) for 2 to 4 weeks. These symptoms suggest a nonspecific viral process, and a provider may not consider HIV in the differential diagnosis. At this point, the asymptomatic infection may continue for a few months to up to 15 years, depending on the viral load. The CD4+ T cells start declining at an average rate of about 50 cells/μL/year.

There are four HIV clinical categories for children with HIV infection, ranging from "not symptomatic" to "severely symptomatic." These categories, paired with the degree of age-specific CD4+ T-lymphocyte count and total lymphocyte percentage, are used to determine the disease stage and management strategies. Newborn examinations are usually normal. Lymphadenopathy is often the first symptom, followed by hepatosplenomegaly. Some children have failure to thrive, chronic or recurrent diarrhea, pneumonia (*Pneumocystis jirovecii* peaks at 3–6 months of age), oral candidiasis, recurrent bacterial infections, chronic parotid swelling, and progressive neurologic deterioration. Those with high HIV loads develop symptoms earlier, including failure to thrive and encephalopathy. Other opportunistic diseases are *Mycobacterium avium* infection, severe CMV after 6 months old, EBV, VZV, disseminated histoplasmosis, RSV, *M. tuberculosis*, and measles, despite vaccination.

After infancy, children generally have more recurrent bacterial infections (20%), parotid gland swelling, lymphoid interstitial pneumonitis, or neurologic deficiencies that can progress to encephalopathy. *S. pneumoniae*, Hib, *S. aureus*, and *Salmonella* organisms are common infections in pediatric AIDS patients. Sinusitis, cellulitis, gingivostomatitis, herpetic zoster, glomerulopathy, cardiac hypertrophy, anemia, CHF, and purulent middle ear infections are common. Malignancies are uncommon in pediatric AIDS.[34]

Diagnostic Studies. With newborn HIV screening, approximately 30% to 40% of those infected in utero are identified within 48 hours of birth and nearly 93% by age 2 weeks. Those infected within the intrapartum period might become positive 2 to 6 weeks after birth.[11] Most infants without other exposure risks (e.g., those breastfed) lose maternal antibodies between 6 and 12 months, but some take as long as 18 or more months to seroconvert. Table 35.5 lists recommended diagnostic tests and suggested timing for use.

Lymphopenia occurs as the disease progresses. There are decreased circulating CD4+ cells (T-suppressor, T-helper cells), and the helper-suppressor ratio is less than one. The CDC identifies the individual as suffering from autoimmune deficiency disease (e.g., AIDS) when their CD4+ T cell count is less than 200/mm^3. Some AIDS patients become seronegative late in the disease because the weakened immune system cannot manufacture antibodies.

Appropriately screen partners and other children of the HIV-infected mother. Perform HIV testing in cases where an infant is adopted or in foster care, and when the HIV status of the mother is unknown. HIV-infected pregnant women are advised to start ART during pregnancy, irrespective of their CD4+ cell counts and

<table>
<tr><td colspan="2">TABLE 35.5   Testing Schedule for Human Immunodeficiency Virus in the Exposed, Nonbreastfeeding Infant[a] in the United States</td></tr>
</table>

Test[b]	Time After Birth
First HIV DNA PCR[c] or HIV qualitative RNA assay[d] from peripheral blood (not cord blood); confirm if positive using the same test on another blood sample	Within 48 hours
Optional, HIV DNA PCR[c] or HIV qualitative RNA assay[d]; confirm if positive	14–21 days (some clinicians prefer this optional testing date)
Second HIV DNA PCR[c] or HIV qualitative RNA assay[d]; confirm if positive	1–3 months
Third HIV DNA PCR[c] or HIV qualitative RNA assay[d]; confirm if positive	4–6 months
Fourth HIV DNA PCR[c] or HIV qualitative RNA assay[d]; confirm if positive	12 and 24 months

[a]Infant is considered infected if two separate samples test positive by HIV DNA PCR or qualitative HIV RNA PCR. Infant greater than 18 months old and nonbreastfeeding is considered *definitely negative* if two negative tests are obtained at ≥1 month and ≥4 months *or* two separate negative tests are obtained at ≥6 months AND no other laboratory or clinical evidence that suggests HIV/acquired immune deficiency syndrome (AIDS).

[b]The following HIV tests are not recommended for use in those younger than 1 month: HIV culture; HIV p24 antigen assay; immune complex dissociated (ICD) p24 antigen assay. Those older than 18 months old can be tested using an HIV antibody assay. Most tests will detect both HIV-1 and HIV-2 infection but will not discern between the two. HIV-2 infection can be confirmed using other tests.

[c]HIV DNA PCR testing may be preferable for infants who are receiving combination antiretroviral treatment (cART) prophylaxis or preemptive treatment because HIV RNA assays may be less sensitive in the presence of such treatment.

[d]The newer qualitative HIV RNA PCR assay detects HIV-1 nontype B or group O strain in infants and is recommended for infants born to mothers from Africa, India, or Southeast Asia or if infection is suspected and the initial HIV DNA PCR assay(s) are negative (HIV DNA PCR has limited sensitivity to this subtype/strain).

[e]This fourth test is an option to document loss of maternal antibodies in infants 12 to 18 months old with prior negative tests; or to definitely exclude or confirm HIV infection in infants 18 to 24 months with prior HIV-antibody positive tests.

DNA, Deoxyribonucleic acid; *HIV,* human immunodeficiency virus; *PCR,* polymerase chain reaction; *RNA,* ribonucleic acid.

Data from US Department of Health and Human Services (USDHHS). Guidelines for the use of antiretroviral agents in pediatric HIV infection: diagnosis of HIV infection in infants and children; 2021. https://clinicalinfo.hiv.gov/en/guidelines/perinatal/diagnosis-hiv-infection-infants-and-children

HIV RNA levels, to help prevent vertical transmission.[36] Before starting a newborn on antiretroviral prophylaxis, a CBC and differential should be obtained because anemia is a side effect of some of the drugs.

If HIV infection is suspected because of a history in a child over 18 months old, screening HIV antibody assays plus a confirmatory antibody test or virologic detection test are warranted. In cases of acute HIV infection or AIDS, antibody tests may be negative and virologic testing is necessary. A pediatric HIV specialist should be consulted.

Differential Diagnosis. The differential diagnosis includes other causes of immunologic deficiency, such as recent immunosuppressive agent use, lymphoproliferative disease, congenital immunologic states, inflammatory bowel disease, DiGeorge syndrome, ITP, chronic allergies, cystic fibrosis, graft-versus-host reaction, congenital CMV, toxoplasmosis, ataxia, or telangiectasia.

Management and Complications. Treatment goals include suppressing viral replication to undetectable levels; restoring/preserving immune function; reducing HIV-associated sequelae; minimizing drug toxicity; promoting normal growth and development; facilitating treatment regimen adherence; and improving quality of life. Information about pediatric HIV and AIDS treatment is subject to change, and the PCP should check with the CDC or clinicalinfo.hiv.gov regarding updated guidelines for diagnosis, treatment, monitoring drug toxicity and adherence, and specific immunization precautions and regimens. Make treatment decisions and laboratory studies in consultation with a pediatric HIV specialist.

Currently recommended drug regimens for ART include at least three oral antiretroviral drugs from at least two drug classes. In general, two nucleoside reverse transcriptase inhibitors plus either a nonnucleoside reverse transcriptase inhibitor or protease inhibitor, often with low-dose ritonavir, are used. Treatment regimens are individualized based on multiple factors such as age, immune status, viral load, clinical categories, viral resistance, potential adherence issues, drug toxicity, and comorbid conditions. Frequent laboratory studies and antiretroviral changes throughout the life of the individual are required.

Established protocols for the HIV-infected mother and her newborn are available on the clinicalinfo.hiv.gov website. The zidovudine prophylaxis protocol (or alternatives) for the HIV-exposed newborn from birth to 6 weeks old can be accessed at the clinicalinfo.hiv.gov and seen in Table 35.5. Ensure bloodwork is done before initiating prophylaxis. Discharge infants from the hospital with the full 6-week course of zidovudine on hand, not just a prescription, and complete administration instructions. This helps ensure greater compliance and prophylaxis continuity. In addition, infants with known HIV exposure whose status remains unknown or who are HIV infected should be prescribed trimethoprim-sulfamethoxazole (TMP-SMX) for prophylaxis against *P. jirovecii* starting at 4 to 6 weeks old and until the child is 1 year old (administered either on 3 consecutive days a week or daily). If the newborn is uninfected with HIV, the prophylaxis can be stopped. Treatment of associated conditions with appropriate medical therapy is indicated using immunoglobulin (IGIV), antifungals, antivirals, antimycobacterials, and nutritional counseling. After delivery, encourage mothers to continue their combination ART (cART), use a reliable method of birth control, and take precautions to prevent sexual transmission of the virus.

Treatment of a child (vs. newborn) infected with HIV also requires collaboration with pediatric HIV specialists because drug regimens are complex and are continually revised. Adolescents present a particular nonadherence risk because of denial and fear of their infection, substance abuse and addiction, misinformation, distrust of and inexperience with the medical system, self-esteem issues, unstable living situations, and/or lack of familial and social support systems. It is important for the PCP to be nonconfrontational yet discuss risk factors and advocate for family planning services and needle exchange programs, PEP regimens, and prompt involvement in new treatments as they become available.

An important role of the PCP in HIV treatment is helping to boost adherence rates. In addition, monitor for side effects closely because many antiretroviral drugs interact with other commonly prescribed medications (including oral contraceptives). The treatment regimens are highly challenging for parents because of complex dosing schedules and the potential unwillingness of children to take the medications. Many preparations are not offered in liquid form or the taste is not appealing to young children. See Chapter 23 for information about addressing and enhancing medication adherence rates in children and adolescents. Untreated HIV becomes a multisystemic illness with multiorgan complications.

Prevention and Reduction of Perinatal Transmission of Human Immunodeficiency Virus. The CDC, WHO, and United Nations AIDS agencies are useful resources for current treatment regimens; recommendations may vary by country. WHO strategies for preventing the transmission of HIV to women and from mother to child include:

- Improve access to ART for HIV-infected women and children. cART use to reduce perinatal HIV transmission is the accepted treatment standard in developed and underdeveloped countries. WHO recommends using a once-daily simplified triple antiretroviral drug regimen for all pregnant and breastfeeding women with HIV, with consideration of lifelong treatment.[30]
- Improve access to testing (<40% of people in United Nations Member States know their HIV status); encourage the use of self-testing kits for early diagnosis and treatment (one is approved by the FDA; others are under development).
- Increase safety education around the topics of blood, tissue, surgery, and injections.
- Expand maternal, newborn, and child health care (to initiate earlier treatment and prevention education).
- Expand sexual and reproductive health education.
- Strengthen infant nutrition support.
- Use cesarean delivery, if indicated.
- Increase the availability of chemoprophylaxis for the neonate and infant until HIV status is known.[30]

In the United States, guidelines for preventing transmission by HIV-infected women include discouraging breastfeeding, even if on cART. Delivery by cesarean is recommended, depending upon the mother's viral load. However, research in developing countries, notably South Africa, demonstrates that a combination of exclusive breastfeeding and cART use by the mother or infant significantly reduces the risk of breast milk HIV transmission. Protection against HIV infection increases if the infant is breastfed exclusively before 6 months with continued breastfeeding to 12 months. HIV-positive women who are treated with cART in developing countries are encouraged to breastfeed their infants.[30]

Because cART is now the standard treatment for HIV-infected pregnant women and their infants, adherence to the recommended postnatal HIV prophylaxis for both the mother and her infant is problematic. A meta-analysis demonstrated that only 73.5% of pregnant women achieved an 80% or greater adherence rate; this rate decreased in the postpartum period.[37] Reasons for the lack of adequate adherence were attributed to the following factors[38]:

- Concern about the safety of ART drugs on the fetus or woman.
- cART dosing frequency.
- Advanced AIDS stage and health-related symptoms of pregnancy (nausea, emesis, fatigue).
- Depression (especially postpartum).
- Physical, economic, and emotional stress.
- Presence of alcohol or drug abuse.
- Lack of social support.

Recent studies reinforced those of Buh and colleagues and found that other mental health issues, age, homelessness, poverty, inconsistent access to ART, and HIV stigma are associated with lower adherence, whereas trust and/or satisfaction with the HIV care provider are correlated with higher adherence.[39] in the United States.

The following is standard knowledge and practice for providers:

- Healthcare providers need to be alert to the potential risk of HIV transmission infection to infants in utero, in the postpartum period, and through human milk. Counsel caregivers against giving premasticated food to infants.
- Document routine HIV education and routine testing with the consent of all adolescents seeking prenatal care; ensure that each adolescent knows her HIV status and the methods available to prevent the acquisition and transmission of HIV to her newborn.
- At the time of delivery, provide education about HIV and complete rapid HIV testing, with consent, if HIV status is unknown.
- Women in the United States diagnosed with HIV infection just before labor or soon after delivery, or those who have known infection risks (e.g., injection drug users) but whose status is unknown at delivery should be advised against breastfeeding. If a woman desires to breastfeed, she can pump (and discard milk) until HIV testing is done and seronegative status is confirmed.
- There are no special precautions for handling expressed breast milk of HIV-infected women. No transmission to another infant has been reported after a single exposure to milk expressed by an HIV-infected mother. Pasteurization and donor screening ensure the safety of human milk banks. The nonprofit Human Milk Banking Association of North America sets standards of testing for all their members' milk banks.
- Counsel adolescents about the risk of HIV transmission (e.g., sexual transmission, needle or syringe sharing) and condom use. Condom use during last intercourse was reported by 53.8% of adolescents, whereas only 9.3% report ever having had an HIV test. Female rates are higher than males.[40]
- School attendance for HIV-infected children: The benefit from school attendance far outweighs the risks. Factors that must be considered include the risk to the immunosuppressed child from "normal germs" from healthy kids and school personnel. Because the casual transmission is unknown, there is no risk to other children if the infected child controls body secretions. Children who display biting behavior or have oozing wounds should be cared for in a setting that minimizes risk to others. The child's PCP is the only person with an absolute need to know the child's primary diagnosis. If the family decides to inform the school, those informed should maintain confidentiality. If the family chooses not to inform the school, parents should get assurance that the school will notify them of any communicable disease outbreaks (e.g., varicella, measles) or physical altercations with others.
- Routine screening of school-age children for HIV antibodies is not indicated.

Preexposure Prophylaxis for Certain High-Risk Individuals. Preexposure prophylaxis (PrEP) is now recommended in the United States and by the WHO for those at ongoing, substantial risk of being infected with HIV. Individuals who qualify for PrEP include those having male-to-male anal sex without a condom or with a diagnosed sexually transmitted disease in the past 6 months; those having sex with an HIV-positive partner; injection drug users who share equipment or who have been in a drug treatment program in the past 6 months; individuals not in a monogamous sexual relationship with partners who have not been recently tested and found to be HIV-negative; or heterosexual men or women who do not use condoms and have sex with high-risk partners (e.g., bisexual males, injection drug users). These risk factors result in HIV transmission rates from 62% to 92%. The clinical practice guideline for PrEP is available on the CDC website (https://www.cdc.gov/hiv/pdf/risk/prep/cdc-hiv-prep-guidelines-2021.pdf).[41] PrEP is recommended for adolescents (weighing at least 35 kg) with sexual or injection behaviors that increase the risk of HIV acquisition. Clinicians should balance risk versus benefit of initiating PrEP with persons under the age of legal adulthood as several studies demonstrate low adherence and persistence rates in adolescents and young adults prescribed PrEP. PCPs considering PrEP for minor persons should also review the laws and regulations regarding PrEP as they differ by jurisdiction.

Postexposure Prophylaxis After Nonoccupational Exposure.
The PCP may need to assess and counsel parents after their child has an accidental exposure (e.g., puncture wound from a needle, bite wound, blood exposure, or sexual abuse). Though transmission is extremely rare, the PCP needs to address the situation with a level of understanding of the risks and CDC recommendations.

All body fluids of an HIV-infected person do not carry the same viral load or risk. For example, exposure to the blood of a known HIV-infected person carries the highest risk, whereas blood-free saliva, semen or vaginal secretions, and human milk carry a low risk; urine, feces, and vomitus are unlikely to transmit the virus. Syringes that might have been used and discarded by an HIV-infected person generate the most parental concern. The following information is useful when counseling parents[30]:
- HIV viability is vulnerable to drying.
- The smaller the needle bore, the more limited the amount of blood present due to a lesser intralumen volume available, and therefore the lower the risk.
- There are no documented HIV transmission cases from an accidently found, discarded needle.
- There is a greater risk of biting an individual who is HIV-positive (saliva contaminated with HIV-infected blood) than from having been bitten by an HIV-positive person (saliva not contaminated with infected blood).

The PCP and parent must weigh the risks and benefits of participating in the PEP regimen against the significant toxicity of the drugs themselves. If instituted, PEP therapy ideally needs to start within 72 hours after exposure and continue for 28 days. Close follow-up for support, medication monitoring (adherence and toxicity), and serial HIV antibody screening are needed (Box 35.1). The CDC provides an algorithm for evaluating and treating possible nonoccupational exposure and makes recommendations as to whether PEP is warranted (http://www.cdc.gov/hiv).

Measles (Rubeola)

Measles (rubeola) is a morbillivirus in the Paramyxoviridae family, is similar to mumps and influenza, and causes serious pediatric illness. There is only one antigenic type. Measles has a characteristic rash, indicating viremia. Worldwide, approximately 20 million people annually are infected with measles with 146,000 deaths. In the United States, annual rates since 2000 ranged from 37 (in 2004) to 668 (in 2014); in 2018 there were 220 reported cases, and in 2021 there were 49 reported cases.[42] Most of the US cases originated in unvaccinated individuals who imported the measles after being in countries with large outbreaks (including, but not limited to England, France, Germany, India, the Philippines, Asia, and Africa). The disease spreads within communities where there

---

• BOX 35.1 **Management After Possible Exposure to Human Immunodeficiency Virus**

1. Treat the exposure site.
   - Wash wounds with soap and water; flush mucous membranes with water. Give Td or Tdap booster if appropriate (see Chapter 19).
2. Evaluate the exposure source if possible to guide need for postexposure prophylaxis.
   - Determine the human immunodeficiency virus (HIV) infection status of the exposure source. If unknown, testing with appropriate consent should be offered if possible.
3. Evaluate the exposed person.
   - Perform HIV serologic testing to identify current HIV infection and hepatitis B and hepatitis C serologic testing as appropriate.
   - Provide or refer for counseling to address stress and anxiety.
   - Discuss prevention of potential secondary HIV transmission.
   - Discuss prevention of repeat exposure, if appropriate.
   - Report the incident to legal or administrative authorities as appropriate to the setting of the exposure and the severity of the incident.
4. Consider postexposure prophylaxis (not to be used for frequent exposures).
   - Explain potential benefits and risks.
   - Discuss issues of drug toxicity and medication compliance.
   - Measure complete blood cell count, creatinine, and alanine transaminase concentration as baseline for possible drug toxicity.
   - Begin postexposure prophylaxis as soon as possible after exposure, preferably within 1 to 4 hours; prophylaxis begun more than 72 hours after exposure is unlikely to be effective.
   - Arrange for follow-up with HIV specialist and psychologist if appropriate.
   - Educate about prevention of secondary transmission (sexually active adolescent should avoid sex, or use condoms, until all follow-up test results are negative).
5. Choose therapy (should contain three [or more] antiretroviral drugs).
   - Consider drug potency and toxicity, regimen complexity and effects on compliance, and possibility of drug resistance in the exposure source.
   - Supply 3 to 5 days of medication immediately, instructing patients to obtain remainder of medication at follow-up visit (for total of 28 days).
6. Follow up.
   - Perform initial follow-up within 2 to 3 days to review drug regimen and adherence, evaluate for symptoms of drug toxicity, assess psychosocial status, and arrange appropriate referrals, if needed.
   - Ensure patient has enough medication to complete 28-day regimen.
   - Monitor for drug adverse effects at 4 weeks with complete blood cell count and alanine transaminase concentration.
   - Evaluate for psychological stress and medication compliance with weekly office visits or telephone calls.
   - Consider referral for counseling if needed.
   - Repeat HIV serologic testing at 6 weeks, 12 weeks, and 6 months after exposure.

From Havens PL, American Academy of Pediatrics Committee on Pediatric AIDS. Postexposure prophylaxis in children and adolescents for nonoccupational exposure to human immunodeficiency virus. *Pediatrics*. 2003;111(6):1475–1489, reaffirmed 2009; Kuhar DT, Henderson DK, Struble KA, et al. Updated US Public Health Service guidelines for the management of occupational exposures to human immunodeficiency virus and recommendations for postexposure prophylaxis. *Infect Control Hosp Epidemiol*. 2013;34(9):875–892; and Center for Disease Control and Prevention (CDC). Post-exposure Prophylaxis (PEP); 2018. https://www.cdc.gov/hiv/basics/pep.html.

are large numbers of unvaccinated or undervaccinated individuals and where herd immunity falls below a critical point.

Humans and primates are the only known infection reservoir. The sources of infection include respiratory secretions, blood, and urine of infected persons. Droplet contact, fomites, and, less likely, aerosol transmission transmit the virus. The peak incidence of infection in susceptible persons occurs during the late winter and spring months. Once exposed, approximately 90% of nonimmune individuals are infected.[42]

The incubation period for measles is 8 to 12 days, and as long as 21 days for modified measles. Modified measles illness presents in children who are passively immunized with immunoglobulin after disease exposure, have residual maternal antibodies, or received an improperly administered measles vaccine. In these cases, the illness is an abbreviated version of the typical disease. The prodrome period can last 1 to 2 days with normal to low-grade fever. URI symptoms are minimal to absent. Koplik spots usually do not appear. The rash is so mild that it is often missed.

A person is contagious 1 to 2 days before symptom onset (3–5 days before the rash) until 4 days after the rash appears, or roughly 14 days (range 7–18 days). There is no carrier state; disease or two vaccinations usually confer lifelong immunity.

Clinical Findings. The clinical manifestations include:
1. Incubation period: There are no specific symptoms.
2. Prodromal period: This first sign of the illness lasts 4 to 5 days and consists of URI symptoms, low to moderate fever (>101°F [38.3°C]), and cough, coryza, and conjunctivitis (the "three C's" of measles). Koplik spots may occur on the oral mucosa opposite the lower molars. They are small, irregular, bluish-white granules on an erythematous background, last 12 to 15 hours, and are pathognomonic of measles infection. They typically disappear 48 hours before the exanthem appears.
3. Rash stage: The rash of unmodified measles usually appears on the third or fourth day of the illness. As the rash appears, the temperature rises, often to 105°F (40.5°C). The rash is maculopapular and first appears behind the ears and on the forehead. Papules enlarge, coalesce, and move progressively downward, engulfing the face, neck, and arms over the next 24 hours. By the end of the second 24 hours, the rash spreads to the back, abdomen, and thighs. As the legs are involved, the face begins to clear. The entire process takes approximately 3 days. Respiratory symptoms are most severe on day 3 of the rash. The more severe the rash, the more severe the illness. It can become hemorrhagic, and this can be fatal because of disseminated intravascular coagulation (DIC). Photophobia generally occurs when the rash begins to spread and worsens. The rash begins to fade after the fourth day. The disease peaks; defervescence occurs. After the rash clears, a residual desquamating light-colored pigmentation occurs, lasting approximately 1 week.

Diagnostic Studies. The single measles IgM antibody level is useful if drawn when symptoms appear; the reactivity is low after more than 30 days. Disease confirmation occurs via viral isolation from urine, blood, throat, or nasopharyngeal secretions, or from serial IgG antibody titers that compare acute and convalescent serum specimens. Measles is a US reportable disease within 24 hours of diagnosis.

Differential Diagnosis and Management. Any viral rash, toxoplasmosis, scarlet fever, Kawasaki syndrome, meningococcemia, Rocky Mountain spotted fever (RMSF), drug rashes, and serum sickness are included in the differential diagnosis.

Treatment is supportive and includes antipyretics, bed rest, adequate hydration, air humidification, and a warm darkened room if photophobia is present. No antiviral therapy is available, although ribavirin has been used off-label to treat severe measles infections and in children who are immunocompromised.[11] Bacterial superinfections (e.g., ear infections, bronchopneumonia,

and encephalitis) are treated with appropriate antibiotics. Manage all children with encephalitis, severe pneumonia, or compromised immune systems in consultation with an infectious disease expert.

Children in the United States and in countries where malnutrition is an issue are at greater risk for measles morbidity or mortality. These children, and those with severe measles, have lower vitamin A levels. The WHO recommends vitamin A for all children with measles regardless of country of residence. Dose once daily for 2 days: under 6 months old, 50,000 international units; 6 through 11 months old, 100,000 international units; 12 months old or older, 200,000 international units.

Care of Exposed Individuals. Administer the measles vaccine within 72 hours of exposure to those who are vaccine eligible. This is the first choice to prevent or modify the infection and may be given to infants 6 to 11 months old. Immune globulin (IVIG) given within 6 days of exposure prevents or modifies the disease in those susceptible such as those without prior measles vaccine, infants younger than 12 months old, pregnant women, and immunocompromised individuals regardless of their measles vaccination status.

Complications. Bacterial superinfection and viral complications manifest as a URI, obstructive laryngitis, otitis, diarrhea, mastoiditis, cervical adenitis, bronchitis, transient hepatitis, and pneumonia, which is the largest cause of death in infants. The causative organism is the measles virus itself or group A beta-hemolytic streptococci (GABHS), pneumococci, *H. influenzae*, or *S. aureus*. Infection can exacerbate underlying tuberculosis (TB). Other complications include myocarditis, purpura fulminans ("black measles") characterized by multiorgan bleeding, encephalitis and other neurologic sequelae, and subacute sclerosing panencephalitis, a fatal complication of wild-type measles. There are usually no complications with modified measles.

Mumps

Mumps is an acute generalized viral disease with painful enlargement of one or more salivary glands, usually the parotid glands. Mumps is in the Paramyxoviridae family. There is only one serotype and humans are the only natural reservoir. The source of infection is contact with the saliva and/or respiratory tract secretions of infected persons. There has been an increase in mumps cases with peak years in 2006, 2016, 2017 (>6000 cases), and 2019 (>3000 cases).[43] Most cases were young adults and college-aged youth and those who had not received two doses of the MMR vaccine. Infection occurs during all seasons but is most common during late winter and spring, and in children younger than 10 years; it affects both sexes equally. Mumps virus crosses the placenta; studies are inconsistent in determining whether infection during the first trimester increases the risk of spontaneous abortion or intrauterine fetal demise. There are demonstrated fetal malformations after prenatal mumps exposure.[11]

The incubation period ranges from 12 to 25 days (usually 16–18 days). Disease communicability is about 1 to 2 days before glandular swelling and up to 5 days after the swelling onset. Some patients are asymptomatic, but the incidence is unknown. Lifelong immunity is usually conferred after one infection; rarely is a second infection seen.

Clinical Findings. There are two clinical stages:
1. *Prodromal stage:* Rare in children but can cause fever, headache, anorexia, neck or other muscular pain, and malaise.
2. *Swelling stage:* Approximately 24 hours after the prodromal stage, 31% to 65% of those affected have painful edema of one or both parotid glands. If both glands are affected, one

generally swells before the other. The gland fills the space between the posterior border of the mandible and mastoid, pushing downward and forward to the zygoma. The ear pushes forward and upward. Edema lasts a few hours to a few days. The enlarged glands usually return to normal size in 3 to 7 days. Rarely, a maculopapular, truncal, pink discrete rash is seen. Pain on the affected side can be elicited by having the patient eat something sour. This is known as the "pickle sign." The Stensen duct is red and swollen.

The Wharton duct is frequently edematous. Fever is usually moderate; 20% are afebrile. Ten percent to 15% of cases involve only the submandibular glands. Submandibular infection is not typically painful; however, the erythema subsides slower. If sublingual salivary glands are involved, there is bilateral edema in the submental region on the floor of the mouth. Edema caused by lymphatic obstruction of the manubrium and upper chest is reported. Orchitis may occur in individuals who contract mumps after puberty.

Diagnostic Studies. This virus is detectable from a buccal swab of Stenson duct exudate, throat washings, saliva, or spinal fluid using RT-qPCR and serologic tests such as mumps-specific IgM antibodies or serial acute/convalescent titers for IgG antibodies. Leukopenia with relative lymphocytosis and an elevated amylase are typical.[11]

Differential Diagnosis, Management, and Complications. Cervical or preauricular lymphadenitis, CMV, HIV, enteroviruses, tumor, suppurative parotitis bacterial (e.g., nontuberculous mycobacterium) or viral (influenza A, coxsackievirus, parainfluenza 1 and 3, EBV) infection, idiopathic recurrent parotitis, parotid ductal obstruction, Mikulicz syndrome, uveoparotid fever, and cancer (especially lymphosarcoma) are included in the differential diagnosis.

Treatment is supportive (antipyretics, bed rest as needed, diet appropriate for chewing discomfort). Corticosteroids or nonsteroidal antiinflammatory drugs (NSAIDs) manage arthritic complications. Manage orchitis with bed rest and scrotal elevation. School and daycare students should be kept home until 9 days after the onset of parotid edema. Use active and passive immunization.

Complications include meningoencephalitis (mostly males older than 20 years), orchitis and/or epididymitis (10% incidence in postpubertal males; sterility is rare), oophoritis (in postpubertal females; fertility is not affected), pancreatitis (rare), thyroiditis (uncommon), myocarditis, deafness (transient or permanent), arthritis (rare), thrombocytopenia, hemolytic anemia (usually self-limited), mastitis, and glomerulonephritis.

Erythema Infectiosum

Erythema infectiosum, or fifth disease, is caused by parvovirus B19. This virus is a member of the Parvoviridae family and is a single-stranded DNA virus that replicates in erythrocyte precursors. It is called *fifth disease* because it was the fifth childhood eruptive rash described historically. These rashes include measles, scarlet fever, rubella, Filatov-Dukes disease, erythema infectiosum, and erythema subitum (roseola infantum, sixth disease). Humans are the only reservoir. Erythema infectiosum is spread via vertical transmission from mother to fetus, by respiratory tract secretions, and percutaneous exposure to blood or blood products. Distribution is worldwide. It is a childhood disease with the highest prevalence in 5- to 15-year-olds, but 5% to 10% of young children, 50% of young adults, and 90% of the elderly population are seropositive. Secondary spread to household contacts is up to 50%.[11] The disease occurs most commonly in late winter and early spring.

The incubation period is approximately 4 to 21 days; the rash and symptoms occur between 2 and 3 weeks after exposure. The highest period of communicability is before the rash, joint pain, or edema (the latter two seen are rare). Chronic infection occurs in those immunocompromised or with most types of hemolytic anemias.

Clinical Findings. The following two phases are seen in erythema infectiosum:
1. *Prodrome:* Consists of mild fever (15–30% of cases), myalgia, headache, malaise, and/or URI symptoms.
2. *Rash:* Appears 7 to 10 days after the prodromal stage and occurs in three stages: it first appears on the face as an intense red eruption on the cheeks (slapped cheek) with circumoral pallor that lasts 1 to 4 days. Next, a lacy maculopapular eruption appears on the trunk and moves peripherally to the arms, thighs, and buttocks. Palms and soles are generally spared. This phase lasts a month. Finally, the rash subsides. Older children may have mild pruritus. There may be periodic recurrences precipitated by trauma, heat, exercise, stress, sunlight, or cold (Fig. 35.4). Children less commonly experience arthralgia (more often in the knees) than adults, who may complain of symmetric polyarthropathy. Arthralgia most commonly resolves in 2 to 4 weeks. Those with hemolytic anemias or who are immunocompromised may have fever, pallor, tachycardia, and symptoms of heart failure.

Diagnostic Studies. Laboratory testing is not generally indicated because it is a clinical diagnosis. Serum B19–specific IgM antibody confirms the presence of infection and persists for 6 to 8 weeks. Anti-B19 IgG confirms past infection. For immunocompromised individuals, PCR assay is the method of choice. Standard cultures are not useful.

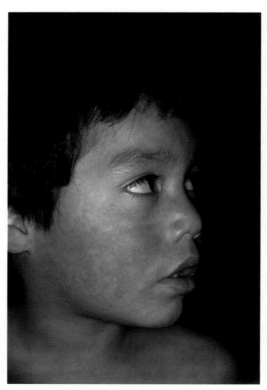

• **Fig. 35.4** Erythema Infectiosum (Fifth Disease).

Differential Diagnosis, Management, and Complications. This is not a difficult disease to diagnose. The differential diagnoses include rubella, enterovirus disease, lupus, atypical measles, and drug rashes.

There is no specific antiviral treatment. Consider transfusion for those with hemolytic anemia or who are immunocompromised. IGIV helps those with immunocompromised conditions. Because there is widespread undetected infection in children and adults, avoidance of known exposure can reduce, but not eliminate, the risk of infection. Children in the rash stage are not contagious and may attend school.

Complications are few and typically not significant in healthy patients; recovery is usually without sequelae. The most frequently reported complications include arthritis (hands, wrists, knees, and/or ankles occurring 2 to 3 weeks after onset of initial symptoms); chronic infection in those immunodeficient; aplastic crisis (more common in those with chronic hemolytic anemias, including sickle cell anemia, thalassemia, hereditary spherocytosis, or other types of chronic hemolysis); thrombocytopenic purpura or neutropenia; myocarditis (rare); papular-purpuric "gloves and socks" syndrome (fever, pruritus, purpura, painful edema, and erythema with a glove-and-sock distribution) followed by petechiae and oral lesions; or fetal hydrops, death, or intrauterine growth retardation if exposed in utero (no reports of congenital anomalies).[44] It is not recommended that pregnant women be excluded from the workplace if there is an outbreak of the parvovirus B19 virus occurring. The American College of Obstetricians and Gynecologists recommends serologic testing to determine susceptibility and evidence of an acute infection for pregnant women exposed to parvovirus B19 infection. Pregnant women with a verified acute parvovirus infection should be monitored closely by their obstetrician.[11] The fetus exposed to the parvovirus B19 virus in utero may develop severe anemia or miscarriage and stillbirth are possible, although this occurs only in 5% of pregnant women who contract the virus and complications are more common in the first trimester.[45]

Parainfluenza Virus

Human parainfluenza virus (hPIV), a paramyxovirus, is similar to influenza and mumps viruses and is an important cause of laryngotracheobronchitis (croup), bronchitis, bronchiolitis, and pneumonia. A small number of parainfluenza cases exacerbate the clinical manifestations of asthma and chronic lung disease, and reinfections occur.[11]

There are four antigenic hPIV types. Types 1 and 2 usually infect children 1 to 5 years old and are usually associated with croup. Outbreaks occur more in summer and fall and in biannual patterns; reinfections occur at any age. Type 3 is endemic, associated more with bronchitis, bronchiolitis, and pneumonia in those younger than 12 months old, results in shorter immunity (a particular problem for immunocompromised patients), and outbreaks peak in the spring and summer (sometimes into fall months). Type 4 infections are less pathologically and clinically understood, may occur year-round, and cause mild to severe respiratory illness. By the time most children are 5 years old, they have been exposed to all hPIV types. An individual typically has repeated infections due to hPIV's immunity is transient and limited.

This virus spreads by direct person-to-person contact through infected nasopharyngeal secretions or from fomite contamination. It replicates in the superficial ciliated epithelial lining the airways of the upper and lower respiratory tract and spreads readily. The incubation period is 2 to 6 days. Healthy children shed virus for 4 to 7 days before symptom onset and up to 7 to 21 days after resolution of symptoms. The virus lives on nonporous surfaces for up to 10 hours.[11]

Clinical Findings. Symptoms may include an acute onset of mild fever, pharyngitis, rhinitis, hoarseness, and cough (including a typical "croup" cough). Lower respiratory involvement symptoms include dyspnea, crackles, wheezing, and hyperaeration. In older children and adolescents, the recurrent infection may manifest as a mild URI.

Diagnostic Studies. Routine testing is not needed. Specific RT-PCR assays are the standard diagnostic test when needed. The virus can be isolated from nasopharyngeal secretions; culture results are usually available within 4 to 7 days (or earlier). Sensitivities vary when rapid antigen identification is performed by IFAs and EIAs. WBC count may be normal or slightly elevated with a mild lymphocyte elevation.

Differential Diagnosis, Management, and Complications. The differential diagnosis includes other viral URIs, allergic croup, laryngotracheitis, bacterial tracheitis, retropharyngeal abscess, epiglottitis, laryngeal diphtheria, foreign body aspiration, or GI reflux.

The treatment is supportive; recovery is uncomplicated in most cases. Reliable studies using ribavirin are lacking; therefore aerosolized ribavirin should only be considered for high-risk patients with severe lower respiratory involvement.[11] With the newer outpatient guidelines for managing croup, few children need hospitalization (see Chapter 32). Use antibiotics when a patient has severe symptoms and a secondary bacterial invasion is suspected (e.g., otitis media, bronchitis, tracheitis, pneumonia). No vaccine is available; intravenous immune globulin is not helpful. Good hand hygiene is important. Complications are infrequent. Immunocompromised individuals are more prone to developing secondary bacterial infections.

Rubella (German or 3-Day Measles)

Rubella is an acute disease caused by an RNA virus of the genus *Rubivirus*, in the Togaviridae family. Humans are the only reservoir; and before widespread use of the rubella vaccine, the disease most commonly occurred in susceptible children. Peak incidence occurred late winter, or early spring with epidemics cycling every 6 to 9 years.[11] Recent outbreaks have occurred outside the United States or in individuals who were underimmunized. The incidence of rubella has decreased by 99% since the introduction of the vaccine.[11] The infection spreads through nasopharyngeal secretions or transplacentally during either apparent or silent infection. It is worldwide in distribution. The virus has been isolated in the blood, breast milk, conjunctival sac, and urine of infected individuals.

One must have prolonged and repeated contact to become infected. The incubation period is 12 to 23 days (mean 17 days). The maximum period of viral shedding (and presumed transmissibility) is believed to be 5 days before to 6 days after the rash appears. Genetic factors may play a role in transmissibility. Infants infected in utero can shed the virus up to 12 months of age.[11] In the United States, disease occurs during late winter and early spring. There is lifelong immunity after naturally occurring disease; however, asymptomatic reinfection can occur in rare situations. Because illness without rash exists, the actual number of reinfections is unknown. Reinfection occurs from wild-type viruses and in those previously immunized.

Routine rubella vaccine uses virtually eliminated endemic rubella infections in the United States and other countries with national immunization programs. Most cases in the United States now occur in those unvaccinated (including infants born to unvaccinated mothers), foreign-born, or immigrants from areas with poor vaccination coverage. Endemic rubella rates have increased and congenital rubella remains high in the Western Pacific, Southeast Asia, and some African regions where vaccination programs are not universal.[11]

If primary maternal rubella infection occurs during the first 12 weeks of pregnancy, there is an estimated 61% risk of congenital defects (ophthalmologic, cardiac, auditory, or neurologic); the risk is 26% if maternal infection occurs in the second trimester. In pregnant women, reinfection rarely results in congenital rubella syndrome. Accidental revaccination of a pregnant woman alone is not a reason for pregnancy termination; surveillance demonstrates signs of infection in the infant but not congenital rubella syndrome.[11]

Clinical Findings. Approximately 25% to 50% of infections are subclinical.[11] Postnatal disease is marked by three stages:

1. *Prodrome:* The mild symptoms of fever (101.5°F [38.6°C]), lower GI upset, pharyngitis, eye pain, arthralgia, malaise, and headache occur about 1 to 5 days before the onset of stage 3 and are occasionally missed.
2. *Lymphadenopathy:* Usually begins within 24 hours but can begin as early as 7 days before the rash appears and lasts for more than 1 week. The postauricular, posterior cervical, and posterior occipital are the primary lymph nodes involved. There is generalized lymph node involvement and at times splenomegaly is noted.
3. *Rash:* An enanthem (known as *Forchheimer spots*) may appear before the general rash, consisting of small rose-colored to reddish spots on the soft palate, but is not pathognomonic. The rubella rash (discrete maculopapules that occasionally coalesce) is often the first obvious sign of illness, typically begins on the face, fades before it spreads to the chest and caudally during the next 24 hours, and usually resolves by the third day. It may be pruritic without a rash or a fine, bran-like desquamation. A low-grade fever may occur during the eruptive phase and continues for up to 3 days. There is no photophobia; anorexia, headache, and malaise are rare. Exanthems occur less often in adolescents and young adults; they may have more pruritus. A facial acneiform rash is more common in adolescents. Paresthesia and tendonitis may be present.[11]

Diagnostic Studies. Diagnosis is usually made by clinical symptoms. Real-time RT-PCR and RT-PCR of nasal or throat (preferred) specimens detect the virus. Serologic testing for disease confirmation or immunity includes EIAs and latex agglutination tests for rubella IgG and IgM antibodies. However, timing is everything; IgM may not be detectable before the fifth day after the rash appears. If the test is conducted earlier and yields negative results, it should be repeated after day 5. To detect IgG antibodies, the specimen should be obtained as soon after symptom onset as possible, and then repeated in 7 to 21 days. IgG antibody levels determine immune status due to natural infection or vaccination. False-positive rubella IgM tests can occur due to the presence of rheumatoid factors or other viral infections. Leukopenia is common.

Differential Diagnosis, Management, and Complications. The disease is difficult to diagnose unless there is an epidemic. The rash is similar to scarlet fever, mononucleosis, enterovirus, roseola, rubeola, erythema infectiosum, EBV, toxoplasmosis, Kawasaki disease, serum sickness, and drug eruptions.

Treatment is supportive (e.g., antipyretics for fever control) unless complications occur. Children with rubella should be kept at home for approximately 1 week after the rash erupts. Use active and passive immunization.

Complications of postnatal rubella are uncommon. These include arthralgia, arthritis, thrombocytopenia, and encephalitis. Arthralgia/arthritis (fingers, knees, wrists) occurs in postpubertal youth with females afflicted more often than males. Onset is about a week after the appearance of the rash and symptoms last 3 to 28 days. Thrombocytopenia or encephalitis can occur within 4 days of the onset of the rash. Manage severe thrombocytopenic purpura with corticosteroid therapy and platelet transfusions. Myocarditis, pericarditis, follicular conjunctivitis, hemolytic anemia, and hepatitis are rare.

Mosquito-Borne Viruses

Zika Virus

Zika is a member of the Flaviviridae family of viruses and is spread by the bite of the infected Aedes mosquito. It is transmitted through sexual encounters, passed from a pregnant woman to her fetus, and through blood transfusions, although this has not been reported in the United States. The virus may impact the growing fetus's brain resulting in microcephaly or other defects. Since 2018 there were no reported local mosquito-borne Zika virus transmissions in the United States; however, the virus is an international threat. A map describing the risk of Zika is available for review before travel.[46]

Clinical Findings. Persons infected with the Zika virus have either asymptomatic or have mild symptoms such as low-grade fever, rash, headache, arthralgia, conjunctivitis, and myalgia that last several days to a week. Current CDC research suggests that Guillain-Barré syndrome is linked with Zika virus; however, only a small proportion of persons with the disease are impacted. Infection is likely protective against future infections.

Diagnostic Studies. The virus' RNA is detectable in blood and urine early in the course of the disease or when individuals are symptomatic. Zika testing is recommended only if patients are symptomatic and traveled to or live in a Zika risk area or had unprotected sex with a partner who lives in or traveled to a Zika risk area. Test pregnant women who are asymptomatic but have ongoing exposure by living or traveling to high-risk areas or who have an abnormal ultrasound.[46]

Differential Diagnosis, Management, and Complications. Mild viral or influenza infection, GI viral infection, and other mosquito-borne diseases are included in the differential diagnosis for mild disease. For these mild cases, supportive treatment is indicated: rest, fever control with acetaminophen, hydration, and nausea/vomiting control. Hospitalization is indicated for those with symptoms of meningitis, encephalitis, severe muscle weakness, paralysis, or dysphagia.

Patient and Family Education. To prevent disease, avoid mosquito bites. Institute mosquito community abatement programs to reduce mosquito breeding grounds. Counseling includes:

- Stay indoors during the mosquitoes' most active times—dawn and dusk; if you must be outdoors during these times, wear light-colored, long-sleeved shirts, and long pants.
- Apply insect repellent with either N,N-diethyl-3-methylbenzamide (DEET), picaridin 5% to 10%, oil of lemon eucalyptus, or soybean oil to exposed skin (permethrin and DEET can be applied to clothing). DEET concentration depends on the time length of expected mosquito or tick exposure: 10% DEET confers approximately 2 hours of protection; 30% about 5 hours. Children over 6 months old may use a concentration of no more than 30% DEET. Apply according to the length of protection needed. Use sparingly and wash DEET off with soap and water when the child is inside.[5]

infects humans. Poorer tropical and subtropical areas of the world experience malaria in epidemic proportions. In the United States, infection is typically acquired from travel or residence abroad, although anopheline mosquitoes are present in temperate regions of the country. Globally, an estimated 198 million cases of malaria were identified in 2013; 500,000 people died of malaria, mostly children in the African region.[53] Infection relapses occur because of dormant liver-stage parasites (hypnozoite) or chronic asymptomatic parasitemia.

Malaria presents as a febrile nonspecific illness without localizing signs from 7 to 30 days after exposure. Malaria should be suspected in a person with a fever who recently traveled to an endemic area. Symptoms typically include high fever with chills, rigor, sweats, and headache, and may appear suddenly and in a 2- to 3-day cyclic pattern. Nausea, emesis, diarrhea, cough, pallor, jaundice, tachypnea, arthralgia, myalgia, abdominal and back pain, and hepatosplenomegaly may occur. The disease progresses in severity and ends in death because of neurologic compromise, renal and respiratory failure, metabolic acidosis, severe anemia, or vascular collapse and shock.

Diagnostic studies may show anemia, thrombocytopenia, elevated bilirubin, and aminotransferases. Diagnosis is confirmed by identifying the parasite microscopically. Negative smears should be retested every 12 to 24 hours during a 72-hour period. PCR, DNA probes, and RNA testing are also used. A rapid test for antigen detection is available.

The choice of treatment is dependent upon the identified species, patterns of drug resistance, and disease severity. Assistance with diagnosis and management is available from the 24-hour CDC Malaria Hotline (770-488-7788). Vaccines and new drugs to combat malaria are under development and in clinical trials.

In malaria-epidemic regions, treatment and preventive efforts involve four measures: (1) case management (diagnosis and treatment), (2) insecticide-treated nets, (3) intermittent preventive treatment of malaria in pregnant women and infants, and (4) indoor residual spraying (IRS). Larval and other vector control, mass drug administration, and mass fever treatment may also be used (see WHO in Additional Resources). The CDC offers useful information regarding traveler risk assessment, antimalarial drug prophylaxis selection for children and adults, a malaria country map, and preventive measures.

Tick-Borne Diseases

Lyme disease (LD), ehrlichiosis, anaplasmosis, Rocky Mountain Spotted Fever (RMSF), tick-borne relapsing fever, babesiosis, tularemia, and African tick bite fever are common tick-borne diseases in the United States. It is important for providers to know the specific tick vectors and vector epidemic geographic areas. Only the first three diseases are discussed here (tularemia is a potential bioterrorism agent). PCPs should be suspicious of and include tick-borne diseases in the differential diagnosis for individuals with influenza-like symptoms (fever, headache, myalgia) during summer (an unusual time for such symptoms), especially if they live and recreate outdoors in endemic areas.

Lyme Disease

Borrelia burgdorferi (Bb), a spirochete, is the causative agent that is transmitted to humans by infected species of *Ixodes* ticks. LD is the most reported vector-borne infection in the United States and Europe. In 2017 in the United States, there were 29,515 confirmed cases with a real concern for significant 10-fold underreporting.[11]

The ticks infected with *Bb* in the United States are predominantly found in the northeast (80% of cases), the mid-Atlantic states, Wisconsin, Minnesota, and Northern California. LD is also endemic in Europe, Scandinavian countries, Mongolia, Eastern Canada, China, Japan, and states of the former Soviet Union.[11] When eastern black-legged deer tick (*Ixodes scapularis*) or western black-legged deer tick (*Ixodes pacificus*) larvae hatch in early summer, they are usually not infected. During their life cycle (nymphal and adult molt stages), the tick feeds on an infected host and becomes infected with *Bb*. In the east, the natural host for *Bb* is the white-footed mouse or deer; in the west, it is the western gray squirrel or western fence lizards, chipmunks, and some bird species (they are poor reservoirs). Tick vectors in Europe include ground-feeding birds and small to medium-sized mammals. The infected tick transmits the organism to humans, more commonly by immature ticks in the nymphal stage. The size of the tick in the nymphal stage is about 1 mm (poppy seed size); in the adult stages from 2.5 to 4 mm (sesame seed size).

There is a varied risk of transmission, depending on the percentage of ticks infected with *Bb*. Coinfection with other tick-borne pathogens must be considered in endemic regions. The risk of human infection after an *Ixodes* tick bite is low, even in endemic areas, and is related to how long the tick feeds. It takes hours for the tick to fully implant its mouth into the host's skin and days to become fully engorged. Many human victims remove the tick before transmission. A high-risk tick bite is identified as an engorged tick that has fed for >72 hours and a low-risk tick bite is defined as having a brief attachment of the tick for <36 hours. It is not recommended to test the tick for spirochete infection, this will yield poor prediction values. Chemoprophylaxis should be considered when the benefits outweigh the risks. Benefits to the prophylaxis occur when the tick is engorged and attached for at least 36 hours and chemoprophylaxis can be initiated as late as 72 hours after the tick removal.[11] The disease is not teratogenic as long as the mother receives the appropriate antibiotic treatment. Most infections occur from June to August and from December through March. The incubation period in the United States begins with the time of the tick bite to the appearance of single or multiple erythema migrans (EM) lesions from 3 to 32 days with a median time of 11 days.[11] There is concern that the current epidemiology statistics for LD in children are inaccurate or incomplete due to the COVID-19 disease.[54]

Clinical Findings. LD presents a variety of symptoms. Classic LD has three stages:

1. *Stage 1 (early localized disease):* In general, within days to weeks after the bite, the classic rash appears at the inoculation site known as *EM*. The EM rash begins as a red, annular macule or papule surrounded by a clear ring and then a larger annular erythematous outer ring. It may appear as a "bull's eye" and needs to be at least 5 cm in size to meet the diagnostic criteria for EM (Fig. 35.5). Multiple lesions may occur in different sites; however, 10% of children do not demonstrate EM. EM typically is painless, warm, and nonpruritic. The rash remains for a few weeks and fades even if untreated. In many cases, the rash does not follow this classic pattern and can be confused with cellulitis; the rapid enlargement of EM assists in distinguishing it. Symptoms that accompany EM include fever, malaise, headache, arthralgia, myalgia, and mild nuchal rigidity.[11] Without treatment, these symptoms, including the rash, become intermittent, lasting for weeks to months.
2. *Stage 2 (early disseminated disease):* Through spirochetemia, the organism disseminates through hematologic or lymphatic

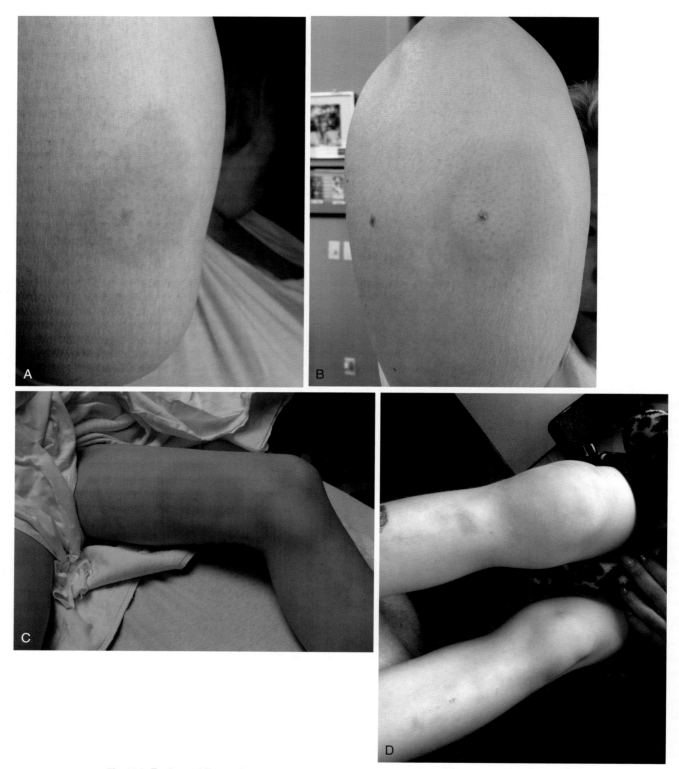

• **Fig. 35.5** Erythema Migrans/Lyme Disease. (A) This 2- to 3-cm lesion is just starting to clear centrally. (B) The central clearing is nearly complete 1 day later, and within the erythematous border, the puncta of a tick bite is evident. (C) Multiple annular lesions of differing sizes and varying degrees of central clearing are seen in this child with Lyme disease. (D) Lyme arthritis is noted in this boy with late onset Lyme disease with a large swollen knee joint without erythema. (From Zitelli BJ, McIntire SC, Nowalk, AJ, et al. *Zitelli and Davis' Atlas of Pediatric Physical Diagnosis*. 8th ed. Elsevier; 2023.)

channels. Multiple secondary annular lesions (1–3 cm) appear that are morphologically similar to, but smaller than, the EM lesion. Symptoms in children with the disseminated disease with or without lesions present with cranial nerve palsies (most common is cranial nerve VII), lymphocytic meningitis, radiculitis, carditis with life-threatening arrhythmias (first, second, and third degree atrioventricular block), and generalized illness (stomachaches, urinary symptoms, migratory musculoskeletal pains). Stage 2 lasts from weeks to 2 years without treatment. Most of the symptoms (including the rash) wax and wane during this time.[11]

3. *Stage 3 (late disease):* Children treated with antibiotic therapy in the early stages do not generally develop the late stage 3 manifestations (late disease). Stage 3 occurs in children that are not treated in stages 1 and 2 and generally manifests as arthritis affecting the large joints, most commonly the knees, cognitive and memory loss, and paresthesia of the hands and feet. Concrete evidence of Lyme arthritis includes the presence of WBCs in the synovial fluid. Untreated, arthritis initially resolves in a few weeks but becomes recurrent and chronic. Adolescents experience more severe arthritis for longer periods of time.[11] Untreated, a late manifestation of the disease appears months to years after the initial infection.

Diagnostic Studies. LD is best diagnosed by clinical and epidemiologic history and physical findings. The presence of EM and plausible geographic exposure is diagnostic; no serologic test is necessary. If the PCP suspects LD without EM, they should keep in mind several factors: first, serologic tests for IgM antibodies become positive 2 to 4 weeks (4–6 weeks for IgG) after a bite. False-positive results are not uncommon and IgM antibodies should not be routinely used for screening. Finally, serologically positive results may indicate prior infection rather than present acute infection because IgM antibodies do not decline until 4 to 6 months after disease onset, and IgG antibodies can remain elevated for several years.[11]

LD requires a two-step approach to diagnostic serologic testing. The first step is EIA (ELISA) or immunofluorescent antibody test. If the results are negative, the second step is not needed. If the first test results are equivocal or positive, a second test using an IgM and IgG Western blot for *Bb* antibodies is done for an individual with symptoms less than 30 days. If symptoms are present for more than 30 days, an IgG Western blot test alone is performed. A positive Western blot test is interpreted as reacting with 5 to 10 scored bands on the IgG assay and 2 to 3 on the IgM assay. The number of bands necessary for the confirmation of LD is controversial. The ELISA produces many false positives because of cross-reactions with other spirochetes, lupus, and varicella organisms. After 4 weeks of symptoms, the IgG result should only be used to support the diagnosis. PCR assay testing is not yet approved for diagnosing LD.[54]

Differential Diagnosis, Management, and Complications. The rash, if present, mimics eczema, tinea, granuloma annulare, cellulitis, or an insect bite. Other differential diagnoses include osteomyelitis, WNV, parvovirus B19, relapsing fever, syphilis, leptospirosis, *Mycoplasma*, septic arthritis, infectious hepatitis, nonresponsive lymphadenopathy, meningitis, multiple sclerosis, amyotrophic lateral sclerosis, juvenile arthritis, Bell palsy, other spirochete-caused diseases, thyroid disease, heavy metal toxicity, and vasculitis. Primary psychiatric disorders should be considered in recalcitrant cases after appropriate Lyme treatment.

Clinical judgment determines clinical management. The earlier in the EM stage that treatment starts, the better the long-term outcome. In suspicious LD cases, delaying treatment until laboratory results are known decreases the chances of successful disease treatment. Antibiotic therapy is not recommended for nonspecific symptoms or asymptomatic seropositivity. The provider should study the literature from the CDC and IDSA or consult with an infectious disease specialist if uncertain about how to proceed.

Give prophylactic doxycycline, amoxicillin, or cefuroxime in children when the history includes the following[11]:

- Tick bite only: The tick is reliably identified as a nymph or adult *I. scapularis* species (providers in endemic areas should have expertise identifying, and most commercial and public health laboratories in endemic areas can make this determination), the tick was attached for at least 36 to 72 hours (as indicated by engorgement size or known exposure time), *and* the tick was acquired in an endemic area. For treatment, see drugs and dosages under early, localized disease or EM.
- Early localized disease (stage 1) or EM usually resolves within several days of starting treatment. The current recommended drugs and dosages are as follows:
  - Children with EM (single or multiple) and for any age: Doxycycline 4.4 mg/kg per day, orally, divided BID, max dose of 200 mg/day for 10 days, *or*
  - Amoxicillin 50 mg/kg per day, orally, divided TID, max dose of 1.5 g/day, for 14 days, *or*
  - Patient unable to take beta-lactam or doxycycline, azithromycin 10 mg/kg per day, orally, daily for 7 days
    - Isolated facial palsy for any age: Doxycycline 4.4 mg/kg per day, orally, divided into 2 doses (max 2 g/day) for 14 days
    - Arthritis: An oral agent as for early localized disease for 28 days; patients younger than 8 years of age should be treated with an oral antimicrobial other than doxycycline. There is limited data on the use of doxycycline for >21 days in children <8 years of age. For patients 8 years and older, all oral options listed earlier can be used, including doxycycline.
    - Persistent arthritis after first course of therapy: Retreat using an oral agent as for first-episode arthritis for 28 days, *or*
    - Ceftriaxone sodium 50 to 75 mg/kg, IV, once per day for 14 to 28 days
    - Atrioventricular heart block or carditis: An oral agent as for early localized disease for 14 to 21 days, *or*
    - Ceftriaxone sodium 50 to 75 mg/kg, IV, once per day (max dose of 2 g/day for 14 to 21 days for a hospitalized patient; oral therapy (using an agent from early localized disease) can be substituted when the patient is stabilized or discharged, to complete the 14- to 21-day course
    - Meningitis: Doxycycline 4.4 mg/kg per day, orally, divided into 1 or 2 doses (maximum dose of 200 mg/day) for 14 days, *or*
    - Ceftriaxone sodium 50 to 75 mg/kg, IV, once per day (maximum dose of 2 g/day) for 14 days[11]
- Early or late disseminated disease: Practice guidelines were developed for the assessment, treatment, and prevention of LD. The guidelines are published by the IDSA. Care of children should follow the earlier treatment recommendations. A consult with a LD specialist should be considered.
- Persistent posttreatment symptoms: A small number of patients diagnosed with LD have prolonged symptoms despite following the guidelines for the treatment of LD. Some providers speculate that this is a chronic form of infection with

its own diagnostic criteria and treatment approaches. In children, lingering fatigue, musculoskeletal pain, or cognitive or short-term memory difficulties occur and may be caused by persistent immune-mediated inflammation rather than continued *Bb* infection. A child with chronic symptoms whose family attributes them to LD should be questioned about prior treatment adherence, reevaluated for reinfection, and referred to appropriate specialists as indicated by symptomatology. A positive serologic finding without other symptoms of clinical disease does not warrant the use of antibiotics.[11]

Complications include Lyme meningitis, myocarditis, myopericarditis, left ventricular dysfunction, or cardiomegaly. Other tick-borne diseases are cotransmitted with LD (human babesiosis and human granulocytic anaplasmosis).

Patient and Family Education. Avoid tick-infested areas whenever possible. If in such areas, follow previously described tick-repellent strategies using DEET. Shower after being outdoors and inspect the entire body carefully every day during the tick season (pay special attention to the armpit, groin, back, and scalp areas). Spray permethrin on clothing and wear light-colored long pants (tucked into socks or shoes), long sleeves, and a hat. Chronic absorption of insecticides can produce toxicity, especially in children; however, when used according to directions, children older than 2 months can safely use DEET. Picaridin (KBR 3023) and plant-based oil of eucalyptus are alternative repellents. Families should know how to remove ticks safely; removed ticks should be saved in a dry container and brought with the child for identification. Pets should be checked each day and ticks removed if found.

Ehrlichiosis and Anaplasmosis

Both ehrlichiosis and anaplasmosis are caused by distinct species of obligate intracellular bacteria carried by the lone star tick (*Amblyomma americanum,* of which two species cause ehrlichial infections) and the black-legged or deer tick (*I. scapularis,* for anaplasmosis). The southeast, south-central, and west Texas are common ehrlichiosis endemic areas in the United States. Anaplasma infections are reported more commonly in the northeast, Midwest states, and the same regions in which LD occurs; the provider must always consider a coinfection with LD or babesiosis and anaplasmosis. Any individual with a history of tick exposure in an endemic area, a nonspecific rapid onset febrile illness from May through October, and some of the following symptoms should be evaluated for ehrlichiosis or anaplasmosis. Children increasingly acquire these diseases, which are most likely underreported.[55] The incubation period for both diseases ranges from 7 to 14 days after a tick bite.

Both infections produce similar acute, systemic symptoms in about half of cases: fever, headache, myalgia, malaise, chills, nausea, and anorexia. Less common symptoms include diarrhea, emesis, weight loss, arthralgia, cough, and mental status changes. A rash occurs in about 60% of infected ehrlichiosis patients and rarely occurs with *Anaplasma.*[55] The rash (petechial, macular, or maculopapular and distinguishable from that of RMSF) varies in appearance, generally involves the trunk, spares the hands and feet, and appears about a week after the onset of other symptoms.

Diagnosis is made using an IFA assay to determine IgG antibody-specific titers on a blood sample tested during the acute and convalescent periods (2–4 weeks apart). Titers are then compared. The gold standard is a fourfold increase in the antibody titer between assays; titers may be negative in the first 7 to 10 days of the illness. DNA by PCR assay titer can also be used. Other laboratory tests show similar results: leukopenia (relative and absolute lymphopenia and a left shift), neutropenia, anemia, or thrombocytopenia with elevated hepatic transaminases in the first week of clinical illness. Pleocytosis with a predominance of lymphocytes and increased total protein is commonly seen in CSF samples.

The differential diagnosis for ehrlichiosis and anaplasmosis include RMSF, LD, other tick-borne illnesses (e.g., babesiosis, Colorado tick fever, relapsing fever, and tularemia), dengue, malaria, enteroviruses, adenoviruses, sepsis, and toxic shock syndrome.

The treatment of choice for both infections, to be started before laboratory confirmation, is doxycycline *for all ages* given the life-threatening nature of these illnesses:

- 100 lb (45.4 kg) or more: 100 mg twice daily PO or IV for 10 to 14 days to cover LD
- Less than 100 lb, 2.2 mg/kg per dose twice daily PO/IV (maximum dose is 100 mg)
  - Data suggest that discoloration of permanent teeth is not significant if doxycycline is taken for 14 days or less.[55] Treatment response should occur within 1 week.
  - Systemic complications include pulmonary infiltrates, bone marrow hypoplasia, respiratory failure, encephalopathy, meningitis, DIC, spontaneous hemorrhage, and renal failure. The mortality rate for ehrlichiosis is about 3%, and anaplasmosis is about 0.5%.[55]
  - Recovery is usually complete after 1 to 2 weeks; some children with the systemic disease have residual neurologic difficulties.
  - Prevention is the same as that for LD. Prophylaxis is not recommended because of the low risk of infection.

Rocky Mountain Spotted Fever

Rickettsia rickettsii, a nonmotile, pleomorphic, weakly gram-negative coccobacillus, is the etiologic agent of RMSF. In the United States, it is the most severe rickettsial disease and the second most common vector-borne disease after LD.[56] Vectors for *R. rickettsii* include the American dog tick *(Dermacentor variabilis)* found in the eastern and central United States, the Rocky Mountain wood tick (*Dermacentor andersoni;* also the vector for Colorado tick fever and tularemia) found in the Rocky Mountain states and west, and the brown dog tick (*Rhipicephalus sanguineus*) recently reported in eastern Arizona. Southwestern Canada, Mexico, and Central and South America also have reported cases.

In the United States, RMSF was historically centered in northern Rocky Mountain states, but it is now found in all contiguous states except Maine and Vermont. Sixty percent of cases occur in North Carolina, Tennessee, Arkansas, Missouri, and Oklahoma.[57] The incidence continues to increase (13 cases per million in 2015[57]). RMSF is most common in spring and summer months when ticks are most active (peak is June and July). The incubation period is 2 to 14 days. The longer the tick is attached, the more likely *R. rickettsii* is to be transmitted. Prompt removal of a tick is important to lower the chance of infection.

Clinical Findings. Symptoms include the following: fever (104°F [40°C]; occurs in up to 98% of children), chills, severe headache, myalgias, malaise, GI upset/tenderness, diarrhea, cough, conjunctival injection, photophobia, and altered mental status. Focal neurologic deficits (e.g., paralysis, transient deafness) appear with disease progression. Most individuals (90%) develop a maculopapular rash, typically 2 to 5 days after fever onset. The rash begins as small, flat, nonpruritic, faintly pink spots on the wrists, forearms, and ankles, then spreads to the trunk (sometimes to palms and soles). It may be easily missed in dark-skinned individuals. On day 6 or later, a petechial rash, a sign of progressive disease, may appear. Only 60% of individuals recall removing a tick.[56]

Diagnostic Studies. The most rapidly available diagnostic aid is immunohistochemical staining or PCR testing performed on a skin biopsy of petechial or macular lesions examining for *R. rickettsii*. The diagnostic gold standard is IFA on paired serologic samples taken in the first week and 2 to 4 weeks later. A fourfold change in IgG-specific antibody titer is typical. However, antibody titers may be negative in the first 7 to 10 days of the illness.

Diagnostic studies show diffuse vascular injury characterized by thrombocytopenia (<150,000 platelets/L), mild to moderate hyponatremia (<130 mEq/mL), leukocytosis as the disease progresses (a left shift), and anemia. Mildly elevated hepatic transaminase levels may be present.

Differential Diagnoses. The differential diagnoses include enteroviral infections, adenoviral infections, meningococcemia, influenza, gram-negative bacterial sepsis, toxic shock syndrome, measles, rubella, secondary syphilis, leptospirosis, typhoid fever, disseminated gonococcal infection, immune thrombocytopenic purpura, thrombotic thrombocytopenic purpura, immune complex vasculitis (e.g., SLE), infectious mononucleosis, hypersensitivity reaction to drugs, murine typhus, rickettsial pox, recrudescent typhus, and sylvatic *R. prowazekii* infection.[55]

Management. It is important to start antibiotic treatment before the onset of the rash and within the first 5 days if other clinical symptoms suggest RMSF, especially because of possible early false-negative serology. Without early treatment, the disease rapidly progresses to death,[55] provide the following guidance:

- If the child appears ill in the summer in an endemic area (with or without a history of exposure to a tick or dog) with an acute fever of fewer than 2 days but without profound malaise/myalgia/headache, obtain a CBC and chemistry panel and monitor the child.
- If the fever progresses to the third day and laboratory studies suggest RMSF, or if the child appears toxic, empiric antibiotics should be started. Although conjunctival injection and peripheral edema may appear at the same time as the rash, their presence points toward a diagnosis of RMSF.
- Treatment consists of doxycycline *for all* ages for 7 to 10 days.
  - Children under 100 lb (45.4 kg): 2.2 mg/kg per dose given twice daily PO or IV
  - Children over 100 lb: 100 mg twice daily PO or IV (maximum dose for all is 100 mg per dose)
  - The benefit of doxycycline therapy outweighs the risk of treatment, even in young children, considering the mortality associated with RMSF.[57]

Complications and Patient and Family Education. Complications include short- or long-term neurologic deficits (e.g., speech and swallowing dysfunction, global encephalopathy, gait disturbances, and cortical blindness). Digit loss due to autoamputation can occur. Untreated, the fatality rate is about 20%; for those treated, the rate is about 5%.[55] For prevention, see the prior discussion under LD.

Bacterial Infections

Although less common than viral diseases, bacterial infections allow for interventions (including antibiotics) that decrease the course of an illness and prevent subsequent complications. Many bacterial infections are diagnosed clinically and treated empirically. A good understanding of the pathophysiology of common bacterial infections, and knowledge of the most likely organisms, allows for efficient and effective treatment. Bacterial infections of the skin and soft tissues, lymphadenitis, osteomyelitis, fasciitis, pneumonia, meningitis, infectious diarrhea, and urinary tract infection (UTI) are discussed in other chapters; fungal infections and parasitic infections are also discussed in other chapters.

Community-Acquired Methicillin-Resistant Staphylococcus Aureus

Methicillin-resistant *Staphylococcus aureus* (MRSA) is a staph infection that is difficult to treat and related to drug resistance. PCPs should know the prevalence of community-acquired methicillin-resistant *S. aureus* (CA-MRSA) to effectively treat severe pneumonia, cellulitis, osteomyelitis, myositis, bacteremia, endocarditis, empyema, meningitis, staphylococcal scalded skin syndrome, toxic shock syndrome, deep tissue abscesses (especially those that come on quickly), spider bites, skin and soft tissue infections, and necrotizing fasciitis. CA-MRSA is often the cause of purulent skin and soft tissue infections in the United States It is increasingly implicated as the causative agent in pneumonia in younger age groups and in those without other underlying risk factors for pneumonia. In the United States, nearly 5% of hospitalized patients are MRSA carriers on the skin or in the nose.[58]

The following history and physical findings place healthy individuals at risk of acquired CA-MRSA infection:

- Boil, furuncle, or abscess without draining pus that is erythematous, warm, or painful; onset may be rapid (key finding).
- Treatment failure with a beta-lactam agent. If an individual has been in contact with a cat, consider cat-scratch disease (CSD) as a differential diagnosis.
- Other family members have similar skin infections.
- Recent history of skin infection, even if it was responsive to a beta-lactam agent.
- Neonate with skin or soft tissue infection.
- Skin lesion looks like a spider bite; larger lesions are suspicious for MRSA.
- Purulence is present.
- History of recurrent small, nontender, nonpruritic maculopapular lesions that become pruritic or painful, multiple lesions present.
- Participation in contact sports (e.g., wrestling, football) where turf burns and abrasions are common, and athletes share lockers, bars of soap, towels, and other equipment.
- Lower socioeconomic status, in the military, homeless, recently incarcerated, living in a crowded environment, using illicit drugs, or participating in high-risk sexual behaviors.
- Nonpregnant or pregnant woman has a breast abscess.
- A history in the past year of hospitalization, surgery, or a percutaneous permanent indwelling medical device placement.
- Attends childcare; is younger than 2 years.
- Cystic fibrosis or progressive respiratory tract infection.
- Head or neck infection (retropharyngeal abscess, mastoiditis, AOM, sinusitis, periorbital and orbital infections), osteomyelitis, myositis, pneumonia with empyema, sepsis, pustulosis in neonates.

PCPs can safely treat many superficial skin lesions, in patients outside of the neonatal period, without obtaining a culture (e.g., impetigo) using topical bacitracin or 2% mupirocin ointment 3 times daily for 7 to 10 days. In all cases, PCPs should assess each case carefully and provide instructions to parents to return if the child is unresponsive to treatment. Anticipate complications and consider the clinical clues previously mentioned for skin and soft-tissue infection. The selection of a drug that covers MRSA should be made based on the community prevalence of MRSA, if the infection was nosocomial, and the severity of the infection.

Recommended management strategies (Fig. 35.6) include:

- Incision and drainage (I&D) with culture is the treatment of choice for any nondraining but fluctuant abscess; antibiotics alone are ineffective (performing I&D before localization of pus is not effective and may promote more serious infection). Antibiotics are not needed after draining the abscess in mild cases. Consider empiric treatment (PO or IV) for MRSA for those with severe local infection, those with signs of systemic toxicity, or those who did not respond to prior oral treatment.[59] Those who are hypothermic or hyperthermic, are tachycardic, or tachypneic with laboratory findings that are concerning, consider consulting an infectious disease specialist. Children that are immunocompromised or at risk for endocarditis may require timely IV antibiotic therapy.
- Send specimens to the laboratory for a Gram stain, culture, sensitivity, and "d-test" (indicates possible inducible clindamycin resistance). Cultures should not be taken from superficial open surface wounds due to contaminating skin bacteria.

- For deep-seated infections without fluid fluctuation and signs of bacteremia (e.g., fever, chills, malaise), the use of warm compresses and oral antibiotics can be considered. The individual should return for further evaluation in 24 to 36 hours for I&D as indicated (providers need to have a way to contact the patient regarding status).
- For uncomplicated soft tissue infection (e.g., bullous and non-bullous impetigo; secondarily infected eczema, ulcers, or lacerations) without fluid fluctuation, empiric topical mupirocin 2% is usually sufficient.
- The use of oral antibiotic treatment for suspected methicillin-sensitive *S. aureus* infection is appropriate under the following circumstances, and providers should contact the child/family within 2 to 3 days to determine treatment response (Table 35.6).
  - Presence of abscesses (one or multiple sites) or rapidly progressing local infection with signs of cellulitis; systemic symptoms; comorbidities or immunosuppression; abscess is in an area difficult to incise/drain (e.g., face, hand, genitalia); or lack of response to I&D. MRSA skin infections can develop into more serious forms of infection and should be monitored very closely.[59]

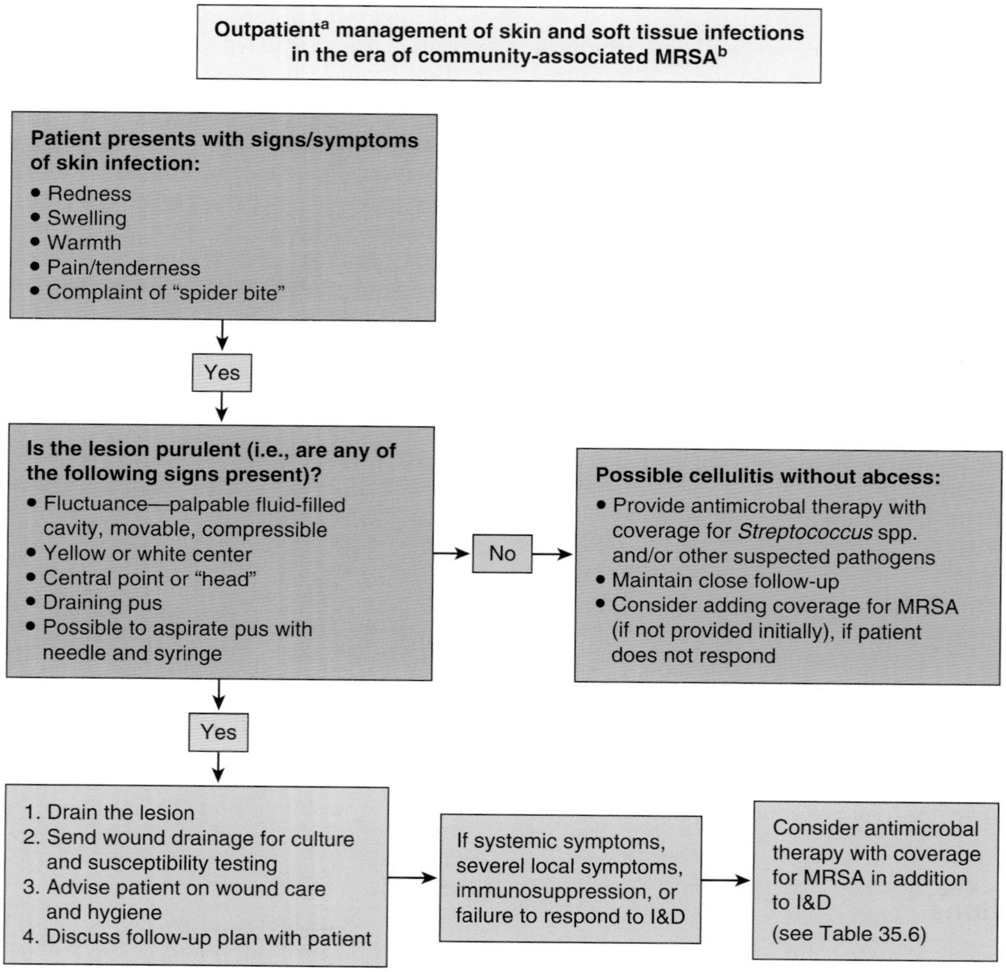

• **Fig. 35.6** Algorithm for Outpatient Management of Skin and Soft Tissue Infections. aSevere infections (appears toxic, has unstable comorbidity or limb-threatening infection; sepsis or life-threatening infection [e.g., necrotizing fasciitis]) require inpatient management; consult an infectious disease specialist. bVisit www.cdc.gov/mrsa for more information. *I&D,* Incision and drainage; *MRSA,* methicillin-resistant *Staphylococcus aureus; SSTI,* skin and soft tissue infection.

TABLE 35.6 Initial Outpatient Treatment Options for Mild to Moderate Suspected Community-Acquired Methicillin-Resistant *Staphylococcus aureus* Infections

Antibiotic[a]	Comments	Precautions
Clindamycin	Treats serious infections (nonpurulent [mild] or purulent) due to *Staphylococcus aureus*. Additional d-test should be done on specimen by lab to ensure clindamycin susceptibility. Resistance seen in deep-seated infections (osteomyelitis, endocarditis, pneumonia) Do not use if local resistance rates exceed 10%–15%	Although uncommon, may cause *Clostridium difficile*-associated disease
Doxycycline	Treats *S. aureus*, but activity against GAS less well known. Use only in children >8 years of age if treatment is >21 days	Can cause photosensitivity; do not use in pregnancy
Minocycline	For children 8 years old and older	Limited recent clinical experience
Linezolid	For complicated skin/soft tissue infections, pneumonia	Is associated with myelosuppression, neuropathy, and lactic acidosis during prolonged therapy. Before using, consult with infectious disease specialist
Trimethoprim-sulfamethoxazole (TMP-SMX)	Limited efficacy data for treating GAS so avoid using for initial treatment of cellulitis	Do not use in infants under 2 months old; do not use in third trimester of pregnancy

Serious systemic symptoms (sepsis), severe local symptoms, immunosuppression, or failure to respond to incision and drainage (I&D) require hospitalization. In typical cases, Gram stain and culture of purulence or exudate from skin lesions of impetigo and ecthyma are recommended to identify *Staphylococcus aureus* and/or a β-hemolytic streptococcus; treatment without these studies is reasonable (Kimberlin et al, 2021).

[a]Treatment recommendations do not apply to neonates. Antibiotic treatment is for 7 days, depending upon response. If response is low, treat for up to 10 to 14 days.

GAS, Group A streptococcus; *PO, per os* (by mouth, orally).

Data from Kimberlin DW, Barnett, ED, et al., eds. *Red Book: 2021 Report of the Committee on Infectious Diseases.* 32nd ed. American Academy of Pediatrics; 2021.

- Prevention measures for athletes and return-to-play guidelines are included in Chapter 18, Box 18.9 and Table 18.18.
- For recurrent MRSA soft tissue infections:
  - Review hygiene and wound care.
  - Institute environmental hygiene measures (clean surfaces in contact with skin [e.g., doorknobs, bathtubs, counters, and toilet seats]).
  - Decolonization techniques should not be used in children with an active infection.[59]

More data are needed regarding the decolonization of MRSA, focusing on the efficacy and identification of beneficial regimens. After treatment of active infections and reinforcing proper preventative measures, consider a consultation with an infectious disease specialist.

Other Emerging Drug-Resistant Bacterial Infections

At least 2.8 million people in the United States acquire a serious bacterial infection that is resistant to one or more antibiotics, and approximately 35,000 deaths are attributed to those infections.[60] Prevention and infection control procedures within the United States reduced the mortality from antibiotic resistance by 18% overall and by 30% in those hospitalized, but these statistics remain too high. Multiple drug-resistant (MDR) gram-negative bacteria and gram-positive bacteria are both major concerns; gram-positive organisms are less concerning for resistance. Resistance to antimalarials, MDR-TB, and extensively drug-resistant tuberculosis (XDR-TB) are increasing. The cost for the treatment of MDR infections is $4.6 billion annually in the United States.[60]

Antibiotics are among the most prescribed drugs for people, with up to 50% of all prescribed antibiotics either dosed ineffectively or unnecessarily.[60] Twenty percent of pediatric visits to ambulatory outpatient settings result in a prescription for antibiotics. Improving antibiotic prescribing/stewardship is an essential part of decreasing antibiotic resistance influenced by inappropriate and/or overuse of antibiotics (see Chapter 23).

Cat-Scratch Disease

B. henselae, a slow-growing, gram-negative bacillus, causes CSD. In 85% to 90% of pediatric infections, CSD presents as a localized cutaneous and regional lymphadenopathy illness. A kitten is 5 times more likely to be the cause than older cats and occasionally, the cause is a dog. The organism is transmitted to humans through a cat or dog bite or scratch from hands contaminated with flea feces that touch an open skin lesion or eye. The infection is most common in fall and winter. There have been no reported cases of person-to-person transmission. The incidence is found greater among children 5 to 9 years of age and the incidence is greater than 22,000 cases annually in the United States. The incubation period between injury and primary skin lesion is 3 to 12 days. Lymphadenopathy occurs after the primary cutaneous lesion appears between 7 to 60 days with a median of 12 days.[61]

Clinical Findings. Systemic illness is present in approximately one-third of cases although most patients are afebrile without constitutional symptoms.[11] The illness typically presents with cutaneous findings and other characteristics that include:

- Erythematous papules (2–5 mm) or pustules arise in two-thirds of individuals approximately 7 to 12 days after inoculation and persist for up to 4 weeks. They follow a linear pattern that parallels the cat scratch. The cutaneous lesions heal spontaneously. Single or multiple lymph nodes may be involved and swell to 1 to 5 cm. Lymphadenopathy may cause tenderness and the skin over the affected lymph nodes may be warm, erythematous, and indurated. The lymph nodes generally affected are the axillary, cervical, submandibular, submental, epitrochlear, and inguinal nodes. The lymphadenopathy should resolve within 4 months. Cellulitis is uncommon, but large nodes may suppurate up to 10% to 20% of the time. Mucous membrane ulcers may occur. A low-grade fever is present in 30% of cases. Other symptoms that may appear are malaise, anorexia, fatigue, and headache.[11]

- A small percentage of children (5%–10%) present with ocular manifestations. Parinaud oculoglandular syndrome (a painful, nonsuppurative conjunctivitis) with preauricular lymphadenopathy, neuroretinitis (unilateral, painless, abrupt visual impairment or loss), and retinal vasculitis are ocular disorders that may occur with CSD.[11]
  - Less common illnesses associated with CSD are culture-negative endocarditis, encephalopathy, osteomyelitis, pneumonia, glomerulonephritis, thrombocytopenic purpura, erythema nodosum, and spleen and liver granulomata.[11]

Diagnostic Studies. Available testing is by IFA and EIA and detecting the IgM and IgG antibodies to antigens of the Bartonella species. *B. henselae* is rarely recovered from cultures and generally takes >10 days to obtain a result. A *Bartonella* DNA PCR can be performed on tissue and body fluids (pleural and CSF) and is highly sensitive and specific in the tissue. CT or ultrasonography identify hepatic or splenic abscesses and granulomas. The CBC may be normal or show mild leukocytosis. The ESR and CRP are elevated early in the disease process but are considered insensitive; hepatic transaminases may increase with systemic disease. Lymph node biopsy may show nonspecific bacilli.[11]

Differential Diagnosis, Management, and Complications. Differential diagnoses include any cause of lymphadenopathy, but primarily include bacterial and viral infections (e.g., streptococci [especially group A-hemolytic], staphylococci, anaerobic bacteria, atypical mycobacteria, tularemia, brucellosis, CMV, HIV, EBV, systemic fungal infections, toxoplasmosis). Malignancy and neck masses from other sources (e.g., cystic hygromas, bronchogenic cysts, tumors) are also in the differential.

Most cases of CSD resolve spontaneously within 2 to 4 months, so symptomatic treatment is usually sufficient. Use antipyretics for moderate fever. Treat painful nodes with moist wraps or needle aspiration. Needle aspiration yields purulent material for diagnostic testing. Avoid I&D of nonsuppurative lesions because of the high risk of chronic draining sinuses. Azithromycin, clarithromycin, TMP-SMX, rifampin (RIF), ciprofloxacin, and doxycycline are commonly used. Antibiotic therapy is not indicated except for cases of CSD found in the immunocompromised population. Therapy can last between 3 to 4 months to prevent relapse.[11]

Discourage children from playing roughly with cats. Wash cat scratches thoroughly with soap and water. Immunocompromised individuals should stay away from cats that scratch or bite and avoid stray cats and cats younger than 1 year. A small percentage of individuals manifest systemic illness. An infectious disease specialist should be consulted in rare cases of culture-negative endocarditis, neuroretinitis, and all immunocompromised children with the illness.[11]

Kingella kingae Infection

K. kingae is an important cause of invasive infections in children younger than 4 years. The organism is part of the normal flora of the pharynx in children (over 6 months old) more than in adults; it is easily transmitted in childcare settings. The onset is usually insidious, which can result in the delay of diagnosis.[11] The history often includes recent or concomitant gingivostomatitis or URI. Suspect *K. kingae* in culture-negative skeletal infections of young children, as it is the most common cause of septic arthritis

in children younger than 3 years.[62] Septic arthritis usually involves the knee, hip, or ankle. Other invasive disease includes osteomyelitis (distal femur is the most common site), endocarditis in those with underlying cardiac disease [HACEK group of organisms (**H**aemophilus spp., **A**ctinobacillus actinomycetemcomitans, **C**ardiobacterium hominis, **E**ikenella corrodens, **K**. kingae)], meningitis, occult bacteremia, and pneumonia. *K. kingae* is the most common cause of spondylodiskitis in the 6 to 48 months age group.[62] The organism is difficult to isolate in solid culture media. Recent studies show PCR dramatically enhances detection in bone and joint fluid samples.[63] The organism is susceptible to many antibiotics (penicillins, aminoglycosides, ciprofloxacin, and erythromycin) but is resistant to vancomycin and 40% of clindamycin isolates showing resistance.[62] Most strains are susceptible to TMP-SMX despite resistance to trimethoprim alone. Standard hygienic preventive measures should be in place in childcare settings to decrease the risk of transmission.[63]

Meningococcal Disease

Many organisms cause meningitis including group B streptococcus, *E. coli*, *Listeria monocytogenes*, enterococci, *S. pneumoniae*, *N. meningitidis*, and *H. influenzae*. The causative organism varies with the patient's age. Only *N. meningitidis* is discussed here (see Chapter 41).

N. meningitidis is a gram-negative diplococcus. It is a common commensal organism in the human nasopharynx. There are 12 confirmed serotypes. Serotype B is responsible for the highest rates of infection, followed by serotypes C, W, and Y. Infants less than 1 year of age and adolescents and young adults 16 to 20 years of age have the highest incidence. The serotypes responsible for 85% of adolescent and young adult cases are B, C, W, and Y; serotype B is responsible for most cases. This is preventable with available vaccines. The organism spreads from person to person via respiratory tract secretions (large droplets) or contact with saliva (kissing). Asymptomatic carriers are the most common source of transmission, as 10% of the population at any given time is a carrier. The disease occurs most often during the winter season in the United States, often 2 to 3 weeks after influenza outbreaks, and peaks in January, February, and March. Epidemics occur in semi-closed communities (e.g., childcare centers, schools, college dormitories [especially among college freshmen], and military barracks). Children or youth with functional or anatomic asplenia, complement deficiencies (e.g., nephritic syndrome, SLE, hepatic failure), or properdin deficiency are at increased risk for invasive or recurring meningococcal disease. The incubation period is 1 to 10 days, generally <10 days for invasive infections. Individuals are contagious until 24 hours after treatment initiation.[11] The mortality rate for invasive infection is 10% and most deaths occur within 48 hours of symptom onset due to septic shock and multi-organ dysfunction. Those presenting with DIC have a mortality rate of >50%.[64]

Meningococcal infection rates decreased beginning in the early 2000s. The potential rationale for the lower incidence is an increase in the administration of influenza vaccines, a decrease in the number of carriage rates, preadolescent and adolescent use of the meningococcal conjugate vaccines, an increase in immunity of the population to meningococcal serotypes not included in vaccines, and a decrease in smoking and exposure to secondhand smoke. All confirmed, suspected and probable cases of meningococcal infection must be reported immediately to the local public health department.[11]

Clinical Findings. Meningococcal disease presentation varies widely from mild viral symptoms with fever to severe disease.

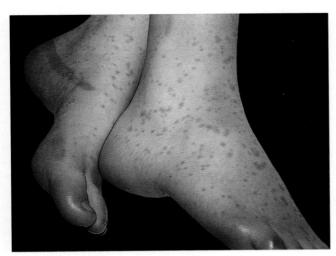

• **Fig. 35.7** Meningococcemia. (From Zitelli BJ, McIntire SC, Nowalk AJ. *Atlas of Physical Diagnosis.* 7th ed. Elsevier; 2018.)

Recognized disease patterns include bacteremia without sepsis, meningococcal sepsis without meningitis, meningitis with or without meningococcemia, meningoencephalitis, and specific organ infection. Presenting symptoms can include:

- Occult bacteremia: This oocurs in a febrile child with URI or GI-like symptoms. There may be a maculopapular rash. Often these children are treated for a viral illness.[11]
- Meningococcemia: Fulminant meningococcemia onset is abrupt, progresses rapidly, and includes initial symptoms of fever, chills, malaise, myalgia, limb pain, macular or maculopapular rash, and some show signs of septic shock. Skin changes are characterized by prominent petechiae (Fig. 35.7) that quickly progress to purpura fulminans and limb ischemia. Other signs are associated with septic shock such as hypotension, DIC, acidosis, adrenal hemorrhage, renal failure, myocardial failure, and coma. In fulminant cases, death can occur within hours of onset despite appropriate therapy. The meningococcal infection leads to septicemia in 35% to 40% of cases and approximately 50% result in meningitis or both.[11]
- Meningococcal meningitis: The most common clinical findings are fever, headache, and stiff neck. Fever and irritability may be the only initial symptoms in young children, whereas fever and headache are more typical in older children and adolescents. Other symptoms include nausea, emesis, photophobia, and altered mental status. Symptoms are indistinguishable from pneumococcal meningitis and in severe cases increased intracranial pressure is a predominant symptom.[11]

Diagnostic Studies. The diagnosis is confirmed with a positive culture or Gram stain from normally sterile sites (blood, CSF, synovial fluid), sputum, or petechial or purpura lesion scraping. Blood and CSF cultures may be negative if the child was pretreated with antibiotics. PCR assays can be used from CSF, serum, and plasma samples to detect meningococcal DNA before the cultures; results are available in 4 to 8 hours. PCR is more sensitive than blood culture and is helpful to detect *N. meningitidis* especially when antibiotics are given before testing and organism growth is suppressed.[11] In a probable case, a positive latex agglutination test of CSF supports the clinical diagnosis of meningitis. However, this test has poor sensitivity and specificity, especially for serogroup B, and is not recommended if the PCR (in addition to culture) is available. Other laboratory findings include leukopenia

or leukocytosis with increased bands and neutrophils, hypoalbuminemia, hypocalcemia, metabolic acidosis with increased lactate, decreased platelets, and elevated ESR and CRP. Decreased prothrombin and fibrinogen and prolonged coagulation times are seen with DIC.

Differential Diagnosis. The list of differential diagnoses is long and includes septicemia caused by other invasive bacteria (e.g., *Pneumococcus* or *H. influenza*), viral meningitis, TB brain abscess, chronic otitis media, and sinusitis. Collagen-vascular diseases, primary hematologic and oncologic disease, erythema nodosa, erythema multiforme, RMSF, *Mycoplasma*, lead encephalopathy, coxsackievirus, echovirus, rubella and rubeola infections, Henoch-Schönlein purpura, ITP, viral exanthems, typhus, typhoid, toxic shock syndrome, rat bite fever, gonococcemia, *S. aureus* endocarditis, and Kawasaki syndrome are also in the differential diagnosis.

Management, Control Measures, and Complications. If the child is suspected of having meningococcemia, hospitalization is mandatory, and IV antibiotics are started pending culture results. A 5- to 7-day treatment course is usually adequate. Empirical treatment includes cefotaxime, ceftriaxone, penicillin G, or ampicillin. For penicillin allergy, consider meropenem. The primary goal for meningococcal infections is the resolution of septic shock and a decrease in intracranial pressure in cases of meningococcal meningitis.[11]

Exposed contacts must be carefully monitored. Household, school, or child contacts who develop a febrile illness must be promptly evaluated for invasive disease. Control measures include:

- Chemoprophylaxis is ideally given within 24 hours of index case identification. Chemoprophylaxis should be prescribed to those in close contact even if the contact received the meningococcal vaccine. Medical staff (unless they performed mouth-to-mouth resuscitation, intubation, or suctioning before antibiotics) are not at high risk and should not receive postexposure chemoprophylaxis. Provide chemoprophylaxis for close contacts within 24 hours after discovering the diagnosis and if it is within 2 weeks of exposure. If therapy other than ceftriaxone or cefotaxime is prescribed for invasive infection, the child should receive chemoprophylaxis to eradicate nasopharyngeal carriage of *N. meningitidis*. Oral RIF or ciprofloxacin are the antimicrobials of choice for infants and children. Azithromycin in a one-time dose is considered second-line therapy.[64] Ciprofloxacin resistance to *N. meningitidis* has been found within the past 15 years. Failure of chemoprophylaxis or antibiotic resistance should be monitored and reported to guide current chemoprophylaxis recommendations.[11]
- Prophylaxis during an outbreak: Vaccination, in conjunction with chemoprophylaxis, is advisable to prevent extended outbreaks only if the identified strain is contained in the vaccine (see Meningococcal vaccine). Vaccines are available for serogroups A, B, C, Y, and W-135.

Complications are caused by inflammation, intravascular hemorrhage, necrosis in multiple organ systems, and shock. Common sequelae include hearing loss, deafness, skin necrosis requiring grafting, amputations, seizures, and ataxia.[64]

Streptococcal Disease

Streptococci are gram-positive spherical cocci that are broadly classified based on their ability to hemolyze RBCs. Complete hemolysis is known as *β-hemolytic*. Partial hemolysis is *α-hemolytic*; nonhemolysis is *γ-hemolytic*. Cell wall carbohydrate differences further subdivide the streptococci into Lancefield antigen subgroups A-H and K-V. Subgroups A-H and K-O are associated with human disease. GABHS is the most virulent, although group B β-hemolytic streptococcus causes bacteremia and meningitis in infants younger than 3 months old (rarely older). Group A streptococcus (GAS) is subdivided into more than 100 subtypes based on their cell surface M protein antigen and fimbriae on the cell's outer edge. The virulence of GAS depends upon their M protein. If the M protein is present, GAS strains resist phagocytosis; if the M protein is weak or absent, the strains are avirulent (e.g., chronic GAS pharyngeal carriers). GAS also produces a variety of enzymes and toxins that stimulate specific antitoxin antibodies for immunity or serve as evidence of past infection but do not confer immunity. There is no cross-immunity between antibodies for different GAS strains (e.g., scarlet fever is caused by three different pyrogenic exotoxins, so the illness can recur). Some general remarks about specific illnesses caused by GAS and non–group A and B streptococcus infection are discussed in this chapter; cross-references to specific chapters are noted for other GAS-caused infections.

Group A Streptococcus. Streptococci usually invade the respiratory tract, skin, soft tissues, and blood. Transmission is primarily through infected upper respiratory tract secretions or, secondarily, through skin invasion. Fomites and household pets are not vectors. Foodborne outbreaks from contamination by food handlers are reported. Both streptococcus pharyngitis and impetigo are associated with crowding, whether at home, school, or other institutions. Streptococcal pharyngitis is rare in infants and children younger than 3 years, but the incidence rises with age, is most common in middle childhood and adolescence, and is most common in the winter and early spring in temperate climates. Carrier rates in asymptomatic children are as high as 25%.[11] By contrast, streptococcus skin infection (impetigo, pyoderma) is more common in toddlers and preschool-age children. Those at increased risk for invasive GAS are individuals with varicella infection, IV drug use, HIV, diabetes, chronic heart or lung disease, infants, and older adults.

The incubation period is 2 to 5 days for pharyngitis and 7 to 10 days for skin infection. In untreated individuals, communicability is from the symptom onset and decreases over a period of weeks.[11] Children are noninfectious 24 hours after the start of appropriate antibiotic therapy.

Clinical Findings and Diagnostic Studies. The following may be seen:

- Respiratory tract infection: Streptococcal tonsillopharyngitis (GABHS) and pneumonia are described in Chapter 32. Peritonsillar abscess, cervical lymphadenitis, retropharyngeal abscess, otitis media, mastoiditis, and sinusitis may be clinical features.
- Scarlet fever: This is caused by an erythrogenic toxin. It is uncommon in children younger than 3 years old. Scarlet fever occurs mostly with pharyngitis and rarely pyoderma, skin, or wound infection. The incubation period is approximately 3 days (the range is 1–7 days). There is an abrupt illness with pharyngitis, emesis, headache, chills, and malaise. Fever reaches 104°F (40°C). Tonsils are erythematous, edematous, and usually exudative. The pharynx is inflamed and may be covered with a gray-white exudate. The palate and uvula are erythematous and edematous, and petechiae are present. The tongue is usually coated and red, desquamation of the coating leaves prominent papillae (strawberry tongue). The typical scarlatina rash appears 1 to 5 days following symptom onset but may be the presenting symptom. The exanthema is red, blanches to pressure, and is finely papular, making the skin feel coarse, with a sandpaper feel. The rash generally begins on the neck,

underarms, or groin, and spreads to the trunk and extremities, becoming generalized within 24 hours. The face may be spared (cheeks may be reddened with circumoral pallor), but the rash is denser on the neck, axilla, and groin. Pastia lines, transverse linear hyperpigmented areas with tiny petechiae, are present in the joint folds (see Fig. 35.3). In severe disease, small vesicles (miliary sudamina) appear on the hands, feet, and abdomen. There is circumoral pallor and the cheeks are erythematous. The rash fades and desquamates after 3 to 4 days, starting on the face and slowly moving to the trunk and extremities, and may include fingernail margins, palms, and soles; this process can take up to 6 weeks. Pharyngitis and constitutional symptoms resolve in approximately 5 to 7 days (average 3–4 days).

- Bacteremia: This occurs after respiratory (pharyngitis, tonsillitis, AOM) and localized skin infections. Some children have no obvious source of infection. Meningitis, osteomyelitis, septic arthritis, pyelonephritis, pneumonia, peritonitis, and bacterial endocarditis are rare but associated with GAS bacteremia. (Neonatal sepsis caused by group B streptococcus is discussed in Chapter 28.)
- Vaginitis and streptococcal toxic shock syndrome (see Chapter 43).
- Perianal streptococcal cellulitis: Symptoms include local itching, pain, blood-streaked stools, erythema, and proctitis. Fever and systemic infections are uncommon. Although infection is usually the result of autoinoculation, sexual molestation should remain among the differential diagnoses.
- Skin infections (see Chapter 37); rheumatic heart disease (see Chapter 33); and necrotizing fasciitis (see Chapter 37).

Differential Diagnosis, Management, and Complications. Many viral pathogens are in the differential for acute pharyngitis including influenza, enterovirus, human metapneumovirus, parainfluenza, rhinovirus, coronavirus, adenovirus, and RSV. EBV is common and is usually accompanied by other clinical findings (e.g., splenomegaly, generalized lymphadenopathy). Other causes of bacterial upper respiratory disease include (although rare) tularemia, *Yersinia*, gonorrhea, *Chlamydia*, and *Mycoplasma*. Staphylococcal impetigo must be differentiated from GABHS pyoderma. Septicemia, meningitis, osteomyelitis, septic arthritis, pyelonephritis, and bacterial endocarditis cause similar symptoms but result from other bacteria.

Antimicrobial therapy is recommended for GABHS pharyngitis to decrease the risk of acute rheumatic fever and illness length, prevent complications, and reduce transmission. See appropriate aforementioned site-specific chapters for recommendations for managing specific infections.

Complications are usually caused by disease spread from localized infection. Upper respiratory complications include cervical lymphadenitis, retropharyngeal abscess, otitis media, mastoiditis, and sinusitis if the primary infection is unrecognized or treatment is inadequate. Acute poststreptococcal glomerulonephritis occurs following skin or upper respiratory GAS infection, whereas acute rheumatic fever only occurs following GAS URIs. Poststreptococcal reactive arthritis occurs following GAS pharyngitis. Skin infection with GAS may progress to cellulitis, myositis, or necrotizing fasciitis. Other complications associated with invasive infections include pneumonia, pleural empyema, meningitis, osteomyelitis, bacterial endocarditis, and streptococcal toxic shock syndrome.

Pediatric acute-onset neuropsychiatric syndrome associated with streptococcal infections is a group of neuropsychiatric disorders thought to result from the production of autoimmune antibodies. Patients with this syndrome demonstrate complex behaviors including obsessive-compulsive behaviors and tics (see Chapter 29).

Non–Group A or B Streptococci. Lancefield group streptococci (principally groups C and G) cause invasive disease in all age groups. They may cause bacteremia, septicemia, UTIs, endocarditis, respiratory disease (upper and lower), skin soft tissue infection, pharyngitis, brain abscesses, pneumonia, septic arthritis, osteomyelitis, pericarditis, toxic shock syndrome, and meningitis in newborns, children, adolescents, and adults. The incubation period and communicability times are unknown. A positive culture from normally sterile body fluids is adequate for diagnosis. Penicillin G is the drug of choice with modification based on culture sensitivities.[11]

Tuberculosis

TB is caused by *M. tuberculosis* and is a very slow-growing organism, taking up to 10 weeks to grow on solid media and 1 to 6 weeks in liquid media. The degree of infectivity depends on the exposure intensity and length and the burden of bacilli carried by the index case. The bacilli are spread primarily by droplet contamination from coughing, sneezing, or talking. Droplets stay suspended in the air for hours. Fomite transmission is uncommon; the portal of entry is most often the respiratory tract from mucus droplets from a person infected with pulmonary TB.[65]

There are two categories of TB infection (TBI), those infected individuals who are asymptomatic and those with infection who experience signs and symptoms of infection.[11] In general, approximately 3% to 4% of those infected with the bacilli progress to active disease during the first year after infection; thereafter, an additional 5% progress to disease.[66] These estimates are based on heavy exposures during disease-prone periods of life.

Globally, one-quarter of the world's population is infected with mycobacteria.[66] Ninety-five percent of active TB cases occur in countries where HIV/AIDS infection is epidemic and health care is poor or inaccessible. Individuals in the United States with the highest incidence of active TB live in urban, low-income areas. Approximately 60% of reported TB cases in the United States are foreign-born, and 80% are among high-risk groups including immigrants, international adoptees, those from or travelers to high-prevalence regions (Asia, Africa, Latin America, and former Soviet Union countries), the homeless, alcoholics, IV drug users, and individuals in correctional facilities or other close communal settings.[11]

Infection is typically detected by a positive Mantoux tuberculin skin testing (TST) or a positive interferon γ release assay (IGRA) in a high-risk child. In certain circumstances, a child may have findings suggestive of TBI and not have a positive TST or IGRA. These tests are reactive within 2 to 10 weeks after initial exposure to an active TB case. The risk of progression to disease is highest in the first 6 months after infection. The risk remains high for the subsequent 2 years after infection, but the infection may remain latent for years before progressing to disease. After treatment starts, infectivity in active cases may cease within days or take several weeks depending on the drugs prescribed, organism response, and other disease characteristics (e.g., for cavitary disease, response takes longer). In children younger than 10 years, there is usually minimal cough and bacilli expulsion and, therefore less contagion. Most pediatric infections are from adults.

In most children and adolescents, initial infection with *M. tuberculosis* is eliminated or contained by host defenses and the person remains asymptomatic. Progression from infection to disease is highest in infants and children 1 to 2 years of age. Children younger than 5 years account for about 60% of American childhood cases; children 5 to 14 years old have the lowest rate of progression to disease.[67] Other factors that make an individual prone to active disease include having another TBI within the prior 2 years; immune status (immunocompromised individuals [from a disease {e.g., HIV} or immunosuppressive drugs] are at higher risk); IV drug use; those with chronic diseases (e.g., Hodgkin disease, lymphoma, diabetes mellitus, chronic renal failure, malnutrition); and those receiving tumor necrosis factor-α antagonists to treat arthritis, inflammatory bowel disease, or other diseases.

Congenital TB is extremely rare. Infants most likely become infected after delivery from contact with an infected person. Exposure in utero occurs from exposure to maternal bacteremia, seeding of the placenta by disseminated (miliary) TB in the fetal circulation, fetal aspiration of amniotic fluid at delivery, or in utero infected amniotic fluid ingestion.[65]

Clinical Findings for Primary Pulmonary Tuberculosis

Table 35.7 describes the clinical findings and interventions for the TB stages. Most children ages 3 to 15 years with primary pulmonary TB are asymptomatic except for a positive TB skin test or IGRA. An effective immune response eliminates most of the bacilli, although small numbers of bacilli spread throughout the body during the bacteremic phase.

Any symptoms in children are generally minor and slightly more evident in infants; up to 50% exhibit radiographic changes but have no physical findings. Most children with the disease first develop hilar lymphadenopathy then focal hyperinflation and atelectasis.[68] Signs and symptoms typically occur 1 to 6 months after infection and include low-grade fever, nonproductive cough, dyspnea (more common in infants), malaise, decreased appetite, weight loss (failure to thrive in infants), night sweats, chills, erythema nodosum, and phlyctenular keratoconjunctivitis (a hypersensitivity reaction marked by elevated clear nodules with surrounding hyperemia near the limbus). Approximately 25% to 35% of children present with extrapulmonary TB symptoms (e.g., meningitis and/or granulomatous inflammation of the lymph nodes, bones, joints, skin, and middle ear and mastoid).[68] Rarely, enlarged lymph nodes compress and obstruct the regional bronchus, causing respiratory distress; this is more commonly seen with infants. Esophageal compression (causing dysphagia or aspiration) and vasoconstriction of major arteries and veins (causing edema) can occur. Recurrent cough, stridor, and wheezing are signs of increasing pulmonary infection.

Screening Tests for Infection

Low-risk groups do not need to be routinely screened for TB. Children are at high risk for TB if they meet any of the following criteria:

- Have close contact with others with suspected or confirmed TB.
- Were born in, or traveled for more than 1 week to, TB-prevalent parts of the world (Asia, Middle East, Africa, Latin America, countries formerly part of the Soviet Union) (it is reasonable to wait 10 weeks after return from areas to screen if the child is well and has no history of exposure).
- Live in an area where there is a rise in TBI.
- Have clinical signs suggestive of TB on chest radiograph or other clinical evidence suggestive of TBI.
- Are HIV positive (beginning at 3–12 months of age), have an immunosuppressive disorder, or are being treated with immunosuppressive drugs.

TABLE 35.7 Characteristics of Tuberculosis in Children

	STAGE		
	Exposure	Infection (LTBI)	Disease
Mantoux skin test or IGRA (for children 3 years and older and in those who have received BCG); use Mantoux if HIV infected	Negative (results not reliable in infants younger than 3 months)	Positive (TST: in 60%–90% of cases)	Positive (TST: in 60%–90% of cases)
Physical examination	Normal	Normal	Usually abnormal[a]
Chest radiograph	Normal	Usually normal[b]	Usually abnormal[c]
Treatment	If <4 years old or with impaired immunity (e.g., HIV)	Always	Always
Number of drugs	One	One (additional regimens available)	Four

[a]More than 50% of infants and children with pulmonary tuberculosis have a normal physical examination.
[b]May reveal healed lesions (calcification in the lungs, hilar lymph nodes, or both).
[c]Some children with extrapulmonary tuberculosis have a normal chest radiograph.

BCG, Bacille Calmette-Guérin vaccine; *HIV*, human immunodeficiency virus; *IGRA*, interferon-gamma release assay; *LTBI*, latent tuberculosis infection.
Data from American Academy of Pediatrics, Kimberlin DW, Barnett, ED, et al., eds. *Tuberculosis, Red Book: 2021 Report of the Committee on Infectious Diseases.* 32nd ed. American Academy of Pediatrics; 2021:786–814; and Hatzenbuehler LA, Starke JR. Tuberculosis *(Mycobacterium tuberculosis).* In: Kliegman RM, et al. *Nelson Textbook of Pediatrics.* 21st ed. Elsevier; 2020.

- Are homeless, reside in correctional or other residential institution, are a member of a migrant farm family.
- Consider in children with Hodgkin disease, diabetes mellitus, chronic renal failure, malnutrition, and those receiving tumor necrosis factor antagonists.

Mantoux Tuberculin Skin Test. TST is based on the delayed hypersensitivity to *M. tuberculosis* antigens. The Mantoux skin test is a purified protein derivative (PPD). If the child becomes infected with TB, the test usually becomes positive 4 to 8 weeks (between 3 weeks and 3 months) after bacilli inhalation.[68] All children with positive TST need quick clinical and radiographic evaluation.

The Mantoux test uses 0.1 mL of 5 tuberculin units (TU) of PPD, is injected intradermally into the volar surface of the forearm and produces a palpable wheal with 6 to 10 mm of induration (crucial for accurate testing). A multipuncture skin test should not be used. Read the Mantoux test 48 to 72 hours later by an experienced healthcare professional. Measure the induration, not the erythema. Sensitivity to the TST persists for years, even after effective antitubercular drug treatment.

Children with prior Bacille Calmette-Guérin (BCG) vaccination can receive the TST and interpretation of the test is the same as for nonrecipients. Prior BCG vaccination produces a mild to severe hypersensitivity reaction, depending on several factors: the age of the BCG vaccine, its quality, the strain of *M. bovis* used, the number of BCG doses received, nutritional status, immunologic factors, infection with environmental mycobacteria, and the frequency of skin testing (boosts the response). The degree of positivity decreases over time, depending on the age at vaccination.

All children with positive TST need quick clinical and radiographic evaluation. A Mantoux skin test is defined as positive for TBI or TB disease if the following reactions occur[11]:
- Induration (5 mm or greater) in children who are in close contact with an individual with active or previously active TB cases, have a chest radiograph consistent with active or previously active TB, clinical TB findings, have an immunosuppressive disorder or HIV infection, or are receiving immunosuppressive drugs.
- Induration (10 mm or greater) in children younger than 4 years with any high-risk factors.
- Induration (15 mm or greater) in children 4 years or older without any risk factors.
- If the skin test shows induration onset after 72 hours, it should be interpreted as positive.
- Skin testing is not always valid and is negative in 10% to 40% of children with positive cultures. Decreased reactivity occurs in immunocompromised children (e.g., with HIV), infants younger than 3 months, those with poor nutrition, or those with other viral infections (notably measles, varicella, and influenza). Ten percent of those with progressive TB (up to 50% with disseminated disease or meningitis) do not react until several months after receiving drug treatment.[11,68] In addition, a poor response to the skin test can occur because of inadequate handling of the Mantoux solution, improper injection technique, or interpretation error. Individuals sensitized to nontuberculous mycobacteria can cross-react and have a less than 10- to 12-mm reaction to TB skin testing.

Interferon γ Release Assays. IGRAs include QuantiFERON-TB Gold In-Tube and T-SPOT.TB. IGRAs are FDA-approved screening tests for detecting T-cell response to specific *M. tuberculosis* antigens. They have the advantage over the Mantoux test of not being affected by prior BCG vaccination. TST is the preferred test for children younger than 2 years. A TST or IGRA can be used in children 2 years and older. Neither TST nor IGRA distinguish between TBI and TB disease. Repeat indeterminate IGRA when clinically indicated. IGRA testing is preferred for the following circumstances[67]: children 2 years or older, especially those that received the BCG vaccine and children of any age who are unlikely to return for the TST reading.

Diagnostic Studies

Chest radiography early in the disease may show only localized, nonspecific infiltrates. Inflammation of lung tissue and hilar lymph nodes continues as the disease progresses; this quickly resolves in most children, but increased hilar adenopathy is usually seen in infants. The hallmark is disproportionately enlarged regional lymph nodes compared with a relatively small pleural focus.[65]

Radiography in older children shows inconspicuous pneumonitis in the lower and middle lung fields. In adolescents, apical or subapical infiltrates are common, often with cavitations, and no hilar adenopathy.[66] Extensive pulmonary infiltrates and cavitation occur if there is erosion and necrosis from disseminated bacilli. Lesions may be the size of millet seeds; hence the name "miliary" TB.

Hilar adenopathy suggests TB, but culture of the organism is essential to establish the diagnosis. Culture specimens may be obtained from gastric aspirates, sputum, bronchial washings, pleural fluid, CSF, urine or other body fluids, or biopsies. However, mycobacteria are isolated in less than 50% of children and 75% of infants with pulmonary TB.[11] Those older than 5 years can be induced to cough to produce sputum with aerosolized hypertonic saline. When age or ability to produce sputum is a factor, early morning gastric aspirates, collected on three separate mornings and analyzed by fluorescent staining is an effective and sensitive testing method. Histologic examination for acid-fast bacilli (AFB) from biopsies is helpful. Solid media cultures can take up to 10 weeks to grow with an additional 2 to 4 weeks for susceptibility testing, whereas liquid cultures take 1 to 6 weeks. Rapid DNA probes or high-pressure liquid chromatography of cultured organisms differentiate between *M. tuberculosis* and *M. bovis* based on PZA resistance that is characteristic of *M. bovis*.

If an isolate from an index case is positive for TB, culture material is not needed from an exposed child. However, a culture is necessary in the following circumstances: the index case is unavailable, the child has HIV infection or is immunocompromised, drug-resistant TB is suspected, or the child has extrapulmonary symptoms.[11] NAAT on respiratory secretions is the standard practice for suspected TB, it does not exclude TB. It aids in the diagnosis of TB when symptoms suggest active TBI, but it does not replace an AFB smear and culture. NAAT results at least 1 week earlier than a culture. Its use expedites the appropriate treatment initiation. Additional research needs to be done before NAATs are approved for use in extrapulmonary or primary TB in children who cannot produce sputum.[11]

Differential Diagnosis

PCPs should consider TB in children with symptoms of basilar meningitis, hydrocephalus, cranial nerve palsy, or stroke. Permanent neurologic dysfunction can result and has a worse prognosis in infants than in older children. The differential diagnosis includes mycotic infections, staphylococcal pneumonia, sarcoidosis, chronic pneumonia, and Hodgkin lymphoma. Differential diagnosis in lymph node diseases includes CSD, tularemia, toxoplasmosis, tumor, brachial cysts, cystic hygroma, and pyogenic infection.

Management

A TB specialist should be consulted when a child has a positive TST, when TB is suspected, or a child has a known TB contact. TB is a reportable infectious disease. After index and contact cases are identified and diagnostic studies are done, the state and/or local health department often initiate treatment and follow-up. The treatment regimens are continually revised based on resistance patterns so consultation with a pediatric TB specialist before initiating treatment is essential. Treatment regimens differ for individuals with concurrent HIV infection.

Antitubercular drug treatment focuses on eradicating the bacilli and inhibiting their multiplication in TBI and early pulmonary disease. Rapid resolution of caseous or granulomatous lesions will not occur. It is imperative to have a strict adherence to drug combinations to minimize drug resistance. This may need to be done under directly observed therapy (DOT). If the treatment regimen is prescribed by a TB specialist or health department, the PCP should know the child's specific antitubercular drug regimen. The first-line drugs are administered orally and include INH, RIF, PZA, and ethambutol. The typical treatment regimens for children/families include[11,65,68]:

- For prophylaxis after contact with a person with TB disease or for TBI: INH, taken once daily or twice weekly for 9 months; RIF, taken once daily for 4 to 6 months; INH and RIF daily for 2 to 3 months; or INH and rifapentine for 12 doses once weekly.
- For pulmonary disease and extrapulmonary disease (except CNS, bone, and joint): all four drugs are taken once daily for 2 months. INH and RIF then continue for 4 months, administered 2 to 3 times a week (duration of treatment with HIV coinfection is 6–9 months or 6 months from sterile sputum culture—whichever is longest).
- For bone, joint infection, and disseminated disease: same as pulmonary except is given for 9 to 12 months.
- For hilar adenopathy only, or no other abnormalities and minimal risk for resistant disease: some experts recommend INH and RIF for 6 months but may need to extend to 9 months if slow improvement or culture is positive 2 months after starting treatment.
- For meningitis: INH, RIF, and PZA are given with either ethionamide, an aminoglycoside, or levofloxacin as the fourth drug. The fourth drug may be stopped if cultures are susceptible to INH and RIF. PZA can be stopped after 2 months if good clinical response. Total treatment time is 9 to 12 months.
- Newborns suspected of having congenital TB: INH, RIF, PZA, and an aminoglycoside are used.

The treatment regimens are continually revised and there are alternative regimens used. Under some alternative regimens, the drugs are administered twice a week under DOT, provide shortened treatment duration, or use different drug combinations depending upon age, drug-resistance, extent of TB infection, and the presence of concurrent infections. The CDC, AAP *Red Book*, and WHO are excellent resources for drug regimens and recommended dosages.

Pregnant women diagnosed with TB disease, who have signs and symptoms, or abnormal findings on chest x-ray consistent with TB should be promptly treated and tested for HIV. If the pregnant woman has TBI and a normal chest radiograph, she should start and remain on TBI treatment for 9 months after the postpartum period and the newborn needs no further evaluation or therapy.[11] If she has active disease, isolation may be recommended, and the newborn should be evaluated for congenital TB disease. If congenital TB is excluded, the infant should be started on treatment for TBI after birth for 3 or 4 months (at which time a Mantoux skin test should be given) even if breastfeeding and the mother is on concurrent therapy.

The exclusively breastfed infant receiving INH should be given pyridoxine, although it is not routinely recommended for children and adolescents. It is also recommended for use in children whose diets are either deficient in meat or milk, if they have HIV, and for pregnant adolescents; the tablets can be pulverized for easier administration. Corticosteroids decrease mortality, neurologic disability, and the inflammation that is detrimental to organ function in children with meningeal, endobronchial, pleural and pericardial effusion, abdominal TB, and miliary TB.

Monitoring Response to Treatment. Index and contact case tracking is under the jurisdiction of state and local health departments. Initial evaluation, drug management, and follow-up may also take place in these centers. However, the PCP plays a crucial role in monitoring response to treatment. The following are general monitoring guidelines[11]:

- See all individuals monthly who are treated for TB. Evaluate for antitubercular drug adherence and side effects, notably for symptoms of hepatitis if on INH (a rare finding in healthy infants, children, and adolescents). Educate patients to call immediately if experiencing signs of hepatoxicity (e.g., emesis, abdominal pain, and jaundice), peripheral neuritis, diarrhea, or GI irritation. Those on PZA may experience hepatoxicity, arthralgia, or GI disturbances. RIF may cause orange secretions in urine, emesis, hepatitis, flu-like symptoms, thrombocytopenia, and pruritus; those on oral contraceptives need to use a backup birth control method.
- Routine lab monitoring is not recommended in children unless they have severe TB disease, meningitis, or disseminated disease. In these cases, check transaminases monthly for the first several months. Other indications for laboratory studies include current or recent liver or biliary disease, use of hepatotoxic drugs (e.g., HIV, seizure medications), clinical evidence of hepatotoxicity, and/or pregnancy or within 12 weeks postpartum.
- Collect sputum for AFB smear and culture after 2 months of drug therapy to evaluate response; if sputum culture is positive after 3 months of therapy, the bacilli need to be rechecked for drug susceptibility.
- If cavitation is present on the initial chest radiograph and a 2-month sputum culture is positive, treatment with INH and RIF should be extended an additional 3 months for a total treatment duration of 9 months.
- Repeat chest radiograph after 2 months; it is good practice to take one after therapy completion as a baseline for comparison against any subsequent films. Hilar adenopathy can persist for 2 to 3 years despite adequate therapy. Residual calcification of the primary focus or regional lymph nodes may be evident on radiograph.
- Extrapulmonary disease: Follow clinical symptoms.
- For those taking ethambutol, ask about the presence of visual disturbances (screen visual acuity and red-green color vision if dosages exceed 20 mg/kg/day or if on more than 2 months of treatment); if unable to test visual acuity, consider an alternate drug.
- Children receive attenuated live-virus vaccines at age-appropriate times, unless they are on high-dose corticosteroids, are severely ill, or have another contraindication.
- If therapy is interrupted, treatment length should be extended. Consult with a TB specialist.

Complications

The following complications with their clinical findings can occur with TB:

- Progressive primary pulmonary disease: Rarely, primary TB progresses and disseminates. This occurs more frequently in infants and children younger than 5 years, a result of their immune systems being immature or unable to eliminate the bacilli. The primary pleural focus enlarges and develops a large caseous center, and liquefaction forms a cavity with large numbers of bacilli. Symptoms in children with progressive disease are more acute and include high intermittent fevers, night sweats, severe cough, and weight loss. Pleural effusion, peritonitis, or meningitis occurs in as many as two-thirds of individuals.[66] In young adults, the infection is usually chronic and the onset is subtle. Nonspecific symptoms include fever, anorexia, weakness, and weight loss. The physical examination should include a careful skin examination, looking for cutaneous eruptions, sinus tracts, scrotal masses, and lymphadenopathy; hepatomegaly, splenomegaly, tachypnea, dyspnea, rales, wheezes, and stridor are often found. Inflamed nodes may erode through the endobronchial wall; fistulas can occur between the lymph node and the bronchial lumen and cause fibrosis, bronchiectasis, and pneumonia.
- Reactivation of pulmonary TB: There is potential for reactivation of pulmonary TB in those who acquire their initial infection when they are older than 7 years. Reactivation is more likely after the child reaches adolescence and presents with either a few symptoms or fever, anorexia, malaise, weight loss, night sweats, productive cough, hemoptysis, and chest pain. These individuals are highly contagious until effective treatment is started, but full recovery is likely with appropriate treatment.[65]
- Miliary disease: During the primary disease's early stages, bacilli disseminate and reach the bloodstream directly from the initial focus or by way of the regional lymph nodes. Before effective drug therapy, miliary disease complication occurred more commonly in infants, children, and adolescents. It now appears more in racial minorities, in those with underlying conditions that may compromise the immune system, and in older adults.[66] Systemic signs such as anorexia, weight loss, and low-grade fever progress over weeks to lymphadenopathy, hepatosplenomegaly, higher fever, dyspnea, cough, rales, wheezing, frank respiratory distress, and pneumothorax or pneumomediastinum. Headache suggests meningitis; abdominal pain suggests tuberculous peritonitis.[68]
- Lymph node disease: This is an extrapulmonary form of TB that affects the superficial lymph nodes also known as *scrofula*. It is caused by drinking raw milk contaminated with *M. bovis* or after initial infection with *M. tuberculosis*. The head, trunk, neck, and inguinal and lower extremity nodes are firm (but not hard), fixed to underlying tissue, and nontender. The lymphadenopathy is usually initially unilateral and progresses to multinode involvement. TST is usually positive; a chest radiograph is normal 70% of the time; cultures from lymph node biopsies reveal mycobacteria in about 50% of cases.[68]
- Pleural effusions: Pleural effusion frequently occurs in primary disease, caused by an extension of the bacillus into the pleural space by subpleural foci or hematogenous spread, or both. It occurs months to years after the primary infection. Symptoms include abrupt onset of low to high fever, shortness of breath, chest pain on deep inspiration, and decreased breath sounds. Response to treatment takes several weeks; radiographic changes can be evident for months following treatment.[65]
- Tuberculous meningitis: Meningitis is the most serious complication of TB. It generally follows primary pulmonary disease in 0.5% to 3% of untreated infants and young children 6 months to 4 years old (rarely in infants younger than 4 months).

Meningeal infection is common in miliary TB. Bacilli migrate to the subarachnoid space. Caseous lesions enlarge, encapsulate, and form a tuberculoma that acts like any other CNS mass. Tuberculomas are rare and usually occur in children younger than 10 years old. Symptoms evolve slowly or rapidly; infants and children generally experience rapid onset. TST is negative in 45% of cases, up to 30% also have negative chest radiographs.[65] Diagnosis is via CSF AFB stain and culture. Symptoms include headache, fever, malaise, irritability, drowsiness, decreased developmental milestones, nuchal rigidity, positive Kernig or Brudzinski signs, hypertonia, emesis, seizures, and other neurologic symptoms. The provider should consider TB in the differential diagnosis for any child who presents with basilar meningitis and hydrocephaly, cranial nerve palsy, or stroke without other apparent cause.

- Cutaneous TB: This variant occurs in 1% to 2% of all TB cases worldwide but is rare in the United States.[68] Individuals at high risk include those with HIV, living in poor sanitary conditions, of low socioeconomic status, and the malnourished.
- Hematogenous spread of TB to other organs or body systems: TB affect all body systems. Spread occurs to endocrine and exocrine glands, urogenital tract, heart, pericardium, skeleton, eyes, abdomen, tonsils, adenoids, larynx, middle ear, and mastoids.
- MDR-TB is resistance to INH and RIF.
- XDR-TB is resistance to INH, RIF, one fluoroquinolone, and at least one aminoglycoside (capreomycin, amikacin, or kanamycin).
- Over the last few years, drug resistance rates in the United States are between 1% and 9%.[65]

Helminthic Zoonoses

Parasitic helminths are poorly studied and not well understood in comparison to viruses and bacteria. These parasites pose considerable threats to humans. With the domestication of animals for companionship and food, the number of parasites shared between humans and animals increased significantly. Zoonotic helminths continue to emerge in human populations and are expected to increase in numbers globally because of livestock trading, climate changes, and an increase in the demand for animal protein for human consumption.[69] Transmission of zoonotic infections occurs by several routes:

- Direct infection by ingestion of eggs or the larvae penetration into the body (infections such as tapeworms and roundworms are acquired from their eggs; hookworms penetrate the skin)
- Indirect infection by ingestion of larvae in food (e.g., fish, meat, snails, freshwater shrimp, land crabs)
- Exposure to an intermediary vector (e.g., mosquitoes, flies, fleas, ticks).

A large percentage of households in the United States have domestic pets. Domesticated dogs, cats, and wild animals (e.g., raccoons) kept as pets can be infected with intestinal helminth parasites. Mild to severe illness results when a helminth transmits to children, most often by fecal contamination. Only toxocariasis larva migrans is discussed here. (See Chapter 34 for a discussion on intestinal parasites.)

Toxocariasis

Toxocariasis, or larva migrans, is caused by parasitic helminth larvae of the roundworm found in dogs (*T. canis*) and cats (*T. catis*). The larvae live for extended periods in human and animal organs and tissues and cause inflammation. The most common clinical syndromes are visceral larva migrans (VLM), ocular toxocariasis (formerly called *ocular larva migrans*), and covert disease. Toxocara VLM occurs most commonly in children 2 to 7 years of age and ocular toxocariasis has a higher incidence in older children and adolescents.[11] They are further classified as *asymptomatic* or *clinically unapparent*. *T. catis* causes less VLM than *T. canis*; *T. canis* causes VLM, OLM, and, in severe cases, neural larva migrans.

Dogs or cats of any age can carry the *Toxocara* roundworm; worldwide, dogs (especially puppies) are a more common vector than kittens. Puppies are infected before birth (not true for kittens) or from their mother's milk. Ingestion of these hardy eggs (they remain viable for months and in inclement weather conditions) occurs from contact with excreta in contaminated soil (e.g., in sandboxes, parks, playgrounds, schoolyards, public places where dogs and cats visit), hands, toys, or in food. Once the eggs are ingested and hatch, the larvae penetrate the intestines and migrate to the liver, lungs, heart, brain, and muscles. With initial or mild infestations, the larvae reach other locations, such as the brain and eye, easier. In humans, the larvae cannot mature into adult worms (as they do in animals), so infected individuals do not pass eggs or larvae in their excreta. The incubation period cannot be determined in an accurate timeline.

Clinical Findings. Symptoms result from the migrating larvae and from the induced eosinophilic granulomatous inflammation of organs and tissues. Symptom severity depends on the number of larvae ingested and the host's inflammatory response. Assess exposure history for pica or geophagia; exposure to dogs, cats, or environments where animals are known to frequent such as parks, sandboxes, and recent travel. In the case of ocular toxocariasis, there may be a history of pica or previous VLM.

Toxocariasis should be considered in any child with a nonspecific history of recurrent abdominal pain, reactive airway disease, and allergies of unknown cause. The clinical history of VLM includes rash, abdominal and/or limb pain, anorexia, nausea, emesis, lethargy, or respiratory symptoms (cough, wheezing). Ocular toxocariasis is usually associated with a history of a "wandering eye" or squinting, light sensitivity, a white pupil, periorbital edema, or eye pain. Neural larva migrans often presents 2 to 4 weeks after larvae ingestion. The child's history includes weakness, incoordination, ataxia, irritability, seizures, altered mental status, stupor, and/or coma.

Physical Examination

- Ocular toxocariasis: Posterior or peripheral subretinal mass, decreased vision, pain, strabismus, or leukocoria
- VLM: Abdominal pain, hepatomegaly, irritability, respiratory symptoms (coughing, wheezing, pneumonia), cervical adenitis, urticaria, pruritic skin lesions or nodules, macular rash
- Neural larva migrans: Neurologic impairment
- Covert larva migrans: Chronic weakness, abdominal pain, allergic signs (asymptomatic eosinophilia or wheezing may be the only indicators of disease).

Diagnostic Studies. Laboratory studies find significant leukocytosis with eosinophilia and on occasion, anemia and hypergammaglobulinemia.

- VLM: CBC reveals leukocytosis, marked eosinophilia (>500/L), hypergammaglobulinemia (IgG, IgM, IgE), and elevated A and B blood group isohemagglutinin titers. *Toxocara* ELISA antibody is confirmatory; it does not, however, distinguish between past and active disease. ELISA testing should be through the CDC rather than commercial laboratories. Liver imaging by ultrasound, CT, or MRI may show diffuse nodular lesions that are <2 cm in diameter. Liver biopsy may identify the larvae but is not sensitive or specific and is rarely indicated.[11]

- Ocular toxocariasis: Serologic VLM testing is not reliable because it is less sensitive. Diagnosis is usually based on the typical clinical findings of retinal scarring or granuloma formation and elevated antibody titers. Vitreous-aqueous fluid *Toxocara* titers are usually higher than serum titers. CT and MRI detect granulomatous lesions.
- Overt larva migrans: May demonstrate eosinophilia and increased IgE.

Differential Diagnosis. Other helminths, hypereosinophilic syndromes, retinoblastoma, autoimmune disease, and allergic conditions are included in the differential diagnoses.

Management and Complications. Pediatric infectious disease referral for evaluation and treatment is indicated for patients with symptomatic VLM, ocular toxocariasis, or CNS disease. Management is based on controlling inflammatory reactions and using appropriate anthelmintic therapy. Albendazole is the drug of choice, mebendazole is an alternative. Longer courses of 3 to 4 weeks are needed to treat disease with CNS and ocular involvement; systemic and intraocular corticosteroid therapy should be considered for ocular toxocariasis (managed by qualified ophthalmologist and infectious disease specialist). A combination of albendazole and corticosteroids should be prescribed in cases of myocarditis.[11] Family pets need an evaluation by a veterinarian. Permanent ocular structural damage may result from ocular toxocariasis. Neural larva migrans may cause acute eosinophilic meningoencephalitis.

Patient and Family Education. Prevention of zoonotic infestations includes identifying possible sources of exposure, encouraging routine helminth testing for pets, decontamination of soiled environments, and further exposure prevention. The last intervention includes education about safe pet fecal cleanup, regular pet deworming, good hand washing, behavioral modification for pica and geophagia, and covering sandboxes when not in use. Communities should be encouraged to promote leash laws and responsible pet ownership (e.g., cleaning up pet fecal waste), to disallow dogs from playgrounds and parks, and to restrict open access to sandboxes.

Infectious Agents Used in Bioterrorism

Agents of biological warfare are categorized by the CDC according to their potential for aerosol transmission, susceptibility of the population, degree of person-to-person transmission, expected high morbidity and mortality rates, the likelihood for delayed diagnosis, and the lack of effective and efficacious treatments. Agents at the highest risk to the populace are known as *category A weapons of bioterrorism*. These include specific bacteria (e.g., *B. anthracis* [anthrax]; *Clostridium botulinum* [botulism]; *Francisella tularensis* [tularemia]; *Y. pestis* [plague]) and viruses (e.g., variola virus [smallpox]; viruses of hemorrhagic fever [Ebola, Marburg, Lassa fever]). Most of these diseases are rarely, if ever, seen in clinical practice settings. Refer to the CDC website (https://emergency.cdc.gov/bioterrorism/) for specific details about agents. The CDC established a Laboratory Response Network to provide standardized diagnostic testing for selected agents and link state and local public health laboratories with other advanced-capacity laboratories (see Additional Resources). Children are at particular risk for exposure to and absorption of biological warfare agents (e.g., anthrax and botulinum toxin). Factors that predispose them to risk include being closer to the ground, and having faster ventilation rates, thinner skin, increased risk of dehydration, and undeveloped cognition that impairs ability to identify and modify risk.

Providers can join other community healthcare providers to develop pediatric readiness plans for large disasters (e.g., storms, earthquakes, acts of bioterrorism). These readiness plans should include triage, isolation and treatment/care facilities, transportation, communication, housing, and the establishment of vaccination clinics on a massive scale for children, especially in communities where health departments and/or emergency departments may not have the procedural skills to address a severely ill pediatric population. PCPs can request email health alerts from the CDC.

Additional Resources

AIDSinfo (US Department of Health and Human Services): https://hivinfo.nih.gov/home-page

Centers for Disease Control and Prevention: www.cdc.gov

American Academy of Pediatrics: www.aap.org

CDC Laboratory Response Network Partner in Preparedness: www.emergency.cdc.gov/lrn/

FluView Interactive: https://www.cdc.gov/flu/weekly/fluviewinteractive.htm

Hepatitis C Laboratory Studies Table: www.cdc.gov/mmwr/preview/mmwrhtml/mm6218a5.htm

Infectious Diseases Society of America (IDSA): www.idsociety.org

Surviving Sepsis Campaign: www.sccm.org/SurvivingSepsisCampaign/Home

Travelers' Health: Malaria Prophylaxis: wwwnc.cdc.gov/travel/yellowbook/2014/chapter-3-infectious-diseases-related-to-travel/malaria#1939

World Health Organization: www.who.int/en/

References

1. National Institute of Health (NIH). Human Microbiome Project. https://commonfund.nih.gov/hmp/.
2. Lloyd-Price J, Mahurkar A, Rahnavard G, et al. Strains, functions and dynamics in the expanded human microbiome project. *Nature.* 2017;550(7674):61–66.
3. Liang G, Bushman FD. The human virome: assembly, composition and host interactions. *Nat Rev Microbiol.* 2021;19(8):514–527.
4. Gilbert JA, Blaser MJ, Caporaso JG, Jansson JK, Lynch SV, Knight R. Current understanding of the human microbiome. *Nat Med.* 2018;24(4):392–400.
5. American Academy of Pediatrics (AAP). Choosing an Insect Repellent for Your Child. www.healthychildren.org/English/safety-prevention/at-play/Pages/Insect-Repellents.aspx.
6. Downes K, Fitzgerald J, Weiss S. Utility of procalcitonin as a biomarker for sepsis in children. *J Clin Microbiol.* 2020;58:e01851-19.
7. Centers for Disease Control and Prevention. National Notifiable Diseases Surveillance System (NNDSS). https://www.cdc.gov/nndss/.
8. Rose E. Pediatric fever. *Emerg Med Clin North Am.* 2021;39(3):627–639.
9. Lapic I, Padoan A, Bozzato D, Plebani M. Erythrocyte sedimentation rate and c-reactive protein in acute inflammation. *Am J Clin Pathol.* 2020;153(1):14–29.
9a. Centers for Disease Control and Prevention. Guideline for Hand Hygiene in Health-Care Settings: Recommendations of the Healthcare Infection Control Practices Advisory Committee and the HICPAC/SHEA/APIC/IDSA Hand Hygiene Task Force. *MMWR.* 2002;51:RR16.

9b. Centers for Disease Control and Prevention. Antibiotic Resistance Threats in the United States, 2019. http://dx.doi.org/10.15620/cdc:82532.

10. Romandini A, Pani A, Scherardi P, Pattarino G, DeGiacomo C, Scaglione F. Antibiotic resistance in pediatric infections: global emerging threats, predicting the near future. *Antibiotics*. 2021;10(4):393.

11. Kimberlin DW, Brady MT, Jackson, Long SS, eds. *Red Book: 2021-2024 Report of the Committee on Infectious Diseases*. 31st ed. American Academy of Pediatrics; 2021.

12. Uprety A, Graf E. Enterovirus infection and acute flaccid myelitis. *Curr Opin Virol*. 2020;40:55–60.

13. Centers for Disease Control and Prevention (CDC). Hepatitis A Questions and Answers for Health Professionals. https://www.cdc.gov/hepatitis/hav/havfaq.htm#A2.

14. Thomas DJ. Infectious gastrointestinal disorders. In: Dunphy LM, Wiland-Brown JE, Porter BO, Thomas DJ, eds. *Primary Care the Art and Science of Advanced Practice Nursing-An Interprofessional Approach*. 5th ed. F.A. Davis; 2019:544–565.

15. Jhaveri R, El-Kamary SS. Hepatitis C virus. In: Cherry JD, Harrison GJ, Kaplan SL, Steinbach WJ, Hotez PJ, eds. *Feigin and Cherry's Textbook of Pediatric Infectious Diseases*. 8th ed. Elsevier; 2019:1723–1728.

16. American College of Obstetricians and Gynecologists (ACOG). Hepatitis B and Hepatitis C in Pregnancy. https://www.acog.org/womens-health/faqs/hepatitis-b-and-hepatitis-c-in-pregnancy.

17. Centers for Disease Control and Prevention. Hepatitis C Questions and Answers for Health Professionals. https://www.cdc.gov/hepatitis/hcv/hcvfaq.htm.

18. Centers for Disease Control and Prevention. Interpretation of Results of Tests for Hepatitis C Virus (HCV) Infection and Further Actions. https://www.cdc.gov/hepatitis/HCV/PDFs/hcv_graph.pdf.

19. Foster MA, Moorman AC, Teshale EH. Hepatitis C virus. In: Long SS, Pickering LK, Prober CG, eds. *Principles and Practice of Pediatric Infectious Diseases*. 6th ed. Elsevier; 2023:1156–1160.

20. American Association for the Study of Liver Diseases. HCV in Children. https://www.hcvguidelines.org/unique-populations/children.

21. Teshale EH, Hepatitis E. virus. In: Long SS, Pickering LK, Prober CG, eds. *Principles and Practice of Pediatric Infectious Diseases*. 6th ed. Elsevier; 2023:1250–1252.

22. American Academy of Pediatrics (AAP). All about Recommended Immunization Schedules. https://www.healthychildren.org/English/safety-prevention/immunizations/Pages/Recommended-Immunization-Schedules.aspx.

23. Centers for Disease Control and Prevention (CDC). Managing People at Risk for Severe Varicella. https://www.cdc.gov/chickenpox/hcp/index.html#high-risk-people.

24. LaRussa PS, Marin M. Varicella-zoster virus infections. In: Kliegman RM, Stanton BF, St. Geme III JW, et al., eds. *Nelson Textbook of Pediatrics*. 20th ed. Elsevier; 2016:1579–1586.

25. Gershon AA. Varicella-zoster virus. In: Cherry JD, Harrison GJ, Kaplan SL, SteinbacJ, Hotez PJ, eds. *Feigin and Cherry's Textbook of Pediatric Infectious Diseases*. 8th ed. Elsevier; 2019:1476–1481.

26. Centers for Disease Control and Prevention (CDC). 2021-2022 U.S. Flu Season: Preliminary In-Season Burden Estimates. Influenza (Flu). https://www.cdc.gov/flu/about/burden/preliminary-in-season-estimates.htm.

27. Centers for Disease Control and prevention (CDC). Overview of Influenza Testing Methods. https://www.cdc.gov/flu/professionals/diagnosis/overview-testing-methods.htm.

28. Centers for Disease Control and Prevention (CDC). Influenza Antiviral Medications: Summary for Clinicians. https://www.cdc.gov/flu/professionals/antivirals/summary-clinicians.htm.

29. Centers for Disease Control and Prevention (CDC). Bird Flu Virus Infections in Humans. https://www.cdc.gov/flu/avianflu/avian-in-humans.htm.

30. World Health Organization (WHO). Influenza: Avian and Other Zoonotic; 2018. http://www.who.int/en/news-room/fact-sheets/detail/influenza-avian-and-other-zoonotic.

31. World Health Organization (WHO). Key Facts HIV; 2022. https://cdn.who.int/media/docs/default-source/hq-hiv-hepatitis-and-stis-library/key-facts-hiv-2021-26july2022.pdf?sfvrsn=8f4e7c93_5.

32. Centers for Disease Control and Prevention (CDC). HIV Surveillance Report. https://www.cdc.gov/hiv/library/reports/hiv-surveillance/vol-33/index.html.

33. Read JS. Epidemiology and prevention of HIV infection in infants, children, and adolescents. In: Long SS, Prober CG, Fischer M, eds. *In Principles and Practice of Pediatric Infectious Diseases*. 6th ed. Elsevier; 2023:681–684.

34. Hayes EV. Human immunodeficiency virus and acquired immunodeficiency syndrome. In: Kliegman RM, St. Geme III, et al., eds. *Nelson Textbook of Pediatrics*. 21st ed. Elsevier; 2020. 1778–1805.

35. Centers for Disease Control and Prevention (CDC). Breastfeeding: Human Immunodeficiency Virus. https://www.cdc.gov/breastfeeding/breastfeeding-special-circumstances/maternal-or-infant-illnesses/hiv.html.

36. Panel on Treatment of HIV During Pregnancy and Prevention of Perinatal Transmission. Recommendations for the Use of Antiretroviral Drugs during Pregnancy and Interventions to Reduce Perinatal HIV Transmission in the United States. https://clinicalinfo.hiv.gov/en/guidelines/perinatal.

37. Fernández-Luis S, Lain MG, Serna-Pascual M, et al. Optimizing the World Health Organization algorithm for HIV vertical transmission risk assessment by adding maternal self-reported antiretroviral therapy adherence. *BMC Publ Health*. 2022;22(1):1312.

38. Buh A, Deonandan R, Gomes J, Krentel A, Oladimeji O, Yaya S. Adherence barriers and interventions to improve ART adherence in Sub-Saharan African countries: a systematic review protocol. *PLoS One*. 2022;17(6):e0269252.

39. Centers for Disease Control and Prevention (CDC). HIV and Prenatal Transmission: Prevention Challenges. https://www.cdc.gov/hiv/group/pregnant-people/challenges.html.

40. Redfield RR, Schuchat A, Dauphin L, et al. Centers for Disease Control and Prevention: youth risk behavior surveillance United States, 2018. *MMWR Surveill Summ*. 2018;67(No. 8):68–103.

41. Centers for Disease Control and Prevention (CDC). Preexposure prophylaxis for the prevention of HIV infection in the United States: 2021 Update. https://www.cdc.gov/hiv/pdf/risk/prep/cdc-hiv-prep-guidelines-2021.pdf.

42. Centers for Disease Control and Prevention (CDC). *Measles Cases & Outbreaks*; 2022. www.cdc.gov/measles/cases-outbreaks.html.

43. Centers for Disease Control and Prevention (CDC). Manual for the Surveillance of Vaccine-Preventable Diseases; Chapter 9: Mumps; 2022. www.cdc.gov/vaccines/pubs/surv-manual/chpt09-mumps.html#hcp-settings.

44. Schuh AM, Marcdante K, Kliegman RM. Infections characterized by fever and rash. In: *Nelson Essentials of Pediatrics*. 9th ed. Elsevier; 2023.

45. Centers for Disease Control and Prevention (CDC). *Pregnancy and Fifth Disease*; 2019. www.cdc.gov/parvovirusb19/pregnancy.html.

46. Centers for Disease Control and Prevention (CDC). Zika Virus. https://www.cdc.gov/zika/.

47. Centers for Disease Control and Prevention (CDC). West Nile Virus. https://www.cdc.gov/westnile/.

48. Rios M. Reducing threats to the blood supply from West Nile virus, dengue virus, and chikungunya virus through development of detection tools and studies of genetic evolution and pathogenesis. US Food & Drug Administration. www.fda.gov/BiologicsBloodVaccines/ScienceResearch/BiologicsResearchAreas/ucm127094.htm.

49. World Health Organization (WHO). *Dengue and Severe Dengue*; 2022. https://www.who.int/en/news-room/fact-sheets/detail/dengue-and-severe-dengue.

50. Chapman LE, Peters CJ, Mills JN, McKee KT. Hantaviruses. In: Cherry JD, Harrison GJ, Kaplan SL, Steinbach WJ, Hotez PJ, eds. *Feigin and Cherry's Textbook of Pediatric Infectious Diseases*. 8th ed. Elsevier; 2019:1854–1866.

51. Centers for Disease Control and Prevention (CDC). Reported Cases of Hantavirus Disease: Hantavirus infection in the United States. www.cdc.gov/hantavirus/surveillance/index.html.

52. Centers for Disease Control and Prevention (CDC). Middle-Eastern Respiratory Syndrome (MERS). https://www.cdc.gov/coronavirus/mers/about/index.html.

53. Centers for Disease Control and Prevention (CDC). Malaria. https://www.cdc.gov/parasites/malaria/index.html.

54. Centers for Disease Control and Prevention (CDC). *Lyme Disease: Resources*; 2022. Retrieved from: www.cdc.gov/niosh/topics/lyme/resources.html.

55. Lantos PM, McKinney R. Rickettsial and ehrlichial diseases. In: Cherry JD, Harrison GJ, Kaplan SLal, et al., eds. *Feigin and Cherry's Textbook of Pediatric Infectious Diseases*. 8th ed. Elsevier; 2019:1963–1975.

56. Reller ME, Dumler JS. Rocky Mountain Spotted Fever (Rickettsia Rickettsii). In: Kliegman RM, Stanton BF, S. Geme III JW, et al., eds. *Nelson Textbook of Pediatrics*. 21st ed. Elsevier; 2020:1619–1627.

57. Centers for Disease Control and Prevention (CDC). Rocky Mountain Spotted Fever (RMSF): Epidemiology and Statistics. www.cdc.gov/rmsf/stats/.

58. Centers for Disease Control and Prevention (CDC). *MRSA: General Information*; 2019. Retrieved from www.cdc.gov/mrsa/community/index.

59. Centers for Disease Control and Prevention (CDC). *MRSA: Healthcare Settings*; 2019. Retrieved from www.cdc.gov/mrsa/healthcare/index.html.

60. Centers for Disease Control and Prevention (CDC). *National Notifiable Diseases Surveillance System: Data & Statistics*; 2021. Retrieved from: www.cdc.gov/nndss/data-statistics/index.html.

61. American Academy of Pediatrics. [*Bartonella henselae (Cat-Scratch disease)*.] In: Kimberlin DW, Barnett ED, Lynfield R, Sawyer MH, eds. *Red Book: 2021 Report of the Committee on Infectious Diseases*. 32nd ed. American Academy of Pediatrics; 2021:226–229.

62. Yagupsky. Kingella species. In: Long SS, Pickering LK, Prober CG, eds. *Principles and Practice of Pediatric Infectious Diseases*. 6th ed. Elsevier; 2023. 962-967.e3.

63. Porsch EA, Geme JF. Kingella kingae. In: Cherry J, Demmler-Harrison GJ, Kaplan SL, et al., eds. *Feigin and Cherry's Textbook of Pediatric Infectious Diseases*. 8th ed. Elsevier; 2019:1222–1228.

64. del Castillo S, Rake A. Infectious disorders. In: Bolick B, Reuter-Rice K, Madden M, Severin P, eds. *Pediatric Acute Care: A Guide to Interprofessional Practice*. 2nd ed. Elsevier; 2021.

65. Chiang SS, Starke JF. Mycobacterium tuberculosis. In: Long SS, Pickering LK, Prober CG, eds. *Principles and Practice of Pediatric Infectious Diseases*. 5th ed. Elsevier; 2018:790–806.

66. Fitzgerald DW, Sterling TR, Hass DW. Mycobacterium tuberculosis. In: Bennett JE, Dolin R, Blaser MJ, eds. *Mandell, Douglas, and Bennett's Principles and Practice of Infectious Diseases*. 9th ed. Elsevier; 2021.

67. Nolt D, Starke JR. Tuberculosis infection in children and adolescents: testing and treatment. *Pediatrics*. 2021;148(6). e2021054663.

68. Cameron LH, Starke JR. Tuberculosis (Mycobacterium tuberculosis). In: Kliegman RM, Stanton BF, St. Geme III JW, et al., eds. *Nelson Textbook of Pediatrics*. 21st ed. Elsevier; 2020:1565–1582.

69. Majewska A, Huang T, Han B, Drake J. Predictors of zoonotic potential in helminths. *Phil Trans*. 2021;376:20200356.

70. Levin MJ, Duchon JM, Swamy GK, Gershon AA. Varicella zoster immune globulin (VARIZIG) administration up to 10 days after Varicella exposure in pregnant women, immunocompromised participants, and infants: Varicella outcomes and safety results from a large, open-label, expanded-access program. *PLoS One*. 2019;14(7):e0217749.

36

Inflammatory Disorders

TASHA LOWERY AND HANA CONLON

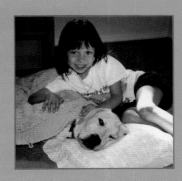

Atopic disorders, rheumatic disorders of childhood, and immunodeficiency disorders share certain characteristics. Inflammation, chronicity, and genetic predisposition are common to these disorders. Inflammatory disorders include atopic, rheumatologic, vasculitis, and immunologic disorders. The most common pediatric atopic disorders that a primary care provider (PCP) is likely to encounter are atopic dermatitis (AD), allergic rhinitis (AR) (or "hay fever"), and asthma. The most common pediatric rheumatic diseases are juvenile idiopathic arthritis (JIA) and systemic lupus erythematosus (SLE). Although the incidence of rheumatic fever has diminished significantly in the United States, cases still occur across the globe. Immunoglobulin A vasculitis (IgAV; formerly known as Henoch Schonlein purpura) is the most common systemic vasculitis syndrome of childhood,[1] and Kawasaki disease (KD) is the most common cause of acquired heart disease.[2] The chapter ends with a synopsis of the more common pediatric primary immune deficiency disorders because as with the other inflammatory disorders, early diagnosis and intervention are critical.

General Principles

Pathophysiology and Defense Mechanisms

Allergic and Atopic Disorders

Allergies are acquired alterations in the body with an immunologic basis. An allergen acts as an antigen that triggers an immunoglobulin E (IgE) response in genetically predisposed individuals. The union of antigen and antibody creates a cascade of biochemical reactions. There are four types of allergic reactions:[3]

- *Type I:* An IgE-mediated reaction, in which the binding region on the IgE (the Fc region) attaches to high-affinity IgE receptors (also known as *FcεRI*) on basophils, mast cells, and eosinophils, resulting in inflammatory mediators and cytokine release.
- *Type II:* A cytotoxic reaction, occurring when IgM or IgG antibodies bind to surface antigens on normal tissue cells activating the complement cascade with resultant inflammation or causing cellular dysfunction or toxicity, leading to cell destruction.
- *Type III:* Immune-complex reactions result from IgG or IgM antibodies-antigen complexes that accumulate in the tissue and circulation, activating the complement cascade. This reaction also attracts granulocytes, which results in tissue damage.
- *Type IV:* Delayed T-cell type reaction (hypersensitivity) involves the activation and proliferations of T cells and their migration to the site of specific antigens. The hypersensitivity reaction is mediated by the T cells and monocytes/macrophages rather than by antibodies. First, there is a local inflammatory and immune reaction at the antigen site that is followed by a secondary cellular response 24 to 72 hours after the initial antigen exposure. Damage to cells and tissues can result from interleukins and other lymphokines secreted by macrophages.

These four types can be easily remembered as type I (A) = **a**llergic, **a**naphylaxis, **a**topy; type II (B) = anti**b**ody; type III (C) = immune **c**omplex; and type IV (D) = **d**elayed. All four types of allergic reactions are mediated by circulating cellular antibodies and generally can occur in any individual. Type I (IgE-mediated) is immediate and involves local and systemic manifestations, resulting in a wide range of clinical manifestations ranging from urticaria and angioedema to anaphylaxis and death. Type II (cytotoxic hypersensitivity or IgG- or IgM-mediated) reactions cause cellular death or dysfunction to target cells by means of IgG and IgM antibody-mediated autoimmunity with or without activation of the entire complement system. IgG and IgM bind to antigens present on cell surfaces with or without subsequent complement fixation. Examples of these reactions include drug-induced hemolytic anemia, immune thrombocytopenia purpura where autoantibodies are directed against platelets, ABO incompatibility transfusion reactions, and hemolytic erythroblastosis fetalis.

In type III (complex-mediated) reactions, immune complexes, normally removed by phagocytic cells, overwhelm the body, resulting in systemic or localized disease. Immune complexes can be deposited in the eye, kidney, skin, joints, and choroid plexus. An example of a local, subacute, type III reaction is an Arthus reaction, which occurs when the body is exposed to a large amount of foreign protein, such as a vaccine. Examples of a systemic reaction include SLE, serum sickness, rheumatic fever, and rheumatoid arthritis. Type IV allergic reaction is a delayed-type hypersensitivity interaction, involving sensitized T-lymphocytic cells. Cytokines are released, which stimulate bone marrow precursors to produce more leukocytes that become macrophages. Examples of type IV reactions are tuberculin skin test reactions and contact dermatitis.

Atopy involves a genetic predisposition to allergic diseases of the epithelial barrier surfaces, commonly affecting the eyes, digestive tract, skin, and respiratory tract.[4] Atopic disorders are immune deviations that likely result from genetic alterations in the immune response possibly from changes in the epigenome due to environmental exposures.[5] Atopy is a form of allergic reactivity that occurs only in certain susceptible individuals. Certain antigens (e.g., cat dander, ragweed) are problematic for atopic individuals, but not for others. Atopic individuals become sensitized to the offending allergen, resulting in an allergic manifestation. Development of one allergic disorder predisposes the child to another disorder, a phenomenon called the *atopic march*.

Development of an allergic response likely results from a combination of genetics, microbial exposure, antibiotic use, environmental and gut microbiome, diet, and lack of breastfeeding. It involves a susceptible individual who is both exposed to an offending antigen and has a predisposition to selective synthesis of IgE when in contact with common environmental antigens. Allergic disease involves the production of IgE, activation of mast cells, eosinophil recruitment, and dysregulated sensory responses leading to pathologic reflexes such as pruritis, airway hyperreactivity, sneezing, and gastrointestinal (GI) discomfort.[4]

In addition, epithelium-derived cytokines, including interleukin (IL)-2, IL-33, and thymic stromal lymphopoietin, activate the immune system from cellular barriers along the GI tract, lung, and skin, calling into play adaptive T helper type 2 (Th2) cells, basophils, eosinophils, mast cells, and innate lymphoid cells. These immune cells help produce type 2 effector cytokines IL-4, IL-5, and IL-13, causing an increase in mucous production, epithelial hyperplasia, and additional inflammatory cells at the epithelial surface. Type 2 cytokines promote the production of IgE from mast cells and basophils. These granulocytes cause the release of proteins and small molecules, including histamine, cytokines, and proteases such as tryptases, which produce not only inflammatory reactions but also activation of the sensory nervous system. Tryptase activates sensory neurons via protease-activated receptors, which causes pruritus. Tissue from atopic patients demonstrates marked increases in sensory innervation at the site of inflammation. Sensory neurons also regulate motility of the immune cells.[4]

Immediate allergic reactions can involve sneezing, hives, wheezing, vomiting, or anaphylaxis. Acute reactions (<30 minutes) can be followed by a late-phase response several hours (2–12) after the initial response. This late-phase response is due to the influx of other inflammatory cells, such as basophils, eosinophils, monocytes, lymphocytes, and neutrophils, and their inflammatory mediators that are recruited to the site of the acute allergic reaction.

The pathogenesis of atopic diseases involves a complex interrelationship of genetic, environmental, and immunologic factors. There are risk factors for development of food allergies and AD at different points in the child's life span. Prenatal factors include genetics, microbial exposure, changes in fetal growth, and antibiotic use. Avoidance of allergic foods during pregnancy does not influence the risk of atopy. In infancy, the microbial environment including alterations in the GI microbiota influences the onset of allergic disease. Breastfeeding may expose an infant to a wide variety of food allergens and, therefore may be protective against allergic disease. There are unanswered questions regarding infant dietary intake combined with a family history of atopy and whether this combination leads to the development of asthma. Exposure to antibiotics in the first 12 months of life alters the intestinal microbiota and may indirectly affect the development of asthma.[6]

Pharmacologic therapy reduces symptoms in the allergic process but does not cure atopic disorders. For example, drugs may be used to control inflammation (corticosteroids), compete with histamine for receptor sites on target tissues (antihistamines), act as a selective leukotriene receptor antagonist (LTRA) (e.g., montelukast), and prevent mast cell degranulation and mediator release (cromolyn sodium). Recent research focuses on the use of pharmacogenomics, epigenomics, and transcriptomics to improve the management of atopic diseases such as asthma.[7]

Rheumatological Disorders

Several rheumatological disorders occur in childhood. In general, they are chronic, autoimmune disorders with multisystem inflammation and circulating autoantibodies directed against the body. Inflammation is a significant factor in these diseases. There are no natural defense mechanisms, and the exact reason why autoimmune diseases develop is not clear. In diseases like SLE, there are circulating autoantibodies, which form immune complexes that lead to complement activation and a cascade of proinflammatory markers that cause tissue damage.

The first-line tests commonly ordered in a child with or suspected of having an autoimmune disease include acute phase reactants, such as C-reactive protein (CRP), erythrocyte sedimentation rate (ESR), serum ferritin, platelets, and procalcitonin; a complete blood count (CBC) with differential; comprehensive, metabolic profile; and urinalysis. Urinalysis is frequently done in rheumatologic disorders known to have renal involvement. Second-line tests include antinuclear antibodies (ANAs), anti-double-stranded deoxyribonucleic acid (DNA), anti-Smith (Sm) antibody, and serum complement levels. The presence of anticyclic citrullinated peptide (anti-CCP) antibody is a surrogate marker, as it is only positive in patients with a positive rheumatoid factor (RF).[8] Table 36.1 describes tests commonly used in the laboratory workup of rheumatic and autoimmune diseases.

Immune Deficiency

The immune system is divided into primitive (innate) immunity and adaptive (acquired) immunity. Both systems rely on effective functioning of leukocytes from the bone marrow.[9] The *innate* immune system involves the natural barriers or surfaces of the body including the skin, mucous membrane, and the cough reflex that protects from invasion of environmental pathogens. The innate immune system includes natural barriers; phagocytes (neutrophils, monocytes, macrophages) and natural killer cells; soluble mediators (complement) and pattern recognition molecules. The complement system attracts cells to the area of inflammation via chemoattractants and enhances phagocytosis. Opsonins are molecules that coat and bind to bacterial surfaces and attract phagocytic cells to engulf or ingest the bacteria. They make the process of phagocytosis more efficient.

The *innate* immune system is responsible for alerting the adaptive immune system to the presence of infection. The adaptive immune system provides a more specific response to the presence of antigens or foreign substances. Lymphocytes, a key player in adaptive immunity, are divided into T cells, B cells, and natural killer cells. T-specific lymphocytes bind with antigens and also trigger a response causing the release of humoral mediators, including cytokines and B-cell–produced immunoglobulins. Antibodies block the binding of antigens to cellular receptors neutralizing microbes and microbial toxins. T cells function as the cellular immune system, whereas the less numerous B cells serve as the humoral immune system. The role of killer cells in host defense involves killer inhibitory receptors that recognize major histocompatibility complex (MHC) antigens; however, their relationship to myeloid cells is not well defined.[10]

General Management Strategies

Atopic and rheumatic disorders and immune deficiencies tend to be chronic conditions with exacerbation and remission of symptoms. Individual management strategies are based on the specific disease process. The following general measures are part of the management of atopic, rheumatoid, and immune deficiency disorders:

- Encourage self-care and learning about one's disease. The use of apps to remind patients about taking their medication can be

TABLE 36.1 Diagnostic Testing in Autoimmune Diseases

Diagnostic Test	What Does It Measure/Significance	Autoimmune Disease
CBC with differential	Looks for anemia of chronic disease, leukopenia/leukocytosis and thrombocytosis/thrombocytopenia	Anemia may be seen in SLE, JIA, other autoimmune diseases Thrombocytosis
Sedimentation rate	Acute-phase reactant Can be falsely low if not measured in a timely fashion	Can be elevated in all autoimmune diseases
C-reactive protein	Acute-phase reactant Produced by the liver More reliable than sedimentation rate Goes up within 6 h and comes down quickly	Can be elevated in all autoimmune diseases
Serum ferritin	Acute-phase reactant	Very elevated (over 5000 ng/mL) in macrophage activation syndrome
Rheumatoid factor	Misnomer; are a measure of autoantibodies that are against the Fc portion of IgG	Elevated most commonly in children with polyarticular JIA
Anticyclic citrullinated peptide (anti-CCP) antibodies	Very specific for JIA but not commonly elevated; not a routine test	More likely to be elevated with severe JIA with irreversible joint damage; found more commonly in polyarticular arthritis
Antinuclear antibody (ANA)	ANAs are measured to determine activity against a variety of nuclear antigens Nonspecific; significant increase is over 1:160 Tend to become positive with age with as many as 5% of healthy adults having a positive ANA	ANA is a nonspecific test; should be done when the history points to SLE
Antidouble-stranded DNA (anti-dsDNA)	Specific antibodies for SLE and are positive in 95% of patients with SLE	Very specific test for SLE; not routinely done as a first-line test
Complement levels	Can be used to monitor disease activity	Second-line test; will be low in SLE and other pediatric vasculitis

CBC, Complete blood count; *IgG*, immunoglobulin G; *JIA*, juvenile idiopathic arthritis; *SLE*, systemic lupus erythematosus.
Modified from Mehta J. Laboratory testing in pediatric rheumatology. *Pediatr Clin North Am.* 2012;59:263–284.

effective.[11] Examples of such include https://medactionplan.com/ and https://safety.smart911.com/mymedschedule

- Address issues associated with living with a chronic disease, such as:
  - Financial burdens associated with the disease
  - School, peer, and family dynamics
  - Body image
  - Pain management as needed
  - Child and adolescent engagement in their care leading to improved adherence
  - Child-parent role in management of a long-term illness or chronic condition
  - Nutrition and avoidance of obesity, if activity is limited, or foods if they are known triggers
  - Social and environmental factors including healthcare disparities, cultural factors, ethnic factors, and healthcare access that may affect the disease process
  - Refer to parent and/or child support groups, professional organizations, and resource groups.

Atopic Disorders

Atopic diseases including asthma, AR, and AD are an important public health concern worldwide with incidence increasing. AR and asthma remain the most common chronic diseases in children.[12] The burden of these diseases on the child's activities of daily living and the social and economic cost point to a need for prevention. Best practices in allergy prevention include feeding peanut food to infants at 4 to 6 months, making sure that vitamin D is appropriately supplemented, and avoiding environmental exposure to allergens to decrease allergies in children. Newer studies examine the effect of supplemental prebiotics, probiotics, and synbiotics on decreasing the emergence of allergens in children.[13,14] The dual allergen hypothesis examines outcomes when an infant is presented with an allergen by different routes. Environmental exposure to peanuts or application of peanut oil on eczematous skin during infancy increases the risk of peanut allergy in children, whereas two significant studies (LEAP and EAT studies) reported that feeding infants peanut-containing food decreased peanut allergies.[12] Viral respiratory infections in infancy also increase the risk of asthma likely through the production of cytokines IL-25 and IL-33 that also interact with inflammatory allergic pathways, inducing Th2-related inflammation.[15]

Among inflammatory disorders, the respiratory disorders are common and can affect about a third of the population. In patients with atopy, the allergic march typically progresses from AD or food allergies to AR and finally asthma. This march can start in young infants, continue through childhood, worsen through adulthood, or ultimately resolve with increasing age. Because patients who are already sensitized have a greater risk of developing more allergies than those without sensitization, prevention of allergy in a patient predisposed to allergy, and avoidance of new sensitization in an individual who already has allergies are key strategies.[16]

Asthma

Asthma is a complex, chronic, multifaceted respiratory disease resulting from inflammation, airway hyperresponsiveness, and airway remodeling. It is characterized by varying degrees of airflow obstruction that presents as coughing, wheezing, chest tightness, breathlessness, and respiratory distress. It can also manifest as a persistent cough without significant wheezing. Asthma is the most common chronic pulmonary disease in children with one out of 12 children ages 0 to 17 years old diagnosed with asthma in 2020. The Centers for Disease Control and Prevention (CDC) reported that in 2020 asthma pathology was higher among boys aged <18 years, non-Hispanic Black (Black) persons, non-Hispanic multiple-race (multiple-race) persons, and Puerto Rican persons. In addition, asthma exacerbations were more prevalent among children, females, and multiple-race persons.[17] Advances in therapy have reduced asthma-related deaths and improved the quality of life for patients with asthma; however, the CDC's report noted that disparities in asthma indicators persist by demographic characteristics, poverty level, and geographic location.[17]

The first contact for many pathogens and environmental irritants is typically the normal airway. Alveolar epithelial cells function to protect the lung against environmental insults and signal immune cells to activate. Alveolar macrophages and neutrophils neutralize foreign particles including pathogens. In airways of patients with asthma, there are eosinophils, degranulated mast cells, lymphocytes, altered goblet cells, and epithelial cell tight junctions. The dendritic T cells present the antigen to native T cells that triggers a Th2 response. The pathophysiology involves the activation of cytokines, which influence T cell differentiation and the intracellular signaling cascade. Toll-like receptor (TLR) and transcription factors, such as nuclear factor kappa light-chain enhancers of activated B cells, play a key role in the pathophysiology of asthma.[18]

Persistent inflammation associated with asthma can result in irreversible changes, such as airway wall remodeling. Inflammation causes acute bronchoconstriction, airway edema, and mucous plug formation. This inflammation can trigger a hyperresponsiveness to a variety of stimuli including allergens, exercise, cold air, and physical, chemical, or pharmacologic agents. This results in bronchospasm that presents as wheezing, breathlessness, chest tightness, and cough that can be worse at night or with exercise. Airflow obstruction is often reversible, either spontaneously or with treatment; however, airway remodeling can occur secondary to persistent fibrotic changes in the airway lining. Fibrosis alters the airway caliber leading to decreased airflow with permanent changes starting in childhood that become recognizable in adults.

Asthma is a disease with multiple phenotypes. Phenotypes can be characterized by age of onset, severity, triggers, comorbidities, and differences in the inflammatory cells responsible for clinical manifestations.[19,20] Identified phenotypes of asthma include childhood allergic vs. nonallergic, adult onset, asthma with air flow restriction and asthma associated with obesity.[20] Allergic asthma starts in childhood and is responsive to typical treatments for asthma such as inhaled corticosteroids (ICS).[20,21] Examples of nonallergic asthma include neutrophilic inflammation–induced asthma and exercise-induced asthma (EIA). Asthma-like symptoms, especially

shortness of breath and cough caused by neutrophilic asthma is largely intractable to standard asthma practices, especially ICS. The airway with neutrophilic inflammation is also characterized by increased bacteria load and decreased biodiversity more like the airway of pediatric patients with cystic fibrosis or adults with chronic obstructive pulmonary disease (COPD). Researchers are investigating biologics as treatment for neutrophilic inflammation related asthma.[21]

Genetics also play a role as patients with 17q21 variants are more likely to have an early onset of asthma. This locus is associated with four genes, but the function of these genes is still unknown. Hereditability of asthma ranges from 55% to 74% in adults and as high as 90% in children.[22] Asthma risk is also related to the type of allergen sensitization with pollen, mold, and staphylococcal enterotoxin associated with severe asthma. Sex hormones have an impact on the immune response as progesterone promotes the T2 response. There is also an association between blood eosinophil counts and eosinophilic phenotype of asthma with an eosinophilic steroid refractory phenotype associated with uncontrolled asthma, despite the use of high-dose steroids. This type of asthma might be seen in older adolescents. In addition, there is a paucicellular asthma phenotype that has a better prognosis and is associated with low-grade inflammatory disease.[23] These phenotypes of asthma are new discoveries and will potentially assist in the development of a personalized medicine approach to the treatment of asthma[22]; however, more research is needed.[20]

The 2020 National Asthma Education and Prevention Program Expert Panel Report (EPR3) continues to classify asthma severity and control in children as intermittent, mild persistent, moderate persistent, or severe persistent depending on symptoms, recurrences, need for specific medications, and pulmonary function (Table 36.2). This stepwise approach remains the foundation for asthma management. Children classified at any level of asthma can have exacerbations with varying degrees of severity. Exacerbations involve progressive worsening of shortness of breath, cough, wheezing, and/or chest tightness. The degree of airway hyperresponsiveness is associated with the severity classification and can change over time.

Allergic asthma exacerbations are biphasic. The immediate, or early asthmatic response (EAR) phase, is characterized by bronchospasm and bronchoconstriction. The pathophysiologic mechanisms involve IgE-mediated degranulation of mast cells with the release of prostaglandin D2, histamine, and cysteinyl leukotrienes leading to smooth muscle contraction and bronchoconstriction. EAR starts within 15 to 30 minutes of mast cell activation and resolves within approximately 1 hour if the individual is removed from the offending allergen. The EAR phase often responds well to inhaled bronchodilator agents. The late-phase asthmatic response is due to inflammatory mediators as well as dendritic cells, eosinophils, neutrophils, helper T cells, and mast cells that cause airway constriction. The late-phase response usually follows the EAR within 6 to 26 hours after exposure to the allergen, is often associated with airway hyperresponsiveness more severe than the EAR presentation and can last from hours to several weeks. This requires the use of corticosteroids as the response to inhaled β-agonist is muted.

Exercise-induced bronchospasm (EIB) describes the phenomenon of airway narrowing during, or minutes after, the onset of vigorous activity. Most people with asthma exhibit airway hyperirritability after vigorous activity and display EIB. For some children, exercise is the trigger for their asthma. Although asthma is

TABLE 36.2 Classification of Asthma Severity in Children: Clinical Features Before Treatment

Classification and Step	Symptoms[a]	Nighttime Symptoms	Lung Function
Step 1: Intermittent	Symptoms 2 times or less per week Asymptomatic and normal PEF between exacerbations Requires SABA 2 days/week Exacerbations brief (few hours or days); varying intensity No interference with normal activity	Two times or less per month	FEV_1 >80% predicted Normal FEV_1 between exacerbations
Step 2: Mild persistent	Symptoms more than 2 times per week but less than 1 time per day Requires SABA more than 2 days/week but not more than one per day Exacerbations may affect activity (minor)	Three to 4 times per month	FEV_1 >80% predicted
Step 3: Moderate persistent	Daily symptoms Daily use of inhaled SABA Some limitations Exacerbations affect activity, 2 times or more per week; may last days	More than 1 time per week but not nightly	FEV_1 >60% but <80% predicted
Step 4: Severe persistent	Continual symptoms Requires SABA several times/day Extremely limited physical activity Frequent exacerbations	Often 7 times per week	FEV_1 <60% predicted

[a]Having at least one symptom in a particular step places the child in that particular classification.

FEV_1, Forced expiratory volume in 1 second; *PEF*, peak expiratory flow; *SABA*, short-acting β₂-agonist.

Modified from National Heart, Lung, and Blood Institute (NHLBI). *Full Report of the Expert Panel: Guidelines for the Diagnosis and Management of Asthma, (EPR-3)*. National Institutes of Health; 2007.

not always associated with an allergic disorder in children, many children with chronic asthma have an allergic component.[24]

The diagnosis of asthma is often delayed in children from 0 to 4 years of age. Instead, they may be diagnosed with reactive airway disease, wheezy bronchitis, or recurrent bronchitis. Asthma is rarely diagnosed before 12 months of age as rates of viral illnesses causing bronchiolitis are high. A diagnosis of asthma should be made with caution in a toddler who only has wheezing associated with viral infections. Using the well-known expression "all that wheezes is not asthma and all asthma does not wheeze," the EPR3 cautions providers about the diagnosis of asthma before age 4 years.

Whether hyperresponsiveness of the airways is present at birth or acquired later in genetically predisposed children is not known. However, the genetic predisposition for the development of an IgE-mediated response to common aeroallergens remains the strongest identifiable predisposing risk factor for asthma.[25] A combination of the genetic predisposition and exposure to certain environmental factors are the necessary components responsible for the pathophysiologic response associated with asthma. Common triggers for asthma exacerbation include viral respiratory infections, environmental allergens, a change in the weather, stress, emotional expression, and exercise as well as comorbid conditions such as sinusitis and gastroesophageal reflex. Global warming, climate change, and air pollution also contribute to allergic asthma.[26]

The majority of children with allergen-induced asthma have hyperresponsive airways that show evidence of sensitization commonly to any of the following inhalant allergens:

- House dust mites, cockroaches, indoor molds
- Saliva and dander of cats and dogs
- Outdoor seasonal molds
- Airborne pollens—trees, grasses, and weeds
- Food allergy, including egg and tree nuts

Overview of Asthma Guidelines and Tools

The 2022 Global Initiative for Asthma (GINA) guidelines[20] recommend careful history taking along with documenting airflow limitations and asking the patient to do a forced expiratory volume in 1 second (FEV_1).

American Academy of Pediatrics (AAP) recommendations clearly advocate for the use of age-specific assessment of asthma control.[27] In a primary care setting, asthma should be monitored using a standardized instrument, which may include the Asthma Control Test (ACT), Asthma Control Questionnaire, Asthma Therapy Assessment Questionnaire, Asthma Control Score, or the Test for Respiratory and Asthma Control in Kids for children 0 to 5 years.[27] The advantage of a standardized questionnaire is that it allows the PCP to assess changes in the patient's asthma and alter the management plan as needed. Because they are self-reporting measures, the use of these tools may underreport the patient's degree of airway inflammation as patients may accept their symptoms as the norm. The ACT, however, has been found to be reliable, valid, and responsive to changes in level of control in patients who are not managed by a specialist.[28] Assessment of quality of life is critical in chronic disease and is frequently used as a measure of efficacy of various asthma treatments.[20] The Pediatric Asthma Quality of Life Questionnaire (PAQLQ) is a validated tool to assess quality of life in children with asthma ages 7 to 17 years. The Pediatric Asthma Questionnaire (PAS) is validated for use with children ages 2 to 5 years.[29] One method to increase provider use of validated tools is to have access to these tools through the electronic medical record (EMR). There is an increase in literature indicating that the more intuitive that tools interface with the EMR, the more likely providers will follow evidence-based practices. Guideline driven care and a written Asthma Action Plan (wAAP) help to decrease pediatric exacerbations (Fig. 36.1).[30]

Objective measures of asthma control include assessment of lung function, airway hyperresponsiveness assessment, and biomarkers. Peak flow is the easiest measure to use but has variable results even when done well. Spirometry is suggested every 1 to 2 years by the EPR3 recommendations. The use of prebronchodilator and postbronchodilator spirometry, otherwise known as the bronchodilator reversibility flow test, can be done to see if there is significant improvement of at least 12% in the FEV_1 following a treatment. Home-based airflow measurement can be done; however, the use of this technology is not widespread.[27]

Airway hyperresponsiveness is assessed by bronchial provocation test done with methacholine or exercise. A 20% reduction in FEV_1 with methacholine or a 10% reduction following exercise shows hyperresponsive airways. In terms of biomarkers, exhaled fractional concentration of nitric oxide (FeNO) is a measure of airway inflammation, and the joint American Thoracic Society (ATS)/European Respiratory Society guidelines for its use are the current standard of care (American Academy of Allergy, Asthma, and Immunology).[31,32] FeNO measures eosinophilic airway inflammation and can be elevated in patients with atopy, but without asthma. While the upper limit of normal is 25 parts per billion (ppb), a change of 20% for values greater than 50 ppb or 10 ppb in values ≤50 ppb is significant.[27] GINA[20] guidelines acknowledge the potential utility of FeNO biomarker testing for moderate to severe intractable asthma. Studies to date, however, have been marred by poor patient adherence to study protocol. GINA recommends resorting to FeNO biomarker testing for atopic type 2 inflammation only after the patient fails to reach adequate control through treatment steps 1–4 in the Stepwise Approach to Managing Asthma.

In primary care and emergency department (ED) settings, patients with acute asthma are assessed based on their respiratory rate, work of breathing, ability to talk in sentences, breathlessness, and alertness. There are apps that can be used in the ED setting (see Resources). The management of an acute exacerbation includes reversal of bronchoconstriction, restoration of oxygen level, and prevention of relapse.[33]

Clinical Findings

History. Critical points to cover in the history include:

- Family history of asthma or other related allergic disorders (e.g., eczema or AR)
- Conditions associated with asthma (e.g., chronic sinusitis, nasal polyposis, gastroesophageal reflux, and chronic otitis media)
- Complaints of chest tightness or dyspnea

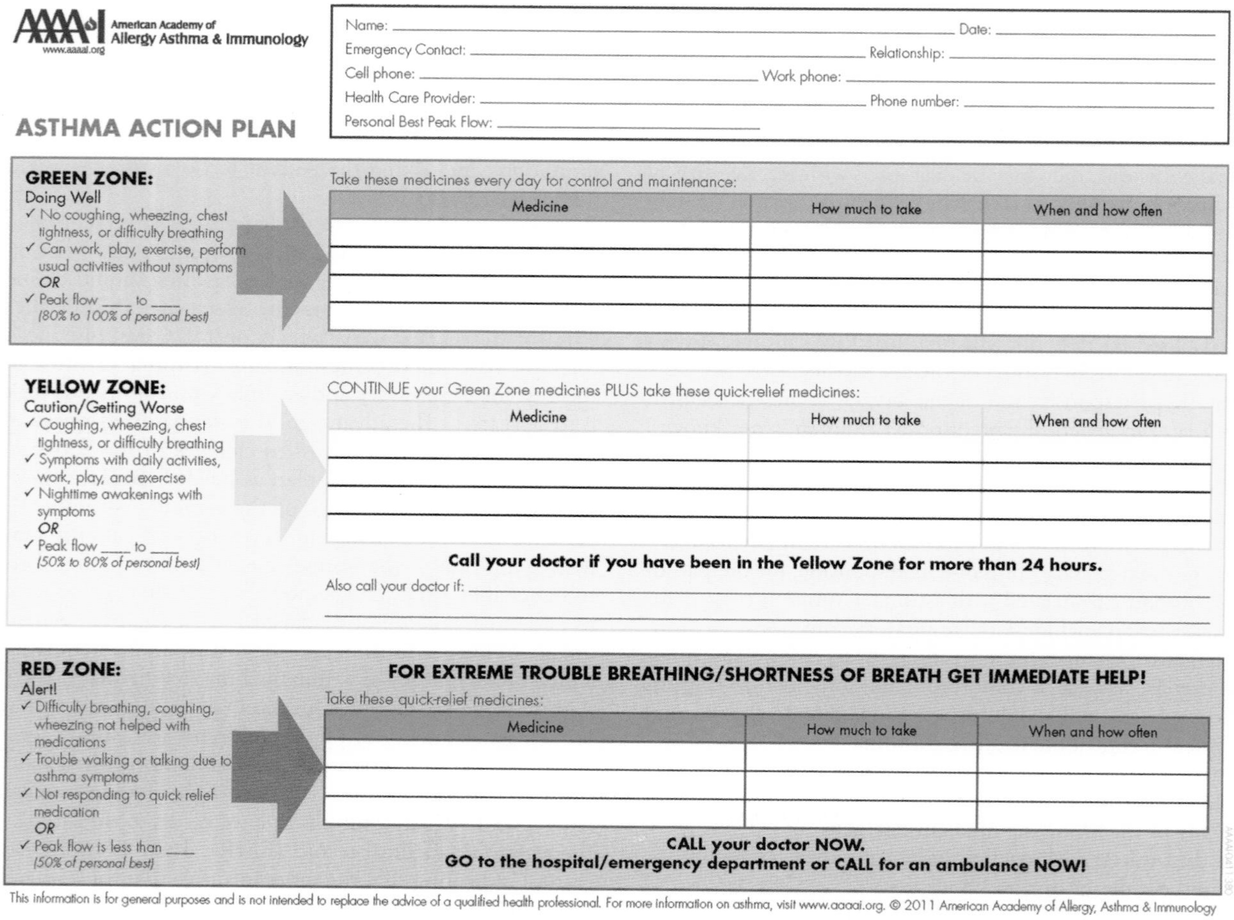

American Academy of Allergy Asthma & Immunology
www.aaaai.org

ASTHMA ACTION PLAN

Name: ______ Date: ______
Emergency Contact: ______ Relationship: ______
Cell phone: ______ Work phone: ______
Health Care Provider: ______ Phone number: ______
Personal Best Peak Flow: ______

GREEN ZONE:
Doing Well
✓ No coughing, wheezing, chest tightness, or difficulty breathing
✓ Can work, play, exercise, perform usual activities without symptoms
OR
✓ Peak flow ____ to ____
(80% to 100% of personal best)

Take these medicines every day for control and maintenance:

Medicine	How much to take	When and how often

YELLOW ZONE:
Caution/Getting Worse
✓ Coughing, wheezing, chest tightness, or difficulty breathing
✓ Symptoms with daily activities, work, play, and exercise
✓ Nighttime awakenings with symptoms
OR
✓ Peak flow ____ to ____
(50% to 80% of personal best)

CONTINUE your Green Zone medicines PLUS take these quick-relief medicines:

Medicine	How much to take	When and how often

Call your doctor if you have been in the Yellow Zone for more than 24 hours.

Also call your doctor if: ______

RED ZONE:
Alert!
✓ Difficulty breathing, coughing, wheezing not helped with medications
✓ Trouble walking or talking due to asthma symptoms
✓ Not responding to quick relief medication
OR
✓ Peak flow is less than ____
(50% of personal best)

FOR EXTREME TROUBLE BREATHING/SHORTNESS OF BREATH GET IMMEDIATE HELP!

Take these quick-relief medicines:

Medicine	How much to take	When and how often

CALL your doctor NOW.
GO to the hospital/emergency department or CALL for an ambulance NOW!

This information is for general purposes and is not intended to replace the advice of a qualified health professional. For more information on asthma, visit www.aaaai.org. © 2011 American Academy of Allergy, Asthma & Immunology

• **Fig. 36.1** Asthma Action Plan. (From American Academy of Allergy, Asthma & Immunology (AAAAI). https://www.aaaai.org/Aaaai/media/MediaLibrary/PDF%20Documents/Libraries/Asthma-Action-Plan_FILLABLE.pdf.)

- Cough and wheezing particularly at night and in the early morning or shortness of breath with exercise or exertion (characteristic of asthma)
- Seasonal, continuous, or episodic pattern of symptoms that may be associated with certain allergens or triggering agents
- Episodes of recurrent "bronchitis" or pneumonia
- Precipitation of symptoms by known aggravating factors (upper respiratory infections, acetaminophen, aspirin).

Physical Examination. Table 36.3 outlines the physical assessment findings correlated with asthma severity. Broadly speaking, the following may be seen on physical examination:

- Heterophonous wheezing (different pitches but may be absent if severe obstruction)
- Continuous and persistent coughing
- Prolonged expiratory phase, high-pitched rhonchi especially at the bases
- Diminished breath sounds
- Altered level of alertness; signs of respiratory distress, including tachypnea, retractions, nasal flaring, use of accessory muscles, increasing restlessness, apprehension, agitation, drowsiness to coma
- Tachycardia, hypertension, or hypotension
- Cyanosis of lips and nail beds if hypoxic
- Possible associated findings include sinusitis, AD, and AR.

Diagnostic Studies. Laboratory and radiographic tests should be individualized and based on symptoms, severity or chronology of the disease, response to therapy, and age. Tests to consider include:

- Oxygen saturation (SaO_2) of hemoglobin by pulse oximetry to assess the percentage of total hemoglobin that is oxygenated to determine severity of an acute exacerbation. This should be a routine part of every assessment of a child with asthma.
- A CBC if secondary infection or anemia is suspected (also check for elevated levels of eosinophils).

TABLE 36.3	Physical Assessment of Asthma and Asthma Severity
Severity of Asthma	**Physical Assessment Findings**
Mild	Wheezing at the end of expiration or no wheezing
	No or minimal intercostal retractions along posterior axillary line
	Slight prolongation of expiratory phase
	Normal aeration in all lung fields
	Can talk in sentences
Moderate	Wheezing throughout expiration
	Intercostal retractions
	Prolonged expiratory phase
	Decreased breath sounds at the base
Severe	Use of accessory muscles plus lower rib and suprasternal retractions; nasal flaring
	Inspiratory and expiratory wheezing or no wheezing heard with poor air exchange
	Suprasternal retractions with abdominal breathing
	Decreased breath sounds throughout base
Impending respiratory arrest	Diminished breath sounds over entire lung field
	Tiring, inability to maintain respirations
	Severely prolonged expiration if breath sounds are heard
	Drowsy, confused

- Routine chest radiographs are not indicated in most children with asthma. Results are typically normal or only show hyperinflation. Imaging should be ordered judiciously with consideration of the long-term risk. However, chest radiographs and imaging are useful in the following situations: selected cases of asthma or suspected asthma or if the child has persistent wheezing without a clinical explanation, and children with hypoxia, fever, suspected pneumonia, and/or localized rales requiring admission. Infants with wheezing during the winter who have clinical bronchiolitis do not need imaging.
- If sinusitis is suspected as the trigger, no diagnostic radiographic testing is needed.
- Allergy evaluation should be considered; however, history and physical examination are key in this consideration. Refer child to pediatric allergist as needed.
- Sweat test should be considered based on history in every patient with asthma.
- Pulmonary function tests:
  - Pulmonary function testing (spirometry) is the best way to evaluate obstructive respiratory pathology.[34] It should be used on a regular basis to monitor, evaluate, and manage asthma. Exercise challenges using spirometry can also be done to evaluate the child with EIA. Spirometry is an underutilized tool worldwide. As previously reviewed, the GINA guidelines[20] recommend spirometry every 1 to 2 years. Children older than 5 years can typically perform spirometry.
  - To evaluate the accuracy of the spirometry, the volume flow loop should have an initial sharp peak with an extension down to the baseline at the end of expiration that is reproducible 3 times.[35] The normal flow-volume is when the horizontal axis shows the vital capacity and the vertical axis shows the peak flow. The US Department of Health and Human Services Publication number 2011-135 reviews how to correct test errors and can be retrieved at https://www.cdc.gov/niosh/docs/2011-135/default.html. While historically spirometry values have been calculated based on the patient's age, height, sex, and race, the use of race as a predictive factor is widely disputed and is no longer considered scientifically sound.[36] Ongoing research seeks to "unwind the race-based evolution of lung function assessment."[36]
- Look at FEV_1, which represents the amount of air exhaled in 1 second. Reversibility with a bronchodilator is an increase in FEV_1 of 12% or more or 100 mL from baseline. Interpretation of percentage predicted is:
  - >75%: Normal
  - 60% to 75%: Mild obstruction
  - 50% to 59%: Moderate obstruction
  - <49%: Severe obstruction
- Forced vital capacity (FVC) represents the amount of air expelled:
  - 80% to 120%: Normal
  - 70% to 79%: Mild reduction
  - 50% to 69%: Moderate reduction
  - <50%: Severe reduction
- FEV_1/FVC represents the amount of air expelled in the first second over the total amount of air expelled and should be greater than 90% of the predicted value. Spirometry testing is done before a breathing treatment and 10 minutes after the treatment. If the child's FEV_1 improves by 12%, asthma is likely because this illustrates hyperresponsiveness.

TABLE 36.4 Abnormal Spirometry Findings in Obstructive and Restrictive Airway Disease

	Obstructive	Restrictive
FVC	Normal or ↓	↓
FEV$_1$	↓	↓
FEV$_1$/FVC	↓	Normal or ↑

FEV$_1$, Forced expiratory volume in 1 second; *FVC,* forced vital capacity.

- Forced expiratory flow (FEF) (FEF$_{25}$ to FEF$_{75}$) reflects the middle portion of the downward limb of the curve and is a good measure of smaller airway function. Interpretation of percentage predicted is:
  - >60%: Normal
  - 40% to 60%: Mild obstruction
  - 20% to 40%: Moderate obstruction
  - <10%: Severe obstruction
- Performing spirometry during well-child checks and sick visits gives the PCP an excellent indication of the amount of inflammation and bronchospasm present in the airway. Table 36.4 identifies abnormal spirometry patterns.
- Consider the use of more sophisticated pulmonary laboratory studies such as FeNO or serum biomarkers for the child with severe asthma.
- Peak flow measurements:
  - If spirometry is not an option, peak expiratory flow (PEF) can be used in children as young as 4 to 5 years old.
  - PEF values are instrument specific; the child's personal best value is the best guide to help detect possible changes in airway obstruction. The predicted range for height and age can be substituted if the child's personal best rate is not available (Table 36.5). Interpretation of PEF reading is as follows if PEF is in the:

- Green zone: More than 80% to 100% of personal best signals good control.
- Yellow zone: Between 50% and 79% of personal best signals a caution.
- Red zone: Between 0% and 50% of personal best signals major airflow obstruction.
- Box 36.1 describes use of peak flowmeter and interpretation of results.

• BOX 36.1 Use of the Peak Flow Meter and Its Interpretation

Steps to follow in using a peak flow meter:
- Have child stand up.
- Make sure that indicator is at the base of the numbered scale.
- Ask child to take a deep breath.
- Have the child place the peak flow meter in the mouth with the lips sealing the mouthpiece. Tell the child not to put his or her tongue in the hole of the mouthpiece.
- Tell the child to blow out as hard and fast as possible.
- Record the rate, but if the child coughs, do not write down that number.
- Repeat steps 2 through 6 two more times.
- Record the highest of the three values.

Peak Expiratory Flow Rate

Maximum flow rate that is produced during forced expiration with fully inflated lungs.

Personal Best Value

Highest value achieved in measuring peak expiratory flow (PEF) rate over a 2-week period when child's asthma is under good control is known as one's *personal best value* or *rate.* Good control is defined as when one feels well without asthma symptoms. To determine personal best, take readings twice daily, in the morning and late afternoon or evening, and 15 to 20 minutes after taking an inhaled short-acting β$_2$-agonist (SABA). Using the personal best value is the most accurate gauge to use to interpret changes in peak flow measurements because the child's own scores are used as the standard for comparison.

TABLE 36.5 Predicted Average Peak Expiratory Flow for Normal Children and Adolescents

Height (Inches)	Males and Females (L/min)	Height (Inches)	Males and Females (L/min)	Height (Inches)	Males and Females (L/min)
43	147	51	254	59	360
44	160	52	267	60	373
45	173	53	280	61	387
46	187	54	293	62	400
47	200	55	307	63	413
48	214	56	320	64	427
49	227	57	334	65	440
50	240	58	347	66	454
				67	467

Modified National Heart, Lung, and Blood Institute (NHLBI). *Executive Summary: Guidelines for the Diagnosis and Management of Asthma, NIH Pub No 94-3042A.* National Institutes of Health; 1994; and Polger G, Promedhar V. *Pulmonary Function Testing in Children: Techniques and Standards.* WB Saunders; 1971.

- Exhaled nitric oxide
  - Fraction of exhaled nitric oxide (FE_{no}) has moderate accuracy when diagnosing children 4 to 5 years and over. It is more accurate in children and in patients who have not been on steroids.[32] Recent studies have shown that repeat measurements during the same visit are not needed.[37]
  - The test measures eosinophilic airway inflammation. The patient must have a constant expiratory flow rate while the FE_{no} is measured. It may support the diagnosis of asthma and can help determine compliance with corticosteroid therapy.
  - A FE_{no} value of more than 35 ppb in children indicates eosinophilic inflammation and likely responsiveness to corticosteroids, whereas values of 25 to 35 ppb should be interpreted with caution.

Differential Diagnosis

Numerous conditions can cause airway obstruction and be incorrectly confused with asthma, especially in young children and infants. Differential diagnoses include acute bronchiolitis; laryngotracheobronchitis; bronchopneumonia; pneumothorax; inhaled foreign body; congenital malformations of the heart; pulmonary abnormalities or bronchopulmonary dysplasia or bronchiectasis; genetic disorders (e.g., cystic fibrosis and α-1-antitrypin deficiency); primary ciliary dyskinesia; tracheal or foreign body compression (e.g., vascular aortic ring, enlarged lymph nodes, or tumors); chronic lower respiratory tract infections caused by immunodeficiency disorders; congenital malformation of the GI system with resultant recurrent aspiration and gastroesophageal reflux disease; vocal cord dysfunction; exposure to toxic substance; and anaphylaxis.

Management

Management strategies are based on whether the child has intermittent, mild persistent, moderate persistent, or severe persistent asthma (see Table 36.2). A stepwise approach is recommended. The National Asthma Education and Prevention Program Coordinating Committee (NAEPPCC) 2020 Focused Updates to the Asthma Management Guidelines introduced alternative treatment plans based upon early or intermittent initiation of ICS and Single Maintenance and Reliever Therapy (SMART) strategies.[37] If control of symptoms is not maintained at a particular step of classification and management, the PCP first should reevaluate for adherence and administration factors. If these factors are not responsible for the lack of symptom control, go to the next treatment step. Likewise, gradual step-downs in pharmacologic therapy may be considered when the child is well controlled for 3 months.[20] ICS may be reduced about 25% to 50% every 3 months to the lowest possible dose needed to control the child's asthma.[38]

Chronic Asthma. Treatment of chronic asthma in children is based on general control measures and pharmacotherapy. Control measures include the following:

- Avoid exposure to known allergens or irritants, especially when mold and pollen counts are at their highest.
- Use air conditioning, close windows and doors, and remain indoors as much as possible during high pollen and mold season.
- Reassure the parent that fever can be controlled with either nonsteroidal antiinflammatory drug (NSAID) or acetaminophen, which will not make the asthma worse unless the child has a known allergic/sensitivity reaction.

- Consider allergen immunotherapy (AIT). Reduction in healthcare cost and improved outcomes associated with allergy immunotherapy are reported.[20,39]
- Treat rhinitis, sinusitis, or gastroesophageal reflux.
- Other pharmacologic agents that may need to be considered include:
  - Anticholinergics: to reduce vagal tone in the airways (may also decrease mucus gland secretion)
  - Cromolyn sodium: to inhibit mast cell release of histamine
  - LTRA: to disrupt the synthesis or function of leukotrienes
  - Long-acting muscarinic antagonists (LAMA): LAMAs are a class of long-acting inhaled bronchodilators. LAMAs are muscarinic antagonist that provide approximately 12 hours of bronchodilation. LAMAs were previously only used in COPD; however, the NAECCPP (2020) found it safe to add a LAMA in addition to an ICS-long-acting beta agonists (LABA) combination for adolescents (>12 years) with uncontrolled asthma. LAMAs were found to improve asthma control and quality of life. The addition of a LAMA, however, has no effect on asthma exacerbations.[38]

Severe Asthma. For severe asthma with an allergic component consider referral to pulmonology for immune modulator treatment. As of 2021, there are two immune modulators US Food and Drug Administration (FDA) approved for children older than 6 years with moderate to severe asthma symptoms: omalizumab and mepolizumab. Benralizumab and dupilumab are FDA approved for adolescents older than 12 years. Omalizumab was the first immune modulator approved and is commonly used when an immune modulator is necessary for asthma or allergic control, such as when asthma symptoms are not controlled by ICS. Omalizumab is a recombinant DNA-derived, humanized IgG monoclonal antibody that binds to human IgE on the surface of mast cells and basophils. The medication is delivered via bi-weekly or monthly injections. Dose is based upon IgE concentration and body weight. Pediatric patients are candidates for anti-IgE monoclonal antibody as a second-line therapy when they have moderate to severe allergy-related asthma, evidence of atopy, reaction to perennial allergens, and an IgE level of >30 IU/mL.[40] Studies show a relevant reduction in exacerbation for children and adolescents with use of this treatment.[20,41] Cost is substantial and therapy presents a risk of anaphylaxis. Pediatric patients who receive omalizumab therapy should also be prescribed an epinephrine autoinjector in the event of delayed anaphylaxis.[4]

- Administer influenza and COVID vaccines at recommended intervals.
- Provide a clear written asthma action plan using a traffic light approach of green, yellow, or red to manage exacerbations. Parents should know what to do when their child has progressed into the yellow (79–50% of best personal peak flow) or red (<50% of personal best peak flow) zone.
- Instruct parent to advance the asthma action plan to the yellow treatment zone if the child has an upper respiratory infection.[26]
- Educate regarding asthma basics, including triggers and prevention with environmental modification, as well as the different treatment modalities including the techniques of administration; dispel any myths regarding asthma medication.
- Address coping and self-management issues. The child and family need to be able to understand their emotions, worries, and uncertainty, as well as when to contact their PCP. Developing and understanding the asthma action plan is an important guide that promotes self-management and provides objective criteria for decision-making.

- Follow up with PCP after an exacerbation requiring ED care.

Pharmacologic management of childhood asthma is based on the severity of asthma and the child's age. The stepwise approach to treatment (Figs. 36.2 and 36.3) is based on severity of symptoms and the use of pharmacotherapy to control chronic symptoms, maintain normal activity, prevent recurrent exacerbations, minimize adverse side effects and achieve nearly "normal" pulmonary function. Within any classification, a child may experience mild, moderate, or severe exacerbations. National Heart, Lung, and Blood Institute guidelines for assessing asthma control and initiating and adjusting asthma therapy for various pediatric age groups are found in Figs. 36.4 and 36.5.

Important considerations to note in the pharmacologic treatment of asthma include:

- Control of asthma should be obtained as quickly as possible by starting at the classification step most appropriate to the initial severity of the child's symptoms or at a higher level (e.g., a course of systemic corticosteroids or higher dose of inhaled corticosteroid). After control of symptoms, decrease treatment to the least amount of medication needed to maintain control. The NAECCPP 2020 Update recommends pediatric patients under 4 years of age who experience at least three episodes of wheezing with viral illness be prescribed a short course (7–10 days) of moderate or high dose of ICS during their upper respiratory illness. This strategy was found to reduce the use of systemic steroids by 33%.[38]

- Systemic corticosteroids may be needed at any time and stepped up if there is a major flare-up of symptoms (e.g., increase symptoms despite use of controller medication and albuterol). Control of inflammation is a key management principle.

- The combination of ICS with a LABA can further control asthma.[42] The NAECCPP 2020 Update describes SMART strategies, which promote the use of a single inhaler of LABA and ICS for maintenance and rescue for patients over 4 years old with moderate to severe, persistent asthma.[37] The studied medications are budesonide/formoterol (Symbicort) and mometasone/formoterol (Dulera). Of note, fluticasone propionate/salmeterol (Advair) is more commonly used in pediatrics; however, this medication was not a part of the SMART trials and is not recommended for use in SMART. The AAP has endorsed the use of SMART strategies; however, neither Dulera or Symbicort is FDA approved as an abortive therapy for asthma exacerbation in the United States.[43]

- Children with intermittent asthma may have long, symptom-free periods; they can also have life-threatening exacerbations, often provoked by respiratory infection. In these situations, a short course of systemic corticosteroids should be used.

A

	Intermittent asthma	Management of persistent asthma in individuals ages 0–4 years				
Treatment	Step 1	Step 2	Step 3	Step 4	Step 5	Step 6
Preferred	PRN SABA and At the start of RTI: Add short course daily ICS^	Daily low-dose ICS and PRN SABA	Daily low-dose ICS-LABA and PRN SABA* or Daily low-dose ICS + montelukast,* or daily medium-dose ICS, and PRN SABA	Daily medium-dose ICS-LABA and PRN SABA	Daily high-dose ICS-LABA and PRN SABA	Daily high-dose ICS-LABA + oral systemic corticosteroid and PRN SABA
Alternative		Daily montelukast* or cromolyn,* and PRN SABA		Daily medium-dose ICS + montelukast* and PRN SABA	Daily high-dose ICS + montelukast* and PRN SABA	Daily high-dose ICS + montelukast*+ oral systemic corticosteroid and PRN SABA

For children age 4 years only, see step 3 and step 4 on management of persistent asthma in individuals ages 5–11 years diagram.

Assess control

- First check adherence, inhaler technique, environmental factors,^ and comorbid conditions.
- **Step up** if needed; reassess in 4–6 weeks
- **Step down** if possible (if asthma is well controlled for at least 3 consecutive months)

Consult with asthma specialist if step 3 or higher is required. Consider consultation at step 2.

Control assessment is a key element of asthma care. This involves both impairment and risk. Use of objective measures, self-reported control, and health care utilization are complementary and should be employed on an ongoing basis, depending on the individual's clinical situation.

^ Updated based on the 2020 guidelines.

* Cromolyn and montelukast were not considered for this update and/or have limited availability for use in the United States. The Food and Drug Administration (FDA) issued a boxed warning for montelukast in march 2020.

• **Fig. 36.2** Stepwise Approach for Managing Asthma in Children 0–4 Years Old (A) and

B

	Intermittent asthma	Management of persistent asthma in individuals ages 5–11 years				
Treatment	Step 1	Step 2	Step 3	Step 4	Step 5	Step 6
Preferred	PRN SABA	Daily low-dose ICS and PRN SABA	Daily and PRN combination low-dose ICS-formoterol^	Daily and PRN combination medium-dose ICS-formoterol^	Daily high-dose ICS-LABA and PRN SABA	Daily high-dose ICS-LABA + oral systemic corticosteroid and PRN SABA
Alternative		Daily LTRA,* or cromolyn,* or nedocromil,* or theophylline,* and PRN SABA	Daily medium-dose ICS and PRN SABA or Daily low-dose ICS-LABA, or daily low-dose ICS + LTRA,* or daily low-dose ICS +theophylline,* and PRN SABA	Daily medium-dose ICS-LABA and PRN SABA or Daily medium-dose ICS + LTRA* or daily medium-dose ICS + theophylline,* and PRN SABA	Daily high-dose ICS + LTRA* or daily high-dose ICS + theophylline,* and PRN SABA	Daily high-dose ICS + LTRA* + oral systemic corticosteroid or daily high-dose ICS + theophylline* + oral systemic corticosteroid, and PRN SABA

Steps 2–4: Conditionally recommend the use of subcutaneous immunotherapy as an adjunct treatment to standard pharmacotherapy in individuals ≥ 5 years of age whose asthma is controlled at the initiation, build up, and maintenance phases of immunotherapy^

Consider omalizumab**^

Assess control

- First check adherence, inhaler technique, environmental factors,^ and comorbid conditions.
- **Step up** if needed; reassess in 2–6 weeks
- **Step down** if possible (if asthma is well controlled for at least 3 consecutive months)

Consult with asthma specialist if step 4 or higher is required. Consider consultation at step 3.

Control assessment is a key element of asthma care. This involves both impairment and risk. Use of objective measures, self-reported control, and health care utilization are complementary and should be employed on an ongoing basis, depending on the individual's clinical situation.

^Updated based on the 2020 guidelines.

* Cromolyn, nedocromil, *LTRAs* including montelukast, and theophylline were not considered in this update and/or have limited availability for use in the United States, and/or have an increased risk of adverse consequences and need for monitoring that make their use less desirable. the Food and Drug Administration (*FDA*) issued a boxed warning for montelukast in march 2020.

** Omalizumab is the only asthma biologic currently *FDA*-approved for this age range.

• **Fig. 36.2, cont'd** 5–11 Years Old (B). Alphabetical order is used when more than one treatment option is listed within either preferred or alternative therapy. *EIB*, Exercise-induced bronchospasm; *ICS*, inhaled corticosteroid; *LABA*, long-acting β_2-agonist; *LTRA*, leukotriene receptor antagonist; *prn*, pro re nata (when necessary); *RTI*, respiratory tract infection; *SABA*, short-acting β_2-agonist. (From Expert Panel Working Group of the National Heart, Lung, and Blood Institute [NHLBI] administered and coordinated National Asthma Education and Prevention Program Coordinating Committee [NAEPPCC]; Cloutier MM, Baptist AP, Blake KV et al. 2020 Focused updates to the asthma management guidelines: a report from the National Asthma Education and Prevention Program Coordinating Committee Expert Panel Working Group. *J Allergy Clin Immunol.* 2020;146[6]:1217–1270.)

- Variations in asthma necessitate individualized treatment plans.
- β_2 agonists can be administered with metered dose inhaler (MDI) therapy via spacer for children with mild and moderate exacerbations of asthma. A nebulizer may be better for children with severe airway obstruction who may have decreased deposition of drug in the base of the lung.[44] A spacer or holding chamber with an attached mask enhances the delivery of MDI medications to a child's lower airways. Spacers eliminate the need to synchronize inhalation with activation of MDI. Older children can use a spacer without the mask. It is important to check technique at every asthma-related visit.

- Dry powder inhalers (DPIs) do not need spacers or shaking before use. Instruct children to rinse their mouth with water and spit afterward. DPIs should not be used in children younger than 4 years old.
- Different ICS are not equal in potency to each other on a per puff or microgram basis. Tables 36.6 and 36.7 compare daily low, medium, and high doses of various ICS used for children. Combination ICS and LABA can be used in children 4 years and older[45] and are the mainstay of SMART strategies.
- For treatment of EIA or EIB:
  - Warm up before exercise for 5 to 10 minutes.
  - As a preventive measure, use an inhaled short-acting β_2 agonist (SABA) 5 to 20 minutes before exercise. A mast cell

Treatment	Intermittent asthma	Management of persistent asthma in individuals ages 12+ years				
	Step 1	Step 2	Step 3	Step 4	Step 5	Step 6
Preferred	PRN SABA	Daily low-dose ICS and PRN SABA or PRN concomitant ICS and SABA^	Daily and PRN combination low-dose ICS-formoterol^	Daily and PRN combination medium-dose ICS-formoterol^	Daily medium-high dose ICS-LABA + LAMA and PRN SABA^	Daily high-dose ICS-LABA + oral systemic corticosteroids + PRN SABA
Alternative		Daily LTRA* and PRN SABA or Cromolyn,* or nedocromil,* or zileuton,* or theophylline,* and PRN SABA	Daily medium-dose ICS and PRN SABA or Daily low-dose ICS-LABA, or daily low-dose ICS + LAMA,^ or daily low-dose ICS + LTRA,* and PRN SABA or Daily low-dose ICS + theophylline* or zileuton,* and PRN SABA	Daily medium-dose ICS-LABA or daily medium-dose ICS + LAMA, and PRN SABA^ or Daily medium-dose ICS + LTRA,* or daily medium-dose ICS + theophylline,* or daily medium-dose ICS + zileuton,* and PRN SABA	Daily medium-high dose ICS-LABA or daily high-dose ICS + LTRA,* and PRN SABA	
		Steps 2–4: Conditionally recommend the use of subcutaneous immunotherapy as an adjunct treatment to standard pharmacotherapy in individuals ≥5 years of age whose asthma is controlled at the initiation, build up, and maintenance phases of immunotherapy^			Consider adding asthma biologics (e.g., anti-IgE, anti-IL5, anti-IL5R, anti-IL4/IL13)**	

Assess control

- First check adherence, inhaler technique, environmental factors,^ and comorbid conditions.
- **Step up** if needed; reassess in 2–6 weeks
- **Step down** if possible (if asthma is well controlled for at least 3 consecutive months)

Consult with asthma specialist if step 4 or higher is required. Consider consultation at step 3.

Control assessment is a key element of asthma care. This involves both impairment and risk. Use of objective measures, self-reported control, and health care utilization are complementary and should be employed on an ongoing basis, depending on the individual's clinical situation.

^ Updated based on the 2020 guidelines.

* Cromolyn, nedocromil, *LTRAs* including zileuton and montelukast, and theophylline were not considered for this update and/or have limited availability for use in the United States, and/or have an increased risk of adverse consequences and need for monitoring that make their use less desirable. The Food and Drug Administration (*FDA*) issued a boxed warning for montelukast in March 2020.

** The AHRQ systematic reviews that informed this report did not include studies that examined the role of asthma biologics (e.g. anti-IgE, anti-IL5, anti-IL5R, anti-IL4/IL13). Thus, this report does not contain specific recommendations for the use of biologics in asthma in steps 5 and 6.

■ Data on the use of *LAMA* therapy in individuals with severe persistent asthma (step 6) were not included in the AHRQ systematic review and thus no recommendation is made.

• **Fig. 36.3** Stepwise Approach for Managing Asthma in Patients ≥12 Years Old and Adults. Alphabetical listing is used when more than one treatment option is listed within either preferred or alternative therapy. *EIB*, Exercise-induced bronchospasm; *ICS*, inhaled corticosteroid; *LABA*, long-acting β_2-agonist; *LAMA*, long-acting muscarinic antagonist; *LTRA*, leukotriene receptor antagonist; *prn*, pro re nata (when necessary); *SABA*, short-acting β_2-agonist. (From Expert Panel Working Group of the National Heart, Lung, and Blood Institute [NHLBI] administered and coordinated National Asthma Education and Prevention Program Coordinating Committee [NAEPPCC]; Cloutier MM, Baptist AP, Blake KV et al. 2020 Focused updates to the asthma management guidelines: a report from the National Asthma Education and Prevention Program Coordinating Committee Expert Panel Working Group. *J Allergy Clin Immunol*. 2020;146[6]:1217–1270.)

stabilizer such as Cromolyn can be added. Combination of both types of drugs is the more effective therapy. Adding an anticholinergic may help if the SABA is not working.[24]

- If a SABA is used daily, a controller therapy should be instituted with either ICS with or without LABA and/or LTRA. Antihistamine should be used for allergic symptoms.

Assessing severity and initiating therapy in children who are not currently taking long-term control medication

A

Components of Severity		Classification of Asthma Severity (0-4 years of age)			
		Intermittent	Persistent		
			Mild	Moderate	Severe
Impairment	Symptoms	≤ 2 days/week	> 2 days/week but not daily	Daily	Throughout the day
	Nighttime awakenings	0	1-2x/month	3-4x/month	> 1x/week
	Short-acting beta$_2$-agonist use for symptom control (not prevention of EIB)	≤ 2 days/week	> 2 days/week but not daily	Daily	Several times per day
	Interference with normal activity	None	Minor limitation	Some limitation	Extremely limited
Risk	Exacerbations requiring oral systemic corticosteroids	0-1/year	≥ 2 exacerbations in 6 months requiring oral systemic corticosteroids, or ≥ 4 wheezing episodes/1 year lasting > 1 day AND risk factors for persistent asthma		
		← Consider severity and interval since last exacerbation. Frequency and severity may fluctuate over time. →			
		Exacerbations of any severity may occur in patients in any severity category.			
Recommended Step for Initiating Therapy (See Fig. 36.3A for treatment steps.)		Step 1	Step 2	Step 3 and consider short course of oral systemic corticosteroids	
		In 2-6 weeks, depending on severity, evaluate level of asthma control that is achieved. If no clear benefit is observed in 4-6 weeks, consider adjusting therapy or alternative diagnoses.			

Notes

- The stepwise approach is meant to assist, not replace, the clinical decisionmaking required to meet individual patient needs.

- Level of severity is determined by both impairment and risk. Assess impairment domain by patient's/caregiver's recall of previous 2-4 weeks. Symptom assessment for longer periods should reflect a global assessment such as inquiring whether the patient's asthma is better or worse since the last visit. Assign severity to the most severe category in which any feature occurs.

- At present, there are inadequate data to correspond frequencies of exacerbations with different levels of asthma severity. For treatment purposes, patients who had ≥ 2 exacerbations requiring oral systemic corticosteroids in the past 6 months, or ≥ 4 wheezing episodes in the past year, and who have risk factors for persistent asthma may be considered the same as patients who have persistent asthma, even in the absence of impairment levels consistent with persistent asthma.

• **Fig. 36.4** Assessing Asthma Severity and Initiating Therapy in Children 0–4 Years Old (A) and

Assessing severity and initiating therapy in children who are not currently taking long-term control medication

B

Components of Severity		Classification of Asthma Severity (5-11 years of age)			
		Intermittent	Persistent		
			Mild	Moderate	Severe
Impairment	Symptoms	≤ 2 days/week	> 2 days/week but not daily	Daily	Throughout the day
	Nighttime awakenings	≤ 2x/month	3-4x/month	> 1x/week but not nightly	Often 7x/week
	Short-acting beta$_2$-agonist use for symptom control (not prevention of EIB)	≤ 2 days/week	> 2 days/week but not daily	Daily	Several times per day
	Interference with normal activity	None	Minor limitation	Some limitation	Extremely limited
	Lung function	• Normal FEV$_1$ between exacerbations • FEV$_1$ > 80% predicted • FEV$_1$/FVC > 85%	• FEV$_1$ = > 80% predicted • FEV$_1$/FVC > 80%	• FEV$_1$ = 60-80% predicted • FEV$_1$/FVC = 75-80%	• FEV$_1$ < 60% predicted • FEV$_1$/FVC < 75%
Risk	Exacerbations requiring oral systemic corticosteroids	0–1/year (see note)	≥ 2/year (see note) ⟶		
		⟵ Consider severity and interval since last exacerbation. ⟶ Frequency and severity may fluctuate over time for patients in any severity category.			
		Relative annual risk of exacerbations may be related to FEV$_1$.			
Recommended Step for Initiating Therapy (See Fig. 36.3B for treatment steps.)		Step 1	Step 2	Step 3, medium-dose ICS option	Step 3, medium-dose ICS option, or step 4 and consider short course of oral systemic corticosteroids
		In 2-6 weeks, evaluate level of asthma control that is achieved, and adjust therapy accordingly.			

Notes

■ The stepwise approach is meant to assist, not replace, the clinical decisionmaking required to meet individual patient needs.

■ Level of severity is determined by both impairment and risk. Assess impairment domain by patient's/caregiver's recall of the previous 2-4 weeks and spirometry. Assign severity to the most severe category in which any feature occurs.

■ At present, there are inadequate data to correspond frequencies of exacerbations with different levels of asthma severity. In general, more frequent and intense exacerbations (e.g., requiring urgent, unscheduled care, hospitalization, or ICU admission) indicate greater underlying disease severity. For treatment purposes, patients who had ≥ 2 exacerbations requiring oral systemic corticosteroids in the past year may be considered the same as patients who have persistent asthma, even in the absence of impairment levels consistent with persistent asthma.

• **Fig. 36.4, cont'd** 5–11 Years Old (B) Who Are Not Currently Taking Long-Term Control Medication. *EIB,* Exercise-induced bronchospasm; *FEV$_1$,* forced expiratory volume in 1 second; *FVC,* forced vital capacity; *ICS,* inhaled corticosteroid; *ICU,* intensive care unit; *SABA,* short-acting β$_2$-agonist. (From US Department of Health and Human Services, National Institutes of Health, National Heart, Lung, Blood Institute. National asthma prevention program: Expert panel report 3: Guidelines for the diagnosis and management of asthma; 2007. https://www.epa.gov/sites/default/files/2014-09/documents/asthgdln.pdf. pp. 307–308.)

• Using a scarf or mask around the mouth in cold weather may decrease EIA.[4]
• High-risk sports for EIB include high-endurance sports, long-distance running, and track and field events.
• Low-risk sports for EIA are those physical activities of short duration: golf, volleyball, gymnastics, baseball, wrestling, football, and short-term track and field events. While some swimming can be a high-endurance event, the warmth and humidity around the pool make breathing easier.[24]

Table 36.8 identifies the usual dosages for long-term control medications (exclusive of ICS) used to treat asthma in children. Quick-relief medications are listed in Table 36.9. Practice

Assessing severity and initiating treatment for patients who are not currently taking long-term control medications

Components of Severity		Classification of Asthma Severity ≥ 12 years of age			
			Persistent		
		Intermittent	**Mild**	**Moderate**	**Severe**
Impairment Normal FEV₁/FVC: 8-19 yr 85% 20-39 yr 80% 40-59 yr 75% 60-80 yr 70%	Symptoms	≤ 2 days/week	> 2 days/week but not daily	Daily	Throughout the day
	Nighttime awakenings	≤ 2x/month	3-4x/month	> 1x/week but not nightly	Often 7x/week
	Short-acting beta₂-agonist use for symptom control (not prevention of EIB)	≤ 2 days/week	> 2 days/week but not daily, and not more than 1x on any day	Daily	Several times per day
	Interference with normal activity	None	Minor limitation	Some limitation	Extremely limited
	Lung function	• Normal FEV₁ between exacerbations • FEV₁ > 80% predicted • FEV₁/FVC normal	• FEV₁ > 80% predicted • FEV₁/FVC normal	• FEV₁ > 60% but < 80 % predicted • FEV₁/FVC reduced 5%	• FEV₁ < 60% predicted • FEV₁/FVC reduced > 5%
Risk	Exacerbations requiring oral systemic corticosteroids	0-1/year (see note)	≥ 2/year (see note) ⟶		
		⟵ Consider severity and interval since last exacerbation. ⟶ Frequency and severity may fluctuate over time for patients in any severity category. Relative annual risk of exacerbations may be related to FEV₁.			
Recommended Step for Initiating Treatment (See Fig. 36.2 for treatment steps.)		Step 1	Step 2	Step 3	Step 4 or 5
				and consider short course of oral systemic corticosteroids	
		In 2-6 weeks, evaluate level of asthma control that is achieved and adjust therapy accordingly.			

Notes:

■ The stepwise approach is meant to assist, not replace, the clinical decisionmaking required to meet individual patient needs.

■ Level of severity is determined by assessment of both impairment and risk. Assess impairment domain by patient's/caregiver's recall of previous 2-4 weeks and spirometry. Assign severity to the most severe category in which any feature occurs.

■ At present, there are inadequate data to correspond frequencies of exacerbations with different levels of asthma severity. In general, more frequent and intense exacerbations (e.g., requiring urgent, unscheduled care, hospitalization, or ICU admission) indicate greater underlying disease severity. For treatment purposes, patients who had ≥ 2 exacerbations requiring oral systemic corticosteroids in the past year may be considered the same as patients who have persistent asthma, even in the absence of impairment levels consistent with persistent asthma.

• **Fig. 36.5** Assessing Asthma Severity and Initiating Therapy in Children ≥12 Years Old and Adults Who Are Not Currently Taking Long-Term Control Medication. *EIB,* Exercise-induced bronchospasm; *FEV₁,* forced expiratory volume in 1 second; *FVC,* forced vital capacity; *ICU,* intensive care unit; *SABA,* short-acting β₂-agonist; *x,* times; *yr,* years. (From US Department of Health and Human Services, National Institutes of Health, National Heart, Lung, Blood Institute. National asthma prevention program: Expert panel report 3: Guidelines for the diagnosis and management of asthma; 2007. https://www.epa.gov/sites/default/files/2014-09/documents/asthgdln.pdf.)

parameters are guides and should not replace individualized treatment based on clinical judgment and unique differences among children. See Fig. 36.6 for one example of how to approach initiation of controller therapy.

Acute Exacerbations of Asthma

Treatment of acute episodes of asthma is based on severity of the episode. Acute episodes are classified as mild, moderate, and severe. Signs and symptoms are summarized in Table 36.10. Early

<table>
<tr><td>TABLE 36.6</td><td colspan="4">Estimated Comparative Daily Dosages for Inhaled Corticosteroids</td></tr>
</table>

Inhaled Corticosteroid	TOTAL DAILY ICS DOSE (mcg)[A]		
	Low	Medium	High
Adults and Adolescents (≥12 Year)			
Beclometasone dipropionate (pMDI, standard particle, HFA)	200–500	>500–1000	>1000
Beclometasone dipropionate (DPI or pMDI, extrafine particle, HFA)	100–200	>200–400	>400
Budesonide (DPI, or pMDI, standard particle, HFA)	200–400	>400–800	>800
Ciclesonide (pMDI, extrafine particle, HFA)	80–160	>160–320	>320
Fluticasone furoate (DPI)	100		200
Fluticasone propionate (DPI)	100–250	>250–500	>500
Fluticasone propionate (pMDI, standard particle, HFA)	100–250	>250–500	>500
Mometasone furoate (DPI)	Depends on DPI device—see product information		
Mometasone furoate (pMDI, standard particle, HFA)	200–400		>400
Children 6–11 Years			
Beclometasone dipropionate (pMDI, standard particle, HFA)	100–200	>200–400	>400
Beclometasone dipropionate (pMDI, extrafine particle, HFA)	50–100	>100–200	>200
Budesonide (DPI)	100–200	>200–400	>400
Budesonide (nebules)	250–500	>500–1000	>1000
Ciclesonide (pMDI, extrafine particle, HFA)	80	>80–160	>160
Fluticasone furoate (DPI)	50		NA
Fluticasone propionate (DPI)	50–100	>100–200	>200
Fluticasone propionate (pMDI, standard particle, HFA)	50–100	>100–200	>200
Mometasone furoate (pMDI, standard particle, HFA)	100		200

[a]Daily doses in this table are shown as metered doses. See product information for delivered doses. ICS by pMDI should preferably be used with a spacer.

For new preparations, including generic ICS, the manufacturer's information should be reviewed carefully, as products containing the same molecule may not be clinically equivalent.

DPI, Dry powder inhaler; *HFA,* hydrofluoroalkane propellant; *ICS,* inhaled corticosteroid; *LABA,* long-acting beta₂-agonist; *LAMA,* long-acting muscarinic antagonist; *NA,* not applicable; *pMDI,* pressurized metered dose inhaler.

From Global Initiative for Asthma, Copyright 2022. www.ginasthma.org.

recognition of warning signs and treatment should be stressed in educating patients, parents, or both.

The initial pharmacologic treatment for acute asthma exacerbations is shown in Fig. 36.7. It consists of inhaled SABAs (albuterol), two to six puffs every 20 minutes for three treatments by way of MDI with a spacer, or a single nebulizer treatment (0.15 mg/kg; minimum 1.25–2.5 mg of 0.5% solution of albuterol in 2–3 mL of normal saline).

If the initial treatment results in a good response (PEF/FEV₁ >70% of the patient's best), the inhaled SABA can be continued every 3 to 4 hours for 24 to 48 hours with a 3-day course of oral steroids at 1 to 2 mg/kg/day in two divided doses to a maximum of 60 mg/day. Reassessment is important to ensure an adequate response and to further assess asthma severity.

An incomplete response (PEF or FEV₁ between 40% and 69% of personal best or symptoms recur within 4 hours of therapy)

is treated by continuing β₂ agonists and adding an oral corticosteroid. The β₂ agonist can be given by nebulizer or MDI with spacer. Parents should be taught to call their PCP for additional instructions. If there is marked distress (severe acute symptoms) or a poor response (PEF or FEV₁ < 40%) to treatment, the child should have the β₂ agonist repeated immediately and should be taken to the ED. Caregivers should call 911 if the distress is severe or the child is agitated and unable to talk. If children experience recurrent acute asthma exacerbations (more than once every 4–6 weeks), adherence to therapy and the treatment plan should be reevaluated.

Although this chapter focuses on the outpatient management of children with asthma, familiarity with other drug options used in more severe asthma exacerbation is important. These include:

- Magnesium sulfate intravenous (IV) is used in EDs to decrease the intracellular calcium concentration. It causes

| TABLE 36.7 | Inhaled Corticosteroids in Children 0–4 Years Old |

This is not a table of equivalence, but instead, suggestions for "low" total daily doses for the ICS treatment recommendations for children aged 5 years and younger, based on available studies and product information. Data on comparative potency are not readily available, particularly for children, and this table does NOT imply potency equivalence. The doses listed here are the lowest approved doses for which safety and effectiveness have been adequately studied in this age group.

Low-dose ICS provides most of the clinical benefit for most children with asthma. Higher doses are associated with an increased risk of local and systemic side-effects, which must be balanced against potential benefits.

Inhaled Corticosteroid	Low Total Daily Dose (mcg)[a]
BDP (pMDI, standard particle, HFA)	100 (ages ≥5 years)
BDP (pMDI, extrafine particle, HFA)	50 (ages ≥5 years)
Budesonide nebulized	500 (ages ≥1 year)
Fluticasone propionate (pMDI, standard particle, HFA)	50 (ages ≥4 years)
Fluticasone furoate (DPI)	Not sufficiently studied in children ≤5 years
Mometasone furoate (pMDI, standard particle, HFA)	100 (ages ≥5 years)
Ciclesonide (pMDI, extrafine particle, HFA)	Not sufficiently studied in children ≤5 years

[a]Age group with adequate safety and effectiveness data.

BDP, Beclometasone dipropionate; *DPI,* dry powder inhaler; *HFA,* hydrofluoroalkane propellant; *ICS,* inhaled corticosteroid; *pMDI,* pressurized metered lose inhaler (nonchlorofluorocarbon formulations); in children, pMDI should always be used with a spacer

From Global Initiative for Asthma, Copyright 2022. www.ginasthma.org.

bronchodilation due to respiratory smooth muscle relaxation. The most significant side effect is hypotension.

- The use of continuous infusion of terbutaline IV is limited to pediatric intensive care settings due to the risk of sinus tachycardia, decreases in systolic and diastolic blood pressure, and myocardial ischemia.[33]
- Theophylline, even at suboptimal doses, improves the lungs' responsiveness to steroids.
- Ketamine, a potent bronchodilator, may be used as an induction agent in critically ill children with asthma and respiratory failure.[33]
- Ipratropium, an anticholinergic bronchodilator, via oral inhalation is used to treat bronchospasms.
- Epinephrine given subcutaneously or intramuscularly is an option in severe asthma where the delivery of medication to smaller airways is limited due to bronchoconstriction.
- Heliox, a mixture of oxygen and helium, can improve drug delivery in obstructed airways because it has a lower density and less airway resistance.[33]

Complications

Complications from asthma can range from mild secondary respiratory infections to respiratory arrest. Poor response to pharmacologic agents can lead to status asthmaticus and ultimately death. Chronic high-dose steroid use can cause growth retardation and other related side effects.

Patient and Parent Education and Prevention

The PCP should support self-care management through in-depth education. Easy-to-understand education must be tailored to reflect cultural beliefs and the individual child and family needs using a "teach back" technique. Correct administration of inhaled medication should be demonstrated during initial training sessions and reevaluated in subsequent visits. Provide instruction on the following:

- Basic understanding of what asthma is, what is effective asthma control, and what is the child's current level of symptomatology.
- Environmental control of allergens or triggers (e.g., smoking and dust).
- Basic understanding of different medications and how to use them. Give clear, written instructions about how to administer, how much and when to give, the need for monitoring side effects, and how long medication should be taken. A written plan is recommended based on either symptoms or peak expiratory flow rate.
- How to use inhalers, spacer devices, or aerosol equipment (Box 36.2) along with proper cleaning of aerosol equipment.
- Identifying asthma symptoms that indicate a need to change therapy or necessitate immediate reevaluation; when and where to seek emergency care.
- Home PEF or symptom monitoring: What to do if symptoms worsen (what medications to add or increase; how frequently to use inhaled medication; specific indications about when to seek additional medical treatment if symptoms worsen).
- Regular physical activity such as walking as tolerated.
- Avoid medications that can exacerbate asthma symptoms (e.g., NSAIDs if this is a known trigger, aspirin).
- Development of a written action/treatment plan with the child or parent (see Fig. 36.1).
- Maintain adequate supply of all medications (including oral corticosteroids) at home and at school or other settings where the child frequents.
- Eat a healthy diet with increased fruits and vegetables; if obese or overweight, discuss diet using motivational interviewing techniques.
- Consider referral to allergist for AIT.
- Discuss asthma action plan with staff at school, camp, or other places away from home.
- Need for regular follow-up every 1 to 6 months and as needed with exacerbations.

Stress that asthma is a chronic disease that can be controlled—the goal of therapy is to maintain normal activity. The absence of symptoms does not mean the disease has disappeared, rather it is well controlled. The child should wear a medical alert bracelet. Acquaint children and parents with local asthma education programs and activities, such as camps for children with asthma. Written instructions and handouts should be provided for other significant individuals in the child's life, including caregivers and school personnel.

Prognosis

Asthma is a chronic disease that, for most children, can be successfully managed with proper pharmacologic therapy, allergen and environmental control, and patient education. Mild asthma

TABLE 36.8 Long-Term Control Medications for the Treatment of Asthma

Medication	Dosage Form	Child Dosage[a]	Adult Dosage[b]	Comments
Inhaled Corticosteroids (see Tables 36.6 and 36.7)				
Systemic Corticosteroids: Applies to All Three Corticosteroids				
Methylprednisolone	2-, 4-, 8-, 16-, 32-mg tablets	0.25–2 mg/kg daily in a single dose in a.m. or every other day as needed for control; 60 mg maximum dose	7.5–60 mg daily in a single dose in a.m. or every other day as needed for control	For long-term treatment of severe persistent asthma, administer single dose in a.m. either daily or on alternate days (alternate-day therapy may produce less adrenal suppression). If daily doses are required, one study suggests improved efficacy and no increase in adrenal suppression when administered at 3 p.m.
Prednisolone	5-mg tablets, 5 mg/5 mL, 1 mg/mL	Same as above	Same as above	
Prednisone	1-, 2-, 5-, 10-, 20-, 50-mg tablets; 5 mg/mL, 1 mg/mL	Short-course "burst": 1–2 mg/kg/day in single or two divided doses a day, maximum 60 mg/day for 3–10 days	Short-course "burst" to achieve control: 40–60 mg/day as single or two divided doses for 3–10 days	Short courses or "bursts" are effective for establishing control when initiating therapy or during a period of gradual deterioration The bursts should be continued until patient achieves 80% PEF rate personal best or symptoms resolve. This usually requires 3–10 days but may require longer treatment. There is no evidence that tapering the dose following improvement prevents relapse
Dexamethasone: Oral, IM, or IV 0.6 mg/kg once a day for 1 or 2 days[18]				
Cromolyn				
Cromolyn	20 mg/ampule for nebulization solution, inhalation	Children ≥2 years: 1 ampule 4 times a day initially; usual dose 3 times a day	1 ampule 3 or 4 times a day; usual dose 3 times a day	≥2 years: Single dose of 20 mg 10–15 min before exercise or allergen exposure provides effective prophylaxis for 1–2 h
Inhaled Long-Acting β₂-Agonists: Should Not Be Used for Symptom Relief or for Exacerbations (Use With Inhaled Corticosteroids)				
Salmeterol	DPI: 50 mcg/inhalation	≥4 years: 1 activation/puff every 12 h	1 activation/puff every 12 h	Use with inhaled corticosteroid only Do not use as a rescue inhaler for symptom relief or for exacerbations
Formoterol	DPI: 12 mcg/single-use capsule	≥5 years: 1 capsule every 12 h apart	1 capsule every 12 h	Do not take orally; must be used with aerolizer Should be used with inhaled steroid
Leukotriene Modifiers				
Montelukast	4- or 5-mg chewable tablet, 10-mg tablet; granules 4 mg/packet	12 months to 5 years: 4 mg a day; 6–14 years old: 5 mg a day	≥15 years: 10 mg a day Prevention of EIB: 6–14 years: 5 mg; ≥15 years old: 10 mg at least 2 h before exercise (no other doses should be given in 24 h)	
Zafirlukast	10- or 20-mg tablet	5–11 years: 10-mg tablet twice a day	>12 years: 20-mg tablet twice a day	Take zafirlukast at least 1 h before or 2 h after meals
Zileuton	600-mg tablet and 600 mg extended release		Give 1 immediate-release tablet 4 times a day or give 2 extended-release tablets 2 times a day	Less desirable because of the need to monitor hepatic enzymes (ALT); used in children older than 12 years
Combined Medication				
Fluticasone/salmeterol	HFA 45, 115, 230 mcg fluticasone/21 mcg salmeterol		HFA: ≥12 years: Two inhalations twice a day of 45 mcg fluticasone/21 mcg salmeterol or 115 mcg fluticasone/21 mcg salmeterol	HFA adult dose not to exceed two inhalations of 230 mcg fluticasone/21 mcg salmeterol twice daily Starting dose dependent on current steroid therapy

TABLE 36.8 Long-Term Control Medications for the Treatment of Asthma—cont'd

Medication	Dosage Form	Child Dosage[a]	Adult Dosage[b]	Comments
	Diskus: 100, 250, or 500 mcg fluticasone/50 mcg salmeterol	Diskus: >4–11 years old: 1 inhalation twice a day of 100 mcg fluticasone/50 mcg salmeterol; dose depends on severity of asthma	Diskus: 1 inhalation twice a day of 100 mcg fluticasone/50 mcg salmeterol; dose depends on severity of asthma	Starting dose based on current steroid therapy
Budesonide/ formoterol aerosol for oral inhalation	Aerosol: 80 mcg *or* 160 mcg budesonide/4.5 mcg formoterol	5–11 years: 2 inhalations twice a day of aerosol 80 mcg/4.5 mcg, not to exceed 4 inhalations/day	≥12 years: 2 inhalations twice a day of aerosol 80 mcg/4.5 mcg, not to exceed 4 inhalations/ day; if not controlled may increase to 160 mcg budesonide/4.5 mcg formoterol inhalation twice daily not exceeding 4 inhalations day	

[a]Infants and children <12 years.

[b]Adult, ≥12 years.

ALT, Alanine amino transferase; *DPI,* dry powder inhaler; *EIB,* exercise-induced bronchospasm; *HFA,* hydrofluoroalkane; *PEF,* peak expiratory flow.

Modified from the National Heart, Lung, and Blood Institute (NHLBI). *Full Report of the Expert Panel: Guidelines for the Diagnosis and Management of Asthma (EPR-3).* National Institutes of Health; 2007; and Taketomo CK, Hodding JH, Kraus DM. *Pediatric Dosage Handbook.* 24th ed. Lexi-Comp; 2019.

TABLE 36.9 Quick-Relief Medications for the Treatment of Asthma

Medication	Dosage Form	Child Dosage[a]	Adult Dosage	Comments
Short-Acting Inhaled β₂-Agonists				
Metered Dose Inhalers				
Albuterol HFA	90 mcg/puff, 200 puffs	Acute exacerbation: 4–8 puffs every 20 min for three doses, then every 1–4 h as needed Maintenance: 0–4 years, 1–2 inhalations every 4–6 h; >5 years, 2 puffs every 4–6 h prn	Acute exacerbation: 4–8 puffs every 20 min for 4 h, then every 1–4 h as needed Maintenance: 2 puffs every 4–6 h prn	Not generally recommended for long-term treatment Regular use on a daily basis indicates the need for additional long-term control therapy
Pirbuterol	200 mcg/INH, 400 INH		Acute exacerbation: 4–8 inhalations every 20 min for up to 4 h, then every 1–4 h as needed Maintenance: 2 inhalations 3 or 4 times/day	
Levalbuterol HFA	45 mcg/puff	Acute exacerbation: 4–8 puffs every 20 min for three doses, then every 1–4 h Maintenance: ≥5 years: 2 inhalations every 4–6 h	Acute exacerbation: 4–8 puffs every 20 min for up to 4 h, then every 1–4 h as needed Maintenance: 2 inhalations every 4–6 h	Not FDA approved for long-term, daily maintenance use Use more than 2 days/week indicates need for long-term control therapy
				Nonselective agents (e.g., epinephrine, isoproterenol, metaproterenol) are not recommended because of their potential for excessive cardiac stimulation, especially at high doses

Continued

Medication	Dosage Form	Child Dosage[a]	Adult Dosage	Comments
Nebulizer Solution				
Albuterol	5 mg/mL (0.5%) 0.63 mg/3 mL 1.25 mg/3 mL	<5 years: 0.63–2.5 mg in 3 mL NS every 4–6 h prn	Adults: 1.25–5 mg in 3 mL of NS every 4–8 h prn	May mix with cromolyn or ipratropium nebulizer solutions; may double dose for mild exacerbations
	2.5 mg/3 mL	>5 years: 1.25–2.5 mg in 3 mL of NS every 4–8 h prn		
Levalbuterol	0.31 mg/3 mL 0.63 mg/3 mL 1.25 mg/3 mL	Acute exacerbation: 0.075 mg/kg (minimum dose 1.25 mg) every 20 min for three doses, then 0.075–0.15 mg/kg (not to exceed 5 mg) every 1–4 h as needed Maintenance: 0–4 years: 0.31–1.25 mg every 4–6 h prn; ≥5 years and adults: 0.31–0.63 mg every 8 h prn	Acute exacerbation: 1.25–2.5 mg every 20 min for three doses, then 1.25–5 mg every 1–4 h as needed Maintenance: 0.31–0.63 mg every 8 h as needed	Use more than 2 days/week indicates need for long-term control therapy
Anticholinergics				
Ipratropium HFA (MDI) Ipratropium (nebulizer solution)	17 mcg/puff, 200-puff canister 0.02% (2.5 mL)	Refer to a pharmacology textbook	Refer to a pharmacology textbook	Evidence is lacking that ipratropium HFA produces added benefit to β_2-agonists in long-term asthma therapy
Systemic Corticosteroids: Dosage Applies to All Three Corticosteroids				
Methylprednisolone	2-, 4-, 8-, 16-, 32-mg tablets	Short-course "burst": 1–2 mg/kg/day in divided doses once or twice daily, maximum 60 mg/day, for 3–10 days	Short-course "burst" to achieve control: 40–60 mg/day as single or two divided doses for 3–10 days	Short courses or "bursts" are effective for establishing control when initiating therapy or during a period of gradual deterioration
Prednisolone	5-mg tablets, 5 mg/5 mL, 15 mg/5 mL			
Prednisone	1-, 2.5-, 5-, 10-, 20-, 50-mg tablets: 5 mg/mL, 5 mg/5 mL			The burst should be continued until patient achieves 80% PEF rate personal best or symptoms resolve; this usually requires 3–10 days but may require longer; there is no evidence that tapering the dose following improvement prevents relapse

[a]<12 years old.

FDA, US Food and Drug Administration; *HFA,* hydrofluoroalkane; *INH,* inhalations; *MDI,* metered dose inhaler; *NS,* normal saline; *PEF,* peak expiratory flow; *prn,* as needed.

Modified from the National Heart, Lung, and Blood Institute (NHLBI). *Full Report of the Expert Panel: Guidelines for the Diagnosis and Management of Asthma (EPR-3).* National Institutes of Health; 2007; and Taketomo CK, Hodding JH, Kraus DM. *Pediatric Dosage Handbook.* 24th ed. Lexi-Comp; 2019.

is more likely to resolve with increasing age than is moderate or severe asthma.

Allergic Rhinitis

AR is a disorder that results in nasal mucosal inflammation due to Th2 cell. More specifically, the antigen uptake by the antigen-presenting cell leads to antigen-specific T cell activation. At the same time proteases lead to epithelia cytokine release, favoring the Th2 cell and basophil activation, releasing Th-2 cytokines that drive B cells to form plasma cells that release IgE. On reexposure to the antigen, the IgE clings to IgE receptors activating mast cells and basophils, leading to the release of cysteinyl leukotrienes and histamine. These substances, along with the local Th2 activation, cause the motor reflex of sneezing and parasympathetic reflex that stimulate vasodilation and nasal secretion. Vascular engorgement leads to obstruction of the nasal passages. Sensory nerves are also hyperresponsive in AR.[47]

There are two phases of the nasal response. The immediate phase occurs 15 to 30 minutes after exposure to an allergen and is due to mast cell mediator release. The late-phase response occurs 6 to 12 hours after exposure and is due to inflammatory

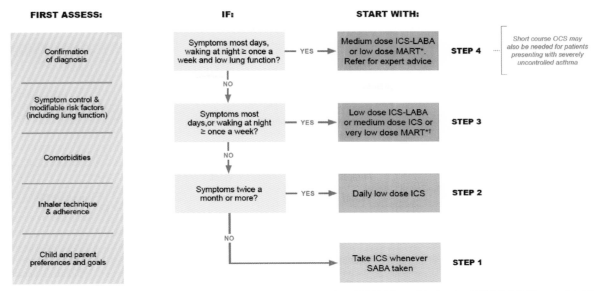

FIRST ASSESS: | **IF:** | **START WITH:**

Confirmation of diagnosis

Symptom control & modifiable risk factors (including lung function)

Comorbidities

Inhaler technique & adherence

Child and parent preferences and goals

Symptoms most days, waking at night ≥ once a week and low lung function? — YES → Medium dose ICS-LABA or low dose MART*. Refer for expert advice — **STEP 4** ... [Short course OCS may also be needed for patients presenting with severely uncontrolled asthma]

NO ↓

Symptoms most days, or waking at night ≥ once a week? — YES → Low dose ICS-LABA or medium dose ICS or very low dose MART*† — **STEP 3**

NO ↓

Symptoms twice a month or more? — YES → Daily low dose ICS — **STEP 2**

NO ↓

→ Take ICS whenever SABA taken — **STEP 1**

*Low dose: BUD-FORM 200/6 mcg; †Very low dose: BUD-FORM 100/6 mcg (metered doses)
MART= maintenance and reliever therapy (ICS-formoterol as both maintenance and reliever)

BUD-FORM: budesonide-formoterol; ICS: inhaled corticosteroid; LABA: long-acting beta₂-agonist; MART: maintenance and reliever therapy with ICS-formoterol; OCS: oral corticosteroids; SABA: short-acting beta₂-agonist. See Box 3-6, p.63 for low, medium and high ICS doses in children.

• **Fig. 36.6** Initiating Controller Therapy Example. (From Global Initiative for Asthma, Copyright 2022. www.ginasthma.org.)

cells (i.e., T lymphocytes, basophils, eosinophils) infiltrating the nasal mucosa.

AR and asthma are increasing in prevalence and are comorbid conditions with up to 40% of individuals with AR also having asthma.[48] The link between upper and lower respiratory disease causes poorly controlled AR to lead to poorly controlled asthma.

Children with AR can have significant symptoms affecting their quality of life and leading to school and work absences. Diagnosis of AR is based on the presence of rhinorrhea, nasal pruritus and congestion, and sneezing. Manifestations can be seasonal or perennial depending on exposure to the offending agent and subsequent sensitization to the offending allergen.[47] There may be a related family or medical history of AD, AR, or asthma.

AR is second only to asthma as the most common atopic disorder. There is an increased incidence in families with an atopic history. Genetic and environmental factors are commonly associated with AR. Repeated exposure to the offending allergen for a period of time is an important contributing factor necessary for sensitizing the immune system to produce an allergic IgE response. Frequently, there is pruritus of the nose, palate, and eyes. The history may also include poor sleep, generalized malaise, and behavioral issues along with impaired school performance.

Mild AR does not impair any of the following four: daily activities, sleep, school, or work activities, and the child is not troubled by the symptoms. The classification can be intermittent if it persists for only 4 weeks or less, or persistent if it is present for longer than 4 weeks. If it is moderate to severe, there are changes in one or more of these four items.[47]

Allergic responses typically take a few years to develop, making AR rare in children younger than 2 years. In a young child with nasal symptoms, consider other differentials.[47] Food allergens occasionally cause rhinitis. AR tends to be seasonal, perennial, or episodic.

Seasonal AR (hay fever or seasonal pollenosis) results from sensitization to airborne allergens, such as tree, grass, and weed pollen (e.g., ragweed) and outdoor molds. There can be geographic variations in seasonal AR depending on climate and when allergens are released into the environment. Perennial AR has year-round signs and symptoms that may be more severe in the winter. Offending substances tend to be indoor allergens, including house dust mites, cockroaches, feathers, allergens, or household pet dander, and indoor mold spores and seasonal pollens. Episodic AR occurs with intermittent exposure to an allergen with a resultant rhinitis and is relates to a distinct event, such as visiting a house where a cat lives.

Clinical Findings

Common symptoms and findings on physical examination include:

- Reduced patency from chronic or recurrent bilateral nasal obstruction as a result of congestion and inflammation
- Mouth breathing, snoring, nasal speech
- Pale to purplish and edema (bogginess) of nasal mucous membranes
- Clear, thin, watery to seromucoid rhinorrhea
- Nasal crease: horizontal crease across the lower third of the nose
- Itching, rubbing of nose, or "allergic salute"
- Nasal stuffiness, postnasal drip, paroxysms of sneezing, congested cough, or night cough
- Allergic shiners, Dennie lines, Morgan fold, or atopic pleats: extra groove in lower eyelid (Fig. 36.8)
- High arched palate; itching of palate, pharynx, nose, or eyes; child may make a palatal click to scratch the palate; enlarged tonsillar and adenoidal tissue
- Repeated sniffling, snorting, coughing, frequent attempts to clear the throat, or hoarseness
- Redness of the conjunctiva, tearing, lid and periorbital edema, infraorbital cyanosis, or allergic shiners (dark periorbital swelling)

TABLE 36.10   Classifying Severity of Asthma Exacerbations

	Mild	Moderate	Severe	Respiratory Arrest Imminent
Symptoms				
Breathless	While walking	While at rest (infant—softer, shorter cry; difficulty feeding)	While at rest (infant—stops feeding)	
	Can lie down	Prefers sitting	Sits upright	
Talks in	Sentences	Phrases	Words	
Alertness	May be agitated	Usually agitated	Usually agitated	Drowsy or confused
Signs				
Respiratory rate	Increased	Increased	Often >30 breaths/min	
Use of accessory muscles; suprasternal retractions	Usually not	Commonly	Usually	Paradoxical thoracoabdominal movement
Wheeze	Moderate, often only end expiratory	Loud; throughout exhalation	Usually loud; throughout inhalation and exhalation	Absence of wheeze
Pulse (beats/min)	<100	100–120	>120	Bradycardia
Functional Assessment				
PEF percentage predicted or percentage personal best	≥70%	Approximately 40–69%	<40% predicted or personal best, or response lasts <2 h	<25%
PaO_2 (on room air) and/or	Normal (test not usually necessary)	>60 mm Hg (test not usually necessary)	<60 mm Hg: possible cyanosis	
PCO_2	<42 mm Hg (test not usually necessary)	<42 mm Hg (test not usually necessary)	≥42 mm Hg: possible respiratory failure	
SaO_2% (on room air) at sea level	>95% (test not usually necessary)	90–95%	<90%	

NORMAL RESPIRATORY AND CARDIAC RATES IN CHILDREN

Breathing When Awake		Pulse	
Age	Rate (Breaths/Min)	Age	Rate (Beats/Min)
<2 months	<60	2–12 months	<160
2–12 months	<50	1–2 years	<120
1–5 years	<40	2–8 years	<110
6–8 years	<30		

The presence of several parameters, but not necessarily all, indicates the general classification of the exacerbation. Many of these parameters have not been systematically studied, so they serve only as general guides.

PaCO₂, Partial pressure of carbon dioxide; *PaO₂*, partial pressure of oxygen in arterial blood; *PEF*, peak expiratory flow; *SaO₂*, oxygen saturation in arterial blood.

From National Heart, Lung, and Blood Institute (NHLBI). *Full Report of the Expert Panel: Guidelines for the Diagnosis and Management of Asthma (EPR-3)*. National Institutes of Health; 2007.

- "Cobblestone" appearance of the pharynx or palpebral conjunctivae (or both) as a result of increased lymphoid tissue
- Chronic mouth breathing can lead to facial changes, dental malocclusions, and snoring
- Sleep disturbances are common in allergic disease with performance problems at school from inadequate sleep.

Diagnostic Studies and Allergy Testing. History, including an evaluation of risk factors, and characteristic clinical findings are the key to diagnosis. Pediatric risk factors include a positive family history, male sex, first-born child, early use of systemic antibiotics, maternal smoking, and exposure to allergens. Diagnostic testing is not always needed. Allergen-specific IgE testing done by skin prick testing is preferred and usually done by an allergist. The presence of eosinophils on nasal smear can help substantiate the diagnosis but is a nonspecific, nonuniversal finding. The presence of nasal eosinophilia often predicts a positive response to nasal corticosteroid

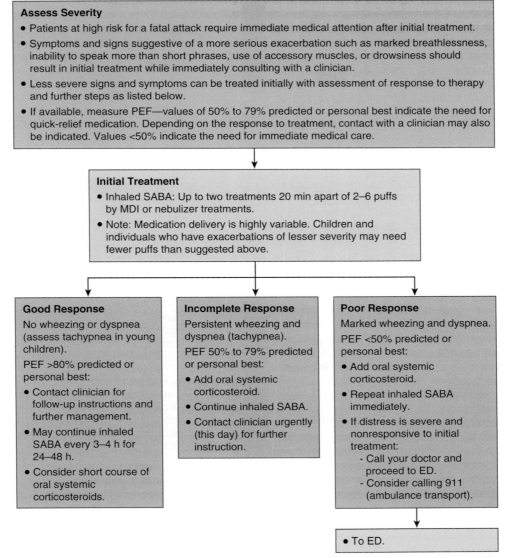

Assess Severity
- Patients at high risk for a fatal attack require immediate medical attention after initial treatment.
- Symptoms and signs suggestive of a more serious exacerbation such as marked breathlessness, inability to speak more than short phrases, use of accessory muscles, or drowsiness should result in initial treatment while immediately consulting with a clinician.
- Less severe signs and symptoms can be treated initially with assessment of response to therapy and further steps as listed below.
- If available, measure PEF—values of 50% to 79% predicted or personal best indicate the need for quick-relief medication. Depending on the response to treatment, contact with a clinician may also be indicated. Values <50% indicate the need for immediate medical care.

Initial Treatment
- Inhaled SABA: Up to two treatments 20 min apart of 2–6 puffs by MDI or nebulizer treatments.
- Note: Medication delivery is highly variable. Children and individuals who have exacerbations of lesser severity may need fewer puffs than suggested above.

Good Response
No wheezing or dyspnea (assess tachypnea in young children).
PEF >80% predicted or personal best:
- Contact clinician for follow-up instructions and further management.
- May continue inhaled SABA every 3–4 h for 24–48 h.
- Consider short course of oral systemic corticosteroids.

Incomplete Response
Persistent wheezing and dyspnea (tachypnea).
PEF 50% to 79% predicted or personal best:
- Add oral systemic corticosteroid.
- Continue inhaled SABA.
- Contact clinician urgently (this day) for further instruction.

Poor Response
Marked wheezing and dyspnea.
PEF <50% predicted or personal best:
- Add oral systemic corticosteroid.
- Repeat inhaled SABA immediately.
- If distress is severe and nonresponsive to initial treatment:
  - Call your doctor and proceed to ED.
  - Consider calling 911 (ambulance transport).

- To ED.

• **Fig. 36.7** Management of Asthma Exacerbations: Home Treatment. *ED,* Emergency department; *MDI,* metered dose inhaler; *PEF,* peak expiratory flow; *SABA,* short-acting β₂-agonist.

sprays. Referrals for skin or serologic testing for IgE antibody to specific allergens should be reserved for children with significant symptoms that do not respond to traditional management.

The American Academy of Allergy, Asthma & Immunology (AAAI)[49] through the Choosing Wisely campaign recommends against ordering large panels of allergen testing and stresses the importance of only doing testing for specific allergens by history. Allergy panel testing can lead to the diagnosis of an allergy that the child does not have, resulting in unnecessary avoidance. It can also result in false reassurance in the face of a negative test, when in fact the child's history is positive for an offending trigger. Neither positive skin testing nor positive allergen-specific IgE blood tests should be the sole basis for telling a family their child is allergic to a particular airborne antigen or food. History is critical to determine the test's accuracy.

Differential Diagnosis

Differential diagnoses are the common cold, purulent rhinitis, sinusitis, adenoidal hypertrophy, foreign body obstruction, nasal polyposis of cystic fibrosis, nasopharyngeal tumors, choanal atresia

or stenosis, and vasomotor rhinitis. Overuse of prescription or over-the-counter topical nasal decongestants can cause drug-induced rhinitis (rhinitis medicamentosa), as can the use of cocaine. Some individuals experience idiopathic rhinitis marked by nasal hyper-responsiveness to nonspecific triggers, such as strong smells (e.g., perfumes, bleach), tobacco smoke, or changes in environmental temperature and humidity. Hormonal rhinitis occurs during pregnancy, puberty, and in hypothyroidism, and food-induced rhinitis is associated with consumption of hot and spicy foods. Patients who have unilateral discharge or blockage, severe headache, or anosmia may have an alternative diagnosis including cerebrospinal fluid rhinorrhea, sinonasal tumors, or chronic rhinosinusitis.[50]

Management

Pharmacologic Therapy. Treatment of patients with AR is tailored to the severity of the disease. For episodic symptoms, oral or nasal H₁ antihistamines with oral or nasal decongestants if needed, can be used. For seasonal or perennial rhinitis with mild symptoms, there is no significant difference between inhaled nasal corticosteroids (INCS), oral or nasal H₁ antihistamine, or

• BOX 36.2 | How to Use a Metered Dose Inhaler

Using an inhaler seems simple, but most patients do not use it correctly.

Steps for Using an Inhaler for Children <5 Years

1. Use of a mask chamber with MDI allows the delivery of inhaled medications even in an uncooperative child.
2. The child should be placed in the parent's lap, and the mask placed around the child's mouth.
3. Press down on the MDI while firmly holding the mask around the child's mouth. The child will eventually take a deep breath and inhale the medication.

Steps for Using an Inhaler for Children ≥5 Years
Getting Ready
1. Take off the cap and shake the inhaler.
2. Breathe out all the way.
3. Hold the inhaler as shown in steps A, B, or C below.

Breathe in Slowly
1. Start breathing in slowly through the mouth, and then press down on the inhaler one time. (If a holding chamber is used, first press down on the inhaler.) Within 5 seconds, begin to breathe in slowly.
2. Keep breathing in slowly, as deeply as possible.

Hold Your Breaths
1. Hold breath for a slow count to 10 if possible.
2. For inhaled quick-relief medicine (β_2-agonists), wait about 1 min between puffs. There is no need to wait between puffs for other medicines.
   A. Hold inhaler 1–2 inches in front of mouth (about the width of two fingers).

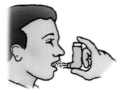

B. Use a spacer/holding chamber. These come in many shapes and can be useful to any patient .

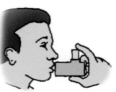

C. Put inhaler in mouth. Do not use for steroids.

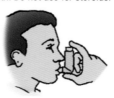

Step A or B is best, but step C can be used if patient has trouble with step A or B.

Clean Inhaler as Needed
Look at the hole where the medicine sprays out from inhaler. If "powder" can be seen in or around the hole, clean the inhaler. Remove the metal canister from the L-shaped plastic mouthpiece. Rinse only the mouthpiece and cap in warm water and let dry overnight. In the morning, put the canister back inside. Put the cap on.

Know When to Replace Inhaler
For medicines taken each day: As an example, a new canister has 200 puffs (number of puffs is listed on canister), and child is told to take 8 puffs/day; 8 puffs/day for 25 days equal 200 puffs in canister. This canister will last 25 days. If child started using this inhaler on May 1, replace it on or before May 25. Write the date on the canister. For quick-relief medicine, take as needed and count each puff. Do not put canisters in water to see if empty. Note if using a Flovent inhaler, you may still feel liquid in the canister and see liquid spray out, the medicine is gone after the total number of puffs has been delivered. The liquid is the leftover propellant and preservative.

MDI, *Metered dose inhaler.*

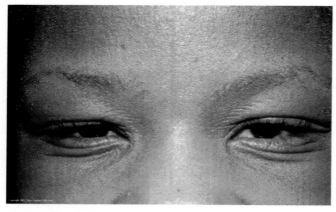

• **Fig. 36.8** Dennie Line or Morgan Line. (From Cohen B. *Pediatric Dermatology.* 5th ed. Elsevier; 2022.)

LTRA and any of the three can be used. For moderate to severe symptoms, INCS are the first-line agents with an alternative of oral H_1 antihistamine plus LTRA for patients who do not tolerate the side effects of INCS or who do not want to use the drug. There is no difference in use of INCS alone or with the use of oral antihistamine plus INCS in children over 12 years.[50] AIT is an option for patients over 12 years who are highly sensitive to multiple allergens; however, the price, is estimated to be greater than $18,000 a year in the United States.[50] AIT can be administered subcutaneously or sublingually (limited to dust mite, northern grasses, and ragweed) in patients who do not respond well to pharmacotherapy. Combination therapy can be offered if patients do not respond well to monotherapy.[50]

Pharmacologic therapy depends on the severity of the symptoms and the ability of the parent or child to adhere to recommendations. INCS reduce inflammation, edema, and mucus production and are typically a key component in long-term therapy to manage AR symptoms. Second- and third-generation antihistamines are frequently used to treat the symptoms of rhinorrhea, sneezing, and nasal and eye pruritus. Pharmacologic agents should be started 1 to 2 weeks before pollen season for children with seasonal AR. Often children with AR benefit from a combination approach; some require only single-line therapy. Antibiotics should only be prescribed for secondary bacterial infections (sinusitis).

Oral Antihistamines
• Oral antihistamines are divided into classes based on the four different types of histamine receptors, each with a varying ability to mediate an allergic response. H_1 and H_2 receptors are

found in a variety of cells and cause the early and late phase of allergic response. H_3 and H_4 receptors cause pruritus as well as a proinflammatory immune response. Different classes of drugs may be more effective for different children (Table 36.11).

- Oral antihistamines are especially helpful in seasonal AR but do little to relieve nasal obstruction. Second-generation antihistamines are particularly effective in relieving symptoms of AR (nasal itching, sneezing, and rhinorrhea) by controlling the release of chemical mediators and are often used to manage this problem.
- Drug dosage may need to be increased until there is relief of symptoms or side effects are experienced.
- Tolerance to a particular antihistamine can develop necessitating the need to rotate drugs.
- If side effects with one antihistamine are experienced, prescribe another antihistamine in a different class or one in the same class but with different actions.
- First-generation antihistamines may interfere with daytime activities and negatively affect school performance; they are no longer recommended for treatment of AR because of impaired safety profile and adverse effects.
- Second- and third-generation antihistamines (e.g., cetirizine, loratadine, fexofenadine) are associated with less sedation effect.

Topical Nasal Antihistamines
- Azelastine is a nasal antihistamine spray approved for use in seasonal AR in children ≥6 months of age. Azelastine acts by competing with histamine for H_1-receptor sites; it has a bitter taste and is associated with sedation. It is available as a combination with fluticasone propionate and approved for children 6 years of age and older.
- Olopatadine is a nasal spray approved for use in children ≥6 years of age. Like nasal azelastine, it is effective in reducing itching, sneezing, rhinorrhea, and congestion.[50]

Decongestants
- Decongestants may help relieve nasal congestion; there is no evidence supporting the use of oral phenylephrine as a decongestant.[50]
- Topical decongestants can cause rebound rhinorrhea (rhinitis medicamentosa) if used for more than 3 to 5 days; errors in administration can cause systemic absorption and side effects of irritability, nervousness, and insomnia among others.
- Children younger than 4 years old should not be given decongestants.

Nasal Cromolyn
- Cromolyn is an intranasal mast cell stabilizer used for seasonal or perennial AR. It is less effective than INCS, and frequent dosing is needed. It is safe for children 2 years and older.

Intranasal Corticosteroids
- These agents are effective in reducing local cytokines and mediator release factors produced by mast cells, basophils, eosinophils, monocytes, and macrophages that lead to inflammation and subsequent nasal obstruction.[47] INCS are considered one of the most effective treatments to manage AR and have been safely used in long-term management of AR to relieve symptoms of nasal congestion, rhinorrhea, itching, and sneezing.
- Clear the child's nasal passages of mucus before use. Table 36.12 lists usual dosages for INCS.
- INCS can take up to 4 weeks before clinical benefit is observed.[47] Side effects include local burning, irritation, sneezing, or soreness (<10% experience these symptoms). Epistaxis is related to improper technique—spraying the nasal septum.

Leukotriene Modifiers
- Montelukast is the only approved LTRA for use in seasonal and perennial AR. It is approved from 6 months to 5 years as a 4-mg packet (granules) once daily. Children 6 to 14 years

TABLE 36.11 Antihistamine Classes

Class	Name	Comments
First-Generation Antihistamines		
Ethanolamine	Diphenhydramine	Sedation, dizziness, thickening of bronchial secretions
	Clemastine	Dry mouth, fatigue, headache, somnolence, bradycardia
	Carbinoxamine	Drowsiness, CNS excitation, and difficulty sleeping
Ethylenediamine	Pyrilamine	Not used in children
Alkylamines	Chlorpheniramine	Drowsiness, sedation, dry mouth, GI symptoms
	Brompheniramine	Palpitations, weight gain, drowsiness, dizziness, headache
Piperazine	Hydroxyzine	Sedation, dizziness, dry mouth
Piperidine	Cyproheptadine	CNS depression or stimulation, weight gain, dry mouth
Second-Generation Nonsedating H_1 Antihistamines		
Nonsedating antihistamines	Loratadine	Dry mouth, fatigue, headache, somnolence Approved for children ≥2 years
	Cetirizine	Dry mouth, fatigue, headache, somnolence Approved for children ≥6 months
	Fexofenadine	Dry mouth, fatigue, headache, somnolence, dysmenorrhea, flulike signs Approved for children ≥6 months for chronic urticaria and ≥2 years for allergic rhinitis

CNS, Central nervous system; *GI*, gastrointestinal.

TABLE 36.12	Intranasal Corticosteroid Preparations Used for Allergic Rhinitis: Usual Dosages	
Drug	**Dosage**	**Age and Dosage**
Beclomethasone, aerosol solution	80 mcg/actuation	≥12 years: 320 mcg once daily (160 mcg/nostril or 2 sprays each nostril of 80 mcg)
Beclomethasone AQ, aqueous suspension	42 mcg/spray	≥6–12 years: Initial, 1 spray/nostril (42 mcg/inhalation) twice a day (total single dose of 84 mcg); increase to 2 sprays/nostril (two 42 mcg inhalations) twice a day (total single dose of 168 mcg) if needed; decreases to 42 mcg (1 spray) each nostril twice a day with control ≥12 years: 84 mcg (1 spray/nostril) or 168 mcg (2 sprays/nostril) twice a day
Budesonide[a]	32 mcg/actuation	≥6 years: Initial, 1 spray/nostril once daily (64 mcg total dose) Maximum dose: <12 years, 2 sprays/nostril once a day (daily maximum dose of 128 mcg) ≥12 years: 4 sprays total/2 sprays each nostril once a day (daily maximum dose of 256 mcg)
Flunisolide	25 mcg/actuation	6–14 years: Initial, 2 spray/nostril twice daily (100 mcg twice a day), or 1 spray/nostril 3 times a day (50 mcg 3 times a day) to a maximum of 4 sprays/nostril daily (200 mcg/day); maintenance dose is 1 spray/nostril daily 15 years: 2 sprays/nostril twice a day (total single dose of 100 mcg) to 2 sprays/nostril 3 times/day (total single dose of 100 mcg); max daily dose of 400 mcg); maintenance 1 spray/nostril daily
Fluticasone propionate (Flonase)	50 mcg/actuation	≥4 years and adolescents: Initial 1 spray/nostril daily; 2 sprays daily if severe or poor response; reduce to 1 spray/nostril/day once symptoms controlled Adult: 2 sprays/nostril daily or 1 spray/nostril twice daily; may reduce to 1 spray/nostril daily once symptoms controlled
Fluticasone furoate (Veramyst)	27.5 mcg/spray	2–11 years: Initial, 1 spray/nostril once a day (total dose of 55 mcg/day), increase to 2 sprays/nostril once a day (total 110 mcg/day); reduce to 1 spray/nostril a day with control ≥12 years and adolescents: 2 sprays/nostril daily (110 mcg/day); reduce to 1 spray/nostril once daily (total 55 mcg/day)
Mometasone	50 mcg/actuation	2–11 years: 1 spray (50 mcg)/nostril daily >12 years: 2 sprays (100 mcg)/nostril daily
Triamcinolone (Nasacort AQ)	55 mcg/spray	2–5 years: 1 spray (55 mcg)/nostril once daily 6–11 years: Initial, 1 spray (55 mcg)/nostril once daily, can increase to 2 sprays (110 mcg)/nostril once daily; maintenance 1 spray (55 mcg)/nostril with control >12 years: 2 sprays (110 mcg)/nostril daily; maintenance dose 1 (55 mcg) spray/nostril daily

[a]Reduce slowly every 2–4 weeks to smallest effective dose.

Data from Taketomo CK, Hodding JH, Kraus DM. *Pediatric & Neonatal Dosage Handbook*. 28th ed. Lexi-Comp; 2021.

should take a 5-mg chewable tablet and teens over 15 years can take the adult dose of 10 mg once a day. Montelukast has a moderate effect when used alone. If patient has AR, administer dose in morning or evening; if patient also has asthma, give the age-appropriate dose in evening. Guidelines suggest the use of INCS for AR as LTRA are not as effective as nasal steroids.[50]

Allergy Immunotherapy and Other Treatments. AIT includes subcutaneous immunotherapy (SCIT), oral immunotherapy (OIT), epicutaneous immunotherapy (EPIT), and sublingual immunotherapy (SLIT). There are limitations to SLIT as only three sublingual tablets are presently FDA approved for use—ragweed, northern pasture grasses like timothy, and dust mites' tablets with clinical trials for peanut allergy ongoing. OIT has the highest rate of allergic side effects. EPIT for peanut and milk allergy is still in the research phase.

AIT is a treatment option for allergic disease including food allergy. In patients with life-threatening reactions to foods or severe allergic asthma, treatment with AIT is the only treatment modality that alters the underlying disease process preventing asthma and offers a potential cure to allergies.[51] AIT has traditionally been administered via SCIT. The FDA has also approved some therapies to be delivered sublingually (SLIT), orally (OIT) and there are FDA trials in progress for EPIT. The goal of AIT is to induce immune tolerance and cause a change in the immune response to specific antigens and also produce longer-lasting benefits without the need for daily medication. The mechanism of action for immunotherapy is centered on modulating the immune response, changing IgE that is allergen specific to IgG4, and to decrease basophil action to allergen cross-linking, causing an increase in regulatory T cells. Desensitization occurs after months of AIT via SCIT or SLIT. EPIT involves putting a small allergen patch to the back or upper arm with daily changes. EPIT proved efficacious in decreasing peanut, milk, and egg allergies. In 2020, after phase III trials, the FDA refused approval citing need for improvements in adhesion of the patch. No safety concerns were found.[52] Unlike SCIT and SLIT, OIT is not curative.

The goal of OIT is to raise the threshold of reaction in patients age 4 to 17 years, so that chance encounters with the substance will not trigger a reaction. Patients who take OIT alone, will still need to carry an EpiPen as complete desensitization to the allergen is not the goal.[53] The goal of AIT is sustained unresponsiveness; however, study results have been mixed as to how often sustained unresponsiveness is achieved. Currently, it is assumed that the majority of patients on OIT will require ongoing measured exposure to allergens.[53]

AIT can induce adverse reactions that can be local, such as tingling following sublingual oral therapy, to systemic reactions that are life-threatening.[51] OIT reactions tend to involve the GI system. Some OIT patients can develop eosinophilic esophagitis, which typically resolves when the OIT is discontinued.[53] The majority of the reactions occur within 30 minutes; therefore the child should be monitored for 30 minutes afterward. AIT should be conducted in a facility that has both the necessary equipment and healthcare professionals prepared to treat anaphylaxis.

Studies investigating the use of omalizumab and other FDA approved biologics in patients older than 12 years with inadequately controlled and significant AR noted significant symptom relief and improved quality of life.[54] Occurrences of adverse reactions were not statistically significant.

Avoidance Strategies. Determine triggering factors if possible and educate the family on the need to avoid exposure to the offending allergen or irritant as much as possible. Allergens causing seasonal rhinitis are more difficult to avoid than are the indoor allergens, such as molds, because pollens are smaller and lighter and thus remain in the air longer. Key avoidance measures for indoor allergens and irritants include the following:

- Control house dust, paying special attention to the child's bedroom.
  - Use dust mite–proof mattress and pillow covers (allergen-impermeable encasement).
  - Wash bed linens in hot water (>130°F [54.4°C]) weekly.
  - Minimize (if possible, eliminate) stuffed toys in child's bedroom.
  - Use vertical blinds instead of horizontal blinds or curtains.
  - Remove carpeting from bedroom.
  - Use plastic or wood furniture instead of cloth or upholstered furniture.
- Eliminate smoking from the child's environment; if household members still smoke despite education, emphasize smoking outside the house and never in the car.
- Consider hairless pets; pet hair collects urine, dander, and saliva; the protein in pet saliva causes the reactivity.
- Reduce mold; avoid damp basements and other sources of moisture in the home environment.
- Indoor humidity should be less than 50%; avoid vaporizers.
- Use dehumidifiers, air conditioners with efficient filters, and air-cleaning devices with an electronic precipitator or with a high-efficiency particulate air (HEPA) filter.
- Eliminate any offending substances; vector control for cockroach elimination.

Complications and Prognosis

Sinusitis may be a complication with AR due to secondary bacterial infection of the swollen sinus mucosal linings. The AAP guidelines on sinusitis and the AAAI do not advise imaging for confirmation of sinusitis.[49] Likewise, eustachian tube dysfunction and its sequel, serous otitis media, are common complications. Malocclusion, the development of a high-arched palate, and the typical allergic facies can result from long-standing AR. Chronic AR may lead to chronic cough and postnasal drip. If a child has both AR and asthma, treatment of the child's AR is essential if the asthma is to be effectively managed.

Perennial AR can be a chronic problem unless offending allergens are identified and eliminated from the environment. If this is not possible, pharmacologic therapy is usually helpful in reducing symptoms. As the child grows and nasal passages increase in size, symptoms may also lessen. Symptoms from seasonal AR often worsen from the adolescent years to mid-adulthood. Moving to a new environment often results in a short respite (1–3 years) from symptoms; however, the child frequently becomes sensitized to new airborne pollens and symptoms of seasonal AR return.

Patient and Parent Education and Prevention

Because AR is often a chronic problem, parents and children need to have specific information about controlling this disorder:

- Instruct on environmental control. Handouts and individualization of information are essential.
- Review pharmacologic therapy, including indications for and changes in medications, frequency of use, and common side effects and contraindications.
- Demonstrate, with return demonstration, how to use intranasal sprays or inhalers if prescribed.

Atopic Dermatitis

AD is a common chronic, pruritic, inflammatory skin disorder of childhood characterized by acute and chronic skin eruptions. The term *atopic eczema* is used interchangeably with *atopic dermatitis*. It is a complex disorder caused by the interaction of genetic susceptibility and micro- and macroenvironment, leading to tissue inflammation in the host. AD manifests a typical morphology and distribution of flexural lichenification or linearity along with acral or hand and feet distribution in adolescents and adults. In school-age children, antecubital and popliteal fossa are common places for AD; in infants, there is facial and extensor involvement. Food allergies are common with children with AD, but the relationship between them is not entirely clear. Certain foods may be a trigger for AD exacerbation. Food allergies may serve as an endotype and a marker for potential AD severity. Pediatric patients with AD are more likely to develop neuropsychiatric disorders including attention-deficit/hyperactivity disorder (ADHD), depression, suicidal ideation, anxiety, and conduct problems. Disruptions with sleep and quality of life are common. There is higher healthcare utilization across the lifespan because AD patients are more susceptible to bacterial and viral skin infections, obesity, coronary artery disease, and other autoimmune diseases.[25]

In AD, the skin's ability to act as a protective barrier is impaired, resulting in xerosis (dry skin), cracking, increased skin markings, lichenification, and susceptibility to bacterial, viral, and fungal infections (Fig. 36.9). Recent studies indicate the need for prevention and the use of daily moisturizer barrier therapy starting in the neonatal period to prevent the onset of AD. The prevention of AD may alter the association between early AD and other allergic manifestations, such as allergic asthma and food allergy.[12,25]

AD affects approximately 15% to 20% of children in the United States and typically develops before 5 years of age in 85% of cases.[25,56] There is no test to determine the diagnosis, but a history of a highly pruritic, relapsing dermatitis with erythematous papules and patches, and periods of exacerbations provides the necessary information for a diagnosis of AD.[57] Children with mild to moderate disease can be managed by PCPs, with severe cases needing referral to dermatology.

The exact etiology is unknown and may vary among individuals. Although many children have high IgE levels, an exact immune mechanism for this disorder is unclear. Studies investigating the pathophysiology of AD point to multifactorial interactions between environmental risk factors, immune deviation, and impaired barrier function. It is a heterogeneous disease with multiple inflammatory pathways. The identification of the filaggrin (FLG) mutation that results in loss of skin function is the strongest risk factor for AD; however, it is only present in a small number of patients.[12] The FLG is produced in the stratum granulosum and contributes to the natural moisture in the stratum corneum as well as corneum hydration and dysregulation of type 1 interferon (INF)-mediated stress response. There is an impairment in the innate immune response in the skin causing increased colonization of microbes; therefore the child is prone to recurrent skin infection. AD is a T cell–driven disease with elevated levels of IL-4 and IL-13, causing IgE elevations. Abnormalities in histamine production (increased in the skin), chemotaxis, monocytes, and cytokines are associated with AD. There is also a decrease in ceramides, reducing the water capacity of the skin and leading to more water loss.[25] Factors that aggravate this condition include harsh soaps, heat, sweating, infections, stress, food allergies, and dry skin.

Sweating increases itching in atopic skin, and transepidermal water loss is increased. A predisposition to the development of pruritus is believed to be a key factor with variability in the extent of the skin involvement and severity of presentation. Pruritus and relapsing eczematous lesions in the typical morphology are essential features in making the diagnosis.[58]

Clinical Findings

The following are commonly seen in AD:
- Pruritus and eczematous changes reflecting typical age-specific morphologic patterns
- History of a chronic or relapsing skin condition
- A positive family history of AD or other atopic disease
- Pityriasis alba, cheilitis, perifollicular accentuation
- Acute manifestations (more common in infants) include:
  - Intense itching and redness
  - Papules, vesicles, edema, serous discharge, and crusts
  - Generalized dry skin (xerosis) with dry hair and scalp; diaper area usually spared
  - Lichenification is typically not seen
- Chronic manifestations (more common in children and adolescents) include:
  - Lichenification—thickened, leathery, hyperpigmented skin; scratch marks
  - Generalized xerosis with flaky and rough skin: Table 36.13 lists characteristics of AD at different ages

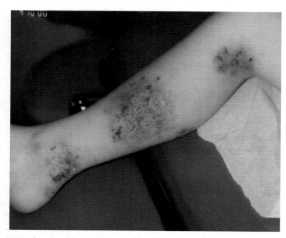

• **Fig. 36.9** Acute Atopic Dermatitis. (Courtesy Peggy Vernon RN, MA, CPNP, DCNP, FAANP, Creekside Skin Care, Centennial, CO.)

TABLE 36.13	Assessment of Atopic Dermatitis	
Onset/Initial Presentation	**Signs and Symptoms**	**Comment/Prognosis**
<3 months	Dry skin first sign	Often not noticed
2–3 months	Itch-scratch-itch cycle starts	
Infantile phase	Acute presentation—common in infants: intense itching; redness, papules, vesicles, edema; serous discharge and crusts Cheeks, forehead, scalp, extending to trunk as symmetric patches or to the extremities; lateral extensor surface of arms and legs; diaper area and groin are spared of lesion	Two-thirds of cases resolve by 2–3 years Generalized xerosis
Childhood phase (starts 2 years to puberty)	Pruritus is severe Lesions are dry and papular with circumscribed scaly patches Involves wrists, hands, popliteal and antecubital fossa; eyebrows thin and broken off with lack of the lateral third of the eyebrow (called *Hertoghe sign*); some only have feet involved; may have allergic-atopic facies and white dermatographism Flexural involvement	One-third continue into teenage years—tendency to be chronic
Adolescent/adult phase	Begins at puberty and can commonly continue into adulthood Often involves the flexural folds (popliteal and antecubital fossae), face, neck, upper arms and back, dorsa of hands, fingers, feet, and toes Dry skin and lichenification are prominent findings Erythematous, dry-scaling papules and plaques with fewer exudates Postinflammatory hypopigmentation or hyperpigmentation that disappears	New or recurrence of a chronic condition

- Other key features of AD:
  - Tendency towards dry skin and a lowered threshold for itching (itch-scratch-itch cycle)
  - Often worsens during dry winter months or with heat in the summer
  - Sweating increases pruritus
  - Chronic AD often secondarily infected with *Staphylococcus aureus* (most commonly) or *Streptococcus pyogenes* (occasionally)
  - Secondarily infection of AD with herpes simplex is called *eczema herpeticum* and is a dermatologic emergency requiring antiviral treatment with acyclovir or valacyclovir (depending on age)
  - Hyperpigmentation may be noted especially in areas of lichenification
- Possible associated features:
  - Atopic pleats—extra groove in lower eyelid called *Dennie lines* or *Morgan fold* (see Fig. 36.8), crease across upper bulb of nose
  - Accentuated palmar and flexural creases; keratoconus
  - Allergic shiners, mild facial pallor, or dry hair
  - Keratosis pilaris—follicular papules occurring on the extensor aspect of the arms, anterior thighs, and lateral aspects of the cheeks
  - Nummular eczema, dyshidrotic eczema, juvenile plantar dermatitis, nipple eczema, or ichthyosis vulgaris
  - White dermatographism (white line following a scratch); some have an associated circumoral pallor (presents as bluish, grey or whitish in color depending on underlying skin color and is thought to be related to local edema and vasoconstriction)

Diagnostic Studies. The diagnosis of AD is based on characteristic clinical findings. A chronic or recurring rash that is pruritic and has a characteristic distribution and appearance, together with a family or personal history of atopy, are key to the diagnosis. Histologic examination of the skin is rarely needed and reserved only for difficult-to-diagnose cases and to exclude other diseases. Skin testing and desensitization are not routinely recommended for children with AD only. If secondary fungal infection is suspected, collect scrapings and use potassium hydroxide (KOH) to look for fungal hyphae.

Differential Diagnosis

Other types of dermatitis, including seborrheic dermatitis, drug reaction, nutritional deficiencies of zinc/biotin, acrodermatitis enteropathica, ichthyosis vulgaris, contact dermatitis, allergic contact dermatitis, nummular dermatitis, psoriasis, and scabies are included in the differential diagnosis. A few genetic conditions are associated with similar skin eruptions (e.g., phenylketonuria, Wiskott-Aldrich syndrome, histiocytosis X, and acrodermatitis enteropathica) as well as primary immunodeficiency diseases, cutaneous T-cell lymphoma, lymphocytic-variant hypereosinophilia syndrome.

Management

Treatment strategy is based on the following key concepts:
- The itch-scratch-itch cycle must be interrupted.
- Dryness of the skin must be corrected by rehydrating the stratum corneum with lubrication as the first-line therapy to enhance skin moisturization. The choice of the moisturizer is dependent on the individual, but should be safe, free of additives, and inexpensive. Application of moisturizer should take

place soon after bath to decrease transepidermal water loss. Start skin barrier protection at birth as it may be protective against the development of AD.
- If moisturization does not control the disease, then topical corticosteroid preparations (TCPs) are used with low-potency corticosteroids for maintenance and higher potency for exacerbations.[59]
- Use of nonsoap surfactants and synthetic detergents, which are more acid, are often recommended but without good supporting evidence.
- Eliminate any known offending agents (irritants and allergic triggers).
- Secondary bacterial or viral infections must be treated.

Management. The American Academy of Dermatology and the AAP published AD guidelines, and there are definite similarities between their guidelines, with variations in recommendations about the frequency and length of certain treatment, such as bleach baths and skin therapy maintenance. Moisturization and topical agents are the mainstay addressed in both guidelines.[54] See Resources section for example of AD action plan. Acute versus chronic care management is also a consideration. The following therapies are key factors in the control of AD.

Teach patients to bathe daily in lukewarm water. Baths should be limited to 5 to 10 minutes. Soaps and shampoos should be dye-free, fragrance free, and hypoallergenic. After the bath, skin should be patted dry and emollients applied within 3 minutes to seal in moisture. In moderate to severe eczema, a twice weekly dilute bleach bath helps to prevent secondary infections through bleach's antiseptic and antistaphylococcal properties. After bathing wet wrap therapy, with emollients and topical steroids, can help to prevent flares in moderate to severe AD.[59]

Emollients are high lipid, low water content moisturizers and are an essential element of daily prevention of AD flares. Chronic emollient use helps to retain and replenish skin moisture, lengthens the time between flares, and reduces flare severity. Studies have not determined a superior over-the-counter or prescription moisturizer. Choice of moisturizer can be left to the patient's preference; however, patients should be educated that ointments have the highest concentration of lipids followed by creams and then lotions. Moisturizers should be applied once to twice a day. In infants with a family history of AD, several randomized clinical trials have demonstrated the utility of emollients alone as primary prevention for AD.[60]

Pharmacotherapy
Steroid Therapy
- Topical TCPs are a mainstay of therapy for flares.[58]
  - TCPs reduce inflammation and pruritus. The classification of the TCP should be known because potent and very potent TCPs are associated with more side effects (e.g., thinning of skin, striae, telangiectasia, generalized hypertrichosis, or adrenal axis suppression) than milder preparations. Most children with AD are controlled with twice-daily application for 2 weeks then doing twice-weekly application of a low-dose TCP for up to 4 months once the lesions are quiet. The rationale for this approach is that the child's skin has a defect in hydration, which can be treated using an intermittent approach.[59]
  - Gels penetrate well and are somewhat more drying, so they are effective in the management of acute weeping or vesicular lesions.
  - Ointments are generally stronger than all other types of preparations.

Ointments penetrate more effectively than creams or lotions and provide occlusion. They are beneficial in the management of dry, lichenified, or plaque-like areas but may occlude eccrine ducts and lead to sweating.

- Application
  - Fingertip method: The amount of steroid to be applied should be a strip of cream from the distal interphalangeal joint to the top of the adult finger for an area equaling two adult palms. Apply a thin layer of TCP to affected areas marked with acute exacerbations twice a day. Some newer TCP formulations require only once a day application.[59]
  - When applied over large areas of dermatitis or if occlusion (covering with plastic wrap) is used, the possibility of significant systemic absorption is greatly increased, especially in infants and young children.
- There are seven classes of steroid with class 1 being very high potency to class 7 being the lowest potency. Greater caution is needed when applying steroids to the face, neck, and skin folds because the skin is thinner and there is higher risk of systemic absorption. Tapering of the strength of the steroids should occur only once the outbreak is fully controlled. The child is then switched to twice-weekly application of a low-dose topical corticosteroid (TCS) at areas of outbreak to reduce the relapse. Baseline moisturizing skin care should continue with a low-strength TCS once to twice a week to reduce inflammation.[59] See Table 37.2 for a listing of TCPs by potency rating.

Phosphodiesterase-4 Inhibitor[61]
- Acts as a mediator in the conversion of cyclic adenosine monophosphate (cAMP) into AMP. In patients with AD, low cAMP levels and high phosphodiesterase (PDE) activity causes inflammatory hyperreactivity.
- Crisaborole (Eucrisa), a topical PDE-4 inhibitor, is an alternative choice in mild to moderate disease.
- Common adverse events include burning and stinging or worsening of AD.

Topical Calcineurin Inhibitors
- Topical calcineurin inhibitors (TCIs)[45,62] are second-line therapy for both acute and chronic AD. Two agents are available—tacrolimus topical (Protopic) ointment 0.03% and 0.1% strengths and pimecrolimus topical (Elidel) 1% cream—and have been shown to be as effective as mid-strength TCS. They can be combined with TCS in the treatment of children whose AD has not responded to TCS. They are considered steroid-sparing agents. Tacrolimus 0.03% and pimecrolimus 1% are approved for use in children ≥2 years, whereas tacrolimus 0.1% is approved in children ≥1years.
- TCIs have black box warnings because of the higher rate of lymphoma in rats given high dosages of these drugs. Most common side effects are itching, stinging, or burning, which starts 5 minutes after the application and can last for an hour but usually decreases after 1 week. Symptoms usually occur during the first several days of administration and in severe cases of AD. TCIs are safe, steroid-sparing agents and work well on thinner skin of the face, neck, groin, and axillae. Sun protection is needed with their use.
- Parents need to be informed of the black box warning and the pros and cons of their use should be discussed. There is an increased theoretical risk of cutaneous viral infections with the use of TCIs.

Other Therapies
- Prescription emollient devices

- Skin barrier repair and treatment: Drugs (i.e., EpiCeram and Eletone) that improve the skin's hydration barrier are available by prescription and are used twice a day. The preparations have unique ratios of lipids that resemble endogenous compositions. They are expensive and not covered by all insurance plans.
- Topical antimicrobials and antiseptics
  - The immune dysregulation in AD results in a tendency for *S. aureus* to colonize the skin in AD, as well as viral infection, including herpes simplex. Reduction of colonization with staphylococcus, as well as treatment of infection, may be equally as important. The use of bleach baths in conjunction with intranasal topical mupirocin for 3 months may be helpful. Dilute bleach baths (⅛ to ¼ cup of chlorine bleach in a full tub of bath water) twice a week, may also be helpful in children with recurrent infection.[59]
  - Topical antibiotic preparations are contraindicated, although the use of mupirocin does reduce colony counts of *S. aureus.*
  - Topical antibacterial scrubs are contraindicated because they dry out the skin and cause irritation.
- Oral antibiotics
  - Short courses of systemic antibiotic agents are essential if secondary skin infection with *S. aureus* or *S. pyogenes* is suspected. First-generation cephalosporins are most commonly used.
  - Be cognizant that the incidence of community-based methicillin-resistant *S. aureus* has rapidly increased.
- Antihistamines and sleep aids
  - Antihistamine agents have little direct effect on pruritus, but sedating doses at night help relieve pruritus, which is worse at night. They have limited effectiveness as monotherapy in AD. The following agents are often used:
  - Hydroxyzine has excellent antihistaminic qualities but can cause drowsiness and behavioral changes. If an antihistamine is needed throughout the day, the usual oral dose of hydroxyzine in children (≤40 kg) is a maximum 2 mg/kg/day divided every 6 to 8 hours with some experts recommending lower daily doses.[45]
  - Diphenhydramine hydrochloride is also a useful antihistamine, especially if sedation is also needed. The usual oral dose of diphenhydramine hydrochloride in children is 5 mg/kg/day divided into 3 to 4 doses with a maximum of 300 mg daily or a fixed dose of 12.5 to 25 mg/dose 3 to 4 times daily.[45]
  - Doxepin is a tricyclic antidepressant with strong antihistamine activity used by dermatologists to treat itching. It is not approved for use in children under 12 years, and the risk of suicidal ideation should be assessed if a child receives this drug.
  - Nonsedating or low-sedating antihistamines may be considered (see Table 36.11).
  - Topical antihistamines are not recommended.
- In patients with AD, nocturnal melatonin levels are lower and may be responsible for sleep disturbances.[63] Melatonin may be considered an alternative to antihistamines.
- Systemic immunomodulating agents
  - Immunomodulating agents (such as cyclosporine, azathioprine, mycophenolate mofetil [MMF], and systemic corticosteroids) can provide help to patients with severe, refractory AD; due to side effect profiles, they should only be used by a specialist after all other options failed.

- Dupilumab, which targets IL-4 and IL-13, is a targeted biologic, and is now approved for the treatment of AD approved for infants 6 months and older with moderate to severe AD
- Nonpharmacologic therapy
- Skin lubrication
  - Emolliate with a moisturizer. Lubricants maintain the skin's hydration, and emollients are the treatment of choice for dry skin.
  - An ointment-based emollient (e.g., Vaseline, petrolatum jelly, vegetable oil, whipped petrolatum, Aquaphor) can be applied just before or just after getting out of bath water while still damp. If the child does not like the greasy feel of an ointment, other topical creams (e.g., Vanicream, CeraVe, Cetaphil) can be used. This is also a good time to apply TCPs, because absorption of the agent is more effective if the skin is hydrated.
  - Emollients can be applied 3 or 4 times a day as needed, such as fragrance-free Eucerin cream, Aveeno, Moisturel, Neutrogena, Dermasil, Curel, or petroleum jelly (an occlusive agent). If a child is sensitive to fragrances, scented creams, such as Nivea and Vaseline Intensive Care, should be avoided. TriCeram is a moisturizer that repairs the stratum corneum barrier function. Like CeraVe, it is a ceramide-dominant, lipid-based emollient. Avoiding products with lanolin and clothing made of wool can be helpful. Urea-containing products, such as Aquacare cream or lotion and Ureacin Crème, soften and moisturize dry skin. Stinging is a side effect when using urea-containing products on fissured or flaring skin.
  - Bathing in lukewarm but not hot water for hydration followed by applying the moisturizer is recommended by the National Institute of Allergy and Infectious Disease. See Resources for AD action plan. If a child experiences stinging when bathing during acute exacerbations, adding 1 cup of table salt into the bath may reduce the stinging sensation.
- Avoidance of triggering factors
  - Avoid common irritating substances, including toiletries, wool, and harsh chemicals.
  - Keep fingernails short to decrease additional skin trauma from scratching.
  - Consider stopping the use of fabric softeners and using a sensitive skin detergent (e.g., All Free and Clear).
  - Evaluate for possible food triggers; if history is positive, testing is not needed. PCPs should *not* do an extensive battery of allergy tests or make recommendations for food elimination based on those tests without a history of food sensitivity.
- Phototherapy: Ultraviolet (UV) narrow-band UVB light treatment may benefit and should only be done by dermatologists; it is rarely used because of the risk of skin cancer.
- Wet wrap therapy (WWT): WWT can be used in significant flares with recalcitrant disease. The usual topical agents are applied followed by a wet layer of tubular gauze or cotton pajama that is applied with a dry outside layer. The child sleeps overnight with the WWT.

Environmental Management
- Decreased environmental humidity and an increase in antigen presentation are key causative factors. Therefore increase environmental humidity and decrease exposure to antigens. Cool temperatures (e.g., through the use of air conditioning) help.

- Eliminate or avoid known or suspected offending agents. These include:
  - Nonbreathable fabrics: nylon or wool; wool is irritating, whereas soft cotton clothing is not. Clothes should be loose fitting.
  - Overheating and overdressing (heat and perspiration are irritant triggers that increase pruritus).
  - Chlorine, turpentine, harsh soaps, fabric softeners, products with fragrances, and bleach.
  - Allergenic agents, such as feather pillows, fuzzy toys, stuffed animals, and pets.
  - House-dust mites: careful attention to the child's bedroom is important (e.g., encasing mattresses and pillows, washing bedding in hot water weekly, frequent vacuuming, removing carpets, or at least frequent cleaning are recommended).

Dietary Management
- In infants, whey-protein partially hydrolyzed infant formula is not hypoallergenic and should not be given to infants who have milk allergy. Dietary restriction should only be done on the basis of a history of food allergy. Food allergens in older children and adults are not common triggers.
- Though pre- and probiotics once held promise, most recent studies have found pre-/probiotics make little to no difference in AD symptoms or patient's quality of life.[64]

Most children with AD can be successfully treated by PCPs. Children who are unresponsive to traditional therapy or have an unusual manifestation should be referred to a pediatric dermatologist.

Complications and Prognosis

Secondary skin infections are a frequent complication of AD caused by *S. aureus,* viruses (eczema herpeticum or disseminated herpes simplex), and fungi (culture or KOH to diagnose). Lichenification, a secondary skin change marked by thickening of the skin, is associated with chronic itching. Keratoconus is occasionally seen and is associated with chronic rubbing of the eyelids. With appropriate treatment, AD can generally be controlled. In two-thirds of children, symptoms of AD become less severe, with complete remission in 20%; however, there is an adolescent and adult stage of AD. Self-image problems may result if AD is severe.

Patient and Parent Education and Prevention

Emphasize that AD is often a recurrent disease that can be controlled. The goal of therapy is to prevent the itch-scratch-itch cycle and hydrate the skin. Specific written instructions and handouts should be provided to the family given the complexity of home management. An action plan for eczema is available (see resources) and can aid in teaching family and child about managing the child's AD. The following should be included:
- The use of medications (when, how much, and how often to use; side effects; and proper application of topical preparations)
- Care of the skin
- Role of environmental controls of allergens or triggers
- What to do if symptoms worsen or signs of secondary skin infection appear and when to seek additional medical treatment
- The need to avoid precipitating factors such as extreme temperatures or humidity, excess sweat, and/or emotional stress; new clothes—wash with mild detergent (with no dyes or perfumes) before wearing them to remove formaldehyde and other chemicals, harsh washing detergents—add second rinse cycle when

washing clothes, wearing coarse clothes; excess soap and water, and cutaneous or systemic infection

Rheumatologic Disorders

Juvenile Idiopathic Arthritis

JIA, formerly known as *juvenile rheumatoid arthritis*, is the term now used to reflect the unknown cause of this condition. The estimated prevalence is 20/100,000 children[65] although the incidence rate varies greatly based on the classification system used. The diagnosis of JIA requires persistent arthritis for more than 6 weeks with onset before 16 years of age. Classification of JIA subtypes is based on presentation of symptoms in the first 6 months of disease. There were two classification methods proposed in the 1970s in the United States and Europe that did not overlap. In the 1990s a newer system was introduced by the International

League of Associations for Rheumatology, which subdivides JIA into seven categories based on symptoms (Box 36.3).

A unified classification nomenclature was helpful from a research perspective; however, it fails to differentiate among chronic arthritides seen in children and adults from those that are unique to childhood. Clear identification of pediatric diseases is an important part of furthering research on therapeutic modalities and highlight that medications approved for adults are not necessarily effective in children, underscoring the need for clinical trials for pediatric treatments.[65] However, minimizing stark differentiation between pediatric and adult arthritis does allow an easier transition from pediatric to adult care and promotes research on care without limitations based on artificially imposed age barriers.[65]

The underlying cause of most forms of JIA is unclear. Proposed triggers include viral infection, vaccinations, vitamin D deficiency, stress, trauma, and environmental factors interfacing with genetic predisposition. Ultimately, how exactly regulatory cells that control

---

• BOX 36.3 Juvenile Idiopathic Arthritis Subtypes and Clinical Joint Characteristics

Oligoarticular (Most Common Type)
- Four or fewer joints with persistent disease never having more than four joints involved
- May present with morning limp
- Up to 70% of children have an ANA, a risk factor for uveitis
- Two subtypes:
  - Persistent oligoarticular lasting >6 months; affecting no more than four joints
  - Extended oligoarticular with ≥four joints after first 6 months

Polyarticular (Up to 30%–35%)
- Arthritis in five or more joints during first 6 months of disease with acute or insidious onset
- May develop rheumatoid vasculitis; resembles adults
- Acute form of uveitis occurs
- Features include slowing of growth, fatigue, a low-grade fever
- Large or small joints involved; typically small joints of hands, feet, ankles, wrists, knees, and cervical spine
- RF negative ANA positive, polyarticular JIA may be mistaken for extended oligoarticular disease
- RF negative or positive; more common in females, with approximately 70% of RF positive cases being females (10–12 years at onset)
- Polyarticular (RF positive)
  - RF positive tests 2–3 months apart
  - Children likely between ages of 8 and 10 years
  - Rapidly progressive arthritis with subcutaneous rheumatoid nodules
  - Adolescent late-onset differs from those with early onset as positive RF and course is similar to adults

Systemic (sJIA)
- Arthritis in more than one joint for 6 weeks and younger than 16 years
- Fever of at least 2 weeks' duration and at least 3 days of daily fever with afternoon spikes up to 104–106°F (40–41.1°C)—a quotidian fever pattern
- May have any of the following:
  - Fleeting salmon-color rash with fever; macules or papules increased in heat areas (axilla and groin)
  - Hepatosplenomegaly, generalized lymphadenopathy, polyserositis manifesting as pericarditis or pleuritis

- High inflammatory markers, marked increase in serum ferritin
- RF and ANA rarely positive
- Usually significant anemia, thrombocytosis, increased acute-phase reactants, elevated transaminase levels
- Potentially fatal complication—MAS with high levels of ferritin above 5000
- Either polyarticular or oligoarticular disease
- A child with chest pain, shortness of breath, change in vocal quality suggesting cricoarytenoid arthritis, signs of MAS, or being treated with an immunosuppressive agent with signs of infection or on NSAIDs with melena and acute anemia will need admission.

Spondyloarthropathy
Enthesitis-related arthritis
- Arthritis and enthesitis or arthritis and enthesitis plus two of the following:
  - Sacroiliac joint involvement with either tenderness or inflammatory lumbosacral pain
  - + HLA-B27
  - Male >6 years with arthritis
  - Acute anterior uveitis
  - First-degree relative with IBS with sacroiliitis, ankylosing spondylitis, reactive arthritis, or acute anterior uveitis
  - Typically, arthritis of lower limbs, especially hips and intertarsal joints with later sacroiliac joints involvement
  - Swelling, tenderness, warmth at insertion of tendons, ligaments, or joint capsules
  - Risk of ankylosing spondylitis (10–15 years later)
  - Occurs in late childhood and adolescence
  - Acute symptomatic uveitis in about 7% of cases

Psoriatic Arthritis
- Asymmetric or symmetric small or large joint arthritis with psoriasis or arthritis with two or more of the following: nail pitting or onycholysis, psoriasis in a first-degree relative, or dactylitis

Undifferentiated
- Arthritis that fails to fulfill one category or fulfills two or more categories

ANA, *Antinuclear antibody;* HLA, *human leukocytic antigen;* IBS, *inflammatory bowel syndrome;* JIA, *juvenile idiopathic arthritis;* MAS, *macrophage activation syndrome;* NSAIDs, *nonsteroidal antiinflammatory drugs;* RF, *rheumatoid factor.*

Modified from Cimaz R. Systemic-onset idiopathic arthritis. *Autoimmun Rev.* 2016;14:931–934; Shenoi S. Juvenile idiopathic arthritis—changing times, changing terms, changing treatments. *Pediatr Rev.* 2017;38(5):221–231; and Siegel DM, Gewanter HL, Sahai S. Rheumatologic diseases. In: McInerny TM, Adam HM, Campbell DE, DeWitt TG, Foy JM, Kamat DM, ed. *American Academy of Pediatrics Textbook of Pediatric Care.* 2nd ed. American Academy of Pediatrics; 2017.

the impact of environmental factors on genetic susceptibility is not well understood.[66] While T cells have long been considered the primary cell involved in triggering an inflammatory response in JIA, there is evidence that T-cell receptor independent CD 31 and IL-17A molecules are expressed in high numbers in synovial fluid of inflamed joints. Fibrocyte-like cells (FLC) express IL-17 receptor A and CD38 is a known ligand for CD31. Stimulation of FLC with IL-17A is also associated with CD38 upregulation and production of cytokines and tissue-destructive molecules.[67]

Systemic juvenile idiopathic arthritis (sJIA) is unique in its absence of autoantibodies and autoreactive T cells. Inflammation is thought to be the result of an autoinflammatory response from the innate immune system, especially macrophage inhibitory factor MIF, tumor necrosis factor alpha and cytokines IL-1, IL-1 receptor, IL-6, and IL-18. The term autoinflammatory disease explains the difference in its pathophysiology versus other forms of JIA. The activation of aberrant phagocytes leads to the production of inflammatory cytokines as well as other inflammatory proteins (S100 A12, S100 A9, and S100 A8). The use of classifying biomarker MRP8/14, S100a12, and IL-18 enables confirmation of disease activity when the child is symptomatic; subclinical disease activity can be evaluated with the same markers.[68] The difference in the pathogenic processes may explain the variances in the clinical presentation of the disease.

JIA is considered an autoimmune disease with alterations in both humoral and cell-mediated immunity. Aside from sJIA, which is considered an autoinflammatory disease, the biomarkers used to classify the disease include ANA, acute-phase reactants, RF, anti-CCP, human leukocyte antigen (HLA)-B27, and MRP8/14.[69] The humoral response is responsible for the release of autoantibodies (especially ANAs), an increase in serum immunoglobulins, and the formation of circulating immune complexes and complement activation. The cell-mediated reaction is associated with a T-lymphocyte response that plays a key role in cytokine production, resulting in the release of tumor necrosis factor-α (TNF-α), IL-1, and IL-6. Activation of B lymphocytes by T-helper cells produces autoantibodies that link to self-antigens. B lymphocytes infiltrate the synovium producing nonsuppurative chronic inflammation of the synovium that can lead to articular cartilage and joint structure erosion.[70]

JIA presents unique challenges to the child, family, and the provider. Approximately 1 in 1000 children are affected with oligoarticular JIA, the most common arthritic subtype. Cytokine production, proliferation of macrophage-like synoviocytes, infiltration with neutrophils and T lymphocytes, and autoimmunity are thought to be the major pathologic processes causing chronic joint inflammation. Although JIA does primarily affect joints, there are other systems that can be affected. Enthesitis is an inflammatory reaction at sites where tendons or ligaments insert into the bone and occurs with several types of JIA. Uveitis is also associated with JIA, is more common with a positive ANA, and can be clinically asymptomatic while potentially causing significant inflammation of the uveal components of the eye.[71] Jaw involvement can also be asymptomatic although it is now thought to be present in the majority of children with JIA and can contribute to significantly impaired jaw function, poor oral health, and quality of life.[72]

The rate of oligoarticular and polyarticular JIA (pJIA) is significantly higher in females than in males unlike systemic arthritis, which is equal across sexes. Oligoarticular JIA has onset in early childhood and early adolescence and typically has knee involvement. It often presents with a morning limp and

a positive ANA in 70% of cases. Polyarticular JIA can be RF positive or negative and peaks at ages 1 to 3 years and during adolescence. The systemic form of JIA occurs at any age and is more complex due to quotidian high fevers, fatigue, erythematous rash, and joint pain. Lymphadenopathy, pericarditis, and hepatosplenomegaly impact less than 40% of patients. It can present with macrophage activation syndrome (MAS) and is often accompanied by weight loss, elevated WBC counts above 30,000 cells/mm³, and platelet counts sometimes elevated to more than 1,000,000/mm³. Ferritin levels of greater than 5000 are common and serum concentrations of MRP8/MRP14 may be useful in differentiating sJIA from infection and other causes of systemic inflammation.[68]

Clinical Findings

History. The major complaints in all forms of JIA involve arthritis characterized by:
- Pain: generally a mild to moderate aching
- Joint stiffness: worse in the morning and after rest; arthralgia may occur during the day
- Joint effusion and warmth
- Younger children may be irritable, refuse to walk or have behavioral regression
- Nonspecific symptoms include decreased appetite, myalgia, nighttime joint pain, inactivity, and failure to thrive.

Systemic symptoms are found more commonly in systemic and polyarticular subtypes and include anemia, anorexia, fever, fatigue, lymphadenopathy, salmon-colored rash (sJIA), and weight loss. Growth abnormalities can result in localized growth disturbances, including premature fusion of the epiphyses, bony overgrowth, and limb-length discrepancies because of increased growth of the affected limb.

Physical Examination. The musculoskeletal examination is key. Examine all joints including the temporomandibular joint and entheses, which are areas where tendons or ligament insert into bones (e.g., Achilles tendon and knees, greater trochanter, metatarsal head, and plantar fascia insertion on the feet). Observe for gait abnormalities using the pediatric Gait, Arms, Legs and Spine Screen (see Resources). Abnormal positioning on the examination table or difficulty getting on and off the table may be noted. Vision screening can be done in office but referral to ophthalmology for uveitis screening is critical (see Chapter 30).

Key musculoskeletal findings include:
- Swelling of the joint with effusion or thickening of synovial membrane, or both, noted on palpation of the joint line
- Heat over inflamed joint and tenderness along joint line
- Loss of joint range of motion and function; holds affected joints in slight flexion; may walk with limp
  Other findings that may be noted:
- Nail pits or onycholysis
- Ciliary injection (note: presence of ciliary injection or an inability to see the optic disc on fundus examination may point to uveitis, which is usually asymptomatic)
- A fleeting salmon-color rash that is more prominent on the trunk.

The classification of the types of arthritis and their characteristic findings are presented in Box 36.3.

Diagnostic Studies. JIA is a diagnosis of exclusion, based on physical findings, and watchful waiting is important as joint pain must be present for greater than 6 weeks. There is no one diagnostic laboratory test for JIA. Most children with oligoarticular arthritis have negative laboratory markers. Those with polyarticular and systemic-onset typically have elevated acute-phase reactants and anemia of chronic disease. A positive result for RF by latex fixation may be present, which occurs in approximately 5% of children with JIA and rarely with sJIA.[73] ANA may be present in up to 50% of children with oligoarticular disease; its presence helps identify children at higher risk for uveitis.

Initial laboratory testing includes a CBC (to exclude leukemia), ESR, and CRP (acute-phase reactants), Lyme testing (enzyme-linked immunosorbent assay [ELISA] followed by Western blot), comprehensive metabolic profile, and liver function tests (creatine phosphokinase, aldolase, and lactate dehydrogenase). Urinalysis and antistreptolysin O (ASO) and anti-DNase B, and complements may be added depending on presenting complaints (see Table 36.1 for a description of these tests). Results may reveal lymphopenia, anemia, elevated transaminases, and hypoalbuminemia; however, laboratory studies may be normal in some children with suspicious findings requiring second-line testing.

Although anti-CCP antibody testing has a high specificity and is more likely to identify children who have more severe JIA with irreversible joint damage, its sensitivity is low (i.e., a negative result does not exclude disease). Therefore it is not a routine first-line test as only children with RF-positive JIA will have anti-CCP antibodies. Imaging studies including radiography, ultrasound, and magnetic resonance imaging (MRI) can help in managing joint pathology. Analysis of synovial fluid is not helpful in diagnosing JIA although recent research has suggested that the neutrophils present in the synovium show an activated profile and may therefore be a helpful tool in the future.[74]

Differential Diagnosis

Various causes of monoarticular arthritis are included in the differential diagnosis. Lyme disease must be excluded as it can present in a similar fashion, and postinfectious conditions, such as poststreptococcal arthritis, rheumatic fever, and reactive arthritis from a variety of bacteria, must be considered. Other autoimmune diseases such as SLE, juvenile dermatomyositis, scleroderma, KD, celiac disease, inflammatory bowel disease, chronic recurrent multifocal osteomyelitis, and IGAV should be considered. Hematologic diseases, such as hemophilia, sickle cell diseases, thalassemia, thyroid disease, serum sickness, and hypertrophic osteoarthropathy can also present with joint pain. Oncologic differentials include tumors (e.g., neuroblastoma) and leukemia. Pigmented villonodular synovitis is a rare uncontrolled cell growth around a joint with destruction of the joint; it does not spread and tends to affect the hip or knee.

Management

Refer children with suspected JIA to pediatric rheumatology. Ophthalmology referral and evaluation is needed for patients with JIA. Those with a positive ANA and oligoarticular JIA, especially females, are at high risk for uveitis, require slit-lamp examination every 3 months for 4 years at which point screening may be spaced out if uveitis never develops. Even if arthritis resolves, regular follow-up with ophthalmology is strongly recommended. ANA-positive JIA patients have a greater risk of uveitis that may not be clinically apparent but can lead to blindness if not detected and treated. Uveitis often does not correspond to the severity of the arthritis (i.e., uveitis may be present despite quiescent arthritis) and needs immediate ophthalmologic management.[75] Specialists in pediatric orthopedics, pain management, and cardiology are consulted as needed. Therapy depends on the degree of local or systemic involvement.

Early and more aggressive pharmacotherapy is now recommended for patients with JIA rather than the previously gradual step-up treatment. Treatment goals are to suppress inflammation, preserve and maximize function, prevent joint deformities, achieve remission, and prevent blindness in those patients with uveitis.[76] Aggressive early treatment to induce a remission is a key consideration in JIA management to prevent deformity and improve outcomes and is the goal of the practice guidelines for both pJIA and sJIA.[77] Aspirin therapy has largely been replaced with the use of NSAIDs. Pharmacologic agents commonly used in the management of JIA include the following[78]:

- NSAIDs: Children with oligoarthritis generally respond well to NSAIDs
  - Ibuprofen: 30 to 40 mg/kg/day three to four divided doses (maximum single dose is 800 mg; maximum daily dose 2400 mg/day)
  - Tolmetin: 15 to 30 mg/kg/day divided in three to four doses (maximum dose is 1800 mg/day)
  - Naproxen: 10 to 15 mg/kg/day in two divided doses (maximum dose is 1000 mg/day)
  - Indomethacin: Older than 2 years old, 1 to 2 mg/kg/day divided in two to four doses (maximum dose is 4 mg/kg/day); adults, 25 to 50 mg/dose 2 or 3 times/day (maximum dose is 200 mg/day)
  - Celecoxib: Older than 2 years and adolescents (≥10 kg to ≤25 kg), 50 mg twice daily; >25 kg, 100 mg twice daily
- Disease-modifying antirheumatic drugs (DMARDs) are managed by pediatric rheumatology.
  - Nonbiologic DMARD treatment: methotrexate, sulfasalazine, leflunomide
  - Biologic DMARD treatment. Initiation of biological agents in JIA is usually done after one nonbiological drug indicated for JIA failed to control the disease after 3 to 6 months. The latest guidelines for JIA management also suggest that biological therapy can be considered first line for patients at higher risk for damage or severe disease (CCP positive or already with erosions). Identification of patients who would most benefit from early initiation of biological therapy is an area of ongoing research.[79] The risk of overwhelming infection is the most common serious adverse event. These agents are administered either subcutaneously or by IV infusion. Agents with FDA approval for use in pediatric patients include tumor necrosis factor inhibitors (TNFi), etanercept (Enbrel) and adalimumab (Humira), to treat pJIA; IL-1 inhibitors, anti-IL-1 anakinra (Kineret), and canakinumab (Ilaris), to treat sJIA; costimulation inhibitor, abatacept (Orencia), for pJIA; and IL-6 inhibitor, tocilizumab (Actemra), approved for sJIA and pJIA.[80]
- Oral glucocorticoids
  - Glucocorticoids are added if there is not a prompt response (typically 1 week) to a biological agent and continued polyarthritis, fever, and rash
  - Steroids are added if MAS or severe serositis
  - Gradual withdrawal of glucocorticoid once symptoms controlled.
- Parenteral agents and intraarticular corticosteroids:
  - Systemic arthritis: anti–IL-1 (anakinra or canakinumab) and anti-IL-6 (tocilizumab).[81]
  - All other types of arthritis: Intraarticular corticosteroid injections are used if there is severe joint involvement. Intraarticular corticosteroid injection with triamcinolone hexacetonide, which is longer acting, can be done either

under anesthesia for younger children or local anesthesia for cooperative older children. Using ultrasound to guide needle placement into the joint is common practice. The need for more than three intraarticular injections per year or extension of the disease requires systemic therapies with DMARDs.[82]

Other treatment modalities include physical therapy—range of motion muscle-strengthening exercises and heat treatments— used for joint involvement and occupational therapy. Rest and splinting are used if indicated.

Complications and Prognosis

Systemic involvement can include iridocyclitis, iritis, uveitis, pleuritis, pericarditis, anemia, fatigue, and hepatitis. Growth failure, leg-length discrepancy, if the arthritis is unilateral, and residual joint damage caused by granulation of tissue in the joint space can occur. Children most likely to *develop* permanent crippling disability include those with hip involvement, unremitting synovitis, or positive RF test.

The course of JIA is variable with no curative treatment. Early aggressive treatment and referral to a specialist are important. After an initial episode, the child may never have another episode, or the disease may go into remission and recur months or years later. The disease process of JIA wanes with age and completely subsides in 85% of children; however, systemic onset, a positive RF, poor response to therapy, and the radiologic evidence of erosion are associated with a poor prognosis. Onset of disease in the teenage years is related to progression to adult rheumatoid disease.

Patient and Parent Education and Prevention

The following education and preventive measures are taken:
- Recommend yearly influenza vaccine as indicated
- 13-valent and 23-valent pneumococcal vaccines in patients with immunocompromising conditions or treatments, and those with functional asplenia as is seen in SLE.[83]
- Offer chronic disease counseling and encourage normal play and recreation.
- Educate about side effects of medications, in addition to splinting, orthotics, and bracing requirements if needed.
- Instruct about need to follow up with an ophthalmologist. Frequency of screening for uveitis is based on subtype of JIA, protocol guidelines, and ophthalmology.
- Confirm family has a plan for giving medications. Instruct about phone reminders using phone applications.
- For children on aspirin therapy (not typically given), educate parents about the risk of Reye syndrome and its signs and symptoms.
- Ensure parent and child understand that physical therapy and occupational therapy are mainstays of treatment for chronic childhood arthritis and should be part of the child's daily routine, including passive, active, and resistive exercises.
- Water therapy and using heat or cold reduce pain and stiffness. Swimming is an excellent activity, except for children with severe anemia and severe cardiac disease; tricycle or bike riding and low-impact dance are other beneficial activities.
- Trampoline use is discouraged because of risk for injury and high impact on joints.
- Refer to the American Arthritis Foundation as a source of information.
- Instruct on the need to involve school personnel in the identification of required school-related services through an individualized education plan (IEP) or a 504.

- Discuss challenges of pain management and its assessment in children with chronic arthritis and encourage parents to advocate for effective pain control for their child.

Systemic Lupus Erythematosus

SLE is a chronic, multisystem autoimmune disease characterized by autoantibodies that cause aberrant immune function with presentation of self-antigens as well as defects in clearance of apoptotic debris. It is a multisystem illness where any organ can be targeted[84] and is associated with inflammatory damage to target organs brought on by autoantibodies attacking self-antigens and immune dysregulation. There is a strong genetic component with more than 80 loci associated with susceptibility of SLE. It is more prevalent in females between puberty and menopause with a 6:1 female to male predilection. The concordance rate is 10-fold higher in monozygotic twins. There is a reported 43.9% heritability with shared environmental factors versus 25.8% to 30.3% with nonshared factors playing a significant role.[85] Environmental factors thought to play a role in its pathogenesis are oral contraceptive use, pregnancy, microbials (viral agents mostly), temperate climates, exposure to UV light, hormonal changes in puberty, and certain drugs (e.g., hydralazine and procainamide). The strongest environmental evidence is for cigarettes and oral contraceptive pills along with exposure to crystalline silica. Emerging research shows that solvent exposure, household and agricultural pesticides, air pollution, and heavy metal may also play a role.[86]

Excess INF production and plasmacytoid dendritic cell activation increase the inflammatory response in multiple organ systems, involving the blood cells, kidneys, nervous system, and skin. Abnormalities of immune function include metabolic derangements, immune cells biochemical defects, and an impaired sensing and repair of DNA damage.[85] B cells are responsible for increased activation of plasma cells with subsequent increases in autoantibody production and T-cell costimulation. This causes immune complexes to form together with recruitment of other immune cells with subsequent tissue injury.

Childhood onset is rare with an incidence of 6 to 30 children per 100,000 children per year. In general, it is more acute and severe in children than in adults. There is a higher incidence in Asians, African Americans, Hispanics, and Native Americans. Males with Klinefelter syndrome and family members with first-degree relatives with SLE have a higher incidence of SLE.[85]

Clinical Findings

The butterfly or malar erythematous facial rash that increases in intensity in sunlight makes the diagnosis more obvious; however, findings vary, making the diagnosis difficult in some patients. Clinical findings depend on organ involvement. Presentation may be abrupt or have a gradual, nonspecific onset. Fever, rash, fatigue, and joint pain are the most typical presentation in children.[84] Box 36.4 outlines the clinical criteria from the Systemic Lupus International Collaborating Clinics.

History. The history may include the following:
- Joint involvement (most common initial finding)
  - Nonerosive arthritis with tenderness, effusion, and swelling
- Arthralgia
- Constitutional and systemic manifestations:
  - Low-grade fever (intermittent or sustained), weight loss, and lymphadenopathy
  - Painless, oral ulcers typically in the mouth or nose
  - Malar or discoid rash; Raynaud phenomenon; alopecia

Must have four criteria with at least one clinical criterion and one laboratory criterion:

1. Acute cutaneous lupus
2. Chronic cutaneous lupus
3. Oral ulcers *or* nasal ulcers (not attributed to another disease)
4. Nonscarring alopecia
5. Synovitis with swelling or effusion or tenderness involving two or more joints
6. Serositis including pleurisy, pericardial effusion, or pain (not attributed to another disease)
7. Renal: red blood cell cast or urine protein to creatinine ratio of 500 mg protein per 24 hours
8. Neurologic—including seizures, psychosis, myelitis, acute confusional state
9. Hemolytic anemia
10. Leukopenia (<4000/mm^3) *or* lymphopenia (<1000/mm^3)
11. Thrombocytopenia (<100,000/mm^3)

Immunologic Criteria

1. ANA level above laboratory reference range
2. Anti-dsDNA antibody level above laboratory reference range
3. Positive anti-Sm: presence of antibody to Sm nuclear antigen
4. Antiphospholipid antibody positivity, as determined by:
   - Positive test for lupus anticoagulant
   - False-positive test result for rapid plasma reagin
   - Medium- or high-titer anticardiolipin antibody level (IgA, IgG, or IgM)
   - Positive test result for anti-2-glycoprotein I (IgA, IgG, or IgM)
5. Low complement (C3, C4, or CH50)
6. Direct Coombs test (in the absence of hemolytic anemia)

ANA, Antinuclear antibody, *Ig,* immunoglobulin.
Modified from Petri M, Orbai AM, Alarcon GS, et al. Derivation and validation of the Systemic Lupus International Collaborating Clinics classification criteria for systemic lupus erythematosus. *Arthritis Rheum.* 2012;64(8):2677–2686.

- Symptoms of organ involvement, typically disorders of the renal, cardiopulmonary, immunologic, neurologic, and hematologic system

Physical Examination. The following may be seen on physical examination[84]:

- Skin manifestations
  - Pallor, livedo reticularis, petechiae, palpable purpura, and digital ulcers
  - Malar or "butterfly" rash—scaly erythematous maculopapular rash covering malar areas extending over the bridge of the nose and cheeks; may spread down the face to the chest and extremities; "butterfly" rash and other lesions can be photosensitive; seen in approximately 95% of those with SLE
  - Mucous membrane manifestations (ulceration) of the mouth and nasal septum
  - Gingivitis, mucosal hemorrhage, erosions, ulcerations
  - Silvery whitening of the vermilion border or thickening, redness, ulceration, or crusting of lips
- Joint tenderness
- Cardiac friction rub caused by pericarditis; pleural friction rubs caused by pleuritis
- Hepatosplenomegaly and lymphadenopathy

Diagnostic Studies. Initial laboratory testing includes CBC, ANA, ESR, CRP, serum chemical analysis (metabolic and protein screen), and urinalysis. The ANA test is positive in more than 97% to 99% of children who have active, untreated SLE and titers above 1:1280 suggest diagnosis; however, ANA specificity is as low as 36% and ANA titer does not correlate with disease activity. A negative ANA makes SLE diagnosis less likely; however, there is always a risk of a rare false-negative test. Recent studies have shown up to 30% of lupus patients screened for clinical trials are ANA negative at time of screening suggesting that the diagnostic value of this particular test may not be as prognostic as previously thought.[87] A positive ANA with clinical findings consistent with SLE should be followed up with testing for double-stranded DNA and the extractable nuclear antigen panel (anti-Smith antibody and anti-RNP antibody) as these are specific for SLE and present in up to 50% of patients with SLE. Anti-Ro (anti-SSA) and anti-La (anti-SSb) antibodies are also associated with SLE.[84]

Leukopenia or lymphopenia, hemolytic anemia, and thrombocytopenia are frequent laboratory findings. Other laboratory and radiographic studies depend on organ involvement and can include a chest radiograph, electrocardiogram (ECG), urine and serologic testing, renal ultrasound, and histopathologic studies. Proteinuria and hematuria are hallmarks of lupus nephritis. Newer biomarkers are in development as a result of advances in genomics, epigenetics, and transcriptomics that will eventually provide greater ability to diagnose SLE and determine a prognosis.

Differential Diagnosis

Differential diagnoses include infection, malignancy, or autoimmune/inflammatory disease. Infectious diseases that resemble SLE include bacterial infections such as brucellosis, leptospirosis, and sepsis; viral infections such as cytomegalovirus, Epstein-Barr virus (EBV), parvovirus, and human immunodeficiency virus (HIV); and other infectious disease such as Q fever (*Coxiella*), tuberculosis, Lyme disease, or toxoplasmosis. Leukemia, lymphoma, neuroblastoma, and Langerhans cell histiocytosis are malignant differentials. Other autoimmune diseases that mimic SLE include acute rheumatic fever (ARF), JIA, Sjögren syndrome, systemic vasculitis, sarcoidosis, hemolytic-uremic syndrome, and autoimmune lymphoproliferative syndrome, and common variable immunodeficiency can also resemble SLE.[84] A temporary, drug-induced lupus can be caused by several pharmacologic agents, including hydantoin compounds, hydralazine, isoniazid, minocycline, procainamide, and sulfonamides. More recent developed drugs associated with drug-induced lupus erythematosus include a number of proton-pump inhibitors and anti-TNFs although these are more associated with autoantibody formation and less than 1% of those who form autoantibodies go on to develop drug-induced lupus.[88]

Management

Children with SLE need an interprofessional approach that includes specialists in rheumatology, nephrology, adolescent medicine, pharmacology, psychiatry, nursing, physical therapy, occupational therapy, and pain management. Other specialist referrals such as cardiology, neurology, ophthalmology, and dermatology are required depending on drug therapy that is prescribed, and organ systems that are involved.

Therapy depends on the degree of local or systemic involvement. Because sunlight is a known trigger of SLE, UVA and B sunscreen is essential both indoors because of daylight fluorescent lighting and outdoors due to sun exposure. Prompt recognition and treatment of disease flares are essential to prevent systemic complications; therefore frequent clinical and laboratory monitoring is important. The following measures also may be helpful:

- NSAIDs are used for relief of musculoskeletal pain, arthritis, arthralgias, serositis, or pain. (If nephritis is present, use with caution and in consultation with the rheumatologist and nephrologist.)

- Antimalarials are used for mild symptoms and maintenance. Regular ophthalmologic follow-up is required for monitoring side effects.
- Oral steroids are prescribed for rapid control; however, the goal is to find a less toxic maintenance therapy. Dosage is adjusted depending on clinical and laboratory findings. Cautious tapering of steroids is often needed.
- Immunosuppressant agents, such as methotrexate and azathioprine (Imuran), may be used as steroid-sparing agents. Methotrexate is used for arthritis, whereas azathioprine is used in treating cytopenias, vasculitic rash, or serositis.[84] MMF or CellCept is used to induce remission in lupus nephritis or for maintenance therapy in other organ diseases. When other agents fail to induce a remission, calcineurin inhibitors such as tacrolimus or cyclophosphamide block T-cell activation via suppression of the calcium/calcimodulin-dependent phosphatase calcineurin. These medications are immunomodulatory but also have the ability to reduce proteinuria via nonimmune mediated mechanisms making them a potentially safer and more attractive therapeutic option.[89]
- Use of other pharmacologic agents or therapies depends on the type and degree of organ system involvement. Rituximab (Rituxan) is a monoclonal antibody that binds and kills active B cells and is used for cytopenias. Belimumab (Benlysta) is a fully human IgG1λ recombinant monoclonal antibody that indirectly targets and decreases B-cell survival and was specifically developed to treat lupus and approved in 2019 for pediatric use in IV form. Anifrolumab, a human monoclonal antibody to type 1 IFN receptor subunit 1 is another monoclonal antibody that is currently only approved in adults.[90]
- Adjunctive treatment includes antihypertensive agents with angiotensin-converting enzyme inhibitors used to reduce proteinuria and anticonvulsive agents prescribed for seizures.
- Estrogen-containing agents for contraception can be used in patients with inactive or stable active SLE, but females with positive antiphospholipid (with or without definite antiphospholipid syndrome) should be discouraged from using estrogen containing contraceptive options. Progestin-only agents should be used instead.[91]
- Parents need education about sun exposure and the use of sunscreen protection as well as the child's need for rest between activities because fatigue is a frequent problem.

There are limited studies demonstrating effectiveness of vitamin D and calcium supplements to prevent or reduce the risk of osteoporosis related to chronic corticosteroid use in children. However, vitamin D deficiency has long been associated with autoimmune disease. Vitamin D inhibits Th17 and Th1 responses, promotes T regulatory cells, and impairs B-cell development and function. Although further research is still needed to elucidate the exact benefit of vitamin D on SLE disease progression, supplementation is recommended for all children with autoimmune disease.[92]

Complications and Prognosis

SLE is a chronic disease with periods of waxing and waning of symptoms; however, complete remission can occur. Children with mild disease do well; those with severe major organ involvement have a poorer prognosis. During disease flares, the child may experience poor sleep and daytime fatigue with decreased cardiovascular conditioning, resulting in increased pain. A diagnosis of SLE in childhood is not always lethal, especially if renal involvement or

cerebritis is not present. Renal failure, central nervous system lupus, myocardial infarction, cardiac failure, and infection are the leading causes of death in children with SLE.[93] There is a higher risk of leukemia in younger children with SLE and a higher risk of lymphoma as well as other cancers in older children.[94] Exposure to UV light may bring out or worsen skin lesions and result in exacerbation of systemic problems. Dermatologic care is often required. Side effects resulting from chronic use of high-dose corticosteroids (e.g., osteoporosis, avascular necrosis) are a complication of treatment.

Juvenile Fibromyalgia Syndrome

Juvenile fibromyalgia is the term used to describe a chronic, idiopathic amplified pain syndrome characterized by widespread, diffuse, nonarticular musculoskeletal pain associated with nonrestorative sleep, unrelenting fatigue, and dysautonomia, anxiety, headaches, and abdominal pain. New information points to an organic problem with the pain processing system, whereas previously JFM was thought to fall under psychosomatic domains. It is estimated that 1% to 2% of pediatric patients have significant JFM. While adolescent onset is typical, and females are more likely to have JFM, it occurs as young as 4 years of age.[95] There is a genetic component with multiple generations affected by the fibromyalgia. JFM can cause significant functional impairment in activities of daily living and interfere with normal adolescent development. Rather than pain at specific trigger points, there is a widespread abnormal sensation.

The pathophysiology of JFM involves abnormal responses to stimuli and changes in the pain mechanism where nociceptive input connects at the level of the dorsal horn. This causes hyperalgesia or increases sensitivity to painful stimuli, allodynia or pain being triggered by touch, or more widespread pain because of receptive field expansion or secondary hyperalgesia. The exact mechanism of pain in this disease is under study.

Pediatric diagnostic criteria were first defined by Yunus and Masi[96] (Box 36.5) but are not validated. Thus, the lack of clearly defined pediatric criteria leads to a delay in diagnosis. The adult 2010 criteria for fibromyalgia evaluate widespread pain criteria and symptom severity (SS) using the Widespread Pain Index and

---

• BOX 36.5 Yunus and Masi Criteria for Juvenile Fibromyalgia

- Pain in at least three areas for more than 3 months without underlying cause and normal laboratory tests
- More than 5 of 18 tender points, which include occiput, low cervical spine, trapezius at the midpoint, supraspinous above the scapula near the medial border, second rib at the costochondral junctions, lateral epicondyle, upper outer quadrants of the gluteal muscle, posterior to greater trochanter prominence, and at the medial fat pad of the knee at the joint line
- Three of 10 minor criteria listed below:
  - Fatigue
  - Poor sleep
  - Irritable bowel syndrome
  - Chronic tension or anxiety
  - Soft tissue swelling
  - Pain affected by weather
  - Paresthesia
  - Pain affected by activity
  - Headache
  - Pain affected by anxiety and/or stress

a SS score.[97] The use of these scales may be helpful in evaluating patients with JFM. Because there are no major organ system abnormalities found, the presentation of JFM can occur as a primary condition or in conjunction with other rheumatologic disorders (secondary fibromyalgia).[95]

Clinical Findings

The finding of 3 months of widespread pain with three of associated symptoms seen in Box 36.5 points to the diagnosis of JFM. The patient may complain of changes in pain with different weather conditions and levels of physical activity. Children with widespread musculoskeletal pain and painful point tenderness may have fibromyalgia and should be referred to a rheumatologist.

History. Pain history is the key finding because early on the associated symptoms of chronic fatigue, depression, or mood disorder may be lacking.[95] Stress may exacerbate the pain; therefore a careful psychosocial history is a critical component to identify triggers. The history may include the following long-standing common symptoms[98]:

- Pain at multiple sites, including muscles and soft tissues around joints
- Pain may awaken from sleep and interfere with routine activities
- Fatigue and malaise, daily tension headache
- Paresthesias, allodynia, hypersensitivity
- Insomnia or prolonged night awakenings
- Depression (a significant number exhibit depressive symptoms) and anxiety
- School absence because of pain is not uncommon; however, the child typically keeps up with schoolwork.

Physical Examination. Typically, there is no evidence of arthritis or muscular weakness. Trigger points around the neck, back, lateral epicondyles, greater trochanter, and knees may provide a gross measure of the patient's discomfort.[95] There is often hypermobility noted, the hypothesis being that hypermobility causes recurrent microtraumas that contribute to pain.[99]

Diagnostic Studies. Laboratory studies are of little benefit in diagnosing JFM but may be helpful in ruling out other diagnoses. Blood count, liver functions, and muscle enzymes are normal. If secondary fibromyalgia is present, order appropriate tests to rule out a different rheumatoid disorder. Children with fibromyalgia can have positive ANA of no clinical significance, as do 20% of children without rheumatoid disorders.

Differential Diagnosis

This syndrome can mimic many other diseases. Primary and secondary fibromyalgia can occur, so the PCP needs to consider that fibromyalgia initially may be mistaken for other rheumatoid disease. It does not, however, have the associated rashes, weight loss, fever, or joint swelling or characteristic laboratory findings associated with other clearly defined diagnoses.[95] Lyme disease is also in the differential, but its course of illness is not characterized by pain.

Management

Children and parents need reassurance that fibromyalgia is not life-threatening, rather it is a chronic condition that can be a lifelong issue. Treatment focuses on relieving symptoms and can include the following:

- Physical therapy for range-of-motion exercises, mild low-impact aerobic exercises (e.g., swimming, bicycling, and walking), and muscle strengthening

- Psychotherapy and relaxation techniques to help cope with this condition
- NSAIDs for pain control; gabapentin can be used to reduce pain sensitivity although providers are encouraged to limit medicalizing patients with amplified pain as this increases their risk for iatrogenic injury and can burden families with unnecessary medical costs.

Prognosis

The outcome of fibromyalgia in children varies, but studies demonstrate the persistence of fibromyalgia into adulthood. Fibromyalgia in children generally has a better prognosis than it does in adults.[95]

Patient and Parent Education

Patients and parents should be educated that fibromyalgia is not a psychosomatic disorder. Guidance should be given about sleep hygiene and the importance of exercise[100] and the possibility that it could be a chronic problem with periods of remissions followed by exacerbations.

Myalgic Encephalomyelitis/Chronic Fatigue Syndrome or Systemic Exertion Intolerance Disease

Myalgic encephalomyelitis/chronic fatigue syndrome (ME/CFS) is a disease with specific characteristics now defined by the Institute of Medicine. Systemic exertion intolerance disease is another term used for this problem. The clinical criteria include a substantial reduction or impairment in the ability to carry out normal activities of daily living persisting for more than 3 months that is accompanied by the new onset of severe, medically unexplained fatigue. This fatigue is not the result of ongoing excessive exertion and does not improve with rest. It is critical to ascertain the frequency and severity not only of the fatigue but also the postexertional malaise and an unrefreshing sleep. In addition to fatigue, unrefreshing sleep, and postexertional malaise, the child must complain of either cognitive impairments or orthostatic intolerance or both. Widespread or migratory myofascial joint, abdominal, or head pain and neuroendocrine (feeling feverish or cold) or immune (flu-like complaints) manifestation may be reported. These symptoms must be different from the way the child was before the onset of the illness. A primary sleep disorder does not make the diagnosis of ME/CFS impossible. The term chronic fatigue does not reflect the seriousness of the condition. There is a recent resurgence in research focusing on diagnosis and management of ME/CFS as an increased number of cases are anticipated as many people continue to be ill for months following the acute phase of COVID-19.[101]

There is convincing evidence for a subset of patients that this is an autoimmune disease with immune dysregulation as well as changes in the cytokine profile and immunoglobulin levels. Decrease in natural killer cell cytotoxicity[102] and changes in the T- and B-cell phenotype[103] were reported. Infections with pathogens such as EBV, human herpesvirus 6 (HHV-6), and parvovirus as well as intracellular bacteria are known triggers. EBV infection is a noninfectious risk factor for various autoimmune diseases. Activation of the nervous system, which causes local inflammation of the nervous system and secondary CNS and peripheral nervous system signaling alteration, is thought to be contributing mechanisms to ME/CFS.[104] Autoantibodies can cause immune activation and dysregulation and cellular metabolic alterations. Enhanced levels of immunoglobulins and alterations in B cells are found in autoimmune diseases such as SLE, JIA, and Sjögren syndrome. As previously described in the SLE pathophysiology, the alteration in autoimmune diseases is multifaceted. Autoantibodies in ME/CFS are directed against neurotransmitters as well as nuclear and membrane structures. There is clinical heterogeneity in the disease onset likely as a result of whether the disease had a noninfectious or infectious trigger.[101] Aggravation of the symptoms with exertion is likely a dysregulation of the autonomic parasympathetic and sympathetic nervous system and includes GI dysfunction, vasomotor instability, and increased pain sensitivity. Depression and mood disorders are often seen as concomitant diagnoses although whether these are a result of having ME/CFS or develop as a result of the same nervous system dysfunction that is thought to trigger ME/CFS development.[106]

Clinical Findings

It is important to evaluate the patient's history carefully as the physical examination findings are limited.

History
- Query about unrefreshing sleep as to how they feel in the morning, the quality of the sleep, need for naps, or problems going to or staying asleep.
- Obtain a history about possible cognitive impairments, ability to multitask, difficulty with complex tasks, or memory issues.
- Question about orthostatic intolerance (e.g., problems with standing, or symptoms when changing positions, need to study on a recliner, or preference for sitting position).
- Questions about pain and systemic manifestations (e.g., feeling feverish or cold, flu-like symptoms).
- Use questionnaires or tools to help clarify symptoms of fatigue pain, orthostatic intolerance, postexertional malaise, or decreases in function (see ME/CFS resources).

Physical Examination. Examination findings may be normal or painful lymph nodes may be present.

Diagnostic Studies. There is ongoing research into potential biomarkers for this disease investigating adenosine triphosphate levels, 5′-adenosine monophosphate-activated protein kinase, skeletal muscle cell acidosis, and a chemical signal for ME/CFS using plasma metabolomics.[102]

Differential Diagnosis

Because ME/CFS is a diagnosis of exclusion, other conditions must be investigated. Care must be taken in diagnosing this disorder in children, because other conditions (e.g., hypothyroidism, sleep apnea, hepatitis B or C, SLE, cancer, alcohol or drug abuse, Lyme disease, and major depressive and other psychiatric disorders) must first be ruled out. The child is best referred to a specialist in CFS for management.

Management

There are no approved treatments for ME/CFS, but pharmacologic and nonpharmacologic methods are under investigation. Most treatment focuses on symptom abatement such as fluid and salt supplementation for orthostatic hypotension and phasing exercise and activities to minimize postexertional malaise.[101] Recent studies with Rituximab in adults showed clinical improvement and further studies are still pending. Initial randomized control trials with intravenous immunoglobulin Ig (IVIG) did not show consistent improvement.[103] It is important to avoid referrals to multiple providers where duplication of laboratory work is done. Although some may not believe this is a real illness, the latest studies point to autoimmune dysfunction and referral to physical activity, which can be helpful in fibromyalgia syndrome, can make patients with ME/CFS significantly worse.[101] The patient's complaints should be taken seriously; referrals to support groups and the CDC website may be helpful. The United States and other governments and major healthcare organizations have withdrawn both cognitive behavioral therapy and graded exercise as recommended therapies for ME/CFS. Instead, it is recommended to focus on symptom management.[101]

Acute Rheumatic Fever

ARF is an exaggerated autoimmune response in a susceptible host to an anaerobic gram-positive coccus, group A streptococcus (GAS). Epitopes, the surface portion of certain subspecies of GAS, are similar to human myosin and to the tissue of the mitral annulus and chordae. These sites act as antigens, which activate the immune response that results in antibody formation and initiation of the antibody/antigen response.[106] Antistreptococcal immunoglobulins, stimulated by repeated streptococcal infections, attack the heart and joints, CNS, and cutaneous tissue. Greater organism virulence is associated with specific M protein types and a more "mucoid" capsule. There appears to be a strong genetic influence for susceptibility to GAS infection, with a family history of rheumatic fever and a lower socioeconomic status as known risk factors.

Group A β-hemolytic streptococci (GABHS) causes several postinfectious, nonsuppurative immune-mediated diseases including ARF, post–streptococcal reactive arthritis (PSRA), pediatric acute-onset neuropsychiatric syndrome, and post-streptococcal glomerulonephritis.[107]

The incidence of ARF has declined in developing countries but is still a significant cause of heart disease worldwide. Echocardiographic techniques allow for a more accurate diagnosis of ARF. Recurrence of ARF following subsequent episodes of GAS pharyngitis (symptomatic or asymptomatic infection) is high. The most commonly affected age group in children is 5 to 15 years.

Clinical Findings and History

The diagnosis of an initial attack of ARF is based on the revised Jones criteria found in Box 36.6. Abdominal pain, malaise, leukocytosis, precordial pain, rapid sleeping pulse rate, and tachycardia out of proportion to the degree of fever is not uncommon. A family history of ARF should also raise the index of suspicion because of an increased frequency in families. The most serious clinical manifestation is carditis that can lead to involvement of the endocardium, which is reflected in valvular dysfunction, or pericarditis due to involvement of the pericardium.[108]

Major Manifestations
- Polyarthritis: Migratory arthritis, involving large joints including the knees, ankle, elbows, and wrist, is the most common manifestation. It responds readily to salicylates and NSAIDs and does not usually last more than 4 weeks, even without treatment. A septic monoarthritis can occur in high-risk populations and can be seen in indigenous Australian populations with ARF in 16% to 18% of patients, but is rarely found in the United States.
- Carditis is common (pancarditis, valves, pericardium, myocardium) and can cause chronic, life-threatening disease (i.e., congestive heart failure [CHF]). ARF is more common in younger children than adolescents. The need to recognize subclinical disease stresses the importance of serial echocardiogram. Symptoms of carditis may be vague and insidious with decreased appetite, fatigue, and pains. When clinically apparent, carditis

• BOX 36.6 Revised Jones Criteria for Rheumatic Fever

Evidence of preceding streptococcal infection by one of the following:
- Increased or rising anti–streptolysin O titer or other streptococcal antibodies (anti-DNASE B) (class I, Level of Evidence B).
  - Rise in titer is better evidence than a single titer result.
- Positive throat culture for group A β-hemolytic streptococci (class I, Level of Evidence B).
- Positive rapid group A streptococcal carbohydrate antigen test in a child whose clinical presentation suggests that the infection is caused by a streptococcal infection

Revised Criteria for Low-Risk Populations (ARF incidence <2 per 100,000 children ages 5–14 years per year or ≤1 per 1000 population/year)
- Major criteria:
  - Carditis (clinical and/or subclinical)
  - Arthritis (polyarthritis)
  - Chorea
  - *Erythema marginatum*
  - Subcutaneous nodules
- Minor criteria:
  - Oligoarthralgia
  - Fever (≥38.5°F)
  - Sedimentation rate ≥60 mm and/or C-reactive protein (CRP) ≥3.0 mg/dL
  - Prolonged PR interval (unless carditis is a major criterion)

Revised Jones Criteria for Moderate- and High-Risk Populations
- Major criteria:
  - Carditis (clinical and/or subclinical)
  - Arthritis (monopolyarthritis or polyarthritis, or polyarthralgia)
  - Chorea
  - *Erythema marginatum*
  - Subcutaneous nodules

- Minor criteria:
  - Fever (≥38.5°F)
  - Sedimentation rate ≥30 mm and/or CRP ≥3.0 mg/dL
  - Prolonged PR interval (unless carditis is a major criterion)
  Doppler findings in rheumatic valvulitis (may be subclinical findings)
- Pathologic mitral regurgitation (all four criteria met)
  - Seen in at least two views
  - Jet length of ≥2 cm in at least one view
  - Peak velocity >3 m/s
  - Pansystolic jet in at least one envelope
- Pathologic aortic regurgitation (all four criteria met)
  - Seen in at least two views
  - Jet length of ≥1 cm in at least one view
  - Peak velocity >3 m/s
  - Pansystolic jet in at least one envelope
  Must have two major criteria, or one major plus two minor criteria for an initial episode of ARF
  High-risk patients who have a history of ARF or rheumatic heart disease (RHD) who get infected with Group A strep
- Two major, one major and two minor, or three minor manifestations may be sufficient for a presumptive diagnosis (class IIb, Level of Evidence C).
- When minor manifestations alone are present, exclusion of other more likely causes of the clinical presentation is recommended before a diagnosis of an ARF recurrence is made (class I, Level of Evidence C). If reinfected with group A streptococci:
- And a reliable past history of ARF or established RHD, and in the face of documented group A streptococcal infection, two major, one major and two minor, or three minor manifestations may be sufficient for a presumptive diagnosis (class IIb, Level of Evidence C).
- When minor manifestations alone are present, the exclusion of other more likely causes of the clinical presentation is recommended before a diagnosis of an ARF recurrence is made (class I, Level of Evidence C).

ARF, Acute rheumatic fever.
From Gewitz MH, Baltimore RS, Tani LY et al. Revision of the Jones Criteria for the diagnosis of acute rheumatic fever in the era of Doppler echocardiography: a scientific statement from the American Heart Association. *Circulation*. 2015;131:1806–1818.

---

presents with tachycardia and a holosystolic murmur heard at the aortic or mitral area with radiation to the infrascapular area. Mitral and aortic valve changes occur in 95% of cases, usually within 2 weeks of RF illness, and can be subclinical. Recurrent episodes of RF lead to worsening valve disease.
- Sydenham chorea is uncommon.
- Erythema marginatum or erythema annulare manifested as nonpruritic, bright pink blanching papules or macules that spread in a serpiginous pattern on the trunk and extremities; it is nonpruritic and an uncommon finding.
- Subcutaneous nodules are painless nodules (0.5–2 cm) that develop on bony prominences or extensor tendons. They usually remain for 1 to 2 weeks and tend to be in groups of three to four nodules. Although this is a major criterion of diagnosis, it is rarely seen in the United States due to low incidence.[109]

Minor Manifestations
- Fever (≥37.5°C or 99.5°F is now the cutoff), arthralgia, history of ARF.

Diagnostic Studies. Diagnostic study findings include an elevated acute-phase reactant (ESR) greater than 30 and a CRP higher than the upper limit of normal, leukocytosis, and a prolonged PR interval on ECG. Additional studies should include an echocardiogram and chest radiograph. Confirmation of streptococcal infection is by culture and serology (ASO titer and anti–deoxyribonuclease B titer) testing. A diagnosis of ARF may be made in two situations without evidence of a preceding streptococcal infection: a child with Sydenham chorea or a child with a chronic, indolent rheumatic carditis.[110] Approximately 80% of children with ARF have an elevated ASO titer. A combination of both DNase-B testing and ASO rising may confirm the recent infection.

Evidence of a prior GAS infection is needed for the diagnosis of a nonsuppurative immune-mediated disease. Confirmation of a GAS infection by throat culture or rapid strep test does not differentiate carrier state from a true infection. Serologic testing for the presence of elevated or increasing antistreptococcal antibody titers (ASO test) or anti-DNase B testing confirms a recent strep infection.[106] The ASO titer and the anti-DNase B levels rise 1 to 2 weeks following an acute GAS infection. The ASO titer peaks in 3 to 6 weeks; anti-DNase B level peaks in 6 to 8 weeks. Both remain elevated for months after GAS infection; increasing titers are the key to the diagnosis.

Differential Diagnosis
Guidelines for echocardiogram findings in patients who present with symptoms and signs of ARF should be closely followed.[111] The differential includes isolated congenital mitral and aortic valve anomalies as well as congenital heart disease (e.g., bicuspid aortic

valve). Infective endocarditis can be mistaken for rheumatic carditis if there are no signs of vegetation and valve damage. Annular dilation from conditions associated with left-sided heart dilation as a result of myocarditis and cardiomyopathy should be considered in the differential diagnosis.[108]

Management

The treatment of ARF includes the following:

- Antibiotic therapy to eradicate GAS infection: Primary prevention requires that a GAS infection be treated within 10 days of onset. Benzathine penicillin G is the drug of choice unless there is an allergic history; erythromycin then becomes the drug of choice. Azithromycin and cephalosporins are also sometimes used.[111] A patient with a history of ARF who has an upper respiratory infection should be treated for GAS whether or not GAS is recovered because an asymptomatic GABHS infection can trigger a recurrence.
- Antiinflammatory therapy: Aspirin usage is falling out of favor due to the risk of toxicity and Reye syndrome. There is increasing use of NSAIDs (naproxen for older patients and ibuprofen for younger patients) to reduce the need for frequent dosing and to provide symptomatic relief for joint symptoms. Some experts recommend the use of corticosteroids in patients with severe carditis, reducing its morbidity and mortality. Yearly influenza immunizations are critical, especially for children on aspirin therapy because of the increased risk of Reye syndrome association with aspirin usage in patients with influenza.
- Chest radiographs, ECG, and echocardiography are indicated; carditis usually develops within the first 3 weeks of symptoms.
- Referral for CHF treatment if needed: medical management and or valve replacement.
- Bed rest is generally indicated only for children with CHF. Children with Sydenham chorea may need to be protected from injury until their choreiform movements are controlled. Steroids in the absence of other symptoms are not useful in the treatment of chorea.
- Children with severe chorea may benefit from the use of antiepileptic agents, such as valproic acid or carbamazepine with the latter being the first-line agent due to liver toxicity with valproic acid.
- Education about the need for prophylaxis is key to prevent further episodes of ARF.

Primary and Secondary Prevention of Acute Rheumatic Fever

- Primary prevention of ARF includes the treatment of GAS pharyngeal infections with appropriate antibiotics, eliminating bacteria before the triggering of an autoimmune response within 9 days of the onset of a sore throat. A 10-day course of oral penicillin or amoxicillin or intramuscular Bicillin can be given.[112] A community-based approach involves identifying a community outbreak and preventing its spread or identifying at-risk children in a community and having resources readily available to screen them for strep throat.
- Secondary prevention involves antibacterial prophylaxis for those with a prior history of ARF because of the greatly increased risk of recurrent ARF with subsequent inadequately treated GAS infections. Intramuscular Bicillin L-A, which slowly releases penicillin to prevent colonization and reoccurrences, can be given every 4 weeks for at least 10 years following ARF and in some cases, lifetime prophylaxis is suggested.[113] This method is more effective than daily penicillin V twice a day; however, adherence to either method is problematic. Pain of injections every 4 weeks is a real problem for children, and globally the quality of Bicillin can vary. In the majority of patients, valvular disease will resolve if they are compliant in taking antibiotic prophylaxis after the first episode of rheumatic heart disease.
- Tertiary prevention is medical and surgical intervention to prevent cardiac damage that occurs from ARF.

Complications

Chronic CHF can occur after an initial episode of ARF or follow recurrent episodes of ARF. Residual valvular damage is responsible for CHF. The risk of significant cardiac disease increases dramatically with each subsequent episode of ARF; therefore prevention of subsequent GAS infections is critical. Family engagement in follow-up is essential to prevent the need for cardiac valvular repair.

Poststreptococcal Reactive Arthritis

PSRA can develop within 7 to 10 days after GABHS pharyngitis and may present with knee, ankle, hip, or wrist arthritis in a patient who does not meet the Jones criteria for ARF.[114] The acute phase reactants are generally not as elevated in PSRA. The most common age in children is 8 to 14 years. There are no specific criteria for PSRA, but a history of recent streptococcal infection documented using the titers discussed earlier is important. In PSRA, the arthritis may occur sooner, be more persistent and cumulative, and involve small joints as well as the more common ones previously mentioned. This form of arthritis is less receptive to NSAID treatment but resolves without joint damage.[114] Although there is no associated cardiac involvement in PSRA, it is suggested that prophylaxis with penicillin to prevent carditis be continued for 1 year after the arthritis occurs.[107]

Pediatric Vasculitis

Pediatric vasculitis represents a complex group of conditions that cause inflammatory changes in the blood vessels. Vasculitis can occur as a primary condition, primarily involving large vessels (Takayasu arteritis), medium-size vessels (childhood polyarteritis nodosa, cutaneous polyarteritis, KD), and small-vessel disease in a granulomatous form (granulomatosis with polyangiitis), eosinophilic granulomatosis with polyangiitis (formerly Churg-Strauss syndrome), or small-vessel disease in a nongranulomatous form (microscopic polyangiitis, IgAV, isolated cutaneous leukocytoclastic vasculitis, hypocomplementemic urticarial vasculitis). Secondary vasculitis can result from infection, malignancy, drugs, or connective tissue disease. The occurrence of primary vasculitis in childhood is approximately 23 per 100,000. Symptoms are variable ranging from skin eruptions to multiorgan failure. Aneurysmal dilations can occur due to neutrophil, lymphocyte, and eosinophilic infiltration.[115] Fever and diffuse pain associated with malaise may be early symptoms, along with elevated acute-phase reactants (ESR, CRP, platelets, ferritin, procalcitonin). As the vasculitis progresses, there may be specific clinical findings, such as organ involvement, purpuric rash, or detection of antibodies known as *antineutrophil cytoplasmic antibodies* (ANCAs). The most common types of vasculitis are IAgV, KD, and Takayasu arteritis involving the aorta and its branches. All of these conditions require pediatric specialist care to prevent significant health problems.

Immunoglobulin A Vasculitis (IgAV)

Immunoglobulin A (IgAV), formerly known as Henoch-Schonlein Purpura, is the most common vasculitis of children and is characterized as an IgA vasculitis. The pathophysiology involves IgA-immune deposits, neutrophil activation and infiltration, and complement factors that produce vascular inflammation.[1] It can occur anytime from infancy (as early as 6 months old) to adulthood. The incidence of the disease is higher in fall and winter, pointing to an environmental trigger including viral infection. While an upper respiratory infection often precedes IgAV, a clear association between an infectious agent and IgAV has not been found although there is evidence that elimination of streptococcal infection can minimize or remove recurrence of IgAV in children.[116] For the majority of children, the prognosis is excellent.

The classic presentation includes abdominal pain, palpable petechial or purpuric rash on the lower extremity, nondeforming arthritis, and colicky abdominal pain. In 30% to 50% of patients, nephritis occurs 4 to 6 weeks after the initial presentation. The most common manifestation of renal disease is microscopic hematuria with or without proteinuria.[117] The abdominal pain is a result of subserosal or submucosal hemorrhage and edema. Intestinal perforation is a rare but life-threatening complication.[118] Neurological involvement (convulsions and confusion) due to vasculitis is not commonly seen.

IgAV is a leukocytic vasculitis with granulocytic infiltration of tissue along with IgA deposition within the vessel walls.[1] Hemorrhage and ischemia are associated findings. With inflammation of the small blood vessels, extravasation of blood occurs into local tissue, resulting in a variety of skin manifestations, including a maculopapular rash or urticarial rash the first 24 hours, followed by purpura, bullae, or necrotic lesions. The rash along with an oligoarticular, self-limiting, and nondestructive arthritis occurs in 80% of children. The lower extremities, typically the ankles and knees, are the most common arthritic sites. The latest Chapel Hill nomenclature describes IgAV as a vasculitis affecting the small blood vessels with IgA1-dominant deposits involving the skin and GI tract, with an accompanying nonerosive arthritis and an associated glomerulonephritis.

Clinical Findings

Clinical findings begin with skin manifestations; one-third of children will have the aforementioned symptoms for 2 weeks, with another third having symptoms up to 1 month and can have reoccurring symptoms for 4 months.[119] Hematuria is the most common renal symptom and usually develops within 4 weeks. Hypertension can be seen at any time from the start of the disease to the recovery phase.[117]

History. The history of a preceding viral illness and the clinical presentation of symptoms listed earlier support the diagnosis of IgAV. It can also present with seizures, stroke, mental status change, hemoptysis due to pulmonary hemorrhage, or edema of the eyes, hands, or scrotum if the child has associated nephrotic syndrome.

Physical Examination.
- Skin rash: Starts as a pinkish maculopapular rash and progresses from red to purple to brown palpable purpura; lower part of the body and lower arm
- Arthritis: Warmth, swelling, and erythema over the joints; periarthritis is common and involves the knees and ankles
- Other findings: Diffuse abdominal pain on palpation, edema of the scrotum, eyes, or hands; hypertension

Diagnostic Studies. The diagnosis of IgAV is based on clinical findings. A urinalysis must be done to check for hematuria and proteinuria (a common sign of nephritis) and needs to be repeated on follow-up due to the risk of renal disease. Other studies include a CBC with differential and platelets, metabolic profile including creatinine and blood urea nitrogen (BUN) to evaluate renal function, and stool guaiac for occult blood as the incidence of GI bleeding is high even in the absence of frank rectal bleeding. IgAV is associated with a nonthrombocytopenic purpura and a normal or high platelet count, as platelet elevation is an acute-phase reactant. Other acute-phase reactants including CRP may be helpful markers of disease activity. If GI obstruction is a consideration, abdominal radiographs should be ordered. Diagnostic studies are useful to identify specific organ system involvement and the severity of complications. Other tests (e.g., chest radiographs, computed tomography [CT] scans, or electroencephalographs) are ordered based on signs and symptoms of complications, such as shortness of breath, seizures, mental status changes, or hypertension. Renal biopsy may be warranted if severe renal involvement.[119]

Differential Diagnosis

Familial Mediterranean fever should be considered in patients with recurrent attacks, especially in patients of Middle Eastern or Mediterranean descent. IgAV must be differentiated from other diseases that cause purpura: immune thrombocytopenic purpura, post–streptococcal glomerular nephritis, hemolytic uremic syndrome, infections, SLE, serum sickness, or hypersensitivity vasculitis. Other types of vasculitis, including microscopic polyangiitis, granulomatosis with polyangiitis, eosinophilic granulomatous polyangiitis (previously Churg-Strauss syndrome), and polyarteritis nodosa, although more common in adults, need to be considered.[119]

Management

Children with IgAV need comanagement with pediatric specialists, depending on organ system involvement. Hospitalization is necessary with moderate to severe GI and renal system involvement or if pulmonary, cardiac, or CNS manifestations are present. The arthritis is generally treated with NSAIDs.[118] Treatment with corticosteroid can improve outcomes, especially in GI complications; however, IVIG, cyclosporine, MMF, methotrexate, cyclophosphamide, and azathioprine can be used as steroid sparing agents in refractory cases.[119] Prophylaxis with corticosteroids does not reduce the incidence of renal disease. In severe, life-threatening cases, treatment with immunophoresis may be instituted. MMF, cyclophosphamide, and azathioprine may be used; persistent proteinuria should be treated with angiotensin-converting enzyme inhibitors or angiotensin-receptor blockers.[117]
- Monitor for GI bleeding via stool guaiac, hematuria and proteinuria, and hypertension.
- Prescribe analgesics and NSAIDs for arthritis.
- Follow up and refer patients with IgAV to nephrologist, cardiologist, and gastroenterologist as complications arise.

Complications and Prognosis

Infrequent complications of IgAV seen in children include myositis, orchitis, hemorrhagic cystitis, pancreatitis, cholecystitis, bowel infarction, perforation or stricture, intussusception, acute renal failure, seizures, ataxia, pulmonary hemorrhage, carditis, anterior uveitis, and episcleritis. Ileoileal intussusception is a complication marked by severe colicky abdominal pain.

The presence of significant nephritis in the initial course of the disease (elevated BUN and persistent high-grade proteinuria) is a potentially serious complication with risk for long-term sequelae, such as hypertension or renal insufficiency. The nephritis can progress to end-stage renal disease in 1% to 7% of children with the disease.[117]

Patient and Parent Education

The provider should educate patients and parents about the illness, its complications, and the risk of recurrence; the need to closely monitor for signs of complications and recurrent disease; and the importance of monitoring blood pressure and follow-up visits to evaluate for renal disease and hypertension.[117]

Kawasaki Disease

KD (also known as *mucocutaneous lymph node syndrome* or *infantile polyarteritis*) presents as an acute febrile illness and is the leading cause of acquired heart disease. It is the second most common childhood vasculitis with a varying incidence from country to country, with Japan having the highest incidence of 264.8 per 100,000 in 2012 in children from 0 to 4 years.[2] In contrast, the rate of KD in the United States has remained stable at 19 per 100,000. Children of Asian/Pacific Islander descent have the highest rate of hospitalization in the United States, pointing to the role genetics play in the disease.[120] In terms of risk factors for coronary artery disease (CAD), the rate is higher at age <6 months or >9 years and in males. Children of Asian, Pacific Islander, and Hispanic descent have poor outcomes. Laboratory parameters, such as a thrombocytopenia, hyponatremia, elevated CRP, neutrophilia, and elevated transaminases, increase the risk of CAD with poor response to IVIG.[121]

The disease is characterized by an acute generalized systemic small and medium vessel vasculitis occurring throughout the body. The infiltration of macrophages in the vasculature is unique to KD. The disease mimics an infectious agent because of seasonal peaks and suggestion of toxin release as the rash resembles an erythroderma. However, the search for an infectious agent has remained elusive. It is proposed that a toxin acts as a superantigen that activates T cells, causing a massive release of cytokines and subsequent inflammation. The present hypothesis is that in genetically susceptible individuals, the infectious agent triggers the inflammatory cascade. No single genetic marker has been found.[120]

There are three vasculopathic processes in the arterial wall. The first phase is an acute arteritis with marked neutrophil infiltration within the lumen of the vessel causing necrosis of all vessel layers. Subacute or chronic vasculitis begins weeks after the fevers and can be seen months or years later. It is closely associated with a third phase marked by luminal myofibroblastic proliferation, which originates in the adventitia and involves cytotoxic T lymphocytes and can result in coronary artery stenosis.[120]

KD exhibits geographic and seasonal outbreaks, in the late winter and early spring. Person-to-person spread is low. The original criteria for KD described in 1967 are still the same and include a persistent fever for at least 5 days plus four of the following: bilateral conjunctival injection, changes of the lips and oral cavity, cervical lymphadenopathy, polymorphous exanthema, and changes in the peripheral extremities (swelling of the hands or feet) or perineal area.

Atypical or incomplete KD should be reserved for children who lack some of the classic findings, have findings that are not usually present in KD, including Kawasaki shock syndrome, and have findings previously listed under clinical findings.[2] Children with atypical or incomplete KD have the same, if not higher, risk of cardiac involvement.

Clinical Findings

The course of the disease is triphasic with an acute phase characterized by conjunctival hyperemia sparing the limbus, erythematous rash, edema of the hands and feet, a polymorphous erythematous rash, and enlarged lymph nodes. The subacute phase begins when the fever, rash, and cervical lymphadenopathy abate. Arthralgias with desquamation of the skin over the tips of the finger, thrombocytosis, and cardiac disease then tend to occur. In the final or convalescent phase, starting at around day 25 of illness, signs of disease are absent but there is still a marked elevation of the ESR. The cardiac findings include abnormalities of the coronary vessels, and myocarditis is almost universal.[120]

In addition to criteria previously mentioned, children, particularly with atypical KD, may have other findings involving the respiratory, musculoskeletal, GI, CNS, and genitourinary systems. They may have peribronchial and interstitial infiltrates or pulmonary nodules on chest radiograph, arthralgia or arthritis as well as diarrhea, vomiting, abdominal pain, hepatitis jaundice, hydrops of the gallbladder, and pancreatitis. CNS findings may include irritability, aseptic meningitis, peripheral facial nerve palsy, and sensorineural hearing loss. There may be a urethritis or meatal redness.[120]

Diagnostic Studies. KD is a diagnosis of exclusion. Results of laboratory investigations are not diagnostic, but rather help rule in another diagnosis. A CBC with differential and platelet count, a comprehensive metabolic profile, ESR, and CRP should be done. It is important to use the laboratory criteria previously mentioned to elucidate the diagnosis of incomplete KD. Laboratory findings include neutrophilia with bands; an elevation of acute-phase reactions such as ESR, CRP, and platelets; elevated serum transaminase levels; hypoalbuminemia; abnormal plasma lipid levels; and anemia and leukocytosis in synovial fluid. Leukopenia and thrombocytopenia in KD may occur in association with the life-threatening MAS.

KD supplemental laboratory criteria were identified to help in diagnosing cases of incomplete KD. The six components that need to be present in a patient with suspected KD but an incomplete diagnosis include (1) albumin ≤3.0 g/dL; (2) urine ≥10 WBC/HPF; (3) platelet count ≥450,000 after 7 days of fever; (4) anemia consistent with age values; (5) total WBC count ≥15,000/mm³; and (6) elevation of alanine aminotransferase.

Differential Diagnosis

Differential diagnoses include viral infections (e.g., measles, adenovirus, EBV, enterovirus, influenza, or roseola); bacterial infections (e.g., cervical adenitis, scarlet fever); toxin-mediated diseases (staphylococcal scalded skin syndrome, toxic shock syndrome), hypersensitivity reactions (drug hypersensitivity reactions, Stevens Johnson syndrome) or acrodynia (mercury toxicity); and sJIA.[120]

Management

- Early diagnosis is essential to prevent aneurysms in the coronary and extraparenchymal muscular arteries. Treatment goals include (1) evoking a rapid antiinflammatory response; (2) preventing coronary thrombosis by inhibiting platelet aggregation; and (3) minimizing long-term coronary risk factors by exercise, a heart-healthy diet, and smoking prevention. The child should be referred for initial treatment that includes the following medications and agents:[121]

- IVIG therapy (a single dose of 2 g/kg over 8–12 hours, ideally in the first 10 days of the illness) to control vascular inflammation. IVIG has immunomodulatory effects that cause downregulation of antibodies and proinflammatory cytokines, augmentation of suppressor T-cell activity, as well as saturation of Fc receptors. Retreatment with immunoglobulin is done when the initial IVIG does not reduce the inflammation.
  - While acetylsalicylic acid has no effect on coronary artery aneurysm (CAA) formation, it does have an antiplatelet effect. The American Heart Association recommends high-dose aspirin be given for its antiinflammatory properties (80–100 mg/kg/day in four divided doses, every 6 hours initially) until afebrile for at least 48 to 72 hours, then lowering the aspirin dose to 3 to 5 mg/kg/day for 6 to 8 weeks with discontinuation if the echocardiogram is normal. If significant coronary artery abnormalities develop and do not resolve, aspirin or other antiplatelet therapy is used indefinitely.
  - If a second treatment of IVIG at 2 mg/kg over 12 hours is not successful, then prednisolone (corticosteroids) has been used (with greater success in Japan than in the United States). Other agents such as cyclophosphamide, anakinra, rituximab, and plasmapheresis may be administered.
  - If coronary aneurysm is present, antiplatelet agents and anticoagulants, such as warfarin or clopidogrel, may be used as an adjuvant to aspirin.[2]
- A baseline echocardiogram should be obtained as soon as the diagnosis is established, with subsequent studies at 2 weeks and 6 to 8 weeks after onset of illness. Cardiac MRI may give a better view of anatomy and cardiac function; CT angiography, while an alternative, involves too much radiation.[121]
- All children on chronic aspirin therapy should receive inactivated influenza vaccination. If varicella or influenza develops, aspirin treatment should be stopped for 6 weeks, and another antiplatelet drug substituted to minimize the risk of Reye syndrome.
- Live virus vaccines should be delayed until 11 months after administration of IVIG (AAP Committee on Infectious Disease) although new research is investigating efficacy of vaccination starting at 6 months post IVIG.[122]
- Children without coronary or cardiac changes should be followed by a cardiologist during the first year after the onset of KD. If there are no cardiac changes during that first year, then the PCP may follow the patient with no activity restrictions imposed at that point.
- Patients with any range of transient coronary artery dilation (including giant aneurysms) should be followed by a cardiologist for years; physical activity limitations may be imposed.
- Follow and counsel all KD patients about a heart-healthy diet.

Complications and Prognosis

The acute disease is self-limited; however, during the initial stage (acute phase), inflammation of the arterioles, venules, and capillaries of the heart occurs and can progress to CAA in 15% to 25% of untreated children (<5% when treated appropriately). The process of aneurysm formation and subsequent thrombosis or scarring of the coronary artery may occur as late as 6 months after the initial illness. Other possible complications include recurrence of KD (<2%); CHF or massive myocardial infarction; myocarditis or

pericarditis, or both (30%); pericardial effusion; and mitral valve insufficiency. Children with a giant CAA can have thrombosis within the CAA as well as stenosis distal or proximal to the CAA calcifications.[123]

Although around 50% of CAA tend to regress after 2 years, there is myointimal thickening and stenosis seen in the segment adjacent to the giant aneurysm and in areas of resolved aneurysms. While the stenosis regresses over years, collateral arteries develop that prevent symptoms. Percutaneous coronary intervention and coronary artery bypass grafting can be used if there is ischemic heart disease.[121] Prompt treatment of chest pain, dyspnea, extreme lethargy, or syncope is always warranted.

Pediatric Primary Immunodeficiency Disorders

Immunodeficiency is a failure of one part of the body's defense mechanism resulting in recurrent infection of variable degrees and associated with morbidity and mortality. Primary immunodeficiency disorder (PIDD) is caused by hereditary or genetic defects. They may be present at birth or in early childhood and affect a single part of the immune system or one or more of its components. These disorders or diseases differ in presentation depending on the type of defect that alters the functions of the body's normal immune system.[124]

There are over 480 inborn errors of immunity.[124] The rapid expansion in this field is due to next-generation sequencing, which has increased the identification of inborn errors of immunity, which underlie the development of PIDDs. A free application can be found as "PID phenotypical diagnosis" or "PID classification" from iTunes and Android app stores (see Additional Resources). New PIDD classifications[124] include immunodeficiencies affecting cellular and humoral immunity, combined immunodeficiencies associated with syndromic features, predominantly antibody deficiencies, diseases of immune dysregulation, congenital defects of phagocyte number or function, defects in intrinsic and innate immunity, autoinflammatory diseases, complement deficiencies, and phenocopies of inborn error of immunity.

Physiology of the Immune System

An understanding of the immune systems is important for understanding the pathophysiology of immunodeficiencies. There are three lines of defense against antigens: *external barriers, innate immunity,* and *adaptive immunity. External barriers* that assist the immune defense system are physical and mechanical and include skin and the epithelial lining of the GI tract, genitourinary tract, and respiratory tract. The biochemical barriers include perspiration, tears, saliva, surfactant, hydrochloric acid in the stomach, and the body's normal bacterial flora.[125]

Innate immunity destroys pathogens. The inflammatory reaction occurs after the pathogen-associated molecular patterns (PAMPS) on immune cells recognize invading antigens. The pattern recognition receptors or PRRs are found on epithelial cells and innate immune cells. PRRs respond without prior exposure and are activated when there is direct contact with specific microbial products, such as lipopolysaccharides, cell wall components, and microbial nucleotides.[126] Innate immunity is utilized by receptors such as the TLR, which cannot discern the cell from the nonself, which trigger defenses that are imprecise and can cause damage to healthy tissue. TLR are germline encoded PRR and play an import role in host cell recognition and response to microbial pathogens. TLR specifically recognize different kinds of antigen components and cause a cascade through adapter molecules, which ultimately leads to a greater inflammatory response.[127] Phagocytes including neutrophils, macrophages, and dendritic cells (DCs) have several PRR that specifically bind to certain PAMPs. Macrophages and DCs act as antigen-presenting cells in *adaptive immunity*.[128]

The complement and cytokines signal specific cellular and humoral immunity to aid in host defenses. Complement amplifies the innate immune response by providing critical factors to enhance phagocytosis via opsonin and attracts white cells to the site of inflammation, thereby acting as chemoattractants. Neutrophils form a first line of defense and ingest the infecting organisms, internalizing the organism into an intracellular compartment and releasing bactericidal products. The role of neutrophils in the early inflammation process is primarily phagocytic, resulting in the creation of pus at the site of infection. Monocytes appear at the site of inflammation 1 to 7 days after the initial neutrophil infiltration and turn to macrophages ingesting and disposing of foreign material, including bacteria.[125] Eosinophils have mild phagocytic activity and help in the regulation of vascular mediators released by mast cells. They play an important role in the hypersensitive allergic response seen in anaphylaxis.[129]

Adaptive immunity is a specific process of recognition in which the host responds specifically to a foreign substance, such as a bacterium antigen. DCs are found all over the body and activate adaptive immunity by packaging antigenic peptides into human leukocyte antigens (MHC proteins). This is presented to the T lymphocyte to optimize T-cell receptor affinity and specificity. DCs also send out signals to allow for full differentiation of the T lymphocyte. The B and T cells play a major role in this system with T lymphocytes forming the cellular arm and B lymphocytes producing specific antibodies or immunoglobulins. In the initial primary exposure, the antigen exposure to B cells results in antibody formation. This reaction stimulates memory T cells to recognize the antigen for future exposures. Antibodies provide protection against bacterial infections and promote the ingestion of bacteria, as well as the neutralization of bacterial toxins and inactivation of virus. There are different classes of antibodies, with IgM and IgG providing protection against systemic infections and IgA providing protection at mucosa surfaces in the GI, genitourinary, and respiratory tract.[125]

Although cytokines primarily act locally, they mediate innate and adaptive immunity and stimulate T-lymphocyte formation. The T-helper cells recognize antigen by binding to the antigenic fragment displayed by the HLA molecules. Th1 cells are the arm of cellular immunity and activate macrophages, enhance cytotoxic T-cell function, produce cytokines, and recognize the infecting agent. Th2 cells enhance antibody formation by B cells, releasing cytokines, increasing IgE production, and mediating eosinophil recruitment and activation.[130]

The soluble protein components of the immune system, aside from antibodies IgA, IgG, and IgM, include cytokines, chemokines, and complement activation products (blood and cell surface proteins that help antibodies clear pathogens). *Cytokines*, such as IL and INF, are critical in the differentiation and maturation of immune cells. ILs are biochemical messengers produced by macrophages and lymphocytes and promote the production of leukocytes, induce leukocyte chemotaxis, and cause alteration of adhesion molecule expression on many cells. IFNs protect against viral infection but do not directly kill the antigen; rather they attempt to prevent further infection. They have no effect on cells

already infected. Other cytokines, such as TNF-α, are secreted by mast cells and macrophages and initiate fever by the production of prostaglandins and other inflammatory serum proteins. *Chemokines* also promote leukocyte chemotaxis.[130]

Primary and Secondary Immunodeficiency Disorders

Immunodeficiency can be a primary or secondary disorder. PIDDs are rare genetic disorders that typically run in families and can result in chronic debilitating disease. Of the primary immunodeficiency diseases, the B-cell line that produces antibodies is the one most commonly associated with these disorders, with IgA deficiency as the most common antibody defect with 1 in 333 to in 18,000 people affected. These patients present with recurrent infections of the respiratory, GI, and urogenital tract.[131] Table 36.14 shows the immune deficiency and the common clinical presentation.

Common PIDDs include selective IgA, IgG subclass deficiencies, transient hypogammaglobulinemia of infancy, and 22q11.2 deletion syndrome (DiGeorge syndrome). Uncommon PIDDs

TABLE 36.14 Selected Pediatric Primary Immunodeficiencies and Their Clinical Presentation

Immunodeficiency	Clinical Presentation
Severe combined immunodeficiency (SCID)	In infancy, persistent thrush, failure to thrive, pneumonia, diarrhea, recurrent difficult-to-treat unusual infections
Wiskott Aldrich syndrome	Thrombocytopenia, bloody stools, draining ears, atopic eczema, recurrent infections with encapsulated organisms, EBV-associated malignancy (Burkitt lymphoma)
Hyper-IgE syndrome	Staphylococcal abscess, pneumatoceles, osteopenia, unusual infection, recurrent otitis and sinusitis, recurrent pneumonias
22q11.2 deletion syndrome	With partial thymic hypoplasia, may have normal course; if no thymus, resemble patients with SCID
Common variable immunodeficiency	Normal or enlarged tonsils, splenomegaly, alopecia areata, thrombocytopenia, sprue-like disease, 438-fold increase in lymphoma
Selective IgA	Infections of respiratory, GI, and genitourinary tracts

EBV, Epstein-Barr virus; *GI*, gastrointestinal; *IgA*, immunoglobulin A; *IgE*, immunoglobulin E.
Modified from Sullivan KE, Buckley RH. Evaluation of suspected immunodeficiency. In: Kliegman RM, St. Geme J, eds. *Nelson Textbook of Pediatrics*. 21st ed. Elsevier; 2020:1097–1103; Buckley RH. Primary defects of antibody production. In: Kliegman RM, Stanton BF, St. Geme JW, et al, eds. *Nelson Textbook of Pediatrics*. 19th ed. Elsevier; 2016:722–728; and Buckley RH. T lymphocytes, B lymphocytes, and natural killer cells. In: Kliegman RM, Stanton BF, St. Geme JW, et al, eds. *Nelson Textbook of Pediatrics*. 19th ed. Elsevier; 2016:722.

include X-linked agammaglobulinemia (XLA), severe combined immunodeficiencies, complement deficiencies, as well as phagocytic disorders like combined granulomatous disease. Secondary immunodeficiencies can occur due to infections, drugs (e.g., corticosteroids), renal failure, HIV, and leukemia and lymphoma.

The first immunodeficiency described was an XLA. The condition causes deficiency of B-cell production that leads to a lack of all types of immunoglobulin. The infant is generally well for the first 1 to 2 months of life, and as maternal antibodies start to wane, the child becomes infected with extracellular pyogenic bacteria. Therefore there is an increased incidence of otitis media, pneumonia, sinusitis, and infections with encapsulated bacteria such as *Haemophilus influenzae* and *Streptococcus pneumoniae*.[132] While children and adults with XLA can develop severe, life-threatening bacterial infections, they are not particularly vulnerable to infections caused by viruses.

Clinical Presentation

History. A history of unusual, frequent, or recurrent infections is crucial to identify children with PIDDs. It is important to remember that these children do not typically have dysmorphology. While children with B-cell disorders have *recurrent* infections, those with defects in T-cell function have a history of *severe* infections. Onset of infection is important and suggests type of cell-line defect: before 6 months of age (T cell); 12 months or later (B cell or a secondary immunodeficiency); and between 6 and 12 months (combined B and T cells or B cell). There may be a sibling who died from sepsis or meningitis, but no workup for immune deficiency was done. A complete family history should be obtained. The child may present with congenital infections but also may present later in infancy, childhood, or adulthood. Box 36.7 contains a list of the 10 warning signs of immunodeficiency.[133]

Physical Examination Findings. The child with an immunodeficiency may not have any distinguishing characteristics. Small or absent cervical lymph nodes, adenoids, and/or tonsils may be a sign of XLA. A child with defects of the great vessels, cleft palate, hypognathia, and low, cupped ears may have 22q11.2 deletion syndrome. Patients with cutaneous telangiectasia may develop ataxia in early childhood and have recurrent infections.[132]

Diagnostic Studies. The child with an immunodeficiency disorder may present with a low lymphocyte count, low neutrophil count, or a low leukocytes count. It is important to calculate the total neutrophil count. A low IgA is likely to be the most common deficiency. The initial workup includes a complete history and physical examination, a CBC with differential and platelet count, and quantitative immunuglobulins, including IgG, IgA, and IgM. Referral to a specialist in immunology may be needed for further testing, including IgG subclass; candida, pneumococcal, and tetanus skin tests; lymphocyte surface markers—CD3, CD4, CD8, CD19, CD15, and CD16—along with a neutrophil oxidation burst and mononuclear lymphocyte proliferation studies. Table 36.14 addresses the more common immunodeficiency disorders and their clinical presentation. Using the 10 warning signs, the PCP can refer to immunology with stage 1 workup already done.[132]

Management

Children with immunodeficiency disorders have a higher risk of oncologic disorders as a result of their treatment, which in some cases requires granulocyte stimulation factor. The role of the PCP is to consider immunodeficiency disorders in children with recurrent, persistent, unusual infections and refer to specialists. These children and their families need coordinated health services in a pediatric healthcare home with providers who will support them and act as their advocate and educator for health supervision and health promotion services. It is also important to recognize that infections in children with immunodeficiency may require consultation due to the unusual nature or more persistent course of the infection.

Additional Resources

Advancing Global Immunology Education: https://www.immunopaedia.org.za/

Mothers of Asthmatics; Allergy and Asthma Network: www.aanma.org

American Academy of Allergy, Asthma, and Immunology: www.aaaai.org

American Academy of Dermatology Atopic Dermatitis Action Plan: https://assets.ctfassets.net/1ny4yoiyrqia/ZPT1WHhZHcxlpbDgq3hZX/3973a527e55d064306e40509d5004bb7/eczema-action-plan.pdf

American Autoimmune Related Diseases Association: www.aarda.org

American College of Allergy, Asthma, and Immunology: www.acaai.org

American Lung Association: www.lung.org

Arthritis Foundation: www.arthritis.org

Asthma and Allergy Foundation of America: www.aafa.org

Centers for Disease Control and Prevention myalgic encephalomyelitis/chronic fatigue syndrome information for healthcare providers: https://www.cdc.gov/me-cfs/healthcare-providers/index.html

Genetic Home Reference: https://ghr.nlm.nih.gov/primer/mutationsanddisorders/predisposition

Jeffrey Modell Foundation Primary Immunodeficiency Resource Center: http://jmfworld.com

Lupus Foundation of America: www.lupus.org

National Asthma Education and Prevention Program: www.nhlbi.nih.gov/about/org/naepp/

National Eczema Association: www.nationaleczema.org

National Heart, Lung, and Blood Institute: www.nhlbi.nih.gov

National Institute of Allergy and Infectious Diseases: www.niaid.nih.gov

National Jewish Health: www.nationaljewish.org/healthinfo

• BOX 36.7 Warning Signs of Primary Immunodeficiency Disorders

- Four or more new ear infections within 1 year
- Two or more serious sinus infections within 1 year
- Two or more months on antibiotics with little effect
- Two or more pneumonias within 1 year
- Failure of an infant to gain weight or grow normally
- Recurrent, deep skin or organ abscesses
- Persistent thrush in mouth or fungal infection on skin
- Need for intravenous antibiotics to clear infections
- Two or more deep-seated infections including septicemia
- Family history of primary immunodeficiency

Courtesy Jeffrey Model Foundation. Education materials. *https://info4pi.org/library/educational-materials/*.

Pediatric Gait Arms and Leg Examination (pGALS): https://geekymedics.com/pgals-paediatric-gait-arms-and-legs-examination-osce-guide/

Primary Immune Deficiency Foundation: https://primaryimmune.org/about-primary-immunodeficiencies

US Environmental Protection Agency (EPA): https://www.epa.gov/asthma

Acknowledgment

The authors acknowledge Rita Marie John for her work on the previous edition.

References

1. Leung AKC, Barankin B, Leong KF. Henoch-Schönlein purpura in children: an updated review. *Curr Pediatr Rev.* 2020;16(4):265–276.
2. Gorelik M, Chung SA, Ardalan K, et al. 2021 American college of rheumatology/vasculitis foundation guideline for the management of Kawasaki disease. *Arthritis Rheumatol.* 2022;74(4):586–596.
3. Huether SE, McCance KL, Brashers V. *Understanding Pathophysiology.* 7th ed. Elsevier; 2020.
4. Oetjen LK, Kim BS. Interactions of the immune and sensory nervous systems in atopy. *FEBS J.* 2018;285(17):3138–3151.
5. Mastrorilli C, Posa D, Cipriani F, et al. Asthma and allergic rhinitis in childhood: what's new. *Pediatr Allergy Immunol.* 2016;27:795–803.
6. Zou Z, Liu W, Huang C, et al. First-year antibiotics exposure in relation to childhood asthma, allergies, and airway illnesses. *Int J Environ Res Publ Health.* 2020;17(16).
7. Farzan N, Vijverber S, Kabesch M, et al. The use of pharmacogenomics, epigenomics, and transcriptomic to improve childhood asthma: where do we stand? *Pediatr Pulmonol.* 2018;53:836–845.
8. Sahai S, Adams M, Kamat D. A diagnostic approach to autoimmune disorders: clinical manifestations: part 1. *Pediatr Ann.* 2016;45(6):e223–e271.
9. Toskala E. Immunology. *Inter Forum Allerg Rhino.* 2018;4(52):S21–S26.
10. Buckley RH. Primary defects of antibody production. In: Kliegman RM, Stanton BF, S.Geme JW, et al., eds. *Nelson Textbook of Pediatrics.* 19th ed. Philadelphia: Saunders/Elsevier; 2016:722–728.
11. Ahmed I, Ahmad NS, Ali S, et al. Medication adherence apps: review and content analysis. *JMIR mHealth uHealth.* 2018;6(3):e62.
12. Brough HA, Lanser BJ, Sindher SB, et al. Early intervention and prevention of allergic diseases. *Allergy.* 2022;77(2):416–441.
13. Fiocchi A, Cabana MD, Mennini M. Current use of probiotics and prebiotics in allergy. *J Allergy Clin Immunol Pract.* 2022;10(9):2219–2224.
14. Trivillin A, Zanella S, Castaldo RJ, et al. Early oral nutritional supplements in the prevention of wheezing, asthma, and respiratory infections. *Front Pediatr.* 2022;10:866868.
15. Mikhail I, Grayson MH. Asthma and viral infections: an intricate relationship. *Ann Allergy Asthma Immunol.* 2019;123(4):352–358.
16. Bawany F, Beck LA, Järvinen KM. Halting the march: primary prevention of atopic dermatitis and food allergies. *J Allergy Clin Immunol Pract.* 2020;8(3):860–875.
17. Pate C, Zahran H, Qin X, et al. *Asthma Surveillance — United States, 2006–2018: MMWR Surveillance Summary 2021.* Centers for Disease Control; 2021:1–32.
18. Mishra V, Banga J, Silveyra P. Oxidative stress and cellular pathways of asthma and inflammation: therapeutic strategies and pharmacological targets. *Pharmacol Ther.* 2018;181:169–182.
19. Pérez de Llano L, Dacal Rivas D, Blanco Cid N, et al. Phenotype-guided asthma therapy: an alternative approach to guidelines. *J Asthma Allergy.* 2021;14:207–217.
20. Global Initiative for Asthma (GINA). *Global Strategies for Asthma Management and Prevention*; 2022. https://ginasthma.org/gina-reports/.
21. Crisford H, Sapey E, Rogers GB, et al. Neutrophils in asthma: the good, the bad and the bacteria. *Thorax.* 2021;76(8).
22. Hernandez-Pacheco N, Pino-Yanes M, Flores C. Genomic predictors of asthma phenotypes and treatment response. *Front Pediatr.* 2019;7:6.
23. Hammad H, Lambrecht BN. The basic immunology of asthma. *Cell.* 2021;184(6):1469–1485.
24. Koya T, Ueno H, Hasegawa T, et al. Management of exercise-induced bronchoconstriction in athletes. *J Allergy Clin Immunol Pract.* 2020;8(7):2183–2192.
25. Yaneva M, Darlenski R. The link between atopic dermatitis and asthma- immunological imbalance and beyond. *Asthma Res Pract.* 2021;7(1):16.
26. Miller RL, Grayson MH, Strothman K. Advances in asthma: new understandings of asthma's natural history, risk factors, underlying mechanisms, and clinical management. *J Allergy Clin Immunol.* 2021;148(6):1430–1441.
27. Dinakar C, Chipps B. Clinical report: guidance for the clinician in rendering pediatric care clinical tools to assess asthma control in children. *Pediatrics.* 2020:41–61.
28. Schatz M, Sorkness CA, Li JT, et al. Asthma Control Test: reliability, validity, and responsiveness in patients not previously followed by asthma specialists. *J Allergy Clin Immunol.* 2006;117(3):549–556.
29. Zhang Y, Clegg JL, Keith S, et al. Content validity of a newly developed observer-reported measure for pediatric asthma in children aged 2-5 years. *J Patient Rep Outcomes.* 2022;6(1):55.
30. Pletta K, Moreno M, Allen G, et al. Electronic Health Record (EHR) quality tools improved and sustained use of asthma action plans for 3 years in a primary care pediatric system. *Pediatrics.* 2019;144:121.
31. American Academy of Asthma, Allergy and Immunology / American College of Allergy, Asthma and Immunology. *Joint Statement of Support on the ATS Clinical Practice Guideline. Interpretation of Exhaled Nitric Oxide for Clinical Applications*; 2012. https://www.aaaai.org/Aaaai/media/MediaLibrary/PDF Documents/My Membership/FeNOJointStatement3-6-12.pdf.
32. Khatri SB, Iaccarino JM, Barochia A, et al. Use of fractional exhaled nitric oxide to guide the treatment of asthma: an official American Thoracic Society Clinical Practice Guideline. *Am J Respir Crit Care Med.* 2021;204(10):e97–e109.
33. Lee MO, Sivasankar S, Pokrajac N, et al. Emergency department treatment of asthma in children: a review. *J Am Coll Emerg Physicians Open.* 2020;1(6):1552–1561.
34. Gallucci M, Carbonara P, Pacilli AMG, et al. Use of symptoms scores, spirometry, and other pulmonary function testing for asthma monitoring. *Front Pediatr.* 2019;7:54.
35. Burrill A, McArdle, Davies B. Lung function in children: a simple guide to performing and interpreting spirometry. *Paediatr Child Health.* 2021;31(7):276–283.
36. Wright JL, Davis WS, Joseph MM, et al. Eliminating race-based medicine. *Pediatrics.* 2022;150(1). e2022057998.
37. Yang SY, Kim YH, Byun MK, et al. Repeated measurement of fractional exhaled nitric oxide is not essential for asthma screening. *J Invest Allergol Clin Immunol.* 2018;28(2):98–105.
38. Cloutier MM, Baptist AP, Blake KV, et al. 2020 focused updates to the asthma management guidelines: a report from the national asthma education and prevention program coordinating committee expert panel working group. *J Allergy Clin Immunol.* 2020;146(6):1217–1270.
39. Miraglia Del Giudice M, Licari A, Brambilla I, et al. Allergen immunotherapy in pediatric asthma: a pragmatic point of view. *Children (Basel).* 2020;7(6).
40. De Keyser HH, Chipps B, Dinakar C. Section on allergy and immunology and section on pediatric pulmonology and sleep medicine. Biologics for asthma and allergic skin diseases in children. *Pediatrics.* 2021;148(5). e2021054270.

41. Henriksen DP, Bodtger U, Sidenius K, et al. Efficacy of omalizumab in children, adolescents, and adults with severe allergic asthma: a systematic review, meta-analysis, and call for new trials using current guidelines for assessment of severe asthma. *Allergy Asthma Clin Immunol.* 2020;16:49.

42. Busse WW, et al. Combined analysis of asthma safety trials of long-acting β. *N Engl J Med.* 2018;379(15):1482.

43. Hendeles L, Blake KV, Galbreath A. A single inhaler combining a corticosteroid and long-acting beta-2 agonist for maintenance with additional doses for reliever therapy (SMART): obstacles for asthma patients in the USA. *Pediatr Allergy Immunol Pulmonol.* 2021;34(2):73–75.

44. Kaur S, Singh V. Asthma and medicines - long-term side-effects, monitoring and dose titration. *Indian J Pediatr.* 2018;85(9):748–756.

45. Taketomo C, Hodding J, Kraus D. *Pediatric and Neonatal Drug Dosage Handbook.* Lexi-Comp; 2021.

46. Caggiano S, Cutrera R, Di Marco A, et al. Exercise-induced bronchospasm and allergy. *Front Pediatr.* 2017;5:1–9.

47. Bousquet J, Anto JM, Bachert C, et al. Allergic rhinitis. *Nat Rev Dis Prim.* 2020;6(1):95.

48. Acevedo-Prado A, Seoane-Pillado T, López-Silvarrey-Varela A, et al. Association of rhinitis with asthma prevalence and severity. *Sci Rep.* 2022;12(1):6389.

49. American Academy of Asthma, Allergy and Immunology. Some Tests and Procedures Are over or Misused to Diagnose and Treat Allergies, Asthma and Immunological Disorders; 2012. https://www.aaaai.org/Aaaai/media/MediaLibrary/PDF%20Documents/Media/Choosing-WiselyT.pdf#:~:text=Don%E2%80%99t%20order%20sinus%20computed%20tomography%20%28CT%29%20or%20indiscriminately,for%20treating%20the%20majority%20of%20acute%20sinus%20infections.

50. Wise SK, Lin SY, Toskala E, et al. International consensus statement on allergy and rhinology: allergic rhinitis. *Int Forum Allergy Rhinol.* 2018;8(2):108–352.

51. Doroudchi A, Imam K, Garcia Lloret M. Allergen immunotherapy in pediatric respiratory allergy. *Curr Treat Options Allergy.* 2021;8:147–160.

52. Scurlock AM, Burks AW, Sicherer SH, et al. Epicutaneous immunotherapy for treatment of peanut allergy: follow-up from the Consortium for Food Allergy Research. *J Allergy Clin Immunol.* 2021;147(3):992–1003.e5.

53. American Academy of Asthma. Allergy and Immunology. The Current State of Oral Immunotherapy; 2020. https://www.aaaai.org/tools-for-the-public/conditions-library/allergies/the-current-state-of-oral-immunotherapy.

54. Chong LY, Piromchai P, Sharp S, et al. Biologics for chronic rhinosinusitis. *Cochrane Database Syst Rev.* 2021;3:CD013513.

55. Davis DMR, Drucker AM, Alikhan A, et al. American Academy of Dermatology Guidelines: Awareness of comorbidities associated with atopic dermatitis in adults. *J Am Acad Dermatol.* 2022;86(6):1335–1336.e18.

56. Chiesa Fuxench ZC, Block JK, Boguniewicz M, et al. Atopic dermatitis in America Study: a cross-sectional study examining the prevalence and disease burden of atopic dermatitis in the US adult population. *J Invest Dermatol.* 2019;139(3):583–590.

57. Abuabara K, Magyari A, McCulloch CE, et al. Prevalence of atopic eczema among patients seen in primary care: data from the Health Improvement Network. *Ann Intern Med.* 2019;170(5):354–356.

58. Ständer S. Atopic dermatitis. *N Engl J Med.* 2021;384(12):1136–1143.

59. Frazier W, Bhardwaj N. Atopic dermatitis: diagnosis and treatment. *Am Fam Physician.* 2020;101(10):590–598.

60. Lowe AJ, Su JC, Allen KJ, et al. A randomized trial of a barrier lipid replacement strategy for the prevention of atopic dermatitis and allergic sensitization: the PEBBLES pilot study. *Br J Dermatol.* 2018;178(1):e19–e21.

61. Yosipovitch G, Gold LF, Lebwohl MG, et al. Early relief of pruritus in atopic dermatitis with crisaborole ointment, a non-steroidal, phosphodiesterase 4 inhibitor. *Acta Derm Venereol.* 2018;98(5):484–489.

62. Eichenfield LF, Stripling S, Fung S, et al. Recent developments and advances in atopic dermatitis: a focus on epidemiology, pathophysiology, and treatment in the pediatric setting. *Paediatr Drugs.* 2022;24(4):293–305.

63. Chang YS, Lin MH, Lee JH, et al. Melatonin supplementation for children with atopic dermatitis and sleep disturbance: a randomized clinical trial. *JAMA Pediatr.* 2016;170(1):35–42.

64. Burks AW, Sampson HA, Plaut M, et al. Treatment for food allergy. *J Allergy Clin Immunol.* 2018;141(1):1–9.

65. Martini A, Lovell DJ, Albani S, et al. Juvenile idiopathic arthritis. *Nat Rev Dis Prim.* 2022;8(1):5.

66. Zaripova LN, Midgley A, Christmas SE, et al. Juvenile idiopathic arthritis: from aetiopathogenesis to therapeutic approaches. *Pediatr Rheumatol Online J.* 2021;19(1):135.

67. Ferguson ID, Griffin P, Michel JJ, et al. T cell receptor-independent, CD31/IL-17A-driven inflammatory axis shapes synovitis in juvenile idiopathic arthritis. *Front Immunol.* 2018;9:1802.

68. Kimura Y, Vastert S. Systemic juvenile idiopathic arthritis. In: Petty RE, Laxer RM, Lindsley CB, Wedderburn LR, Mellins ED, Fuhlbrigge RC, eds. *Textbook of Pediatric Rheumatology.* 8th ed. Philadelphia, PA: Elsevier; 2021:1046–1058.

69. Mahmoud SA, Binstadt BA. Autoantibodies in the pathogenesis, diagnosis, and prognosis of juvenile idiopathic arthritis. *Front Immunol.* 2019;9:3168.

70. Moura RA, Fonseca JE. B Cells on the stage of inflammation in juvenile idiopathic arthritis: leading or supporting actors in disease pathogenesis? *Front Med (Lausanne).* 2022;9:851532.

71. Sen ES, Ramanan AV. Juvenile idiopathic arthritis-associated uveitis. *Clin Immunol.* 2020;211:108322.

72. Stoustrup P, Twilt M, Resnick CM. Management of temporomandibular joint arthritis in JIA: tradition-based or evidence-based? *J Rheumatol.* 2018;45(9):1205–1207.

73. Hinks A, Marion MC, Cobb J, et al. Brief report: the genetic profile of rheumatoid factor-positive polyarticular juvenile idiopathic arthritis resembles that of adult rheumatoid arthritis. *Arthritis Rheumatol.* 2018;70(6):957–962.

74. Metzemaekers M, Malengier-Devlies B, Yu K, et al. Synovial fluid neutrophils from patients with juvenile idiopathic arthritis display a hyperactivated phenotype. *Arthritis Rheumatol.* 2021;73(5):875–884.

75. Angeles-Han ST, Ringold S, Beukelman T, et al. 2019 American College of Rheumatology/Arthritis Foundation Guideline for the screening, monitoring, and treatment of juvenile idiopathic arthritis-associated uveitis. *Arthritis Care Res (Hoboken).* 2019;71(6):703–716.

76. Crayne CB, Beukelman T. Juvenile idiopathic arthritis: oligoarthritis and polyarthritis. *Pediatr Clin.* 2018;65(4):657–674.

77. Ong MS, Ringold S, Kimura Y, et al. Improved disease course associated with early initiation of biologics in polyarticular juvenile idiopathic arthritis: trajectory analysis of a childhood arthritis and rheumatology research Alliance consensus treatment plans study. *Arthritis Rheumatol.* 2021;73(10):1910–1920.

78. Funk RS, Balevic S, Cooper JC, et al. Therapeutics. In: Petty RE, Laxer RM, Lindsley CB, Wedderburn LR, Mellins ED, Fuhlbrigge RC, eds. *Textbook of Pediatric Rheumatology.* 8th ed. Philadelphia, PA: Elsevier; 2021:708–855.

79. Ringold S, Angeles-Han ST, Beukelman T, et al. 2019 American College of Rheumatology/Arthritis Foundation guideline for the treatment of juvenile idiopathic arthritis: therapeutic approaches for non-systemic polyarthritis, sacroiliitis, and enthesitis. *Arthritis Care Res (Hoboken).* 2019;71:717–734.

80. Brunner HI, Ruperto N. Therapeutics: biologics and small molecule. In: Petty RE, Laxer RM, Lindsley CB, Wedderburn LR, Mellins ED, Fuhlbrigge RC, eds. *Textbook of Pediatric Rheumatology.* 8th ed. Elsevier; 2021:856–951.

81. Ruperto N, Brunner HI, Ramanan AV, et al. Subcutaneous dosing regimens of tocilizumab in children with systemic or polyarticular juvenile idiopathic arthritis. *Rheumatology (Oxford)*. 2021;60(10):4568–4580.

82. Li S, Zhang W, Lin Y. Application of intra-articular corticosteroid injection in juvenile idiopathic arthritis. *Front Pediatr*. 2022;10:822009.

83. Centers for Disease Control and Prevention (CDC). Use of 13-valent pneumococcal conjugate vaccine and 23-valent pneumococcal polysaccharide vaccine among children aged 6-18 years with immunocompromising conditions: recommendations of the Advisory Committee on Immunization Practices (ACIP). *MMWR Morb Mortal Wkly Rep*. 2013;62(25):521–524.

84. Klein-Gittelman MS, Beresford MW. Systemic lupus erythematosus, mixed-connective tissue disease, and undifferentiated connective tissue disease. In: Petty RE, Laxer RM, Lindsley CB, Wedderburn LR, Mellins ED, Fuhlbrigge RC, eds. *Textbook of Pediatric Rheumatology*. 8th ed. Elsevier; 2021:1489–1699.

85. Harry O, Yasin S, Brunner H. Childhood-onset systemic lupus erythematosus: a review and update. *J Pediatr*. 2018;196:22–30.e2.

86. Woo JMP, Parks CG, Jacobsen S, et al. The role of environmental exposures and gene-environment interactions in the etiology of systemic lupus erythematous. *J Intern Med*. 2022;291(6):755–778.

87. Pisetsky DS, Lipsky PE. New insights into the role of antinuclear antibodies in systemic lupus erythematosus. *Nat Rev Rheumatol*. 2020;16(10):565–579.

88. He Y, Sawalha AH. Drug-induced lupus erythematosus: an update on drugs and mechanisms. *Curr Opin Rheumatol*. 2018;30(5):490–497.

89. Peleg Y, Bomback AS, Radhakrishnan J. The evolving role of calcineurin inhibitors in treating lupus nephritis. *Clin J Am Soc Nephrol*. 2020;15(7):1066–1072.

90. Fanouriakis A, Tziolos N, Bertsias G, Boumpas DT. Update on the diagnosis and management of systemic lupus erythematosus. *Ann Rheum Dis*. 2021;80(1):14–25.

91. Andreoli L, Bertsias GK, Agmon-Levin N, et al. EULAR recommendations for women's health and the management of family planning, assisted reproduction, pregnancy and menopause in patients with systemic lupus erythematosus and/or antiphospholipid syndrome. *Ann Rheum Dis*. 2017;76(3):476–485.

92. Yamamoto EA, Jørgensen TN. Relationships between vitamin D, gut microbiome, and systemic autoimmunity. *Front Immunol*. 2020;10:3141.

93. Trindade VC, Carneiro-Sampaio M, Bonfa E, et al. An update on the management of childhood-onset systemic lupus erythematosus. *Paediatr Drugs*. 2021;23(4):331–347.

94. Song L, Wang Y, Zhang J, et al. The risks of cancer development in systemic lupus erythematosus (SLE) patients: a systematic review and meta-analysis. *Arthritis Res Ther*. 2018;20(1):270.

95. Weiss JE, Kashikar-Zuck S. Juvenile fibromyalgia. *Rheum Dis Clin N Am*. 2021;47(4):725–736.

96. Yunus MB, Masi AT. Juvenile primary fibromyalgia syndrome: a clinical study of thirty-three patients and matched normal controls. *Arthritis Rheum*. 1985;28(2):138–145.

97. Wolfe F, Clauw DJ, Fitzcharles MA, et al. The American college of rheumatology preliminary diagnostic criteria for fibromyalgia and measurement of symptom severity. *Arthritis Care Res (Hoboken)*. 2010;62(5):600–610.

98. Weiss JE. *Pediatr Rheumatol Online J*. 2019;17(1):51.

99. Coles ML, Weissmann R, Uziel Y. Juvenile primary fibromyalgia syndrome: epidemiology, etiology, pathogenesis, clinical manifestations and diagnosis. *Pediatr Rheumatol Online J*. 2021;19(1):22.

100. Sherry DD. Amplified pain-a helpful diagnosis. *JAMA Pediatr*. 2022;176(1):10–11.

101. Bateman L, Bested AC, Bonilla HF, et al. Myalgic encephalomyelitis/chronic fatigue syndrome: essentials of diagnosis and management. *Mayo Clin Proc*. 2021;96(11):2861–2878.

102. Tomas C, Newton J. Metabolic abnormalities in chronic fatigue syndrome/myalgic encephalomyelitis: a mini-review. *Biochem Soc Trans*. 2018;46(3):547–553.

103. Sotzny F, Blanco J, Capelli E, et al. Myalgic encephalomyelitis/chronic fatigue syndrome: evidence for an autoimmune disease. *Autoimmun Rev*. 2018;17(6):601–609.

104. Rasa S, Nora-Krukle Z, Henning N, et al. Chronic viral infections in myalgic encephalomyelitis/chronic fatigue syndrome (ME/CFS). *J Transl Med*. 2018;16(1):268.

105. Komaroff AL, Lipkin WI. Insights from myalgic encephalomyelitis/chronic fatigue syndrome may help unravel the pathogenesis of post-acute COVID-19 syndrome. *Trends Mol Med*. 2021;27(9):895–906.

106. Lahiri S, Sanyahumbi A. Acute rheumatic fever. *Pediatr Rev*. 2021;42(5):221–232.

107. Maness D, Martin M, Mitchell G. Poststreptococcal illness: recognition and management. *J Amer Fam Physician*. 2018;97(8):517–522.

108. Méndez Eirín E, Suárez Ouréns Y, Guerra Vázquez JL. Cardiac manifestations of rheumatic diseases. *Med Clin (Bare)*. 2021;156:615–621.

109. Heard MA, Green MC, Royer M. Acute rheumatic fever: a review of essential cutaneous and histological findings. *Cureus*. 2021;13(1):e12577.

110. Alsaeid K, Uziel Y, Weiss PF. Reactive arthritis. In: Petty RE, Laxer RM, Lindsley CB, Wedderburn LR, Mellins ED, Fuhlbrigge RC, eds. *Textbook of Pediatric Rheumatology*. 8th ed. Elsevier; 2021:3185–3891.

111. Arvind B, Ramakrishnan S. Rheumatic fever and rheumatic heart disease in children. *Indian J Pediatr*. 2020;87(4):305–311.

112. American Academy of Pediatrics Committee of Infectious Diseases. In: Kimberlin D, Barnett E, Lynfield R, Sawyer M, eds. *Red Book: 2021–2024 Report of the Committee on Infectious Diseases*. 32nd ed. American Academy of Pediatrics; 2021.

113. Karthikeyan G, Guilherme L. Acute rheumatic fever. *Lancet*. 2018;392(10142):161–174. Erratum *Lancet*. 2018;392:820.

114. Bawazir Y, Towheed T, Anastassiades T. Post-streptococcal reactive arthritis. *Curr Rheumatol Rev*. 2020;16(1):2–8.

115. Cabral DA, Ozen S, Morishita KA. Vasculitis and its classification. In: Petty RE, Laxer RM, Lindsley CB, Wedderburn LR, Mellins ED, Fuhlbrigge RC, eds. *Textbook of Pediatric Rheumatology*. 8th ed. Elsevier; 2021:2341–2360.

116. Fan GZ, Li RX, Jiang Q, et al. Streptococcal infection in childhood Henoch-Schönlein purpura: a 5-year retrospective study from a single tertiary medical center in China, 2015-2019. *Pediatr Rheumatol Online J*. 2021;19(1):79.

117. Dyga K, Szczepańska M. IgA vasculitis with nephritis in children. *Adv Clin Exp Med*. 2020;29(4):513–519.

118. Du l, Wang P, Liu C, Li S, Yue S, Yang Y. Multisystemic manifestations of IgA vasculitis. *Clin Rheumatol*. 2021;40(1):43–52.

119. Brogan P, Nott KA. Immune complex small-vessel vasculitis. In: Petty RE, Laxer RM, Lindsley CB, Wedderburn LR, Mellins ED, Fuhlbrigge RC, eds. *Textbook of Pediatric Rheumatology*. 8th ed. Elsevier; 2021:2361–2421.

120. Rife E, Gedalia A. Kawasaki disease: an update. *Curr Rheumatol Rep*. 2020;22(10):75.

121. Dionne A, Burns JC, Dahdah N, et al. Treatment intensification in patients with Kawasaki disease and coronary aneurysm at diagnosis. *Pediatrics*. 2019;143(6). e20183341.

122. Morikawa Y, Sakakibara H, Kimiya T, Tokyo Pediatric Clinical Research Network, et al. Live attenuated vaccine efficacy six months after intravenous immunoglobulin therapy for Kawasaki disease. *Vaccine*. 2021;39(39):5680–5687.

123. Ae R, Maddox RA, Abrams JY, et al. Kawasaki disease with coronary artery lesions detected at initial echocardiography. *J Am Heart Assoc*. 2021;10(7):e019853.

124. Tangye SG, Al-Herz W, Bousfiha A, et al. Human inborn errors of immunity: 2022 update on the classification from the international union of immunological societies expert committee. *J Clin Immunol*. 2022;42(7):1473–1507.

125. McComb S, Thiriot A, Akache B, et al. Introduction to the immune system. *Methods Mol Biol*. 2019;2024:1–24.

126. Carty M, Guy C, Bowie AG. Detection of viral infections by innate immunity. *Biochem Pharmacol*. 2021;183:114316.

127. Fitzgerald KA, Kagan JC. Toll-like receptors and the control of immunity. *Cell*. 2020;180(6):1044–1066.

128. Metur SP, Klionsky DJ. Adaptive immunity at the crossroads of autophagy and metabolism. *Cell Mol Immunol*. 2021;18(5):1096–1105.

129. Mishra V, Banga J, Silveyra P. Oxidative stress and cellular pathways of asthma and inflammation: therapeutic strategies and pharmacological targets. *Pharmacol Ther*. 2018;181:169–182.

130. Saravia J, Chapman NM, Chi H. Helper T cell differentiation. *Cell Mol Immunol*. 2019;16(7):634–643.

131. Amaya-Uribe L, Rojas M, Azizi G, et al. Primary immunodeficiency and autoimmunity: a comprehensive review. *J Autoimmun*. 2019;99:52–72.

132. Russell TB, Schiller JH. Immunologic assessment. In: Schuh AM, Marcdante KM, Kliegman RM, eds. *Nelson Essentials of Pediatrics*. 9th ed. Elsevier; 2022:301–324.

133. Modell V, Orange JS, Quinn J, et al. Global report on primary immunodeficiencies: 2018 update from the Jeffrey Modell Centers Network on disease classification, regional trends, treatment modalities, and physician reported outcomes. *Immunol Res*. 2018;66(3):367–380.

37
Dermatologic Disorders

TAMI B. BLAND

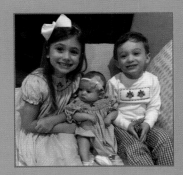

The skin is the body's largest organ with the primary purpose of protection and thermoregulation. It is important to note that skin varies from one part of the body to another and that alterations in skin appearance not only reflects overall health but also gives clues to underlying conditions.

Anatomy and Physiology

The skin is composed of two layers with an underlying subcutaneous layer (Fig. 37.1). The *epidermis*, a thinner outer layer, functions as a protective barrier between the body and the environment and is composed of five layers of stratified squamous epithelium. Most epidermal cells are keratinocytes, which produce *keratin*, a protective protein and the structural protein of hair and nails. New keratinocytes mature and are shed approximately every 28 days. The outer layer of the epidermis is called the *stratum corneum,* or *horny layer.* It is composed of keratin and is responsible for much of the barrier protection against microorganisms and irritating chemicals. It also facilitates the exchange of fluids and electrolytes with the environment and provides strength for the skin. Ambient moisture influences the epidermal barrier, with either excess or inadequate amounts contributing to micro- and macroscopic breaks. Melanocytes, produced in the basal layer of the epidermis, contribute to the color of the skin, eyes, and hair. They protect the epidermis from ultraviolet (UV) light irradiation. It is important to note that differences in skin color are not caused by differences in the number of melanocytes, but the variation in the number, size, and distribution of melanosomes, or pigment granules, within the melanocytes.[1]

The *dermis* is the thicker middle layer that contributes strength, support, and elasticity to the skin. It is a tough, leathery mechanical barrier that also regulates heat loss, provides host defenses of the skin, and aids in nutrition and other regulatory functions. The dermis is primarily composed of collagen, which is the major structural protein for the entire body. It includes mast cells, inflammatory cells, blood and lymph vessels, and cutaneous nerves that elicit sensations. These specialized receptors are a defense mechanism to protect the skin surface from environmental trauma.

Underlying the dermis is subcutaneous tissue primarily composed of adipose tissue. It contains arteries and arterioles that assist in skin thermoregulation. The subcutaneous tissue insulates and cushions the body from trauma, provides energy, and metabolizes hormones.

Skin appendages include the hair, sebaceous glands, nails, and sweat glands. *Hairs* are threads of keratin. Hair follicles are found over the entire body except for the palms, soles, knuckles, distal and interdigital spaces, lips, glans and prepuce of the penis, and areolae and nipples of the breast. Two types of hair can be found on the body. Terminal hair is thick, visible, and found on the scalp, axillae, and pubis. Very fine vellus hair is found over the remainder of the body. The visible portion of the hair is the shaft. The hair root is embedded in the dermis as a pilosebaceous unit, consisting of a hair follicle and a sebaceous gland. The hair shaft may be straight, wavy, helical, or spiral. *Sebaceous glands* are usually attached to hair follicles. They are distributed over the entire body except the soles, palms, and dorsa of the feet and are most abundant on the scalp and face. These glands secrete a lipid called *sebum* when stimulated by androgen and function to prevent excessive water evaporation, minimize heat loss, lubricate the skin and hair, and are thought to have some antimicrobial properties. *Nails* are epidermal cells composed of keratin and grow continually. They serve in grasping, protection of fingertip, and sensory function. The nailbed, underneath the nail plate, is composed of layers of epidermis and dermis, which serve as structural support. The nail root lies just under the epidermis. There are three types of sweat glands. *Eccrine glands* secrete sweat and are distributed over most of the entire body. They help maintain fluid and electrolyte balance and body temperature. *Ceruminous glands* are in the external ear canal and secrete a waxy pigmented substance called *cerumen.* *Apocrine glands* are located primarily in the axillary, genital, and periumbilical areas. They open into hair follicles, require androgens to stimulate their secretions, and are thought to be responsible for body odor.

Pathophysiology and Defense Mechanisms

Disruption of the skin and subcutaneous tissue can result from:
- Bacterial, fungal, and viral infections
- Allergic and inflammatory reactions
- Infestations
- Vascular reactions
- Papulosquamous/bullous eruptions
- Congenital lesions
- Hair and nail disorders

There are three cutaneous reactions to trauma, infection, or inflammation. *Pigment lability* occurs as postinflammatory hypo- or hyperpigmentation. If superficial, with changes in the epidermis only, original pigmentation returns in about 6 months (e.g., in diaper rash, seborrhea, tinea, pityriasis alba). If dermal changes happen, dermal tattooing may occur, causing long-term or permanent changes (e.g., excoriated acne, impetigo, varicella, contact dermatitis). A *follicular response* results in prominent papule and follicle formation, especially with atopic dermatitis, pityriasis rosea, syphilis, or tinea versicolor. A *mesenchymal* response, which

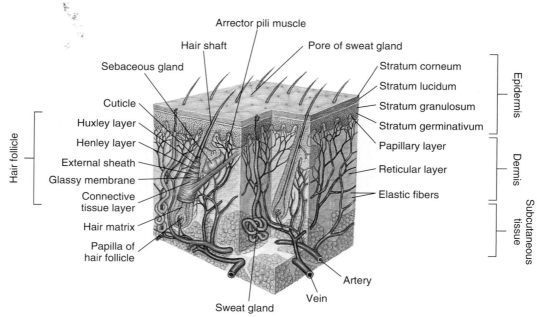

Arrector pili muscle
Hair shaft
Pore of sweat gland
Sebaceous gland
Stratum corneum
Stratum lucidum
Stratum granulosum
Stratum germinativum
Epidermis
Cuticle
Huxley layer
Henley layer
External sheath
Glassy membrane
Connective tissue layer
Hair matrix
Papilla of hair follicle
Hair follicle
Papillary layer
Reticular layer
Elastic fibers
Dermis
Subcutaneous tissue
Artery
Vein
Sweat gland

• **Fig. 37.1** Structure of the Skin. (From Ball JW, Dains JE, Flynn JA, Solomon BS, Stewart RW. *Seidel's Guide to Physical Examination.* 10th ed. Elsevier; 2022.)

often follows varicella, ear piercing, burns, or any surgical procedure may cause scars and/or keloids. *Keloids* are scars that thicken and extend beyond the margins of the initial injury.

Assessment of the Skin and Subcutaneous Tissue

History and Clinical Findings

The history should include:
- Onset and duration of present or recent skin condition
- Related concerns (e.g., pruritus, scaling, cosmetic appearance)
- Symptom analysis
  - Timing: how long has the skin condition been present?
  - Appearance/progression
    - What did the skin condition originally look like?
    - How has it changed in appearance?
    - Is the way it looks today typical of its appearance?
    - Where did the eruption first begin?
    - Has the rash or lesion spread to other locations (pattern of spread)?
    - Has it blistered, bled, or had discharge?
    - Distribution/parts of the body not affected (e.g., face, soles, palms).
    - Does it come and go?
    - Associated systemic symptoms (e.g., fever, malaise, pain, pruritus).
- Factors that alleviate, trigger, or worsen skin symptoms
- Exposures
  - Foods, animals, plants, new substances, people with similar symptoms or illness, soaps, hair products, lotions, detergents
  - Allergies to things that could cause skin reactions
  - Medication or products (prescription and over the counter [OTC]) taken over the past few days, including creams, ointments, powders, or lotions (Note: It is

helpful to have individuals bring in medications/products they have used.)
- Historical context
  - Prior incidents of a similar skin condition
  - Recent travel
- How much is the problem affecting your life or feelings about yourself?
  The review of systems should include:
- Usual state of health and recent illnesses
- Skin, hair, and nails: Skin type (dry/oily), recent and long-term changes, previous skin condition(s)/disease(s)
- Eyes, ears, nose, and throat: Swelling, itching, crusting, discharge or circles around eyes, nasal mucus discharge, patency or irritation, dry mouth, lesions, or pain
- Chest: Wheezing, coughing, or respiratory difficulty
  The past medical history should include:
- Chronic illnesses with related dermatologic findings
- Family review of systems
  - Any family member with similar symptoms
  - Skin/atopy disorders (e.g., asthma, seasonal/drug allergies, atopic dermatitis)
  - Chronic illnesses with dermatologic findings

Physical Examination

The dermatologic examination includes a thorough look at the skin, scalp, hair, palms and soles, nails, and anogenital region. It is important to remember that the entire body, not just exposed skin, needs to be examined. Be sensitive to thermoregulation in infants and potential embarrassment in older children and adolescents. A well-lit room is essential with natural daylight being optimal. A hand lens and lighting with goose neck lamp, otoscope, or dermatoscopic head on an otoscopic handle is also effective. Portable dermatoscopic lights (Fig. 37.2) are now easily obtained and give a better view of skin structures. A glass slide gently pressed on the skin (diascopy) also allows viewing of the skin with and without capillary filling. A Wood's lamp is used to examine

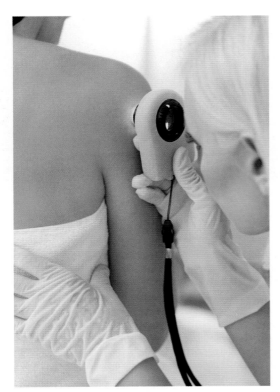

• **Fig. 37.2** Examination With a Handheld Dermascope. (Copyright Zoranm iStock.com.)

fluorescent-positive fungal infections and depigmenting skin disorders (e.g., vitiligo). Note: A Wood's lamp is no longer of use for tinea capitis examination, since the most common organism in the United States, the *Trichophyton* species, does not fluoresce.[2]

Essential documentation includes:
- Location and type of lesion
- Color/color changes, size, and shape
- Arrangement (e.g., isolated, grouped, linear, annular, zosteriform)
- Pattern (e.g., sun-exposed area, symmetry)
- Distribution (e.g., regional, generalized, crops)
- Border (e.g., indistinct, well circumscribed)
- Consistency (e.g., firm, soft, mobile)

Darker-skinned individuals vary in several ways from lighter-skinned individuals due to different genetic backgrounds and customs.
- Erythema may be difficult to see in Black patients. It typically appears more purplish (Fig. 37.3).
- Some inflammatory disorders (e.g., atopic dermatitis, pityriasis rosea) can have a follicular pattern in Black individuals.
- Darker-skinned patients have more significant postinflammatory hypo- and hyperpigmentation.
- Darker skin may burn but sunburn and chronic sun-induced diseases found in adulthood have a low incidence in Black and Hispanic patients.
- Café-au-lait spots are more common in darker-skinned individuals, but the presence of six or more should still raise a concern for neurofibromatosis.
- Dermal melanocytosis is more commonly found in those of African and Asian descent.
- Typical physiologic changes seen in darker-skinned patients:
  - Increased pigmentation in tongue and gums

- Nails with pigmented streaks
- Voigt-Futcher lines are often found in patients with darker skin. These are lines of pigmentary demarcation along lateral edges separating darker posterior surfaces and lighter anterior surfaces. This is generally more pronounced on distal extremities.[3]

Primary skin lesions (Box 37.1) arise from previously normal skin. *Secondary* skin lesions (Box 37.2) result from changes in primary skin lesions. Other useful descriptive dermatological terms are listed in Box 37.3.

Diagnostic Studies

Proper sample procurement is important. Lesions can be scraped with a metal blade. The scrapings can be obtained from the edges of skin lesions, plucked hair (getting the root is essential), the nail plate, or subungual debris. The scrapings, scales, or debris are then placed on a glass slide or in culture material. For tinea lesions, an endocervical brush or moistened swab is more effective for scales and broken hair. A surgical blade is useful for draining blisters. It is important to scrape under scabs to access organisms present. (Note: Moistening the lesion may facilitate this).

Laboratory tests can include:
- Complete blood count (CBC) and differential; C-reactive protein (CRP) or erythrocyte sedimentation rate (ESR)
- Microscopic examination of skin scrapings:
  - Potassium hydroxide (KOH) for fungal disorders (hyphae or spores; Fig. 37.4)
  - Mineral oil, dotted on lesions, may reveal scabies mites, eggs, or feces
- Wright, Giemsa, or Wright-Giemsa stains for bacteria, white cells, and multinucleated giant cells (or Tzanck cells found in viral lesions, such as herpes, varicella, or zoster)
- Microbial culture of lesions for bacteria, viruses, or fungi
- Referral for patch/skin testing for allergic/contact reactions
- Referral for skin biopsy (punch or shave method)

Management Strategies

Hydration and Lubrication

Adequate skin hydration is essential to prevent and treat skin conditions. If the skin is overhydrated, the bonds between cells at the stratum corneum loosen. If the skin is too dry, it cracks. Both involve breaking the skin barrier. Excessive (greater than 90%) or deficient (less than 10%) humidity can cause disruption of the skin. Macerated skin benefits from less humidity, while pruritic, dry skin is often relieved by increasing ambient humidity (e.g., use of vaporizer or humidifier). In hot temperatures, pruritis can be alleviated by air conditioning.

Bathing and Moisturizers

Moisturizers and lubricants treat chronic dryness and inflammation of the skin by retaining water in the skin. Bathing, by itself, does little to hydrate skin. Applying emollients or moisturizers immediately after a bath may help to retain the skin moisture and increased frequency of moisturizer use may be more beneficial in most children.[4] Regular bathing reduces scale and debris, cleanses, and eradicates causative organisms of many skin infections, including staphylococcus, which is commonly found in individuals with atopic dermatitis. Baths containing baking soda

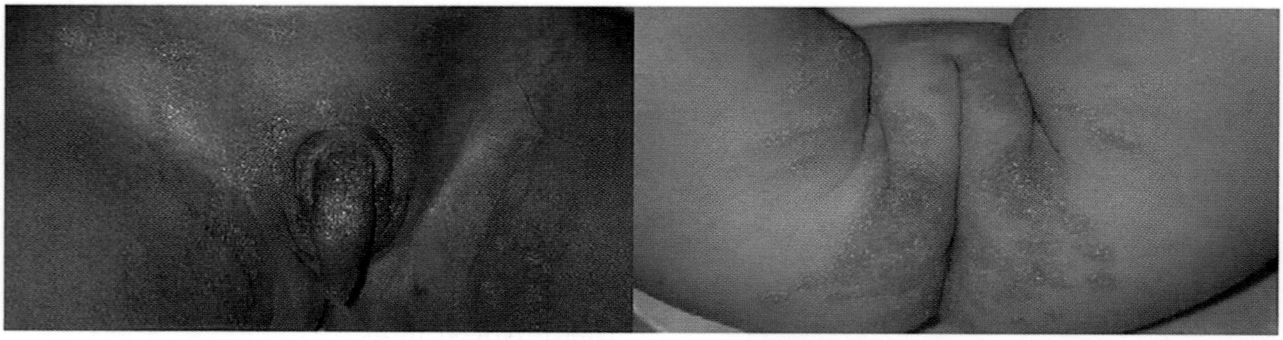

• **Fig. 37.3** Effect of Pigmentation on Erythema. Note irritant diaper dermatitis presentation in skin of different pigmentation. (From Jothishanker G, Stein S. Impact of skin color and ethnicity. *Clin Dermatol.* 2019;37[5]:418-429.)

• **BOX 37.1   Primary Skin Lesions**

Macule: Flat, nonpalpable, discolored lesion, 1 cm or smaller

Patch: Macule, >1 cm

Papule: Solid, sharply circumscribed, flat, raised lesion of varied color, ≤1 cm

Angioma or hemangioma: Papule made of blood vessels

Plaque: Solid, raised, lesion with distinct borders, >1 cm

Nodule: Firm, movable lesion in the dermis or subcutaneous fat, ≤2 cm

Tumor: Large nodule, may be firm or soft

Purpura: Red-purple macule or papule of extravasated blood, does not blanch

Ecchymosis: Hemorrhagic patch or plaque, purple to brown, varied in size and shape

Hematoma: Collection of extravasated blood larger than 1cm

Telangiectasia: Collection of macular or raised dilated capillaries

Vesicle: Blister filled with clear fluid

Bulla: Vesicle >1 cm

Wheal: Evanescent, irregularly shaped, elevated, pruritic lesion, often pale at center

Comedone: Plug of keratin and sebum in hair follicle, open (blackhead), closed (whitehead)

Cyst: Palpable lesion with definite borders filled with liquid or semisolid material

Milia: White, small cysts with epidermal keratin

• **BOX 37.2   Secondary Skin Lesions**

Scales: Dry and/or greasy fragments of epidermis

Desquamation: Peeling sheets of scale

Pustule: Raised lesion filled with pus, frequently erythematous, often in hair follicle or sweat pore

Crusts: Dried exudate of varied color from ruptured vesicles/pustules comprised of serum, dried blook, scales, and/or pus

Erosion: shallow well-defined loss of superficial epidermis

Ulcer: Deeper than erosion; open lesion extending into dermis

Excoriation: Abrasion or removal of epidermis; scratch

Fissure: Linear, wedge-shaped cracks extending into dermis

Scar: Healed lesion of connective tissue, permanent change from destruction of epidermis and dermis

Keloid: Healed lesion of hypertrophied connective tissue

Lichenification: Skin lines with visible furrows from thickening of skin from rubbing

Atrophy: Thinning skin, may appear translucent and shiny

Striae: Fine pink or silver lines in areas where skin has been stretched

---

• **BOX 37.3   Descriptive Terms for Dermatologic Lesions**

Acral: Involving extremities (hands, feet, ears, and so on)

Annular: Ring-shaped

Arcuate or arcuate: Arc-shaped configuration

Confluent: Running together

Contiguous: Touching or adjacent

Dermatomal or zosteriform: localized to a dermatome or one or more dorsal ganglia

Diffuse or generalized: Scattered, widely distributed

Discrete: Distinct and separate

Eczematous: Inflamed, dry skin with thickening oozing crust, vesicles or crusts

Grouped or clustered: Arranged in sets

Guttate: Small, drop-like

Herpetiform: Referring to grouped vesicles resembling those of herpes

Iris: Arranged in concentric circles, one inside the other

Linear: Arranged in a line

Localized: In a limited area

Multiform: More than one variety or shape of cutaneous lesion

Nummular or circinate: Coin-shaped or circular

Pedunculated: Having a stalk

Polycyclic: Oval with more than one ring

Reticular: Netlike

Serpiginous: Snakelike, creeping

Symmetric: Balanced on both sides

Target or iris: Erythematous papule or plaque characterized by a red to violet dusky center surrounded by a raised, edematous pale ring and red periphery

Telangiectatic: Referring to dilated terminal vessels

Umbilicated: Depressed or shaped like a navel

Universal: widespread affecting the entire skin

Verrucous: Wartlike

---

or colloidal oatmeal may relieve pruritus. Bathing and other heat exposures can make a rash seem worse temporarily. Nonallergic, mild soaps or soap substitutes are best. Known irritants (e.g., bubble bath solutions) should be avoided.

Other Considerations

• Common irritants and sensitizing agents (i.e., wool, sweat, saliva) should be avoided.

• Children with food allergies are more likely to experience eczematous skin manifestations than the general population.[4]

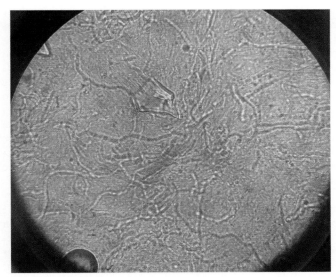

• **Fig. 37.4** Fungal Elements (Broad Septate Hyphae) as Seen on Microscopic Examination of a Potassium Hydroxide (KOH) Preparation. (From Long SS. *Principles and Practice of Pediatric Infectious Diseases.* 6th ed. Elsevier; 2023.)

Dressings

Wet Dressings

For acute oozing, crusting, or pruritis, wet dressings help dry the skin, decrease itching, and remove crusts. Thin cloths, such as diapers, handkerchiefs, or strips of sheets, make the best wet dressings. Dressings should be moderately wet but not dripping, with lukewarm water and applied for 10 to 20 minutes 2 to 4 times daily over a period of 48 to 72 hours. Alternative solutions include saline (1 teaspoon salt with 1 pint of water) or Burow's solution (1 Domeboro tablet [i.e., aluminum acetate/calcium acetate] with 1 pint of cool or tepid water). Topical medications applied following wet dressings are absorbed more effectively. Short-term (up to 10 days) topical corticosteroids under the dressing may alleviate pruritus or burning sensations. Care must be taken to prevent excessive steroidal absorption by focused application of steroid only to the affected areas.[3]

Occlusive Dressings

Occlusive dressings decrease water evaporation from the skin and enhance hydration and absorption of topical medications. Plastic wrap is placed over the affected area after hydrating the skin and/or applying cream/ointment; these dressings should not be left on longer than 8 hours. Ointments, oils, urea compounds, and propylene glycol used alone may be considered occlusive. Lichen simplex chronicus, dyshidrotic eczema, and psoriasis benefit from occlusion.

Sun Protective Agents

Sunscreen and sunblock protect the skin from UV radiation. Longer wavelengths (UVA) are only weakly phototoxic; most of the sun's damage is done by the shorter wavelength

---

• BOX 37.4 Preparations of Topical Medications

Aerosols: Mechanism of action like lotions and gels; easy dispersion over the skin; particularly useful on the scalp

Creams: Contain more water than oil and therefore are less occlusive; can be drying so better used with less dry skin, in high-humidity areas, in summertime, and on parts of body that naturally cause occlusion (body folds); often accepted better by patient but require more frequent application

Gels: Liquefy on contact and leave a uniform film on drying; alcohol-based gels can burn on application; primarily used for acne and in hairy areas

Lotions: Mixtures of powder and water, useful for drying, cooling, and soothing actions; *emulsion lotions* contain some oil, so are not as drying as lotions; lotions come in suspension or solution

Oils: Fluid fats that hold medication to the skin as barriers or occlusive agents

Ointments: Best used with dry skin; composed primarily of oil with little or no water; provide most potent concentration of medication because of their occlusive action on skin; generally, need to be used only every 12 h; fewer allergic or irritation reactions because fewer additives or preservatives are needed; tend to leave a greasy feeling; not favored by older children and adolescents; can cause heat retention from decreased evaporation

Pastes: Made of a combination of powder and oil, which makes them somewhat difficult to apply and remove, but effective in providing dryness and protection for skin, particularly diaper area

Powders: Absorb moisture and reduce friction, provide cooling, decrease itching, increase evaporation; especially useful in intertriginous areas

Shampoos: Liquid soaps or detergents for cleaning the hair and skin (e.g., tar for psoriasis or seborrhea, antifungal shampoos for tinea versicolor or tinea corporis); short contact method of therapy and more useful when longer contact is irritating

Foam: Gaseous form with one or more active substances; inert substances evaporate with body heat and active medication is left on the skin; shown to have effective drug delivery; well accepted by most patients and increasing in use

---

UVB. Both wavelengths contribute to premature skin aging, eye damage (including cataracts), skin cancers, and immune system suppression. Sunscreens are graded by their ability to provide sun protection. Because skin damage from the sun begins in childhood and is cumulative, daily application of a fragrance-free sunscreen with a sun protection factor (SPF) of 30 is recommended for individuals 6 months of age and up. Newborns and infants should be kept out of direct sun exposure.[5]

Sunscreen is never a substitute for sensible sun protection, which includes limiting exposure to intense sun rays. Other protective strategies include wearing protective clothing, hats with visors, and sunglasses with UV protection. Water resistant sunscreens should be applied 30 minutes before exposure to the sun to allow binding of the agents to the stratum corneum. Reapply sunscreens after swimming, excessive periods of perspiration, or after washing or showering.

Medications

General Considerations

Thought must be given not only to the medication, but also to its preparation vehicle (Box 37.4) including stabilizers, preservatives, and perfumes. Occasionally, an individual is sensitive to a medication vehicle or preparation, and symptoms are aggravated rather than relieved. Common agents that increase sensitization include ethylenediamine, lanolin, parabens, thimerosal, diphenhydramine, propylene glycol, topical anesthetics, and neomycin. The following guidelines for use of preparations may be helpful:

- Acute inflammation—wet dressings, powders, suspension lotions, alcohol- or water-based lotions, aerosols, or foams
- Chronic inflammation—creams, oil-based lotions or gels, ointments, or foams
- Individual's tolerance for and willingness to use certain vehicles
- Individual's environment (dry or humid)

All topical medications, except powders, have enhanced absorption if applied to skin immediately after it has been saturated with water. Occlusion enhances absorption (see previous discussion). Application of the topical medication is best done in one direction, preferably along the hair follicles, without rubbing, applied with a single motion. Use an adequate, but not excessive amount.

Antibacterial Agents

Soap and topical antiseptics thoroughly cleanse the skin and reduce the number of bacteria on the skin. Topical antibiotics are applied to treat minor skin infections. Antibacterial agents are either bacteriostatic (e.g., erythromycin, clindamycin), which inhibit growth and replication of bacteria or bactericidal (e.g., bacitracin, polymyxin B), which kill bacteria directly. When possible and practical, a culture should be obtained before starting therapy.[6] Products containing neomycin should be avoided because of the high incidence of contact sensitization. Oral antibiotics may be necessary to treat more significant bacterial skin infections. If methicillin-resistant *Staphylococcus aureus* (MRSA) is suspected, obtain a culture and sensitivity of the drainage (see Chapter 35).

Antifungal Agents

Many topical antifungals are OTC medications. Oral antifungals are used for hair and nail infections or refractory skin infections. Because of concerning side effects and minimal clinical experience in children, oral antifungals should be used with caution in children; many of these drugs are not US Food and Drug Administration (FDA) approved for pediatric use

Antiviral Agents

Topical antivirals are used to control cutaneous herpes infections. Oral antivirals, such as acyclovir, can shorten the course of the infection and can be used in children with acute or recurrent herpetic skin infections.

Wart therapy agents destroy keratinocytes. These agents include salicylic acid and lactic acid collodion, salicylic plaster, salicylic solution, liquid nitrogen, cantharidin, podophyllum, and trichloroacetic acid.

Antiinflammatory Agents

Topical glucocorticoids are the most commonly prescribed antiinflammatory agents. They are also used to decrease pruritis and promote vasoconstriction. They are subdivided into three categories: high potency (Class I–II), moderate potency (Class III–V), and low potency (Class VI–VII) and classified as fluorinated or nonfluorinated. Nonfluorinated steroids are less potent and have fewer side effects. The key to topical steroids is to be familiar with a few low-, medium-, and high-potency steroids and use them consistently. Note: It is important to note that %'s listed do NOT reflect the product's strength (e.g., a 0.01% Class I topical steroid is far more potent than a 3% Class VII steroid. Ointments are more potent than creams, creams are more potent than lotions, and foams are more effective in hairy areas. Absorption is enhanced in areas that are traumatized or denuded (Table 37.1).

Primary care providers (PCPs) should use the lowest potency available, use them sparingly, and for the shortest length of time possible. Further, only low-potency steroids should be used on the face, buttocks, groin, and axillae. High-potency topical steroid preparations are rarely used in pediatrics. See Table 37.2 for suggested strengths of topical steroids when initiating treatment. Potential side effects of prolonged topical steroid use include skin atrophy, striae, increased fragility of the skin, hypopigmentation, secondary infection, acneiform eruption, folliculitis, miliaria, hypertrichosis, telangiectasia, and purpura. Oral glucocorticoids (e.g., prednisone) are used only in acute situations and are limited to short courses.[7] Intralesional steroid injections may be used by dermatology to control localized eczema, lichen planus, or psoriasis.

Antipruritic Agents

Topical antihistamines, especially diphenhydramine HCl and topical anesthetic medications, should be used with caution because of burning and/or stinging. Oral antihistamines are frequently used to relieve itching. Nonsedating antihistamines (e.g., hydroxyzine, cetirizine, fexofenadine) have the added benefit of helping in patients with an allergic component. Sedating antihistamines (e.g., diphenhydramine HCL) may be more effective at night to control pruritis and improve sleep.[7]

Immunomodulators

This class of immunosuppressive, nonsteroidal antiinflammatory topical medication is used for short- or intermittent long-term treatment of atopic dermatitis and pruritis when conventional therapy is inadvisable, ineffective, or not tolerated. They do not cause atrophy or hypopigmentation but commonly cause burning and itching. Immunomodulators are expensive, are pregnancy category C, and cannot be used in young children under age 2 years.

Scabicides and Pediculicides

These agents are toxic to mites and lice. Spinosad, permethrin, and malathion are used in children but should be used with precise instructions on application due to potential toxicity. Lindane is no longer recommended for use in any child as there are safer medications available to treat these conditions.

Hair and Scalp Preparations

Antimicrobial, tar, keratolytic, and detergent shampoos are used on the hair and scalp when needed for infection, psoriasis, dandruff, dermatitis, or general cleansing.

TABLE 37.1	Potency of Topical Corticosteroids	

Potency/Strength	Generic Name	Trade Name
1. High potency ↑↑↑↑	Betamethasone dipropionate augmented 0.05%	Diprolene O/L/G
	Clobetasol proprionate 0.05%	Clobex L/S/Sp, Cormax O/S, Olux F, Olux-E F, Temovate C/O/G/S, Temovate-E C,
	Halobetasol propionate 0.05%	Ultravate C/O
	Fluocinonide 0.1%	Vanos C
	Flurandrenolide 4mcg/cm^2	Cordran tape
	Diflorasone diacetate 0.05% O	
2. ↑↑↑	Amcinonide 0.1% O	
	Betamethasone dipropionate 0.05%	Diprolene AF C, Diprolene C
	Diflorasone diacetate 0.05%	ApexiCon E C
	Halcinonide 0.1%	Halog C/O
	Fluocinonide 0.05% C/O/G/S	
	Desoximetasone 0.25%	Topicort EC/O
	Desoximetasone 0.05%	Topicort G
	Mometasone furoate 0.1%	Elocon C/O/L
	Triamcinolone acetonide 0.5% O	
3. ↑↑	Fluticasone proprionate 0.05%	Cutivate C/L
	Fluticasone proprionate 0.005%	Cutivate O
	Betamethasone valerate 0.1% C/O/L	
	Betamethasone valerate 0.12%	Luxiq F
	Amcinonide 0.1% C/O/L	
	Triamcinolone acetonide 0.1% C/O/L	
	Triamcinolone acetonide 0.5% C	
	Desoximetasone 0.05% C	
	Fluradrenolide 0.05%	Cordran C/L
4. ↑	Fluradrenolide 0.025%	Cordran C
	Triamcinolone acetonide 0.1%	Kenalog C
	Triamcinolone acetonide 0.2%	Kenalog Sp
	Desoximetasone 0.05% C	
	Fluocinolone acetonide 0.025%	Synalar O
	Hydrocortisone valerate 0.2% O	
	Mometasone furoate 0.1%	Elocon C/L
5. ↓↑	Fluocinolone acetonide 0.025%	Synalar C
	Clocortolone pivalate 0.01%	Cloderm C
	Hydrocortisone valerate 0.2% C	
	Hydrocortisone butyrate 0.1%	Locoid C/O/L/S
	Hydrocortisone probutate 0.1%	Pandel C
	Prednicarbate 0.1%	Dermatop O/C
	Traimcinolone acetonide 0.1% L	
6. ↓↓	Desonide 0.05%	Verdeso F, Desowen O/L, Desonide G, Tridesilon C
	Hydrocortisone 2.5% C/O/L	
	Fluocinolone acetonide 0.01%	Dermotic Oil, Synalar S, Derma-Smooth/FS oil
	Alclometasone dipropionate 0.05% C/O	
7. ↓↓↓	Triamcinolone acetonide 0.025% C	
	Hydrocortisone 1.0% C/O	
8. Low potency	Hydrocortisone 0.5% C	

Delivery modes: *C,* cream; *EC,* emollient cream; *L,* lotion; *O,* ointment; *G,* gel; , solution; *Sp,* spray; *F,* foam.
From Cohen BA. *Pediatric Dermatology,* ed 4. Elsevier; 2013:11; Bolognia JL, Schaffer JV, Duncan KO, Ko CJ. *Dermatology Essentials.* Elsevier; 2014:985; Paller, AS, Mancini, AJ. *Hurwitz Clinical Pediatric Dermatology,* ed 5. Elsevier; 2016:51; and Karch AM. *Lippincott nursing drug guide.* Wolters Kluwer Health; 2015.

<table>
<tr><td>TABLE 37.2</td><td colspan="3">Suggested Strength of Topical Steroids to Initiate Treatment in Selected Diseases</td></tr>
</table>

Class I–II	Class III–V	Class VI–VII
Psoriasis	Atopic dermatitis	Dermatitis (eyelids)
Lichen planus	Nummular eczema	Dermatitis (diaper area)
Severe hand eczema	Seborrheic dermatitis	Mild dermatitis (face)
Poison ivy (severe)	Intertrigo (brief course)	Mild anal inflammation
Hyperkeratotic eczema	Tinea (brief to control inflammation)	Mild intertrigo
Chapped feet	Scabies (after scabicide)	
Nummular eczema (severe)		
Alopecia areata		

From Dinulos JGH. *Habif's Clinical Dermatology: A Color Guide to Diagnosis and Therapy.* 2nd ed. Elsevier; 2021.

Bacterial Infections of the Skin and Subcutaneous Tissue

Diagnosis and treatment of common bacterial infections are listed in Table 37.3.

Impetigo

Impetigo is a very common pediatric bacterial infection of the superficial layers of the skin. Primary impetigo is from a direct bacterial infection of previously normal skin and secondary is where an infection occurs due to a break in the skin, such as eczema. It has two classifications: the more common nonbullous, with honey-colored crusts on superficial lesions, and bullous, with larger bullae or blisters that can continue to develop for days (Fig. 37.5). Impetigo is typically caused by *S. aureus* or *Streptococcus pyogenes* with *S. aureus* being a much more common pathogen. Bullous and secondary lesions are almost always *S. aureus.*[7]

Impetigo bacterial strains are highly contagious, and colonization of the skin often occurs several days to months before lesions

TABLE 37.3 Diagnosis and Treatment of Common Bacterial Infections

	Causative Organism	Presentation	Area of Involvement	Treatment	Prevention
Impetigo	*Staphylococcus aureus* or *Streptococcus pyogenes*	Honey-colored crust on erythematous base, or blisters that rupture, leaving varnish-like coat	Superficial layers of skin (epidermis)	Topical antibiotic if minor; oral antibiotics (amoxicillin/clavulanate, cephalexin, dicloxacillin, cloxacillin, or clindamycin) if more significant infection	Moisturize skin; thoroughly cleanse any break in skin
Cellulitis	Most commonly group A beta-hemolytic streptococcus or *S. aureus*	Erythema, swelling, tenderness; irregular borders with significant induration	Dermis and subcutaneous tissue	Oral antibiotic depending on likely organism; amoxicillin clavulanate, cephalexin, or clindamycin	Same as above
Folliculitis, furuncle, carbuncle	Noninfectious; most common is *S. aureus, P. aeruginosa*	Pruritus, erythematous papule or pustule at hair follicle; deeper with furuncle; multiple with carbuncle	Hair follicle; swimming suit area if associated with hot tub use	Warm compresses, topical keratolytics, topical antibiotics, or antistaphylococcal antibiotic if severe; treat for *Pseudomonas* if associated with hot tub use	Same as above; good hygiene and antibacterial soap; keep hot tub maintained well
Paronychia	*S. aureus, Streptococcus,* or *Pseudomonas; Candida* if chronic	Tenderness, drainage	Nailfold	Warm water soaks, drainage, oral antistaphylococcal antibiotics if severe	Appropriate nail hygiene; prevent persistent moist environment

Data from Paller AS, Mancini AJ. *Hurwitz Clinical Pediatric Dermatology: A Textbook of Skin Disorders of Children and Adolescence.* 6th ed. Elsevier; 2022; and Cohen BA, editor. *Pediatric Dermatology.* 5th ed. Elsevier; 2022.

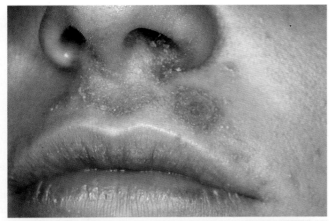
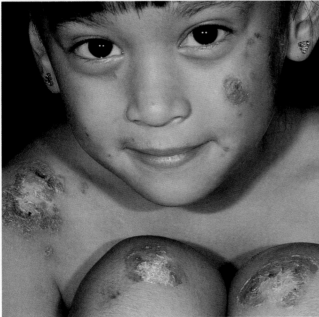

• **Fig. 37.5** (A) Nonbullous Impetigo. (B) Bullous Impetigo. (From Dinulos JGH. *Habif's Clinical Dermatology: A Color Guide to Diagnosis and Therapy.* 7th ed. Elsevier; 2021.)

appear; the organism usually spreads from autoinoculation via hands, towels, clothing, nasal discharge, or droplets. Impetigo occurs more frequently with poor hygiene; during the summer months; in warm, humid climates; and in lower socioeconomic groups. Most impetigo will resolve spontaneously in 2 to 3 weeks with no treatment. Lesions heal with hyperpigmentation in Black patients. Streptococci that cause pharyngitis rarely cause impetigo and vice versa. Poststreptococcal glomerulonephritis is a rare complication of certain strains of *S. pyogenes,* but treatment of impetigo probably does not prevent this sequela.[7]

Clinical Findings

History
- Pruritus, spread of the lesion to surrounding skin, and earlier skin disruption at the site.

- Systemic symptoms are infrequent.
  Physical Examination. The following can be found:
- Nonbullous impetigo—begins as 1- to 2-mm very thin vesicles that rupture, leaving moist, honey-colored, crusty lesions on mildly erythematous, eroded skin; less than 2 cm in size; little pain but rapid spread.
- Bullous impetigo—vesicle that quickly evolves to bullae that rupture, leaving thin varnish-like coating or scale; periphery may form fluid-filled rim that eventually forms a scaling border; center of lesion moist erythematous base that oozes serum.
- Lesions are most common on face, hands, neck, extremities, or perineum; satellite lesions may be found near the primary site, although they can be anywhere on the body.
- Regional lymphadenopathy.
  Diagnostic Studies. Gram stain and culture are ordered if identification of the organism is needed in recalcitrant or severe cases.

Differential Diagnosis

Herpes simplex, varicella, nummular eczema, contact dermatitis, tinea, kerion, and scabies are included in the differential diagnoses.

Management

Management involves the following:
- Topical antibiotics are preferred if the impetigo is superficial, nonbullous, or localized to a limited area. Mupirocin (3 times/day) and retapamulin (2 times/day) are considered best choices for topical treatment. Removal of crust before application of antibiotic is important. Treatment of a local lesion does not treat evolving lesions at another site.
- Oral antibiotics are recommended for multiple lesions or nonbullous impetigo, infection in multiple family members, childcare groups, or athletes. Use an antibiotic that is active against β-lactamase–producing strains of *S. aureus* and treat for 7 to 10 days.[7]
  - Cephalexin
  - Amoxicillin/clavulanate
  - Dicloxacillin
  - Clindamycin (choice for penicillin-allergic patients)
- Severe disease and/or infants with bullous impetigo: use parenteral beta-lactamase–resistant antistaphylococcal penicillin, such as methicillin, oxacillin, or nafcillin.
- If there is no response in 7 days, swab beneath the crust, and obtain Gram stain, culture, and sensitivities. Community-acquired MRSA should be considered. This organism is more susceptible to clindamycin and trimethoprim-sulfamethoxazole (TMP-SMX) (see Chapter 35).
- Educate regarding cleanliness, hand washing, and spread of disease.
  - Washing the affected area with antibacterial soap twice a day may be helpful.
  - Washing the entire body with antibacterial soap daily during treatment may prevent spread of infection.
- Exclude from day care or school until treated for 24 hours.
- Schedule a follow-up appointment in 48 to 72 hours if not improved.

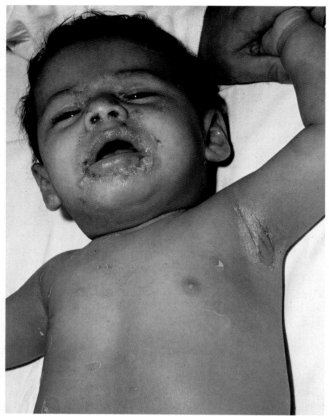

• **Fig. 37.6** Staphyloccocal Scalded Skin Syndrome. (From Dinulos JGH. *Habif's Clinical Dermatology: a Color Guide to Diagnosis and Therapy.* 7th ed. Elsevier; 2021.)

Complications

- Cellulitis, an infection of the subcutaneous tissue, may occur with nonbullous impetigo and present in the form of *erysipelas* (i.e., infection involving the dermis only). Lymphangitis, suppurative lymphadenitis, guttate psoriasis, erythema multiforme, scarlet fever/scarlatina, or glomerulonephritis may occur following infection with some strains of *Streptococcus.* Acute rheumatic fever is a rare complication of streptococcal skin infections.
- Staphylococcal scalded skin syndrome (SSSS), or Ritter disease, is a blistering disease that results from circulating epidermolytic toxin–producing *S. aureus.* It is most common in neonates, infants, and children younger than 5 years. It manifests abruptly with fever, malaise, lethargy, poor feeding, and tender erythroderma, especially in the neck folds, conjunctivae, throat, and nares. A sandpaper-like rash, similar to scarlet fever, is common. Nikolsky sign (i.e., peeling of skin with a light rub to reveal a moist red surface) is a key finding (Fig. 37.6). Children under 5 years are at the highest risk for the disease; treatment may include hospitalization and parenteral antibiotics. Antibiotics of choice are intravenous (IV) or oral dicloxacillin, a penicillinase-resistant penicillin, first- or second-generation cephalosporins, or clindamycin. Corticosteroids are contraindicated because of immune system suppression. Quicker healing without scarring results with minimal handling of the skin, and ointments and topical mupirocin at the infection site.[7] Severe cases may need treatment similar to extensive burn care.

Patient and Family Education

- Thorough cleansing and use of triple antibiotic ointment for any breaks in the skin helps prevent impetigo.
- Keep skin moisturized to prevent any breaks in the skin.
- Postinflammatory pigment changes can last weeks to months.
- The individual should not return to school or day care until 24 hours of antibiotic treatment is completed.

Cellulitis

Cellulitis is a localized bacterial infection involving the dermis and subcutaneous layers of the skin. It is commonly seen following a disruption of the skin surface such as an insect or animal bite, trauma, tinea, or a penetrating wound. Cellulitis is more common in children with diabetes and immunosuppression (see Chapter 39).

In children, cellulitis is often periorbital, perivaginal, perianal, buccal, or it involves a joint or an extremity. *S. aureus* and *group A beta-hemolytic streptococcal* (GABHS) are the most common causes. Buccal cellulitis, limited to infants, is almost always caused by *Haemophilus influenzae* but the incidence has decreased since the introduction of the *H. influenza* vaccine.[8] Erysipelas, a superficial (dermis and epidermis) variant of cellulitis typically has systemic symptoms before appearance of skin lesions and is most often associated with *S. pyogenes* or other β-hemolytic streptococci. MRSA associated cellulitis often has pus accumulation. Rarely, other aerobic, anaerobic, and fungal organisms can cause cellulitis in immunocompromised individuals.

Clinical Findings

History

- Chronic skin conditions or previous skin disruption at the site. Note that edema that occurs within 24 hours of an insect bite is most likely to be inflammatory, whereas edema that occurs between 48 and 72 hours is more likely to be infectious.
- Fever, pain, malaise, irritability, anorexia, vomiting, and chills can be reported.
- Recent sore throat or upper respiratory infection.
- Anal pruritus, stool retention, constipation, and blood-streaked stools.

Physical Examination

- Erythematous, indurated, tender, swollen, warm areas of skin with poorly demarcated borders.
- Buccal cellulitis often appears with a blue to purple tinge and is rarely associated with *H. influenza.*
- Regional lymphadenopathy.
- Infants and young children may present with well-demarcated perianal erythema up to 2 cm around the anus; vulvovaginitis is common in females and balanoposthitis in males.
- Erysipelas presents with rapidly advancing lesions that are painful, bright red, have sharp margins and an "orange peel" look and feel.

Diagnostic Studies. Most cellulitis cases are treated empirically. CBC and blood culture are done if the child is febrile, appears ill or toxic, or is younger than 1 year. Leukocytosis is common. Positive blood cultures are less common. Perform Gram stain and culture of the erythematous area if unusual organisms are suspected, pus is present (more typical of MRSA), or the individual looks toxic. An aspirate at the point of maximum inflammation is more likely to yield a causative organism than one taken from the leading edge, although the bacterial counts tend to be low with either method.[4]

Differential Diagnosis

Pressure erythema, giant urticaria, contact dermatitis, popsicle panniculitis (reaction to cold exposure), early erythema nodosum, subcutaneous fat necrosis, herpetic whitlow, and diaper dermatitis are included in the differential diagnoses.

Management

Immediate antibiotic therapy is required.

- Hospitalization is recommended if the child is a neonate or febrile infant, is acutely ill or toxic, or has facial/periorbital cellulitis.
  - Infants younger than 3 months with cellulitis require a full septic workup and initiation of empiric therapy with parenteral antibiotics.[3]
- Antibiotic therapy
  - As noted earlier, prompt administration of antibiotics is essential.
  - Empiric coverage for GABHS and *S. aureus* appropriate in most routine cases, except facial involvement. If concerned about high community rates, ensure coverage against MRSA:
    - Cephalexin
    - Dicloxacillin
    - Penicillin VK
    - Amoxicillin/clavulanate
    - Trimethoprim-sulfamethoxazole (more effective against MRSA)
    - Clindamycin (for serious infections and/or more effective against MRSA)
- Follow up in 24 hours to assess response and observe toxicity. Continue daily visits until child is recovering. Counsel parents to call the PCP immediately or return for an urgent visit if the infection is not improving or is getting worse.

Complications

Recurrent perianal streptococcal infection, septicemia, necrotizing fasciitis, and toxic shock syndrome (TSS) are possible complications, and all require immediate referral for care and hospitalization.

- Necrotizing fasciitis is not common in children and while most often associated with GABHS, may be polymicrobial in nature. This disease, commonly referred to as *flesh-eating strep* or *gangrene,* is an acute, rapidly progressing necrotic invasion through the skin and subcutaneous tissue to the fascial compartments. It is more common in individuals with decreased local resistance (i.e., surgery, varicella), malnutrition, or chronic disease. Necrotizing fasciitis begins as cellulitis (usually on the leg or abdomen in infants) with severe pain, edema, fever, and bullae on an erythematous surface. It quickly progresses to ulcer, eschar and gangrene, shock, and altered mental status within 2 days. Prompt treatment may be lifesaving with hospitalization, surgical debridement, and fluid management, IV antibiotic treatment, and, in cases of GABHS, intravenous immunoglobulin (IVIG). The overall mortality rate is reported to be about 25% (Fig. 37.7).[3]
- TSS is an acute febrile illness with rapid onset that causes significant fever, vomiting and diarrhea, engorged mucous membranes, hypotension, a diffuse macular or sunburn-like rash, conjunctival injection, and multiple organ system involvement. *S. aureus* or *S. pyogenes* (group A streptococci) are the causative agents associated with TSS, and incubation can be as little as 14 hours. Both organisms can be associated with

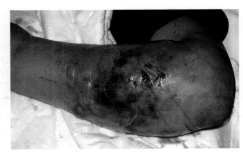

• **Fig. 37.7** Necrotizing Fasciitis. (Courtesy Luis Requena, MD. From Bolognia JL, Schaffer JV, Duncan KO, et al. *Dermatology Essentials.* 2nd ed. Elsevier; 2022.)

invasive infection (e.g., pneumonia, osteomyelitis, bacteremia, or endocarditis) or focal tissue invasion that is rapidly progressive. Initially recognized in menstruating adolescents, but now found in all ages, particularly under 2 years, and often associated with varicella, surgical packing, and cutaneous infections. Treatment is intensive, requires hospitalization, and consists of fluid management, antibiotics, and other supportive measures. The mortality rate of all TSS in patients 0 to 18 years is 5% to 10%.[9] It is a reportable disease in all states (Fig. 37.8).

Patient and Family Education

- Thoroughly cleanse any break in the skin to help prevent cellulitis.
- Keep bites, scrapes, and rashes clean and bandaged until healed to prevent them from being infected by staphylococcal bacteria.
- Frequent hand washing is essential.
- Immunize against *H. influenzae.*
- Perianal spread can occur through shared bath water.
- See Chapter 35 regarding treatment of children and families with MRSA infection.

Folliculitis, Furuncle, and Carbuncle

A superficial bacterial inflammation of the hair follicle is called *folliculitis;* an abscess involving a hair follicle is called a *furuncle* (i.e., boil). A *carbuncle* involves multiple, adjacent follicles.

Obstruction and damage (acne, waxing, shaving) of the follicular orifice is the most important factor contributing to the development of folliculitis, but a moist environment, maceration, poor hygiene, occlusive emollients, and prolonged submersion in contaminated water are also factors. Noninfectious folliculitis is most common, but *S. aureus* is the common causative organism, and this is the most common presentation of MRSA. Irritant folliculitis may follow a topical medication or rubbing of thighs with jeans. *Pseudomonas aeruginosa* may be found with hot-tub folliculitis (Fig. 37.9). Gram-negative organisms are often associated with acne and significantly oily skin.

Clinical Findings

History

- Pruritus with folliculitis; tenderness with furuncle
- Hot-tub exposure
- Irritating surface agent
- Occasional fever, malaise, or lymphadenopathy

Physical Examination. The individual is often asymptomatic, but the following can be seen:

- Discrete, erythematous 1- to 2-mm papules or white/creamy pustules on an inflamed base centered around a hair follicle

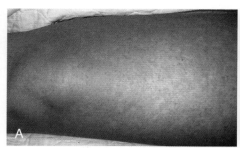
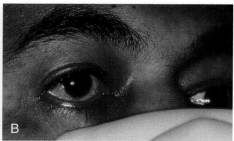

• **Fig. 37.8** Toxic Shock Syndrome. (A) Blotchy erythema on thigh. (B) Hyperemia of the conjunctiva. (From Bolognia JL, Schaffer JV, Duncan KO, et al. *Dermatology Essentials.* 2nd ed. Elsevier; 2022.)

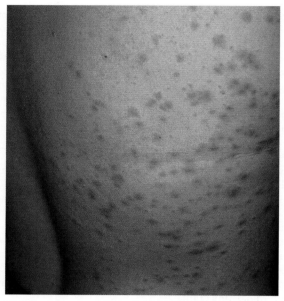

• **Fig. 37.9** Pseudomonas "Hot Tub" Folliculitis. (From Bolognia JL, Schaffer JV, Duncan KO, et al. *Dermatology Essentials.* 2nd ed. Elsevier; 2022.)

- Involvement of face, scalp, extremities (typically thighs and upper arms), buttocks, and back
- Nodules with larger areas of erythema and tenderness (furuncle)
- Pruritic papules, pustules, or deep red to purple nodules, most dense in areas covered by swimsuit 8 to 48 hours after exposure (e.g., hot-tub folliculitis)
- Systemic symptoms not common

Diagnostic Studies. Gram stain and culture are occasionally ordered. In the case of persistent or difficult-to-treat folliculitis, consider the possibility of MRSA.

Differential Diagnosis

Cellulitis, *Candida* infection, tinea infection, acne vulgaris, rosacea, and chemical folliculitis constitute the differential diagnoses.

Management

The following steps are taken:
- Warm compresses after washing with soap and water several times a day.
- Weekly to twice weekly benzoyl peroxide (BP), chlorhexidine, or bleach baths.

- Topical keratolytics, such as BP 5% to 10% twice/day for 5 days, especially if chronic or recurrent.
- Fluctuant lesions should be incised and drained, which may be sufficient for many lesions.
- For bacterial lesions:
  - If lesion is superficial, topical antibiotic, such as mupiricin or clindamycin, twice a day for 10 to 14 days.
  - Antistaphylococcal β-lactamase–resistant antibiotics, such as dicloxacillin or cephalexin in severe or widespread cases.
- For "hot-tub" folliculitis:
  - In general, self-limiting in immunocompetent patients.
  - May need oral quinolone for severe cases.
  - Keep hot tub well maintained.
- Review of personal hygiene habits; avoid shaving until resolved.
- Follow-up treatment in 1 week for folliculitis, in 1 day for furuncle or abscess, which may need incision and drainage.
- Identify and eliminate predisposing factors.
- If recurrent, look for nasal or skin carrier state of gram-positive organisms.

Complications

Deep abscess formation or carbuncles can occur. *Sycosis barbae* occurs on the chin, upper lip, and jaw, especially in adolescent Black males.

Patient and Family Education

Good personal hygiene and an antibacterial soap minimize spread to other household members. Hot-tub folliculitis resolves in 5 to 14 days but can recur up to 3 months after exposure.

Paronychia

Paronychia is a chronic or acute inflammation and infection around a fingernail or toenail (Fig. 37.10). It is a common disorder in childhood and adolescence caused by bacteria (often *S. aureus,* occasionally *Streptococcus* or *Pseudomonas*), *Candida* (in infants with thrush or thumb sucking or when hands are frequently immersed in water), or herpes. It is more common with tight shoes, or when nails are misaligned or cut too short or with rounded edges.

Clinical Findings

History. Tenderness, drainage, and discomfort (especially with walking) are reported.

Physical Examination
- Proximal nailfold is erythematous, swollen, and tender; if chronic, may not be tender
- Purulent exudate expressed

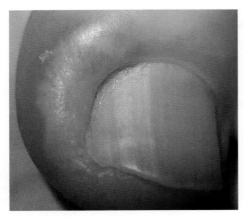

• **Fig. 37.10** Paronychia. (From Bolognia JL, Schaffer JV, Duncan KO, et al. *Dermatology Essentials*. 2nd ed. Elsevier; 2022.)

- Cuticle broken or absent in chronic condition
- Nontender erythema and edema with thickened, disrupted nail (*Candida* infection, often with secondary bacterial infection)

Diagnostic Studies. A culture of the exudate is occasionally done.

Differential Diagnosis

Herpetic whitlow (i.e., grouped vesicles on an erythematous base) and eczematous inflammation should be ruled out.

Management

Management includes the following:
- Frequent warm soaks, after which cotton pledgets are inserted beneath the nail to lift it.
- Systemic oral antibiotic if acute infection; coverage for staphylococcal infection should be considered.
- In *Candida* cases, antifungals rarely lead to a cure. Topical corticosteroids can decrease the inflammation and allow for tissue repair.
- If purulent exudate is present, loosen cuticle from nail with a No. 11 blade or 22- to 24-gauge needle to allow exudate to escape.
- If condition is recurrent, refer for surgical removal of lateral portion of nail.
- Do a follow-up visit in 1 month, as recurrent infection is possible.

Complications

Acute paronychia typically resolves easily but can become chronic if proper nail care is not followed or hands are not protected in a chronically moist environment. Rarely, long-term antibiotic therapy is needed. Horizontal ridges may appear at the base of the nail in chronic paronychia. Deep tissue infections and cellulitis are rare.

Patient Education

- Instruction on proper trimming of nails and care of toenails:
  - Wear wide-toed shoes.
  - Trim nails straight across and not too short.
- If condition is chronic and associated with hands frequently in water, wear cotton gloves under rubber/plastic gloves to keep hands dry.

Fungal Infections of the Skin

Diagnosis and treatment of common fungal infections are listed in (Table 37.4).

Candidiasis (Moniliasis)

Candidiasis is a fungal infection of the skin or mucous membranes commonly called a *yeast infection* or *thrush*. See Chapter 43 for discussion of vaginal candidiasis.

Candida albicans, a yeast-like fungus, is commonly found on skin and oral, vaginal, and intestinal mucosal tissue. Although *Candida* is part of the normal flora, overgrowth and penetration of inflamed skin or mucous membranes can occur with chronic moisture, an impaired immune response (e.g., diabetics, immunocompromised), or the use of antibiotics, steroids, or contraceptives. Oral candidiasis is common in otherwise healthy newborns and infants. Systemic infection with candidiasis is not discussed in this text.

Clinical Findings

History. The history often includes:
- Antibiotic, steroid, or inhaled corticosteroid use over the previous weeks
- Occurrence of a rash in a moist, warm area such as the diaper area
- Maternal yeast infection in the breastfeeding infant
- Rash is often pruritic

Physical Examination
- Mouth—friable, adherent white plaques resembling cottage cheese on an erythematous base on the mucous membranes (i.e., thrush); cracked lips (i.e., cheilitis); fissured and inflamed corners of the mouth (i.e., angular cheilitis) (Fig. 37.11).
- *Intertrigo*—involvement of skin folds (e.g., neck, axillae, abdominal creases, interdigital spaces, flexural folds, or groin) displaying as bright erythema in the folds (Fig. 37.12).
- Diaper area—moist, beefy-red macules and papules on sharply marked borders with satellite lesions; erosions may also be present (Fig. 37.13).
- Vulvovaginal area—thick, cheesy, yellow discharge; erythema; edema; and itching
- *Balanitis*—erythematous and scaly patches on penis. Papules and vesicles might also be present.
- Nail plates—transverse ridging of the nail plate, loss of cuticle, and mild proximal lateral periungual erythema (chronic paronychia)

Diagnostic Studies. If treatment failure or questionable diagnosis occurs, KOH-treated scrapings of satellite lesions or mucosa reveal yeast cells and pseudohyphae.

Differential Diagnosis

The differential diagnoses include erythema toxicum, miliaria, staphylococcal infection, neonatal herpes simplex, psoriasis, seborrheic dermatitis, and congenital syphilis.

Management

The following steps are taken:
- Thrush
  - Infants: Oral nystatin suspension by dropper in each cheek 4 times/day 1 to 2 days after white adherent patches are gone. If breastfeeding, the mother should put the solution on her nipples to eliminate reinfection. A second course is

TABLE 37.4	Diagnosis, Treatment, and Prevention of Common Fungal Infections				
Infection	**Causative Organism**	**Presentation**	**Area of Involvement**	**Treatment**	**Prevention**
Candidiasis, thrush	*Candida albicans*	Moist, bright-red rash with sharp borders, satellite lesions; white plaques in mouth, tongue, mucous membranes	Mouth, diaper area, intertrigal folds	Topical or oral antifungal, generally nystatin	Diaper area hygiene
Tinea capitis	*Trichophyton tonsurans, Microsporum canis*	Different presentations with hair loss and breakage, scaly lesions, pustular lesions and/or kerions	Scalp and hair shaft	Oral antifungals for extensive time; topicals are ineffective	Avoiding contaminated contacts; good grooming practices (frequent shampooing, no tight hair traction, minimize greasy pomades)
Tinea corporis	*Trichophyton mentagrophytes, Trichophyton rubrum, Microsporum canis*	Pruritic, slightly erythematous circular lesion with a slightly raised border and central clearing; well demarcated	Skin other than scalp, palms, soles, groin	Topical antifungals; identify and treat source; exclude from day care until treated for 24 hours; use oral medications for resistant cases	Identify and treat contacts; avoid chronic moist environment
Tinea cruris	*Epidermophyton floccosum, T. rubrum, T. mentagrophytes*	Erythematous, sharply marginated plaques, raised border of scaling lesions or pustules	Groin, upper thighs, perianal area	Same as for tinea corporis; loose clothes, absorbent medicated powder	Avoid tight, chafing clothing; keep area dry, especially in hot, humid weather
Tinea pedis	*T. rubrum, T. mentagrophytes*	Vesicles and erosions; fissure between toes with scaling and erythema; onychomycosis	Instep and sides of foot; between toes; toenails	Same as for tinea corporis; absorbent medicated powder	Cotton socks; open-toed shoes; keep feet dry; protect from contaminated surfaces (showers, locker rooms) moisturize feet to avoid splitting and cracking
Tinea versicolor	*Malassezia furfur fungus*	Multiple scaly, discrete oval macules in guttate or raindrop pattern; hypopigmented to hyperpigmented areas; fail to tan in summer	Trunk, upper extremities, face	Selenium shampoo; ketoconazole shampoo; oral itraconazole or fluconazole for severe or recurrent disease (use with caution)	Repeat treatments as prophylaxis for recurrence (recurrence is common)
Onychomycosis (tinea unguium)	*T. rubrum, T. tonsurans, Candida*	Opaque white or silvery nail that becomes thick and yellow	Finger and toenails; feet are more common in pediatrics	Topical ciclopirox if over 12 years; oral antifungals for extended time; monitor liver function tests	Antifungal foot powders, frequent nail clipping, breathing socks and shoes; foot protection in common areas e.g., locker rooms

sometimes needed to clear the infection. If resistant to treatment, oral fluconazole.[3]
- Children: Cheilitis, and angular cheilitis: nystatin or clotrimazole troche.
- Cutaneous
  - Topical antifungals (e.g., nystatin, miconazole, clotrimazole, ketoconazole, ciclopirox, econazole) applied to skin at every diaper change until the rash is gone plus an additional 1 to 2 days.[3] Avoid antifungal/corticosteroid combination medications.
  - If inflammation is severe, 1% hydrocortisone can be applied simultaneously to the diaper area for 1 to 2 days.

- Keep area dry and cool. Minimize skin irritation:
  - Discontinue oral antibiotics and steroids when possible.
  - Educate about avoiding underlying predisposing factors (e.g., lip licking).
  - Add topical or oral antibiotic if secondary infection is suspected.
- Nail involvement (i.e., chronic paronychia) can be treated with topical application of antifungal cream twice daily, but it will take several months for the nail plate to grow out normally; oral fluconazole may be needed for severe or resistant involvement.

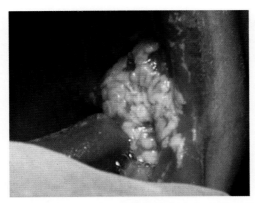

• **Fig. 37.11** Oral Candidiasis. (From Zitelli BJ, McIntire S, Nowalk AJ, et al. (Eds). *Zitelli and Davis' Atlas of Pediatric Physical Diagnosis*. 8th ed. Elsevier; 2023.)

Complications

Chronic mucocutaneous candidiasis resulting from immunologic deficit can occur and is heralded by widespread involvement (e.g., oral, skin, nails). Paronychia may occur with thumb sucking.

Patient and Family Education

Emphasize good hand washing. Treatment failure is usually due to lack of compliance.
- Frequent diaper changes.
- Leave diaper area open to air as much as possible.
- Blow-dry with warm air (low setting) for 3 to 5 minutes at diaper change (especially helpful in intertriginous areas in infants and obese children).
- Avoid rubber pants.
- Use mild soap and water; rinse well; avoid diaper wipes.
- Avoid other medications not prescribed.
- Powder may help maintain dryness.
- Discard or sterilize pacifiers.

Tinea Capitis

This dermatophyte infection invades the scalp and hair shaft, causing an inflammatory response and hair shaft fragility. *Trichophyton tonsurans* is responsible for most cases but pet exposure (especially cat) can lead to infection with *Microsporum canis*. Tinea capitis occurs mainly in the pediatric population and the incidence is higher in Black individuals. Many children are asymptomatic carriers and *T. tonsurans* is transmitted by fomites when humans share hats, combs, and brushes, or by cats, dogs, or rodents. This common fungal infection of the head or body is a superficial skin infection also known as "ringworm."

Tinea from *T. tonsurans* manifests itself as : (1) diffuse fine scaling without obvious hair breaks and with subtle to significant hair loss (Fig. 37.14A); (2) discrete areas of hair loss with stubs of broken hairs (black-dot ringworm) (Fig. 37.14B); (3) "classic" patchy hair loss and scaly lesions with raised borders (Fig. 37.14C); and (4) scaly, pustular lesions, or kerions (Fig. 37.14D–E). *M. canis* infections are typically more inflammatory, popular, have loose and broken hairs, and develop tender boggy kerions. The incubation period is up to 4 days and new lesions can appear for months if not treated.[1]

Clinical Findings

History. Hair loss, pruritis, and contact with another person or pet with ringworm are sometimes reported.

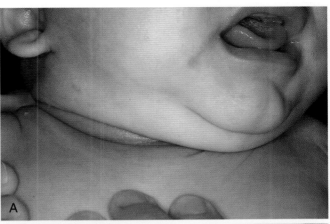

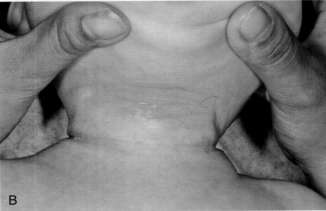

• **Fig. 37.12** (A) Candida Intertrigo. (B) Streptococcal Intertrigo. Note the absence of satellite papules that are characteristic of candida intertrigo. (From Paller AS, & Mancini AJ. *Paller and Mancini: Hurwitz Clinical Pediatric Dermatology*. 6th ed. Philadelphia: Elsevier; 2022.)

Physical Examination
- Scaling, erythema, or crusting usually occurs.
- Bald patches or areas of broken hairs are noted.
- *T. tonsurans* manifests as black-dot tinea, with tiny black dots that are the remainder of hair that has broken off at the shaft; no scalp scale is present (most common).
- *M. canis* leaves the hair broken and lusterless with a fine gray scale on the scalp.
- Occipital or posterior cervical adenopathy may be significant.
- A kerion is a boggy, inflamed mass filled with pustules. It results from a delayed inflammatory reaction. There may be regional lymphadenopathy, fever, and leukocytosis.

Diagnostic Studies. A clinical diagnosis is typically accurate with no further testing needed, especially if cervical or occipital lymphadenopathy is present. Examine hair scrapings as follows:
- Wood's light fluoresces yellow-green (positive with *M. canis*; negative with *T. tonsurans*).
- KOH examination of scraped hair: Wait 20 to 40 minutes for warming after application of KOH to examine. If Wood's light is positive, under microscopy the KOH-prepared outer surface of hair is coated with tiny mats of spores; if Wood's light is negative, hyphae and spores are present in hair shaft.
- Fungal culture of a completely plucked hair with its root using a Kelly clamp is most reliable.

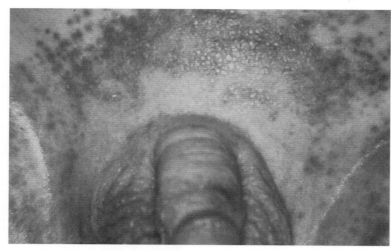

• **Fig. 37.13** Diaper Candidiasis. Note involvement of intertriginous areas. (From Zitelli BJ, McIntire S, Nowalk AJ, et al. (Eds). *Zitelli and Davis' Atlas of Pediatric Physical Diagnosis*. 8th ed. Elsevier; 2023.)

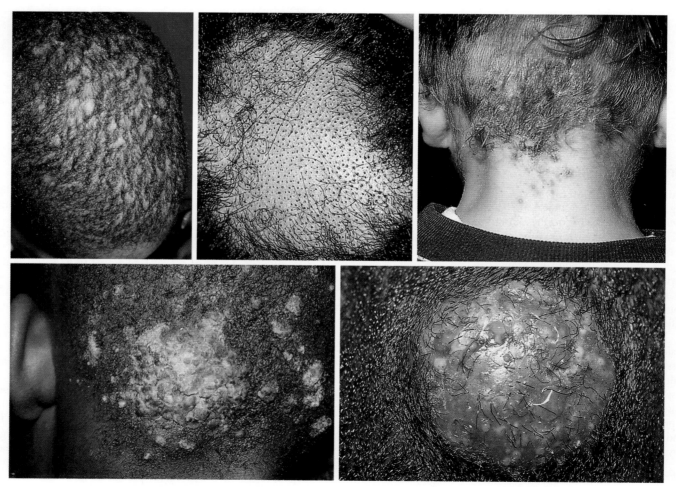

• **Fig. 37.14** Tinea Capitis. (From Zitelli BJ, McIntire S, Nowalk AJ, et al. (Eds). *Zitelli and Davis' Atlas of Pediatric Physical Diagnosis*. 8th ed. Elsevier; 2023.)

Differential Diagnosis

Traumatic alopecia, alopecia areata, hypothyroid and hyperthyroid hair loss, seborrhea, atopic dermatitis, psoriasis, impetigo, and folliculitis are included in the differential diagnoses.

Management

Topical antifungals are ineffective. Antibiotic treatment is not indicated. The following steps are taken:

- Griseofulvin taken with fatty food, to enhance absorption. Treatment should be continued 6 to 8 weeks or for at least 2 weeks after clinical and mycologic cure.
- Terbinafine is increasingly being used in patients over 4 years of age.
- Fluconazole is also approved but has been shown to be less effective. Oral itraconazole is effective but concerns about heart safety limit its use. In addition to oral antifungal therapy, shampoo with selenium sulfide 2.5% or econazole or ketoconazole 2% (2–3 times per week for 4 weeks) to decrease spore viability and keep other household members from being infected.
- If a long-standing kerion with severe inflammation is present, give prednisone for 5 to 14 days and consider systemic antibiotics for secondary bacterial infection.
- Asymptomatic carriers are common so consider culturing family members or pets if recurrence is a concern.
- A follow-up visit should be scheduled after 2 weeks to evaluate response to treatment. Medication should be continued until 2 weeks after culture is negative. Follow-up should be continued every 2 to 4 weeks until new hair growth is evident.
- Monitoring of CBC, liver function tests (LFTs), and renal function is no longer required in children treated with oral griseofulvin due to its favorable safety profile; however, if extended therapy with the medication, over 8 weeks, laboratory evaluation may be considered.[1]

Complications

An interface dermatitis *(id)* reaction to the fungus, not to the medication, can occur. It manifests either as a red, superficial edema or as scaly, red plaques and papules on the scalp and is treated with 1 to 2 weeks of topical or systemic steroids. Permanent hair loss and scarring can occur with an untreated kerion.[1]

Patient and Family Education

- Identify source of infection (*M. canis,* animal source; *T. tonsurans,* human source) and treat the source.

- Side effects of medication should be explained and monitored; griseofulvin typically may result in gastrointestinal disturbances, photosensitivity, skin eruptions, and headache.
- Hair regrowth is slow (3–12 months) and, if a kerion was present, hair loss can be permanent.
- Laundering sheets and clothes in a hot water wash and hot dryer cycle and vacuuming may decrease spread in the family.
- Grooming practices (e.g., hair traction, greasy pomades, infrequent shampooing) may be predisposing factors.
- There is a high rate of asymptomatic carriers; culture is the only definitive means of identification.

Tinea Corporis

Tinea corporis, or "ringworm," is a superficial fungal skin infection involving the body other than the scalp, palms, soles, and groin. It is also identified by the part of the body affected (e.g., tinea manuum [hand], tinea faciei [face]). Tinea corporis is most commonly caused by the dermatophytes *M. canis, Tricophyton rubrum,* or *T. mentagrophytes.* Transmission comes as the stratum corneum is invaded following direct contact with infected humans, animals, or fomites. Contact sports (especially wrestling), hot and humid climates, crowded living conditions, day care, school settings, and immunosuppression increase the risk of tinea corporis. Autoinoculation accounts for spreading lesions.[1]

Clinical Findings

History. Localized and systemic symptoms are not common. Known contact with a person or animal with tinea is sometimes reported.

Physical Examination

- Classical appearance of lesions: Annular, oval, or circinate with one or more flat, scaling, mildly erythematous circular patches or plaques with red, scaly borders (Fig. 37.15).
- Lesions spread peripherally and clear centrally or may be inflammatory throughout with superficial pustules.
- Often prominent over hair follicles.
- Multiple secondary lesions may merge into a large area several centimeters in diameter.
- Lesions on the face may not be annular.

Diagnostic Studies. If treatment failure or questionable diagnosis occurs:

- Definitive diagnosis is KOH-treated scrapings of border of lesion that reveal hyphae and spores (see Fig. 37.4).
- Fungal culture of the lesion.

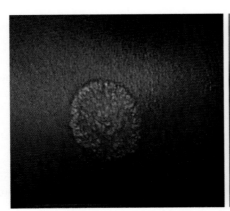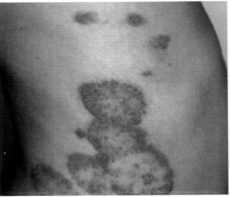

• **Fig. 37.15** Tinea Corporis. (From Zitelli BJ, McIntire S, Nowalk AJ, et al. (Eds). *Zitelli and Davis' Atlas of Pediatric Physical Diagnosis.* 8th ed. Elsevier; 2023.)

Differential Diagnosis

Pityriasis rosea herald patch, impetigo, nummular eczema, psoriasis, seborrhea, contact dermatitis, tinea versicolor, granuloma annulare, and Lyme disease are in the differential diagnoses.

Management

- For superficial or localized tinea corporis, topical antifungals, such as miconazole or clotrimazole (see Table 37.4), are generally effective. Antifungal and steroid combinations should be avoided. Apply cream to the lesion, including a zone of normal skin, twice a day until clinical resolution, which can take 1 to 4 weeks. Prescription antifungals (e.g., econazole, ciclopirox) penetrate the skin more effectively, but are more expensive.[1]
- Tinea faciei and tinea corporis gladiatorum (associated with wrestling teams) may require oral medication.
- Extensive infection, immunosuppression, coexisting tinea infections on scalp or nails, or infection that is unresponsive to topical treatment may require systemic treatment. Griseofulvin (see Table 37.4) is the systemic drug of choice for children older than 2 years old. Treatment typically lasts for 2 to 4 weeks for areas other than the scalp. Griseofulvin should be taken with fatty foods for better absorption.

Complications

Tinea incognito is a dermatophyte infection that has been altered by the use of topical calcineurin inhibitors (e.g., tacrolimus and pimecrolimus) or steroid creams, either alone or in combination with a topical antifungal. The lesions improve, but there is a rapid relapse when the creams are stopped, and chronic infection persists. A hypersensitivity response, *id,* may also occur.[1]

Patient and Family Education

- Find the source of infection and treat or eliminate it to prevent recurrence. Keep skin dry following application of antifungal.
- Identify and treat contacts.
- Educate about communicability of lesions and length of treatment.
- Exclude from day care or school until 24 hours after treatment has begun.
- Follow up in 2 weeks or sooner if lesions are not responding. If unresponsive, diagnosis is incorrect, or resistance is possible. Culture to confirm diagnosis and change class of antifungal used.

Tinea Cruris

Tinea cruris, commonly called "jock itch," is a superficial fungal skin infection found on the groin, upper thighs, and intertriginous folds. Caused by the dermatophyte *Epidermophyton floccosum, T. rubrum,* or *T. mentagrophytes,* tinea cruris rarely occurs before adolescence and is more common in males, obese individuals, or those with hyperhidrosis or experiencing chafing from tight clothes or moisture. It is extremely common in warm, moist climates.[1]

Clinical Findings

History

- Hot, humid weather, tight clothing, vigorous physical activity and chafing, or contact sport, such as wrestling.
- Often associated with tinea pedis.

Physical Examination

- Erythematous to slightly brown, sharply marginated plaques with a raised border of scaling, pustules, or vesicles; central clearing may be present.

- Usually bilateral and symmetric, but not always.
- Occurs on inner thighs and inguinal creases; penis, scrotum, and labia majora generally spared.
- May spread to perianal region and/or thighs.
  Diagnostic Studies. If treatment failure or questionable diagnosis occurs:
- KOH-treated scraping reveals hyphae and spores
- Fungal culture

Differential Diagnosis

Psoriasis, candidiasis, contact dermatitis, seborrhea, intertrigo, and erythrasma are in the differential diagnoses.

Management

Management is the same as for tinea corporis. Duration of topical treatment is usually 4 to 6 weeks. Steroid use is to be avoided.[1]

Complications

Appropriate treatment and care rarely result in complication. Steroid use can result in atrophy and/or tinea incognita, complication of advanced crusty lesions with boggy granuloma and follicles distended with purulent material.[1]

Patient and Family Education

- Reduction of perspiration and moisture is important. Advise the patient to wear cotton underwear and loose clothing and to use absorbent antifungal powder.
- Plain talcum powder or antifungal powder may be helpful.
- Often spread similarly to other forms of tinea so practice good hygiene, especially after wrestling or sporting events.

Tinea Pedis

Tinea pedis is the most common fungal disease found on the feet and is commonly called *athlete's foot.* Caused by the dermatophytes *T. rubrum* or *T. mentagrophytes,* tinea pedis is less common in preadolescent patients and is more common in males. *T. rubrum* is a relatively noninflammatory infection with dull erythema and silvery scaling on the sole and sides of the foot. *T. mentagrophytes* presents with three different appearances: (1) vesicles and erosions on the instep of one or both feet and heels; (2) an occasional fissure between the toes with surrounding erythema and desquamation; and (3) onychomycosis (Fig. 37.16A–B).[8]

Tinea pedis is typically acquired through direct contact with contaminated surfaces (e.g., warm moist environment of showers and locker room floors) and often occurs with tinea cruris.

Clinical Findings

History

- Sweaty feet
- Use of nylon socks or nonbreathable shoes
- Exposure in family or at school
- Pruritis, intense burning, stinging, foul odor
- Microtrauma to feet: cracks, abrasions, nicks, cuts
- Contact with damp areas (e.g., swimming pools, locker room, showers).

Physical Examination

- Red, scaly, cracked rash on soles or interdigital spaces and instep, especially between the third, fourth, and fifth toes
- Infection initially presents as white peeling lesions becoming erythematous, vesicular, macerated, fissured, and scaly
- Occasionally spreads to dorsum of foot

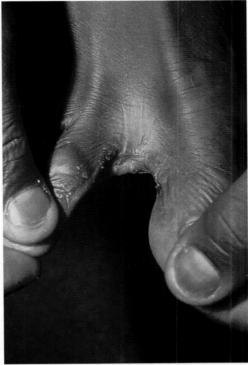

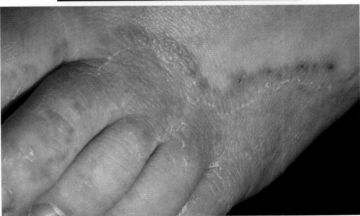

• **Fig. 37.16** Tinea Pedis. (From Zitelli BJ, McIntire S, Nowalk AJ, et al. (Eds). *Zitelli and Davis' Atlas of Pediatric Physical Diagnosis.* 8th ed. Elsevier; 2023.)

• Chronic infection manifested by diffuse scaling (e.g., plantar hyperkeratosis) and mild erythema
Diagnostic Studies. Laboratory studies are the same as those for tinea corporis.

Differential Diagnosis

Contact dermatitis, atopic dermatitis, dyshidrotic eczema, psoriasis, pitted keratolysis, and juvenile plantar dermatosis (e.g., red, dry fissures of weight-bearing surface) are in the differential diagnosis.

Management

• Management is the same as that for tinea corporis. Antifungal medication should be applied 1 cm beyond the borders of the rash twice daily until 7 days after clearing. Usual treatment is 3 to 6 weeks.

• In rare cases, griseofulvin may be required, and treatment for 6 to 8 weeks is usually recommended.
• Aluminum chloride (Drysol, Certain Dri, Xerac AC, or Arrid Extra Dry antiperspirant sprays) may be used for hyperhidrosis.[1]

Complications

A secondary bacterial infection, indicated by foul odor, can occur. An *id* response may also occur.

Patient and Family Education

• Advise patient to keep feet dry, use absorbent antifungal powder or sprays, wear cotton socks, avoid scratching, and wear shoes that allow the feet to breathe or go barefoot when home. Thoroughly dry feet and between toes after using a commercial showering facility.

- For maceration between toes, cotton/foam inserts between the toes may speed recovery.
- Rinse feet with plain water or water and vinegar; dry carefully, especially between the toes. Moisturize and protect feet to prevent splitting and cracking.
- Acute vesicular lesions can be treated with wet compresses 2 to 4 times daily for 10 to 15 minutes in addition to application of topical antifungals.
- Tinea pedis may need the addition of a keratolytic agent (lactic acid or urea) with the application of antifungals.
- Tennis shoes may be washed in the machine with soap and bleach. Hot water is required to kill fungal spores.
- Physical education or sports may be continued. Use care to prevent spreading of disease.
- Follow up in 2 to 3 weeks or sooner if lesions are not responding.

Onychomycosis

Onychomycosis is a fungal infection of the nail(s) that is typically caused by *T. rubrum*, *T. tonsurans*, or *Candida*. When the nail infection is due to a dermatophyte, it is often called *tinea unguium*. One or two nails are often involved. The infection may be superficial, hypertrophic (i.e., onychauxis), or cause separation of the nail plate from the tissue (i.e., onycholytic).[1]

The infecting organism invades the nail, proliferates, and destroys the nail integrity, causing separation of the nail plate from the nailbed (Fig. 37.17). In most cases, infection originates at the distal edge of the nail. A yellowish discoloration spreads proximally, looking like a streak in the nail; spreading occurs and eventually the nail becomes brittle and separates from the nail bed. Onychomycosis caused by *candida* causes destruction of the nail and hyperkeratosis of the nail bed. It is uncommon during the first 2 decades of life, limited most commonly to adolescents and adults. When it occurs in children, there is often a concurrent tinea pedis or tinea manuum. There may be a relationship to the use of occlusive shoes.

Clinical Findings

History. The patient may report a thickened, discolored nail. The condition is usually asymptomatic.

Physical Examination
- Opaque white or silvery nail that becomes thick, yellow, with subungual debris.
- Toenails are involved more often than fingernails with tinea.

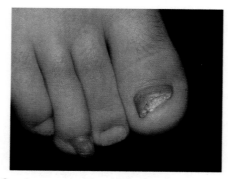

• **Fig. 37.17** Onychomycosis. (From White GM, Cox NH, editors. *Diseases of the Skin: a Color Atlas and Text*, ed 2. Elsevier; 2006.)

- *Candida* infections are more common in infants and fingernails are involved more often than toenails.
- Seldom symmetric; it may be one to three nails on one extremity.
  Diagnostic Studies. Typically, this is a clinical diagnosis, but KOH preparations and fungal cultures of the material under the nail are helpful in confirming the diagnosis.

Differential Diagnosis

Psoriasis (involves all nails and includes pitting), hereditary nail defects, dystrophy secondary to eczema or chronic paronychia, lichen planus, and trauma are the differential diagnoses.

Management

1. Topical treatment with ciclopirox may provide cure in 75% of patients but medication is limited to those over 12 years of age and must be used for up to 48 weeks.
2. Oral medication has proven to be more successful:
   - Itraconazole for 12 weeks or as pulse therapy for 1 week each month for 3 months. In general, 2 to 3 pulses are commonly needed for fingernails and 3 to 4 pulses for toenails. May have lower recurrence rates.
   - Terbinafine treatment is generally 6 weeks for fingernails and up to 12 weeks for toenails.
   - Fluconazole has slower resolution time (6–9 months for fingernails and 8–18 months for toenails).
3. Follow-up visits at 1-month intervals for LFTs are recommended; long-term follow-up every 6 months is suggested.

Complications

The disease itself rarely causes any kind of complication, other than a worsening of the appearance of the nail as the infection progresses. There are potential side effects to medications and monitoring for these is an important part of management.

Patient and Family Education

Communicate that a cure may be difficult to obtain, and relapse is common.
- Preventative measures include antifungal foot powders, frequent nail clipping, breathable socks and shoes.
- Avoid reexposure in locker rooms and other damp communal locations.
- Shoes should be discarded or treated with disinfectants and antifungal powders.[6]

Tinea Versicolor (Pityriasis Versicolor)

Tinea versicolor is caused by the *Malassezia* fungus. Scaly macules typically present in the summer but tend to be persistent throughout the year. Tinea versicolor occurs predominantly on the trunk and upper extremities and occurs more commonly in adolescents, but breastfeeding infants can acquire the organism from their mother and exhibit facial lesions.[1]

Clinical Findings

History. The infection is associated with warm, humid weather. Occasional mild itching may occur.

Physical Examination. Multiple, annular, scaling, discrete macules or patches, ranging from hypopigmented in dark-skinned individuals to hyperpigmented (salmon-colored to brown) in light-skinned individuals, are seen on the neck, shoulders, upper back and arms, chest midline, and face (especially in infants). They tend to have a guttate or raindrop pattern. (Fig. 37.18A–C).

Diagnostic Studies. KOH scrapings, though not necessary, reveal short, curved hyphae and circular spores ("spaghetti and meatballs"). Scrapings fluoresce yellow-green under Wood's lamp.

Differential Diagnosis

Pityriasis alba, pityriasis rosea, vitiligo, postinflammatory hypopigmentation or hyperpigmentation, seborrhea, and secondary syphilis are included in the differential diagnoses.

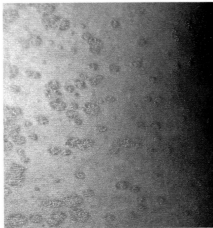
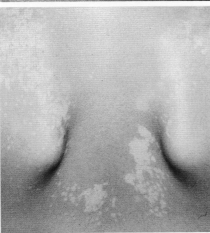
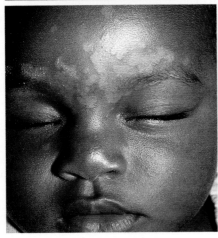

• **Fig. 37.18** Tinea Versicolor. (From Cohen BA, editor. *Pediatric Dermatology*. 5th ed. Elsevier; 2022.)

Management

The following steps are taken:
- Selenium sulfide 2.5% lotion or 1% shampoo (OTC) applied in a thin layer several hand-widths beyond lesions for 10 minutes daily before rinsing for 1 to 2 weeks followed by monthly applications for 3 months to help prevent recurrences.
- Older adolescents can use ketoconazole 2% shampoo as a single application or daily for 3 days.
- Topical antifungal creams, which may be effective, are not practical given the extensive coverage area.
- Resistant or severe cases in older adolescents sometimes require oral antifungal treatment. Itraconazole and ketoconazole have been found to be effective, but caution must be taken due to potential for liver toxicity and cardiac damage.[3]
- Follow up in 1 month.

Patient and Family Education

- Sun exposure makes lesions appear hypopigmented as the surrounding skin tans.
- Repigmentation takes several months.
- Relapse is likely if prophylaxis is not done occasionally.
- Skin irritation occurs with overnight application.
- Absence of flaking when skin is scraped is a sign of effective treatment.

Viral Infections of the Skin

Herpes Simplex

Herpes simplex virus (HSV) infections are very contagious and very common in all populations. HSV-1 and HSV-2 primarily infect the epidermis and mucosal surfaces. Upon exposure and initial acute infection, the virus replicates and establishes a latent infection in regional nerve ganglia. Incubation takes days to weeks and the primary HSV infection may be asymptomatic. Reactivation occurs with triggering factors (e.g., stress, menses, illness, sunburn, dental procedures, windburn, and fatigue).

HSV-1 usually affects the oral mucosa, pharynx, lips, and occasionally, the eyes, causing a herpes labialis infection, commonly called *cold sores* or *fever blisters* (Fig. 37.19). Gingivostomatitis is most common between the ages of 10 months and 5 years. HSV-2 infection commonly occurs in neonates through maternal-fetal transmission (see Chapter 28) or herpetic vulvovaginitis (see Chapter 43). HSV-1 can also be found in the genital area and Type 2 can be found on the lips and mouth, primarily due to oral-genital contact. Genital HSV infection in a non–sexually active adolescent is a concern and the question of sexual abuse should be investigated. *Herpetic whitlow,* occurring on a finger or thumb, resembles paronychia. It can be HSV-1 or 2 and primarily occurs through autoinoculation on the fingers of thumb-sucking patients with gingivostomatitis, herpes labialis, or genital HSV infection.[3] Herpetic keratoconjunctivitis is discussed in Chapter 30; other information may be found in Chapter 35.

Clinical Findings

History. In the first clinical presentation of HSV, fever, malaise, sore throat, and decreased fluid intake can occur. Gingivostomatitis is often accompanied by fever, drooling, difficulties eating and drinking, foul breath odor, and irritability. Initial presentations of genital HSV are associated with painful vesicles in genital areas. In recurrent HSV infection, there is often a painful prodrome of burning, tingling, paresthesia, and itching at the involved site.

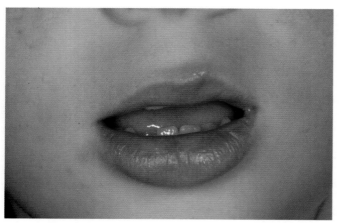

• **Fig. 37.19** Herpes Labialis. (From Paller AS, & Mancini AJ. *Paller and Mancini: Hurwitz Clinical Pediatric Dermatology.* 6th ed. Elsevier; 2022.)

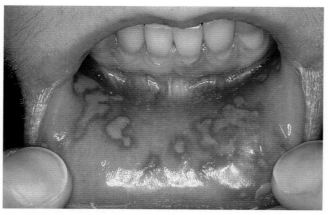

• **Fig. 37.20** Herpetic Gingivostomatitis. (From James WD, Elston DM, Treat JR, et al. *Andrews' Diseases of the Skin.* 13th ed. Elsevier; 2020.)

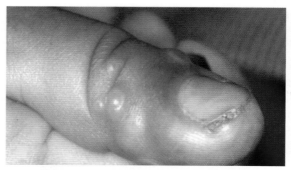

• **Fig. 37.21** Herpetic Whitlow. (From Cohen BA, editor. *Pediatric Dermatology.* 5th ed. Elsevier; 2022.)

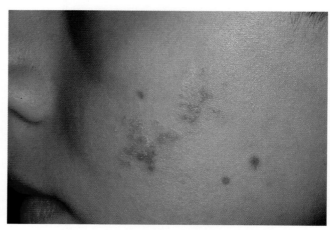

• **Fig. 37.22** Cutaneous Herpes Simplex. (From Paller AS, Mancini AJ, editors. *Hurwitz Clinical Pediatric Dermatology.* 5th ed. Elsevier; 2016.)

Recent acute febrile illness or sun exposure may be reported with all types of recurrent HSV.

Physical Examination. The following are seen on physical examination:

- HSV-1
  - Gingivostomatitis: Pharyngitis with grouped vesicles on an erythematous base that ulcerate and form white plaques on mucosa, gingiva, tongue, palate, lips, chin, and nasolabial folds; lymphadenopathy and halitosis are present (Fig. 37.20).
  - Herpes labialis: Localized cluster of small, clear, tense vesicles with an erythematous base that become weepy and ulcerated, progressing to crustiness, usually only on one side of the mouth and on the vermillion border—a classic cold sore.
  - Herpetic whitlow: Deep-appearing, painful vesicles or bullae with erythema distal finger(s) (Fig. 37.21).
  - Cutaneous HSV: Can occur anywhere on the body and may be misdiagnosed as impetigo or herpes zoster (HZ). Erythema always present but may lack typical vesicles[3] (Fig. 37.22).
- HSV-2
  - Grouped vesicopustules and ulceration with edema.
  - First clinical lesions on vaginal mucosa, labia, or perineum in females and on the penile shaft or perineum in males;

females may have cervical involvement; oral lesions are possible.
  - Recurrent lesions on labia, vulva, clitoris, or cervix in females and on the prepuce, glans, or sulcus in males; generally, less severe cutaneous lesions.
  - Regional lymphadenopathy.

Diagnostic Studies. Most often, these are clinical diagnoses. A Tzanck smear can be done on fluid from the lesions to identify epidermal giant cells; however, it does not distinguish HSV-1 from HSV-2. Viral cultures are the gold standard for definitive diagnosis. Direct fluorescent antibody tests, enzyme-linked immunosorbent assay (ELISA) serology, and polymerase chain reaction (PCR) tests are usually only used with severe forms of HSV infection.

Differential Diagnosis

Differential diagnoses include aphthous stomatitis, coxsackie virus or hand-foot-and-mouth disease, varicella, impetigo, folliculitis, and erythema multiforme.

Management

Management is directed by presentation and patient-specific factors (e.g., age, area and extent of involvement, and immune status) (Table 37.5). Treatment includes:

- Herpes labialis and gingivostomatitis
  - Disease is often self-limited over 10 days to 2 weeks. May treat if symptoms are severe, younger patients have decreased oral intake, or there are underlying conditions

	Presentation	Clinical Findings	Treatment	Education
TABLE 37.5	**Diagnosis and Treatment of Herpes Simplex and Herpes Zoster**			
Herpes simplex	Gingivostomatitis as primary infection; herpes labialis or herpes facialis as recurrent infection	Pharyngitis with erythematous vesicles, near, on, and/or in mouth; small, clear vesicles on erythematous base progressing to crusting	Burow solution; observation of self-resolution preferred; acyclovir in underlying disorder; antibiotics if secondary infection; oral anesthetics; supportive care	Degree and duration of contagion; triggers to infection
Herpes zoster	Reactivation of latent varicella virus, especially after mild cases or in infants younger than 1 year old or immunocompromised host	Two or three clustered groups of vesicles on erythematous base, especially over 2nd cervical to 2nd lumbar and 5th–7th cranial nerve dermatomes; does not cross the midline; pain (can be severe), itch, tingle is minimal in children	Burow solution; antihistamine; drying lotions; possible acyclovir; antibiotics if secondary infection	New vesicles occur for up to 1 week; takes 2–3 weeks to resolve; contagious until lesions stop erupting and are crusted over

such as immunosuppression, underlying skin disease, significant systemic symptoms.[7]

- Topical antiviral creams have not shown to be much benefit but can be tried in patients over 12 years: acyclovir 5% for 4 days. Start with onset of symptoms.
- Oral antivirals for patients over 2 years. Best if started in first 3 days.
  - Ages 2 to 11 years: acyclovir for 5 to 10 days
  - Ages 12 years and up:
- Valacyclovir twice/day for 1 day.
- Acyclovir for 7 to 10 days (maximum length of treatment is 10 days).
- For recurrent episodes, treat at onset of symptoms with acyclovir for 5 days. For significant recurrence problem (6 or more episodes a year): acyclovir for up to 12 months.[7]
- Herpetic whitlow.
  - Typically resolve with treatment
- If severe pain or underlying skin disease, oral acyclovir for 5 to 10 days may speed healing.
- Antibiotics for secondary bacterial (usually staphylococcal) infection:[3]
  - Mupirocin: topically for 5 days
  - Erythromycin: for 10 days
  - Dicloxacillin: for 10 days
- Oral anesthetics for comfort; use with caution in children. Note: Child needs to be able to rinse and spit:
  - Viscous lidocaine 2% topical
  - Liquid diphenhydramine alone or combined with aluminum hydroxide or magnesium hydroxide as a 1:1 rinse (maximum of 5 mg/kg/d diphenhydramine in case it is swallowed); it can also be applied to the lesions with cotton-tipped swabs.
- Newborn infant, immunosuppressed child, child with infected atopic dermatitis, or child with a lesion in the eye or on the eyelid margin; consult with or refer to an appropriate provider.
- Offer supportive care, such as antipyretics, analgesics, hydration, and good oral hygiene.
- Exclude from daycare only during the initial course (gingivostomatitis) and if the child cannot control secretions.

Complications

Pharyngitis can develop from orolabial lesions. Eczema herpeticum or Kaposi varicelliform eruption is discussed in Chapter 35. Secondary

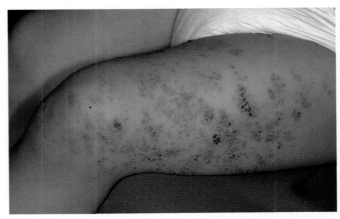

- **Fig. 37.23** Herpes Zoster. (From Paller AS, & Mancini AJ. *Paller and Mancini: Hurwitz Clinical Pediatric Dermatology.* 6th ed. Elsevier; 2022.)

bacteremia with GABHS, *S. aureus*, or other organisms may occur. HSV has also been implicated as a possible cause of erythema multiforme and Stevens-Johnson syndrome (SJS). HSV can lead to sepsis and/or meningitis in neonates and immunocompromised individuals.

Patient and Family Education

- Cool compresses and lubricants can help with lesion discomfort.
- Contagiousness of lesions and oral secretions must be understood, and avoidance measures should be discussed.
- Triggers can include physical and psychological stress, trauma, fever, exposure to UV light, illness, menses, medical and dental procedures that traumatize oral tissue, and extreme weather. Describe symptoms of recurrence and possible outbreak prevention treatment when recurrence is common.
- Explain the course of initial disease symptoms, with fever lasting up to 4 days and lesions taking at least 2 weeks to heal. Initial presentation is more severe than recurrence.
- Use of daily sunblock on lips may prevent recurrence.

Herpes Zoster

HZ is a recurrent varicella infection commonly called *shingles* (Fig. 37.23). Caused by reactivation of the latent varicella zoster infection from the sensory root ganglia, HZ occurs in 10% to 20% of all individuals, is rare in childhood, and occurs more frequently with increasing age (three times more common in adolescents than preschoolers). HZ is more common following mild cases of varicella infections before 1 year old (3–20 times increased risk) and in immunocompromised children. There is still conflicting evidence as to whether individuals vaccinated for varicella have a lower incidence of HZ later in life.[3]

Clinical Findings

History. Burning, stinging pain, tenderness to light touch, hyperesthesia, or tingling precedes eruption by about 1 week, although this is less common in children. The lesions can be extremely itchy and painful.

Physical Examination
- Two or three clustered groups of macules and papules progress to vesicles on an erythematous base. These vesicles become pustular, rupture, ulcerate, and crust.
- Lesions develop over 3 to 5 days and last 7 to 10 days. Lesions may develop for up to 1 week followed by crusting and healing during the next 2 weeks. In children, delayed chronic pain, known as *postherpetic neuralgia,* is rare.
- Lesions commonly follow the dermatomes of the second cervical to lumbar nerves and the fifth to seventh cranial nerves with scattered lesions outside these areas.
- Lesions do not cross midline (key to diagnosis); sharp demarcation at the midline with occasional contralateral involvement.
- Lymphadenopathy may occur.

Diagnostic Studies. The diagnosis is usually clinical. Viral culture can be used but takes up to a week for results. The most sensitive confirmation testing is PCR using a swab taken from vesicular lesions. Bacterial culture or Gram stain can be used to distinguish from impetigo.

Differential Diagnosis

Local cutaneous HSV infection and impetigo are differential diagnoses.

Management

Management steps include the following[10]:
- Refer for immediate ophthalmologic examination if eyes, forehead, or nose is involved.
- Refer for involvement of ear involvement (e.g., Ramsay Hunt syndrome).
- Antihistamines for itching.
- Analgesics for discomfort; Note: Do not use salicylates.
- Antiviral medications are not recommended for otherwise healthy children with HZ. Acyclovir or valacyclovir may be considered for those at risk: immunocompromised persons, chronic cutaneous disease, long-term salicylate therapy.
- Observe for secondary bacterial (usually staphylococcal) infection. Topical Mupirocin twice daily is generally effective. Oral antibiotics are rarely needed.

Complications

Complications are rare except in immunocompromised persons. Occasionally, HZ is the initial finding in acquired immunodeficiency syndrome (AIDS), especially if more than one dermatome is involved. Eczema herpeticum may occur. Postherpetic neuralgia pain is rare in the pediatric population. Secondary skin infections are the most common complication.

Patient and Family Education

- New vesicles appear for up to 1 week and take 2 to 3 weeks to resolve. Illness is usually mild.
- Comfort measures: Burow's solution compressions 3 times daily; warm, soothing baths; ointment (e.g., Aquaphor, Vaseline) to moisturize the lesions and decrease itching.
- The child is contagious for varicella until lesions are crusted. If the lesions can be covered, the child does not need to be excluded from school or childcare. If the lesions cannot be covered, the child should avoid contact with others until the lesions are crusted.[10]

Molluscum Contagiosum

A benign common childhood viral skin infection with little health risk, molluscum contagiosum often disappears on its own in a few weeks to months and is not easily treated. This poxvirus replicates in host epithelial cells. It attacks skin and mucous membranes and is spread by direct contact, by fomites, or by autoinoculation (typically scratching). It is commonly found in children and adolescents. The incubation period is about 2 to 7 weeks but may be as long as 6 months. Infectivity is low but the child is contagious, as long as lesions are present.

Clinical Findings

History
- Itching at the site
- Possible exposure to molluscum contagiosum

Physical Examination
- Lesions begin as very small smooth, dome-shaped, white to flesh-colored discrete papules. Papules progressing to become umbilicated (may not be evident) with a cheesy core; keratinous contents may extrude from the umbilication (Fig. 37.24A).
- Face, trunk, axillae, extremities, and occasionally pubic and genital areas are the most commonly involved areas; palms, soles, and scalp are spared.
- Single papule to numerous papules; most often numerous clustered papules and linear configurations.
- Sexually active or abused children can have genitally grouped lesions, but genital area may be infected through autoinoculation (Fig. 37.24B).
- Children with eczema or immunosuppression can have severe cases; those with human immunodeficiency virus (HIV) infection or AIDS can have hundreds of lesions.

Diagnosis. The diagnosis of molluscum is generally a clinical one.

Differential Diagnosis

Warts, closed comedones, small epidermal cysts, blisters, folliculitis, and condyloma acuminatum are included in the differential diagnoses.

Management

- Untreated lesions usually disappear within 6 months to 2 years but may take up to 4 years to completely disappear. The decision to treat may be based on discomfort, reduction of itching, minimization of autoinoculation, limitation of transmission, and for cosmetic reasons. Genital lesions may need to be treated to prevent spread to sexual partners.
- Dermatology specialists can assist the family in determining the best treatment option based on pain and side effects of treatment and known efficacy in the molluscum presentation.

- Hypoallergenic surgical adhesive tape
- Laser therapy
- Salicylic acid
- KOH
- Cantharidin

Complications

Molluscum dermatitis, an inflammatory, scaly, erythematous, hypersensitive reaction, can occur and will respond to moisturizer; avoid hydrocortisone because it causes molluscum to flare. Impetiginized lesions, inflammation of the eyes or conjunctiva, and scarring can occur.

Patient and Family Education

Wait and see approach is usually appropriate since spontaneous clearing generally occurs. Keeping nails short and lesions covered will help prevent autoinoculation. Patients are contagious, but there is no need to exclude them from day care or school. Scarring is unusual.[7]

Warts

Warts are common childhood skin lesions characterized by a proliferation of the epidermis and mucosa infected by the human papillomavirus (HPV). There are over 100 HPV types, and each one produces characteristic lesions in specific locations (e.g., verruca vulgaris, verruca plana, verruca plantaris, and condyloma acuminatum). The 9-valent HPV vaccine protects against most oncogenic and nononcogenic HPV types and while proven to reduce the incidence of cervical cancer, it may be proving useful in the prevention of anogenital warts. Though most common on the extremities, warts can occur anywhere on the body, including the face, scalp, and genitalia. Trauma promotes inoculation of the HPV (Koebner phenomenon); as a result, most warts are on the hands, fingers, elbows, and plantar surfaces of the feet.

The transmission of warts from person to person depends on viral and host factors, such as quantity of virus, location of warts, preexisting skin injury, and cell-mediated immunity. Transmission is from fomites or skin-to-skin contact, and autoinoculation is frequent. Incubation is from 1 to 6 months, possibly years.

Although a large percentage of all warts resolve spontaneously within 3 to 5 years, there is a high recurrence rate. Cutaneous warts are rarely a serious health concern but present cosmetic problems for children and their families.[2]

Clinical Findings

History. The history typically is gradual development of lesion and occasionally, a knowledge of known exposure to someone with warts.

Physical Examination

- Common warts (verruca vulgaris) are usually elevated flesh-colored single papules with scaly, irregular surfaces and occasionally, black pinpoints, which are thrombosed blood vessels. They are usually asymptomatic and multiple and are found anywhere on the body, although most commonly on the hands, nails, and feet. They may be dome shaped, filiform, or exophytic (Fig. 37.25). Filiform warts project from the skin on a narrow stalk and are usually seen on the face, lips, nose, eyelids, or neck. Periungual warts are common among nail biters, occurring around the cuticles of the fingers or toes.[8]
- Flat warts (verruca plana or juvenile warts) are seen commonly on the face, neck, and extremities. They are small, slightly

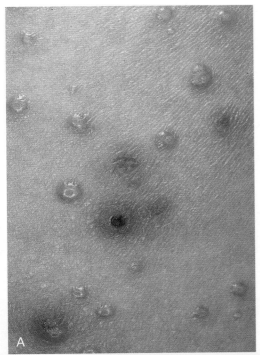

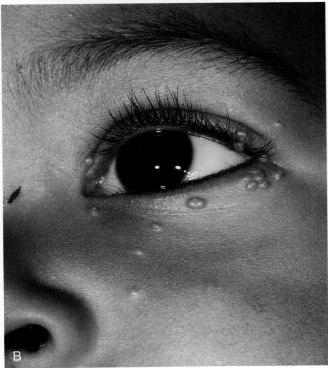

• **Fig. 37.24** (A) Molluscum contagiosum. (B) Autoinoculation around the eye of molluscum contagiosum. (From Dinulos JGH. *Habif's Clinical Dermatology: A Color Guide to Diagnosis and Therapy.* 7th ed. Elsevier; 2021.)

The most common treatment modality is mechanical (e.g., curettage, forceps), but topical treatments are becoming more common. Current treatment options with larger supporting controlled studies include[7]:

- Curettage
- Forceps
- Cryosurgery

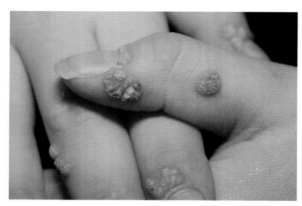

• **Fig. 37.25** Common Warts. (From Zitelli BJ, McIntire S, Nowalk AJ, et al, editors. *Zitelli and Davis' Atlas of Pediatric Physical Diagnosis.* 8th ed. Elsevier; 2023.)

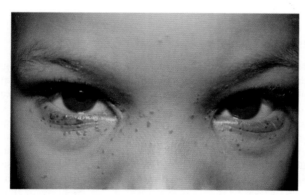

• **Fig. 37.26** Flat Warts. (From Zitelli BJ, McIntire S, Nowalk AJ, et al, editors. *Zitelli and Davis' Atlas of Pediatric Physical Diagnosis.* 8th ed. Elsevier; 2023.)

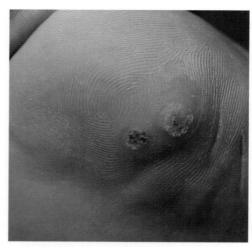

• **Fig. 37.27** Plantar Warts. (From Zitelli BJ, McIntire S, Nowalk AJ, et al, editors. *Zitelli and Davis' Atlas of Pediatric Physical Diagnosis.* 8th ed. Elsevier; 2023.)

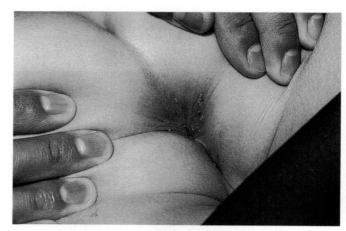

• **Fig. 37.28** Condylomata Acuminata. (From Paller AS, & Mancini AJ. *Paller and Mancini: Hurwitz Clinical Pediatric Dermatology.* 6th ed. Elsevier; 2022.)

elevated papules and number from few to several hundred (Fig. 37.26). Frequently spread by picking and scratching and thus may be found spread across the face or extremities.

• Plantar warts (verrucae plantaris or mosaic) are commonly found on weightbearing surfaces of the feet. They grow inward and disrupt skin markings (Fig. 37.27). When the lesion becomes larger and deeper, it can become painful for the patient to walk.

• Condylomata acuminata on genital mucosa and adjacent skin are multiple, confluent warts with irregular surfaces, light color, and cauliflower-like appearance (Fig. 37.28).

Differential Diagnosis

Differential diagnoses include calluses, corns, foreign bodies, moles, comedones, and squamous cell carcinoma. Plantar warts can be distinguished by their interruption of the skin lines and characteristic black dots.

Management

There is no single effective treatment for warts. The recurrence rate is high; they typically do not resolve with just a single treatment. No treatment is necessary if the warts are asymptomatic. The decision to treat should be based on location, number and size of lesions, discomfort, and whether they are cosmetically objectionable. Treatment should not be harmful, and scarring should be avoided. Genital warts found in young children or in adolescents who are not

sexually active should create suspicion of sexual abuse. While most PCPs recommend against treatment specific options are outlined in (Box 37.5). Follow up in 2 to 3 weeks to evaluate response.

Complications

Removal of warts can cause scarring. A ring of satellite warts may develop at the edge of the blister following treatment with destructive agents. Immunocompromised hosts can have extensive involvement.

Patient and Family Education

A blister, sometimes hemorrhagic, may form 1 to 2 days after liquid nitrogen treatment. Redness and itching may herald regression of a wart. Parents and patients must be warned that multiple or prolonged treatment is often necessary.

Infestations of the Skin

Pediculosis (Lice)

Lice are dependent on humans for existence, needing human blood for their sustenance. They feed by pressing their mouth

• BOX 37.5 Treatment Options for Warts

- Keratolytics eliminate the wart by causing an inflammatory response and topical peeling. They are often available over the counter, cause little pain, and are low in cost and risk, but they are slow to work.
  - Salicylic acid paints with a concentration of greater than 20% are applied with an applicator once or twice a day for 2–12 weeks. On thick skin, a combination of 16.7% salicylic acid and 16.7% collodion is more effective. This method is useful for common or periungual warts, but it is not effective with warts larger than 5 mm in diameter. Both products may be more effective if combined with duct tape occlusion.
  - Salicylic acid plasters cut to size and taped in place. Depending on the product, either: Apply plaster and repeat every 48 hours as needed, or apply plaster at bedtime, leave in place for at least 8 hours, remove plaster in the morning, and repeat every 24 hours as needed. After the plaster is taken off, the area should be soaked for 45 min and the dead epidermis removed. A new plaster is then applied. Treatment can last 2–12 weeks. This method is especially useful for plantar warts.
  - Retinoic acid gel 0.025–0.1% applied at bedtime causes mild erythema with scaling. It may take months to resolve. This method is useful for flat warts, but it does not work for common, plantar, or periungual warts.
- Occlusion with duct tape: Place on for 12 h a day for 6 days in a row, followed by soaking and scraping of epidermis; is easy, painless, and inexpensive.
- Destructive agents eliminate the wart by causing necrosis and blister formation. Most techniques are painful and require patient cooperation.
  - Cryotherapy: Liquid nitrogen, available over the counter as well as for in-office use, is applied for 2–10 days until an area 1–3 mm beyond the wart turns white or patient complains of pain; goal is to induce blister formation above the dermal-epidermal junction. This method often results in a ring of warts around the area that was treated. Take care not to freeze the wart too vigorously. Caution should be used when freezing warts over joints and the lateral aspects of digits. This method is uncomfortable and often not tolerated by children. Retreatment is often necessary.
  - Podophyllum 25% solution in compound benzoin tincture is applied to the wart with a toothpick; it should be washed off in 4 h; may be repeated in 1 week. Podofilox, available over the counter for home use, is applied twice a day for 3 days. After a 4-day rest period, the 3-day cycle may be repeated as necessary. This technique is useful for common or genital warts. Using this medication for other than anogenital warts is not FDA approved.
  - Surgical excision of warts can lead to scarring that can be more painful than the wart itself but can be highly effective for large individual warts. Surgery by snipping with scissors, not scalpel, is useful for filiform warts.
  - Laser treatments are often as effective as cryosurgery but can be painful and require several treatments for complete resolution.
- Condylomata therapy should usually start with watchful waiting, especially in young children. Refer for treatment if extensive or symptomatic.
- Immunotherapy modalities stimulate an immune response to HPV. These newer treatment modalities do not have controlled studies evaluating their effectiveness and are not approved under the age of 12 years.
  - Oral cimetidine, a histamine 2–receptor-blocking agent, may improve immunity to HPV. It is used in conjunction with other modalities at a dose of 20–30 mg/kg divided twice a day for 3–4 months.
  - Contact sensitization and interferon injection are methods used by dermatologists, usually in adult patients.

FDA, US Food and Drug Administration; HPV, human papillomavirus.

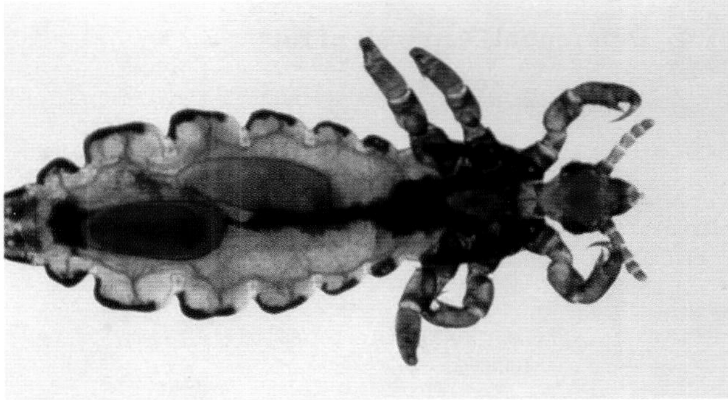

• **Fig. 37.29** Head Louse. Note the elongated body, three pairs of legs, and nits within the body. (From Paller AS, Mancini AJ. *Paller and Mancini: Hurwitz Clinical Pediatric Dermatology.* 6th ed. Elsevier; 2022.)

against the skin, piercing the skin, and injecting an anticoagulant to promote blood flow during feeding. Pediculosis (lice infestation) can affect the scalp (most common), body, or pubic area (commonly considered a sexually transmitted disease). The three species of lice are: *Pediculus humanus capitis* (head lice), *Pediculus humanus* corporis (body lice), and *Phthirus pubis* (pubic or "crab" lice). Lice are small but visible to the naked eye. They have translucent, grey/brown bodies with six legs and no wings. The body and head lice are longer bodied with three pair of claw-like legs (Fig. 37.29). The pubic louse has a short body and resembles a crab.

Lice egg cases are called *nits*, which are attached to the hair shaft with a cement. These waterproof shells are grey to white in color and appear like specks less than 1 mm in size. Nits incubate for about 1 week, hatch and grow into adult lice over another 1 to 2 weeks, then begin laying eggs. Head lice live approximately 30 days on a host and lay up to 10 eggs/day. Transmission is by direct or indirect contact, often by sharing hairbrushes, caps, clothing, or linen or through close living quarters, or sexual activity (pubic lice). Lice can crawl but not jump.

Pediculosis capitis is common in children. Head lice are not considered a health hazard, because they do not spread disease. All socioeconomic groups are affected, but lice are most common in school-age children, with the peak season occurring from August to November. Lice are less common in Black individuals, perhaps because the different nature of the hair shaft makes it difficult for the louse to grasp the shaft.[3]

Pediculosis corporis is left often seen in childhood and is typically associated with homeless individuals, refugees, and those living in crowded situations. The louse is rarely seen on the body; rather it attaches to clothing and intermittently pierces the skin. It is the louse that most commonly carries human disease (e.g., epidemic typhus and trench fever).

Pubic lice may involve the scalp, eyebrows, or eyelashes but primarily are found in the pubic area. Clothing and bed linens are a source of residence. If pediculosis pubis is found in a child, sexual abuse must be considered.

Clinical Findings
History
- A history of infestation in a family, friend, or daycare contact.
- Dandruff-like substance in the hair.
- Itching, scratching, and irritability if infestation has been present for a few weeks.
- Reports of a crawling sensation in the scalp.

TABLE 37.6	Differential Diagnosis of Nits
Diagnosis	**Comment**
Nits	Firmly adherent to hair shaft; not easily removed with fingers
Seborrheic dermatitis (dandruff)	Diffuse scalp scaling; scales occasionally adhere to hair but easy to remove; scalp erythema may be present
Hair casts	Keratin protein that encircles hair shaft; easily removed
Piedra	Fungal infection of hair; firm nodules attached to hair shafts, white or black in color
Psoriasis	Thick silvery scales, often present overlying red plaques on the scalp
Hair products	Hairspray, mousse, gel, etc.

From Paller AS, Mancini AJ. *Hurwitz Clinical Pediatric Dermatology: A Textbook of Skin Disorders of Children and Adolescence.* 6th ed. Elsevier; 2022.

Physical Examination

- Head lice:
  - Lice and nits can be visualized. Nits are usually laid within 2 mm of the scalp; as the hair grows, the nits and empty shells are found farther from the scalp, indicating more long-term infestation. Nits found further from the scalp are more likely to be nonviable.
  - Care must be taken to differentiate hair casts, epithelial cells, and other debris from nits (Table 37.6).
  - Common sites are the back of the head, nape of the neck, and behind the ears; eyelashes can be involved. Scalp excoriations and occipital or cervical adenopathy can be present.
- Body lice:
  - Excoriated macules or papules may be present. A secondary bacterial infection of the skin may hide the original bite lesions.
  - Belt line, collar, and underwear areas are common sites.
  - A hemorrhagic gray-blue macule may be seen where the louse extracted blood.
  - Axillary, inguinal, or regional lymphadenopathy can be present.
- Pubic lice:
  - Live lice and nits are usually seen.
  - Excoriation and small bluish macules and papules may be present.
  - Eyelashes can be involved; spread to other short-haired areas (thighs, trunk, axillae, beard) may occur.

Diagnostic Studies

- Microscopic examination of a hair shaft can more clearly identify nits.
- Test for other sexually transmitted infections if pubic lice found; specifically gonorrhea and syphilis.

Management

Correct diagnosis is imperative to effective management. Treatment is recommended when live lice and viable nits are observed, because nonviable nits, which do not necessarily indicate the presence of lice, can persist on the hair shaft for several months.

Treatment options are varied and controversial. Treatment failure is common, whether because of poor technique or because of increasing drug resistance to available pharmacologic treatment options in children who have been treated multiple times. Pyrethroid insecticides have documented widespread resistance. The increasing treatment failure has led to the trial of many alternative treatments such as OTC medications, and dangerous substitutes (e.g., kerosene) may be used by parents. It is recommended that PCPs follow local resistance patterns when determining treatment.

Pediculicides are a first-line treatment option. They are toxic substances, however, and should be used only as directed and with care. Proper pediculicide application is key to success. Before use, do not use a shampoo that contains conditioner or cream rinse, or petrolatum products on the hair or scalp. Keep the pediculicide out of the eyes. If applying to damp hair, make sure the hair is damp, not wet as it dilutes the pediculicide. Do not rewash the hair for 1 to 2 days following treatment. Most treatments call for reapplication in 7 to 10 days with 9 days being the optimal interval based on the life cycle of lice.[3]

- Permethrin 1% cream rinse (OTC) is the treatment of choice for head lice because of its safety (can be used with infants 2 months and older), efficacy, and 10-day residual. Hair should be shampooed and towel dried (damp), permethrin applied, left on for 10 minutes, and then rinse. Hair should not be rewashed for at least 24 to 48 hours. Resistance to permethrin 1% has been reported but prevalence is unknown. Reapplication is recommended.
- Spinosad (Rx) is approved for use in patients 6 months of age and older. Superiority of spinosad over permethrin has been well documented. It is applied to dry hair and left on for 10 minutes before rinsing. Reapplication is recommended only if live lice are seen.
- Pyrethrin (OTC), a natural extract from the chrysanthemum plant, is effective as a pediculicide but not as an ovicide. Pyrethrin is formulated with piperonyl butoxide to form a 10-minute shampoo or mousse that is applied to dry hair, with a repeat reapplication in 7 to 10 days. Pyrethrin is contraindicated in patients with allergy to ragweed or chrysanthemum. Because pyrethrin does not kill both lice and eggs, treatment failures are more common than with permethrin. Highly variable resistance is found with pyrethrin.
- Topical ivermectin lotion (Rx) is a single-dose, 10-minute application to dry hair. It is approved for patients 6 months old and older. Caution is advised for use during pregnancy. Repeat application is not necessary as the lice of treated eggs are not viable.
- Malathion lotion 0.5% (Rx) is an organophosphate with a pine-needle–oil base. It is a potent lice killer that binds to the hair shaft for 4 weeks and, while it is not a first-line therapy, it is considered the most effective therapy for killing lice and nits. It is not recommended in individuals younger than 2 years old. The drug is flammable, and if ingested causes severe respiratory distress. A single application is adequate for most patients but a repeat application in 7 to 10 days is appropriate if live lice are seen.[8]
- Benzyl alcohol 5% lotion (Rx) is a nonneurotoxic product for use in patients 6 months and older. This agent kills lice through blockage of their respiratory mechanism. It is not ovicidal and repeat treatment is recommended.

Many PCPs and families choose to forgo the use of pediculicides in favor of a manual removal of lice and nits. Although combing may not always be necessary, this step is usually taken to remove nits after a pediculicide is used. Proper technique is the key to success. A good light, a magnifying glass, and tweezers are useful. A wide-toothed comb may be used initially to straighten the hair, but a fine-toothed nit-removal comb is necessary to remove nits. There are now lice-removal salons across the United States that offer manual nit removal and treatment.

- Some products claim to dissolve the substance (cement) that attaches the nit to the hair to facilitate removal; however, there are no effective agents for this purpose.[3] Use a proper nit-removal comb with fine teeth (included in most pediculicide kits).
- Comb damp hair for a minimum of 20 to 30 minutes, working from close to the scalp down in 1-inch sections. Pay special attention to the nape of the neck and behind the ears.
- If eyelashes are involved, coat with petroleum jelly 2 or 3 times a day for 8 to 14 days and manually remove nits.
- Comb-outs and inspection should be repeated every night for 2 to 3 weeks to ensure cure.

An important step in lice treatment is thorough cleansing of the environment.

- Examine family members, friends, school, and daycare contacts. Only those with signs of infestation or those who share a bed with the index patient need to be treated because of the emergence of treatment-resistant lice and pediculicide toxicity.[3]
- Launder sheets, towels, clothing, and headgear in hot water and machine dry on hot cycle for 20 minutes, iron, or dry clean.
- Although rarely needed, any other item in close contact with others that cannot be washed or dry-cleaned should be stored in a plastic bag for 2 weeks.
- Soak brushes, combs, and hair accessories in pediculicide or rubbing alcohol for 1 hour, followed by washing in hot soapy water.
- Spraying or fumigating the house is not recommended.

Alternative treatments include herbal or essential oils and occlusive methods such as olive oil, pine oil, tea-tree oil, margarine, mayonnaise, styling gels, and petroleum jelly, all of which suffocate and kill the lice. Further evidence-based studies are needed regarding these practices. Avoid wrapping the hair in plastic and putting the child under a hair dryer and warn about the dangers of washing the hair with gasoline or kerosene.

Treatment failure is not unusual. Common mistakes that lead to recurrence of lice include dilution of pediculicide by applying to wet, not damp hair; use of a shampoo with conditioner or cream rinse before treatment; inadequate combing techniques; not cleansing personal care items; and not screening and treating family members and close contacts. However, with proper use of a pediculicide, if lice reappear, reinfection from contact with an untreated individual is a more likely cause. Resistance to pediculicide products is not well understood and appears to be regional. There are neither formal recommendations nor FDA approval for dealing with resistance. Some methods for treating resistant lice include the following:

- Benzoyl alcohol 5% if the child is older than 6 months
- Malathion 0.5% if the child is older than 2 years
- Manual removal by wet combing
- Occlusive method with careful technique for two to four lice life cycles.

Body lice are treated by deinfestation of bedding and clothing. Treatment with permethrin may be helpful for the occasional louse that remains. Pubic lice are treated as pediculosis capitis[3]

Complications

Secondary bacterial infection can occur.

Patient and Family Education

Items for discussion include the following:

- Daily to weekly checks or combing for lice or nits should be carried out at home.
- Educate family members about the expected course that lice infestation is not a social disease, and about the need to avoid excessive or unnecessary retreatment. Do not use extra amounts; do not treat more than three times with the same medication without being seen by a care provider; do not mix pediculicides.
- Children should not be excluded or sent home from school because of lice. Parents should be notified and informed that the child should be treated. The American Academy of Pediatrics discourages "no-nit" policies in schools, because such policies have been ineffective in controlling head lice transmission and result in excessive lost school and workdays.[8]
- Rinse topical pediculosides in sink rather than shower to reduce skin exposure and in warm water rather than hot water to reduce absorption through vasodilation.

Scabies

Scabies is caused by the mite *Sarcoptes scabiei*, which is an obligate human parasite that burrows into the epidermis and causes intense itching. Scabies is a highly contagious infestation spread through close contact and shared clothing or linen. It takes approximately 15 minutes for transmission of the mites from one person to another. The female mite burrows into the skin, laying up to three eggs a day as she travels. The eggs hatch in about 3 to 4 days and mature into adult mites in 10 to 14 days. The female mite has a life span of 15 to 30 days. Sensitization, which causes intense itching, occurs approximately 3 weeks after infestation.

Scabies occurs in all socioeconomic groups and in all age groups. Females and children, the immunocompromised, mentally or physically challenged, and HIV patients are at increased risk for scabies. Closed communities and institutions have a higher endemic rate.

Animal-transmission scabies is most commonly a canine form of scabies (*S. scabei* var. *canis*). The dog afflicted with sarcoptic manage usually presents with patchy loss of hair with scaling. These animals are most often undernourished and heavily parasitized. The canine scabies mite cannot reproduce on humans and the infestation is usually self-limited, clearing spontaneously over several weeks.

Clinical Findings

History

- Key finding: Itching, worse at night, initially mild but progressively more intense. Often presents before clinical signs are present.
- Fitful sleep, crankiness, or rubbing of hands and feet (infants).

Physical Examination

- Complaints are significantly greater than examination findings. Excoriation is commonly found.
- Characteristic lesions include curving S-shaped burrows, especially on webs of fingers and sides of hands, folds of wrists and armpits, forearms, elbows, belt line, buttocks, genitalia, or proximal half of foot and heel (Fig. 37.30C). Genital lesions are common.

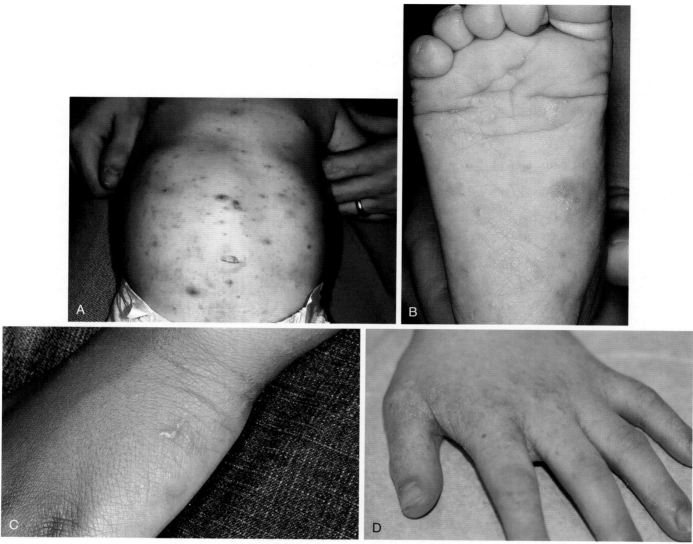

• **Fig. 37.30** Scabies. (A) Scabies—erythematous papules and crusting. (B) Scabies—erythematous papules and linear burrows. (C) Scabies—curvilinear burrow of the lateral hand. (D) Crusted scabies—scaly papules or plaques that are eczema like in appearance. (From Paller AS, Mancini AJ. *Paller and Mancini: Hurwitz Clinical Pediatric Dermatology.* 6th ed. Elsevier; 2022.)

- Vesiculopustular lesions tend to be found in infants and young children (Fig. 37.30A–B). They classically have vesicular lesions on palms, soles, scalp, face, posterior auriculae, and axillae, concentrated in the folds; head and neck lesions typically are red-brown vesicopustules or nodules. However, any child younger than 2 years old can have an unusual manifestation.
- Secondary lesions include itchy papules, red-brown nodules from significant hypersensitivity response, crusting, excoriation, and other signs of secondary infection. Scabies nodules may persist for months.
- Infants classically have dozens of lesions; older children may have fewer than 10.
- Crusted, or Norwegian scabies, presents as scaly papules or plaques and is more often found in immunocompromised and mentally or physically challenged patients. The lesions may be heavily crusted and hyperkeratotic. This form of scabies has large numbers of mites and is much more contagious (Fig. 37.30D). It may be less pruritic and mimic atopic dermatitis, psoriasis, or drug reaction.
- Animal-transmitted scabies tends to spare interdigital webs and genitalia and the burrows are absent.
  Diagnostic Studies.
- Microscopic examination of scrapings in mineral oil can reveal eight-legged mite, eggs, or feces. Do not use KOH because it dissolves the mites, eggs, and feces. Burrows and fresh papules are best for specimen collection.

Differential Diagnosis

Papular urticaria; atopic, seborrheic, or contact dermatitis; insect bites; folliculitis; lichen planus; and dermatitis herpetiformis are included in the differential diagnoses.

Management

Resistance to medication is not common and continued infestation is usually due to treatment failure rather than resistance. Reasons for treatment failure include an incorrect diagnosis, not applying medication to the whole body, or not treating all members of the household. The patient may develop postscabetic eczema that can be misdiagnosed as treatment failure. Evaluate and treat with topical corticosteroids. Management involves the following:

- Pharmacologic treatment begins with applying a thin layer of scabicide to the entire body, from the neck down. Areas of special importance are under the fingernails, the scalp, behind the ears, all folds and creases, and the feet and hands. A second application of the scabicide should be reapplied in 7 days on all symptomatic patients, but studies suggest a relatively high cure rate after one application.
  - Permethrin 5% cream remains the drug of choice for the treatment of scabies. Despite frequent use over the past 2 decades, there is no clear evidence of resistance to permethrin 5% cream for the treatment of classic scabies.[3] It is indicated for use in patients as young as 2 months old. Unlike adults and older children, infants generally present with lesions on the head, include the scalp as an area of treatment.
  - Ivermectin orally is an off-label use and should only be considered for severe infections and crusted scabies. Because it is not ovicidal, a second treatment 1 to 2 weeks after the first is often recommended. Ivermectin is often used in conjunction with full body application of permethrin 5% cream. Ivermectin is not recommended for children younger than 5 years.[3]
- Antihistamines (e.g., hydroxyzine, diphenhydramine) or topical 1% hydrocortisone can be helpful for itching, which can last for several weeks after successful treatment.
- Systemic antibiotic therapy should be given for any secondary bacterial infection.
- Simultaneous treatment of family members, friends, and school and daycare contacts, even if asymptomatic, is essential.
- At time of treatment, linens and any clothing worn during the past 48 hours should be washed with hot water, put into a hot dryer for 20 minutes, or dry-cleaned. The house should be vacuumed.
- Store nonwashable items in sealed plastic bags for 1 week. Mite survival when separated from the human host is only a few days.

Complications

A secondary bacterial infection, most often from *S. aureus* or GABHS, is possible and should be treated. Postscabetic syndrome is common, with visible lesions and pruritus persisting for days to weeks following treatment; nodular lesions can persist for weeks to months.

Patient and Family Education

- Educate family on proper application of a thin layer of cream to the entire body from the neck down and rinsing after 8 to 14 hours.
- Ensure the family understands the course of disease. Rash and itching persist for up to 3 weeks following treatment.
- Avoid overbathing and further irritation of the skin.
- The patient will be infectious and cannot return to school or day care until 24 hours after treatment.

Allergic and Inflammatory Skin Conditions

Acne Vulgaris

Acne is the most common skin disorder in the United States and affects 80% to 85% of individuals between 11 and 30 years of age.[3] It usually begins at the onset of puberty, occurring earlier in females (12–13 years old) than males (14–15 years old). Although not a serious physical disorder, acne has been associated with psychosocial morbidity and decreased emotional wellbeing. The severity of acne is directly related to the extent psychological impact. It has even been shown that patients with mild to moderate acne demonstrate higher rates of depression and suicidal ideation.[3] For these reasons, it is important to note that the benefits of acne therapy may be far more significant than the dermatological improvement of the patient.

Acne is an inflammatory disorder of the pilosebaceous unit (the hair follicle and sebaceous gland (see Fig. 37.1). The three components of acne formation are: increased sebum production, hyperkeratosis, and bacterial proliferation. Acne lesions start with the formation of a microcomedone, which is caused by the obstruction of a hair follicle with keratin, an increase of sebum production by the sebaceous gland, and an overgrowth of normal skin flora. The occluded pilosebaceous unit enlarges due to stimulation of the sebaceous gland by androgens. A common skin flora, *Propionibacterium acnes*, leads to pustule formation. The microcomedones enlarge into open (blackheads) or closed (whiteheads) comedones. The black appearance may be due to the oxidation of the keratinous material.

Although rarely a serious disorder, acne lesions can become inflamed (e.g., papules, pustules, nodules) and may cause permanent scarring and decreased self-esteem, and occasionally heralds underlying disease. It tends to improve in the summer and worsens with menses and stress. The pathogenesis of acne is multifactorial; sex, age, neuroendocrine regulation, genetic factors, and environment are significant factors. The role of diet remains controversial. Acne may be associated with a high-glycemic diet.

Clinical Findings

History
- Family history of acne
- Stage of pubertal development (sexual maturity rating—see Chapter 13) and menstrual history
- Facial and hair products used, especially occlusive products or pomades
- Oral and topical prescription medication, especially oral contraceptives, antibiotics, or steroids
- Current or previous acne treatment and results
- Sports participation, especially if wearing football pads, helmets, headbands, or other protective devices
- Jobs, such as cooking at a fast-food grill or working at a gas station
- Other medical conditions, such as those affecting the hypothalamic-pituitary-adrenal axis, which result in an increase in androgens

Physical Examination.
Lesions are most commonly found on the face, back, and chest.
- Noninflammatory lesions:
  - Microcomedone—a follicular plug as a result of obstruction of the pilosebaceous unit (hair follicle and sebaceous gland) typically localized on the face and trunk.
  - Open comedone (i.e., blackhead)—a noninflammatory lesion or papule, firm in consistency, caused by blockage at the mouth of the follicle and occurring on the face, upper back, shoulders, and chest. The black color is thought to come from oxidized keratinous material at the follicular opening. This is the main lesion in early adolescence.

TABLE 37.7	Treatment Algorithm for the Management of Acne			
	Mild (Comedonal)	**Mild (Inflammatory/Mixed)**	**Moderate (Inflammatory/Mixed)**	**Severe (Inflammatory/Mixed)**
First-line treatment	• BP • Topical retinoid • Salicylic acid cleanser	• BP/retinoid combo • BP/antibiotic combo • Antibiotic/retinoid combo + BP	• BP/retinoid combo • BP/antibiotic combo ± topical retinoid • Antibiotic/retinoid combo + BP ± oral antibiotic	• BP/retinoid combo + oral antibiotic • BP/antibiotic combo + topical retinoid + oral antibiotic • Antibiotic/retinoid combo + BP + oral antibiotic
Alternative treatment (topical dapsone may be considered in place of topical antibiotic)	• Add topical retinoid or BP (if not on already) • BP/antibiotic combo • BP/retinoid combo • Antibiotic/retinoid combo	• Substitute another combo product • Add missing component (e.g., topical retinoid, BP, topical antibiotic) • Change type, strength, or formulation of topical retinoid	• Substitute another combo product • Add missing component (e.g., topical retinoid, BP, topical antibiotic, oral antibiotic) • Change type, strength, or formulation of topical retinoid • Consider hormonal therapy for female patients • Consider oral isotretinoin	• Consider change in oral antibiotic • Consider isotretinoin • Consider hormonal therapy for female patients
Maintenance therapy	• Topical retinoid • BP/retinoid combo	• Topical retinoid • BP/retinoid combo	• Topical retinoid • BP/retinoid combo	• Topical retinoid • BP/retinoid combo

BP, Benzoyl peroxide.

If combination products are unavailable, consider separate prescriptions for individual components.

From Paller AS, Mancini AJ. *Hurwitz Clinical Pediatric Dermatology: A Textbook of Skin Disorders of Children and Adolescence.* 6th ed. Elsevier; 2022.

- Closed comedone (i.e., whitehead)—a noninflammatory lesion, semisoft in consistency, caused by blockage at the neck of the follicle. This is a precursor to inflammatory acne.
- Inflammatory lesions occur secondary to rupture of noninflamed lesions into the dermis and can include papules, pustules, excoriation, lesion crusting, nodules, cysts, scars, and sinus tracts (confluent nodules likely to scar).

The severity of acne is determined by the quantity, type, and spread of lesions. It is helpful to use a diagram of the face or a grading graph to identify the number and type of lesions to allow more precise patient follow-up. If only open and closed comedones are found, the disorder is called *comedonal acne.* Most adolescents have a combination of comedones, red papules, and pustules called *papulopustular acne,* which can be mild or severe. *Nodulocystic acne* is the most severe form and requires more intensive intervention. Specific types of acne include *frictional,* occurring from rubbing of bras, tight clothes, or headbands; *pomadal,* along the temple and forehead, as a result of pomades or oil-based cosmetics; *athletic,* on forehead, chin, or shoulders, caused by helmets and pads; and *hormonal,* with a beard distribution.

Differential Diagnosis

Cosmetic, mechanical, environmental, or drug-induced acne; rosacea; flat wart; milia; perioral dermatitis; and folliculitis are included in the differential diagnoses.

Management

The goals of acne management are to (1) reduce the excess production of sebum, (2) counteract the abnormal desquamation of epithelial cells, (3) decrease the proliferation of *P. acnes,* and (4) prevent or decrease scarring. Choice of treatment depends on the extent, severity, and duration of disease; type of lesions; and psychological effects the adolescent is experiencing. Table 37.7 shows the treatment algorithm. Box 37.6 lists some of the common medications used. Medications used in treatment of acne vary by action, route of administration, and strength. They include topical and systemic preparations; keratolytic or comedolytic agents; those with antibacterial or antibiotic effects; hormonal agents; and preparations that have a combination of actions.

- Topical keratolytic or comedolytic agents, used to minimize follicular obstruction and break up microcomedones, are the first line of acne treatment. While benzoyl peroxide is still a very effective therapy, retinoids have become the mainstay of first-line therapies. Tretinoin has been shown to be effective alone over a 12-week period in 63% of cases.[11] If keratolytics are not effective alone, they may be dispensed in a combination form with a topical antibacterial agent. Many strengths and forms are available, the strongest being the gels, if tolerated; creams are the least drying. A general rule is to start low in strength and slowly in frequency and advance as tolerated or needed. A useful technique to decrease the incidence of irritation is to start therapy only for 3 nights a week and slowly increase to a nightly application over a few weeks. A minimum of 4 to 6 weeks of treatment is required before improvement is seen. Each topical therapy works by a different mechanism and can be used together and interchangeably. Retinoids may degrade significantly when mixed with benzoyl peroxide, therefore preformulated combination products are preferred. If using individual agents, they should be applied at different times. Combination products appear to increase compliance when compared to individual applications.[11] Dryness, erythema, irritation, and scaling can occur with these products, and the strength and frequency of use must be adjusted for this. A pea-sized application should be made after washing the face; initially, every other night and advancing to every night.

• BOX 37.6 Medications Commonly Used in Treating Acne

Topical Keratolytic or Comedolytic Agents

Retinoids:
   Tretinoin: 0.01–0.025% gel; 0.025–0.1% cream; 0.1% microgel
   Tazarotene: 0.05–0.1% cream or gel
   Adapalene: 0.1% gel or cream; 0.3% gel; 0.1% lotion
   Trifarotene: 0.005% cream
Benzoyl peroxide: 2.5%, 5%, 8%, 10% gel; 5%, 10% cream; 5%,10% lotion;
   2.5%, 4%, 5%, 6%, 7%, 10% wash
Azelaic acid: 20% cream
Salicylic acid: 0.5–2% lotion, cream, cleanser, pads, solution, or toner

Topical Antibiotics

Clindamycin: 1% solution, lotion, gel, pledget, foam
Erythromycin: 1.5–2% solution, 2% gel or swabs
Dapsone: 5%, 7% gel
Minocycline: 4% foam

Combination Topical Agents

Clindamycin/benzoyl peroxide: 1%, 2.5%, 5% gel
Erythromycin/benzoyl peroxide: 3%, 5% gel
Adapalene/benzoyl peroxide: 0.1%, 0.3%, 2.5% gel
Clindamycin/tretinoin: 0.025%, 1.2% gel

Oral Antibiotics

Tetracycline
Minocycline
Doxycycline
Erythromycin

Combination Oral Contraceptives

Ethinyl estradiol/norgestimate
Ethinyl estradiol/norethindrone acetate/ferrous fumarate
Ethinyl estradiol/drospirenone
Ethinyl estradiol/drospirenone/levomefolate

From Zaenglein AL, Pathy AL, Schlosser BJ, et al. Guidelines of care for the management of acne vulgaris. *J Am Acad Dermatol.* 2016;74(5):945–973.

Retinoids can cause photosensitivity and sunscreen should be used. Teratogenicity is controversial but should be considered, and most avoid their use in pregnancy. There have been no studies comparing efficacy of retinoids so strength, side effects, and cost of products should be considered when using.

- Tretinoin is a vitamin A derivative and is the oldest medication in this class. It is the only retinoid that can be used down to age 10 years (all others are for 12 years and older). Sensitivity to tretinoin is worst in the first 2 weeks of use and decreases thereafter.
- Adapalene is the second retinoid approved for acne use and the 0.1% gel is the only FDA-approved formulation available OTC. It seems to cause less irritation and less photosensitivity.
- Tazarotene is a retinoid that is also available in a foam if patient prefers that formulation.
- Trifarotene is the only FDA-approved medication for chest and back acne.
- BP, the most frequently used topical preparation for acne, is used once or twice a day, depending on the severity of acne and dryness of skin. It is a powerful antimicrobial with comedolytic and antiinflammatory effects. Use in combination with topical antibiotics causes less antibiotic resistance.

- Salicylic acid and BP are the two most common agents found in OTC acne treatments. It reduces sebum and comedones.
- Azelaic acid is an antibacterial and keratolytic. It is useful in individuals with sensitive or dark skin and is also effective in treating acne rosacea. May work better at decreasing hyperpigmentation.[11]
- Topical antibiotics are used to control the inflammatory process and reduce bacterial colonization of the skin and follicles, usually most helpful in moderate inflammatory acne. They are also used to maintain control after treatment with oral antibiotics, and are applied to the entire skin surface, not just to problem areas. They should not be applied within 30 minutes of shaving. Because of developing bacterial resistance, topical antibiotics are not recommended as monotherapy.
- Topical clindamycin with BP and erythromycin with BP are combination products that are more effective than either drug alone and have less resistance from *P. acnes.* This combination is especially effective in mild to moderate inflammatory acne or as an adjunct to oral therapy.[3]
- Topical dapsone is a newer topical antibiotic that may have greater antiinflammatory action.
- Oral antibiotics are used in addition to topical agents to decrease the concentration of *P. acnes* and to decrease the degree of inflammation if there is no response to topical agents. Systemic antibiotics should be used for the shortest time possible, no longer than 3 to 4 months, and often require 3 to 4 weeks to see improvement. Once improvement is noted, the dose should be tapered to a daily dose, and then discontinued. Combination use with BP or retinoid is recommended with continuation of topical medication after stopping the oral antibiotic. The tetracycline class of antibiotics and the second-generation tetracyclines (minocycline, doxycycline) are considered first-line oral antibiotic therapy.[11]
- Tetracyclines can be teratogenic and are to be avoided in pregnancy. They are also known to stain the teeth in those under 9 years. Photosensitivity reactions can occur. Doxycycline appears to have an increased incidence of these side effects. Minocycline is increasingly common as an oral antibiotic for acne treatment, but many consider doxycycline to be safer due to the increased risk for severe side effects with minocycline.[3]
- Erythromycin use should be limited to those who cannot take tetracycline because of increasing resistance to erythromycin. Erythromycin can be taken with food, but gastrointestinal upset is common, and vulvovaginal candidiasis can be problematic.
- Hormonal and other therapies: Hormonal associated acne can be distinguished by association with menstrual cycles, menstrual irregularities, large and deep-seated nodular lesions in the anterolateral neck regions, or signs of polycystic ovarian syndrome. Any concerns about illness associated with an androgen excess should be referred to an endocrinologist. Hormonal therapies can be used in females to oppose effects of androgen on sebaceous glands. Oral contraceptive pills (OCPs) are the only FDA-approved hormonal therapeutic in children and have proven to be very effective at reducing inflammatory lesions. OCPs contain both an estrogen and a progestin, and those with a lower progestin activity are FDA approved (see Box 37.6).
- Isotretinoin in an oral retinoid used for severe, recalcitrant nodulocystic acne. This pregnancy Category X drug is known for

its teratogenic effect and requires evaluation by a dermatologist before use. It is known to be associated with inflammatory bowel disease and an association with depression and suicide is controversial. The usual course is 20 weeks; there are many side effects, and LFTs, serum cholesterol, triglycerides, human chorionic gonadotropin, and urinalysis for pregnancy must be monitored every month while the patient is taking the medication.

- The iPledge program creates a registry for all patients being treated with isotretinoin. The FDA requires healthcare providers, female patients, and pharmacists to access the iPledge website monthly after office visits and before filling their prescription for documentation regarding pregnancy, blood donation, and contraceptive counseling.[3]
- Dermatologists may use intralesional steroid therapy for large cysts or nodules; resurfacing lasers and dermabrasion are used for acne scarring.
- Noncomedogenic moisturizers can be used for dryness, which is common with treatment. Noncomedogenic makeup is also available and helpful in treating these patients.

Complications

Failure can be due to lack of patient motivation, lack of education, inappropriate treatments, initial treatment that was too strong, or expectations of a quick fix. Psychological effects include decreased self-esteem and poor body image, problems with interpersonal relationships, self-consciousness, embarrassment, depression, and decreased athletic participation, especially in gymnastics, swimming, and wrestling. Resistance of *P. acnes* to tetracycline, erythromycin, and minocycline is increasing.

Patient and Family Education

- When prescribing treatment, it is important to keep the regimen as simplified as possible and to be sure that the patient and family understand the therapy. Give the plan in a written form to ensure better adherence. Also consider psychological comorbidities that may be associated with the course of acne and resulting cosmetic appearance. Encourage open discussion regarding possible acne-associated stressors and self-perceptions of the patient.
- Education is the priority. The adolescent must have realistic expectations and understand the pathophysiology and the process of treatment, including the fact that the acne often worsens before improving. Reading materials about acne and its treatment provide support for self-management efforts.
- Wash face twice a day with a mild soap (e.g., Dove, Neutrogena, Aveeno Cleansing Bar). Avoid scrubbing, rubbing, picking, and squeezing. Medication should be applied lightly.
- Use of a comedone extractor can cause scarring and should be discouraged. Hot soaks applied to pustules may help their resolution.
- All products used on the face should be labeled as *noncomedogenic*.
- Identify and discontinue use of aggravating substances, such as oil-based cosmetics, pomades, hair spray, mousse, and face creams.
- Identify possible aggravating factors, such as stress; hot, humid weather; and jobs involving frying oil or grease.
- Limited evidence supports a strong connection between foods and acne; however, a well-balanced diet is important to maintaining healthy skin.
- Discuss psychosocial concerns and provide support.
- Remind the adolescent that results take months and that adherence to treatment is essential to improvement.
- Sun exposure helps clear acne for some adolescents but may worsen it for others. Sunscreen use is recommended, and

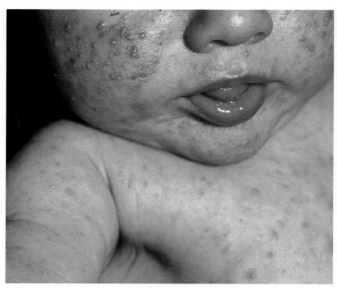

• **Fig. 37.31** Typical Papules and Pustules of Neonatal Acne. (From Paller AS, Mancini AJ. *Paller and Mancini: Hurwitz Clinical Pediatric Dermatology.* 6th ed. Elsevier; 2022.)

caution about sun exposure should be given if a medication that increases photosensitivity is being used.

- Follow-up visits should occur at least every 4 to 6 weeks until control is established, defined as when lesions clear or only a few new lesions appear every 2 weeks. Refer to a dermatologist for nonresponsive or severe cases.
- *Neonatal acne* (Fig. 37.31) presents in the first weeks of life and is best treated with a plan of watchful waiting and gentle daily cleansing with soap and water. Oils, lotions, and ointments typically aggravate the condition, and it generally resolves in 3 to 6 months. If the condition is more severe or persistent, the mild 2.5% BP can be sparingly used.
- *Infantile acne* presents between 1 and 12 months. The lesions may appear not only on the face but chest and back as well. Because of possible scarring, most experts recommend treatment with combination of BP, topical antibiotics, and/or topical retinoids (if comedonal acne is present). Careful examination for growth and signs of precocious puberty or androgen excess is warranted.[3]
- *Mid-childhood acne* presents between 1 and 7 years and is considered abnormal. Acne at this age is most likely related to an underlying endocrine disorder and a referral to pediatric endocrinology should be considered. Treatment for the acne is like that for infantile acne.

Atopic Dermatitis

See Chapter 36 for a discussion of Atopic Dermatitis.

Contact Dermatitis

Contact dermatitis is an acute or chronic inflammation resulting from a hypersensitive reaction to a substance (either irritants or allergens). Although it occurs at any age, contact dermatitis is extremely common in children.

Common types of contact dermatitis include the following[12]:
- Irritant contact dermatitis is not an allergic process. There is damage to the skin because of repeated and/or cumulative exposure to the offending agent.

- Dry skin dermatitis caused by extremely low humidity (less than 30%), excess soap or cleansing cream use, or inadequate rinsing of soap products.
- Lip-licker dermatitis caused by frequent lip licking, most often in dry, cold weather.
- Phytophotodermatitis from sun exposure following contact with plants or juices (e.g., limes, lemons, carrots, celery, figs, parsnips, dill) manifests as a blistered lesion on an erythematous base and may be confused with a burn.
- Allergic contact dermatitis is seen only after sensitization to an allergen has occurred and a subsequent type IV-delayed hypersensitivity response has activated an immune cascade. Sometimes the cause is obvious; often no specific cause can be identified.
  - Nickel dermatitis from contact with jewelry, belts, snaps, or eyeglasses.
  - Plant oleoresins, such as poison ivy, oak, or sumac; contact can be direct or indirect (exposure to burning plant material); oils may be inhaled, causing damage to lung tissue. Urushiol, the oil-based allergen in poison ivy, oak, and sumac can remain on contaminated items, such as clothing, animal hair, toys, and sports equipment resulting in sequential outbreaks due to reexposures. It is the recurrent contact with the urushiol causing the dermatitis and not a "spreading" of the rash itself. Poison ivy (rhus dermatitis) is the most common allergic contact dermatitis in the United States.
  - Topical medications such as neomycin, bacitracin, and benzocaine can cause a significant reaction. Remember that these medications are often combined with other medications such as antifungals and corticosteroids.
  - Latex dermatitis, associated with the use of products containing latex (e.g., gloves).
  - Other common allergens include dyes, lanolin, and preservatives found in skin care products, household cleansers, and the resins in plastic and clothing. These substances can even be found in skin care products and personal wipes.

Clinical Findings

History. Diagnosis of contact dermatitis can be challenging and often the source of the skin reaction is not found. A thorough history is critical including:
- Contact with any new or unusual substances
- History of any known food, environmental, or contact allergies
- Family allergy history since there is a genetic component to allergies
- Home and routine activities
- Repeated exposure to any substance or item
- Location and pattern of eruption

Physical Examination. The area of involvement offers clues to the causative agent. Often, the rash is localized to one area and has sharp borders (Fig. 37.32). The severity of the rash depends on the length of exposure and the concentration of the irritant. Minimal contact may produce only mild erythema, whereas prolonged or concentrated contact may produce significant erythema, edema, and blistering with possible crusting and secondary infection. Irritant reactions tend to be immediate, whereas allergic ones are delayed.
- Location of the rash may be your biggest clue. A linear-type rash can be secondary to the vine of a plant or wearing a necklace or bracelet. Circular areas can be seen from snaps on clothing. Inflammation of the earlobes (from jewelry) or as a reaction pattern on the toes and dorsum of the foot (from shoes) or post-auricular and wrist area reactions (from perfume) can be seen.
- A chafed appearance with shiny, mild to severely erythematous, peeling, or dry, fissured skin or red patches and plaques with secondary scales may be seen if the reaction is due to an irritant (e.g., dorsum of the hand may exhibit the aforementioned characteristic appearance with frequent hand washing with irritating soaps).
- Erythema, vesicles, and weeping may be present in the acute stage of allergic contact dermatitis. The lesions are pruritic.
- Hyperpigmentation and lichenification, often mimicking atopic dermatitis, are seen in chronic conditions.

Differential Diagnosis

Differential diagnoses include atopic dermatitis, impetigo, herpes simplex, psoriasis, and seborrhea.

Management

Appropriate skin care, recognizing and eliminating offending agents, and treating inflammation are key to managing contact dermatitis successfully. If possible, identify and avoid the substance (irritant or allergen) causing the dermatitis. Since 1999, the Mayo Clinic Contact Dermatologist Group has been a part of the website SkinSAFE (see Additional Resources) that helps people avoid ingredients that may cause reaction to skin allergies. Users can search for products using a known allergen and a list of suitable and avoidable products are given. General treatment measures for contact dermatitis include:
- Burow solution soaks or oatmeal baths and cool compresses (1 teaspoon salt/pint water) applied for 20 minutes every 4 to 6 hours to soothe vesicular rashes.
- Water and emollients applied to the skin to restore moisture to areas of dryness and chafing. Lanolin-and-petrolatum–based emollients should not be used if there is inflammation.
- Topical corticosteroids used 2 to 3 times daily give relief in 2 to 3 days, although it may take 2 to 3 weeks for complete healing. Taper systemic oral corticosteroids for a 2- to 3-week period if the area of allergic involvement exceeds 10% of the skin surface, involves extensive parts of the face, eyelids, genitals, or intense inflammation and pruritis in the hands.[2]
- Oral antihistamines are helpful if itching and scratching are problems.

Refer to a dermatologist or an allergist for patch testing if the dermatitis worsens, fails to respond, or recurs. Allergic contact dermatitis can develop into chronic dermatitis if left untreated. Psoralen and UVA treatment, narrow-band UVB treatment, systemic treatment with immunomodulators, and targeted biologic therapy may be considered if unresponsive to other measures.

Complications

Secondary bacterial or candida infections are common. A generalized *id* reaction can develop to an allergen, which presents as a secondary or "sympathy" rash distant from the primary site of exposure (Fig. 37.33).

Patient and Family Education

- Resolution may take 2 to 3 weeks. Continue therapy until completely resolved.
- Wash all clothing and pets that may have been in contact with the plant from rhus dermatitis. Thorough bathing after known exposure may help as well.

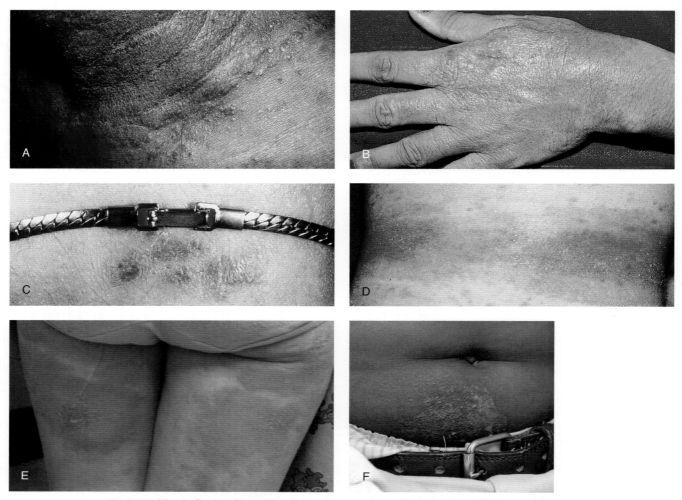

• **Fig. 37.32** Allergic Contact Dermatitis. Benzocaine reaction on (A) the neck and (B) the top of the hand. Nickel allergy on (C) the wrist. Elastic waistband reaction in (D). The itchy dermatitis in (E) was secondary to school toilet seat. Chronic contact dermatitis from a nickel belt buckle (F). (From Cohen BA, editor. *Pediatric Dermatology*. 5th ed. Elsevier; 2022.)

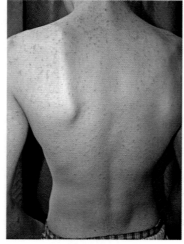

• **Fig. 37.33** Widespread Itchy Eczematous Popular Eruption, Id Reaction, 2 Days After Exposure to Poison Ivy. (From Cohen BA, editor. *Pediatric Dermatology*. 5th ed. Elsevier; 2022.)

- To prevent phytophotodermatitis, wash hands after handling citrus fruits and other known causative foods, especially if sun exposure is expected.
- Do not use flavored lip creams in cases of lip-licker dermatitis. Emollient lotions and petroleum-based emollients can moisturize the skin and discourage lip licking because of their bad taste.
- Encourage use of SkinSAFE website to avoid known allergens.
- Keep affected dermatitis areas well moisturized.

Diaper Dermatitis

Diaper dermatitis is the most frequent contact dermatitis seen in children and one of the most common skin disorders of infants (Table 37.8 and Fig. 37.34). The initial rash is termed *irritant contact diaper dermatitis. Jacquet dermatitis,* a severe form manifested by perianal erosions and lesions primarily on the labia and buttocks, is especially prone to secondary infection.

Factors contributing to diaper dermatitis include the following:
- Cleansing method with harsh soaps or irritant detergents.

TABLE 37.8	Diagnosis and Treatment of Diaper Dermatitis			
Type	**Cause**	**Presentation and Location**	**Other Characteristics**	**Treatment**
Irritant contact dermatitis	Related to wearing diapers; contact with urine and feces	Chapped, shiny, erythematous, parchment-like skin with possible erosions on convex surfaces; creases spared	May progress to involve creases; skin may be dry	Frequent diaper changes, gentle cleansing; greasy lubricant; sitz bath, air-dry; 0.5%–1% hydrocortisone for severe inflammation
Candidiasis	Related to wearing diapers; a superinfection with *Candida*	Shallow pustules, fiery-red scaly plaques on convex surfaces, skin folds, labia, and scrotum	Satellite lesions, oral thrush; recent antibiotic or diarrhea	Antifungal cream plus same measures as for contact dermatitis
Miliaria or intertrigo	Related to wearing diapers; a result of heat and occlusion	Discrete vesicles or papules (miliaria); erythematous, scaly, maceration in skinfolds	Sweat retention or friction associated	Self-limited (miliaria); avoid precipitating factors; care as for contact dermatitis
Seborrhea	Exaggerated by wearing diapers; overgrowth of *Malassezia* yeast in areas of sebaceous gland activity	Greasy, erythematous scales, well circumscribed in creases of skin, groin; spared convex surfaces	Typically, also occurs on scalp, face, or body; often superinfected with *Candida*	Ketoconazole and/or hydrocortisone is treatment of choice
Atopic dermatitis (AD)	Exaggerated by wearing diapers; exact cause unknown	Increased number of lines in skin; areas of excoriation in folds and convex surfaces and buttocks; less widespread	AD in other areas; usually begins in first year of life; scratches skin with diaper change; hyperlinear skinfolds with diffuse borders	Skin care as for contact dermatitis and as indicated for AD (see Chapter 36); antibiotics for bacterial infection
Psoriasis	Exaggerated by wearing diapers; psoriasis evolves in response to chronic trauma	Greasy silvery yellow, well-defined sharp, scaly plaques on convex surfaces and inguinal folds; less widespread; often indistinguishable from seborrheic dermatitis	Psoriasis may not affect other places; May persist for months in the diaper area	Treatment often required for weeks or until toilet trained; steroids; ketoconazole if *Candida* present
Bacterial dermatitis	Usually caused by staphylococcal or streptococcal infection	Red, denuded areas or fragile blisters; crusting and pustules in suprapubic area and periumbilicus	Frequent complication of irritant dermatitis	Oral and topical antibiotics are frequently needed

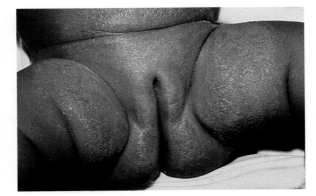

• **Fig. 37.34** Diaper Dermatitis. Note sparing of intertriginous creases. (From Zitelli BJ, McIntire S, Nowalk AJ, et al, editors. *Zitelli and Davis' Atlas of Pediatric Physical Diagnosis.* 8th ed. Elsevier; 2023.)

• Chemical irritation caused by prolonged contact with skin products, urine, feces, or breakdown products. Feces and its breakdown products are the major factors.
• Mechanical irritation from diapers or skinfolds.
• Occlusion of skin with plastic or rubber pants.

• Other skin dermatoses aggravated by wearing diapers (e.g., seborrhea, atopic dermatitis, psoriasis).
• In the diaper area around the anus, the rash is often due to diarrhea; if the skin is affected but the folds are spared, urine is often responsible.

Clinical Findings

History
• Type of diapers and diaper covering used; recent change in brand or laundering products
• Frequency of wet diapers and stools
• Frequency of diaper changes and methods of cleansing used
• Any new infant care products used
• Medication taken (particularly antibiotics) or used on rash
• Present or recent use of antibiotics.

Physical Examination. Erythema, edema, and vesiculation are typically the first characteristic changes observed. Irritant contact dermatitis commonly appears as shiny, peeling, erythematous macular or papular rash that is confluent in the diaper area, sparing folds. The skin at the edges of diapers or diaper covers may be erythematous, macerated (acute) or dry (chronic), and/or hyperpigmented. Chronic changes include scale, lichenification, and increased/decreased pigmentation.

Differential Diagnosis

Differential diagnoses include contact dermatitis; bacterial, viral, or monilial infection; atopic dermatitis; psoriasis; seborrhea; scabies; and congenital syphilis.

Management

- Use a protective barrier ointment or cream, such as Desitin (cod liver oil with zinc oxide), A&D Ointment, Aquaphor, petrolatum, or zinc oxide at the first sign of irritation.
- Sitz baths in warm water for 10 to 15 minutes 4 times a day.
- Burow solution soaks or compresses four times a day if skin is weepy.
- Hydrocortisone 0.5% to 1% applied as a thin layer three times a day for no more than 5 days, especially if skin is dry, for moderate to severe diaper dermatitis. Do not use fluorinated steroids. Combination corticosteroid antifungal preparations are discouraged because the strength of the steroid is often higher than desired.
- Any recalcitrant rash should be referred to a dermatologist.
- Reassess if not improved in 2 to 3 days.

Complications

Secondary infection with bacteria, viruses, or fungi can occur (see previous sections). Note: Red flags that could indicate systemic disease or require consultation with dermatology include severe erosions or ulcers; bullae or pustules; large papules or nodules; purpura, or petechiae; and redness or scaliness over entire body.

Patient and Family Education

The best treatment is prevention!
1. Keep diaper area dry, clean, and aerated.
2. Frequent diaper changes are essential; during the healing period, every 1 to 2 hours is recommended with one change at night and a minimum of eight changes in a 24-hour period for infants. Cleanse the area well with water at every diaper change and use mild soap, rinsing well following a stool. Avoid vigorous cleansing because this can worsen matters. Avoid using wipes during healing and consider hypoallergenic wipes at other times.
3. In addition to frequent changes, use thick or absorbent diapers.
4. Cloth diapers should be soaked, prerinsed, washed in a mild soap, double rinsed with cup of vinegar, and dried in the sun if possible. Consider hypoallergenic laundry detergent.
5. Disposable diapers must be large enough not to bind and should never be worn with rubber pants.
6. Expose diaper area to air by leaving diaper off or by blow-drying with low heat three or four times per day.
7. Increase intake of fluids to dilute urine.

Seborrheic Dermatitis

Seborrhea is a chronic inflammatory dermatitis characterized by a symmetrical, red, scaling eruption that is most often found in hair-bearing, intertriginous areas. In infants, it is commonly found on the scalp and called *cradle cap*. In older patients, it is known as *dandruff* and can be found on scalp as well as eyebrows. The condition is thought to be related to overproduction of sebum because it commonly occurs in areas with large numbers of sebaceous glands. It is more common in neurologically impaired individuals and those with an immunodeficiency. The pathogenesis is not well understood, but an overgrowth of *Malassezia ovalis*, a saprophytic yeast, is thought to be the causative organism. Seborrhea

occurs most often in early infancy and adolescence, is associated with blepharitis, and is more common in spring and summer.

Clinical Findings

History. Diagnosis is usually based on clinical presentation.

Physical Examination. In infants, erythematous, flaky to thick crusts of yellow, greasy (waxy appearance) scales occur predominantly on the scalp, but also on the face, behind the ears, on the neck and trunk, and in the diaper area (Fig. 37.35). Scalp lesions may be difficult to differentiate from psoriasis. In older children, there are mild flakes with some erythema and yellow, greasy scales on the scalp, forehead, nasal bridge, and eyebrows; behind the ears; on the face and flexural surfaces; and in intertriginous areas. The dermatitis is not pruritic and has no pustules.

Differential Diagnosis

Atopic dermatitis, psoriasis, *Candida* infection, contact dermatitis, tinea, scabies, and pityriasis rosea are included in the differential diagnoses.

Management

Three categories of agents may be helpful in the treatment of seborrheic dermatitis in both infants and adolescents. These include antifungal agents, antiinflammatory agents, and keratolytic agents:
- Antifungal: Azoles, selenium sulfide
- Antiinflammatory: Topical steroids, topical calcineurin inhibitors
- Keratolytic (remove excess scale): Topical salicylic acid, urea

Cradle cap in infants may be self-limited, typically resolves spontaneously in the first year of life.[10] Mineral oil may be applied to the scalp for 5 to 10 minutes before shampooing with a mild shampoo. Scales can be removed with a soft brush or toothbrush. Frequent shampooing is generally effective. There are no medicated or prescriptive shampoos approved for children under 2 years old.

Scalp involvement in older children can be treated with shampoo containing ketoconazole, zinc pyrithione, selenium sulfide, or salicylic acid. Many of these are available OTC. Shampoo should be left on the scalp for 5 to 10 minutes before scrubbing crusts and then rinsing.

Other areas of seborrheic dermatitis can be managed with ketoconazole and ciclopirox shampoo or cream. More involved cases may require intermittent use of twice daily low-potency topical corticosteroids. Topical corticosteroids added weekly for recalcitrant dermatitis.

Complications

Secondary infection with bacteria or Candida can occur. Severe, generalized seborrhea is commonly found in persons infected with HIV.

Family and Patient Education

Treatment can take weeks or months to be effective. It is important to continue treatment for a few days after resolution. Repeat treatment at the first sign of recurrence to prevent progression of disease. Frequent washing of the hair may help prevent recurrence. Return to office for reevaluation if problem becomes persistent.

Reactive Erythema

These disorders are characterized by erythematous patches, plaques, and nodules. There is a wide variation in size, shape, and

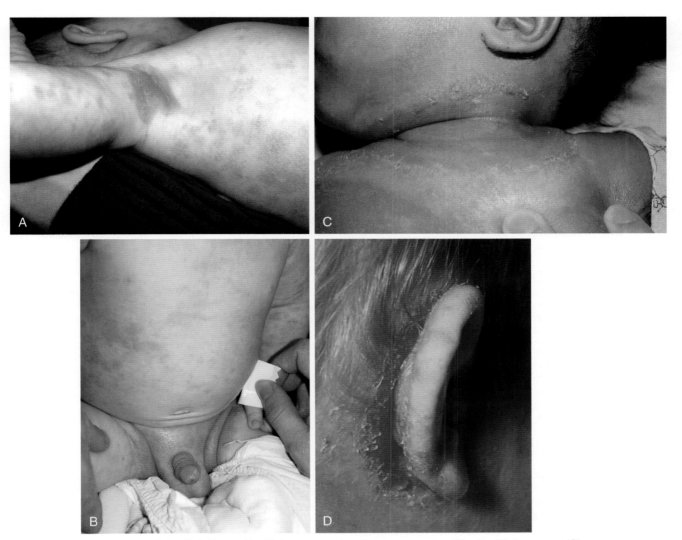

• **Fig. 37.35** Seborrheic Dermatitis. Note greasy, red, scaling appearance on (A) axilla, (B) diaper area, (C) intertrigal space of neck, and (D) postauricular area. (From Zitelli BJ, McIntire S, Nowalk AJ, et al, editors. *Zitelli and Davis' Atlas of Pediatric Physical Diagnosis.* 8th ed. Elsevier; 2023.)

distribution and they can be triggered by environmental or internal factors. Due to this wide variety of skin reactions, diagnosis can be difficult (Table 37.9).

Morbilliform Drug Eruptions

The morbilliform rash, an *exanthematous reaction* manifested by erythematous macules and/or papules (often measles-like), is the most common allergic skin reaction to a drug. While almost any drug can be a trigger, the most common drugs causing reactions are antibiotics (penicillins, cephalosporins, sulfonamide antibiotics), nonsteroidal antiinflammatory drugs (NSAIDs), antiseizure medications, and oral antifungal drugs.[2,3] Exanthematous rashes typically have their onset within 1 to 2 weeks of starting a new medication and can occur after the medication has been stopped. Repeated exposure can lead to faster reactions and progress to anaphylaxis.

Clinical Findings

History
- Medication taken within the past 3 weeks

- Recent illness: The risk of this type of eruption is increased if the child also has a viral infection (e.g., the rash that appears after giving penicillin to a child with Epstein-Barr virus [EBV])
- Varying degrees of itching that can be intense
- Rash worsens even after medicine is discontinued for up to 5 days
- Possible low-grade fever

Physical Examination. Findings include the following:
- Condition often begins as a symmetric, macular erythematous rash that becomes papular and confluent.
- Patches of normal skin are scattered throughout areas of involvement.
- Rash begins on the trunk, where it is a brighter red, more confluent, and extends distally to the extremities, including the palms and soles.
- Rash may turn brownish red and desquamate in 7 to 14 days.
- The face often has confluent areas of erythema.
- Mucous membranes are typically spared.

Diagnostic Studies. The following are ordered if necessary for differential diagnosis: CBC, monospot test, CRP, antinuclear antibodies, anti–streptolysin O (ASO), cold agglutinins.

TABLE 37.9	Drug Eruptions, Urticaria, and Erythema Multiforme		
	Drug Eruption	**Urticaria**	**Erythema Multiforme**
Etiology	Reaction to medication, especially penicillin, cephalexin, erythromycin, sulfa drugs, NSAIDs, barbiturates, isoniazid, carbamazepine, phenytoin	Hypersensitive reaction; immunologic antigen-antibody response to release of histamines; often unknown cause; possible reaction to food, drug, insect bite or sting, pollen; possible reaction to infection, especially streptococcal, sinus, mononucleosis, hepatitis	Immune-mediated hypersensitivity reaction often to infection, especially HSV; also to many other agents
Clinical findings	Symmetric, macular, erythematous to papular, confluent morbilliform rash; intense itching; patches of normal skin throughout; begins on trunk, extends distally, including palms and soles; face with confluent erythema	Key finding: Appears suddenly, fades in 20 minutes to 24 hours Family history of hives; possible atopy; intense itching; mild erythema, annular, raised wheals with pale centers; lesions scattered or coalesced; blanch with pressure; associated edema of eyelids, lips, tongue, hands, feet	Key finding: Target or iris lesions: lesions fixed, symmetric, typical distribution on hands, feet, elbows, knees, also face, neck, trunk History of infection, especially herpes labialis; variety of lesions on skin and mucous membranes—macules, papules, vesicles, early lesions, such as, urticaria; possible oral mucous membrane involvement
Treatment	Stop drug and label as allergen to the child; give antihistamine, antipruritic, prednisone if severe; lubricate skin; rash can last 7–14 days; use medical alert bracelet	Quick resolution; identify and remove offending agent if possible and treat; stop antibiotic; give oral antihistamines; topical antipruritics; epinephrine or prednisone if anaphylactic, angioedema, or refractory; refer if >6-week duration	Identify, treat, discontinue trigger if possible; treat infection; supportive measures for hydration, prevention of secondary infection, relief of pain; oral antihistamines, cool compresses; oral lesions—mouthwash, topical anesthetics; lesions last 5–7 days, recur in batches over 2–4 weeks, resolve without scarring or sequelae

HSV, Herpes simplex virus; *NSAIDs,* nonsteroidal antiinflammatory drugs.

Differential Diagnosis

Viral exanthem; measles; toxic erythema, such as in scarlet fever, staphylococcal scarlatina, or Kawasaki disease; TSS; roseola; and erythema infectiosum are included in the differential diagnoses. A patient who presents with this exanthematous rash but also has fever, facial swelling, and/or lymphadenopathy may have drug reaction with eosinophilia and systemic symptoms (DRESS) syndrome (see later). Although not described in this chapter, other drug-related dermatologic reactions include acute generalized exanthematous pustulosis, drug hypersensitivity syndrome, serum sickness-like reaction, vasculitis, fixed drug eruption, acneiform eruptions, and SJS.

Management

Decisions about whether a drug is to be implicated depend on the patient's previous history of taking the drug, the experience of the general population with the drug, the morphology and timing of the rash, and other possible explanations for the rash (e.g., viral illness). Patients may show rash resolution despite continuation of drug. The following steps are taken:

1. Treatment is typically supportive.
2. Discontinuation of the suspected drug is generally recommended with the understanding that viral exanthems may often present in the same manner.
3. Label the patient's medical record with the *potential* allergen.
4. Prescribe antihistamines if itching is present; recommend a lubricant and antipruritics as adjuncts.
5. Systemic steroids are not usually indicated in a morbilliform drug eruption. Topical steroids may be helpful if pruritis is severe.[2]
6. Schedule follow-up visit as determined by severity of reaction and other illness.

Refer to an allergist for skin testing to confirm allergy if there are limited or no alternative medications, for desensitization, to clarify drug allergy, for severe parental anxiety, or if symptoms are severe and life threatening.

Complications

Progression of the rash if medicine is continued can lead to toxic epidermal necrolysis (TEN) or SJS (see EM, SJS, TEN section) or allergic interstitial nephritis.

Patient and Family Education

- The rash can last 7 to 14 days with itching, and it may worsen before getting better.
- There is potential risk from further exposure to that drug or related ones; alternative therapies should be explained.
- Identification and communication of the individual's allergy are imperative. If allergy is life-threatening, wearing a medical alert bracelet or necklace is essential.

Drug Reaction With Eosinophilia and Systemic Symptoms (DRESS Syndrome)

Also known as *drug hypersensitivity syndrome,* this drug reaction may begin with cervical lymphadenopathy and pharyngitis. Most patients progress to an exanthematous drug reaction that accompanied by fever, facial swelling, edema, conjunctivitis, arthritis, and lymphadenopathy. The rash progresses cephalocaudally. It may present as much as 6 weeks after the offending medication is begun. Organ involvement is frequent with the liver being the most common and can lead to death. Not well understood, this reaction may have a genetic connection with an inability to metabolize medication metabolites. The most common medications involved are trimethoprim-sulfamethoxazole and antiseizure medications.[2,3]

Clinical Findings

History
- Medications started within the past 1 to 2 months
- Symptoms of fever, pharyngitis, arthralgia
- Rash that may have started on the face

Physical Findings
- Exanthematous rash that may have begun on the face
- Other physical findings include cervical lymphadenopathy, facial edema, conjunctivitis, and erythema spreading caudally
- Patient often appears ill

Diagnostic Studies. The following are helpful with diagnosis: CBC, hepatic transaminases, serum creatinine level, and urinalysis. Elevated eosinophils and liver/renal involvement are common.

Differential Diagnosis

Morbilliform drug eruption, viral exanthem; measles; toxic erythema, such as in scarlet fever, staphylococcal scarlatina, or Kawasaki disease; TSS; roseola; and erythema infectiosum are included in the differential diagnosis. Although not described in this chapter, other drug-related dermatologic reactions include acute generalized exanthematous pustulosis, drug hypersensitivity syndrome, serum sickness-like reaction, vasculitis, fixed drug eruption, acneiform eruptions, and SJS.

Management

Patients with a considered diagnosis of DRESS syndrome should be immediately referred to hospital-based care. Discontinuation of offending medication and systemic corticosteroids are critical in the management of the reaction.

Complications

Organ involvement is common with DRESS syndrome, particularly the liver and kidney. There is as much as a 10% mortality rate with internal involvement.[2] Thyroiditis can present months after presentation and can persist for months.

Patient and Family Education

- Follow-up with specialist care as directed.
- There is an ongoing risk from further exposure to that drug or related ones; alternative therapies should be explained.
- Be sure to discuss all new medications with PCP as cross-reactions are common.
- Identification and communication of the child's allergy are imperative. Wearing a medical alert bracelet or necklace is essential.

Urticaria and Angioedema

Urticaria (commonly called *hives*) and angioedema are hypersensitivity reactions (usually a type I reaction—immunoglobulin E [IgE] mediated) (Fig. 37.36). Urticaria involves the superficial dermis; in contrast, angioedema involves the deeper dermis and subcutaneous tissue. Urticaria and angioedema are more common in younger patients than adults, and about 50% of patients with urticaria also have angioedema. Urticaria occurs sometime in the lives of about 15% of the population. Transient or acute urticaria lasts less than 6 weeks; chronic, recurrent, or persistent urticaria lasts more than 6 weeks.

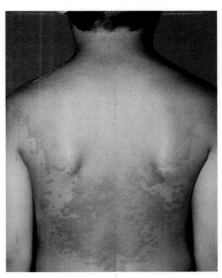

• **Fig. 37.36** Urticaria. (From Paller AS, Mancini AJ. *Paller and Mancini: Hurwitz Clinical Pediatric Dermatology.* 6th ed. Elsevier; 2022.)

Urticaria and angioedema are the result of a complex interplay of immunologically mediated antigen-antibody responses to the release of histamine from mast cells and other vasoactive mediators, such as leukotrienes and prostaglandins. Vasodilation and increased vascular permeability cause erythema and the characteristic wheal of urticaria. Onset is usually rapid, and resolution occurs within a few days of onset. A small number of patients can develop chronic urticaria, lasting from 6 weeks to years. This is typically idiopathic but can be associated with an autoimmune disease. Dermatographia (skin writing) is a relatively rare variant of physical urticaria and refers to hives triggered by rubbing or scratching of skin.

Possible causative factors of urticaria include the following:
- In younger children, infections (most often viral), are the most common cause. However, almost every infectious agent has been associated with urticaria.[3]
- Reactions to foods (e.g., nuts, eggs, seafood, strawberries, tomatoes), stings.
- Insect bites and stings, parasites, food additives, and physical stimuli (e.g., heat or cold, sun, or water) are less common.
- Reaction to drugs, with penicillins being the most common. It is important to note that only a small percentage of patients are allergic to penicillins when skin prick testing is done. Other antibiotics, antiseizure medications, monoclonal antibodies, and NSAIDS are also common.[3]
- Reaction to skin contact with antigens, such as chemicals, latex, fish, or caterpillars.
- Genetic origin.
- Approximately 50% of urticarial is idiopathic or unknown.

Angioedema is a part of the spectrum of urticaria and is an extension of the reaction into the subcutaneous tissue. It results from vasodilation, increased tissue permeability, and subsequent interstitial edema. The most common areas affected are the eyelids, hands, feet, genitalia, lips, tongue, airway, and gastrointestinal tract.[3] Angioedema may be a component of anaphylactic reactions. These histamine responsive reactions have similar triggers as urticaria.

Clinical Findings

History

- Family or previous history of hives, angioedema, connective tissue disease, autoimmune disease including juvenile arthritis.
- Possibility of atopy.
- Intense itching and scratching.
- Ingestion (within 4 hours) of nuts, shellfish, chocolate, berries, spices, egg white, milk, fish, sesame.
- Ingestion or injection of medicines (e.g., penicillin, sulfa drugs, sedatives, diuretics, analgesics, acetylsalicylic acid), additives, or preservatives.
- Injection of diagnostic agents, vaccine, insect venom, blood.
- Infection with upper respiratory infectious agent, virus, streptococcus, mononucleosis; hepatitis; parasites.
- Inhalation of allergens (animal dander, pollen, dust, smoke, or aerosols).
- Flea or mite bites.
- Cold, heat, exercise, sun, water, pressure, or vibration.
- Inflammatory bowel disease (enlarged lips may be confused with chronic angioedema).

Physical Examination. Location of lesions may help determine the cause (e.g., a lesion around the mouth or tongue is likely due to an ingested agent). Findings can include the following:

- Urticaria is seen as mildly erythematous, annular, raised wheals or welts with pale centers from 2 mm to several centimeters in diameter; however, they can be of various shapes. Such lesions typically:
  - Are scattered or coalesced but generalized.
  - Appear suddenly as individual lesions and fade in anywhere from 20 minutes to less than 24 hours, reappearing in other areas later; if fixed more than 48 hours, it is not urticaria.
  - Blanch with pressure.
  - Seem to be intensified with heat.
  - Occur most commonly as papulovesicular lesions with central punctate lesion and wheals in toddlers (papular urticaria).
  - Can appear as large, blotchy, erythematous lesions with 1- to 3-mm central wheals (cholinergic urticaria).
  - Test for dermatographism by stroking the skin, for cholinergic urticaria by applying heat or observing immediately after exercising, for cold urticaria by applying cold packs, for pressure urticaria by applying weighted bands for several minutes, and for water urticaria by applying wet compresses.
- Angioedema is seen as asymmetric, localized, nondependent, and transient edema.
  - Typically, less pruritic than urticaria
  - May involve the upper airway and progress to life-threatening obstruction
  - Can cause associated edema of eyelids, lips, tongue, hands, feet, and genitalia

Diagnostic Studies. In most cases, allergy testing and laboratory evaluations are not needed. If urticaria with possible anaphylaxis from an insect bite is suspected, refer to an allergist for testing and hyposensitization. If fever is present, evaluate for underlying disease.

Differential Diagnosis

Contact dermatitis, atopic dermatitis, scabies, erythema multiforme (lesions are fixed with dusky centered target-like lesions that appear within 72 hours (Fig. 37.37); mastocytosis, reactive erythemas, vasculitis, psoriasis, and juvenile arthritis are also included in the differential diagnoses (see Table 37.9).

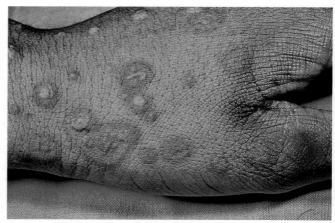

• **Fig. 37.37** Erythema Multiforme. (From Cohen BA, editor. *Pediatric Dermatology*. 5th ed. Elsevier; 2022.)

Management

Control of symptoms is the main goal of treatment. The following steps are taken:

1. Identify and remove the offending substance if possible. Stop all antibiotics. Avoid any possible food or environmental trigger.
2. Administer medications as indicate:
   - Oral antihistamines until itching and urticaria are resolved. Nonsedating antihistamines are less effective. Urticaria is less likely to recur if the antihistamine is continued for 1 to 2 weeks after resolution.
   - Topical antipruritics may be helpful.
   - Epinephrine may be needed if anaphylaxis or significant angioedema with swelling of the face, mucous membranes, and airway is present. Referral to emergency center if epinephrine is needed.
   - Oral corticosteroids with rapid taper only if refractory to other measures or if angioedema is present with swelling of lips and face.
3. Follow-up visit if not improved within 24 to 48 hours.

Chronic urticaria persisting longer than 6 weeks needs evaluation for infection or systemic causes or referral for further evaluation. An emergency epinephrine kit should be prescribed for children after the first episode or with recurrent episodes of life-threatening urticaria or angioedema.

Complications

Angioedema or anaphylaxis occurs by the same mechanism as urticaria:

- Anaphylactic symptoms require emergency intervention.
- Serum sickness begins with hives, but has other systemic symptoms (e.g., fever, arthralgias, malaise, lymphadenopathy, or proteinuria).
- If urticaria is from a drug reaction, rechallenge with the drug is more likely to cause anaphylaxis.

Patient and Family Education

The following are needed:

- Explanation of causes (often unknown), course, and treatment. The entire episode usually resolves in 24 to 48 hours, rarely extending beyond 3 to 4 weeks. Further evaluation is needed only if urticaria lasts longer than 8 weeks.
- Papular urticaria hypersensitivity often declines within 6 to 12 months.

- Physical urticarias last 2 to 4 years in most cases, but occasionally persist into adulthood.
- Occasionally, macular blue-brown lesions are found on resolution of urticaria.
- Avoid allergen if known; wear a medical alert bracelet in case severe reaction occurs. Refer for hyposensitization if life-threatening symptoms occur.
- Carry an epinephrine kit, if indicated.

Erythema Multiforme, Stevens-Johnson Syndrome, Toxic Epidermal Necrolysis

In the past, erythema multiforme minor, SJS (also known as *erythema multiforme major*), and TEN were thought to be related disorders. However, erythema multiforme minor is a distinct disorder that does not progress to SJS or TEN. Erythema multiforme is an acute, usually benign, self-limited eruption characterized by target lesions and minor mucosal involvement (papules and varying bullae); it is rarely associated with complications.

Erythema multiforme usually follows an infection, with approximately 80% of cases of classic erythema multiforme attributed to HSV, in particular, herpes labialis or progenitalis lesion(s). The herpetic lesion may have healed or had a subclinical presentation but led to an immune response in the body. Erythema multiforme tends to be recurrent as do herpes lesions. Erythema multiforme may also be associated with other viruses, such as EBV, cytomegalovirus, and other herpesviruses.[3]

SJS and TEN are variants of the same hypersensitivity disorder. Patients may be diagnosed with SJS initially and then progress to TEN. The differentiation between these two conditions is the degree of involved skin and the systemic involvement. SJS may be drug-induced (sulfonamides, penicillins, phenobarbital, carbamazepine, and lamotrigine) but in children is more typically due to *Mycoplasma* and occasionally HSV. TEN is almost always associated with a drug reaction. Both conditions are associated with significant risk of morbidity and mortality.

Clinical Findings

History
- With erythema multiforme:
  - Recent or current infection with herpes virus (herpes labialis or progenitalis)
  - Exposure to UV light or trauma to area
  - Typically a primary lesion without a prodromal period
- With SJS or TEN:
  - MAY present with a prodrome of high fever, cough, sore throat, vomiting, diarrhea, chest pain, and arthralgia that usually lasts 1 to 3 days (but can last from 1–14 days) followed by the onset of lesions.
  - Recent use of medication known to be associated with SJS and TEN.
  - Recent respiratory infection.
- With TEN:
  - ALWAYS presents with a prodrome of high fever, cough, sore throat, vomiting, diarrhea, chest pain, and arthralgia that usually lasts 1 to 3 days (but can last from 1–14 days) followed by the onset of lesions.

Physical Examination. It is important to differentiate the clinical findings of erythema multiforme from SJS and TEN.
- In erythema multiforme:
  - Lesions vary from patient to patient, within a single episode, and with recurrence.

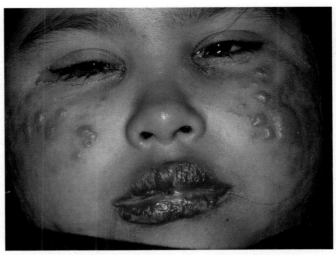

- **Fig. 37.38** Stevens-Johnson Syndrome (SJS). (From Paller AS, Mancini AJ. *Paller and Mancini: Hurwitz Clinical Pediatric Dermatology.* 6th ed. Elsevier; 2022.)

- Lesions initially appear dusky, as red macules or edematous papules that evolve into target lesions with multiple, concentric rings of color change.
- Lesions are fixed (another diagnostic clue), tend to be symmetric, and have a typical distribution predominantly on the face, extensor surface of the arms and legs, dorsum of the hands and feet, and the palms and soles.
- The oral mucosa is commonly involved, and 50% of children will present with shallow oral lesions.[3]
- Systemic symptoms (low-grade fever, malaise, myalgia, arthralgia) are not always present and are usually mild.
- In SJS (Fig. 37.38):
  - Dusky red macular, targetoid, bullous lesions form.
  - Hemorrhagic blisters form quickly. Bullae rupture easily leaving ulcerations that are soon covered with exudate.
  - Lesions are scattered and isolated and may be confluent on the trunk and face.
  - Prominent mucosal involvement of eyes, nose, and mouth.
- In TEN:
  - Rapidly coalescing target lesions and widespread bullae that become full-thickness epidermal peeling or sloughing within 24 hours.
  - Nikolsky sign (peeling of skin with a light rub that reveals a moist red surface) is present.
  - Conjunctivae, urethra, rectum, oral and nasal mucosa, larynx, and tracheobronchial mucosa may or may not be involved.

Diagnostic Studies. Studies are ordered as indicated by the clinical condition of the child.

Differential Diagnosis

Urticaria can be differentiated by lack of itching, lability of lesions, and shorter-lasting hives that are pale centrally, not target or iris lesions (see Table 37.9). Viral exanthems are more centrally located, confluent, and less erythematous. Purpura is present in vasculitis. In SSSS, the skin peels superficially (not full thickness) and is significantly red. Kawasaki disease and lupus erythematosus are also included in the differential diagnoses.

Management

Care for erythema multiforme is generally supportive because the condition is self-limited.

- Symptomatic and supportive care: Maintain hydration, prevent secondary infection, and relieve pain:
  - Mild analgesics, cool compresses, and oral antihistamines (e.g., diphenhydramine).
  - Soothing mouthwashes or topical anesthetics (e.g., Kaopectate or Maalox, mixed in equal parts with diphenhydramine).
  - Topical intraoral anesthetics (e.g., dyclonine liquid, viscous lidocaine), are sometimes used in older children and adolescents; however, with caution.
  - Wound care.
  - IV fluids if oral hydration is not adequate.
  - Systemic antihistamines, analgesics, and antimicrobials as needed.
- Treatment of herpes simplex:
  - Avoid sun exposure and use sunscreen and protective clothing.
  - Prophylaxis for recurrent erythema multiforme with oral acyclovir for a 6- to 12-month trial with periodic stopping to reassess.
  - Acyclovir during an acute episode of erythema multiforme does not alter its course.

SJS and TEN are potentially life-threatening diseases. Children are typically admitted to the pediatric intensive care unit or burn unit for wound care, management of hydration and electrolyte issues, nutritional support, and pain control.

Complications

SJS and TEN are associated with significant morbidity including pneumonitis, sepsis, gastrointestinal bleeding, renal disease, keratitis, and other ophthalmologic disorders. In SJS, mortality is as high as 25% with septicemia being the leading cause.[3] Fluid and electrolyte losses contribute so that the mortality rate is higher with TEN.

Patient and Family Education

Erythema multiforme lesions can erupt in crops that last 1 to 3 weeks, but resolve without scarring or sequelae, except for transient desquamation, scaling, or hyperpigmentation. Recurrence of erythema multiforme is common. Most patients with SJS and TEN do recover. Scarring may develop when secondary infection occurs. Ongoing ophthalmologic care is needed after severe conjunctival and corneal involvement.

Papulosquamous Eruptions of the Skin

Pityriasis Rosea

Pityriasis rosea is a common, benign, self-limited papulosquamous disease (Fig. 37.39). The etiology of pityriasis rosea is

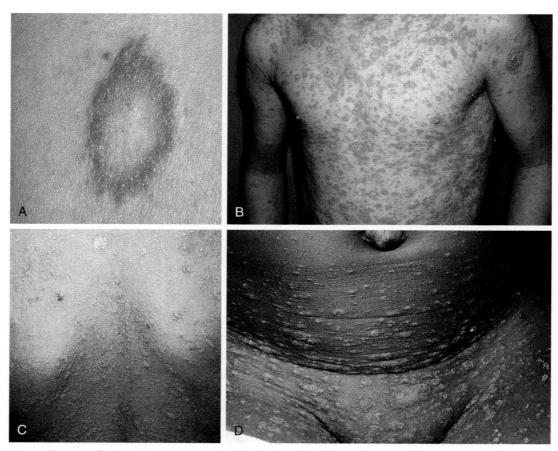

• **Fig. 37.39** Pityriasis Rosea. (A) Herald patch, which is often mistaken for tinea corporis. (B) Numerous oval lesions on chest of white teenager. (C) Christmas tree pattern on the back of a black adolescent. (D) Small, papular lesions as well as larger scaly patches most prominent on abdomen and thighs of 5-year-old female. (From Cohen BA, editor. *Pediatric Dermatology*. 5th ed. Elsevier; 2022.)

controversial. It is thought to be caused by human herpesvirus 6 or 7 (HHV-6 or HHV-7) since it is minimally contagious and occurs most commonly in the fall, early winter, and spring in temperate climates. Fifty percent of all cases occur before 20 years old, most commonly in adolescence, with males and females equally affected. Approximately 98% of cases result in lifelong immunity.[13]

Clinical Findings

History. Although most are otherwise well, a small percentage (5%) of patients experience a prodrome of mild symptoms including malaise, pharyngitis, lymphadenopathy, and headache before onset of rash. Those that have prodromal symptoms tend to have a more florid rash. Approximately 25% of patients report some pruritis.

Physical Examination
- Herald spot or patch (key finding in 70% of presentations): a 2- to 5-cm solitary, ovoid, slightly erythematous lesion with a finely scaled slightly elevated border that enlarges quickly with central clearing); typical locations for the herald patch include the trunk, upper arm, neck, or thigh. Patient often presents after herald patch has resolved and this sign is unable to be determined.
- Secondary generalized lesions appear that are symmetric, small macular to papular, thin and round to oval. The lesions have thin scales centrally with thicker scales peripherally ("collarette" scales surround the lesions). They are also pale pink; more common on trunk and proximal extremities from neck to knees; typically spare the face, scalp, and distal extremities; and usually occur 2 to 21 days after the appearance of the herald patch.
- Christmas tree pattern—rash, especially on back, follows dermatome skin lines with oval lesions running parallel and wrapping around the trunk horizontally.
- Oral lesions have punctate hemorrhages, erosions or ulcerations, erythematous macules, or annular plaques; such lesions occur in about 16% of patients.
- An atypical presentation, limb-girdle pityriasis rosea, can occur with lesions involving areas that are usually spared (e.g., the face, axilla, groin). The face and neck are frequent areas of involvement in young children, especially Black children.[3]

Diagnostic Studies. If needed, a KOH preparation of a skin scraping is done to rule out tinea.

Differential Diagnosis

Include psoriasis, guttate psoriasis, nummular eczema, scabies, tinea (especially the herald patch), secondary syphilis, drug eruptions, or viral exanthems in the differential diagnoses.

Management

The following steps are taken:
- Application of calamine lotion (or other lotions containing menthol and/or camphor or pramoxine), tepid baths with Aveeno, antihistamines, and emollients may provide relief from itching.
- The role of topical/oral steroids and oral erythromycin in hastening resolution is controversial.[3]

Complications

Postinflammatory hypo- or hyperpigmentary changes may occur, especially in dark-skinned individuals.

Patient and Family Education

Pityriasis rosea is a benign, self-limited, and noncontagious disease that has three cycles (emerging, persisting, and fading) with spontaneous resolution in 6 to 12 weeks. Resolution may take as long as 6 months. Minimal sun exposure can help lesions resolve more quickly. Prevent sunburn.

Psoriasis

Psoriasis is an immune-mediated disorder associated with genetic predisposition and environmental risk factors. Though the exact cause is unknown, it has been linked to the histocompatibility complex on the sixth chromosome. More than one-third of patients have a family history of psoriasis.[3] Psoriasis occurs at all ages; 30% of cases have onset in childhood and it is more common in white children. The disease results from keratinocyte proliferation and dermal vascular abnormalities. Trigger factors include infection (particularly streptococcal and staphylococcal), local trauma, stress (physical and emotional), and certain drugs (corticosteroids, lithium, β-blockers, NSAIDs). Guttate psoriasis, often triggered by a group A beta-hemolytic strep (GABHS) infection, may be the first sign of psoriasis in children.[2] The list of comorbidities for psoriasis is evolving. It has been shown to frequently coexist with obesity and metabolic syndrome, cardiovascular disease, dyslipidemia, inflammatory bowel disease, and depression. In fact, obesity appears to be a risk factor for psoriasis.[14]

Psoriasis is characterized by thick silvery scales, varied distribution patterns, and an isomorphic (Koebner phenomenon) response (Fig. 37.40). Subtypes of psoriasis include chronic plaque, guttate (often triggered by a streptococcal infection), erythrodermic, and pustular psoriasis. Typical locations include diaper area psoriasis, inverse psoriasis (involves flexural regions typically spared), facial psoriasis (more common in pediatric patients than adults), scalp psoriasis (often the initial site), genital involvement (more common in older children), nail involvement, and other more severe but much less common manifestations. Pustular and erythrodermic are less common in the pediatric population. Psoriatic arthritis is rare in children but when it occurs, it is often a presenting symptom before the rash is seen.[14]

Clinical Findings

History
- Family history of psoriasis
- Streptococcal infection of the oropharynx or perianal area before onset (guttate)
- Skin trauma before onset
- Medication use
- Itching (variable)

Physical Examination
- Common areas and types of psoriasis[3]:
  - Plaque psoriasis: Discrete, initially erythematous, symmetric, well-marginated rash becoming papular with silver scales that may be trivial to widespread.
  - Guttate (teardrop) psoriasis: Widespread, symmetric, round, or oval 0.5- to 2-cm lesions occurring primarily on the trunk and proximal extremities, occasionally on the face, scalp, and ears and rarely on the palms or soles. There is less scaling than in psoriasis vulgaris.
  - Psoriasis vulgaris: Well-circumscribed, erythematous plaques with thick, silvery white scales concentrated on elbows, knees, scalp, and hairline, but also seen on eyebrows, around ears, and in intergluteal fold and genital area.

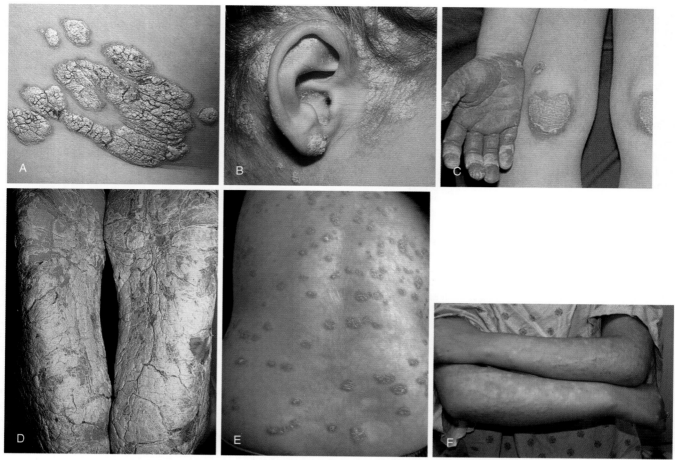

• **Fig. 37.40** Psoriasis. (A) Typical erythematous plaques with silver scale. (B) Scalp psoriasis extending to forehead, neck, and ears. (C) Thick, painful plaques on palms and knees. Soles and elbows were also involved (not shown here). (D) Severe plantar keratoderma. (E) Guttate lesions following streptococcal pharyngitis. (F) Disseminated guttate lesions after an upper respiratory infection. (From Cohen BA, editor. *Pediatric Dermatology.* Philadelphia: Elsevier; 2022.)

- Facial psoriasis: Periorbital area is the most commonly affected and lesions often mistaken for atopic dermatitis. Geographic tongue is a form of this psoriasis.
- Scalp psoriasis: Typically well-demarcated, erythematous plaques with thick, adherent silvery scales. May be greasy and salmon-colored and easily confused with seborrheic dermatitis. Seborrheic dermatitis generally stays inside hairline where psoriasis can spread beyond hair to forehead, ear, and neck regions.
- Koebner phenomenon (isomorphic response): Psoriatic lesions occur in areas of local injury, such as scratches, surgical scars, or sunburns.
- Auspitz sign: Bleeding occurs when a scale is removed.
- Nail signs: Nails have "ice pick" pits and ridges, are thick and discolored (yellowing), can have splinter hemorrhages or subungual hyperkeratosis, and can be separated from the nailbed.
- Napkin or diaper area psoriasis: Appears eczematous with sharply defined plaques, bright red coloration, shiny with large drier scales, affecting inguinal and gluteal folds. In general, due to trauma of urine and feces and improves when toilet trained.

Diagnostic Studies
- ASO if guttate pattern
- KOH-treated scrapings and culture to rule out fungal infection
- Venereal Disease Research Laboratory (VDRL) to rule out secondary syphilis.

Differential Diagnosis

Pityriasis rosea, lichen planus, drug eruptions, seborrhea, Candida infection, contact or irritant dermatitis, atopic dermatitis, tinea, dyshidrosis, secondary syphilis, HSV, and other nail-pitting conditions such as tinea, onychomycosis, and trauma.

Management

In children, treatment should be as conservative as possible. Medications and treatments should be rotated for best effectiveness. For all but mild cases, a dermatology referral is appropriate. The following are treatment options:

- Topical steroids are the mainstay of therapy. Apply class II to IV steroids (see Table 37.2) twice per day with ointments being the preferred formulation due to better penetration. They should be used intermittently but not discontinued spontaneously, because worsening can occur. Monitoring the child during use is important. Severe plaques and larger areas may need a referral for higher-potency steroid. Systemic steroids are not indicated and may worsen the condition, causing pustular flare.[3]
- Sun exposure in moderate amounts alleviates lesions. Prevent sunburn.

- Emollient creams (such as petrolatum, Eucerin, Aquaphor, or Cetaphil) for dry skin can minimize trauma and subsequent psoriasis and may improve psoriasis.
- Follow up every 2 weeks until psoriasis is controlled and during exacerbations and then as needed. Refer to dermatologist when exacerbations are frequent.
  Dermatology management may include:
- Keratolytic agents to reduce thick, unresponsive plaques. Tar or keratolytic shampoos (ketoconazole, anthralin, salicylic acid) can be used on the scalp to soften and remove scales. This can be followed with a steroid oil, foam or solution.
- Ultraviolet treatments under controlled supervision may be more effective for older children.
- Vitamin D_3 topical products are effective for mild to moderate plaque psoriasis. Available in cream, ointment, and lotion, it is safe, effective, and well tolerated for short- and long-term treatment. Hypercalcemia is reported with application of excessive quantities over large areas. Dual therapy with high-potency steroids is frequently used.[14]
- Retinoids may be effective in management of pustular psoriasis but are often too irritating for use in childhood psoriasis and need to be combined with other treatment modalities.
- Topical calcineurin inhibitors are the treatment of choice for facial and intertriginous psoriasis in children.
- Anthralin, a quinone, is effective topically and should be used before UV light and systemic therapy.[14]
- UV light therapy may be used for disseminated, chronic, or recalcitrant disease. Narrowband UVB light therapy is preferred in children due to safety and efficacy. Salicylic acid blocks UVB and should not be used in combination with phototherapy.
- Cyclosporine and methotrexate are systemic therapies used for recalcitrant and severe disease.
- Other treatment options include psoralens, intralesional steroids, retinoids, cyclosporine, biologic therapy, and immunotherapy.

Complications

The following complications are possible and require referral to dermatology:
- *Candida* infection: May be a secondary infection in the diaper area.
- Erythrodermic and pustular psoriasis: Unusual in childhood; characterized by generalized or local multiple 1- to 2-mm pustules with erythema and scaling also involving palms and soles; accompanied by malaise, fever, electrolyte and fluid imbalances, temperature instability, and leukocytosis; can be fatal.
- Exfoliative erythroderma: Rare manifestation, including desquamation and loss of hair and nails with previous history of psoriasis.
- Psoriatic arthritis: An inflammatory arthritis that is rare but increasing in frequency, most common in females 9 to 12 years old. Prognosis is good but should be referred to rheumatology.

Patient and Family Education

Emotional support and education are the most important aspects in dealing with psoriasis. Areas for discussion include the following:
- Psoriasis is chronic and involves unpredictable spontaneous remissions and exacerbations. Control and relief are sought, but cure is not available. Treatment may require up to 1 month to determine effectiveness.
- Guttate psoriasis often resolves with antibiotic treatment for streptococcal infection. Psoriasis vulgaris may persist for months to years.
- Lifestyle changes help prevent recurrence. These include avoiding cutaneous injury, streptococcal infection, sunburn, stress, itching, bites, tight clothes and shoes, some medications (e.g., oral steroids, NSAIDs), and occlusive dressings. Good skin care, including regular use of emollients and avoiding irritating underarm deodorants and harsh soaps, may improve psoriasis and minimize recurrences. With nail involvement, avoid long fingernails or toenails and use of nail polish. Do not vigorously brush or comb hair if scalp area is affected.
- Psoriasis tends to improve during summer and with increased sunlight.
- Psoriasis is considered stable if there are either no new plaques or if existing plaques are not enlarging.
- Refer patients to the National Psoriasis Foundation (see Additional Resources).

Lichen Striatus

Lichen striatus (LS) has a peak incidence in school-aged children and is characterized by flat-topped papules in a linear pattern, often along embryonic lines, or lines of Blaschko. Although the etiology is unknown, it is thought to be related to a cutaneous defect from an embryologic mutation of somatic cells that is triggered by a viral infection or trauma. It affects females 2 to 3 times more than males. LS is typically located on the extremities, upper back, or neck, but can be found on the palms, soles, nails, genitals, or face. Lesions spontaneously disappear after 3 to 12 months, but they may last up to 3 years. Short relapses occur on occasion.

Clinical Findings

History. Lesions appear spontaneously without prodrome. There is some evidence of a family inheritance.

Physical Examination
- Linear, erythematous to hypopigmented or flesh-colored, flat-topped papules with adherent scale.
- Limited to one extremity, initially lesions coalesce in a linear distribution down an extremity.
- Lesions involving a nailbed result in nail deformity.
- Rarely are lesions noted on the face.
- May be asymptomatic or may be intensely pruritic.
- May resolve with hypopigmentation that lasts several months.

Differential Diagnosis

The unilateral linear lesions are characteristic. However, differential diagnoses include lichen planus, lichen nitidus, flat warts, linear epidermal nevi, psoriasis, epidermal birthmarks, and linear Darier disease.

Management

Lesions generally resolve without treatment in 1 to 2 years. Lubricants and topical steroids do not hasten resolution but can reduce scaling and pruritis.[3]

Complications

Resolution often results in an area of hypopigmentation, which may eventually disappear.

Patient and Family Education

LS is a benign, self-limited, noncontagious disorder that results in complete resolution. Recurrence can occur but is rare.

Keratosis Pilaris

Keratosis pilaris is a common skin condition that is a result of follicles becoming blocked by keratin plugs. The etiology is unknown but patients with the condition tend to have dry skin and sometimes atopic dermatitis. The erythematous papules are typically found on the extensor aspects of the extremities, buttocks, and the cheeks.

Clinical Findings

History. Keratosis pilaris appears spontaneously without prodrome. It is usually asymptomatic, although most patients are bothered by the appearance and seek treatment.

Physical Examination
- Rough, dry skin on the posterior upper arms, anterior thighs, buttocks, and cheeks
- Small papules with follicular plugs of stratum corneum
- Variable degree of erythema surrounding the papule
- Occasional diffuse eruption with small sterile pustules

Diagnostic Studies. Skin biopsy reveals inflammation outside the hair follicle; however, this is typically not needed because the diagnosis is easy to determine.

Differential Diagnosis

Microcomedones of acne, molluscum contagiosum, warts, milia, and folliculitis are often confused with keratosis pilaris.

Management

It is important to recognize keratosis pilaris as a benign disorder to avoid detrimental treatment. Management includes the following:
- In mild cases, lubricants and emollients to moisturize skin are sufficient for improvement.
- Topical keratolytics combined with lactic acid 12%, salicylic acid, urea creams, retinoids, and lubricants are applied several times daily.
- Severe cases may be referred to dermatology for laser therapy.
- Antibiotics active against *S. aureus* are useful for folliculitis.

Patient and Family Education

The chronic but benign nature of keratosis pilaris should be stressed. Treatment takes weeks to months, and recurrence is common. Be sure to recognize the cosmetically distressing nature of the condition.

Vascular Disorders and Pigmented Nevi

Vascular abnormalities, frequently called "birthmarks," are common lesions categorized into two categories: tumors and malformations. Vascular tumors are subdivided into benign, locally aggressive/borderline, and malignant forms. Hemangiomas, the most common vascular tumor, fall into the benign category and are much more common in White patients (up to 10%), females, and premature infants. *Infantile hemangiomas* are absent at birth or appear as a red macule or barely visible telangiectasia. Over the first 6 to 9 months, the lesion enlarges and becomes raised. This is followed by a slow involution, most of which occurs before the age of 4 years.[8] *Congenital hemangiomas* are fully formed hemangiomas found at birth and may not involute as is seen in typical infantile hemangiomas. Large, deep hemangiomas can cause cardiovascular complications, disseminated intravascular coagulation, or compression of internal organs.

Common vascular malformations include simple capillary changes found in *salmon patches* (nevus simplex) and *port-wine stains* (nevus flammeus). Salmon patches, the most common vascular lesion of infancy, is found in 30% to 40% of infants.[3] These innocent lesions, seen at birth, do not usually need any further investigation. Port-wine stains, which may resemble early infantile hemangiomas, are typically found at birth but do not proliferate. Port-wine stains occur in 0.2% to 0.3% of newborns.[2] They typically do not resolve but darken with age and may thicken and become raised later in life. These lesions are almost always unilateral and may be an isolated lesion or be associated with a syndrome (e.g., Sturge-Weber).

Pigmented lesions are the most common neoplasms in children, with melanocytic nevi being extremely common. *Melanocytic nevi* are caused by an alteration in the melanocyte cells that produce melanin and transfer it to keratinocytes, giving a brown pigment to skin and hair. These nevi can be congenital or acquired. Acquired nevi appear after infancy and increase in number with age. They are associated with sun exposure (UV light) and fair skin types, race, and genetic predisposition increase the risk of development. Congenital melanocytic nevi are less common (1%–2% of newborns), frequently have hair, and have a very small risk for the development of malignant melanoma. *Congenital dermal melanocytosis* (found in up to 90% of Black and Native American, 62%–86% of Asian, 70% of Hispanic, and less than 10% of White individuals) is present at birth and fades over the first 3 years.[3] *Café-au-lait spots* (found in up to 40% of healthy children) are pigmented macules or patches that typically have no significance. The presence of six or more, diameter of 0.5 cm before puberty or 1.5 cm after puberty or the presence of axillary or inguinal freckling should raise suspicion for neurofibromatosis type 1 (see Chapter 41).[10] *Lentigines* typically start and increase in number throughout childhood. Their color is not affected by sunlight. There is an inherited patterned lentiginosis that is an autosomal dominant disorder of darker-skinned individuals. Although found with some genetic disorders, most affected individuals are otherwise healthy. Atypical nevi, also called *dysplastic nevi,* are potential precursors for malignant melanoma. Dysplastic nevi are uncommon before age 18 years but have a higher incidence in melanoma-prone families.[3]

Another common skin lesion, *granuloma annulare*, is characterized by annular eruptions whose pigmentation is not due to changes in melanocyte production. Granuloma annulare is common in the pediatric population, especially in school-age children. The cause is not well understood, and the lesions are easily confused with tinea corporis. Subcutaneous lesions are also a common sign; they may present alone or with the typical cutaneous lesions.[2]

The lesion rings begin as nodules, may be up to 4 cm in diameter and often overlap to form plaques. There is often some redness or hyperpigmentation.

Clinical Findings

- Presence from birth, or age first noted
- Progression of lesion
- Familial tendencies for similar nevi, especially for history of melanoma
- Genetic diagnosis and family history

• BOX 37.7 Common Vascular and Pigmented Lesions

I. Vascular malformations
   A. Salmon patch or nevus flammeus: Light pink macule of varying size and configuration. Commonly seen on the glabella, back of neck, forehead, or upper eyelids.
   B. Port-wine stain: Purple-red macules that occur unilaterally and tend to be large. Usually occur on face, occiput, or neck, although they may be on extremities.
   C. Hemangiomas
      1. Superficial ("strawberry") hemangiomas are found in the upper dermis of the skin and account for the majority of hemangiomas.
      2. Deep cavernous hemangiomas are found in the subcutaneous and hypodermal layers of the skin; although like superficial hemangiomas, there is a blue tinge to their appearance. With pressure, there is blanching and a feeling of a soft, compressible tumor. Variable in size, they can occur in places other than skin.
      3. Mixed hemangiomas have attributes of both superficial and deep hemangiomas.
II. Pigmented lesions
   A. Dermal melanocytosis: Blue or slate gray, irregular, variably sized macules. Common in the presacral or lumbosacral area of dark-skinned infants; also on the upper back, shoulders, and extremities. Most of the pigment fades as the child gets older and the skin darkens. Solitary or multiple, often covering a large area.
   B. Café-au-lait spots: Tan to light brown macules found anywhere on the skin; oval or irregular shape; increase in number with age.
   C. Acquired melanocytic nevi are benign, light brown to dark brown to black, flat, or slightly raised, occurring anywhere on the body, especially on sun-exposed areas above the waist.
      1. Junctional nevi represent the initial stage, with tiny, hairless, light brown to black macules.
      2. Compound nevi—a few junctional nevi progress to more elevated, warty, or smooth lesions with hair.
      3. Dermal nevi are the adult form, dome shaped with coarse hair.
      4. Atypical nevi usually appear at puberty, have irregular borders, variegated pigmentation, are larger than normal nevi (6–15 mm); usually found on trunk, feet, scalp, and buttocks.
      5. Halo nevi appear in late childhood with an area of depigmentation around a pigmented nevus, usually on trunk.
      6. Spitz nevi occur primarily in children and are smooth, pink to brown, and dome-shaped papules. They are often found on the head and neck (see Fig. 37.44).
      7. Nevus spilus often begin like café-au-lait patches but develop into light-brown speckled lentiginous nevus that have darker papules.
   D. Lentigines are small brown to black macules 1–2 mm in size appearing anywhere on the body in school-age children. They are larger than a freckle but smaller than a café-au-lait spot (Fig. 37.45).
   E. Freckles: 1–5 mm light brown, pigmented macules in sun-exposed areas.

Physical Examination

Findings include the following (Box 37.7):
- Most but not all vascular malformations have some finding at birth.
- Hemangiomas (Fig. 37.41) are classified as superficial, deep (cavernous), or mixed. They range in size from a few millimeters to several centimeters. Occasionally they may cover an entire limb, resulting in asymmetric limb growth. Rapidly growing lesions may ulcerate. Involution is heralded by gray areas in the lesion followed by flattening from the center outward. Most hemangiomas appear as normal

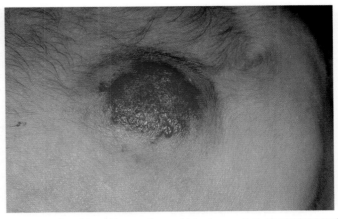

• **Fig. 37.41** Combined Hemangioma. Note: larger, deep component and the bright red, superficial component of this combined lesion. (From Paller AS, Mancini AJ. *Paller and Mancini: Hurwitz Clinical Pediatric Dermatology.* 6th ed. Elsevier; 2022.)

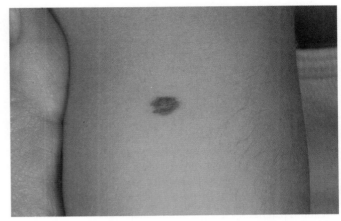

• **Fig. 37.42** Atypical Nevus With Irregular Borders. (From Paller AS, Mancini AJ. *Paller and Mancini: Hurwitz Clinical Pediatric Dermatology.* 6th ed. Philadelphia: Elsevier; 2022.)

skin after involution, but others may have residual changes, such as telangiectasias, atrophy, fibrofatty residue, and scarring.[3]
- Pigmented nevi may be present at birth or acquired during childhood.
- Atypical nevi (Fig. 37.42) are larger than acquired nevi; have irregular, poorly defined borders; and have variable pigmentation.
- The lesion rings of granuloma annulare (Fig. 37.43), which begin as nodules, may be up to 4 cm in diameter and often overlap to form plaques. There is often some redness or hyperpigmentation. It is most common on the distal extremities, especially the dorsal surfaces of hands and feet.

Differential Diagnosis

Hematomas or ecchymoses of child abuse are occasionally confused with some nevi and hemangiomas. It is important to differentiate between benign nevi and those that are at increased risk for progression to melanoma. Granuloma annulare and tinea corporis are similar in appearance.

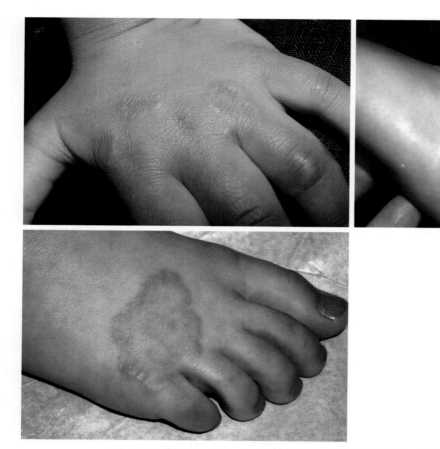

• **Fig. 37.43** Granuloma Annulare. (From Zitelli BJ, McIntire S, Nowalk AJ, et al, editors. *Zitelli and Davis' Atlas of Pediatric Physical Diagnosis.* 8th ed. Elsevier; 2023.)

Management

1. Salmon patches: Fade with time, usually by 5 to 6 years old; no treatment is needed.
2. Port-wine stains: A permanent defect that grows with the child, so cosmetic covering is often used. If forehead and eyelids are involved, there is potential for multiple syndromes (e.g., Sturge-Weber, Klippel-Trenaunay-Weber, Parkes Weber). Neurodevelopmental and ophthalmologic follow-up is needed. Referral to dermatology for possible laser treatment or cosmesis is required.
3. Hemangiomas:
   - Monitor closely, especially during the proliferation phase.
   - If the lesions are strategically placed (e.g., eye, lip, oral cavity, ear, airway, diaper area, lumbosacral), ulcerating, multiple, very large, or grow very quickly, prompt referral to dermatology is indicated because early treatment is most effective.
   - Management is directed at preventing or reversing complications, disfigurement, psychosocial stress, and/or ulceration that can lead to infection, pain and scarring. Education with anticipatory guidance and support is an appropriate therapy in most cases. Sequential photographs showing improvement can be helpful.
   Current standard of care for infantile hemangiomas is the β-blocker propranolol. Treatment is the most effective in the proliferation phase but may help in later stages. Potential side effects include hypotension, bradycardia, bronchospasm, hypoglycemia, and hypothermia.[3]

   - Steroids (intralesional and oral) and subcutaneous interferon-α, may also be used in cases of nonresponsive and severe treatment-resistant or life-threatening lesions.
   - Involution (without treatment) occurs at a rate of 10% per year. Scarring may be present if ulceration occurs; fibrofatty masses, atrophy, and telangiectasis can occur following involution. Laser therapy is effective management for residual telangiectasias.[3]
4. Dermal melanocytosis: Document to distinguish from bruise; fade with time, usually no traces by adulthood.
5. Café-au-lait spots:
   - If six or more lesions larger than 5 mm in diameter are present in children younger than 15 years old and more than 1.5 cm in diameter for older individuals, or if axillary freckling (Crowe sign), neurofibromas, or iris hamartomas are present, refer child to evaluate for neurofibromatosis type 1 (see Chapter 41).
   - Other possible diagnosis for abnormal café-au-lait spots include McCune-Albright syndrome, tuberous sclerosis, LEOPARD syndrome, epidermal nevus syndrome, Bloom syndrome, ataxia-telangiectasia, and Silver-Russell syndrome.
6. Acquired melanocytic nevi: Most are benign but should be watched for possible development of melanoma. Giant nevi (e.g., bathing trunk nevus) have an increased risk of developing melanoma and need referral to a dermatologist.
7. Atypical nevi appear most commonly in adolescents and require regular follow-up because of increased risk for melanoma. Melanoma often manifests with new lesions rather than from

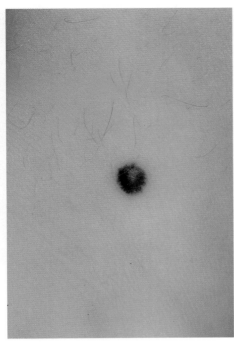

• **Fig. 37.44** Spitz Nevus. (From Paller AS, Mancini AJ. *Paller and Mancini: Hurwitz Clinical Pediatric Dermatology*. 6th ed. Elsevier; 2022.)

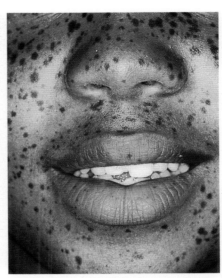

• **Fig. 37.45** Lentiginous Lesions in a 13-Year-Old With LEOPARD Syndrome. (From Cohen BA, editor. *Pediatric Dermatology*. 5th ed. Elsevier; 2022.)

transformation of current ones. A halo nevus, a depigmented ring around a pigmented nevus, has a low risk for melanoma development. However, a spitz nevus (Fig. 37.44) (smooth, pink to brown, dome-shaped papule often occurring on head and neck) and nevus spilus (light-brown speckled lentiginous nevus with darker papules) should be evaluated frequently due to an increased melanoma risk. Guidelines for when a child with a nevus should be referred to a dermatologist are listed in Box 37.8.

8. Granuloma annulare typically resolve spontaneously but topical steroids may be used if nodules or lesions are bothersome. The required length of use can produce dermal thinning, so observation is generally preferred.

Complications

Ulceration, infection, platelet trapping, airway or visual obstruction, or cardiac decompensation can occur with large vascular lesions. Kasabach-Merritt syndrome occurs when thrombocytopenic hemorrhage occurs in a large, deep hemangioma. Melanoma is a possible complication of many nevi. Familial atypical multiple mole melanoma, an autosomal dominant syndrome, has been identified genetically. Children with multiple atypical nevi and family members with melanoma are at risk for childhood melanoma.

Patient and Family Education

- Reassurance is important for lesions that just need time for resolution. Assure the family that the lesions are not a result of anything that the parents have done. See Resources for websites offering support for families.
- Teaching the family to watch nevi for any changes is important. Changes of particular concern are development of an off-center

---

• BOX 37.8   When to Refer Nevi to Dermatology

- Suspicious-appearing nevus (ABCDE: asymmetry, border, color, diameter, evolving)
- Rapidly growing or changing nevus
- More than 50 nevi
- One or more atypical nevi
- History of one or more first-degree relatives with melanoma
- Presence of a giant or large congenital nevus
- Signs of excessive sun exposure (increased nevi/freckles in exposed areas)
- History of immunosuppression and multiple nevi on examination

---

nodule or papule, color change, bleeding, persistent irritation, erosion, ulceration, and rapid growth.
- Encourage follow-up specialty care as needed for any lesion comorbidity.

Cutaneous Manifestations of Underlying Disease

Acanthosis Nigricans

Acanthosis nigricans is not a skin disease per se; rather it is typically a sign of an underlying problem. It may be related to:
- Obesity: This is more commonly seen in darker-pigmented individuals and has a higher incidence (in descending order) in Native American, Black, and Hispanic individuals.[3]
- Endocrine disorders: Insulin resistance and diabetes mellitus are the most common endocrine associations. Others include polycystic ovarian syndrome, hypothyroidism, hyperandrogenic states, and Cushing syndrome.
- Heredity: This autosomal dominant trait has no association with obesity. It may appear at birth or during childhood with proliferation during adolescence.

760 UNIT III Disease Management

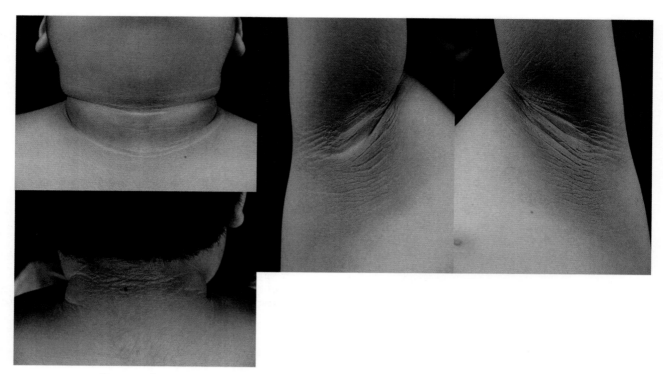

• **Fig. 37.46** Acanthosis Nigricans. (From Karadag AS, You Y, Denarti R, et al. Acanthosis nigricans and the metabolic syndrome. *Clin Dermatol.* 2018;36[1]:48–53.)

- Associated syndromes: There are many syndrome associations, including Prader-Willi, Bloom, lupus erythematosus, scleroderma, and FGFR3 mutation syndromes (including Crouzon syndrome, hypochondroplasia, and achondroplasia).
- Medications: Commonly associated medications include oral contraceptives, niacin, corticosteroids, and stilbestrol.
- Malignancy: This cause of acanthosis nigricans is rare in children but it may be associated with adenocarcinoma, Wilms tumor, and less commonly lymphoma.

Acanthosis nigricans may occur as a benign condition unassociated with any underlying pathology. The majority of acanthosis nigricans is associated with obesity, insulin resistance, and diabetes mellitus. All but the malignant form of acanthosis nigricans result in papillary hypertrophy and hyperkeratosis, not an increase in pigment from melanocytes. Malignant cases of acanthosis nigricans may involve mucous membranes. There is no sex predominance.

Clinical Findings

History
- Past medical history including endocrine disorders
- Medications

Physical Examination. Acanthosis nigricans is characterized by symmetric, brown thickening of the skin (Fig. 37.46). Initially it appears as "dirty" skin that will not wash clean. As time progresses, the skin develops a velvety, leathery, warty, or papillomatous surface. It is primarily found in intertriginous areas (e.g., axillae, neck, groin) and over bony prominences (e.g., knuckles, elbows, knees). In areas of maceration, odor or discomfort from secondary infection may be reported.

Differential Diagnosis

Terra firma-forme dermatosis, a condition believed to be a disorder of keratinization that results in the retention of melanin and sebum within the epidermis, can occur anywhere on the body.

Although it can look like dirt, terra firma-forme dermatosis is not related to hygiene and cannot be washed off with soap and water. Unlike acanthosis nigricans, however, the darkened skin plaques of terra firma-forme dermatosis can be removed with vigorous rubbing with isopropyl alcohol.[15] It is important to diagnose terra firma-forme dermatosis to avoid an extensive and expensive workup for an endocrine or metabolic disorder. Other differential diagnoses include Addison disease, pellagra, erythrasma, and confluent and reticulated papillomatosis.

Management

Treatment consists of addressing the underlying causes. This most commonly includes diet changes, weight loss, and correction of metabolic abnormality (hyperinsulinemia). It is important to screen for associated comorbidities (e.g., hyperlipidemia, hyperglycemia). In nonoverweight individuals, an underlying malignancy must be considered. The skin lesions themselves are benign, usually asymptomatic, and do not require intervention. While response may be poor, topical or oral retinoids, lactic acid-containing emollients, or topical keratolytic agents (salicylic acid, urea) may provide some improvement.

Patient and Family Education

It is important for patients to understand that acanthosis nigricans may be a cutaneous marker for an underlying condition such as insulin resistance and type 2 diabetes in obese individuals or for a malignancy. Addressing the problem may prevent other weight and diabetes comorbidities. Acanthosis nigricans generally improves with adequate treatment of the underlying disorder.

Hypopigmentation Disorders

Decreased skin pigmentation, leaving white or light-colored areas, can be a result of either genetic or acquired disorders. Genetic

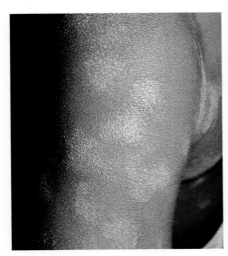

• **Fig. 37.47** Pityriasis Alba. Note poorly demarcated, hypopigmented, scaley areas. (From Cohen BA, editor. *Pediatric Dermatology*. 5th ed. Elsevier; 2022.)

disorders include albinism, piebaldism, and tuberous sclerosis. The reader is encouraged to look beyond this text for information on these less common conditions. Acquired hypopigmentation disorders include vitiligo, postinflammatory hypopigmentation, *pityriasis alba*, and tinea versicolor (previously discussed).

Vitiligo is presumed to be an autoimmune disorder. A patterned pigmentation loss with great variation in location, size, and shape of individual lesions, vitiligo occurs in 1% to 2% of the population worldwide, with 50% of cases appearing before 20 years of age. Generalized vitiligo is the most common subtype in children followed by focal and segmental vitiligo. Focal and segmental vitiligo may progress to the generalized form. While not common, patients with vitiligo have other autoimmune disorders, most commonly alopecia areata and hypothyroidism.[3]

Hypopigmentation can follow inflammation or injury to the melanocytes in the skin resulting from diseases such as atopic dermatitis, psoriasis, or pityriasis rosea. It may follow conditions with significant hyperpigmented inflammation such as abrasions, burns, or sever atopic dermatitis. It is generally self-limited and is cosmetically more obvious in darker skinned individuals. Pityriasis alba (Fig. 37.47) is a specific form of hypopigmentation that is predominantly seen in ages 3 to 16 years. The lesions have scales and are more commonly seen with atopic dermatitis, psoriasis, and contact dermatitis.[3]

Clinical Findings

History
- Family history of vitiligo or markedly premature graying of the hair
- History of halo nevus
- Onset of depigmentation (birth or more recent)
- Presence of any systemic or skin diseases
- Any recent trauma to the skin; Koebner phenomenon noted in about 15% of children with vitiligo

Physical Examination
1. Vitiligo:
   - Vitiligo is frequently found with halo nevus (one or more).
   - The generalized form is bilateral, typically symmetrical, and most frequently begins on exposed areas such as dorsal surfaces of the hands, neck, and face. Flat milk-white macules or papules with scalloped, distinct borders of varied size.
   - Segmental vitiligo can be symmetric or asymmetric and may follow a nerve segment.
   - Focal vitiligo presents as few to multiple lesions, seen most commonly on face and trunk.
2. Postinflammatory hypopigmentation:
   - Macules and patches are frequently seen with irregular mottling and borders. They can be linear or patterned depending on inflammatory cause of hypopigmentation.
   - Lesions may be associated with previously hyperpigmented areas but may be seen in conjunction with hyperpigmented areas.
3. Pityriasis alba:
   - Lesions may be 1 cm to several centimeters in diameter. They may begin as hyperpigmented areas and become sharply demarcated with scales in addition to the hypopigmentation.
   - The face, neck, and arms are most commonly affected.

Diagnostic Studies. For vitiligo, a skin biopsy and CBC, fasting glucose, thyroid function and antithyroid antibodies, early-morning serum cortisol, and VDRL are sometimes indicated when other autoimmune disorders are being considered. A Wood's light may be helpful in fair-skinned individuals to delineate a contrast between the normal and depigmented skin.

Differential Diagnosis

Pityriasis rosea, tinea versicolor, and albinism (which is seen at birth and affects eye color) are included in the differential diagnoses.

Management

The following steps are taken:
- Vitiligo
  - No treatment option will be completely successful.
  - Broad-spectrum sunscreens are used to decrease the tanning of normal skin.
  - Cover-up agents, such as skin dyes and walnut oil, may be used for cosmetic improvement.
  - Mild to moderate steroids and topical calcineurin inhibitors are first-line therapy. Some 40% to 90% of pediatric patients show a response to these treatments within a 6-month period.[3]
  - Phototherapy is the treatment of choice when topical therapy is ineffective.
  - Referral to dermatology is appropriate for these patients.
- Inflammatory hypopigmentation and pityriasis alba
  - No treatment is necessary as the condition is generally self-limited.

Complications

Patients are at risk for severe sunburn. Vitiligo patients rarely have involvement of eye pigment but referral to ophthalmology for examination is appropriate. Hypopigmentation disorders, especially extensive cases, can have a profound effect on psychological and quality of life issues.

Parent and Patient Education

- Due to the nature of autoimmune disorders, families should be alert for other immune disorders both in the patient and in family members.

	TABLE 37.10 Diagnosis and Treatment of Alopecia		
	Etiology	**Clinical Findings**	**Treatment**
Tinea capitis	*Trichophyton tonsurans* 90%–95%; *Microsporum canis;* others	Fine diffuse scaling with hair loss and discrete stubs of broken hair; patchy hair loss with scaling and raised borders to lesions; pustular lesions or kerions	Griseofulvin taken with fatty food until 2 weeks after negative culture; prednisone if kerion present; culture family members; sporicidal shampoo; follow up in 2 weeks; launder sheets, clothes, vacuum house
Telogen effluvium	Emotional or physical stress (severe illness, chemo, major surgery)	Typically thinning but not complete hair loss. Hair part may appear wider	Resolution is usually spontaneously. It is important to address any associated illness or emotional stress. This condition rarely progresses to patches of complete hair loss.
Traumatic alopecia	Chemical, thermal, traction (hairstyling) Infants often lose hair on the occipital scalp due to friction while lying on their back Trichotillomania is behavioral (pulling and twisting of hair)	Traumatic: Incomplete hair loss with varying lengths Traction: Erythema and pustules, hair thins and breaks in certain areas, especially linear Trichotillomania: Circumscribed hair loss with irregular borders and broken hair of varied lengths, no erythema or scarring, especially frontal, parietal, or temporal	Will self-resolve with cessation of causative trauma. A short course of antibiotics is prescribed if pustules are present. Traction: Avoid hairstyles that precipitate; use mild shampoo, gentle brushing; short course of antibiotics if pustules are present. Trichotillomania: Discussion with parents, counseling, behavioral modifications.
Alopecia areata	Possible autoimmune mechanism	Single or multiple round or oval patches of complete or near-complete hair loss, primarily in frontal or parietal areas. There is no erythema or scaling. Scalp may be smooth with fine new hair growth, Nail ridging or pitting often seen. Occasional loss of eyelash, eyebrow, body, or pubic hair.	Discussion and support are critical. If only one or two patches are present, reassure that regrowth will occur. If extensive, refer to dermatologist for alternative treatments; supportive care; prescription for wig; refer to National Alopecia Foundation.

- Connection to support groups is helpful because hypopigmentation can be a highly disfiguring condition, especially for those with dark complexions.
- Complete repigmentation in vitiligo is rare, but partial repigmentaion is common, especially in the summer months.
- Repigmentation can be expected with inflammatory hypopigmentation (including pityriasis alba), generally within months.

Hair Loss

Alopecia, hair loss from areas of skin that normally produce hair, can be limited to one area or scattered over the scalp. It can be complete or leave residual hairs of differing lengths. Scarring alopecia is not common in children and is associated with several disorders, both congenital and acquired. Nonscarring alopecia is the primary type of hair loss in children. The four main causes of nonscarring hair loss are tinea capitis, traumatic alopecia, telogen effluvium, and alopecia areata (Table 37.10).

Traumatic alopecia, characterized by incomplete hair loss with hair of varying lengths, can be due to chemical exposure, thermal damage, traction, or friction. It is a benign problem and the hair will typically grow back. The most common forms are traction alopecia (Fig. 37.48) and *trichotillomania*. *Traction* alopecia, commonly seen in Black females, is due to hair styling. Common causes are cornrows, ponytails, or braids; tight curlers; or excessive brushing. *Trichotillomania* is a common disorder seen in children of all ages after infancy. Hair loss is varied and is caused by repeated pulling and/or excessive twisting of hair with fracturing of the longer hair shafts. Etiology is multifactorial, including genetic predisposition and environmental and behavioral variables. In early childhood, it is associated with habitual behaviors

and situational stress. Trichotillomania most commonly occurs in adolescence and is classified as an obsessive-compulsive disorder and is often accompanied by other obsessive behaviors (e.g., nail biting, skin/lip picking).[3]

Telogen effluvium (Fig. 37.49) is the most common type of alopecia in children.[3] It occurs when the normal cycle of hair growth (anagen phase) and rest (telogen phase) is disrupted. There is often a history of a stressful event that interrupts the anagen phase 2 to 4 months before diagnosis. Some common triggers are acute illness, major trauma, surgery, thyroid dysfunction, anemia, malnutrition, and emotional distress.

Alopecia areata is an asymptomatic, complete hair loss occurring primarily in frontal or parietal areas (Fig. 37.50). The cause of alopecia areata is unknown but a family history of autoimmune disorders is common. It most commonly occurs in adolescence and young adulthood. Onset before puberty has a poorer prognosis. There is an association with atopic dermatitis, which is stronger in younger patients. Appearance of patches has a sudden onset occurring over just days.

Clinical Findings

History

- Timing of the hair loss, including shedding
- Recent illness
- Chronic diagnosis (e.g., thyroid disease, autoimmune disorders)
- Nutritional history
- Various methods of hair styling with tight pulling of hair
- Habits, such as nail biting, finger sucking, or hair twirling
- Recent life changes or stressors

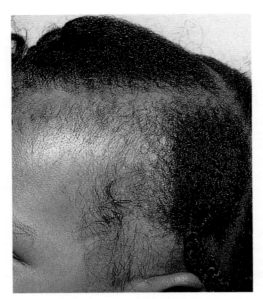

• **Fig. 37.48** Traction Alopecia. (From Zitelli BJ, McIntire S, Nowalk AJ, et al, editors. *Zitelli and Davis' Atlas of Pediatric Physical Diagnosis*. 8th ed. Elsevier; 2023.)

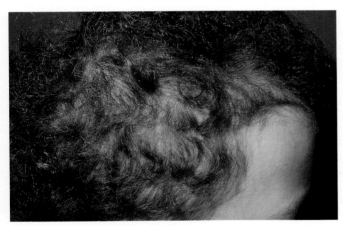

• **Fig. 37.49** Telogen Effluvium Occurring 3 Months After Pneumococcal Sepsis. (From Paller AS, Mancini AJ. *Paller and Mancini: Hurwitz Clinical Pediatric Dermatology*. 6th ed. Elsevier; 2022.)

- Medications (e.g., antiseizure medications, antithyroid medications, β-blockers, isotretinoin, lithium, oral contraceptives, vitamin A supplements, warfarin)
- Excess time spent lying supine.

Physical Examination
- Erythema, pustules, and/or scarring indicates possible infectious cause or more systemic illness
- Absence of erythema, scaling, and broken hairs typically rules out trauma or infection

Diagnostic Studies
The following can be obtained:
- KOH examination or fungal culture, to rule out tinea
- Skin biopsy
- Thyroid screening, as alopecia areata can be associated with autoimmune thyroiditis

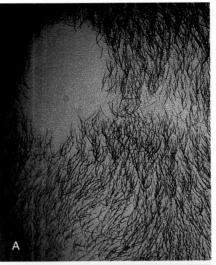

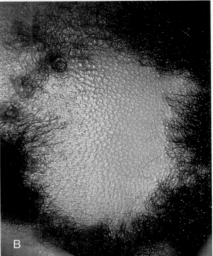

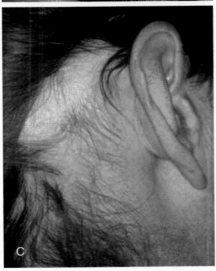

• **Fig. 37.50** Alopecia Areata. (A) Round patch of alopecia. (B) Shiny, round patch of complete alopecia. (C) Patches of smooth nonscarring alopecia from behind the ears to occipital scalp. Note no inflammation or skin changes. (From Cohen BA, editor. *Pediatric Dermatology*. 5th ed. Elsevier; 2022.)

Differential Diagnosis

Differential diagnoses include tinea capitis, trichorrhexis nodosa, and neonatal occipital alopecia. It is also important to rule out child abuse, confirming who is pulling out the hair.

Management

1. Trichotillomania
   - In very young children, trichotillomania is usually benign and resolves spontaneously. Positive reinforcement and substitution therapy can help resolution.
   - Older children and adolescents usually require individual and family therapy. Attempt to relieve stress and cope with any traumatic events. Cognitive-behavioral therapy and/or pharmacologic therapy with anxiolytics may be indicated if behavior modification strategies prove unsuccessful.
   - Referral to dermatology is usually appropriate.
2. Alopecia areata
   - If extensive involvement, refer to dermatology for treatment options. Treatment options include topical corticosteroids, local irritants, topical minoxidil, topical sensitizers, and UV light therapy.[2]

Complications

Prolonged traction alopecia can lead to scarring and permanent hair loss. Trichobezoars (i.e., hairballs) can occur with trichotillomania and often lead to gastrointestinal symptoms. Self-esteem issues are common and some children with trichotillomania have extensive psychopathologic conditions.

Patient and Family Education

The cause of the hair loss must be discussed, and support offered to resolve issues. A straightforward discussion and ongoing support of the individual and family are essential.
- Traumatic hair loss
  - Avoid any hairstyle or device that causes traction on the hair, including cornrows, ponytails, braids, and curlers. Use only mild shampoo, shampoo infrequently, use wide-toothed combs with rounded ends, and brush gently.
  - Management of trichotillomania is difficult and often requires convincing the individual/family the origin of the hair loss as many deny the behavior. A strong relationship between the PCP, mental health team, and the individual/family is important for a successful change in behavior.
- Telogen effluvium
  - Reassurance that regrowth should occur if causative factor can be identified and resolved.
- Alopecia areata
  - All families should be put in touch with the National Alopecia Areata Foundation (NAAF), a national support group for affected children and families. The condition is self-limited in most children and adolescents. Full recovery, often within 1 year, is more likely if three or fewer areas are involved and if onset is in late childhood; however, the greater the hair loss, the longer it takes for regrowth. Approximately one-third of patients have a recurrence within months to years, with a worsening prognosis with each episode. Camouflaging the affected area with hats, headbands, and altered hair styles may be successful. Individuals may consider wearing a wig, depending on the severity of involvement; prescribing the wig as a medical treatment helps defray the cost. Locks of Love is an organization that provides hairpieces to financially disadvantaged children younger than 21 years, and NAAF also offers support (see Resources).

Body Modifications: Tattoos, Body Piercing, and Scarification

A tattoo is an indelible mark fixed on the body by inserting pigment under the skin. Body piercing is the creation of a hole anywhere in the body (e.g., ear, eyebrow, lip, naris, tongue, navel, nipple, genitalia) to insert jewelry. Scarification is the practice of intentionally irritating the skin to cause a permanent pattern of scar tissue. All are considered forms of *body modification,* which has been practiced throughout the ages in many cultures as rites of passage.

Body modifications are a mainstream trend, but there are limited data on the prevalence of tattoos and piercing in those under 18 years. In a 2002 survey of youth 12 to 22 years of age, 10% to 23% had a tattoo and 27% to 42% had a body piercing other than in the earlobe.[17] A 2016 Harris Poll survey found approximately 33% of US adults had at least one tattoo, with a higher tattoo rate in younger versus older cohorts.[18] Body piercing rates (beyond ear lobe piercing in females) are also higher. Across all ages, females have a higher prevalence in tattooing and piercing. There is a lack of studies in the United States to indicate the prevalence of scarification. While often associated with high-risk behaviors in the past, the scientific link between tattooing and high-risk behaviors is less consistent today.

Many states have legislation that prevents tattooing or piercing of minors or requires parental consent before a procedure is done. The National Conference of State Legislatures maintains a website detailing each state's body art laws (see Additional Resources). When not legally available, many adolescents seek out unlicensed tattoo artists or social contacts. Studies have shown that young people are often unaware of the risks associated with piercings and tattoos (e.g., HIV, hepatitis B, hepatitis C, tetanus).[17]

While scarification is often self-performed, there are also increasing numbers of body artists. Common techniques include hot and cold branding, cutting with a scalpel, and laser branding. Few states have any regulations for this activity.

Clinical Findings

History

Questions to discuss include the following:
- When and where the body art was obtained
- Location and care of site
- Complications
- Immunization status

Physical Examination

Look for signs/symptoms of infection, erythema, crusting, or scabs.

Differential Diagnosis

Nonsuicidal self-injury is an impulsive or compulsive behavior with the intent of self-harm and without suicidal intent. It is often associated with mental health disorders, with most individuals seeking relief from emotional pain. Those who practice ongoing body modifications should receive a careful psychosocial assessment.

Management

1. Aftercare for tattoos:
   - Antiseptic and a bandage are applied immediately after the tattoo and not removed for 24 hours. After 24 hours, leave tattoo open to air.
   - A moderate amount of oozing and local swelling is normal for 48 hours. Keep skin moist with antibiotic ointment, thick skin cream, or vitamin E.
   - Scab should be left alone except for the application of antibiotic ointment.
   - Protect from rough surfaces that can traumatize; protect from sunburn.
   - Tattoos generally take 2 weeks to heal.
   - Review signs and symptoms of infection.
2. Aftercare for body piercings:
   - Wash hands before touching; cleanse area twice a day with antibacterial soap.
   - A moderate amount of oozing and swelling is normal; if crusts appear, remove with wet swab.
   - Tongue:
     - Use ice to minimize swelling.
     - Rinse mouth 10 to 12 times a day with half-strength Listerine, twice a day with carbamide peroxide.
     - No deep kissing for 48 hours; once healed, use dental dams for dental work, and avoid smoking.
   - Navel:
     - Slowest to heal, most likely area to reject jewelry.
     - Cleanse twice a day with antibacterial soap.
     - Avoid handling; avoid clothing that rubs for up to 1 year.
   - Nipples and genitalia:
     - Cleanse twice a day with antibacterial soap.
     - Avoid manipulation and tight garments; cotton clothes are ideal.
     - Use latex barriers with sexual activity. Note: Jewelry may compromise barrier contraceptive methods.
3. Healing times are variable and should be considered. A tattoo may take 2 to 3 weeks to heal. Body piercing, depending on the site, can take from 4 to 8 weeks for ears to 6 to 12 months for navel and genital piercings (Table 37.11).
4. Infection can be treated with dicloxacillin. The decision to remove jewelry during an infection should be based on whether leaving it in place will provide a route for drainage, become an obstacle to healing, or be an ongoing source of infection.
5. Always screen for high-risk behaviors.
6. Discuss the need to remove dangling ornaments during contact sports.

Complications

Common complications of tattooing or body piercing include infections, allergic reactions to the dyes or jewelry, and the transmission of bloodborne diseases, primarily hepatitis B and C but potentially HIV. Other reported complications of tattoos include skin neoplasms, syphilis, leprosy, cutaneous tuberculosis, tetanus, hyperplasia, and granuloma annulare. Complications of piercings also include excessive bleeding, nerve damage, keloids, dental fracture, soft-tissue damage, and speech impediments.

Patient and Family Education

Provide information and encourage teenagers to thoroughly research and consider the idea of getting a tattoo or body piercing. Almost one-fourth of individuals regret getting a tattoo. Removing tattoos is expensive, not necessarily completely successful, and fraught with complication (e.g., scarring, rashes) (Box 37.9). Maintaining an open, nonjudgmental attitude when discussing the options and caring for adolescents who have body art is essential. Alternatives to discuss include temporary stick-on tattoos and use of henna or other body paints.

TABLE 37.11 Healing Time for Body Piercings

Type of Piercing	Time to Heal
Navel	4 weeks–12 months
Ear cartilage	6 weeks–9 months
Nostril	6 weeks–4 months
Earlobe and eyebrow	4–8 weeks
Nipple	6 weeks–9 months
Lip	6–8 weeks
Tongue	3–8 weeks
Outer labia	4 weeks–4 months
Inner labia	2–8 weeks
Clitoris	2–10 weeks
Male genitalia	2 weeks–4 months

Data from Hoover CV, Rademayer CA, Farley CL. Body piercings: motivations and implications for health. *J Midwifery Women Health*. 2017;62:521–530.

• BOX 37.9 Getting a Tattoo or Body Piercing

Make an Informed Decision
- Be sure equipment/needles have been sterilized and dye was not previously used on another individual to decrease risk of infections, hepatitis, or possibly even HIV.
- The law in many states prohibits the tattooing of minors.
- Asking a friend to apply a tattoo may ruin a friendship if the tattoo does not look like you thought it would.
- Tattoos and permanent makeup are not easily removed and, in some cases, may cause permanent discoloration.
- Tattoo removal is very expensive. Blood donations cannot be made for 1 year after getting a tattoo, body piercing, or permanent makeup.

Before You Get a Tattoo or Body Piercing: Think Carefully
- *First:* Talk to your friends or others who have been tattooed or pierced. Ask them about their experience, the cost, pain, healing time, and so on. Ask them what they would do if they had a chance to do it over again.
- *Second:* Understand that you do not have to tattoo or pierce your body to belong. Remember that you are directly involved in decisions that affect your health and body. You can always change your mind or wait if you are not sure.
- *Third:* Because of potential complications, if you decide to get a tattoo or body piercing, never tattoo or pierce your own body or let a friend do it.

Continued

• BOX 37.9 Getting a Tattoo or Body Piercing—Cont'd

Health Risks to Consider Before You Act

- Both tattooing and piercing involve puncturing the skin to introduce a foreign material, jewelry, or ink, and the procedures carry similar risks. The primary health concern is introducing bloodborne germs or viruses into your body.
- Bloodborne illnesses, such as hepatitis B and C, tetanus, tuberculosis, and HIV infection, can lead to serious health problems or death.
- Make sure you have had the three series hepatitis B vaccination and a tetanus booster within the past 10 years.
- Localized infections, such as *Staphylococcus* or *Pseudomonas*, can lead to illness, deformity, and scarring.
- Tattoo troubles: *Tattoos are open wounds that may become infected.* Keep the new tattoo clean and moist with an ointment to prevent a scab from forming. If you are allergic to the inks in the tattoo, the site will not heal, and scarring may occur.
- Piercing problems: Complications depend on the location of the piercing. Navel infections are the most common; it takes approximately 1 year for navel piercings to heal. Ear cartilage heals slowly. Tongue piercings may lead to tooth and enamel damage from biting on the jewelry and jewelry knocking against a tooth, partial paralysis if the jewelry pierces a nerve, and extreme inflammation during the first few days.

HIV, Human immunodeficiency virus.

Selecting a Tattoo Artist or Piercer

- Visit several piercers or tattooists. The work area should be kept clean and have good lighting. If they refuse to discuss cleanliness and infection control with you, go somewhere else.
- Consent forms (which the customer must fill out) should be handled before tattooing. Reputable piercing and tattoo studios will not serve a minor without signed consent from parents. Check the laws in your state about tattooing of minors if you are younger than 18 years old.
- The tattooist or piercer should have an *autoclave*—a heat sterilization machine used to sterilize equipment between customers.
- Packaged, sterilized needles should be used only once and then disposed of in a biohazard container.
- Immediately before tattooing or piercing, the tattooist or piercer should wash and dry his or her hands and wear latex gloves. These gloves should be worn at all times while the tattoo or piercing is being done. If the tattoo artist or piercer leaves or touches other objects, such as the telephone, new gloves should be put on before the procedure continues.
- Only jewelry made of a noncorrosive metal, such as surgical stainless steel, niobium, or solid 14-karat gold, is safe for a new piercing.
- Leftover tattoo ink should be disposed of after each procedure. Ink should never be poured back into the bottle and reused.

Additional Resources

American Academy of Dermatology: www.aad.org

Association of Professional Piercers: www.safepiercing.org

Dermatology Online Journal: https://escholarship.org/uc/doj

Electronic Textbook of Dermatology: www.telemedicine.org/stamfor1.htm

FIRST: Foundation for Ichthyosis and Related Skin Types: www.firstskinfoundation.org

International OCD (Obsessive-Compulsive Disorder) Foundation: https://iocdf.org

iPledge Program: www.ipledgeprogram.com

Locks of Love: https://locksoflove.org

Loyola University Dermatology: www.meddean.luc.edu/lumen/meded/medicine/dermatology/melton/title.htm

National Alopecia Areata Foundation: www.naaf.org

National Organization for Albinism and Hypopigmentation: www.albinism.org

National Pediculosis Association, Inc.: www.headlice.org

National Psoriasis Foundation: www.psoriasis.org

National Vitiligo Foundation, Inc.: www.vrfoundation.org

Nevus Network: www.nevusnetwork.org

Prevent Cancer Foundation: www.preventcancer.org

Skin Cancer Foundation: www.skincancer.org

SkinSafe: https://www.skinsafeproducts.com/

Tattooing And Body Piercing:| State Laws, Statutes, and Regulations: http://www.ncsl.org/research/health/tattooing-and-body-piercing.aspx

Trichotillomania Learning Center (TLC): https://rarediseases.org/organizations/trichotillomania-learning-center

Tuberous Sclerosis Alliance: https://www.tscalliance.org

Vitiligo Support International: https://vitiligosupport.org

References

1. James WD, Elston DM, Treat JR, et al. *Andrews' Diseases of the Skin: Clinical Dermatology.* 13th ed. Elsevier; 2020.
2. Cohen BA, ed. *Pediatric Dermatology.* 5th ed. Elsevier; 2021.
3. Paller AS, Mancini AJ. *Hurwitz Clinical Pediatric Dermatology: A Textbook of Skin Disorders of Children and Adolescence.* 6th ed. Elsevier; 2022.
4. Lebwohl MG, Heymann WR, Coulson IH, Murrell DF, eds. *Treatment of Skin Disease.* 6th ed. Elsevier; 2022.
5. Rigel DS, Taylor SC, Lim HW, et al. Photoprotection for skin of all color: consensus and clinical guidance from an expert panel. *J Am Acad Dermatol.* 2022;86(3):S1–S8.
6. Bolognia JL, Schaffer JV, Duncan KO, et al. *Dermatology Essentials.* 2nd ed. Elsevier/Saunders; 2022.
7. Dinulos JGH. *Habif's Clinical Dermatology: A Color Guide to Diagnosis and Therapy.* 2nd ed. Elsevier; 2021.
8. From Zitelli BJ, McIntire S, Nowalk AJ, et al., eds. *Zitelli and Davis' Atlas of Pediatric Physical Diagnosis.* 8th ed. Elsevier; 2023.
9. Silvestre C, Vyas H. Toxic shock syndrome: diagnosis and management. *Paediatr Child Health.* 2022;32(6):226–228.
10. Marcdante KJ, Kliegman RM, Schuh AM. In: *Nelson Essentials of Pediatrics.* 9th ed. Elsevier; 2023.
11. Eichenfield DZ, Sprague J, Eichenfield LF. Management of acne vulgaris: a review. *JAMA.* 2021;326(20):2055–2067.
12. Kellerman RD, Rakel D, KUSM-W Medical Practice Association (2022). *Conn's Current Therapy.* Elsevier; 2022.
13. Van Ravenstein K, Edlund BJ. Diagnosis and management of pityriasis rosea. *Nurs Pract.* 2017;42(1):8–11.
14. Menter A, Cordoro KM, Davis DM, et al. Joint American Academy of dermatology–national psoriasis foundation guidelines of care for the management and treatment of psoriasis in pediatric patients. *J Am Acad Dermatol.* 2020;82(1):16–201.
15. Leung AKC, Barankin B, Lam JM. Terra firma-forme dermatosis. *J Pediatr.* 2018;195:302–302.e1.
16. Breuner CC, Levine DA. AAP Committee on Adolescence Adolescent and young adult tattooing, piercing, and scarification. *Pediatrics.* 2017;140(4):96–111.
17. Shannon-Missal L. Tattoo takeover: three in ten Americans have a tattoo, and most don't stop at one. *Harris Poll No.* 2016;12. http://www.theharrispoll.com/health-and-life/Tattoo_Takeover.html.
18. Mayers LB, Chiffriller SH. Body art (body piercing and tattooing) among undergraduate university students: "then and now". *J Adolesc Health.* 2008;42(2):201–203.

38

Hematologic Disorders

DEANNA SCHNEIDER

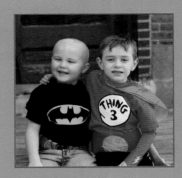

The hematologic system is a massive fluid organ that permeates the entire body, acting as the body's transport system for nutrients and other vital elements. Essential body functions carried out by blood include the transfer of respiratory gases, hemostasis, phagocytosis, and the provision of cellular and humoral agents to fight infection. Abnormalities of blood cells are seen in various disease states and with alterations in nutrition. The use of diagnostic hematologic studies is necessary to differentiate common nutritional deficiencies with straightforward treatments from oncologic or rare diseases with a genetic or chronic component.

Anatomy and Physiology

Blood is composed of cellular components, each with specialized functions, and a fluid component called *plasma,* which serves as the transport medium. The cells that comprise whole blood are categorized as *erythrocytes,* or red blood cells (RBCs); *leukocytes,* or white blood cells (WBCs); and *thrombocytes,* or platelets (Fig. 38.1).

Plasma, the clear yellow fluid in which proteins are the major solutes, plays an essential role in holding heat in the body and maintaining intravascular volume. Plasma proteins (e.g., albumins, globulins, fibrinogen) are synthesized by the liver and are the largest components of the blood, which makes them essential to maintaining intravascular volume. They also contribute to coagulation, serve as the main cells responsible for humoral immunity, and are important in acid-base balance.

The complete blood count (CBC), which provides an assessment of all cell categories, is commonly used in routine health evaluations. Abnormally high or low counts in any cell category can indicate or provide insight into the presence of many conditions; however, because different conditions present at different ages, values must be interpreted using age-appropriate, pediatric hematologic parameters (Table 38.1). It is also important to remember that hematologic values in neonates differ significantly from those in older children and adults—a reflection of the developmental changes during fetal hematopoiesis that correlate with gestational age.[1] Blood formation in the human embryo begins in the yolk sac during the first several weeks of gestation. During the second trimester, blood is formed primarily in the fetal liver, spleen, and lymph nodes. In the last half of gestation, hematopoiesis shifts from the fetal liver and spleen to the bone marrow where, by birth, most blood formation is taking place.[2]

Erythrocytes

Erythropoietin, produced primarily by renal glomerular epithelial cells, regulates the production of RBCs. In response to a decrease in the number of circulating RBCs or a decrease in the oxygen pressure of arterial blood (Pao_2), erythropoietin stimulates the bone marrow to convert certain stem cells to proerythroblasts. Substances essential for RBC formation include iron, vitamin B_{12}, folic acid, amino acids, and other nutrients.

The RBC matures in stages: proerythroblast, erythroblast, normoblast, reticulocyte, and erythrocyte. As cellular differentiation occurs, the nucleus present in the early forms of the cell is extruded and replaced by hemoglobin (Hgb). The RBC assumes its characteristic anucleated biconcave disk shape, which enables it to pass through small capillaries and sinuses without being destroyed. The large surface-to-volume ratio of the semipermeable membrane facilitates rapid gas exchange.

The youngest circulating RBCs are the reticulocytes (e.g., blast forms are typically seen only in the bone marrow). Once released from the bone marrow, reticulocytes are in circulation for 1 to 2 days before becoming mature RBCs. A mature RBC survives about 120 days before it is destroyed through phagocytosis in the spleen, liver, or bone marrow. The *reticulocyte count* is about 4% to 6% for the first 3 days of life, which reflects the relatively greater amount of erythropoiesis that occurs in the fetus. This increase is followed by a sudden drop, a second surge around 2 months, and a slow decline to 0.5% to 1.5% by 1 year of age, which remains the norm for the rest of the individual's life. Although it is not a routine component of the CBC, a reticulocyte count can be used to assess hematologic stress and/or the effectiveness of the body's early response to treatment (e.g., a tracking response to iron therapy for anemia).

Hemoglobin

Hgb is the oxygen-carrying protein molecule in the RBC and makes up approximately 99% of the protein content of the RBC (Fig. 38.2). Production of Hgb requires circulating iron, the synthesis of a protoporphyrin ring, and the production of globin. Each Hgb molecule comprises two pairs of polypeptide chains. The globin portion contains protein in a precise sequence of amino acids coded by genes located on chromosomes 11 and 16. Normal Hgb contains two alpha (α) and two beta (β) chains, which attach to heme groups; large iron-containing disks; and porphyrin, a nitrogen-containing organic compound.

Each of the four iron atoms in the Hgb molecule combines reversibly with an atom of oxygen to form oxyhemoglobin. The percentage of oxyhemoglobin is the arterial oxygen saturation (Sao_2), which is measured indirectly through pulse oximetry (Spo_2) or directly through arterial blood gas determination (Pao_2). When the oxygen concentration is lower (as in the tissues), oxygen is released from Hgb to meet cellular demands.

Structural Variations

Normal adult Hgb contains two alpha (α) and two beta (β) chains. Equal numbers of each chain are essential for normal cell function.

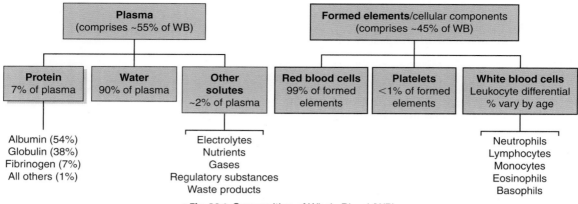

• **Fig. 38.1** Composition of Whole Blood (WB).

TABLE 38.1 Age-Specific Blood Cell Indices

Age	Hgb (g/dL)[a]	HCT (%)[a]	MCV (fL)[a]	MCHC (g/dL RBC)[a]	Reticulocytes	WBCs (×10³/mL)[b]	Platelets (10³/mL)[b]
26–30 weeks' gestation[c]	13.4 (11)	41.5 (34.9)	118.2 (106.7)	37.9 (30.6)	—	4.4 (2.7)	254 (180–327)
28 weeks	14.5	45	120	31.0	(5–10)	—	275
32 weeks	15.0	47	118	32.0	(3–10)	—	290
Term[d] (cord)	16.5 (13.5)	51 (42)	108 (98)	33.0 (30.0)	(3–7)	18.1 (9–30)[e]	290
1–3 days	18.5 (14.5)	56 (45)	108 (95)	33.0 (29.0)	(1.8–4.6)	18.9 (9.4–34)	192
2 weeks	16.6 (13.4)	53 (41)	105 (88)	31.4 (28.1)	—	11.4 (5–20)	252
1 month	13.9 (10.7)	44 (33)	101 (91)	31.8 (28.1)	(0.1–1.7)	10.8 (4–19.5)	—
2 months	11.2 (9.4)	35 (28)	95 (84)	31.8 (28.3)	—	—	—
6 months	12.6 (11.1)	36 (31)	76 (68)	35.0 (32.7)	(0.7–2.3)	11.9 (6–17.5)	—
6 months–2 years	12.0 (10.5)	36 (33)	78 (70)	33.0 (30.0)	—	10.6 (6–17)	(150–350)
2–6 years	12.5 (11.5)	37 (34)	81 (75)	34.0 (31.0)	(0.5–1.0)	8.5 (5–15.5)	(150–350)
6–12 years	13.5 (11.5)	40 (35)	86 (77)	34.0 (31.0)	(0.5–1.0)	8.1 (4.5–13.5)	(150–350)
12–18 Years							
Male	14.5 (13)	43 (36)	88 (78)	34.0 (31.0)	(0.5–1.0)	7.8 (4.5–13.5)	(150–350)
Female	14.0 (12)	41 (37)	90 (78)	34.0 (31.0)	(0.5–1.0)	7.8 (4.5–13.5)	(150–350)
Adult							
Male	15.5 (13.5)	47 (41)	90 (80)	34.0 (31.0)	(0.8–2.5)	7.4 (4.5–11)	(150–350)
Female	14.0 (12)	41 (36)	90 (80)	34.0 (31.0)	(0.8–4.1)	7.4 (4.5–11)	(150–350)

[a]Data are mean (−2 SD).

[b]Data are mean (±2 SD).

[c]Values are from fetal samplings.

[d]1 month, capillary hemoglobin exceeds venous: 1 hour: 3.6-g difference; 5 day: 2.2-g difference; 3 weeks: 1.1-g difference.

[e]Mean (95% confidence limits).

HCT, Hematocrit; *Hgb*, hemoglobin; *MCHC*, mean cell hemoglobin concentration; *MCV*, mean corpuscular volume; *RBC*, red blood cell; *WBC*, white blood cell.

Data from Forestier F, Dattos F, Galacteros F, et al. Hematologic values of 163 normal fetuses between 18 and 30 weeks of gestation. *Pediatr Res.* 1986;20:342; Oski FA, Naiman JL. *Hematological Problems in the Newborn Infant.* WB Saunders; 1982; Nathan D, Oski FA. *Hematology of Infancy and Childhood.* WB Saunders; 1998; Matoth Y, Zaizor K, Varsano I, et al. Postnatal changes in some red cell parameters. *Acta Paediatr Scand.* 1971;60:317; and Wintrobe MM. *Clinical Hematology.* Williams & Wilkins; 1999.

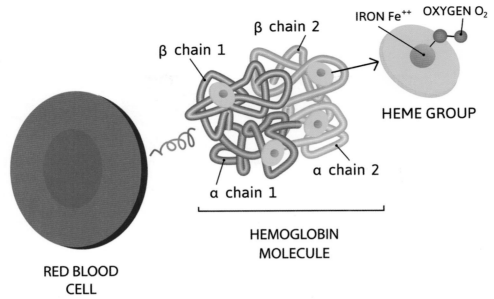

• **Fig. 38.2** Structure of Hemoglobin in Red Blood Cell. (Copyright Anastasila Krasavina/iStock.com.)

An imbalance of the chains damages and destroys RBCs, thereby producing anemia. At birth, approximately 70% of Hgb is made up of fetal hemoglobin (Hgb F), which is composed of two alpha and two gamma (γ) chains and has a high affinity for oxygen. By 12 months of age, the percent of Hgb F is less than 2%, whereas adult Hgb A_1 is 95%. Hgb A_2 is another adult Hgb, which consists of two α and two delta (δ) chains. Hgb A_2 normally makes up only 2.5% of the total Hgb; however, it may be increased in certain conditions such as β-thalassemia. Hgb Bart, which consists of four γ chains and has a very high affinity for oxygen, is present in the developing embryo and typically decreases before birth but may be present in some cases of α-thalassemia.

Among the most commonly occurring Hgb variants are Hgb S (sickle), Hgb C, Hgb E, persistence of Hgb F, and Hgb H. The incidence of these Hgb types tends to peak within certain geographic/regional populations. Atypical combinations of Hgb variants can occur, each with its own resulting condition or problems. *Hemoglobin electrophoresis,* which separates each Hgb out on a gel medium, is the diagnostic test used to differentiate the Hgb variants from Hgb A, thus aiding in the diagnosis of specific hemoglobinopathies. Other hemoglobinopathies occur because of diminished production of one of the two subunit chains, the most common being one of the *thalassemias.* Another Hgb variant is an altered state, as occurs with methemoglobin. In this condition, the ferrous form of iron oxidizes to the ferric state, causing the *heme* to be incapable of carrying oxygen. If reduced Hgb levels exceed 5 g/dL (i.e., 5 g/L not transporting oxygen), serious tissue hypoxia and cyanosis can occur. Methemoglobinemia can be congenital or caused by exposure to certain drugs and chemicals.

Normal Values

Hgb increases with increased gestational age. In the full-term newborn, Hgb levels are typically high ($\geq$14 g/dL) as a result of increased tissue oxygenation and reduced production of erythropoietin. Hgb levels begin to drop shortly after birth, reaching a low point (11 g/dL) at about 6 to 9 weeks. This drop represents a *physiologic* anemia caused by the shortened survival of fetal RBCs and the rapid expansion of blood volume during this period. A decrease in Hgb, or anemia, can also develop secondary to a decrease in RBC production, blood loss, or increased RBC destruction. Owing to the effect of these processes, oxygen transport to the tissues is adversely affected, and the individual can become clinically anemic, as manifested by pallor and, with further deterioration, heart failure or shock.

Antigenic Properties of Red Blood Cells (Blood Type)

RBCs are classified into different types according to the presence of antigens on the cell membrane. The antigenicity is genetically determined, representing contributions from both parents. The most common antigens are designated A, B, and Rh. A person inherits either A or B antigen (type A or B blood), both antigens (type AB blood, making that person a universal recipient), or neither antigen (type O blood, making that person a universal donor). The A and B antigens are sugars, whereas Rh antigens are proteins (Fig. 38.3). The antigens expressed in the RBCs determine an individual's blood type. These distinctions become especially important when blood transfusions are necessary or in the assessment of maternal-fetal blood incompatibilities. Individuals belong to one of eight different blood types: A Rh+, A Rh–, B Rh+, B Rh–, AB RH+, AB Rh–, 0 Rh+, or 0 Rh–, each having different combinations of *antigens* on the surface of the RBCs.

Leukocytes

Leukocytes, or WBCs, are larger and fewer in number than erythrocytes. The primary function of WBCs is to protect the body from invasion by foreign organisms (e.g., viruses, bacteria, parasites, and fungi) and to distribute antibodies and other immune response components. When the WBC count reaches a critically low level, the individual is at risk for infection. Conversely, an elevated WBC count typically indicates that an infection or serious disease, such as leukemia, exists. The WBC count has two components: (1) the total number of WBCs and (2) the differential, which indicates the percentage of each type of WBC present in the same specimen. An increase in the percentage of one type of WBC means a decrease in the percentage of the other, and vice versa.

There are five types of WBCs: neutrophils, lymphocytes, monocytes, eosinophils, and basophils (Table 38.2). WBCs can

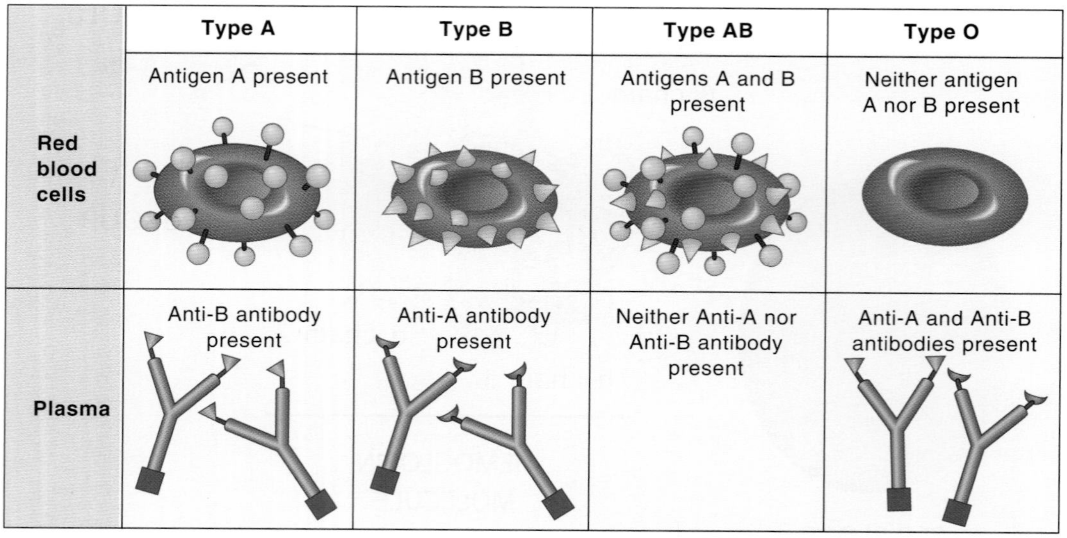

• **Fig. 38.3** Red Cell Antigenicity. (From Patton KT, Bell F, Thompson T, et al. *Anatomy & Physiology*, ed 11. Elsevier; 2022.)

be grouped into two broad classifications: (1) granulocytes and (2) agranulocytes. Table 38.3 provides normal leukocyte and differential counts by age.

Granulocytes: Neutrophils, Basophils, and Eosinophils

In children, granulocytes typically make up 40% to 70% of all WBCs. Granulocytes are further divided into neutrophils (also known as *polymorphonucleocytes*, or *polys*), eosinophils, and basophils.

Neutrophils. The major function of *neutrophils* is the phagocytosis or destruction of harmful particles and cells, particularly bacterial organisms. Neutrophils evolve as they mature in the bone marrow and are released into the blood from myeloblasts; they include—in the order of degree of maturity—promyelocytes, myelocytes, metamyelocytes, bands, and segmented neutrophils. A relative increase in the number of circulating immature neutrophils (bands) is referred to as a *left shift* and typically signifies the presence of an acute bacterial infection or inflammatory process.

Basophils. *Basophils*, or mast cells, typically account for less than 3% of WBCs present in blood. Although they do not respond to bacterial or viral infection, they are involved in the phagocytosis of antigen-antibody complexes. The cytoplasm of basophils contains heparin, histamine, and serotonin. A decrease in basophils (baso*penia*) can occur with acute allergic reactions and hyperthyroidism as well as stress, ovulation, and pregnancy. An increase in basophils (baso*philia*) can occur with allergic rhinitis/seasonal pollenosis, nephrosis, ulcerative colitis, and hypothyroidism.

Eosinophils. *Eosinophils*, which typically make up only 1% to 2% of WBCs, are similar to basophils in that they are involved in the phagocytosis of antigen-antibody complexes and are not responsive to bacterial or viral infections. They are also helpful in evaluating the severity of asthma. An elevation in eosinophils (eosino*philia*) can occur in allergic reactions, atopic dermatitis, asthma, and autoimmune disorders, as well as parasitic infections and malignancies. A decrease in eosinophils (eosino*penia*) may occur with increased adrenosteroid production.

Agranulocytes: Lymphocytes and Monocytes

Lymphocytes. *Lymphocytes* (or immunocytes) make up 25% to 35% of WBCs. They originate in the bone marrow but differentiate in lymphoid tissues (e.g., spleen, liver, thymus, lymph nodes, intestines). Thymus-dependent lymphocytes (T cells) are part of the cell-mediated immune response whereby cytotoxic agents and macrophages are synthesized. There are three types of T cells: cytotoxic (killer T cells), helper T cells, and regulatory T cells. Lymphocytes that remain in the bone marrow (B cells) are precursors that can recognize antigens and transform into plasma cells, which release immunoglobulins or antibodies into the bloodstream.

Monocytes. *Monocytes* constitute 4% to 6% of WBCs. After briefly circulating in the peripheral vascular system, monocytes migrate to the tissues to mature and become part of the monocyte/histiocyte/immune cell system. Their primary function is the phagocytosis of bacteria and cellular debris; they serve as a backup system to the granulocytes, which are the body's first line of defense.

Platelets and Coagulation Factors

The smallest cellular components in blood are the platelets, or thrombocytes, which are essential to hemostasis and clot formation. When a blood vessel is injured, platelets adhere to the inner surface of the vessel and form a hemostatic plug. As platelets degrade, a series of at least 13 clotting factors or proteolytic enzymes are released; these bring about the clotting process in a cascading sequence of successive reactions (Fig. 38.4). Age-specific coagulation values exist for each aspect of the coagulation process and should be referenced for proper assessment and treatment management (Table 38.4).

Pathophysiology

Hematologic problems are generally classified as disorders of RBCs, WBCs, and platelets and/or coagulation function. These three broad categories of function are further divided into disorders of blood cell production, maturation, or destruction.

Assessment of Hematologic Disorders

History

A comprehensive history and physical examination are essential to unravel the mystery behind any suspected hematologic disorder,

TABLE 38.2   White Blood Cell Differential and Key Characteristics

Major Division of White Blood Cells	Differential	Description
Granulocytes (50–75%)	Neutrophils	Primary defense against bacterial infection and mediating stress Elevated with bacterial or inflammatory disorders
	Bands (<1%)	Immature neutrophils released from the bone marrow
	Eosinophils (2–4%)	Associated with antigen-antibody response Elevated with exposure to allergens or inflammation of skin, parasites
	Basophils (1–2%)	Phagocytes: contain heparin, histamines, and serotonin Increased in leukemia, chronic inflammation, hypersensitivity to food, radiation therapy
Agranulocytes (30–40%)	Lymphocytes (25–35%)	Primary components of the immune system; B-cells and T-cells Elevated with viral infections, leukemia, radiation exposure Decreased with diseases affecting the immune system
	Monocytes (<2%)	Elevated in infections and inflammation, leukemia Decreased with some bone marrow injury, leukemias

keeping in mind that many hematologic disorders have a genetic basis. To discern inheritable disorders, it is necessary to obtain a detailed family history. Certain erythrocyte disorders—such as thalassemia, sickle cell anemia (SCA), and glucose-6-phosphate dehydrogenase (G6PD) deficiency—occur with greater frequency in individuals whose ancestors came from specific geographic regions. A three-generation pedigree can provide visual clues to patterns of heritability and may help to narrow down the diagnostic

TABLE 38.3	Normal Leukocyte and Differential Counts			
	12 Months Old	4 Years Old	10 Years Old	21 Years Old
Leukocytes, total	11.4 (6.0–17.5)	9.1 (5.5–15.5)	8.1 (4.5–13.5)	7.4 (4.5–11.0)
Neutrophils, total	3.5 (1.5–8.5) (31%)	3.8 (1.5–8.5) (42%)	4.4 (1.8–8.0) (54%)	4.4 (1.8–7.7) (59%)
Neutrophils, band forms	0.35 (3.1%)	0.27 (0–1.0) (3.0%)	0.24 (0–1.0) (3.0%)	0.22 (0–0.7) (3.0%)
Neutrophils, segmented	3.2 (28%)	3.5 (1.5–7.5) (39%)	4.2 (1.8–7.0) (51%)	4.2 (1.8–7.0) (56%)
Eosinophils	0.30 (0.05–0.70) (2.6%)	0.25 (0.02–0.65) (2.8%)	0.20 (0–0.60) (2.4%)	0.20 (0–0.45) (2.7%)
Basophils	0.05 (0–10) (0.4%)	0.05 (0–0.20) (0.6%)	0.04 (0–0.20) (0.5%)	0.04 (0–0.20) (0.5%)
Lymphocytes	7.0 (4.0–10.5) (61%)	4.5 (2.0–8.0) (50%)	3.1 (1.5–6.5) (38%)	2.5 (1.0–4.8) (34%)
Monocytes	0.55 (0.05–1.1) (4.8%)	0.45 (0–0.8) (5.0%)	0.35 (0–0.8) (4.3%)	0.30 (0–0.8) (4.0%)

Values are expressed as cells ×10^3/μL. Mean values are given; ranges are in parentheses. Percentage values are for mean values.

From Altman PL, Dittmer DS, eds. *Blood and Other Body Fluids.* Washington, DC: Federation of American Societies for Experimental Biology; 1961.

possibilities. In particular, the primary care provider (PCP) should ask about family members with a history of anemia, jaundice, and/or splenomegaly (or history of splenectomy), as well as gallbladder disease/gallstones (or history of cholecystectomy), bleeding tendencies, and/or chronic illnesses as these may suggest a heritable erythrocyte disorder. Family history of childhood malignancy or immune disorders may also suggest a predisposition to development of oncologic conditions involving the hematologic system.

A comprehensive review of each child's medical and social history as well as a thorough review of systems is fundamental. Particular attention should focus on the following:

- Birth history, including gestational age/weight, presence of neonatal jaundice, use of phototherapy, blood transfusion history, birth/neonatal complications.
- Alterations in growth and/or development.
- Behavioral changes—irritability, lethargy, fatigue, school issues.
- Presence of pallor, petechiae/bruising, extremity pain/swelling, epistaxis, bleeding from gums, prolonged or abnormal bleeding for associated injury.
- Nutritional history with focus on key nutrient intake (iron, folate, vitamin B_{12}), milk intake in infants and young children.
- Gastrointestinal (GI) disorders.
- Bone fractures or other trauma.
- Recent acute infections/illness, history of frequent infections and/or enlarged lymph nodes.
- Presence of fevers, night sweats.
- Drug/environmental/toxin exposures and/or history of pica.
- International travel.
- Surgical history, including any abnormal bleeding with procedures.
- Menstrual history, heavy menses, if appropriate.

In addition, for infants, the newborn screening panel results must be reviewed. In the United States, sickle cell disease (SCD) is the most common genetic disease identified through the state-mandated screening programs.[3] If rounding in the nursery, the PCP should validate home address and phone while doing newborn rounds to make sure that there is correct information to contact the family if abnormal results are noted. The PCP must also verify and document the results in the child's medical record. More information about newborn screening can be found at https://www.cdc.gov/newbornscreening/.

Physical Examination

The physical examination should be comprehensive, including vital signs and growth documentation. The following positive signs are particularly important to identify owing to their association with specific problems:

- Pallor (conjunctivae, buccal mucosa, palmar creases), jaundice, petechiae/bruising, hyperpigmentation
- Retinal hemorrhages, glossitis, and/or bleeding from mucous membranes
- Lymphadenopathy, hepatosplenomegaly
- Frontal bossing and/or prominent maxilla
- Joint or extremity pain, spoon nails
- Heart murmurs (typically a systolic ejection murmur), tachycardia, distended neck veins

Initial Diagnostic Evaluation

The initial laboratory evaluation of a suspected hematologic disorder includes a CBC with WBC differential and RBC indices, reticulocyte count, and review of peripheral blood smear, which identifies abnormal morphology and/or staining. Table 38.5 notes the common components of the CBC and what the reported value measures or reflects.

A knowledge of which tests to order and how to interpret laboratory data are integral to analyzing the information gleaned from the hematopoietic system. It is important to evaluate a CBC in an organized fashion and look at all three reported components: RBCs, WBCs, platelets. As previously stated, proper interpretation of these values requires the PCP to take developmental norms into account (see Tables 38.1 and 38.3). In addition, laboratory norms vary slightly with the individual lab, so it is important to evaluate the child's results in accordance with local laboratory norms and to check whether the local lab uses pediatric normal reference ranges.

The PCP should evaluate the RBCs first by looking at the Hgb and hematocrit (Hct) for anemia. If anemia is present, as evidenced by decreased Hgb and/or Hct, examine the RBC count

Normal PT and PTT
- von Willebrand disease (type 2B)
- Platelet dysfunction
- Thrombocytopenia
- Vascular abnormalities
- Factor XIII deficiency
- Fibrinolytic disorders

Prolonged aPTT and normal PT
- Factor VIII, IX, XI, XII
  deficiency or inhibitor
- Lupus anticoagulant
- von Willebrand disease
- Heparin

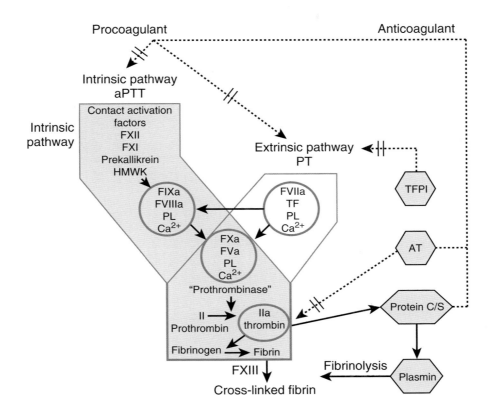

Prolonged PT and aPTT
- Normal TT:
  - Liver disease
  - Vitamin K deficiency (late)
  - Factor II/V/X deficiency or inhibitor
  - Combined factor deficiencies
  - Lupus anticoagulant
- Prolonged TT
  - DIC
  - Low fibrinogen
  - Dysfibrinogenemia

Prolonged PT and normal aPTT
- Factor VII deficiency or inhibitor
- Mild liver disease
- Vitamin K deficiency (early)
- Warfarin

• **Fig. 38.4** The Clotting Cascade and Differential Diagnosis of Bleeding Disorders. *aPTT*, Activated partial thromboplastin time; *DIC*, disseminated intravascular coagulation; *PT*, prothrombin time; *TT*, thrombin time. (Modified from Rodriguez V and Warad D. Pediatric coagulation disorders. *Pediatr Rev.* 2016:37[7]:279-290.)

and RBC indices in detail. Classification and diagnosis of anemia are discussed later in this chapter. Further diagnostic studies may be indicated to delineate the type of anemia.

Evaluation of the WBC portion of the CBC is frequently used to diagnose and manage infection and inflammatory disorders, in addition to hematopoietic malignancies, myelopoietic disorders, drug effects, and response to cytotoxic agents. Review the WBC to make sure that all five cell lines are present in the differential

and then evaluate, or calculate if necessary, the absolute neutrophil count (ANC). ANC is calculated by multiplying the total WBC count by the total neutrophil count (including segmented and banded forms). Finally, the platelet count should be evaluated to assess for the presence of thrombocytosis (elevated) or thrombocytopenia (decreased) and the mean platelet volume (MPV) evaluated for platelet size. Further discussion and interpretation of these values is discussed later in the chapter.

TABLE 38.4 Age-Specific Coagulation Values

Coagulation Test	Preterm Infant (30–36 weeks), Day of Life 1[a]	Term Infant, Day of Life 1	Day of Life 3	1 Month–1 Year	1–5 Years	6–10 Years	11–16 Years	Adult
PT (s)	13.0 (10.6–16.2)	15.6 (14.4–16.4)	14.9 (13.5–16.4)	13.1 (11.5–15.3)	13.3 (12.1–14.5)	13.4 (11.7–15.1)	13.8 (12.7–16.1)	13.0 (11.5–14.5)
INR		1.26 (1.15–1.35)	1.20 (1.05–1.35)	1.00 (0.86–1.22)	1.03 (0.92–1.14)	1.04 (0.87–1.20)	1.08 (0.97–1.30)	1.00 (0.80–1.20)
aPTT (s)[b]	53.6 (27.5–79.4)	38.7 (34.3–44.8)	36.3 (29.5–42.2)	39.3 (35.1–46.3)	37.7 (33.6–43.8)	37.3 (31.8–43.7)	39.5 (33.9–46.1)	33.2 (28.6–38.2)
Fibrinogen (g/L)	2.43 (1.50–3.73)	2.80 (1.92–3.74)	3.30 (2.83–4.01)	2.42 (0.82–3.83)	2.82 (1.62–4.01)	3.04 (1.99–4.09)	3.15 (2.12–4.33)	3.1 (1.9–4.3)
Bleeding time (min)[a]					6 (2.5–10)	7 (2.5–13)	5 (3–8)	4 (1–7)
Thrombin time (s)	14 (11–17)	12 (10–16)[a]		17.1 (16.3–17.6)	17.5 (16.5–18.2)	17.1 (16.1–18.5)	16.9 (16.2–17.6)	16.6 (16.2–17.2)
Factor II (U/mL)	0.45 (0.20–0.77)	0.54 (0.41–0.69)	0.62 (0.50–0.73)	0.90 (0.62–1.03)	0.89 (0.70–1.09)	0.89 (0.67–1.10)	0.90 (0.61–1.07)	1.10 (0.78–1.38)
Factor V (U/mL)	0.88 (0.41–1.44)	0.81 (0.64–1.03)	1.22 (0.92–1.54)	1.13 (0.94–1.41)	0.97 (0.67–1.27)	0.99 (0.56–1.41)	0.89 (0.67–1.41)	1.18 (0.78–1.52)
Factor VII (U/mL)	0.67 (0.21–1.13)	0.70 (0.52–0.88)	0.86 (0.67–1.07)	1.28 (0.83–1.60)	1.11 (0.72–1.50)	1.13 (0.70–1.56)	1.18 (0.69–2.00)	1.29 (0.61–1.99)
Factor VIII (U/mL)	1.11 (0.50–2.13)	1.82 (1.05–3.29)	1.59 (0.83–2.74)	0.94 (0.54–1.45)	1.10 (0.36–1.85)	1.17 (0.52–1.82)	1.20 (0.59–2.00)	1.60 (0.52–2.90)
vWF (U/mL)[a]	1.36 (0.78–2.10)	1.53 (0.50–2.87)			0.82 (0.47–1.04)	0.95 (0.44–1.44)	1.00 (0.46–1.53)	0.92 (0.5–1.58)
Factor IX (U/mL)	0.35 (0.19–0.65)	0.48 (0.35–0.56)	0.72 (0.44–0.97)	0.71 (0.43–1.21)	0.85 (0.44–1.27)	0.96 (0.48–1.45)	1.11 (0.64–2.16)	1.30 (0.59–2.54)
Factor X (U/mL)	0.41 (0.11–0.71)	0.55 (0.46–0.67)	0.60 (0.46–0.75)	0.95 (0.77–1.22)	0.98 (0.72–1.25)	0.97 (0.68–1.25)	0.91 (0.53–1.22)	1.24 (0.96–1.71)
Factor XI (U/mL)	0.30 (0.08–0.52)	0.30 (0.07–0.41)	0.57 (0.24–0.79)	0.89 (0.62–1.25)	1.13 (0.65–1.62)	1.13 (0.65–1.62)	1.11 (0.65–1.39)	1.12 (0.67–1.96)
Factor XII (U/mL)	0.38 (0.10–0.66)	0.58 (0.43–0.80)	0.53 (0.14–0.80)	0.79 (0.20–1.35)	0.85 (0.36–1.35)	0.81 (0.26–1.37)	0.75 (0.14–1.17)	1.15 (0.35–2.07)
PK (U/mL)[a]	0.33 (0.09–0.57)	0.37 (0.18–0.69)			0.95 (0.65–1.30)	0.99 (0.66–1.31)	0.99 (0.53–1.45)	1.12 (0.62–1.62)
HMWK (U/mL)[a]	0.49 (0.09–0.89)	0.54 (0.06–1.02)			0.98 (0.64–1.32)	0.93 (0.60–1.30)	0.91 (0.63–1.19)	0.92 (0.50–1.36)
Factor XIIIa (U/mL)[a]	0.70 (0.32–1.08)	0.79 (0.27–1.31)			1.08 (0.72–1.43)	1.09 (0.65–1.51)	0.99 (0.57–1.40)	1.05 (0.55–1.55)
Factor XIIIs (U/mL)[a]	0.81 (0.35–1.27)	0.76 (0.30–1.22)			1.13 (0.69–1.56)	1.16 (0.77–1.54)	1.02 (0.60–1.43)	0.97 (0.57–1.37)
d-dimer		1.47 (0.41–2.47)	1.34 (0.58–2.74)	0.22 (0.11–0.42)	0.25 (0.09–0.53)	0.26 (0.10–0.56)	0.27 (0.16–0.39)	0.18 (0.05–0.42)
FDPs[a]								Borderline titer = 1:25–1:50 Positive titer <1:50

Coagulation Inhibitors

ATIII (U/mL)[a]	0.38 (0.14–0.62)	0.63 (0.39–0.97)			1.11 (0.82–1.39)	1.11 (0.90–1.31)	1.05 (0.77–1.32)	1.0 (0.74–1.26)
α₂-M (U/mL)[a]	1.10 (0.56–1.82)	1.39 (0.95–1.83)			1.69 (1.14–2.23)	1.69 (1.28–2.09)	1.56 (0.98–2.12)	0.86 (0.52–1.20)
C1-Inh (U/mL)[a]	0.65 (0.31–0.99)	0.72 (0.36–1.08)			1.35 (0.85–1.83)	1.14 (0.88–1.54)	1.03 (0.68–1.50)	1.0 (0.71–1.31)
α₂-AT (U/mL)[a]	0.90 (0.36–1.44)	0.93 (0.49–1.37)			0.93 (0.39–1.47)	1.00 (0.69–1.30)	1.01 (0.65–1.37)	0.93 (0.55–1.30)
Protein C (U/mL)	0.28 (0.12–0.44)	0.32 (0.24–0.40)	0.33 (0.24–0.51)	0.77 (0.28–1.24)	0.94 (0.50–1.34)	0.94 (0.64–1.25)	0.88 (0.59–1.12)	1.03 (0.54–1.66)
Protein S (U/mL)	0.26 (0.14–0.38)	0.36 (0.28–0.47)	0.49 (0.33–0.67)	1.02 (0.29–1.62)	1.01 (0.67–1.36)	1.09 (0.64–1.54)	1.03 (0.65–1.40)	0.75 (0.54–1.03)

Fibrinolytic System[a]

Plasminogen (U/mL)	1.70 (1.12–2.48)	1.95 (1.60–2.30)			0.98 (0.78–1.18)	0.92 (0.75–1.08)	0.86 (0.68–1.03)	0.99 (0.7–1.22)
TPA (ng/mL)					2.15 (1.0–4.5)	2.42 (1.0–5.0)	2.16 (1.0–4.0)	4.90 (1.40–8.40)
α₂-AP (U/mL)	0.78 (0.4–1.16)	0.85 (0.70–1.0)			1.05 (0.93–1.17)	0.99 (0.89–1.10)	0.98 (0.78–1.18)	1.02 (0.68–1.36)
PAI (U/mL)					5.42 (1.0–10.0)	6.79 (2.0–12.0)	6.07 (2.0–10.0)	3.60 (0–11.0)

[a]Modified from Monagle P, Barnes C, Ignjatovic V, et al. Developmental haemostasis. Impact for clinical haemostasis laboratories. *Thromb Haemost.* 2006;95;362-372; and Calihan J. Hematology. In: Kleinman K, Mcdaniel L, Molloy M, eds. *Harriet Lane Handbook.* 22 ed. Elsevier; 2021: chap 14.

[b]aPTT values may vary depending on reagent.

α2-AP, α2-Antiplasmin; α2-AT, α2-antitrypsin; α2-M, α2-macroglobulin; aPTT, activated partial thromboplastin time; ATIII, antithrombin III; FDPs, fibrin degradation products; HMWK, high-molecular-weight kininogen; INR, international normalized ratio; PAI, plasminogen activator inhibitor; PK, prekallikrein; PT, prothrombin time; TPA, tissue plasminogen activator; VIII, factor VIII procoagulant; vWF, von Willebrand factor.

TABLE 38.5 Common Components of the Complete Blood Count (CBC)

CBC Component	What It Measures or Reflects
Leukocytes	
White blood cell count (WBC)	• Number of all WBCs per mL of blood • Unit: x10³/mL
Differential: • Lymphocytes • Neutrophils • Monocytes • Eosinophils • Basophils	• Percentage of each type of WBC present in the blood • Might include immature cells (e.g., banded or segmented neutrophils)
Absolute neutrophil count (ANC)	• Total number of neutrophils in the blood, including immature cells
Erythrocytes	
Hemoglobin (Hgb)	• Amount of Hgb (by weight) in the blood • Unit: g/dL • Assesses the O₂-carrying capacity of the RBC
Hematocrit (Hct)	• Percentage of volume of blood occupied by RBCs • Typically 3 times the Hgb • Calculated value
Red blood cell count (RBC)	• Number (in millions) of RBCs per μL of blood
Mean corpuscular volume (MCV)	• Size or volume of the average RBC
Mean corpuscular hemoglobin (MCH)	• Amount of Hgb in each RBC
Mean corpuscular hemoglobin concentration (MCHC)	• Amount of Hgb in the average RBC in comparison to its size
Red cell distribution width (RDW)	• Variability in RBC size
Platelets	
Platelet count	• Number of platelets per μL of blood • Unit: ×10³/μL
Mean platelet volume (MPV)	• Size or volume of the average platelet

Erythrocyte Disorders

Anemia

Anemia is a reduction in circulating RBCs. Affecting approximately 40% of children worldwide, it is the most common hematologic abnormality seen in infants and children.[4] It can occur due to a decrease in RBC production, abnormalities of RBCs, a shortened RBC life span, RBC destruction, or an acute/ongoing loss from bleeding. Anemia is not a specific disease entity in and of itself but represents a heterogenous group of pathologic conditions. It may be due to an intrinsic hematologic disorder or be a manifestation of acute or chronic disease. Diagnostic evaluation should be directed accordingly.

Classification of Anemias

Anemias are often categorized on the basis of RBC size, which is reflected in the mean corpuscular volume (MCV), and appearance, which is reflected in the mean corpuscular Hgb (MCH). RBC size is typically defined as either *normocytic* (within age-appropriate norms), microcytic (small), or macrocytic (large). Appearance is defined as normochromic (within age-appropriate norms), *hypochromic* (pale), or *hyperchromic* (darker or concentrated). Examination of the peripheral smear can also reveal nuances in RBC appearance, which can, in turn, help to narrow diagnostic categories (e.g., basophilic stippling may suggest lead poisoning). Variations in RBC morphology (Box 38.1) can also provide clues and/or help to distinguish between disorders.

RBC indices (e.g., MCV, MCH, mean cell Hgb concentration [MCHC]) provide insight regarding the cell size (MCV) and/or color (MCH and MCHC), which in turn, provides an organizing framework in approaching anemias. For instance, common causes of microcytic (reduced MCV), hypochromic (reduced MCH) anemia are iron deficiency (ID), lead poisoning, and thalassemia trait, whereas common causes of macrocytic (increased MCV) anemia include exposure to certain medications (e.g., anticonvulsants), deficiencies in vitamin B_{12} or folate, liver disease, and hypothyroidism. RBC indices are therefore helpful in narrowing the diagnostic possibilities, especially because anemia can generally be classified on the basis of the MCV and MCH. Evaluating the RBC distribution width (RDW) can also be helpful in differentiating anemias (Box 38.2). Additional laboratory findings that further differentiate the microcytic anemias are presented in Table 38.6.

The reticulocyte count also helps to distinguish disorders associated with hemolysis (RBC destruction) or bleeding (RBC loss) from those with bone marrow depression (decreased RBC production). In the case of hemolysis or bleeding, reticulocyte counts typically increase as the bone marrow attempts to compensate from the loss of RBCs. In the case of bone marrow depression, however, reticulocyte counts decrease due to the lack of production. Fig. 38.5 provides a schematic for classifying the most common forms of anemia based upon reticulocyte response and RBC indices.

Another classification system to describe anemia reflects RBC production, maturation, or destruction (Fig. 38.6). *Hypoproliferative* anemias result from a failure in RBC production and tend to be normocytic, normochromic anemias with a decreased reticulocyte count, making it seem that the body is not responding to the anemia. *Maturational* anemias reflect a defect in nuclear maturation, typically caused by nutritional deficiencies or a chemical/toxic exposure. The third category, *hemolytic anemias*, refers to anemias that result from increased cell destruction. The hemolysis may be caused by defects in the red cell membrane, hemoglobinopathies, or congenital enzyme defects (e.g., G6PD deficiency).

Microcytic Anemia: Iron Deficiency Anemia

Iron deficiency anemia (IDA) is the most common nutritional disorder and hematologic condition in the world, with rates highest in South Asia and Africa and lowest in Australasia and high-income areas of North America.[4] In the United Sates, 8% to 14% of children between the ages of 13 and 36 months are iron

• BOX 38.1   Peripheral Blood Morphologic Findings in Various Anemias

Microcytes
Iron deficiency
Thalassemias
Lead toxicity
Anemia of chronic disease

Macrocytes
Newborns
Vitamin B_{12} or folate deficiency
Diamond-Blackfan anemia
Fanconi anemia
Aplastic anemia
Liver disease
Down syndrome
Hypothyroidism

Spherocytes
Hereditary spherocytosis
Immune hemolytic anemia (newborn or acquired)
Hypersplenism

Sickled Cells
Sickle cell anemias (SS disease, SC disease, $S\beta^+$ thalassemia, $S\beta^0$ thalassemia)

Elliptocytes
Hereditary elliptocytosis
Iron deficiency
Megaloblastic anemia

Target Cells
Hemoglobinopathies (especially hemoglobin C, SC, and thalassemia)
Liver disease
Xerocytosis

Basophil Stippling
Thalassemia
Lead intoxication
Myelodysplasia

Red Blood Cell Fragments, Helmet Cells, Burr Cells
Disseminated intravascular coagulation
Hemolytic uremic syndrome
Thrombotic thrombocytopenic purpura
Kasabach-Merritt syndrome
"Waring blender syndrome"
Uremia
Liver disease

Hypersegmented Neutrophils
Vitamin B_{12} or folate deficiency

Blasts
Leukemia (ALL or AML)
Severe infection (rarely)

Leukopenia/Thrombocytopenia
Fanconi anemia
Aplastic anemia
Leukemia
Hemophagocytic histiocytosis

Howell-Jolly Bodies
Asplenia, hyposplenia
Severe iron deficiency

ALL, Acute lymphocytic leukemia; *AML,* acute myeloid leukemia.
From Kliegman, RM, Lye PS, Bordini BJ, et al. *Nelson Pediatric Symptom-Based Diagnosis.* Elsevier; 2018.

---

deficient, and approximately 30% of these will go on to develop IDA. The incidence of IDA among children in the United States has been declining slightly during the past 4 decades, although the prevalence remains high among children living at or below poverty level. Other risk factors include childhood obesity and a history of prematurity or low birth weight.[5] While it can be present throughout childhood, the disease peaks at three timepoints: the neonatal period, in preschool-aged children, and adolescence (particularly in menstruating females and athletes).[6]

Iron is an important micronutrient for humans and plays a key role in many physiologic processes including RBC formation, energy metabolism, myoglobin production, neurotransmitter production, collagen development, and immune system function. Approximately 75% of the iron in the body is functional and contained in Hgb and other tissues. Approximately 0.1% is bound to transferrin for transport around the body. The remaining excess iron is stored as ferritin in the liver, intestinal epithelium, bone marrow, and spleen. Iron is both absorbed from nutritional intake in the proximal duodenum and recycled within the body. As there is no physiologic mechanism for iron excretion, its levels are tightly regulated.[7–9]

ID typically occurs as the result of inadequate oral intake (e.g., restrictive diets, overuse of cow's milk or other milk substitutes),

• BOX 38.2   Red Blood Cell Distribution Width in Common Anemias of Childhood

Anemia	MCV
Elevated RDW (Nonuniform Population of RBCs)	
Hemolytic anemia with elevated reticulocyte count	High
Iron deficiency anemia	Low
Anemias resulting from red blood cell fragmentation: DIC, HUS, TTP	Low
Megaloblastic anemias: vitamin B_{12} or folate deficiency	High
Normal RDW (Uniform Population of RBCs)	
Thalassemias	Low
Acute hemorrhage	Normal
Fanconi anemia	High
Aplastic anemia	High

DIC, Disseminated intravascular coagulation; *HUS,* hemolytic uremic syndrome; *MCV,* mean corpuscular volume; *RBC,* red blood cell; *RDW,* red blood cell distribution width; *TTP,* thrombotic thrombocytopenic purpura.
From Kliegman, RM, Lye PS, Bordini BJ, et al. *Nelson Pediatric Symptom-Based Diagnosis.* Elsevier; 2018.

TABLE 38.6	Differentiating Features of Microcytic Anemias		
Test	**Iron Deficiency Anemia**	**Thalassemia Minor[a]**	**Anemia of Inflammation[b]**
Serum iron	Low	Normal	Low
Serum iron-binding capacity	High	Normal	Low or normal
Serum ferritin	Low	Normal or high	Normal or high
Marrow iron stores	Low or absent	Normal or high	Normal or high
Marrow sideroblasts	Decreased or absent	Normal or increased	Normal or increased
Free erythrocyte protoporphyrin	High	Normal or slightly increased	High
Hemoglobin A_2 or F	Normal	High β-thalassemia; normal α-thalassemia	Normal
Red blood cell distribution width[c]	High	Normal	Normal or increased

[a]α-Thalassemia minor can be diagnosed by the presence of Bart hemoglobin on newborn screening.

[b]Usually normochromic; 25% of cases are microcytic.

[c]Red blood cell distribution width quantitates the degree of anisocytosis (different sizes) of red blood cells.

Modified from Marcdante, KJ, Klieg RM, Schuh AM. *Nelson Essentials of Pediatrics.* 9th ed. Elsevier; 2023.

inadequate absorption (e.g., Celiac disease, inflammatory bowel disease), excessive blood loss (e.g., GI losses, menstruation), or increased iron demand (e.g., periods or rapid growth, pregnancy). ID develops on a continuum; first the body depletes its iron stores, which then progresses to deficiency and eventually results in anemia.[9]

Screening for Iron Deficiency Anemia

The minimal laboratory screening for ID is the Hgb level. Often the simplest and most cost-effective measurement is a CBC, which includes the Hgb, Hct, MCV, and RDW. The American Academy of Pediatrics (AAP) Committee on Nutrition recommends universal Hgb screening for anemia at 12 months of age.[10–12] This screening should include an assessment of risk factors for ID and IDA such as iron poor diets, prematurity, heavy menses, among others (Box 38.3). Screening Hgb can be performed on children younger than 1 year of age when risk factors warrant it. According to the Centers for Disease Control and Prevention (CDC), adolescent females should also be screened every 5 to 10 years during routine examinations, and yearly if risk factors or previous history of IDA are present.[13]

When IDA screening or any other routine health screening recommendation is being implemented, it is important to keep in mind that screening is not just a one-time test; the effectiveness of treatment must be determined through follow-up testing. Thus, after routine 12-month and adolescent female Hgb testing, risk assessment for anemia should be performed at all preventive pediatric healthcare visits, with follow-up blood testing if positive. If children are at risk for IDA, a repeat Hgb should be performed as often as indicated.

While current AAP guidelines recommend screening for IDA based on anemia, there has been recent movement towards using serum ferritin levels to screen for ID before the development of anemia.[14,15] Iron deficient states in the first few years of life, both anemic and nonanemic, have been associated with negative neurodevelopmental outcomes that can last well into adulthood.[16] Several organizations, including the World Health Organization (WHO) and the United States Preventive Services Task Force,[17,18]

now recommend using serum ferritin to screen for ID. The WHO recommends using a serum ferritin value of <12 mcg/mL to define ID in children aged 0 to 59 months.[17] While a serum ferritin level is helpful because it reflects current stores of iron, it must be interpreted carefully because ferritin is an acute-phase reactant and may be increased with inflammatory conditions. Obtaining a C-reactive protein level as a marker of inflammation can assist in evaluating serum ferritin levels.[6,19]

Clinical Findings

When assessing for ID and IDA, it is important to conduct a detailed history and complete physical examination. A thorough history may be sufficient to determine etiology and guide treatment, especially in the case of inadequate oral intake or excessive blood loss. ID can present with or without anemia and children with moderate to severe anemia can be asymptomatic. Common symptoms and clinical findings associated with ID and IDA can be seen in Table 38.7.

Diagnostic Studies. IDA is frequently identified in routine screenings of Hgb level via capillary sampling. Capillary samples rely on proper technique. Excessive squeezing of the finger may produce inaccurate results; therefore venous sampling is the most reliable indicator. IDA is likely if there is a low Hgb level for age (typically in the range of 8–11 g/dL), a history of low iron intake, and no concern about other possible causes for the anemia or the possibility of another hemoglobinopathy. If the age of the child and the dietary patterns are consistent with ID and there is microcytosis with a mild anemia (Hgb ≥ 9 g/dL), many clinicians begin a trial of iron supplementation for 4 to 6 weeks without further diagnostic testing and then follow the child's Hgb and reticulocyte counts.

Although a low Hgb level is sufficient to diagnose IDA, additional diagnostics may be helpful for both diagnosis and management. Serum ferritin can be ordered to evaluate for iron stores, which would be low. Transferrin saturation can be measured to assess the percentage of iron-binding sites on transferrin that are occupied, which would also be low. Total iron binding capacity (TIBC), which measures the availability

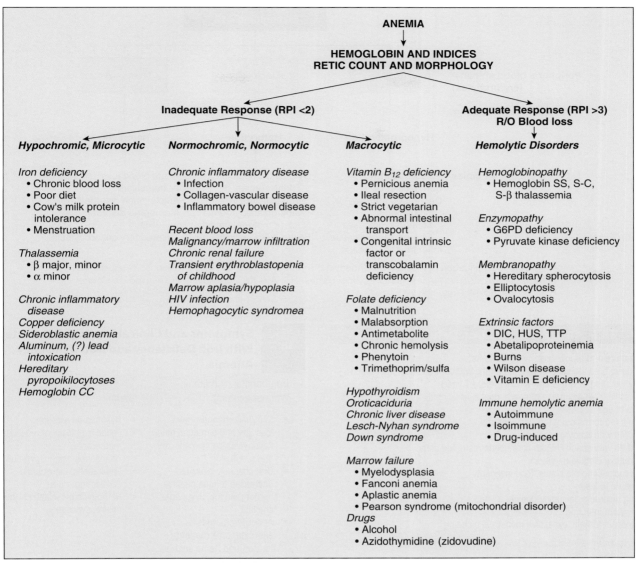

• **Fig. 38.5** Use of the Complete Blood Count, Reticulocyte Count, and Blood Smear in the Diagnosis of Anemia. *DIC,* Disseminated intravascular coagulation; *G6PD,* glucose-6-phosphate dehydrogenase; *HUS,* hemolytic uremic syndrome; *R/O,* rule out; *RPI,* reticulocyte production index; *TTP,* thrombotic thrombocytopenic purpura. (Modified from Marcdante, KJ, Klieg RM, Schuh AM. *Nelson Essentials of Pediatrics.* 9th ed. Elsevier; 2023.)

of iron-binding sites on transferrin, would therefore be high. RBC indices on a CBC are also useful and typically show the following[6,20,21]:
- Microcytic, hypochromic RBCs
- Low or normal MCV; low to normal RBC number
- High RDW (>14%)
- Mentzer index greater than 13 (Box 38.4)

As ID progresses in stages, so do laboratory results. First iron stores deplete, which is reflected in a decreased serum ferritin. This is followed by a decrease in transferrin saturation and increase in TIBC. Anemia develops when Hgb decreases, resulting in an increase in RDW and decrease in MCV. Once treatment begins, this process is reflected on laboratory studies in reverse.[21]

Differential Diagnosis

For those children with low Hgb/Hct who do not have a history suspicious for IDA, the investigation must expand to include less

common sources for the anemia. In addition, careful consideration should be given when there is no response to iron therapy within 1 month and there is confidence that iron supplements, the mainstay of treatment of IDA, are being given correctly.[6] A more extensive evaluation would include a CBC with differential, platelet count, RBC indices, reticulocyte count, and a lead level. A peripheral blood smear should be examined to assess the number and morphology of RBCs, WBCs, and platelets. The differential diagnosis for anemia can then be determined on the basis of whether RBC production is adequate or inadequate and whether the cells are microcytic, normocytic, or macrocytic to further guide diagnosis and management.

Anemia caused by ID should be differentiated from other microcytic, hypochromic anemias such as lead poisoning, thalassemias, anemia of chronic disease (also known as *anemia of inflammation*), and hereditary sideroblastic anemia. A peripheral smear may be helpful as the presence of basophilic stippling suggests lead poisoning. β-thalassemia is indicated by elevations in Hgb A₂

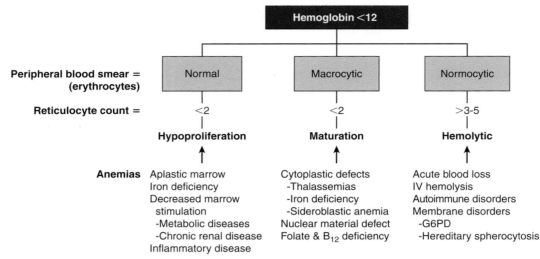

• **Fig. 38.6** Classification of Anemia by Underlying Erythrocyte Disorder. *G6PD*, Glucose-6-phosphate dehydrogenase; *IV*, intravenous. (Modified from Hillman RS, Ault KA, Rinder HM. *Hematology in Clinical Practice*. 4th ed. McGraw-Hill; 2005.)

• **BOX 38.3** **Risk Factors for Iron Deficiency Anemia**

- Premature and/or low-birth-weight infants
- Exclusive breastfeeding beyond 6 months without iron supplementation
- Early weaning to whole cow's milk (before 1 year)
- Excessive (>25 oz) intake of cow's, goat's, or soy milk in children 1–5 years of age
- Infants fed formula not fortified with iron
- Children with feeding problems
- Children with special health care needs/restricted diets
- Alternative diets (e.g., vegan)
- Low socioeconomic status, food insecurity
- Exposure to lead
- Eating disorders, including obesity
- Hookworm infection
- Adolescent female, excessive menstrual bleeding

---

on electrophoresis and a Mentzer index of less than 13. Anemia of inflammation presents with normal-to-high serum ferritin and elevated TIBC.[9]

Children with extremely low Hgb, abnormal vital signs, and/or associated red flags (Box 38.5) should be seen immediately. The presence of co-occurring neutropenia, thrombocytopenia, nucleated RBCs, or immature myeloid elements is particularly concerning. When abnormalities in all elements—erythrocytes, platelets, and leukocytes—are found, a bone marrow disorder is probable. Referral to a pediatric hematologist-oncologist, and in some cases hospitalization, is warranted.

Other causes of anemia, such as blood loss with occult rectal bleeding, should be considered in children with a low Hgb level who eat a normal diet with adequate servings of iron-rich foods. Stool guaiac should be checked for occult blood loss. Additional investigation is warranted in children younger than 6 months of age or older than 18 months or who demonstrate no response to treatment after 2 to 4 weeks.

Iron Deficiency Anemia and Lead Poisoning

Lead poisoning (plumbism) has long been known as a common comorbid condition to IDA.[22] Lead molecules inhibit essential

---

TABLE 38.7 **Symptoms and Clinical Findings Associated With Iron Deficiency and Iron Deficiency Anemia**

Iron Deficiency (With or Without Anemia)	Anemia
• Skin/hair changes: hair loss, dry and damaged hair, koilonychia/spoon nails, dry and rough skin • Oral changes: glossitis, decreased tongue papillae, burning tongue, dysphagia, cheilitis • Appetite changes: anorexia, pica (appetite for nonfood items such as paper, dirt, and clay) and pagophagia (the desire to ingest ice) • Behavioral changes: fatigue, sleep disorders, irritability, malaise • Sensitivity to cold • Breath-holding spells • Restless leg syndrome	• Dyspnea on exertion • Pallor, especially of mucous membranes • Headaches, tinnitus, vertigo • Palpitations, tachycardia, cardiac murmurs • Hemodynamic instability, heart failure, syncope

Modified from Mattiello V, Schmugge M, Hengartner H, von der Weid N, Renella R. Diagnosis and management of iron deficiency in children with or without anemia: consensus recommendations of the SPOG Pediatric Hematology Working Group. *Eur J Pediatr.* 2020;179(4):527–545.

• **BOX 38.4** **Mentzer Index**

Mentzer index = MCV/RBC. If the ratio is < 13, the anemia is more likely to be thalassemia trait; if the ratio is > 13, the anemia is more likely to be due to iron deficiency.

• BOX 38.5 Red Flags During an Anemia Evaluation

Anemia Accompanied by

- Abnormal vital signs (tachycardia, hypotension, hypertension)
- Neutropenia and/or thrombocytopenia
- High MCV with normal RDW
- Blasts on the peripheral smear
- Firm adenopathy
- Bruising or bleeding
- Weight loss, failure to thrive
- Shortness of breath, fatigue
- Fever
- Hypoxia
- Organomegaly
- Edema
- Oliguria-anuria
- Bloody diarrhea
- Red urine (hemoglobinuria)
- Family history of anemia

MCV, Mean corpuscular volume; *RDW,* red blood cell distribution width.
From Kliegman, RM, Lye PS, Bordini BJ, et al. *Nelson Pediatric Symptom-Based Diagnosis.* Elsevier; 2018.

mitochondrial membrane and enzyme function, which prevents iron from binding to protoporphyrin, an essential building block in heme synthesis. This results in increased levels of protoporphyrin, reflected as elevated free electrolyte protoporphyrin on laboratory studies, and anemia.

Lead primarily enters the body through ingestion, therefore children are at an increased risk of exposure at periods of development with increased hand-to-mouth activity.[23] Accordingly, children should be screened for lead exposure between 6 and 12 months of age, which conveniently coincides with screening for IDA. They should again be screened between 18 and 24 months. An estimated 99% of lead-poisoned children are identified through screening procedures rather than clinical recognition. Additional screening should be based on at-risk status.[11,12] There is no "safe" blood lead level. At present, the CDC use a blood lead level of 3.5 mcg/dL or greater on a single visit to identify children with higher levels of lead in their blood than most children.[24] Local health departments determine the prevalence of lead poisoning in their area and issue additional guidelines related to blood lead screenings for targeted children in their catchment areas. The CDC is also an excellent resource for guidance on prevention, sources of exposure, interpretation of blood lead levels, and available programs for prevention throughout the country.[25]

Management

ID is associated with a serum ferritin level of <15 ng/mL. Mild IDA is considered with Hgb levels of ≥9 g/dL but less than the lower limit of normal for age. Moderate IDA is characterized by Hgb levels of 7 to <9 g/dL, and severe <7 g/dL. Children with severe cases should be carefully evaluated as to whether the child needs referral to hematology; levels less than 4 g/dL necessitate consultation. Most forms of IDA can be initially treated with oral forms of iron, but intravenous formulations may be used in some cases.[21]

For infants and children, the treatment for IDA primarily consists of iron supplementation, typically in the form of an iron salt such as ferrous sulfate.[26] Dosages should be calculated in elemental iron. Standard treatment is 3 mg/kg/day of elemental iron,[21]

although dosages up to 6 mg/kg/day have been used.[27] In adolescents, the daily maximum of elemental iron is 200 mg.[28]

To evaluate effectiveness of treatment, a reticulocyte count should be reassessed within 1 week as reticulocytosis may be seen within a few days of treatment. Hgb should return to a normal level within 4 to 6 weeks. If a therapeutic response is observed (Hgb increase of >1 g/dL or >3% increase in Hct), iron supplementation should continue to normalize Hgb, then continue for 2 to 3 months to replete iron stores. Serum ferritin levels should be rechecked 6 months after iron supplements are stopped to determine resolution of the anemia and adequacy of iron stores.[21] If there is no response to iron supplementation, both alternative diagnoses and barriers to treatment adherence should be explored.

Prevention

It has long been established that the best management for ID is prevention through adequate nutritional intake. This begins for the fetus during pregnancy and continues throughout life. Full-term infants accumulate almost 80% of their iron stores during the last trimester of pregnancy, highlighting the importance of maternal iron supplementation during pregnancy.[29] Delayed clamping of the umbilical cord also ensures that newborns receive the maximal transfusion to begin life. Along with prematurity, maternal anemia, maternal hypertension with intrauterine growth retardation, and/or gestational diabetes can result in less iron transferred to the fetus. In the case of preterm births, the decreased iron stores are depleted rapidly, and the normal physiologic nadir occurs earlier, aggravated by a smaller total blood volume at birth and poor GI absorption. The use of erythropoietin to prevent and treat anemia of prematurity also increases the risk of ID. Because of these risk factors, in general, preterm (<37 weeks' gestation) and low-birth-weight infants require an oral supplement of elemental iron. The most recent guidelines from the AAP recommend dosages of 2 to 4 mg/kg/day from 2 weeks through 12 months of age,[10] but recent systematic reviews highlight the paucity of evidence to support dosage and duration of supplementation.[30]

Breast milk provides an average iron content of 0.35 mg/L with a high bioavailability. Based on the average intake of the exclusively breastfed infant, this results in approximate adequate daily iron intake of 0.78 L/day or 0.27 mg/day for infants from birth to 6 months. Recommended dietary allowance for iron for children between 7 and 12 months of age is 11 mg/day.[31] Infants fed with standard infant formulas receive a sufficient iron intake of 12 mg/dL; however, because there is large variation in the iron content in human milk, the content of maternal milk may not always provide for the needs of the growing infant.[10] Infants born at term typically have sufficient iron stores until 4 to 6 months of age. Therefore it is recommended that the exclusively breastfed term infant receive elemental iron supplementation of 1 mg/kg/day (15 mg maximum) beginning at 4 months of age and continuing until iron-containing complementary foods are introduced and taken in adequate quantities. This same iron supplementation recommendation holds for the partially breastfed infants who receive more than half of their daily feeding as human milk.[10] However, there is a paucity of data as to whether this duration of supplementation is sufficient given that there are no current data on the prevalence of ID with or without anemia in infants between 4 and 12 months of age. Recent studies have noted that infants aged 6 to 12 months continue to be iron deficient, despite these recommendations.[32]

As the rate of growth decreases in early childhood, so does the nutritional requirement of iron, down to 7 mg/day between 1 and 3 years of age.[31] While nutritional needs may be met by iron fortification of various foods, developmental challenges related to food choice in this age may make adequate intake challenging. Liquid supplementation for this age group is appropriate until 36 months of age. Chewable multivitamins with iron can be used for children older than 3 years of age, but the supplement formulation must be evaluated for adequate replacement.

Patient and Family Education

Parents or caretakers should be counseled to increase iron-rich foods in their child's diet. Exclusively breastfed term infants should be started on iron supplementation at 4 months of age and iron-fortified cereal and/or pureed meats added to the child's diet after 6 months of age. Whole cow's milk should be avoided in infants younger than 12 months of age due to its low iron content and the possibility of insensible GI blood loss. After 12 months of age, cow's milk ingestion should be limited to 24 oz/day. Goat's milk should not be the sole diet of a child, not only because of its lack of iron but also its lack of folic acid. For preterm infants, supplementation with oral iron drops should begin no later than 1 month of age. Education for older children taking iron supplements includes advising parents to avoid giving iron with meals or milk that vitamin C juice enhances absorption, and that the child's stools will probably turn black. Foods containing soy can inhibit the absorption of iron. Any dental staining associated with taking iron can be removed with dental cleaning. Parents should also be cautioned to keep the medication safely out of reach to prevent accidental ingestion.

Thalassemias

Adult Hgb is composed of two alpha and two beta polypeptide chains. Thalassemias are a group of genetic disorders affecting production of the globin chains in Hgb. They are categorized into two types: alpha (α) and beta (β), based on the affected globin chain. The α chain is coded for four genes (two from each parent) on chromosome 16 and the β chain is coded for two genes (one from each parent) on chromosome 11. Abnormality in, or absence of, any of these genes results in an imbalance in the α/β globin-chain-ratio and a spectrum of clinical disease related to the quantity of globin that is produced.

In the carrier of α-thalassemia, only one α gene is affected, which enables the production of adequate amounts of Hgb with few or no symptoms. Disease severity increases as more genes are affected. When all four genes are affected, and there are no α chains, the β-globulin subunits cluster into groups of four. These β tetramers are incapable of carrying oxygen, and the affected fetuses die in utero (hydrops fetalis). In the carrier of β-thalassemia, only one gene is affected and there are sufficient β chains to bind with the abundant α chains and create functional Hgb molecules; however, a resultant asymptomatic mild microcytic anemia is present. In β-thalassemia disease, when both genes are affected, the absence of β chains causes α chains to not bind with each other, but rather degrade; ongoing degradation results in severe anemia and the need for ongoing transfusions.[33]

Categorizing the thalassemias is less straightforward than with many anemias because although the heterozygous disease is hypochromic and microcytic, the homozygous diseases are also hemolytic. There is a wide spectrum of clinical features. Previous terminology classified various disease states as "minor," "intermedia," and "major" based on clinical manifestations, but this was simplified to better reflect the spectrum of disease and help guide management. The preferred terminology now characterizes the thalassemias, particularly those involving β globin-chains, instead by their clinical dependence on transfusion (transfusion-dependent and non–transfusion-dependent).[34]

Regardless of the category, thalassemias that present clinically involve some degree of anemia and increased erythropoiesis. The erythropoiesis results in bone marrow expansion, but the pathogenesis of this is not fully understood. The presence of focal osteomalacia and delayed bone maturation are at least partially explained by suboptimal blood transfusions and iron overload. Furthermore, the marrow expansion results in frontal bossing and hyperplasia of the maxillary bones, leading to typical facies. The possibility of thalassemia increases if the onset of anemia and symptoms occurs before 3 to 6 months of age and there is a prior family history of thalassemia or a family history of anemia, miscarriage, or fetal demise or jaundice, gallstones, anemia, or splenomegaly.[33]

α-Thalassemias

The α-thalassemias are composed of several variant hemoglobins that are responsible for the various presentations. Current nomenclature often refers to the subtypes by including an indication of the number of α globin genes affected. Gene deletions cause complete or partial absence of globin chains while nondeletional mutations cause reduced production or structurally abnormal globin chains. The severity of symptoms increases as more genes are affected.[33]

The most severe form of α-thalassemia involves the deletion of four genes, which results in hydrops fetalis and is not compatible with extrauterine life. The most clinically significant form of α-thalassemia is Hgb H disease, which occurs when there are deletions of three α genes. Initial presentation may occur in the neonatal period with hypochromic, microcytic anemia with hyperbilirubinemia in the setting of hemolysis.[20] In older children, PCPs may see hepatosplenomegaly, jaundice, and sometimes thalassemia-like bone changes. Children may also experience delayed growth. These children are typically not transfusion-dependent, but during times of physiologic stress they may require RBC transfusion.[33–35]

There are two different carrier states of α-thalassemia. In α-thalassemia trait, where two genes are affected, the child exhibits microcytosis and hypochromia but has normal percentages of Hgb A_2 and Hgb F. The other trait state, where only one gene is affected, is referred to as a *silent carrier state* but can have either a silent hematologic phenotype or present with microcytic hypochromia and some erythropoiesis.[33] One can see how important it is to differentiate α-thalassemia conditions from IDA, which can be done through calculating Mentzer's index (see Box 38.4).

Management. Hgb H disease exacerbations may necessitate occasional transfusion during hemolytic or aplastic crises. No treatment is indicated for the carrier trait expressions of disease, and the microcytosis seen in these expressions requires that serum iron studies should be done before starting any iron supplements. The α-thalassemia syndromes occur most frequently in those of Southeast Asian descent. Those carrying the α-thalassemia trait alleles require careful genetic counseling because there are complex patterns of inheritance that could affect the phenotype of such individuals' offspring.[34]

β-Thalassemia Trait/Minor

Inheritance of a single heterozygous mutation for a β-globin gene results in β-thalassemia trait, also known as *minor* or *minima*. Children are typically asymptomatic, but can demonstrate mild microcytic, hypochromic anemia on CBC. Elevated levels of Hgb A_2 are usually seen on Hgb electrophoresis in β-thalassemia, which can aid in diagnosis.[33] Typically, these children do not require treatment. β-thalassemia trait may be confused with ID or lead poisoning; the condition is often identified after a trial of oral supplementation shows no improvement in anemia.[20] It is particularly important to diagnose this condition correctly to avoid iron overload. Calculating a Mentzer index (see Box 38.4) when evaluating anemia is a simple way to differentiate between IDA and thalassemias.

Non–Transfusion-Dependent β-Thalassemia.
Previously known as *β-thalassemia minima disease*, non–transfusion-dependent β-thalassemia (NTDT) is a wide clinical spectrum of disease severity. The condition results from inheritance of two β-globin gene mutations, typically heterozygous, associated with a mild phenotype.[20] The first clinical presentation of NTDT is often symptomatic anemia with infection early in life, often after 2 years of age; however, many children do well and are diagnosed with NTDT later in life with routine screening or after experiencing complications related to hemolysis.[34]

Clinical Findings. Like all thalassemias, a CBC demonstrates microcytic, hypochromic anemia; baseline Hgb can range from mildly decreased at 7 to 10 g/dL to severely decreased at 4 to 5 g/dL depending upon the various Hgb variants. Owing to the wide spectrum of disease severity in NTDT, physical examination findings can vary. Those on the more severe end of the spectrum, without adequate treatment, may have growth delays, marked pallor with jaundice, and moderate-to-severe hepatosplenomegaly. Less severe phenotypes may have few symptoms with only anemia and mild splenomegaly. It is important to evaluate for thalassemia-associated complications including delayed puberty, cardiac murmurs, and abnormal skeletal changes such as frontal bossing, maxilla hyperplasia, and flat nasal bridge.[34]

Management. Treatment for NTDT is patient-specific and based on severity. In general, these patients do not require regular transfusions for survival, but they may require occasional transfusions when under physiologic stress (e.g., infection). Children with mild-to-moderately severe chronic anemia can go on to require more transfusions later in life.[20] Additional guidelines for treatment are available.[36] The PCP should consider engaging the pediatric hematologist for assistance in managing this condition, particularly if a more severe phenotype is suspected. Primary emphasis should be on the education of all family members; genetic testing and counseling should be offered.

Transfusion-Dependent β-Thalassemia.
Inheritance of two β-globin gene mutations that are severe, whether in a compound heterozygous or homozygous manner, results in the most severe thalassemias. Homozygous β-thalassemia major (or Cooley anemia) is associated with severe anemia resulting from the decreased or absent production of Hgb A and hemolysis caused by the precipitation of excess α chains in the RBCs.[33] This results in ineffective hematopoiesis and, if untreated, patients can develop the classic thalassemic facies, pathologic bone fractures, growth failure, and significant hepatosplenomegaly.[20]

Clinical Findings. Affected infants usually become symptomatic in the first year of life as fetal Hgb levels decline. These infants present with pallor, failure to thrive, hepatosplenomegaly, irritability, and a severe microcytic, hypochromic anemia with steady-state Hgb <5 g/dL. RBC morphology reveals significant microcytosis, poikilocytosis, hypochromia, target cells, and nucleated RBCs. Hgb electrophoresis is diagnostic and reveals elevated Hgb A_2 and Hgb F levels may be up to 100%.[34]

Management. Proper management of the child requires collaboration with a pediatric hematologist. Standards of care for thalassemia patients should be followed.[37] Regular RBC transfusions are usually necessary to achieve the goal of maintaining a pretransfusion Hgb level of 9.5 to 10.5 g/dL and suppressing intra- and extramedullary hematopoiesis. To help with future cross matching, the provider should obtain a complete typing of the patient's erythrocyte profile before the first transfusion (phenotyping). This helps to decrease difficulties with subsequent transfusions. Splenectomy may also be indicated.[37] Hematopoietic stem cell transplantation is the only curative modality for β-thalassemia major. This has been most successful in children younger than 15 years without excessive iron overload and hepatosplenomegaly who have sibling-matched human leukocyte antigen (HLA) allogeneic hematopoietic transplantation.[38] Gene therapy[39] and other novel therapeutics[40] are being investigated and hold promise for those with this major disorder.[37]

Iron chelation is a mainstay of treatment for these patients. Repeated transfusions create a hyperferric state and chelation is necessary to prevent complications primarily affecting the heart, liver, and endocrine system. Iron overload can develop even without the use of blood transfusions because of the increased iron absorption associated with high rates of erythropoiesis and red cell destruction. Monitoring for iron stores should be done on a regular basis. Chronic iron chelation therapy is necessary to remove the excess iron resulting from frequent transfusions.[37]

Iron chelation therapy should be employed to maintain serum ferritin concentrations <1000 mcg/L. Iron levels can also be evaluated using magnetic resonance imaging (MRI) with T_2 imaging to evaluate iron loading in critical organs such as the liver and the heart, with iron typically depositing in the liver before the heart. In the United States, deferasirox is now the first-line treatment for iron overload. It is administered orally, with lower dosages used in NTDT when chelation is indicated. The previous initial treatment, deferoxamine, may also still be used; however, it is administered parenterally or subcutaneously, is time-consuming, and associated with pain and has therefore fallen out of favor. All chelators stabilize the ferritin levels, thus achieving a negative iron balance. Iron excretion through chelation is further aided by the ingestion of vitamin C. Because the iron is excreted through the kidneys, hydration and monitoring of renal status are vital.[37]

Complications. If the condition is left untreated, bone marrow expansion causes the characteristic facies of frontal bossing and maxillary overgrowth. Other complications of disease and treatment include osteopenia, thrombolytic symptoms, cardiopulmonary problems, asplenia secondary to splenectomy, cholelithiasis, and extramedullary hematopoiesis.[20,33]

Medications used to chelate iron have additional side effects. Deferasirox, the daily oral agent, commonly produces headache, nausea, vomiting, joint pain, and fatigue. It has a black box warning of GI hemorrhage in addition to kidney and liver failure. Deferoxamine has risks associated with the administration of intravenous medication (infection) and vision and hearing loss.[37] In addition, there are the inherent risks and complications of transfusion including transfusion reaction, fever, and, although rare, hepatitis or human immunodeficiency virus (HIV) infection.

The disease, its complications, and treatments are painful for the child and monopolize a large portion of these patients' and their and families' lives. Families need professional support, education, such as information that can be found through the resources of the Thalassemia Support Foundation or Cooley's

Anemia Foundation, as well as interaction with other families affected by this disorder.

Macrocytic Anemia

Macrocytic (megaloblastic) anemias are characterized by macrocytic RBCs, hypersegmented polymorphonuclear leukocytes in the peripheral blood, and megaloblasts in the bone marrow. Relatively rare in the pediatric patient, macrocytic anemias result from impaired DNA synthesis due to a lack of the necessary building blocks—typically folic acid, vitamin B_{12}, or both. These anemias may develop if the diet (e.g., goat's milk, strict vegetarian) lacks these two substances or if the gastric intrinsic factor necessary for the absorption of vitamin B_{12} is absent.[20]

Clinical Findings

History. Suspicion should be high if there is a history of young infants being fed a diet of powdered cow's milk products and/or alternative milk sources, such as goat's milk, as these are deficient in folic acid and vitamin B_{12}. Of equal concern are older children who have strict vegetarian or vegan diets and those with signs of severe nutritional deficiencies, absorption problems, or tapeworm infestations. Children with folic acid deficiency tend to be irritable and have inadequate weight gain and chronic diarrhea. Children with diseases of the upper small intestine, such as Celiac disease and inflammatory bowel disease, are also at increased risk for developing the condition.[20,41]

Physical Examination. Physical findings relate to the severity of the anemia but can include weakness, pallor, and a beefy-red, smooth sore mouth and tongue.

Diagnostic Studies. A CBC, peripheral smear, reticulocyte count, and vitamin levels are useful in diagnosing the condition, with results typically showing the following[20,41]:
- Elevated MCV (>100 fL) and decreased reticulocyte count.
- Blood smear showing nucleated RBCs and macro-ovalocytes with anisocytosis and poikilocytosis; basophilic stippling may be seen in B_{12} deficiency.
- Normal WBC and platelet counts, but possibly decreased in more severe cases.
- Large and hypersegmented neutrophils.
- Thrombocytopenia or possible large platelets.

In folic acid deficiency, serum levels <3 ng/mL suggest deficiency, but levels of RBC folate are a better reflection of chronic deficiency with a normal level being 150 to 600 ng/mL of packed cells. If measured, iron and vitamin B_{12} levels are normal-to-elevated. Vitamin B_{12} deficiency is typically identified by measuring total levels or levels bound in the blood, although false negatives and false positives are common. Evaluating methylmalonic acid and total homocysteine levels, which would be elevated in the case of B_{12} deficiency, may be helpful.[41,42]

Management

Management of folic acid deficiency and juvenile pernicious anemia (caused by a lack of vitamin B_{12}) is typically best done in consultation with a pediatric hematologist. Treatment is dietary supplementation and correction of the underlying disorder (e.g., infection) if possible.

In folic acid deficiency confirmed by measurement of the RBC folate level, folic acid may be administered in a dose of 0.5 to 1 mg/day for 3 to 4 weeks until complete hematologic recovery. Maintenance therapy with a multivitamin containing 0.2 mg of folate is sufficient. In Vitamin B_{12} deficiency, treatment is dictated by the underlying cause. Supplementation is available in parenteral, intramuscular, subcutaneous, oral, and intranasal formulations.[41] Dosages vary to achieve the desired physiologic requirement of 1 to 3 mcg/day.[41,42]

Normocytic Anemias

Anemias that have an RBC size within the normal range are termed *normocytic*. Normocytic anemias tend to coincide with chronic illness, traumatic blood loss, early stages of acute anemia, or pregnancy. They are not common in children. Final determination of the etiology extends beyond blood cell indices and includes further chemistry laboratory tests such as blood urea nitrogen (BUN), creatinine, serum glutamic-oxaloacetic transaminase, alkaline phosphatase, bilirubin, erythrocyte sedimentation rate, urinalysis, and thyroid profile. Outside of trauma, GI microscopic blood loss and dysmenorrhea are common causes of blood loss, therefore stool evaluation for occult blood and a menstrual history can also be helpful.[20]

Transient Erythroblastopenia of Childhood

Idiopathic or transient erythroblastopenia of childhood (TEC) is a benign disorder of unknown cause that occurs in children during the first few years of life, usually after the first year of life. It is characterized by anemia, reticulocytopenia, and erythroid hypoplasia of the bone marrow. The cause of this transient suppression of erythropoiesis with resultant decreased RBC production is not clear, although it frequently follows a viral infection. The most commonly associated viruses are parvovirus B19, human herpes virus type 5, and echovirus type 11, although these viruses are often not detected. TEC is associated with a temporary failure of erythropoiesis caused by probable viral suppression or as a result of an immunoglobulin (Ig) G, IgM, or cell-mediated autoimmune response.[43]

Clinical Findings

History. TEC occurs mainly in previously healthy children between 6 months and 3 years of age, with most children at least 12 months of age.[44] The child may have a history of a preceding infection. Diagnosis is often delayed and, given that the lifespan of the RBC is approximately 120 days, it might take some time to clinically manifest. Symptoms of anemia may prompt presentation, although it may be identified incidentally during routine laboratory evaluation for an unrelated concern.[43]

Physical Examination. Children have symptoms of anemia, typically a gradually increasing pallor. Parents may report noticing decreased energy levels or fatigue in their child. Pallor and fatigue develop over a course of days or weeks and are often associated with viral symptoms, although no specific virus has been implicated. Tachycardia, tachypnea, and a systolic ejection murmur may be present in the setting of marked anemia. The presence of lymphadenopathy and hepatosplenomegaly are rare and should prompt additional evaluation.[43] Breath-holding spells have also been associated with TEC.[45]

Diagnostic Studies. The following are seen in TEC[43,44]:
- Moderate-to-severe anemia
- Markedly low reticulocyte count
- MCV characteristically normal for age
- WBC count usually normal but some degree of neutropenia can occur in up to 20%
- Platelet count normal or elevated

- High-serum iron level reflecting decreased utilization
- Bone marrow aspiration indicating erythroid hypoplasia

Differential Diagnosis

The syndrome can be differentiated from congenital hypoplastic anemia (Diamond-Blackfan syndrome) by the normal size of the RBCs; Diamond-Blackfan syndrome typically presents with normochromic, macrocytic anemia. Children with Diamond-Blackfan syndrome typically present between 2 and 6 months of age and approximately 50% of children will have craniofacial abnormalities, among other skeletal, genitourinary, and cardiac abnormalities.[46] Children with TEC have a normal physical examination. The peak incidence of TEC coincides with that of IDA, but the differences in MCV should help differentiate between these diagnoses.[44]

Management

TEC is self-limited, with recovery taking place 1 to 2 months after diagnosis. Treatment is supportive and no specific treatment is indicated, although transfusions may be required for severe anemia.[43] A referral to a hematologist may be needed.

Hemolytic Anemias

Hemolytic anemias are caused by premature destruction of RBCs and increased marrow production of reticulocytes. They can be classified as either hereditary or acquired and should be suspected in cases of an elevated reticulocyte count in the absence of bleeding or heparin therapy. In particular, the hereditary and congenital anemias manifest in infancy and early childhood. They may be due to a variety of hemoglobinopathies or defects in the red cell membrane. Determining the etiology of hemolysis necessitates careful history taking, including family medical history, child's medical history, diet, medication intake, and environmental exposures. Confirmation of the diagnosis comes from Hgb electrophoresis, Heinz body stain, and osmotic fragility test.

Sickle Cell Anemia, Disease, and Trait

SCD describes a group of complex, chronic disorders characterized by hemolysis, unpredictable acute complications that may become life-threatening, and the possible development of chronic organ damage. The replacement of the normal Hgb A with Hgb S, which carries the amino acid valine instead of glutamic acid and modifies the β-globin chain, is responsible for the condition. Hgb S tends to polymerize or come out of solution at low Pao_2, low pH, low temperature, and low osmolality. This process collapses the RBC, giving it a "sickled" shape and producing chronic hemolytic anemia. The new shape is rigid and clogs small blood vessels, producing ischemia, pain, and other vaso-occlusive problems. Children who have homozygous inheritance receive Hgb S from both parents have SCA or Hgb SS. The spectrum of disease can also include heterozygous inheritance patterns where the genes coding for the β-globin can include the sickle variant in addition to another variant such as Hgb C, β-thalassemia, or others; this is termed *SCD syndrome*. Patients with SCA, or Hgb SS, typically have Hgb S as >90% of their Hgb, while those with SCD typically have Hgb S as >50% of all Hgb.[47]

Hgb SS has an autosomal recessive inheritance pattern. It is found most often in people of African descent but is also detected among ethnic groups from the Mediterranean, the Caribbean, Central and South America, and India. Owing to migration, it now occurs worldwide. Sickle cell trait/carrier, where the patient produces mostly Hgb A and a small amount of Hgb S (HgbAS), occurs in approximately 1 in every 13 African Americans births.[48] This incidence exceeds that of most other serious genetic disorders in children, including cystic fibrosis and hemophilia. Routine neonatal screening identifies most infants with SCD born in the United States because such screening is mandated in all states and the District of Columbia.[47,49] It is still important to obtain a careful family medical history because many adults do not realize that they are carriers.

Clinical Findings

The clinical findings in sickle cell conditions are multisystemic and chronic, necessitating vigilant care to minimize the occurrence of crises and complications. Children with Hgb SS tend to have the most severe presentation, with findings including the following[49]:

- Fatigue and anemia, abdominal pain, and pain crises
- Dactylitis (swelling and inflammation of the hands and/or feet) and arthritis
- Bacterial infections, leg ulcers
- Eye damage, lung and heart injury, aseptic necrosis, and bone infarcts
- Priapism, splenic sequestration (sudden pooling of blood in the spleen), and liver congestion

Children with sickle cell trait (HgbAS) essentially have a benign clinical course. Their RBCs contain only 30% to 40% Hgb S, and sickling does not occur under most conditions. It is only in rare instances of hypoxia, such as in shock, while flying in unpressurized aircraft, or traveling to high elevations that signs of vaso-occlusion can appear. However, the presence of sickle cell trait has been implicated as a causative factor in the sudden deaths of young military recruits, college football players, and some teens. Extreme exercise, typically to exhaustion; dehydration; and relative hypoxia (altitude) are major confounding factors. Reproductive and genetic counseling is important for these patients.[50]

Physical Examination. SCA symptoms typically begin to emerge in the second 6 months of life as the amount of Hgb S increases and Hgb F declines. Thereafter, painful vaso-occlusive crises occur. Owing to the multisystemic nature of complications these children need prompt, detailed evaluation and intervention. After 5 years of age, splenomegaly usually disappears because of autoinfarction of the organ. Rates of height and weight gain usually slow after 7 years of age, and puberty may be delayed by 3 to 4 years.

Diagnostic Studies. The following laboratory results are seen in SCD:

- Hct of 20% to 29%
- Hgb 6 to 10 g/dL (severe)
- Reticulocyte count elevated: 5% to 15%
- Normal to increased WBCs and platelets
- MCV greater than 80 fL; MCHC greater than 37 mg/dL
- Hgb electrophoresis (after infancy), isoelectric focusing, or high-performance liquid chromatography showing a predominance of Hgb S and no Hgb A
- Morphology: irreversibly sickled cells or chronic elliptocytes, Howell-Jolly bodies, nucleated RBCs

Hgb electrophoresis results in a newborn with sickle cell trait will be Hgb FAS, and Hgb FS for a child with either SCA or sickle β-0 thalassemia. Normal results of Hgb electrophoresis are Hgb FA.

Differential Diagnosis

Chronic hemolytic anemia should be included in the differential diagnosis. Other syndromes characterized by hemolytic anemia and vaso-occlusion are Hgb SC disease, SCA, and a combination of Hgb S with α- or β-thalassemia. These diseases may be differentiated through electrophoresis and family testing if necessary. Hgb SC disease is typically less severe than Hgb SS; the course of sickle cell β-thalassemia can be severe or mild depending on the amount of β globin; sickle cell α-thalassemia is associated with milder anemia. Prenatal genetic testing is available in instances of high suspicion; otherwise, mandated newborn screening provides the diagnosis in most cases before symptoms present.

Management

Management of the child with SCA is complicated and should be done in consultation with a pediatric hematologist. Remarkable progress in the care of children with SCA can be directly attributed to the development of standards of care and anticipatory guidance. The National Heart, Lung, and Blood Institute (NHLBI) developed the most recent evidence-based clinical practice guidelines for the management of SCA in 2014.[51]

Children with SCD need regular primary care services and coordinated consultative services and information. Growth is closely monitored, immunizations must be done on time, parents require support, and communication with specialty services should be coordinated (e.g., an annual ophthalmologic examination by a retinal specialist). Care is comprehensive, spanning normal well-child issues through acute crises and hospitalization. The AAP issued guidelines for health supervision for children with SCA and SCD in 2002 and reaffirmed them in 2021.[52] Some of the key aspects of care for the child with SCA and SCD are as follows:

- Hydration, illness prevention, and pain management are fundamental aspects of disease management. Nonsteroidal anti-inflammatory drugs (NSAIDs) or acetaminophen may be adequate for mild to moderate pain, but opioids should be used when these are not adequate for management. (As in the case of anyone taking opioids, abuse and addiction issues must be considered. Consultation with a pediatric pain specialist maybe warranted.)
- The CBC and reticulocyte count are monitored every few months.
- All the usual immunizations of childhood are to be administered on time, including annual influenza and COVID-19 vaccination. PCPs should follow CDC guidelines and pay special attention to footnotes that provide special instructions for patients with sickle cell.[53] Nearly all patients with sickle cell will infarct their spleen during their lifetime. (Typically, by 12 months in SCA and by adolescence in SCD.) PCPs should therefore pay special attention to, and prioritize *Haemophilus influenzae* type b (Hib), pneumococcal, and meningococcal vaccines.[54,55]
- Functional asplenia increases the risk of bacteremia/sepsis from encapsulated bacteria and is a leading cause of morbidity and mortality in sickle cell patients. Penicillin VK prophylaxis (125 mg PO twice daily) is initiated at diagnosis. At 3 years of age, the dose is increased to 250 mg PO twice daily and continued at least until the fifth birthday or until the child has received two doses of pneumococcal polysaccharide vaccine 23.[51] Adherence to this regimen should be revisited at every visit as this has been shown to encourage compliance.[54]
- Folic acid supplementation at 1 mg/day is typically given to adults to prevent folate deficiency due to hemolysis. This is not standard therapy for children unless a folic acid deficiency is suspected; it should be individualized for each patient.

- Aggressive treatment of infections and maintenance of hydration and body temperature are used to prevent hypoxia and acidosis; volume replacement may be necessary to prevent circulatory collapse.
- Coexisting medical problems associated with lower oxygen saturations, such as asthma and obstructive sleep apnea, must be treated.
- In children with severe SCA, hydroxyurea is used to reduce the number of painful crises and the incidence of acute chest syndrome (a leading cause of death in adolescents with SCA). It is a preventive medication and not effective during the acute crisis. Hydroxyurea use is associated with a lower need for blood transfusions and fewer hospital visits by reducing the frequency and severity of painful events and episodes of acute chest syndrome. It increases Hgb F levels within cells, which decreases Hgb S levels, increases RBC water content, and alters the adhesion of RBCs to endothelium. There is some early evidence suggesting that it helps to improve growth and preserves organ function, and it is recommended in the NHLBI guidelines. Despite these benefits, side effects do occur, including an increased risk of serious infection. As always, the practitioner must carefully weigh all risks and benefits before integrating this medication into the treatment plan.
- Annual stroke prevention screening of major intracranial vessels with transcranial Doppler ultrasound evaluation should start around 2 years of age and continually annually until 16 years. A reading of greater than 170 cm/s time-averaged mean maximal velocity indicates a high risk for stroke and requires prompt specialist referral.[51,54]

Children with SCD are usually comanaged by their PCPs and specialists in hematology. Emergency admission or referral is necessary in the presence of the following[54]:

- Fever (to evaluate for sepsis) greater than 101°F (38.3°C)
- Pneumonia, chest pain, or other pulmonary symptoms concerning for acute chest syndrome
- Sequestration crisis as evidenced by splenomegaly with decreased Hgb or Hct
- Aplastic crisis as evidenced by decreased Hct and reticulocyte count
- Severe painful crisis, priapism
- Unusual headache, visual disturbances, neurologic changes

Consultation is also necessary for the chronic sequelae of persistent bone pain or leg ulcers, pregnancy, and contraception. Stem cell transplantation may be a consideration in children with significant disease and, if successful, is curative. Gene therapy is under investigation and has shown some success as have new medications.[54]

Complications

Because of functional asplenia, the greatest concern is febrile illness, indicating infection and possible sepsis. In view of the serious threat of pneumococcal sepsis in children younger than 5 years of age, all complaints of fever, poor feeding, lethargy, and irritability should be clinically evaluated. The consequences of hemolysis may include chronic anemia, jaundice, cholelithiasis, and delayed growth and sexual maturation. Vaso-occlusion and tissue ischemia may result in acute and chronic injury to virtually every organ system, with stroke being a major concern.[49] Even patients without stroke or elevated transcranial Doppler studies can experience cognitive dysfunction due to chronic hypoxemia. The role of toxic stress associated with having a chronic illness and its effect on patient, caregivers, and the entire family cannot be discounted. Psychological support services may be warranted in addition to early intervention services, neuropsychological testing and services, individualized education plans, and other forms of support.[54]

Patient and Family Education

The parents of children with sickle cell conditions need a great deal of support in raising a child with a genetically transmitted chronic illness. Clear patterns of communication should be established between the family and the PCP using a partnership model. Initial education includes the genetics and pathophysiology of the disease and the importance of regular health maintenance visits. Discussion should emphasize the need for early evaluation and treatment of febrile illness, acute splenic sequestration, aplastic crisis, and acute chest syndrome. Parents can be taught to palpate their child's spleen. Any downward displacement or enlargement of the spleen below the left costal margin should be evaluated by a healthcare professional and the blood counts monitored for increasing anemia. As the child grows, the family should be educated about other potential clinical complications, such as stroke, enuresis, priapism, cholelithiasis, delayed puberty, retinopathy, avascular necrosis of the hip and shoulder, and leg ulcers.

Preventive care measures also include the following:
- Timely administration of routine immunizations, including pneumococcal and meningococcal vaccines, and yearly influenza vaccine
- Prophylactic antibiotics
- Genetic counseling for those with sickle cell trait
- Support groups
- Educating adolescents with the trait about their status and the risk of disease transmission
- Hematopoietic stem cell transplant (the only intervention that can cure SCD with strict inclusion criteria identified for transplant eligibility)

Hereditary Spherocytosis

Hereditary spherocytosis (HS) is a hemolytic anemia characterized by a deficiency or abnormality of key proteins in the RBC membrane, akyrin-1, β-spectrin, band 3, α-spectrin, and protein 4.1R. These abnormalities reduce the cell surface area causing the RBCs to assume a more spherical shape and making them more likely to be sequestered and prematurely destroyed in the spleen. HS causes a spectrum of disease from mild chronic hemolysis to severe transfusion-dependent anemia.[20] HS has a prevalence of approximately 1 in 2000 to 5000 persons of mainly northern European ancestry.[56]

Clinical Findings

HS has a wide spectrum of clinical manifestations. Most exhibit mild-to-moderate hemolytic anemia, although compensated hemolysis without anemia can be seen in mild cases. Severe cases may be transfusion-dependent.[20] Jaundice usually appears in the newborn period, and it may be difficult to differentiate HS from hyperbilirubinemia caused by ABO incompatibility. The manifestations of chronic hemolysis may be apparent on examination including chronic fatigue, malaise, abdominal pain, and splenomegaly may also be noted. Splenomegaly is usually present by 2 years of age. A family history is often suggestive of an inherited hemolytic anemia.[56]

Diagnostic Studies. Diagnosis of HS is usually straightforward as a positive history, physical examination, and basic laboratory studies are sufficient to make the diagnosis. Laboratory findings in HS include the following:[56]
- Chronic anemia with reticulocytosis
- MCV is low-normal to decreased, MCHC is usually increased
- Evidence of hemolysis including indirect hyperbilirubinemia, decreased haptoglobin, elevated lactate dehydrogenase (LDH)
- On peripheral smear, a small proportion of the RBCs is spherocytic and smaller than normal and lacks the central pallor of the usual biconcave disk-shaped cell.
- Osmotic fragility of the cells is increased, as is the rate of autohemolysis of incubated blood.

Management

The treatment of HS is generally supportive. Infants born to a parent with known HS should be monitored carefully for hyperbilirubinemia. Some may require transfusions until they are able to compensate for hemolysis, usually between 6 and 12 months of age. Children with mild disease may require nothing but monitoring for complications. Those with severe HS who require multiple transfusions may need a splenectomy (often in combination with removal of the gallbladder), which usually produces a clinical cure. It should be deferred until after 6 years of age because of the increased risk of encapsulated bacterial infection before that age. Risks associated with splenectomy are postsplenectomy sepsis, penicillin-resistant pneumococcal infection, pulmonary hypertension, and ischemic heart disease and stroke. Pneumococcal and meningococcal vaccines should be given before splenectomy and subsequent postsplenectomy prophylaxis regimens should be initiated. Children with moderate HS and active hemolysis should receive folic acid supplementation to support erythropoiesis, which can be discontinued if they undergo splenectomy.

Complications

Aplastic crisis (often indicated by fever, fatigue, abdominal pain, and jaundice) associated with parvovirus and other viral infections is the most serious complication during childhood. Febrile illnesses should be vigorously treated. A child who is postsplenectomy and has a temperature greater than 101.5°F (>38.5°C) without an obvious source of infection should be hospitalized and treated with intravenous antibiotics until blood cultures are negative. Gallstone formation can occur as a result of chronic hemolysis, and an ultrasound should be performed beginning at 4 years and every 3 to 5 years thereafter, or as indicated for increased abdominal symptoms.[56]

Glucose-6-Phosphate Dehydrogenase Deficiency

A drug-induced hemolytic anemia can be caused by genetic deficiency of the G6PD enzyme in the RBC. Symptoms are generally associated with infections or exposure to oxidant metabolites of certain drugs that cause the precipitation of Hgb, injury to the red cells, and rapid hemolysis. The *G6PD* gene is found on the X chromosome. G6PD deficiency is transmitted as an X-linked recessive trait and is the most common metabolic abnormality of the RBC, affecting more than 400 million people worldwide. It frequently affects those of African, Italian, Greek, Mediterranean, Middle Eastern, and Asian descent.[20,57]

Clinical Findings

History. Most are asymptomatic until they are exposed to a triggering substance. Patients generally have a history of recent infection or oxidant ingestion via drug—specifically, aspirin-containing antipyretics, sulfonamides, antimalarials, antihelmintics, naphtha quinolones—or fava beans. The degree of hemolysis is dependent on the amount ingested and the extent of enzyme deficiency.[57]

Physical Examination. Patients typically present with fever, nausea, abdominal pain, diarrhea, jaundice, and dark urine within 48 hours of ingestion. Hallmarks of hemolysis, including hepatosplenomegaly and pallor, may be appreciated.[20]

Diagnostic Studies. In episodes of acute hemolysis, a normocytic normochromic anemia is evident on CBC and other studies, such as haptoglobin and free Hgb, are consistent with acute hemolysis. For diagnostic purposes, several dye reduction tests are available. Screening tests to measure a deficiency of G6PD should be used in high-risk groups. Only a few states include G6PD in their routine newborn screening panels; these tests measure G6PD enzyme activity in the RBC. After a hemolytic crisis, however, screening may produce a false-negative result because the younger blood cells that remain after hemolysis may show normal enzymatic activity. This is thought to be associated with higher G6PD activity taking place in reticulocytes. As is such, enzyme assay should be obtained 2 to 3 months after an episode for accurate diagnosis.[20,57]

Management

Prevention is key as there is no specific treatment available. In the cases of severe anemia, treatment is supportive and RBC transfusion may be indicated. Keeping the child well hydrated and monitoring for renal failure are also important during a hemolytic crisis.

Patient and Family Education

Patients and caregivers should be counseled to avoid the offending foods and drugs—the most common being fava beans, foods containing menthol and sulfites, aspirin, sulfonamide antibiotics, and antimalarials.

Platelet and Coagulation Disorders

Clinicians should evaluate for bleeding disorders in children before undergoing extensive surgery and in children with petechiae, frequent nosebleeds, mucous membrane bleeding, or excessive bleeding from minor trauma. Evaluation of these complaints includes a family history of bleeding or platelet disorders and a thorough bleeding history. Initial laboratory studies should include a CBC, platelet count, prothrombin time (PT), and activated partial thromboplastin time (aPTT). The most common diagnoses that can be differentiated with these tests are idiopathic thrombocytopenic purpura (ITP), hemophilia, von Willebrand disease, and leukemia. The coagulation cascade provides a mechanism for understanding the interconnectedness of all the factors involved in coagulation (see Fig. 38.4).

Bleeding History

The first step in assessing for disordered coagulation is a thorough history. In addition to family history of abnormal bleeding, it is important to evaluate for use of medications that can cause bleeding (e.g., nonsteroidal medications, aspirin), bleeding or easy bruising following mild traumas (e.g., falls) or significant bleeding after dental procedures or losing baby teeth. Asking about frequent or prolonged nose bleeds may also be helpful. In the adolescent female, asking about period length, number of pads or tampons used, and issues with bleeding through pads or tampons on a regular basis may also be helpful.[58,59] Standard bleeding assessment tools are available and can be helpful. The

International Society on Thrombosis and Hemostasis Bleeding Assessment Tool (ISTH-BAT) (https://bleedingscore.certe.nl/) is easy to use; a score of more than 2 is considered positive in children.[60] The Pediatric Bleeding Questionnaire (PBQ) was initially developed to screen children for von Willebrand disease,[61] but can also be used to assess bleeding in pediatric patients.

Overview of Diagnostic Studies

A platelet count, PT, and aPTT are usually sufficient screening tests to evaluate for disordered hemostasis. Additional diagnostic evaluation can be based upon those results.[62] The common studies and normal results are listed subsequently:

- Platelet count (normal range is 150,000–450,000/mm^3)
- PT (normal range is 11.5–14 seconds)
- aPTT is the method used to determine PTT, although it is commonly still referred to as the PTT (normal range is 25–40 seconds)
- Specific coagulation factor assays determine which clotting factors are absent
- Platelet function tests, such as platelet function analysis (PFA)

The PT and aPTT measure all of the clotting factors except factor XIII. PT measures the function of the extrinsic and common pathways; aPTT measures the function of the intrinsic and common pathways. If the platelet count is normal and either the aPTT or PT is prolonged or both, then a coagulation factor deficiency is possible. The typical laboratory findings of hemophilia are normal PT and PFA and an abnormal aPTT.[63]

If the PT and aPTT are elevated in association with thrombocytopenia, the probable diagnosis is disseminated intravascular coagulation (DIC), which is a syndrome secondary to a severe systemic disease process such as sepsis, malignancy, toxins, or liver failure; it is frequently accompanied by shock. In DIC, there is a systemic activation of the coagulation process. Extensive, ongoing activation of coagulation results in the depletion of platelets and coagulation factors, which leads to bleeding and thrombosis.

Immune Thrombocytopenia

Immune thrombocytopenia (ITP) is the most common acute onset of thrombocytopenia in otherwise well children, affecting 1.9 to 6.4 per 100,000 children per year.[59] Previously called *idiopathic thrombocytopenic purpura*, the terminology changed due to increased understanding of the pathophysiology. Furthermore, the word "purpura" is no longer used as many patients with the condition may not bleed. ITP is now the preferred name for the condition. Although there is not a complete understanding of the underlying pathophysiology, it results from an autoimmune response in which circulating platelets are destroyed and usually occurs after viral illnesses. Most cases occur between 1 and 4 years of age. The vast majority of cases are considered *newly diagnosed* and resolve within 6 months even without treatment. ITP that last 3 to 12 months is considered *persistent*, and longer than 12 months is termed *chronic* ITP.[64]

Clinical Findings

The classic presentation of ITP is a well-appearing young child with acute onset of mucosal bleeding, bruising, and petechiae. These symptoms typically do not manifest until the platelet count is less than 20,000/mm^3. Additional findings include the following:

- Bruising may be most prominent over the legs.
- A preceding viral illness 1 to 4 weeks before onset is common; vaccination, allergic reaction, and insect bites have also been implicated.[59]
- Mucosal bleeding can be most prominent from the gums and lips.
- Nosebleeds that can be severe and difficult to control
- Menorrhagia in an adolescent female
- Absence of enlarged liver, spleen, and lymph nodes
- Bone pain and pallor are rare.

Patients who present with thrombocytopenia and constitutional symptoms such as weight loss, fever, hepatosplenomegaly, or lymphadenopathy require evaluation for an underlying disorder such as leukemia, reactions to medications (e.g., quinine, heparin), lupus erythematosus, cirrhosis, HIV, hepatitis C, congenital conditions such a X-linked thrombocytopenia, autosomal macrothrombocytopenia, Wiskott-Aldrich syndrome, and von Willebrand factor (vWF) deficiency.[65]

Diagnostic Studies. There is no specific test that is diagnostic of ITP. Thrombocytopenia is the hallmark finding on CBC, but other causes must be eliminated with a thorough history and physical examination, or additional laboratory investigations. Laboratory findings in ITP include:

- Low platelet count (<150,000/mm^3) with an otherwise normal CBC.
- Severe thrombocytopenia with a platelet count less than 20,000/mm^3 is common and platelet size is normal or increased.
- Normal PT and aPTT and normal WBC and RBC counts.
- Megathrombocytes on the peripheral smear.
- Hgb may be decreased if there is a history of significant nose or menstrual bleeding, but the MCV remains normal.

Differential Diagnosis

Many conditions are associated with thrombocytopenia and a careful and thorough evaluation should be conducted to exclude particularly worrisome conditions. If the peripheral smear shows fragmented RBCs, BUN and creatinine levels should be measured to evaluate for hemolytic uremic syndrome. Abnormal coagulation studies suggest a factor deficiency or other bleeding disorder. The presence of abnormalities on the CBC outside of thrombocytopenia (anemia, neutropenia, leukocytosis, etc.), abnormal cells on peripheral smear, bone pain, hepatosplenomegaly, or congenital anomalies should prompt referral to a pediatric hematologist for possible bone marrow aspiration to evaluate for hematologic malignancies and other disorders.[65] In a sick, febrile child with isolated thrombocytopenia, petechiae, or purpura, the major diagnosis to consider first is meningococcemia. These children should also be referred, hospitalized, and treated for presumed sepsis.

Management

The prognosis for most patients with ITP is excellent, with spontaneous recovery in the majority of pediatric cases within the first 6 months. Most cases can be managed on an outpatient basis with an "expectant watch-and-wait" approach[65]; however, children must limit activity to prevent trauma and bleeding, which can have significant impacts on quality of life.

Deciding to treat ITP requires consideration of multiple factors including bleeding symptoms, platelet count, and quality of life issues. Completion of an ITP-designated bleeding score, as provided by the American Society of Hematology in the Updated International Consensus Report on the Investigation and Management of Primary Immune Thrombocytopenia,[65] can help guide the clinician in treatment decisions. Initial therapy consists of a short course of corticosteroids. Careful consideration should be given to obtaining a bone marrow evaluation before initiation of steroid treatment, particularly in the presence of any other abnormal findings, as steroids are a mainstay of treatment for many hematologic malignancies. Intravenous immunoglobulin (IVIG) as a single dose is also given to children with active severe bleeding and those who have contraindications for steroid use; WinRho (Anti-D) is given intravenously or subcutaneously with the dose depending on Hgb level; Rh(D) immune globulin is useful only in Rh-positive individuals. Splenectomy, immunosuppressive therapy, and anti-CD20 antibody are options for those children with refractory or chronic ITP. New agents that stimulate thrombopoiesis, such as romiplostim and eltrombopag, are also available options and approved by the US Food and Drug Administration for use in children ≥1 year of age with chronic ITP. Treatment guidelines updated in 2019 are readily available to further guide diagnosis and treatment.[65]

Complications

The most serious complication of ITP is intracranial hemorrhage, which occurs in less than 1% of newly diagnosed cases. Risk factors for intracranial hemorrhage include low platelet count (<10,000/mm^3), head trauma, other signs of bleeding. Complaints of significant headache necessitate a careful neurologic evaluation. Increased rates of *Helicobacter pylori* infection have been seen in children with chronic ITP. Treatment of the infection can improve ITP disease course in some cases.[65]

Patient and Family Education

In newly diagnosed cases, if the platelet count is greater than 20,000/mm^3 and no bleeding is observed, children and parents should be advised to avoid contact sports, aspirin and other NSAIDs, and any other herbal or pharmacologic agents that interfere with platelet function; they should also notify the practitioner of any excessive bleeding. Epistaxis can be treated with local measures.

Hemophilia A and B and von Willebrand Disease

Inherited coagulation deficiencies are described according to the absent coagulation factor. Most result in abnormal bleeding. Hemophilia results from a deficiency of factor VIII (hemophilia A) or factor IX (hemophilia B). In hemophilia A and B, absence or deficiency of the coagulation factor results in prolonged bleeding either spontaneously from small vessels or as a result of trauma. A rough guide to gauge the severity of hemophilia is the percentage of function of the factor levels with 100% (100 U/dL) equal to the function of factor found in 1 mL of normal plasma. The clotting factor levels with percentage of factor activity associated with severity of bleeding are as follows: less than 1 U/dL (<1%), severe; between 1 and 5 U/dL (1–5%), moderate; and more than 5 U/dL (>5%), mild.[66] Definitive diagnosis is usually made by measurement of these factors in association with an aPTT test. Genetic testing may be done in severe cases.[67]

In plasma, factor VIII binds with vWF, which is a specific circulatory protein and acts as a carrier protein. von Willebrand disease (also known as *vascular hemophilia*) is a heterogeneous group of hereditary bleeding disorders caused by a quantitative or qualitative abnormality of vWF protein (Table 38.8). In type I, the protein is quantitatively reduced; in type II, it is qualitatively abnormal; and it is absent in type III.[68]

TABLE 38.8 Comparisons of Hemophilia A, Hemophilia B, and von Willebrand Disease

	Hemophilia A	Hemophilia B	von Willebrand Disease
Inheritance	X-linked	X-linked	Autosomal dominant
Factor deficiency	VIII	Factor IX	VWF, factor VIII
Bleeding site(s)	Muscle, joint, surgical	Muscle, joint, surgical	Mucous membranes, skin, surgical, menstrual
Prothrombin time (PT)	Normal	Normal	Normal
Activated partial thromboplastin time (aPTT)	Prolonged	Prolonged	Prolonged or normal
Bleeding time	Normal	Normal	Prolonged or normal
Factor VIII coagulant activity (VIIIC)	Low	Normal	Low or normal
von Willebrand factor antigen (vWF: Ag)	Normal	Normal	Low
von Willebrand factor activity (vWF: Act)	Normal	Normal	Low
Factor IX	Normal	Low	Normal
Ristocetin-induced platelet agglutination	Normal	Normal	Normal, low, or increased at low-dose ristocetin
Platelet aggregation	Normal	Normal	Normal
Treatment	DDAVP[a] or recombinant VIII	Recombinant IX	DDAVP[a] or vWF concentrate

[a]Desmopressin (DDAVP) for mild to moderate hemophilia A or type I von Willebrand disease.

Modified from Marcdante, KJ, Klieg RM, Schuh AM. *Nelson Essentials of Pediatrics.* 9th ed. Philadelphia: Elsevier; 2023.

Because the genes for the coagulation factors are sex linked (carried on the X chromosome) and recessive, hemophilia A and B affect primarily males. Females are generally only carriers of the disorder. According to the CDC, about 1 in 5000 males is affected with hemophilia A; each year about 400 babies are born with hemophilia A; hemophilia A is approximately 4 times more common than hemophilia B.[69] von Willebrand disease occurs in both sexes affecting approximately 1% of the general population. It is the most common inherited bleeding disorder and is associated with either a qualitative or quantitative defect in vWF.[70] The primary sites of bleeding differ depending on whether the problem is hemophilia A or B or von Willebrand disease.

Clinical Findings

Table 38.8 provides comparisons of hemophilia A, hemophilia B, and von Willebrand disease. Additional findings associated with hemophilia include the following[66]:
- A positive family history in the vast majority of cases
- Excessive bruising
- Prolonged bleeding from mucous membranes after minor lacerations, immunizations, circumcision, or during menstruation (menorrhagia)
- Hemarthrosis characterized by pain and swelling in the elbows, knees, and ankles
- A greatly prolonged aPTT

A specific assay for factor VIII or IX activity confirms the diagnosis.

Additional findings associated with von Willebrand disease include the following[68]:
- Mucous membrane bleeding (epistaxis, menorrhagia), easy bruising, and excessive posttraumatic or postsurgical bleeding.
- History of ecchymosis of trunk, upper arms, and thighs.
- Factor VIII clotting activity usually decreased.
- vWF antigen usually decreased and decreased vWF. Normal platelet count but isolated decreased platelet count associated with type 2B.

Management

Treatment of hemophilia consists of prevention of trauma and replacement therapy to increase factor VIII or factor IX activity in plasma. Plasma-derived and recombinant factor concentrates are available for replacement, with recombinant factor preferred.[71] Special consideration is given to the newborn with suspected hemophilia, who should receive newborn care including vitamin K.[72] Hemarthrosis is the leading form of significant local bleeding. Local measures include the application of cold and pressure to affected painful joints. As with all bleeding disorders, aspirin and other NSAIDs should be avoided. Anticipatory guidance should be directed at avoiding high-risk behaviors and contact sports and the importance of wearing a bike helmet. Physical therapy may be needed to assist with decreased mobility caused by hemarthrosis and joint scarring.

Ideally most children with hemophilia should be enrolled in a comprehensive hemophilia treatment center to facilitate a collaborative, interdisciplinary approach to management. The PCP should remain central to the care of the child. Owing to the risk of bleeding, education and anticipatory guidance with a focus on injury prevention are essential. Immunizations should be given either subcutaneously with a 26-gauge needle when possible or intramuscularly with a 25-gauge needle followed by firm pressure, without rubbing, and ice at the site for several minutes. Iron replacement may also be necessary in children with severe bleeding disorders. The National Hemophilia Foundation recommends that prophylaxis therapy be considered optimal treatment for children with severe hemophilia and is usually initiated with the first joint bleed. This is often in the first year of life as mobility increases. Additional guidelines for treatment and management of hemophilia can be found in the World Federation of Hemophilia Guidelines for the Management of Hemophilia, 3rd edition.[71]

von Willebrand disease is treated depending on the type and severity of the bleeding. The treatment for von Willebrand disease is desmopressin (DDAVP) and factor VIII-vWF concentrates. Local measures to control bleeding may also be part of the treatment plan. Adjunctive therapy (e.g., estrogen and/or aminocaproic acid) depends on the type of von Willebrand disease (type 1, 2A, 2B, 2M, 2N, or 3), which is determined by the level of qualitative or quantitative factor deficiency. The use of aminocaproic acid, an antifibrinolytic agent, is sometimes recommended for dental extraction and nosebleeds.[68]

In patients where DDAVP is not an option, most patients with von Willebrand disease are now given lifelong prophylaxis or treatment to prevent spontaneous bleeding and preserve joints.[73] Additional guidelines for the treatment of von Willebrand disease can be found through the National Hemophilia Foundation.[73]

For patients with bleeding disorders, a written treatment plan tailoring replacement product dosage based on the location of the bleed should be in the electronic health record (EHR) and given to the parents to carry with them. For those living in remote areas, arrangements should be made to ensure factor replacement is available at local institutions for treatment of bleeding episodes if required. The child should also wear a medical alert bracelet or necklace.

Complications

In patients with hemophilia A and B, bleeding is understandably the primary complication. Continued hemorrhage results in anemia and eventually hypovolemic shock. Bleeding is particularly concerning when it occurs in closed areas, such as in the joints or intracranially. Hemarthrosis can affect mobility and function by causing degenerative joint disease. Injury prevention is essential, but strategies must be employed to foster quality of life and allow children to develop a healthy musculoskeletal system. Psychosocial intervention may be needed to help families avoid overprotectiveness or permissiveness.

Thrombophilia

Thrombophilia refers to the increased ability to form blood clots and may result from either acquired and/or inherited risks factors. Thrombotic events (venous thromboembolism [VTE] and stroke) are rare in healthy children but have been increasingly recognized in tertiary pediatric centers. Advances in treating critically ill children—coupled with increased awareness of inherited factors, improved imaging to identify thrombosis, and the prothrombotic lifestyle choices in society today—have led families to seek testing in healthy children. Screening for inherited thrombophilia in children with VTE is controversial, but the testing of healthy children who have a family history of thrombosis or thrombophilia is even more controversial.[74]

The most common inherited thrombophilias are factor V Leiden mutation, prothrombin 20210 mutation, antithrombin deficiency, and protein C or S deficiency. Also to be considered are factors that may be either inherited or acquired and are helpful in identifying patients who have multiple prothrombotic risk factors and may need testing; these would include antiphospholipid antibodies, elevated fasting homocysteine levels, and elevated factor VIII.[74]

Most causes of thrombosis in children are iatrogenic, such as the presence of a central (indwelling) venous catheter, or factors involving an underlying disease such as surgery, trauma, immobilization, infection, systemic lupus erythematosus, structural venous anomalies, and cancer.[74] Oral contraceptive use has also long been associated with an increased risk of thrombosis.[75] Typically, testing for thrombophilia in these situations is not warranted.

Testing for thrombophilia should be considered when a child develops a clot without any clear risk factors, or when there is a significant family history. Children with two or more inherited thrombophilia traits have been shown to be at increased risk for VTE. Those with potential benefits from screening and testing are children with a strong family history of thrombophilia, such as a VTE in a first-degree relative younger than 40 years. Identifying these children has the benefit of counseling adolescent females who may be considering the use of oral contraceptives and targeted thromboprophylaxis in high-risk situations (femoral fracture in an obese teen who also has inherited thrombophilia). Educating patients about signs and symptoms of VTE, which could lead to earlier diagnosis, may also be useful. Counseling should revolve around lifestyle modifications including avoiding a sedentary lifestyle, overweight or obesity, and smoking.[74] Additional guidance can be found via the American Society of Hematology's evidence-based guidelines for management of pediatric VTE.[76]

Pancytopenia

Pancytopenia is marked by a decrease in all three formed elements of the blood—erythrocytes, leukocytes, and platelets. A child usually presents with clinical findings of infection or bleeding rather than anemia because of the longer life span of RBCs compared with platelets and WBCs. As such, it is not a single disease but results from a combination of disease processes. Pancytopenia is caused by one of the three following processes:

- Production failure (e.g., aplastic anemia)
- Sequestration (e.g., hypersplenism)
- Increased peripheral destruction of mature cells (e.g., certain infections/known medications)

The child should be referred to a pediatric hematologist for treatment focused at correcting the underlying mechanism, such as hematopoietic stem cell transplantation (failure of production), splenectomy, or other treatments aimed at reducing peripheral destruction of cells or sequestration.

Leukocyte Disorders

White Blood Cell Count

The WBC count is used as an indicator of infection or illness; the percentages of the different types of cells also provide useful diagnostic information. The WBC count is automated and is a routine part of the CBC. The WBC differential is obtained on a smear of blood one cell layer thick, usually with a Wright stain procedure that contains both basic and acidic dyes. The ANC is calculated from the results of the differential: If WBCs = 3600/mm³, percentage of segmented neutrophils = 20, percentage of band neutrophils = 5, lymphocytes = 60, monocytes = 10, and eosinophils = 5, then ANC = 3600 × 0.25 (sum of % segs and bands) = 900.

White Blood Cell Dysfunction

The WBC count and differential are useful diagnostic guides in the management of a variety of childhood illnesses. The normal range of granulocyte and lymphocyte counts varies throughout childhood. Leukocytosis is an increase in the number of circulating leukocytes, primarily with a neutrophilic response particularly to bacterial infections. A relative increase in the number of circulating immature neutrophils (bands), or "left shift," is a defensive mechanism in response to an inflammatory process or acute bacterial infection. Multiple abnormalities in WBC indices should raise suspicion of a malignant disorder.

Alterations of Granulocytes

Neutropenia is defined as a decrease in the number of circulating neutrophils and bands in the peripheral blood. Determining neutropenia requires calculation of the ANC, which is done by multiplying the entire WBC by the total neutrophil count, including the segmented and band forms. Evaluation of the ANC must be done in reference to developmental norms. Neutrophils predominate in the newborn and then rapidly decrease in the infant. By 5 years of age, neutrophil and lymphocytes are equivalent. Adult levels, where neutrophils are approximately 70% of all WBCs, are reached by puberty.[77] There are also racial differences, with those of African, Middle Eastern, and West Indian descent having lower numbers at baseline when compared to White individuals; a condition termed *benign ethnic neutropenia*.[78] Neutropenia is classified as mild (ANC of 1000–1500/mm³), moderate (ANC of 500–1000/mm³), or severe (ANC <500/mm³). Those with severe neutropenia in particular are at a substantially increased risk for developing infections from their own endogenous flora and nosocomial infections.[77]

Neutropenia results from decreased cellular production (as in various hematologic diseases, infections, drug-induced states, and nutritional deficiencies), increased peripheral destruction (as in autoimmune disorders), or peripheral pooling (as in bacterial infections, hemodialysis, and cardiopulmonary bypass). Most cases of neutropenia are discovered during evaluation of the WBC count in a child with an acute febrile illness and are often transient and typically follow viral infections, such as parvovirus B19, human herpes virus 6, hepatitis A and B, respiratory syncytial virus, influenza A and B, Epstein-Barr virus (EBV), and cytomegalovirus. The general management of neutropenic patients includes careful identification and prompt treatment of any suspected or proven infections.[77]

While some neutropenia is acquired related to infections, the largest group of neutropenic patients includes children who are receiving chemotherapy. They are at risk for developing severe, life-threatening bacterial infections depending on the degree and duration of neutropenia. Despite improvements in supportive care and treatment with granulocyte colony–stimulating factor (G-CSF), bacterial and fungal infections remain a major cause of morbidity and mortality in these patients. The standard of care for febrile neutropenic children with cancer is hospitalization for empiric administration of broad-spectrum antibiotics.[79]

Qualitative abnormalities of granulocytes are usually related to defects of phagocytosis. Although individually rare, these defects may be genetic or acquired. Malnutrition, sepsis, diabetes, and leukemia are acquired disorders related to defects in leukocyte function, particularly phagocytosis and microbicidal activity. Granulomatous diseases are relatively rare disorders of granulocytes, particularly neutrophils, in which the enzymes necessary for bactericidal activity are lacking. Such diseases result in severe, recurrent infections of the skin, lymph nodes, lungs, liver, and bone. Children with these conditions present early in life with frequent infections and are typically diagnosed before 5 years of age. Treatment includes treatment and prevention of infections, hematopoietic stem cell transplantation, and recent advances in gene therapy, which show promise.[80]

Lymphocytosis

Lymphocytosis is most commonly produced by viral illnesses, including mumps, measles (rubeola), rubella, varicella, mononucleosis, hepatitis, and EBV. EBV infection is also characterized by large, atypical lymphocytes seen on peripheral smear, which can also be seen in toxoplasmosis infection. Lymphocytosis is uncommon in bacterial infections, except in *Bordetella pertussis* infection in which a marked lymphocytosis is characteristic. Infection with the *Toxoplasma gondii* parasite is also associated with lymphocytosis and atypical lymphocytes. Pronounced, prolonged lymphocytosis in the pediatric patient should prompt the practitioner to consider an oncologic process.

Cancer

Childhood cancer is uncommon and often presents with symptoms of a benign illness. The signs and symptoms are variable and nonspecific and can include continued unexplained weight loss; headaches (typically in the early morning); swelling or persistent pain in bones, joints, back, or legs; lumps or masses; excessive bruising, bleeding, or rash; constant infections; night sweats; persistent nausea or vomiting without nausea; persistent fatigue; vision changes; and/or recurrent or persistent fevers of no known etiology. Many different types of cancer can occur in young people, including cancers seen in adults as well as cancers unique to children. More than 15,000 cases of pediatric cancer are diagnosed in the United States each year, the most common being leukemia, lymphoma, and brain cancer; however, the rate of childhood cancers in the United States varies by state and region.[81,82] According to the most recent United States statistical data:[82]

- Overall, pediatric cancer rates are highest in males, those aged 0 to 4 years and 15 to 19 years, and in White individuals.
- The Northeast had the highest rate of child/adolescent cancer, whereas the South had the lowest rate.
- Children and teens who lived in a city and/or in prosperous counties had higher rates of cancer than those living outside cities and/or in poorer counties.
- The highest incidence of leukemia is seen in the West.
- The highest incidence of lymphoma and brain tumors is seen in the Northeast.

In contrast to adult cancers, only a small percentage of all childhood cancers have a known preventable cause. Development of cancer is thought to be multifactorial potentially involving the interplay of environmental exposures including infections and genetic susceptibility traits. Ionizing radiation is a well-recognized risk factor,[83] and healthcare providers are encouraged to limit the use of computed tomography (CT) scans in children and pregnant women to those situations with a defined clinical indication; then the lowest possible radiation dose should be used. Numerous epidemiologic studies have investigated potential environmental causes of childhood cancer, but few strong or consistent associations have been found.

Leukemias

Leukemias are a group of malignant hematologic diseases in which normal bone marrow elements are replaced by abnormal, poorly differentiated lymphocytes known as *blast cells*. Genetic abnormalities in hematopoietic cells take over, resulting in the unregulated clonal proliferation of malignant cells. Leukemias are classified according to cell type involvement (e.g., lymphocytic or nonlymphocytic) and by cellular differentiation (e.g., B-cell, T-cell).

The leukemias are the most common form of childhood cancer, accounting for up to 30% of all pediatric cancers. The majority of childhood leukemia cases are acute lymphoblastic/lymphocytic leukemia (ALL) with a peak incidence between 2 and 5 years of age. ALL accounts for approximately 75% of all leukemias in children from birth to 14 years, and 46% of leukemias in those 15 to 19 years of age.[81] Overall, rates of ALL are highest in Hispanics.[84] Acute myeloid/myelogenous leukemia (AML) is less common in children than ALL and accounts for approximately 14% of leukemias in children from birth to 14 years of age, but 30% of leukemias in those 15 to 19 years of age.[81] The remainder of cases include chronic variations, leukemias affecting myelomonocytes, and others that do not fit classic definitions.

In addition to ionizing radiation, including therapeutic exposure to irradiation for cancer treatment, additional risk factors for development of leukemia include genetic conditions such as Down syndrome and neurofibromatosis type 1. Familial monosomy 7 and previous exposure to chemotherapeutic agents also increase the risk of developing AML.

Although there have been dramatic improvements in survival for ALL over the past 4 decades, with outcomes approaching 90% in the latest studies, progress has been slower for myeloid leukemia and certain subgroups such as infant ALL, adolescent/young adult ALL, and relapsed ALL.[81] Recent advances include the recognition of molecularly defined subgroups, which continues to inform precision medicine approaches.

Clinical Findings

Most of the clinical signs and symptoms of leukemia are related to leukemic replacement of the bone marrow and the absence of blood cell precursors. History frequently reveals repeated infections, fever, and weight loss. Reports of prolonged fatigue, irritability, and decreased energy are common. Children are often more prone to bleeding as evidenced by epistaxis, gum bleeding, and easy bruising. They may also complain of bone and joint pain as leukemic cells rapidly multiply in the bone marrow. Physical examination often demonstrates pallor, lymphadenopathy, hepatosplenomegaly, and petechiae. The child may be pale, listless, irritable, or chronically tired. Rarely, children may present with headache and evidence of increased intracranial pressure suggesting leukemic involvement in the central nervous system (CNS). All these symptoms may be vague or nonspecific; therefore providers must maintain a high index of suspicion for cancer.

Diagnostic Studies. The following are used to diagnose leukemia:

- CBC with differential, WBCs, platelet, and reticulocyte counts. Thrombocytopenia and anemia are present in most cases. The WBC count may be elevated, normal, or low with varying levels of neutropenia.
- A peripheral smear may demonstrate malignant cells.
- Bone marrow examination frequently shows an infiltration of blast cells replacing normal elements of the marrow.
- Cerebral spinal fluid examination can reveal infiltration of leukemic cells.

Chromosomal and genetic abnormalities are found in the leukemic cells of most children with leukemia. These genetic alterations may include changes in the number of chromosomes and a structure with recurrent translocations and deletions, which provide important information for prognosis and treatment. Further classification regarding cell type, morphologic characteristics, and cell surface markers is generally made at the cancer treatment center to which the child is referred. Diagnostic studies play a key role in staging disease, determining treatment course, and evaluating response to therapy. For children with suspected cancer, referral to a pediatric cancer center for a thorough diagnostic evaluation is warranted.

Management

Approximately 90% of children diagnosed with ALL can now be cured; they are considered cured after 10 years in remission. The treatment program for most types of acute leukemia involves 4 to 6 weeks of induction therapy, with the goal of removing the leukemic cells from the body (remission) and restoring normal hematopoiesis. This is followed by a consolidation phase of therapy lasting several months and then a maintenance phase for 2 to 3 years. Mainstays of therapy include systemic and intrathecal chemotherapy administration and systemic administration of corticosteroids. Although a component of treatment for high-risk patients in the past, the use of cranial irradiation as part of therapy is significantly decreasing. Children undergo repeat diagnostic studies at regular intervals to determine response to treatment.

For children with ALL who relapse and are unable to achieve remission, the need for hematopoietic stem cell transplantation may be considered; for some children with certain chromosomal rearrangements or those who are considered at high risk for relapse, transplantation might be considered sooner. Chimeric-antigen receptor (CAR) T-cell therapy is approved for treating advanced B-cell ALL or extremely resistant ALL but not other leukemias or pediatric cancers. It is an immunotherapy using a patient's T cells and genetically modifying them to target and bind to CD19, a B-cell surface cell protein/antigen found on cancerous B cells. Research on this prescription mode of treatment is promising.

Compared to ALL, patients with AML have a poorer prognosis; therefore treatment is more aggressive and consists of induction chemotherapy, CNS treatment (whether prophylactic or disease-directed), and postremission therapy. Hematopoietic stem cell transplantation, ideally from an HLA-matched sibling or parent, might be considered in the first complete remission for children with high-risk disease.

Long-term sequelae of cancer therapy for leukemias have been identified in research studies and include effects on cognition, neuropsychologic functioning, growth deficiencies, and an increased risk for second malignancies, such as AML or lymphoma. CNS irradiation is linked to learning disabilities and impaired IQ, especially in children younger than 5 years who also received intrathecal therapy. As a result, cranial radiation dosages have been reduced, and earlier neuropsychologic testing is recommended.

Other documented potential late effects of ALL treatment include congestive heart failure, avascular necrosis, and osteoporosis.

The role of the PCP is crucial to facilitate proper referrals and effective interdisciplinary communication and to assist the family in their coping and adaptation processes. Special attention should be paid to siblings whose lives can be particularly disrupted. Regular health supervision visits are also important and should not be overlooked. Immunizations should be given as appropriate depending on the stage of treatment and the child should be monitored for failed remission or metastasis, with common sites including the CNS and testicles, and late childhood cancer effects.

Lymphomas

Lymphomas are hematologic malignancies that originate in the lymphatic and reticuloendothelial systems. Behind leukemias and brain tumors, they are the third most common malignancy diagnosed in children. Lymphomas are among the most common malignancies diagnosed in adolescents.[81] Broadly, they are defined as Hodgkin and non-Hodgkin lymphoma (NHL).

Hodgkin Lymphoma

Hodgkin lymphoma (HL) is classically characterized by the presence of large, binucleate, or multinucleate neoplastic cells known as *Hodgkin Reed-Sternberg cells*. HL usually originates in a cervical lymph node and spreads to other lymph node regions; if left untreated, it will spread to organ systems including the liver, spleen, bone, bone marrow, and brain. Involvement of the bone marrow and CNS is rare. Disease staging is done via physical examination and imaging to determine the bulk and degree of disease spread.[85] Due to advances in treatment over the years, the prognosis for HL is quite good with 5-year survival rates of 98% to 99%.[81]

Most cases of HL are diagnosed in adolescents and young adults (AYA) between the ages of 15 and 30 years.[85] HL accounts for 12% of all cancers in children between 15 and 19 years of age.[81] The risk of developing HL, particularly in AYAs, is higher in areas of economic development and in those with higher socioeconomic status. Exposure to infections in early childhood is thought to be protective; however, a history of EBV infection correlates with some forms of HL. Development of HL has been noted in immunocompromised persons, including those with HIV. Clusters of cases in families also suggest a genetic predisposition.[86]

Clinical Findings. The most common manifestations of HL include the following[85]:

- Painless enlargement of the lymph nodes, usually in the cervical area. Nodes are often rubbery, firm, matted together, nontender to palpation.
- Hepatosplenomegaly may be present.
- Chronic cough can be present, suggesting tracheal compression by a large mediastinal mass.
- "B symptoms" such as fever, decreased appetite, weight loss of 10% or more of total body weight within 6 months of diagnosis, and drenching night sweats, which play an important role in disease staging.

Diagnostic Studies. Initial diagnostic evaluation when HL is suspected includes chest radiography to evaluate for the presence of a large mediastinal mass. Laboratory studies to consider, with results suggestive of HL, include the following:

- CBC with anemia and elevated or depressed leukocytes or platelets
- Elevated sedimentation rate and C-reactive protein

- Elevated serum copper and ferritin level
- Comprehensive metabolic plan demonstrating abnormal liver function test results
- Urinalysis showing proteinuria

Excisional lymph node biopsy is recommended for pathologic evaluation, and bone marrow evaluation studies may be warranted. Imaging studies are essential for staging, with positive emission tomography (PET), MRI, and CT playing a role. Interpretation by a radiologist with experience in HL is important as there are many nuances and accurate staging is critical to determining therapy.[85]

Management. The child should receive treatment at a comprehensive pediatric oncology center in collaboration with the PCP. Multiple treatment agents allow different mechanisms of action to avoid overlapping toxicities. Optimal results are obtained through irradiation, chemotherapy with numerous agents, or a combination of both. Treatment regimens developed by groups such as Children's Oncology Group (COG) and the European Network for Pediatric Hodgkin Lymphoma are frequently used. Before initiation of treatment, consideration should be given to fertility preservation and discussion of options with a specialist as infertility associated with treatment is possible.[85]

Although successful treatment of HL is common, follow-up after completion of HL treatment is imperative. Approximately 75% of children who survive HL go on to have chronic medical conditions and impaired health-related quality of life. Secondary cancers (especially breast, thyroid, and nonmelanoma skin cancer), cardiac and pulmonary toxicities, thyroid dysfunction, and reproductive issues are seen. Fatigue, decline in cognitive performance, and sexual dysfunction can greatly impact quality of life; therefore regular screening for late effects should be monitored regularly by the oncologist and PCP.[85]

Non-Hodgkin Lymphomas

The NHLs are a diverse group of neoplasms in the lymphatic tissues that result from malignant proliferation of T cells, B cells, or indeterminate lymphocyte cells. From a pathophysiologic standpoint, these malignancies arise from abnormalities that can occur at various points in the complex hematopoiesis process, which results in a great deal of diversity and challenges with classification. In pediatrics, the most common types of NHL are lymphoblastic lymphoma, anaplastic large cell lymphoma, and mature B-cell lymphoma; the last of which is further divided into Burkitt lymphoma and diffuse large B-cell lymphoma.

NHLs account for 6% of cancer diagnoses in children from birth to 14 years and 7% in those aged 15 to 19 years. Compared to HLs, their prognosis is poorer with 5-year survival rates of 90% and 89%, respectively.[81] Incidence rates and distribution of most subtypes of NHL differ by age, race, and geographical region. Generally speaking, NHLs occur more frequently in boys than in girls. They are most frequently diagnosed in children during the second decade of life and infrequently in children younger than 4 years.[87] NHLs are also a frequent malignancy in children with inherited or acquired immunodeficiency syndromes; they are also associated with Epstein-Barr, human immune, and cytomegalovirus infections.[88]

Clinical Findings. Owing to the heterogenicity of disease, clinical presentation in NHL varies; any organ, tissue, or anatomic area can be involved. NHLs typically present with rapidly enlarging masses (Burkitt lymphoma, in particular, grows rapidly) with the most common initial sites including the abdomen, head and neck, and mediastinum; involvement of the bone, skin, CNS, and kidneys is also seen. Physical examination can reveal abdominal pain, distention, fullness, and constipation; nontender lymph node enlargement is also common. Duration of symptoms before a diagnosis is made is typically 1 month or less. Rapid progression can result in conditions that require immediate intervention including[89]:

- Airway obstruction, superior vena cava syndrome, or pleural effusion arising from anterior mediastinal mass.
- Intestinal obstruction, intussusception, inferior vena cava syndrome, ureteral obstruction, and postrenal failure resulting from abdominal masses.
- Cranial nerve palsies, spinal cord compressions, meningitis-like symptoms from CNS lymphoma.
- Critical electrolyte abnormalities due to rapid cellular breakdown in the setting of altered renal function, also known as *tumor lysis syndrome.*

Diagnostic Studies. Diagnostic studies are ordered depending on the location of the lymphoma and symptoms. They include CBC with differential, which may be normal at diagnosis; liver function tests; LDH; uric acid; and electrolyte levels. Unexplained anemia, thrombocytopenia, or leukopenia can be due to bone marrow infiltration, and elevated electrolytes and LDH may indicate rapidly proliferating tumors and tumor lysis syndromes. Imaging studies such as chest radiography, ultrasound, CT or MRI scan, or PET scan of the area in question may demonstrate masses and/or lymphadenopathy in the neck, chest, or abdomen. Staging the extent of the disease is mandatory before beginning treatment and may include gallium and/or bone scans, bone marrow aspirates and biopsies, and lumbar puncture with cerebrospinal fluid analysis.[89,90]

Management. Optimal therapy involves a multidisciplinary approach from the time of diagnosis. Because of rapid developments in treatment and the importance of careful histologic evaluation, these children should be referred to a comprehensive pediatric oncology center for care. NHLs are sensitive to chemotherapy; radiation is used infrequently. Hematopoietic stem cell transplantation is done in some cases of relapse or more aggressive disease.[90] Advances in immunotherapy and gene therapy also show great promise.[91]

Role of the Primary Care Provider in Care of the Child With Cancer

PCPs must be knowledgeable of symptoms suggesting an oncologic process and evaluate appropriately with initial diagnostic studies. If a neoplasm is suspected, a phone call to the nearest comprehensive pediatric oncology/hematology center enables the child to be seen quickly and prevents a delay in diagnosis by waiting for insurance authorization. Staff in these centers can obtain authorization quickly based on clinical findings. As part of coordinated care, the PCP must maintain a relationship with the patient and family and follow the child for well-child care when the disease process is stabilized by (1) securing basic information on the type of cancer, stage, location, and histology; (2) treatments (i.e., chemotherapy, radiation, surgery); (3) listing potential or at-risk late effects and monitoring needs; (4) any psychological issues; and (5) implementing preventive strategies (e.g., immunizations, exercise, diet). A strong collaborative relationship between the PCP and pediatric oncologist is essential. Children with cancer diagnoses may require behavioral health and preventative care, which is frequently best delivered in the primary care setting. In

some settings, PCPs may be asked to provide episodic care for children receiving cancer-directed treatment in conjunction with the pediatric oncologist. Providers should seek education and support from appropriate resources to ensure that patients and families receive optimal care.

Childhood cancer diagnosis is a chronic illness with effects reaching across families and communities. The PCP's established, trusting relationship with patients and families places them in a unique supportive role for families in the face of a childhood cancer diagnosis. Some families have reported a preference for such a diagnosis to be disclosed by their PCP.[92] Throughout the illness course, the PCP plays an essential role in providing sibling support, educating families and communities on childhood cancer, and ensuring referrals are made for appropriate family support. The National Institutes of Health National Cancer Institute has excellent materials for health professionals, parents, and children regarding childhood cancer (www.cancer.gov/types/childhood-cancers).

Late Effects of Childhood Cancers

Remarkable advances have been made in the treatment of childhood cancer. Overall survival rates are now above 80%[81]; however, as survival rates have improved, so has the number of childhood cancer survivors. As a consequence of treatment exposures, many survivors carry an increased risk for late morbidity and mortality including organ system complications, increased risk of secondary malignancies, and social and financial burdens. The PCP plays an essential role in providing focused surveillance for these complications and by facilitating early detection and treatment to preserve health and promote quality of life for this special population.

Any adverse effect or problem that does not resolve after completion of therapy is labeled a late effect of childhood cancer. Late effects can be attributed to radiation therapy, chemotherapy, surgery, hematopoietic stem cell transplant, or combinations of treatments; they can also be associated with the location of the cancer itself, age and development of the child at diagnosis, preexisting conditions in the child before their cancer diagnosis, and other factors. While the chance of developing late effects increases over time, they can occur shortly after treatment, with puberty, or with aging. Research has identified common problems and identified routine surveillance recommendations for patients. Table 38.9 provides a list of therapy-related late effects by organ system.

After treatment is completed, visits with the pediatric oncologist decline. Some survivors may have access to survivorship and late effects clinics at comprehensive pediatric cancer centers, but PCPs also assume care, which includes monitoring for late effects. Providers must be aware of survivors' prior treatment modalities, their associated late effects, risk of occurrence, and standards for risk-based monitoring for such problems. COG created guidelines to assist clinicians in providing comprehensive long-term follow-up for childhood, adolescent, and AYA cancer survivors that are readily available at http://www.survivorshipguidelines.org/. The documents provide resources for obtaining an oncologic history, recommended surveillance based on treatment history, and relevant counseling and educational resources for both the provider and the survivor.

Recent research has also demonstrated the significant impact childhood cancer has on the mental health, social milestones, socioeconomic attainment, and engagement in risky behaviors, and overall health-related quality of life for survivors.[93] PCPs

TABLE 38.9	Potential Therapy-Related Late Effects by Organ System
Organ System	Late Effects
Psychological/Behavioral	Anxiety, depression, risky behaviors, fatigue
Neurocognitive	Attention deficits, impaired executive function, learning difficulties
Auditory	Hearing loss
Ocular	Cataracts, xeropthalmia, retinitis, optic nerve injury
Dermatologic	Fibrosis, altered pigmentation
Cardiovascular	Cardiomyopathy, coronary artery disease, pericarditis
Pulmonary	Pulmonary fibrosis, interstitial pneumonitis
Gastrointestinal	Esophageal stricture, bowel obstruction, bladder fibrosis
Urinary tract	Renal insufficiency, hemorrhagic cystitis, bladder fibrosis
Musculoskeletal	Reduced bone mineral density, osteonecrosis, scoliosis/kyphosis, limb length discrepancy, hypoplasia
Neurologic	Peripheral neuropathy, stroke, leukoencephalopathy
Reproductive	Infertility, gonadal dysfunction
Endocrine/metabolic	Overweight/obesity, growth hormone deficiency, hypothyroidism, precocious puberty, diabetes mellitus
Immune	Functional hyposplenism, chronic infection

Modified from information presented in Landier W, Skinner R, Wallace WH, et al. Surveillance for late effects in childhood cancer survivors. *J Clin Oncol.* 2018;36(21):2216–2222, and Children's Oncology Group. *Long-Term Follow-up Guidelines for Survivors of Childhood, Adolescent and Young Adult Cancers*, Version 5.0. Children's Oncology Group; 2018.

are in an ideal position to monitor and evaluate for physical late effects and provide anticipatory guidance, education, support, and encouragement. A focus on healthy lifestyle choices and dietary practices; avoidance of sun, alcohol, recreational drugs, and tobacco should always be stressed.

Additional Resources

American Childhood Cancer Organization: www.acco.org/
Cooleys Anemia Foundation: https://www.thalassemia.org/
Children's Oncology Group: Survivorship Guidelines: http://www.survivorshipguidelines.org/
CureSearch: National Childhood Cancer Foundation: www.curesearch.org
Leukemia and Lymphoma Society: https://www.lls.org/

National Cancer Institute: Surveillance, Epidemiology, and End Results (SEER) Program.: http://seer.cancer.gov/csr/1975_2014/
National Hemophilia Foundation: https://www.hemophilia.org/
National Institutes of Health: Childhood Cancer: www.cancer.gov/types/childhood-cancers
National Newborn Screening Information: www.cdc.gov/newbornscreening/
Sickle Cell Disease Association of America (SCDAA): www.sicklecelldisease.org

References

1. Scholkmann F, Ostojic D, Isler H, Bassler D, Wolf M, Karen T. Reference ranges for hemoglobin and hematocrit levels in neonates as a function of gestational age (22-42 weeks) and postnatal age (0-29 days): mathematical modeling. *Children (Basel)*. 2019;6(3).
2. Chou ST. Development of the hematopoietic system. In: Kliegman RM, St. Geme JW, Blum NJ, Shah SS, Tasker RC, Wilson KM, eds. *Nelson Textbook of Pediatrics*. 21st ed. Elsevier; 2020.
3. Sontag MK, Yusuf C, Grosse SD, et al. Infants with congenital disorders identified through newborn screening - United States, 2015-2017. *MMWR Morb Mortal Wkly Rep*. 2020;69(36):1265–1268.
4. Safiri S, Kolahi AA, Noori M, et al. Burden of anemia and its underlying causes in 204 countries and territories, 1990-2019: results from the global burden of disease study 2019. *J Hematol Oncol*. 2021;14(1):185.
5. Rothman JA. Iron-deficiency anemia. In: Kliegman R, St. Geme JW, Blum NJ, Shah SS, Tasker RC, Wilson KM, eds. *Nelson Textbook of Pediatrics*; 2020.
6. Mattiello V, Schmugge M, Hengartner H, et al. Diagnosis and management of iron deficiency in children with or without anemia: consensus recommendations of the Spog Pediatric Hematology Working Group. *Eur J Pediatr*. 2020;179(4):527–545.
7. Dev S, Babitt JL. Overview of iron metabolism in health and disease. *Hemodial Int*. 2017;21 suppl 1(suppl 1):S6–S20.
8. Yiannikourides A, Latunde-Dada GO. A short review of iron metabolism and pathophysiology of iron disorders. *Medicines (Basel)*. 2019;6(3).
9. Witmer CM. Hematologic manifestations of systemic disease (including iron deficiency, anemia of inflammation and DIC). *Pediatr Clin North Am*. 2013;60(6):1337–1348.
10. Baker RD, Greer FR, et al. Diagnosis and prevention of iron deficiency and iron-deficiency anemia in infants and young children (0–3 years of age). *Pediatrics*. 2010;126(5):1040–1050.
11. Hagan JF, American Academy of P, Shaw JS, et al. *Bright Futures: Guidelines for Health Supervision of Infants, Children, and Adolescents*. 4th ed. American Academy of Pediatrics; 2017.
12. American Academy of Pediatrics. Recommendations for Preventive Pediatric Health Care. https://www.aap.org/periodicityschedule.
13. Sekhar DL, Murray-Kolb LE, Wang L, et al. Adolescent anemia screening during ambulatory pediatric visits in the United States. *J Community Health*. 2015;40(2):331–338.
14. Oatley H, Borkhoff CM, Chen S, et al. Screening for iron deficiency in early childhood using serum ferritin in the primary care setting. *Pediatrics*. 2018;142(6).
15. Mei Z, Addo OY, Jefferds ME, et al. Physiologically based serum ferritin thresholds for iron deficiency in children and non-pregnant women: a US National Health and Nutrition Examination Surveys (NHANES) Serial Cross-Sectional Study. *Lancet Haematol*. 2021;8(8):e572–e582.
16. Georgieff MK. Iron assessment to protect the developing brain. *Am J Clin Nutr*. 2017;106(suppl_6):1588S–1593S.
17. Guidelines Review Committee on Nutrition and Food Safety. *Who Guideline on Use of Ferritin Concentrations to Assess Iron Status in Individuals and Populations*; 2020.

18. Kemper AR, Fan T, Grossman DC, Phipps MG. Gaps in evidence regarding iron deficiency anemia in pregnant women and young children: summary of US preventive services task force recommendations. *Am J Clin Nutr*. 2017;106(suppl_6):1555S–1558S.

19. World Health Organization (WHO). Monitoring Nutrition Status and Food Safety Events. *C-reactive Protein Concentrations as a Marker of Inflammation or Infection for Interpreting Biomarkers of Micronutrient Status: Vitamin and Mineral Nutrition Information System*; 2014. https://www.who.int/publications/i/item/WHO-NMH-NHD-EPG-14.7.

20. Gallagher PG. Anemia in the pediatric patient. *Blood*. 2022.

21. Powers JM, O'Brien SH. How I Approach iron deficiency with and without anemia. *Pediatr Blood Cancer*. 2019;66(3):e27544.

22. Clark M, Royal J, Seeler R. Interaction of iron deficiency and lead and the hematologic findings in children with severe lead poisoning. *Pediatrics*. 1988;81(2):247–254.

23. Markowitz M. Lead poisoning: an update. *Pediatr Rev*. 2021;42(6):302–315.

24. Ruckart PZ, Jones RL, Courtney JG, et al. Update of the blood lead reference value - United States, 2021. *MMWR Morb Mortal Wkly Rep*. 2021;70(43):1509–1512.

25. Centers for Disease Control and Prevention. *Childhood Lead Poisoning Prevention Program*; 2022. https://www.cdc.gov/nceh/lead/default.htm.

26. Powers JM, Buchanan GR, Adix L, et al. Effect of low-dose ferrous sulfate vs iron polysaccharide complex on hemoglobin concentration in young children with nutritional iron-deficiency anemia: a randomized clinical trial. *JAMA*. 2017;317(22):2297–2304.

27. Powers JM, Buchanan GR. Diagnosis and management of iron deficiency anemia. *Hematol Oncol Clin North Am*. 2014;28(4):729–745, vi-vii.

28. Camaschella C. Iron deficiency. *Blood*. 2019;133(1):30–39.

29. Means RT. Iron deficiency and iron deficiency anemia: implications and impact in pregnancy, fetal development, and early childhood parameters. *Nutrients*. 2020;12(2).

30. McCarthy EK, Dempsey EM, Kiely ME. Iron supplementation in preterm and low-birth-weight infants: a systematic review of intervention studies. *Nutr Rev*. 2019;77(12):865–877.

31. Institute of Medicine (US) Panel on Micronutrients. *Dietary Reference Intakes for Vitamin A, Vitamin K, Arsenic, Boron, Chromium, Copper, Iodine, Iron, Manganese, Molybdenum, Nickel, Silicon, Vanadium, and Zinc*. The National Academies Press; 2001.

32. Abrams SA, Hampton JC, Finn KL. A substantial proportion of 6- to 12-month-old infants have calculated daily absorbed iron below recommendations, especially those who are breastfed. *J Pediatr*. 2021;231:36–42.e2.

33. Kwiatkowski J. Thalassemia syndromes. In: Kliegman R, St. Geme JW, Blum NJ, Shah SS, Tasker RC, Wilson KM, eds. *Nelson Textbook of Pediatrics*. 21st ed. Elsevier; 2020.

34. Viprakasit V, Ekwattanakit S. Clinical classification, screening and diagnosis for thalassemia. *Hematol Oncol Clin North Am*. 2018;32(2):193–211.

35. Farashi S, Harteveld CL. Molecular basis of A-thalassemia. *Blood Cells Mol Dis*. 2018;70:43–53.

36. Vichinsky E, Musallam K, Cappellini MD, eds. *Guidelines for the Management of Non Transfusion Dependent Thalassaemia (NTDT)*. 2nd ed. Thalassaemia International Federation; 2017.

37. Cappellini MD, Cohen A, Porter J, Taher A, eds. *2021 Guidelines for the Management of Transfusion Dependent Thalassaemia (TDT)*. 4th ed. Thalassaemia International Federation; 2021.

38. Strocchio L, Locatelli F. Hematopoietic stem cell transplantation in thalassemia. *Hematol Oncol Clin North Am*. 2018;32(2):317–328.

39. Thompson AA, Walters MC, Kwiatkowski J, et al. Gene therapy in patients with transfusion-dependent B-thalassemia. *N Engl J Med*. 2018;378(16):1479–1493.

40. Motta I, Bou-Fakhredin R, Taher AT, Cappellini MD. Beta thalassemia: new therapeutic options beyond transfusion and iron chelation. *Drugs*. 2020;80(11):1053–1063.

41. Thornburg CD. Megaloblastic anemias. In: Kliegman R, St. Geme JW, Blum NJ, Shah SS, Tasker RC, Wilson KM, eds. *Nelson Textbook of Pediatrics*. 21st ed. Elsevier; 2020.

42. Green R, Allen LH, Bjørke-Monsen AL, et al. Vitamin B(12) deficiency. *Nat Rev Dis Primers*. 2017;3:17040.

43. Burns RA, Woodward GA. Transient erythroblastopenia of childhood: a review for the pediatric emergency medicine physician. *Pediatr Emerg Care*. 2019;35(3):237–240.

44. Thornburg CD. Acquired pure red blood cell anemia. In: Kliegman R, St. Geme JW, Blum NJ, Shah SS, Tasker RC, Wilson KM, eds. *Nelson Textbook of Pediatrics*. 21st ed. Elsevier; 2020. chap 477.

45. Hellström Schmidt S, Tedgård U, Pronk CJ. Breath-holding spells occur disproportionately more often in children with transient erythroblastopenia. *Acta Paediatr*. 2016;105(9):1088–1093.

46. Thornburg CD. Congenital hypoplastic anemia (Diamond-Blackfan anemia). In: Kliegman R, St. Geme JW, Blum NJ, Shah SS, Tasker RC, Wilson KM, eds. *Nelson Textbook of Pediatrics*. 21st ed. Elsevier; 2020.

47. Smith-Whitley K. Hemoglobinopathies, sickle cell disease. In: Kliegman R, St. Geme JW, Blum NJ, Shah SS, Tasker RC, Wilson KM, eds. *Nelson Textbook of Pediatrics*. 21st ed. Elsevier; 2020.

48. Centers for Disease Control and Prevention. Data & Statistics on Sickle Cell Disease. https://www.cdc.gov/ncbddd/sicklecell/data.html.

49. Kato GJ, Piel FB, Reid CD, et al. Sickle cell disease. *Nat Rev Dis Prim*. 2018;4:18010.

50. Pecker LH, Naik RP. The current state of sickle cell trait: implications for reproductive and genetic counseling. *Blood*. 2018;132(22):2331–2338.

51. National Heart, Lung, and Blood Institute. *2014 Expert Panel Report on the Evidence-Based Management of Sickle Cell Disease*; 2014. https://www.nhlbi.nih.gov/sites/default/files/media/docs/sickle-cell-disease-report%20020816_0.pdf.

52. Section on Hematology/Oncology Committee on Genetics. Health supervision for children with sickle cell disease. *Pediatrics*. 2002;109(3):526–535.

53. Centers for Disease Control and Prevention. Child and Adolescent Immunizations Schedule. https://www.cdc.gov/vaccines/schedules/hcp/imz/child-adolescent.html.

54. Kimrey S, Saving KL. Sickle cell disease: a primer for primary care providers. *Pediatr Ann*. 2020;49(1):e43–e49.

55. Lee GM. Preventing infections in children and adults with asplenia. *Hematol Am Soc Hematol Educ Program*. 2020;2020(1):328–335.

56. Merguerian MD, Gallagher PG. Hereditary sperocytosis. In: Kliegman R, St. Geme JW, Blum NJ, Shah SS, Tasker RC, Wilson KM, eds. *Nelson Textbook of Pediatrics*. 21st ed. Elsevier; 2020.

57. Brandow AM. Enzymatic defects, glucose-6-phosphate dehydrogenase deficiency and related deficiencies. In: Kliegman R, St.Geme JW, Blum NJ, Shah SS, Tasker RC, Wilson KM, eds. *Nelson Textbook of Pediatrics*. 21st ed. Elsevier; 2020.

58. Rodeghiero F, Pabinger I, Ragni M, et al. Fundamentals for a systematic approach to mild and moderate inherited bleeding disorders: an EHA Consensus Report. *Hemasphere*. 2019;3(4):e286.

59. Haley KM. Platelet disorders. *Pediatr Rev*. 2020;41(5):224–235.

60. Elbatarny M, Mollah S, Grabell J, et al. Normal range of bleeding scores for the Isth-Bat: adult and pediatric data from the Merging Project. *Haemophilia*. 2014;20(6):831–835.

61. Casey LJ, Tuttle A, Grabell J, et al. Generation and optimization of the self-administered pediatric bleeding questionnaire and its validation as a screening tool for Von Willebrand disease. *Pediatr Blood Cancer*. 2017;64(10).

62. Scott JP, Flood VH, Raffini LJ. Hemostasis, clinical and laboratory evaluation of hemostasis. In: Kliegman R, St. Geme JW, Blum NJ, Shah SS, Tasker RC, Wilson KM, eds. *Nelson Textbook of Pediatrics*. 21st ed. Elsevier; 2020.

63. Rodriguez V, Warad D. Pediatric coagulation disorders. *Pediatr Rev*. 2016;37(7):279–291.

64. Kühne T. Diagnosis and management of immune thrombocytopenia in childhood. *Hämostaseologie*. 2017;37(1):36–44.

65. Provan D, Arnold DM, Bussel JB, et al. Updated international consensus report on the investigation and management of primary immune thrombocytopenia. *Blood Adv.* 2019;3(22):3780–3817.

66. Scott JP, Flood VH. Factor Viii or factor Ix deficiency (hemophilia a or B). In: Kliegman R, St. Geme JW, Blum NJ, Shah SS, Tasker RC, Wilson KM, eds. *Nelson Textbook of Pediatrics.* 21st ed. Elsevier; 2020.

67. Berntorp E, Fischer K, Hart DP, et al. Haemophilia. *Nat Rev Dis Prim.* 2021;7(1):45.

68. Scott JP, Flood VH. Von Willebrand disease. In: Kliegman R, St. Geme JW, Blum NJ, Shah SS, Tasker RC, wilson KM, eds. *Nelson Textbook of Pediatrics.* 21st ed. Elsevier; 2020. chap 504.

69. Centers for Disease Control and Prevention National Center on Birth Defects and Developmental Disabilities. Data and Statistics on Hemophilia. https://www.cdc.gov/ncbddd/hemophilia/data.html.

70. Centers for Disease Control and Prevention National Center on Birth Defects and Developmental Disabilities. Data and Statistics on Von Willebrand Disease. https://www.cdc.gov/ncbddd/vwd/data.html.

71. Srivastava A, Santagostino E, Dougall A, et al. WFH guidelines for the management of hemophilia, 3rd Edition. *Haemophilia.* 2020;26(suppl 6):1–158.

72. Moorehead PC, Chan AKC, Lemyre B, et al. A practical guide to the management of the fetus and newborn with hemophilia. *Clin Appl Thromb Hemost.* 2018;24(9_suppl):29s–41s.

73. Connell NT, Flood VH, Brignardello-Petersen R, et al. Ash isth NHF WFH 2021 guidelines on the management of von Willebrand disease. *Blood Adv.* 2021;5(1):301–325.

74. Raffini LJ, Scott JP. Hereditary predisposition to thrombosis. In: Kliegman R, St. Geme JW, Blum NJ, Shah SS, Tasker RC, Wilson KM, eds. *Nelson Textbook of Pediatrics.* 21st ed. Elsevier; 2020.

75. Teal S, Edelman A. Contraception selection, effectiveness, and adverse effects: a review. *JAMA.* 2021;326(24):2507–2518.

76. Monagle P, Cuello CA, Augustine C, et al. American Society of Hematology 2018 guidelines for management of venous thromboembolism: treatment of pediatric venous thromboembolism. *Blood Adv.* 2018;2(22):3292–3316.

77. Michniacki TF, Walkovich KJ. Leukopenia. In: Kliegman R, St. Geme JW, Blum NJ, Shah SS, Tasker RC, Wilson KM, eds. *Nelson Textbook of Pediatrics.* 21st ed. Elsevier; 2020.

78. Atallah-Yunes SA, Ready A, Newburger PE. Benign ethnic neutropenia. *Blood Rev.* 2019;37:100586.

79. Kebudi R, Kizilocak H. Febrile neutropenia in children with cancer: approach to diagnosis and treatment. *Curr Pediatr Rev.* 2018;14(3):204–209.

80. Yu HH, Yang YH, Chiang BL. Chronic granulomatous disease: a comprehensive review. *Clin Rev Allergy Immunol.* 2021;61(2):101–113.

81. Siegel RL, Miller KD, Fuchs HE, et al. Cancer statistics, 2021. *CA Cancer J Clin.* 2021;71(1):7–33.

82. Siegel DA, Li J, Henley SJ, et al. Geographic variation in pediatric cancer incidence - United States, 2003-2014. *MMWR Morb Mortal Wkly Rep.* 2018;67(25):707–713.

83. Asselin BL. Epidemiology of childhood and adolescent cancer. In: Kliegman R, St. Geme JW, Blum NJ, Shah SS, Tasker RC, Wilson KM, eds. *Nelson Textbook of Pediatrics.* Elsevier; 2020. chap 518.

84. Siegel DA, Henley SJ, Li J, et al. Rates and trends of pediatric acute lymphoblastic leukemia - United States, 2001-2014. *MMWR Morb Mortal Wkly Rep.* 2017;66(36):950–954.

85. Flerlage JE, Hiniker SM, Armenian S, et al. Pediatric hodgkin lymphoma, version 3.2021. *J Natl Compr Canc Netw.* 2021;19(6):733–754.

86. Connors JM, Cozen W, Steidl C, et al. Hodgkin lymphoma. *Nat Rev Dis Primers.* 2020;6(1):61.

87. National Cancer Institute. *NCCR Explorer: An Interactive Website for NCCR Cancer Statistics*; 2022. https://Nccrexplorer.Ccdi.Cancer.Gov/.

88. Goldman SC, Hochberg J, Cairo MS. *Lymphoma. Nelson Textbook of Pediatrics.* 21st ed. Elsevier; 2020.

89. Buhtoiarov IN. Pediatric lymphoma. *Pediatr Rev.* 2017;38(9):410–423.

90. Barth M, Xavier AC, Armenian S, et al. Pediatric aggressive mature b-cell lymphomas. *J Natl Compr Canc Netw.* 2022;20(11):1267–1275.

91. Derebas J, Panuciak K, Margas M, et al. The new treatment methods for non-Hodgkin lymphoma in pediatric patients. *Cancers (Basel).* 2022;14(6).

92. Wharton B, Beeler DM, Cooper S. The "Day Zero Talk": the initial communication of a pediatric oncology diagnosis by primary care physicians and other primary care providers. *J Cancer Educ.* 2020;18:18.

93. Brinkman TM, Recklitis CJ, Michel G, et al. Psychological symptoms, social outcomes, socioeconomic attainment, and health behaviors among survivors of childhood cancer: current state of the literature. *J Clin Oncol.* 2018;36(21):2190–2197.

39

Endocrine and Metabolic Disorders

BETH HEUER

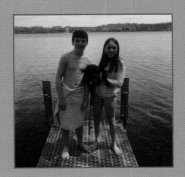

Endocrine and metabolic disorders affect many pediatric patients and range from relatively common (e.g., type 1 and type 2 diabetes mellitus, hypothyroidism) to extremely rare. Many children with endocrine and/or metabolic disorders are comanaged by primary care providers (PCPs) in collaboration with specialists including endocrinologists, geneticists, and adolescent medicine providers. Although a great degree of overlap happens in these disorders, distinctive processes occur in each. As such, specific conditions will involve different approaches to assessment and management. Endocrine and metabolic diseases also include processes such as osteoporosis and genetic disorders including cystic fibrosis; these disorders are covered elsewhere in this text. This chapter begins with an overview of the anatomy, physiology, and pathophysiology of the endocrine and metabolic system and general issues related to the assessment and management of the disorders.

Anatomy and Physiology

The endocrine system regulates growth, pubertal development and reproduction, homeostasis of the individual, and the production, storage, and utilization of energy. While the endocrine system was previously understood to function via hormones produced in glands with action at a distant site, hormones may also act in a *para*crine fashion affecting target cells *near* the cells that produce them, or in an *auto*crine fashion in which the target cells of the hormones are the *same* cells that produce them (Table 39.1).

Many endocrine glands are controlled by the hypothalamic-pituitary axis. The hypothalamus is critical in the maintenance of homeostasis and is modulated in part by hormones that operate using both positive and negative feedback loops. The hypothalamus then regulates the pituitary gland by releasing factors formed in hypothalamic neurosecretory neurons. The pituitary gland responds through positive and negative feedback of hormones and by paracrine and autocrine factors of the pituitary itself. Many of the hormones of the hypothalamic-pituitary axis (or molecules that share structural similarity to such hormones) are made in other body tissues. The hypothalamic-pituitary axis also links to the adrenal glands (hypothalamic-pituitary-adrenal axis) and regulates stress responses among other bodily functions, and into the gonads (hypothalamic-pituitary-gonadal axis) to regulate the reproductive system.

An example of a feedback loop that is hormonally activated is that thyrotropin-releasing hormone (TRH) from the hypothalamus stimulates pituitary thyrotropin (thyroid-stimulating hormone [TSH]) secretion, which in turn stimulates thyroid hormone production (triiodothyronine [T_3] and thyroxine [T_4]). Thyroid hormone levels provide feedback to the hypothalamus and pituitary, thereby suppressing TRH and TSH secretion so that a balance is reached (Fig. 39.1) In a similar fashion, the adrenal glands secrete corticosteroids, and the gonads produce progesterone, androgens, and estradiol, all of which influence hypothalamic and pituitary hormone production. For some systems, the hormone secretion set point changes as individuals develop.

Hormone secretion can be regulated by nerve cells and by factors important in the immune system (e.g., cytokines interact with hormones that influence weight homeostasis). Other hormones are released within body tissues, such as adiponectin and leptin, which are released from adipose tissue. Adiponectin helps with insulin sensitivity and inflammation, and low adiponectin levels are associated with type 2 diabetes, obesity, and metabolic syndrome. Leptin helps to regulate hunger and control energy expenditure to help maintain a consistent weight. Obesity results in leptin resistance, which reduces the body's sensation of feeling full or satiated.

Metabolic function in the body involves complex biochemical processes to transform essential amino acids, carbohydrates, and lipids into substances or energy that can be used at the cellular level to perform essential cell functions. These biochemical processes or metabolic pathways are driven by enzyme activity. Any disruption along these pathways, whether congenital or acquired, can lead to multisystemic dysfunction.

Pathophysiology

Endocrine abnormalities occur when an alteration in the regulation of the normal feedback system results in the hyposecretion or hypersecretion of one or more hormones. Multiple factors cause alterations in hormone production. These factors include tumors, trauma, infection, systemic disease, genetic disorders, congenital malformation or agenesis of an endocrine gland, idiopathic causes, and iatrogenic causes (e.g., medications). The defect or problem can originate at the pituitary-hypothalamic level, because of organ abnormalities, or for

TABLE 39.1	Common Hormones and Their Role in the Endocrine System	
Source of Production	**Hormone Secreted**	**Hormone Function**
Adrenal glands	Aldosterone	Regulate water, salt, blood pressure
	Corticosteroids	Maintain blood glucose & blood pressure; regulate salt and water balance; role in antiinflammation; enhances muscle strength
	Epinephrine	Increase blood flow, O_2 consumption, heart rate
	Norepinephrine	Maintain blood pressure
	Dehydroepiandrosterone (DHEA)	Substrates for placental estrogen biosynthesis, then increase at onset of adrenarche
	Dehydroepiandrosterone sulfate (DHEAS)	
Pituitary gland	Antidiuretic hormone (vasopressin)	Control blood pressure; affects water retention in the kidneys
	Adrenocorticotropic hormone (ACTH)	Production of estrogen in women and testosterone in men; oogenesis and spermatogenesis
	Growth hormone (GH)	Growth and development; fat distribution; protein production
	Luteinizing hormone (LH) and follicle stimulating hormone (FSH)	Production of estrogen in women and testosterone in men; oogenesis and spermatogenesis
	Oxytocin	Stimulates milk production in the breast and contraction of the uterus
	Prolactin	Initiates/maintains milk production in the breast; impacts sex hormone levels
	Thyroid-stimulating hormone (TSH)	Stimulates production and secretion of thyroid hormones
Hypothalamus	Growth hormone-releasing hormone (GHRH)	Regulates release of GH in the pituitary gland
	Gonadotropin releasing hormone (GnRH)	Regulates production of LH/FSH in the pituitary gland
	Corticotropin releasing hormone (CRH)	Regulates adrenocorticotropin hormone release in the pituitary gland
Thymus	Humoral factors	Assists in development of the lymphoid system
Thyroid gland	Thyroid hormone	Regulates metabolism; affects growth, maturation, and nervous system activity
Parathyroid gland	Parathyroid hormone (PTH)	Regulation of blood calcium levels
Kidneys	Renin and angiotensin	Regulates aldosterone production from the adrenal glands; control of blood pressure
	Erythropoietin	Red blood cell production
Pancreas	Glucagon	Increase blood glucose levels
	Insulin	Lower blood glucose levels; stimulate metabolism of fat, glucose, and protein
Ovaries	Estrogen	Development of female sexual characteristics and reproductive development; function of breasts and uterus; bone health
	Progesterone	Stimulates uterine lining development; prepare breasts for milk production
Testes	Testosterone	Development of male secondary sexual characteristics; increases bone and muscle mass
	Estradiol	Modulates libido, erectile function, and spermatogenesis
Pineal gland	Melatonin	Regulation of circadian rhythms

unknown reasons that lead to unresponsiveness to the endogenous hormones. Hypothyroidism and hyperthyroidism are examples of disease entities in which the interrelationships of the hypothalamic-pituitary-thyroid axis may be altered at any one of these sites.

Metabolic diseases are typically related to inborn errors of metabolism (IEMs), where a genetic mutation leads to disrupted biochemical functioning. Acquired metabolic disorders arise from external factors (such as excessive caloric intake or poor physical activity) and may occur as complications of severe diseases or illnesses (such as renal failure or toxic ingestions).

Assessment

Endocrine and metabolic disorders cause constitutional symptoms and multisystemic organ dysfunction. Assessment requires a thorough family history, physical examination, and specific diagnostic testing for the suspected disorder.

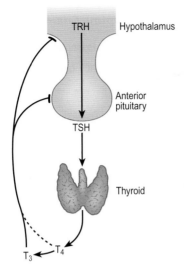

• **Fig. 39.1** Hypothalamic-Pituitary-Thyroid Axis. Thyrotropin-releasing hormone (TRH), from the hypothalamus, stimulates the release of thyroid-stimulating hormone (TSH) from the anterior pituitary. The TSH stimulates the thyroid gland to release T_3 and T_4, which exert a negative feedback inhibitory effect on the hypothalamus and pituitary gland. (From Naish J, Syndercombe Court D. *Medical Sciences*. 3rd ed. Elsevier; 2019.)

History

- Maternal complications or exposures during pregnancy
- Growth pattern since birth
- Recent alterations in growth pattern
- Use of medications, including herbs and supplements that could affect endocrine or metabolic function
- Presence of any unusual odors, recurrent vomiting, or unexplained lethargy
- Age when secondary sexual characteristics began to develop
- Diet and exercise history
- Parental and sibling heights and ages at onset of puberty
- Family history of endocrine, autoimmune, or metabolic disorders (e.g., diabetes mellitus, thyroid disease)
- Obtain a family history of at least three generations and (if applicable) consanguinity and ethnicity

Physical Examination

A detailed examination should include the following:
- Measure stature (length/height).
  - Supine *length* (also referred to as *recumbent height*) is preferred for children younger than 2 years old or until walking well. *Height* is measured using a stadiometer for children older than 2 years and walking well.
  - Plot height, weight, and head circumference on a standardized growth chart appropriate to the child's age and sex. The Centers for Disease Control and Prevention (CDC) recommends that the World Health Organization (WHO) growth charts be used to monitor growth in children younger than 2 years.[1] CDC growth charts are used for children from 2 to 20 years of age. Serial measurements are critical to assess growth patterns over time. In addition, growth charts are available for children with certain genetic conditions, such as trisomy 21 (Down syndrome) and Turner (45, X0) syndrome, and should be used to assess growth patterns of children with these conditions.

- Check for proportionate appearance: measure sitting and standing heights for upper to lower segment (US:LS) ratio and arm span.
- Assess *height age* (the age corresponding to the child's height when plotted at the 50th percentile on a growth chart) and *growth velocity* (linear growth in centimeters or inches over the past year).
- Inspect the child's genitalia for signs of typical or atypical genitalia.
- Identify the stage of sexual development using sexual maturity rating (Tanner staging).
- Note facial, axillary, and pubic hair for presence, distribution, and texture. Note male-pattern alopecia in females.
- Examine the skin for presence of striae and/or acanthosis nigricans of the neck, axilla, breast, knuckles, and skin folds.
- Palpate the thyroid gland for symmetry and size, noting enlargement or presence of nodules and/or prelaryngeal lymph nodes (located anterior to the larynx), known as *Delphian nodes*.
- Assess for presence of dysmorphic features.
- Examine the abdomen noting any organomegaly.
- Complete general neurologic examination.

Acquired endocrine disorders are often due to either hyposecretion or hypersecretion of a specific hormone or combination of hormones, and the child may or may not appear ill. Signs of dehydration and tachycardia are physical findings associated with endocrine pathology. Newborns with metabolic disorders may initially appear well, but physical signs develop with postnatal metabolic activity. Characteristic physical findings associated with specific disease entities are presented later in this chapter. Diagnostic testing depends on presenting symptoms and practice guidelines and will be discussed in more detail with each disease presentation.

Management Strategies

General Measures

Clinical consequences for the child affected by an endocrine or metabolic disorder vary from mild to severe. If undiagnosed and untreated, some disorders may lead to irreversible intellectual or physical disability, neurologic or end-organ damage, and/or death. Early detection, accurate diagnosis, and timely intervention are necessary to achieve favorable outcomes. Chronic disease sequelae and their effects on lifestyle must also be addressed and include family, school, peer, and emotional adjustment; body image, self-esteem, and social competence; disease understanding, acceptance, and self-care; and regimen adherence. A successful outcome depends on the patient and family receiving support and encouragement in self-care, learning about the disease, and understanding the patient-parent role in managing a long-term illness or chronic condition. See disease entities for specific management strategies.

Genetic Counseling

Genetic testing is an indispensable component of the comprehensive endocrine diagnostic evaluation[2] and genetic counseling is often necessary. Implications are significant for the family of a child with endocrine or metabolic disorders that are genetically linked, such as Turner syndrome, Prader-Willi syndrome, familial hyperinsulinemic hypoglycemia, maturity-onset diabetes of the young (MODY), and others.

General Medication Considerations

Pharmacologic therapy, including hormone replacement, whether temporary or lifelong, is often essential. Short, clear instructions about medications are important; how much to give, when and how to administer, possible side effects, and when to adjust medication are key messages to convey. Long-term adherence to medications can become problematic with chronic illnesses and requires constant vigilance on the part of providers who interact with the child.

Dietary Considerations

Certain endocrine and metabolic diseases (e.g., diabetes, phenylketonuria) require strict adherence to dietary plans and restrictions. Parents, patients, caregivers, and school personnel must be aware of the dietary needs and restrictions and the effect of diet on the disease process. Families must also be given support to adjust to the economic, social, and psychological demands created by such restrictions.

Patient and Family Education

Close supervision and frequent follow-up are necessary for children with metabolic and endocrine disorders. These children are best evaluated both initially and over time by an interprofessional team with expertise in pediatric endocrinology and metabolism or clinical genetics. Parent and patient education should include:
- Nature of the disorder, treatment plan, and possible complications.
- Plan for long-term follow-up, including the timing and process of transition to adult care services.
- Family-based disease management strategies and appropriate level of self-management responsibility for the child based on age and developmental stage.

The PCP, as part of the interprofessional team, is in an ideal position to reinforce the patient's plan of care and provide ongoing support. In addition, essential primary healthcare needs and anticipatory guidance cannot be overlooked.

Endocrine Disrupting Chemicals

There is growing public awareness about possible adverse effects in humans from exposure to chemicals that can interfere with the endocrine system. Endocrine disrupting chemicals (EDCs) are chemicals that interfere with the way the body's hormones work.[3] These substances are found in industrial chemicals (which can then leach into the soil and enter the food chain), pesticides, fungicides, plastics, manufactured goods, and personal care products including cosmetics. Some EDCs mimic hormones and "trick" the body into thinking that it should respond to the influence of the chemical. Other EDCs block natural hormones from doing their jobs. EDCs have been linked with neurodevelopmental disorders, increased cancer risk, and immune and reproductive dysfunction. There remains an ongoing concern for sustained exposure to EDCs in infants and children who mouth toys made from plastics that contain these chemicals.[4] See Table 39.2 for a list of EDCs.

Disorders of Endocrine Function

The most common endocrine pathologies of childhood may be grouped into the following areas:

TABLE 39.2	Endocrine Disrupting Chemicals
Chemicals	**Examples**
Pesticides	DDT, Chlorpyrifos, Atrazine, 2,4-D, Glyphosate
Antibacterials	Triclosan
Industrial solvents and lubricants and their byproducts	Polychlorinated biphenyls (PCBs), dioxin
Electronics and building materials	Brominated flame retardants, PCBs
Plastics and food storage materials	Bisphenol A (BPA), phthalates, phenols
Personal care products, medical tubing	Phthalates, parabens, UV filters
Children's products	Cadmium, lead, phthalates
Clothing, textiles	Perfluorochemicals

- Growth disorders
- Differences in sex development
- Disorders of pubertal development
- Adrenal conditions
- Thyroid conditions
- Diabetes mellitus, types 1 and 2
- Posterior pituitary gland dysfunction

Growth Disorders

Children grow in a predictable way, and deviation from a normal growth pattern can be the first sign of an endocrine disorder. Accurate and reliable serial growth measurements must be collected to assess a pattern of growth and current growth velocity. A child's predicted growth potential is based on genetic potential and may change with altered nutritional status and illness patterns. An estimate of the child's expected stature (±2 standard deviations where 1 standard deviation equals 2 inches) can be made by calculating a sex-adjusted mid-parental target) height:
- Boys: [(father's height in inches) + (mother's height in inches)/2] + 2.5 inches
- Girls: [(father's height in inches) + (mother's height in inches)/2] − 2.5 inches

Growth disorders may be classified as primary or secondary. *Primary* growth disorders include skeletal dysplasias, chromosomal abnormalities (e.g., Turner syndrome), and genetic short stature. *Secondary* growth disorders may result from poor nutrition, chronic disease, an endocrine disorder, and idiopathic constitutional growth delay (CGD) (Box 39.1). The following discussion focuses on growth hormone deficiency (GHD) and CGD. Table 39.3 reviews the characteristics of GHD and CGD.

Growth Hormone Deficiency

Growth hormone (GH) is an anterior pituitary hormone released in response to sleep, exercise, and hypoglycemia. Secretion of GH occurs in a series of irregular and pulsatile bursts throughout the day and night with most GH activity occurring during sleep. GH

• BOX 39.1 **Chronic Illnesses Contributing to Growth Failure**

Gastrointestinal disease
- Celiac disease
- Inflammatory bowel disease
- Cystic fibrosis

Cardiovascular disease
- Cyanotic heart disease
- Congestive heart failure

Renal disease
- Uremia
- Renal tubular acidosis

Hematologic disorders
- Chronic anemia

Inborn errors of metabolism

Chronic infection

Anorexia nervosa

---

stimulates insulin-like growth factor (IGF) secretion and action. In addition, insulin-like growth factor binding proteins (IGFBPs) extend the serum half-life of IGFs and transport them to target cells.[5] The GH–insulin-like growth factor (IGF)-I axis is a key endocrine mechanism regulating linear growth in children.[6] Of note, low IGF-1 levels are also associated with chronic disease states, hypothyroidism, diabetes, renal disease, and poor nutrition, thus IGF-1 measurement is not a reliable screening test for short stature in youth with these conditions.[5] GHD can be either congenital or acquired, and individuals may also be resistant to GH.

Clinical Findings

History. A history obtained to evaluate the short or slowly growing child should include:
- Details of pregnancy, delivery, and newborn period
  - Mother's health during pregnancy
  - Labor and delivery course and presence of complications
  - Birth length, weight, and head circumference
  - Neonatal course, including a history of prolonged jaundice, hypoglycemia, and/or presence of micropenis (often diagnostic of congenital GHD)
  - Dysmorphic features, especially midline facial defects or eye abnormalities
- Parents' and siblings' height, weight, and growth pattern (calculate mid-parental height)
- Age at which growth was first noted to decelerate
- Presence of chronic illness(es)
- Symptoms of hypothyroidism or other known pituitary hormone deficiency
- Trauma or insult to the central nervous system (CNS)
- Treatment with cranial radiation
- Nutritional status

Physical Examination. Physical examination of the child with concerns for growth delay should include:
- Identification of dysmorphic features associated with GHD including frontal bossing, "cherubic" facial features, and delayed tooth eruption.[7]
- Presence of midline defect (e.g., cleft palate, single central incisor) suggests the possibility of a growth-hormone axis abnormality.
- Evaluation of the fundi for signs of increased intracranial pressure.

- Palpation of the thyroid gland for the presence of a goiter or nodules.
- Development of secondary sexual characteristics with the evaluation of sexual maturity rating (Tanner stage).
  - In boys, the testicular volume should be measured using a Prader orchidometer
- Measurement of body proportions include:
  - Recumbent length or height.
  - Arm span—the distance between the tips of the fingers when the patient holds both arms outstretched horizontally while standing against a solid surface.
  - Upper-to-lower (U/L) body segment ratio—determined by subtraction of the measurement from the symphysis pubis to the floor (known as the lower segment) from the total height. Interpretation of the U/L body segment ratio is dependent on the age of the child.
    - Body proportion varies during childhood. The U/L ratio is approximately 1.7 at birth; 1.3 at 3 years old; 1:1 at 10 years old; and 0.89 to 0.95 in postpubertal children.
- Neurologic signs of an intracranial lesion.

Diagnostic Studies. If growth velocity is subnormal (including when prior heights are not available), initial evaluation should include:
- Serum glucose (hypoglycemia or hyperglycemia)
- Complete blood count (CBC) and erythrocyte sedimentation rate (ESR)
- Urinalysis and chemistry panel
- Screening for gastrointestinal disorders as appropriate (e.g., celiac disease screening [tissue transglutaminase immunoglobulin A or tTG-IgA], irritable bowel disease [ESR, stool for ova and parasites)
- Growth factors (IGF-1) and insulin-like growth factor–binding protein 3 [IGFBP-3])
- Thyroid function tests: Free T_4 and TSH should be obtained to exclude both pituitary TSH deficiency and primary hypothyroidism
- Bone age radiograph of left wrist and hand
  - Delayed bone age in a small-stature child with decreased growth velocity may suggest the possibility of malnutrition, chronic illness, endocrine disorders, or possibly psychosocial causes of growth failure.[8]
- Karyotype to rule out Turner syndrome in girls
  - Girls with Turner mosaicism may not manifest the typical clinical findings of Turner syndrome (e.g., cubitus valgus, webbing of the neck), thus highlighting the importance of karyotyping all females presenting with short stature.
- As indicated, other genetic testing to rule out syndromic causes of short stature, such as Russell-Silver syndrome, Noonan syndrome, and Prader-Willi syndrome.
- Measurement of GH production may be necessary. Because the secretion of GH is pulsatile, random serum measurement of the hormone is inappropriate. GH stimulation testing (using agents such as arginine, levodopa, clonidine, and/or glucagon) is needed to accurately assess GH production. The most recent guidelines (2016) from the Pediatric Endocrine Society note that providers should not rely on the results of a GH stimulation test as the sole diagnostic criterion of GH deficiency.[9]

Differential Diagnosis

Pediatric patients with short stature often have multiple factors contributing to their stature. Many chronic illnesses can slow linear growth, likely through a variety of mechanisms including

TABLE 39.3　Characteristics of Growth Hormone Deficiency and Constitutional Growth Delay in Children

Condition	Etiology	Onset	Presentation	Endocrine/Metabolic Disturbance
Growth hormone deficiency (GHD)	Idiopathic (most common) Pituitary or hypothalamic disease Trauma Minor organic hypothalamic lesion Infection Radiation	Congenital or acquired	Slow growth rate with normal birth weight Signs and symptoms of increased intracranial pressure Microphallus Proportional short stature Delayed bone age	Deficiency or impairment in secretion of growth hormone–releasing hormone
Constitutional growth delay (CGD)	Variation of normal growth Not a disease	First years of life with impaired growth	Growth velocity is normal after 3 years of age Delayed puberty with pubertal growth spurt Delayed bone age Positive family history	None—final height is appropriate for parents' height

---

• BOX 39.2　US Food and Drug Administration–Approved Indications for Growth Hormone Therapy

- Chronic kidney disease
- Growth hormone deficiency
- Idiopathic short stature
- Noonan syndrome
- Prader-Willi syndrome
- *SHOX* gene haploinsufficiency or mutation
- Small for gestational age without catch-up growth
- Turner syndrome

---

malnutrition, acidosis, anorexia, and deficiencies of minerals (e.g., zinc, iron) and vitamins necessary for growth (see Box 39.1). Typically, children with poor growth because of chronic illness are underweight for their height; their weight gain slows before growth deceleration. Deficiency of thyroid and/or sex hormones is characterized by subnormal growth velocity, normal to increased weight for height, and delay in bone age.

Management

Children should be referred to a pediatric endocrinologist for further assessment and testing if hypothyroidism, low IGF-1, and IGFBP-3, or other hormone deficiency is confirmed or for unexplained persistent slow growth without evidence of chronic illness. Treatment with GH is strongly recommended in children and adolescents with GHD to accelerate growth rate and foster attainment of normal adult height.[10] The US Food and Drug Administration (FDA) has currently approved eight indications for GH therapy (Box 39.2), including in children born small for gestational age with no catch-up growth in early life, idiopathic short stature, and several genetic disorders associated with poor linear growth. Initial dosing of GH (somatropin) is based on a child's body weight, with doses ranging from 0.16 to 0.24 mg/kg/week (22–35 mcg/kg/day) and then subsequent dosing is individualized. Children receiving GH should have their height monitored several times per year and IGF-1 levels should be monitored at least annually.[8]

There are concerns about the long-term safety of GH use, especially in patients with specific risk factors (e.g., certain genetic syndromes such as Noonan syndrome, and those with obesity or a family history of cardiac disease). There appears to be no increased

risk of cancer development related to GH administration in children who have idiopathic GHD, idiopathic short stature, or those who were small for gestational age. There can be an increased risk of diabetes due to the effects of GH on glucose metabolism.[11] Additional reported side effects of GH include headache, arthralgia, scoliosis, and injection-site reaction.[12]

The timely initiation of GH therapy is instrumental in allowing children to achieve their genetic height potential. Adherence to the GH treatment injection regimen in patients with GHD is necessary, especially during the first 2 years of treatment. Research has shown that each missed injection per week in the first 2 years resulted in 0.11 standard deviations less height gain.[13] An individualized treatment approach should be taken to decide whether to discontinue pediatric dosing before the attainment of this growth velocity.

Constitutional Growth Delay

Constitutional delay of growth and puberty is a variant of normal growth and should not be considered a disease entity. When the child has no evidence of chronic illness, has a delay in bone age, and is growing at a normal rate for bone age, the likely diagnosis is CGD. These children generally reach normal adult height, although they may be slightly shorter compared with other family members.

Clinical Findings

History. The history may include the following:
- Normal length and weight at birth
- Slowed linear growth between 1 and 3 years old and then normal growth velocity; normal height velocity is the most critical factor in diagnosing CGD
- Height ≤ third percentile on standardized growth charts
- Delayed pubertal development
- History of similar growth patterns in other family members: often there is a family history of at least one family member with a delayed onset of puberty and/or growth than what would be expected

Physical Examination. Findings on physical examination include:
- Delayed bone age with growth velocity normal for bone age
- Final height prediction based on bone age within a range of calculated target height
- Neurologic examination within normal limits

Diagnostic Studies. The same screening tests used to evaluate GHD are performed to rule out pathologic conditions. A bone age radiograph can often be helpful in distinguishing between CGD and idiopathic short stature. A delayed bone age along with a family history of delayed puberty in at least one parent can help confirm the diagnosis of constitutional growth delay.[14] A child with idiopathic short stature will have a bone age consistent with his or her chronologic age.

Management

Reassurance and support should be provided to the child and family regarding ultimate height and development. An endocrine referral may be necessary to differentiate CGD from GHD and for possible hormone replacement therapy. The most current International Pediatric Guidelines recommend priming with sex steroids before GH stimulation testing for prepubertal boys older than 11 years or prepubertal girls older than 10 years to prevent unnecessary GH treatment in children in whom a diagnosis of constitutional delay of growth and puberty may be likely.[15] In females, priming is typically accomplished using oral 17β-estradiol or stilbestrol for two to seven evenings preceding the test. In males, intramuscular (IM) testosterone is administered 1 week before the test.[16]

Growth Excess

In contrast to those with CGD, some children are tall as young children, compared to family members, and enter puberty early, yet ultimately reach a height within the normal range for their family. Rarely will this accelerated growth require referral to a pediatric endocrinologist. Tall stature in comparison with parents' height or rapid growth velocity in childhood may represent an underlying abnormality. These include:

- Primary skeletal abnormalities, such as Marfan syndrome, Klinefelter syndrome (47, XXY), and other overgrowth syndromes such as Beckwith-Wiedemann and Sotos syndromes.
- Overnutrition that advances the bone age and the timing of puberty: In these children, weight gain occurs first, and the weight percentile is further above the growth curve than the height percentile.
- Excess adrenal androgens or gonadal steroids: These children have physical examination findings of early puberty.

Diagnostic Testing

A bone age study should be obtained. Normal bone age in a tall child growing in concordance with their genetic potential is reassuring, and laboratory testing is not routinely required in cases of familial/constitutional tall stature. Baseline laboratory testing includes IGF-1, IGFBP-3, TSH, free T_4, and karyotype if indicated.[17] Additional testing may include evaluation of gonadotropins and sex hormones, glucose suppression test, and brain magnetic resonance imaging (MRI) to rule out pituitary pathology.

Management

Treatment strategies are dependent on the underlying etiology. Patients with precocious puberty are tall during childhood. If left untreated, however, these children develop short stature into adulthood due to premature closure of the growth plates. Providers should consider referring for endocrine consultation for the following:

- Growth velocity significantly higher than expected for age and pubertal status.

- Tall stature with inappropriate pubertal status for age.
- Height prediction corrected for bone age places at a much higher percentile than mid-parental height.
- Concern for abnormal body proportions or dysmorphology with tall stature.
- When a diagnosis of familial/constitutional tall stature cannot be confidently made.

Differences in Sex Development

Differences of sex development otherwise referred to as *disorders of sex development* (DSDs), are congenital conditions in which the development of chromosomal, gonadal, or anatomic sex is abnormal.[18] Abnormalities of sexual differentiation are usually present in the neonatal period or early infancy with atypical genitalia. These disorders may also be diagnosed prenatally with ultrasound and/or amniocentesis. Some disorders are not diagnosed, however, until the pediatric patient experiences atypical pubertal development or when fertility issues are discovered. Physical findings include clitoromegaly (with or without a common urogenital sinus), female-appearing external genitalia with a notable labial or inguinal mass, posterior labial fusion, micropenis, hypospadias, and nonpalpable testes.[19] DSDs occur when the XX fetus is exposed to excess androgen in utero, the XY fetus is unable to produce or respond to androgens, or, rarely, true hermaphroditism. True hermaphroditism, in which the infant has both ovarian and testicular tissue, is rare and the phenotypic appearance may be those of either sex.[20]

One of the most common causes of DSD is congenital adrenal hyperplasia (CAH) (see section later). The presence of CAH exposes an XX fetus to excess androgens during fetal life. Less common virilizing conditions include aromatase deficiency or presence of a virilizing tumor in the mother.

Androgens play a critical role in male development and are particularly important in utero, and masculinization of the fetus is dependent on androgen action within a narrow window of development.[21] In an XY fetus, DSD can present as a spectrum of undervirilization[19] and result from inadequate androgen production or partial androgen insensitivity. Infants with 46, XY chromosomes who have an androgen receptor defect with complete androgen insensitivity will have genitalia that appears female; these children are not detected in the newborn period unless a karyotype is performed for some other reason. Children with complete androgen insensitivity may not be identified until the time of an inguinal hernia repair when a testis is discovered or during the teen years when pubic hair or menstruation fails to develop.

Approach to Management

An experienced multidisciplinary team provides optimal care to patients with DSDs. Each patient requires an individualized, holistic approach, and family counseling should begin immediately. An essential component of the evaluation and treatment is providing emphasis to the family that karyotypic sex is not "equivalent" to sex.[19] During evaluation in the neonatal period, it is important to avoid prematurely designating sex or using gendered pronouns.[21] The Society for Endocrinology UK also suggests that the term "atypical" genitalia be used instead of "ambiguous."[22]

Clinical Findings

All infants should receive a complete genital examination before discharge from the nursery. The initial laboratory evaluation of

• BOX 39.3 Laboratory Evaluation for Differences of Sexual Development

- Karyotype
- FISH
- Electrolytes
- Glucose
- 17-hydroxyprogesterone (17-OHP)
- Dehydroepiandrosterone-sulfate (DHEAS)
- Androstenedione
- Testosterone
- Dihydrotestosterone (DHT)
- FSH
- LH
- Anti-Müllerian hormone (AMH)
- Additional testing (as needed)
- Renin
- Aldosterone
- Urine electrolytes and creatinine
- Urine protein: creatinine ratio
- ACTH stimulation test
- hCG stimulation test
- Imaging studies
- Ultrasound (abdomen, pelvis, gonads, adrenals)
- Genitogram (assesses contour of the urethra and its connection to vagina, presence of uterus, rectovaginal fistula)

ACTH, Adrenocorticotropic hormone; *FISH*, fluorescence in situ hybridization; *FSH*, follicle-stimulating hormone; *hCG*, human chorionic gonadotropin; *LH*, luteinizing hormone.
From Stambough K, Magistrado L, Perez-Milicua G. Evaluation of ambiguous genitalia. *Curr Opin Obstet Gynecol.* 2019;31(5):303–308.

an infant with atypical genitalia should be directed by a pediatric endocrinologist and includes:

- A formal karyotype must be completed, but these results are typically available in 1 to 2 weeks. A rapid fluorescence in situ hybridization test with X and Y chromosome probes will provide results within 48 hours.
- Adrenal steroid testing
  - In XY infants, LH, FSH, anti-Müllerian hormone, inhibin B, testosterone, and dihydrotestosterone should be measured as first-line studies to evaluate testicular function.[23]
  - In XX infants, serum 17-hydroxyprogesterone (OHP) is necessary to establish a diagnosis of 21-OH deficiency. Plasma glucose and electrolytes are also essential to evaluate for CAH.
- Abdominal, pelvic, and scrotal/soft tissue ultrasound can determine the presence of gonads, uterus, and/or vagina.
- Ultrasound of the adrenal glands may be useful in cases of suspected CAH (Box 39.3).

Management

The PCP who addresses the initial concern for a DSD must document the abnormality and refer to a specialist team that includes a pediatric endocrinologist, medical geneticist, pediatric urologist, and psychology support. Any initial studies should be sent with the referral. The specialist team should meet with families and educate them about the normal process of genital development, the cause of their child's abnormality, the evaluation process, and the determination of gender for childrearing. Female is the appropriate sex of rearing for XX infants with CAH and for infants with complete androgen insensitivity. Determining the sex assignment for childrearing in incompletely masculinized XY infants

is complicated and waiting to assign the sex of rearing until the evaluation is complete is imperative. Early surgical intervention for undescended testicles is recommended.[22] Initiation of treatment of the underlying cause, if known (e.g., CAH), is essential.

Disorders of Pubertal Development

The physical changes of puberty occur in response to production of sex steroids by the ovaries or testes. Hypothalamic gonadotropin-releasing hormone (GnRH) regulates the release of luteinizing hormone (LH) and follicle-stimulating hormone (FSH) from the pituitary gland, which in turn stimulates gonadal hormone secretion.

By mid-gestation the fetal hypothalamic-pituitary-gonad (HPG) axis is intact; at term, GnRH, LH, and FSH are produced at low levels. When placental and maternal hormones are removed at delivery, unrestrained production of these hormones may occur in the newborn, with the infant experiencing a "mini puberty" between 2 weeks and 3 months of postnatal life. After infancy, the hypothalamic GnRH pulse generator is more sensitive to feedback inhibition from the brain, and by 1 year of age, LH and FSH decrease to the prepubertal range, and the child enters a "latency" period, which will continue until the time of puberty. Puberty occurs when feedback inhibition is released, and GnRH is again produced. The timing of the release correlates better with bone age than chronologic age.

Testosterone levels increase dramatically throughout childhood and adolescence in males, although there can be significant variability.[21] Boys normally begin puberty anywhere from 9 years old to 14 years old. The first sign of puberty is increased testicular volume in 85% of boys. Clinicians should be concerned when puberty presents early or is delayed as well as if it occurs out of sequence.

Precocious Puberty

Precocious puberty (PP) is defined as the appearance of secondary sex characteristics before the age of 8 years in girls and the age of 9 years in boys because of early activation of the HPG axis. Precocious puberty is categorized as either complete or central PP (also known as *CPP* or *true precocious puberty*) or incomplete. Incomplete PP is further divided into three subcategories: premature thelarche, premature adrenarche, and isolated menarche.[24]

Premature thelarche, isolated breast development without any other features of puberty, occurs in infant and toddler girls and is sometimes present at birth. This breast development, likely due to increased sensitivity of breast primordia to estradiol, transient estradiol secretion from ovarian cysts, dietary estrogen intake, or transient activation of the HPG axis, has been proposed as a possible mechanism, resolves over time, and rarely progresses to true precocious puberty. It is important to note that for infants and toddlers with suspected premature thelarche, growth acceleration is not present, bone age is consistent with chronologic age, and there are no other signs of puberty. There is a marked indication of younger median ages of thelarche, possibly due to increased body mass index (BMI) in the pediatric population and the presence of endocrine-disrupting chemicals.[25]

Adrenarche represents the peripubertal maturation of the adrenal cortex.[26] Premature adrenarche is the early onset of pubic or axillary hair in either boys (before 10 years old) or girls (before 8 years old) not associated with other features of true puberty. Bone and height age may be slightly advanced in relation to chronologic

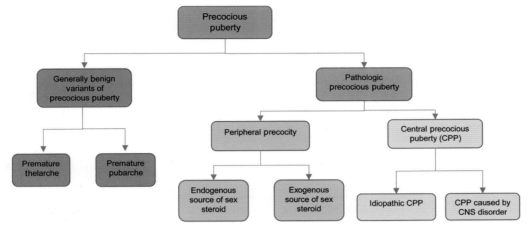

• **Fig. 39.2** Classification of Precocious Puberty. *CNS*, Central nervous system. (Data from Rosenfield RL, Cooke DW, Radovick S. Puberty and its disorders in the female. In: Sperling MA, ed. *Pediatric Endocrinology*, 4th ed. Elsevier; 2014; Kaplowitz P, Bloch C. Evaluation and referral of children with signs of early puberty. *Pediatrics*. 2016; 137(1):1–6; and Klein A, Emerick JE, Sylvester JE, et al. Disorders of puberty: an approach to diagnosis and management. *Am Fam Physician*. 2017;96(9):590–599.)

age in children with premature adrenarche. Premature adrenarche may be caused by a mild form of CAH, exposure to topical testosterone, or rarely, an adrenal tumor. Most often, the condition is idiopathic. Premature adrenarche affects more females than males at a ratio of 10:1. Females with idiopathic premature adrenarche are at increased risk for polycystic ovary syndrome and metabolic syndrome.[27]

Isolated menarche is an uncommon condition in which girls have one to a few episodes of vaginal bleeding without breast development. This diagnosis should be considered if vaginal bleeding is isolated or cyclical and without evidence of other secondary sex characteristics. In this condition, sexual abuse, vaginal tumor, vulvovaginitis, urethral prolapse, genital injury, foreign body, and primary hypothyroidism all need to be excluded.[28]

True precocious puberty refers to the onset of multiple features of puberty earlier than the typical range (Fig. 39.2). The most widely accepted definition of precocious puberty is the onset of thelarche in girls less than 8 years old and the onset of testicular enlargement in boys less than 9 years old.[29] Features of precocious puberty may include accelerated linear growth, breast development, testicular or penile enlargement, and pubic hair development. Depending on the duration of symptoms, bone age may be advanced. Precocious puberty can be divided into two broad categories: (1) central, gonadotropin dependent; or (2) peripheral, gonadotropin independent (Box 39.4).

Prolonged exposure to exogenous sex hormones (accidental ingestion of combined oral contraceptive pills, transdermal delivery of testosterone gel from skin-to-skin contact) and exposure to endocrine-disrupting chemicals can cause peripheral precocious puberty. Other exogenous hormone sources can include hormone-containing hair products, and both topical lavender oil and tea tree oil (which have estrogenic activity in vitro) has been linked to premature thelarche in young girls.[30]

In the United States, the incidence of precocious puberty is estimated to be 1:5000 to 1:10,000 children.[31] Precocious puberty is more common in females compared with males and in Black children compared with White children. CPP is more common in females and is usually idiopathic. Boys with CPP are 40% to 50% more likely to have an associated CNS pathology including tumor, infection, or hemorrhage.[32]

• **BOX 39.4 Disorders of Puberty**

Central Precocious Puberty
Idiopathic (most frequent cause; more common in girls)
Central nervous system (CNS) tumors
• Hamartoma
• Craniopharyngioma
Post-CNS radiation
CNS infection
CNS trauma
Congenital adrenal hyperplasia

Peripheral Precocious Puberty
Girls
• Ovarian cyst or tumor
• Estrogen secreting ovarian or adrenal tumor
• McCune-Albright syndrome
Boys
• Testicular tumor
• Testotoxicosis (activating mutation of the luteinizing hormone receptor)
Both sexes
• Human chorionic gonadotropin (HCG)-secreting tumor (rare; more common in boys)
• Hypothyroidism

Normal Variants of Puberty
Premature adrenarche
Premature thelarche

Clinical Findings

Many children who present with features of early puberty do not require treatment. However, all children who exhibit signs of puberty at a younger than typical age should have an evaluation to determine the etiology. Those children who start to develop signs of puberty at the early end of the typical range should be evaluated if they have either rapid progression of pubertal signs resulting in a bone age more than 2 years ahead of chronologic age or new CNS-related findings (e.g., headaches, seizures, and/or focal neurologic defects).

History. Evaluation includes the following:
- Age of onset and pattern of growth
- Type, duration, and order of progression of pubertal symptoms (i.e., breast tissue, pubic hair, phallic/testicular enlargement, acne, body odor). Asynchronous order of Tanner stage development suggests increased likelihood of a pathological cause.[33]
- Any symptom suggestive of a CNS lesion (e.g., headache, vision disturbance)
- Family pattern of pubertal onset
- Exposure to topical estrogens or testosterone, oral estrogens, or environmental hormone disruptors (endocrine disruptors)

Physical Examination. Physical examination should include:
- Assessment of stature and growth velocity
- Description of the child's sexual maturity rating (Tanner stage):
  - Presence of pubic and/or axillary hair and breast development: breast development should be evaluated by palpation, not just inspection to differentiate between the presence of true breast tissue versus fat deposition.
  - Presence of pubic and/or axillary hair and increase in penile length and/or testicular volume (boys). A Prader orchidometer should be used to measure testicular volume.

Diagnostic Studies. Diagnostic studies should include:
- Premature thelarche: No laboratory studies are necessary in the infant or toddler girl unless other pubertal features are present or continued increase in breast size.
- Premature adrenarche: Serum 17-OHP to exclude CAH and a 24-hour urine collection for 17-ketosteroids or imaging of the adrenal glands to exclude an adrenal tumor.
- Isolated menarche: Thyroid function tests to exclude primary hypothyroidism, and pelvic ultrasound to rule out the presence of an ovarian cyst or pelvic tumor.
- True precocious puberty:
  - Bone age radiograph of left wrist and hand
  - LH, FSH, and estradiol or testosterone: use a laboratory with a sensitive assay that will detect early pubertal values at the lower end of the range.
    - If LH and FSH are high (in the pubertal range: indication of central etiology), order an MRI to exclude CNS tumor.
    - If LH and FSH are low (in the prepubertal range: indication of peripheral puberty), complete a GnRH stimulation test to distinguish central from peripheral puberty.
  - If the etiology is peripheral puberty:
    - Pelvic ultrasonography of girls
    - Testicular ultrasonography of boys
    - Serum 17-OHP to rule out a severe form of CAH
- In children with a family history of CPP, genetic testing is indicated.
- MKRN2 mutation is the most common monogenetic cause of CPP. DLK1 deletions are also reported.

In males, there is a high risk of intracranial pathology associated with CPP, and CNS imaging is indicated. In females older than age 6 years with no neurologic symptoms, brain MRI as a diagnostic tool is more controversial. In a metaanalysis of MRI findings in children with CPP, only 9% of MRIs detected CNS lesions (including incidental findings such as benign cysts), and only 1.6% of those lesions required interventions.[34]

Management

Treatment of early puberty depends on the etiology and should always be done with the guidance of a pediatric endocrinologist. Management is important to help increase final adult height and

depends on the underlying disorder, age of the child, degree of advancement of the bone age, and the child's and family's emotional response to the condition. Patients and families also choose to postpone menarche to reduce potentially negative psychosocial impacts.[33] Radiation, surgery, and/or chemotherapy may be indicated in the case of CNS tumors.

GnRH agonists bind to and activate the GnRH receptor in the pituitary gland, which causes an initial increase of LH and FSH. Within several weeks, however, the pituitary gland becomes desensitized and pauses the natural hormone production for the duration that the medication is taken. GnRH agonists bring serum sex steroids to prepubertal levels. Monthly and 3-month depot leuprolide injections, triptorelin 6-month depot injections, and subcutaneous histrelin implants are all available and have reasonable safety and tolerability profiles.[35] During early therapy, patients and families need to be educated that the initial stimulatory effects of GnRH agonists will cause gonadotropin and sex steroid levels to rise above baseline, leading to a transient increase in pubertal symptoms (which can include vaginal bleeding).

Delayed Puberty

Delayed puberty in females is defined as the absence of thelarche at the age of 13 years.[24] Puberty is considered delayed when a male 14 years old or older or a female 13 years old or older has no clinical features of puberty on physical examination or if puberty has not progressed within a timely basis. Females should progress to menarche within 5 years of breast budding; males should attain sexual maturity rating stage 5 pubertal development within 4.5 years of initiation of puberty. If puberty is either delayed or has failed to progress, the child should be referred to an endocrinologist for evaluation of hypogonadism. Of note, many females with Turner syndrome start puberty and then stall, and approximately 10% of these patients have spontaneous menarche.[36]

Any chronic condition that delays bone age may cause delayed puberty because the timing of puberty correlates better with bone age than chronologic age. In addition, failure of any part of the HPG axis may also delay puberty (Box 39.5). The most common cause of delayed puberty is CGD.

Clinical Findings

History and Physical Examination. History and physical examination should focus on clinical clues indicating a chronic illness, symptoms of hypothyroidism (discussed later in this

---

BOX 39.5 Etiology of Delayed Puberty

Chronic Illness
- Gastrointestinal with poor weight gain
- Chronic renal failure
- Anorexia nervosa or bulimia
- Chronic anemia
- Respiratory or cardiac disease
- Medication-induced poor weight gain

Constitutional Growth Delay
- Endocrine diseases associated with delayed bone age
- Hypothyroidism

Growth Hormone Deficiency
- Failure of the hypothalamic-pituitary-gonadal axis

chapter), prior history of CNS insult, or new CNS symptoms suggesting hypopituitarism. A review of systems should include questions about the pattern of growth, especially growth velocity, loss of sense of smell (anosmia) is associated with Kallmann syndrome, a type of hypogonadotropic hypogonadism characterized by delayed or absent puberty in males[37] and galactorrhea (suggestive of pituitary tumor). Physical examination should include height, weight, waist circumference, and body proportions, assessment of Tanner stages, and evaluation for signs and symptoms of hypogonadism.

Diagnostic Studies. Laboratory testing should begin with an assessment of LH, FSH, and estradiol in girls and LH, FSH, and testosterone in boys. If there is suspicion of Turner or Klinefelter syndrome, the karyotype is also essential.[36] Diagnostic testing should also include focused screening for acute or chronic illness or nutritional disorders.

- CBC, ESR, C-reactive protein, liver enzymes, electrolytes, blood urea nitrogen, creatinine
- Free T_4 and TSH
- IGF-1 and IGFBP-3, if GHD is suspect
- Serum prolactin
- LH and FSH (elevated LH and FSH is indicative of primary hypogonadism)
- Celiac screening with tTG-IgA
- Karyotype as indicated
- Bone age radiograph (left hand and wrist)

Management

A referral to a pediatric endocrinologist is necessary to determine the etiology and necessary treatment. Hormonal replacement with recombinant GH is the treatment of choice for children with hypogonadism. In males, consideration can be made for use of testosterone as either IM injection or via topical gel. Human recombinant FSH and LH have also been used in children with hypogonadotropic hypogonadism.[38] While youth with CGD can be reassured that puberty will occur spontaneously, albeit later compared with some peers, it is important to understand that genetic variations leading to CGD can cause significant variations in the timing of pubertal onset.[39]

Gender-Affirming Hormonal Transition in Transgender and Gender-Diverse Youth

Gender is a multifactorial construct representing the interaction of social, environmental, cultural, and behavioral factors and choices that influence a person's self-identity and health. *Gender-diverse youth* are individuals who identify as transgender, who may be questioning their gender identity; or who identify as agender, fluid, or nonbinary.[40] *Transgender* is a term used to describe a person whose gender identity differs from the sex assigned at birth. One's sexual orientation, the attraction to any gender, is not synonymous with one's gender identity.

Although the exact prevalence of transgender youth is not known, The Trevor Project estimates that 1.5% of adolescents identify as transgender.[41] This number may be grossly underestimated considering that young people may not feel comfortable identifying or disclosing that they are transgender. Therefore it is likely that PCPs will not only encounter but also assist in the planning and coordination of the interprofessional (mental health, endocrine, primary care) care needed by these youth. While recognizing the need for a multidisciplinary approach to care for these youth, this discussion is limited to hormonal interventions for

transgender adolescents, specifically pubertal suppression at the onset of puberty for youth experiencing a significant increase in gender dysphoria and prescription of cross-sex hormones to assist with the transition to their affirmed gender. Research continues to emphasize that transgender and gender-diverse youth need to be cared for in a way that affirms their gender identities while also minimizing the negative physical and psychosocial outcomes that may be associated with pubertal development.[42]

In 2017 the Endocrine Society published clinical practice guidelines for the endocrine treatment of gender-dysphoric persons.[43] Protocols from the World Professional Association for Transgender Health (WPATH) and the Endocrine Society describe a combined approach that includes psychological support and medical intervention. Treatment is structured in three phases: (1) diagnostic phase without medical interventions; (2) extended diagnostic phase, characterized by puberty-blocking with GnRH agonists; and (3) induction of puberty that is congruent with gender identity.[44]

Pubertal Suppression

Gender-diverse youth often experience heightened gender dysphoria (distress caused by the difference between one's assigned and affirmed gender) at or near the onset of puberty. The timing of endocrine therapy can have a significant impact on the mental health of youth with gender dysphoria. Being at an older age and later pubertal stage at the time of presentation for gender-affirming care are associated with increased rates of psychoactive medication use and increased rates of depression and anxiety.[45]

Current research on the use of puberty-blocking hormones suggests that clinicians follow the guidelines from WPATH and the Endocrine Society to enhance the positive outcomes associated with the use of these medications.[42] WPATH criteria for considering pubertal suppression in adolescents are presented in Box 39.6. The input of a qualified mental health professional regarding the youth's diagnosis of gender dysphoria and readiness for suppression of puberty is essential in making the decision. In addition,

---

• BOX 39.6 Minimum Criteria for Puberty Suppressing Hormones

- The adolescent meets the diagnostic criteria of gender incongruence as per the ICD-11 in situations where a diagnosis is necessary to access health care.
- The experience of gender diversity/incongruence is marked and sustained over time.
- The adolescent demonstrates the emotional and cognitive maturity required to provide informed consent/assent for the treatment.
- The adolescent's mental health concerns (if any) that may interfere with diagnostic clarity, capacity to consent, and gender-affirming medical treatments have been addressed.
- The adolescent has been informed of the reproductive effects, including the potential loss of fertility and the available options to preserve fertility, and these have been discussed in the context of the adolescent's stage of pubertal development.
- The adolescent has reached Tanner stage 2 of puberty for pubertal suppression to be initiated.

Modified from World Professional Association for Transgender Health. Standards of Care for the Health of Transsexual, Transgender, and Gender Nonconforming People 2022. https://www.tandfonline.com/doi/pdf/10.1080/26895269.2022.2100644; and Coleman E, Radix AE, Bouman, WP, et al. Standards of care for the health of transgender and gender diverse people, Version 8. *Int J Transg Health.* 2022;23(1):S1–S259.

adolescents are considered for pubertal suppression when they achieve a sexual maturity (Tanner) rating of ≥2.

GnRH agonists medications (which include leuprorelin, triptorelin, or histrelin), while more commonly used to delay pubertal progression in children with central precocious puberty, are a reversible intervention that leaves the body in a neutral pubertal state. Fisher et al.[44] describe that treatment with GnRH agonists effectively suspends pubertal development, allowing adolescents the time to explore their gender identity without the distress derived by the undesired body changes (including breast development, menarche, increased testicular size, voice deepening, and virilizing hair patterns).

Monitoring for adequate pubertal suppression of the HPG axis includes LH, FSH, and total testosterone for youth with testes and LH, FSH, and estradiol in those with ovaries with adjustments in GnRH agonist dosing as needed.[44] During this time, youth should be assessed regarding their desire to continue to the next phase of treatment. If gender identification changes, pubertal suppression regimens are reversible. Upon cessation of therapy, the normal pubertal process will resume.[46] It is also important to monitor for negative effects of delayed puberty, including halted growth spurt and impairment in bone mineral accumulation. The Endocrine Society clinical practice guidelines[43] recommend monitoring clinical pubertal development every 3 to 6 months and laboratory parameters every 6 to 12 months during sex hormone treatment.

Induction of Puberty Congruent With Gender Identity. The Endocrine Society guidelines support the initiation of gender-affirming hormonal treatment at the age of 16 years, and earlier in selected cases after a thorough evaluation by a multidisciplinary team with expertise in gender identity development.[44] This stage of treatment induces secondary sexual characteristics consistent with the affirmed gender, and some of these changes are irreversible.

Induction of male puberty in transgender males involves the use of testosterone via IM injection. At the implementation of testosterone therapy, the GnRH analog used to suppress puberty will often be continued to maintain suppression of the hypothalamic-pituitary axis and suppression of menses. Virilization occurs in the first 3 to 6 months, including the growth of facial and body hair, deepening of the voice, muscular development (particularly in the upper body), and clitoral enlargement.

Induction of female puberty in transgender females consists of oral or transdermal estrogen formulations. A GnRH analog may be continued and/or an antiandrogen such as spironolactone can be added to reduce testosterone production and unwanted hair growth. Feminizing physical changes include breast development (starting within 3 months), an increase in hip circumference, and a decrease in waist circumference.

Use of Gender-Inclusive Language and Pronouns. Care providers need to have awareness of and sensitivity to the myriad gender identities and expressions that exist to help capture people's rich diversity of experiences. The language around gender continues to grow and change, and it is important to understand what one's gender-related words mean to each person.[47] Pronouns can be gender binary or gender neutral. It is essential that the PCP always ask what pronoun and name the individual uses. The term "preferred pronoun" should be avoided, as it suggests a degree of flexibility or invalidity.[48] Pronouns are also contextual, and individuals may use different names and different pronouns depending on the situation. If a pronoun is used incorrectly, it is best to apologize, say what pronoun was meant to be used, and continue

forward. Refer to Chapter 7 for further information on binary and gender-neutral pronouns.

Polycystic Ovary Syndrome

Polycystic ovary syndrome (PCOS) is a complex endocrine disorder characterized by hyperandrogenemia, progressive hirsutism, oligomenorrhea, irregular menses cycle, and enlarged polycystic ovaries. The incidence of PCOS ranges from 3% to 15% based on genetic background, race, and diagnostic criteria. PCOS is more typically found in females of reproductive age who are overweight or obese; however, not all females with PCOS carry excess body weight and this finding is not a diagnostic criterion.[49] Metabolic comorbidities include insulin resistance and impaired glucose tolerance, type 2 diabetes, nonalcoholic fatty liver disease (NAFLD), and metabolic syndrome.[25] Approximately 70% of females with PCOS are reported to be accompanied by insulin resistance, which results in long-term reproductive and metabolic complications.[50] PCOS is a diagnosis by exclusion, and international treatment guidelines have been established for the diagnosis and management of PCOS.[51]

Clinical Findings

- Irregular menstrual cycle—missed or fewer periods (<8 in a year), periods every 21 days or more often, or absent menses
- Hirsutism (presence of hair on the face, chin, or on the body where males typically have hair)
- Severe acne
- Thinning hair or male-pattern alopecia
- Obesity (central) or unexpected weight gain or difficulty losing weight
- Acanthosis nigricans (darkening of skin in neck creases, groin, underneath breasts)
- Skin tags

Diagnostic Testing. A thorough physical examination should be performed to rule out any other underlying conditions. See Table 39.4 for diagnostic testing for PCOS. Basic studies include cholesterol and glucose testing (see the section on type 2 diabetes) as well as androgen and testosterone levels. To evaluate insulin resistance and glucose metabolism, the oral glucose tolerance test (OGTT) and insulin tolerance test are the gold standards. Venous plasma glucose and insulin levels are assessed in a fasting state and 1 and 2 hours after administering oral glucose solution.[50]

Recent guidelines note that pelvic ultrasound should not be used for the diagnosis of PCOS in those who are <8 years postmenarche because there is a high incidence of multifollicular ovaries in adolescents. Ovarian size has been positively associated with total testosterone, androstenedione, LH, and LH:FSH ratio.[52]

Anti-Müllerian hormone (AMH) levels are not recommended for PCOS diagnosis.[51] AMH is secreted by ovarian cells, with the highest level of secretion occurring during folliculogenesis. While AMH levels would elevate as the ovaries create multiple cysts, there is currently a lack of standardized assays and appropriate normative ranges.

Differential Diagnosis

It is important to rule out other causes of menstrual irregularities and/or hyperandrogenism. Late-onset CAH, androgen-secreting ovarian or adrenal tumors, Cushing disease, hypothyroidism, and hyperprolactinemia should be included in the differential diagnosis.

TABLE 39.4	Diagnostic Testing for Polycystic Ovary Syndrome
Laboratory Test	**Indication**
Beta-hCG	Rule out pregnancy
TSH	Rule out thyroid dysfunction
17-OH progesterone	Rule out nonclassic CAH
Total testosterone, free testosterone	Quantify level of hyperandrogenism
Androstenedione	Rule out androgen-secreting tumor
Dehydroepiandrosterone sulfate (DHEAS)	Rule out nonclassic CAH or androgen-secreting tumor
Prolactin	Rule out hyperprolactinemia with amenorrhea
FSH, LH, estradiol	Rule out premature ovarian failure in patients with amenorrhea (high FSH, low estradiol)
Fasting blood glucose, HgbA1c, lipid panel	Metabolic syndrome

CAH, Congenital adrenal hyperplasia; *FSH,* follicle stimulating hormone; *hCG,* human chorionic gonadotropin; *LH,* luteinizing hormone; *TSH,* thyroid stimulating hormone.

Modified from Ibáñez L, Oberfield SE, Witchel S, et al. An international consortium update: pathophysiology, diagnosis, and treatment of polycystic ovarian syndrome in adolescence. *Horm Res Paediatr.* 2017;88(6):371–395; and Witchel SF, Burghard AC, Tao RH, Oberfield SE. The diagnosis and treatment of PCOS in adolescents: an update. *Curr Opin Pediatr.* 2019;31(4):562–569.

Management

Referral to an endocrinologist is needed for optimal management. See the section in this chapter on the treatment of obesity, type 2 diabetes, and dyslipidemia. Nonpharmacologic treatment of overweight and obese young females involves multicomponent lifestyle interventions for a healthy diet, increased physical activity, and behavioral strategies.

Pharmacologic treatment may include one or a combination of the following agents: metformin, thiazolidinediones, combination oral contraceptives (lower-dose preparation preferred), and orlistat. In PCOS, the use of metformin therapy has been associated with improvements in lipid profiles, glucose tolerance, and insulin sensitivity, along with decreased serum androgen levels and induction of ovulation.[53] Long-term therapy with metformin treatment of overweight-obese females with PCOS and normal baseline blood glucose resulted in a reduction of body mass, improvements in menstrual frequency and androgen laboratory values, and low conversion rate to type 2 diabetes.[54]

A combination of oral contraceptives with estrogen and progestin is used to help regulate menses and provide endometrial protection from high unopposed levels of circulating estrogen during cycles of anovulation. The estrogen content in these products also lowers serum androgens by increasing the hepatic production of sex hormone–binding globulin and suppressing LH.[49] The antiandrogens spironolactone and flutamide are sometimes used to address clinical hyperandrogenism symptoms, although neither medication is approved by the FDA for hyperandrogenism. Refer to dermatology for hair removal products and procedures (such as laser hair removal), as well as treatment for severe or refractory acne symptoms.

Comorbid conditions such as depression, anxiety, eating disorders, negative body image, and psychosexual dysfunction are reported in patients with PCOS. Therefore appropriate screening and management of these symptoms (including cognitive behavioral therapy and psychopharmacologic therapy) is essential and may improve adherence to therapy recommendations.[55]

Complications

PCOS is associated with an increased risk of type 2 diabetes, hypertension and cardiovascular disease, NAFLD, obstructive sleep apnea, depression and anxiety, endometrial hyperplasia and endometrial cancer, and infertility.

Adrenal Disorders

Anatomy and Physiology

Adrenal gland steroid production is under the control of the hypothalamic-pituitary axis. The hypothalamus secretes corticotropin-releasing hormone (CRH) in a pulsatile fashion, which stimulates the production and secretion of adrenocorticotropic hormone (ACTH) by the pituitary gland. ACTH regulates adrenal glucocorticoid (cortisol) and androgen production. Cortisol levels are highest in the morning, low in the afternoon and evening, and lowest at midnight. Secreted in response to hypoglycemia, hypotension, pain, or other stressful events, cortisol has negative feedback on the synthesis and secretion of CRH, vasopressin, and ACTH.

The adrenal gland also produces mineralocorticoid hormones including aldosterone, which regulates electrolyte and extracellular volume homeostasis. Aldosterone is regulated by renal production of renin interacting with angiotensinogen, to create angiotensin. In addition to electrolyte homeostasis (especially sodium balance), the renin-angiotensin system is involved in the regulation of blood pressure, and renal blood flow.[56] Aldosterone production also occurs in enzymatic steps, many of which are common to the cortisol production pathway.

Adrenal Insufficiency

Adrenal insufficiency is characterized by adrenal hypofunction, leading to deficits in glucocorticoids (especially cortisol), mineralocorticoids (most often aldosterone), and adrenal androgens.[57] This insufficiency can be primary, secondary, or tertiary depending on the underlying etiology. In *primary* adrenal insufficiency (adrenal gland hypofunction), glucocorticoid (cortisol), *and* mineralocorticoid (aldosterone) hormones are deficient. The gland hypofunction can be due to abnormalities in the development of the adrenal glands, progressive adrenal destruction, impaired steroidogenesis, or resistance to ACTH action.[58] In *secondary* adrenal insufficiency, pituitary hypofunction leads to a reduction in ACTH, causing a deficit in glucocorticoid. In *tertiary* adrenal insufficiency, the hypothalamus produces an insufficient amount of CRH, leading to a downstream reduction in glucocorticoids and androgens. This insufficiency can result from long-term glucocorticoid drug therapy.

Among those with primary adrenal insufficiency, there are two forms of "classic" CAH. In *simple virilizing* CAH, there is normal aldosterone biosynthesis. In the salt-wasting form of CAH, there is impaired aldosterone production.[59] The incidence of classic CAH[60] in most populations is between 1:14,000 and 1:18,000.

• BOX 39.7 Adrenal Insufficiency

Deficiency of Corticotropin-Releasing Hormone or Adrenocorticotropin
Isolated deficiency
  Congenital
  Acquired due to hypophysitis (pituitary gland inflammation)
Multiple pituitary hormone deficiencies
  Congenital (e.g., septo-optic dysplasia, midline defects)
  Acquired (e.g., CNS trauma, infection, tumor, radiation)

Primary Adrenal
Congenital
  CAH (most common 21-OH deficiency)
  Adrenal hypoplasia (X-linked, autosomal recessive, ACTH receptor
    defect)
Acquired
  X-linked adrenoleukodystrophy
  Autoimmune (Addison disease)
  Infection

21-OH, 21-Hydroxylase; *ACTH,* adrenocorticotropin; *CAH,* congenital adrenal hyperplasia; *CNS,* central nervous system.

Those with impaired aldosterone deficiency are at risk for lethal salt-wasting crises (hyponatremia, hyperkalemia, acidosis, and dehydration) in the neonatal period if left undiagnosed/untreated. However, 10% of individuals with simple virilizing CAH also risk having a salt-wasting crisis during excessive physical stress.

Primary adrenal insufficiency may be due to an inability to produce cortisol secondary to an enzyme defect in the adrenal steroid pathway (e.g., CAH), hypoplasia of the adrenal gland, or an acquired defect (Box 39.7). Infants born extremely prematurely (24–28 weeks' gestation) sometimes demonstrate symptoms of adrenal insufficiency because the hypothalamic-pituitary-adrenal axis has not yet matured.

Secondary adrenal insufficiency can occur because of ACTH deficiency, as one of the multiple hypothalamic-pituitary deficiencies, or rarely as an isolated problem. Most often, the infant or child has a syndrome known to be associated with hypopituitarism (e.g., septo-optic dysplasia), has also been discovered to have GHD, or has a destructive lesion of the hypothalamus or the pituitary (e.g., tumor) or a history of prior radiation to the brain or CNS trauma. Exogenous steroid use also suppresses the hypothalamic-pituitary-adrenal axis and can lead to adrenal insufficiency.

CAH is caused by a group of autosomal recessive disorders affecting cortisol biosynthesis. From 95% to 99% of cases of CAH are due to 21-hydroxylase (21-OH) deficiency, which results from mutations in the *CYP21A2* gene.[60,61] Approximately 75% of children with CAH caused by 21-OH deficiency will also have aldosterone deficiency. In addition to interrupting normal cortisol production, 21-OH deficiency causes shunting of cortisol precursors to the androgen pathway, which results in excessive adrenal androgen production.

In all 50 states, newborn screening programs test for the presence of CAH caused by 21-OH deficiency. Early detection of CAH is essential to avoid potentially life-threatening adrenal and salt-wasting crises in affected infants. In addition, screening reduces the delay of correct sex assignment in those females with significantly virilized genitalia. Female infants born with classic CAH typically have virilization of the external genitalia (e.g., clitoral enlargement and/or labial fusion) from excessive androgen exposure in utero. The uterus, fallopian tubes, and ovaries are, however, unaffected by androgen exposure. Male infants have normal external genitalia and no other physical signs of CAH at birth.[60]

X-Linked Adrenoleukodystrophy

X-linked adrenoleukodystrophy disease (ALD) is an X-linked peroxisomal disorder that leads to adrenal insufficiency in up to 90% of affected individuals. As with many X-linked disorders, males are most often affected. Females may be carriers and have milder forms of the disease. The incidence is estimated at 1:17,000 and ALD screening is part of newborn screening in many states. It is caused by mutation at the ABCD1 transporter, which helps channel very long chain fatty acids to the peroxisome so that they can be oxidized (broken down). See Inborn Errors of Metabolism in this chapter for additional information about peroxisomal disorders.

Clinical Findings

History
- Symptoms of cortisol deficiency include a history of poor appetite, failure to thrive, weight loss, weakness, and vomiting.
- Symptoms of aldosterone deficiency include vomiting, poor feeding, lethargy, and dehydration.

Physical Examination. The following signs are often seen:
- Dehydration and hypotension
- Excessive pigmentation of the skin and mucous membranes (present only with primary adrenal insufficiency)
- An adrenal crisis in a conscious pediatric patient presents with hypoglycemia, hypotension, altered mental status, abdominal pain, and vomiting.[56]

Diagnostic Studies. Diagnostic evaluation of adrenal disorders includes initial screening, biochemical evaluation, and molecular genetic testing (Table 39.5). Among the diagnostic study results, serum glucose will identify hypoglycemia. Blood gases and bicarbonate levels will quantify metabolic acidosis. Electrolytes will reveal low sodium and elevated potassium with aldosterone deficiency. A serum cortisol value greater than 20 mcg/dL indicates adrenal sufficiency; a value less than that must be interpreted in the clinical context in which the sample was drawn.

Often an ACTH stimulation test, performed in collaboration with a pediatric endocrinologist, is needed to conclusively diagnose both primary and secondary adrenal insufficiency. Serum ACTH is elevated in primary adrenal insufficiency. Serum renin level is elevated, and aldosterone level is low in aldosterone deficiency. Plasma renin and aldosterone levels are interpreted best if they are drawn when serum sodium levels are low. Prenatal diagnosis can be performed when both parents are known carriers of CYP21A2 mutations. Carrier status is often diagnosed when parents have a previous child with 21-OH deficiency.

Management

The successful management of CAH requires excellent parent and patient knowledge of the disorder and adherence to treatment strategies. Treatment of adrenal insufficiency includes hormone replacement and is best managed by a pediatric endocrinologist. All infants affected with classic CAH benefit from treatment with both a glucocorticoid and an adjunctive mineralocorticoid for at least the first year of life. Oral fludrocortisone and sodium chloride are prescribed for salt-wasting CAH, although sodium chloride is generally only needed during infancy and the fludrocortisone dosing is often reduced before adulthood.[62]

TABLE 39.5 Diagnostic Evaluation of Adrenal Disorders

Disorder	Symptoms	Supporting Labs	Etiologies	Diagnostic Tests for Confirmation of Etiology
Primary adrenal insufficiency (PAI)	Dehydration Hypotension Hyperpigmentation Abdominal pain Fever Fatigue	↓ 8 a.m. cortisol ↑ 8 a.m. ACTH ↓ glucose ↓ Na ↑ K ↑ Renin	Addison disease	21-hydroxylase antibodies
			CAH	↑ 8 a.m. 17-OHP *Classic:* 17OHP usually >3500 ng/dL, always >1000 ng/dL *Nonclassic:* 17OHP >1000 ng/DL If 17OHP 200–1000 ng/dL, proceed with high-dose ACTH stimulation test For borderline cases or genetic counseling of CAH test for *CYP21A2* genotype
			X-linked adrenoleuko-dystrophy	↑ VLCFA level *ABCD1* gene analysis Brain MRI if elevated VLCFA or ABCD1 mutation found
Secondary adrenal insufficiency (SAI)	Fatigue Weakness Abdominal pain Vomiting Fever Same as PAI without hyperpigmentation and symptoms of mineralocorticoid deficiency	↓ 8 a.m. cortisol ↓ 8 a.m. ACTH	Hypopituitarism Septo-optic dysplasia Growth hormone deficiency Hypothalamic or pituitary tumor Prior brain radiation CNS trauma Exogenous steroid use	Low-dose ACTH stimulation test

17OHP, 17-Hydroxyprogesterone; *ACTH,* adrenocorticotropic hormone; *CAH,* congenital adrenal hyperplasia; *CNS,* central nervous system; *MRI,* magnetic resonance imaging; *VLCFA,* very long chain fatty acid.

Modified from Chovel-Sella A, Halper A. Adrenal insufficiency. *Endocr Condit Pediatr.* 2020:285–288; and Rose SR, Wassner AJ, Wintergerst KA, et al; AAP Section on Endocrinology, AAP Council on Genetics, Pediatric Endocrine Society, American Thyroid Association. Congenital hypothyroidism: screening and management. *Pediatrics.* 2023;151(1):e2022060420.

Practice guidelines for diagnosis and treatment of primary adrenal insufficiency include management and prevention of adrenal crisis.[63] Adrenal crisis is a medical emergency requiring prehospital IM hydrocortisone, admission for intravenous (IV) hydrocortisone and fluids, with blood glucose monitoring. IV stress doses of hydrocortisone succinate vary with age: 25 mg in children younger than 3 years; 50 mg in children 3 to 12 years; and 100 mg in children older than 12 years, administered every 6 hours. Parents should be instructed regarding the need for stress doses of hydrocortisone succinate when their child has a febrile illness, surgery, or trauma. They should also be taught how to administer hydrocortisone via IM injection in case the child is vomiting or otherwise unable to swallow or retain oral medication. This injection allows parents extended time to seek further medical advice or intervention.

Parent/caregiver education should include indications for increasing hydrocortisone doses when the child has a "sick day" (including fever, gastroenteritis with dehydration, trauma, or need for surgery) and how to administer the appropriate dose of hydrocortisone succinate IM. This information should be reviewed with parents and/or caregivers on an annual basis. Not only must IM hydrocortisone always be available, but the child's additional caregivers (such as teachers) must also know appropriate administration details and techniques.[62] Families must also communicate with providers that a hydrocortisone stress dosing protocol is necessary when the child undergoes any type of surgical procedure or experiences physical trauma.

Maintenance therapy for classic CAH includes oral corticosteroid (hydrocortisone) in replacement doses of 10 to 15 mg/ m^2 (typically divided 3 times per day).[60] Children with CAH tend to have higher hydrocortisone needs. The mineralocorticoid (aldosterone) deficiency is treated with daily oral fludrocortisone acetate. In addition, salt supplementation (1–2 mg/day of sodium chloride) is given to infants up to 8–12 months of age who require mineralocorticoid replacement because: (1) the kidneys have decreased responsiveness to mineralocorticoid supplementation at this age, and (2) there is low salt content in breast milk and formulas.[64]

Treatment of CAH requires a fine balancing act to replace steroids, thereby preventing androgen overproduction. Excess steroid intake can lead to delayed growth, whereas not enough steroids contribute to bone age advancement and ultimately short stature. Individual treatment plans are essential to meet the specific needs of individual children. The PCP should be familiar with the medical endocrinology treatment plan and reinforce it at routine well- and sick-child visits.

At the pubertal onset, females with CAH that is well controlled typically experience normal menarche. Those who are not well controlled can experience symptoms including irregular menses, acne, hirsutism, male pattern alopecia, and reduced fertility. Affected males with suboptimal control can have reduced testicular volume and can develop benign testicular adrenal rest tumors (known as TARTs).

Hyperadrenal States

Cushing syndrome results from prolonged exposure to excess corticosteroids, and can be iatrogenic or exogenous, caused by glucocorticoid treatment for an illness (e.g., serious asthma, to prevent rejection after a transplant, or as part of chemotherapy protocols). Endogenous Cushing syndrome is uncommon in pediatrics, with an incidence of 0.7 to 2.4 per million in the general population per year,[65] but can have serious consequences if not identified and treated. Endogenous cortisol excess may be due to a pituitary tumor producing ACTH, an adrenal tumor, or ectopic production of ACTH from a nonpituitary tumor (rare in children).

Clinical Findings

History and Physical Examination. Features of cortisol excess include weight gain, growth failure, osteopenia, hypertension, plethora (hypervolemia), and delayed puberty. In addition, acne, striae, and hirsutism are common skin findings. Compulsive behaviors may be reported.

Diagnostic Studies. In situations where growth is slow or growth data are missing and cortisol excess needs to be excluded by laboratory evaluation, a 24-hour urine collection for free cortisol or a late evening serum or salivary cortisol is the best screening test.

Differential Diagnosis

Obesity is a differential diagnosis, but almost all children with simple obesity are tall for their age, and cortisol excess can be excluded on physical examination alone.

Management

Pediatric providers must avoid prescribing prolonged courses of corticosteroids whenever possible. When children receive glucocorticoids for underlying illness for longer than 7 to 10 days, the steroid dose should be weaned rather than abruptly discontinued to allow the hypothalamic-pituitary-adrenal axis to recover normal function and sometimes to prevent a flare-up of the underlying disease. Procedures for tapering the dose are empiric, but in general, the longer the child has been on glucocorticoids, the longer the taper. Withdrawal plans are based on the goal of treating the child with the lowest possible dose of glucocorticoids to avoid long-term adverse effects while avoiding potential adrenal insufficiency during withdrawal. Decreasing the dose to a physiologic dose while monitoring the cortisol level is one method of weaning. A morning cortisol value of 20 mcg/dL indicates that the hypothalamic-pituitary axis is intact, and it is safe to wean further and ultimately discontinue the steroid.

Thyroid Disorders

Anatomy and Physiology

Genetics plays an early role in the development of thyroid disorders. In utero, gene transcription errors can impact normal thyroid gland development and function. The hypothalamic-pituitary-thyroid axis begins functioning in the second trimester of pregnancy.[66] The hypothalamus produces TRH, which in turn stimulates pituitary production of TSH. TSH stimulates the thyroid gland to secrete primarily T_4. Approximately 80% of the TH secreted by the normal thyroid is T_4, with T_3 comprising the remaining 20%. T_4 is converted in peripheral tissues to T_3. Both T_3 and T_4 bind to thyroid-binding proteins, primarily thyroid-binding globulin (TBG). The free, unbound form of T_3 and T_4 is biologically active. T_4 inhibits hypothalamic TRH and pituitary TSH secretion. The TH has an important role in growth

---

• BOX 39.8 **Medications That May Alter Thyroid Levels**

Alter Thyroid Hormone Secretion
- Iodine, lithium—decrease thyroid hormone secretion
- Amiodarone—decrease or possibly increase thyroid hormone secretion
- Tyrosine kinase inhibitors—unknown
- Immune check point inhibitors—induce thyroiditis

Decrease TSH Secretion
- Glucocorticoids, dopamine agonists, somatostatin analogs—inhibit TSH release
- Immune check point inhibitors—induce hypophysitis

Decrease T_4 Absorption
- Calcium carbonate
- FeSO4 (iron) supplements
- Soy-based infant formula
- Proton pump inhibitors
- Aluminum hydroxide antacids

Alter T_3 and T_4 in Serum
- Estrogen—increase thyroid binding globulin (TBG)
- Androgens, glucocorticoids—decrease TBG
- Heparin, NSAIDs, furosemide, phenytoin—displace T_4 from binding proteins

Increased Hepatic Metabolism
- Phenobarbital
- Phenytoin
- Carbamazepine

NSAID, Nonsteroidal antiinflammatory drug; T_4, thyroxine; *TSH,* thyroid stimulating hormone.
From Bauer AJ, Wassner AJ. Thyroid hormone therapy in congenital hypothyroidism and pediatric hypothyroidism. *Endocrine.* 2019;66(1):51–62.

---

and development, basal metabolic activity, oxygen consumption, brain development, and metabolism of lipids, carbohydrates, and proteins. There are medications that can alter thyroid function (Box 39.8), leading to hypothyroidism or hyperthyroidism.

Hypothyroidism

Primary hypothyroidism (caused by a problem in the thyroid gland itself) is categorized as either congenital or acquired, depending on the underlying etiology and age at presentation.[66] In the United States, the incidence of congenital hypothyroidism (CH) is approximately 1 in 3000 to 4000 births, varying by geographic location and race/ethnicity.[67] Female infants are more commonly affected, as are preterm infants, those from multiple gestation births, and infants whose mothers are of advanced maternal age. Infants born with Down syndrome are at higher risk for CH, with males and females equally affected.

CH results from abnormal thyroid gland development (dysgenesis is characterized as dysplasia, aplasia, or ectopia) or from an issue with thyroid hormone synthesis. Thyroid dysgenesis accounts for approximately 85% of cases of CH. Less frequently, CH may result from an abnormality at the level of the pituitary or hypothalamus (affecting 1 in 25,000–1 in 50,000 live births). CH is the most common cause of preventable intellectual disability, with newborn screening detecting many of these cases. Recent studies indicate, however, that delayed TSH elevations despite initial newborn screening are more common and more severe

BOX 39.9 Causes of Acquired Primary Hypothyroidism

Etiology
- Chronic lymphocytic thyroiditis (Hashimoto thyroiditis)
- Drug induced
- Thyroidectomy
- I[131] ablation
- Infiltrative and storage disorders (histiocytosis X, cystinosis)
- Subacute thyroiditis
- Cranial/spinal radiation

BOX 39.10 International Classification of Inherited Metabolic Disorders

- Amino acid metabolism
  - Peptide and amine metabolism
  - Carbohydrate metabolism
  - Fatty acid and ketone body metabolism
  - Energy substrate metabolism
  - Metabolite repair/proofreading
  - Lipid metabolism
  - Lipoprotein metabolism
  - Nucleobase, nucleotide, and nucleic acid metabolism
  - Tetrapyrrole metabolism
  - Organelle biogenesis, dynamics, and interactions
  - Vitamin and cofactor metabolism
  - Trace elements and metals
- Mitochondrial disorders include issues with cofactor biosynthesis, DNA maintenance and replication, mtDNA-related disorders, gene expression, and "other disorders of mitochondrial dysfunction"
- Nuclear-encoded disorders of oxidative phosphorylation
- Miscellaneous disorders of intermediary metabolism
- Congenital disorders of glycosylation
- Neurotransmitter disorders
- Endocrine metabolic disorders

Data from Ferreira CR, Rahman S, Keller M, et al. An international classification of inherited metabolic disorders (ICIMD). *J Inherit Metab Dis.* 2021;44(1):164–177.

than previously thought.[68] Untreated CH leads to developmental delays from irreversible brain damage, variable degrees of growth failure, deafness, and neuromuscular abnormalities. Proper identification and aggressive treatment of CH are essential to optimize developmental outcomes. The prognosis for normal neurologic development is excellent when appropriate treatment with levothyroxine (LT4) is instituted within the first month of life.[69]

CH screening in newborns will also identify infants with TBG deficiency. While the deficiency itself does not cause any health problems, it is important to diagnose and understand TBG deficiency to avoid unnecessary treatments. Although this is not a condition that requires treatment, newborn screening tests will reveal a low level of thyroid hormone (T_4) with low, normal, or slightly elevated thyrotropin (TSH) levels. Since the level of TH is dependent on the availability of binding proteins, those newborns with TBG deficiency have a low level of TBG. The physical examination is within normal limits and there is no history (e.g., midline defect) to suggest central hypothyroidism. Laboratory testing for infants with suspected TBG deficiency includes assessment of free T_4 and TBG levels. The free T_4 will be within normal limits because its level does not depend on binding proteins; the TBG level will be low, which confirms TBG deficiency.[69,70]

The most common cause of acquired hypothyroidism in children in the Western world is Hashimoto thyroiditis, an autoimmune condition leading to the destruction of the thyroid gland. While the exact etiology is not fully understood, Hashimoto disease is associated with T–lymphocytic infiltration of the thyroid gland and follicular destruction. Those with this diagnosis have detectable antibodies specific to thyroid antigens.

Worldwide, iodine deficiency is the main cause of acquired primary hypothyroidism and has led to salt iodination as a public health measure in many countries. Hypothyroidism can also be due to a TSH deficiency that is secondary to pituitary disease or dysfunction of the hypothalamus (central hypothyroidism). Other causes of acquired hypothyroidism are listed in Box 39.9. Children with type 1 diabetes and/or other autoimmune conditions are at increased risk for Hashimoto thyroiditis.

Pediatric patients can also present with subclinical hypothyroidism, where the TSH values are above the upper limit of the reference range but free T_4 levels are within normal limits. This may be benign and can go into remission, but the risk of progression to overt thyroid dysfunction depends on the underlying condition.[71]

Clinical Findings

History. Growth failure, goiter, delayed or arrested puberty, delayed tooth eruption, weight gain, fatigue, dry skin, hyperlipidemia, a decline in school performance, and menorrhagia can be present in the child with hypothyroidism. A family history of thyroid disease or other autoimmune conditions is frequently present. A history of risk factors for hypopituitarism (e.g., CNS insult, frequent headaches, midline defects such as cleft palate) is useful information when assessing the risk for TSH deficiency.

Physical Examination. The clinical manifestations of primary hypothyroidism vary with the age of the child.
- At birth, the newborn may appear completely healthy, thus the importance of newborn screening programs for early identification of hypothyroidism. The most common neonatal signs are prolonged jaundice, constipation, and umbilical hernia. Infants with CH may also have large anterior and posterior fontanelles with a higher incidence of delayed closure, macroglossia, decreased muscle tone, and poor feeders. Some infants develop respiratory distress and poor peripheral circulation with cool, cyanotic skin in the extremities.
- Older children who present with acquired hypothyroidism may exhibit delayed growth or subnormal growth velocity, goiter, weight gain, and delayed return of the deep tendon reflexes. Children with central hypothyroidism (thyroid deficiency secondary to pituitary or hypothalamus dysfunction) may show poor growth, increased weight for height, and features suggestive of hypopituitarism, such as midline facial or eye abnormalities.

Diagnostic Studies. For primary hypothyroidism:
- The diagnosis of CH is usually made within 7 to 10 days of birth, detected by newborn screening tests using a filter paper blood spot card sent to a contracted screening laboratory. The initial blood spot sample should be obtained at least 24 hours after delivery to avoid false-positive results due to a physiologic postnatal TSH surge.[66,72]
  - The screening laboratory measures TSH and T_4 (thyroxine). If the blood spot results indicate a low T_4 and elevated TSH, this suggests CH. The screening labs are then confirmed by the PCP with a follow-up venous blood sample (typically

free T_4 and TSH). If the free T_4 is low and TSH is elevated, this confirms a CH diagnosis.

- TSH (normal range 0.5–5.5 mIU/L) is the most sensitive marker of inadequate TH levels. An increase in TSH to between 5.5 and 10 mIU/L is considered subclinical hypothyroidism and a level of >10 mIU/L is considered overt hypothyroidism.[66]
- A low T_4 or free T_4 in the setting of an elevated TSH may further distinguish a condition where LT4 replacement would be beneficial.

For central hypothyroidism:
- Free serum T_4 is low with a normal TSH.
- For children with TBG deficiency: Total T_4 will be low, but free T_4 and TSH will be normal. TBG level should be measured to quantify TBG deficiency.[69]

Management

The goal of treatment for primary hypothyroidism is a normalization of the TSH level. The treatment aim in central hypothyroidism is to achieve serum T_4 or free T_4 concentrations in the upper half of the age-specific normal range. Hypothyroidism is treated with replacement doses of LT4, which is typically initiated when TSH is >10 mIU/L. *In infants whose whole blood TSH is ≥40mIU/L, LT4 should be initiated as soon as the confirmatory serum sample is obtained, without awaiting the results.*[66]

Liquid suspensions of LT4, while not previously available in the United States, were recently approved by the FDA,[68] but data on the use of this medication form remains limited. Parents have been traditionally instructed to crush the tablet and administer the medication via a spoon with a few drops of water, breast milk, or formula. Compounded LT4 solutions do not provide reliable dosing and should not be used. Limited data suggest brand-name LT4 may be superior to generic in children with severe CH, but not in those with equally severe acquired hypothyroidism.[66] Dosing of LT4 (mcg/kg) varies by age and weight (Table 39.6). Because of the long half-life of LT4, if a single dose is missed, the dose can be doubled the next day. Children and adolescents needed higher weight-based doses of TH replacement than adults, most likely due to a shorter half-life of both T_3 and T_4 in children. However,

these weight-based dose requirements decrease as they moved into adulthood.[66] Anticipatory guidance is necessary regarding dose timing and medication adherence.

Ongoing laboratory monitoring and follow-up are also age dependent. Because normal thyroid function in the first 3 years of life is critical for normal cognitive development, more frequent monitoring is necessary for young infants and young children. Once on medication, thyroid levels are monitored every 1 to 2 weeks until normal, and then every 1 to 2 months during the first year of life and every 2 to 4 months during the second and third year of life.[66] Children older than 3 years should be monitored every 3 to 6 months to see if dose adjustments are needed as the child grows.[73] In transient CH, a thyroid ultrasound should be performed before any trial off LT4 to confirm a normal thyroid gland.

In general, an elevated TSH (in primary hypothyroidism) or low free T_4 (in central hypothyroidism) indicates the need to increase the dose of medication. Following an adjustment in TH replacement, thyroid function testing should be repeated in 4 weeks to be sure that the new dose is adequate.

Hyperthyroidism

Hyperthyroidism occurs in childhood when the thyroid gland overproduces TH or when a child is given too large a dose of TH replacement. While autoimmune Graves disease is the most common cause of hyperthyroidism, only 1% to 5% of all patients with Graves disease are children.[74] In this condition, thyroid-stimulating immunoglobulin binds to the TSH receptor, resulting in excessive thyroid hormone production.

Infants born to females with a current or past history of Graves disease may present with neonatal Graves disease, secondary to the placental transmission of maternal TSH receptor antibodies (TRAb), which stimulate the fetal thyroid gland. Although neonatal Graves disease is self-limiting with the dissipation of maternal antibodies by approximately 3 months of age, early identification and management are critical because these infants are at risk for significant morbidity and mortality.[74] Some children with Hashimoto thyroiditis will have a short (6–18 months) phase of hyperthyroidism (Hashimoto thyrotoxicosis) at the onset of the disease. Other causes of hyperthyroidism include congenital activating mutations of the TSH receptor gene, autonomous thyroid nodules, selective pituitary resistance to thyroid hormones, and pituitary tumors that secrete TSH.[74]

Clinical Findings

History. The history of a child with hyperthyroidism may include:
- Palpitations
- Tremor
- Increased appetite often accompanied by weight loss
- Loose bowel movements
- Fatigue, muscle weakness, and myopathy
- Poor sleep
- Behavioral changes or declining academic performance

Physical Examination. Often observed findings in hyperthyroidism include:
- Goiter
- Thyroid bruit may be present, as well as a palpable thrill due to increased blood flow through the gland.
- Tachycardia, wide pulse pressure
- Brisk reflexes, tremor

TABLE 39.6	Thyroid Hormone Dosing
Age	Levothyroxine Sodium (L-Thyroxine/LT4) mcg/kg/day (Once Daily)
0–3 months	10–15
3–12 months	6–10
1–3 years	4–6
3–10 years	3–5
10–16 years	2–4
>16 years	1.7

Modified from Bauer AJ, Wassner AJ. Thyroid hormone therapy in congenital hypothyroidism and pediatric hypothyroidism. *Endocrine.* 2019;66(1):51–62; and Rose SR, Wassner AJ, Wintergerst KA, et al; AAP Section on Endocrinology, AAP Council on Genetics, Pediatric Endocrine Society, American Thyroid Association. Congenital hypothyroidism: screening and management. *Pediatrics.* 2023;151(1):e2022060420.

- Underweight for height, warm moist skin
- Eye orbitopathy/exophthalmos, caused by enlargement of the extraocular muscles and an increase in the orbital fat volume (approximately 50% of children with Graves disease have exophthalmos).
- In addition to the aforementioned, additional presenting symptoms of neonatal Graves disease include: hyperexcitability, staring with or without eyelid retraction, advanced bone age, a small anterior fontanel, and splenomegaly or hepatomegaly.

Diagnostic Studies. Clinical diagnosis is straightforward and confirmed with laboratory testing. Free T_4 and total T_4 levels are elevated and the TSH is suppressed below the sensitivity of the assay. In rare cases, serum-free T_4 may be near normal, whereas serum T_3 is selectively elevated (T3 toxicosis). Measuring a T_3 level is helpful in hyperthyroidism because it may be more dramatically elevated than the T_4 and be a better marker to monitor. The presence of TRAb levels is specific for Graves disease because of its autoimmune nature.

A thyroid ultrasound is performed to assess for parenchymal abnormalities or focal lesions.[75] In hyperthyroidism, the ultrasound will typically reveal diffuse, often homogeneous, thyroid gland enlargement.

Management

Children with hyperthyroidism should be referred to a pediatric endocrinologist for discussion of treatment options (i.e., medical therapy using antithyroid drugs, radioactive iodine, or consideration for total or near-total thyroidectomy) and ongoing management.[76] Treatment with the drug methimazole is considered first-line therapy for children with Graves disease. Minor adverse reactions to methimazole are reported in 5% to 25% of patients and include rashes, urticaria, gastrointestinal problems, and joint pain.[74] Propylthiouracil, another antithyroid drug option, has been associated with adverse effects including hepatotoxicity, agranulocytosis, and skin rash. Effective drug therapy normalizes serum thyroid levels within a month. Improvements in metabolic rates, growth velocity, and body weight are typically seen within 3 months, and serum TSH levels are generally detectable after 2 to 4 months of treatment.

Less than 30% of children achieve remission after initial treatment with antithyroid medication, and radioactive iodine (RAI) is considered a safe, effective alternative treatment when there is a lack of remission, poor compliance, adverse effects, or relapse with daily medication.[77] The goal of RAI is complete thyroid ablation, and specialists can consider this treatment in children over the age of 5 years. In children, less than 5 years of age or for those with a large goiter and notable orbitopathy, total or near-total thyroidectomy is the preferred treatment.[78]

Parathyroid Disorders

The four parathyroid glands, located just posterior to the thyroid gland, have the sole purpose of maintaining the body's calcium and phosphate homeostasis. While parathyroid disease is relatively rare in pediatric populations, it is important to understand the causes and treatments related to abnormal parathyroid function.

Anatomy and Physiology

The parathyroid glands secrete parathyroid hormone (PTH) to control calcium and phosphate metabolism in the kidneys, intestine, and long bones.[79] Low-ionized calcium levels stimulate the release of PTH while increased serum calcium levels exert a negative-feedback signal on the parathyroid glands to stop the release of PTH. In the kidneys, PTH increases calcium reabsorption and facilitates the synthesis of vitamin D (calcitriol, known as *1,25-dihydroxy vitamin D*). In long bones, PTH stimulates osteoblast differentiation into osteoclasts, which then deconstruct bone through the process of resorption. Bone demineralization causes the release of ionized calcium and phosphate into the bloodstream. In the small intestine, PTH works in conjunction with vitamin D to absorb calcium from food intake.

Hypoparathyroidism

Primary hypoparathyroidism can be caused by congenital malformations and by surgical parathyroid removal or devascularization during anterior neck operations (such as lymph node removal or thyroidectomy). DiGeorge syndrome is the most common genetic cause of hypoparathyroidism, representing approximately 60% of pediatric patients with this disorder.[80] Autoimmune disease can also cause destruction of the parathyroid gland.[79]

Pseudohypoparathyroidism

Pseudohypoparathyroidism is associated with a group of metabolic disorders in which proximal renal tubular resistance to PTH leads to hypocalcemia and hyperphosphatemia. An example of a condition associated with pseudohypoparathyroidism is Albright hereditary osteodystrophy.[81] Features of this and related disorders include brachydactyly, ectopic ossification (bony formations in the skin and muscle tissue), early-onset obesity, and short stature.[82]

Transient Hypoparathyroidism

Infants born to mothers with hypercalcemia and hyperparathyroidism can experience transient hypoparathyroidism due to suppression of fetal PTH release. Treatment consists of close monitoring of ionized calcium levels and treatment of hypocalcemia, typically with calcium carbonate. Spontaneous resolution of hypoparathyroidism typically occurs within a few months.[83]

Clinical Findings

Clinical findings in hypoparathyroidism are related to hypocalcemia. These symptoms include:

- Muscle cramps
- Tetany
- Weakness
- Paresthesia
- Laryngospasm
- Seizure-like activity

Physical Examination. Clinicians assess for hypocalcemic tetany by attempting to elicit the Trousseau sign (carpal spasms exhibited when arterial blood flow to the hand is occluded for 3–5 minutes with a blood pressure cuff inflated to 15 mm Hg above systolic blood pressure) and the Chvostek sign (facial spasms produced by lightly tapping over the facial nerve just in front of the ear).

Diagnostic Studies. Laboratory tests will reveal low PTH with a concomitant low calcium level. Measurement of 25-hydroxy vitamin D is important to exclude vitamin D deficiency as a cause of hypocalcemia. Serum magnesium measured as hypomagnesemia may cause PTH deficiency and subsequent hypocalcemia. Serum phosphorus levels are also obtained because low PTH will cause hyperphosphatemia.

Management

Treatment of patients with hypoparathyroidism involves correcting hypocalcemia by administering calcium and vitamin D supplements. It is essential to avoid symptomatic hypocalcemia, maintain serum calcium at or slightly below the lower range of normal, maintain normal serum magnesium levels, and keep the serum phosphate as close to normal as possible.[80] For chronic/severe hypoparathyroidism, recombinant PTH has become an important component of hypoparathyroidism management, but standards for its use in the management of pediatrics have not been developed. A calcium-rich diet is also recommended. Severe tetany or seizures resulting from hypocalcemia are treated emergently with IV calcium gluconate given slowly over 10 minutes with electrocardiogram monitoring for bradycardia.

Hyperparathyroidism

Hyperparathyroidism, while uncommon in pediatric patients, has been associated with parathyroid adenomas or hyperplasia. Primary hyperparathyroidism is characterized by abnormal regulation of PTH secretion, leading to hypersecretion of PTH relative to the serum calcium concentration. Neonatal primary hyperparathyroidism presents at birth or during the first 6 months of life. Familial primary hyperparathyroidism is associated with multiple endocrine neoplasia syndromes and genetic mutations that cause hypocalciuric hypercalcemia.

Secondary hyperparathyroidism is seen in chronic kidney, liver, and bowel diseases, where lower ionized calcium levels cause excess secretion of PTH. Patients with chronic kidney disease develop hyperphosphatemia, vitamin D deficiency, and hypocalcemia, causing excess secretion of PTH. Tertiary hyperparathyroidism can occur due to the autonomous secretion of PTH in patients with chronic kidney disease.[84]

Clinical Findings

Physical Examination. In infants with neonatal primary hypoparathyroidism, presenting symptoms include respiratory distress, hypotonia, failure to thrive, hypercalcemia, and metabolic bone disease. In older pediatric populations, symptoms may include:
- Fatigue
- Depression
- Confusion
- Loss of appetite
- Polydipsia
- Vomiting
- Constipation
- Arthralgias
- Bone pain
- Kidney stones
- Polyuria
- Pathological bone fractures
- Acute pancreatitis

Diagnostic Studies. In primary hyperparathyroidism, laboratory testing reveals increased PTH, increased serum calcium, decreased serum phosphorus, and normal to increased alkaline phosphatase. In secondary hyperparathyroidism, calcium may be normal or slightly decreased.

Management

Treatment strategies include managing hypercalcemia and resulting hypophosphatemia and addressing the underlying cause, such as adenoma. Primary hyperparathyroidism may be definitively treated by subtotal or total parathyroidectomy, although calcimimetic drugs (such as cinacalcet and etecalcitide) are used to reduce serum PTH and calcium levels. Secondary hyperparathyroidism related to chronic kidney disease includes dietary phosphorus restriction and use of phosphate binders, vitamin D supplementation, and calcimimetics.[84]

Diabetes Mellitus

Diabetes mellitus, one of the most common chronic diseases in childhood, is a group of conditions characterized by inadequate insulin secretion, insulin resistance, or both. These dynamics lead to defective metabolism of carbohydrates, protein, and fat and subsequent hyperglycemia. According to the CDC,[85,86] >11% of the US population is diagnosed with diabetes, and the incidence in youths <20 years of age is ~35 per 10,000.

The seminal SEARCH for Diabetes in Youth study in 2009 revealed that 3.4 million youth were diagnosed with type 1 diabetes and 1.7 million youth were diagnosed with type 2 diabetes in the United States.[87] Females and males were affected in equal numbers. The prevalence of type 1 diabetes varied by race and ethnicity and was highest among non-Hispanic White youth (2.55/1000 children). Native American children had a much lower prevalence of type 1 diabetes (0.35/1000 children), and only 32% of diabetes among Native American children was type 1. Within the last decade, the annual incidence of diagnosed diabetes in youth was estimated at 18,200 with type 1 diabetes, and 5800 with type 2 diabetes. In 2019 about 244,000 children and adolescents were diagnosed with type 1 diabetes.[85]

Additional pediatric diabetes disorders include MODY, diabetes-related to chronic conditions (e.g., cystic fibrosis, posttransplantation of solid organs) or correlated with genetic disorders (e.g., Down syndrome), and hyperglycemia and diabetes induced by chronic medication use (e.g., steroids). New cases of type 1 diabetes are more frequently diagnosed during the autumn and winter months. The incidence of both type 1 and type 2 diabetes continues to increase worldwide.[88]

Type 1 Diabetes

Type 1 diabetes is a multifactorial disease that is associated with genetic predisposition and autoimmune destruction of pancreatic β-cells in the islets of Langerhans. The onset of diabetes symptoms is thought to be triggered by a preceding environmental event in susceptible individuals. This destruction of β-cells results in an absolute deficiency in insulin secretion reduced biologic effectiveness, or both. Normal metabolic function depends upon the availability of enough circulating insulin. Insulin deficiency results in uninhibited gluconeogenesis and a blockage in the use and storage of circulating glucose. Hyperglycemia is the result of the defective metabolism of carbohydrates, proteins, and fats.

Pancreatic autoantibodies have been identified for five specific β-cells antigens: insulin (IAA), glutamate decarboxylase 65 (GADA), islet antigen-2 (IA-2A), zinc transporter 8 (ZnT8A), and tetraspanin-7 (Tspan7A). These autoantibodies can be identified by age 6 months, with peak incidence occurring in early childhood. Pediatric research indicates that the presence of ≥2 autoantibodies is associated with a 70% risk of developing diabetes within 10 years of follow-up.[89]

Because of the autoimmune dysfunction associated with type 1 diabetes, patients should also be evaluated for concomitant autoimmune disorders. These include Hashimoto thyroiditis (most common), adrenal insufficiency, Graves disease, juvenile idiopathic arthritis, systemic lupus erythematosus, psoriasis, Sjögren disease, and celiac disease.[90] Of note, there is also a small cohort of patients with type 1 diabetes without a known etiology. These patients have permanent insulinopenia and are prone to diabetic ketoacidosis (DKA) but have no evidence of β-cells autoimmunity.

Clinical Findings

Although the onset of type 1 diabetes is gradual with the destruction of pancreatic islet cells over time, children may become ill quite suddenly once symptoms manifest. As diabetes develops, the symptomatology reflects the decreasing degree of β-cell mass, increasing insulinopenia and hyperglycemia, and increasing ketoacids.

History. The patient's recent history may reveal the onset of a viral infection, cold, or flu; parents may notice increased urination and thirst during the recovery period, with additional signs and symptoms appearing over a period of days or weeks. The following early symptoms are often reported:
- Polydipsia, polyphagia, polyuria
- Nocturia
- Blurred vision
- Weight loss or poor weight gain
- Fatigue and lethargy
- Vaginal moniliasis

Over 30% of children with new-onset type 1 diabetes either present with or have an episode of DKA near the time of diagnosis. The prevalence[91] of DKA at or near type 1 diabetes diagnosis increased by 2% annually from 2010 to 2016, following the high but stable prevalence observed from 2002 to 2010. Younger age, female sex, ethnic/race minority status, lower socioeconomic status, and lack of private health insurance are risk factors for presenting in DKA at diabetes onset.[92]

Physical Examination. Although children typically have polyuria, polydipsia, and weight loss, the physical examination of children with new-onset type 1 diabetes may be remarkably benign. Findings can range from benign to severe and can include:
- Dehydration (child may not look clinically dehydrated unless actively vomiting)
- Weight loss or slow weight gain
- Muscle wasting
- Tachycardia
- Vaginal yeast, thrush, or other infection

Presentation in Diabetic Ketoacidosis. Pediatric patients may present in a hyperosmolar hyperglycemic state or in DKA. Hyperglycemia results from decreased glucose utilization due to insulinopenia and increased glucose production from the liver. Without insulin, the body's ability to break down fats (lipolysis) is not suppressed, leading to ketoacid development. The hyperglycemic state also causes osmotic diuresis, with dehydration and electrolyte imbalances, with significant depletion of sodium and phosphorus.[93]

If ketoacidosis develops, symptoms include:
- Flushed cheeks and face
- Fruity-smelling breath
- Altered mental status
- Dehydration with an inability to take fluids orally
- Kussmaul breathing (starts as slow and shallow respiration, but progresses to rapid, labored, deep breathing) as a response to acidosis

Diagnostic Studies. Urine testing and blood glucose measurements are generally sufficient to make the diagnosis:

- Urine for glucose and ketones.
- Metabolic screen for acid-base status to exclude DKA.
- Hemoglobin A$_{1c}$ (HbA$_{1c}$), which correlates with average blood glucose concentrations over the previous 3 months.
- Blood glucose.
- Pancreatic autoantibody panel (GAD65, IA2/ICA512, IAA, and, in selected cases, ZnT8) to confirm the diagnosis of type 1 diabetes, particularly in those cases where there may be uncertainty regarding type. While autoantibody prevalence often decreases as diabetes duration increases, autoantibodies may persist for many years.[94]
- C-peptide, which is an insulin secretion biomarker, is helpful for assessing insulin-producing β-cell residual function.[95]
- To determine the presence of ketoacidosis in the emergency setting, beta-hydroxybutyrate level and venous blood gas are obtained.
- Initial management of new-onset diabetes also includes screening for concomitant associated autoimmune conditions, including hypothyroidism and celiac disease. The American Diabetes Association (ADA) and the International Society for Pediatric and Adolescent Diabetes recommend testing for thyroid function (free T$_4$, TSH), thyroid antibodies, and tTG-IgA soon after diagnosis.[96] Thyroid function should be repeated every 1 to 2 years while tTG IgA should be tested within 2 and 5 years. Hashimoto thyroiditis and/or celiac disease may be present at the initial diagnosis of type 1 diabetes.

Staging and Diagnostic Criteria for Diabetes

Screening for Type 1 Diabetes in Family Members. When one member of a family is diagnosed with type 1 diabetes, other family members require screening as well. The risk for people in the general population is about one in 300, but for those who have a family member with type 1 diabetes, the risk is one in 20, or 15x greater. Families concerned about the risk to other family members should be directed to the Type 1 Diabetes TrialNet[97] website (www.diabetestrialnet.org) where free screening can be obtained either at home or from worldwide risk screening and study locations as part of an international clinical study. Children younger than 18 years old who test negative for the presence of antibodies associated with type 1 diabetes can be retested each year to determine if the risk has changed. If antibodies are present, information will be provided regarding eligibility for participation in a diabetes prevention study.

The latent phase, or stage I diabetes, is characterized by normal glucose levels but having two or more autoantibodies present. In stage II diabetes, the child exhibits impaired glucose tolerance and one or more of the following: HbA$_{1c}$ between 5.7% and 6.4%, an impaired fasting glucose between 100 and 126 mg/dL, or an impaired glucose tolerance indicating a 2-hour plasma glucose between 140 and 200 mg/dL. Stage III diabetes diagnostic criteria includes an HbA$_{1c}$ of 6.5% or greater, or a fasting plasma glucose of 126 mg/dL or greater, or 200 mg/dL plasma glucose result following an oral glucose test, or 200 mg/dL random plasma glucose in conjunction with polyuria and weight loss.[98]

Differential Diagnosis. Type 1 diabetes must be distinguished from stress-induced hyperglycemia, which in some studies occurs in up to 4% of normal children during a serious illness. MODY (described later) may be misdiagnosed as type 1 diabetes.

Management

The treatment goals for children with type 1 diabetes are to achieve normal growth and development, optimal glycemic control, and positive psychosocial adjustment to diabetes while minimizing acute or chronic complications. Identified risk factors for hospital admission related to diabetes include uncontrolled HbA_{1c}, at least one previous admission for hyperglycemia with ketosis of DKA within the last 12 months, and patient coverage with noncommercial insurance were risk factors for hospital admission.[92]

Management of new-onset type 1 diabetes involves determining the insulin regimen and dose best suited to the individual child, the target range for blood glucose levels, and the best methods to manage the child's diet. Children and families must learn how to inject insulin and then use insulin pumps, monitor blood glucose levels, quantify the number of carbohydrates in the food, prevent hypoglycemia, manage diabetes during illness, and adjust insulin dose or carbohydrate intake for strenuous activities. Diabetes education should be structured based on the child's age and developmental tasks, family management priorities, and family health literacy status. The child should be incorporated into the educational experience as soon as they are developmentally ready. These children and families need ongoing access to certified pediatric diabetes educators, pediatric registered dietician nutritionists, and psychologists or social workers when necessary. Telemedicine and virtual coaching have become essential components of diabetes education and management. Each component of the treatment regimen is discussed in the following sections.

Initial Management. A critical concept in the management of diabetes is that control of glucose levels to near normal reduces the risk of long-term complications.[98] All children with type 1 diabetes should be started on insulin at diagnosis. Children with ketoacidosis should be admitted to the hospital for IV insulin treatment, fluid replacement, and careful monitoring to prevent cerebral edema that, although rare, can cause significant morbidity or mortality.

Whenever possible, children should be referred for ongoing care provided at a children's diabetes center for initiation of insulin therapy and diabetes education. Institutional protocols vary about whether well-appearing children without ketones who have newly diagnosed type 1 diabetes require hospital admission or can be managed with outpatient treatment.[92] Outpatient management at the initial diagnosis of type 1 diabetes has no disadvantages regarding glycemic control, complications, psychosocial factors, or total costs. Technology is lessening the burden of managing diabetes. Research showed that high-tech devices and communication helped to lessen the impact of COVID-19 lockdowns on children with type 1 diabetes.[99]

Monitoring Blood Glucose Levels. Frequent monitoring of blood glucose levels is required to dose insulin and prevent hypoglycemia/hyperglycemia. Children and families are taught to self-monitor blood glucose (SMBG) before meals, at bedtime, and sometimes in the middle of the night and during symptoms of hypoglycemia/hyperglycemia. Blood glucose meters have benefited from continued advances in technology; many blood glucose meters provide results within 5 seconds and automatically store and categorize blood glucose values by time of day or relation to meals.

Continuous glucose monitors (CGMs) are different from traditional glucose meters in that they measure glucose in the interstitial fluid rather than blood glucose. Typically, there is a 5-minute lag between interstitial glucose readings and blood glucose readings. In 2017 the FDA approved the use of the Dexcom G5 CGM for insulin dose calculations instead of the need for a fingerstick blood glucose measurement. CGMs have three components: a sensor (small wire) that is placed in subcutaneous tissue,

a transmitter that rests on the skin, and a receiver that displays the data. More recent systems have replaced the need for stand-alone receivers and instead display real-time interstitial glucose levels and trend graphs on mobile phones. Glucose data can be shared through the Cloud in real-time to alert family members of their child's glucose level. Alarms warn of low- and high-blood glucose levels, using individually determined preset blood glucose ranges. Some CGMs are also integrated into insulin pumps as described later.

Providers must be aware of social and ethnic disparities that have been identified in the use of CGM; research has indicated lower rates of initiation and sustained use of CGM in those with noncommercial insurance, and in non-Hispanic Black children.[99,100] In addition, the costs of Smartphone technology may be prohibitive to some pediatric patients and their families.[101]

Recent research indicates that the use of CGMs can be effective in lowering HbA_{1c} and reducing hypoglycemia, but that children and adolescents are less likely than adults to continue its use.[102] Although those who use CGMs report satisfaction, many barriers exist including "alarm fatigue" from frequent alarms, cost, and variability of accuracy.[103]

Insulin. In general, the goal of insulin therapy is to achieve optimal glycemic control. The treatment goals must be individualized and reassessed over time. A HbA_{1c} of <7% is considered appropriate for many pediatric patients but should be modified in those with frequent hypoglycemia or hypoglycemia unawareness.[104] Individualized insulin dosing is multifactorial and includes consideration of the patient's age, weight, pubertal stage, the duration and phase of diabetes, the integrity of injection sites, nutritional intake and patterns, exercise, and daily routine, along with blood glucose and HgbA1c results. Adjustments are also made for intercurrent illness.[105] Frequently used insulin preparations are listed in Table 39.7.

The selection of an insulin regimen depends on the age of the child, family preferences and lifestyle, the family's social and educational resources, and the clinician's comfort level. All children require medical nutrition therapy/dietary recommendations that match the insulin schedule.

To achieve glycemic targets, exogenous insulin replacement that mimics physiologic insulin behavior is preferred for most children. In children without diabetes, the pancreas secretes a small amount of background or basal insulin throughout the day and a larger amount of bolus insulin when a meal is consumed. Intensive basal-bolus insulin therapy attempts to match this. In general, basal insulin doses should be less than bolus insulin doses.[105]

Intensive basal-bolus insulin therapy can be delivered using either multiple daily injections (MDIs) or continuous subcutaneous insulin infusion (CSII) using an insulin pump based on patient and family preferences. MDI regimens can be implemented using a long-acting insulin analog administered typically once a day to provide a steady basal insulin replacement with boluses of rapid-acting insulin at meal and snack times. This regimen requires a minimum of four injections per day. Many insulin analogs are available in pen delivery systems.

The use of insulin pumps is considered safe and efficacious even when used with young children and is a popular way to deliver insulin to children with type 1 diabetes. The use of CSII has been shown to modestly lower HbA_{1c}.[106] In CSII therapy, the pump infuses rapid-acting insulin into the subcutaneous tissue through a small, flexible, soft cannula. The cannula is replaced in a new site by the wearer or the family every 2 or 3 days. Basal insulin replacement is achieved by the delivery of small doses

TABLE 39.7   Insulin Products

Type of Insulin	Brand Name	Generic Name	Onset	Peak	Duration
Ultra-fast acting	Fiasp	Insulin aspart	8–10 min	~ 1 h	3–5 h
Rapid acting	Novolog	Insulin aspart	15 min	30–90 min	3–5 h
	Aprida	Insulin glulisine	15 min	30–90 min	3–5 h
	Humalog	Insulin lispro	15 min	30–90 min	3–5 h
Short-acting	Humulin R	Regular (R)	30–60 min	2–4 h	5–8 h
	Novolin R				
Intermediate-acting	Humulin N	NPH (N)	1–3 h	8 h	12–16 h
	Novolin N				
Long-acting	Levemir	Insulin detemir	1 h	Peakless	20–26 h
	Lantus	Insulin glargine			
Ultra-long acting	Tresiba	Insulin degludec	30–90 min	Peakless	Up to 42 h
Premixed NPH (intermediate-acting) and regular (short-acting)	Humulin 70/30 Novolin 70/30	70% NPH and 30% regular	30–60 min	Varies	10–16 h
	Humulin 50/50	50% NPH and 50% regular	30–60 min	Varies	10–16 h
Premixed insulin lispro protamine suspension (intermediate-acting) and insulin lispro (rapid-acting)	Humalog Mix 75/25	75% insulin lispro protamine and 25% insulin lispro	10–15 min	Varies	10–16 h
	Humalog Mix 50/50	50% insulin lispro protamine and 50% insulin lispro	10–15 min	Varies	10–16 h
Premixed insulin aspart protamine suspension (intermediate-acting) and insulin aspart (rapid-acting)	NovoLog Mix 70/30	70% insulin aspart protamine and 30% insulin aspart	5–15 min	Varies	10–16 h

of rapid-acting insulin continuously throughout the day. These doses can be tailored to the child's physiologic requirements over a 24-hour period. Many pediatric patients eat small meals and snacks frequently, and pump users can administer bolus-dosing insulin as often as needed without additional injections. Bolus doses are calculated by the pump if the user enters the amount of carbohydrate to be eaten and/or their blood glucose. Pump dose calculations are based on personalized settings and then modified depending on insulin still working from prior doses, referred to as "insulin on board".

CSII via an insulin pump is particularly useful for delivering small bolus doses of insulin and varying the dose of basal insulin delivered over a 24-hour period. Challenges associated with the use of CSII include accessibility, lack of long-acting insulin injection, the time required for education, troubleshooting, technology reliance, and having to continually wear a device.[101] Insulin pumps may inadvertently put the child at risk for ketosis if the infusion catheter kinks or becomes obstructed or if the pump malfunctions. Finally, if a device or app is malfunctioning or misplaced, the user will still need to perform calculations manually. Education about managing device failure is critical for patients and families.

In 2020 the FDA approved a hybrid closed-loop diabetes management device (MiniMed 770G system)[107] for use by individuals ages 2 to 6 years with type 1 diabetes. This device provides continuous glucose monitoring and continuous basal insulin delivery, and gives insulin boluses with minimal input from patients or their caregivers. This delivery system adjusts background insulin every

5 minutes and utilizes Bluetooth technology to alert patients and caregivers of any changes via Smartphone. Systems have features to pause basal insulin when the child's blood glucose is low. Hybrid closed-loop systems still require an attentive user to frequently monitor blood glucose, count carbohydrates, bolus for meals, and/or elevated blood glucose, and troubleshoot system errors.

Both MDI and CSII allow unreliable eaters to match their carbohydrate intake with insulin; children may be flexible with the timing of meals and snacks. Families learn to use a carbohydrate-to-insulin ratio (to cover the carbohydrate content of the meal/snack) and a blood sugar correction formula (if the blood glucose is above the target range) to determine each quick-acting insulin dose. If families either find MDI and/or CSII too demanding or need support to maintain the regimen during the school day, other insulin regimens may be considered including sliding scale dosing, although their use is waning.

Another technological advance is the Smart Insulin Pen (SIP) technology. The SIP is described as a reusable injector pen that features a Smartphone interface with a tracking application (app). The app includes a calculator function, which determines insulin doses based on personalized settings, and automatically tracks patient data.[101]

The usual sites for insulin injection or infusion are the legs, arms, abdomen, hips, and buttocks. Young children with minimal subcutaneous abdominal fat may have difficulty with the abdominal site. Rotation of injection and infusion sites is necessary to prevent the thickening of tissue around injection sites (lipohypertrophy) and poor absorption of insulin.

In some pediatric patients with new-onset type 1 diabetes, not all pancreatic β-cells have been completely destroyed. After insulin treatment has been started, children may enter a "honeymoon period" because the remaining functional β-cells seem to recover function with insulin treatment. When this occurs, the exogenous insulin requirements decrease and there is a period of stable blood glucose control, often with nearly normal glucose concentrations. This period usually starts in the first weeks of therapy, often continues for 3 to 6 months, and can last up to 2 years. Close follow-up after beginning insulin therapy is necessary to prevent hypoglycemic episodes. In general, insulin dose adjustments are based on the blood glucose patterns over several days. In general, the insulin dose would be decreased if any unexplained severe hypoglycemic events occur. To manage hypoglycemic episodes, there are now improved formulations of glucagon for autoinjection or nasal administration.[98]

To further improve the science of glycemic control, ongoing research involves the development of ultra-rapid insulins and glucose-responsive "smart" insulins that "turn on" and "turn off" in response to a hypo-or hyperglycemia.[88]

Adjusting Insulin Dosages. Parents and teens can be educated to make insulin adjustments based on blood glucose patterns. They analyze what time of day the blood glucose is consistently outside of the target range (either too low or too high) and adjust the insulin dose that most directly is related to the problematic blood glucose pattern. Usually, parents can safely make up to a 10% adjustment to the basal or bolus insulin dose. With practice and guidance, many families eventually feel comfortable adjusting the insulin dose independently; others may feel more comfortable conferring with their diabetes care provider.

Medical Nutrition Therapy. Nutrition is an essential component of diabetes management. Diets should be healthy and daily calories spread over three meals and snacks. Caloric requirements are based on the child's age, body weight, and activity level. Calories are distributed between protein (15%), carbohydrates (55%), and fat (less than 30% of caloric intake with less than 7% in the form of saturated fats) and account for food preferences, including those pertaining to culture. Carbohydrates such as legumes, whole grains, vegetables, fruits, and dairy products (with emphasis on foods that are higher in fiber and have a lower glycemic index) are preferred over other sources, especially those containing added sugars.[108] The meal plan for a child with diabetes should include the same healthy foods recommended for all pediatric patients. The goal is to balance food intake with insulin dose and activity to maintain blood glucose levels within the target range and to prevent both hyperglycemic and hypoglycemic episodes.

A pediatric dietician/nutritionist is essential to provide ongoing guidance to the child and family. Carbohydrate counting is an approach that allows greater flexibility for children using basal-bolus insulin regimens. Children with diabetes can safely eat sugary treats on occasion by including those treats within their prescribed carbohydrate allotment. Low-calorie (e.g., saccharin, aspartame, sucralose, and acesulfame potassium) sweeteners are safe in moderation. Monitoring intake when eating out can be a challenge. Dieticians may help families to identify effective mobile phone applications that can be used to determine appropriate intake.

Exercise. Exercise is encouraged in all children, including those with diabetes, to promote cardiovascular fitness, control weight, and enhance social interaction and self-esteem. Other benefits of exercise include improved glycemic control and lipid profiles, improved quality of life, and decreased total daily dose of insulin in pediatric patients with type 1 diabetes.[109] Youth with type 1

diabetes should not be excluded from participation in sports activities, including competitive sports. Any restrictions placed on an individual would be necessary only when optimal glycemic control cannot be maintained or if complications or comorbidities are not compatible with the activity. Physical activity should include 60 minutes of moderate- to vigorous-intensity aerobic activity daily, along with vigorous muscle- and bone-strengthening activities at least 3 days per week.[104] Research indicates that pediatric patients with diabetes who engaged in 60 min of activity ≥3 days a week had significantly lower HbA$_{1c}$ compared to those who exercised less than 3 days a week.[110]

Control of the child's blood glucose level during exercise, especially rigorous exercise such as athletic competition, is a challenge. It requires ongoing blood glucose monitoring (before, during, and after exercise), careful planning of meals and carbohydrates, snacks around the time of exercise, and adjustment of insulin dosing to counterbalance the effect of exercise on blood glucose levels.

During physical exercise, the body's metabolic demands increase, causing increased uptake of glucose into the tissues and a reduction in blood glucose. Skeletal muscle also relies on stores of glycogen, triglycerides, free fatty acids, and glucose production, largely from the liver. For athletes without diabetes, hormonal mediators maintain normal blood glucose levels even under high athletic conditions. In these individuals, exercise leads to decreased plasma insulin levels and increased glucagon that trigger hepatic glucose production. However, in youth with type 1 diabetes, this hormonal pathway is interrupted. Thus, if the level of insulin is too low, exercise can trigger the release of high levels of glucose and ketone bodies, leading to hyperglycemia and eventually, if unchecked, to DKA. Conversely, if too much exogenous insulin is administered, the feedback loop for increased glucose mobilization is interrupted, and hypoglycemia results.

Glucose levels can vary by the type, duration, and intensity of exercise performed. Aerobic exercise reduces blood glucose by raising glucose uptake. Short high-intensity or anaerobic exercise increases blood glucose by prolonging insulin action. This effect can last for up to 24 hours after short intense activities.[111] Therefore to compensate for the effect of exercise on blood glucose levels, children and families are taught to decrease prandial insulin dosing for the meal/snack before exercise and/or increase their food intake. In addition, patients on insulin pumps can lower basal rates by 10% to 50% or more or suspend for 1 to 2 hours during exercise.[104] Anaerobic exercise requires conservative blood glucose correction for higher glucose levels following exercise, as hypoglycemia can still occur later in the day. Because exercise can affect blood glucose levels for as long as 24 hours after exercise has occurred, parents need to be aware of the risk of nocturnal hypoglycemia on active days and monitor blood glucose levels more frequently including overnight.

It is generally recommended that young athletes with type 1 diabetes have a medical team participating in their health care, ideally including an endocrinologist and nutritionist who specialize in diabetes and are familiar with the energy requirements of the individual's sport. Depending on the level of athletic endeavor, an exercise physiologist may also be part of the team. It is essential that coaches, trainers, or other athletic staff be aware of the young athlete's diabetes care plan and be trained in aspects of care.

Ongoing Management. Children with type 1 diabetes should be seen for follow-up every 3 to 4 months, with the visit tailored by age and developmental stage and careful attention paid to diabetes management including:

- Self-monitoring blood glucose results
- Frequency of hypoglycemia

- HbA$_{1c}$
- Physical activity level
- Emotional adjustment to the disease
- Social issues, such as peer pressure
- Eating issues: Young females and males with diabetes may attempt to lose weight by withholding or decreasing insulin dosages to lose weight.[112] Providers should have a high index of suspicion for disordered eating in youth with elevated BMIs and HbA$_{1c}$ levels.
- Periodic screening for the development of additional autoimmune conditions (which can include later-presenting diagnoses such as myasthenia gravis, autoimmune hepatitis, and Addison disease).[104]
- A physical examination that focuses on:
  - Growth and weight gain
  - Blood pressure
  - Stage of puberty
  - Injection site assessment for lipodystrophy
  - Clues for another autoimmune disease (thyroiditis and celiac disease)

Ongoing management of type 1 diabetes also includes the following referrals:

- Dietician consultations for nutritional review.
- Collaboration with school nurses, teachers, and administrators to ensure treatment regimens are followed in the school or daycare setting.
- Continued well-child health supervision and appropriate immunizations (e.g., annual influenza vaccination).
- Long before it becomes medically necessary, providers should begin to discuss and guide patients through the process of transitioning to adult care. Many diabetes centers have structured programs in place to ameliorate the process, and providers frequently begin these discussions when patients are in early puberty.[113]

Complications

Morbidity and mortality in type 1 diabetes come from metabolic derangements and from long-term complications that affect the small and large blood vessels. Chronic hyperglycemia has been shown to cause long-term complications of microvascular disease (retinopathy, nephropathy, neuropathy, depression, and cognitive defects) and macrovascular disease (arterial obstruction and ischemic heart disease). Microvascular complications, including diabetic kidney disease, affect approximately 25% of young persons with a duration of type 1 diabetes of >10 years.[114] Complications can be prevented, or their rate of progression slowed by improving glycemic control through the use of intensive insulin regimens consisting of MDI or CSII. A multidisciplinary approach includes referral to other subspecialties depending on the presence of comorbid conditions. Recommendations for screening and treatment of complications and comorbid conditions are listed in Table 39.8.

Depression and anxiety rates are high in youth with type 1 diabetes.[115] Appropriate screenings and referrals for psychological counseling, ideally by providers knowledgeable of the tasks required for diabetes management, are recommended.

In caring for pediatric populations with type 1 diabetes, the PCP ensures well-child annual care, administration of vaccines (including annual influenza vaccine and appropriate pneumococcal vaccine), compliance with dilated eye examinations, and screening for microalbuminuria.[93]

Patient and Family Education

Providing families and children with information that helps them to gain control of a very difficult disease is crucial. Education of the child, family, and caregivers should include insulin therapy, self-monitoring of glucose, nutrition, and meal planning (including carbohydrate counting), exercise, managing sick days, school issues, coping skills, and prevention of complications. Those with diabetes should always wear a form of medical identification. School personnel must be informed of the plan of care and must implement an individualized care plan for the child. The ADA stresses that starting at puberty, preconception counseling must be incorporated into diabetes clinic visits for all females of childbearing potential.[53] During the transition to adult care, patients require additional education and support, as a loss to follow-up is associated with worsening glycemic control and with avoidable hospitalizations.[113]

Prediabetes and Type 2 Diabetes

Both prediabetes and type 2 diabetes in youth are serious and growing public health problems.[116] Approximately one in five adolescents ages 12 to 18 years carried the diagnosis of prediabetes during the years 2005 to 2016. *Prediabetic* refers to patients who exhibit abnormal carbohydrate metabolism but whose glucose levels do not meet the criteria for diabetes. Prediabetes is associated with cardiometabolic risk and is more commonly seen in males and in children and adolescents with obesity.

The incidence of type 2 diabetes is also rising: from 2002 to 2015, the incidence rose from 9.0 cases per 100,000 children and adolescents to 13.8 cases per 100,000 in the same population. The Diabetes Report Card published by the CDC[117] estimates that >5000 new cases/year of type 2 diabetes are diagnosed among US youth younger than age 20 years. There is a higher prevalence of type 2 diabetes in females, but it remains unclear whether more females are screened secondary to concerns for obesity than their male counterparts.[118] Most of the increase in incidence is among non-White and non-Asian children and adolescents.[119] There are also social and ethnic disparities related to both initial presentation and comorbidities associated with type 2 diabetes. Compared to non-Hispanic White youth, non-Hispanic Black, and Hispanic youth with type 2 diabetes present with worse metabolic control and tend toward persistently worse HbA$_{1c}$ trajectories.[120] The overall prevalence rates may be underreported, especially because children may have no symptoms or mild symptoms for a long period of time. Children usually are diagnosed during the preteen and teenage years, between 10 and 19 years old, with a peak age for presentation at mid-puberty (around age 14 years).

Type 2 diabetes begins with increased tissue resistance to insulin, resulting in hyperinsulinemia and hyperglycemia. As hyperglycemia creates increased insulin demand, there is a progressive deterioration in pancreatic β-cell insulin secretion. The increasing demand for insulin over time causes the pancreas to lose its ability to effectively secrete insulin. Unlike in type 1 diabetes, autoimmune destruction of pancreatic β-cell does not typically occur.

During the pubertal growth spurt, GH secretion causes an approximately 30% reduction in insulin sensitivity.[121] Adolescents with normally functioning pancreatic β-cells secrete additional insulin to compensate for this puberty-related effect. However, if β-cells do not function properly, metabolic decompensation begins, leading to prediabetes with eventual progression to type 2 diabetes. In addition, the glucagon-like peptide (GLP-1) receptor

TABLE 39.8   Recommendations for Screening and Treatment of Complications and Comorbid Conditions in Type 1 Diabetes

	Thyroid Disease	Celiac Disease	Hypertension	Dyslipidemia	Nephropathy	Retinopathy	Neuropathy
Method	TSH, consider antithyroglobulin and antithyroid peroxidase antibodies	tTG-IgA if total IgA normal; IgG tTG and deamidated gliadin antibodies if IgA deficient	Blood pressure monitoring	Lipid profile (nonfasting is acceptable initially)	Albumin-to-creatinine ration; random sample acceptable initially	Dilated fundoscopy or retinal photography	Foot exam with pedal pulses, pinprick, 10-g monofilament sensation tests, vibration, and ankle reflexes
When to start	Soon after diagnosis	Soon after diagnosis	At diagnosis	Soon after diagnosis; preferable after glycemia is improved and child ≥2 years	Puberty or >10 years, whichever is earlier and diabetes duration of 5 years	Puberty or ≥11 years, whichever is earlier, and diabetes duration of 3–5 years	Puberty or ≥10 years, whichever is earlier, and diabetes duration of 5 years
Follow-up frequency	Every 1–2 years if thyroid antibodies (–); more often is symptoms develop or presence of thyroid antibodies	Within 2 years and then at 5 years after diagnosis; sooner if symptoms develop	Every visit	If LDL ≤100 mg/dL, repeat at 9–11 years; then if <100 mg/dL, every 3 years	If normal, annually; if abnormal, repeat with confirmation in 2 of 3 samples over 6 months	If normal, every 2 years; consider less frequently (every 4 years) if HbA$_{1c}$ < 8% and eye professional agrees	If normal, annually
Target	N/A	N/A	<90th percentile for age, sex, and height; if ≥13 years, 120–120/80 mmHg)	LDL <100 mg/dL	Albumin-to-creatinine ratio <30 mg/g	No retinopathy	No neuropathy
Treatment	Appropriate treatment of underlying thyroid disease	After confirmation, start gluten-free diet	Lifestyle modification and ACE inhibitor or ARB for hypertension (≥95th percentile for age, sex, and height or, if ≥13 years, ≥130/80 mmHg)	If abnormal, optimize glucose control and medical nutrition therapy; if after 6 months LDL >160 mg/dL or >130 mg/dL with cardiovascular risk factor(s), initiate statin therapy (for those >10 years)	Optimize glucose and blood pressure control; ACE inhibitor if albumin-to-creatinine ratio is elevated in 2 of 3 samples over 6 months	Optimize glucose control; treatment per ophthalmology	Optimize glucose control; referral to neurology

ACE, Angiotensin-converting enzyme; *ARB*, angiotensin receptor blocker; *HbA$_{1c}$*, Hemoglobin A$_{1c}$; *IgA*, immunoglobulin A; *LDL*, low-density lipoprotein; *TSH*, thyroid-stimulating hormone; *tTG-IgA*, tissue transglutaminase antibody-IgA.

From American Diabetes Association. Children and adolescents: standards of medical care in diabetes—2022. *Diabetes Care.* 2021;45(Suppl1):S208–S231.

protein in the pancreas is often found in insufficient levels in type 2 diabetes patients, and medications that can target this protein offer a promising therapeutic option.

Type 2 diabetes is strongly associated with environmental factors such as obesity, sedentary lifestyles, and high-caloric, fatty foods. Additional risk factors for the development of type 2 diabetes include having been born to a mother with gestational diabetes, being small for gestational age at birth (sign of intrauterine undernutrition), being overweight and/or obese, or having a family history of type 2 diabetes. Type 2 diabetes appears to be more aggressive in pediatric populations, with a faster rate of deterioration of β-cell function than seen in adults.[122]

Clinical Findings

Screening Guidelines for Prediabetes and Type 2 Diabetes in Children and Adolescents. Screening for diabetes is equally important in both males and females, yet research indicates that male adolescents were less likely to undergo HbA_{1c}-based screening due to differential ordering practices.[118] According to the US Preventive Services Taskforce (USPSTF) and the ADA,[123] risk-based screening for pediatric prediabetes and type 2 diabetes should be considered in children and adolescents after the onset of puberty or 10 years of age, whichever occurs earlier, with overweight (BMI ≥85th percentile) or obesity (BMI ≥95th percentile) and one or more additional risk factors for diabetes:

- Family history of type 2 diabetes in either a first- or second-degree relative
- Native American, Hispanic, Asian American, Pacific Islander, or Black ethnicity/race
- Maternal history of gestational diabetes or maternal history of type 2 diabetes
- Signs of or conditions associated with insulin resistance such as acanthosis nigricans, dyslipidemia, polycystic ovary disease, or small for gestational age at birth.

If risk-based screening tests are normal, repeat every 3 years, and more frequently if BMI is increasing. The following tests are considered appropriate for screening: fasting plasma glucose, 2-hour plasma glucose during an OGTT, and HbA_{1c}. Panel testing for pancreatic autoantibodies is recommended in all individuals with clinically suspected type 2 diabetes to help to differentiate it from type 1 diabetes.[88]

The symptoms of type 2 diabetes may be absent or subtle, so pediatric patients at risk should be screened per the recommendations from the ADA 2022 Standards of Medical Care in Diabetes:[104]

- Screen if overweight (BMI is greater than 85th percentile for age and sex, or weight is greater than 120% of ideal weight), plus any two of the following risk factors:
  - Family history of type 2 diabetes in first- or second-degree relative
  - Race/ethnicity (Native American, Black, Hispanic, Asian American, Pacific Islander)
  - Signs of insulin resistance or conditions associated with insulin resistance (e.g., acanthosis nigricans, PCOS, hypertension, dyslipidemia)
  - Maternal history of diabetes or gestational diabetes during pregnancy with this child
- Screen every 3 years.
- Use fasting plasma glucose test following diagnostic criteria for diabetes discussed earlier.
- Use clinical judgment to screen for type 2 diabetes in high-risk patients who do not meet these guidelines.

History. The history and presenting symptoms of type 2 diabetes may include:

- Polydipsia, polyphagia, polyuria
- Nocturia or bedwetting
- Blurred vision
- Obesity, especially central
- Report of hyperpigmented, velvetlike thickening in skin folds
- Frequent or slow-healing infections
- Fatigue, symptoms of sleep apnea
- History of premature adrenarche
- Family history of type 2 diabetes

Physical Examination. The physical examination should include an assessment of height, weight, stage of pubertal development, and blood pressure. The following findings may be present:

- Dehydration
- Overweight (BMI greater than 85th percentile for age and sex) or obesity
- Weight loss (less common)
- Acanthosis nigricans noted in the axilla, and in neck, groin, and other skin folds
- Vaginal yeast, thrush, other infection
- PCOS symptoms (e.g., acne, hirsutism)
- Hypertension
- Children may have ketoacidosis if they have gone undiagnosed for a long time

Diagnostic Studies. Early diagnosis may enable clinicians to treat children and adolescents with type 2 diabetes more effectively without requiring insulin. Providers must remain cognizant that comorbidities may already be present at the time of diagnosis of type 2 diabetes, and screening should also include evaluation for these diagnoses. Screening should be conducted in all high-risk children without symptoms (see earlier screening guidelines) and should include:

- Urine for glucose and albumin
- Fasting blood glucose
- HbA_{1c}
- Lipid panel
- TSH and free T_4
- Insulin level

Laboratory findings consistent with prediabetes are fasting plasma glucose level of 100 to 125 mg/dL (5.6–6.9 mmol/L), an HbA_{1c} level between 5.7% and 6.4%, or a 2-hour postload glucose level of 140 to 199 mg/dL (7.8–11.0 mmol/L).[104]

Laboratory findings consistent with a diagnosis of type 2 diabetes are: fasting plasma glucose level ≥126 mg/dL (7.0 mmol/L), an HbA_{1c} level ≥6.5%, or a 2-hour postload glucose level ≥200 mg/dL (11.1 mmol/L) with OGTT.

Differential Diagnosis

Some obese children have type 1 diabetes and may be misdiagnosed as type 2. The presentation of type 1 diabetes can be of slower onset in older children and adults. A diagnosis of MODY (described later) should also be considered.

Management

SMBG is an essential component of type 2 diabetes, and the frequency of SMBG should be individualized, with consideration to how those values will be used to adjust therapy, the burden to patient and family, and the risk of hypoglycemia.[53] Adherence to SMBG is noted to lessen over time in adolescents. In the longitudinal Treatment Options for Type 2 Diabetes in Adolescents and Youth study, SMBG adherence of ≥80% was associated with a

≥1% reduction in HbA_{1c} at 6 and 12 months. Low SMBG adherence was common, more frequently noted >1 year after diagnosis, and was associated with higher HbA_{1c}.[124]

According to the USPSTF, lifestyle interventions to enhance weight loss and increased physical activity are the first-line therapies for preventing the progression of prediabetes to diabetes and treating type 2 diabetes.[119] Goals include improving nutritional practices and physical activity behaviors to facilitate weight loss. However, in the United States, fewer than 10% of children with type 2 diabetes are successful in achieving glycemic control with diet and exercise alone. If lifestyle changes are not successful in normalizing blood glucose levels, pharmacologic agents should be added to the treatment regimen.

Pharmacologic agents approved for the use of type 2 diabetes in the pediatric population were metformin and insulin. More recently, several injectable GLP-1 receptor agonists (liraglutide and extended-release exenatide) have been approved for pediatric patients. Other GLP-1 agonists such as dulaglutide are also being studied in children and adolescents. These medications improve glycemic control by creating the same effects in the body as the GLP-1 receptor protein in the pancreas: increasing insulin secretion, decreasing glucagon secretion, and slowing gastric emptying. These medications continue to expand in the adult population to include both injectable and oral forms. Other medications are approved in adults with type 2 diabetes but are not yet FDA-approved for children and adolescents.[114] These include sodium-glucose cotransporter 2 inhibitors, which are shown to reduce the progression of cardiovascular and kidney disease, and dipeptidyl peptidase-4 inhibitors, which also inhibit glucagon release upstream of GLP-1.

As with type 1 diabetes, the treatment plans for children with type 2 diabetes must be individualized. The treatment goal of both type 1 and type 2 diabetes is the same—the normalization of blood glucose values through the achievement of optimal glycemic control (HbA_{1c} in the 6.5% to ≤7.5% range, depending on hypoglycemia risk, as noted in the section on Type 1 diabetes). This typically requires:

- Daily self-monitoring by the child: If the child is treated with multiple insulin injections or continuous pump therapy, check blood glucose levels three or more times each day; there remains insufficient evidence for the ADA to recommend how often testing should be completed by youth with type 2 diabetes not on insulin therapy. For those on less-frequent insulin injections, oral medication, or medical nutrition therapy alone, a daily check may be adequate.
- HbA_{1c} and plasma glucose levels are monitored every 3 to 4 months for those whose therapy has changed or who are not meeting glycemic goals. Children who are meeting goals and have stable glycemic control can be monitored every 6 months.
- Follow-up every 3 to 4 months on lifestyle, nutrition, and other complications of obesity, discussed in more detail later.
- Screening and successful control of the associated complications, such as hypertension and hyperlipidemia, are important. See Table 39.8 for screening recommendations, which parallel those for type 1 diabetes.

Lifestyle Changes: Nutrition and Exercise. When diagnosed early, type 2 diabetes may respond to lifestyle changes, such as alterations in diet and exercise. A family-centered approach to dietary changes and increased physical activity is recommended. Medical nutrition therapy is an important part of the treatment plan. Referral to a registered pediatric dietician nutritionist is essential, with the goals of weight loss and regulating nutritional

intake. A low-fat diet, self-monitoring of weight, and being physically active are important components of nutrition therapy. Successful weight management may consist of weight maintenance rather than weight loss depending on the child's age and BMI. Changes in family eating patterns can contribute to weight maintenance or loss that may normalize insulin levels. Nutrition counseling should be provided both at the time of diagnosis of type 2 diabetes and as part of ongoing clinical management and should be consistent with the guidelines of the Academy of Nutrition and Dietetics. It is essential that diabetes self-management education be presented in a way that is culturally competent and supportive.[53]

Inactivity and the increasing obesity epidemic are directly related to the escalating incidence of type 2 diabetes in young people. Physical activity is not only one of the major type 2 diabetes prevention messages, but it is also a critical component of treatment. Youth with type 2 diabetes, like all children and adolescents, are encouraged to participate in at least 60 minutes of moderate to vigorous physical activity daily (with muscle and bone strength training at least 3 days/week).[104]

Overweight or obese youth may initially have poor physical conditioning with reduced endurance. Activity and exercise plans should allow for a gradual and safe buildup in intensity and length. A nutritionist can be helpful in ensuring adequate calories for performance needs, as well as for safe weight loss. Overweight or obese adolescents may lack self-esteem or motivation to participate in school sports activities but may be willing to walk as a form of exercise. Wireless fitness trackers that monitor activity, caloric expenditure, heart rate, and fitness may have utility in the management of diabetes in children and adolescents.[125]

The benefits of regular physical exercise for youth with type 2 diabetes include improved insulin sensitivity, positively altered skeletal muscle proteins and enzymes associated with glucose metabolism and insulin signaling, weight control, reduced risk of cardiovascular disease (CVD) and dyslipidemia, and improved self-confidence and self-esteem.[126] Glycemic control during exercise is generally not difficult to maintain. For adolescents who are taking oral hypoglycemic medication or insulin for type 2 diabetes, the benefits of improved insulin sensitivity through regular exercise participation may enable them to reduce medication.

Pharmacotherapy. Both metformin and insulin have been shown to improve β-cell function. There is a growing body of evidence on the use of hypoglycemic agents in children. Metformin is currently the only oral agent approved by the FDA for use in children with type 2 diabetes. Many other medications prescribed for adults with type 2 diabetes are used off-label in pediatrics. Metformin decreases the amount of glucose produced by the liver and increases insulin sensitivity of the liver and muscles.

The recommended approach to starting metformin is at a dose of 500 to 1000 mg/day, with gradual escalation every 1 to 2 weeks, depending on patient tolerability, to a recommended therapeutic dose of 1000 mg b.i.d. Metformin rarely causes hypoglycemia, so blood glucose needs to be checked only before breakfast and 2 hours after dinner. Mild gastrointestinal side effects (mild abdominal pain, bloating, loose stools) may occur with metformin use but are usually self-limiting. In adults, metformin users can experience vitamin B_{12} deficiency probably secondary to malabsorption, especially with higher doses and longer use. The prevalence of vitamin B_{12} deficiency among pediatric patients treated with metformin has shown a great deal of variation,[127] but providers should have an index of suspicion for vitamin B_{12} deficiency if clinical signs appear (e.g., pallor, fatigue, decreased appetite, "pins and needles" sensations). Because metformin is contraindicated in patients with liver disease, liver function tests should be monitored.

If the pediatric patient does not respond to metformin alone, a combination of two oral agents may be used under the guidance of a pediatric endocrinology specialist. Two other newer medication options, the GLP-1 receptor agonists liraglutide and exenatide, are also FDA-approved in children older than 10 years and are given via injection.

The ADA also recommends that when a child or adolescent has marked hyperglycemia (blood glucose ≥250 mg/dL and/or HbA_{1c} ≥8.5%) without acidosis at diagnosis but who is symptomatic (polyuria, polydipsia, nocturia, and/or weight loss) should be treated initially with basal insulin while concurrently initiating and titrating metformin.[53] Typically, the insulin needs are higher than in children with type 1 diabetes because of insulin resistance. Following the stabilization of blood glucose levels, it may be possible to gradually wean the insulin. Over time, the natural course of type 2 diabetes can result in the body's inability to produce sufficient endogenous insulin, making treatment with oral agents ineffective. If this occurs, insulin replacement using long- and/or rapid-acting insulin will be necessary. Other indications for use of insulin in youth with type 2 diabetes include metformin intolerance or renal insufficiency.

Medication may also be needed to control hypertension (see Chapter 33) and dyslipidemia (discussed later in this chapter), which are two frequent comorbidities in youth with type 2 diabetes.

Complications

Complications of type 2 diabetes are like those of type1 diabetes and include hyperglycemia, insulin resistance, hypertension, and dyslipidemia. Microvascular and macrovascular changes can lead to serious health consequences in adulthood, including cardiovascular disease, retinal changes, macular edema, and neuropathy.[114] Nephropathy is a more common complication in those with type 2 than type 1 diabetes. NAFLD and eventual dependence upon insulin for control can occur. There is emerging data on additional therapeutic strategies for the management of pediatric type 2 diabetes complications, including dyslipidemia.

Patient and Family Education

Youth with type 2 diabetes require much of the same education as those with type 1 diabetes: information about the nature of the disease; strategies and techniques to manage the physical disease (e.g., medication, insulin, nutrition, exercise); networks, support, and skills to cope with emotional and psychological issues; collaboration with school personnel; and wearing a form of medical identification. As with patients with type 1 diabetes, preconception counseling must start at puberty and be incorporated into diabetes clinic visits for all females of childbearing potential.[53]

Maturity-Onset Diabetes of the Young

Maturity-onset diabetes of the young, also known as *monogenic-MODY*, is a group of inherited disorders of nonautoimmune diabetes that may clinically resemble type 1 or type 2 diabetes. MODY is characterized by impaired insulin secretion without significant defects in the action of insulin. To date, at least 15 genetic loci on different chromosomes have been identified as being linked to MODY.[128] This disorder should be suspected in typically nonobese youth with mild to moderate, nonketotic-prone hyperglycemia and a strong family history of diabetes.[129] The

family history may reveal multiple family members with diabetes not characteristic of type 1 or type 2 diabetes. On average, children with monogenic MODY present with symptoms younger, are less likely to be overweight or obese, and are less likely to be from an ethnic minority group compared with children presenting with new-onset type 2 diabetes. In comparison with patients with type 1 diabetes, those with MODY typically do not have pancreatic autoimmunity and have fewer insulin requirements.

Diagnostic Studies

In addition to baseline testing as outlined for type 1 and type 2 diabetes, genetic testing is performed to determine the subtype of monogenic-MODY and can facilitate a prediction of the clinical course and prognosis.

Management

Management for patients with MODY is tailored to the underlying genetic mutation, with options including insulin therapy, sulfonylureas, off-label medications used in the treatment of adult diabetes, or no treatment at all. Patients require ongoing monitoring of micro- and macrovascular complications.

Posterior Pituitary Gland Disorders

The abnormal posterior pituitary function is uncommon in pediatrics. The two hormones associated with the posterior pituitary are vasopressin and oxytocin. Vasopressin, also known as *antidiuretic hormone (ADH)* or *arginine vasopressin* is the body's main regulator of water homeostasis. The two disorders associated with vasopressin dysfunction are the syndrome of inappropriate antidiuretic hormone secretion (SIADH) and diabetes insipidus (DI).

Syndrome of Inappropriate Antidiuretic Hormone Secretion

SIADH is characterized by the presence of hyponatremia (sodium <135 mEq/L) with inappropriately concentrated urine (>100 mOsm/kg) in the setting of normal hydration status or mild hypervolemia. SIADH is caused by the unsuppressed release of vasopressin (ADH) from the pituitary gland or from nonpituitary sources, and its excessive action on the vasopressin receptor in the kidney. There are numerous causes of SIADH, including cerebral disorders (i.e., hemorrhage, infections such as meningitis, trauma, and psychosis), the abnormal release of ADH from the pituitary, tumors, pulmonary diseases such as pneumonia, specific medications (e.g., carbamazepine, several selective serotonin reuptake inhibitors, methotrexate, and lamotrigine), surgery (up to 1 week postoperatively), general anesthesia, and systemic infections.[130]

Diagnostic Studies

Serum electrolytes will reveal decreased sodium and chloride levels, while urinary sodium and urine-specific gravity will be elevated. Serum osmolality will be low (<250 mOsm/kg) while urine osmolality will be excessively concentrated (>100 mOsm/kg).

Management

Treatment of SIADH is coordinated with pediatric endocrinology or nephrology and involves restricting fluid intake to generate a negative fluid balance.[131] Hypertonic saline is sometimes used to treat hyponatremia in the inpatient setting. Pharmacologic treatment may include the use of loop diuretics such as furosemide, urea, and/or medications known to cause nephrogenic DI, such as lithium carbonate.[132]

Diabetes Insipidus

DI presents with hypernatremia and inappropriately dilute urine in the setting of mild hypovolemia. Polyuria and polydipsia may also be present. In more severe cases, patients can present with severe dehydration, vomiting, constipation, fever, irritability, nocturia, failure to thrive, and growth retardation.[133] *Central* DI results from decreased ADH secretion from the posterior pituitary. *Nephrogenic* DI occurs when there is ADH resistance at the collecting tubules of the kidney.

Diagnostic Studies

Laboratory testing includes a comprehensive metabolic panel and serum osmolality. Normal serum glucose and calcium rule out diabetes or hypercalcemia-induced nephrogenic DI. Normal serum potassium excludes hypokalemia-induced nephrogenic DI. Normal blood urea nitrogen (BUN) also makes renal disease etiology less likely.

A water deprivation test determines the body's ability to concentrate urine, with urine osmolality and specific gravity markers aiding in diagnostic decision-making. If central or nephrogenic DI is present, the urine osmolality will be low, the plasma osmolality rises, urine specific gravity will be <1.005 and the urine-to-plasma osmolality ratio is <2. A vasopressin test is then done following the water deprivation test to differentiate between central and nephrogenic DI. In central DI, the urine volume will decrease, the specific gravity will be ≥1.010, and the urine osmolality increases by 200% or more in response to vasopressin administration. In nephrogenic DI, there are no changes to urine volume, osmolality, or specific gravity.

Genetic testing in patients with suspected inherited central DI should be considered if there is a positive family history of DI or with early-onset idiopathic disease. Brain MRI is used to evaluate the pituitary gland in pediatric patients and identify a cause for central DI.

Management

Desmopressin is the first-choice drug in patients with central DI. Pediatric patients receive a fixed dose of desmopressin 2 to 3 times/day orally and are given subsequent dosing if polyuria develops (>5 mL/kg/h). To prevent hyponatremia, patients should be instructed to avoid drinking more fluids than the amount necessary to quench thirst.

Metabolic Disorders

Metabolic disorders can be congenital (IEMs) or acquired.

Obesity, dyslipidemia, and metabolic syndrome are three acquired metabolic disorders that have increased prevalence in pediatric populations. The focus of this section is on these disorders, as early recognition and treatment can decrease morbidity in children and adolescents.

Obesity

Obesity is a chronic disease whose prevalence has dramatically increased in children and adults worldwide.[134] Obesity in childhood is defined as a BMI greater than or equal to the 95th percentile. This definition has been further expanded into three classes.[135]

Class I obesity is defined as a BMI between the 95th percentile to 120% of the 95th percentile. Class II is defined as a BMI of 120% of the 95th percentile to 140% of the 95th percentile. Class III is defined as a BMI greater than 140% of the 95th percentile.

The diagnoses of overweight and obesity are typically associated with an imbalance between calories consumed and calories burned. From an endocrine perspective, the mechanisms of weight homeostasis are complex, regulated by neurohormonal pathways that control hunger and satiety, and metabolism. Regulation involves the hypothalamus (as evidenced by the obesity associated with children who develop craniopharyngiomas), hormones produced by adipocytes (e.g., leptin), and the gut (e.g., ghrelin). In most children, hormone deficiency or excess does not explain obesity. Although several classic hormonal imbalances (such as hypothyroidism, cortisol excess, and GHD) may be associated with overweight or obesity, youth with these endocrine conditions are likely to be either of short stature or growing at a subnormal growth velocity. Obesity is also associated with over 25 genetic syndromes, with Prader-Willi syndrome being the most common. Additional causes of obesity include medications (e.g., corticosteroids, antiepileptic, antidepressants, and antipsychotic drugs) and cerebral injuries affecting the hypothalamic centers associated with weight regulation.[136]

Obesity in children and adolescents is associated with impaired glucose tolerance and type 2 diabetes, hypertension, dyslipidemia, early/subclinical atherosclerotic changes, obstructive sleep apnea, gastroesophageal reflux disease (GERD), NAFLD, and musculoskeletal disease.[116] There is a strong correlation between the youth's obesity grade and risk secondary to CVD. Children with BMI >95th percentile have a three- to fivefold increased risk of CVD mortality by age of 50 years.[137] As pediatric obesity rates have continued to rise, there has been a parallel increase in pediatric NAFLD prevalence,[138] making it the leading cause of liver disease in children. The long-term risks associated with NAFLD include progression to nonalcoholic steatohepatitis, cirrhosis, or hepatocellular carcinoma.

An additional overriding issue for youth who are overweight or obese is the mental health cost of these conditions. Issues include depression, eating disorders, school adjustment problems, bullying, and low self-esteem.[139] Stigmatization of obesity occurs within peer groups and the general public as well as among healthcare professionals. Mental health assessment and treatment can be a life-changing component in the holistic care of this patient population.

Evaluation

The American Academy of Pediatrics (AAP) has recommended that pediatric health care providers screen children and adolescents ≥ age 6 years annually for obesity, based on BMI percentile, and offer referral for intensive, family-based behavioral treatment to improve weight status.[134] Due to the asymptomatic nature of prediabetes and early type 2 diabetes and their association with overweight/obesity, screening is necessary to identify at-risk patients (see diagnostic criteria for type 2 diabetes). Consistent with clinical practice guidelines developed jointly by the European Society of Endocrinology and the Pediatric Endocrine Society, pediatric patients with a BMI greater than the 85th percentile for age and sex should be screened for comorbidities and associated cardiovascular risk factors.[140] Providers will evaluate for the following:

- Dyslipidemia with fasting lipid panel
- Prehypertension and hypertension with a blood pressure measurement

- Nonalcoholic fatty liver disease with liver enzyme alanine aminotransferase (ALT)
- Obstructive sleep apnea by a history of snoring, and daytime somnolence. If history is positive, refer to a pediatric pulmonologist/sleep specialist for a nocturnal polysomnography.
- PCOS with a free and total testosterone level (if symptomatic with irregular menses, acne, or hirsutism)

Psychological issues by a history of low self-esteem, behavior problems, or depression. If history is positive, refer a to mental health specialistThe AAP has recently added additional screening recommendations for comorbid conditions including slipped capital femoral epiphysis, Blount Disease, and idiopathic intracranial hypertension.[134]

Management

The updated AAP clinical practice guidelines on obesity focus on the multilevel contributors to obesity, including policy factors (e.g., food insecurity, marketing of unhealthy foods), neighborhood and community factors (e.g., food deserts with lack of access to healthy foods), individual factors (e.g., prenatal and postnatal risks, genetic factors, and childhood illnesses), and family/environmental home factors (e.g., psychosocial stressors, sedentary behaviors and screen time).[134]

Children with type 2 diabetes, PCOS, or other metabolic or endocrine disorders associated with obesity should be followed in concert with a pediatric endocrinologist. The Pediatric Endocrine Society has recommended against routine evaluation for endocrine conditions in children with obesity unless the youth's stature is inconsistent with his/her genetic potential or growth velocity is inconsistent with what is expected at the child's pubertal stage.[141] If there is an underlying cause of obesity, identification can improve personalized treatment.[136] All overweight and/or obese youth should be evaluated for potential comorbidities.

Per the AAP, Intensive Health Behavioral and Lifestyle Treatment (IHBLT) is considered the foundational approach to management of obesity in children.[134] The AAP has outlined components of Comprehensive Obesity Treatment (COT) for children and adolescents, which include:

- Intensive, long-term treatment through the medical home
- A non-stigmatizing, individualized approach to treatment
- Attention to social drivers of health that impact holistic patient care
- Use of motivational interviewing to address nutrition, physical activity, and health behavior change for weight reduction and health promotion
- Development of collaborative treatment goals that are not limited to BMI stabilization or reduction. Goals may reflect improvement or resolution of comorbidities, self-image, quality of life, and more
- Use of interdisciplinary strategies including intensive health behavior and lifestyle treatment, with pharmacotherapy and metabolic and bariatric surgery as indicated

Ideally, COT is provided through partnership of primary care teams and pediatric weight management specialty teams.[134] The magnitude of weight loss necessary to improve cardiovascular risk factors among youth has not been fully determined.[140]

Screening should be offered in the primary care setting and a treatment plan established with the family for nutritional counseling and ongoing support to achieve a more active lifestyle. In general, the goal is weight maintenance, not loss, in the overweight child without any complications; it is expected that these children will eventually grow into their weight and achieve a BMI less than the 85th percentile. For children with an overweight-related complication, weight loss of 1 pound per month would be an appropriate goal; more rapid weight loss in children who have not yet reached their growth potential may be associated with a slowing in linear growth.

Consensus is lacking as to the most effective way to manage childhood obesity. Goals for reducing calories consumed and increasing daily exercise must be made within the context of each family (Table 39.9). Success is more likely to be achieved if the entire family participates in lifestyle changes. Providers must work closely with families to ensure consistent follow-up, assess the effectiveness of interventions, and modify the treatment strategy if necessary.

Evidence-based guidelines recommend a multifactorial lifestyle intervention approach for pediatric weight management including diet, exercise, and behavior modification.[142]

Lifestyle changes may not be adequate treatment for those youth with severe obesity. More intensive approaches to obesity management include antiobesity pharmacotherapy and bariatric surgery. Very few medications (Phentermine, Liraglutide, Orlistat) are approved by the FDA for use in adolescent obesity and have shown only modest weight loss results.[142] Off-label use of medications including bupropion/naltrexone, topiramate or phentermine/topiramate extended-release, metformin, semaglutide, and lisdexamfetamine have been investigated in pediatric patients.[143]

Bariatric Surgery

Bariatric surgery is consistently associated with clinically significant, durable weight loss. Surgical procedures include the Roux-en-Y gastric bypass and the increasingly preferred vertical sleeve gastrectomy. Suggested indications for bariatric surgery in children and adolescents include failure of lifestyle interventions to produce weight loss and continued or worsening comorbidity.[135,142] The 2019 American Academy of Pediatrics policy statement defining the eligibility criteria for metabolic and bariatric surgery (MBS) notes that a BMI >40 (or 140% of the 95th percentile), or a BMI >35 (or 120% of the 95th percentile), along with just one obesity-related comorbidity, greatly increases the risk of morbidity/mortality from obesity.[144] MBS is recommended for youth with Class III obesity, a BMI of >140% of the 95th percentile, or a BMI >40, whichever is lower. MBS is additionally recommended for those with Class II obesity with a BMI of 120% of the 95th percentile or a BMI greater than 35 with obesity-related comorbidity (including type 2 diabetes, hyperlipidemia, obstructive

TABLE 39.9	Facilitating Factors for Effective Lifestyle Modification for Obesity
Setting	Within the medical home, under the guidance of pediatric-focused clinician
Delivery	Individual *and* family-based
Characteristics	Interaction and support within a safe space Nonjudgmental, empathetic, non-stigmatizing Motivational interviewing
Timing, frequency and intensity	Prompt, upon identification of problem Longitudinal, due to chronicity of the disease At the needed level of intensity- greater contact hours associated with greater treatment effect
Expectations	Aligned with patient and family needs

sleep apnea, GERD, NAFLD, among others).[135] More research is needed regarding the long-term (≥5 years) safety and efficacy of bariatric surgery in pediatric patients.

A multidisciplinary approach to the youth undergoing MBS is essential, with a team including a psychologist, the PCP, a bariatric and/or general pediatric surgeon, a dietician, and a nurse care coordinator. Social workers, Child Life specialists, and physical therapists are also valued members of the care team.

Dyslipidemia: Hypercholesterolemia and Hyperlipidemia

Dyslipidemias, which affect approximately 20% of pediatric patients ages 6 to 19 years, are metabolic disorders that result in elevated levels of total cholesterol, low-density lipoprotein (LDL) cholesterol, triglycerides, and/or decreased levels of high-density lipoprotein (HDL) cholesterol. These lipoprotein abnormalities can occur in any combination.[145] Dyslipidemias can be genetic (primary) or acquired (secondary). Pediatric dyslipidemias are associated with premature atherosclerosis and an increased risk of cardiovascular events at an earlier adult age.

Primary dyslipidemias are a heterogeneous group of diseases, with familial hypercholesterolemia (FH) being the most common of these disorders. FH is a genetically linked disorder of lipoprotein metabolism that results in dyslipidemia early in life. This disease is caused by pathogenic variants in one or more of the three main genes responsible for LDL-cholesterol clearance. The most commonly affected gene, accounting for >90% of cases, involves the LDL receptor,[146] making this an important target for novel treatment approaches. The two types of FH are heterozygous FH and homozygous FH. Homozygous hypercholesterolemia is characterized by extremely high LDL levels (e.g., ≥600 mg/dL) and a poor outcome if the patient does not have extremely aggressive early treatment. Even with treatment, atherosclerotic vascular disease is common by 30 years of age. Other rarer types of primary hyperlipidemia include familial hypertriglyceridemia, apolipoprotein A-1 deficiency, familial hypoalphalipoproteinemia, familial dysbetalipoproteinemia, and polygenic hypercholesterolemia.

Secondary hyperlipidemias result from exogenous factors, such as obesity, drugs (e.g., isotretinoin, oral contraceptives, antipsychotics), endocrine or metabolic disorders (e.g., hypothyroidism, diabetes); metabolic storage diseases (e.g., glycogen storage disease); obstructive liver disease (e.g., biliary atresia); and other causes, such as anorexia nervosa.

Clinical Findings

Hyperlipidemia itself is an asymptomatic condition and does not typically present as a clinical illness in children. Diagnoses are often made later in life after a significant burden of cardiovascular sequelae becomes apparent. Although not all children with dyslipidemia will have cardiovascular problems as adults, screening of children at risk is important to identify those with hyperlipidemia and hypercholesterolemia and to intervene to reduce CVD complications in the future.[147]

History. Risk factors for hypercholesterolemia and hyperlipidemia in the pediatric patient include the presence of diabetes, hypertension, or a BMI ≥95th percentile as well as youth who smoke cigarettes. The family history may also reveal early CVD (males ≤55 years old; females ≤65 years old) or a parent with a total cholesterol level ≥240 mg/dL or higher or known dyslipidemia.[147] Monogenic primary dyslipidemias should also be considered if there is a personal or family history of recurrent or very early pancreatitis.

Physical Examination.[147] The child may have no clinical signs or symptoms or may have:
- Tendon or cutaneous xanthomas (aggregates of lipid materials) at any age. These are most common in the finger extensor tendons and the Achilles tendon.
- Arcus cornea (deposition of cholesterol, triglycerides, or phospholipids forming an arc on either the top or bottom side of the iris, within the cornea) seen before ages younger than 4 or 5 years.
- Tuberous xanthomas (firm skin nodules) or xanthelasma (yellow fatty deposit plaques on the eyelid).

Diagnostic Studies. When the family history is positive for hypercholesterolemia or early CVD, screening should be considered by 2 years old. Selective screening should be performed on children/adolescents over 2 years of age with family or individual risk factors (overweight/obesity, hypertension, or diabetes) as soon as these factors are identified. Universal screening with a fasting lipid profile or nonfasting non-HDL cholesterol testing should be considered between 9 and 11 years of age and again after the pubertal stage development (17–21 years old). Fasting lipid profiles should be obtained on two separate occasions and the results averaged.[148] Between ages 12 and 16 years, screening can be inaccurate with a falsely low result due to decreased lipid synthesis during puberty.[147]

Management

The goal of treatment is to reduce the cumulative cholesterol exposure time through early diagnosis and effective combination therapies.[146] Components of treatment involve ongoing screening, lifestyle modifications, and drug therapy. Comprehensive treatment for these disorders is best coordinated through multidisciplinary pediatric lipid clinics, where available.

Lifestyle Changes. Prevention and/or control of hypercholesterolemia through lifestyle changes is a primary intervention. Dietary change has been the first step in the treatment of children older than 2 years with hypercholesterolemia (LDL >110 mg/dL with total cholesterol of at least 200 mg/dL) and, combined with other lifestyle changes, remains a critical component of treatment. For those presenting with FH, dietary treatment of hypercholesterolemia is not indicated in children <2 years of age due to the increased need for dietary fats because of the rapid growth and development of the nervous system.[147]

The National Lipid Association (NLA) encourages individuals to change lifestyle patterns, including diet alterations. Educational materials related to this approach are available on the NLA website (see Additional Resources). Many issues arise with dietary changes in children (e.g., increasing dietary fiber may cause early satiety and increase the risk of poor nutrient intake in children), so consultation with a pediatric dietitian nutritionist is essential to ensure that children receive adequate nutrition. Diet intervention is based on increased consumption of fruit, vegetables, and whole grains compared to the percentage of ingested fat.[149]

Pharmacotherapy. The following guidelines are recommended for medication therapy in pediatric populations.[150]

In children <10 years of age who present with:
- Homozygous FH with LDL typically above 400 mg/dL—at detection
- CVD within the first 2 decades of life/postcardiac transplantation

TABLE
39.10 **Treatment Options for Dyslipidemia**

Medication	Starting dose	Maximum dose	Approved Starting Age (Years)	Indication	Precautions
Statin Drugs					
Simvastatin	10 mg/day	40 mg/day	10	Heterozygous familial hypercholesterolemia after failure of an adequate trial of diet therapy	• Consultation with lipid specialist recommended • Avoid concomitant gemfibrozil administration • Monitor liver function and creatine kinase • No long-term use data available in pediatrics • Myopathy is the most common adverse effect • Contraception must be used in adolescent females due to teratogenicity
Atorvastatin	10 mg/day	20 mg/day	10		
Lovastatin	10 mg/day	40 mg/day	10		
Pravastatin	8–13 years old: 20 mg/day 14–18 years old: 40 mg/day	80 mg/day	8		
Rosuvastatin	5 mg/day	20 mg/day	8		
Fluvastatin	20 mg/day	80 mg/day	10		
Pitavastatin	1 mg/day	4 mg/day	8		
Other Drugs					
Bile acid sequestrants	• Consultation with lipid specialist is recommended • No pediatric indications are FDA approved • No pediatric dosing recommendations				
Fibrates					

FDA, US Food and Drug Administration.

Data from Food and Drug Administration. https://www.accessdata.fda.gov/scripts/cder/daf.

- LDL ≥190 mg/dL + positive family history, *or* one high-risk factor/condition, *or* two moderate risk factors/conditions

Children ≥10 years of age presenting with:
- LDL ≥190 mg/dL
- LDL ≥160 mg/dL + positive family history, *or* one high-risk factor/condition, *or* two moderate risk factors/conditions
- LDL ≥130 mg/dL + two high-risk factors/conditions, *or* one high-risk factor/condition and two moderate risk factors/conditions, *or* clinical CVD

High-risk conditions are type 1 or 2 diabetes, chronic renal disease or end-stage renal disease/postrenal transplant, postorthotopic heart transplant, and Kawasaki disease with current aneurysms. *High-risk factors* are hypertension requiring drug therapy (blood pressure ≥99th percentile + 5 mm Hg), current smoking, and BMI ≥97th percentile. *Moderate risk conditions* are Kawasaki disease with regressed coronary aneurysms, systemic lupus erythematosus, juvenile rheumatoid arthritis, human immunodeficiency virus infection, and nephrotic syndrome. *Moderate risk factors* are hypertension not requiring drug therapy, BMI ≥95th percentile but <97th percentile, and HDL <40 mg/dL.

The use of HMG-CoA reductase inhibitors (statins) can be considered if the child has severe hypercholesterolemia. The statins function by inhibiting the rate-limiting enzyme in the synthesis of cholesterol (Table 39.10). The introduction of statins into a comprehensive treatment plan may occur as early as age 8 to 10 years but is considered after the failure of aggressive lifestyle modification. There are no long-term safety data about the use of statins in pediatric patients.[144] Other medications used in the adult population, including fibrates and nicotinic acid, are not approved for use in children. Research is ongoing for targeted gene therapies that impact lipid synthesis and metabolism, including monoclonal antibodies and small interfering ribonucleic acid therapy.[146] While omega-3 fatty acid supplements are sometimes recommended by providers, there are no pediatric dosing guidelines and efficacy has not been well-established in children. Because of the side effects of drugs and the uncertainty about their long-term use in the pediatric population, children who require drug therapy should be referred to a specialized pediatric lipid center for treatment. In severe cases, liver transplantation may be considered a treatment option.

Metabolic Syndrome

Metabolic syndrome describes a constellation of cardiometabolic risk factors including insulin resistance, elevated blood pressure, elevated triglyceride levels, reduced HDL levels, and abdominal obesity.[151,152] With the rising prevalence in overweight and obesity, the incidence of metabolic syndrome in young people has also increased. The prevalence of metabolic syndrome in pediatric populations worldwide ranges from 0.3% to 26.4%.[137,149] An accepted diagnostic definition of metabolic syndrome in children and adolescents has not been uniformly adopted, thus absolute prevalence has been difficult to calculate.[151] In the pediatric population, criteria such as waist circumference and BMI, elevated blood pressure and dyslipidemia are characterized using age- and sex-specific percentiles and pediatric thresholds. There are variations in metabolic characteristics and anthropomorphic measures based on sex, race/ethnicity, and geographic location. With these considerations, a single definition of metabolic syndrome may misrepresent or underrepresent the prevalence of this syndrome.

Long-Term Implications of Metabolic Syndrome

The endocrine abnormalities associated with metabolic syndrome create chronic inflammation and the development of oxidative stress.[153] Oxidative stress, defined as an imbalance in the production and degradation of reactive oxidative species, is closely associated with metabolic syndrome and leads to obesity, diabetes, and CVD. It is also associated with carcinogenesis and the development of NAFLD.

Management

Treatment strategies are targeted at managing obesity and treating the cluster of cardiometabolic risk factors. See sections on the management of obesity and dyslipidemia for details. Those children who remain hypertensive despite lifestyle modifications, or who have symptomatic hypertension, stage 2 hypertension without a clearly modifiable factor (such as obesity), or any stage of hypertension associated with type 1 diabetes or chronic kidney disease can be started on antihypertensive drug monotherapy. Appropriate pharmacologic treatment choices are angiotensin-converting enzyme inhibitors or angiotensin II receptor blockers, long-acting calcium channel blockers, or thiazide diuretics.[137]

Inherited Metabolic Disorders

Most inherited metabolic disorders are caused by a defined or presumed genetic mutation that alters the function of a single enzyme or its cofactor, resulting in an altered function of a metabolic pathway. This leads to dysfunction in either generating energy or breaking down waste by-products. There are multiple classifications for inherited metabolic disorders, including a new proposed International Classification of Inherited Metabolic Disorders (Box 39.11).

Inborn Errors of Metabolism

IEMs are a heterogeneous group of inherited disorders with alterations of specific biochemical reactions. These disorders can present as early as a few hours after birth but may take several weeks to present as metabolic demands increase in the neonate.

Individual IEM are rare, with most having an incidence of <1 per 100,000 births. Globally, it is estimated that the birth prevalence of all-cause IEMs is 50.9 per 100,000 live births, with the highest rates of IEMs in the Eastern Mediterranean region, where there are higher rates of parental consanguinity. Collectively, however, the incidence may approach 1 in 800 to 1 in 2500 births.[154] Clinical consequences for the affected individual vary from mild to severe. Early detection, accurate diagnosis, rapid intervention, and patient/family education in managing the child's disorder are necessary to reduce morbidity, as treatments may prevent irreversible intellectual disability, physical disability, neurologic damage, or death; and reduce the long-term financial burden and overall quality of life.

One of the most common IEMs is phenylketonuria, an autosomal recessive disorder where the body is deficient in the enzyme phenylalanine hydroxylase and cannot metabolize phenylalanine. Left untreated, clinical manifestations include severe intellectual disability, epilepsy, and behavioral, psychiatric, and movement problems. Patients also develop a musty odor, eczema, and develop light pigmentation of skin, eyes, and hair.[155]

This section briefly reviews the classification and pathophysiology of IEMs, describes newborn screening strategies, includes common clinical presentations and emergency management of conditions found in the newborn period; and presents a brief overview of the diagnosis and treatment of a few more common disorders.

Pathophysiology

Fig. 39.3 provides an overview of the major metabolic pathways. Most defects are caused by a single gene mutation encoding a specific enzyme whose function is to facilitate the conversion of various substances (substrates, [e.g., foodstuffs]) into others (metabolic products, [e.g., urea]). The block in the pathway variably leads to accumulation of substrate proximal to the block (e.g., lysosomal storage disorders); accumulation of toxic metabolites (e.g., galactose byproducts in galactosemia); deficiency of a product distal to the block (e.g., tyrosine in phenylketonuria [PKU]); feedback inhibition or activation by the metabolite; or some combination thereof. Loss of enzyme function varies by degree, altering the clinical phenotype, the clinical course, and the response to treatment among individuals with the same diagnosis.

Assessment of Inborn Errors of Metabolism

IEMs are rare but should be included in the differential diagnosis of any critically ill neonate, as well as infants, children, adolescents, and adults, presenting with symptoms that are progressive or otherwise unexplained. The timing of symptom onset in relation to the initiation of feedings can be an important clue. Infants with IEM commonly appear normal at birth with effects of the disease becoming apparent over the course of days to months. As substrates or toxic metabolites accumulate, such as in organic acidemias, nonspecific symptoms that may be indistinguishable from sepsis typically appear. However, finding a cause of symptoms does not necessarily rule out the possibility of an IEM (e.g., electrolyte

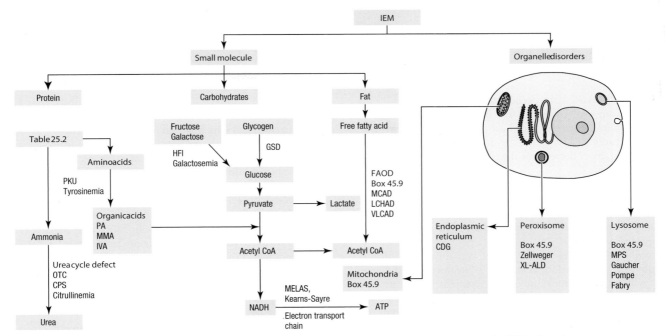

• **Fig. 39.3** Overview of Major Metabolic Pathways. *Acetyl CoA,* Acetyl coenzyme A; *ATP,* adenosine triphosphate; *CDG,* congenital disorders of glycosylation; *CPS,* carbamoyl phosphate synthetase I deficiency; *FAOD,* long-chain fatty acid oxidation disorders; *GSD,* glycogen storage disease; *HFI,* hereditary fructose intolerance; *IEM,* inborn errors of metabolism; *IVA,* isovaleric acidemia; *LCHAD,* long-chain 3-hydroxyacyl-coenzyme A dehydrogenase deficiency; *MCAD,* medium-chain acyl-coenzyme A dehydrogenase deficiency; *MMA,* methylmalonic acidemia; *MPS,* mucopolysaccharidosis; *NADH,* nicotinamide adenine dinucleotide; *OTC,* ornithine transcarbamylase deficiency; *PA,* phosphatidic acid; *PA,* propionic acidemia; *PKU,* phenylketonuria; *VLCAD,* very long-chain acyl-coenzyme A dehydrogenase deficiency; *XL-ALD,* X-linked adrenoleukodystrophy. (From Krueger, C, Ejaz, R, & Sondheimer, N. Metabolic disease. In: Schonfeld, D, Silver, S, Diskin, C, et al, eds. *The Hospital for Sick Children Handbook of Pediatrics.* 12th ed. Elsevier; 2022.)

abnormalities diagnosed as renal Fanconi syndrome may be caused by an underlying accumulation of the amino acid cysteine).

Clinical Findings

History. A thorough family and individual history are important to identify possibilities of IEMs. Details in a family and patient history that should raise suspicion include:
- Consanguinity, family history of IEM, siblings with an unexplained infant or neonatal death
- Decompensation when ill greater than anticipated for the nature of the illness
- Developmental delay, psychomotor retardation, or loss of previously acquired milestones
- Failure to thrive
- Symptoms concurrent with a change in diet
- Unusual odor (sweat, urine, or cerumen)

Physical Examination. A complete examination is essential, with attention to dysmorphia, muscle tone, ocular symptoms, organomegaly, and respiratory function. Box 39.11 provides an overview of signs and symptoms suspicious of inborn metabolic errors at various ages.

Diagnostic Studies. Effective intervention for IEMs depends on the ability to identify the disorder before the onset of symptoms. Screening for the presence of IEMs allows the provider to identify the condition and, if possible, begin treatment before physiologic damage has occurred. However, not all IEMs are amenable to treatment, and in some cases, supportive or palliative care

may be the only option. As a result, all 50 US states have instituted screening programs for newborn infants. Newborn screening occurs between 24 hours and 72 hours after birth and is done via dried blood spot testing. Results are available within 7 to 10 days. The limitations of newborn screening include the potential for false-negative and false-positive results, and confirmatory testing is required.[156]

Technological advances have allowed screening for a wide array of disorders. Further laboratory studies are generally necessary for the diagnosis of IEM; however, determining what studies to perform may not always be straightforward. Testing for common (i.e., nonmetabolic) causes of presenting symptoms should not be sacrificed for metabolic testing, but it is not always prudent to wait for all routine tests to be performed and for the results known before submitting samples for metabolic disease testing. This additional step facilitates workup should the patient be referred to a metabolic specialist. When the ill child has signs and symptoms of what could be an IEM, the PCP should consult immediately with a metabolic specialist, rather than wait for the results of tests. For chronic presentations, after common etiologies are ruled out, refer to a metabolic specialist for testing beyond routine analysis.

Initial laboratory studies for the neonate with a suspected IEM include:
- Newborn screening on any significantly ill neonate, unless proof of prior collection is obtained
- A second newborn screening at 10 to 14 days of age if the ill neonate was discharged early (before 24 hours of age)

- CBC with differential and urinalysis
- Blood glucose
- BUN and creatinine
- ALT, aspartate aminotransferase, bilirubin
- Coagulation studies
- Blood gases
- Serum electrolytes with special attention to anion gap
- Plasma ammonia: collected free flowing (no tourniquet, no heel stick) immediately placed on ice and analyzed within 45 to 60 minutes
- Plasma lactate: collected free flowing
- Creatine kinase
- Plasma quantitative amino acids, plasma acylcarnitine profile, and plasma carnitine levels
- Ketones (if acidotic and hypoglycemic), organic acids, and mucopolysaccharides and oligosaccharides if storage disease is suspected.

If newborn screening results are not available, the clinical history, physical examination, screening laboratories, and imaging results will provide important clues to patient stabilization and management.[157] Metabolic screening panels vary between laboratories. Some laboratories offer a metabolic screening panel, typically on urine; however, some laboratories prefer urine and blood. Diagnostic testing may also consist of biochemical or nuclear deoxyribonucleic acid (DNA) analysis obtained from blood. Mitochondrial DNA testing can be prioritized if there is a family history of mitochondrial disorders in siblings or maternal relatives, as mitochondrial DNA is almost exclusively inherited from the mother.[158]

Other more invasive tests may be needed, including a lumbar puncture (cerebral spinal fluid for lactate, amino acids, glucose) or biopsy from skin, liver, or muscle (enzyme assays). In addition, for the child with chronic encephalopathy, brain MRI and magnetic resonance spectroscopy are used to assess for structural anomalies and biochemical dysfunction. Familiarity with the appropriate methods of specimen collection and handling (before and during shipment of the samples to the laboratory) is important because inappropriate practices alter the quality of the sample, potentially leading to unreliable results and thus either missed or erroneous cases.

Metabolic Emergencies

There are numerous physiologic stressors such as infection and dehydration that can begin a cascade of catabolism of protein and energy reserves. This is referred to as a *metabolic crisis*. Emergency management of many metabolic disorders requires hospital admission and specialist care. The goal of emergency management is twofold: (1) to prevent catabolism and (2) to remove toxic substrates or metabolites. Aggressive management is necessary to avert or reduce neurologic sequelae. This acute care management may require IV medications (including glucose to halt catabolism), diet restriction, hemodialysis, or advanced life support.[157]

General Management Strategies

Management of metabolic disorders varies depending on the specific condition, its severity, and whether it is an acute or chronic presentation. Caregivers of children with a known diagnosis of inborn errors become very astute at early recognition of symptoms in their child and are crucial partners in the healthcare team. Most families should have emergency protocol letters, sick day protocols, and 24-hour on-call contact information.

The variability of IEMs requires individual management tailored to the patient's specific diagnosis and phenotype. However, the following strategies provide several broad categories from which treatments are drawn:
- Control substrate accumulation:
  - Restrict dietary intake.
  - Control endogenous production of the substrate (e.g., give high-calorie, no-protein feeds during illness to prevent catabolism, which would release amino acids).
  - Accelerate removal of the substrate (e.g., administer sodium benzoate/phenylacetate in urea cycle disorders [UCDs] to increase elimination of waste nitrogen through an alternate pathway).
- Dietary supplementation:
  - Replace or supplement the diet with products that become deficient distal to the metabolic block or if the diet is medically restricted (e.g., arginine or citrulline in UCD).
- Vitamin and cofactor replacement:
  - Increase the supply of certain vitamins or cofactors (e.g., vitamin E, Coenzyme Q-10 [ubiquinol], biotin) to improve cellular function and reduce oxidative stress.
- Enzyme replacement therapy (ERT):
  - ERT (an IV infusion of enzyme replacement given every 1–2 weeks) is widely available in the clinical setting for certain lysosomal storage diseases.
- Bone marrow or organ transplant:
  - Allogeneic stem cell transplantation (using exogenous bone marrow or cord blood) is clinically available for some disorders, but it is in the early stage of widespread clinical use.
  - Organ transplant can essentially "cure" some metabolic diseases by transplanting an organ in which the mutant genes are expressed.

There are multisystemic complications in many of the IEMs, including intellectual disability, developmental delays, cardiac disease, renal failure, hypertension, spinal cord compression, and bone or joint abnormalities.

Specific Metabolic Disorders in Children

Disorders of Carbohydrate Metabolism

This group of disorders is caused by the inability to metabolize the monosaccharides (glucose, galactose, and fructose) and the polysaccharide glycogen. Aberrant glycogen synthesis or disorders of gluconeogenesis also contribute to faulty carbohydrate metabolism.

Glycogen storage diseases are genetic disorders that result in enzymatic defects affecting the synthesis or breakdown of glycogen. Glycogen is a glucose polymer stored in muscle and the liver, and deficiency of any enzyme involved in the metabolic pathway of glycogen can affect the biosynthesis or degradation of glycogen in the organ in which the enzyme is expressed. These defects result in a variety of disease presentations (Table 39.11). Signs and symptoms may include cardiomegaly, hepatosplenomegaly, hypoglycemic seizures, lactic acidosis, ketosis, hyperlipidemia, elevated transaminases, easy fatigability, hypotonia, and muscle weakness. Treatment is aimed at maintaining normal blood glucose levels and may require continuous feedings through a gastrostomy tube, frequent feedings, and/or ingestion of uncooked cornstarch or glycoside (long-acting cornstarch) slurry at regular intervals throughout the day. Parents and children must be aware of the symptoms of hypoglycemia, and home glucose monitoring is recommended.

TABLE 39.11 Primary Underlying Pathophysiology in Select Metabolic Disorders

Disorder	Deficiency	Accumulation of Toxic Compound	Result
Hypoglycemic Disorders			
Glycogen Storage Disease	↓ glucose to prevent fasting hypoglycemia	Glycogen resulting in storage in liver, muscle, heart	Risk of hypoglycemic brain injury and dysfunction of tissue with storage
Medium-chain fatty acid oxidation defects	Fat for energy		Use of glucose with consequent hypoglycemia
Long-chain fatty acid oxidation defects	Fat for energy		Use of glucose with consequent hypoglycemia; mitochondrial dysfunction in liver, heart, etc., leading to organ dysfunction
Ketone utilization disorders	Fat for energy	Ketones	Risk of hypoglycemic brain injury; profound metabolic acidosis and reversible neurologic dysfunction Cyclic vomiting
Galactosemia		Galactose-1-phosphate Galactitol	Elevated galactose leads to severe hepatic dysfunction, neurologic injury, and impaired immune response
Encephalopathic Disorders			
Urea cycle defects		Ammonia	Central nervous system dysfunction, probably mediated through glutamine
Phenylketonuria	Tyrosine	Phenylalanine	Impairment of tryptophan metabolism leading to serotonin deficiency; defective neurotransmission and white matter damage
Maple syrup urine disease		Leucine	Leucine toxicity leading to cerebral edema
Propionic acidemia, methylmalonic acidemia, other organic acidemias		Organic acids	Systemic or local impairment of mitochondrial function; impaired neurotransmission; impairment of urea cycle
Cellular Component Disorders			
Mitochondrial disease	Deficiency of ATP (energy) in affected tissues		Failure of affected tissues to carry out normal functions (e.g., muscle weakness, failure of relaxation of blood vessel muscles); lactate accumulation; cardiomyopathy
Peroxisomal disorders	Defect in peroxisomal β-oxidation; Deficiency of steroid hormones necessary for signaling	Accumulation of the saturated very long-chain fatty acids	Aberrant embryonic patterning and hormone deficiency, defects in maintenance of myelin and white matter
Lysosomal storage disorders		Tissue-specific accumulation of compound not metabolized by lysosome	Cell type–specific damage and dysfunction as a result of lysosomal failure and reaction to waste product buildup
Other			
Disorders of creatine biosynthesis	Deficiency of cerebral creatine	Accumulation of guanidinoacetate in AGAT deficiency leads to seizures	Global brain energy defect leads to severe cognitive delays and seizures
Cholesterol biosynthesis disorders	Deficiency of steroid hormones		Endocrinopathies; disordered cellular signaling leading to aberrant organogenesis

AGAT, Arginine:glycine amidinotransferase deficiency; *ATP*, adenosine triphosphate.

From Neil E. Metabolic assessment. In: Nelson WE, Kliegman RWJ, et al. *Nelson Textbook of Pediatrics*. Elsevier, 2020.

Galactosemia results from a disorder of galactose metabolism. Infants with classic galactosemia appear normal at birth but demonstrate clinical manifestations after milk feeding. Although galactosemia is typically discovered during newborn screening, neonates may show clinical signs before the results of the screening are known. Clinical manifestations of severe, untreated galactosemia include poor weight gain, lethargy, jaundice, tubular kidney dysfunction, vomiting, coagulopathies, and *Escherichia coli* sepsis. Treatment in classic galactosemia consists of eliminating dietary galactose and ensuring that the child is receiving appropriate calcium supplementation.

Urea Cycle Disorders

A defect in any enzyme of the urea cycle results in hyperammonemia secondary to the body's inability to detoxify waste nitrogen through its normal conversion to urea. As an end product of amino acid catabolism, ammonia is highly toxic to the CNS. Five enzymes are required for the conversion of ammonia to urea, and deficiency in any of these enzymes results in disease. In infants, symptoms related to the effects of hyperammonemia start after protein ingestion and include vomiting, lethargy, irritability, malaise, and potential seizures and coma. Older children may exhibit ataxia, confusion, agitation, irritability, and combativeness. Treatment of acute hyperammonemia is completed by acute care staff with the goal being to establish a source of glucose and rapidly decreasing ammonia levels. Patients are maintained on a protein-restricted diet to minimize the nitrogen load that must be metabolized.[159] Care is supervised closely by a metabolic dietician. Despite appropriate treatment, children with UCD are vulnerable to metabolic decompensation, mild to moderate mental retardation, and premature death.

Amino Acid Metabolism Disorders

More than 30 defects of amino acid metabolism are attributed to enzyme or cofactor defects. Although all these disorders result from defects in amino acid metabolism, they are generally classified as aminoacidopathies or organic acidurias, or acidemias, depending on whether amino acids or organic acids are detected in urine or plasma. The most common aminoacidopathy is PKU. Other diseases in this category include maple syrup urine disease, tyrosinemias, and homocystinuria.

Phenylketonuria

Classic PKU is the most common form of PKU and results from a deficiency of the enzyme phenylalanine hydroxylase, which converts phenylalanine to tyrosine. PKU is detected during newborn screening. Untreated PKU leads to elevated phenylalanine concentrations in the blood and brain, resulting in CNS damage that causes profound intellectual disability (see Table 39.11). No clinical manifestations are noted at birth, and the effects of high phenylalanine levels may not be apparent in the first few months, by which time, if untreated, irreversible brain damage has occurred. Treatment for PKU involves limiting the dietary intake of phenylalanine, although it is an essential amino acid that cannot be eliminated entirely because patients need to receive enough to meet growth needs. The diet is supplemented with a medically modified formula, free of phenylalanine. Over the child's first few years of life, parents are educated on the phenylalanine content of foods; the child's phenylalanine level is frequently monitored, and a phenylalanine "allowance" is established based on the child's dietary tolerance. The current recommendation is a "diet for life" to prevent long-term cognitive and neurologic sequelae.

Disorders of Fatty Acid Oxidation

Fatty acids are an important energy resource for the body, used during times of fasting and stress when glycogen stores become depleted. Defects can occur at any point in fatty acid transport or the mitochondrial beta-oxidation pathway, yielding more than 20 disorders in which individuals are unable to metabolize fatty acids. The more common fatty acid oxidation disorders are medium-chain acyl-coenzyme A dehydrogenase (MCAD) deficiency,

very-long-chain acyl-coenzyme A dehydrogenase deficiency, and long-chain 3-hydroxy acyl-coenzyme A dehydrogenase deficiency.

Individuals with MCAD deficiency may be asymptomatic for a lifetime or have a premature death. Fasting, stress, or illness may lead to hypoketotic hypoglycemia, hypotonia, muscle weakness, lethargy, and vomiting progressing to seizures, coma, encephalopathy, and death. Any increase in energy demand may tip the balance and result in a metabolic crisis as vital organs are deprived of fuel. Treatment varies and may include fasting avoidance and carnitine supplementation to correct secondary carnitine deficiency. For individuals with MCAD deficiency, avoidance of fasting is the mainstay of treatment. The most serious consequence of this group of disorders is the inability to use fatty acids for energy production and the lack of ketone production (burned for energy) during times of fasting, which may result in death.

Lysosomal Storage Disorders

Lysosomal storage disorders are caused by an accumulation (storage) of glycoproteins, glycolipids, or glycosaminoglycans (e.g., mucopolysaccharide storage [MPS] diseases) within lysosomes and various tissues, which leads to the various clinical presentations and symptoms. Symptoms vary depending on the site of storage and the specific disorder and may include hepatosplenomegaly, coarse facies, corneal clouding, developmental regression, intellectual disability, thrombocytopenia, bone pain, abnormal liver function studies, respiratory problems, hydrocephalus, and cardiomyopathy. Enzymatic assay and mutation analysis are available for most disorders. Initial diagnostic testing for mucopolysaccharidosis consists of screening urinary glycosaminoglycans (urine MPS screen), but a normal screen does not rule out the diagnosis. Treatment varies from symptom management to enzyme replacement therapy with varying degrees of success.

Additional Resources

Academy of Nutrition and Dietetics: www.eatright.org

Adrenal Insufficiency Coalition: https://www.adrenalinsufficiency.org/

Association of Diabetes Care & Education Specialists (ADCES): www.diabeteseducator.org

American College of Medical Genetics and Genomics: www.acmg.net

American Diabetes Association: www.diabetes.org

American Thyroid Association: www.thyroid.org

Barbara Davis Center for Diabetes: University of Colorado Anschutz Medical Campus: www.barbaradaviscenter.org

Child Growth Foundation: www.childgrowthfoundation.org

Children with Diabetes: www.childrenwithdiabetes.com

Children's Diabetes Foundation: http://www.childrensdiabetesfoundation.org

Endocrine Society: www.endocrine.org

GeneReviews: www.ncbi.nlm.nih.gov/books/NBK1116/

National Library of Medicine Genetics Home Reference: https://ghr.nlm.nih.gov/

Human Growth Foundation: www.hgfound.org

Juvenile Diabetes Research Foundation (JDRF): www.jdrf.org

Magic Foundation: www.magicfoundation.org

National Heart, Lung, and Blood Institute: www.nhlbi.nih.gov

National Institutes of Health: www.nih.gov

National Institute of Diabetes and Digestive and Kidney Diseases: www.niddk.nih.gov/health-information/diabetes

National Lipid Association: www.lipid.org
Online Mendelian Inheritance in Man (OMIM): www.omim.org
Pediatric Endocrinology Nursing Society: www.pens.org
UCSF Center of Excellence for Transgender Health: https://prevention.ucsf.edu/transhealth
Standards of Care for the Health of Transgender and Gender Diverse People, V8: www.tandfonline.com/doi/pdf/10.1080/26895269.2022.2100644

References

1. Centers for Disease Control and Prevention. *Growth Charts*; 2019. https://www.cdc.gov/growthcharts/.
2. Eggermann T, Elbracht M, Kurth I, et al. Genetic testing in inherited endocrine disorders: joint position paper of the European reference network on rare endocrine conditions (Endo-ERN). *Orphanet J Rare Dis.* 2020;15(1).
3. Endocrine Society. Endocrine Disrupting Chemicals (EDCs). https://www.endocrine.org/patient-engagement/endocrine-library/edcs.
4. Kirchnawy C, Hager F, Osorio Piniella V, et al. Potential endocrine disrupting properties of toys for babies and infants. *PLoS One.* 2020;15(4). :e0231171.
5. Savgan-Gurol E. Growth factors. In: Stanley T, Misra M, eds. *Endocrine Conditions in Pediatrics.* Switzerland: Springer; 2020:145–147.
6. Blum WF, Alherbish A, Alsagheir A, et al. The growth hormone–insulin-like growth factor-I axis in the diagnosis and treatment of growth disorders. *Endocr Connect.* 2018;7(6):R212–R222.
7. National Organization for Rare Disorders. *Growth Hormone Deficiency*; 2015. https://rarediseases.org/rare-diseases/growth-hormone-deficiency/.
8. Escobar O, Perez-Garcia EM. Decreased growth velocity and/or short stature. In: Stanley T, Misra M, eds. *Endocrine Conditions in Pediatrics.* Switzerland: Springer; 2020:3–10.
9. Grimberg A, DiVall SA, Polychronakos C, et al. Guidelines for growth hormone and insulin-like growth factor-I treatment in children and adolescents: growth hormone deficiency, idiopathic short stature, and primary insulin-like growth factor-I deficiency. *Horm Res Paediatr.* 2016;86(6):361–397.
10. Smyczyńska J. Inclusion and withdrawal criteria for Growth Hormone (GH) therapy in children with idiopathic GH Deficiency—towards following the evidence but still with unresolved problems. *Endocr.* 2022;3(1):55–75.
11. Cianfarani S. Safety of pediatric rhGH therapy: an overview and the need for long-term surveillance. *Front Endocrinol.* 2021;12.
12. Sävendahl L, Polak M, Backeljauw P, et al. Long-term safety of growth hormone treatment in childhood: two large observational studies: NordiNet IOS and ANSWER. *J Clin Endocrinol Metab.* 2021;106(6):1728–1741.
13. van Dommelen P, Koledova E, Wit JM. Effect of adherence to growth hormone treatment on 0–2 year catch-up growth in children with growth hormone deficiency. *PLoS One.* 2018;13(10). :e0206009.
14. McGill D. Bone age. In: Stanley T, Misra M, eds. *Endocrine Conditions in Pediatrics.* Switzerland: Springer; 2020:215–218.
15. Galazzi E, Improda N, Cerbone M, et al. Clinical benefits of sex steroids given as a priming prior to GH provocative test or as a growth–promoting therapy in peripubertal growth delays: results of a retrospective study among ENDO–ERN centres. *Clin Endocrinol.* 2020;94(2):219–228.
16. Hage C, Gan HW, Ibba A, et al. Advances in differential diagnosis and management of growth hormone deficiency in children. *Nat Rev Endocrinol.* 2021;17(10):608–624.
17. Viswanathan P, Pinto B. Increased growth velocity and/or tall stature. In: Stanley T, Misra M, eds. *Endocrine Conditions in Pediatrics.* Switzerland: Springer; 2020:11–15.
18. Krausz C, Rosta V. Genetics and alterations in the development of male reproductive system: diagnosis and clinical management. *Pediatr Adolesc Androl.* 2021:1–27.
19. Stambough K, Magistrado L, Perez-Milicua G. Evaluation of ambiguous genitalia. *Curr Opin Obstet Gynecol.* 2019;31(5):303–308.
20. Mohammad Hossein RS, Reza AH. Abnormal sex determinism: true hermaphrodite (TH). *J Clin Transl Endocrinol Case Rep.* 2020;18:100070.
21. Mason KA, Schoelwer MJ, Rogol AD. Androgens during infancy, childhood, and adolescence: physiology and use in clinical practice. *Endocr Rev.* 2020;41(3).
22. Ahmed SF, Achermann J, Alderson J, et al. Society for Endocrinology UK Guidance on the initial evaluation of a suspected difference or disorder of sex development (Revised 2021). *Clin Endocrinol.* 2021;95(6):818–840.
23. León NY, Reyes AP, Harley VR. A clinical algorithm to diagnose differences of sex development. *Lancet Diabetes Endocrinol.* 2019;7(7):560–574.
24. Sultan C, Gaspari L, Maimoun L, et al. Disorders of puberty. *Best Pract Res Clin Obstet Gynaecol.* 2018;48:62–89.
25. Eckert-Lind C, Busch AS, Petersen JH, et al. Worldwide secular trends in age at pubertal onset assessed by breast development among girls. *JAMA Pediatr.* 2020;174(4). :e195881.
26. Witchel SF, Pinto B, Burghard AC, et al. Update on adrenarche. *Curr Opin Pediatr.* 2020;32(4):574–581.
27. Panayiotopoulos A, Bhangoo A, Khurana D, et al. Glucocorticoid resistance in premature adrenarche and PCOS: from childhood to adulthood. *J Endocr Soc.* 2020;4(9).
28. Ng SM, Apperley LJ, Upradrasta S, et al. Vaginal bleeding in prepubertal females. *J Pediatr Adolesc Gynecol.* 2020;33(4):339–342.
29. Elchuri SV, Momen JJ. Disorders of pubertal onset. *Prim Care Clin Off Pract.* 2020;47(2):189–216.
30. Eugster EA. Treatment of central precocious puberty. *J Endocr Soc.* 2019;3(5):965–972.
31. Mucaria C, Tyutyusheva N, Baroncelli GI, et al. Central precocious puberty in boys and girls: similarities and differences. *Sexes.* 2021;2(1):119–131.
32. Shim YS, Lim KI, Lee HS, et al. Long-term outcomes after gonadotropin-releasing hormone agonist treatment in boys with central precocious puberty. *PLoS One.* 2020;15(12). :e0243212.
33. Bradley SH, Lawrence N, Steele C, et al. Precocious puberty. *BMJ.* 2020:l6597.
34. Cantas-Orsdemir S, Garb JL, Allen HF. Prevalence of cranial MRI findings in girls with central precocious puberty: a systematic review and meta-analysis. *J Pediatr Endocrinol Metab.* 2018;31(7):701–710.
35. Eugster EA. Update on precocious puberty in girls. *J Pediatr Adolesc Gynecol.* 2019;32(5):455–459.
36. Stanley T, Misra M. Delayed or stalled pubertal development. In: Stanley T, Misra M, eds. *Endocrine Conditions in Pediatrics.* Switzerland: Springer; 2020:67–70.
37. Acién P, Acién M. Disorders of sex development: classification, review, and impact on fertility. *J Clin Med.* 2020;9(11):3555.
38. Alsaleem M, Saadeh L. Micropenis. StatPearls. https://www.ncbi.nlm.nih.gov/books/NBK562275/.
39. Jonsdottir-Lewis E, Feld A, Ciarlo R, et al. Timing of pubertal onset in girls and boys with constitutional delay. *J Clin Endocrinol Metab.* 2021;106(9):e3693–e3703.
40. Sanders RA, Fields EL. The LGBTQ+ patient: the pediatric provider plays a role in supporting sexual minority and gender-diverse youth. *Contemp Pediatr.* 2021;38(6):20+.
41. The Trevor Project. *Data on Transgender Youth*; 2022. https://www.thetrevorproject.org/research-briefs/data-on-transgender-youth/.
42. Rew L, Young CC, Monge M, et al. Review: puberty blockers for transgender and gender diverse youth—a critical review of the literature. *Child Adolesc Ment Health.* 2021;26(1).

43. Hembree WC, Cohen-Kettenis PT, Gooren L, et al. Endocrine treatment of gender-dysphoric/gender-incongruent persons: an Endocrine Society clinical practice guideline. *J Clin Endocrinol Metab.* 2017;102(11):3869–3903.

44. Fisher A, Senofonte G, Cocchetti C, et al. Gender dysphoria: management in the transition age. In: Jannini E, Foresta C, Lenzi A, Maggi M, eds. *Pediatric and Adolescent Andrology.* Switzerland: Springer Nature; 2021:255–264.

45. Sorbara JC, Chiniara LN, Thompson S, et al. Mental health and timing of gender-affirming care. *Pediatrics.* 2020;146(4). :e20193600.

46. Mitzi M. Puberty blockers: a review of GnRH analogues in transgender youth. Transfeminine Science. https://transfemscience.org/articles/puberty-blockers/.

47. Millington K, Williams C. Transgender care. In: Stanley T, Misra M, eds. *Endocrine Conditions in Pediatrics.* Switzerland: Springer; 2020:357–363.

48. Pronouns.org. Resources on Personal Pronouns. https://pronouns.org/.

49. Conlon JL, Malcolm S, Monaghan M. Diagnosis and treatment of polycystic ovary syndrome in adolescents. *J Am Acad Physician Assist.* 2021;34(10):15–22.

50. Li X, Yang D, Pan P, et al. The degree of menstrual disturbance is associated with the severity of insulin resistance in PCOS. *Front Endocrinol.* 2022;13.

51. Peña AS, Witchel SF, Hoeger KM, et al. Adolescent polycystic ovary syndrome according to the international evidence-based guideline. *BMC Med.* 2020;18(1).

52. Rackow BW, Vanden Brink H, Hammers L, et al. Ovarian morphology by transabdominal ultrasound correlates with reproductive and metabolic disturbance in adolescents with PCOS. *J Adolesc Health.* 2018;62(3):288–293.

53. Arslanian S, Bacha F, Grey M, et al. Evaluation and management of youth-onset type 2 diabetes: a position statement by the American Diabetes Association. *Diabetes Care.* 2018;41(12):2648–2668.

54. Jensterle M, Kravos NA, Ferjan S, et al. Long-term efficacy of metformin in overweight-obese PCOS: longitudinal follow-up of retrospective cohort. *Endocr Connect.* 2020;9(1):44–54.

55. Benson J, Severn C, Hudnut-Beumler J, et al. Depression in girls with obesity and polycystic ovary syndrome and/or type 2 diabetes. *Can J Diabetes.* 2020;44(6):507–513.

56. Heath C, Siafarikas A, Sommerfield A, et al. Peri–operative steroid management in the paediatric population. *Acta Anaesthesiol Scand.* 2021;65(9):1187–1194.

57. Hahner S, Ross RJ, Arlt W, et al. Adrenal insufficiency. *Nat Rev Dis Prim.* 2021;7(1).

58. Kirkgoz T, Guran T. Primary adrenal insufficiency in children: diagnosis and management. *Best Pract Res Clin Endocrinol Metab.* 2018;32(4):397–424.

59. Wiener JS, Huck N, Blais AS, et al. Challenges in pediatric urologic practice: a lifelong view. *World J Urol.* 2020;39(4):981–991.

60. Claahsen-van der Grinten HL, Speiser PW, Ahmed SF, et al. Congenital adrenal hyperplasia—current insights in pathophysiology, diagnostics, and management. *Endocr Rev.* 2021;43(1):91–159.

61. Ekbom K, Strandqvist A, Lajic S, et al. Assessment of medication adherence in children and adults with congenital adrenal hyperplasia and the impact of knowledge and self–management. *Clin Endocrinol.* 2021;94(5):753–764.

62. Prentice P. Guideline review: congenital adrenal hyperplasia clinical practice guideline 2018. *Arch Dis Child Educ Pract Ed.* 2020. edpract-2019-317573.

63. Rushworth RL, Torpy DJ, Falhammar H. Adrenal crisis. *N Engl J Med.* 2019;381(9):852–861.

64. Chovel-Sella A, Halper A. Adrenal insufficiency. In: Stanley T, Misra M, eds. *Endocrine Conditions in Pediatrics.* Springer; 2020:285–288.

65. Ferrigno R, Hasenmajer V, Caiulo S, et al. Paediatric Cushing's disease: epidemiology, pathogenesis, clinical management and outcome. *Rev Endocr Metab Disord.* 2021;22(4):817–835.

66. Bauer AJ, Wassner AJ. Thyroid hormone therapy in congenital hypothyroidism and pediatric hypothyroidism. *Endocrine.* 2019;66(1):51–62.

67. Bowden SA, Goldis M. Congenital Hypothyroidism. StatPearls. https://www.ncbi.nlm.nih.gov/books/NBK558913/.

68. Cherella CE, Wassner AJ. Update on congenital hypothyroidism. *Curr Opin Endocrinol Diabetes Obes.* 2020;27(1):63–69.

69. Rose SR, Wassner AJ, Wintergerst KA, et al. AAP section on endocrinology, AAP Council on genetics, pediatric endocrine society, American thyroid association. Congenital hypothyroidism: screening and management. *Pediatrics.* 2023;151(1). :e2022060420.

70. Leung AKC, Leung AAC. Evaluation and management of the child with hypothyroidism. *World J Pediatr.* 2019;15(2):124–134.

71. Salerno M, Improda N, Capalbo D. Management of endocrine disease: subclinical hypothyroidism in children. *Eur J Endocrinol.* 2020;183(2):R13–R28.

72. Draznin M, Borgohain P, Kanungo S. Newborn screening in pediatric endocrine disorders. *Endocr.* 2022;3(1):107–114.

73. Barker JM, Triolo TM. Hypothyroidism. In: Stanley T, Misra M, eds. *Endocrine Conditions in Pediatrics.* Switzerland: Springer; 2020:243–246.

74. Léger J, Carel JC. Diagnosis and management of hyperthyroidism from prenatal life to adolescence. *Best Pract Res Clin Endocrinol Metab.* 2018;32(4):373–386.

75. Park JE, Hwang SM, Hwang JY, et al. The relationship between ultrasound findings and thyroid function in children and adolescent autoimmune diffuse thyroid diseases. *Sci Rep.* 2021;11(1).

76. Mooij CF, Cheetham TD, Verburg FA, et al. 2022 European Thyroid Association guideline for the management of pediatric Graves' disease. *Eur Thyr J.* 2022;11(1).

77. Kaplowitz PB, Vaidyanathan P. Update on pediatric hyperthyroidism. *Curr Opin Endocrinol Diabetes Obes.* 2020;27(1):70–76.

78. Delshad H, Takyar M. Long-term antithyroid treatment in pediatric and juvenile Graves' disease. *Int J Endocrinol Metab.* 2020;18(Suppl).

79. Jamshidi R, Egan JC. Pediatric parathyroid disease. *Semin Pediatr Surg.* 2020;29(3). :150923.

80. Bilezikian JP. Hypoparathyroidism. *J Clin Endocrinol Metab.* 2020;105(6):1722–1736.

81. Stefanko N, Grant S. Disorders of parathyroid bone and mineral endocrinology. In: Marcdante K, Kliegman R, Schuh A, eds. *Nelson Essentials of Pediatrics.* Elsevier; 2023:685a–686a.

82. Linglart A, Levine MA, Jüppner H. Pseudohypoparathyroidism. *Endocrinol Metab Clin N Am.* 2018;47(4):865–888.

83. Boddu SK, Kharidehal N, Balla KC. Refractory yet transient neonatal hypocalcemia due to hitherto undiagnosed asymptomatic maternal hyperparathyroidism: a case report. *J Neonatol.* 2021;35(4):238–241.

84. Khalatbari H, Cheeney SHE, Manning SC, et al. Pediatric hyperparathyroidism: review and imaging update. *Pediatr Radiol.* 2021;51(7):1106–1120.

85. Centers for Disease Control and Prevention. National Diabetes Statistics Report. https://www.cdc.gov/diabetes/data/statistics-report/index.html.

86. Centers for Disease Control and Prevention. Prevalence of Diagnosed Diabetes. https://www.cdc.gov/diabetes/data/statistics-report/diagnosed-diabetes.html.

87. Pettitt DJ, Talton J, Dabelea D, et al. Prevalence of diabetes in U.S. youth in 2009: the SEARCH for Diabetes in Youth study. *Diabetes Care.* 2013;37(2):402–408.

88. Shah AS, Nadeau KJ. The changing face of paediatric diabetes. *Diabetologia.* 2020;63(4):683–691.

89. Misra S. Pancreatic autoantibodies: who to test and how to interpret the results. *Pract Diabetes.* 2017;34(6):221a–223a.

90. Vakharia M, Kim G. Deeper Dive into "Other" Endocrine Pathologies in Children/adolescents with Diabetes Mellitus. Presented at: NAPNAP 43rd National Conference on Pediatric Health Care; March 2022.

91. Jensen ET, Stafford JM, Saydah S, et al. Increase in prevalence of diabetic ketoacidosis at diagnosis among youth with type 1 diabetes: the SEARCH for Diabetes in Youth Study. *Diabetes Care*. 2021;44(7):1573–1578.

92. Mejia−Otero JD, Adhikari S, White PC. Risk factors for hospitalization in youth with type 1 diabetes: development and validation of a multivariable prediction model. *Pediatr Diabetes*. 2020;21(7):1268–1276.

93. Sonawalla A, Jafri R. Type 1 diabetes mellitus. In: Stanley T, Misra M, eds. *Endocrine Conditions in Pediatrics*. Switzerland: Springer; 2020:307–311.

94. Long AE, George G, Williams CL. Persistence of islet autoantibodies after diagnosis in type 1 diabetes. *Diabet Med*. 2021;38(12).

95. Jamiołkowska-Sztabkowska M, Głowińska-Olszewska B, Bossowski A. C-peptide and residual β-cell function in pediatric diabetes – state of the art. *Pediatr Endocrinol Diabet Metab*. 2021;27(2):123–133.

96. Kochummen E, Marwa A, Umpaichitra V, et al. Screening for autoimmune thyroiditis and celiac disease in minority children with type 1 diabetes. *J Pediatr Endocrinol Metabol*. 2018;31(8):879–885.

97. Diabetes TrialNet. Type 1 Diabetes Facts. https://www.trialnet.org/t1d-facts.

98. American Diabetes Association. Classification and diagnosis of diabetes: standards of medical care in diabetes—2019. *Diabetes Care*. 2018;42(Supplement 1):S13–S28.

99. Choudhary A, Adhikari S, White PC. Impact of the COVID-19 pandemic on management of children and adolescents with type 1 diabetes. *BMC Pediatr*. 2022;22(1).

100. Lai CW, Lipman T, Willi SM, et al. Early racial/ethnic disparities in continuous glucose monitor use in pediatric type 1 diabetes. *Diabetes Technol Ther*. 2021;23(11):763–767.

101. Ilkowitz J, Wissing V, Gallagher MP. Pediatric Smart Insulin Pen use: the next best thing. *J Diabetes Sci Technol*. 2021. :193229682110413.

102. Sethuram S, Rapaport R. Update: pediatric diabetes. *J Diabetes*. 2020;12(10):769–771.

103. CGM Alarm Fatigue. Children with Diabetes. https://children-withdiabetes.com/clinical-director/cgm-alarm-fatigue/.

104. American Diabetes Association. Children and adolescents: standards of medical care in diabetes—2022. *Diabetes Care*. 2021;45(suppl 1):S208–S231.

105. Danne T, Phillip M, Buckingham BA, et al. ISPAD clinical practice consensus guidelines 2018: insulin treatment in children and adolescents with diabetes. *Pediatr Diabetes*. 2018;19(suppl. 27):115–135.

106. Dos Santos TJ, Donado Campos J de M, Argente J, et al. Effectiveness and equity of continuous subcutaneous insulin infusions in pediatric type 1 diabetes: a systematic review and meta-analysis of the literature. *Diabetes Res Clin Pract*. 2021;172:108643.

107. Medtronic. MiniMed, MiniMed 770G System. https://www.medtronicdiabetes.com/minimed-770g-system-kids/.

108. Chiang JL, Maahs DM, Garvey KC, et al. Type 1 diabetes in children and adolescents: a position statement by the American Diabetes Association. *Diabetes Care*. 2018;41(9):2026–2044.

109. Moser O, Riddell MC, Eckstein ML, et al. Glucose management for exercise using continuous glucose monitoring (CGM) and intermittently scanned CGM (isCGM) systems in type 1 diabetes: position statement of the European Association for the Study of Diabetes (EASD) and of the International Society for Pediatric and Adolescent Diabetes (ISPAD) endorsed by JDRF and supported by the American Diabetes Association (ADA). *Pediatr Diabetes*. 2020;21(8):1375–1393.

110. King KM, Jaggers JR, Della LJ, et al. Association between physical activity and sport participation on Hemoglobin A1c among children and adolescents with type 1 diabetes. *Int J Environ Res Publ Health*. 2021;18(14):7490.

111. Absil H, Baudet L, Robert A, et al. Benefits of physical activity in children and adolescents with type 1 diabetes: a systematic review. *Diabetes Res Clin Pract*. 2019;156:107810.

112. Lee Tracy E, Berg CA, Baker AC, et al. Health-risk behaviors and type 1 diabetes outcomes in the transition from late adolescence to early emerging adulthood. *Child Health Care*. 2018;48(3):285–300.

113. Butalia S, McGuire KA, Dyjur D, et al. Youth with diabetes and their parents' perspectives on transition care from pediatric to adult diabetes care services: a qualitative study. *Health Sci Rep*. 2020;3(3).

114. TODAY Study Group. Long-term complications in youth-onset type 2 diabetes. *N Engl J Med*. 2021;385(5):416–426.

115. Rechenberg K, Koerner R. Anxiety and depressive symptoms in adolescents with type 1 diabetes. *J Pediatr Health Care*. 2022;36(4):396.

116. Andes LJ, Cheng YJ, Rolka DB, et al. Prevalence of prediabetes among adolescents and young adults in the United States, 2005-2016. *JAMA Pediatr*. 2019:e194498.

117. Centers for Disease Control and Prevention. *Diabetes Report Card*; 2021. https://www.cdc.gov/diabetes/library/reports/reportcard.html.

118. Vajravelu ME, Lee JM, Amaral S, et al. Sex−based differences in screening and recognition of pre−diabetes and type 2 diabetes in pediatric primary care. *Pediatr Obes*. 2020;16(2).

119. Jonas D, Vander Schaff E, Riley S. *Screening for Prediabetes and Type 2 Diabetes Mellitus in Children and Adolescents: An Evidence Review for the U.S. Preventive Services Task Force. Evidence Synthesis No. 216*. AHRQ Publication No. 21-05288-EF-1. Agency for Healthcare Research and Quality; 2021.

120. Bacha F, Cheng P, Gal RL, et al. Racial and ethnic disparities in comorbidities in youth with type 2 diabetes in the Pediatric Diabetes Consortium (PDC). *Diabetes Care*. 2021;44(10):2245–2251.

121. Savic Hitt TA, Katz LEL. Pediatric type 2 diabetes: not a mini version of adult type 2 diabetes. *Endocrinol Metab Clin N Am*. 2020;49(4):679–693.

122. Barrett T, Jalaludin MY, Turan S, Novo Nordisk Pediatric Type 2 Diabetes Global Expert Panel, et al. Rapid progression of type 2 diabetes and related complications in children and young people-A literature review. *Pediatr Diabetes*. 2020;21(2):158–172.

123. United States Preventive Services Taskforce. Draft Recommendation: Prediabetes and Type 2 Diabetes in Children and Adolescents: Screening. https://www.uspreventiveservicestaskforce.org/uspstf/draft-recommendation/prediabetes-type2-diabetes-children-adolescents-screening#fullrecommendationstart.

124. Weinstock RS, Braffett BH, McGuigan P, et al. Self-monitoring of blood glucose in youth-onset type 2 diabetes: results from the TODAY study. *Diabetes Care*. 2019;42(5):903–909.

125. Jaggers JR, McKay T, King KM, et al. Integration of consumer-based activity monitors into clinical practice for children with type 1 diabetes: a feasibility study. *Int J Environ Res Publ Health*. 2021;18(20):10611.

126. Anderson E, Durstine JL. Physical activity, exercise, and chronic diseases: a brief review. *Sports Med Health Sci*. 2019;1(1):3–10.

127. Taş Ö, Kontbay T, Dogan O, et al. Does metformin treatment in pediatric population cause vitamin B12 deficiency? *Klin Pädiatr*. 2022;234(4):221–227.

128. Broome DT, Pantalone KM, Kashyap SR, et al. Approach to the patient with MODY-monogenic diabetes. *J Clin Endocrinol Metab*. 2021;106(1):237–250.

129. Urakami T. Maturity-onset diabetes of the young (MODY): current perspectives on diagnosis and treatment. *Diabetes Metab Syndr Obes*. 2019;12:1047–1056.

130. Bardanzellu F, Marcialis MA, Frassetto R, et al. Differential diagnosis between syndrome of inappropriate antidiuretic hormone secretion and cerebral/renal salt wasting syndrome in children over 1 year: proposal for a simple algorithm. *Pediatr Nephrol*. 2021;37(7):1469–1478.

131. Castellanos LE. Sodium, osmolality, and antidiuretic hormone. In: Stanley T, Misra M, eds. *Endocrine Conditions in Pediatrics.* Springer; 2020:171–173.

132. LynShue KA, Yau M, Sperling MA. Critical care endocrinology. *Pediat Crit Care.* 2021:1317–1349.

133. Patti G, Napoli F, Fava D, et al. Approach to the pediatric patient: central diabetes insipidus. *J Clin Endocrinol Metab.* 2022;107(5):1407–1416.

134. Hampl SE, Hassink SG, Skinner AC, et al. Clinical practice guideline for the evaluation and treatment of children and adolescents with obesity. *Pediatrics.* 2023;151(2).

135. Steinhart A, Tsao D, Pratt JSA. Pediatric metabolic and bariatric surgery. *Surg Clin N Am.* 2021;101(2):199–212.

136. Kleinendorst L, Abawi O, van der Voorn B, et al. Identifying underlying medical causes of pediatric obesity: results of a systematic diagnostic approach in a pediatric obesity center. In: Buchner DA, ed. Plos ONE; Vol. 15. ; 2020(5):e0232990..

137. Calcaterra V, Cena H, Pelizzo G, et al. Bariatric surgery in adolescents: to do or not to do? *Children.* 2021;8(6):453. https://doi.org/10.3390/children8060453.

138. Mitsinikos T, Mrowczynski-Hernandez P, Kohli R. Pediatric non-alcoholic fatty liver disease. *Pediatr Clin N Am.* 2021;68(6):1309–1320. https://doi.org/10.1016/j.pcl.2021.07.013.

139. Kang NR, Kwack YS. An update on mental health problems and cognitive behavioral therapy in pediatric obesity. *Pediatr Gastroenterol Hepatol Nutr.* 2020;23(1):15.

140. de Ferranti SD, Steinberger J, Ameduri R, et al. Cardiovascular risk reduction in high-risk pediatric patients: a scientific statement from the American Heart Association. *Circulation.* 2019;139(13).

141. Styne DM, Arslanian SA, Connor EL, et al. Pediatric obesity—assessment, treatment, and intervention: an Endocrine Society clinical practice guideline. *J Clin Endocrinol Metab.* 2017;102(3):709–757.

142. Alman KL, Lister NB, Garnett SP, et al. Dietetic management of obesity and severe obesity in children and adolescents: a scoping review of guidelines. *Obes Rev.* 2020;22(1).

143. Singhal V, Sella AC, Malhotra S. Pharmacotherapy in pediatric obesity: current evidence and landscape. *Curr Opin Endocrinol Diabetes Obes.* 2020;28(1):55–63.

144. Armstrong SC, Bolling CF, Michalsky MP, et al. Pediatric metabolic and bariatric surgery: evidence, barriers, and best practices. *Pediatrics.* 2019. e20193223.

145. Buterbaugh JS. Pediatric dyslipidemia and screening recommendations. *J Nurse Pract.* 2021;17(10):1178–1182.

146. Brandts J, Ray KK. Familial hypercholesterolemia. *J Am Coll Card.* 2021;78(18):1831–1843.

147. Mosca S, Araújo G, Costa V, et al. Dyslipidemia diagnosis and treatment: risk stratification in children and adolescents. In: Suzuki T, ed. J Nutr Metab; Vol. 2022. ; 2022:1–10.

148. Rohrs, H. What are the NHLBI guidelines on pediatric lipid screening? https://www.medscape.com/answers/1825087-189832/what-are-the-nhlbi-guidelines-on-pediatric-lipid-screening.

149. Stewart J, McCallin T, Martinez J, Chacko S, Yusuf S. Hyperlipidemia. *Pediatr Rev.* 2020;41(8):393–402.

150. Sunil B, Ashraf AP. Dyslipidemia in the pediatric population. In: Stanley T, Misra M, eds. *Endocrine Conditions in Pediatrics.* Springer; 2020:339–347.

151. Reisinger C, Nkeh-Chungag BN, Fredriksen PM, et al. The prevalence of pediatric metabolic syndrome—a critical look on the discrepancies between definitions and its clinical importance. *Int J Obes.* 2020;45(1):12–24.

152. Felix A, John RM. Pediatric metabolic syndrome. *Nurse Pract.* 2019;44(7):25–26.

153. Xu H, Li X, Adams H, et al. Etiology of metabolic syndrome and dietary intervention. *Int J Mol Sci.* 2018;20(1).

154. Waters D, Adeloye D, Woolham D, et al. Global birth prevalence and mortality from inborn errors of metabolism: a systematic analysis of the evidence. *J Glob Health.* 2018;8(2).

155. van Spronsen FJ, Blau N, Harding C, et al. Phenylketonuria. *Nat Rev Dis Prim.* 2021;7(1).

156. Marsden D, Bedrosian CL, Vockley J. Impact of newborn screening on the reported incidence and clinical outcomes associated with medium- and long-chain fatty acid oxidation disorders. *Genet Med.* 2021;23(5):816–829.

157. Strauss KA. Metabolic crises. *Pediatr Crit Care.* 2021:1351–1396.

158. Heuer B. Mitochondrial DNA: unraveling the "other" genome. *J Am Assoc Nurse Pract.* 2021;33(9):673–675.

159. Matsumoto S, Häberle J, Kido J, et al. Urea cycle disorders—update. *J Hum Genet.* 2019;64(9):833–847.

40

Musculoskeletal Disorders

LESLIE N. RHODES

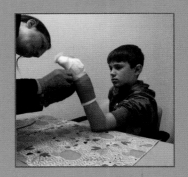

Primary care providers (PCPs) play a vital role in the early detection and appropriate management of musculoskeletal conditions in pediatrics. Common musculoskeletal disorders include athletic injuries, back pain, foot injuries, knee disorders, shin splints, and fractures. Congenital problems include spinal deformities, hip and foot anomalies, growth disorders and developmental delay, metabolic disorders, and neuromuscular disorders ranging from cerebral palsy to muscular dystrophy. A variety of other conditions can cause musculoskeletal findings, including intentional and unintentional injury, cancer, and juvenile idiopathic arthritis. Iatrogenic deformities can result from cultural practices, such as using a cradleboard, or from fetal position and intrauterine compression, which can also cause deformities. Disorders of the musculoskeletal system present unique problems because growth and development of this system contribute to the evolution of pathologic conditions over time. Limited mobility, pain, and deformity can interfere with the child's lifestyle. Pediatric patients with functional disabilities may not be able to fully participate in all activities with peers and family or meet the physical requirements of various occupations. They may also face challenges related to self-esteem. PCPs must be vigilant and seek to help pediatric patients and their families prevent these problems.

PCPs assess development of the musculoskeletal system, identify problems requiring early intervention, focus on lifestyle assessment and injury prevention, and monitor the long-term outcomes of orthopedic care. They are often the first to refer to specialists for early diagnosis and treatment. When necessary, they help families integrate orthopedic care within daily living activities at home and school and help families to cope with the issues of disability, deformity, and long-term care.

Anatomy and Physiology

Limb formation occurs early in embryogenesis (4–8 weeks of gestation); primary ossification centers are present in all the long bones of the limbs by the 12th week of gestation. Development of the skeletal system begins around the fourth week of gestation, with ossification of the fetal skeleton beginning during the fifth month of gestation. The clavicles and skull bones are the first to ossify, followed by the long bones and spine. The epiphyses of the newborn's long bones are composed of hyaline cartilage. Soon after birth, the cartilage along the epiphyseal plate begins secondary ossification. The shape of the lateral spine also changes from a C shape at birth to an S curve by late adolescence. As the child starts to walk, the lateral lumbar curve develops. The sacrum starts out as five separate bones at birth, becoming fused as one large bone by 18 to 20 years of age.[1]

Bone age, measured by radiographs of the left hand and wrist, is used to quantitatively determine somatic maturation and serves as a mirror that reflects the tempo of growth. In adolescents, the skeletal growth spurt begins at about Tanner stage 2 in females and Tanner stage 3 in males. Growth peaks around stage 4 and then ends with stage 5. The growth spurt lasts longer in males than in females. The pelvis widens early in pubescent females. In both sexes, the legs usually lengthen before the thighs broaden. The shoulders then widen and the trunk completes its linear growth. Bone growth ends when the epiphyses close.

Long bones have a growth plate, or physis, at each end that separates the epiphysis from the diaphysis or shaft. Openings through this plate allow blood vessels to penetrate from the epiphysis. In the growth plate, chondrocytes produce cartilage cells, dead cells are absorbed, and the calcified cartilage matrix is converted into bone. The entire growth plate area is weaker than the remaining bone because it is less calcified. Because blood supply to the growth plate comes primarily through the epiphysis, damage to epiphyseal circulation can jeopardize the survival of the chondrocytes. If chondrocytes stop producing, growth of the bone in that area stops (Fig. 40.1).

There are two ways that pediatric bones grow. Longitudinal growth occurs in the ossification centers; changes in bone width and strength take place via intramembranous ossification. The length of long bones comes from growth at the epiphyseal plates, whereas their diameter increases as a result of deposition of new bone on the periosteal surface and resorption on the surface of the medullary cavity. Growth of the small bones, hip, and spine comes from one or more primary ossification centers in each bone. Apophyses are the sites for connection of tendons to bone. In pediatrics, these sites, which are similar to epiphyses, allow for growth and are weaker than bone. These sites can become inflamed with overuse, as occurs in Osgood-Schlatter disease.

The development of bones and muscles is influenced by use. In infants and the first years of early childhood, the legs straighten and lengthen with the stimulus of weight bearing and independent walking. The infant is born with the full complement of muscle fibers. Growth in muscle length results from lengthening of the fibers, and growth in bulk comes from hypertrophy. Length of muscles is related to growth in length of the underlying bone. If a limb is not used, it grows minimally. If muscles and bones are not used in their intended typical manner, as occurs with spastic diplegia, the forces for development tend to stimulate growth in abnormal patterns. Thus scoliosis can develop or limb length inequality may increase in severity. Muscle contractures occur if muscles are not used regularly and put through their full range of motion. The growth of fibrous tissue, tendons, and ligaments is also dependent on mechanical demands.

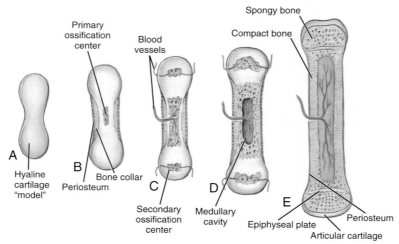

• **Fig. 40.1** Growth Plates and the Transition From Cartilage to Bone at the Epiphyseal Plate. (A) Hyaline cartilage "model." (B) Periosteum and bone collar form. (C) Blood vessels and osteoblasts infiltrate primary ossification centers. (D) Osteoclasts form the medullary cavity. (E) Ossification is complete. Hyaline cartilage remains as articular cartilage and in the epiphyseal plate. (From Giss, K, Chan, C. Musculoskeletal system. In: Duderstadt, KG, Keeton, VF eds. *Pediatric Physical Examination: An Illustrated Handbook.* 4th ed. Elsevier; 2023.)

Nutritional, mechanical, and hormonal factors during the growth process influence the thickness of bones and the health of the marrow. Adequate protein, calcium, and vitamin D in the diet are key nutritional elements that affect the growth and development of the pediatric musculoskeletal system.

The muscle structures originate from the embryonic mesoderm. Muscle fibers are developed by the fourth or fifth month of gestation and grow in tangent with their respective bones. The rate of muscle growth (muscle mass and cell sizes) speeds up dramatically around 2 years of age, with females exhibiting a greater rate of growth than males until this sex difference is reversed at puberty.[1] Tendons are associated connective tissues; they are tough, flexible fibrous bands connecting muscles to bones. Ligaments are composed of fibrous connective tissue that joins bones to each other.

Pathophysiology and Defense Mechanisms

Pathophysiology

Muscles and bones can be affected by localized or systemic problems. An initial orthopedic problem can be symptomatic of a larger problem (e.g., juvenile arthritis). Tendon and ligament injuries that result in sprains and strains or apophysitis are the result of traumatic injury or overuse.

Systemic Problems

Musculoskeletal presentation in pediatrics can be a feature of potentially life-threatening conditions (such as sepsis, malignancy, or nonaccidental injury) or chronic pediatric conditions (such as inflammatory bowel disease, cystic fibrosis, and juvenile idiopathic arthritis).

Systemic problems can include chronic conditions such as hemophilia, sickle cell disease, and arthritic diseases; neurologic problems, such as cerebral palsy; and various cancers, including osteosarcoma and leukemia. Pediatric patients with metabolic problems, such as vitamin D–resistant rickets, have bony deformities. Acute systemic disorders can also affect the musculoskeletal system. For example, viruses and bacteria can infect joints and bones. In developing countries, tubercular infections of bones are common and devastating. PCPs must assess patients from a broad perspective, obtain a thorough history to include other body systems, and order appropriate laboratory studies that identify systemic problems.

Genetic Disorders

Many genetic problems have an orthopedic component. Osteogenesis imperfecta (OI) is a genetic disorder characterized by decreased levels of collagen, the major protein of the body's connective tissue. Mutations in genes encoding type 1 collagen (*COL1A1* or *COL1A2* genes) account for approximately 85% to 90% of OI cases.[2] Pediatric patients with OI have bones that break easily, even from minor trauma.

Down syndrome results in hypotonia and the possibility of loose joint capsules and ligaments. Pediatric patients with Down syndrome have a higher incidence of atlantoaxial instability, scoliosis, dislocation of the hip, Legg-Calvé-Perthes disease (LCPD), instability of the patella, and pes planus (flat feet).

Marfan syndrome presents with longer than normal fingers, low muscle tone, and lax joints that are prone to dislocate. Severe scoliosis may develop in pediatric patients with neurofibromatosis, Turner syndrome, and Noonan syndrome. Females with Turner syndrome may present with webbed neck, short stature, valgus deformity of the elbow, and short fourth metacarpal deformity. Noonan syndrome can present with webbed neck, pectus carinatum or excavatum, clumsiness, poor coordination, and motor delay (see Chapter 27).

Many orthopedic problems have a multifactorial inheritance pattern. If one child in a family has a dislocated hip or scoliosis, the risk for these conditions increases for the other siblings. The pediatric PCP must understand the genetic disorder to monitor related orthopedic problems, consider the genetic implications, and provide families with appropriate genetic information or refer them for genetic counseling.

Intrauterine Compression Deformations

The developing fetus moves its body parts frequently, which influences musculoskeletal development. When the fetus fills the uterine space, movements are restricted and body parts begin to assume the shape in which they are fixed. Because of in utero positioning, joint and muscle contractions can develop and are generally considered physiologic in nature. Fetal movement is required for proper development of the musculoskeletal system, and anything that restricts fetal movement can cause deformation from intrauterine molding.

Two major intrinsic causes of deformations are neuromuscular disorders and maternal oligohydramnios. Extrinsic causes are related to fetal crowding that restricts fetal movement. Infants with deformations caused by extrinsic causes (e.g., breech position) have an excellent prognosis with corrections occurring spontaneously. Because much of the bony structure is cartilaginous, molding occurs with relative ease. Intrauterine positioning issues can result in tibial bowing and 20 to 30 degrees of hip flexion. Occasionally, a foot may be turned awkwardly (clubfoot, metatarsus adductus [MA], congenital vertical talus, cavovarus foot deformity), legs might be fixed straight up with the feet near the ears (congenital knee dislocations), or the neck may be tipped to one side (torticollis). Such positioning issues are outside the range of normal and the outcomes are deformities in various degrees. The longer the position is maintained, the more severe the problems will be. In general, there is a tendency for bowing and late deformations to straighten; however, the effects related to in utero positioning may not fully abate until the child is 3 to 4 years of age. More severe deformities (e.g., rigid MA) must be referred to orthopedics for treatment as soon as they are identified. A softer skeleton is easier to realign toward typical anatomical position.

Injuries

Unique differences in the pediatric skeletal system predispose pediatric patients to injuries unlike those seen in adults. The important differences are the presence of periosseous cartilage, physes, and a thicker, stronger, more osteogenic periosteum that produces new bone, called *callus,* more rapidly and in great amounts.

Sports- and recreation-related injuries account for a significant number of emergency department visits each year for pediatric patients ranging in age from 5 to 14 years. Physeal fractures in preadolescent children are the most common musculoskeletal injuries seen. Clavicular fractures are seen at all ages ranging from a newborn birth injury to trauma in adolescence. Injury to the clavicle is usually sustained by a fall on an outstretched hand or by direct force; approximately 90% of pediatric clavicle fractures occur in the middle third of the clavicle.[3] Fractures of the wrist and forearm account for nearly half of all fractures in pediatric patients.

Tendinosis may occur in the young athlete in the rotator cuff from throwing motions and swimming, in the iliopsoas in dancers, and in the ankle of dancers, gymnasts, and figure skaters. Shoulder injuries can be acute or may result from chronic overuse. Overuse injuries are common chronic injuries in pediatrics;

they are related to repetitive stress on the musculoskeletal system without sufficient time to recover. Apophysitis is an overuse injury unique to the skeletally immature active child or athlete. Tensile loading and stress to the apophysis—which is a secondary growth center at the insertion of the tendon—cause irritation, inflammation, and microtrauma affecting muscles, ligaments, tendons, bones, and growth plates.[4]

The possibility of nonaccidental trauma should always be considered when orthopedic injuries, especially fractures, are present. PCPs should have a high index of suspicion if an injury is unexplained or unwitnessed, if the severity of injury is incompatible with the history, or if the injury is inconsistent with the child's developmental capabilities. Rib fractures, metaphyseal fractures, multiple fractures in various stages of healing, and complex skull fractures should be carefully evaluated. The management of traumatic injuries is discussed in Chapter 25. Assessment of nonaccidental trauma is discussed in Chapter 22.

Defense Mechanisms

Fracture Healing

One of the major differences between adult and pediatric bones is that the periosteum in pediatric patients is very thick. The major reason for increased healing speed of pediatric fractures is the periosteum, which contributes to the largest part of new bone formation around a fracture. Pediatric patients have significantly greater osteoblastic activity in this area because bone is already being formed beneath the periosteum as part of normal growth. This already active process is readily accelerated after a fracture. Periosteal callus bridges a fracture in pediatric patients long before the underlying hematoma forms cartilage anlagen that go on to ossify. Once cellular organization from the hematoma has passed through the inflammatory process, repair of the bone begins in the area of the fracture. In most pediatric patients, by 10 days to 2 weeks after a fracture, a rubber-like bone forms around the fracture and makes it difficult to manipulate. As part of the reparative phase, cartilage formed as the hematoma organizes; it is eventually replaced by bone through the process of endochondral bone formation. The more growth potential the child has, the more remodeling will occur. Remodeling power is highest near the physes.

Growth Plate Fractures. Fractures of the long bones can produce permanent deformities in pediatric patients if the fracture occurs through the growth plate. The outcome depends on the fracture location and type, age of the child, status of the blood supply to the physis, and treatment. The Salter-Harris classification is based on the mechanism of injury, relationship of the fracture line to the layers of physis, and prognosis with respect to subsequent growth disturbance. There are five classifications (Fig. 40.2). Type I involves a fracture through the zone of hypertrophic

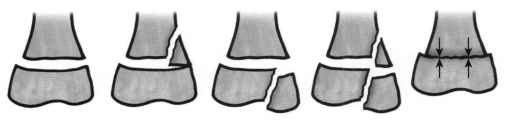

• **Fig. 40.2** Salter-Harris Classification of Physical Fractures, Types I to V. (From Baldwin KD, Shah AS, Wells L, et al. Pediatric fracture patterns. In Kliegman RM, St. Geme JW, Blum NJ et al., eds. *Nelson Textbook of Pediatrics.* 21st ed. Elsevier; 2020.)

cells of the physis with no fracture of the surrounding bone. Type II fractures, the most common type of growth plate fracture, are similar to type I except that a metaphyseal fragment is present on the compression side of the fracture. Growth disturbances are less likely in types I and II.

Type III fracture involves physeal separation with fracture through the epiphysis into the joint and requires anatomic reduction, occasionally through an open approach. Type IV fracture involves the metaphysis, physis, and epiphysis. Type V fracture involves a compression or crushing injury to the physis. Type V fractures are rare and are difficult to diagnose initially due to the lack of radiologic signs. Types IV and V require anatomic reduction to prevent articular incongruity and osseous bridging across the physis. Certain growth plates are more prone to growth disturbances. Pediatric patients should be reevaluated intermittently for 1 year after healing to assess possible growth or functional disturbances.

Shaft Fractures. The mechanism of injury is an important part of the history in evaluating a child for a traumatic injury. Closed pediatric fractures are often caused by low-energy activities and play; open fractures are generally caused by more force.

There are a variety of shaft fractures. In children between 9 months and 6 years of age, torsion of the foot may produce an oblique fracture of the distal aspect of the tibial shaft without a fibular fracture. These fractures are usually the result of tripping while walking or running, stepping on a ball or toy, or falling from a modest height. The child is typically seen due to failure to bear weight, a limp, or pain when asked to stand on the involved extremity. Physical findings may be minimal, and radiographs may show the characteristic faint oblique fracture line crossing the distal tibial diaphysis and terminating medially. Treatment is immobilization. Fractures of the forearm in pediatric patients most often result from a fall on an outstretched hand. This results in forceful axial loading with resultant bony failure in compression and bending of the arm. These forces generally cause torus or greenstick fractures. The rotational malalignment may not be identified and may be undertreated. During physical examination, PCPs should check for soft tissue injury, subtle rotational deformities, and neurovascular involvement and compare the injured limb with the contralateral one. Anteroposterior (AP) and lateral radiographs as well as oblique views of the wrist and forearm should be obtained if the physical examination suggests a fracture or dislocation. It is important to examine the entire arm and consider radiographic views of the joints above and below suspected fractures. Failure to diagnose and treat rotational malalignment is the most common cause of loss of forearm rotation in pediatrics.

Assessment of the Orthopedic System

History

History of Present Illness

- *Onset:* Appearance of first symptoms, insidious or sudden, association with injury or strain, accompanied by any constitutional symptoms or signs (e.g., fever, malaise, swelling, ecchymosis)
- *Pain:* Onset, location, duration and characteristics, course of radiation, severity, extent of disability produced, effect of various activities including weight bearing, relief measures, changes from day to night or from day to day, child's refusing to move the painful part or assuming a pain-relieving position, effects of previous treatment, presence of pain or discomfort in other parts of the body

- *Deformity:* Character (swelling, inflammation, contracture, joint stiffness, unusual positioning, appearance), first appearance and who noted it, association with injury or disease, rate of change, extent of disability, a cosmetic problem or a cause of embarrassment
- *Injury:* How, when (time and date), and where; mechanism or manner in which injury was produced; involvement in organized or competitive sports
- *Altered function:* Weakness, limp, decreased range of motion, loss or decrease sensation, or alteration in perfusion that may be associated with circumferential swelling
- *Altered gait patterns:* Toe walking, in-toeing or out-toeing, limping, shortened single-limb stance phase, Trendelenburg gait, steppage gait (associated with footdrop), or Gower sign
- *Other factors or constraints:* Type of shoe worn; use of backpack and amount of weight in backpack, amount of time spent at repetitive tasks or at computer station; aggravating factors: dominant hand; use of complementary or alternative modalities
- Medication use: Steroids, antiinflammatories, analgesics

Family History

- Identify any family members with musculoskeletal problems; many orthopedic problems have a genetic component.

Medical History

- *Pregnancy history and birth history:* Breech delivery, shoulder presentation, multiple births, oligohydramnios, asphyxia at birth; maternal alcohol or substance abuse.
- *Development history:* Milestones met at appropriate age, such as first walking and sitting; delays in achieving gross or fine motor developmental milestones.
- *Illnesses, accidents, or surgeries:* Trauma, meningitis, juvenile arthritis, chronic diseases; especially those affecting nutritional status (e.g., inflammatory bowel disease, sickle cell disease).

Review of Systems

Obtain a history of any infections, constitutional diseases, or congenital problems that might have an orthopedic component. Any history of fractures, joint pains, strains or sprains? Any limitation in physical activity or sports participation?

Physical Examination

Orthopedic examination techniques specific to pediatrics are described in the following sections and should be completed in addition to the normal orthopedic examination maneuvers.

Inspection and Palpation

Inspection of the skin—noting the skin color, presence of swelling or atrophy, erythema, ecchymosis, scars, or unusual pigmentation—is essential. Palpate skin for differences or inconsistencies in temperature and perfusion and palpate bone and joints to ascertain tenderness, prominence, indentations, and crepitus.

Range-of-Motion Examination

Observe the child's posture while sitting, standing, and walking as well as assess and evaluate the proportion of upper extremities to lower extremities. Evaluation of symmetry as well as range of motion, muscle size, strength, and tone should be a part of a musculoskeletal examination. Range of motion is the normal range, flexion, extension, and rotation of a joint. Joint hypermobility is the ability of the joint to move beyond its normal range. Hypermobility of joints generally does not cause problems, although there is a slight increase in dislocation and sprain of the involved joint. Normal joint motion is age related (e.g., external hip rotation is greatest in early infancy). Passive range of motion, in which the examiner moves the joint, provides information about joint mobility and stability. It can also provide information about the limits of contracted tendons and muscles. Active range of motion, in which the child moves the joint, provides information about both muscle and bony structures working together for functional movement.

Limited range of motion can be the result of mechanical problems, swelling, muscle spasticity, pain, infection, injury, or arthritis. Note pain, stiffness, limitations or deviations, and rigidity.

Gait Examination

Ambulation typically begins between 8 and 18 months of age. The development of a typical gait is dependent on progressive neurologic maturation. Initially, a child's gait is characterized by a short stride length, a fast cadence, and slow velocity with a wide-based stance. The gait undergoes developmental changes. Walking velocity, step length, and duration of the single-limb stance increase with age, whereas the number of steps taken per minute decreases. A mature gait pattern is well established by 3 years of age. Typical neurologic maturation results in efficiency and smoothness of gait; by 7 years of age, the gait characteristics are similar to those of an adult.[5] A typical gait cycle consists of the stance phase, during which the foot is in contact with the ground, and the swing phase, during which the foot is in the air. The stance phase is further divided into three major periods: the initial double-limb support, followed by the single-limb stance, and then another period of double-limb support.

Observe the child walking without shoes and with minimal covering. Compare stance and swing phases in both legs, and the range of motion of each joint should be evaluated. Inspect from the front, side, and back as the child walks normally, on his or her toes, and then on the heels. The gait should be smooth, rhythmic, and efficient. Ankle, knee, and hip movements should be symmetric and full with little side-to-side movement of the trunk.

Limping is a disturbance in the normal pattern of gait. Abnormal gait can be antalgic or nonantalgic. An antalgic gait is characterized by a shortening of the single-limb stance phase to prevent pain in the affected leg. Painful or antalgic gaits serve to reduce stress or pain at the affected area. The trunk shifts to the opposite side to keep balance and reduce stress; the stance phase and stride length are shortened as compensatory mechanisms. Causes of a painful gait include infection, trauma, or acquired disorders. A nonantalgic gait may be caused by general weakness, spasticity, muscular disorders, or leg-length discrepancies. Gait disturbances may become more apparent with fatigue. When there is a concern regarding sensory or motor deficits, the PCP should assess and evaluate the child's spinal nerves and deep tendon reflexes.

Posture

To assess posture adequately, the child should be examined undressed to their underwear. The examiner must look at the child from the front, side, and back.

- Pelvis and hips should be level. Place hands on the iliac crest to test for a pelvic tilt caused by limb-length discrepancy.
- Legs should be symmetric in shape and size. Patellae should be straight ahead.
- The feet should point straight ahead, with an imaginary line from the center of the heel through the second toe. There

should be an arch (except in babies, in whom a fat pad obscures the arch) and straight heel cords.
- The spine should be straight, and the back should look symmetric, with shoulder and scapular heights and waist angles equal. There should be slight lordotic curves at the cervical and lumbar areas.

Hip Examinations

Barlow Maneuver. The Barlow maneuver assesses the potential for dislocation of a nondisplaced hip in an infant during the first month of life (Fig. 40.4A), looking for laxity and instability. With hip instability, the femoral head slips/drops out of the acetabulum or can be gently pushed out of the socket; this is termed a *positive Barlow sign*. The dislocation is palpable as this maneuver is performed. The maneuver must be performed gently in a noncrying neonate/infant to keep from damaging the femoral head. Examine the hips one at a time. The hip generally relocates spontaneously after release of the downward (posterior) force. A video of the Barlow maneuver video is available at https://www.youtube.com/watch?v=lqtLIhNnJUw.

Ortolani Maneuver. The Ortolani maneuver is the reverse of the Barlow maneuver (Fig. 40.4B). It reduces a posteriorly dislocated hip and is performed gently to reduce a recently dislocated hip. A palpable clunk as the femoral head is relocated is considered a positive Ortolani sign.[6] A click is a common sound and is not considered a positive Ortolani sign. Positive Barlow and Ortolani maneuvers may be achieved only during the first few months of life. Dislocations can occur later in infancy; PCPs must test the hips using other strategies and note limited abduction in older infants until they are walking independently (Fig. 40.5). A video of the Ortolani test is available at https://youtu.be/Nuxk5BSUj08.

Galeazzi Maneuver. The Galeazzi sign can signal conditions that cause leg-length discrepancies. The Galeazzi maneuver includes flexing the hips and knees while the infant or child lies supine, placing the soles of the feet on the table near the buttocks, and then looking at the knee heights for equality (Fig. 40.3A). The Galeazzi sign is positive if the knee heights are unequal. However, it is not reliable in pediatric patients with dislocatable but not presently dislocated hips or in pediatric patients with bilateral dislocation.

Klisic Test. The Klisic test provides an observational sign of hip placement. The PCP places the tip of the third finger of one hand over the greater trochanter and the index finger of the same hand on the anterosuperior iliac spine. An imaginary line is drawn between the index and third fingers. Typically, the imaginary line points to the umbilicus. If the hip is dislocated, the trochanter is elevated and the imaginary line points halfway between the umbilicus and the pubis (i.e., the line points below the umbilicus). This sign is another physical assessment marker of hip dislocation (Fig. 40.6).[7]

Trendelenburg Sign. The Trendelenburg test can be used to identify conditions that cause weakness in the hip abductors. It is elicited by having the child stand and then raise one leg off the ground. If the pelvis (iliac crest) drops on the side of the raised leg, the sign is positive and indicates weak hip abductor muscles on the side that is bearing the weight. It may or may not be painful as it involves muscle weakness around the hip joint. Typically, the muscles around a stable hip are strong enough to maintain a level pelvis if one leg is raised (Fig. 40.3C). With bilaterally dislocated hips, a wide-based Trendelenburg limp is noted.

Internal and External Rotation. The child is placed prone, and the knees are flexed 90 degrees. Internal rotation is measured as

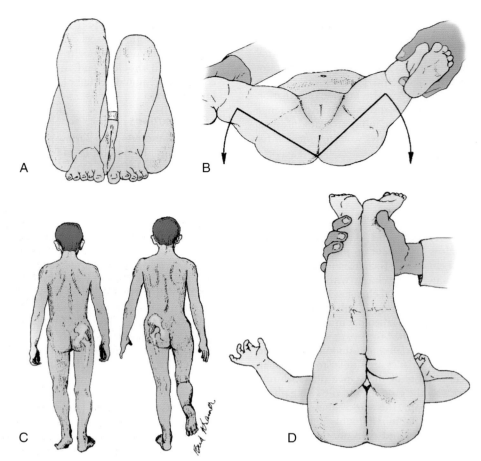

• **Fig. 40.3** Physical Findings in Congenital Hip Dislocation. (A) Leg-length inequality is a sign of unilateral hip dislocation (Galeazzi sign). (B) Limitation of hip abduction is often present in older infants with hip dislocation. Abduction of greater than 60 degrees is usually possible in infants. Restriction or asymmetry indicates the need for careful radiologic examination. (C) Trendelenburg sign. In single-leg stance, the abductor muscles of the normal hip support the pelvis. Dislocation of the hip functionally shortens and weakens these muscles. When the child attempts to stand on the dislocated hip, the opposite side of the pelvis drops. (D) Thigh-fold asymmetry is often present in infants with unilateral hip dislocation. An extra fold can be seen on the abnormal side. However, the finding is not diagnostic. It may be found in typical infants and may be absent in pediatric patients with hip dislocation or dislocatability. (From Scoles P. *Pediatric Orthopedics in Clinical Practice*. 2nd ed. Mosby; 1988.)

the legs are allowed to fall apart as far as possible, using gravity alone or with light pressure. The angle between vertical (0 degree) and the leg position is the internal rotation. It is measured for each leg (Fig. 40.7A). Asymmetric hip rotation is abnormal. External rotation is measured by allowing the legs to cross while the child is still prone. The angle between vertical and the leg position is measured for each leg (Fig. 40.7B). Again, asymmetric hip rotation is abnormal. By 1 year of age, a typical child has approximately 45 degrees of internal and external hip rotation.

Back Examination

Adams Test. The Adams forward bend test looks for asymmetry of the posterior chest wall on forward bending and allows for the evaluation of structural scoliosis. The child bends at the waist to a position of 90 degrees back flexion with straight legs, ankles together, and arms hanging freely or with palms together (in a diving position) but not touching the toes or floor (Fig. 40.8). The back is then inspected for asymmetry of the height of the curves on the two sides or rib hump; the PCP inspects the child's back by looking at it from the rear and side positions. The examiner

should be seated or standing in front of the child to best scan each level of the spine visually. If a rib hump is present, a scoliometer, if available, can be used to measure the angular tilt of the trunk. A spinal rotation greater than 10 degrees measured by placing the scoliometer at the peak of the curvature indicates the need for further evaluation.[1]

Diagnostic Studies

Radiographs are an important diagnostic tool for the musculoskeletal system. Imaging should begin with standard radiographs of the area of concern. AP and lateral views of the affected area, bone, or joint are typically ordered to analyze the anatomic structures with oblique views added when joints are involved. Views of both extremities may be ordered for comparison. Computed tomography (CT) scans augment radiographs to detail specific areas of the body. CT is useful in detailing the relationship of bones to their contiguous structures. Magnetic resonance imaging (MRI) provides excellent visualization of joints, soft tissues, cartilage, and medullary bone. It can distinguish between various physiologic changes that

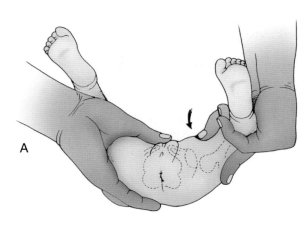

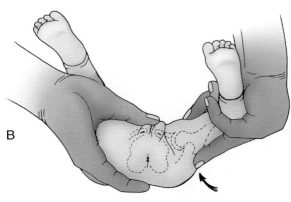

• **Fig. 40.4** Barlow (Dislocation) Test and Ortolani (Reduction) Test. (A) The "stabilizing hand" is positioned with the thumb on the symphysis and the fingers on the sacrum. The thumb of the abducting hand is placed on the inner aspect of the thigh and gives lateral pressure to the adductor region, while the hand (wrapped around the knee with the index finger on the lateral side of the thigh) provides gentle downward pressure. If there is hip instability, dislocation is palpable as the femoral head slips out of the acetabulum. Diagnosis is confirmed with the Ortolani test. (B) With the infant relaxed on a firm surface, the hips and knees are flexed to 90 degrees. The infant's thigh is grasped with the middle finger over the greater trochanter and the thigh is lifted to bring the femoral head from its dislocated posterior position to opposite the acetabulum. Simultaneously, the thigh is gently abducted, reducing the femoral head in the acetabulum. In a positive finding, the examiner senses reduction by a palpable, nearly audible "clunk." Test one hip at a time for both of these tests. (From Marcdante KJ, Kliegman RM, Jenson HB, et al., eds. *Nelson Essentials of Pediatrics*. 6th ed. Elsevier; 2011.)

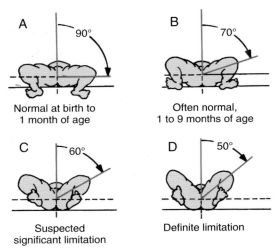

• **Fig. 40.5** Hip Abduction Test. The child is placed supine and the hips are flexed 90 degrees and fully abducted. Although the normal abduction range is quite broad (A and B), one can suspect hip disease in any patient who lacks more than 35 to 45 degrees of abduction (C suspicious and D abnormal). (From Chung SMK. *Hip Disorders in Infants and Children*. Lea & Febiger; 1981.)

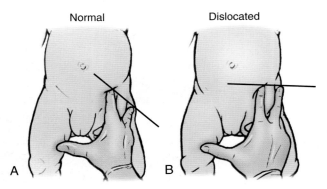

• **Fig. 40.6** The Klisic Test. (From Kliegman RM, Stanton BF, St. Geme JW, et al, eds. *Nelson Textbook of Pediatrics*. 19th ed. Elsevier; 2011.)

occur in bone marrow related to age and disease process. Ultrasonography can provide information about cartilaginous areas or tissues not visible on radiograph and is highly sensitive for detecting effusion of the hip joint. Bone scans (scintigraphy) are more sensitive than radiographs, demonstrate bone metabolism, and are useful in detecting causes of obscure skeletal pain. Although CT scanning and radiographs offer tremendous benefits in diagnosing and guiding care for pediatric patients with musculoskeletal problems, PCPs must be mindful of the cost and amount of radiation a child is exposed to and weigh the risks versus benefits of their use.

Laboratory studies can help to identify systemic disease, infection, or inflammation. Erythrocyte sedimentation rate (ESR), C-reactive protein (CRP), complete blood count (CBC), blood cultures, rheumatoid factor, and antinuclear antibodies are hematologic tests that can assist in the diagnosis and management of bone disorders. Other laboratory tests also provide an understanding of muscle metabolism (e.g., carnitine, lactic acid, leptin, pyruvates). Some bony lesions and joint effusions of muscle tissue may have to be biopsied.

Management Strategies

Counseling

Counseling for orthopedic problems involves several components. The family should understand and have time to ask questions about all of the following issues: the pathologic condition, including possible etiologies; treatment plan; prognosis with and without treatment; any genetic implications of the diagnosis; and long-term care issues. Counseling helps families cope with a poor, chronic, or challenging diagnosis and its short- and long-term implications. Congenital problems are often identified prenatally, at birth, or shortly thereafter. Families must be given the diagnosis truthfully, humanely, and as soon as possible. Issues of etiology must be discussed to address parents' feelings of guilt for causing the problem and to discuss genetic implications, if any. A plan of care that is mutually agreed on by the family and the PCP must be developed before the infant is discharged from the hospital or clinic.

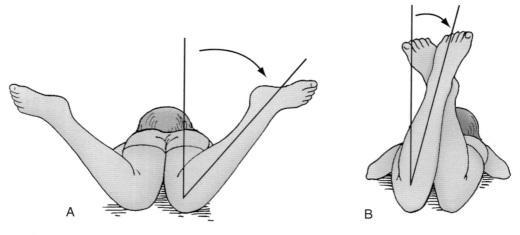

• **Fig. 40.7** Hip Rotation in Extension. (From Thompson GH. Gait disturbances. In: Kliegman RM, ed. *Practical Strategies in Pediatric Diagnosis and Therapy*. Saunders; 1996.)

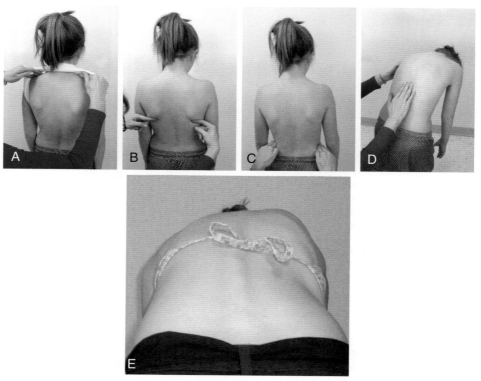

• **Fig. 40.8** Assessment of the Spine. (A) Testing shoulder symmetry. (B) Scapular symmetry. (C) Iliac crest symmetry. (D) Beginning Adams forward bend test. (E) Positive rib hump on forward bend. (From Skirven T, Osterman A, Dedorczk J, et al. *Rehabilitation of the Hand and Upper Extremity*. 6th ed. Elsevier; 2012; Duderstadt KG, ed. *Pediatric Physical Examination: an Illustrated Handbook*. Elsevier; 2014:277.)

Anticipatory Guidance: Musculoskeletal Development

Families are sometimes concerned about problems that PCPs believe are within normal limits and do not require an orthopedic referral. PCPs should provide the child's family with a description of the child's predicted musculoskeletal development. Timelines and milestones that parents can use to monitor their child's development are particularly helpful in allowing families to understand their child's pattern of growth. Misperceptions about the implications of minor variations must be clarified, and the family should

always be given the opportunity to return for further assessment or discussion if concerns remain. Examples of common developmental concerns are flat feet in infants and early childhood and bowlegs or knock knees in early childhood.

Shoes

The use of therapeutic shoes to correct orthopedic problems is controversial as these shoes typically do little to correct deformities. Shoes for the average child should keep the feet warm and protected from injury. Shoes should be selected to fit properly and comfortably with room for growth. High-top shoes in early childhood may have the advantage of staying on more securely, but they do not provide additional support.

Features of a good shoe are as follows:

- Flexible sole—to allow as much free motion as possible; for young children, test to see if the shoe can be flexed in the parent's hand.
- Flat—do not allow high heels in early and middle childhood.
- Foot shaped—avoid pointed toes or other shapes that do not conform to the normal configuration of the foot.
- Fitted generously—better to be too large than too small.
- Friction similar to skin—the soles should have the same friction as skin so that they are not slippery.

Well-cushioned, shock-absorbing shoes are helpful in the child or adolescent athlete to decrease the chances of developing overuse syndrome. Shoe modifications may be needed in certain conditions. Shoe lifts are needed if limb-length differences exceed 2.5 cm. Orthotics can also be used in certain orthopedic situations to distribute pressure on the sole of the foot more evenly and facilitate function.

Care of Pediatric Patients in Casts and Splints

Casts and splints are applied to immobilize a limb, promote healing, maintain bone alignment, diminish pain, protect the injury, and help compensate for surrounding muscular weakness. Splints are noncircumferential immobilizers that accommodate swelling. Splints are used in orthopedic conditions where swelling is anticipated—that is, in acute fractures or sprains and for initial stabilization of reduced, displaced, or unstable fractures before orthopedic intervention. Casts are circumferential immobilizers. They provide superior immobilization but are less forgiving than splints and have a higher rate of complications. The use of casts and splints is generally limited to a short period of time. If prolonged immobilization is required, joint stiffness and muscle atrophy may occur, occasionally warranting physical or occupational therapy to regain function.

The child's cast should be kept cool, clean, and dry. Cover it with plastic wrap or a plastic bag when the child bathes or is in a situation where the cast may get wet. Cast covers can also be purchased that allow full submerging of the cast while keeping the cast dry. If the cast becomes wet, a hair dryer set on cool setting can be used for drying small areas. If the cast becomes soiled, clean it with a slightly damp washcloth and cleanser.

Teach the family how to do a circulatory inspection to check the function of nerves and blood vessels. Casts can be perceived by pediatric patients to be itchy, and they may insert small toys or long thin objects that cannot be seen externally in attempt to relieve the itching. These objects or an area of swelling may impede the blood flow or neurologic innervation. It is very important to educate the child and the family not to put any objects in the cast. The child's toes or fingers below the cast should be pink and warm to the touch. The child should be able to feel all sides of his or her fingers or toes when touched and be able to wiggle all of the fingers or toes. Skin care following cast and splint removal is imperative. For the first few days following splint and cast removal, the skin will be delicate and sensitive. It may appear pale yellow and will be flaky. The family should be instructed to soak and gently cleanse the skin, pat it dry, and avoid rubbing or peeling excess skin.

The family must know when to call the PCP—that is, if the toes or fingers are cold to the touch and appear pale or blue, complaints of tingling or numbness, inability to move fingers or toes, and excessive swelling. Additional problems with casts (i.e., foul smell, breakage, or loosening) and/or alteration in skin integrity following the removal of a cast or splint must be reported.

Physical and Occupational Therapy

Pediatric patients with developmental delays, cerebral palsy, spinal disorders, and torticollis should be referred for physical and/or occupational therapy. Treatments focus on improving gross and fine motor skills, balance and coordination, strength and endurance, as well as cognitive and sensory processing. Structured physical therapy after orthopedic injury can be helpful.

Orthopedic Conditions Specific to Pediatrics

Annular Ligament Displacement

Annular ligament displacement, previously described as a subluxation of the radial head and frequently called *nursemaid's elbow,* is a frequent injury that occurs in children 6 months to 5 years of age with most cases occurring between 1 and 3 years. The injury typically occurs when traction is applied to the arm of a young child, which is most often the result of pulling a child by the hand or grasping a child's hand to prevent a fall. This motion causes the annular ligament to slide over the head of the radius, where it becomes entrapped in the radiohumeral joint when the distal traction is released (Fig. 40.9A).[8]

Clinical Findings

History. Often the history is nonspecific, and the parent may not have been aware of when the injury occurred. Alternatively, a parent will commonly report that the child cried, complaining of arm pain after being pulled up by his or her arm or swung by the arms. The parent typically reports that since the incident, the child has refused to use the affected arm, crying out in pain if the arm is moved, particularly the elbow.

The injury produces immediate pain and limited supination. Swelling and ecchymosis are not always present. Pain may be present with movement but not on palpation. Following the injury, a toddler typically will resist moving his or her arm and can be observed holding the affected arm in pronation and slight flexion against their body.[8]

Diagnostic Studies. Radiographs are not routinely recommended when the history and clinical presentation are classic. If obtained, radiography of the elbow is normal. If the history of the injury is not consistent with a mechanism expected to cause angular ligament displacement or if the physical examination leads to the possibility of additional injury, radiographs are indicated.

Differential Diagnosis

Annular ligament displacement has a classic history and presentation. If the child does not improve after the reduction procedure (see next section), a fracture of the elbow or clavicle should be considered. The clinical presentation of a fracture may be similar to that of an angular ligament displacement injury and therefore must be ruled out. Consider maltreatment if presentation is atypical, recurrent dislocations with unclear mechanism of injury, or other symptoms or signs are present.

Management

Two techniques can be used to reduce the radial head: supination and flexion or hyperpronation and extension. Do not attempt either procedure if epitrochlear tenderness is present because this may be indicative of a more serious injury (e.g., fracture).

The steps to correct the angular ligament displacement are as follows:

- Approach the child in a slow, nonthreatening way, and distract him or her by talking or other diversionary tactics.
- Use either the supination and flexion technique as illustrated in Fig. 40.9B, or the hyperpronation technique. With the pronation maneuver, the PCP gently extends the elbow to pronate (palm down) the child's forearm and continues to gently rotate the child's forearm (hyperpronate) until thumb faces downward.[8] Once hyperpronation and extension are achieved, the

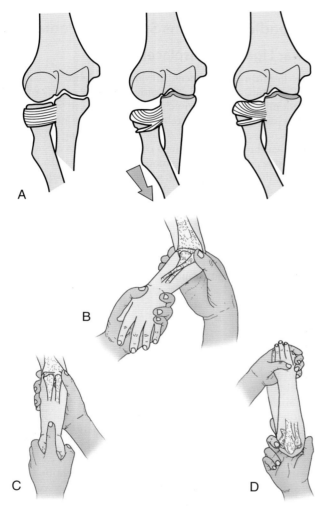

• **Fig. 40.9** (A) Annular ligament displacement, formerly known as *subluxation of the radial head.* The pathology of nursemaid's elbow or pulled elbow. The anterior ligament is partially torn when the arm is pulled. The radial head moves distally, and when traction is discontinued, the ligament is carried into the joint. (B and D) Reduction of radial head subluxation by supination and flexion technique. (B) The palm of the child's hand is grasped as if to shake it. Axial traction is applied to the forearm with the wrist adducted to the ulnar side. Pressure is also applied directly over the radial head of the elbow. (C) The forearm is supinated while axial traction and pressure are maintained over the forearm and radial head. (D) The elbow is flexed to the shoulder while supination and pressure are maintained over the radial head. (A, From Rang M. *Children's Fractures.* 2nd ed. PhilJB Lippincott; 1983:193; Kliegman RM, Stanton BF, St. Geme JW, et al., eds. *Nelson Textbook of Pediatrics.* 19th ed. Saunders; 2011. B–D, From Shah B. Reduction of radial head subluxation. In: Finberg L, Kleinman RE, eds. *Saunders Manual of Pediatric Practice.* 2nd ed. Saunders; 2002:1162.)

PCP then releases the forearm and elbow and evaluates if the attempt at reduction was successful.

- A palpable or audible "pop" or "click" usually signals successful reduction. Typically, the child begins reaching for objects again with the affected arm within 15 minutes of reduction. If reduction is successful, no further treatment is necessary.

Complications

Several attempts (up to three at reduction) may be necessary before the patient resumes normal use of the arm. If normal use does not follow reduction attempts, immobilization using a sling with prompt orthopedic follow-up is indicated. This injury is associated with a high rate of recurrence. Education and anticipatory guidance should be provided to caregivers to prevent reinjury.

Patient and Parent Education

Key points to cover include instructing caregivers not to lift or pull the child by the hand or elbow and to lift the child from the axillae.

Brachial Plexus Injuries

The brachial plexus is a network of nerves in the shoulder arising from the spinal cord; it enables movement and sensation in the shoulders, arms, and hands. Injury to the shoulder and brachial plexus during the birthing process is known as *obstetric brachial plexus palsy* or *neonatal brachial plexus palsy.* Brachial plexus injury types I through IV are typically classified using the Narakas criteria (Table 40.1). Most injuries affect the upper brachial plexus (C5 and C6 nerve roots), resulting in weakness or paralysis of the shoulder and upper arm; they are known as *Erb-Duchenne (or Erb) palsy.* More severe injuries involving the lower plexus (C7, C8, and T1 nerve roots) impair hand function and cause ipsilateral ptosis and miosis; they are known as *Dejerine-Klumpke (or Klumpke) palsy.*[9]

Neonatal brachial plexus injury, although uncommon, is as a result of a complication during delivery. The association with brachial plexus injuries and shoulder dystocia cannot be interpreted as causation even though they have shared risk factors. These risk factors include maternal diabetes, maternal weight gain, multiparity, fetal macrosomia, fetal malposition, induced labor, labor abnormalities,

TABLE 40.1	Brachial Plexus Injury Using the Narakas Classification	
Name	**Nerves and Muscles Involved**	**Prognosis**
Narakas type I	C5 and C6; shoulder and biceps	Recovery is usually complete.
Narakas type II	C5–C7; shoulder, biceps, and forearm extensors	Recovery is usually complete.
Narakas type III	C5–T1	Variable with complete paralysis of limb; shoulder and biceps recovery is fair to poor with hand recovery variable.
Narakas type IV	C5–T1	Complete paralysis of the limb and Horner syndrome; shoulder and biceps recovery is fair to poor with hand recovery variable.

operative vaginal delivery, and history of previous pregnancy complicated by shoulder dystocia or neonatal brachial plexus palsy.[10]

Clinical Findings

History. History should include obstetric history, mode of delivery, and postnatal health of the infant.

Physical Examination. A thorough head-to-toe examination is required to identify any deformations or other injuries that may have occurred in utero or during delivery. Assess passive range of motion, and newborn reflexes should be tested to identify neurologic deficits. Findings may include:

- Erb palsy, presenting with an adducted arm, which is internally rotated at the shoulder: the wrist is flexed, and fingers are extended, resulting in a characteristic "waiter's tip" posture.
- Absent bicep reflex with asymmetric Moro and tonic neck reflex on the affected side.
- Limp wrist and hand with absent grasp reflex (lower plexus involvement).
- Horner syndrome (ipsilateral ptosis, miosis, enophthalmos, anhidrosis) if the sympathetic fibers of the T1 nerve root are involved.
- Occasionally, hand paralysis with normal shoulder movement, which is a rare occurrence of an isolated C8 through T1 injury.
- Limited neck movement due to damage to the sternocleidomastoid muscle; skull fracture.
- Impaired respiratory effort as a result of diaphragmatic paralysis and flaccidity.
- Ruptured intraabdominal structures, especially the liver and spleen, which require careful abdominal examination.

Diagnostic Studies. Radiologic examination, electrophysiologic studies, and MRI are useful to confirm a clinical diagnosis and the extent of injury. Radiographs of the chest and upper limbs are important because they reveal associated injuries, such as rib, transverse process, and clavicular/humeral fractures. A chest radiograph is necessary to rule out phrenic nerve injury. Electrodiagnostic studies with electromyography and nerve conduction velocities are used to determine the severity of the neural lesion.

Differential Diagnosis

The differential diagnosis of upper extremity paralysis in a newborn includes epiphyseal separation of the humeral head, fracture of the clavicle or humerus, septic arthritis, acute osteomyelitis of the upper extremity, spinal cord injury, cervical cord lesions, and congenital malformations of the plexus and upper limb.[11]

Management

An interprofessional team approach is ideal, with referral to providers who specialize in treating brachial plexus injuries. Referral should be made in the first week of life. The initial goal of therapy is to maintain passive range of motion, supple joints, and muscle strength. Indications for surgical exploration and reconstruction of the brachial plexus include failure of recovery of elbow flexion and shoulder abduction from the third to the sixth months of life. The spectrum of nerve surgery includes neurolysis, neuroma resection, nerve grafting, and nerve transfers.

Complications

Late sequelae include internal rotation contractures, hypoplasia of the arm, altered sensibility, flexion contractures of the elbow, dislocation of the radial head, and psychologic and social consequences.

Prognosis

Recovery can occur spontaneously and is highly dependent on the level and extent of nerve injury. Paralysis of the upper portion of the arm generally has a better prognosis than does paralysis of the lower part. If the paralysis is due to edema surrounding the nerve fibers (neurapraxia), spontaneous full recovery within a few weeks is likely; if it is due to disruption of the nerve fibers (axonotmesis), function generally returns in a few months. More severe injuries, total disruption of the nerves (neurotmesis), and root avulsion require surgery with partial or complete recovery observed over several years. Fortunately, 50% of plexus injuries occur at the upper nerve roots (C5–C6), involve neurapraxia and axonotmesis, and heal spontaneously.[12]

Clavicular Fracture

Clavicular fractures seen in newborns result from birth trauma. In young children, they can result from accidental or nonaccidental trauma, or as a result of a direct hit or indirect trauma and are most commonly associated with a fall. Approximately 90% of these fractures occur in the middle third of the clavicle. The clavicle is the first bone to ossify and the last physis in the body to close, usually not until age 22 to 25 years.[3]

Clinical Findings

History. History varies depending on the age of the child. In the neonate, it may include:
- Difficult delivery, high birth weight, midforceps delivery, and shoulder dystocia
- Irritability when infant is moved or lifted

In the older child, it may include:
- History of fall or trauma with focus on mechanism of injury; typically, the fall is on an outstretched hand

Physical Examination. In all children, look for the following:
- Pain with shoulder movement
- Decreased arm movement on affected side (asymmetric spontaneous arm movements) or absent Moro reflex
- Swelling, bony abnormality, discoloration, and/or crepitus elicited over the fracture site
- Callus felt over the fracture site within a few days
- Spasm of the sternocleidomastoid muscle on the affected side
- An associated Erb palsy

Diagnostic Studies. Imaging studies are recommended. Radiography with routine clavicular views is sufficient.

Differential Diagnosis

Brachial plexus palsy, shoulder dislocation, or other bony problems should be considered.

Management

Management of the neonate involves:
- Incomplete fractures that do not cause pain need no treatment.
- Immobilization of the shoulder is an option when movement results in a painful arm (usually with a complete fracture). Pin the sleeve of the infant's arm to the front of the shirt for 1 to 2 weeks.

Management of the older child involves:
- Sling immobilization for comfort to support the affected extremity is often sufficient. In general, sling immobilization can be discontinued at 3 to 4 weeks.
- A figure-eight clavicular brace can be used if displacement results in a decreased shaft length. However, it is uncomfortable to wear, and its effectiveness is questionable.
- Protection for 4 to 5 weeks is generally sufficient because union requires about 4 weeks of healing.

- An older child may need analgesics or a nonsteroidal antiinflammatory drug (NSAID) for pain.
- The need for surgical intervention is uncommon with clavicular fractures. Surgery may be needed in the case of open fractures, neurovascular compromise, multiple traumas, rib cage fractures, and fractures with greater than 100% displacement with severe skin tenting.

Prognosis

The prognosis is excellent. Often the injury in neonates is identified only at later primary care visits when the callus lump is palpated, although the child may be irritable until the fracture is stable. The infant is usually asymptomatic within 7 to 10 days. Parents need information and emotional support. In older children, general healing time is 6 to 8 weeks with average return to noncontact sports in 4 to 6 weeks and contact sports in 8 to 12 weeks. Bony callus appears approximately 10 days after injury as a painless firm "lump."

Costochondritis and Sternochondritis

Costochondritis is a common cause of chest pain in pediatrics. The condition is characterized as an inflammatory process of one or more of the costochondral cartilages that causes localized tenderness and pain in the anterior chest wall. Trauma to the area and unaccustomed physical effort (lifting heavy objects or coughing) are factors known to cause costochondritis; however, most cases are idiopathic. Inflammation is the underlying problem.

Clinical Findings

History. Pain localized to the costosternal or costochondral junction is the major symptom. It often presents with tenderness over more than one rib as a result of referred pain. The primary rib that is inflamed and usually responsible for the symptoms is most often the one that exhibits the greatest sensitivity to palpation. Characteristics of the pain include the following:

- Acute or gradual onset; typically insidious, occurring over several days or weeks
- Sharp, darting, or dull quality
- Radiation from chest to upper abdomen or back
- Occasional complaints of a feeling of tightness caused by muscle spasm
- Exacerbating factors may include coughing, sneezing, deep inspiration, movement of the upper torso and upper extremities

Physical Examination. Palpation reveals tenderness over the costochondral junction. The tenderness is localized and most common at the sternocostal cartilage of the second through seventh ribs. The presence of pain increased on palpation, swelling (a unique bulbous enlargement of the joint commonly noted over a single upper costochondral junction) with or without redness, and tenderness at the costal cartilage are referred to as the *Tietze syndrome*. Ecchymosis may be seen in cases of trauma. Respiratory effort and auscultation of the lungs, heart, and abdomen are normal.

Diagnostic Studies. No diagnostic studies are needed because history and physical findings are diagnostic. Chest radiography may exclude other possible causes but offers no diagnostic value. A CT scan can demonstrate swelling of the costal cartilage.

Differential Diagnosis

Rib fractures are the key differential diagnosis if pain is associated with an injury. Childhood rheumatic diseases can also produce complaints similar to those of costochondritis but generally have other characteristic physical findings. Costochondritis is one of the differential diagnoses of pediatric chest pain (see Chapter 33).

Management

Treatment consists of using mild analgesia and NSAIDs to relieve discomfort and avoiding strenuous activity. Cough suppressants may be beneficial if cough is an aggravating factor. Stretching exercises and the application of ice to the area are useful. Parents and children must be reassured that this is a benign, self-limited condition and is not related to cardiac disease.

Back Pain

Young children do not commonly complain of severe back pain. Most episodes of back pain in pediatric patients are brief, with nonspecific findings and history. Back pain that warrants immediate attention includes complaints from children younger than 4 years of age, persistent symptoms, self-imposed activity limitations, systemic symptoms, increasing discomfort, persistent nighttime pain, neurologic symptoms, history of tuberculosis or cancer, and back pain accompanied by unexplained weight loss.[13] Younger children who have such complaints should be carefully evaluated for occult pathologic conditions, and the PCP's index of suspicion about underlying pathologic conditions should be raised.

The older the child or adolescent, the more likely it is that the back pain is musculoskeletal in origin. The young athlete is especially susceptible to back injury. Intense training can cause repetitive microtrauma. Back pain can result from sprains of the ligaments or muscles (or both) of the back due to injury.

Clinical Findings

History. Onset, location, duration, characteristics, aggravating and relieving factors, frequency, and intensity of the pain are key questions to ask in forming an initial impression. In addition, it is important that PCPs differentiate between mechanical and inflammatory causes. The history should include questions related to the timing of back pain and aggravating or relieving factors. Specifically, the back pain reported with morning stiffness or prolonged rest is associated with inflammatory causes, whereas back pain reported with activity is associated with mechanical causes.

The following findings should alert the pediatric PCP to possible pathologic conditions:

- Pain that prohibits play or activities, persists or worsens, or occurs at night
- History of trauma (vertebral fracture)
- Positive neurologic or musculoskeletal signs on examination
- Systemic signs, such as fever, chills, weight loss, and malaise
- Presence of any radicular symptoms, gait disturbances, muscle weakness, altered sensation, and changes in bowel and/or bladder function

In school-age children and adolescents, back pain can be associated with a history of the following:

- Muscle strain as a result of "overuse syndrome" from excessive muscular exertion, usually related to sports, commonly in sedentary children who have recently increased their activity level
- Wearing high heels
- Neck/shoulder, low back, and arm pain in relation to computer or video game use; excessive TV watching

Physical Examination. The examination should include a complete musculoskeletal and neurologic assessment with the child adequately exposed for the clinical examination. Inspect for any changes in alignment in the frontal or sagittal plane; range of motion should be assessed in flexion, extension, and lateral bending. Younger children may be asked to pick an object up off the floor to assess spinal flexion. Palpation reveals any areas of tenderness and/or muscle spasm. Palpate the top of the iliac crests while the child is standing to assess leg lengths. A careful neurologic examination should be performed.

Diagnostic Studies. A CBC with differential, ESR, and CRP are useful tests for infectious conditions; rheumatoid factor and antinuclear antibodies are useful tests for suspected rheumatologic disorders. Initially, AP and lateral radiographs of the involved region of the spine are recommended. With lumbar back pain, right and left oblique views are also recommended. MRI is most helpful for viewing soft tissue and intraspinal detail, and CT is superior for assessing bone involvement.

Differential Diagnosis

Occult pathologic conditions should be ruled out. Discitis, vertebral osteomyelitis, vertebral fracture, or tumor can cause significant back pain in toddlers. Older children can experience these same problems in addition to intervertebral disc herniation, vertebral endplate fractures, low back stress fracture, and spondylosis/spondylolisthesis. Back pain is a commonly reported symptom in children with somatization. Athletes with a history of low back pain lasting more than 1 month deserve careful evaluation. A low back stress fracture or spondylosis must be included in the differential diagnoses as well as spondylolisthesis.

Management

Treatment is determined by findings on history and physical examination and can include referral for radiographs (AP and lateral views) and imaging studies or referral to a pediatric orthopedist. If the back pain is due to injury, pain management and physical therapy may be part of the treatment plan.

Scoliosis

Scoliosis is a three-dimensional deformity most commonly described as a lateral curvature of the spine in the frontal plane. There are two types of scoliosis: nonstructural and structural. Nonstructural, also known as *functional scoliosis*, involves a curve in the spine without rotation of the vertebrae. The curve is reversible, because it is caused by conditions such as poor posture, muscle spasms, pain, or leg-length discrepancy. Structural scoliosis involves a rotational element of the spine and has various classifications depending on the cause. The remaining discussion pertains to structural scoliosis.

The diagnosis is based on a curvature of more than 10 degrees using the Cobb method, in which the angle between the superior and inferior end vertebrae (tilted into the curve) is measured (see Diagnostic Studies). In most pediatric cases, the etiology is unknown and is termed and classified as *idiopathic*. Other classifications include congenital, in which vertebrae fail to form (e.g., hemivertebrae), and neuromuscular (e.g., cerebral palsy, neurofibromatosis, Marfan syndrome). Kyphosis, which results from disorders of sagittal alignment (such as postural kyphosis and Scheuermann disease). Kyphosis, commonly termed *round back*, is discussed following scoliosis.

- *Idiopathic:* Etiology is unknown and is likely multifactorial. It is the most common type of scoliosis. There are three types classified by age at onset:
  - Infantile (0–3 years of age)
  - Juvenile (3–10 years of age)
  - Adolescent (11 years of age and older)
- *Congenital:* A structural anomaly present at birth (e.g., hemivertebrae) often associated with other congenital abnormalities, such as renal and cardiac anomalies; progression of curvature can worsen rapidly, particularly during periods of rapid growth (e.g., first 2–3 years of life and adolescence).
- *Neuromuscular:* Most common in nonambulatory patients. Secondary to weakness/imbalance/spasticity of the muscles of the trunk caused by primary neuromuscular problems (e.g., cerebral palsy or muscular dystrophy). In contrast to idiopathic and congenital scoliosis, curves caused by neuromuscular disorders can continue to progress after skeletal maturity.

Adolescent idiopathic scoliosis is the most common type. Its etiology is unknown, but it often has a familial or genetic pattern. The overall incidence of adolescent idiopathic scoliosis is approximately 2% to 3% with between 0.3% and 0.5% of pediatric patients with scoliosis having curves greater than a 20-degree Cobb angle on radiography and less than 0.1% demonstrating curves greater than 40 degrees.

Hormonal changes and sexual maturity play a role in the disease process, and a rapid growth period is believed to be a significant factor in the progression of the curvature associated with adolescent idiopathic scoliosis. In addition, the risk of curve progression depends on the amount of growth remaining, the magnitude of the curve, and sex. Although the incidence of adolescent idiopathic scoliosis is nearly equal in females and males, females have a much higher risk of developing curves greater than 30 degrees.[13] The most common type of idiopathic scoliosis is found in adolescents, and it is the major focus of the remaining discussion.

Small to moderate scoliotic curves (10–30%) usually do not increase significantly after skeletal growth is complete but they bear watching, particularly during periods of rapid growth. More severe curves are more likely to progress during the growth years. For a given child, however, it is difficult to predict progression because even small curves (10–25%) can progress to severe deformity. Regular monitoring of any curve in a skeletally immature child by the PCP is important (Table 40.2).

The female-to-male ratio increases with increasing curve magnitude. For curves less than 20 degrees, the risk for progression is low; these curves generally need only to be observed. However, for curves between 20 and 45 degrees, the risk for progression is high during growth, and early intervention is of paramount importance. In pediatric patients with curves greater than 50 degrees, the spine loses its ability to compensate, and progression is expected. Young premenarchal females with large curves are a vulnerable group because their spines are skeletally immature, with growth remaining. The majority of adolescents with idiopathic scoliosis have a right thoracic, left lumbar curve.

Clinical Findings

History. Scoliosis is generally painless and insidious onset is typical. In general, there is no significant history. The PCP should assess the following:
- Family history of scoliosis
- Age of menarche
- Etiologic factors related to the various causes of structural scoliosis

The presence of pain with a lateral curvature of the spine can suggest an inflammatory or neoplastic lesion as the cause of the scoliosis. Some pediatric patients with idiopathic scoliosis complain of mild pain that is activity related. Severe, constant, or night pain and point tenderness can be indicative of other pathologic

TABLE 40.2 Scoliosis, Kyphosis, and Lordosis

	Curve	Etiology	Clinical Findings	Radiographs	Management
Scoliosis	Lateral	Classifications: idiopathic (most common); neuromuscular; constitutional; secondary; congenital; miscellaneous; functional (leg-length discrepancy—not scoliosis)	History: positive family history; related to etiologies (classifications); painless curvature; typically have right thoracic curve	AP and lateral standing views to identify degree of curve; >10 degrees abnormal; may have one curve (C) or two curves (S); vertebrae show lateral deviation and rotation	Referral to orthopedic surgeon; brace or surgery; need to monitor progression of curve Most curves do not increase after growth is complete; females with idiopathic scoliosis more likely to have curve progression and need close monitoring
Kyphosis	AP curve of thoracic spine	Familial (Scheuermann disease); secondary to tumor, trauma, etc.; congenital; postural, not true kyphosis	Postural round back	Narrow disk space and loss of normal anterior height of vertebrae	Postural: PT, dancing, and swimming can be helpful If structural, refer to an orthopedic surgeon for observation, bracing, or surgery
Lordosis	AP curve of lumbar spine	As a result of hip contractures; physiologic; family and racial groups; before puberty	Abdomen and buttock protuberant; if result of hip contractures, lordosis disappears when sitting	Standing lateral views	If lumbar spine flattens and lordosis disappears when child bends forward, it is physiologic and no treatment is needed; if fixed, refer to an orthopedist

AP, Anteroposterior; *PT,* physical therapy.

conditions (e.g., metastatic tumor or stenosis) and warrants further investigation.

Physical Examination. Children of all ages should be evaluated in the standing position, from both the front and the side, to identify any asymmetry. Looking primarily at the straightness of the spine can be misleading because scoliosis involves both rotation and misalignment of the vertebrae. The Adams forward bend position accentuates the rotational deformity of scoliosis. Asymmetries to look for include:
- Unequal shoulder height.
- Unequal scapular prominences and heights: Note that the muscle masses may be somewhat unequal, especially if the child uses one shoulder more than the other, as in carrying books. Look for bony, not muscular, prominence.
- Unequal waist angles: The hip touches one arm and the contralateral arm hangs free.
- Unequal rib prominences and chest asymmetry.
- Asymmetry of the elbow-to-flank distance and some deviation of the spine from a straight head-to-toe line.
- Unequal rib heights when the child stands in the Adams forward bend position (see Fig. 40.8E).
- During the Adams test, the examiner looks for asymmetry of the posterior chest wall on forward bending, the earliest abnormality seen. Rotation of the vertebral bodies toward the convexity results in outward rotation and prominence of the attached ribs posteriorly. The anterior chest wall may be flattened on the concavity due to inward rotation of the chest wall and ribs. Associated findings may include elevation of the shoulder, lateral shift of the trunk, and an apparent leg-length discrepancy.

Congenital scoliosis may be visible in the infant lying prone; it is sometimes more prominent if the infant is suspended prone. Inspect for skin abnormalities, sacral dimple, and hairy patches.

The physical examination should also include the following:
- Observation for equal leg lengths
- Examination of the skin for hairy patches, nevi, café-au-lait spots, lipomas, dimples
- Neurologic examination checking for weakness or sensory disturbance
- Cardiac examination with diagnosis of Marfan syndrome

Diagnostic Studies. Standing PA and lateral radiographs of the entire spine are recommended at the initial evaluation of patients with clinical findings suggestive of a spinal deformity. On the PA radiographs, the degree of curvature is determined by the Cobb method. An MRI is helpful when an underlying cause of the scoliosis is suspected based on age (infantile and juvenile curves), abnormal findings in the history or physical examination, and atypical radiographic features. The latter include uncommon curve patterns, such as the left thoracic curve, double thoracic curves, high thoracic curves, widening of the spinal canal, and erosive or dysplastic changes in the vertebral body or ribs. On the lateral radiograph, an increase in thoracic kyphosis or absence of segmental lordosis may be suggestive of an underlying neurologic abnormality.

Differential Diagnosis

Structural scoliosis must be differentiated from functional scoliosis. The latter disappears when the child is placed in the Adams forward bend position, whereas the former is enhanced in this position. Persistent functional scoliosis to one side in a child with a neuromotor problem can eventually become structural and must be managed with physical therapy or other means to prevent progression. Consider systemic problems (e.g., neurofibromatosis, cerebral palsy, multiple sclerosis, Rett syndrome, rickets, tuberculosis, and tumor).

Management

The primary aim of scoliosis management is to stop the progression of curvature. Treatment options include observation, bracing, and surgery. The management presented in this text addresses adolescent idiopathic scoliosis. Observation is always indicated for curves less than 20 degrees. Bracing or surgery may be indicated for larger curves. Brace treatment may reduce the need for surgery, restore the sagittal profile, and change vertebral rotation. Indications for bracing are a curve between 25 and 45 degrees. Additional indications for brace therapy include skeletally immature patients with curves of 20 to 25 degrees that have shown more than 5 degrees of progression. Studies show brace treatment to be effective in preventing progression; however, it has been found that the success of treatment is proportional to the amount of time that the patient wears the brace. Various historic brace treatment protocols suggest wearing a brace as much as 23 hours per day although high quality evidence supports wearing the brace at least 13 hours a day; therefore compliance is a significant factor for this treatment modality.[14] Surgical treatment is indicated for pediatric patients who do not respond to bracing and/or for those with curvature exceeding 45 to 50 degrees.[14] There are various surgical procedures; all aim to control progressive curvatures.

Referral to an orthopedist or a center that specializes in working with infants and children with scoliosis is essential. Support must be given to the child and family through the diagnostic and treatment phases, considering school and peer factors. PCPs must help the child with psychological adjustment issues that arise if bracing or surgery is recommended and instituted. Some specific concerns of the child can include self-esteem problems, managing hostility and anger, learning about the disease and its care, wondering about the long-term prognosis, and concerns about clothing and participation in sports and other activities.

Complications

Progressive scoliosis can result in a severe deformity of the spinal column and cause deformities so severe that they impair both respiratory (see Chapter 32) and cardiovascular function, limit physical activities, and impair comfort. The psychological consequences of an untreated scoliosis deformity can be immense.

Prevention

Prevention is not possible; however, screening and early identification of pediatric patients with scoliosis may help avoid more expensive, invasive care and prevent the potential long-term consequences of the disorder. However, screening is effective only if the identified pediatric patients are referred for care. Parents must be notified, a referral arranged, and follow-up ensured.

Kyphosis

The thoracic spine typically has between 20 and 45 degrees of posterior curvature, which is considered physiologic. *Kyphosis* describes the condition when the normal posterior curvature of the thoracic spine becomes excessive or exaggerated and is outside the physiologic range of normal. With kyphosis, there is an AP forward curve of the thoracic spine with the apex posterior (i.e., the back is prominent). The most common clinical type of kyphosis is postural (postural round back). The curvature of the spinal column points backward and, when viewed from the side, gives the appearance of a humpback. In postural kyphosis, the Adams forward bend test demonstrates normalization of the lateral spine profile when viewed from the side (see Table 40.2) and the child can reverse the round-back appearance with active extension. Postural kyphosis is the most common type and is more often seen in females than males. It rarely causes pain and the curvature is flexible.

Scheuermann kyphosis is an osteochondrosis that presents as an abnormality of the vertebral epiphyseal growth plates. Onset generally occurs in adolescence. The kyphosis is rigid; the pain is located over the deformity and is worse at the end of the day. Scheuermann kyphosis is defined by vertebral wedging of 5 degrees or more on three adjacent vertebral bodies visualized on a standing lateral radiograph of the thoracic and lumbar spine. Associated radiographic findings include irregularities of the vertebral end plates, disk-space narrowing, and herniation of the intervertebral disk penetrating into the vertebral body.

Management

Depending on the cause and severity of the kyphosis, there are a variety of treatment options. Postural kyphosis may be improved with an exercise and physical therapy program that strengthens the supporting muscles. Activities (such as, dancing or swimming) that require a full range of motion of the shoulders, back, and arms can be helpful. Adolescent kyphosis may be treated with a combination of a back brace, exercise, and physical therapy. Surgery may be required in children with structural problems that cause kyphosis and in adolescents with curvature of the back that exceeds 50 to 60 degrees. Kyphosis caused by infections or tumors may also require surgery.

Lumbar Lordosis

Lumbar lordosis, or hyperlordosis, is an AP curve of the lumbar area of the spine (i.e., the child stands with the abdomen and buttocks protuberant). It is the least common of the congenital spinal deformities and is often associated with kyphosis or scoliosis. Congenital lordosis deformity is usually progressive. Lordosis can be a secondary result of a hip problem in which full extension is limited by hip flexion contractures or from lumbosacral deformities.

Management

If lumbar lordosis is suspected, examine the child in a forward-bending position. If the lumbar spine flattens and the lordosis disappears, this indicates that the spine is flexible and the lordosis is only physiologic. This child should be seen for follow-up in 6 to 12 months, and the examination should be repeated to make sure that continued physiologic findings are obtained. If the lordosis persists in the forward bending position, this indicates a fixed structural deformity and needs referral to an orthopedist. Lordosis resulting from hip flexion contractures is absent while sitting; it is commonly seen in children with cerebral palsy, spina bifida, and developmental dysplasia of the hip (see Table 40.2).

Developmental Dysplasia of the Hip

Developmental dysplasia of the hip (DDH) represents a spectrum of anatomic abnormalities in which the femoral head and acetabulum are in improper alignment and/or grow abnormally. This includes dysplastic, subluxated, dislocatable, and dislocated hips. Dysplasia is characterized by a shallow, more vertical acetabular socket with an immature hip/acetabulum. In subluxation, the hip is unstable, and the head of the femur can slide in and out of the acetabulum. DDH occurs congenitally or develops in infancy or childhood. Dysplasia may be diagnosed many years after the new-born period.

The incidence of DDH is estimated to range from 1.5 to 20 per 1000 live births in the United States. It is found more commonly with breech births and is four times more common in females than males. A positive family history (genetic risk factors) increases the risk of having a child with this problem. Other risk factors associated with DDH that are seen in infants include oligohydramnios, torticollis, and lower limb deformities (e.g., clubfoot, MA, and dislocated knee).

Physiologic, mechanical, and genetic factors are implicated in DDH. Physiologic factors include the hormonal effect of maternal estrogen and relaxin, which are released near delivery and produce a temporary laxity of the hip joint. Mechanical factors include constant compression in utero with restriction of movement late in gestation if the fetal pelvis becomes locked in the maternal pelvis. This is seen with first pregnancy, oligohydramnios, and breech presentation.

In the unstable hip, the femoral head and acetabulum may not have a normal tight, concentric anatomic relationship, which can lead to abnormal growth of the hip joint and result in permanent disability. In the newborn, the left hip is most often involved because this hip typically is the one in a forced adduction position against the mother's sacrum.

The hip can dislocate noncongenitally or in utero in pediatric patients with certain muscular or neurologic disorders that affect the use of the lower extremities, such as cerebral palsy, arthrogryposis, or myelomeningocele. Dislocation results from the abnormal use of the extremity over time.

Clinical Findings

History. Risk factors for DDH include female sex positive family history, high birth weight, breech positioning in the third trimester, and tight lower extremity swaddling. Of note, only 30% to 40% of patients with DDH have a recognized risk factor.[15]

Physical Examination. A hip examination should be performed on pediatric patients as part of their well-child supervision until the child begins to walk. Findings of DDH include the following:

- Routine examinations of the hips and lower extremities until the infant is walking. The Barlow and Ortolani tests are used to screen for DDH in neonates. Once an infant reaches the second and third months of life, the soft tissue surrounding the hips begins to tighten and the Barlow and Ortolani tests are less reliable. The Klisic and Galeazzi tests are used to screen older infants. Routine ultrasonography is not recommended; however, an ultrasound should be obtained if there is a high index of suspicion of dysplasia based on a positive clinical examination.
- Some 60% to 80% of abnormal hips of newborns identified by physical examination resolve by 2 to 8 weeks.
- In the older infant 6 to 18 months of age:
  - Limited abduction of the affected hip and shortening of the thigh (unequal leg lengths) are reliable signs (see Figs. 40.3 and 40.5).
  - Normal abduction with comfort is 70 to 80 degrees bilaterally. Limited abduction includes those cases with less than 60 degrees of abduction or unequal abduction from one side to the other (see Fig. 40.5).
  - There should be a positive Galeazzi sign unless bilateral (see Fig. 40.5A).
- Other findings include asymmetry of inguinal or gluteal folds (thigh fold asymmetry is not related to the disorder [see Fig. 40.5D]) and unequal leg lengths, shorter on the affected side.

In the ambulatory child who was not diagnosed earlier or was not corrected, the following might also be noted:
- Short leg with toe walking on the affected side
- Positive Trendelenburg sign (see Fig. 40.3C)
- Marked lordosis or toe walking
- Painless limping or waddling gait with child leaning to the affected side

If the hips are dislocated bilaterally, asymmetries are not observed. Limited abduction is the primary finding on examination (see Fig. 40.5). Also in subluxation of the hip (not frankly dislocated), limited abduction again is the primary indicator. A waddling gait may also be noted.

Diagnostic Studies. Ultrasound is superior to radiographs for evaluating cartilaginous structures and is recommended when the infant reaches 6 weeks of age. Ultrasound is used to assess the relationship of the femur to the acetabulum and provides dynamic information about acetabular development and stability of the hip. Radiologic evaluation of the newborn to detect and evaluate DDH is recommended once the proximal epiphysis ossifies, usually by 6 months. Radiography earlier than this is unreliable, because so much of the hip joint is cartilaginous in the young infant. AP radiographs of the pelvis are indicated.

Management

The goal of management is to restore the articulation of the femur within the acetabulum. Most neonatal hip instability findings resolve spontaneously by 6 to 8 weeks. However, close observations of these infants is recommended. Any infant with persistently abnormal findings on physical examination requires prompt referral to an orthopedist.

- Refer infant to an orthopedist if the newborn examination is positive. Follow up the newborn examination again at 2 weeks of age with a thorough hip examination to check for DDH. If the examination is positive or inconclusive, refer the infant to an orthopedist.
- Refer infant if limited or asymmetric hip abduction is noted.
- Ultrasonography is an option for: infants less than 6 months of age with a normal DDH examination and a history of breech presentation in the third trimester, previous clinical hip instability, improper swaddling, or a positive family history (including a close relative with hip replacement for dysplasia at <40 years of age), or parental concern.[16]
- Most neonatal hip instability resolves spontaneously by 6 to 8 weeks of age. Close observation of these children is recommended.
- The treatment of choice for persistent subluxation and reducible dislocations identified in the early phase is a Pavlik harness. The harness is applied with hips having greater than 90 degrees of flexion and with adduction of the hip limited to a neutral position. Radiographic or ultrasound documentation can be used during treatment to verify the position of the hip. If the infant does not respond to treatment with the harness, surgical treatment may be needed.
- The earlier treatment is started with the Pavlik harness, the better the prognosis for a successful outcome. The harness is worn 23 hours a day except for bathing. The infant with a Pavlik harness should be seen frequently to make sure that it fits properly, to identify complications associated with the use of the harness (e.g., avascular necrosis and femoral nerve palsy), and to ensure that the femur is properly seated in the socket. Ultrasonography can be performed while the Pavlik harness is worn to assess hip reduction and acetabular development. The length of time the

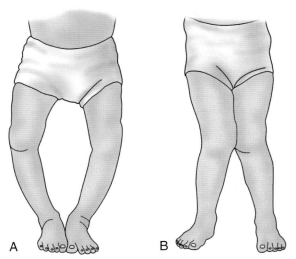

• **Fig. 40.12** Genu Varum and Genu Valgum. In genu varum (A), the knees are tilted away from the midline; the intercondylar (knee) distance with the ankles together is then measured. In genu valgum (B), the knees are tilted toward the midline; the intermalleolar distance with the knees approximated is then measured. (From Scoles P. *Pediatric Orthopedics in Clinical Practice.* Chicago: Year-Book Medical Publishers; 1982.)

growth plate can result in later genu varum as growth across the plate progresses unevenly.

With Blount disease, there is abnormal growth of the medial aspect of the proximal tibial epiphysis that results in progressive varus angulation of the tibia. Blount disease is rare, but it can occur in infancy, early childhood, middle childhood, or adolescence. It is seen more frequently in African American populations, is associated with obesity and early walkers, and commonly has a positive family history. Onset in infancy presents the highest risk for greatest deformity.[19]

Clinical Findings

History. Family history is important because certain heritable conditions—Marfan syndrome, OI, or vitamin D–resistant rickets—may predispose a child to this condition. Additional history may include progression since birth. Increasing deformation is problematic.

Physical Examination
- Tibial-femoral angle greater than 16 degrees
- Associated internal tibial torsion
- Lower extremity length discrepancy
- Intercondylar (knees) distance with the ankles together—measurement greater than 4 to 5 inches suggests the need for additional evaluation
- Joint laxity of lateral collateral ligaments in older children

Diagnostic Studies. The standard radiograph for the older child is a weight-bearing AP of the lower extremities with the patellae facing forward and a lateral radiograph of the involved extremity. Note the femur and tibia length and diaphyseal deformities. In physiologic bowing, the deformity is gentle and symmetric, with a metaphyseal-diaphyseal angle less than 11 degrees and normal appearance of the proximal tibial growth plate. In Blount disease, the bowing is asymmetric, abrupt, and with sharp angulation; the metaphyseal-diaphyseal angle is greater than 11 degrees; and there is medial sloping of the epiphysis and widening of the physis.[20]

Differential Diagnosis

Physiologic, persistent, and pathologic genu varum, metabolic (rickets), neurologic problems, Blount disease, infections, tumor,

osteochondrodysplasias, and internal tibial torsion should be ruled out.

Management

In physiologic genu varum (no increasing deformity), the following apply:
- No active treatment; spontaneous resolution is expected. Corrective shoes and splinting are unnecessary.
- Reassure parents; provide information about the natural progression of the problem.
- Observe the child's condition every 3 to 6 months to be sure the problem is resolving, especially during the second year of life. Serial photographs of the legs can be helpful.

Indications for orthopedic evaluation of genu varum include the following:
- Family history of pathologic bowing
- Asymmetric deformity: unilateral bowing, gait abnormalities, leg-length discrepancy
- Blount varus angulation/increasing deformity
- Progressive varus deformity[20]

In pathologic genu varum (increasing deformity), the following apply:
- Blount disease may be treated with bracing in children younger than 3 years. Bracing is effective and can prevent progression. In children older than 4 years, operative intervention is necessary.
- Monitor to be sure braces are used consistently, with good fit.
- Observe to be sure the problem is not worsening.

Complications

Knee degeneration and deformity result if pathologic genu varum is not treated. Early identification and referral reduce the complexity and expense of treatment and residual deformities.

Genu Valgum

Genu valgum also referred to as *knock knees* (see Fig. 40.12), is a common orthopedic condition in pediatrics. Lower extremity alignment goes through a predictable progression from varus to valgus over the first 6 years of life. Causes of genu valgum include physiologic and pathologic processes. Physiologic genu valgum improves spontaneously between 4 and 6 years of age. Pathologic conditions leading to valgus are rickets, renal osteodystrophy, skeletal dysplasia, posttraumatic physeal arrest, tumors, and infection.

Clinical Findings

History
- Progression of the deformity
- Joint pains or stiff gait
- Older child may report knee pain due to the stretching of the medial aspect of the knee

Physical Examination
- Bilateral tibial-femoral angle less than 15 degrees of valgus in the child up to 6 years of age is considered normal; a valgus angle greater than 15 degrees is outside the range of normal
- Unilateral deformity
- Awkwardness of gait
- Subluxating patella
- Intermalleolar (ankles) distance with knees together: measurement greater than 3 inches suggests the need for additional evaluation
- Short stature: genu valgum associated with short stature should be referred

Diagnostic Studies. No radiographic studies are needed unless a pathologic condition is suspected. Long-length AP radiographs of the leg in a weight-bearing stance are used for preoperative planning.

Differential Diagnosis

Rule out pathologic conditions of genu valgum.

Management

Physiologic genu valgum resolves spontaneously over time. Pediatric patients under the age of 10 are treated with observation and reassurance. Management of pathologic genu valgum is based on the underlying pathologic cause. Surgical intervention is reserved for those with residual deformity after being optimized medically.

Tibial Torsion

Tibial torsion is a common problem in pediatrics that is characterized by internal rotation of the tibia. Medial tibial torsion, also known as *internal tibial torsion,* consists of abnormal medial or internal rotation, resulting in in-toeing of the feet. Lateral tibial torsion, also known as *external tibial torsion,* consists of abnormal lateral or external rotation resulting in out-toeing.

Tibial torsion may be congenital, developmental, or acquired. Internal tibial torsion is the most common cause of in-toeing during the second year of life and is often noted around 6 to 12 months of age when children begin to walk. In most cases, it is a physiologic condition resulting from in utero positioning. Internal tibial torsion gradually resolves on its own by the time the child reaches 8 years of age. External tibial torsion is a cause of out-toeing in late childhood and is usually an acquired deformity. Contracture of the iliotibial band is the underlying problem.

Clinical Findings

Physical Examination. Observe the child's gait for in-toeing. The thigh-foot angle (TFA) is used to assess tibial rotation. With the child prone and the knees flexed 90 degrees, the foot and thigh are viewed from directly above (looking downward at the angle of the thigh and foot). The foot should be relaxed. Internal tibia

torsion exists if the TFA is negative by more than 10 to 20 degrees (–10 to –20 degrees), bearing in mind the child's age. In-toeing is expressed in negative values (Fig. 40.13). The typical range at 13 years of age is –5 to +30 degrees. Abnormal lateral or external torsion is associated with forward-pointing patellae and outward-pointing feet. A TFA measurement of greater than 30 degrees indicates abnormal external tibial torsion.

Diagnostic Studies. Radiographs are usually not necessary.

Differential Diagnosis

Differential diagnoses include genu varum (the knee has an abnormal tibial-femoral angle), femoral torsion (femoral anteversion), adducted great toe, and MA. All of these produce in-toeing gaits. Adducted great toe (the searching toe) is a benign condition that resolves spontaneously. Lateral femoral torsion (femoral anteversion) also causes an out-toeing gait. Screening for associated hip dysplasia and neurologic disorders (e.g., cerebral palsy [see Chapter 41]) is recommended.

Management

- Internal tibial torsion should be referred to an orthopedist if the problem is significant (TFA more than –20 degrees by 3 years of age). Surgical intervention may be needed for severe cases that persist into late childhood and cause significant functional problems.
- Special shoes are ineffective for the treatment of internal tibial torsion.
- External tibial torsion with TFA greater than +30 degrees should be referred to an orthopedist because it usually worsens with growth and does not correct spontaneously.

Complications

Tibial torsion (the TFA is outside the acceptable range of normal) can lead to significant functional problems in severe cases.

Osgood-Schlatter Disease

Osgood-Schlatter disease is a common cause of knee pain in adolescents. It is caused by microtrauma in the deep fibers of the patellar

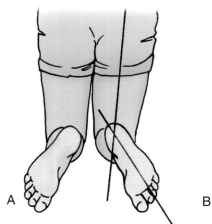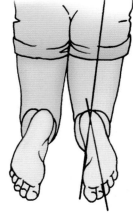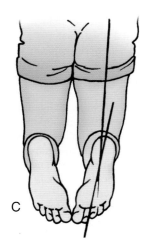

• **Fig. 40.13** Thigh-Foot Angle. (A) External tibial torsion produces excessive outward rotation. (B) Normal alignment is characterized by slight external rotation. (C) Internal tibial torsion produces inward rotation of the foot and a negative angle. (From Thompson GH. Gait disturbances. In Kliegman RM, Nieder ML, Super DM, eds. *Practical Strategies in Pediatric Diagnosis and Therapy.* Saunders; 1996.)

tendon at its insertion on the tibial tuberosity. The diagnosis is usually based on history and physical examination. The quadriceps femoris muscle inserts on a relatively small area of the tibial tuberosity and naturally high tension exists at the insertion site. In pediatric patients, additional stress is placed on the cartilaginous site with vigorous physical activity (overuse), leading to traumatic changes at insertion. Osgood-Schlatter disease is often seen in the adolescent years after the patient has undergone a rapid growth spurt the previous year. It occurs more frequently in males than in females, typically between 13 and 14 years in males and 11 years in females.

Clinical Findings

History
- Recent physical activity (such as, running track, playing soccer or football, or surfboarding) commonly produces the condition
- Pain increases during and immediately after the activity and decreases when the activity is stopped for a while
- Running, jumping, kneeling, squatting, and ascending/descending stairs exacerbate the pain
- Pain is bilateral in 20% to 50% of cases
- Approximately 25% of patients give a history of precipitating trauma

Physical Examination. Characteristic findings include the following:
- Pain may be reproduced by extending the knee against resistance, stressing the quadriceps, or squatting with the knee in full flexion
- Focal swelling, heat, and point tenderness found at the tibial tuberosity
- May palpate a bony prominence over the tibial tuberosity
- Full range of motion of knee

Diagnostic Studies. The diagnosis is based on history and physical examination. Radiographs are not needed unless another pathologic condition is suspected.

Differential Diagnosis

Other knee derangements, tumors (osteosarcoma), and hip problems with referred pain should be considered. The referred pain of hip problems is diffuse across the distal femur without point tenderness at the tibial tubercle.

Management

Osgood-Schlatter disease is a self-limiting condition, with symptom management the key consideration. The following steps are taken:
- Avoid or modify activities that cause pain until the inflammation subsides.
- Use ice or other cold therapy to reduce pain and inflammation.
- Once the acute symptoms have subsided, quadriceps stretching exercises, including hip extension for complete stretch of the extensor mechanism, may be performed to reduce tension on the tibial tubercle. Stretching of the hamstrings may also be useful.
- Use of NSAIDs is debatable. Because this condition may last up to 2 years, the chronic use of NSAIDs may be problematic.
- A neoprene sleeve over the knee may help to stabilize the patella.
- A patellar tendon strap that wraps around the joint just below the knee reduces strain on the tibial tuberosity.
- Cylinder casting or bracing with limited weight bearing for 2 to 3 weeks may be used in severe cases.

- Overuse is to be avoided and balanced training with adequate warm-up before physical activity/sports participation should be encouraged.
- Use of knee pads may help protect the tibial tuberosity from direct injury for those who engage in sports that result in knee contact.

Complications

In the postpubertal child, a residual ossicle in the tendon next to the bone may cause persistent pain. Surgical removal is indicated and relieves the pain.

Knee Injuries

Chapter 18 presents a further discussion of sport-related injuries and issues related to the musculoskeletal examination and common sports. Table 40.3 outlines the etiology, assessment, management, and differential diagnosis of common knee injuries seen in pediatric patients and young adults.

Pes Planus

There are three types of pes planus (flat feet): a flexible flatfoot, a flexible flatfoot with a tendo-Achilles contracture, and a rigid flatfoot. Flexible flatfoot is often familial, common, and benign. Physiologic or flexible flatfoot is common in infants and early childhood. It is typically due to a fat pad in the arch that makes the appearance of the arch seem flat or due to physiologic ligamentous laxity. The arch is seen when the foot is suspended but flattens with weight bearing. This generally resolves by 3 years of age. Flexible flat feet persisting into adolescence are usually associated with familial ligamentous laxity, as it is hereditary. Flatfoot can also be associated with certain syndromes (Marfan and Down syndromes), myelodysplasia, cerebral palsy, and obesity. Flat feet may be secondary to muscle imbalance or weakness, a bony abnormality, or shortened heel cords. Rigid flatfoot is pathologic.

Clinical Findings

History. Onset is noticed with weight bearing. The flexible flatfoot is painless and asymptomatic. Examine the shoes to see if there is abnormal wear on the inner side.

Physical Examination. Clinical manifestations include the following:
- There is a normal longitudinal arch when examined in a non–weight-bearing position, but the arch disappears when standing.
- On standing, the hindfoot collapses into valgus and midfoot sag becomes evident.
- Generalized ligamentous laxity is commonly observed.
- Subtalar motion is normal in flexible flatfoot.

Differential Diagnosis

Congenital vertical talus should be considered if the foot is rigid and no arch can be molded or if the foot has a rocker-bottom appearance. Calcaneovalgus foot might also be considered.

Management

Management involves the following:
- Symptomatic feet and rigid flatfoot should be treated; refer to an orthopedist
- For painful, flexible flatfoot, a removable longitudinal arch support may be recommended

TABLE 40.3   Characteristics of Various Types of Knee Injuries and Conditions

Condition	History, Mechanism of Injury	Clinical Findings	Management	Differential Diagnosis, Prognosis, and Comments
Quadriceps contusion	Typically a sports injury that results in bruising/contusion of the quadriceps muscle Injury can sometimes result from minor trauma or indirectly from tensile overload	Acute pain, swelling, and restriction of active and passive range of motion of hip and knee; tenderness over quadriceps	RICE: not to exceed 48 hours Progressive leg and gravity-assisted ROM after rest Flexion of the knee is the last function to return to normal, so it is a good indicator for return to sport NSAID for pain relief	In teens, rule out rhabdomyosarcoma of the quadriceps, Ewing sarcoma, and osteosarcoma if there is swelling and pain in the thigh without a clear history of trauma
Meniscal tear (torn cartilage)	Associated with a significant injury in a youth; results from axial loading with rotation Tear of a normal meniscus is rarely seen in children <12 years of age Congenitally abnormal cartilage (discoid) can tear at any age	Pain, swelling, and limping Joint-line tenderness and positive McMurray sign Patient may report a sensation of clicking or catching in the knee or locking of the knee Can be isolated or may occur in combination with ACL or MCL injuries	RICE initially; MRI if suspected tear; arthrography with MRI to rule out nerve injury with a prior tear; pain management Surgical intervention: meniscectomy generally relieves symptoms	Some 75% of patients develop degenerative articular changes on radiograph by 30 years of age A small percentage of youths develop degenerative changes 3–5 years after injury Chondral fractures and injuries to articular cartilage have similar histories and physical findings
Sprain of the ACL	Acute injury; typically, there is a twisting or hyperextension while the foot is planted and knee extended Report of a "popping" feeling and knee shifting or pulling apart	Swelling/effusion and pain Instability with lateral movement Positive Lachman test	Following the injury, a knee brace or immobilizer is used until swelling and pain subside ACL reconstruction Pain management Neuromuscular training to prevent injury	Associated with MCL and meniscal tears
Sprains of the MCL	Most commonly injured ligament of the knee due to valgus stress to an extended knee Patient reports tearing sensation with medial pain, swelling, stiffness	Instability with lateral movement and medial knee pain Tenderness over the MCL If tenderness extends along the distal femoral physis, suspect physeal fracture	RICE, splint, or hinged knee brace to protect against valgus stress Pain management Plain radiographs to look for physeal and epiphyseal fractures in skeletally immature children Surgical repair on an isolated collateral ligament is not beneficial; nonoperative treatment is the standard of care	Combined ACL and MCL injuries are common Physeal fractures are more common than MCL sprains in youths
Osteochondritis dissecans	Juvenile and adolescent types common in 10- to 15-year-olds; boys more common than girls Isolation and sometimes sequestration of an osteochondral fragment without significant trauma May be caused by microtrauma or trauma or may involve metabolic or genetic factors Pain increased with activity and diminished with rest and intermittent effusions Locking and catching are unusual findings but may be present if bone fragments are detached	Activity-related pain and swelling Tenderness of the femoral condyle	Plain radiographs or MRI; 4–6 weeks of immobilization and non–weight bearing if <12 years of age Youths >12 years: Arthroscopic surgery Eliminate high-impact activities; non–weight bearing for several weeks until symptoms abate About 50% heal spontaneously with rest and protected weight bearing Surgical intervention if still symptomatic despite 6–12 months of conservative treatment, symptomatic loose body, or nonunion	Mimics symptoms of a torn meniscus Articular cartilage transplantation for selected patients

TABLE 40.3 **Characteristics of Various Types of Knee Injuries and Conditions—Cont'd**

Condition	History, Mechanism of Injury	Clinical Findings	Management	Differential Diagnosis, Prognosis, and Comments
Dislocation of the patella	Associated with patellar malalignment Most cases involve lateral dislocation with pain and swelling Most occur in youths <20 years Family history in 20–30% More frequently seen in girls than in boys	Massive and tense effusion Tenderness at the medial border of the patella and medial retinaculum Guarding with gentle pressure on the medial patella with lateral displacement	Nonoperative management: 2–3 weeks of joint rest with splint or knee immobilizer (patella-stabilizing sleeve), then intensive rehabilitation Isometric exercises, especially of quadriceps. Some 80–85% of cases are successfully managed with nonoperative treatment Surgical correction for recurrent dislocations or chronic instability	Outcomes with nonoperative therapy vs. acute surgery are similar Patellar dislocation tends to recur (recurrence is more frequent in a younger child) but decreases over time Degenerative arthritis with recurrent dislocations is common with or without surgery

ACL, Anterior cruciate ligament; *MCL,* medial collateral ligament; *MRI,* magnetic resonance imaging; *NSAID,* nonsteroidal antiinflammatory drug; *RICE,* rest, ice, compression, and elevation; *ROM,* range of motion.

Data from Anderson SJ. Lower extremity injuries in youth sports. *Pediatr Clin North Am.* 2002;49:627–641; Hosalkar HS, Wells L. The knee. In: Kliegman RM, Behrman RE, Jenson HB, et al., eds. *Nelson Textbook of Pediatrics.* 18th ed. Saunders; 2007; Landry GL. Management of musculoskeletal injury. In: Kliegman RM, Behrman RE, Jenson HB, et al., eds. *Nelson Textbook of Pediatrics.* 18th ed. Saunders; 2007; McMahon P, ed. *Current Diagnosis and Treatment: Sports Medicine.* Lange Medical Books/McGraw-Hill; 2007; and Staheli LT, ed. *Pediatric Orthopaedic Secrets.* 2nd ed. Hanley and Belfus; 2003.

- If the Achilles tendon is tight, passive stretching may be helpful
- Routine radiographs are not indicated unless pathologic flatfoot is suspected

Complications

Some cases of flatfoot are symptomatic in adulthood; in severe cases, the bones of the feet adapt to their abnormal position with pronation and the possible development of bunions, which may require surgery. Congenital vertical talus is a complication in childhood and should be identified early and referred for treatment.

Patient Education

Parents must understand that arch supports may relieve pain but do not help the foot to "grow" an arch.

Metatarsus Adductus

MA involves adduction of the forefoot relative to the hindfoot where the forefoot is supinated and adducted. The most common cause is intrauterine molding; the deformity is bilateral in 50% of cases. A nonflexible foot, especially with heel valgus, or persistence may indicate a more serious problem.

Clinical Findings

History. There can be a family history of MA.
Physical Examination
- The forefoot is adducted, whereas the midfoot and hindfoot are normal.
- The lateral border of the foot has a convex shape, with the base of the fifth metatarsal appearing prominent. Normally, this border should look straight. Sometimes spreading of the toes is noted with a wider space between the first and second toes.
- The foot should normally be straight. If one draws a line from the middle of the heel, it should pass through the second toe or between the second and third toes. In MA, the forefoot has an increased angle (>15 degrees) or resists stretching (Fig. 40.14).

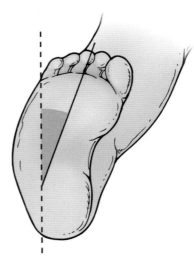

Fig. 40.14 Metatarsus Adductus (MA) Angle. An angle (created by the intersecting lines) that is greater than 15 degrees indicates MA.

- To determine whether the foot is flexible or rigid, the heel is grasped with one hand while the forefoot is abducted with the other. In flexible MA, the forefoot can be abducted past midline.
- A careful hip examination should be performed to rule out associated DDH.
   Diagnostic Studies. Radiographs are not performed routinely. AP and lateral weight bearing are indicated in toddlers or older children with residual deformities. The AP radiographs demonstrate adduction of the metatarsals at the tarsometatarsal articulation and an increased intermetatarsal angle between the first and second metatarsals.

Differential Diagnosis

Consider congenital vertical talus, which will be rigid, or clubfoot, in which the foot is inverted and in the pointed-toe position.

Management

Management is based on the rigidity of the deformity; most pediatric patients respond to nonoperative treatment.

- For the flexible foot that can be brought past midline, the soft tissues can be stretched by the parents with each diaper change. Instruct parents to hold the hindfoot in one hand and stretch the midfoot to overcorrect the deformity to the count of five and repeat five times. The soft tissues should blanch with each stretch. Be sure that the parent is not just pushing on the great toe. Feet that correct just to the neutral position may benefit from stretching exercises. If there is no improvement in 4 to 6 weeks, serial plaster casts may be considered. Surgical treatment is controversial but may be considered in the small subset of pediatric patients with symptomatic residual deformities that have not responded to conservative treatment.
- For the nonflexible foot:
  - Refer to orthopedics.
  - Educate the family that the treatment for infants may include serial short-leg casts or braces to stretch the foot (two or three casts for 2 weeks per cast) or other management if the bones of the foot are more severely affected. If the child is older than 2 to 3 years, surgery may be needed to correct the problem.
  - Surgical treatment is controversial but may be considered in patients with symptomatic residual deformities that have not responded to conservative treatment.

Talipes Equinovarus

Talipes equinovarus (clubfoot) has three elements: the ankle is in equinus (the foot is in a pointed-toe position), the sole of the foot is inverted as a result of hindfoot varus or inversion deformity of the heel, and the forefoot has the convex shape of MA (forefoot adduction). At birth, the foot cannot be manually corrected to a neutral position with the heel down.

The etiology is thought to be multifactorial and likely involves the effects of environmental factors in a genetically susceptible host. Clubfoot may be idiopathic or hereditary, neurogenic (as seen with myelomeningocele), or associated with syndromes (e.g., arthrogryposis and Larsen syndrome). It varies in severity, with uterine positioning a factor in mild clubfoot. The incidence is 1 to 2 per 1000 live births, with approximately 30% to 50% of cases being bilateral, and it is more common in male infants.[21] The problem is congenital and can be identified in neonates.

Clinical Findings

History. Clubfoot is present at birth, but the parents may not note curvature.

Physical Examination. Note the inflexibility of sole of the foot. It is inverted as a result of hindfoot varus or inversion deformity of the heel, and the forefoot has a convex shape with forefoot adduction. It can be bilateral. A complete physical examination should be performed to rule out coexisting musculoskeletal and neuromuscular problems.

Diagnostic Studies. AP and lateral radiographs are sometimes recommended, often with the foot held in a maximally corrected position. A common radiographic finding is "parallelism" between lines drawn through the axis of the talus and the calcaneus on the lateral radiograph, indicating hindfoot varus. Radiographs are not required in an infant to diagnosis the anomaly.

Management

The following steps are taken:

- Refer to orthopedics upon diagnosis, ideally shortly after the infant is born, because the joints are most flexible in the first hours and days of life. Nonoperative treatment should be initiated as soon as possible after birth. Treatments include taping and strapping, manipulation, and serial casting. The Ponseti method of clubfoot treatment involves a specific technique for manipulation and serial casting. Weekly cast changes are performed; 5 to 10 casts are usually required. Up to 90% of pediatric patients will need a percutaneous tenotomy of the heel cord as an outpatient followed by a long leg cast with the foot in maximal abduction and dorsiflexion. This is followed by a full-time bracing program for 3 months and then nightly bracing for 3 to 5 years. For older pediatric patients with untreated clubfeet or for those who have residual deformity, osteotomies, although rare, may be required in addition to the soft tissue surgery.[21]
- Stiffness remains a concern at long-term follow-up. Although pain is uncommon in childhood and adolescence, symptoms may appear during adulthood.

Complications

With growth, the abnormality can become increasingly distorted, making correction more difficult. Calf hypoplasia and a shorter than normal foot can occur even with correction.

Overriding Toes

Overriding toes are generally identified at birth. Efforts to tape them into a correct position or otherwise modify their position are usually futile. Overriding of the second, third, and fourth toes generally resolves with time. Occasionally, if severe, they can be surgically improved. Shoe fit can be a problem.

In-Toeing and Out-Toeing Rotational Problems

When a child has an in-toeing or out-toeing gait, the degree of rotation and source of the rotational deformity must be assessed (Fig. 40.15). These conditions include internal femoral torsion (femoral anteversion), internal tibial torsion, and MA. The causes of in-toeing usually are physiologic, are related to age, and resolve as the child grows (Table 40.4). In addition, in-toeing in pediatrics can vary with activities and from step to step.

Clinical Findings

History

- This should include onset, progression, functional limitations, previous treatment, evidence of neuromuscular disorder, and significant family history.

Physical Examination

- Observe the gait. Note that the slightly older child may consciously or unconsciously improve or worsen the gait for the examiner. Observing the child running may also be helpful.
- Lay the child prone on the examining table.
- Examine for femoral anteversion (medial and lateral rotations).
- Examine for internal or external tibial torsion (TFA).
- Examine for MA or other deformity.

The child may have a combination of any or all of the aforementioned problems.

Management

See management of underlying causes for management strategies.

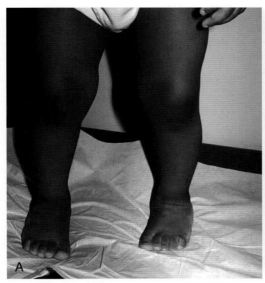
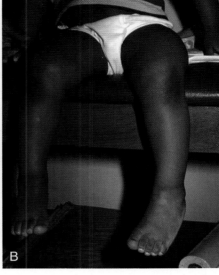

• **Fig. 40.15** Internal Tibial Torsion. (A) On weight bearing, the hip, thigh, and knee are normally oriented and the patella faces anteriorly, but the lower leg and foot turn inward. The deformity results in prominent in-toeing on walking, which may cause the child to trip frequently. (B) In this view of the child while sitting, it is easy to appreciate that the lateral malleolus is positioned anteriorly to the medial malleolus. This shifts the ankle mortise and foot to a medially oriented position. (From Zitelli BJ, McIntire SC, Nowalk AJ, et al. *Zitelli and Davis' Atlas of Pediatric Physical Diagnosis*. 8th ed. Elsevier; 2023.)

TABLE 40.4 Typical Cause of In-Toeing and Out-Toeing Rotational Problem

Cause	Possible Diagnoses	Typical Finding	Age at Manifestation
In-toeing	Clubfoot	Equinovarus, plantar foot flexion, forefoot adduction, and hindfoot varus	At birth
	Metatarsal adductus	Curved foot: refer if not flexible	Birth–6 months
	Abducted great toe	Searching toe: resolves spontaneously	Toddler period
	Internal tibial torsion	Refer if thigh-foot angle (TFA) more than −10 to −20 degrees	12–18 months
	Internal femoral torsion	Refer if >70 degrees medial and <10 degrees lateral hip rotation	2–5 years
Out-toeing	Physiologic infantile out-toeing	Feet may turn out when infant is positioned upright: resolves spontaneously	Early infancy
	External tibial torsion	Refer if TFA ≥30 degrees	Late childhood
	Lateral femoral torsion	Refer if >2 standard deviations of the mean	Late childhood

Toe Walking

Some young pediatric patients initially stand on their toes until they establish the heel-toe pattern, usually within the first 6 months of walking. Consistent toe walking is frequently associated with neurologic problems, such as cerebral palsy. Autistic children or those with early muscular dystrophy may toe walk. Pediatric patients with tight heel cords may toe walk. Unilateral toe walking can be associated with a short leg, as found with a dislocated hip. Toe walking also can be a habit, especially in pediatric patients who used walkers or jumpers. In these pediatric patients, toe walking generally resolves before 3 years of age and is not associated with musculoskeletal deformity. It is important to differentiate between the idiopathic toe walker and the child who toe walks because of a neuromusculoskeletal condition associated with tight heel cords and contractures.

Clinical Findings

History. The PCP should assess onset of walking, use of walker or jumper, severity of toe walking, any other developmental delays, or associated neurologic conditions.

Physical Examination. The examination should include the following:
- Looking at shoe wear and heel wear to assess extent of toe walking
- Assessing for tight heel cords. The foot should be brought beyond a 90-degree angle
- Conducting a neurologic assessment
- Measuring leg lengths and examining hips

Management. Management depends on etiology. Orthopedic management is needed for tight heel cords, unequal leg lengths, and hip problems.

Leg Aches of Childhood

Extremity pain, often referred to as *growing pains* by the layperson, is a frequent clinical presentation. The pain is usually nonarticular; in two-thirds of pediatric patients, it is described as being located in the shins, calves, thighs, or popliteal fossa. It is almost always bilateral. The pain appears late in the day or is nocturnal, often waking the child. The pain lasts from minutes to hours. By morning, the child is almost always pain-free. Because it occurs late in the day and is often reported on days of increased activity, it may represent a local overuse syndrome; it may also be associated with low vitamin D levels and decreased bone strength. Leg aches of childhood are generally not associated with serious organic disease, have a peak incidence between 3 and 12 years of age, and usually resolve by late childhood; with the prevalence of 2.6% to 49.6% of school-age children who experience intermittent leg aches.[22] However, it is important to differentiate these pains from more serious pathologic conditions. Restless legs syndrome, also known as *periodic limb movement disorder*, is a more recently recognized common source of nocturnal leg pains in pediatrics.

Clinical Findings

History. Pain or leg aches are typically described as:
- Occurring characteristically in the evening or late in the day; may wake the child up from sleep
- Pain gone in the morning with no limitation of activity
- Poorly localized and bilateral
- Occurring commonly in the front of the thighs, in the calves, and behind the knees
- Transient and occurring over a period of time as long as several years
- Not associated with a limp or disability
- Without reported fevers or swelling
- Without report of recent or remote trauma

Physical Examination
- Have the child stand on tiptoes and heels.
- Measure leg lengths.
- Evaluate range of motion.
- Assess for swelling, erythema, and tenderness.
- Observe for limping.

Findings include normal physical examination with no joint pain or tenderness, guarding, swelling, erythema, or reduced range of motion.

Diagnostic Studies. There is no single diagnostic test. It is a diagnosis of exclusion.

Differential Diagnosis

Restless legs syndrome, neoplastic lesions, leukemia, sickle cell anemia, juvenile arthritis, and subacute osteomyelitis apophysitis must be ruled out.

Management

Reassure parents that these common complaints have a benign etiology and generally resolve spontaneously. Symptomatic treatment with massage, heat, and analgesia may be of benefit. Stress the need for parents to bring the child in for reevaluation if there is a change in symptoms or other signs emerge. Refer the child if the pain is localized to one region, is associated with swelling or other constitutional symptoms, is increasing in severity, or alters gait.

Limps

Deviations from the normal age-appropriate gait pattern can be caused by a wide variety of conditions. A limp is usually mild and self-limited and caused by contusion, strain, or sprain. In some cases, the cause can be a sign of a serious inflammatory or infectious process. Age is an important factor in diagnosing the many causes of limping. Table 40.5 describes the various types of limps commonly seen in pediatrics.

Clinical Findings

History. A careful history is needed, including:
- Presence of pain
- History of trauma, past medical history
- Presence of fever, night sweats
- Weight loss or anorexia
- Type of limp (Table 40.6)
- Interference with activities
- Review of systems

Physical Examination
- The child should be in a diaper or underwear during examination.
- Observe for areas of erythema, swelling, atrophy, and deformity.
- Observe each limb segment.
- Identify limp type; have the child walk and run while distracted.

TABLE 40.5 Types of Limp

Type of Limp	Cause	Characteristics	Examples
Antalgic	Pain: typically due to infection, fracture, or trauma	Walking on a painful extremity results in an attempt to get weight quickly off affected side; gait has shortened stance phase[a]	Sore knee: patient walks with fixed knee Sore toe: patient tries not to roll off toe at toe-off phase of the stride Appendicitis causes slight slumping posture and shortened stride on the right side due to psoas muscle irritation
Trendelenburg gait/abductor lurch	Hip problems: typically developmental, congenital, or muscular disorders	Tilts over affected hip to decrease mechanical stresses; unaffected leg is off the ground during swing-through phase of gait	Hip dysplasia; LCPD
Equinus/toe-to-heel gait	Neurologic incoordination	Unsteady wide-based gait	Cerebral palsy: toe-to-heel sequence to gait during stance phase due to heel-cord contractures
Circumduction	Functionally longer leg; knee or ankle stiffness	Longer leg progresses forward in swing motion	Leg-length inequality, knee injury with hyperextension, ankle problems

[a]Stance phase: represents 60% of the gait cycle; swing about 40%.

LCPD, Legg-Calvé-Perthes disease.

TABLE 40.6   Differential Diagnosis of Limping

Condition	Age	Pain (±)	Historical Findings	Clinical Findings	Causative Factors	Management
Developmental dysplasia of the hip	Infant, toddler, child, adolescent	−	Breech delivery; MA; torticollis; poor treatment outcomes if not diagnosed at birth or shortly thereafter	Limited abduction; Trendelenburg; radiography at 2–3 months old; shortening of leg; acetabular dysplasia	Familial; joint laxity, positioning, maternal hormones	Newborn: no triple diapers Pavlik harness to hold hips in flexion and abduction; after 6 months of age, closed versus open reduction; after 18 months of age, osteotomy
Leg-length inequality	Toddler, child, adolescent	−	None	Circumduction gait; joint contracture; >1 cm discrepancy in leg lengths	Congenital; neurogenic; vascular; tumor; trauma; infection	Shoe lifts; epiphysiodesis (fusion of growth plate to arrest growth of the opposite side) if discrepancy 2–6 cm
Neuromuscular (NM) disease	Toddler, child, adolescent	−	Depends on cause	Depends on cause; equinus or abductor gait	Cerebral palsy, muscular dystrophy, and other NM diseases	Referral to appropriate specialists
Discitis	Toddler, child, adolescent	+	Varied: fever, malaise, unwilling to walk, backache.	Stiff back, ↑ ESR; positive radiograph within 2–3 weeks—narrow disk space, irregular vertebral body endplate; bone scan, CT, MRI show early findings; early bone scan has typical findings	Bacterial infection in disk space (Staphylococcus aureus) or inflammatory response	Immobilization and antistaphylococcal antibiotic therapy
Septic arthritis	Toddler, child, adolescent	++	Moderate to high fever, malaise, arthralgias; irritability; progressive course	Redness, warmth, and swelling of joint—knee or hip; limited hip motion; ESR >25 mm/h	S. aureus likely organism	Appropriate antibiotic coverage (7 days, IV; 3–4 weeks total)
Acute hematogenous osteomyelitis	Toddler, child, adolescent	+	Varied: malaise, low-grade to high fever; may have severe constitutional symptoms; toxicity	Refusal to walk or move limb; point tenderness; limp; 7–10 days to see radiographic bony changes; 25% ↑ WBCs; ↑ CRP	S. aureus likely organism	Appropriate antibiotic coverage (generally 7 days, IV; 4–6 weeks total or until ESR is normal)
Neoplasm	Toddler, child, adolescent	+	Depends on type of neoplasm	Varied	Neoplasm—benign or malignant	Referral to oncologist
Trauma	Toddler, child, adolescent	+	Depends on type (fractures, strains, sprains)	Varied	Varied	Rule out physical abuse if discrepancy related to developmental capabilities, injury history, and type of injury
Occult trauma: toddler fracture	Toddler	+	Well child	Commonly radiograph (oblique view) shows spiral fracture of tibia; refusal to walk, mild soft tissue swelling	Trauma	See Trauma, earlier

Continued

TABLE 40.6	Differential Diagnosis of Limping—Cont'd					
Condition	**Age**	**Pain (±)**	**Historical Findings**	**Clinical Findings**	**Causative Factors**	**Management**
Transient synovitis	3–8 years	+	Mild to moderate fever, mild irritability; resolves within 1 week	Limited hip motion; ESR <25 mm/h	Inflammatory reaction; unknown etiology; often URI (50%) prior	Rest
Juvenile arthritis (JA)	Childhood until 16 years	+	Fever, rashes, ↑ WBCs; some iritis; joint stiffness and swelling; S and S >3 months	Mono-/polyarticular arthropathy; + ANA (25–88%); ↑ ESR in moderate/severe JA	Unknown; genetic (HLA) or environmental	Treat with NSAIDs initially; may need sulfasalazine, methotrexate, corticosteroids; joint replacements when older
Slipped capital femoral epiphysis (SCFE)	9–15 years	+	>90th percentile weight; African American; male	Limited abduction and extension; external rotation of thigh if hip flexed	Multifactorial: mechanical; endocrine; trauma; familial	Needs immediate surgery; non–weight bearing with crutches until admitted; bilateral involvement does occur
Legg-Calvé-Perthes disease (LCPD)	3–12 years	+	Acute or chronic onset; pain in hip, groin, knee; stiffness; male	+ Trendelenburg, shortening; ↓ abduction, internal rotation, hip extension; + radiographs but not early	Familial; breech birth; prior trauma (17%)	In female, tends to be more serious problem; bracing and surgery may be needed; bilateral involvement does occur

ANA, Antinuclear antibody; *CRP,* C-reactive protein; *CT,* computed tomography; *ESR,* erythrocyte sedimentation rate; *HLA,* human leukocyte antigen; *IV,* intravenous; *MA,* metatarsus adductus; *MRI,* magnetic resonance imaging; *NSAID,* nonsteroidal antiinflammatory drug; *PT,* physical therapy; *S and S,* signs and symptoms; *URI,* upper respiratory infection; *WBC,* white blood cell.

- Stance and swing phase should be compared in both legs.
- Range of motion of each joint should be evaluated, especially the hip.
- Complete a neurologic examination, including strength, reflexes, balance, and coordination.
- Assess Trendelenburg sign for hip stability.

Diagnostic Studies. A CBC with differential and measurement of ESR and CRP levels should be obtained to rule out infection, inflammatory arthritis, or malignancy. Imaging should include radiographs of the area of concern. When imaging the hip, frog-leg lateral views should be obtained. Ultrasound may be used to detect effusion of the hip joint. If radiographs and ultrasound are positive, a CT scan or MRI may be indicated.

Differential Diagnosis

Fracture, DDH, LCPD, SCFE, tumor, infection, juvenile arthritis, and others should be considered (see Table 40.6).

Management

Refer the patient to an orthopedist immediately unless the etiology is a mild strain or a local lesion that can be managed conservatively by the PCP.

Overuse Syndromes of Childhood and Adolescence

Overuse injuries, overtraining, and burnout among child and adolescent athletes are growing problems. It is estimated that about 60% to 70% of US children and adolescents participate in some form of sport activity.[23] An overuse injury is microtraumatic damage to a bone, muscle, or tendon that has been subjected to repetitive stress without sufficient time to heal or undergo the natural reparative process. *Apophysitis* refers to the irritation, inflammation, and microtrauma of the apophysis. The risk of overuse injuries is more serious in the pediatric population because the growing bones cannot handle as much stress as the mature adult bone. Typical overuse injuries of childhood are varus overload of the elbow ("Little League elbow"), Osgood-Schlatter disease, calcaneal apophysitis (Sever disease), proximal humeral epiphysiolysis ("Little League shoulder"), patellofemoral pain syndrome, shin splints, and stress fractures (Table 40.7).

Clinical Findings

History. An in-depth history of the sport played, activities performed (e.g., pitching, kicking, swinging), and hours played per week, including games and practice, must be determined. The PCP must ask specific questions related to the child's pain. For example, what makes the pain better or worse? Further history and discussion with the child and adolescent should include questions such as the following related to the timing of the pain as it relates to the child's activity:

- Is there pain in the affected area after physical activity?
- Is there pain during the activity without restricting performance?
- Is there pain during the activity that restricts activity?
- Is there chronic, unremitting pain even at rest?

TABLE 40.7   Overuse Injuries of Childhood: Characteristic Features and Their Treatment

Condition	Clinical Findings	Treatment	Comments
Osgood-Schlatter disease	Swelling and tenderness/pain over tibial tubercle	NSAIDs, knee pad, knee immobilizer if severe pain for 1–2 weeks	Most resolve with time (12–18 months); radiographs only if pain persists (shows soft tissue swelling and possible residual ossicle)
Patellofemoral pain syndrome	Anterior knee pain	Rest, NSAIDs, retraining, and strengthening of quadriceps muscles	Arthroscopic surgery only if recurring problems
Proximal humeral epiphysiolysis ("Little League shoulder")	Shoulder pain—gradual onset; pain ↑ with throwing, especially curve ball	Modify activity; gradual restart, but limit intensity and frequency of throwing with retraining and muscle strengthening	Seen in skeletally immature children; radiographs show widening proximal humeral physis
Sever disease, calcaneal apophysitis	Swelling/tenderness/pain posterior aspect of the heel Pain with forced dorsiflexion of the ankle	Activity modification; limit running, jumping, and specific sport that causes pain Heel cushions, arch supports Pre-/postsport icing Gentle heel cord stretching exercises	Most resolve with rest and return to previous level of activity/sport within 2 months Radiograph evaluation is not diagnostic or prognostic Radiographic evaluation should be used for exclusion of other causes of heel pain
Shin splints	Pain along medial border of tibia; child has a history of prolonged running.	NSAIDs; ice after running; retraining and muscle strengthening after inflammation ↓; gradual return to running.	Associated with poor running technique, hard running surface, muscle weakness; inadequate running shoes; sudden increase in running; is an inflammatory response; may need to consider exertional compartment syndrome
Stress fractures	Tenderness and swelling at site	Reduce or eliminate activity that caused injury for 10–14 days; may need to cast	Caused by microtrauma; most commonly seen in active teens but can occur during childhood; proximal tibia most common site
Varus overload of the elbow ("Little League elbow")	Elbow pain with activity; locking and ↓ extension of elbow; medial humeral epicondylar tenderness	Rest; NSAIDs; ice; when pain-free, gradual return to activity with retraining; surgery if elbow instability. Enforce pitch count restrictions	Leads to osteochondral lesions and stress fractures if severe; radiographs reveal widening proximal physis; also seen in gymnasts

NSAID, Nonsteroidal antiinflammatory drug.

Physical Examination. The examination is dependent on the joint or limb involved. Check for deformity, warmth, swelling, range of motion, and ecchymosis. Observe for guarding of an extremity or limping.

Differential Diagnosis

Depending on the presenting symptoms, a plain film, CT, MRI, or bone scan may be indicated.

Management

Most of the injuries can be managed conservatively with proper and timely diagnosis. Treatment often involves resting and icing the extremity or joint, doing retraining and strengthening exercises, gradually reintroducing activities, and using analgesics. NSAIDs help reduce the inflammatory component of the trauma. Patient and parent education is important to prevent further injury and disability and to allow the child to return to safe sport participation. If not managed properly and effectively, overuse injuries can affect normal physical growth and maturation. PCPs can be instrumental in educating the active child, parents, and coaches in developing strategies to prevent overuse injuries. These include careful monitoring of training workload, especially during growth spurts; providing time for prepractice neuromuscular training to enhance strength and conditioning; and frequent evaluation of proper use and sizing of sporting equipment.[23]

Muscle Dystrophies

The muscular dystrophies are a group of hereditary disorders of skeletal muscle that produce progressive degeneration of skeletal muscle, leading to weakness. The muscular dystrophies are autosomal-dominant, X-linked, and can appear in several children in a family. The X-linked dystrophies are the most common, with the most common dystrophy being Duchenne muscular dystrophy (see also Chapter 41). The prevalence of Duchenne muscular dystrophy is estimated at 1 in every 3500 to 1 in 5000 live male births.[24]

Clinical Findings

History
- Disease becomes evident between 2 and 6 years of age.
- There is usually a family history of muscle disease.
- Failure to achieve motor milestones, especially independent ambulation, is noted.
- Toe walking is commonly seen.
- Loss of motor skills, such as the ability to climb stairs easily, is typical.
- Easy fatigue with physical activity is reported.
- A history of good days and bad days in relation to ability to accomplish physical activities is common.
- There is increasing difficulties with motor activities.

Physical Examination

- Toe walking
- Large firm calf muscles
- Fibrotic or "doughy" feel to the muscles
- Widely based lordotic stance
- Waddling Trendelenburg gait
- Lower extremities showing early weakness of gluteal muscle strength
- Positive Gower sign: this sign is obtained by asking the child to get up off the floor without help. The sign is positive if the child uses his or her arms to push off from the legs, gradually standing in a segmented fashion.

Diagnostic Studies. See Chapter 41 for details related to diagnostic studies.

Management

Referral to a multidisciplinary neuromuscular team for management. These teams typically consist of providers specializing in neurology, orthopedics, pulmonary, nutrition, and physical therapy. Social services and nursing care are vital. Genetic counseling may be necessary depending on the diagnosis.

The use of chronic oral steroids has been found to delay motor disability and improves longevity. Physical therapy is used to promote mobility and prevent contractures. Supportive care including proper bracing and supportive equipment are necessary. Surgery may be needed for severe contractures and scoliosis.

Patient and family support is needed. Muscle diseases are chronic and debilitating; some are fatal conditions. Helping the child to lead as normal a life as possible while coping with his or her condition is a major task for parents and caregivers.

Popliteal Cysts

Popliteal cysts, or Baker cysts, are due to the egress of fluid through a normal communication of a bursa or may be caused by herniation of the synovial membrane through the joint capsule. Baker cysts appear much less frequently in pediatrics than in adults.

Clinical Findings

Findings include swelling behind the knee with or without discomfort. Cysts are generally located at or below the joint line.

Diagnostic Studies. Ultrasonography can distinguish between a fluid-filled cyst and solid tumor. Radiographs will show if there is soft calcification in the mass.

Differential Diagnosis

Lipomas, xanthomas, vascular tumors, and fibrosarcomas must be ruled out.

Management

Observation is the treatment of choice. The cyst usually resolves in 10 to 20 months. Ice and NSAIDs are used to promote comfort and relieve pain. Surgical incision is indicated only when symptoms are severe and limiting.

Ganglions of the Hands

Ganglions are the most common benign lesions of soft tissue in pediatrics (see Popliteal Cysts). A ganglionic cyst is an acquired, mucinous, fluid-filled painless lesion that originates from the synovial-lined space. A ganglion grows out of a joint. It rises out of the connective tissues between bones and muscles.

Clinical Findings

Ganglions of the hand are hard, fixed masses commonly found on the wrist (commonly dorsal) and flexor aspects of the finger. The etiology of these cysts is unknown. Transillumination of the cyst with an otoscope or examination by ultrasonography plus findings on physical examination are keys to the diagnosis.

Management

Ganglionic cysts in pediatrics are rarely symptomatic and usually regress spontaneously. The likelihood of recurrence with any form of treatment is higher in pediatrics than in adults with such lesions. Conservative care with rest and splinting can be tried. If conservative care fails to result in partial or complete resolution, refer for needle aspiration or surgical excision, which is the most reliable method to eliminate a ganglion because the tract that extends into the joint is removed. Steroid injections are not advised.

Additional Resources

American Academy of Orthopaedic Surgeons (AAOS): www.aaos.org

AAOS Ortho Info: http://orthoinfo.aaos.org

Backpack Safety Tips: http://orthoinfo.aaos.org/topic.cfm?topic=A00043

Muscular Dystrophy Association (MDA): www.mda.org

Ortho Bullets Pediatrics High-Yield Topics: http://www.orthobullets.com

Pediatric Orthopaedic Society of North America (POSNA): https://posna.org/Physician-Education/Study-Guide (provides physician education study guides)

Scoliosis Research Society (SRS): www.srs.org

STEPS: www.steps-charity.org.uk (National charity in the United Kingdom for those affected by a lower limb condition)

United Brachial Plexus Network: www.ubpn.org (Erb palsy support and information network)

Acknowledgment

The author acknowledges the contributions of Cynthia Marie Claytor, the chapter author in the previous edition.

References

1. Giss K, Chan C. Musculoskeletal system. In: Duderstadt KG, Keeton VF, eds. *Pediatric Physical Examination: An Illustrated Handbook.* 4th ed. Elsevier; 2023.
2. Tournis S, Dede AD. Osteogenesis imperfecta: a clinical update. *Metabolism.* 2018;80:27–37.
3. Jasty N, Study Group F, Heyworth B. Evaluation and management of mid-shaft clavicle fractures in adolescents: current concepts review. *JPOSNA.* 2020;2(3).
4. Locke L, Rhodes L. Management of musculoskeletal disorders. In: Kyle T, ed. *Primary Care Pediatrics for the Nurse Practitioner a Practical Approach.* Springer Publishing Company, LLC; 2022:595–616.
5. Hallemans A, Verbecque E, Dumas R, et al. Developmental changes in spatial margin of stability in typically developing children relate to the mechanics of gait. *Gait Posture.* 2018;63:33–38.
6. Williams N. Improving early detection of developmental dysplasia of the hip through general practitioner assessment and surveillance. *Aust J Gen Pract.* 2018;47(9):619–623.
7. Marcdante KJ, Kliegman RM, Schuh AM. Hip. In: Marcdante KJ, Kliegman RM, Schuh AM, eds. *Nelson Essentials of Pediatrics.* 9th ed. Elsevier; 2022:758a–762a.

8. Ulici A, Herdea A, Carp M, et al. Nursemaid's elbow - supination-flexion technique versus hyperpronation/forced pronation: randomized clinical study. *Indian J Orthop.* 2019;53(1):117–121.

9. Marcdante KJ, Kliegman RM, Schuh AM. Assessment of the mother, fetus and newborn. In: Marcdante KJ, Kliegman RM, Schuh AM, eds. *Nelson Essentials of Pediatrics.* 9th ed. Elsevier; 2022:227a–245a.

10. Johnson GJ, Denning S, Clark SL, et al. Pathophysiologic origins of brachial plexus injury. *Obstet Gynecol.* 2020;136(4):725–730.

11. Oishi S, Chris S, Lake A. Disorders of the upper extremity. In: Herring JA, ed. *Tachdjian's Pediatric Orthopaedics: From the Texas Scottish Rite Hospital for Children.* 6th ed. Elsevier; 2022:300–421.

12. Selcen D. In: Post TW, ed. *Neonatal Brachial Plexus Palsy.* UpToDate; 2022.

13. Marcdante KJ, Kliegman RM, Schuh AM. Spine. In: Marcdante KJ, Kliegman RM, Schuh AM, eds. *Nelson Essentials of Pediatrics.* 9th ed. Elsevier; 2022:769a–775a.

14. Shannon BA, Mackenzie S, Hariharan AR, et al. Update in nonoperative management of adolescent idiopathic scoliosis to prevent progression. *J Pediatr Orthop Soc North Am.* 2021;3(4):1–9.

15. Reidy M, Collins C, MacLean JGB, et al. Examining the effectiveness of examination at 6-8 weeks for developmental dysplasia: testing the safety net. *Arch Dis Child.* 2019;104(10):953–955.

16. D'Alessandro M, Dow K. Investigating the need for routine ultrasound screening to detect developmental dysplasia of the hip in infants born with breech presentation. *Paediatr Child Health.* 2019;24(2):e88–e93.

17. Nigrovic PA. In: Post TW, ed. *Approach to Hip Pain in Childhood.* UpToDate; 2022.

18. Kienstra AJ, Macias CG. In: Post TW, ed. *Evaluation and Management of Slipped Capital Femoral Epiphysis (SCFE).* UpToDate; 2022.

19. Marcdante KJ, Kliegman RM, Schuh AM. Lower extremity and knee. In: Marcdante KJ, Kliegman RM, Schuh AM, eds. *Nelson Essentials of Pediatrics.* 9th ed. Elsevier; 2022:762–766.

20. Robbins CA. Deformity reconstruction surgery for Blount's disease. *Children.* 2021;8(7):556.

21. Cady R, Hennessey TA, Schwend RM. Diagnosis and treatment of idiopathic congenital clubfoot. *Pediatrics.* 2022;149(2):e2021055555.

22. Pavone V, Vescio A, Valenti F, Sapienza M, Sessa G, Testa G. Growing pains: what do we know about etiology? A systematic review. *World J Orthop.* 2019;10(4):192–205.

23. Hergenroeder AC. In: Post TW, ed. *Sports Participation in Children and Adolescents: The Participation Physical Evaluation.* UpToDate; 2022.

24. Ricotti V, Selby V, Ridout D, et al. Respiratory and upper limb function as outcome measures in ambulant and non-ambulant subjects with Duchenne muscular dystrophy: a prospective multicentre study. *Neuromuscul Disord.* 2019;29(4):261–268.

41

Neurologic Disorders

DANIEL CRAWFORD AND LAUREN SIEBRASE-WILKES

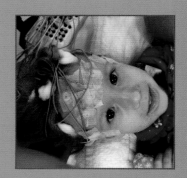

Neurologic disorders can present in a variety of ways and degrees. No other body system has as much influence on a child's overall development and the function of other organ systems. The challenges for primary care providers (PCPs) are to be able to screen for and identify neurologic disorders, know when to appropriately refer to specialists, facilitate the coordination of resources or case management services, and support families and children in coping with challenges associated with neurologic disorders. Early detection and intervention are essential for many neurological disorders and require PCPs to understand basic neurologic function to screen for and identify these problems. Routine examination and assessment by the PCP are pivotal in establishing a baseline and when concerns arise and/or abnormal findings are detected.

Anatomy and Physiology

The nervous system is a complex network of nerves and cells that transmits information between the brain and the rest of the body. It is made up of two main sections: the central nervous system (CNS) and the peripheral nervous system (PNS) (Table 41.1; Figs. 41.1 and 41.2). The CNS consists of the brain and spinal cord and is primarily responsible for receiving and processing information and initiating a response or action. It is sometimes discussed by regions: *hind-* (lower brainstem), *mid-* (central brainstem), and *fore-* (cerebral hemispheres) brain; however, it is more commonly discussed by section: *brainstem* (autonomic processes), *cerebellum* (balance/coordination), and *cerebral hemispheres* (motor control, sensory perception, language, cognition, memory, and decision-making).

The PNS consists of nerves that branch off from the spinal cord and brain and extend throughout the body. It is responsible for delivering information between the CNS and body. The PNS can be further subdivided into two subsystems: autonomic and somatic nervous system. The autonomic nervous system can be further subdivided into the sympathetic and parasympathetic systems (Box 41.1). The somatic nervous system is responsible for motor and sensory function through a network of nerves that send information to the brain (afferent nerves) and out to the body (efferent nerves).

The nervous system functions through a complex network of specialized cells that send electrical signals via nerve pathways between the nervous system and organs. These electrical signals are mediated through chemical transmission across synaptic junctions. The chemicals involved in this process are called *neurotransmitters* (Table 41.2). The cranial nerves extend through the face, head, and neck and can have sensory functions and/or motor functions, while the spinal nerves extend throughout the body, providing sensory and/or motor functions. Throughout the nervous system, the *gray* matter is primarily composed of neurons and glial cells, whereas *white* matter is primarily composed of axons.

Pathophysiology and Defense Mechanisms

The nervous system is intimately related to the functioning of the entire body; problems in any part of the system can have clinical implications. Examples include the uncontrolled firing of cerebral neurons (seizures), the inability of cerebral neurons to fire or the inability of the CNS to process stimuli and respond accordingly (coma), or the inability of peripheral nerves to respond to or receive signals through the pyramidal system of afferent and efferent nerves (paralysis). Other problems occur when specific areas of the nervous system or individual nerves are damaged. Additional causative factors for CNS disorders include:

- *Systemic* disorders can occur as the brain is extremely sensitive to changes in physiology anywhere in the body. Thus, any metabolic change, whether from external or internal factors (autoimmune, inflammatory, and/or infectious causes), may affect the CNS. Examples include delirium from toxins, diabetic coma, meningitis, ataxia, and chorea.
- *Neurodegenerative* disorders result from a loss of structure or function of neurons in the brain or spine, including death of neurons. Most neurodegenerative diseases are caused by genetic mutations.
- *Inherited* disorders, such as chromosomal and gene duplications and deletions, can directly affect the nervous system (see Chapter 27). Some single-gene defects can have direct neurologic effects (e.g., neurofibromatosis), whereas others can have indirect effects via the abnormal metabolites released (e.g., phenylketonuria).
- *Structural* defects: Because the CNS is structurally complex, there are many opportunities for defects to occur in utero (e.g., cortical migration defects, hydrocephalus, anencephaly, and myelomeningocele [MMC]).
- *Trauma*: Head and spinal cord injuries can have profound short- and long-term consequences in pediatrics. Recovery from head trauma can be lengthy and require extended rehabilitation. Even then, return to baseline does not always occur. Peripheral nerves can regenerate if conditions are optimal; however, the axons of injured neurons cannot regrow within the spinal cord. Outside the cord, if the cut ends are reconnected with special attention to the myelin sheath, regeneration of the injured nerve begins at the proximal end of the neuron soon after injury.

TABLE 41.1 Anatomic Units of the Nervous System and Functions

Anatomic Unit	Function
I. Central Nervous System	
A. Brain	
1. Forebrain—cerebrum	
a. Cortex (gray matter)	
(i) Frontal lobe	Anterior—decision-making, emotions, memory, judgment, ethics, abstract thinking Posterior—motor control Broca area—speech
(ii) Parietal lobe	Sensory processing and integration, language, reading, writing, pattern recognition
(iii) Temporal lobe	Memory storage, auditory processing, olfaction Wernicke's area—language comprehension
(iv) Occipital lobe	Visual processing
b. Diencephalon	
(i) Thalamus	Receives/sorts sensory input, modulates motor impulses from cortex
(ii) Hypothalamus	Integrates autonomic functions
2. Midbrain	Connects brain with cerebellum, pons, medulla; (CN III, IV)
3. Hindbrain	
a. Pons	Bridges cerebellum, medulla, midbrain; (CN V, VI, VII, VIII)
b. Medulla	Proximal end of spinal cord; contains reticular system—arousal; (CN IX, X, XI XII)
c. Cerebellum	Coordination and movement; balance; smooth movements
B. Spinal cord	
1. Dorsal roots	Afferent sensory fibers
2. Ventral roots	Efferent motor fibers
II. Peripheral Nervous System	
A. Cranial nerves	Sensory and motor components; olfaction; vision; hearing; facial, tongue, pharyngeal, eye, shoulder movements
B. Spinal nerves	Transmit motor, sensory, and autonomic signals

CN, Cranial nerve.

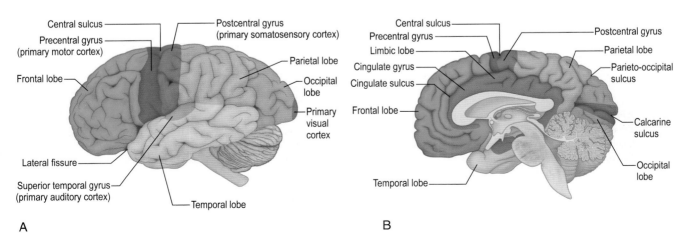

• **Fig. 41.1** Principal Gyri, Sulci, and Functional Areas of the Cerebral Cortex. (A) Lateral aspect. (B) Medial aspect. (From Crossman AR, Neary D. *Neuroanatomy: An Illustrated Colour Text*, ed 6. Elsevier; 2020.)

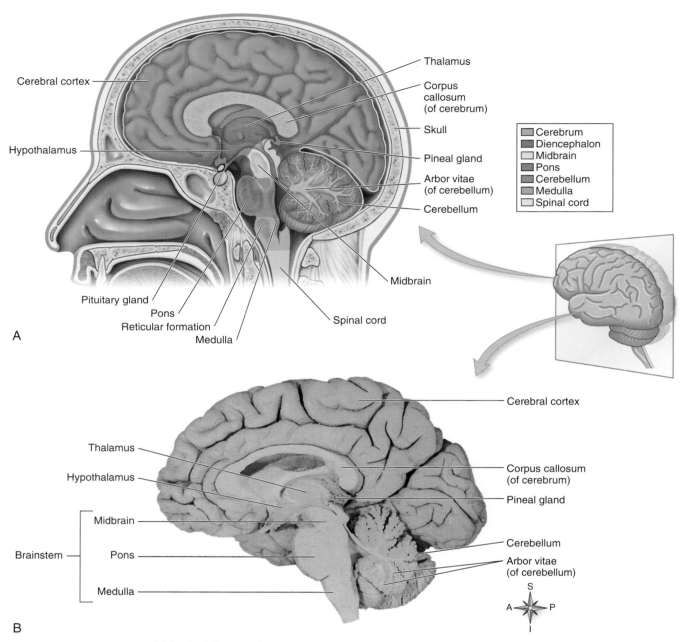

• **Fig. 41.2** Midsagittal Section of the Brain Showing the Major Portions of the Diencephalon, Brainstem, and Cerebellum. (From Patton K, Bell F, Thompson T, et al. *The Human Body in Health & Disease*, 8th ed. Elsevier; 2024.)

• *Benign or malignant tumors* evolve when there is a problem with cellular division, which can cause unrestricted growth. Problems with the body's immune system can also lead to such tumors.
• *Neurotransmitter dysfunction* (deficiencies and/or excess) can result in seizures, ataxia, hypotonia, oculomotor dyspraxia, and developmental delay.

Assessment of the Nervous System

Assessment of the nervous system requires a careful history from the child and family and a detailed physical examination to determine if a neurologic disorder is present. For children with neurologic problems, it is important to establish a thorough understanding about social, environmental, developmental, and family issues that may exist. If neurologic disorder is suspected, the provider should try to localize the findings through determining the suspected location and pattern of impairment. Historical information from children older than 3 years and from one or more family members provides the most accurate picture. Imaging, diagnostic testing, or laboratory studies may be required. See Chapter 29 for guidelines on neurodevelopmental assessments of children.

• BOX 41.1 Autonomic Nervous System: Parasympathetic and Sympathetic Functions

Parasympathetic System
- Pupil constriction
- Increased watery saliva
- Lacrimal gland vasodilation
- Coronary vessel vasoconstriction
- Bronchial muscle constriction
- Stomach and colon peristalsis
- Genitalia vasodilation
- Urinary bladder constriction
- Skin vessel dilation

Sympathetic System
- Pupil dilation
- Increased viscous/thick saliva
- Coronary vessel vasodilation
- Bronchial muscle relaxation
- Stomach and colon constriction
- Adrenaline secretion
- Sphincter relaxation or constriction
- Genitalia vasoconstriction
- Urinary bladder relaxation
- Skin vessel constriction

History

History of Present Illness

- Onset: When did the first symptoms appear? Was the onset insidious or sudden? Was it associated with another event (e.g., illness, injury, surgery, poisoning, ingestion)? If yes, describe the event. Was the onset accompanied by any constitutional symptoms? How have the symptoms evolved?
- Duration: How long have the symptoms been present? If intermittent, how long do symptoms last when they are present, and how frequently do they occur?
- Pain: Location and character, path of radiation, severity, extent of disability produced, effect of various activities or stimuli (e.g., light/sound sensitivity), aggravating or alleviating factors (e.g., change in position, time of day), effects of previous treatment, and/or presence of pain or discomfort in other parts of the body. Note: Morning awakening with headaches, vomiting, double vision, and/or balance problems require immediate referral.
- Sensory deficits: Changes in hearing, vision, taste, or smell; loss of pain sensation; vertigo; dizziness; numbness; and/or tingling.
- Injury: How, when (date/time), why, where? Mechanism or manner in which the injury was produced: accidental or nonaccidental? Immediate treatment provided? If past injury(ies), at what age(s) did the injury(ies) occur?
- Reflexive responses: Vomiting, coughing, persistence/return of primitive reflexes, tics, and/or clonus.
- Behavioral changes: Irritability, stupor, changes in appetite, lack of attention, random activity (e.g., lip smacking, emotional lability, changes in school performance).
- Motor and coordination changes: Ataxia, spasticity, and/or increased or decreased tone.
- Review of systems

Medical History

- Prenatal history: Maternal/paternal ages, alcohol, drug ingestion, environmental toxins exposure, radiation exposure, nutrition, prenatal care, injuries, smoking, human immunodeficiency virus (HIV) or other infectious disease exposure, maternal illness, bleeding, preeclampsia, diabetes, previous abortions and stillbirths, other complications during pregnancy.
- Birth/neonatal history: Unusual circumstances around the birth, vaginal or cesarean birth, complications, labor and delivery, birth weight/length, occipital frontal (head) circumference (OFC), resuscitation, APGAR scores, trauma, congenital anomalies, feeding history (reflux, colic, frequent formula changes), jaundice, seizures, infection, gestational age, sleep disturbances, multiple birth. Note: Premature, low birth weight, and infants who are small for gestational age (SGA) face particular challenges regarding future development.
- Injuries/infections: Meningitis, encephalitis, head injuries, frequent musculoskeletal injuries that can suggest coordination disturbance or impulsive behavior.
- Cardiovascular/respiratory disorders
- Environmental exposure to toxins (e.g., lead exposure).
- Metabolic disorders: Diabetes mellitus, thyroid disease.
- Past neurologic disease(s)/testing: Tics, hydrocephalus, seizures (type, description, frequency, onset, medications); genetic testing, or imaging studies.
- Psychiatric disorders: Hallucinations, delusions, illusions.
- Drug/other ingestions: Lead poisoning, dietary/herbal supplements, substances of abuse.
- Renal disease: Uremic syndrome manifests with confusion, convulsions, coma.
- General: Allergies, immunizations, hearing, vision, dental, skin integrity, behavior, nutritional status (including eating disorders).
- Medications: Over the counter, prescription, recreational drug use.
- Other: Health conditions, treatments, providers, or resources involved with patient.

Family History

- Family members with similar symptoms/features or inherited disorders.
- Obtain a three-generation pedigree (see Chapter 27), including consanguinity, neurologic disorders (e.g., migraine, epilepsy, neurodegenerative disorder), intellectual functioning of family members.

Developmental, Functional Health, and Social History

- Developmental history: Age at which major milestones were achieved in all domains, history of developmental concern, need for therapies, or developmental regression.
- Cognition and school performance: At grade for age? Standardized assessment results? If concerns are identified, further evaluation with a neuropsychologist or provider with special expertise in child neurology or developmental pediatrics can be considered.
- Inquire about the effects of symptoms on all areas of health promotion and safety, nutrition, elimination, activity, communication, role relationships, values and beliefs, sexuality, sleep, family coping and resilience (management style), and stress tolerance, temperament, and self-concept. Note: Neurobiology, epigenetics, protective factors, and developmental timing may

TABLE 41.2 **Examples of Neurotransmitters**

Neurotransmitter	Location[a]	Function[a]
Small-Molecule Transmitters		
Class I		
Acetylcholine (ACh)	Junctions with motor effectors (muscles, glands); many parts of brain	Excitatory or inhibitory; involved in memory
Class II: Amines (derived from amino acids)		
Monoamines (contain one amino group)		
Serotonin (5-HT[b])	Several regions of the CNS	Mostly inhibitory; involved in moods and emotions, sleep
Histamine	Brain	Mostly excitatory; involved in emotions and regulation of body temperature and water balance
Catecholamines (Contain a Catechol Ring and One Amino Group)		
Dopamine (DA)	Brain; autonomic system	Mostly inhibitory; involved in emotions and moods and in regulating motor control
Epinephrine (Epi)	Several areas of the CNS and in the sympathetic division of the ANS	Excitatory or inhibitory; acts as a hormone when secreted by sympathetic neurosecretory cells of the adrenal gland
Norepinephrine (NE)	Several areas of the CNS and in the sympathetic division of the ANS	Excitatory or inhibitory; regulates sympathetic effectors; in brain, involved in emotional responses
Class III: Amino Acids (contain an amine group, carboxylic acid group, and a specific R group)		
Glutamate (glutamic acid, Glu)	CNS	Excitatory; most common excitatory neurotransmitter in CNS
Gamma-aminobutyric acid (GABA)	Brain	Inhibitory; common inhibitory neurotransmitter in brain
Glycine (Gly)	Spinal cord	Inhibitory; common inhibitory neurotransmitter in spinal cord
Class IV: Other Small Molecules		
Nitric oxide (NO)	Several regions of the nervous system	May be a signal from postsynaptic to presynaptic neuron
Purines (Contain Adenine, A Double-Ring Purine Structure)		
Adenosine triphosphate (ATP)	Autonomic ganglia, brain	Regulation of autonomic signaling; regulates nerve repair; glia-neuron communication
Adenosine (ADO)	Brain	May be involved in regulating sleep
Large-Molecule Transmitters		
Neuropeptides (chains of amino acids)		
Vasoactive intestinal peptide (VIP)	Brain; some ANS and sensory fibers; retina; gastrointestinal tract	Function in nervous system uncertain
Cholecystokinin (CCK)	Brain; retina	May be involved in memory, learning, mood
Substance P	Brain, spinal cord, sensory pain pathways; gastrointestinal tract	Mostly excitatory; transmits pain information
Enkephalins	Several CNS regions; retina; intestinal tract	Mostly inhibitory; opioids that modulate pain
Endorphins	Several CNS regions; retina; intestinal tract	Mostly inhibitory; opioids that modulate pain
Dynorphins	Several CNS regions	Mostly inhibitory; opioids that modulate pain
Neuropeptide Y (NPY)	Brain, some ANS fibers	Variety of functions including enhancing blood vessel constriction by ANS, regulation of energy balance, learning, and memory

[a]These are examples only; most of these neurotransmitters are also found in other locations, and many have additional functions.

[b]5-Hydroxytryptamine (synonym for serotonin).

ANS, Autonomic nervous system; *CNS,* central nervous system.

From Patton KT, Bell F, Thompson T, et al. *Anatomy & Physiology,* ed 11. Elsevier; 2022.

play a role in resilience in children, ranging from the micro (how they function in their day-to-day lives) to the macro (their response to global threats and surprises).

- Inquire about the family composition, including critical family events, additions or losses of family members, military deployment, incarceration; home, neighborhood, and school environment; culture and ethnicity; exposure to violence, adverse childhood experiences, or other stressors; strengths; resources; childcare; social determinants of health; identified social supports (e.g., family, friends, health professionals); and community agencies involved with the family and child.

Physical Examination: General

The following elements of the general physical examination should be noted:
- Growth pattern, including length/height, weight, body mass index (BMI), and OFC, sexual maturity rating.
- Abnormalities of the skin (e.g., café au lait macules, angiomas, neurofibromas, ash leaf spots, or other pigmentation changes).
- Dysmorphic features (see Chapter 27).
- Cardiovascular system (including blood pressure, femoral pulses).
- Musculoskeletal system: Gowers' sign (child unable to rise from seated position on floor without "walking" hands up legs to get to standing position), calf muscle hypertrophy, muscle atrophy, and muscular function (strength/range of motion).
- Hearing/vision: Including cataract, corneal clouding, cherry-red spot, change of vision.
- Abdominal masses/organomegaly.

Neurologic Examination

The neurologic examination moves from the highest level of functioning to the lowest. Cerebral function is tested first and is followed by

evaluation of the cranial nerves (CNs), motor function, sensory function, coordination, and reflexes. The neonate's neurologic functioning is largely subcortical; therefore the examination is more limited than in an older infant or child. An infant's cry should be assessed and can be an indicator of several diseases (e.g., high pitched with increased intracranial pressure, a cat's meow with cri du chat syndrome, hoarse with hypothyroidism). In infants and children, watching them carefully while collecting the history and engaging with them in an age-appropriate manner can provide a significant portion of the neurologic examination data. A ball, some small toys (e.g., a small car), a bell, and something that attracts attention (e.g., a pinwheel) are useful for completing the examination in young children.

Behavior and Mental Status

Test the following cortical functions:
- Responsiveness
- Orientation
- Judgment
- Thought/cognition
- Language and speech (receptive, expressive, written); speech flow, voice quality, organization of thoughts
- Memory and concentration
- General knowledge
- Ability to relate to others: parents versus strangers
- Mood and affect

Cranial Nerve Function

The assessment of CN function typically includes CN II–XII because CN I (olfactory) is not functional until the infant is 5 to 7 months old and is difficult to assess in children. Details for age-specific CN assessment techniques can be found in Table 41.3.

Motor Examination

Fine motor coordination, gait, posture, strength, muscle symmetry, quality of movement, and tone are aspects of the motor examination.

TABLE 41.3 Cranial Nerve Assessment in the Young vs. Older Child

	Young—Infancy and Early Childhood	Older—Middle Childhood and Adolescence
CN I	Difficult to assess, typically not present before 5–7 months of age; grossly assess by observing grimace/response to strong odors	Differentiation of smells
CN II	Recognition of objects introduced into visual fields; funduscopic exam if tolerated	Visual acuity, visual fields, funduscopic exam
CN III, IV, VI	Pupillary response to light, extraocular movements with tracking object of interest, ptosis	Pupillary response to light, extraocular movements, ptosis
CN V	Grossly assess by noting response to light facial touch	Sensation to light facial touch, temporalis and masseter strength
CN VII	Note symmetry of facial expressions	Symmetry of smile and rise of eyebrows, orbicularis oculi strength, strength with cheeks puffed out
CN VIII	Response to soft sounds made outside of visual fields, observe for lateralization of sounds	Weber and Rinne; can use whisper test
CN IX, X	Symmetrical rise of soft palate, gag reflex	Symmetrical rise of soft palate, gag reflex
CN XI	Difficult to assess if unable to follow directions but can evaluate symmetry of sternocleidomastoid (SCM) movements	Turns head against resistance, shoulder shrug
CN XII	Tongue lies and/or protrudes midline	Tongue protrudes midline

CN, Cranial nerve.

- Fine motor coordination: Fine motor coordination is tested by having the child pick up small pieces, write, stack blocks, copy pictures, turn book pages, put puzzles together, or do other hand activities. In older children, assessment of their handwriting appropriateness for their age should be observed.
- Muscle strength/size: Look at muscle size, contour, and symmetry. Have the child stand from seated on the floor. Look for Gowers sign. Ask the child to move extremities against resistance and grip your fingers hard. Note strength and symmetry; grade strength using same standardized scale, also noting muscular hypertrophy, hypotrophy, or atrophy.
- Muscle tone (resting strength): Is the trunk control and/or extremities floppy, rigid, or somewhat stiff when the child is resting or active? How difficult is it to move body parts passively? Tone may be increased or decreased all over or differ between the legs and the trunk and arms. Symmetry of muscle tone should be noted.
- Involuntary movements: Tremors are fine involuntary movements. Chorea or choreiform movements are large, irregular jerking and writhing movements. Athetoid movements are slow writhing movements, especially of the hands and feet. Dystonia is an uncontrolled change in tone characterized by contraction of the affected muscles.
- Infant-specific motor examination: Motor testing should include observation for symmetry of movements, consistent fisting of the hands, opisthotonos, scissoring, abnormal tone, tremors, presence/reappearance of primitive reflexes, and absent later-onset infant reflexes (e.g., Landau, parachute reflexes).

Sensory Examination

Evaluate functioning of the spinothalamic tract and dorsal column. The spinothalamic tract can be assessed by evaluating sharp/dull sensation and/or temperature sensation. The dorsal column can be assessed by evaluating joint position sense, and/or vibratory sensation. If an abnormality is identified, the examiner should attempt to localize the abnormality. Note: Examination is limited in infants and young children.

Reflexes

- Deep tendon reflexes (biceps, brachioradialis, triceps, patellar, Achilles [ankle jerk] reflex).
- Superficial reflexes (upper/lower abdominal, cremasteric, gluteal, plantar).
- Primitive reflexes (sucking, rooting, asymmetric tonic neck, grasp, trunk incurvation, stepping (Note: they may be absent or decreased in a satiated or sleepy infant).
- In older children and adults, a positive Babinski is an important sign of upper motor neuron disease.

Coordination

Gait should be assessed with the patient walking, and if indicated, running, walking on their toes, then on their heels. For children 5 years of age and older, tandem gait (e.g., ability to walk heel to toe, one foot in front of the other) should also be assessed. For younger children balancing on each foot independently, hopping on each foot or jumping can be considered. The Romberg test should be performed as a part of the balance assessment. Coordination of movements should be assessed using a developmentally appropriate combination of finger-to-nose, rapid alternating, and heel-to-shin movements. Abnormalities with the coordination examination such as ataxia, poor coordination and/or balance,

dysmetria or dysdiadochokinesia, should be noted and require further evaluation.

Cranium Examination

The neurologic examination should always include assessment of head shape and OFC until the child is 2 years old (American Academy of Pediatrics Bright Futures) or until 36 months old, per the Centers for Disease Control and Prevention (CDC), and if it appears abnormally large or small in an older child. Inspect the skull for symmetry and shape. Auscultation over the skull or above the eyes may reveal a cranial bruit. Percussion of the skull can give a sound resembling a cracked pot when the sutures are separated, as with increased intracranial pressure. The anterior fontanel should be slightly depressed with very faintly perceived pulsations until its closure between 18 and 24 months.

Autonomic Nervous System

Alterations in blood pressure, sweating, or temperature can be indicators of autonomic nervous system problems.

Meningeal Signs

Evidence of meningeal irritation, such as with meningitis, includes positive Kernig and Brudzinski signs. A Kernig sign is positive if resistance and head or neck pain are elicited when the patient bends over from the waist and touches fingers to toes. In an infant, the Kernig sign can be tested by extending the leg at the knee with the infant lying supine. A positive sign can be as subtle as facial grimacing. A positive Brudzinski sign is evidenced by the patient spontaneously flexing the hip and knees after the examiner passively flexes the neck.

Diagnostic Studies

- Advanced imaging: Computed tomography (CT) scans display differences in density of the intracranial tissues and structures and have a limited spectrum of use as routine study given the large amount of radiation exposure and evidence suggesting risk for neoplasia because of repeated exposure. Magnetic resonance imaging (MRI) provides a higher quality image without radiation exposure and can provide additional information related to structure of the neurologic system (e.g., CNS or spinal cord malformations, tumors). There may be a medical need to order more specific tests, such as a magnetic resonance angiogram/venogram (used to detect blood vessel stenosis and aneurysms), magnetic resonance spectroscopy (used to detect metabolic changes in an isolated location of the brain), functional MRI (used to detect subtle metabolic changes in the brain that indicate how certain parts of the brain are working), or a positron emission tomography scan to assess blood flow, oxygen use, and sugar (glucose) metabolism. A neurologic consultant can advise the best approach.
- Laboratory studies provide indicators of systemic disease, infection, or inflammation. For children taking certain neurologic medications, routine therapeutic drug levels or monitoring for systemic side effects may be needed.
- Genetic testing can be a valuable diagnostic tool for evaluation of etiology of various neurologic disorders (see Chapter 27, Table 27.6).
- Lumbar puncture (LP) provides information about intracranial pressure, metabolism, neurotransmitters, infections, and trauma.

- Electroencephalography (EEG) provides information about the electrical activity of the CNS, which is important in assessing cortical function, risk for seizure, and evaluating for brain death.
- Ultrasonography can be useful in infants to evaluate for intracranial hemorrhage or hydrocephalus.
- Other studies can include polysomnography (helps assess narcolepsy, apnea of infancy, certain movement disorders, nocturnal seizures, obstructive or central sleep apnea and other sleep-related symptoms); electromyography (EMG; tests muscle activity); nerve conduction studies; evoked responses (brainstem—auditory, somatosensory, and visual); electronystagmography (measures eye movements to assess vertigo and postconcussion symptoms); and cerebral arteriography (visualizes cerebral blood vessels to evaluate vascular anomalies and tumors). These studies are typically coordinated in conjunction with specialty care.

Management Strategies

One of the greatest challenges for the PCP is when families remain concerned about a child's development when the PCP findings are within normal limits. When no neurology referral is necessary, the family needs to be reassured, providing them with the anticipated pattern of neurologic development, including timelines and markers that they can use to monitor their child's development. The family should always be given the opportunity to return for further assessment or discussion if concerns remain. The temperament of the child and the child's learned social behavior versus pathologic symptoms may need to be addressed (e.g., breath holding vs. seizures), as well as the presence of an underlying parental issue not being shared (e.g., unreported injury).

Educational Needs

Management strategies should always consider the educational needs of the child. When a neurologic disorder is present, it often affects learning, although neurologic problems are not synonymous with intellectual disability. Sensory problems may affect the child's ability to receive the input necessary for learning. Motor problems may affect both the child's ability to interact with the environment and the ability to communicate. Special infant or preschool early intervention educational programs can assist the child to learn by using the most appropriate learning modalities. Teachers often need assistance in understanding the limitations and strengths of the child. An Individualized Education Program (IEP) or 504 plan may need to be established to support academic success. Parents should be encouraged to develop close communication with the educational staff because this relationship is mutually beneficial for optimizing the learning experience of the child.

Referrals for Other Key Assessments

Many neurologic conditions are inherited conditions. Genetic implications are best communicated through formal genetics counseling. Physical therapy can be useful to help restore or maintain function or to teach new motor skills. The physical therapist should be accustomed to dealing with children. Physical therapy services are often combined with occupational and speech therapy to promote maximal development. For children where concerns about possible cognitive problems exist, referral to neuropsychology for formal cognitive functioning evaluation should be considered. Referral for social services should be considered when this may benefit the child's health, academic success, or wellbeing. Children and families with children who experience multiple comorbidities frequently have ongoing issues with coping, monitoring, and management of medical and financial resources. Medical social workers, public health nurses, and case managers can provide invaluable assistance for these families for continuity and coordination of care.

Medications

A variety of medications are used to control the effects of neurologic problems. Yet, many of these medications are used off-label in children. Most medications require time for the effects to become apparent, need dosage adjustments, and are affected by the metabolism of the individual child. Periodic measurement of therapeutic drug levels is needed for some medications either for dosing decisions or treatment monitoring. Some medications also require monitoring for potential side effects, which need to be weighed against their beneficial effects. Many medications require tapering of dosages when treatment is to be discontinued.

Selected Neurologic Disorders

Headaches

Headache is one of the most common neurologic complaints to present in pediatric primary care or to result in a referral to specialty practices. It is estimated that at least 30% of children experience recurrent headaches and the incidence rate of headaches in children tends to increase as they age.[1] Migraine headaches are the most common type of pediatric headache followed by tension-type headaches.[1] Children with headaches often initially present to the PCP for evaluation, and many of these headaches can be managed in that setting. Since headaches can be indicative of a disorder, a symptom of acute illness, or a musculoskeletal problem, it is imperative for PCPs to have an adequate knowledge related to diagnosing and managing headaches. The exact etiology and physiologic mechanisms remain unknown. What is known is that headaches occur when there is neuronal and perineuronal hyperexcitability of the sodium and calcium channels that leads to a neuroinflammatory response. Pain occurs when intracranial structures experience vasodilation, inflammation, or traction-displacement. Intracranial structures that sense pain include blood vessels and the basal dura mater. The extracranial structures that sense pain include the nerves (e.g., trigeminal nerve), blood vessels, muscles (e.g., trapezius), and the sinuses.

There is strong familial predisposition, as most children with headaches have at least one parent with a history of migraine headaches. Before 10 years of age, the incidence of headache is higher in males than females. During adolescence, females have a higher incidence, with hormonal influences likely playing a role. It is also common for recurrent headaches of any etiology, to become more frequent during adolescence. All children will experience a headache at times; however, headaches that warrant referral to neurology are more commonly seen in middle childhood and adolescence.

Headaches can be considered acute or chronic, based on frequency or duration of symptoms, and are classified into the following categories:
- Primary headache—intrinsic to the brain (migraine, tension-typed headaches, trigeminal cephalalgia)

- Secondary headache—extrinsic to the brain (trauma, infection, vascular, psychiatric)
- Chronic neuropathies (trigeminal neuralgia).

This standardized classification was developed by the International Headache Society. This most current edition of this classification system is the International Classification of Headache Disorders 3rd edition (ICHD-3) and is globally considered to be the most accurate set of guidelines used by clinicians when diagnosing headaches. An overview of the most common types of primary headaches seen in children is listed in Box 41.2.[2] For a more comprehensive overview of headache classification, see the ICHD-3 guidelines (https://ichd-3.org/wp-content/uploads/2018/01/The-International-Classification-of-Headache-Disorders-3rd-Edition-2018.pdf)

History. A thorough history is the single most crucial step when assessing a pediatric patient for headaches and determining the appropriate ICHD-3 headache classification. This history should include:

- Onset—When did the headaches first begin? Does the pain start suddenly or gradually increase? Is there a specific time of day, or day of the week that the headache(s) occur(s), or does this vary?
- Location—Have the child identify where specifically the pain is located. Does the pain always occur in the same place? Ask about radiation. Is it unilateral or bilateral? **NOTE:** Bilateral pain is more commonly reported by younger children versus unilateral pain in adolescents.
- Duration—Inquire about how long the headaches last and about periods without pain between headaches.
- Quality/severity—Have the child describe the nature of the pain using their own words. Frequent headache pain descriptors include throbbing, pulsing, stabbing, aching, squeezing, and sharp. Note: Young children are often unable to precisely describe the quality of pain.
- Frequency—How often are the headaches occurring? Determine if there is any pattern. Has the frequency/pattern increased or how has it changed?
- Associated symptoms—Inquire about what, if any, symptoms occur with the headache, including aura symptoms before the headache. Common associated symptoms include photophobia, phonophobia, nausea, vomiting, dizziness, and blurred vision. Less common associated symptoms that require further inquiry include gait changes, confusion/altered mental status, and hemiplegia.
- Aggravating/alleviating factors—What has the child/family noticed makes the symptoms worse/more likely to occur? What makes them better when they occur? Inquire about medications or other remedies that the family has tried.
- Disability—The level of effect on normal activities should be determined. Questions centered on the number of days the child has missed school or social functions should be included. Standardized tools to assess disability (e.g., Pediatric Migraine Disability Assessment [PedMIDAS]) are available to help gather an accurate picture of the effects on daily life.

Directly eliciting responses from the child during the interview, separate from the parent/caregiver, can be difficult; however, there is great value in doing this. It is important to engage directly with the child and to ask open-ended questions or use drawings to gather the necessary history data. Headache diaries can be helpful.

Lifestyle factors, including:

- Hydration—Inquire about the amount of water/nonwater beverages the child drinks in a day. It is also helpful to inquire about caffeine intake.

• BOX 41.2 Most Common Types of Primary Headaches Seen in Primary Care Settings

Diagnostic Criteria Based on History

Pediatric Migraine Headache

A. More than five attacks fulfilling features of B through D
B. Duration: 2–72 h
C. At least two of the following features:
   1. Bilateral or unilateral (commonly bilateral in young children; unilateral pain usually emerges in late adolescence or early adult life)
      a. Usually frontal/temporal
      b. Occipital location is unusual and should be carefully evaluated (occipital headache in children whether unilateral or bilateral is rare and calls for diagnostic caution; many cases are attributable to structural lesions)
   2. Pulsating quality
   3. Moderate to severe intensity aggravated by routine physical activity
   4. At least one of the following:
      a. Nausea and/or vomiting
      b. Photophobia and phonophobia (can infer from behavior)
   5. Not attributed to another disorder

Infrequent Episodic Tension Type Headache

A. At least 10 episodes occurring on <1 day per month on average (<12 days/year) and fulfilling criteria B through D
B. Headache lasting from 30 min to 7 days
C. Headache has at least two of the following characteristics:
   1. Bilateral location
   2. Pressing/tightening (nonpulsating) quality
   3. Mild or moderate intensity
   4. Not aggravated by routine physical activity, such as walking or climbing stairs
D. Both of the following:
   1. No nausea or vomiting (anorexia may occur)
   2. No more than one of photophobia or phonophobia
E. Not attributed to another ICHD-3 diagnosis

Chronic Tension Headache

A. Headache occurring on 15 days per month on average for >3 months (180 days/year) and fulfilling criteria B through D
B. Headache lasts hours to days or may be continuous
C. Headache has at least two of the following characteristics:
   1. Bilateral location
   2. Pressing/tightening (nonpulsating) quality
   3. Mild or moderate intensity
   4. Not aggravated by routine physical activity such as walking or climbing stairs
D. Both of the following:
   1. No more than one of photophobia, phonophobia, or mild nausea
   2. Neither moderate or severe nausea nor vomiting
E. Not attributed to another ICHD-3 diagnosis

ICHD-3, International Classification of Headache Disorders, 3rd edition.
Modified from Headache Classification Committee of the International Headache Society (IHS) The International Classification of Headache Disorders, 3rd edition. *Cephalgia.* 2018;38(1):1–211.

- Nutrition—A detailed dietary assessment should be completed looking at number of meals eaten in a day, frequency of eating, and nutritional patterns. It can also be helpful to assess risk for diet-related nutritional deficiency and the presence of any restrictive dietary practices.
- Sleep—Inquire about the time the child goes to bed, how long it takes to fall asleep, any waking from sleep, and time the child

wakes in the morning. Specific questions about snoring, tonsillar size, and sleep apnea should be asked. Variation between days (e.g., weekday vs. weekend) should be assessed. The child should be asked whether they feel tired or rested upon waking and asked questions about daytime sleepiness. Sleep hygiene practices, including access to or use of technology devices before sleep should be assessed (see Chapter 16).

- Screen time—Inquire about the amount of time spent in front of a screen during the day. Include nondiscretionary (e.g., school-related work) and discretionary (e.g., phone use, video games, TV) screen time per day.
- Psychologic—Stress and other psychological factors can manifest as physical symptoms and should be included in the assessment. The PCP can consider the use of standardized screening tools for depression and anxiety if warranted.

Physical Examination. A complete physical and neurological examination should be performed. Specific attention should be paid to the following:

- Blood pressure, length/height, weight, and OFC
- Head—general assessment of range of motion and symmetry; palpate and assesses for tenderness/pain of scalp, neck muscles—including at the occipital nerve insertion site, jaw—particularly for temporomandibular joint dysfunction
- Eyes—Check for papilledema and/or painful eye movements
- Sinuses—Ethmoid/maxillary (present at birth); frontal (develops at approximately age 7 years); sphenoid (develop in adolescence)
- Thyroid gland/Delphian node
- Cranial nerve function
- Gait and Romberg
- Deep tendon reflexes

Diagnostic Studies. Neuroimaging with brain MRI or head CT and diagnostic testing, such as an EEG, are not typically indicated for the initial evaluation in most children with headaches; however, imaging should be considered in children who also have a focal neurological deficit on examination, altered mental status with or between headaches, headaches waking the child from sleep, a rapid progression of symptoms, a headache only present with certain body positions, no return to baseline between headaches, or any red flag criteria (Boxes 41.3 and 41.4). Neuroimaging might also be considered in children that have not seen improvement using abortive therapies or at least one prophylactic medication (if clinically indicated) following lifestyle modification. If studies are warranted, a brain MRI is the gold standard provided more urgent imaging evaluation is not needed. Lumbar puncture is typically only necessary in the setting of symptomatic papilledema or suspected infectious etiology, such as meningitis, and warrants urgent evaluation in an appropriate emergency setting, preferably a children's hospital, if available. Imaging should be completed before performing lumbar puncture in these cases. EEG should be considered if there is concern for or suspicion of seizures. Laboratory studies can evaluate for other underlying etiologies (e.g., thyroid dysfunction, iron deficiency anemia).

Differential Diagnosis. It is important that the PCP determine the appropriate headache type based on ICHD-3 criteria, as these criteria guide treatment. In most cases, a thorough history and examination will differentiate between primary and secondary etiologies and further headache subtypes. For primary headache disorders, the ICHD-3 criteria (see Box 41.2) are foundational for headache type differentiation; however, it can be difficult to differentiate between migraine and tension-type headaches in children, particularly in children who are unable to describe the

---

• BOX 41.3 Red Flags Suggestive of Secondary or Pathologic Headaches

- Headache upon awakening from sleep that then fades; increases in frequency and severity over a period of only a few weeks; is persistent and unilateral
- First or worst headache
- Pain that awakens the child from sleep
- Vomiting but not nauseated that may relieve the headache, or intractable vomiting
- Visual disturbances, diplopia, edema of the optic disc (papilledema)
- Increased pain with straining, sneezing, coughing, defecation, or changes in position
- Occipital region and neck pain
- Educational, mental, personality, or behavioral alterations; irritability
- New onset seizures or facial or extremity numbness
- Unsteadiness or dramatic changes in balance, gait abnormalities
- Fever with or without nuchal rigidity
- Family history of neurologic disorders (e.g., brain tumors, neurofibromatosis, vascular malformations)
- Child has a history of a ventriculoperitoneal shunt, meningitis, hydrocephalus, tumor, or prior history of malignancy

From Kacperski, J, Kabbouche MA, O'Brien HL, Weberding JL. The optimal management of headaches in children and adolescents. *Ther Adv Neurol Disord.* 2016;9(1):53–68.

---

nature of their pain. The primary location of the pain (frontal/temporal with migraine vs. occipital/band-like with tension-type) can be helpful. There are certain precursors to migraine headaches that may also be noted in the history, including cyclic vomiting or abdominal migraine (see Chapter 34), benign paroxysmal vertigo, and motion sickness. Children with tension-type headaches may also report sore muscles in the neck and shoulders or have tenderness with palpation of these regions on examination. If the diagnosis remains unclear and the symptoms do not respond to initial intervention, referral to pediatric neurology is the next step.

There are numerous secondary causes of headaches to consider that can be narrowed significantly based on the clinical presentation. Brain lesions are uncommon in pediatric patients presenting with headache as the sole symptom; however, the presence of red flag symptoms (see Boxes 41.3 and 41.4) should prompt further evaluation. Idiopathic intracranial hypertension (IIH), also called *pseudotumor cerebri*, is characterized by headaches in the presence of increased intracranial pressure. This condition is more commonly seen in adolescents and the incidence is higher in females and individuals who are obese. IIH typically presents with headache, vision disturbances, and papilledema on funduscopic examination. Note: Papilledema without other symptoms should be evaluated by ophthalmology with a dilated funduscopic examination to determine the clinical significance.

Children with chronic hypertension may also have headaches, which requires comanagement to see optimal results. Sleep apnea can be contributing factor for headaches and should be of particular concern for children who have snoring or notable pauses in breathing during sleep. Headaches associated with sleep apnea commonly occur upon waking; however, they rarely awaken the child. Tonsillar hypertrophy and/or obesity are risk factors for obstructive sleep apnea (see Chapter 16). Referral to an ENT or sleep medicine specialist should be considered if concern for sleep apnea exists. Medication-overuse headaches result from the overuse of medication used for abortive treatment of headaches, including acetaminophen, nonsteroidal antiinflammatory drugs (NSAIDs), and over-the-counter combination headache

• BOX 41.4 **Red Flags Suggestive of Intracranial Structural Pathology by Age**

Infants
- Full anterior fontanelle
- Open metopic and coronal sutures
- Poor growth
- Impaired upward gaze
- Abnormal head growth
- Shrill cry
- Lethargy
- Vomiting

Children
- Headache described as severe, excruciating of recent onset, unlike any previously experienced headache, no period of normal functioning between episodes, *or* persistent and unilateral
- Papilledema or abnormal eye movements (or one or both eyes suddenly turn in)
- Ataxia, hemiparesis, or abnormal deep tendon reflexes
- Cranial bruits
- Personality changes

medications (e.g., Excedrin), especially when used over 15 days per month. Over time, individuals with medication overuse headache will experience increasing headache symptoms combined with increased medication use. Anxiety and depression are common comorbidities seen in children with headaches. Screening for anxiety and depression can be used to guide clinical decision making; if either are present, referral to a mental health provider to initiate appropriate treatment should be considered as this typically improves clinical outcomes.

Management. Lifestyle modification is central to the management of chronic migraine and tension-type headaches in children. Elements that must be addressed in this modification plan include hydration, nutrition, sleep, technology use, exercise, and stress management. These lifestyle modifications, along with the avoidance of headache triggers, must be in place to allow for further pharmacologic and nonpharmacologic interventions to be effective.

Medications. Medication management can be divided into two categories, abortive and preventive, and is determined by headache frequency and severity. In most cases, abortive therapy is appropriate. It includes nonpharmacologic and pharmacological interventions that should be able to be implemented as soon as the child or parent recognizes the need, wherever the child is (e.g., school, work, extracurricular activities). For the best results, medication should be taken at the onset of the headache or aura symptoms. Medications that are commonly used for abortive therapy are outlined in Table 41.4. NSAIDs, particularly naproxen sodium, tend to be preferable to acetaminophen for first-line abortive therapy, given the increased risk for medication-overuse headache associated with acetaminophen. The use of these medications should be limited to no more than 3 days per week to avoid developing medication-overuse headaches. If these first-line abortive medications are not effective for individuals with migraine headaches, the use of triptans can also be considered. Triptans are not typically prescribed for abortive treatment of tension-type headaches. The provider should factor in patient-specific information and formulary availability when determining the most appropriate triptan to prescribe. In severe cases, the child may need to come into the emergency department to be given IV fluids and medication to stop the headache.

Daily preventive medication is recommended for children who have already made the recommended lifestyle modifications yet continue to have more than four headaches per month. It may also be considered for those who do not respond to abortive therapy or those whose headaches are accompanied by other neurologic symptoms, such as vision loss or hemiplegia. Medications that are commonly used for preventative treatment of migraine headaches are outlined in Table 41.5. Many of these same medications are used to treat tension-type headaches. Despite being commonly used, these medications tend to have lower than typical response rates when compared to placebo and carry the risk for undesirable side effects associated with them.[3] More recent advances in medication therapy for pharmaco-resistant migraine headaches in children include the use of Botox injections and calcitonin gene-related peptide receptor monoclonal antibodies.

Nonpharmacologic Management. There have been recent studies to support the use of nutraceuticals (i.e., products derived from food sources that provide both nutrition and medicinal benefits) in the treatment of pediatric migraine headache daily as a preventative treatment. Magnesium (200–400 mg/day) is a common nutraceutical used for headaches. It is often given in conjunction with other supplements, including riboflavin, coenzyme q10, or butterbur or in combination nutraceuticals (e.g., Migrelief). For children who have difficulty with sleep, melatonin can be considered. Individuals with chronic headaches, particularly those with tension-type headaches, may see improvement in symptoms with massage therapy. Other evidence-based nonpharmacologic therapies include relaxation, biofeedback, mindfulness, meditation, yoga, hypnosis, and cognitive behavioral therapy.[4]

Patient and Parent Education. Education is key to migraine and chronic headache management. A self-administered rescue plan, headache hygiene, and/or lifestyle modifications are essential to maximizing care. Areas to consider include:
- Headache plan: Develop a step-by-step plan for acute headache management and headache hygiene. This plan should include school management. Examples may include ice, rest, or a dark environment.
- Headache diary: Helpful for identifying triggers/monitoring patient progress. Paper and online versions are available (e.g., smartphone app).
- Triggers: Every person's triggers are different, so identify and avoid them as much as possible. Consider dietary (less common in children), physiologic, and environmental possibilities. Physiologic triggers include hormonal changes, emotional anxiety, irregular eating or sleep, and stress. Environmental triggers include weather changes, altitude, lighting, sun exposure, odors, motion, or activity (too little or too much).
- Nutrition: Stress the importance of eating breakfast, three meals a day at regular hours, and not skipping meals. Every meal should contain a protein and be high-fiber and low fat to keep sugar and sodium levels normal.
- Fluid intake: Adequate hydration is imperative. A rule of thumb for hydration should be 1oz water per kilogram of body weight per day plus additional water when physically active. Caffeine should be avoided. Sports drinks without caffeine may help during a headache.
- Sleep: Get plenty of regular sleep (8–12 hours at night) but do not oversleep. Try to go to bed and wake up every day near the same time. Turn off all electronic devices 1 to 2 hours before bedtime. Do not keep phone in bedroom.

TABLE 41.4 Therapies for Acute Pediatric Headache

Drug	Dosage	Side Effects and Comments
Medications (These Should Be Tried First in Acute Management)		
Acetaminophen (gel capsule)	10–15 mg/kg PO every 4 h up to 500 mg every 4 h	For mild to moderate pain, acetaminophen has faster onset of action than ibuprofen
Ibuprofen	7.5–10 mg/kg/dose PO every 6–8 h; maximum daily dose of 2400 mg	Use at onset of attack. Greater headache resolution than acetaminophen (rebound headache can occur) Take with food
Naproxen sodium	Children >2 years old: 5–7 mg/kg PO every 8–12 h Adolescents: 400 mg as initial dose; 200 mg PO every 8–12 h (maximum 1000 mg/24 h)	Safe and effective. Take with food
Ondansetron (Zofran)	Ages 4–11 years old, one 4-mg tablet *or* ODT tablet *or* 5 mL	For vomiting associated with headaches
Migraine-Specific Abortive Acute Medications		
Sumatriptan	Nasal spray: 5 mg/spray; 5 mg for children <40 kg, 10–20 mg for children >40 kg Subcutaneous (self-administered): 0.1 mg/kg for children <40 kg, 4–6 mg for children >40 kg Oral: 12.5–25 mg for children <40 kg, 50–100 mg for children >40 kg	**Children >12 years old with no response to NSAIDs. Tablets are FDA approved for ages 12–17 years.** Other formulations may be used off label. If the first dose is given in the outpatient setting, the patient should be monitored for 1 hour. Do not use in basilar-type and hemiplegic migraine or in those with cardiovascular disease, uncontrolled hypertension, or who have used MAOI in prior 2 weeks. Use with caution in patients who have migraine with aura.
Rizatriptan	Tablet or ODT: 5 mg for children <40 kg, 10 mg for children >40 kg	**FDA approved for children ages 6–17 years.** Do not use in basilar-type and hemiplegic migraine or in those with cardiovascular disease, uncontrolled hypertension, or who have used MAOI in prior 2 weeks. Use with caution in patients who have migraine with aura.
Zolmitriptan	Nasal spray: 2.5 mg for children <40 kg, 5mg for children >40 kg Tablet: Same weight-based dose	**Nasal spray is FDA approved for children ages 12–17 years.** Tablets may be used off label. Do not use in basilar-type and hemiplegic migraine or in those with cardiovascular disease, uncontrolled hypertension, or who have used MAOI in prior 2 weeks. Use with caution in patients who have migraine with aura.
Almotriptan	Tablet: 6.25 mg for children <40 kg, 12.5 mg for children >40 kg	**FDA approved for children ages 12–17 years.** Do not use in basilar-type and hemiplegic migraine or in those with cardiovascular disease, uncontrolled hypertension, or who have used MAOI in prior 2 weeks. Use with caution in patients who have migraine with aura.

FDA, US Food and Drug Administration; *MAOI*, monoamine oxidase inhibitor; *ODT*, orally disintegrating tablet.

- Exercise: Aerobic activity 30 to 60 minutes with increased heart rate and 5 to 10 minutes of stretching most days. Note: Weightlifting does not count toward the aerobic activity goal.
- School: Headaches can result in significant loss of school attendance, but attendance should be mandatory. Develop a home/school headache plan. A quiet rest period may be allowed at school if needed, and school nurses can be helpful in developing a plan. If the child remains home, activities should be restricted to bed and all homework completed. The child should be returned to school if the pain improves during the school day. Minimize attention to the headache.
- Electronic use: Limit discretionary use of devices/screen time (TV, movies, videogames, computer, phones). Use night mode/lowlight setting on devices in the later hours of the day.
- Stress: Plan activities to avoid overcrowded schedules and stressful situations. The child and parents should be taught pain and

stress management techniques, as well as relaxation exercises, including progressive muscle relaxation. If there are issues with posture and neck muscle tension, massage, or warm compresses before stretching can decrease tightness. Rolling the neck area with a tennis or racquetball may also help tight muscles. Referral to a physical therapist is often helpful. Establish a plan as needed for use of other nonpharmacologic management.

Head and Traumatic Brain Injury

Traumatic brain injury (TBI) involves tissue damage to the brain and its surrounding structures. Injury can range from mild to severe and be open or closed. This section focuses on mild TBI and primary care management. Mechanisms for TBIs in children include both the primary injury and secondary injury related to acceleration-deceleration or rotational forces. Injuries are

TABLE 41.5 Prophylactic Therapies for Pediatric Migraine

Drug	Dosage	Side Effects and Comments
Antidepressants		
Amitriptyline	0.25 mg/kg/day PO at bedtime; may increase dose by 0.25 mg/kg/day every 2 weeks; maximum dosage 1 mg/kg/day	One of the most widely used agents, but off-label. **Use with caution in children <12 years old** and with immediate family history or patient risk for bipolar disorder. Order ECG if dosage exceeds 25 mg/day. Adverse effects: somnolence, dry mouth, dysrhythmia.
Antiseizure Medications		
Divalproex sodium	Dosage depends on preparation and age—consult pharmacology reference	**Not for use in children younger than 3 years.** Adverse effects: weight gain, tremor, hair loss, dizziness. Risk for hepatotoxicity and bone marrow suppression
Topiramate	Adolescent/adult immediate release oral preparation: initially 25 mg once daily (in evening); may increase weekly by 25 mg daily up to 100 mg daily	Extended-release formulations available may reduce side effects if present with standard formulation. Adverse effects: weight loss, episodes of paresthesia, cognitive slowing, loss of appetite, dizziness, irritability; monitor any change in school/cognitive performance.
Antiserotonergic Agents		
Cyproheptadine	Not recommended <2 years old ≥3 years and adolescents: 0.2–0.4 mg/kg/day divided in two equal doses; can also be given as a once daily dose at bedtime	**Most effective in children ages 3–12 years.** Adverse effects: weight gain (due to appetite stimulation), dry mouth and somnolence; sedation more problematic at doses higher than 4–8 mg/24 h.
Antihypertensives		
Propranol	35 kg: 10–20 mg 3 times a day >35 kg: 20–40 mg 3 times a day Adults: 80 mg/day divided every 6–8 h with a maximum of 160–240 mg/day in divided doses every 6–8 h	May take several weeks to a month to be effective. Do not use in children with history of asthma; use with caution in children with depression. Adverse effects: lowers blood pressure, depressive effects or exercise-induced asthma.

Maintain use for at least 4–6 months and then wean slowly.

5-HT, 5-Hydroxtryptamine; *ECG,* electrocardiogram; *PO,* per os (by mouth, orally); *prn,* as needed.

Data from Chawla J. Migraine headache medication, Medscape; 2021. http://emedicine.medscape.com/article/1142556-medication#2; Hershey AD. Migraine. In: Kliegman RM, Stanton BF, St. Geme JW, et al., eds. *Nelson Textbook of Pediatrics.* 21st ed. Elsevier; 2019:2040–2045; and Taketomo CK, Hodding JH, Kraus DM. *Pediatric & Neonatal Dosage Handbook.* 21st ed. Lexi-Comp; 2014.

characterized by damage to the vasculature, cortex, white matter and/or the deep cerebral structures. Typically, open head trauma produces more focal injuries, while closed head trauma causes multifocal or diffuse damage. Secondary effects of trauma may include hypoxia, ischemia, hypotension, brain swelling, hemorrhage, contusion, and seizures.

Common causes of TBI include falls, sports-related injuries, motor vehicle accidents, assault, and being struck by or against objects. There are higher incidence rates of TBI among males. Varying degrees of disability result from TBI. Influencing factors that may correlate with degree of disability include severity of injury, recurrence of injury, mechanism of injury, and access to care following injury.

One determinant of brain injury severity is the Glasgow Coma Scale (GCS) score (Table 41.6). When using GCS to estimate severity of injury, typically a GCS of 13 to 15 is considered mild TBI (mTBI), 9 to 12 considered moderate TBI, and 8 or less considered severe TBI. Other clinical factors should be considered in evaluating the overall clinical picture when determining brain injury severity (Table 41.7). The most common type of mTBI is concussion, which is often managed in the primary care setting.

History. Symptoms of mTBI can mimic those of other medical conditions, thus making the diagnosis challenging. An evidence-based assessment tool (see Chapter 18) should be used. These tools include:

- History of how injury occurred, cause, body part affected, forces, and circumstances. If injury involved a fall, the height from which the child fell.
- Specific symptoms occurring at the time of injury, including loss of/alteration in consciousness
- Any physical, cognitive, emotional, or sleep (Table 41.8) changes.

Nonaccidental trauma should be suspected when a head injury is present without a history of a fall or with a history of a fall from a relatively low height (less than 4 feet). It is also recommended that a skeletal survey be obtained in children younger than 3 years, because younger children are at higher risk for skeletal trauma as well (see Chapter 22).

Physical Examination.

- Assess vital signs. Changes may indicate more significant systemic or neurologic involvement.
- Perform a thorough physical examination, including a careful neurologic examination that includes level of consciousness, mental status, motor function (both gross and fine motor), sensory function, CN functioning, and reflexes.
- Calculate the GCS score (see Table 41.6).

TABLE 41.6	**Pediatric Glasgow Coma Scale**		

	>1 Year	<1 Year	Score[a]
Eye opening	Spontaneously	Spontaneously	4
	To verbal command	To shout	3
	To pain	To pain	2
	No response	No response	1
Motor response	Obeys	Spontaneous	6
	Localizes pain	Localizes pain	5
	Flexion-withdrawal	Flexion-withdrawal	4
	Flexion-abnormal (decorticate rigidity)	Flexion-abnormal (decorticate rigidity)	3
	Extension (decerebrate rigidity)	Extension (decerebrate rigidity)	2
	No response	No response	1

	>5 Years	2–5 Years	0–23 Months	
Verbal response	Oriented	Appropriate words/phrases	Smiles/coos appropriately	5
	Disoriented/confused	Inappropriate words	Cries and is consolable	4
	Inappropriate words	Persistent cries and screams	Persistent inappropriate crying and/or screaming	3
	Incomprehensible sounds	Grunts	Grunts, agitated, and restless	2
	No response	No response	No response	1

[a]Total score = (E+M+ V); max = 15; min = 3.

TABLE 41.7	**Classification of Head Injuries Based on Key Characteristics**			

Classification	Glasgow Coma Scale[a]	Neurologic Focal Deficit[b]	Loss of Consciousness	Other Neurologic Findings
Mild	13–15	No	No or brief loss (<30 min)	May have linear skull fractures
Moderate	9–12	Focal signs	Variable loss	May have depressed skull fracture or intracranial hematoma
Severe	≤8	Focal signs	Prolonged loss	Often have depressed skull fractures and intracranial hematoma

[a]Either initial or subsequent scores.
[b]Neurologic focal deficit (e.g., hemiparesis, reflex asymmetry, Babinski sign, abnormal cranial nerve findings).

- Evaluation of concussion symptoms. Standardized assessments (e.g., Sport Concussion Assessment Tool [SCAT5]) offer guidance for assessment of some of these symptoms; particularly those in the physical and cognitive domains.
  Child SCAT5 (ages 5–12 years): https://bjsm.bmj.com/content/bjsports/early/2017/04/26/bjsports-2017-097492childscat5.full.pdf
  SCAT5 (ages 13+ years):
  https://bjsm.bmj.com/content/bjsports/early/2017/04/26/bjsports-2017-097506SCAT5.full.pdf
- Examine for other signs of trauma, such as neck injury, internal abdominal injuries, or bone fractures. **NOTE:** Periorbital hemorrhage ("raccoon-eyes"), ecchymosis behind the ear ("Battle's sign"), blood behind the eardrum, and bleeding from the ears or nose indicate a basilar skull fracture and warrant immediate attention in an Emergency Department (ED).

Diagnostic Studies. The severity of trauma dictates the need for diagnostic studies. When considering imaging, algorithms can help direct decision making (e.g., PECARN Algorithm).[5] Other than severity, indications for neuroimaging include:
- Penetrating trauma, depressed skull fracture, or signs of basilar injury
- Amnesia about the injury
- Focal neurologic signs or deficit
- Persistent vomiting or seizures
- History of coagulopathy.

TABLE 41.8 **Mild Traumatic Brain Injury (Concussion) Symptoms**

Physical	Cognitive	Emotional	Sleep
Headache	Confusion	Abnormal irritability	Drowsiness
Nausea/vomiting	Altered concentration	Feelings of sadness or being "emotional"	Insomnia or hypersomnia
Difficulty with balance	Mental torpor	Abnormal feelings of being nervous	Difficulty falling asleep
Changes in vision	Altered memory		
Dizziness	Forgetfulness (especially conversations or recent events)		
Light or sound sensitivity	Needs to repeat or slowly answer questions		
Paresthesias			
Feelings of being dazed or stunned			

Modified from Centers for Disease Control and Prevention (CDC). Heads up: facts for physicians about mild traumatic brain injury (MTBI). https://www.cdc.gov/headsup/partners/index.html.

CT is the preferred imaging technique for emergency situations, because it can be obtained rapidly, and the child can be monitored easily. Acute hemorrhage is more easily detected by CT (without contrast) than by MRI. If CT is ordered after several days (3 or more days past injury), it should be done both with and without contrast to pick up extravasated blood if present. CT can reveal brain edema, midline displacements, hydrocephalus, loss of brain tissue, and most skull fractures. The greatest risk with head CT, particularly with repeated imaging, is concentrated radiation exposure. In nonemergent settings, MRI can be considered if more detailed visualization is needed of intracranial structures; however, young children typically require sedation for this test. It is not uncommon to find incidental findings, so the PCP must be confident in determining which findings correlate clinically with the patient's presenting symptoms.

Differential Diagnosis. Differentiating minor head trauma that will resolve on its own from more extensive brain injury is challenging, as mild nonspecific clinical signs are of limited predictive value. Most children with headache, lethargy, or vomiting after mTBI do not have demonstrable intracranial injury, but the PCP must assess for symptoms of more significant head injury. Symptoms and/events that precede the injury may provide clues for underlying etiology.

Management. With mTBI, the level of consciousness is a key determinant of next steps. Prompt identification of a deteriorating level of consciousness and access to emergent medical or surgical evaluation and intervention are essential components of the management plan. Initial observation in a primary care setting, urgent care, or ED setting, followed by home observation under the care of a parent/caregiver who understands what urgent signs and symptoms to observe for and can quickly access emergency medical services if needed is recommended. Most children will see symptom improvement within 1 to 6 weeks following injury if managed appropriately. This initial management typically will include restrictions on both physical activity and activities with increased cognitive demand. Once symptoms resolve, return to activity is allowed following a stepwise return-to-play plan (see Chapter 18). Symptoms may be more prolonged in subsequent head injuries. At any point, if symptoms deteriorate or become more suggestive of more severe injury, urgent evaluation in an emergency or specialty care area should be completed. Symptoms that persist beyond 6 weeks following injury should be evaluated by a specialist. Additional details related to mTBI management can be found in Chapter 18.

Complications. Initial complications can include posttraumatic seizures, cerebral contusion, epidural hematoma, subdural hematoma, intracerebral hematoma, subarachnoid hemorrhage, acute brain swelling, and structural damage secondary to penetrating injuries. Second impact syndrome (SIS) occurs when the brain swells catastrophically after a person sustains a second mTBI before resolution of symptoms from a previous injury. The second impact can occur any time after an initial mTBI and can lead to catastrophic results. Intracranial lesions, particularly epidural hematomas, are life-threatening and require urgent intervention. Features indicative of serious injury include prolonged loss of consciousness, persistent vomiting, altered level of consciousness, seizures, unequal pupil size, focal neurologic examination findings, severe headache, and GCS less than 15. While mTBI generally has no residual physical deficit, subtle cognitive, emotional, or sleep deficits may persist from weeks to months. A neuropsychological evaluation may be helpful to plan appropriate educational and behavioral management for selective cases of mTBI, especially when symptoms persist. Collaboration between the healthcare team and school can be beneficial. The treatment plan must be communicated to school personnel and should identify a gradual stepwise return to school and activities, with any modifications clearly defined.

Patient and Parent Education. It can be helpful to provide parents/caregivers with written education materials and make every effort to ensure they understand instructions for postinjury care and the indications for immediate follow-up (Box 41.5). Parents should also be advised that symptoms typically occur within the first 3 days following injury, but some symptoms may not become more noticeable for days or weeks. Long-term complications following mTBI may be present in any of the primary symptom domains. Any symptom that lasts longer than 6 weeks should be evaluated by a specialist. Neuropsychological prescreening should be completed as a baseline measure before participation in sports or other activities that may result in head injury. This allows for subsequent comparative evaluation of neurocognitive functioning following head injury.

Prevention.

- Use appropriate seat restraints when riding in motor vehicles.
- Protect children from falls in the home or from playground equipment. Advise families of risks associated with residential trampolines.
- Wear helmets when using bicycles, skateboards, scooters, motorcycles, inline skates, snowboarding, skiing, and when appropriate for sports participation. The proper fitting/upkeep of helmets are important.
- Ensure that sports teams and trainers use appropriate helmets and training equipment to help prevent head injury and follow state laws regarding mTBI prevention.

Epileptic Paroxysmal Events

Epilepsy

Epilepsy is a neurologic disorder characterized by recurrent unprovoked seizures. A seizure is an event caused by an abnormal electrical signal arising from within the cerebral cortex. Seizures can present in many ways, but the two primary types of seizures are generalized (arising across the cortex) and focal (arising from one specific area of the cortex). The International League Against Epilepsy (ILAE) created a system for classification of seizure types and presentation (Fig. 41.3)[6] and PCPs should be familiar with them. The diagnostic criteria for epilepsy is a single unprovoked seizure with a known increased risk for future provoked seizures OR two unprovoked seizures that occur greater than 24 hours apart OR diagnosis of an epilepsy syndrome.[7] The ILAE has also published a classification of the different types of epilepsies (Fig. 41.4).[8] It is important for providers to remember that epilepsy is a clinical diagnosis based on the aforementioned criteria. Although diagnostic studies can be of great value, the diagnosis itself is most often based on historical and physical findings.

History. Questions should include:

- Description of the seizure: Focal or generalized (if known), semiology (presentation characteristics of the seizure), loss of consciousness, aura, length of postictal sleep or confusion, duration of the episode, history of prior seizures and associated illness or injury.
- Underlying or concurrent medical diagnosis (e.g., diabetes, renal disease, cardiovascular disorder).
- Previous CNS infection or head trauma.
- Intrauterine infection, birth trauma, bleeding.
- Toxic exposure(s) or drug use/abuse.
- Antiseizure medication adherence (stopped abruptly, doses missed); changes in drug manufacturer, change to generic from name brand.
- Family history of seizures.
- History of developmental or learning delay or regression.

Physical Examination. The following elements should be determined:

- Weakness or focal abnormalities on the neurologic examination.

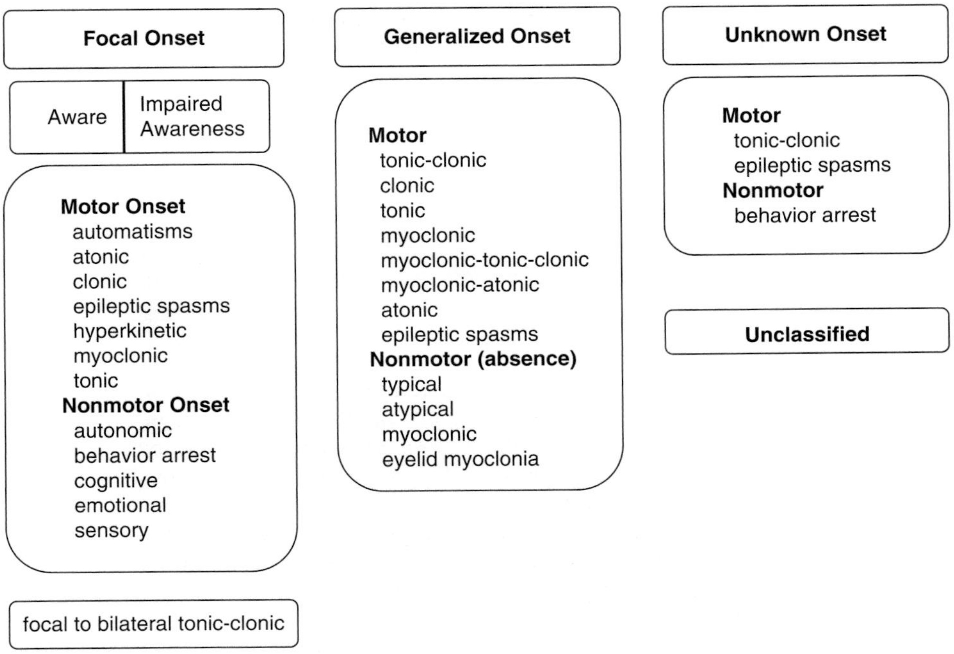

• **BOX 41.5** **Head Injury Education Key Points for Parents**

Contact the PCP or take the child to an ED if the following symptoms are observed:

- Increased drowsiness, sleepiness, inability to wake up, unconsciousness
- Vomiting more than twice
- Neck pain
- Watery or bloody drainage from ear or nose
- Seizures or fainting
- Unusual irritability, personality change, confusion, or any unusual behavior
- Headache that gets worse or lasts more than a day
- Unequal pupils, blurred vision, abnormal or changing hearing, or speech
- Gait abnormality (e.g., clumsiness or stumbling), weakness of any muscle of arms, legs, or face

---

Focal Onset	Generalized Onset	Unknown Onset
Aware / Impaired Awareness	**Motor** tonic-clonic clonic tonic myoclonic myoclonic-tonic-clonic myoclonic-atonic atonic epileptic spasms **Nonmotor (absence)** typical atypical myoclonic eyelid myoclonia	**Motor** tonic-clonic epileptic spasms **Nonmotor** behavior arrest
Motor Onset automatisms atonic clonic epileptic spasms hyperkinetic myoclonic tonic **Nonmotor Onset** autonomic behavior arrest cognitive emotional sensory		**Unclassified**

focal to bilateral tonic-clonic

• **Fig. 41.3** ILEA 2017 Classification of Seizure Types. (From Fisher RS. An overview of the 2017 ILAE operational classification of seizure types. *Epilepsy Behav.* 2017;70:271–273.)

- Presence of seizure activity during the examination.
- Hypertension.
- Signs of systemic disease or cardiovascular disorder.
- Skin findings suggestive of neurocutaneous syndromes (i.e., café-au-lait macules, ash leaf spots, hypopigmented macules, or facial hemangiomas).
- Signs of head trauma.
- Transillumination of the skull in infants.
- For children presenting with "staring spells" that are questionable for childhood absence epilepsy (CAE), the PCP can perform 2 to 3 minutes of hyperventilation using a pinwheel or similar object, which will often provoke a seizure, which is diagnostic for CAE. Note: Appropriate safety precautions should be taken before performing this, and the child and family should also be informed of the intent before proceeding.

Diagnostic Studies. The most common diagnostic studies include:

- Complete blood count (CBC), including platelets.
- Liver function tests (LFTs)—useful for diagnostic purposes or as a baseline before antiseizure medication (ASM) therapy is started.
- Metabolic screen, including blood glucose.
- Urine/serum toxicology—only if illicit drug exposure is suspected.
- Genetic testing—expanding use in epilepsy assessment (see Chapter 27; Table 27.6).
- LP—when child is younger than 6 months; at any age for child with persistent changes in mental status or failure to return to baseline functioning; at any age for child with meningeal signs.
- EEG—standard in all children after first unprovoked seizure. An abnormal EEG supports the diagnosis and can be useful in differentiating the type of epilepsy; however, a normal EEG when the child is not seizing does not rule out epilepsy. Video electroencephalogram (VEEG) over 1 to 6 days is an option to help characterize events concerning for seizures.
- MRI—imaging studies are not routinely indicated for generalized seizures provided the seizure is followed by a normal neurologic examination and return to baseline mental status. Imaging is recommended: (1) following a focal seizure or if the EEG reveals focal electrographic abnormality; (2) if the patient demonstrates cognitive changes after several hours and postictal focal dysfunction (signs of increased intracranial pressure, such as found with tumors, abscesses, strokes, or vascular malformations); (3) if the seizure lasted more than 15 minutes; (4) in infants younger than 6 months old; and (5) if any new onset of focal neurologic deficit has occurred.
- CT scan—used only in emergent cases of marked cognitive, motor, or neurologic dysfunction of unknown etiology.
- Polysomnography can be useful to assess symptoms occurring during sleep.

Differential Diagnosis. Among the differential, the PCP should consider breath-holding spells, inattentive staring, benign movements (e.g., sleep myoclonus, infant jitteriness), self-stimulation, tantrums, cyclic vomiting, benign paroxysmal vertigo (BPV), syncope, migraine headaches, gastroesophageal reflux, night terrors, conversion disorder, nonepileptic seizures, metabolic problems, tumors, other CNS problems, or a cardiovascular problem. Tics are involuntary, spasmodic, nonrhythmic, repetitive movements, but not associated with impaired consciousness and can be suppressed by the patient.

Management. If the PCP suspects epilepsy, refer to a provider with expertise in child neurology for further workup, diagnosis, and initiation of treatment. The PCP can then collaborate as a member of the interprofessional team, providing ongoing monitoring, managing ASM renewal, monitoring laboratory studies, and case management.

Medications. Medication is generally the first-line treatment with the goal being no seizures and no side effect (Table 41.9). ASM selection should be individualized based on type of epilepsy but should also account for potential side effects, medical history, sex, and age. Medication information, including potential side effects, should be reviewed with the patient and family before initiating therapy. For children who do not respond to treatment with two ASMs (achieving maximum therapeutic dose with continued seizures), their epilepsy is intractable. Exploring additional nonpharmacologic treatment options should be considered for intractable epilepsy.

Therapeutic considerations include medication adherence, the presence of side effects, and therapeutic drug level when appropriate. Key points to consider include:

- Some children can be controlled with subtherapeutic blood levels, while others experience seizure control and freedom from side effects at levels beyond the therapeutic range.

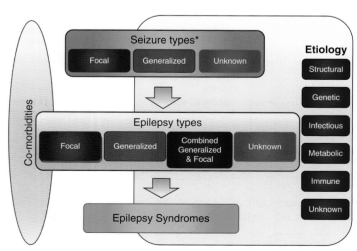

• **Fig. 41.4** Framework for the Classification of Seizures. *Denotes onset of seizures. (From Scheffer IE, Berkovic S, Capovilla G, et al. ILAE classification of the epilepsies: position paper of the ILAE Commission for Classification and Terminology. *Epilepsia*. 2017;58:512–521.)

TABLE 41.9	Common Antiseizure Medications Used in Children				
Medication	**Seizure Type**	**Metabolism**	**Drug Level**	**Common (Severe) Adverse Effects**
Levetiracetam	Focal, generalized	Enzymatic hydrolysis	6–20 mg/L	Mood changes, headache, **significant aggression or depression**
Lamotrigine	Focal, generalized	Liver	1–15 mg/L	Somnolence, headache, dizziness, **Stevens-Johnson syndrome (SJS)**
Oxcarbazepine	Focal	Liver	13–28 mg/L	Hyponatremia, dizziness, ataxia, drowsiness, **SJS, blood cell count changes**
Topiramate	Focal, generalized	Liver	2–25 mg/L	Paresthesia, weight loss, cognitive change, renal stones, **glaucoma, metabolic acidosis**
Lacosamide	Focal, generalized	Liver	5–10 mcg/mL	Dizziness, headache, vision change, ataxia, **syncope, arrhythmia, suicide**
Valproic acid	Focal, generalized	Liver	50–100 mcg/mL	Weight gain, tremor, hair loss, liver toxicity, pancreatitis, bone marrow suppression
Ethosuximide	Childhood absence epilepsy	Liver	40–100 mcg/mL	Upset stomach, headache, weight gain, **blood cell count changes, SJS**
Carbamazepine	Focal	Liver	4–12 mcg/mL	Tiredness, dizziness, photosensitivity reaction, **SJS, hypersensitivity**
Phenobarbital	Neonatal seizures, status epilepticus	Liver	15–40 mcg/mL	Sleep change, sedation, gastrointestinal symptoms, **irreversible cognitive change, blood cell count changes, SJS**

NOTE: **bold** denotes severe effects.

- Half-lives can be longer when new ASMs are introduced or when other non-ASMs (e.g., antibiotics, contraceptives) are being taken. Steady state concentrations (and elimination) of the drug are achieved at five half-lives.
- If gastrointestinal side effects occur, consider changing to an enteric-coated pill or taking the medication after eating. Decreasing the dosage, while increasing the frequency may help; however, administration of ASMs no more than twice daily can achieve better adherence.
- The first signs of toxicity usually include sedation, as well as changes in behavior, cognition, and/or balance. Note: Some children may exhibit these changes yet have drug levels within the normal range.
- Metabolites of the drugs can cause hypersensitivity side effects.
- Monitor routine drug levels, with trough levels for some ASMs (e.g., valproic acid).
- Some herbal products (e.g., kava kava) may interfere with seizure control.

For many children, it may be possible to taper medication if the child is able to go 2 years without a seizure. Historically, child neurology providers obtain an EEG before medication withdrawal, but recent literature suggests that this test may not be necessary. Some children are not considered candidates for ASM withdrawal based on type of epilepsy, etiology, or examination/diagnostic findings, but the decision is very individual. Most ASMs can be tapered for withdrawal over a period of 6 to 8 weeks, but timing should be reviewed before beginning taper.[9] Only one ASM should be withdrawn at a time. If seizures recur, which is most likely within the first 6 months, ASM therapy is resumed, typically the same medication and dose before withdrawal. Epilepsy can be considered resolved when a child is able to go for 10 years without a seizure, and 5 of those 10 years being off medication.[7]

Nonpharmacologic Options: Ketogenic Diet. The ketogenic diet should be considered for children with intractable epilepsy, particularly if they are not a surgical candidate, or as a first-line treatment for specific types of epilepsy, such as GLUT1 transporter deficiency. It is a rigid diet that allows for high ratios of fat to protein plus carbohydrates to transform the body's primary source of energy from glucose to ketones (ketosis). The traditional ketogenic diet ratio is 4:1, but more recently, lesser ratios have been implemented successfully. Strict adherence to the prescribed ratio is necessary as deviation can result in breakthrough seizures. The ketogenic diet is typically comanaged with a pediatric neurologist and a dietician with special knowledge related to the ketogenic diet. Children must be screened for growth and nutritional status before starting the ketogenic diet and many centers also screen families to determine if they have the capability and resources to follow the diet. Accordingly, the ketogenic diet is typically initiated in the hospital setting to allow for more extensive education and monitoring, but outpatient initiation is possible under the right conditions. Side effects of the ketogenic diet include potential vitamin and mineral deficiencies (e.g., calcium, vitamin D, magnesium, phosphorous), abdominal pain, constipation or diarrhea, fatigue, slowed growth, and renal stones.

Surgical Interventions. Surgical intervention can be another effective nonpharmacologic treatment option for intractable epilepsy and is now considered earlier in the treatment process than it was in the past. There are a variety of surgical options that can be considered and are individualized based on the patient. These can range from resection of a seizure focus or hemisphere, which is sometimes curative, to more palliative procedures that disrupt pathways in the brain, such as with a corpus callosotomy or multiple subpial transection. Laser ablation is an emerging option available at select centers and can provide exceptional outcomes for appropriate candidates. Postoperatively, some children will be able to reduce the number of ASMs they are taking, but this is not always the case.

An additional surgical option is implantation of a vagus nerve stimulator (VNS). This option can be considered for intractable epilepsies, particularly for those that may not be candidates for other surgical intervention. The VNS is an implanted device where the generator is typically placed in the left anterior chest wall inferior to the clavicle. A wire lead is then run from the device and coiled around the ipsilateral vagus nerve. While the mechanism is not entirely well understood, electrical impulses are sent regularly from the generator up the vagus nerve to the brain. Many patients with a VNS see improvement in seizure control and some decrease ASM use. The VNS also has a magnet that can be swiped across the generator in case of a prolonged seizure to function as a rescue option that stops the seizure. Device programming can be done in the office setting and standard dosing increments are available from the device manufacturer.

Counseling. It is important that family members understand the diagnosis, treatment, plan for follow-up and prognosis. For the child, information should be presented in an age-appropriate manner. Children can experience psychosocial stress surrounding their diagnosis, and all providers should assess the stress level and the child's coping skills. Parents are encouraged to treat the child as they normally would. Support groups or similar resources can be helpful to both children and their families. Many ASMs are teratogenic; therefore contraception education is essential for females of childbearing age. It is equally important to consider and counsel patients about potential effects of ASMs on contraceptives and vice versa.

Safety. Uncontrolled seizures can present safety hazards. The child and family need to consider situations that the child will be in and be sure that someone knows what to do if a seizure occurs, including school personnel. Seizure first aid should be taught to family members. Swimming alone is never recommended, but swimming, contact sports, and climbing are allowed if the child is well controlled and there is supervision. Children should wear a helmet any time they are riding anything with wheels (e.g., bike, skateboard, scooter, skates). If falls and head injury occur frequently, safety helmets worn at all times are sometimes warranted. While driving laws vary by state, it is generally recommended that adolescents be restricted from driving until they have been seizure-free for 6 months.

Immunizations. For the PCP, consultation with the child's neurology provider is advised, as the CDC recommends deferring Diphtheria-Tetanus-Pertussis vaccine (DTaP) until a child's neurologic status is clarified and stabilized from a known progressive neurologic disorder, such as infantile spasms, uncontrolled epilepsy, or progressive encephalopathy. This vaccine is contraindicated in children who have experienced encephalopathy (e.g., coma, decreased level of consciousness, or prolonged seizures) not attributable to another identifiable cause within 7 days of administration of a previous dose of DTaP.[10]

Complications. Status epilepticus (SE) refers to a seizure that lasts for greater than 30 minutes or multiple seizures without recovery between events. It is classified as *convulsive* or *nonconvulsive* SE based on clinical presentation. A child who has convulsive SE is at increased risk for morbidity and mortality due to lack of oxygenation, decreased cerebral perfusion, metabolic acidosis, hypoglycemia, hyperkalemia, lactic acidosis, increased temperature, and increased intracranial pressure. Such an occurrence needs to be handled as a medical emergency. It can be

triggered by an acute brain infection, progressive neurologic disease, medication failure or nonadherence, electrolyte imbalance, or rarely, a febrile seizure in an otherwise healthy child without other risk factors. Other adverse outcomes can include behavioral problems, acquired intellectual disability, focal deficits, and death. Administration of a rescue medication in the prehospital setting is recommended. Medications that are commonly used for this purpose include rectal diazepam, intranasal midazolam, or buccal clonazepam. Most children with epilepsy should have a rescue medication prescribed to be given by parents/caregivers (including school personnel) for prolonged or clustered seizures in the prehospital setting. Patients who are given a rescue medication should be evaluated by a healthcare provider following administration.

Sleep-Related Epilepsy

Some children present with seizures that appear to occur during sleep. While a complete clinical history can distinguish seizures from parasomnias, there is one sleep-associated epilepsy that can be challenging to differentiate from parasomnias—sleep-related hypermotor epilepsy (SHE). SHE can be inherited (autosomal dominant) or occur sporadically, and the events can be more complex than typical seizures with vocalizations, complex automatisms, and ambulation. Routine EEG and MRI often show no abnormality and the events can often mimic parasomnias. The patient typically wakes up fully after the event, has recollection of the event, and often experiences academic decline, which is not consistent with parasomnias where the patient has amnesia and sleeps through the event. The Frontal Lobe Epilepsy and Parasomnias scale can be adapted for use in children to help differentiate SHE from parasomnias.[11]

Febrile Seizures

Febrile seizures are the most common type of seizures in childhood and occur in up to 5% of children. It is a seizure that occurs in conjunction with a fever. The fever is typically defined as 38°C and can appear before or after the seizure. Febrile seizures typically occur between the 6 and 60 months of age. Seizures with fever outside these age parameters warrant further evaluation. Febrile seizures can be classified as either simple or complex. *Simple* febrile seizures present as generalized seizures and last for less than 15 minutes. *Complex* febrile seizures present with generalized or focal seizures, lasting more than 15 minutes, and/or with clustering of seizures (i.e., multiple seizures without recovery between). In rare cases, children may experience febrile status epilepticus (i.e., seizure lasting >30 minutes), which rarely stops spontaneously and requires prompt intervention. Children in febrile SE warrant prompt attention and often require medications to end the seizure. The etiology of febrile seizures is unclear and excludes seizures that are caused by intracranial illness or are related to an underlying CNS problem. The risk is higher in children with a family history for febrile seizures or in those with predisposing factors (e.g., neonatal intensive care unit [NICU] stay more than 28 days, developmental delay, daycare attendance). Nearly two-thirds of children with febrile seizure will experience one isolated febrile seizure without recurrence. Risk factors for recurrence include: first febrile seizure before 18 months of age, low degree of temperature at time of the seizure, fever does not present until after the seizure, or family history of febrile seizures.

History. The history should include:
- Description of seizure, type (generalized vs. focal), duration, frequency in 24 hours
- Relationship of the seizure to a febrile episode and degree of temperature

- Any abnormal neurologic findings noted *before* the seizure (not consistent with febrile seizure)
- Family history of seizures, include febrile seizures
- Maternal smoking in the perinatal period
- Prematurity or neonatal hospitalizations for more than 28 days
- Parents' perception of development of child

Physical Examination. The physical examination is the same as for epilepsy.

Diagnostic Studies. Diagnostic studies include:
- EEG should be performed for all *complex* febrile seizures; not typically indicated for simple febrile seizures.
- MRI for *complex* febrile seizure or for focal examination findings
- LP if history and physical examination (H&P) suggest acute bacterial meningitis or other CNS infection
- No standard laboratory studies; however, age, sex, and findings from the H&P should direct decision-making.

Differential Diagnosis. Consider sepsis, meningitis, metabolic or toxic encephalopathies, hypoglycemia, anoxia, trauma, tumor, and hemorrhage. Febrile delirium and febrile shivering can be confused with seizures. Breath-holding spells can mimic febrile seizures; however, breath-holding is always provoked by crying or tantrums. Epileptic seizures are unprovoked but may occur during an illness.

Management. Routine *seizure first aid* should be initiated as follows:
- Protect the airway, breathing, and circulation if the seizure is still occurring. Place the child in a side-lying position to prevent aspiration or airway obstruction.
- Do not put anything into the child's mouth during the seizure.
- Time the duration of the seizure. For seizures lasting greater than 5 minutes, call 911.

Fever management:
- Reduce the fever with acetaminophen or ibuprofen (oral or suppository) after the seizure has stopped, although the use of antipyretics will not necessarily prevent another febrile seizure. Prophylactic pharmacologic management is not indicated.

Providers can prescribe a rescue medication to be used for prolonged febrile seizures or clusters of febrile seizures in the prehospital setting. Antipyretics can reduce the discomfort associated with a fever, but there is no conclusive evidence to suggest that these alter the risk of having another febrile seizure.

Patient and Parent Education. Families need information about febrile seizures, risks, seizure first aid, and management. Education should include risk factors for recurrence, reassurance that nothing can be done to prevent the seizures, and that no long-term consequences are associated with simple febrile seizures and most complex febrile seizures. The PCP can reassure parents that simple febrile seizures are adequately managed in the primary care setting; however, with complex febrile seizures, further evaluation and/or referral may be warranted.

Complications. Persisting motor intellectual/learning deficits and/or death do not occur in patients with febrile seizures outside of febrile SE. Children with complex febrile seizures may have a slightly increased risk to develop epilepsy later in life.

Nonepileptic Paroxysmal Events

Psychogenic Nonepileptic Seizures

Psychogenic nonepileptic seizures (PNES), a common manifestation of conversion disorder in children, may be difficult to distinguish from epileptic seizures, even with direct observation. Further, children with PNES often have an existing diagnosis of epilepsy, making the diagnostic evaluation process much more complicated. In such cases, PNES can serve as attention-seeking behaviors for the child who misses the attention gained before seizure control was achieved with their epilepsy diagnosis. PNES is most commonly seen in adolescent females.[12] Psychosocial stressors and/or traumatic events are often revealed when obtaining a comprehensive history. Distinguishing characteristics of PNES include:
- Uni- or bi-laterally coordinated motor activity (e.g., thrashing, jerking, scissor-like movements), rather than characteristic tonic-clonic movements.
- No aura or malaise; positive for heart palpitations or feeling like choking before seizure.
- Occur *only* before a witness; most often at home; do not interrupt play, may occur at school; situation specific.
- On physical examination: pupils equal, round, reactive to light and accommodation (PERRLA); no associated tongue biting or injury.
- Gradual onset, with abrupt recovery—no postictal state.
- Discomfort/distress expressed; occasional ataxia/fumbling; consciousness may be impaired, but the patient is not unconscious.
- No incontinence.
- No EEG changes, even during episodes.

If suspected, but the history is unclear, a VEEG or admission to an Epilepsy Monitoring Unit (EMU) may be helpful. No ASMs are used in the case of children who do not have an underlying epilepsy diagnosis. Treatment for PNES is generally directed by psychology/psychiatry and often involves cognitive behavioral therapy or other therapy-based approaches. Most instances of PNES improve or cease after the diagnosis is made and interventions are in place.

Benign Paroxysmal Vertigo

Benign paroxysmal vertigo (BPV) is a syndrome characterized by episodic vertigo. It is one of the most common causes of episodic vertigo in children.[13] Symptoms generally present before the child is 4 years of age and more common with a family history of migraine headaches and/or the development of migraine headaches later in childhood. The history may include rapid onset of an attack (vertigo, disequilibrium, nausea) that lasts seconds to minutes, daily attacks that occur in clusters over several days and then may not recur for weeks or months, and a possible history of motion sickness. Symptoms are likely to have resolved by the time the child is examined. BPV is not associated with hearing loss, tinnitus, or loss of consciousness. The physical examination findings consist of:
- Acute unsteadiness: The child may fall or refuse to walk or sit; the child may grab on to a parent or object for steadiness.
- Nystagmus may be present within but not between attacks.
- Vomiting and nausea may be present and be quite prominent.
- Child appears frightened and/or pale.
- Child may be lethargic or drowsy; some children may sleep and return to normal activities on awakening.
- Neurologic examination is essentially negative except for abnormal vestibular function. Note: If the child also presents with a history suggestive of migraine headaches, consider vestibular migraine as a possible differential diagnosis.

Because the symptoms of BPV can appear to mimic cranial neuropathies, MRI of the brain will often be ordered to assess for structural abnormality. An MRI of the brain would be essential if abnormalities were identified during the neurologic examination between episodes.

One possible diagnostic study involves ice water caloric testing to detect abnormal vestibular function. However, this test is rarely done due to the intense discomfort that it produces. Other diagnostic studies are available if questions about the diagnosis persist. Referral to a vestibular specialist should be considered to pursue additional diagnostic testing.

Typically, pharmacologic intervention is not indicated, given the short duration of the attacks.[14] Once a diagnosis is made, parental reassurance is key. Spontaneous resolution of symptoms associated with BPV typically occurs by 8 to 10 years of age.

Narcolepsy

Narcolepsy is a disorder characterized by excessive daytime sleepiness, fragmented nocturnal sleep, signs of rapid eye movement (REM) intrusion, and cataplexy. It is an imbalance among wakefulness, REM, and slow wave sleep (SWS) states that can range from mild to severe. Other manifestations of narcolepsy include sleep paralysis and hypnogogic hallucinations. *Hypnogogic hallucinations* are vivid dreamlike visual, tactile, or auditory hallucinations that occur as the patient is falling asleep. Children may complain of feeling someone whispering in their ear or breathing on their neck. Rarely can the patient decipher the whispering. *Sleep paralysis* is the total inability to move any muscles (except respiratory muscles) when falling asleep or waking up. Sleep paralysis occurs outside of narcolepsy, due to sleep deprivation or sleep disordered breathing, and those conditions need to be ruled out before considering narcolepsy.

Narcolepsy typically occurs between 10 and 25 years of age; however, it is seen in children as young as 5 years of age. The *HLA-DQB1*06:02* gene allele has been identified in most patients with narcolepsy; yet, diagnosing narcolepsy is complex, and a referral to a sleep specialist is warranted. Medication management is the core therapy for narcolepsy with cataplexy. Cataplexy, a brief sudden loss of skeletal muscle tone, is typically brought on by laughter but can also be stimulated by other strong emotions. Neck, facial, and knee weakness are common cataplexy symptoms. Respiratory muscles are not affected. During cataplexy events, individuals retain consciousness, which can help to differentiate it from seizures (particularly atonic seizures). Excessive daytime sleepiness and weight gain tend to present before cataplexy in children.[15]

Narcolepsy with cataplexy is caused by a deficiency of hypothalamic hypocretin (or orexin) and this can be measured in the cerebral spinal fluid. It occurs in 200 to 500 per 1 million people in North American and European populations.[15] There is a low prevalence of familial cases.

Disorders of Muscle Tone

Cerebral Palsy

Cerebral palsy (CP) is a chronic, nonprogressive motor disorder that is the result of damage to the areas in the brain that control motor function. It can be congenital or acquired (posttrauma, infection, etc.). There are three major types of CP: (1) spastic, (2) athetoid (or dyskinetic), and (3) ataxic (Table 41.10). The prevalence of CP is to be between 1.3 and 2.9 per 1000 live births.[16,17] The current diagnostic criteria for CP are motor dysfunction and either abnormal neuroimaging or risk factors for CP.[17]

Symptoms of *congenital* CP appear within the first few years of life. Early detection is important because it allows for early treatment, which can have a significant impact on long-term outcomes. Depending on the area affected and the extent of damage, children with CP can also have disturbances in sensation, perception, cognition, communication, and behavior. In addition, epilepsy, or musculoskeletal problems secondary to the motor impairment, may occur. The degree of brain injury is individual, and the degree of impairment is not always directly associated with the degree of injury. CP was once believed to be caused only by birth complications (neonatal or perinatal asphyxia or trauma); however, it is now believed that there are a wide range of factors that may contribute to the development of CP. More recent evidence suggest that some cases of CP are of genetic etiology.[16] The etiology remains unknown in a large percentage of cases.

History. The history should include assessment for the presence of associated comorbid, developmental, and functional health problems, as well as risk factors (Box 41.6).

Additional items include:
- Prenatal/birth history risk factors.
- Hearing and/or vision/ocular problems (e.g., strabismus, nystagmus, optic atrophy).
- Change in growth parameters, especially decreased OFC.
- Early head injury, meningitis, or seizures.
- Muscle tone: hypotonic/hypertonic. Note: In CP, tone can be hypotonic before 6 months old, then become hypertonic in the affected extremities.
- Developmental milestones (particularly motor) may be delayed but should still be attained, depending on the extent of CP.
- Persistent primitive reflexes are common (e.g., Moro, asymmetric tonic neck).
- Hand preference before 1 year old is highly suspect.
- Oral-motor coordination problems (e.g., feeding history of regurgitating through the nose, inability to coordinate suck/swallow/advance the diet to textured foods).
- Irritability, depressed affect, including unusual sleepiness, as a neonate.
- Difficulty with movement, grasp/release, self-feeding, and head control; inability to change position per developmental level.
- Communication problems (e.g., speech, language).

Physical Examination.
- Development: Assess gross motor, fine motor, language, and personal social skills. Motor milestones are commonly delayed. Note quality of movements (e.g., smoothness of gait, grasping, and clarity of speech). Standardized tools to assess motor dysfunction should be used within the appropriate age groups, including the Hammersmith Infant Neurological Examination (ages 2–24 months) and the Gross Motor Function Classification System Extended and Revised (GMFCS). It should be noted that the GMFCS score is more reliable in children over the age of 2 years.[17]
- Feeding: Note a reversed swallow wave; (i.e., tongue thrust swallowing) uncoordinated suck and swallow; decreased tone of the lips, tongue, and cheeks; increased gag reflex; involuntary tongue and lip movements; increased sensitivity to food stimuli; poor occlusion; and delayed inhibition of the suck reflex.
- Diet: Evaluate the diet for adequate nutrition, assess length/height, weight, and BMI.
- Skin: Dermatologic signs of other syndromes should be identified (e.g., neurocutaneous syndrome).
- Orthopedic: Scoliosis, contractures, and/or dislocated hip(s).
- Neurologic examination: The following may be seen:
  - Asymmetric or abnormal deep tendon reflexes and movement
  - Ankle clonus, no fasciculations

TABLE 41.10	Terms Used to Describe Abnormal Motor Examination	
Term	**Description**	**Associated Impairments**
Movement Type		
Spastic	Inability of a muscle to relax	Often evident after 4–6 months; delayed speech; convergent strabismus; toe-walking; flexed elbows; delayed walking until 18–24 months; one-third have seizures
Athetoid	Inability to control muscle movement (continuous, writhing movements)	Infant has difficulty feeding as a result of tongue thrust, is initially hypotonic with head lag; increasing tone with rigidity over time; speech delay
Ataxic	Problems with balance and coordination	Tremors
Body Part Involved		
Diplegic	Affects both legs more than both arms	Most have limited use of legs; can walk often with aids; walk typically scissor-like with knees bent in and crisscross over each other
Hemiplegic	Affects one side of the body (upper extremity more than the lower extremity)	Often not detected at birth; right side often more affected than left; 50% develop seizures; growth arrest of affected limb(s); individuals usually able to walk
Tetraplegic/ quadriplegic	Affects all four extremities, trunk and head	Affects upper extremities more than lower; 50% with grand mal seizures; IQ impairment can be severe; most unable to walk or stand
Specific Problems With Movement or Function		
Dystonia	Involuntary, slow, sustained muscle contraction	Abnormal posture, writhing motion of arms, legs, trunk
Choreic	Disorganized tone	Uncontrollable jerky movements fingers/toes
Tremor	Involuntary, rhythmic movements of opposing muscles; can affect extremities, head, face, vocal cords, trunk	
Ballismus	Violent, jerky movements; may affect only one side of body	
Rigidity	Stiffness	

IQ, Intelligence quotient.

• BOX 41.6 Risk Factors for Cerebral Palsy

Congenital
- Maternal vaginal bleeding between the sixth and ninth month of pregnancy.
- Severe proteinuria late in pregnancy; preeclampsia.
- Antepartum hemorrhage, maternal stroke, seizure.
- Maternal hyperthyroidism and/or maternal intellectual disability.
- Maternal/intrauterine infection exposure (evidenced by chorioamnionitis).
- Labor and delivery complications; breech presentation; traumatic delivery.
- Fetal distress; APGAR score of less than 3 at 10 min.
- Small for gestation age; low birth weight (<1000 g); prematurity, postmaturity.
- Multiple births; microcephaly; intrauterine drug exposure.
- Intracranial hemorrhage; neonatal seizure; coagulopathy in fetus or newborn.

Acquired
- Meningitis, encephalitis.
- Head trauma, nonaccidental trauma, motor vehicle accident, falls, near drowning.

- Tone increased although tone is occasionally decreased; hypotonia before 6 months of age is common; tone may also be mixed
- Minimal muscle atrophy
- Persistent primitive reflexes (e.g., asymmetric tonic neck and Moro after 6 months of age)
- Delayed reflexes (e.g., parachute reflex remains absent after 9–10 months of age; protective reflexes remain absent after 5 months of age)
- Preferred handedness before 1 to 2 years of age

Diagnostic Studies.
- Imaging: MRI of the brain aids in visualizing potential structural abnormalities of the brain and should be done for all children suspected of having CP.
- Genetic and metabolic studies can be done to identify genetic or metabolic causes of CP but are not routinely indicated in diagnosis unless clinically indicated.

Differential Diagnosis. The first and main requirement is to differentiate central from peripheral disorders. CP is always a central disorder. Many other conditions can have CP-like motor involvement, including organic causes (e.g., sepsis from intrauterine infections), fetal alcohol syndrome, hydrocephalus, tumors, agenesis of the corpus callosum or other brain malformations, Tay-Sachs disease, phenylketonuria, Lesch-Nyhan syndrome, spinal

• BOX 41.7 **Problems Associated With Cerebral Palsy**

Cognitive: learning disabilities, intellectual disability
Seizure disorders: various types
Language and speech disorders: articulation, vocal strength and quality, language processing
Vision: refractive errors, strabismus, amblyopia, cataracts, retinopathy of prematurity, cortical blindness, homonymous hemianopsia (hemiplegia)
Hearing: conductive and/or sensorineural disorders
Other sensory: tactile hypersensitivity or hyposensitivity, dyspraxia, balance and movement problems, proprioceptive difficulties, stereognosis
Motor: prolonged primitive reflexes, absence of protective reflexes, delayed motor milestones, hip subluxation and dislocation, scoliosis, contractures
Feeding and eating problems: chewing, sucking, and swallowing deficits, drooling, hypoxemia, fatigue, underweight and overweight, gastroesophageal reflux, aspiration
Bowel: constipation, encopresis
Urinary: bladder control, urinary retention, urinary tract infections
Dental: malocclusions, enamel deficits and caries, gum hyperplasia (with phenytoin)
Pulmonary: respiratory infections, pneumonia
Skin: pressure ulcers, latex allergy
Behavioral and emotional: behavioral disorders, attention-deficit disorder with and without hyperactivity, self-injurious behaviors, depression, autism, growth failure

cord injury, hypothyroidism, neuromuscular diseases, movement disorders, seizures, genetic and metabolic disorders (e.g., cerebral folate deficiency), or *acquired* causes (e.g., severe TBI).

Management. Management requires balancing multiple associated problems (Box 41.7). The care can serve as a model for the management of children with a variety of neurologic problems.

- Referral: Children with CP should be evaluated and cared for at centers that have an established interdisciplinary team, including providers with expertise in developmental pediatrics, gastroenterology, orthopedics, neurology, nursing and/or advanced practice nursing, speech pathology, physical and occupational therapy, education and psychology, and social work. Care may also involve an ophthalmologist, feeding clinic and nutritionist services, and genetic counseling, as needed.

- Family education: Families need to understand two main concepts. First, CP is nonprogressive, but without intervention, the child's motor dysfunction may progressively worsen. Second, the extent of brain damage does not always correlate to the level of disability. Children who receive special services—physical therapy, occupational therapy, speech therapy, and other interventions—have better outcomes than children who do not, and early intervention typically leads to better outcomes. See United CP (https://ucp.org/) for educational materials and available services.

- Family support: In general, families grieve when given the diagnosis of CP and need support during this time. Support groups or opportunities to meet other families with affected children are often helpful. The emotional needs of siblings must not be overlooked. A social worker can be helpful to families.

- Financial resources: CP services are long-term and expensive and adaptive equipment, such as leg braces and wheelchairs, need maintenance and replacement. Many children will be eligible for Supplemental Security Income or state program benefits for the severely disabled. The Individuals with Disabilities Education Act of 1997 requires children with disabilities be assessed for and instructed in the use of assistive devices along with appropriate referrals to regional centers. Medical social workers and public health nurses can help in connecting families to appropriate services. Respite care may be available.

- Nutrition: Children with CP may be at risk for inadequate nutrition if they have oral-motor coordination problems. In addition, children with *athetosis* may need as much as 50% to 100% more calories to support the constant writhing movements. Children with *spasticity*, on the other hand, may need fewer calories because of their decreased movements. Feeding clinics are often helpful as feeding therapy, modified positioning during feedings, and special feeding devices can help. Occasionally, oral-motor coordination problems are so severe that a gastrostomy and/or fundoplication to prevent reflux and aspiration are needed.

- Elimination: Constipation is common because of lack of exercise, inadequate fluid and fiber intake, medications, poor positioning, and low abdominal muscle tone, especially in children with significant motor impairment. Stool softeners (e.g., docusate sodium), may help and laxatives (e.g., senna concentrate, milk of magnesia) may be useful but should not be used long term. Osmotic agents can be used (e.g., polyethylene glycol). Bladder control, urinary retention, and increased risk for urinary tract infections (UTIs) are common. Most children with CP achieve bladder control between 3 and 10 years old. For some, toilet training may be difficult, especially for those with intellectual disability.

- Dentistry: A diligent dental care program is necessary. Orofacial muscle tone can contribute to malocclusion. Problems with oral mobility make daily dental hygiene difficult, leading to gum disease. For children with CP and epilepsy, the side effects of some seizure medications can include swollen gums and tooth decay.

- Drooling: Inability to manage oral secretions results in drooling. Drooling can lead to social isolation, wet clothing, skin excoriation, malodorous breath, and discomfort. It can also lead to choking, gagging, and aspiration. The anticholinergic glycopyrrolate is approved for use in those 3 to 16 years old with chronic excessive drooling. Oral dosage is 20 mcg/kg/dose 3 times a day initially, with increases of 20 mcg/kg dose every 5 to 7 days if needed; maximum dosage is 100 mcg/kg/dose 3 times daily, not exceeding 1500 to 3000 mcg/dose. Oral solutions should be given 1 hour before or 2 hours after meals. Side effects may be problematic (e.g., dry mouth, vomiting, constipation, flushing, urinary retention, nasal congestion). Clinical improvement resulting in a reduction in drooling has been demonstrated with this treatment. Surgical intervention is a last resort and commonly involves removing the submandibular gland or nerves or cutting/ rerouting the salivary duct.

- Respiratory: Positioning problems, an increase in gastroesophageal reflux, and difficulty in clearing secretions create higher risk for respiratory problems, notably pneumonias (especially from aspiration). The duration of respiratory symptoms with upper respiratory infections (URIs) may be increased in these children because they may have sleep-related obstruction or other positioning difficulties, with slow respiratory return to baseline. A tracheotomy may be necessary in severe cases of upper airway obstruction or difficulty. Suctioning equipment may be required.

- Skin: The skin in sedentary children is more likely to break down and cause a pressure ulcer(s). Further, significant spasticity may lead to the development of skin lesions over bony prominences. Note: There is an increased incidence of skin latex allergies with CP.
- Movement and mobility: Functional mobility, including positioning and seating, standing, transportation, bathing, dressing, play, and mobility in the school setting are important to assess and manage. Involvement of occupational and physical therapists is key as families need help incorporating strategies into their daily lives and environment. The goals of therapy are to improve physical conditioning and gain maximal independence in mobility, fine motor activities, self-care, and communication by promoting efficient movement patterns, inhibiting primitive reflexes, and achieving isolated extremity movements. Bracing, postural support and seating systems, adaptive devices, and early intervention programs beginning in infancy are important. Open-front walkers, quadrupedal canes, gait poles, wheelchairs, and motorized wheelchairs are beneficial in helping children explore their environment more efficiently. Although the condition is not progressive in terms of the brain lesion, contractures, scoliosis, dislocated hips, and other deformities can develop if the child is allowed to maintain abnormal positions for long periods of time. Accordingly, range-of-motion exercises are a long-term need.
- Medications: Antispasmodic medications (e.g., baclofen, tizanidine, diazepam, dantrolene) may be used to minimize contractures and spasticity. Baclofen is the most used and can be delivered via oral route or intrathecal pump. These medications are appropriate for children needing a mild decrease in their muscle tone or in those with widespread spasticity. For optimal results, dosages often need to be high, and side effects can result (e.g., drowsiness, upset stomach, high blood pressure, possible liver damage with chronic use). *Botulinum toxin A* injections are used as treatment for spasticity, which can be helpful with improving function, decreasing pain, or reducing contractures. Although botulinum toxin A has become standard treatment for spasticity in children, it is used off-label. Its use is dependent on the evaluation recommendations made by providers with expertise in pediatric physiatry, pediatric neurology, or pediatric orthopedic surgery. Input from the child's therapy team and family should also be factored into this decision. Botulinum toxin A is injected directly into muscles (sometimes guided by an electromyogram or electrical stimulation). The child may experience mild flulike symptoms and transient worsening of spasticity. Injections are most effective when used in conjunction with an appropriate therapy regimen that helps strengthen the antagonist and agonist muscles. The dosage administered depends on which muscles are being selected and muscle size. Results are generally seen within 5 to 7 days and last 3 to 4 months. Botulinum toxin A has been safely used in infants older than 1 month. Resistance can occur because neutralizing antibodies can develop. Therefore only the smallest possible effective dose must be used and at least 3 months must lapse between injections.
- Communication: With the difficulty in oral-motor control, speech therapy may be of assistance. Augmentative devices, such as computers with voices, can allow for language development and communication of needs for children with severe speech impairment. Hearing deficits need to be identified and managed by an audiologist.
- Vision: Visual acuity, eye tracking, and binocularity are key factors to be assessed by a provider with expertise in pediatric ophthalmology/optometry.
- Osteopenia: Individuals with CP are at risk of bone density loss secondary to their inability to ambulate. Monitoring of calcium and vitamin D should be strongly considered and supplemental vitamin D prescribed if levels are low. Concerns for osteopenia should be referred to an orthopedic and/or endocrinology specialist for evaluation.
- Pain: Spastic muscles, strain on compensatory muscles, and frequent or irregularly occurring muscle spasms can cause chronic and acute pain. Gabapentin, diazepam, and complementary therapies (e.g., distraction, biofeedback, relaxation, therapeutic massage) can help with pain management.
- Special education: Early intervention and specialized educational programs through school systems should be considered and engaged early on, if appropriate.
- Surgery: At times, surgery is used to release contractures or to sever overactivated nerves (e.g., selective dorsal root rhizotomy). An implantable pump can be used to deliver intrathecal baclofen (antispasmodic). It is programmable with an electronic telemetry wand. Pumps have been successfully implanted in children as young as 3 years of age, but carry a few risks (e.g., surgical risks, catheter migration/defects, toxicity). However, the pump averts the significant CNS depression associated with the administration of large oral doses of baclofen. Selective dorsal root rhizotomy (of spinal nerves) plus intrathecal baclofen decrease spasticity and increase range of motion of affected limbs. Intense physical therapy is an instrumental adjunct treatment.
- Strength training can help with balance and weakness. Functional electrical stimulation, which involves insertion of a microscopic wireless device into specific muscles or nerves, can activate and strengthen muscles.[18]

Complications. Children who receive no intervention have poor functional abilities, make less progress developmentally, and are at risk for unnecessary contractures and deformities (see Box 41.7).

Hypotonic Infant

Muscle tone reflects the muscle's resistance to passive movement. Normal muscle tone requires an intact central and peripheral nervous system. The infant with hypotonia, or low muscle tone, is often referred to as a "floppy infant." Hypotonic infants present with flaccid extension of the arms and abduction of the legs ("frog-leg" appearance) if the hypotonia is severe. Less significant signs of hypotonia include poor head control, prolonged head lag when pulling the infant to a sitting position from supine, or a feeling of poor resistance when lifting the infant from a seated or lying position. Systemic illness, medication, level of alertness, and gestational age can influence tone and the PCP should note these influencing factors. Physical examination techniques that can help with assessment include the pull to sit test, scarf sign, measurement of the popliteal angle, vertical suspension, or ventral suspension (Demonstrations available at https://neurologicexam.med.utah.edu/pediatric/html/newborn_ab.html). If hypotonia is noted, the PCP should look for other abnormal neurologic examination findings, with particular attention to dysmorphic features, abnormal deep tendon reflexes, delayed developmental milestones, ptosis, muscle atrophy, or fasciculations.

Hypotonia can result from ischemic or hemorrhagic brain insults, congenital brain malformations, inherited disorders, neuromuscular disease, metabolic disorders, and prematurity. In some cases, it can be idiopathic. Additional diagnostic testing may include creatine kinase levels, thyroid function tests, genetic testing, and laboratory studies to evaluate for metabolic disorder (see Chapter 39), MRI of the brain, electromyogram with nerve conduction studies, and muscle biopsy. Referral to neurology should be considered for all hypotonic infants; referral to other specialties, such as genetics, cardiology, or pulmonology, depends on clinical presentation and testing. Many conditions that present with hypotonia require long-term management with physical and occupational therapies to support attaining maximal developmental potential. Prognosis is dependent on the underlying cause.

Neuromuscular Disorders

Neuromuscular diseases in pediatrics are largely genetic in etiology and originate from dysfunction in the peripheral nervous system. This includes disorders of the anterior horn cell (e.g., spinal muscular atrophy), peripheral nerve (e.g., Charcot-Marie-Tooth disease), the neuromuscular junction (e.g., congenital myasthenic syndrome), and the muscle (myopathies and muscular dystrophies). Progression and severity vary depending on where the motor unit is affected and age of onset. Most children with neuromuscular diseases present with chronic signs and symptoms related to muscle weakness. Historically, pediatric neuromuscular diseases have been associated with lifelong morbidities resulting in severe disability and shortened lifespan. Advocacy related to early diagnosis has resulted in many states adding neuromuscular disorders to newborn screening and genetic testing panels. Current therapies have slowed disease progression and improved the quality of life in children with certain neuromuscular diseases.

A thorough and detailed H & P are essential for evaluating any child with suspected neuromuscular disease. A stepwise approach starts with obtaining a detailed birth, neonatal, past medical, developmental, and family history (including three-generation pedigree). A focused neuromuscular history is then obtained, which includes symptom onsets, gait and functional disturbances, sensory deficits, endurance level and associated gastrointestinal, respiratory, and cardiovascular concerns. The physical examination should be thorough and include a comprehensive, age-appropriate neurologic and musculoskeletal examination. Particular attention should be given to muscle tone, strength, muscle development (atrophy/hypertrophy), musculoskeletal deformities, developmental milestones, and cardiopulmonary status.

Spinal Muscular Atrophy

Spinal muscular atrophy (SMA) is one of the most common neuromuscular disorders seen in children and is characterized by motor neuron degeneration. SMA occurs in approximately one in 11,000 live births and is the leading inherited cause of infant mortality.[19] It is caused by mutations to the *SMN1* and *SMN2* genes found on the long arm (q) of chromosome 5. There are five types of SMA (0–IV) each with a different phenotype related to milestones achieved and life expectancy. Clinical manifestations include weakness, hypotonia, progressive muscle atrophy and decreased/absent reflexes. Disease progression is often rapid at the onset, slowing in later stages. Diagnosis is made with genetic testing early on during prenatal screening, through newborn screening (state dependent), or as part of the workup in a suspected infant or child. Molecular and gene replacement therapies have been developed with promising results. Corticosteroids (e.g., prednisone) are often given in conjunction with other therapies. It

is important to monitor for effects of chronic steroid use. Children with SMA typically require multidisciplinary management, care coordination, and psychosocial support services.

Duchenne Muscular Dystrophy

Duchenne muscular dystrophy (DMD) is the most common type of muscular dystrophy seen in children. DMD is an X-linked recessive disorder caused by a mutation of the gene responsible for the production of dystrophin. While DMD is an X-linked disorder, mothers of affected boys, as well as some female offspring, are carriers and can have mild symptoms. History and physical examination findings are reviewed in Chapter 40, but one distinctive finding is the appearance of muscular calves in early childhood accompanied by the inability to hop. The initial diagnostic evaluation when DMD is suspected includes serum creatine kinase (CK), aldolase, aspartate aminotransferase, and LFTs. Serum CK is elevated before the development of symptoms, peaking by age 2 years with levels often 10 to 20 times above normal. CK levels will decrease with disease progression due to muscle being replaced by fat and fibrosis tissue. This active muscle breakdown causes elevated LFTs levels. Muscle biopsy, EMG, and genetic testing can be used to confirm diagnosis. There is no cure for DMD, and treatment is primarily focused on maintaining function (see Chapter 40). Disease progression is accompanied by cardiac and respiratory involvement presenting in the second or third decade of life, which ultimately leads to premature death.

Congenital Malformations

Congenital malformations can occur in the brain, spinal cord, and skull, which directly alter nervous system development—structurally and functionally. It is important for PCPs to have a basic understanding of these malformations as there are often overlapping clinical features, genetic or molecular pathways that result in specific neurologic disorders.

Neural Tube Defects

Neural tube defects (NTDs) are the second leading type of all congenital defects and are a result of complex interaction of genes and environmental conditions that alter neural tube development in early pregnancy (neural tube typically closes within the third to fourth week of gestation). Defects lead to malformations of the brain or spine, which are divided into two main subtypes: closed and open. Severity of the condition and prognosis varies depending on location of the defect. In the United States, approximately one per 1200 births are affected each year, with rates as high as 5 per 1000 births in other parts of the world.[20] The CDC's Birth Defects COUNT is a global initiative to reduce neural tube defects with implementation of preventive measures, such as folic acid fortification of foods. The CDC also urges females of reproductive age to take 400 mcg of folic acid each day.

Despite these efforts, NTD incidence has not significantly changed within these nonmodifiable risk groups: race/ethnicity, female sex of the neonate, and family history of NTD in a first- or second-degree relative. Hispanic females have a higher risk compared to non-Hispanic White and Black females. Differences in genetic and environmental factors between racial/ethnic groups remain unknown; however, it has been suggested that gene mutations may differ amongst these populations. Independent risk factors include obesity, diabetes—type 1 or 2, and females with epilepsy. For females with epilepsy, certain ASM have a higher yield of teratogenicity (e.g., valproic acid, carbamazepine) and are contraindicated during pregnancy. Females with epilepsy need to discuss their medication with their neurology provider before conception and or as soon as they discover they are pregnant. While ASM, such as valproic acid, does not reduce folate levels, it is thought to interfere with its metabolism.

Gene variants in the methylenetetrahydrofolate reductase (MTHFR) enzyme, have been identified in females who have had a pregnancy complicated by NTD. MTHFR is an enzyme that regulates folate and homocysteine levels, therefore females that carry a homozygous gene mutation have lower folate concentrations. Alpha-fetoprotein (AFP) is another biomarker measured throughout pregnancy to evaluate the risk of NTD in the fetus. It is a protein produced by the developing fetus. Elevated levels have been associated with a higher risk of NTD, whereas low levels have been associated with trisomy 21 (Down syndrome). It is recommended that AFP levels be evaluated during weeks 15 to 20 of pregnancy.

MMC or spina bifida, is the most complex NTD. MMC includes the protrusion of both the spinal cord nerve roots *(myelo)* and the three layers of membranes *(meninges)* that cover the spinal cord through this spinal defect. At times, the protruding dural sac may contain only the meninges or both meninges and nerve roots. The location and extent of involvement is directly correlated with the severity of the neurologic sequalae. The majority of MMC occur in the lumbosacral cord; however, MMC originating from the thoracic cord tend to be more complex and result in more serious complications. Additional details related to MMC can be found in Chapter 28. Other types of NTD include:

- Meningocele—protrusion of sac of fluid without spinal cord contents.
- Spina bifida occulta—opening in the spinal cord without sac protrusion.
- Encephalocele—protrusion of brain tissue and meninges through opening in the skull.
- Anencephaly—lack of development of forebrain and skull (Note: Anencephaly is not compatible with life, and neonates with this condition typically die shortly after birth).

Severity of symptoms and complexity of the treatment plan is typically related to severity of the defect with some (e.g., spina bifida occulta) not requiring any intervention and others (e.g., encephalocele) requiring advanced intervention.

Clinical Features of Neural Tube Defects.

- Physical presence of sac-like protrusion along the spine (contents vary) and/or lack of bone structure (skull) in severe forms.
- Sacral dimple/tuft of hair in mild cases.
- Lower extremity paralysis with varying degrees of spasticity.
- Sensory loss: lack of response to pain, touch, temperature.
- Bladder/anal sphincter dysfunction.
- Absence of selected deep tendon reflexes.
- Other clinical physical anomalies that can accompany any NTD include cleft lip/palate, omphalocele, diaphragmatic hernia, tracheoesophageal fistula, congenital heart disease, hydronephrosis, orthopedic abnormalities, and imperforate anus.

Management and Complications. Surgical closure is the recommended treatment and can be performed prenatally or in the neonatal period (typically within the first week of life). Surgical closure within 48 hours of delivery is the most common approach with the goal of preventing meningitis and reducing the severity of neurologic deficits. Empirical antibiotic treatment is often initiated and keeping site clean and moist are critical should surgery not be able to be performed immediately after delivery. Intrauterine surgical repair is available, but not everywhere, and only if the diagnosis is made before 25 weeks' gestation.

Ultrasounds (cranial/abdominal), urodynamic studies, and neuroimaging to assess structural involvement of spinal cord and brain are common in the neonatal period. Hydrocephalus is present in 70% to 90% of neonates, so shunt placement is often required during this time. Secondary conditions (e.g., seizures, urinary and bowel dysfunction, lower extremity spasticity, tethered cord, scoliosis, leg and foot weakness, shunt management) require ongoing and multidisciplinary care. The PCP's role is critical for interim assessments, treatment of acute illnesses (e.g., UTI), providing caregiver education about home management, and coordinating services between involved specialists.

Prognosis. Advancements in medical and surgical management have improved the survival rate. The child's mobility and function correspond to the anatomic level of the defect and long-term management (e.g., mobility devices, medication, splinting, etc.) focuses on optimal quality of life. Intermittent urinary catheterization and bowel training is often lifelong, although other interventions may change over time. Individuals with NTD often have normal intelligence; however, specific cognitive and or language disabilities can be present that could alter independent living later in life. (More information regarding the level of spina bifida function can be found at https://www.spinabifidaassociation.org/wp-content/uploads/how-sb-lesions-impact-daily-function1-1-1-1.pdf.)

Prevention. As noted earlier, folic acid supplementation (400 mcg/day) with a daily multivitamin is helpful in preventing neural tube defects and should be taken by all females of childbearing age. For females who have had a previous pregnancy resulting in NTD, supplementation at markedly higher levels (e.g., 4000 mcg/day) might be recommended.

Tethered Cord

The spinal cord is attached to the base of the brain and free at the caudal end, allowing for freedom of movement during growth, activities, and skeletal changes (e.g., scoliotic curves). With tethered cord, the caudal end is fixed by a ropelike strand of fibrous tissue (filum terminale) at or below the L2 level, causing abnormal stretching and damage to nerve cells, fibers, and blood vessels. A tethered cord is often associated with a congenital spinal anomaly, such as spina bifida (90%), but tethering can also result from bony protrusions, tough membranous bands, lipomas, tumors, cysts, scarring, and trauma in the cauda equina.

Not all tethering leads to clinical symptoms. If symptoms do occur, they manifest as functional deficits to nerves that emanate from the area of the cauda equina. In children, findings may include lesions, hairy patches, dimples, or fatty tumors on the lower back; foot and spinal deformities; weakness in the legs; low back pain; scoliosis; and incontinence. Tethered spinal cord syndrome appears to be the result of improper growth of the neural tube during fetal development and is closely linked to spina bifida. Symptoms are not always evident in infancy, and it may go undiagnosed until adulthood, when pain, sensory and motor problems, and loss of bowel and bladder control emerge. Skin changes are often seen later and include dimples above the gluteal cleft or within the cleft spinal hair tufts, a deviated gluteal fold, spinal fatty deposits, midline birthmarks, and sacral sinuses or tracts (Fig. 41.5). Note: Dimples at the coccyx are generally benign.

When the PCP suspects a tethered cord, an MRI of the spine is the gold standard for viewing the parenchymal anatomy. A referral to a pediatric neurosurgeon is also indicated for further evaluation of surgical suitability. Surgery is usually the treatment of choice and can halt and prevent further neurologic dysfunction. Earlier

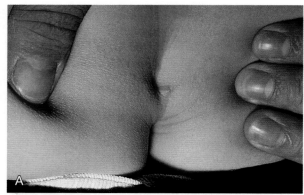

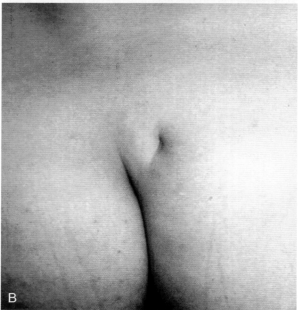

• **Fig. 41.5** (A) Deep sacral dimple above the gluteal crease. Most sacral dimples that fall within the gluteal crease are normal. Dimples that are deep, large (>0.5 cm), located in the superior portion or above the gluteal crease (>2.5 cm from the anal verge), or that are associated with a deviated gluteal crease or other cutaneous markers should be radiologically imaged. (B) Buttocks of teenage male with tethered cord secondary to lipomeningocele. Note sacral dimple and deviation of gluteal fold to the left.

surgical intervention tends to improve long-term functional outcomes.[21] If a child has reached full skeletal height with minimal symptoms, monitoring is all that is often done; however, the PCP should be watchful for retethering in children who have had surgery for tethered cord, as it can occur as the child gets older. In addition, any child with a history of repaired spina bifida must be closely monitored for early symptoms of tethered cord.

Chiari Malformation

Chiari malformations are uncommon congenital spinal cord anomalies, which are subdivided into four primary types (I–IV). *Type I* malformation is the most common type and involves the downward displacement of the caudal end of the cerebellar vermis 5 mm or more below the foramen magnum. The incidence rate is between 1% and 3.6% of children.[22] *Type II* malformation is less common and characterized by a downward displacement of hindbrain below the foramen magnum. It occurs in children with

a history of MMC and can be discovered on prenatal ultrasound. Types III and IV are more severe and rare.

Many children with type I malformations are asymptomatic, and the malformation is discovered as an incidental finding on neuroimaging related to other neurologic symptoms or events. type I malformation can cause headache, neck pain, atrophy and decreased reflexes in the lower extremities, sensory losses, and scoliosis. Any child with a MMC should be suspected of having type II malformation. Symptoms of type II include symptoms seen with type I malformations, as well as hydrocephalus, respiratory distress, syncope, poor feeding, vomiting, dysphagia, tongue paralysis, and cardiopulmonary failure. Diagnosis is made with MRI of the brain. In higher-grade or symptomatic malformations, consideration should be given to completing an MRI of the spine to evaluate for syringomyelia. Many patients with Chiari malformation type I do not require intervention. Children with Chiari malformations should be referred to neurosurgery for evaluation. Surgery for type I malformations is typically reserved for children who are symptomatic or with syringomyelia.[22] Surgical decompression and its risk must be weighed against symptom severity at presentation. For these children, surgical decompression of the posterior fossa may be considered. Ventriculoperitoneal shunt may be considered in children who are symptomatic and with hydrocephalus.

Note: Because of the risk of brainstem herniation, an LP should never be attempted in a child with a Chiari malformation.

Hydrocephalus

Congenital hydrocephalus is discussed in Chapter 28. *Acquired* hydrocephalus has different etiologies, pathologies, and diagnostic criteria. It can be subdivided into transitional (diagnosed as a child), longstanding ventriculomegaly or chronic congenital hydrocephalus, identifiable etiology (e.g., hemorrhage, cerebral trauma, infection, mass), or idiopathic normal pressure hydrocephalus. Early recognition is imperative. Investigation and intervention are required to avoid morbidity and mortality. Box 41.4 presents red flags for increasing intracranial pressure in infants and children.

A cardinal feature of acute hydrocephalus is increased intracranial pressure, which is associated with a well-recognized pattern of symptoms that include: an altered level of consciousness, headaches, nausea, and vomiting (which is worse in the morning). Other signs and symptoms may include a new onset of esotropia, or horizontal diplopia associated with abducens nerve palsy or other cranial neuropathies. New onset of a gait disturbance may also be present. These findings indicate the need for urgent evaluation in an emergency setting by a neurologist or neurosurgeon. Diagnosis can be further investigated with neuroimaging. MRI of the brain is the preferred imaging modality, but CT of the head may be appropriate in emergent settings. Hydrocephalus may require surgical intervention, such as placement of a ventriculoperitoneal shunt, which needs to be followed long-term by neurosurgery. For PCPs caring for children with ventriculoperitoneal shunts, it is beneficial to develop an understanding of signs and symptoms of shunt malfunction and other issues that may arise in this population.

Disorders of Head Size or Shape

The size and shape of the skull are related to the volume of its contents, including brain, cerebrospinal fluid (CSF), and blood. While variations in size and shape of the skull can be seen in neurotypical infants and have a benign etiology, it can also give indication of underlying conditions. External forces (positional) can also influence skull shape during infancy. The skull is measured by obtaining OFC, with the infant/child upright (see Chapter 5). Measurements that are 2 or more standard deviations (SD) lower or higher than the mean for age/sex, as well as a trend that does not follow the child's established OFC curve, should raise concern. As with other growth measures, gestational age of preterm infants should be considered when evaluating head circumference.

Macrocephaly

Macrocephaly is defined as an OFC more than 2 standard deviations above the mean for age/sex or an OFC that is increasing rapidly. Heads that appear large may be familial and not clinically significant; however, the initial evaluation should include measuring parents' OFCs. Benign familial macrocephaly may occur as a part of, or related to, an inherited disorder, such as Soto syndrome (cerebral gigantism) or neurofibromatosis type 1 (NF1). Macrocephaly can also be attributed to hydrocephalus, megalencephaly (enlarged brain), subdural hematoma, tumor, and thickening of the skull. Infants with anatomic megalencephaly have macrocephaly at birth; however, those with a metabolic etiology are normocephalic at birth. It is possible that macrocephaly is associated with benign causes, such as benign extraaxial fluid or benign enlargement of the subarachnoid spaces. MRI of the brain is the preferred imaging modality. To avoid anesthesia exposure that may be required with a complete MRI of the brain, an axial T2 MRI can be easily completed without sedation in young children. Head ultrasounds are another option for infants with an open anterior fontanel. This method is noninvasive and quick, providing immediate evaluation. It can be particularly helpful when other imaging is not available in an appropriate timeframe. CT scan of the head can be considered in emergent situations but should be limited due to concern for radiation exposure with repeat imaging.

Microcephaly

Microcephaly is defined as an OFC 2 standard deviations below the mean for age/sex, or when growth decelerates from the normal pattern. The skull may appear to be normally shaped; however, palpation may reveal overriding suture lines. Microcephaly can result from conditions in which the brain never formed correctly (small brain), which are typically apparent from birth (e.g., congenital Zika syndrome). A decreasing or plateauing OFC curve may start after the infant reaches 3 to 6 months of age. Any infant with microcephaly has an increased risk for developmental delay, disorders of tone, and seizures based on underlying etiology (Box 41.8). Management of microcephaly is supportive, often involves an interdisciplinary team directed toward optimizing functionality from resulting deficits. Referral to a neurology provider should be made for diagnostic purposes and an MRI of the brain can provide details related to intracranial structures.

Craniosynostosis

Craniosynostosis occurs when there is premature closure of one or more cranial sutures—resulting in an abnormally shaped skull (Fig. 41.6). It occurs in approximately one in every 2500 births and is believed to be associated with a variety of genetic and intra- and extrauterine environmental factors.[23] Primary craniosynostosis results from atypical bone or suture development, while secondary craniosynostosis results from atypical brain growth. Craniosynostosis can also suggest underlying genetic disorder (e.g., Apert syndrome, Crouzon syndrome).

> ### • BOX 41.8   Conditions Causing Microcephaly
>
> **Primary Microcephaly**
> - Chromosomal disorders
> - Defective neurulation
>   - Anencephaly
>   - Encephalocele
> - Defective prosencephalization
>   - Agenesis of the corpus callosum
>   - Holoprosencephaly (arrhinencephaly)
> - Defective cellular migration
> - Microcephaly vera (genetic)
>
> **Secondary Microcephaly**
> - Intrauterine disorders
>   - Infection
>   - Toxins
>   - Vascular
> - Perinatal brain injuries
>   - Hypoxic-ischemic encephalopathy[a]
>   - Intracranial hemorrhage
>   - Meningitis and encephalitis[a]
>   - Stroke
> - Postnatal systemic diseases
>   - Chronic cardiopulmonary disease
>   - Chronic renal disease
>   - Malnutrition
>
> [a]Denotes the most common conditions and the ones with disease modifying treatments.
> From Pina-Garza JE, James KC: *Fenichel's Clinical Pediatric Neurology*, 8th ed. Philadelphia: Elsevier; 2019.

Physical Examination. Visual inspection and palpation of the head, including all sutures, is a critical aspect of any pediatric examination. An absent "soft spot" (anterior fontanel), raised, firm edges along suture lines, and facial asymmetry may be a sign of craniosynostosis. Plotting the OFC can alert the PCP when there is slow or no growth. Symmetry of neck rotation should also be included in the examination to rule out torticollis as a contributing factor. Infants with torticollis typically have some limitation of neck rotation away from the side of their occipital flattening and may require physical therapy for symptom management and parental education. Hydrocephalus occurs frequently in craniosynostosis. In nonsyndromic craniosynostosis, the only clinical feature is an abnormal head shape, such as plagiocephaly (Fig. 41.7). In cases in which syndromic craniosynostosis is of concern, physical anomalies in the hands/fingers and feet/toes are often present.

Diagnostic Studies. A CT scan is standard for evaluating skull shape deformity and suture lines. Three-dimensional CT scans are also becoming more available and aid in this diagnosis. Deformational plagiocephaly does not require imaging studies when the H & P are diagnostic. Consider further neuroimaging with MRI, if the neurologic examination is abnormal.

Differential Diagnosis. In about 5% of young infants, the frontal metopic suture may be prominent. This can be mistakenly identified as frontal bossing or metopic synostosis. However, this prominence is not clinically significant and does not require intervention. If the PCP has concerns (e.g., prominent metopic suture vs. metopic synostosis, positional plagiocephaly vs. lambdoid synostosis), refer to neurosurgery for evaluation.

Management. If craniosynostosis is suspected, referral to pediatric neurosurgery or craniofacial plastic surgeon is

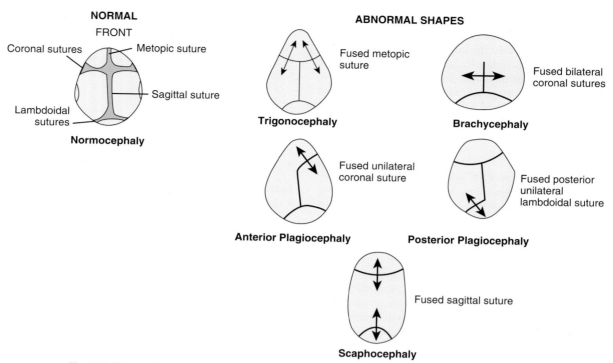

• **Fig. 41.6** Characteristics of Skull Deformities Seen With Craniosynostosis. (Modified from Cohen MM Jr. Craniosynostosis update 1987. *Am J Med Genet Suppl.* 1988;4:99–148.)

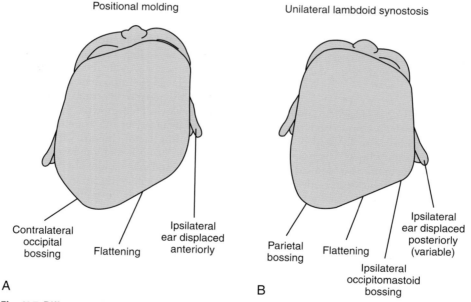

• **Fig. 41.7** Differences Between Positional Molding (A) and Unilambdoid Synostosis (B). (From Gruss JS, Ellenbogen RG, Whelan MF. Lambdoid synostosis and posterior plagiocephaly. In: Lin KY, Ogle RC, Jane JA, eds. *Craniofacial Surgery: Science and Surgical Technique.* Saunders; 2002.)

needed for further evaluation. Treatment is often surgical, but in some cases reassurance and education, repositioning, exercises for any associated torticollis, and clinical follow-up are sufficient. If the condition is inherited, management needs to be planned according to the problems associated with the syndrome, including genetic counseling and long-term follow-up.

PCPs can help limit deformational plagiocephaly by counseling parents to: (1) lay infant down in supine Back-to-Sleep position for sleep, alternating left and right occiputs, (2) place infants prone for "tummy time" or in a side position for play, (3) avoid holding an infant in a manner that puts pressure on a flattened part of the skull, and (4) have infants spend minimal time in car seats or other upright devices that maintain supine positioning.

With positional plagiocephaly, improvement should occur over a 2- to 3-month period if interventions are instituted early; particularly after the child is able to sit independently. Monitor head shape during all well-child visits. The majority of positional plagiocephalies are self-limited; sometimes physical therapy is indicated in recalcitrant cases (e.g., torticollis). Helmet therapy for significant plagiocephaly can be considered.

Inherited Disorders

Neurofibromatosis Type 1

NF1 affects multiple organ systems and results from a genetic mutation on the long arm (q) of chromosome 17 responsible for tumor suppression. It has an autosomal dominant pattern of inheritance, but approximately 50% of cases are de novo (spontaneous) mutations. NF1 is the most common neurocutaneous syndrome and affects about 1:3000 people worldwide.[24] Historically, NF1 was called *von Recklinghausen disease* and was first described in 1882. More recently, diagnostic criteria for NF1 have been developed. NF1 should be suspected in an individual with two (or more) of the following findings:
- Six or more café-au-lait macules, greater than 5 mm in diameter (prepubertal) and greater than 15 mm in diameter (postpubertal)
- Two or more neurofibromas of any type OR one plexiform neurofibroma
- Freckling in the axillary or inguinal regions
- Optic glioma
- Two or more Lisch nodules (iris hamartomas)
- A distinctive osseous lesion (e.g., sphenoid dysplasia, tibial pseudarthrosis)
- A first-degree relative (parent, sibling, offspring) with NF1.

NF1 carries the risk for other comorbid diagnoses, including malignancy (CNS and non-CNS), skeletal deformities (e.g., osteopenia, scoliosis), cardiovascular abnormalities (e.g., congenital heart disease, vasculopathies, hypertension), and neurocognitive deficits.

Nervous system malignancies include optic pathway or brainstem gliomas, which occur in about 15% to 20% of the NF1 population, glioblastomas, and malignant peripheral nerve sheath tumors. Non-CNS malignancies may include breast cancers, leukemia, and lymphoma, pheochromocytoma, rhabdomyosarcoma, and GI tumors.

The following evaluations are recommended to determine the extent of the disease and individual needs:
- Medical history with particular attention to features of NF1.
- Physical examination with particular attention to the skin, skeleton, cardiovascular system, and neurologic systems. Measurement and assessment of changes in neurocutaneous features. Serial blood pressure measurements.
- Ophthalmologic evaluation, including slit lamp examination of the irises and infrared reflectance imaging or optical coherence tomography of the fundus.
- Developmental assessment.
- Routine head MRI scanning in asymptomatic individuals is controversial because of the requirement for sedation in small children and is typically done at the time of diagnosis.
- Other studies as indicated based on clinically apparent signs or symptoms.
- Consultation with a clinical geneticist and/or genetic counselor to obtain a thorough family history with particular attention to NF1 features.

The PCP must be familiar with diagnostic criteria and monitoring and be able to coordinate needed services with specialists or a neurofibromatosis center. Management of NF1 includes referrals to specialists for routine assessment of various body systems that may become involved including the eyes, skin, CNS or PNS, cardiovascular system, endocrine system, or musculoskeletal system. Surgical interventions to remove disfiguring or uncomfortable neurofibromas is considered if clinically indicated. Treatment of optic gliomas is generally unnecessary unless symptomatic (most are not). Frequently, the PCP is the initial contact and the source on ongoing monitoring. Attention-deficit/hyperactivity disorder is a common finding in children with NF1. Other neurodevelopmental findings may include speech delay, autism spectrum disorder, and learning disabilities. A small percentage of children with NF1 will have intellectual disability. Many children with NF1 are at risk for anxiety and social challenges because of social stigma related to physical appearance. The combination of these issues may make school particularly challenging for these children. Early recognition and intervention are critical for optimal school performance (see Chapter 29).

Infectious and Immune-Mediated Neurologic Conditions

Central Nervous System Infections

Infections of the CNS can manifest acutely (over 1–24 hours) or chronically (over 1–7 days or more). Bacteria, viruses, fungi, spirochetes, protozoa, and parasites can all cause CNS infection. The meninges, superficial cortical structures, blood vessels, and brain parenchyma can be involved. The most common microbes are:
- In infants: *Escherichia coli* (42%), followed by group B *Streptococcus* (23%). Streptococcus pneumoniae is more likely in older infants.[25]
- In children: *Streptococcus pneumoniae*.[26] There has been a decrease in *Haemophilus influenzae* type B and *Neisseria meningitidis* cases since the introduction of vaccination for those pathogens.[26]
- Infants/children with immune deficiencies: *Pseudomonas aeruginosa*, *Staphylococcus aureus*, coagulase-negative staphylococci, *Salmonella* spp., and *Listeria monocytogenes*.

Pathology generally includes colonization of the nasopharynx by adhesion to the mucosa via various mechanisms, followed by invasion of the mucosa and penetration into the bloodstream between or through epithelial cells. Eventually, bacteria invade the blood-brain barrier (BBB), multiply in the CSF, and trigger an inflammatory response, which results in increased permeability of the BBB. The poorest end results lead to cerebral edema, derangements of cerebral metabolism, neuronal damage, strokes, and severe impairment or death.

History. The following may be reported:
- Upper respiratory tract or gastrointestinal symptoms accompanied by fever.
- Increasing lethargy and irritability or behavioral change.
- Recent head injury or neurosurgical procedure.
- Immunocompromised host.
- History of travel, sick contact, insect bites, animal contacts.

Physical Examination. Findings on physical examination include:
- Systemic signs—fever, malaise, and/or impaired heart, lung, or kidney function, ill-appearing infant or child.
- CNS signs—headache; stiff neck and spine; nausea and vomiting; fever or hypothermia; changes in mental status, ranging from irritability to lethargy or coma; seizures; and focal or sensory deficits in CNs, notably CN III, CN IV, and CN VI.

- Meningeal irritation—positive Kernig or Brudzinski signs (may be absent in younger infants).
- Bulging fontanel and/or increasing OFC in a young infant.
- Papilledema—late finding in older children or adolescents. By age, the most common findings are as follows:
- 0 to 3 months old: fever, hypothermia, lethargy, irritability, poor feeding, apnea, focal seizures, enteric or respiratory symptoms, nuchal rigidity, and a bulging fontanel.
- 3 months to 5 years old: petechial rash, localized CNS signs as described earlier.
- From 6 to 18 years old: petechial rash, CN VII palsy (Lyme disease), sinusitis symptoms, localized CNS signs.

Diagnostic Studies. CSF culture remains the gold standard for diagnosis of CNS infection. In addition, blood cultures, CBC with differential, urinalysis, and chemistry panel are done. Enterovirus meningitis and herpes simplex virus rapid tests are available. EEG and/or brain biopsy may be needed. Imaging may include head CT without contrast to rule out space-occupying lesions, hemorrhage, or trauma. An MRI of brain and spine should be done if there is a concern for myelitis/encephalitis, abscess, or inflammation. Cerebral edema is often not demonstrated on scans.

Management and Complications. Outcomes are typically based on the type of infectious agent and severity of initial infection, age of the child (the younger, the worse the outcome), length of symptoms before the diagnosis and initiation of treatment, and antibiotic and dosage. The PCP needs to refer all children with potential CNS infection as rapidly as possible. Hypovolemia, hypoglycemia, hyponatremia, acidosis, septic shock, increased intracranial pressure, and other complications occur quickly and need aggressive management. Hearing loss can occur in all forms of meningitis and all children with meningitis merit postinfection auditory evaluation. Blindness, hydrocephalus, CP, seizures, and global developmental delays can also occur depending on the type of organism involved.

Bell Palsy

Bell palsy is an acute unilateral paralysis or weakening of the facial nerve that may include individual or all branches of the facial nerve (CN VII). Symptoms are attributed to edema and venous congestion in areas of the nerve canal. Viral etiology is suspected, but the exact mechanism or etiology remains unknown.[27] Bell palsy can occur across the lifespan, but it is seen most frequently in adolescents.

History. The child may initially experience localized pain or tingling in one ear and then experience sagging of the facial features corresponding to the affected branches of the facial nerve on the affected side. Onset is rapid and can progress to maximal intensity within hours. If there is a history of severe preceding pain, this should prompt the provider to consider other differential diagnoses. The history often reveals a viral illness or symptomatology within the 2 weeks preceding onset.

Physical Examination. A neurologic assessment of facial nerve function may be difficult in children; it is not critical to make an accurate diagnosis. All other CNs should be assessed for dysfunction in an age-appropriate manner. The PCP should observe for:

- Unilateral motor changes in the forehead, cheek, and perioral area; face muscles pull to the "normal" side when the child makes facial expressions.
- Normal BP.
- Dribbling/drooling from the weak side; eating and drinking are more difficult.
- Hypersensitivity to loud noises.

- Eyelid fails to close on the affected side, complete blinking may be absent and exposure keratitis may be present; lacrimation may be impaired.
- Taste anterior two-thirds of tongue and salivation may be impaired.
- No limb weakness.
- Any skin lesions on the affected side of the face indicate active viral infection (e.g., herpes) of the nerve or its motor neurons.
- Potential ear infection—otoscopic examination.

Diagnostic Studies. Diagnostic testing is not indicated unless other cranial neuropathies or focal abnormalities are present on neurologic examination, the patient does not improve over a 6-week period, or other neurologic symptoms occur.

Differential Diagnosis. Included in the differential diagnosis are:

- Ramsay Hunt syndrome (herpes zoster or shingles that includes unilateral rash near or over ear with ipsilateral facial weakness).
- Guillain-Barré syndrome (GBS)—includes an additional symptom of absent tendon reflexes of limbs.
- Congenital hypoplasia of depressor angularis oris muscle.
- Trauma—forceps used during delivery can cause a facial nerve compression neuropathy that spontaneously resolves within a few days to weeks.
- Melkersson-Rosenthal syndrome (involves recurrent facial palsies with swollen lips, tongue, cheeks, or eyelids).
- Möebius syndrome (rare birth defect caused by the absence or underdevelopment of CN 6 and 7, with the potential involvement of other CNs).
- Other—acute otitis media, poliomyelitis, histiocytosis X, varicella, facial nerve tumors, neurofibroma, infiltration of facial nerves with leukemic cells, rhabdomyosarcoma of the middle ear, hypertension, and brainstem infarcts.

Management. Symptoms often resolve without intervention, but there are instances where treatment is indicated. If eyelid closure is incomplete, prescribe methylcellulose eye drops or ocular lubricant to the affected eye several times daily and patch the eye when outdoors, during active play, and when sleeping. The American Academy of Neurology and the American Academy of Otolaryngology agree that steroids should be used in newly diagnosed patients (oral prednisone is dosed at 1 mg/kg/day for 1 week, then tapered for 1 week; starting within the first 3–5 days).[28,29] In those who do not experience full recovery, facial retraining has been explored as a possible treatment, but evidence is limited.

Complications. Approximately 85% of children recover spontaneously within 3 weeks while the remaining children may take up to 5 months. If recovery is incomplete, lack of salivation in response to food, lack of lacrimation, facial contractures, and tics may occur. A small percentage of children experience recurrence.

Reye Syndrome

Reye syndrome is an encephalopathy process, which is associated with a viral infection and primarily affecting those under 18 years of age. A decline in incidence has been associated with the decreased use of salicylates in pediatrics. It may also be related to improvements in the diagnosis of underlying inborn errors of metabolism. Fatty changes of the liver and sudden, acute cerebral edema are hallmarks of Reye syndrome, along with elevated liver enzymes and hyperammonemia. After the initial prodromal symptoms of the illness, the clinical course proceeds in predictable stages, beginning with severe vomiting and progressing to irrational behavior, stupor and coma, apnea, fixed pupils, decorticate posturing with increasing brain edema, and death. Immediate admission to a hospital equipped for tertiary supportive care is needed. Treatment includes respiratory support and methods to control cerebral edema and reduce ammonia levels. Survivors of Reye syndrome may have severe neurologic sequelae. Infants are more severely affected than older children.

Guillain-Barré Syndrome

Guillain-Barre Syndrome (GBS) is an acute polyradiculoneuropathy that primarily affects peripheral nerves. It is characterized by progressive weakness and diminished or absent reflexes that follows a respiratory (e.g., *Mycoplasma pneumoniae*) or gastrointestinal (e.g., *Campylobacter jejuni* or *Helicobacter pylori*) infection by approximately 10 days. Infection with Epstein-Barr virus has also been implicated, but it is linked to a milder form of GBS. Recently, there have been case reports of GBS secondary to SARS-CoV-2 infection.[30] Additional studies may include CSF examination and nerve conduction studies. Most diagnoses include acute demyelinating neuropathy. Known variants include acute motor axonal degeneration (as evidenced by ophthalmoparesis, ataxia, and areflexia) and acute sensory neuropathy.

History. The following are common:
- Fever
- Nonspecific viral infection (gastrointestinal or respiratory) occurring within recent past
- Weakness or neurologic changes in sensory, motor, or visual system
- Paralysis onset is gradual, progressing in an ascending order (*Landry ascending paralysis*), starting in the lower extremities, and progressing to the bulbar muscles over days or weeks; maximum weakness reached within 2 to 3 weeks.

Physical Examination.
- Tenderness and pain in muscles with palpation
- Irritability
- Inability or refusal to walk due to flaccid tetraplegia or quadriplegia
- Paresthesia may or may not be present.
- Respiratory insufficiency (may occur later as progression of the disease)
- Dysphagia, facial weakness
- Papilledema and visual acuity changes may be seen; extraocular muscle involvement is rare.
- Miller-Fisher syndrome (acute external ophthalmoplegia, ataxia, areflexia) may be seen.
- Signs of viral meningitis or meningoencephalitis
- Urinary retention or incontinence (20% of cases; usually transient in nature)
- Bradycardia, postural hypotension, asystole

Diagnostic Studies.
- CSF studies: elevated CSF protein (usually greater than twice upper limit of normal); normal glucose, no pleocytosis (fewer than 10 white blood cells/mm^3)
- Negative blood cultures; viral cultures rarely conclusive
- Normal/mildly elevated creatine kinase (CK) level
- Antiganglioside antibodies (against GM1, GD1) may be elevated in axonal neuropathy form of the disease.
- Decreased motor nerve conduction velocities; slowed sensory nerve conduction; EMG: shows acute denervation of muscle.

Differential Diagnosis. Bickerstaff brainstem encephalitis, meningitis, meningoencephalitis, spinal muscle atrophy, HIV, metabolic diseases, and West Nile virus are included in the differential diagnoses.

Management. Hospitalization is paramount for observation and for handling complications of respiratory muscle paralysis. Intravenous immunoglobin (IVIG) for 5 days is standard protocol. In some cases, a second course of IVIG may be used due to the severity of neurologic deterioration; however, 97% of children have a monophasic disease course. Plasmapheresis and/or immunosuppressive drugs may be used in cases unresponsive to IVIG, but conflicting evidence exists related to these therapies.[30] Care is supportive and includes respiratory support, prevention of decubitus, and treatment of secondary bacterial infections. Rehabilitative therapy should begin early. Children with GBS may have neuropathic and nociceptive pain, which may be severe. NSAIDs may not provide adequate relief, and opioids may exacerbate autonomic symptoms. Chronic pain must be addressed during treatment and rehabilitation therapy.

Complications. Chronic varieties of GBS can occur, as evidenced by recurrence or lack of improvement of symptoms over months or years. Unresolved weakness, flaccid tetraplegia or quadriplegia, and bulbar and respiratory muscle compromise may linger or remain and last longer than 2 months, which is then referred to as chronic inflammatory demyelinating radiculopathy.

Myasthenia Gravis

Myasthenia Gravis (MG) is a neuromuscular disorder that is also classified as an autoimmune disorder. It produces an immune-mediated neuromuscular blockade or neuromuscular junction disorder that originates when circulating receptor-binding antibodies decrease the number of available acetylcholine receptors (AChRs) on the postsynaptic muscle membrane or motor endplate, leaving the motor endplate less responsive than normal.

It can occur anytime between infancy and adulthood. *Ocular* MG primarily experience symptoms that primarily affect the eyes and face, while generalized MG has a broader effect and can affect breathing, speaking, and is more likely to cause limb weakness. Children with MG can also experience other autoimmune diseases (e.g., systemic lupus erythematosus, thyroiditis, rheumatoid arthritis, and/or diabetes mellitus). *Congenital* MG is a subtype of the disorder that involves multiple genes, although mutations in the *CHRNE* gene (17p13.2) are responsible for more than half of all cases. Symptoms of congenital MG start at or close after birth and persist. Mothers with MG may have infants with a transient neonatal myasthenic syndrome because of the transfer of placental anti-AChR antibodies. Once the infant's own receptors regenerate and reinsert into synaptic membranes, the symptoms resolve.

Physical Examination. The key findings include:
- Ptosis/extraocular muscle weakness (usually the first symptom): Older children may complain of double vision; younger children may try to hold their eyelids open with their fingers. The ocular signs may be asymmetric.
- Dysphagia: Infants commonly have feeding problems; older children fatigue when chewing. There may be slurred speech/snarling appearance when trying to smile.
- Muscular weakness of neck flexor muscles (infants), limb-girdle, and distal muscles of hands: Limb weakness is not a common symptom of onset, and symptoms do not include muscle fasciculations, myalgias, or sensory symptoms. The weakness may be so mild as to only occur after exercise.
- Rapid muscular fatigue as evidenced by inability to:
  - Hold an upward gaze for 30 to 90 seconds
  - Sustain a chin to chest position while supine
  - Maintain arm abduction for more than 1 to 2 minutes

- Sustain rapid hand-fisting movements for long periods of time

Diagnostic Studies.

- A short-acting cholinesterase inhibitor (e.g., edrophonium chloride) is given as a clinical test; it should cause spontaneous improvement of ptosis and ophthalmoplegia within seconds; other muscles should fatigue less rapidly.
- EMG is more diagnostic than a muscle biopsy.
- AChR antibody testing should be performed; however, it is often inconclusive; only one-third of adolescents and an occasional prepubertal child exhibit these antibodies.
- Other tests can include serologic antinuclear antibodies and immune complexes; thyroid profile; CK level (normal with MG); chest radiograph (any enlarged thymus needs to be followed up with a tomography or CT scan of the anterior mediastinum); electrocardiography (should be normal); muscle biopsy may be considered.

Differential Diagnosis. Hypothyroidism (Hashimoto thyroiditis), polymyalgia rheumatica, multiple sclerosis (MS), progressive external ophthalmoplegia, GBS, Möbius syndrome, congenital ptosis, congenital myopathies, myotonic dystrophy, and glycogen-storage disease are in the differential.

Management. Treatment of MG is influenced by subtype of the disorder, but typically requires treatment with anticholinesterase therapy. Pyridostigmine is often preferred over neostigmine due to a more favorable side effect profile. The ability to discontinue pyridostigmine can be an indicator that the patient has met treatment goals and may guide the tapering of other therapies. The initial dosage is age and weight dependent. It is then titrated upward until the patient responds, side effects are controlled, or until increases are no longer effective. Corticosteroids, cytotoxic agents (e.g., azathioprine, cyclosporine), or thymectomy may also be considered to achieve treatment goals if symptoms are severely debilitating (bulbar or respiratory involvement). Plasmapheresis, high-dose steroids, and IVIG may be considered for acute management of respiratory symptoms.

Complications. Complications include poor growth secondary to steroid use and possible immunodeficiency in adulthood after thymectomy. Long-term therapy with anticholinergics may lead to cholinergic crises that are present similarly to myasthenic crises.

Neurodegenerative Disorders

Multiple Sclerosis

MS is a chronic, relapsing disorder of the CNS that involves demyelination of the brain, spinal cord, and optic nerves. It is estimated that only 3% to 10% of individuals with MS experienced the onset of symptoms before adulthood, but rarely before 10 years of age.[31] Two to 3 times as many females as males are affected. It is widely believed that MS is an autoimmune inflammatory neurodegenerative disorder, but the underlying cause of MS is thought to be multifactorial. Macrophages, activated T-lymphocytes, and other destructive molecules are stimulated by events that are not fully understood. These inflammatory cells cause both CNS demyelination and axon damage within the white matter of the brain, including the optic nerve. No specific virus has been isolated, although some research findings suggest the Epstein-Barr virus may play a role in disease development.

The clinical course is variable but is typified by the *initial relapse and remittance* and *secondary progression*. Episodes of focal neurologic dysfunction can last weeks, or months followed by partial or complete recovery. Pediatric patients have acute exacerbations

---

• **BOX 41.9**   **Symptoms of Multiple Sclerosis**

- Unilateral weakness, ataxia or other cerebellar symptoms (frequent presenting symptom).
- Symptoms that last for more than 24 hours.
- Headache (may be severe, prolonged, generalized).
- Motor symptoms (vague paresthesias of lower extremities, distal portions of hands, feet and face).
- Visual disturbance (diplopia, blurred vision, or sudden loss of vision as a result of optic neuritis).
- Vertigo, dysarthria, and sphincter disturbances uncommon; neurogenic bladder may present in acute transverse myelitis.
- Repeated episodes frequently preceded by fever, nausea, vomiting, and lethargy; may occur within months or years of each other.

From Boesen MS, Sellebjerg F, Blinkenberg M. Onset symptoms in paediatric multiple sclerosis. *Dan Med J.* 2014;61(4):A4800.

---

3 times as frequently as adults. Frequent relapses early in the disease process may lead to a more rapid progression to irreversible disability; however, once irreversible disability begins, the rate of progression is independent of the frequency of relapses. Most symptoms in children are the same as for all other ages (Box 41.9); however, seizures and mental status changes (lethargy) are seen in children but not typically seen in adults. A diagnosis of MS is typically made in children after two episodes of demyelinating events, lasting longer than 24 hours, separated by more than 30 days, involving a distinct CNS region(s) and with no other plausible diagnosis.[32]

Diagnostic studies include:

- Neuroimaging: An MRI (gadolinium enhanced) early in the course of the disease can be important in predicting the clinical future. In children, demyelination of white matter presents as well defined and perpendicular to the corpus callosum. Evidence of disturbance of the BBB is thought to be a better predictor than the number of T2 white matter lesions for developing inflammatory MS lesions and atrophy. Gray matter lesions may also be present but can be more difficult to detect with conventional imaging.
- Other studies may include an LP (may show oligoclonal bands) and visual-evoked potentials.

Once diagnosed, treatment for MS includes the use of disease modifying therapies and the use of high-dose methylprednisolone for acute symptom management. Yet, because of the frequency of other childhood conditions and disorders with similar presentations and symptoms, determining a diagnosis of MS may be challenging. Differential diagnoses may include acute disseminated encephalomyelitis (ADEM), other demyelinating disorders, brain tumor, focal encephalitis, nonviral infections with focal cerebritis or abscess formation, cerebrovascular diseases, leukodystrophies, systemic vasculitis, mitochondrial disorder, vitamin B_{12} deficiency (with macrocytic anemia), and spinal cord disorders. If MS is suspected, prompt referral for evaluation to pediatric neurology should be initiated.

Rett Syndrome

Rett syndrome is a genetic neurodevelopmental disorder characterized by developmental arrest and regression and multisystem comorbidities. The gene mutation most commonly associated with Rett syndrome is a mutation in the gene encoding *methy-CpG-binding protein-2* on the X chromosome (Xq28), and is usually inherited in an X-linked dominant manner. Other genes that are associated with this disorder include *CDKL5* (Xp22.13) and *FOXG1* (14q13). Despite this being a genetic disorder, inheritance of the gene mutation is uncommon with most cases representing de novo mutations. These mutations alone are not sufficient to make a Rett diagnosis; therefore clinical criteria for diagnosis remains key. Standardized diagnostic criteria for Rett syndrome exist.[33]

Rather than cause brain degeneration, Rett syndrome arrests maturation of certain areas of the brain. This syndrome most commonly affects females, although males can also be affected. The typical age where the onset of symptoms occurs is between 5 and 18 months old. Children with Rett syndrome typically experience developmental regression, including partial or complete loss of purposeful hand skills and partial or complete loss of acquired spoken language, followed by a plateau of developmental milestones. They often develop bruxism, apraxia, gait abnormalities, and stereotypic hand movements (e.g., wringing/squeezing, clapping/tapping, hand-mouthing or biting, and handwashing/rubbing automatisms). Head growth deceleration is an early red flag. Rett syndrome can affect many body systems potentially including respiratory dysregulation, gastrointestinal dysfunction, scoliosis, sleep disturbance, and less commonly prolonged QTc interval. Neurologic comorbidities may include seizures and spasticity, which are often late developments in the syndrome, therefore arrangement of a screening EEG is advised for children with this diagnosis.

Physical, occupational, and speech therapies and seizure management are important to preserve functional abilities. As with all neurodevelopmental problems, families need significant support and social services. Life expectancy varies depending on complicating factors. Differential diagnoses include CP, autism, psychosis, other neurodevelopmental disorders, genetic disorders, or other neurodegenerative diseases.

References

1. Merison K, Victorio MCC. Approach to the diagnosis of pediatric headache. *Semin Pediatr Neurol.* 2021;40:100920.
2. Headache classification committee of the international headache society (IHS) the international classification of headache disorders, 3rd edition. *Cephalgia.* 2018;38(1):1–211.
3. Powers SW, Coffey CS, Chamberlin LA, et al. Trial of amitriptyline, topiramate, and placebo for pediatric migraine. *N Engl J Med.* 2017;376(2):115–124.
4. Rastogi RG, Arnold TL, Borrero-Mejias C, et al. Non-pharmacologic and mindful-based approaches for pediatric headache disorders: a review. *Curr Pain Headache Rep.* 2021;25(12):78.
5. Kuppermann N, Holmes JF, Dayan PS, et al. Identification of children at very low risk of clinically-important brain injuries after head trauma: a prospective cohort study. [published correction appears in Lancet. 2014;383(9914):308] *Lancet.* 2009;374(9696):1160–1170.
6. Fisher RS, Cross JH, D'Souza C, et al. Instruction manual for the ILAE 2017 operational classification of seizure types. *Epilepsia.* 2017;58(4):531–542.
7. Fisher RS, Acevedo C, Arzimanoglou A, et al. ILAE official report: a practical clinical definition of epilepsy. *Epilepsia.* 2014;55(4):475–482.
8. Scheffer IE, Berkovic S, Capovilla G, et al. ILAE classification of the epilepsies: position paper of the ILAE Commission for Classification and Terminology. *Epilepsia.* 2017;58(4):512–521.
9. Moosa ANV. Antiepileptic drug treatment of epilepsy in children. *Continuus (Minneap Minn).* 2019;25(2):381–407.
10. Kroger AT, Duchin J, Vazquez M. *General best practice guidelines for immunization: best practices guidance of the Advisory Committee on Immunization Practices* (ACIP). https://www.cdc.gov/vaccines/hcp/acip-recs/general-recs/downloads/general-recs.pdf.
11. Maytum J, Garcia J, Leighty D, Belew J. Utility of the frontal lobe epilepsy parasomnia scale in evaluation of children with nocturnal events. *J Neurosci Nurs.* 2021;53(1):34–38.
12. Operto FF, Coppola G, Mazza R, et al. Psychogenic nonepileptic seizures in pediatric population: a review. *Brain Behav.* 2019;9(12):e01406.
13. Davitt M, Delvecchio MT, Aronoff SC. The differential diagnosis of vertigo in children: a systematic review of 2726 cases. *Pediatr Emerg Care.* 2020;36(8):368–371.
14. Gelfand AA. Episodic syndromes of childhood associated with migraine. *Curr Opin Neurol.* 2018;31(3):281–285.
15. Bassetti CLA, Adamantidis A, Burdakov D, et al. Narcolepsy: clinical spectrum, aetiopathophysiology, diagnosis and treatment. *Nat Rev Neurol.* 2019;15(9):519–539.
16. Lewis SA, Shetty S, Wilson BA, et al. Insights from genetic studies of cerebral palsy. *Front Neurol.* 2021;11:625428.
17. Michael-Asalu A, Taylor G, Campbell H, Lelea LL, Kirby RS. Cerebral palsy: diagnosis, epidemiology, genetics, and clinical update. *Adv Pediatr.* 2019;66:189–208.
18. Novak I, Morgan C, Fahey M, et al. State of the evidence traffic lights 2019: systematic review of interventions for preventing and treating children with cerebral palsy. *Curr Neurol Neurosci Rep.* 2020;20(2):3.
19. Nicolau S, Waldrop MA, Connolly AM, et al. Spinal muscular atrophy. *Semin Pediatr Neurol.* 2021;37:100878.
20. Avagliano L, Massa V, George TM, et al. Overview on neural tube defects: from development to physical characteristics. *Birth Defects Res.* 2019;111(19):1455–1467.
21. Lu VM, Niazi TN. Pediatric spinal cord diseases. *Pediatr Rev.* 2021;42(9):486–499.
22. Albert GW. Chiari malformation in children. *Pediatr Clin North Am.* 2021;68(4):783–792.
23. Yilmaz E, Mihci E, Nur B, et al. Recent advances in craniosynostosis. *Pediatr Neurol.* 2019;99:7–15.
24. Miller DT, Freedenberg D, Schorry E, et al. Health supervision for children with neurofibromatosis type 1. *Pediatrics.* 2019;143(5):e20190660.
25. Ouchenir L, Renaud C, Khan S, et al. The epidemiology, management, and outcomes of bacterial meningitis in infants. *Pediatrics.* 2017;140(1):e20170476.
26. Davis LE. Acute bacterial meningitis. *Continuum (Minneap Minn).* 2018;24(5 Neuroinfectious Disease):1264–1283.
27. Zhang W, Xu L, Luo T, et al. The etiology of Bell's palsy: a review. *J Neurol.* 2020;267(7):1896–1905.
28. Schwartz SR, Jones SL, Getchius TS, et al. Reconciling the clinical practice guidelines on Bell's palsy from the AAO-HNSF and the AAN. *Neurology.* 2014;82(21):1927–1929.
29. Madhok VB, Gagyor I, Daly F, et al. Corticosteroids for Bell's palsy (idiopathic facial paralysis). *Cochrane Database Syst Rev.* 2016;7(7):CD001942.
30. Shahrizaila N, Lehmann HC, Kuwabara S. Guillain-Barré syndrome. *Lancet.* 2021;397(10280):1214–1228.
31. Brenton JN, Kammeyer R, Gluck L, et al. Multiple sclerosis in children: current and emerging concepts. *Semin Neurol.* 2020;40(2):192–200.
32. Duignan S, Brownlee W, Wassmer E, et al. Paediatric multiple sclerosis: a new era in diagnosis and treatment. *Dev Med Child Neurol.* 2019;61(9):1039–1049.
33. Banerjee A, Miller MT, Li K, et al. Towards a better diagnosis and treatment of Rett syndrome: a model synaptic disorder. *Brain.* 2019;142(2):239–248.

42

Genitourinary Disorders

AMBER WETHERINGTON

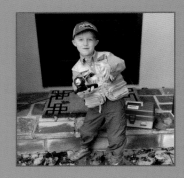

The genitourinary (GU) system is a critical center for metabolism that is responsible for regulating water and electrolytes (sodium, potassium, chloride, calcium, phosphate, and magnesium), excreting waste products (urea, creatinine, poisons, and drugs), and regulating acid-base and hormone secretion (vitamin D, renin, erythropoietin, and prostaglandins). In addition to regulating water and electrolytes, excretion, and acid-base balance, the male GU system also has reproductive and excretory functions. GU problems in infants, children, and adolescents range from commonly occurring, easily treated diseases to significant congenital or acquired conditions. Pediatric primary care providers (PCPs) play a significant role identifying problems, managing disorders, maintaining optimal function, and providing education and support to children and families related to GU function. Primary care management of GU conditions includes assessment, diagnosis and management of disorders, provision of continuity of care, and referral to and collaboration with pediatric urologists and nephrologists.

Standards of Care

Hypertension in infants and young children is usually secondary to another disease process and is most commonly renal in origin. Older school-age children and adolescents may present with primary hypertension due to obesity; however, GU disorder must be considered. Routine blood pressure (BP) screening is recommended at every preventive health care visit beginning at 3 years old.[1] The management and treatment of hypertension is discussed in Chapter 33. The American Academy of Pediatrics (AAP) and the Bright Futures Practice Guidelines do not recommend screening for asymptomatic bacteremia or chronic kidney disease with a urine dipstick or complete urinalysis (UA) at any age.[1]

Anatomy and Physiology

The renal system is composed of two kidneys, two ureters, a bladder, and a urethra. The kidneys are positioned posteriorly on the abdominal wall. The main structures of the kidney are the cortex, the medulla, and the collecting system. The renal medulla and nephrons are present at birth, but the peripheral tubules are small and immature. By adolescence, the kidneys are adult size and weight. The ureters are muscular tubes that move urine from the kidneys to the bladder by peristaltic contractions. The bladder is a muscular reservoir that collects urine, lies close to the anterior abdominal wall in early childhood, later descends into the pelvis as the child grows, and changes shape from cylindrical to pyramidal.

As the bladder fills to capacity, nerves signal the brain of the need to urinate. When urination occurs, the sphincter between the bladder and urethra opens and bladder contractions create pressure that forces urine out the urethral meatus. The male urethra is significantly longer than the female urethra; it leaves the bladder in the lower pelvis, passes through the prostate, has openings for the release of bulbourethral gland fluids and semen during sexual activity, extends the length of the penile shaft, and exits at the tip of the glans. The female urethra descends from the bladder and exits the body inside the labia minora, midline, just posterior to the clitoris.

Physiologically the kidneys filter, clear, reabsorb, and secrete substances essential to metabolism. The urinary system begins forming and excreting urine at 3 months of gestation. Glomerular filtration and renal blood flow increase at birth and stabilize by 1 to 2 years old. In infants, total extracellular fluid volume is significantly greater than adults, and fluid composition has lower bicarbonate concentration. Normal urine excretion is 1 to 2 mL/kg/h. The kidneys mature throughout infancy and kidney function approaches adult values between 6 and 12 months old.

Pathophysiology and Defense Mechanisms

Urinary system disorders occur anywhere from the kidneys to the urethral meatus. Upper tract disorders involve the kidneys and ureters, while lower tract disorders involve the bladder, urethra, or meatus. This differentiation is difficult because disorders in one part of the system frequently affect the entire system, and present silently or symptomatically. The main GU pathologic mechanisms are infection, inflammatory response, congenital malformation, or injury.

The urinary tract is normally sterile. The bladder's mucosal lining inhibits bacterial growth and adherence, urine's acidic pH further protects the urinary system by inhibiting bacterial growth, and urine flow out of the bladder provides mechanical defense by its flushing action.

Assessment of the Genitourinary System

History and Clinical Findings

- History of the present illness
  - Symptom onset and pattern (e.g., acute, chronic, cyclic)
  - Fever
  - Abdominal pain
  - Flank pain

- Preceding injury or illness, especially streptococcal infection
- Vomiting
- Voiding pattern: Stream force and direction, dribbling or discharge, enuresis or incontinence, dysuria, urinary urgency or hesitancy
- Color, odor, frequency, and urine volume
- Bowel patterns or chronic constipation
- Sexual activity or abuse
- Family history
  - Renal disease, deafness, hypertension, GU structural abnormalities, or GU syndromes
  - Past history of urinary tract infection (UTI), hematuria, proteinuria, syndromes associated with GU abnormality

Physical Examination

- Growth parameters: Failure to thrive (FTT) is associated with UTI, renal tubular acidosis (RTA), and chronic renal failure in infants. Unusual weight gain is associated with nephrotic syndrome or acute renal failure.
- BP: Often elevated with nephritis and nephrotic syndrome
- Edema or pallor
- Ear position and formation: Congenital renal disorders are associated with low-set or abnormal ears
- Abdominal masses, ascites, flank (including costovertebral) or suprapubic tenderness
- External genitalia abnormalities
- Unusual facial features associated with syndromes that include renal disease

Diagnostic Studies

Order diagnostic studies as indicated. Proper urine collection, transport, and storage is essential to obtain accurate results. Normal urine composition varies considerably during a 24-hour period. Most reference values are based on analysis of the first morning voided urine. This specimen is preferred because it has a uniform volume and concentration and lower pH, which preserves the formed elements. Evaluate urine within 30 minutes and keep it refrigerated (below 39.2°F or 4°C) if stored. Use preservative-containing containers for specimens that require extended storage (e.g., overnight).[2]

Obtain a UA to assess the following:

- Physical characteristics: Color, clarity, odor, specific gravity, and osmolality
- Specific gravity measures hydration and renal concentration ability and varies from 1.003 to 1.030. A first-voided urine specimen specific gravity of 1.010 or higher indicates normal renal concentration function. Urine with a specific gravity greater than 1.030 is concentrated.
- Chemical characteristics: Urine dipsticks are Clinical Laboratory and Improvement Amendments of 1988 (CLIA) waived and used widely to determine pH, specific gravity, and the presence of glucose, ketones, protein, bile pigments, hemoglobin, nitrites, and leukocyte esterase. For correct results, strips must remain in their original containers and not be exposed to moisture, light, cold, or heat until used. Urine must be fresh, warmed to room temperature if refrigerated, and read at correct time intervals for each test strip (Table 42.1). Urine pH varies from 4.6 to 8 based on acid-base balance. Blood indicates the presence of hemoglobin; intact erythrocytes cause spotty changes on the dipstick, and free hemoglobin or myoglobin cause uniform color change. Leukocyte esterase indicates white blood cells

(WBCs) in the urine (pyuria) and warrant further investigation. Nitrites are an indirect measure of bacteriuria and the most specific infection marker. Common urinary pathogens contain enzymes that reduce nitrate in urine to nitrite. There is an increased risk of false negative results for leukocyte esterase and nitrite in children younger than 3 years; however, new research supports UA dipstick testing alone as statistically reliable.[3]

Obtain a urine culture for children with UTI symptoms, the risk criteria for UTIs (during infancy, potty training, in sexually active adolescent girls and with bladder and bowel dysfunction) are met, the child has a high fever without a source, or following a urine sample positive for nitrites or leukocyte esterase. The combination of leukocyte esterase and nitrites is highly predictive of a positive urine culture. Negative leukocyte esterase and nitrites reasonably rule out a UTI; however, a culture is still indicated for both negative and positive urine dipstick findings, especially if patient previously voided within 4 hours. Specimens obtained early in the morning or when the patient has not voided for several hours are ideal as it allows time for the nitrates to convert to nitrites.[4]

Microscopic urine examination: Performed on centrifuge-spun and unspun urine with consideration of collection method. Urine that is positive for blood or protein on dipstick should be validated by UA with reflexive microscopy.

- Red blood cells (RBCs): In general, more than 2 to 5 per high-power field (HPF; ×40) in unspun urine or more than 2 to 10 per HPF in spun urine is abnormal. If cells are dysmorphic, the blood's origin is most likely renal.
- WBCs: Fewer than two WBCs per HPF is normal. More than 10 WBCs indicates an infection. Leukocytes found in unspun urine are associated with bacterial colony counts of greater than 100,000.
- Bacteria: The presence of any bacteria is abnormal.
- Casts: RBCs, hyaline, waxy, epithelial, leukocyte, or fatty casts are present in various disease states.
- Crystals: Are amorphous and are not of clinical significance.

Depending on the results of the UA and/or clinical symptoms, other tests may be indicated, including:

- Gram stain: Bacteria on the Gram stain indicate the presence of infection.
- Urine culture and sensitivities: Culture remains the gold standard for diagnosing and identifying the best treatment for UTIs. Urine specimens unrefrigerated for 2 hours or more are subject to bacterial overgrowth, pH change, and RBC and WBC casts dissolution.
- A 24-hour urine collection: A 24-hour urine sample is needed to determine total calcium excretion, the calcium-creatinine ratio, and total protein excretion.
- Blood urea nitrogen (BUN) estimates the urea concentration in blood and measures toxic metabolites that cause uremic syndrome.
- Serum creatinine and creatinine clearance estimate the glomerular filtration rate (GFR), a measure of kidney function.
- Serum electrolytes and acid-base status help detect renal tubular abnormalities.
- Ultrasonography is a noninvasive method if identifying GU structures.
- Dimercaptosuccinic acid (DMSA) scanning is the most sensitive tool to detect acute pyelonephritis and renal scarring. DMSA is appropriate when there is concern for scarring or when serum creatinine is elevated.[5]

TABLE 42.1	Chemical Characteristics of Urine		
Constituent	**Positives Indicate**	**Cause of False Positive**	**Cause of False Negative**
Glucose	Metabolic problem (e.g., diabetes), recent high glucose intake, oral corticosteroids, galactosemia	Antibiotics, delay in reading, myoglobin, oxidizing contaminants	Ascorbic acid intake, ketones, high specific gravity
Ketones	Dehydration, starvation, missed breakfast, strenuous exercise, stress, fever, metabolic problems (e.g., diabetes)	Irrigating solution, highly pigmented urine	If urine left standing, acetone evaporates
Protein	Renal disease, orthostatic proteinuria	Exercise, fever, dehydration, alkaline or concentrated urine (specific gravity >1.02), semisynthetic penicillin, oxidizing, cleansing agents	Dilute or acidic urine
Blood (hemoglobin)	If concurrent microscopic examination is negative for RBCs: free hemoglobin secondary to chemicals, illness, or drugs; myoglobin secondary to burns, muscle trauma, physical child abuse, myositis, strenuous exercise If concurrent microscopic examination is positive for RBCs: external excoriation, renal problems	Menses, oxidizing cleansing agents, dilute urine, myoglobinuria, strenuous exercise	Ascorbic acid, dipstick exposed to air, pH of urine <5.1
Nitrite	Bacteria causing urinary tract infection	Rare	Common; urine should be in bladder at least 4 h, dilution of nitrate in urine
Leukocyte esterase	Pyuria (white blood cells in urine); inflammation from irritation or infection of vulva, vagina, or urethra; bladder or kidney inflammation with or without infection	Oxidizing agents	Immunocompromised, proteinuria, vitamin C in the urine, technical error related to time at reading dipstick
Urobilinogen	Hemolytic disease; hepatic disease	Sulfonamides, presence of phenazopyridine	Exposure to light, urine remains at room temperature too long
Bilirubin	Hepatic disease; biliary obstruction	Presence of phenazopyridine	Urine remains at room temperature too long

RBC, Red blood cell.

From Riley RS, McPherson RA. Basic Examination of urine. In: *Henry's Clinical Diagnosis and Management by Laboratory Methods.* 24th ed. Elsevier; 2022:468–509.

- Voiding cystourethrogram (VCUG) is the most reliable method to detect vesicoureteral reflux (VUR). Indications for VCUG in a child with a UTI are limited to febrile UTIs after an abnormal ultrasound or DMSA scan, or when there is a second febrile UTI.[6]

Management Strategies

Education and Counseling

Education and counseling are essential components in the management of GU disorders. Inform parents and children about the pathologic condition, etiology, treatment, prevention strategies, and prognosis with and without treatment. The PCP and family must decide on an agreeable plan of care. Urinary problems occur any time during infancy, childhood, or adolescence and vary in severity, chronicity, and disability.

Referral

Referral to a pediatric urologist, nephrologist, or surgeon may be required. When a referral is made, the PCP retains the essential role of case manager for the child and provides care continuity. The PCP is often the person the family knows best and is most comfortable with when discussing concerns, potential plans, and long-term management.

Genitourinary Tract Disorders

Urinary Tract Infection and Pyelonephritis

There are three kinds of UTI in children: (1) asymptomatic bacteriuria, (2) cystitis, and (3) pyelonephritis. Young children may have limited or unusual symptoms; therefore a high degree of suspicion must be maintained to diagnose UTI. Inflammation and infection occur at any point in the urinary tract, so a UTI must be identified according to location. *Asymptomatic bacteriuria* is bacteria in the urine without other symptoms, is benign, and does not cause renal injury. *Cystitis* is an infection of the bladder that produces lower tract symptoms but does not cause fever or renal injury. *Pyelonephritis* is the most severe type of UTI and involves the renal parenchyma or kidneys and must be readily identified and treated because of the potential irreversible renal damage. Clinical signs consistent with pyelonephritis include fever, irritability, and vomiting in an infant, and urinary symptoms associated with fever, bacteriuria, vomiting, and renal tenderness in older children. In a child younger than 24 months of age, pyelonephritis is the most common significant bacterial infection when fever with an unknown etiology is present.[7] A *complicated UTI* is a UTI with fever, toxicity, and dehydration, or a UTI occurring in a child younger than 3 to 6 months old. UTIs are classified based on their association with other structural or functional abnormality such as VUR, obstruction, dysfunctional voiding, or pregnancy. In addition, a UTI must be identified as a first occurrence, recurrent (within 2 weeks with the same organism or any reinfection with a different organism), or chronic (ongoing, unresolved, often caused by a structural abnormality or resistant organism). Age and sex of the pediatric patient are important factors in determining the evaluation method and the course of treatment.

The organism most commonly associated with UTI is *Escherichia coli* (70%), although other organisms (e.g., *Klebsiella, Enterococcus, Proteus, Staphylococcus,* and *Pseudomonas*) cause infection. UTI secondary to group B streptococcus is more common in neonates. Several factors contribute to the etiology of UTIs. Most UTIs are ascending (i.e., the infection begins with colonization of the urethral area and ascends the urinary tract). If the infection progresses to the kidney, intrarenal reflux deep into the kidneys can lead to scarring. However, the most important risk factor for the development of pyelonephritis in children is VUR, which is detected in 10% to 45% of young children who have symptomatic UTIs. Furthermore, reflux of infected urine from the bladder increases the risk of pyelonephritis. Renal damage occurs in the compound papillae, located in the upper and lower poles of the kidney and the usual site of scarring, which have wide and gaping openings allowing intrarenal reflux.

Host resistance factors and bacterial virulence factors are also important in the etiology of UTIs. Bacterial adherence allows organisms to ascend the urinary tract. Virulence is the toxicity of substances released by bacteria, the greater the virulence, the greater the damage to the urinary tract. Both of these factors enhance colonization of the urinary tract and aid in bacterial persistence and effect. Host factors include the presence of a structural abnormality, dysplasia (such as VUR, obstruction, or other anatomic defect), or functional abnormalities (such as dysfunctional voiding or constipation). Other host factors affecting risk include female sex (due to short urethra), poor hygiene, irritation, sexual activity or sexual abuse, and pinworms. Several bacterial factors are known, but the two most important ones are adherence and bacterial virulence. Bacteria that have fimbriae or pili adhere to the bladder mucosa surface, which allows the bacteria to resist the bladder's defensive cleansing flow of urine and causes tissue inflammation and cell damage.

UTIs are common in children, with most febrile UTIs occurring before 1 year of age. Uncircumcised males less than 1 year old are much more likely to develop a febrile UTI, but there is a greater propensity for females to be diagnosed with UTIs overall. During the first year of life the male to female ratio is 2.8:5.4, after 1 year old this increases to 1:10. The risk of UTI is greatest during infancy, the potty-training transition period, and in sexually active adolescent girls. Bladder and bowel dysfunction (see Chapter 17) increases risk for UTI in all ages. Children may ignore an urge to urinate for a variety of reasons, most commonly holding in favor of playing or refusing to go to the bathroom at school. Incomplete bladder emptying and urinary stasis, combined with a high-pressure environment and turbulent urine flow, provides an ideal setting for bacterial growth. The risk of recurrence within the first year after an initial infection is common.[7]

History and Clinical Findings

The following information should be obtained:
- Family history of VUR, recurrent UTI, or other kidney problems

- Prenatally diagnosed renal abnormality
- Previous infection: Request records from the past infection evaluation and diagnostic studies
- Circumcision
- Risk factors for infants 2 to 24 months old with no other source of infection[6]
  - Age
  - Temperature of 39°C or higher for 24–48 hours or longer.
- Voiding patterns: Frequency, abnormal stream, complete emptying, dribbling, enuresis, holding urine, incomplete emptying, and bathroom avoidance
- Constipation
- Irritants, such as nylon underwear or clothing (spandex, tight pants or shorts that rub); bubble bath or sitting in soapy bath water
- Hypertension
- Sexual activity, masturbation, or sexual abuse
- Other infection: Pinworms, diaper rash

Physical Examination. See Table 42.2 for age-related symptoms.
- General appearance (toxic appearing?)
- Vital signs: Temperature, BP
- Growth parameters: Growth may be decreased with chronic UTI or renal insufficiency, especially in infants
- Flank pain or costovertebral angle (CVA) tenderness
- Abdominal examination: Suprapubic tenderness, bladder distention or a flank mass (obstructive signs), mass from fecal impaction
- Genitalia: Vaginal erythema, edema, irritation, or discharge; labial adhesions; uncircumcised male, urethral ballooning; weak, dribbling, thread-like stream

TABLE 42.2 Clinical Findings of Urinary Tract Infection in Children of Various Ages

Neonatal	Infancy	Early Childhood	Middle Childhood and Adolescence
Jaundice	Malaise, irritability	Altered voiding pattern	"Classic dysuria" with frequency, urgency, and discomfort
Hypothermia	Difficulty feeding	Malodor	
Failure to thrive (FTT)	Poor weight gain	Abdominal/flank pain[a]	Malodor
Sepsis	Fever[a]	Enuresis	Enuresis
Vomiting or diarrhea	Vomiting or diarrhea	Vomiting or diarrhea[a]	Abdominal/flank pain[a]
Cyanosis	Malodor	Malaise	Fever/chills[a]
Abdominal distention	Dribbling	Fever[a]	Vomiting or diarrhea[a]
Lethargy	Abdominal pain/colic	Diaper rash	Malaise

[a]Findings increase likelihood of pyelonephritis.

- Neurologic examination (if voiding is dysfunctional): Perineal sensation, lower extremity reflexes, sacral dimpling, or cutaneous abnormality

Diagnostic Studies. Clinical guidelines for the contemporary management of UTI in children were published in 2021.[6] The method used to collect urine has an effect on the results' interpretation. Bagged urine specimens, even after cleaning the external genitalia before placement, produce a high incidence of false-positive UA results due to contamination and thus must not be used to determine UTI. If antimicrobial therapy must be initiated due to an ill-appearing child, catheterization and urine culture must be obtained before administering antibiotics.[6] Older children who can void on command should be able to obtain a clean-catch void. Having the female child sit with knees apart, feet supported, and torso leaned forward while on the toilet separates the labia and decreases contamination.

Urine culture is essential to confirm the diagnosis. UTIs cause cultures with greater than 100,000 colonies of a single pathogen in a clean catch urine specimen, or greater than 50,000 in a catheterized or suprapubic specimen.[7]

- UA should be used only to raise or lower suspicion. Suspicious findings include foul odor, cloudiness, nitrites, leukocytes, alkaline pH, proteinuria, hematuria, pyuria, and bacteriuria.
- Leukocyte esterase chemical tests detect pyuria, but pyuria may arise from causes other than UTI.
- Consider obtaining a laboratory UA with reflexive Gram stain and microscopy if dipstick findings are positive.
- Bacterial identification and determination of sensitivities are necessary in patients who appear toxic or could have pyelonephritis, have relapses or recurrent UTI, or are nonresponsive to medication.
- Complete blood count (CBC) (elevated WBC count), erythrocyte sedimentation rate (ESR), C-reactive protein, BUN, and creatinine should be done if the child is younger than 1 year old, appears ill, or if pyelonephritis is suspected.
- Blood culture should be done if sepsis is suspected (see Chapter 24).

Differential Diagnosis

The differential diagnoses include urethritis, vaginitis, viral cystitis, foreign body, sexual abuse, dysfunctional voiding, appendicitis, pelvic abscess, and pelvic inflammatory disease. Any child who has acute fever without a focus, FTT, chronic diarrhea, or recurrent abdominal pain should be evaluated for UTI.

Management

Goals of treatment are to quickly identify the extent and level of infection; to eradicate infection; to provide symptomatic relief; to find and correct anatomic or functional abnormalities; and to prevent recurrence and renal damage.[6] When deciding on a treatment plan, the child's age, sex, symptoms, the suspected location of the UTI, and antibiotic resistance patterns in the community must be considered. Fig. 42.1 outlines treatment of UTIs in the pediatric patient.

Infants and Early Childhood. To diagnose UTI, the infant or early childhood child should have both a UA suggesting infection (positive leukocyte and/or nitrite tests) and urine culture from a sterile catheterization or suprapubic aspiration with at least 50,000 cfu/mL. Risk factors have been identified to help the clinician determine appropriate management. Higher risk factors for girls include age younger than 12 months, fever of at least 102.2°F (39°C), fever lasting at least 2 days, and absence of another source of infection. Higher risk factors for boys include fever of at least 102.2°F (39°C), fever lasting more than 24 hours, and absence of another source of infection.[8]

Asymptomatic Bacteriuria. Bacteriuria that occurs without pyuria does not require treatment.

Uncomplicated Cystitis. Use regional antibiotic resistance patterns and culture and sensitivity results when choosing antibiotics. Short-term (3–5 days) antibiotics may be as effective in treating nonfebrile bladder infections as standard 7- to 10-day dosing with no increased risk of recurrence.[7] Children 2 to 24 months old and febrile children should have 7 to 14 days of antibiotics. Additional specific recommendations for the febrile young child are found in the contemporary guidelines[6] and include that febrile infants and young children should undergo renal and bladder ultrasonography with further evaluation conducted if there is a recurrence of a febrile UTI or abnormal findings on the ultrasonography.

Recommended oral medications include the following[9]:

- Trimethoprim-sulfamethoxazole (TMP-SMX): More than 2 months old—8 to 12 mg/kg TMP component in two divided doses; adolescents, 160 mg TMP component every 12 hours.
- Amoxicillin: Younger than 3 months—20 to 30 mg/kg/day in two divided doses every 12 hours; older than 3 months old (consider increased risk of bacterial resistance)—25 to 50 mg/kg/day in two divided doses; adolescents, 250 to 500 mg every 8 hours or 875 mg every 12 hours.
- Cephalexin: 50 to 100 mg/kg/day divided in four doses and given every 6 hours (maximum dose of 4 g/day).
- Nitrofurantoin: Older than 1 month—5 to 7 mg/kg/day divided every 6 hours (maximum 400 mg/24 hours); adolescents—50 to 100 mg/dose every 6 hours (macrocrystals) or 100 mg twice a day (monohydrate macrocrystals dual release).
- Recurrent UTI: Further evaluation required. Prophylactic antibiotic use (Box 42.1) is controversial and should be used selectively.[10] Consult with urology or nephrology for antibiotic prophylaxis consideration.
- Acute pyelonephritis: Oral therapy is equally as effective as parenteral therapy in treating pyelonephritis and preventing kidney damage if the child is not vomiting.
- Hospitalization is required based on symptom severity—dehydrated, vomiting, or not drinking. Children 1 month old and younger should be admitted and provided a parenteral regimen.
- Treat infants over 1 month and children with uncomplicated pyelonephritis (well hydrated, no vomiting, no abdominal pain) with cephalexin or amoxicillin clavulanate.
- Treat adolescents with uncomplicated pyelonephritis with either amoxicillin clavulanate (875/125 mg twice a day) or ciprofloxacin (500 mg twice a day or extended release 1000 mg once a day).
- Follow-up cultures are not recommended. However, follow-up urine culture should be done 48 to 72 hours after initiating treatment if symptoms persist or if high community organism resistance is present.
- If the culture is not sterile or if there is no clinical improvement after 48 to 72 hours, change antibiotic based on sensitivity report. Obtain bacterial identification and sensitivity studies if not performed initially and use an alternative broad-spectrum antibiotic pending those results. Repeat culture after 48 to 72 hours if response to therapy limited.

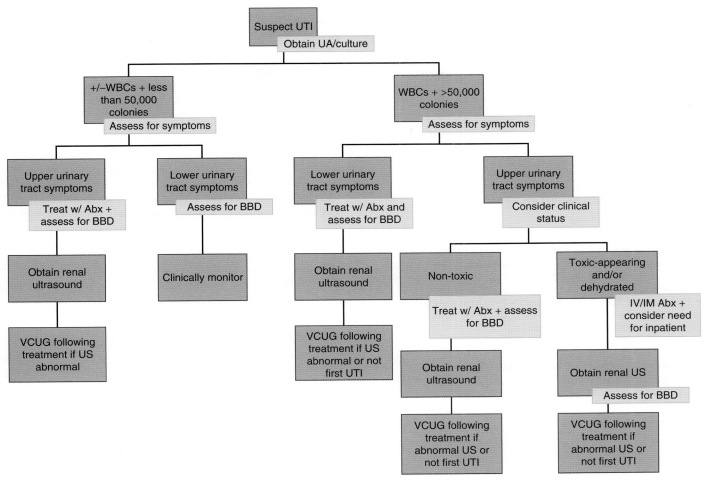

• **Fig 42.1** Suspect Urinary Tract Infection (UTI) Algorithm. Lower urinary tract symptoms include bladder symptoms (urinary frequency/urgency/incontinence/dysuria); upper urinary tract symptoms include fever, flank pain, gross hematuria, vomiting, malaise), abnormal renal ultrasound includes findings such as hydronephrosis, renal scarring, abnormal renal size. *BBD*, Bowel and bladder dysfunction; *IM*, intramuscular; *IV*, intravenous; *UA*, urinalysis; *US*, ultrasound; *VCUG*, voiding cystourethrogram; *WBCs*, white blood cells. (Data from Mattoo TK, Shaikh N, Nelson CP. Contemporary management of urinary tract infection in children. *Pediatrics.* 2021;147[2]:e2020012138.)

• Give phenazopyridine at 12 mg/kg/day for 6- to 12-year-olds and 200 mg for those older than 12 years old, 3 times a day for dysuria.
• Radiologic evaluation (Table 42.3) is recommended to identify structural or functional abnormalities of the urinary tract and renal scarring or damage.
  • Children younger than 2 years with the first UTI should have a renal and bladder ultrasound as soon as the urine is sterile or when the prescribed antibiotic is completed. In addition, all children with fever, diagnosed with pyelonephritis, or with recurrent UTIs should have a renal and bladder ultrasound. VCUG does not need to be done routinely with first febrile UTI. However, if ultrasound reveals hydronephrosis, scarring, or other atypical or concerning findings, VCUG should be utilized.[5]
  • DMSA scan ordered by the urologic specialist may be obtained when renal scarring is suspected or when diagnosis of pyelonephritis is uncertain.[5]

Patient and Family Education, Prevention, and Prognosis

Discuss the following with parents and/or patients:
• Clearly explain the cause, potential complications, and overall treatment plan, including short- and long-term plans.
• Frequently and completely void and increase fluid intake, especially water. Schedule voiding times, voiding with knees spread apart, or double voiding (voiding and then immediately attempting to void again) is helpful.
• Treat perineal inflammation to help prevent UTI.
• Treat constipation.
• Treat pinworms.
• Encourage sexually active females to drink water before intercourse and void immediately afterward.
• Decrease intake of bladder irritants, such as the "four Cs" (caffeine, carbonated beverages, chocolate, citrus), aspartame (NutraSweet), alcohol, and spicy foods.
• Seek prompt medical attention with fever recurrence and/or fever duration for more than 48 hours, especially if younger than 24 months.

• BOX 42.1 Radiologic Workup and Prophylaxis for Urinary Tract Infections

Why Do a Radiologic Workup?
- To identify any structural or functional abnormality of the urinary tract
- To identify any renal scarring or damage

Who Requires a Workup?
- Order a renal and bladder ultrasound on children with the first positive urine culture and with fever and systemic illness. In children with one or more infections of the lower urinary tract (dysuria, urgency, frequency, suprapubic pain), renal and bladder ultrasound may be considered; however, assessment and treatment of bladder and bowel dysfunction is most important.
- If the renal ultrasound is abnormal, voiding cystourethrogram is indicated.

What About Prophylaxis?
- There is controversy about if and when prophylaxis should be used. If a decision to use prophylaxis is made and depending on the source, between one-quarter to one-half of the treatment dose of antibiotic may be given at bedtime.
- Nitrofurantoin: Older than 2 months old: 1–2 mg/kg as a single daily dose; expensive; liquid form poorly tolerated; consider sprinkling capsules over applesauce, yogurt, pudding
- TMP-SMX: TMP 2 mg/kg as a single daily dose or 5 mg/kg twice per week (based on TMP component) if older than 1 month
- Cephalexin: 10 mg/kg as a single daily dose
- Amoxicillin: 10 mg/kg as a single daily dose; can be used for a newborn or premature infant; not used past the first 2 postnatal months; shelf life for liquid is 14 days

TMP-SMX, Trimethoprim-sulfamethoxazole.

Vesicoureteral Reflux

VUR is retrograde regurgitation of urine from the bladder into the ureters, and potentially the kidney. The major concern with VUR is the exposure of the kidney to infected urine, which may cause pyelonephritis. Primary VUR is the most common type and typically involves an abnormally short ureter and ineffective vesicoureteral valve. Secondary VUR is caused by either functional or structural bladder outlet obstruction. It is graded according to the International Reflux Study (IRS) Classification (Fig. 42.2). Grade I does not reach the renal pelvis; grade II extends up to the renal pelvis without dilation; grade III describes reflux to the renal pelvis with mild to moderate dilation of the ureter and the renal pelvis; grades IV and V (high grade) include definite ureter and renal pelvis distension and can include hydronephrosis or reflux into the intrarenal collecting system.[11]

VUR is the most common anatomic abnormality found in young infants and children with UTI. Approximately 30% to 40% of children with affected siblings have reflux, and 50% of children with affected mothers have reflux.[11] A metaanalysis identified a positive correlation with recurrent UTIs, voiding dysfunction, and renal scarring.[5]

History and Clinical Findings

The history may be positive for a previous UTI, abnormal voiding pattern or dysfunction, unexplained febrile illness, chronic constipation, prenatal high-grade hydronephrosis, and/or UTI symptoms. The family history may be positive for VUR.

Diagnostic Studies
- Ultrasonography, although it may be normal even in the presence of reflux.

TABLE 42.3 Radiologic Studies Done for Evaluation of Urinary Tract Conditions

Study	Cost	Advantages	Disadvantages	Use
Ultrasound	Least expensive	Shows structure, shape, and growth. Detects structural abnormality, obstruction, pyelonephritis, large scars. Painless, low risk, no radiation, noninvasive, available	Does not detect small scars of VUR. Poor visualization of ureters. Does not measure renal function or transient injury to kidney	Initial evaluation with first UTI and follow-up
Voiding cystourethrogram (VCUG) (radiographic)	Least expensive	Detects and grades VUR if high or low pressure, high or low bladder volumes, during voiding, during early or late bladder filling. Visualizes bladder and urethra (especially in males) and diverticula	Does not detect obstruction, pyelonephritis, scars. Greater radiation than with scan. Requires intravesical administration of contrast	Indicated in infants and children with abnormal ultrasound
Dimercaptosuccinic acid (DMSA) renal scan (nuclear)	Most expensive	Detects acute inflammation, scars, and obstruction. Earlier detection of parenchymal damage—large or small scars, permanent or focal—than with IVP (1–3 years old)	Does not detect VUR or measure renal function. Does not evaluate calyces, ureters, bladder, or urethra	Follow-up for fever of unknown origin and negative ultrasound in neonates. To diagnose acute pyelonephritis. To detect renal scars
Computed tomography (CT) (contrast)	Expensive	Detects obstruction, pyelonephritis, large scars	Does not detect small scars or VUR Risk of allergic reaction, acute renal failure	Trauma

IVP, Intravenous pyelogram; *UTI,* urinary tract infection; *VUR,* vesicoureteral reflux.

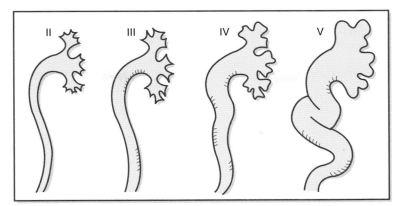

• **Fig 42.2** Grading of Vesicoureteral Reflux. Grade I: Vesicoureteral reflux (VUR) into a nondilated ureter. Grade II: VUR into the upper collecting system without dilation. Grade III: VUR into dilated ureter and/or blunting of calyceal fornices. Grade IV: VUR into a grossly dilated ureter. Grade V: massive VUR, with significant ureteral dilation and tortuosity and loss of the papillary impression. (From Elder JS. Vesicoureteral reflux. In: Kliegman RM, St Geme JW, et al, eds. *Nelson Textbook of Pediatrics*. 21st ed. Elsevier; 2020:2796–2800.)

TABLE 42.4   Management of Primary Vesicoureteral Reflux in Children

	Monitor Clinically	Treat BBD	CAP	Yearly Renal Ultrasound + VCUG	Surgical Correction
Grade I	Yes	Yes	Avoid	Avoid	Avoid
Grade II	Yes	Yes	Consider	Consider	Consider
Grade III	Not alone	Yes	Yes	Yes	Consider
Grade IV–V	Not alone	Yes	Yes	Yes	Consider

BBD, Bowel bladder dysfunction; *CAP*, continuous antibiotic prophylaxis; *VCUG*, voiding cystourethrogram.

- VCUG establishes the presence of reflux and determines the grade.
- DMSA scan assesses for renal scarring if renal ultrasound is abnormal.
- BP and serum creatinine if bilateral renal abnormalities are found.
- UA, and subsequent urine culture if UA suggests UTI.

Management

In 2010, the American Urological Association created guidelines for the management of VUR and reaffirmed those guidelines in 2017.[5] The treatment goal is infection and subsequent scarring prevention. Early identification and appropriate treatment of infection achieve this goal (Table 42.4).

- Most children outgrow their reflux as their ureter intramural length increases. Grades I and II reflux resolve spontaneously in up to 85% of children, grade III reflux resolves spontaneously in 50%. Factors associated with decreased chance for resolution include grades IV and V reflux, bilateral reflux, and older children who present with reflux. Very few children with low-grade VUR require surgery.[11]
- Treat underlying comorbidities, such as constipation and dysfunctional voiding.
- Prophylactic antibiotics to prevent UTI, pyelonephritis, renal injury, and other sequelae may be used when a child has VUR. Prophylaxis is recommended for children with history of a febrile UTI, VUR grades III–V, or for children younger than 1 year

old.[5] Recently, a number of other studies questioned the efficacy of prophylactic antibiotics for both VUR and recurrent UTI. There are no set guidelines for prophylaxis in children over 1 year of age, and management should consider the presence of bowel and bladder dysfunction (BBD), VUR grade, renal scarring, and parental choice. Untreated BBD can increase incidence of breakthrough UTIs while on continuous antibiotic prophylaxis.[5]

- Perform interval urine cultures with symptoms of unexplained illness.
- Repeat VCUG once every 12 to 24 months after diagnosis. Use the 24-month interval in patients with less chance for spontaneous resolution, such as high-grade or bilateral VUR or presence of BBD. Obtain annual BP and growth measurement. VCUG is optional if parents choose an observation-only approach, which is appropriate in the absence of UTIs or BBD.
- Surgical correction includes endoscopic injection of a bulking agent at the ureteral orifice and open surgical correction (ureteral reimplantation).[5]

Patient and Family Education, Prevention, and Prognosis

- VUR does not cause scarring, infection does; but VUR is a risk factor for pyelonephritis and subsequent scarring. Ensure prompt treatment of UTI. Emphasize the necessity of urine culture with any suspicious symptoms. The potential for untreated, chronic UTI leading to chronic renal disease must be explained. BP and growth should be monitored.
- Treatment of BBD improves surgical outcomes.

- Siblings are no longer routinely screened for presence of VUR.[5]
- Prophylactic medicines are best given at night because of urinary stasis while asleep. Recommended medications used for prophylaxis are listed in Box 42.1.
- Review the education discussed in the UTI section.

Hematuria

Hematuria is the presence of five or more RBCs per HPF in three consecutive, fresh, centrifuged specimens obtained over several weeks.[12] The number of RBCs per HPF considered to be abnormal ranges from one to more than five per HPF in unspun urine, and more than five to 10 per HPF in spun urine. In this text, *hematuria* is defined as more than two RBCs per HPF in unspun urine or five per HPF in spun urine. The term *gross hematuria* is blood seen in the urine by the naked eye. The color helps identify the location of the disorder. Brownish, tea-colored urine with casts or protein is usually glomerular in origin. Blood clots and red-to-pink urine with isomorphic RBCs but no protein usually originates from the lower tract. Factors causing hematuria can occur anywhere in the urinary system, from the urinary meatus to the kidneys. A false positive urine dipstick can occur in the presence of myoglobinuria or hemoglobinuria, in which case no RBCs are seen on microscopic examination; so dipstick hematuria should be confirmed by microscopy. Hematuria can be microscopic or macroscopic. Microscopic hematuria may be either persistent or transient.

Microscopic hematuria is common in childhood and may be present in up to 5% of healthy children on a screening UA. Upon rescreening, only 1% to 2% of those children are found to have persistent microhematuria. Careful history taking and physical examination is key, as it is important to rule out symptoms that may accompany the microscopic hematuria and lead to a diagnosis that is clinically significant.[12] The causes of macroscopic hematuria include hypercalciuria, immunoglobulin A (IgA) nephropathy, glomerulonephritis (GN), UTI, hydronephrosis, tumor, cystitis cystica, polyps, or epididymitis. The incidence of hematuria is 0.5% to 2% when confirmed with repeat UA. However, 50% of children with gross hematuria have UTIs.[12,13]

History and Clinical Findings

- Previous medical history of cystic kidney disease, sickle cell disease, systemic lupus erythematosus (SLE), malignancy
- Family or previous history of hematuria, nephrolithiasis, cystic kidney, hemoglobinopathy, sickle cell disease or trait, SLE, hypertension, congestive heart disease, malignancy, deafness, renal failure
- Preceding illness: Viral or streptococcal pharyngitis, impetigo
- Onset, duration, pattern, and timing of hematuria; color of urine
- Dysuria, urgency, frequency, or enuresis
- Presence of pain (back, abdominal, or flank) with voiding
- Straining or squatting with urination (tumor)
- Strenuous exercise or trauma (including bladder catheterization)
- Trauma, foreign body
- Sexual activity or abuse
- Current menstruation
- Edema, rash, pallor, or arthralgias
- Certain drugs (sulfonamides, nitrofurantoin, salicylates, phenazopyridine, toxins [lead, benzenes]), and foods (food color, beets, blackberries, rhubarb, and paprika) can discolor the urine but will not result in RBCs in the urine.[12]
- Symptoms related to chronic renal disease (Box 42.2)

BOX 42.2 Seven Red Flags for Chronic Renal Failure

1. Failure to thrive (poor growth, fatigue, anorexia, nausea, gastroesophageal reflux, vomiting)
2. Chronic anemia (normochromic, normocytic, nonresponsive to medication)
3. Complicated enuresis (daytime frequency, urgency, incontinence, chronic constipation, encopresis, infrequent voiding, straining to void, recurrent urinary tract infection)
4. Prolonged, unexplained vomiting or nausea (especially in the morning), anorexia, weight loss without diarrhea
5. Hypotension
6. Unusual bone disease (e.g., rickets, valgus deformity, fracture with minor trauma)
7. Poor school performance (e.g., headache, fatigue, inattention, withdrawal from activities)

Physical Examination

- Growth parameters: FTT or falling growth curves (chronic renal insufficiency or long-standing acidosis)
- Vital signs, especially BP
- Malformed ears (congenital renal disease)
- Oliguria or anuria
- Edema, hypertension, and proteinuria, which are suggestive of glomerular disease
- Flank pain, which is suggestive of an upper tract disorder
- Abdominal or flank mass, which suggests an obstruction such as Wilms tumor, cystic disease, or posterior valves
- External genitalia: Excoriation, bleeding, foreign body, abuse

Diagnostic Studies

- Urine dipstick analysis for pyuria, proteinuria, hematuria, and concentration
- If greater than 1+ hematuria by dipstick (which equals three RBCs/HPF or 0.02 mg/dL hemoglobin), microscopic examination for RBCs is needed to differentiate RBCs from hemoglobinuria or myoglobinuria.
- The most significant differentiating factor is the presence of proteinuria. If present, rapid evaluation and early referral to nephrology are essential. See section on Nephrotic Syndrome.
- Microscopic examination of the urine includes RBCs, size and shape of the cells, casts, crystals, and WBCs.
- Distorted, misshapen RBCs of different sizes suggest glomerular disease.
- Crystalluria is most commonly caused by hypercalciuria.
- Urine culture
- 24-hour urine collection
- First morning UA on first-degree relatives
- Renal ultrasound is most useful when evaluating hematuria accompanied by pain. Spiral helical computed tomography (CT) scan is the most sensitive modality for diagnosing nephrolithiasis, but there is a large radiation exposure.[12]
- If there are systemic symptoms (e.g., edema, hypertension, changes in urine output), consider further evaluation as described in the Nephritis and Glomerulonephritis section.
- Renal biopsy is recommended for recurrent gross hematuria and coexisting nephritic syndrome, hypertension, renal insufficiency, systemic illness, and parent anxiety.[12]
- Cystoscopy, which is invasive and costly, rarely used, and done if other results are inconclusive and symptoms persist.

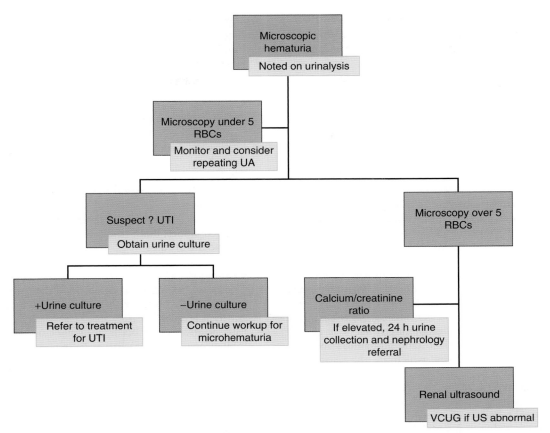

• **Fig 42.3** Management of Asymptomatic Microscopic Hematuria. *RBC*, Red blood cells; *UA*, urinalysis; *US*, ultrasound; *UTI,* urinary tract infection; *VCUG*, voiding cystourethrogram.

Differential Diagnosis

Categories of hematuria to be considered in the diagnostic workup of hematuria are[12,13]:

- Gross hematuria.
  - Urine color is red or tea-colored; microscopic examination shows RBCs.
  - Common causes are poststreptococcal glomerulonephritis (PSGN), renal disease, UTI, trauma, coagulopathy, crystalluria, and nephrolithiasis. Recurrent episodes of gross hematuria are rare.
  - Consider Henoch-Schönlein purpura (HSP) when there is gross hematuria in the presence of abdominal pain, with or without bloody stools, arthralgias, and purpuric rash (see Chapter 38).
  - Consider IgA nephropathy with gross hematuria in the presence of acute illness or strenuous exercise.
  - Sickle cell disease and trait can cause recurrent gross hematuria (mostly males, unilateral kidney).
  - Rhabdomyosarcoma causes gross hematuria and voiding dysfunction.
- Attention and methodical approach are required as history and physical examination guide the workup.
- Renal disease is more likely if microscopic hematuria is accompanied by proteinuria on a first morning sample.
- Other nonspecific symptoms (fever, malaise, weight change), extrarenal symptoms (malar rash, purpura, arthritis, headache, dysuria, abdominal or flank pain, edema, oliguria) may be present.
- Asymptomatic microscopic hematuria rarely indicates significant renal disease.
- Family history is important to assess for benign familial hematuria.
- Hypercalciuria is commonly associated with asymptomatic microscopic hematuria and symptomatic urolithiasis. The diagnosis is made when spot first morning specimen urine calcium-creatinine ratio is elevated more than 0.2, or the 24-hours urinary calcium is more than 4 mg/kg/day. Hypercalciuria is associated with immobilization, diuretics, vitamin D intoxication, hyperparathyroidism, and sarcoidosis.[12,13]
- Regularly monitor for hypertension and proteinuria.
- Asymptomatic hematuria with proteinuria is worrisome for renal disease and further evaluation for renal problems is required.
- Consider evaluating for orthostatic proteinuria (see Proteinuria section). Persistent proteinuria is indicative of a glomerular process.
- Hematuria caused by external irritation of the urinary meatus will resolve with removal of the irritant (diaper rash, soaps, bubble bath, lotions) or avoidance of the offending behavior (e.g., scratching, masturbation, sexual activity).

Management

Undertake a progressive approach to evaluating hematuria with the goal of not overlooking serious, treatable, progressive conditions while avoiding unnecessary studies (Fig. 42.3). Referral is indicated for gross hematuria with unclear cause, symptomatic microscopic hematuria, or persistent asymptomatic hematuria and proteinuria as renal biopsy may be indicated.[12,13]Asymptomatic hematuria requires periodic evaluation every 1 to 2 years to reevaluate for coexisting conditions or proteinuria, and to revisit family history of hematuria or hearing deficits.

Patient and Family Education, Prevention, and Prognosis

Patient education should stress the importance of follow-up for hematuria evaluation. Prognosis depends on the cause of the hematuria.

Proteinuria

Proteinuria originates from problems with glomerular filtration, tubular reabsorption or secretion, or both. The incidence of proteinuria is cited at 30% to 55% in middle childhood. It persists, however, in up to 6% of children when four consecutive urine specimens are tested.[14]

Protein in the urine is commonly detected by dipstick. It may be transient, recurrent, or fixed. Proteinuria can be a disease symptom, or it can reflect a benign, self-limited condition. The quantity of protein and the timing of its presence determine its significance. Qualitative protein in urine, as tested by dipstick, is a positive result if it registers 1+ (30 mg/dL) or more in urine with a specific gravity of less than 1.015. Quantitative protein is tested by measuring a volume of urine over a set period. A level of less than 4 mg/m^2/h is considered normal, 4 to 40 mg/m^2/h is abnormal, and greater than 40 mg/m^2/h indicates nephritic disease.

Four groups of proteinuria exist: (1) isolated, (2) transient or functional, (3) glomerular, and (4) tubulointerstitial.

- Isolated proteinuria includes orthostatic proteinuria and persistent asymptomatic proteinuria, which are the most common.
- Orthostatic proteinuria accounts for up to 60% (75% in adolescents) of proteinuria cases.[14] In this condition, the child excretes abnormal amounts of protein when upright but normal amounts when lying down. Orthostatic proteinuria is diagnosed by assessing a first morning void as described in the Diagnostic Studies section.
- Persistent asymptomatic proteinuria is a common, transient phenomenon in an otherwise healthy child who has a normal clinical and laboratory workup and abnormally high proteinuria.
- Transient or functional proteinuria is usually caused by some type of stress.
- At least 75% of asymptomatic patients with proteinuria in a single urine specimen have normal urine on repeated testing.
- Exercised-induced proteinuria is documented by collecting a urine sample, having the patient exercise vigorously for several minutes, and then collecting another sample. The postexercise sample is usually strongly positive or +2 or higher on the urine dipstick.
- Fever-induced proteinuria accompanies any febrile state and usually subsides with fever resolution. Other stress-related causes include cold exposure, infection, congestive heart failure, and seizures. This type of proteinuria usually resolves in 1 to 2 weeks, and if resolution is verified, no further workup is required.
- Glomerular proteinuria and tubulointerstitial proteinuria are the least common types and characterized by high proteinuria levels or +4 on the urine dipstick. Some authorities believe that children with persistent proteinuria, even at low levels, should be followed with a high index of suspicion for an underlying, progressive renal disorder.

History and Clinical Findings

Most infants, children, and adolescents with proteinuria are asymptomatic but if proteinuria is significant enough to cause hypoproteinemia edema is present. Other history and physical findings include:

- Family history of deafness, visual problems, and renal disease
- Recent strenuous exercise or febrile illness
- Polydipsia or polyuria
- Vague symptoms, such as malaise, fatigue, or pallor
- Symptoms related to chronic renal disease (see Box 42.2)

Physical Examination
- Growth and development parameters (poor weight gain or FTT with chronic disease; weight gain with nephrotic syndrome)
- BP (hypertension), pulse, respiratory rate
- Edema, especially periorbital edema, or symptoms of fluid retention
- Abdominal examination to determine the presence of a mass, enlarged kidney, fluid, tenderness

Diagnostic Studies
- UA (repeated 3 times over 1–2 weeks), preferably done on a first-voided specimen.
- 1+ protein (30 mg/dL) is significant if the specific gravity is less than 1.015; 2+ protein (100 mg/dL) is significant if the specific gravity is greater than 1.015.
- False-positive results occur in highly concentrated or alkaline (pH greater than 5.5) urine. False-negative results occur in dilute or acidic urine.
- Compare a first void urine sample collected immediately after arising with a specimen collected after several hours of activity to rule out orthostatic etiology. Have the child void before sleep to obtain accurate results. A typical result yields negative to trace amounts on the first morning specimen, but 1+ or greater on the second specimen. If the result is equivocal, evaluate back-to-back urine samples (from arising to bedtime and bedtime to arising) for quantitative protein.
- Microscopic urine: RBCs or WBCs (or both), casts, bacteria, oval fat bodies, or other abnormalities are present in most pathologic conditions.
- A urine protein-to-creatinine ratio on a first morning voided sample. Normal values are less than 0.5 mg/dL in children younger than 2 years and less than 0.2 mg/dL in children older than 2 years; greater than 2 mg/dL is considered nephritic. An abnormal urine protein-to-creatinine ratio requires further testing.[14]
- When evaluating proteinuria, a 12- or 24-hour timed urine collection for creatinine (normal: 14–20 mg/kg/24 hours) and protein excretion (normal: less than 4 mg/m^2/h) is requested to evaluate kidney function.
- If protein in urine is greater than 4 mg/m^2/h, check the CBC, electrolytes, BUN, creatinine, albumin/total protein, C3, C4, cholesterol, liver functions, and urine culture and refer to nephrology. A renal specialist may obtain ultrasonogram, VCUG, and radionuclide scans to evaluate for systemic disease as indicated (e.g., antinuclear antibody [ANA], antistreptolysin O [ASO], streptozyme, hepatitis B, human immunodeficiency virus [HIV], tuberculosis).

Differential Diagnosis

Pseudoproteinuria can be caused by semisynthetic penicillins or antiinflammatory agents.

Management

The persistence, quantity, and presence of other abnormalities (e.g., hematuria) are key in evaluating proteinuria (Fig. 42.4).

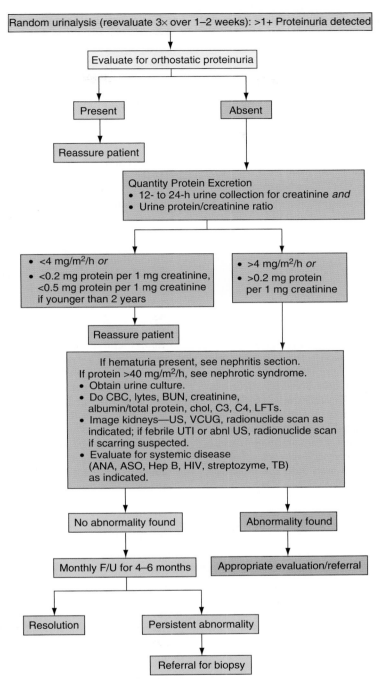

Random urinalysis (reevaluate 3× over 1–2 weeks): >1+ Proteinuria detected

Evaluate for orthostatic proteinuria

Present → Reassure patient

Absent →

Quantity Protein Excretion
• 12- to 24-h urine collection for creatinine *and*
• Urine protein/creatinine ratio

• <4 mg/m²/h *or*
• <0.2 mg protein per 1 mg creatinine, <0.5 mg protein per 1 mg creatinine if younger than 2 years

• >4 mg/m²/h *or*
• >0.2 mg protein per 1 mg creatinine

Reassure patient

If hematuria present, see nephritis section.
If protein >40 mg/m²/h, see nephrotic syndrome.
• Obtain urine culture.
• Do CBC, lytes, BUN, creatinine, albumin/total protein, chol/C3, C4, LFTs.
• Image kidneys—US, VCUG, radionuclide scan as indicated; if febrile UTI or abnl US, radionuclide scan if scarring suspected.
• Evaluate for systemic disease (ANA, ASO, Hep B, HIV, streptozyme, TB) as indicated.

No abnormality found

Abnormality found

Monthly F/U for 4–6 months

Appropriate evaluation/referral

Resolution

Persistent abnormality

Referral for biopsy

• **Fig 42.4** Evaluation of Proteinuria Algorithm. *abnl,* Abnormal; *ANA,* antinuclear antibody; *ASO,* antistreptolysin O; *BUN,* blood urea nitrogen; *C3,* complement 3; *C4,* complement 4; *CBC,* complete blood count; *chol,* cholesterol; *F/U,* follow-up; *Hep B,* hepatitis B; *HIV,* human immunodeficiency virus; *LFT,* liver function test; *lytes,* electrolytes; *TB,* tuberculosis; *US,* ultrasound; *UTI,* urinary tract infection; *VCUG,* voiding cystourethrogram. (Modified from Norwood VF, Peters CA. Disorders of renal functional development in children. In: Wein AJ, Kavoussi LR, Partin AW, et al., eds. *Campbell-Walsh Urology.* Elsevier; 2016:2849–2872.)

• If protein by dipstick is trace or 1+ and specific gravity is greater than 1.015, offer reassurance; recheck urine monthly for 4 to 6 months. If protein is persistent, refer the patient to nephrology.
• If protein by dipstick is greater than 1+, evaluate the child for orthostatic proteinuria (see Diagnostic Studies).

• If first morning urine protein is 1+ or 2+, perform either a quantitative 12- to 24-hour urine protein excretion test or a random urine total protein-creatinine ratio and UA with microscope. Proceed as shown in Fig 42.4.
• If protein by dipstick is greater than 2+, evaluate for nephrotic syndrome (see later section).

- If hematuria is present, evaluate for nephritis (see later section).
- Follow-up is important to monitor for any change in status.
- Refer to a nephrologist if persistent unexplained nonorthostatic proteinuria, any hematuria or RBC or WBC casts, polyuria or oliguria, nephrotic protein levels, elevated BUN or creatinine, elevated BP, systemic complaints (e.g., joint pain, rashes, or arthralgias), or a child with a family history of renal failure, GN, sensorineural hearing loss, or kidney transplantation.

Patient and Family Education, Prevention, and Prognosis

Patient education should stress the importance of follow-up to evaluate the cause of proteinuria. Children with mild asymptomatic proteinuria who have a normal first morning specimen do not require extensive testing for kidney disease but should be monitored annually.

Nephrotic Syndrome

Nephrotic syndrome is due to excessive protein excretion in urine as a result of alterations in the integrity of the glomerular filtration barrier. The main mechanism of the protein loss is increased glomerular permeability. The loss can be selective (albumin only) or nonselective (including most serum proteins), and such selectivity is an important diagnostic distinction. The classic definition of nephrotic syndrome is significant proteinuria (3–4+ protein with UA, greater than 40 mg/m^2/h or a protein:creatinine ratio on a first morning void of greater than 2–3:1), hypoalbuminemia (<2.5 g/dL), edema, and hyperlipidemia. Edema formation results from a plasma oncotic pressure decrease due to a loss of serum albumin, which causes water to extravasate into the interstitial space. This leads to decreased intravascular volume with decreased renal perfusion and activation of the renin-angiotensin system.[15] With protein loss, the liver increases its protein synthesis causing concurrent hyperlipidemia and lipiduria. In addition, the reduced intravascular volume stimulates antidiuretic hormone, which enhances the reabsorption of water.

Nephrotic syndrome is a chronic disease characterized by periods of remission (when both the urinary protein excretion and serum albumin normalize) and relapses (recurrence of proteinuria and hypoalbuminemia after complete remission). Ninety-five percent of the children with minimum change nephrotic syndrome (MCNS) are "steroid responders," they have remission with steroid treatment. Steroid responsiveness is the best prognostic indicator for nephrotic syndrome.[15] The nonresponders are usually steroid resistant and a small number are partial responders, with minimal steroid response, or steroid-dependent and require high prednisone doses with frequent relapses.

Nephrotic syndrome occurs as a result of genetic, immune, systemic, nephrotoxic, allergic, infectious, malignant, vascular, or idiopathic processes. Despite significant research, histopathology is better understood than the pathogenesis. The primary mechanism is believed to be immunologic.[15]

History and Clinical Findings

- History of allergy in up to 50% of children with MCNS.
- Edema is the cardinal clinical feature, especially periorbital edema, dependent areas (tight shoes or underwear), and lax tissues (puffy eyes).
- Low urine production.

- Gastrointestinal symptoms: anorexia, paleness, listlessness, diarrhea, vomiting, abdominal pain (right upper quadrant).
- Respiratory difficulties secondary to ascites, effusion, pneumonia in advanced disease.

Physical Examination
- Edema initially in tissues of low resistance and dependent areas: periorbital, scrotal, and labial. If generalized, can progress to involve the whole body (anasarca)
- Anorexia, irritability, fatigue, abdominal discomfort, and diarrhea
- Muscle wasting, malnourishment, growth failure if prolonged
- If the disease is progressive, hydrothorax with respiratory difficulty
- Hypertension; normal BP if hypovolemic
- Chronically ill-appearing

Diagnostic Studies
- UA and microscopic examination (protein 2+ or greater, hyaline and fine granular casts, microhematuria [in 33%], elevated specific gravity, fat bodies, and casts in urine).
- Quantitative urine protein excretion (24-hour collection or protein-creatinine ratio on a random first morning urine).
- CBC, electrolytes, BUN, creatinine, calcium, serum albumin (less than 2 g/dL), total protein; liver enzymes, triglycerides, lipoproteins, cholesterol, C3 and C4 (normal), ANA, varicella antibody test if exposure while on corticosteroids.
- Venereal Disease Research Laboratory (VDRL), hepatitis B surface antigen, HIV, malaria, purified protein derivative (PPD) as indicated by history.
- Neonatal or infant nephrotic syndrome requires a karyotype as intersex is associated with Denys-Drash syndrome.
- Referral with possible kidney biopsy is recommended if MCNS criteria are not met, systemic disease is present, hypertension and hematuria are present, hypocomplementemia or nonselective proteinemia is present, patient is older than 7 years, patient is nonresponsive to steroids, or if relapses are frequent.

Differential Diagnosis

Infants (newborn to 1 year old) usually have congenital renal problems, children 7 years old and older are likely to have focal glomerulosclerosis or mesangial proliferative GN, and teens usually have membranous nephropathy. The differential diagnosis includes hypoproteinemia from starvation, liver disease, and protein-losing enteropathy; none of these conditions has associated proteinuria. GN should be considered in the differential diagnosis.

Management

Nephrotic syndrome is a complex, often chronic disorder that responds to careful management with a gratifying long-term positive outcome. The diagnosis is made with 95% certainty on clinical impressions. A major goal is to control edema while awaiting definitive remission.

- Consultation with and/or referral to nephrology should occur because the strategies for managing these children change often.
- Hospitalization may be necessary initially if disease is severe.
- Prednisone (2 mg/kg/day; maximum 60 mg) to induce remission, which can occur as early as 14 days, as evidenced by diuresis. Continue steroids for at least 4 to 6 weeks.[15] Treat relapses with a short steroid course and wean the patient as soon as the proteinuria resolves.

- Noncorticosteroid medications (cyclophosphamide and cyclosporine) are used by nephrologists if the child is steroid-dependent, steroid-resistant, or relapses frequently.[15]
- Activity and diet recommendations: No limitation is placed on activity. During active disease, salt may be restricted by nephrology. At other times, a diet appropriate for age is recommended.
- Diuretics and albumin replacement are sometimes used in the acute phase. Home BP monitoring may be recommended.
- Daily home proteinuria testing may be recommended to monitor the child and promptly identify exacerbations. Relapses are identified by persistent proteinuria greater than 2+ every day for 3 days.

Children with nephrotic syndrome are susceptible to pneumococcal, *E. coli, Pseudomonas,* and *Haemophilus influenzae* infection because of fluid stasis; these infections manifest as peritonitis, pneumonia, cellulitis, or septicemia. Hypertension or hypotension are a possibility. Thromboembolism is possible due to hypercoagulability. Protein losses and compromising edema are also potential complications.

Patient and Family Education, Prevention, and Prognosis

Patient education should stress the importance of continued, regular care to monitor renal function and the early treatment of the disease or concurrent infections. Families must be educated to know that relapses are to be expected. An understanding of the disease process, side effects of steroids, recognition of infection, and the importance of monitoring proteinuria for relapses is crucial. If chronic steroid treatment is needed, the patient and family must understand the medication's side effects. The prognosis is good in steroid responders, with relapses that decrease in frequency as the child ages, typically without residual renal dysfunction. It is important for families to understand that idiopathic nephrotic syndrome should not be classified as a chronic illness, and patients should fully participate in all age-appropriate activities and resume an unrestricted diet during periods of remission.[15]

Nephritis and Glomerulonephritis

Nephritis is a noninfectious, inflammatory kidney response characterized by varied degrees of hypertension, edema, proteinuria, and hematuria that is either microscopic or macroscopic with dysmorphic RBCs and casts. Nephritis is classified as acute, intermittent, or chronic. Primary GN occurs when the glomerulus is the original and predominant structure impaired. Secondary GN occurs when renal involvement is secondary to systemic disease (e.g., SLE, HSP, primary vasculitis, Goodpasture syndrome, or drug hypersensitivity reactions). Involvement occurs in the glomerulus, the interstitium, is localized in one part of the kidney, or generalized throughout. GN refers to inflammation primarily in the glomeruli; interstitial nephritis refers to inflammation in the interstitium, it is primarily caused by drug reactions. PSGN is the classic form of GN.

Acute nephritis most commonly occurs as PSGN, which is characterized by a history of streptococcal infection within the prior 2 weeks and an acute onset of edema, oliguria, hypertension, and gross hematuria. Consider an alternative diagnosis if the following findings are present: nephrotic protein levels, lack of evidence for a postinfection mechanism, rapidly deteriorating renal function, or clinical or laboratory findings suggesting other forms of GN (e.g., rash, positive ANA).

Intermittent gross hematuria and proteinuria syndromes include the following:

- IgA nephropathy, or Berger disease, is the most common chronic GN in children of European or Asian descent and is uncommon in African Americans. It is more common in males than females (2:1). This condition is immunologic and causes recurrent gross and microscopic hematuria, and often proteinuria. It is present in about one-third of persons biopsied for persistent microscopic hematuria. It is often precipitated by viral infections or strenuous exercise, and each episode lasts less than 72 hours. BP is normal, no edema is present, and C3 is normal. Definitive diagnosis is made by biopsy. The prognosis is good in the absence of elevated serum creatinine or nephrotic-range proteinuria, although progression to chronic renal insufficiency can occur.[13–15]
- Hereditary or familial nephritis involves many disorders, but the best known is Alport syndrome. More common and severe in males, with onset before 15 years old, this condition is inherited as an X-linked dominant trait 75% of the time. The initial manifestation is isolated, persistent, microscopic hematuria with intermittent macrohematuria and variable proteinuria, occurring with an upper respiratory infection or exercise. Laboratory abnormalities are variable; biopsy verifies the diagnosis. Extrarenal abnormalities, including neurogenic deafness, ocular abnormalities, and macrothrombocytopenia are common. Vision and hearing screening are essential, and PCPs should refer if abnormalities are noted. Severe forms of the disease can lead to end-stage renal disease, which is often heralded by hypotension.
- Familial or benign recurrent nephritis, also known as *thin basement membrane disease,* is a disorder inherited as an autosomal dominant trait with unknown etiology. Episodes are characterized by macroscopic and microscopic hematuria and mild proteinuria, often precipitated by upper respiratory tract infection. Laboratory values other than UA are normal. The diagnosis is confirmed by biopsy, which may not be needed if the disease is mild and confirmed in relatives. In the absence of notable proteinuria, deafness, ocular defects, renal failure, and with normal biopsy findings, the prognosis is excellent.

Chronic nephritis is most commonly known as *membranoproliferative GN* and is distinguished by four types: I, II, III are idiopathic and the fourth is secondary to infectious or immune diseases. Differentiation of type is based on a renal biopsy. Chronic nephritis occurs after acute nephritis or in individuals with nonspecific complaints, such as anorexia, intermittent vomiting, and malaise. It manifests by diminished renal function that ultimately has detrimental effects on other organ systems. Types I and II may respond to steroids, but the overall prognosis is guarded.

The inflammatory kidney response results from various causes such as infection, an immunologic response, drugs, toxins, and vascular or systemic disorders. PSGN is an immune response by the host to a group A beta-hemolytic skin or pharyngeal streptococcal infection, whereas acute postinfectious glomerulonephritis (APGN) is caused by bacterial, fungal, viral, parasitic, or rickettsial agents.

PSGN is the most common form of nephritis in childhood, occurs most often between 5 and 12 years old, occurs more often in males (2:1), and is unusual in children younger than 3 years. The incidence of APGN is difficult to determine because of the large number of patients with subclinical cases.[13–15]

History and Clinical Findings

- Streptococcal skin (more likely) or pharyngeal infection within the past 2 to 3 weeks (PSGN). A latent period of 7 to 10 days elapses between infection and symptom onset; if fewer than 5 days or more than 14 days, consider other causes.
- A respiratory tract infection may precede the diagnosis in half of the patients.
- Abrupt onset of gross hematuria
- Reduced urine output (with diuresis in 5–7 days)
- Lethargy, anorexia, nausea, vomiting, abdominal pain
- Chills, fever, backache (pyelonephritis)

Physical Examination

- Hypertension that is transient and resolves in 1 to 2 weeks
- Edema, especially periorbital edema, or abrupt onset with weight gain
- Circulatory congestion—dyspnea, cough, pallor, pulmonary edema if severe
- Ear malformations
- Flank or abdominal pain or a mass (in polycystic kidney or malignancy [e.g., Wilms tumor])
- Costovertebral angle tenderness (in pyelonephritis)
- Rashes or arthralgias (with SLE, HSP, or impetigo)
- Evidence of trauma or abuse

Diagnostic Studies

- UA with microscopic examination—tea color; elevated specific gravity; macrohematuria and microhematuria; proteinuria not exceeding the amount of hematuria; pyuria in PSGN; granular, hyaline, WBC, or RBC casts; and dysmorphic RBCs.
- Serum C3 or C4 (low early in disease, returning to normal in 6–8 weeks), total protein and albumin (elevated).
- CBC, ESR, ASO titer (elevated), streptozyme test (positive), antideoxyribonucleic acid antibody titer.
- Electrolytes, BUN, creatinine, and cholesterol.
- Fluorescent antinuclear antibody (SLE), hepatitis titers, sickle cell or hemoglobin electrophoresis, tuberculin PPD, and fluorescent treponemal antibody absorption (syphilis).

Differential Diagnosis

Acute nephritis also occurs as part of systemic illnesses, such as SLE, HSP, hemolytic-uremic syndrome, vasculitis, or as a reaction to drugs or irradiation.

Management

Consultation with nephrology is recommended in all cases (Fig. 42.5).

PSGN treatment is supportive because resolution occurs spontaneously 95% of the time. The course is not affected by

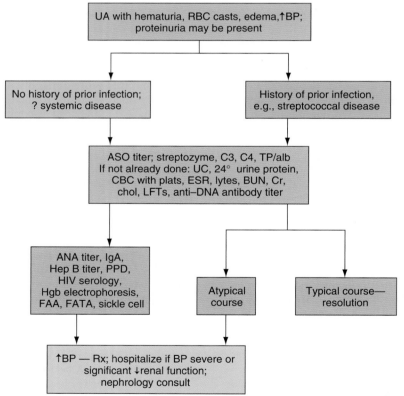

• **Fig 42.5** Evaluation of Nephritis Algorithm. *ANA*, Antinuclear antibody; *ASO*, antistreptolysin O; *BP*, blood pressure; *BUN*, blood urea nitrogen; *C3*, complement 3; *C4*, complement 4; *CBC*, complete blood count; *chol*, cholesterol; *Cr*, creatinine; *DNA*, deoxyribonucleic acid; *ESR*, erythrocyte sedimentation rate; *FAA*, fluorescent antinuclear antibody; *FATA*, fluorescent treponemal antibody absorption; *Hep B*, hepatitis B; *Hgb*, hemoglobin; *HIV*, human immunodeficiency virus; *IgA*, immunoglobulin A; *LFT*, liver function test; *lytes*, electrolytes; *plats*, platelets; *PPD*, purified protein derivative; *RBC*, red blood cell; *Rx*, prescribe; *TP/alb*, total protein/albumin; *UA*, urinalysis; *UC*, urine culture.

corticosteroids, immunosuppression, or other treatment modalities. During the peak of oliguria and hypertension, in the first few days of illness, hospitalization may be required with fluid and sodium limitation and diuretic, antihypertensive, and antibiotic treatment if cultures are positive. Resolution occurs once diuresis begins. Gross hematuria persists for 1 to 2 weeks, urine can be abnormal for 6 to 12 weeks, and microscopic hematuria can persist for up to 2 years. Complement levels return to normal in 6 to 8 weeks.[13–15]

- Acute nephritis—possible hospitalization with treatment as described previously.
- IgA nephropathy—annual follow-up with BP, UA, and determination of renal function.
- Benign familial or hereditary nephritis—perform audiometry and review family medical history. Hereditary markers are being developed for this disease.
- Benign recurrent nephritis—monitor UA and renal function every 1 to 2 years.
- Chronic nephritis—a team approach is required to adequately provide care.

Prolonged oliguria and renal failure can occur if acute nephritis progresses. Hypertensive encephalopathy or congestive heart failure can occur secondary to PSGN. Irreversible parenchymal damage causes hypertension and renal insufficiency.

Patient and Family Education, Prevention, and Prognosis

Patients with PSGN may have macrohematuria or microhematuria for up to 6 to 12 months, but the long-range outcome is excellent. Thin-basement-membrane disease has a good outcome. IgA nephropathy with severe histologic findings has a poor outcome, especially if the child is African American. Patient education should stress the importance of continued, regular care to monitor renal function.

Myoglobinuria

Myoglobin in the urine is associated with acute tissue injury, or rhabdomyolysis. Myoglobinuria is often confused with hematuria as it is associated with a red- or rust-colored pigment in the urine and causes a positive blood test on a urine dipstick. Myoglobin is released into the bloodstream with muscle damage. Myoglobin breaks down into byproducts that are harmful to the kidneys, resulting in acute renal injury. As long as renal injury is prevented and rhabdomyolysis does not occur, myoglobinuria is not associated with long-term effects or high mortality.[16]

History and Clinical Findings

- Crushing injury to the muscle, such as with traumatic injury
- Red or dark-colored urine
- Myalgias or weakness
- Drug abuse, toxins, or exposure to snake venom
- Strenuous exercise
- Metabolic disorder such as severe hyperkalemia or diabetic ketoacidosis
  Physical Examination
- Thorough examination of body surface area to assess for muscle injury
- Areas of pressure necrosis or ischemia
  Diagnostic Studies
- UA
- Microscopic urine analysis with few or no red blood cells; centrifuged urine remains pigmented

- Markedly elevated serum creatinine kinase level; serum CK of over 1000 is usually seen in patients with rhabdomyolysis
- Serum complete metabolic panel. Acute renal insufficiency elevates BUN and creatinine. Creatinine elevation occurs due to the creatinine leakage from damaged muscles. Comprehensive metabolic panel reveals hyperkalemia, hyperphosphatemia, or hypocalcemia.
- Increased levels of other muscle enzymes (aldolase, lactic acid dehydrogenase [LDH], aspartate aminotransferase [AST])

Differential Diagnosis

Myoglobinuria must be differentiated from gross hematuria, other metabolic disorders, and other local causes of muscle pain and weakness.

Management

The primary management goal is to prevent acute renal insufficiency, requires nephrology consultation, possible inpatient management, and treats underlying fluid and electrolyte abnormalities. Normal saline administration and diuresis induction are therapy mainstays. Urine alkalinization with sodium bicarbonate reduces the breakdown of myoglobin in the bloodstream. In patients with crush injuries, treatment of soft tissue injury and prevention of compartment syndrome are essential. Discontinuation or reversal of drugs, venoms, or other toxins in the system may be necessary.

Patient and Family Education, Prevention and Prognosis

Families must understand that long-term therapy may include hemodialysis or peritoneal dialysis in severe cases that result in acute renal disease. Myoglobinuria generally clears or improves within a couple of weeks. Discharge criteria from the hospital should include confirmation of serum CK, UA normalizing, and absence of rhabdomyolysis clinical signs.[16]

Renal Tubular Acidosis

Dysfunction of renal tubule transport capability results in a condition known as *renal tubular acidosis* (RTA). There are several types, type I, classic or distal RTA (dRTA), occurs with distal tubule defects. Proximal tubule defects are the most common type and result in proximal RTA (pRTA), type II, or *bicarbonate-wasting RTA*. Type III is a subtype of type I that occurs primarily in preterm infants. Type IV, also known as *hyperkalemic RTA*, occurs with problems in the aldosterone functioning most commonly following obstructive uropathy relief.[17]

RTA is often an isolated, idiopathic, and primary problem. It is usually found in children evaluated for growth failure and when illness, dehydration, or starvation stresses a child. RTA is more common in males than females.

History and Clinical Findings

- Failure to gain weight (especially) and height—the most common symptoms
- Polyuria and polydipsia
- Muscle weakness (caused by hypokalemia)
- Irritability before eating, satiation after eating, vomiting, diarrhea, or constipation in dRTA
- Preference for liquids over solid foods, poor appetite, or anorexia, especially with type IV

Physical Examination

- Arrested growth curve toward the end of the first year with prior consistent growth
- Normal physical examination and development

Diagnostic Studies. Studies include serum electrolytes, including carbon dioxide (CO_2) (hypokalemia, hyperchloremic metabolic acidosis), renal function tests (BUN, creatinine), calcium, phosphorus, alkaline phosphatase, and UA (first morning void) for glucose and pH.

If any of the laboratory findings are abnormal, consider the following:

- 24-hour creatinine clearance to establish the normal GFR, calcium (normal less than 4 mg/kg/24 hours), and calcium-creatinine ratio
- Renal ultrasonography to determine the anatomy and rule out nephrocalcinosis, nephrolithiasis, hydronephrosis, obstructive uropathy, and parenchymal damage

Differential Diagnosis

Primary RTA must be differentiated from secondary RTA, which can be due to many disease states or conditions, such as other causes of growth failure (e.g., FTT), hypothyroidism, and systemic acidosis.

Management

Management goals include correcting the acidosis, maintaining normal bicarbonate (greater than 20 mEq/L), restoring growth, and minimizing complications.

- Oral alkalizing medications are given to achieve these goals. Common agents include Bicitra (sodium citrate and citric acid), Polycitra (sodium, potassium citrate, and citric acid), sodium bicarbonate, and baking soda. The dose must be titrated to the child's response based on weight and laboratory results (CO_2 and electrolytes). Initiate medication at 3 mEq/kg/day, and check laboratory results in a few days. Titrate the dose until a serum bicarbonate level of 20 to 22 mEq/L is achieved.[17] Doses should be given frequently throughout the day (with meals) and as late as possible at night (at bedtime).
- The medication response helps confirm the diagnosis and RTA type. dRTA rapidly responds to treatment, and normal bicarbonate levels are maintained with little difficulty. pRTA requires higher doses to normalize bicarbonate and is less easily maintained. Type IV RTA requires mineralocorticoid treatment if aldosterone is deficient.
- Maximizing caloric intake to enhance growth is accomplished by emphasizing solid foods for all meals and snacks and avoiding water and noncaloric foods. Providing nutritional supplements is also ideal.
- Meticulous follow-up is imperative. Weight and laboratory results should be monitored biweekly to monthly until weight gain is established and CO_2 stabilizes. Measure weight on the same scale.
- Avoid pseudoephedrine because it is minimally excreted in alkalinized urine and may cause toxicity.
- Referral to a pediatric nephrologist is necessary for any child who is not growing well despite treatment, whose laboratory values are not normalizing with treatment, has unusual laboratory results, has type IV RTA, or has any RTA complications.

Patient and Family Education, Prevention, and Prognosis

It is rare to have complications with pRTA. Hypercalciuria can occur with dRTA, leading to nephrocalcinosis, nephrolithiasis, renal parenchymal destruction, and occasionally, renal failure. Rickets sometimes occurs in type IV RTA. Patient education should stress the importance of continued, regular care to monitor renal function and growth. Isolated pRTA responds quickly to treatment, with children "catching-up" growth and reaching normal maximum height. pRTA resolves spontaneously without symptom recurrence, often within 1 to 2 years, but may take up to a decade.[17] dRTA usually lasts a lifetime; type IV resolves with underlying problem correction.

Nephrolithiasis and Urolithiasis

Urinary stones (nephrolithiasis) happen anywhere in the urinary tract. In North America, urinary stones children have are found most frequently in the kidneys; bladder stones occur in less than 10% of the pediatric cases and are most often related to urologic abnormalities. Bladder stones are endemic to other parts of the world and are likely related to diet.

The prevalence of urinary stones varies by region, with a higher incidence in the Southeast United States and in White individuals, and slightly more often in males than females. Seventy-five percent of children who have nephrolithiasis are predisposed to stone formation. Metabolic risk factors account for more than 50% of cases, structural abnormalities account for 32%, and infections account for 4%. Hypercalciuria is the most common metabolic cause (accounts for 30–60%) of urinary calculi and there are many other causes including renal tubular dysfunction, endocrine disturbances, bone metabolic disorders, UTI, familial idiopathic hypercalcemia, and medications.[18] Hyperoxaluria is found in up to 20% of children with nephrolithiasis. Hyperuricosuria has been documented in 2% to 10% of children with stone formation.

History and Clinical Findings

- Family history of nephrolithiasis, arthritis, gout, or renal disease
- Stones or fragments passed in urine
- Dietary history high in protein, sodium, calcium, and oxalate intake
- Infant colic
- History or symptoms suggestive of a UTI in a preschooler

Physical Examination

- Abdominal, flank, or pelvic pain (occurs at all ages, but present in 94% of adolescents)

Diagnostic Studies

- UA shows gross or microscopic hematuria (90%) and 20% of children also have a UTI.[18]
- Hypercalciuria is diagnosed by a 24-hour urinary calcium excretion greater than 4 mg/kg. Screening may be performed on a random urine specimen by measuring the calcium (mg/dL)-to-creatinine (mg/dL) ratio. Greater than 0.2 suggests hypercalciuria in an older child; normal ratios may be as high as 0.8 in infants younger than 7 months.[18]
- Unenhanced spiral CT of the abdomen and pelvis is 96% specific in diagnosing a stone. However, it is important to consider that the amount of radiation a patient is exposed to in a CT is the equivalent of about three plain x-ray films. A negative abdominal radiograph, combined with a negative renal and

bladder ultrasound are adequate alternatives for ruling out stones, especially for nonemergent cases or when CT technology is unavailable.[19]

- Analyze stone composition to aid in the diagnosis of the metabolic abnormality, which presents in up to 75% of children.[19]

Differential Diagnosis

Other diagnoses causing flank pain should be considered (e.g., UTI, pyelonephritis, or trauma). Slightly more than half of preschool children with nephrolithiasis have flank pain or other afebrile illnesses, including gastrointestinal viral syndromes and early appendicitis, chronic recurrent abdominal pain of no known cause, and emotional stress.

Management

Increased fluid intake is the first line of therapy regardless of the cause. In adolescents, a goal of 2 L of urine output per day is helpful. Consult and refer to urology as stone removal may be required if the stone is not passed, and severe symptoms continue for more than 24 to 48 hours or pain is intolerable. Extracorporeal shockwave lithotripsy (ESWL) is safe in children; follow-up studies show it does not cause long-term kidney damage.[20] Skin bruising and hematuria are almost universal side effects of ESWL. Stones may also be removed by using rigid or flexible endoscopes passed through the urethra into the bladder or ureter. Percutaneous removal with open surgical lithotomy is still an option if other techniques fail.

Refer to a dietician. Dietary restrictions control stone formation and renal injury in most metabolic disorders contributing to stone formation.

Patient and Family Education, Prevention, and Prognosis

Recurrence rates are high if left untreated, and patients with hyperuricosuria may have symptomatic or asymptomatic calculi. Despite an excellent response to therapy, children with nephrolithiasis require long-term follow-up with nephrology because of the potential for renal insufficiency and end-stage renal disease.

Wilms Tumor

Wilms tumor, the most common malignancy of the GU tract, is typically found as a firm, smooth mass in the abdomen or flank. This malignancy manifests as a solitary growth in any part of either or both kidneys. There are approximately eight cases of Wilms tumor per million in children younger than 15 years with 500 new cases every year. Most Wilms tumors occur in children between ages 2 and 5 years. The peak incidence and median age at diagnosis is 3.5 years old.[21] About 1% to 2% of children with Wilms tumor have a family history of Wilms, and the tumor is inherited in an autosomal dominant manner. An important feature of Wilms tumor is the occurrence of associated congenital anomalies including renal abnormalities, cryptorchidism, hypospadias, duplication of the collecting system, ambiguous genitalia, hemihypertrophy, aniridia, cardiac abnormalities, and Beckwith-Wiedemann, Denys-Drash, and Perlman syndromes. Wilms tumor occurs with equal frequency in both sexes although males are usually diagnosed younger. There is a higher frequency in African Americans and a lower frequency in Asians. It is staged as follows:

- Stage I: The tumor is limited to the kidney and can be completely excised with the capsular surface intact.
- Stage II: The tumor extends beyond the kidney but can still be completely excised.
- Stage III: There is postsurgical residual nonhematogenous extension confined to the abdomen.
- Stage IV: There is hematogenous metastasis, most frequently to the lung.
- Stage V: There is bilateral kidney involvement.

History and Clinical Findings

- The most frequent finding is increasing abdominal size or an actual palpable mass.
- Pain is reported if the mass has undergone rapid growth or hemorrhage.
- Fever, dyspnea, diarrhea, vomiting, weight loss, or malaise may be reported.

Physical Examination

- A firm, smooth abdominal, or flank mass that does not cross the midline may be noted.
- BP is elevated if renal ischemia is present (rare).
- A left varicocele is found in males if the spermatic vein is obstructed.
- A careful examination is needed to rule out congenital anomalies.

Diagnostic Studies

- Chest and abdominal radiography are performed to differentiate neuroblastoma, which is usually calcified.
- Abdominal ultrasonography is used to differentiate a solid from a cystic mass or hydronephrosis and multicystic kidney.
- UA demonstrates hematuria in 25% to 33% of children.
- Obtain a CBC, reticulocyte count, and liver and renal chemistry studies.
- A CT scan of the chest, abdomen, and pelvis to stage the disease and bone marrow aspirate is done by the oncology team.

Differential Diagnosis

Neuroblastoma is the main differential diagnosis (the mass often crosses the midline). Multicystic kidney, hydronephrosis, renal cyst, or other renal malignancies are additional conditions to consider.

Management

Diagnostic workup is the initial urgent priority, with concurrent referral to a pediatric cancer center for treatment. Surgery removes the affected kidney and possibly the ureter and adrenal gland, and combined chemotherapy and radiotherapy are instituted if the disease is advanced or has unfavorable histologic findings. Coordinate close follow-up with the cancer team. The lungs and liver are the most common sites of metastasis. Hypertension is possible because of renal ischemia and occasionally leads to cardiac failure.

Patient and Family Education, Prevention, and Prognosis

The prognosis is determined by the histology of the neoplasm, the patient's age (the younger the better), the size of the tumor, the number of positive nodes, and, most significantly, the disease staging. The cure rate is about 80% to 90% for infants with stage 4S; reoccurrence of the disease has a less than 50% response to alternative chemotherapeutic agents.[21] Pediatric urology should determine if a child should be allowed to participate in sports. Kidney protector use is highly recommended during sports. The National Wilms Tumor Study (see Additional Resources) is a good reference for information about management, sequela, and prognosis.

Chronic Genitourinary Conditions in Males: Hypospadias

Hypospadias is a common congenital abnormality in which the urethral meatus is located anywhere from the proximal glans to the perineum on the ventral surface (underside) of the penis. Chordee, a ventral bowing of the penis, occurs when a tight band of fibrous tissue pulls on the penis. *Torsion* refers to rotation of the penis to the right or left.

The etiology of hypospadias is unknown. It is believed that the endocrine system probably has an important role, but it remains unclear. The primitive gonad in the eighth week of embryonic development differentiates into male or female. As the genital tubercle enlarges, developmental arrest occurs along the line of urethral fusion and causes hypospadias.

Hypospadias occurs in 1 in 250 male infants with an increased risk if family members have hypospadias. Ten percent of affected boys also have undescended testicles, inguinal hernia, or hydrocele.[22]

History and Clinical Findings

- A family history of a male relative with GU problems may be reported.
- There is report of an unusual direction, particularly downward, to the urine stream.
- Other findings include inguinal hernia or undescended testicles (10%), and/or chordee.[22]

Physical Examination. In a newborn, the classic finding is a dorsally hooded foreskin. It is essential to visualize the urethral meatus, which is facilitated by pulling the ventral shaft skin in a downward and outward direction. The deformity is described by location—glandular, coronal, subcoronal, penoscrotal, scrotal, and as distal (60%), mid-shaft (25%), or proximal (15%).

Differential Diagnosis

The differential diagnosis includes intersex abnormalities.

Management

The goal of surgical repair is to have a functional penis that appears normal. Historically, circumcision was avoided because the foreskin was used in the surgical repair. However, newer surgical techniques that do not require the use of skin flaps change this standard of care. Physiologic phimosis may prevent visualization of a urethral anomaly during a well-child examination, especially with a mild form of hypospadias. Surgical success is not compromised in these cases. Refer to pediatric urology at birth or at detection of the anomaly. Surgery to correct hypospadias is best done around 6 to 12 months old. Repair is usually accomplished in a one-stage outpatient procedure unless it is a complex defect.

With unrepaired hypospadias, peer taunting, problems with erections, abnormal urine stream, and ultimately potential for ineffective sperm delivery are possible complications. Intersex abnormalities are possible if associated with cryptorchidism.

Patient and Family Education, Prevention, and Prognosis

Provide education and reassurance regarding the etiology, repair, and outcome. Carefully assess newborns when hypospadias is

reported in a family member. Hypospadias is usually an isolated anomaly, but it requires further workup to assess the anatomy of the urinary system for other anomalies.

Cryptorchidism (Undescended Testes)

Cryptorchidism is a testis that does not reside in and cannot be manipulated into the scrotum. A retractile testis is out of the scrotum but can be brought into the scrotum and remains there. A gliding testis can be brought into the scrotum but returns to a high position in the scrotum once released. An ectopic testis lies outside the normal path of descent. An ascended testis is one that has fully descended, but spontaneously reascended and lies outside the scrotum. A trapped testis is one dislocated after herniorrhaphy. Any testis that is not in the scrotum is subject to progressive deterioration. Undescended testes is a common disorder that often causes great anxiety for parents.

Testes develop in the abdomen and descend in the seventh fetal month to the upper part of the groin, subsequently progressing through the inguinal canal into the scrotum. Failure of the testes to descend can be caused by mechanical lesions or secondary to hormonal, chromosomal, enzymatic, or anatomic disorders.

This condition is the most common GU disorder in males, occurring in 3.4% of term newborns. Testicular descent occurs at 7 to 8 months gestation, so it is therefore more common in preterm (30%), low birth weight, and twin infants. A great majority of undescended testes descend spontaneously during the first 3 months of life but after 6 months old it is rare (0.8%) for them to descend. Cryptorchidism is bilateral in 10% of cases. Retractile testes are bilateral and most common in males 5 to 6 years old.[23]

History and Clinical Findings

- Family history of undescended testes or testicular malignancy
- Testes not consistently descended during the infant's bath/warm environments
- Risk factors include prematurity, hypospadias, congenital hip subluxation, low birth weight, Down syndrome, Klinefelter syndrome
- Other congenital, endocrine, chromosomal, or intersex disorders

Physical Examination. Having the child sit cross-legged or frog-legged, squatting or standing can facilitate testicle descent and palpation.
- Scrotal rugae less fully developed
- Bilateral or unilateral absence of a testicle
- Ascending testicle, when the testicle is descended at birth but moves out of normal scrotal position as the child ages, usually between 4 and 10 years of age. This is often associated with a history of retractile testes.
- Retractile testes move between the scrotum and external ring but can be manipulated to the lower part of the scrotum and remain there. Retraction is especially common with tactile stimulation of the area or cold in children 3 months old through puberty. This is not associated with an increased risk of malignancy or fertility issues.
- Gliding testes lie between the scrotum and external ring and be manipulated to the lower part of the scrotum but return to the high position.
- Location of the testis is described as prescrotal (at the external inguinal ring); canalicular, high or low (between the external and internal rings), the most common type; ectopic (superficial

inguinal, femoral, or perineal); or intraabdominal (above the internal inguinal ring), and nonpalpable, occurring in less than 15% of males with undescended testes.

Diagnostic Studies. None are indicated except in newborns with potential sex abnormalities, hypopituitarism, Down syndrome, or congenital adrenal hyperplasia. The risk of intersex abnormality is 27% if hypospadias and unilateral or bilateral cryptorchidism are present.

Differential Diagnosis

Anorchism and chromosomal abnormalities are the differential diagnoses.

Management

The goals of treating undescended testes are to improve fertility, decrease malignancy risk, and minimize the psychological stress associated with an empty scrotum. Management is surgical intervention between 9 and 15 months old. Hormonal therapy is not effective in stimulating testicular descent. Surgery at 6 months old is appropriate if orchiopexy is performed by a skilled pediatric urologist or surgeon with an attendant and pediatric anesthesiologist. In a child younger than 6 months, regular examination to assess the position of the testes should be performed at every well-childcare visit. If the testes remain undescended, referral to a pediatric urologist or surgeon should occur by age 6 months. Referral should occur if a retractile testis does not retain scrotal residence. If undescended testes are found after 1 year old, the child should be immediately referred to a pediatric urologist or surgeon for treatment. Poor testicular development, infertility, malignancy, vulnerability to trauma, testicular torsion, and inguinal hernia are possible complications of undescended testicles.

Patient and Family Education, Prevention, and Prognosis

Histologic changes occur in an undescended testis as early as 6 months old, with irreversible changes shown by 2 years old that contribute to infertility and are associated with malignancy. Infertility as a complication of cryptorchidism has been reported in as many as 15% of men with unilateral undescended testes and 35% to 50% if bilateral.[23] Testicular malignancy in males with cryptorchidism is two to four times higher than the general population. Correction of undescended testes does not diminish the incidence of testicular cancer, although an increased incidence in testicular tumors has been observed if orchiopexy is done at later ages. Malignancy is more common with an intraabdominal testis. A testicular neoplasm in one child mandates examination of his male siblings.[23] Testicular self-examination should be taught to these select young men.

Undescended testes do not resolve with puberty; retractile testes generally settle into the scrotum by puberty. Open discussion of the problem, management, and potential complications is essential. The AAP Council on Sports Medicine and Fitness does not include an absent testicle as a condition to discourage sports participation.[24]

Hydrocele

A common cause of painless scrotal swelling is a hydrocele, a serous fluid collection in the scrotal sac. Incomplete closure of the processus vaginalis through which the testes descend into the scrotum allows a hydrocele to develop. Incidence is 0.5% to 2% in neonates.[25] A noncommunicating hydrocele has fluid collecting in the scrotum only. If the processus vaginalis remains patent so that fluid moves from the abdomen to the scrotum, it is called a *communicating hydrocele* and is more likely to be associated with a hernia (Fig. 42.6).

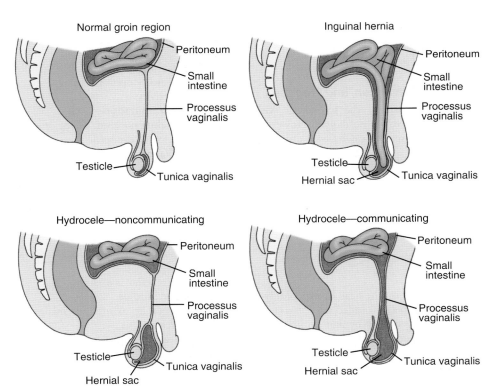

• **Fig 42.6** Hydroceles and Hernias. (From Katz A, Richardson W. Surgery. In: Zitelli BJ, McIntire SC, Nowalk AJ, eds. *Zitelli and Davis' Atlas of Pediatric Physical Diagnosis*. 2018:616–657.)

History and Clinical Findings

Hydroceles that persist beyond 1 year old are assumed to be in conjunction with a hernia. In older children, they also occur after trauma, with an inflammatory illness, or neoplasm.

- Intermittent or constant bulge or lump in the scrotum, often more distally placed. Scrotal size increases with activity and decreases with rest.
- Overlying skin may be tense.
- Bluish discoloration in the area of bulge
- No distress or vomiting
  Physical Examination
- Asymmetry or a scrotal mass present; if swelling is present in the inguinal area, a hernia is probable; swelling is usually unilateral.
- Testes descended
- Cremasteric reflex present
- Noncommunicating hydrocele—scrotal sac tense, slightly blue tinged, fluctuant, and does not reduce; no swelling in the inguinal region.
- Communicating hydrocele—fluid in the scrotal sac comes and goes (probably flat in the morning, swollen later in the day).
- In general, physical examination is the preferred method of diagnosis. Scrotal ultrasound may be helpful in ruling out other etiologies of scrotal swelling but could potentially miss a communicating hydrocele due to fluid fluctuation.

Differential Diagnosis

Hernia, undescended testicle, retractile testicle, and inguinal lymphadenopathy are the differential diagnoses.

Management

- Noncommunicating hydrocele: Fluid is generally absorbed spontaneously; no treatment is indicated unless the hydrocele is so large that it is uncomfortable or persists longer than 1 year.
- Communicating hydrocele: Many communicating hydroceles will resolve without surgery and deserve observation.[25] If the hydrocele persists for more than 1 year, referral for surgical intervention is recommended.

Patient and Family Education, Prevention, and Prognosis

Reassure parent that the increased size of the scrotal sac will resolve, usually by 1 year old, and involves no danger. However, if a hernia is present, this will not resolve on its own and will require surgical correction. Families should be assured that the risk of incarceration is low, and childhood hernias are not usually painful. Surgery is generally performed on an outpatient, nonemergent basis. Signs of hernia must be explained, and parents must be alerted to observe and report any abnormal findings. It is often helpful for the parent to document any scrotal swelling with a digital image/photograph.[25]

Spermatocele

A benign, painless scrotal mass or cyst on the head of the epididymis or testicular adnexa containing sperm is called a *spermatocele*. A spermatocele is an uncommon, generally benign finding and occurs in the mature male or older adolescents.

History and Clinical Findings

- Scrotal swelling but otherwise asymptomatic
- Painless, mobile cystic nodule usually less than 1 cm in size, superior and posterior to the testicle

- No change in size with the Valsalva maneuver
- An ultrasound may be ordered if large and bothersome or painful

Differential Diagnosis

A varicocele, mass, and an epididymal cyst (identical in appearance but not containing sperm) are the differential diagnoses.

Management

No treatment is required unless the cyst is large and bothersome or painful in which case referral to a urologist is recommended.

Patient and Family Education, Prevention, and Prognosis

Any pain or discomfort should be reported. Testicular self-examination assists in early detection of this disorder in later adolescence.

Varicocele

A varicocele is a benign enlargement or dilation of testicular veins causing a painless scrotal mass of varying size that may feel like a "bag of worms." It is usually found on the left side.

The etiology of varicoceles is probably multifactorial, with the physiologic changes associated with puberty playing some role. A varicocele is caused by valvular incompetence of the spermatic vein resulting in dilated or varicose veins. Varicoceles are rare before 10 years old, present in 5% of adolescent males, and 15% of adult males. Up to 85% to 95% arise on the left side because the left spermatic vein drains into the left renal vein and arterial compression of the renal vein obstructs blood flow from the vein. In contrast, the right spermatic vein drains into the vena cava. Only 2% of varicoceles occur bilaterally.[23]

History and Clinical Findings

- Usually, a painless swelling is noted in the left side of the scrotum, occasionally a "dull ache" or "heavy" feeling if large.
- Scrotal swelling with prolonged standing causes pain; swelling and pain resolve upon reclining. Pain can occur with strenuous physical activity.
  Physical Examination
- In the standing position, a "bag of worms" can be felt posterior and superior to the testis that collapses on lying and enlarges with the Valsalva maneuver.
- Measure and compare the size of both testes (length, width, and depth) using a standard orchidometer.
- Grade 3 varicocele, the classic "bag of worms," is larger than 2 cm and easily visualized; grade 2 varicocele is 1 to 2 cm in diameter and is easily palpable when the adolescent stands but is not visible; grade 1 varicocele is the most common, very small, and difficult to palpate (the Valsalva maneuver may help).
- Cremasteric reflex is present.
  Diagnostic Studies
- Ultrasonography to rule out malignancy in children younger than 10 years.
- Serial ultrasonography to measure testicular size every 6 to 12 months.

Differential Diagnosis

Varicoceles must be differentiated from other testicular masses, such as lipoma, hernia, hydrocele, spermatocele, and tumors.

Management

Asymptomatic grade 1 varicocele with normal testicular volumes usually does not require intervention in adolescence but involves ultrasonographic monitoring of testicular size every 12 months.[26] Any change in comfort level should be reported. Referral to a surgeon or urologist should be made if the varicocele is grade 2 or 3, if the varicocele is painful, if the difference in testicular volume is marked (>2 mm by ultrasound), if the varicocele is right sided or bilateral, or if testicular growth slows over a 6- to 12-month period.[23] Ligation is the usual procedure, completed on an outpatient basis with few complications. Laparoscopy for varicocelectomy gained popularity amongst urologists in recent years.

Atrophy or testicular growth arrest, as noted by a discrepancy in testicular size, can occur. Lower fertility rates with decreased sperm concentration and motility occur and are factors in an aggressive surgical approach for the adolescent male with grade 2 or 3 varicocele. Hydrocele may be an insignificant, self-limiting complication following surgery.

Patient and Family Education, Prevention, and Prognosis

A varicocele is the most common cause of infertility. Because of this, early identification is essential. All patients should be counseled about the long-term risks to fertility. Correction of testicular atrophy and an improved sperm count and fertility are noted in 80% to 90% of those undergoing surgery in early adolescence.[23] Testicular self-examination assists in early detection of this disorder.

Inguinal Hernia

An inguinal hernia is a scrotal or inguinal swelling (or both) that results in bulging of abdominal contents through a weakness in the abdominal wall (see Fig. 42.6). In females, inguinal hernias cause swelling in the inguinal area and labia majora. Incomplete closure of the processus vaginalis, through which the testes descend into the scrotum, allows the presence of abdominal contents in the inguinal canal or scrotum. Males who are obese, weightlifters, or have a family history of undescended testes are at high risk for hernias. Having a sibling with an inguinal hernia increases one's risk, and 11.5% of patients have a family member with a history of inguinal hernia.[25]

Inguinal hernias are much more common in males than in females (8–10:1), occurring in 1% to 5% of males. Premature infants are at increased risk (7–30% of males, 2% of females). More than 50% of hernias are diagnosed during the first year of life, with the peak incidence in the first 3 months of life. Bilateral hernias are common (10–20%). Unilateral hernias are more likely to occur on the right side (50–60%) than the left (30%).[25] Indirect hernias are a congenital condition and are the most common type in children. Direct hernias are rare in childhood and normally are the result of straining and weakened abdominal muscles.

History and Clinical Findings

- Family or personal history of undescended testes.
- Swelling in the inguinal area, scrotum, or both that comes and goes and increases with crying or straining.
- Prematurity, weightlifting, or obesity.
  Physical Examination
- Swelling is found in the inguinal area, scrotal area (labia majora in females), or both.

- The hernia is reducible with pressure on the distal end.
- Direct hernias push outward through the weakest point in the abdominal wall.
- Indirect hernias push downward at an angle into the inguinal canal.
- The child is fussy and has a distended abdomen if the hernia is incarcerated.
- Silk glove sign: A sensation of two surfaces rubbing against each other while one palpates the spermatic cord as it crosses the pubic tubercle.

Diagnostic Studies. An abdominal radiograph is helpful if air is present below the inguinal ligament. Ultrasonography differentiates a hernia from a hydrocele and is especially helpful if an incarcerated hernia is suspected.

Differential Diagnosis

Hydrocele, undescended testes, and inguinal lymphadenopathy are included in the differential diagnosis.

Management

If a child is seen with a hernia, an attempt should be made to reduce it, and the child should be referred to a surgeon or urologist for repair within 1 to 2 weeks. Even if no swelling is seen at the visit but is elicited by the history, the child should be referred to a surgeon or urologist. Inguinal hernias do not resolve spontaneously. Premature infants should have the hernia repaired before discharge. If the hernia is not easily reduced; if it is painful; or if a hard, tender, or red mass is present, refer immediately. If reduction is difficult and ischemia is ongoing, hospitalization and surgical repair within 24 to 48 hours are indicated.

Incarceration and strangulation of a hernia cause pain, irritability, erythema, vomiting, and abdominal distention. The overall incidence of incarceration is 12% to 17%, and two-thirds of incarcerated hernias occur during the first year of life.[25] Both of these conditions are surgical emergencies. Bowel ischemia is of immediate concern, and testicular injury occurs from torsion as a result of the direct pressure of the incarcerated hernia or as a result of ischemia from cord compression. Because of the 40% to 60% contralateral occurrence of hernias in children, bilateral exploration is usually done at the time of surgery in infants younger than 1 year old.

Patient and Family Education, Prevention, and Prognosis

If surgery is deferred, parents must be aware of the signs and symptoms of incarceration (tenderness, redness, crying, nausea, vomiting, abdominal distention) and be cautioned to seek immediate evaluation by a healthcare provider should they occur.

Testicular Masses

A mass located on the testicle is most often a malignancy. Testicular tumors can occur at any age; 35% of prepubertal testicular tumors are malignant. Most of the tumors are yolk sac tumors; however, rhabdomyosarcoma and leukemia can appear in this age group; 98% of painless testicular tumors in adolescents are malignant.[23]

History and Clinical Findings

- Family history of testicular cancer.
- Sensation of fullness or heaviness.

- Possibly no complaints because testicular masses cause little or no pain and are often small.
- Cryptorchidism, trauma, and atrophy.
  Physical Examination
- A hard, painless testicular mass.
- There may be an associated hydrocele.
- The abdomen and supraclavicular areas should be assessed for any palpable nodes.
  Diagnostic Studies
- Serum levels of alpha-fetoprotein, β-human chorionic gonadotropin, and lactate dehydrogenase if tumor is suspected.
- Scrotal sonography establishes the location of the mass and differentiates a cystic from a solid mass.
- CT scan is indicated to evaluate for metastasis and ordered by specialists.

Differential Diagnosis

Intratesticular masses, which are almost always malignant, must be differentiated from extratesticular masses, such as hernia, varicocele, hydrocele, or spermatocele.

Management

Any child or adolescent with a testicular mass must be referred immediately for further evaluation. Treatment is dependent on the stage and type of tumor and includes orchiectomy, irradiation, and/or chemotherapy.

Patient and Family Education, Prevention, and Prognosis

Metastasis may occur before the initial tumor is noticed. Pay attention to complaints about back or abdominal pain, unexplained weight loss, dyspnea (pulmonary metastases), gynecomastia, supraclavicular adenopathy, urinary obstruction, or a "heavy" or "dragging" sensation. Early detection and therapeutic intervention can lead to a 90% survival rate; 90% of relapses occur in the first 12 months after treatment. Testicular examination should be routinely done during physical examinations.

Acute Male Genitourinary Conditions

Scrotal Trauma

Trauma to the scrotum most often occurs as a result of sports participation or play, usually from direct blows to the scrotum and straddle injuries. In a prepubertal child, the testicle is often spared damage because of the small size and mobility of the testes. Damage occurs when the testicle is forcibly compressed against the pubic bones. Significant symptoms (swelling, discoloration, and tenderness) from minor trauma suggest an underlying tumor.

History and Clinical Findings

- Pain after injury; older children and adolescents usually report a specific mechanism of injury, time, and place.
- Scrotal swelling, discoloration, ecchymosis, and tenderness are common.
- Clear transillumination is compromised if a hematoma is present.
- Ultrasound differentiates the degree and type of injury and assesses for testicular rupture.

Differential Diagnosis

Urethritis, epididymitis, orchitis, and prostatitis should all be included in the differential diagnosis. Degrees of injury include the following:

- Traumatic epididymitis: Inflammation, but no infection. Pain and tenderness with scrotal erythema and edema and a tender indurated epididymis develop within a few days after injury. UA and Doppler ultrasonographic findings are normal. The course is usually acute but short-lived.
- Intratesticular hematoma
- Hematocele with contusion and ecchymosis of the scrotal wall with severe scrotal injury
- Testicular torsion

Management

Nonsteroidal antiinflammatory drugs (NSAIDs), cool compresses, scrotal support or elevation, and bed rest are modalities used to help relieve pain. An enlarging scrotum merits immediate surgical exploration, as does hematocele.

Patient and Family Education, Prevention, and Prognosis

On rare occasion, testicular rupture can occur and manifest with massive swelling and ecchymosis. Prevention is the best approach to this disorder; wear an athletic cup when participating in sports where injury could occur.

Testicular Torsion

Testicular torsion is the result of twisting of the spermatic cord with subsequent compromise of the testicular blood supply. In general, there is a 6-hour window before significant ischemic damage and alteration in spermatic morphology and formation occurs.[23] Normal fixation of the testis is absent, so the testis rotates and blocks blood and lymphatic flow. Torsion occurs after physical exertion, trauma, or on arising, and at any age but is most common in adolescence and is uncommon before 10 years old. The left side is twice as likely to be involved because of the longer spermatic cord.

History and Clinical Findings

- Sudden onset of unilateral, unrelenting scrotal pain, often associated with nausea and vomiting.
- History of intermittent testicular pain. Prior episodes of transient pain are reported in about half of patients.
- Minor trauma, physical exertion, or onset of acute pain on arising is possible.
- May be described as abdominal or inguinal pain by the embarrassed child.
- Fever is minimal or absent.
  Physical Examination
- Ill-appearing and anxious male, resisting movement
- Gradual, progressive scrotal edema with erythema, warmth, and tenderness
- The ipsilateral scrotum can be edematous, erythematous, and warm
- Testis larger than opposite side, elevated, lying transversely, exquisitely painful
- Spermatic cord thickened, twisted, and tender
- Slight elevation of the testis increases pain (in epididymitis it relieves pain)
- The cremasteric reflex is absent on the side with torsion

- Neonate—hard, painless, mass with edema or discolored scrotal skin
  Diagnostic Studies
- UA is usually normal; pyuria and bacteriuria indicate UTI, epididymitis, or orchitis.
- Doppler ultrasound or testicular flow scan considered if Doppler ultrasound normal and time allows.

Differential Diagnosis

Epididymal appendage torsion, acute epididymitis (mild to moderate pain of gradual onset), orchitis, trauma (pain is better within an hour), hernia, hydrocele, and varicocele are included in the differential diagnosis.

Management

Testicular torsion is a surgical emergency, and identification with prompt surgical referral critical. Occasionally, manual reduction can be performed, but surgery should follow within 6 to 12 hours to prevent retorsion, preserve fertility, and prevent abscess and atrophy. Contralateral orchiopexy may be done because of a 50% occurrence of torsion in nonfixed testes. Rest and scrotal support do not provide relief.

Patient and Family Education, Prevention, and Prognosis

Testicular atrophy, abscess, or decreased fertility and loss of the testis as a result of necrosis occurs if the torsion persists more than 24 hours.

Torsion of the Appendix Testis

Torsion of the appendix testis is a common cause of acute scrotal pain and is often misdiagnosed. It commonly occurs in the prepubertal age group and may be a response to hormonal stimulation. Once the appendix torses, it falls off and is resorbed by the body. Recurrence in another appendix, such as the appendix epididymis, occurs but is not associated with prior appendix testis torsion. This condition is the most common cause of testicular pain in males 2 to 10 years old.[23]

History and Clinical Findings

- Gradual onset of scrotal pain.
- "Blue dot" sign, which is a subtle blue mass visible through the scrotal skin: Early in the process there may be a 3- to 5-mm tender indurated mass on the upper pole.[23]
- Doppler ultrasonography or testicular flow scan considered if Doppler ultrasound within normal and time allows.
- Cremasteric reflex present.

Differential Diagnosis

Testicular torsion, acute epididymitis, orchitis, trauma, hernia, hydrocele, and varicocele are included in the differential diagnosis.

Management

Appendix testis torsion is a self-limited condition; inflammation resolves in 3 to 5 days. Management includes NSAIDs, limited activities or bed rest until pain is gone, and warm compresses. Surgery is rarely indicated but might be necessary if testicular torsion cannot be ruled out or if symptoms do not resolve spontaneously in a few days.

Epididymitis

Epididymitis is an inflammation of the epididymis that is painful, acute, and commonly caused by *Neisseria gonorrhoeae* or *Chlamydia trachomatis* in the sexually active adolescent, often co-occurring with infection in the urethra or bladder. However, it can be caused by a viral, coliform bacterial, or tubercular infection; chemical irritation; GU tract anomalies; or dysfunctional voiding. It is rare before puberty, but it occurs in younger boys from *E. coli* infection. It may occur in children younger than 2 years with GU tract abnormalities.[23]

History and Clinical Findings

- Trauma or sexual encounters within past 45 days
- Painful scrotal swelling, usually gradual but may be acute
- Dysuria and frequency, or obstructive voiding
- Fever, nausea, vomiting
  Physical Examination
- Scrotal edema and erythema are noted.
- The epididymis is hard, indurated, enlarged, and tender; the spermatic cord is tender.
- The testis has normal position and consistency.
- The cremasteric reflex is normal (not present in older adolescents).
- Elevation of testis may relieve pain (in torsion it increases pain).
- Hydrocele may be present due to inflammation.
- Urethral discharge may be present: purulent in gonorrhea, and scant and watery in chlamydial infection.
- Rectal examination reveals prostate tenderness and produces urethral discharge.
  Diagnostic Studies
- UA: Pyuria and occasional bacteria may be present.
- CBC: Elevated WBC count
- Urethral culture and Gram stain: Urine nucleic acid amplification tests for gonococci and *Chlamydia*
- Other sexually transmitted infections (STIs) and HIV testing if there is a history of sexual activity
- Doppler ultrasonography to differentiate torsion of the testis
- If the above tests are not diagnostic, refer to urology to identify urogenital problems with evaluation by VCUG, ultrasonography, or both in prepubertal children and in those who deny sexual activity.

Differential Diagnosis

The differential diagnosis includes testicular torsion, hernia, hydrocele, varicocele, spermatocele, trauma, tumor, or concomitant urethritis. Testicular cancer has been confused with epididymitis.

Management

Management involves symptom relief and causative organism treatment. Bed rest, scrotal support, and elevation are indicated. Apply ice packs as tolerated. Sitz baths and analgesics or NSAIDs relieve pain. Antibiotic treatment includes the following[27]:
- First line: Ceftriaxone (500 mg intramuscularly one time) plus doxycycline (100 mg twice a day for 10 days).
- Alternative treatments: Ceftriaxone (500 mg intramuscularly one time) plus ofloxacin (300 mg twice a day for 10 days) or levofloxacin (500 mg once a day for 10 days).

- Referral to urology is indicated if a solitary testicle is involved, if a prompt response to treatment does not occur, or if a question about the diagnosis remains. Treatment of sexual partner(s) from the past 60 days is indicated if caused by an STI. Intercourse should be avoided until cured. Follow-up is needed within 3 days if no improvement or if symptoms recur after treatment. Follow-up after antibiotics is recommended to ensure that no palpable mass remains.

Patient and Family Education, Prevention, and Prognosis

Infertility, abscess formation, testicular infarction, and late atrophy are possible but rare complications. Because epididymitis is usually caused by an STI, partners must be evaluated and treated. Patients must understand the sexually transmitted etiology of this disease. Pain and edema usually resolve within 1 week. For additional differentiation of scrotal pain see Table 42.5.

Phimosis and Paraphimosis

Phimosis refers to a foreskin that is too tight to be retracted over the glans penis. Physiologic or primary phimosis occurs over the first 6 years of life when the glans does not completely separate from the epithelium. Pathologic or secondary phimosis occurs after puberty or when the foreskin cannot be retracted after previously being retracted. Paraphimosis is a retracted foreskin that cannot be reduced to the normal position.

Phimosis can be congenital or acquired from infection and foreskin inflammation. Paraphimosis causes penis constriction and results in pain, glans edema, and possible necrosis. Paraphimosis is most common in adolescents and can follow masturbation, sexual activity, or forceful retraction.

History and Clinical Findings

- May be a history of infection or inflammation of the penis
- Retraction of the foreskin with an inability to reduce it (paraphimosis)
- Pain and dysuria
- Signs of urinary obstruction—ballooning of the foreskin with urination and/or abnormal intermittent urinary stream

Physical Examination

- Phimosis—a tight, pinpoint opening of the foreskin with minimal ability to retract the foreskin; foreskin flat and effaced
- Pathologic phimosis—thickened rolled foreskin
- Paraphimosis—edema and bluish discoloration of the glans and foreskin

Management

- Phimosis: Normal cleansing with gentle stretching of the foreskin until resistance is felt. Most foreskins are retractable by 5 or 6 years old. Never forcefully retract the foreskin. Circumcision is indicated if urinary obstruction or infection is present. Persistent phimosis can be treated with 0.05% betamethasone cream twice daily for 2 to 4 weeks. This frequently allows successful retraction of the foreskin, promotes awareness of improved hygiene, and offers an alternative to circumcision.[22]
- Paraphimosis: Reduction may be accomplished by lubricating the foreskin and glans, simultaneously compressing the glans, and placing distal foreskin traction. If this technique is not successful, surgical release of the constricting band must be done to prevent necrosis of the glans. Paraphimosis is a surgical emergency.[22] Investigation of events leading to the paraphimosis is needed to rule out sexual abuse.

Patient and Family Education, Prevention, and Prognosis

Infection and urinary obstruction can occur with phimosis; however, a tight foreskin in uncircumcised males is normal and usually resolves by 6 years old. It is not an indication for circumcision. Necrosis of the penis is possible with paraphimosis. The foreskin of infants and children should never be forcibly retracted.

Balanitis and Balanoposthitis

Balanitis is an inflammation of the glans; *balanoposthitis* is an inflammation of the foreskin and glans penis occurring in uncircumcised males or those with phimosis. Debris accumulation under the foreskin, probably resulting from poor hygiene, irritates the foreskin and glans and leads to infection. If purulent discharge

TABLE 42.5	**Evaluation of the Acute Scrotum**							
Condition	**Pain**	**Examination**	**Age of Onset**	**Urinalysis**	**Ultrasound**	**Cremasteric Reflex**	**Treatment**
Testicular Torsion	Acute, random, Severe	Entire testis swollen, possible abnormal lie	Puberty	Negative	Yes, confirm Doppler flow	Absent	Attempt to manually detorse, scrotal exploration
Torsion of Appendix Testis	Gradual onset	"Blue dot sign" may be visible at upper pole	Prepubertal	Negative	Yes, may show increased flow	Present	Rest and scrotal elevation
Epididymitis	Usually gradual, can be acute	Epididymal tenderness and induration	Adolescence, if younger may indicate urinary tract abnormality	Positive	Yes, confirm epididymal swelling	Present	Antibiotics, NSAIDS, rest

NSAIDs, Nonsteroidal antiinflammatory drugs.

with fiery-red erythema and moist translucent exudates are present, consider streptococcal etiology. Normal skin flora is the usual cause of infection, but gram-negative bacteria are possible. If a urethral discharge is present, an STI must be considered. Occasionally, trauma or allergy can be the cause.

History and Clinical Findings

- A fussy infant or pain and dysuria in an older child. Edema and inflammation are noted on the foreskin and glans.
- Cultures may help determine infectious causes.

Management

Prescribe oral and topical antibiotics as directed by the cultures, along with warm bathtub soaks. Depending on the swelling, topical steroids might also be prescribed.

Patient and Family Education, Prevention, and Prognosis

Paraphimosis can occur with severe infections; however, avoid forcible foreskin retraction. A review of proper hygiene and the removal of irritants is needed. Occurrence is not an indication for circumcision.

Additional Resources

American Association of Kidney Patients: www.aakp.org
IgA Nephropathy Support Network: www.igansupport.org
National Cancer Institute: Wilms Tumor and Other Childhood Kidney Tumors Treatment: www.cancer.gov/types/kidney/patient/wilms-treatment-pdq
National Institute of Diabetes and Digestive and Kidney Diseases: www.niddk.nih.gov/health-information/health-topics/kidney-disease/Pages/default.aspx
National Kidney Foundation: www.kidney.org
Society of Urologic Nurses and Associates: www.suna.org
Testicular Cancer: https://www.cancer.org/cancer/testicular-cancer/about/what-is-testicular-cancer.html
Urology Care Foundation: The Official Foundation of the American Urologic Association: www.urologyhealth.org

References

1. Hagan JF, Shaw JS, Duncan PM, eds. *Bright Futures: Guidelines for Health Supervision of Infants, Children and Adolescents*. 4th ed. American Academy of Pediatrics; 2017. Recommendations for preventative pediatric health care. https://downloads.aap.org/AAP/PDF/periodicity_schedule.pdf.
2. Quest Diagnostics. *Urine Collection*; 2022. https://www.questdiagnostics.com/healthcare-professionals/test-directory/specimen-handling/urine-collection.
3. Tzimenatos L, Mahajan P, Dayan PS, et al. Accuracy of the urinalysis for urinary tract infections in febrile infants 60 days and younger. *Pediatrics*. 2018;141(2).
4. Dean AJ, Lee DC. Bedside laboratory and microbiological procedures. In: *Roberts and Hedges' Clinical Procedures in Emergency Medicine and Acute Care*. 7th ed. Elsevier; 2019:1442–1469.
5. American Urological Association (AUA). *Management and Screening of Primary Vesicoureteral Reflux in Children: AUA 2010 Guideline*;
6. 2017. https://www.auanet.org/guidelines-and-quality/guidelines/non-oncology-guidelines/pediatric-urology.
7. Mattoo TK, Shaikh N, Nelson CP. Contemporary management of urinary tract infection in children. *Pediatrics*. 2021;147(2):e2020012138.
8. Jerardi KE, Jackson EC. Urinary tract infections. In: Kliegman RM, S.Geme JW, eds. *Nelson Textbook of Pediatrics*. 21st ed. Elsevier; 2020:2789–2795.
9. Roberts KB. Revised AAP Guideline on UTI in febrile infants and young children. *Am Fam Physician*. 2012;86(10):940–946.
10. Lee CKK. Drug dosages. In: Hughes HK, Kahl LK, eds. *The Harriet Lane Handbook: Handbook for Pediatric House Officers*. 21st ed. Elsevier; 2018:732–1109.
11. Mattoo TK, Shaikh N, Nelson CP. Contemporary management of urinary tract infection in children. *Pediatrics*. 2021;147(2).
12. Elder JS. Vesicoureteral reflux. In: Kliegman RM, S.Geme JW, eds. *Nelson Textbook of Pediatrics*. 21st ed. Elsevier; 2020:2796–2800.
13. Flores XF. Clinical evaluation of the child with hematuria. In: Kliegman RM, S.Geme JW, eds. *Nelson Textbook of Pediatrics*. 21st ed. Elsevier; 2020:2718–2720.
14. Brown DD, Reidy KJ. Approach to the child with hematuria. *Pediatr Clin North Am*. 2019;66(1):15–30.
15. Flores XF. Conditions associated with proteinuria. In: Kliegman RM, S.Geme JW, eds. *Nelson Textbook of Pediatrics*. 21st ed. Elsevier; 2020:2750–2752.
16. Erkan E. Nephrotic syndrome. In: Kliegman RM, S.Geme JW, eds. *Nelson Textbook of Pediatrics*. 21st ed. Elsevier; 2020:2752–2760.
17. Harmelink MM. Rhabdomyolysis. In: Kliegman RM, Toth H, eds. *Nelson Pediatric Symptom Based Diagnosis*. 2nd ed. Elsevier; 2023:619–629.
18. Dixon BP. Renal tubular acidosis. In: Kliegman RM, S.Geme JW, eds. *Nelson's Textbook of Pediatrics*. 21st ed. Elsevier; 2020:2761–2766.
19. Elder JS. Urinary lithiasis. In: Kliegman RM, S.Geme JW, eds. *Nelson Textbook of Pediatrics*. 21st ed. Elsevier; 2020:2835–2840.
20. Desai R. Nephrology. In: Hughes HK, Kahl LK, eds. *The Harriet Lane Handbook: A Manual for Pediatric House Officers*. 21st ed. Elsevier; 2018:516–547.
21. Lucena LB, Bautista BF, Hernánde AP, et al. Minimally extracorporeal shock wave lithotripsy and combined therapy in children: efficacy and long-term results. *Front Pediatr*. 2021;9:609664.
22. Daw NC, Nehme G, Huff VD. Wilms tumor. In: Kliegman RM, S.Geme JW, eds. *Nelson's Textbook of Pediatrics*. 21st ed. Elsevier; 2020:2681–2685.
23. Elder JS. Anomalies of the penis and the urethra. In: Kliegman RM, S.Geme JW, eds. *Nelson Textbook of Pediatrics*. 21st ed. Elsevier; 2020:2821–2826.
24. Elder JS. Disorders and anomalies of the scrotal contents. In: Kliegman RM, S.Geme JW, eds. *Nelson Textbook of Pediatrics*. 21st ed. Elsevier; 20202827–20202833.
25. Miller SM, Peterson AR. The sports preparticipation evaluation. *Pediatr Rev*. 2019;40(3):108–128.
26. Aiken JJ. Inguinal hernias. In: Kliegman RM, S. Geme JW, eds. *Nelson Textbook of Pediatrics*. 21st ed. Elsevier; 2020:2064–2070.
27. Macey MR, Owen RC, Ross SS, et al. Best practice in the diagnosis and treatment of varicocele in children and adolescents. *Ther Adv Urol*. 2018;10(9):273–282.
28. Centers for Disease Control and Prevention (CDC). Sexually transmitted diseases treatment guidelines. *MMWR (Morb Mortal Wkly Rep)*. 2021;70(4):98–101.

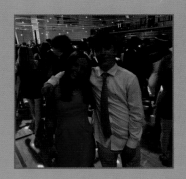

43

Gynecology and Reproductive Health

ELIZA BUYERS

Pediatric and adolescent gynecology provides the primary care provider (PCP) with varied and interesting challenges. Knowledge, sensitivity, and comfort with this topic gives providers the ability to work with children, adolescents, and parents to offer education about issues that may be considered personal or embarrassing. Establishing and maintaining an open relationship with both parents and their children helps ease the transition to adulthood as adolescents take an increasingly larger role in determining their own care. Gynecologic issues include concerns about vulvar, vaginal, menstrual, and breast health, as well as broader sexual and reproductive health topics. PCPs who understand the anatomy and physiology of the reproductive system will offer guidance and support that can empower adolescents throughout their entire life.

The most common gynecologic concerns for prepubertal children are vulvovaginal issues, which overwhelmingly respond to general measures that reduce irritation. The onset of puberty introduces the presence of endogenous estrogen and dramatically changes the anatomy and physiology of the reproductive system. The menstrual cycle is the hallmark of puberty for individuals with ovaries and can be understood as an additional vital sign reflecting overall pubertal status and insight into other factors affecting health and wellbeing. Concerns about the menstrual cycle should be discussed, evaluated, and treated when indicated. Sexual health, including discussions of healthy relationships, sexual and gender identities, family planning, contraception, and counseling for the prevention of sexually transmitted infections (STIs) is another fundamental aspect of primary care for adolescents.

Anatomy, Physiology, and Assessment of the Female Reproductive System

The fetus is sexually undifferentiated for the first 6 weeks of gestation, having two bipotential gonads and bipotential paramesonephric (müllerian) and mesonephric (wolffian) ducts. Testes-determining factor on the Y chromosome causes testicular differentiation. The production of anti–müllerian hormone by the Sertoli cells in the male gonad inhibits müllerian duct development, and the wolffian duct differentiates into the epididymis, vas deferens, and seminal vesicle. Without the influence of the Y chromosome, the gonads develop into ovaries by about 8 weeks' gestation and reach maturity by 20 weeks' gestation. The müllerian ducts develop into the fallopian tubes, uterus, cervix, and the superior portion of the vagina. Differentiation of the external genitalia and the lower third of the vagina, including the hymen, occurs with the development of external urologic structures.

In utero, maternal estrogen thickens and enlarges the female genital structures and also stimulates the lining of the uterus. Mucus produced by the cervix results in physiologic leukorrhea of the newborn period. After birth, maternal hormones are withdrawn, resulting in endometrial shedding; this may cause a small amount of vaginal bleeding.

The External Genitalia and Vagina Before Puberty

By 8 weeks after birth, without the influence of maternal or endogenous estrogen, the labia majora flattens and the labia minora thins. Because of the absence of estrogen, the genital epithelium of the vaginal opening is atrophic, erythematous, and easily traumatized (Fig. 43.1 and Table 43.1). There are several different normal hymenal configurations, with annular and crescent being the most common (Fig. 43.2).

The microbiology of the prepubertal vagina reflects the hypoestrogenic atrophic epithelium with a pH of 6.5 to 7.5. Normal flora includes lactobacilli, common aerobic, anaerobic, and enteric organisms. If done, a routine bacterial culture of the prepubertal vagina will demonstrate a broad variety of organisms, including skin and fecal flora. The presence of these organisms does not in itself signal disease or infection and must be correlated with clinical concerns.

When the prepubertal child is in a frog-leg position, the labia are open and allow for a visual examination of the vulva and lower vagina. Although special attention will be paid to the external genitalia when the child or parent has a specific concern, a brief inspection of the external genitals should be a part of all complete physical examinations in prepubertal children. There are a variety of positions in which to examine the external genitalia: the "frog-leg" position is usually comfortable and easily incorporated into part of a complete physical examination (Fig. 43.3).

A brief and routine genital examination as one element of a complete physical evaluation demonstrates to the child and parents that the external portion of the urinary, gastrointestinal, and reproductive systems are important and normal parts of the body. It can be tempting to skip over the genital examination, especially if a child or parent is anxious or uncooperative. However, it is important to be able to attest to the normal appearance (vs. a

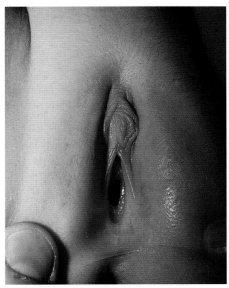

• **Fig. 43.1** Prepubertal Vulva. (From Montano GT, Torres OA. Pediatric and adolescent gynecology. In: *Zitelli and Davis' Atlas of Pediatric Physical Diagnosis,* 8th ed. Elsevier; 2023.)

TABLE 43.1	Prepubertal External Genitalia, Normal Findings
Finding	**Typical Appearance/Description**
Pubic hair	Absent (Tanner 1)
Labia majora	Flat, no fat pads
Labia minora	Thin
Clitoris	Not enlarged (<3 mm length or width)
Hymen and vaginal epithelium	Tissue hypoestrogenic: thin, erythematous, fragile
Anus and perianal region	Without lesions or skin changes

postpubertal or diseased state) of the vulva and vaginal opening in the prepubertal child. The examination also provides context for any questions or concerns and allows for the discussion of topics that may not otherwise be brought up, such as:

- Explain that an external examination of the genitalia in children is an important part of a full health examination, just like checking the heart, lungs, throat, etc.
- Explain that the examination is visual only and looks at the outside of the body.
- Explain that the parent/guardian gives permission for the examination and is present with the child (unless sexual abuse is a consideration).
- Use the examination as an opportunity to label body parts with correct anatomic terms such as vulva, vaginal opening, and labia and discuss socially appropriate language and behaviors when in public.
- Discuss basic hygiene.
- Discuss safety, privacy, and body boundaries.
- Encourage questions and discussion with child and parent, acknowledging the medical office as the appropriate place for such discussions.
- Allow for further evaluation if abnormal findings are observed.

In addition, a complete external examination, along with a breast examination, is needed to accomplish pubertal staging, which allows for anticipatory guidance regarding the physical changes of puberty and to assess for premature or delayed development.

External Genitalia and Vagina After the Onset of Puberty

The sexual maturity rating (SMR) is discussed in Chapter 13. The vulva and vagina of the postpubertal female vary significantly from the prepubertal state (Fig. 43.4 and Table 43.2). Some adolescents choose to remove some or all of their pubic hair, which can make staging for pubic hair more difficult. As pubic hair grows on the mons pubis and labia majora, so do the fat pads in these areas, which serve to protect the vulva and vaginal opening. At the time of puberty, the labia minora also enlarge and grow to adult size. Normal labia minora are varied in size, shape, color, and appearance. Asymmetry in the size of the labia minora is very common

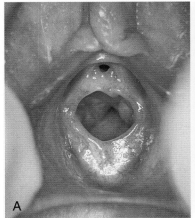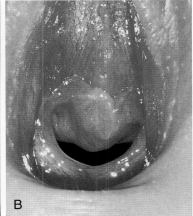

• **Fig. 43.2** Normal Hymenal Configurations. (A) Annular. (B) Crescent. (From Montano GT, Torres OA. Pediatric and adolescent gynecology. In: *Zitelli and Davis' Atlas of Pediatric Physical Diagnosis,* 8th ed. Elsevier; 2023.)

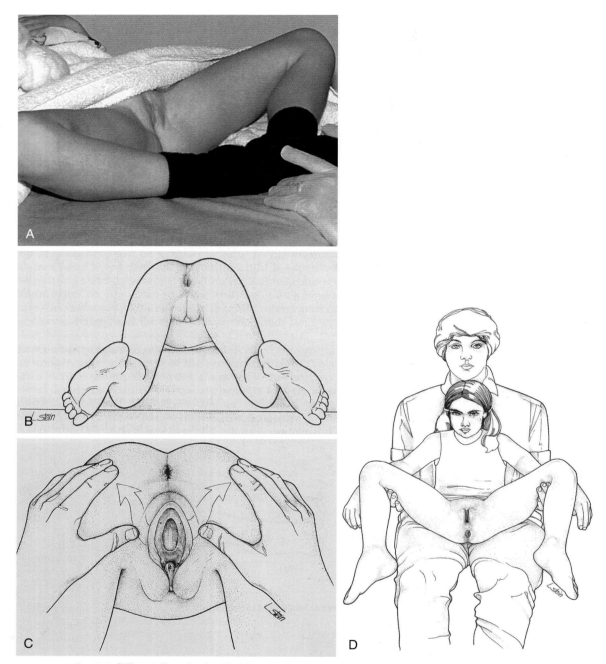

• **Fig. 43.3** Different Examination Positions for Performing a Gynecologic Examination on a Child. (A) Frog leg position. (B) Knee chest position. (C) Prone position. (D) Sitting on parent's lap. (A, From McCann JJ, Kerns DL. *The Anatomy of Child and Adolescent Sexual Abuse: A CD-ROM Atlas/Reference.* Inter-Corp; 1999. B–D, From Finkel MA, Giardino AP, eds. *Medical Examination of Child Sexual Abuse: A Practical Guide.* 2nd ed. Sage; 2002.)

and considered a normal variant. The minora may or may not extend past the labia majora.

Once ovarian estrogen production has begun, which will first be noted by thelarche, or breast budding, inspection of the vaginal opening will now reveal that the tissue, including the hymen, is more estrogenized and thickened. Over the next 1 to 2 years preceding menarche, the vaginal tissue will become more stretchy, and most postmenarchal preteens and teens can comfortably place and use internal feminine hygiene products (e.g., tampons, menstrual cup) without difficulty. Postpubertal vaginal secretions occur

daily; small amounts of clear or cloudy fluid are produced, the amount and color of the discharge changing normally throughout the menstrual cycle or due to other factors such as clothing, bathing, and dietary habits. Education about the normalcy of vaginal discharge after thelarche but even before the onset of menarche helps reassure children, adolescents, and parents who may be surprised by its presence.

Estrogen increases the glycogen content in vaginal epithelial cells, encouraging the colonization of lactobacilli, production of lactic acid, and a decrease in vaginal pH to less than 4.7. The

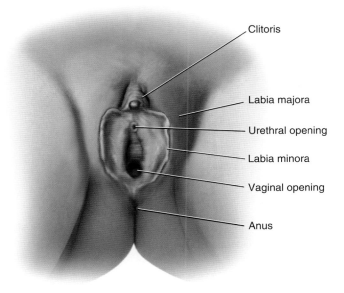

Clitoris

Labia majora

Urethral opening

Labia minora

Vaginal opening

Anus

Normal

• **Fig. 43.4** Postpubertal Vulva. (From Montano GT, Torres OA. Pediatric and adolescent gynecology. In: *Zitelli and Davis' Atlas of Pediatric Physical Diagnosis,* 8th ed. Elsevier; 2023.)

TABLE 43.2 Postpubertal External Genitalia, Normal Findings

Finding	Typical Appearance/Description
Pubic hair and labia majora	Mons pubis and labia majora develop fat pads. Tanner stage 4–5, but hair may be partially or completely removed
Labia minora	May or may not be symmetric. Size and shape may be different. Normal variant may extend past labia majora. Reassure that all labia lengths are normal
Hymen, vaginal epithelium	Tissue is estrogenized, moist. Discharge may be clear, white, thin or thick. Mild to no odor with adequate hygiene
Anus and perianal region	Normal examination without lesions or skin changes

• BOX 43.1 General Recommendations for Hygiene and Self-Care for the Vulva and Vagina

- For any itching or irritation, baths in plain water (without any additives) are recommended 2–3 times per day.
- In general, gently wash with plain water. Avoid bubble baths and sitting in water with soap or shampoo, as this removes moisture and causes dryness and itching.
- When bathing, gently wipe away any debris from the labial folds if needed. Avoid scrubbing with washcloth or scrubby brush.
- Gently dry off the vulva after washing. If desired, a hair dryer on the cool setting may be used for drying.
- Always wipe from front to back after a bowel movement.
- Cool compresses can be used if needed to soothe itching or irritation.
- Limit the use of "commercial" wipes only to remove visible debris. All wipes contain chemicals that cause dryness and possible irritation.
- Wear white cotton underwear. Certain colors contain dyes that cause irritation and noncotton materials are less breathable.
- Wear loose-fitting and breathable clothing. Thong underwear, spandex, Lycra, and tight pants can cause irritation.
- Change promptly out of wet swimsuits and sweaty exercise clothes.
- Sleep without underwear or wear only very loose pajama pants. Avoid tight sleepers or "onesies" that do not allow air to circulate.
- Avoid scented pads and tampons.
- Some individuals wear a pad or panty liner every day to absorb normal vaginal discharge. Educate patients about the physiologic and protective role of discharge and offer the option of changing underwear more often if the moisture is bothersome.
- Avoid sprays, washes, vaginal douches, and other products marketed for "feminine hygiene."
- If irritation occurs, soak in plain water a few times each day; also wear looser clothes and no underwear when possible.
- If irritation occurs, wash underwear separately from other clothes. Use a small amount of laundry soap and double rinse. Do not use fabric softeners.

normal vaginal flora in the postpubertal patient remains heterogeneous, including lactobacillus and other components of the vaginal flora, such as *Gardnerella vaginalis, Escherichia coli,* group B streptococci, genital mycoplasma, and *Candida albicans.*[1] Detection of these organisms on culture or on deoxyribonucleic acid (DNA) testing does not signal infection and must be correlated with clinical concerns.

When a formal inspection of the vulva is indicated in the adolescent, many recommend that the patient be given a handheld mirror while the PCP, using a moistened cotton swab, points out the major anatomic structures. Preteens and teens often have questions about the vulva, and this offers a perfect opportunity to educate them and reassure them of their normalcy.

General principles of vulvar and vaginal self-care that are helpful for people of all ages are included in Box 43.1. When needed,

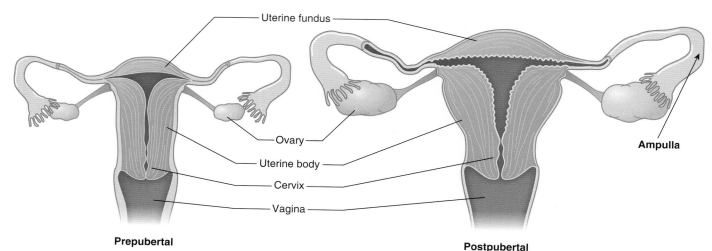

• **Fig. 43.5** Prepubertal and Postpubertal Cervix, Uterus, and Ovaries. Note 1:1 ratio of cervix to uterus, atrophic endometrium, and small ovaries in prepuberty. Estrogen induces growth of the uterus in proportion to the cervix (1:3), thickens endometrium, and reproductive-age ovarian size.

plain warm-water baths are best, with the avoidance of baking soda or any other additives. Products labeled and marketed for "feminine hygiene" are unnecessary and in some cases can be harmful.

Internal Reproductive Organs

The size and growth of the internal reproductive organs correlate with the stage of pubertal development. The prepubertal cervix and uterus are small and approximately of equal size; the endometrium is atrophic owing to the absence of estrogen-induced stimulation; the ovaries are small (1–3 cm3). With exposure to endogenous estrogen, the internal reproductive structures grow significantly and reach adult size once menarche has occurred (Fig. 43.5).

An internal pelvic examination is not indicated or recommended as part of routine health screening. Recommended screening for STIs in sexually active adolescents can be done via urine sample, or a self-collected vaginal swab. When to initiate screening for cervical cancer should be based on current recommendations. At the time of this publication, the USPTF (2018) recommends cervical cytology alone (pap smear) starting at age 21 years, however, this guidance is likely to shift to human papillomavirus (HPV) testing alone starting at age 25 years based on new recommendations from the American Cancer Society.[2]

When an internal pelvic examination is indicated in a postpubertal adolescent (indications discussed later), it is usually well tolerated as long as the teen understands the reasons for the examination, how it will be performed, and agrees to participate. A moistened cotton swab can be used to explore the vaginal opening, hymenal configuration, and confirm vaginal patency when needed. If an internal bimanual examination is indicated, a small lubricated gloved finger can palpate the vagina and cervix. When visual inspection of the upper vagina and cervix is indicated, a small, lubricated speculum can be used (Fig. 43.6). Internal examinations are often not necessary and should only be done when specific information needs to be obtained. For example, a careful vulvar inspection and a vaginal swab may be the only steps necessary in a young, non sexually active patient reporting vaginal discharge.

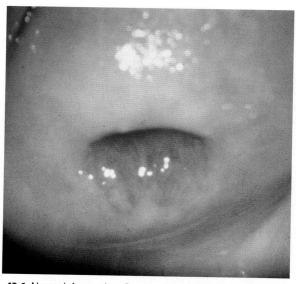

• **Fig. 43.6** Normal-Appearing Cervix of an Adolescent Female During Speculum Examination. (From Montano GT, Torres OA. Pediatric and adolescent gynecology. In: *Zitelli and Davis' Atlas of Pediatric Physical Diagnosis,* 8th ed. Elsevier; 2023.)

Female Pubertal Development and the Menstrual Cycle

Ovarian estrogen production initiates pubertal changes associated with secondary sex characteristics in children with ovaries, and the menstrual cycle is the hallmark event. Educating children and their families reduces anxiety and encourages communication with the PCP. Based on Tanner staging of the breast, providers can offer anticipatory guidance on the timing of the first menstrual period, or menarche, as well as practical education about how to record its frequency, duration, and amount, and then encouraging patients to bring their data to each appointment. Smartphone apps offer an accurate and appropriate way of collecting this information.

• BOX 43.2 Physiology of an Ovulatory Cycle in Brain, Ovaries, and Endometrium

Brain

- Early in follicular phase, increasing gonadotropin-releasing hormone (GnRH) pulsations from the hypothalamus signal the anterior pituitary to secrete follicle stimulating hormone (FSH). FSH also stimulated by lower levels of estrogen noted at the end of the menstrual cycle.
- Later in follicular phase, increasing levels of estrogen produced by ovary causes FSH suppression and luteinizing hormone (LH) secretion and surge.
- During luteal phase, LH production continues.
- During menstrual phase, FSH levels increase again.

Ovaries

- Early in follicular phase, ovarian follicles stimulated by FSH to develop a dominant follicle.
- FSH stimulates granulosa cells to increase production of estrogen. Increasing estrogen production feeds back to anterior pituitary causing LH surge in the later follicular phase.
- LH surge stimulates rupture of the dominant follicle, also called *ovulation*.
- During luteal phase, follicle remains become the corpus luteum. Its theca lutein cells secrete progesterone.
- If pregnancy does not occur, the corpus luteum decays and stops secreting progesterone after 10 days.

Endometrium

- During first part of an ovulatory cycle, the endometrium is exposed to estrogen alone causing proliferation of the glands and arteries of the endometrium (proliferative phase).
- After ovulation, the endometrium is exposed to a combination of estrogen and progesterone. Progesterone stops endometrial proliferation and causes the lining to change to a secretory phase (secretory phase).
- With demise of the corpus luteum, progesterone levels drop and endometrium sheds, resulting in menstrual bleeding (menstrual phase).
- Menstrual fluid leaves the uterus through the cervix and exits the body through the vagina.

Physiology of Menstrual Bleeding

Menstrual bleeding occurs due to a complex interaction between the hypothalamus, anterior pituitary gland, ovary, and endometrium. Box 43.2 and Fig. 43.7 describe and illustrate the physiology of a normal ovulatory cycle at the level of the brain, ovaries, and uterus.

Ovulatory and Anovulatory Menstrual Cycles

Ovulatory menstrual cycles are regular in frequency, duration, and blood loss. This is due to ovulation, which causes release of progesterone by the corpus luteum; in the absence of pregnancy, progesterone levels drop 10 days after ovulation resulting in a concerted shedding of the endometrial lining known as the menstrual period. In anovulatory cycles, there is an absence of progesterone produced by the corpus luteum and the endometrium therefore is stimulated by estrogen alone and becomes thickened and fragile. Anovulation can result in no periods at all (amenorrhea) or can result in bleeding that is unpredictable and chaotic. Immaturity of the hypothalamic-pituitary-ovarian (HPO) axis is the most common cause of anovulation in early adolescence, although other causes must be considered and are discussed in the sections on amenorrhea and abnormal uterine bleeding (AUB). Despite the frequency of anovulation among adolescents, most cycles still align with the norms listed in Box 43.3. Further evaluation is warranted in individuals who are more than 1-year postmenarchal

and have repeated erratic menstrual cycles or the absence of periods for longer than 90 days.

Coagulation Pathway and the Menstrual Cycle

During the menstrual phase, blood vessels within the endometrium are rapidly repaired due to interactions of platelets and clotting factors. Inherited or acquired conditions (e.g., Von Willebrand disease, platelet dysfunction disorders) that affect the coagulation system may result in heavy, prolonged bleeding and associated blood loss. Further evaluation is needed when cycles are outside of the norms given in Box 43.3. A complete blood count (CBC) and iron levels are essential to accurately assess blood loss, and further testing is indicated if anemia is detected.

Early Pregnancy: Key Concepts and Physiology

For adolescents, a prerequisite to making responsible and informed decisions about pregnancy is medically accurate information on sexual health and human reproduction. PCPs play a critical role in teaching and discussing these issues. Clinicians can educate adolescent patients and their families in the clinic setting and advocate for scientifically accurate information to be taught in school as well as at home.[3]

Understanding human reproduction allows PCPs to offer scientifically accurate information to their patients, families, and community. Reviewing the physiology of early pregnancy is also the easiest way to understand the mechanism of various contraceptive methods and the evaluation for early pregnancy.

When a male ejaculates inside the vagina, active sperm travel through the cervix, uterus, and fallopian tubes to the ampulla, where they remain active and capable of fertilization for 5 days following intercourse (Fig. 43.8). Fertilization only takes place in the ampullar portion of the tube and can only occur when an egg is released (ovulation) with sperm already present. Fertilization is a complex process and does not always occur even when both egg and sperm are present. Implantation occurs 5 to 6 days after fertilization when the fertilized egg, now called a *blastocyst*, implants inside the uterine wall. Some pregnant females will have bleeding with implantation, which can be mistaken for a short menstrual period. Due to a wide range of genetic, environmental, and other factors, over half of fertilized eggs in normal, healthy couples fail to implant inside the uterus and therefore pregnancy does not occur. When implantation does occur, the placenta is formed and begins to produce human chorionic gonadotropin (hCG), which can be detected in the blood and urine as soon as a few days after implantation. Urine hCG testing is considered a highly accurate confirmation of pregnancy, although home test instructions can be confusing and a repeat test in the clinic is always warranted. However, it may take 14 to 17 days from intercourse for a urine pregnancy test to become positive.

During pregnancy, hCG, estrogen, and progesterone levels increase. Box 43.4 lists common symptoms of early pregnancy. It is appropriate to screen for pregnancy when adolescents present with these concerns even if sexual contact is not reported. It may be necessary to reassure families and patients that pregnancy screening is part of the diagnostic evaluation and does not mean that the provider suspects sexual activity.

Vulvar and Vaginal Concerns

Vulvar and vaginal concerns are common among children and adolescents. Vaginitis is the spectrum of conditions that cause vulvovaginal

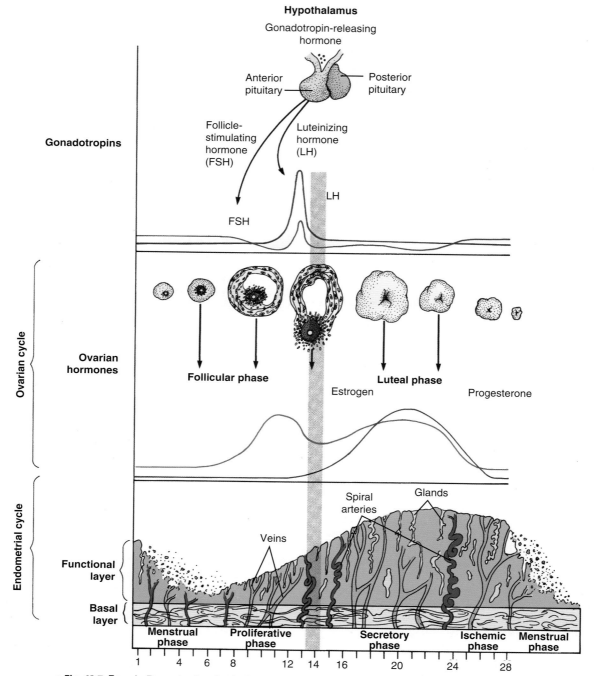

Hypothalamus

Gonadotropin-releasing hormone

Anterior pituitary — Posterior pituitary

Gonadotropins

Follicle-stimulating hormone (FSH)

Luteinizing hormone (LH)

LH

FSH

Ovarian cycle

Ovarian hormones

Follicular phase

Luteal phase

Estrogen

Progesterone

Endometrial cycle

Spiral arteries

Glands

Veins

Functional layer

Basal layer

| Menstrual phase | Proliferative phase | Secretory phase | Ischemic phase | Menstrual phase |

1 4 6 8 12 14 16 20 24 28

• **Fig. 43.7** Female Reproductive Cycle Showing Changes in Hormone Secretion, the Ovary, and the Uterine Endometrium. *FSH*, Follicle stimulating hormone; *LH*, luteinizing hormone.

• **BOX 43.3** **Norms for the Menstrual Cycle in Adolescent Girls**

Median age at menarche: between 12 and 13 years
Normal interval range: 21–45 days (mean: 34 days)
Flow length: ≤7 days
Product use: 3–6 pads or tampons per day

symptoms such as a change in vaginal discharge, pruritus, burning, irritation, erythema of the vulvar tissues, dysuria, and spotting. Vulvar skin conditions may cause similar symptoms and must be considered.

Evaluation

Evaluation of vulvar and vaginal concerns includes a focused history with special attention to the quality, location, and duration

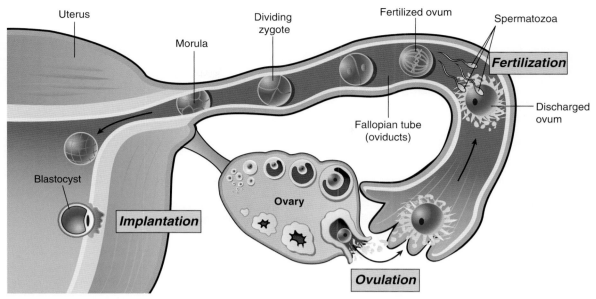

• **Fig. 43.8** Ovulation, Fertilization, and Implantation. (From Salvo SG. *Massage Therapy*. 5th ed. Elsevier; 2015.)

• BOX 43.4   Common Symptoms in Early Pregnancy

- Late or skipped menstrual period
- Abnormal bleeding
- Painful or swollen breasts
- Nausea with or without vomiting
- Fatigue

---

of symptoms. Ask patients about hygiene practices and materials and products that come in contact with the vulva and vagina. The physical examination includes an assessment of the external genitalia for the presence or absence of clinical findings, including patient identification of the area that is causing discomfort. The majority of concerns can be addressed without an internal pelvic examination; however, a speculum examination may be indicated in certain adolescents who have concerns about vaginal discharge and are agreeable to evaluation. Testing for STIs can be done via urine, or self-collected vaginal swab if preferred.[1]

A saline-moistened swab can be used to collect vaginal discharge for culture in the prepubertal child with a suspected acute bacterial infection. When nonspecific causes are suspected, a bacterial culture may not be helpful because of the broad range of organisms, including skin and fecal flora, found in the hypoestrogenic and alkaline prepubertal vagina. Common causes of vaginitis in postpubertal individuals, such as yeast, are extremely uncommon in prepubescent children.

In postpubertal adolescents, vaginal discharge can be collected by inserting a cotton-tipped swab inside the vagina or collected at the time of a speculum examination. Measurement of vaginal pH is helpful in the diagnosis of vaginal discharge. An elevated pH suggests bacterial vaginosis (pH >4.5) or trichomoniasis (pH 5–6) and helps to exclude candidal vulvovaginitis (pH remains normal at 4–4.5). Narrow-range pH paper (4–5.5) should be applied directly to the vaginal secretions; false elevation in pH can occur due to cervical mucus, blood, and semen. Microscopy can be performed by mixing the swab with one to two drops of saline on one

slide and adding one drop of 10% potassium hydroxide (KOH) to a smear on a second slide. A bacterial culture is typically not helpful in adolescents given the heterogeneity of the normal vaginal flora. Commercial diagnostic testing [rapid antigen and nucleic acid amplification tests (NAATs)] are available for identifying bacterial vaginosis, candidiasis, and trichomoniasis and may improve diagnostic accuracy. In sexually active adolescents or when sexual abuse may be suspected, a NAAT may be used to screen for gonorrhea and chlamydia. Yeast culture is helpful if clinical suspicion is high for candidal infection, but microscopy is negative or not available.

Prepubertal Vulvar and Vaginal Concerns

Prepubertal Vulvovaginitis

This is one of the most common gynecologic concerns. Atrophic vaginal epithelium and absence of labial fat pads and pubic hair predispose to vulvar trauma and irritation. "Nonspecific" vaginitis causes as many as 75% of vulvovaginal symptoms and occurs as a result of poor hygiene—especially noted around the time of toilet training—or the use of soap, detergent, or cream. Symptoms due to nonspecific causes tend to be bothersome but are usually not severe and may come and go over weeks or months.

Vulvovaginal infections resulting from specific bacterial causes are less common than nonspecific causes and usually have an acute onset with visible discharge. Infectious causes include group A streptococci and *Haemophilus influenzae* as well as enteric organisms. STIs must be considered. Yeast infections are rare in prepubertal children, as a high vaginal pH does not allow for growth of *Candida* species. Other causes of vulvar and perianal itching include pinworms and lichen sclerosis. A foreign body usually causes odor, discharge, and possibly bleeding but is less likely to cause vulvar symptoms. Consider sexual abuse with all vulvovaginal concerns. Ask patients about other systems and screen for urinary tract infection (UTI), constipation, and bowel and bladder dysfunction.

Advise all patients with vulvovaginal symptoms to stop the use of all products, even those deemed "hypoallergenic," and follow

TABLE 43.3	Characteristics, Evaluation, and Treatment of Prepubertal Vulvovaginitis		
Cause and Characteristics		**Evaluation**	**Treatment**
Nonspecific Vulvovaginitis • Discharge may be clear, yellow, green, malodorous • With or without itching; less commonly, dysuria • Vulvar erythema, may extend to anus and there may be excoriations • May have contact dermatitis concurrently		• Careful history and exam with attention to hygiene practices • If vaginal culture is done, it will likely reveal diverse flora	See Box 43.1
Irritant or Contact Dermatitis • Vulvar soreness and itching • History of bubble bath, sandbox, prolonged contact with urine/feces • May develop after prolonged exposure to commercial products (e.g., perfumes, clothing dyes) • May occur after use of topical agent to treat vulvovaginal symptoms		• Careful history and exam with attention to hygiene practices • Attention to products used in vulvar area (e.g., soaps, detergents, underwear)	See Box 43.1
Specific Bacterial Infections • Acute onset, with pain, possible itching and bleeding • "Beefy red" appearance with group A strep infection • Respiratory pathogens may be associated with current or recent respiratory infection • Enteric pathogens may be associated with recent or current diarrhea		• Culture confirms pathogen • Respiratory: Streptococcus pyogenes (Group A β-hemolytic streptococcus), Staphylococcus aureus, Haemophilus influenzae, Streptococcus pneumoniae, other flora • Enteric: Shigella, Yersinia, other flora	• Specific to pathogen, e.g., S. pyogenes: penicillin V, amoxicillin • Shigella: trimethoprim-sulfamethoxazole, ampicillin
Pinworms (*Enterobius vermicularis*) • Itching including perianal areas, especially at night • Excoriations and erythema but no discharge		• Tape test reveals eggs • Treatment indicated if other family members infected or symptoms suggestive of infection	• Single dose of mebendazole or albendazole, repeated in 2 weeks
Candidal Diaper Dermatitis • Itching and erythema in groin and labial skin folds • Beefy red areas, vesicles and pustules at periphery • Vaginal involvement unlikely before puberty		• KOH prep shows budding yeast and pseudohyphae	• Topical nystatin or miconazole; fluconazole orally • Dryness and frequent diaper changes necessary
Infections Resulting From Sexual Abuse • Gonorrhea, chlamydia, trichomoniasis, herpes simplex, human papillomavirus		• Treat for STI if sexual abuse suspected and/or suspicious clinical findings	• See CDC treatment guidelines for sexually transmitted infections • Report to child protection services; exam as indicated
Foreign Body • Malodorous discharge, minimal vulvar symptoms, possible bleeding • Tissue paper most common • Patient/parent may report item inserted into vagina		• Can attempt removal with warm irrigation fluid after introitus treated with a topical anesthetic • Exam under anesthesia and vaginoscopy may be needed	• Try general self-care measures if symptoms mild • Refer if symptoms increased

CDC, Centers for Disease Control and Prevention; *KOH*, potassium hydroxide; *STI*, sexually transmitted infection.

the hygiene measures outlined in Box 43.1. For nonspecific causes and dermatitis, symptoms should improve greatly or resolve within 2 to 3 weeks. When patients have persistent complaints despite treatment or the provider is unsure about the diagnosis, referral to a specialist with expertise in the diagnosis and treatment of prepubertal vaginitis is indicated. Examination under anesthesia along with vaginoscopy may be indicated to assess for a foreign body (most commonly tissue paper) or a cervical or vaginal lesion as the cause (Table 43.3).

Lichen Sclerosis

Patients who have lichen sclerosis report intense itching and soreness; they may also report bleeding. Diagnosis is made clinically by visualizing white, atrophic skin along with ulcerations and subepithelial hemorrhages on the genitalia, perineum, or perianal area. The clitoris has a normal appearance but the labia minora are flattened and may be scarred (Fig. 43.9). Left untreated on or near the vulva, the labia shrink and the opening to the vagina may be scarred. Treatment is with clobetasol propionate 0.05%

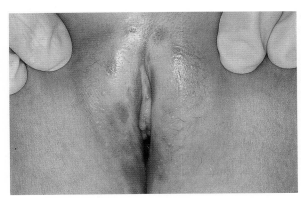

• **Fig. 43.9** Lichen Sclerosis. (From Montano GT, Torres OA. Pediatric and adolescent gynecology. In: *Zitelli and Davis' Atlas of Pediatric Physical Diagnosis,* 8th ed. Elsevier; 2023.)

to the affected area once to twice each day for 2 weeks. Treatment continues until the child is asymptomatic and the disease is not visible, followed by tapering of the medication. Referral to a specialist such as a pediatric gynecologist or dermatologist should be made if there is any uncertainty about diagnosis and/or treatment.

Prepubertal Vaginal Bleeding

Bleeding in the first week of life secondary to withdrawal from maternal hormones is physiologic. Other prepubertal vaginal bleeding is not normal and should be promptly evaluated with a careful history and physical examination. Local causes of vaginal bleeding include vaginitis, lichen sclerosis, retained foreign body, condyloma, trauma (including sexual abuse), urethral prolapse, and other benign or rare growths. Endometrial causes include precocious puberty, other endocrine abnormalities, and functional estrogen-producing ovarian cysts or tumors. Patients with thrombocytopenia or bleeding disorders may have other signs such as epistaxis, petechiae, and hematomas. Referral to a specialist in pediatric gynecology should be made if the cause of bleeding is not identified.

Labial Adhesions

Adhesions of the labia minora are a common finding and occur primarily in children 3 months to 6 years of age due to the hypoestrogenic state of the vulva. This finding is usually not symptomatic but discovered on routine examination; adhesions may be partial or appear to completely occlude the vaginal opening (Fig. 43.10). A careful history should be obtained for functional concerns with voiding (such as postvoid dribbling or recurrent UTIs), trauma, and inadequate hygiene. Treatment in asymptomatic patients is conservative, with careful attention to vulvar hygiene and reassurance without the use of any topical agents. In symptomatic patients, topical estrogen and/or steroid cream applied to the adhesion with gentle pressure is usually curative, although recurrence is not uncommon. Use of a bland emollient to the separated labia may help prevent recurrence until endogenous estrogen is present with the onset of puberty.

Imperforate Hymen

Occasionally, imperforate hymen is diagnosed in the newborn when uterovaginal secretions due to maternal estrogen accumulate in the vagina (i.e., hydrocolpos) (Fig. 43.11). A careful examination will differentiate imperforate hymen from labial adhesions. Associated complications of imperforate hymen in the newborn are rare and treatment is usually delayed until after the onset of puberty but before the onset of menarche. Findings of an imperforate hymen warrant consultation with a pediatric gynecologist to

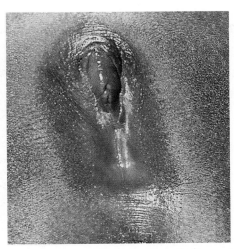

• **Fig. 43.10** Labial Adhesions. (From Montano GT, Torres OA. Pediatric and adolescent gynecology. In: *Zitelli and Davis' Atlas of Pediatric Physical Diagnosis,* 8th ed. Elsevier; 2023.)

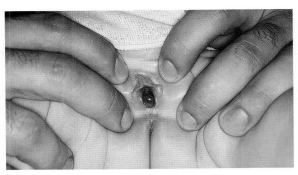

• **Fig. 43.11** Imperforate Hymen (Bulging). (From Kaefer M. Management of abnormalities of the genitalia in girls. In: *Campbell-Walsh-Wein Urology,* 12th ed. Elsevier; 2021.)

discuss precautions and plan for future management. Imperforate hymen is also a cause of primary amenorrhea; affected adolescents present with otherwise normal pubertal development however are still amenorrheic 3-years following thelarche. Due to accumulated menstrual fluid, they may have cyclic pelvic pain and a bulging hymen on examination. Excision of the hymen by an experienced surgeon is indicated. Imperforate hymen is not typically associated with other congenital anomalies.

Postpubertal Vulvar and Vaginal Concerns

The vulva and vagina of the postpubertal child vary significantly from the prepubertal state, primarily due to the presence of endogenous estrogen. Physiologic discharge can cause concern and warrants evaluation and then reassurance when indicated. Vulvovaginitis is more likely to be caused by a specific infection in postpubertal than in prepubescent patients; however, it can still be exacerbated or entirely due to noninfectious processes.

Vulvovaginitis in Adolescents

Initial diagnostic evaluation of acute symptoms should include testing for candidiasis, bacterial vaginitis, and trichomoniasis, which account for over 90% of infection-related vaginitis episodes. Table 43.4 lists common causes and characteristics of vaginitis and vulvar complaints following puberty.

TABLE 43.4 Common Causes of Vaginitis and Vulvar Complaints in Postpubertal Adolescents

	Discharge	Cause and Diagnosis	Acuity, Additional Symptoms/History	Treatment[a]
Physiologic Discharge	White or transparent Thick or thin Usually no odor, may have slight odor Gradual onset as occurs because of estrogen and changes in hormones during menstrual cycle Reports discharge on and off for weeks, months, or years	Endocervical secretions and vaginal cells sloughing Mediated by normal, healthy production of estrogen, and may change in midmenstrual cycle with ovulation Diagnostic testing negative Wet prep reveals numerous epithelial cells without inflammation	Weeks to months of concern, may get heavier and lighter No vulvar symptoms or minimal pain and itching Concerns about wetness of underwear and feels the need to wear panty liners, which may cause irritation	Reassure and educate about protective functions of physiologic discharge Review best practices for hygiene and self-care (Box 43.1)
Contact Dermatitis	Normal to increased discharge Thick or thin Usually no odor: may have slight odor	Soaps, perfumes/sprays, pads, panty liners, laundry detergents and fabric softeners, OTC creams marketed to treat vaginal itching and/or yeast, baby wipes Due to excessive cleaning or poor hygiene Diagnostic testing negative	Usually, chronic symptoms; can have acute flares Obtain careful history about all habits	Stop using all possible irritants Soak in plain water bath 1–3 times a day, use cool compresses as needed Wear loose-fitting and breathable clothes, avoid Lycra and thongs Skip underwear when not needed (e.g., sleeping at night)
Candidiasis	Discharge scant or thick, white, and curd-like Usually no odor Itching, pain, and swelling dominant concern, not discharge itself	80% of infections due to *Candida albicans* Vaginal pH normal (4–4.5). Wet prep KOH slide reveals budding pseudohyphae and yeast forms DNA probe test available Consider yeast culture if no response to treatment	Acute inflammatory symptoms of itching and soreness, redness, external dysuria, and swelling of vulva. Candida part of normal, vaginal flora. Correlate with findings/symptoms if lab test positive	OTC intravaginal agents in creams and suppositories: clotrimazole, miconazole, tioconazole Prescription intravaginal: butoconazole 2% cream, 5 g in one application Orteroconazole 0.4% cream 5 g for 7 days Prescription oral: fluconazole 150 mg PO once
Bacterial Vaginitis	Thin, gray, or yellow; malodorous; "fishy smelling" Fishy odor may increase after intercourse when semen mixes with discharge	Vaginal pH elevated (>4.5) Wet prep shows "clue cells," epithelial cells studded with coccobacilli and rare leukocytes Fishy, amine odor after applying KOH to wet mount DNA probe test available for *Gardnerella vaginalis* and vaginal fluid sialidase activity	Minimal irritation or inflammation. No vulvar symptoms *G. vaginalis* is part of normal, vaginal flora Correlate with findings/symptoms if positive lab test	Metronidazole 500 mg PO bid for 7 days Ormetronidazole gel 0.75%, 5 g intravaginally daily for 5 days Orclindamycin cream 2%, 5 g intravaginally at bedtime for 7 days
Trichomoniasis	Thin, frothy, green-yellow, purulent, malodorous	Vaginal pH is elevated (5–6). Motile trichomonads on wet prep (only 60% of patients) Strongly consider DNA probe test or other diagnostic test if patient is sexually active or infection suspected	May have burning, itching, dysuria	Metronidazole 2 g PO once Ormetronidazole 500 mg PO bid for 7 days Ortinidazole 2 g PO once
Acute cervicitis (caused by chlamydia or gonorrhea)	May be yellow May cause no symptoms or minimal symptoms	Numerous white cells (>10 per high power field) on wet prep NAAT testing diagnostic; done via urine, self-collected vaginal swab, or endocervical swab	May have dysuria, increased discharge, spotting, pelvic pain	See the CDC's STI treatment guidelines for updated recommendations

[a]Treatments are recommended by the Centers for Disease Control at www.cdc.gov.

DNA, Deoxyribonucleic acid; *KOH*, potassium hydroxide; *NAAT*, Nucleic acid amplification test; *OTC*, over the counter; *STI*, sexually transmitted infection.

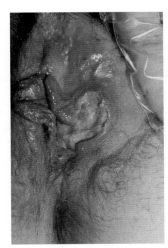

• **Fig. 43.12** Vulvar Ulcers. (From Montano GT, Torres OA. Pediatric and adolescent gynecology. In: *Zitelli and Davis' Atlas of Pediatric Physical Diagnosis*, 8th ed. Elsevier; 2023.)

Nonsexual Genital Ulcers

The condition of nonsexual genital ulcers (NSGUs), or vaginal aphthosis, is poorly understood. Vulvar ulcers are unusual, painful, and distressing, particularly in young teens who have never been sexually active. Patients report intense vulvar pain, extreme external dysuria, and have ulcerated vulvar lesions that measure 1 to 3 cm in diameter and can appear necrotic; they may also have significant labial edema (Fig. 43.12). The vast majority of patients recall systemic signs and symptoms of a viral illness (fever, malaise, headache, gastrointestinal symptoms) preceding the symptom onset. NSGU has been associated with many systemic viral illnesses, including Coronavirus infection[4] as well following vaccination. Diagnosis is made by a careful history excluding sexual abuse and a complete examination (including inspection of the mouth for additional ulcers). Providers may consider polymerase chain reaction (PCR) testing of the lesion to rule out herpes simplex; however, classic NSGU are much larger in appearance than herpetic vesicles. Other causes of ulcers—such as syphilis, Crohn disease, systemic lupus erythematosus, and other immune diseases—should be considered. The primary goal of treatment is pain relief and the prevention of superimposed infection. Comfort measures include plain water baths, topical anesthetics (viscous xylocaine), voiding in the tub to reduce external dysuria, and acetaminophen or ibuprofen for pain. Local and systemic steroids may also be indicated. Significant pain may be present for 10 to 14 days, with complete resolution in 3 weeks. Recurrence is not unusual, but symptoms are usually less severe. PCPs not familiar with this condition should consult with a specialist in adolescent gynecology.

Concerns About Labial Appearance

The trend to remove pubic hair and increased access to stereotypical images are likely contributing factors to concerns about labial appearance. At the time of puberty, the labia minora enlarge and grow to adult size. Despite conventional images and diagrams of female genitalia, normal labia minora are endlessly varied in size, shape, color, and appearance. Asymmetry in the size of the labia minora is common and considered a normal variant. The labia minora may or may not be extended past the labia majora and there is no definition of "labial hypertrophy" as all labial lengths and widths are considered normal.[5] If there is irritation, the PCP can offer solutions such as the application of emollients

and changing the type of clothing worn so as to stop irritation. Many are unaware of normal variations in the labia minora and may need additional education and reassurance. Labiaplasty is not recommended for adolescents and female genital surgery based on concerns about appearance is not warranted.[6]

Menstrual Concerns

Amenorrhea

Amenorrhea is the absence of menstrual periods and can be temporary or permanent due to central, gonadal, or peripheral dysfunction. PCPs should use their understanding of the normal physiology of the menstrual cycle (see Box 43.2 and Fig. 13.2) to evaluate amenorrhea and oligomenorrhea in a stepwise fashion that avoids unnecessary testing and reduces anxiety for the patient and family. An adolescent who has not started breast growth by 13 years of age warrants evaluation. Causes of pubertal delay are discussed in Chapter 39, although there is significant overlap between the causes of pubertal delay and amenorrhea. *Primary amenorrhea* describes the failure to have a period within 3 years of breast development or menarche by age 15 years. *Secondary amenorrhea* is no menstrual period for three menstrual cycles (~90 days) or the absence of menstrual periods for at least 6 months if patient has had at least one period. *Oligomenorrhea* describes infrequent menstrual periods as occurring greater than every 45 days, or fewer than 6 to 8 per year.

History and Physical

A careful history, physical examination, and pregnancy testing are the first steps in the evaluation of all cases of amenorrhea. Historical items to discuss with patients and families are listed in Table 43.5. Physical finding to note include:

- External genital examination to confirm that vagina is present; confirm that hymen is patent. Vaginal tissue can be observed to see if atrophic or estrogenized.
- SMR of breasts given that menstrual periods usually occur when breasts are at SMR IV and rare before SMR III.
- Physical signs of an eating disorder: Anorexia/dehydrated; low pulse, blood pressure, and temperature; dry skin; lanugo; bulimia-swollen cheeks (parotid glands), calluses on hands/fingers, enamel erosion and/or stains on teeth (see Chapter 14).
- Signs of androgen excess: Cystic or severe acne, excess hair on face or body, male pattern (temporal) baldness.
- Body changes suggestive of hyperinsulinemia: Central adiposity, acanthosis nigricans, striae.

  If an individual with primary amenorrhea is found to have an abnormal genital examination, such as imperforate hymen or absence of a vaginal opening with otherwise normal labia and hymenal tissue (e.g., müllerian agenesis and androgen insensitivity syndrome), a pelvic ultrasound should be done to confirm the presence of an upper vagina, cervix, uterus, and ovaries as well as to assess for any obstruction of menstrual flow. Any abnormalities warrant consultation for further evaluation and management with a gynecologist, endocrinologist, or other provider experienced at diagnosing and treating primary amenorrhea.

Additional Testing

Laboratory testing for causes of amenorrhea can be expensive and confusing (Box 43.5). After performing a pregnancy test, the tests that are most helpful initially include follicle stimulating hormone (FSH), estradiol, thyroid stimulating hormone, prolactin, and a

TABLE 43.5 Patient History for Evaluating the Cause of Amenorrhea

History	Significance of Positive Finding
Age of thelarche (onset of puberty, noted as breast budding)	Normal age of thelarche 8–13 years, average age 10 years. Menarche (first period) usually 2–3 years after thelarche
Menstrual history: age of first period, length between cycles, and days of bleeding	Need to distinguish between primary and secondary amenorrhea, as 15% of primary cases have abnormal findings on pelvic exam/ultrasound Menstrual history can suggest previously ovulatory (regular) or anovulatory (chaotic) cycles
Pubertal and menstrual timing for both parents and all siblings	Familial or constitutional delay—the most common reason for delayed onset of puberty; menarche should occur 2–3 years after thelarche
Height and weight growth curves	Menarche typically occurs after the most rapid pubertal growth spurt, with growth slowing after menarche Obesity and/or rapid weight gain can cause anovulation; it may be associated with polycystic ovarian syndrome (PCOS) and/or eating disorders or other conditions Weight loss or being underweight can cause hypothalamic amenorrhea/anovulation or suggest restrictive eating and/or eating disorders
Patient involvement in competitive athletics Screening for female athlete triad, usually characterized by frequent exercise, high stress and perfectionism, restrictive or "very healthy" eating habits	Intense activity can cause pubertal delay and amenorrhea Female athlete triad can cause functional hypothalamic amenorrhea/anovulation due to inadequate energy intake
Anxiety, depression, self-harm, obsessive thoughts about diet, exercise, and/or body image Consultation with parent and during one-on-one interview with adolescent	Stress can induce hypothalamic amenorrhea. Mental health concerns associated with eating disorder or poor energy intake
Concerns about severe acne, excess facial hair, male-pattern baldness	Androgen excess conditions such as PCOS can cause anovulation
Autoimmune disorders (e.g., Graves disease, celiac disease)	Certain autoimmune conditions associated with primary ovarian insufficiency
Previous surgeries	Previous dilation and curettage (D&C) can cause scarring of uterine lining
Congenital anomalies and/or syndromes	Renal, skeletal, abdominal wall, and anorectal anomalies associated with Müllerian anomalies Turner syndrome (XO) associated with ovarian hypofunction or premature ovarian failure
Previous malignancy treated with radiation, chemotherapy, surgery	May cause damage to reproductive system Brain lesions may cause damage to pituitary
Family history of fragile X syndrome	Female carriers of fragile X premutation have increased risk of primary ovarian insufficiency
Current use of hormonal contraception *During one-on-one interview, ask about all medications used, and specifically contraceptive use. Teens may initiate and use contraception confidentially.*	Hormonal methods may induce amenorrhea. After negative pregnancy test, reassure this is an expected side effect and benefit of many hormonal methods.
History of sexual contact *During one-on-one interview, ask about any type of intimate contact. Do not use the term "sexually active."*	Hormonal methods may induce amenorrhea. After negative pregnancy test, reassure this is an expected side effect and benefit of many hormonal methods.

sensitive testosterone assay. PCPs, who are not comfortable with the interpretation of these labs, should refer patients to a gynecologist, endocrinologist, or adolescent medicine provider. Additional follow-up testing such as chromosomal analysis and brain magnetic resonance imaging (MRI) may be indicated after evaluation by the specialist.

Causes of Amenorrhea

There are four major causes of amenorrhea: pregnancy, hypogonadotropic conditions, ovarian dysfunction, and structural causes. The most common cause of amenorrhea during the reproductive years is pregnancy, which can occur even before the onset of the

first menstrual period. Parents and patients may have to be reassured that pregnancy testing, usually via urine hCG, is part of the standard, evidence-based protocol for the evaluation of amenorrhea. Further testing should be delayed until a negative pregnancy test has been documented.

Central causes of amenorrhea include hypothalamic or pituitary gland dysfunction; altered pulsatility of gonadotropin-releasing hormone in hypothalamic causes or depressed production of gonadotropins (FSH and luteinizing hormone [LH]) in pituitary causes, result in inadequate stimulation of the ovary, low estrogen levels, and anovulation. The history often suggests these conditions, and laboratory testing confirms low or low-normal estrogen

• BOX 43.5 Tests for Evaluating Amenorrhea

Pregnancy test: Done via urine sample. Explain to patient and family that this must be done in all cases of amenorrhea, even when earlier sexual contact seems very unlikely.

Follicle stimulating hormone (FSH): An elevated FSH suggests premature, primary ovarian insufficiency, which warrants referral to endocrinology and/or gynecology for additional testing for a chromosomal abnormality, possible associated conditions, counseling about future fertility, and hormonal replacement therapy when indicated.

Thyroid Studies (TSH and T4): Hypothyroidism and hyperthyroidism can cause amenorrhea as well as other medical complications. Detection of central hypothyroidism warrants evaluation for deficiency of other pituitary hormones.

Prolactin: An elevated prolactin should be repeated fasting and before 8 a.m. when possible. Hyperprolactinemia, due to a tumor or other causes, can cause hypothalamic dysfunction leading to amenorrhea. A slight elevation in prolactin can be associated with the use of certain medications and can also occur when a patient has PCOS. Hyperprolactinemia warrants consultation with an endocrinologist or another provider (gynecologist, adolescent medicine) who is familiar with causes and treatment.

Estradiol: This test can be helpful when a patient is being assessed for hypothalamic causes of amenorrhea. A normal level of estradiol is reassuring that the ovary is producing adequate levels of estrogen. A low level of estradiol is seen when there is primary ovarian insufficiency or when hypothalamic suppression of the ovaries is significant, as seen in girls with anorexia.

Luteinizing hormone (LH): May sometimes be included in the initial evaluation of amenorrhea but is more useful when central causes are being considered. A low LH is consistent with a hypogonadotropic process.

Total and free testosterone: Total serum testosterone is useful in assessing for an androgen-secreting tumor when a patient presents with hirsutism in addition to amenorrhea. A very sensitive calculated free testosterone is needed to assess for biochemical hyperandrogenism in evaluation of PCOS (see Chapter 39). Serum testosterone is also useful in assessing patients with primary amenorrhea who are found to have absent reproductive organs. It will be at male levels when androgen-insensitivity is the cause but at normal female levels with mullerian agenesis.

DHEA-S and androstenedione: These are androgens that may be assessed when considering causes of amenorrhea that also cause hirsutism and may be elevated in PCOS.

17-OH progesterone (17-OHP): Used to evaluate for nonclassic congenital adrenal hyperplasia, which needs to be ruled out before diagnosing PCOS.

Pelvic Ultrasound: Assesses for the presence or absence of internal reproductive organs and obstruction of menstrual blood flow if this cannot be done adequately by pelvic examination. In cases of secondary amenorrhea, a pelvic ultrasound is usually not indicated.

Chromosomal analysis: Some patients with amenorrhea should have this testing—for example, those who are found to have primary ovarian insufficiency (elevated FSH, low estradiol) and when androgen-insensitivity syndrome is possible.

Pituitary magnetic resonance imaging: Imaging of the pituitary to assess for tumor or mass effect is indicated when there are concerns about a central cause of amenorrhea. Examples include significantly elevated prolactin, central hypothyroidism, low FSH and LH suggestive of pituitary hormone deficiency.

PCOS, Polycystic ovarian syndrome; *T4*, thyroxine; *TSH*, thyroid stimulating hormone.

---

pituitary include tumors, prolactinomas, pituitary infarction, and previous irradiation or surgery.

Ovulatory dysfunction in adolescence is common and is usually due to immaturity of the HPO axis. It can take 6 to 8 years following menarche for consistent ovulatory cycles to be present. Despite this, after the first menstrual year, bleeding that occurs more often than every 21 days or does not occur at least every 45 days warrants attention. Many adolescents experience anovulation for several years following their first period; this may result in erratic bleeding or no bleeding at all. This condition generally accompanies a normal history, physical examination, and laboratory testing. Treatment is based on the individual needs of the patient and at a minimum should involve close monitoring of the patient and menstrual periods, which should return to a normal frequency of at least every 45 days.

Ovarian insufficiency is marked by a low serum estradiol and elevated FSH (typically above 40 mIU/mL). In these cases, chromosomal analysis should be obtained, and management coordinated with a genetics specialist when abnormal. The most common genetic cause of gonadal failure is Turner syndrome (XO, or mosaic with FXO). Other causes of ovarian insufficiency include previous chemotherapy or radiation therapy, fragile X carriers, and autoimmune causes. However, many causes of primary ovarian insufficiency are unknown.[7]

Polycystic ovarian syndrome (PCOS) is one of the most common causes of amenorrhea and oligomenorrhea. Diagnosis of PCOS in adolescents requires both ovulatory dysfunction and clinical and/or biochemical hyperandrogenism. PCOS is a diagnosis of exclusion and, as such, laboratory testing is required to rule out other causes of anovulation and hyperandrogenism. Ovarian morphology is not used to diagnose PCOS in adolescents; polycystic-appearing ovaries on ultrasound should be considered a normal variant until at least 8-year postmenarchal.[8] PCOS is due to combination of genetic and environmental factors, but a clear etiology is unknown. One of the most common features of PCOS is insulin resistance leading to metabolic complications (see Chapter 39). Congenital anomalies of the reproductive system causing primary amenorrhea include imperforate hymen, transverse vaginal septum, and partial or complete absence of the vagina and uterus. Girls with an imperforate hymen may have cyclic abdominal pain because of the buildup of trapped menstrual blood. Referral to a gynecologist is needed for surgical correction of this condition. Patients with müllerian agenesis have an abnormal external genital examination or pelvic ultrasound, otherwise normal growth and development, normal 46 XX karyotype, and a normal female hormonal profile.[9] When a congenital anomaly is discovered, referral to an adolescent gynecologist or other specialist familiar with this condition is essential.

In postmenarchal adolescents, anatomic causes of amenorrhea are unlikely. However, if a uterine procedure such as curettage has been done, there may be scarring of the uterine lining, which would prevent normal growth of the endometrium.

Abnormal Uterine Bleeding

Menstrual flow outside of normal volume, duration, regularity, or frequency of the cycle is called AUB. Irregularity in menstrual cycles is common and expected during adolescence but may warrant further evaluation (Box 43.6). AUB can be a presenting symptom of anovulation or of a bleeding disorder. The evaluation

---

levels and low or low-normal LH and FSH levels. Functional causes include chronic diseases and illnesses, stress, competitive athletics, and eating disorders. Structural causes of dysfunction of the hypothalamus include Kallmann syndrome and of the

- Heavy or prolonged menstrual bleeding that causes anemia or has been ongoing since menarche.
- History of surgery-related bleeding or bleeding associated with dental work.
- Two or more of the following: bruising 1–2 times per month, epistaxis 1–2 times per month, frequent gum bleeding, or a family history of excessive bleeding.
- Family history of a known bleeding disorder.

TABLE 43.6 Causes of Abnormal Uterine Bleeding in Adolescents

Cause	Clinical Considerations
Pregnancy	Test all patients with abnormal uterine bleeding (AUB) even when sexual contact has not been reported
Bleeding disorders (von Willebrand disease, platelet dysfunction disorders, acquired disorders)	Screen if there is anemia or other concerning symptoms or signs
Anovulation • Immaturity of hypothalamic-pituitary-ovarian (HPO) axis • Hyperandrogenic anovulation (PCOS) • Anovulation due to thyroid disease, or primary pituitary disease • Primary ovarian insufficiency (will usually present with oligomenorrhea or amenorrhea)	Anovulation allows for a disordered endometrium, which can result in chaotic and heavy bleeding Consider lab testing for TSH, FSH, and androgens when indicated
Medications: hormonal therapy, contraception, anticoagulation therapy	
Cervicitis due to sexually transmitted infections (STIs)	Test for chlamydia, gonorrhea
Benign structural causes (fibroids, polyps)	Uncommon in adolescents
Rare tumors (estrogen- and/or androgen-secreting tumors, rhabdomyosarcoma)	Uncommon, rare cause

FSH, Follicle stimulating hormone; *TSH,* thyroid stimulating hormone.

and management of vaginal bleeding due to trauma or pregnancy is discussed elsewhere.

Heavy Menstrual Bleeding

Adolescents who report more than 7 days of bleeding each menstrual period, frequent episodes of bleeding, excessive product use, large clots, and repeated flooding onto clothes should be assessed with a CBC and ferritin level to look for anemia and iron deficiency. Patients who are found to be anemic from their menstrual bleeding, or have other risk factors, should have screening for a bleeding disorder.

Adolescents with heavy and/or prolonged bleeding patterns should have a pregnancy test, CBC with platelets and ferritin (to screen for iron deficiency). Patients who are actively bleeding and found to have significant anemia, or who exhibit symptoms of hemodynamic instability such as hypotension and tachycardia should be sent to an emergency department (ED) for evaluation and management, including assessment for a bleeding disorder, blood type, screen and crossmatch with potential blood administration. If unable to tolerate oral medication, intravenous (IV) estrogen therapy is used to stop acute bleeding. Those with significant anemia, who require hospitalization, or who have a compelling history of a bleeding disorder should be screened for a coagulopathy (see Chapter 38). As many as 20% of this population will be found to have a coagulopathy, and consultation with hematology and gynecology and close follow-up as an outpatient is warranted. Ongoing concerns about anemia or excessive bleeding also warrant referral to a hematologist for further evaluation and treatment.

Causes of Abnormal Uterine Bleeding

Most adolescents with AUB do not have a bleeding disorder; they have AUB resulting from anovulation. Anovulation causes the lining of the endometrium to become disordered and fragile, resulting in chaotic bleeding patterns. Table 43.6 lists causes of AUB in adolescents and should be considered and evaluated by laboratory testing when indicated. Given that structural causes are very rare in this population, a pelvic ultrasound is not typically indicated in the initial evaluation for bleeding in adolescence. A pelvic examination in not warranted unless there is a history of trauma; anesthesia should be offered if an examination would be uncomfortable for the child or adolescent.

Treatment of Abnormal Uterine Bleeding

The treatment of AUB depends on the severity of the condition, its cause, and the preference of the patient and her family. Hormonal therapy (Boxes 43.7 and 43.8) is the mainstay of treatment. Iron supplementation is indicated for anemia or low iron stores with new evidence that better absorption is achieved with

every-other-day dosing.[10] Treatment should be continued until abnormal bleeding patterns have resolved for 3 months and laboratory values have normalized. IV iron may be indicated in patients who continue to have low iron levels despite months of oral therapy.

For patients who have only mild symptoms, nonsteroidal antiinflammatory drugs (NSAIDs) such as ibuprofen or naproxen are one option. In addition to reducing pain, these medications decrease associated menstrual blood loss. If iron stores are depleted, iron supplementation is indicated. Patients should track their menstrual bleeding and alert their PCP about any concerns. Bleeding patterns should be reviewed periodically, and the evaluation repeated when indicated. Patients with mild symptoms should be educated that hormonal therapy is an option if desired, or if medical or functional concerns increase.

Patients with moderate symptoms need iron supplementation and hormonal therapy to reduce further blood loss. Patients should have a repeat CBC and ferritin in 3 months to ensure that anemia and iron deficiency are improved or resolved. Iron supplementation should continue for 3 months after hemoglobin and ferritin levels have normalized. Hormonal therapy should continue for a minimum of 3 to 6 months and possibly longer based on patient and family preference.

Patients with severe anemia require immediate treatment for their bleeding in an ED setting. Iron supplementation and hormonal therapy will control and prevent further bleeding. Patients should be seen within 5 to 7 days after leaving the hospital to assess hemoglobin status. Increased bleeding as an outpatient

---

• BOX 43.7 Overview of Hormonal Therapy

Common Indications for Hormonal Therapy
- Abnormal uterine bleeding
- Dysmenorrhea
- Chronic pelvic pain
- Endometriosis
- Premenstrual syndrome
- Menstrual migraines
- Seizures associated with the menstrual cycle
- Acne
- Hirsutism
- Menstrual suppression
- Patient preference

Mechanism of Action
- All methods contain progestin, which induces endometrial atrophy and results in less bleeding and cramping. Progestin effect on endometrium allows for a safe way to reduce or eliminate periods.
- Combined hormonal methods (oral contraceptive pill [OCP], skin patch, vaginal ring) contain progestin and estrogen. Estrogen increases sex-hormone binding globulin (SHBG), which results in lower free testosterone and therefore fewer androgenic concerns like acne and hirsutism. Takes 3–6 months or longer of use for full effects.
- Systemic methods (OCP, skin patch, vaginal ring, depot medroxyprogesterone acetate [DMPA], implant) prevent ovulation, which may be a trigger for pain, premenstrual syndrome (PMS), and other concerns in some adolescents.

Key Counseling Points
- Methods are labeled as "birth control," but this should not be a barrier to use in preteens or adolescents who would greatly benefit from these medications. Can reassure patients and families that there is no change in sexual behavior/interest when adolescents initiate these methods for medical reasons.
- Do not negatively affect future fertility and do not cause cancer.
- There are many different kinds of hormonal therapy. If one option does not meet a patient's/family's needs, another option can be tried.
- During the first 3–6 months of hormonal therapy, breakthrough bleeding is common and should be expected. Unplanned bleeding can be minimized by using the method correctly (e.g., pill must be taken at the same time each day; expect breakthrough bleeding if a pill is missed.)

• BOX 43.8 Common Types of Hormonal Therapies

- Combined hormonal contraception (OCPs, skin patch, vaginal ring)
- Oral progesterone (e.g., norethindrone acetate)
- Depot medroxyprogesterone acetate
- Levonorgestrel IUD
- Subdermal implant

If concerns about safety given an adolescent's medical conditions, providers can refer to the U.S. Medical Eligibility Criteria (USMEC) for evidence-based guidance.

IUD, Intrauterine device; *OCPs,* oral contraceptive pills.

---

should prompt the patient or family to call their PCP and return to the ED if necessary. Hormonal therapy should be continued for a minimum of 6 to 9 months. Consultation with gynecology or adolescent medicine is indicated to ensure appropriate evaluation, management, and follow-up. Patients with a suspected or diagnosed bleeding disorder should be referred to hematology.

Most commonly, AUB in adolescents is due to anovulation caused by immaturity of the HPO axis. AUB due to this cause may warrant treatment; however, the underlying condition will resolve as the endocrine system matures. For adolescents found to have medical conditions (e.g., PCOS, thyroid dysfunction), treatment of the underlying condition along with hormonal therapy may be needed.

Pelvic Pain

There are many causes of pelvic pain in adolescents. Pain is a response to distention, stretching, compression, irritation, and ischemia and can be referred from another site. The clinical neuroanatomy of the female pelvis is complex, with several organ systems sharing visceral and somatic innervation. Stress and overall sense of health and wellbeing greatly affect an individual's response to pain and ability to cope with it.

Acute Pelvic Pain

Common gynecologic causes of acute pain in adolescents include pelvic inflammatory disease (PID), ovarian cysts, ovarian torsion, ectopic pregnancy, and an acute exacerbation of chronic pelvic pain (Box 43.9). Nongynecologic causes of acute, severe pelvic pain include appendicitis, kidney stones, and UTI. Evaluation of acute pain must include a careful history, physical examination, and pregnancy testing. Other testing includes pelvic ultrasound to assess for ovarian causes, imaging for appendicitis, urinalysis, pregnancy test, and screening for STIs. An adolescent with acute pelvic pain should receive immediate attention at a medical center that can provide aggressive evaluation and treatment for gynecologic and nongynecologic causes (Box 43.10). *Ovarian or fallopian*

• BOX 43.9 Gynecologic Causes of Pelvic Pain in Adolescents

Serious, Requiring Urgent Intervention
- Ectopic pregnancy
- Rare obstetric emergencies (abruption, uterine rupture)
- Ovarian or fallopian tube torsion

Common
- Dysmenorrhea
- Mittelschmerz
- Pelvic inflammatory disease with or without tubo-ovarian abscess
- Ovarian and paratubal cysts
- Acute exacerbation of chronic pelvic pain
- Vulvovaginitis

Other
- Pregnancy
- Endometriosis
- Vaginal foreign body
- Müllerian anomalies causing obstruction
- Leiomyoma (fibroids)
- Vaginismus
- Pelvic floor dysfunction

tube torsion describes the twisting of the adnexa, resulting in partial or complete tissue ischemia. The onset of pain is acute, sharp, and associated with nausea and vomiting. Surgical intervention is necessary to detorse the adnexa and prevent necrosis and loss of the ovary. Removal of the adnexa is rarely indicated. Patients with suspected torsion should be sent to an ED and surgical consultation obtained.

Chronic and Recurrent Pelvic Pain

The initial evaluation of mild to moderate, recurrent, or chronic pelvic pain is best done with a comprehensive approach to the patient and symptoms (see Chapter 24). In addition to the gynecologic causes of pain listed in Box 43.9, there are gastrointestinal, urinary, musculoskeletal, neurogenic, and psychological causes that must be considered (see Box 43.10). History, including a confidential interview to screen for social and emotional concerns, and a physical examination are the first steps in evaluation. Common causes of chronic or recurring gynecologic pain are discussed next.

Dysmenorrhea

Dysmenorrhea is painful menstruation. Pain usually begins with the onset of menses but can occur 1 to 2 days before the onset

> ### • BOX 43.10 Differential Diagnosis of Pelvic Pain in Adolescents, Nongynecologic Causes
>
> **Gastrointestinal (see Chapter 34)**
> - Constipation
> - Appendicitis
> - Irritable bowel syndrome
> - Functional abdominal pain syndrome
> - Celiac disease
> - Lactose intolerance
> - Gastroenteritis
> - Hernia
> - Inflammatory bowel disease
> - Intestinal obstruction
>
> **Urinary (see Chapter 42)**
> - Urinary tract infection (UTI), pyelonephritis
> - Renal calculi
> - Urethral syndrome
> - Interstitial cystitis
>
> **Musculoskeletal (see Chapter 40)**
> - Trauma
> - Joint pain or injury
> - Inflammation of muscles and ligaments
>
> **Neurogenic (see Chapter 41)**
> - Nerve compression due to injury
> - Neuropathic pain
>
> **Psychologic**
> - Physical and/or sexual abuse (current or previous)
> - Depression and/or anxiety
> - Eating disorder
> - School avoidance
> - Substance use/abuse
> - Fear of pregnancy

of bleeding in some adolescents. There may be associated nausea, vomiting, diarrhea, headaches, dizziness, and back pain. Primary dysmenorrhea refers to recurrent, menstrual-related pain in the absence of pelvic pathology and is thought to be due to the release of prostaglandins from the endometrium. Secondary dysmenorrhea describes painful menstruation in the presence of pelvic pathology such as endometriosis, ovarian cysts, or infection. The evaluation of dysmenorrhea in adolescents starts with a detailed medical and menstrual history. Typical characteristics of dysmenorrhea are listed in Box 43.11. The physical examination should be normal, and pelvic ultrasound is not routinely indicated.

Treatment for dysmenorrhea starts with education about the condition, tracking the menstrual cycle, and basic self-care before and during menstrual periods. Over-the-counter and prescription NSAIDs are effective in many cases due to their antiprostaglandin effect. Preloading with medication before the onset of menses is most effective to block prostaglandin production before the onset of severe pain. Ibuprofen 400 to 800 mg every 8 hours or naproxen 550 mg every 12 hours are commonly used. Acetaminophen is unlikely to be helpful in relieving dysmenorrhea. Hormonal therapy, which causes the endometrial lining to become more atrophic, therefore releasing less prostaglandin, is another treatment option for adolescents who do not respond to initial treatment. Options include combined hormonal methods (oral contraceptive pills [OCPs], skin patch, vaginal ring) given in extended or continuous fashion and progesterone-only treatments (evonorgestrel intrauterine device [IUD], etonogestrel subdermal implant, depot medroxyprogesterone acetate [DMPA], and oral progestin). Patients who continue to have pain following several months of treatment should be referred to a gynecologist for additional evaluation.[11]

Mittelschmerz

The term mittelschmerz refers to the pain caused by normal ovarian function at the time of ovulation. It occurs during the middle of the menstrual cycle, is typically unilateral and mild to moderate in severity, and lasts for a few hours to several days. If needed, treatment is with an OTC pain medication; hormonal therapies that block ovulation are another option.

Ovarian Cysts

Ovarian cysts during the reproductive years are common and may not cause any pain or may cause pain of wide-ranging severity. Ultrasound is the preferred method of imaging for ovarian cysts and describes location, size, and cyst complexity. Severe pain caused by an ovarian cyst may be due to stretching of the ovarian capsule or leakage of fluid onto the peritoneum. Severe pain

> ### • BOX 43.11 Characteristics of Primary Dysmenorrhea in Adolescents
>
> - Onset of severe cramps usually 1 to 2 years after the onset of menses but can be anytime.
> - Pain is in the lower or midabdomen. May radiate to back or thighs.
> - Character is crampy and stabbing at times. May be severe.
> - NSAIDs and heat usually helpful but may not alleviate pain.
> - Missing of school and activities not uncommon if pain is severe.
> - Absence of pain outside menstruation.
> - Can be associated with nausea, vomiting, dizziness, and fatigue.
> - Physical examination is normal.
>
> *NSAIDs,* Nonsteroidal antiinflammatory drugs.

associated with nausea and vomiting should be addressed immediately given the risk of ovarian torsion.

Ovarian cysts in adolescents are often due to normal physiologic functions and resolve on their own. Supportive care with OTC pain medications, heat, and rest may be helpful. Pain from an ovarian cyst should gradually improve over the days to weeks following its onset, with complete resolution of symptoms within 1 to 2 months. A repeat ultrasound done 8 to 12 weeks following initial imaging is recommended to confirm that the cyst has resolved. Cysts that do not resolve in 3 months are less likely to be functional and may represent a neoplasm, such as teratoma, cystadenoma, or paratubal cyst. Ovarian cancer is rare in adolescents but must be considered. Patients who have ovarian or adnexal findings that suggest a solid or complex cyst, or do not resolve within 3 months should be referred to a gynecologist for possible removal. Patients who are unable to perform normal functions or have increasing pain should be referred sooner.

Endometriosis

Endometriosis is the presence of endometrial glands and stroma outside their normal location within the lining of the uterus. Historically, endometriosis was considered a disease of adult females only. However, current studies show that at least two-thirds of teens with chronic pain or dysmenorrhea that does not respond to hormonal therapies and NSAIDs will have endometriosis found at diagnostic laparoscopy.[11] The most common symptoms are cyclic as well as noncyclic pelvic pain, gastrointestinal pain, and urinary symptoms. The cause of endometriosis is multifactorial, with several theories about its origins. A family history of endometriosis is correlated with a higher risk of the condition. NSAIDs and hormonal therapy may help to resolve symptoms, but if there is no response to therapy within 3 months, referral to a gynecologist is warranted.

Premenstrual Syndrome

Premenstrual syndrome (PMS) includes a cluster of emotional and physical symptoms that occur in cyclic fashion about 1 to 2 weeks before the menstrual period and resolve with the onset of menses. Common PMS symptoms include bloating, breast pain, headache, food cravings, anxiety, fatigue, irritability, and depression. Premenstrual dysphoric disorder (PMDD) is a severe form of PMS defined in the American Psychological Association's *Diagnostic and Statistical Manual of Mental Disorders,* fifth edition. The diagnosis of PMS is made with the patient's prospective recording of her symptoms for 2 to 3 months (Box 43.12). Depression and anxiety can overlap or mimic PMS, so screening for underlying mental health concerns due to PMS or PMDD is important. Mild and moderate PMS symptoms often improve with lifestyle changes, such as increased aerobic exercise, relaxation techniques,

---

• BOX 43.12 Premenstrual Syndrome

Symptoms attributable to premenstrual syndrome:
- Present during the 5 days before the period
- Occur for at least 2 menstrual cycles in a row
- End within 4 days after period starts
- Interfere with some normal activities

Exclude depression, anxiety, and social-emotional stressors, which can mimic premenstrual syndrome but will not occur in a cyclic pattern that align with the menstrual cycle.

---

adequate sleep, and avoidance of foods high in fat, salt, sugar, and caffeine. Hormonal therapy used to prevent ovulation and the subsequent fluctuations in hormone levels can also be used to treat PMS, along with other evidence-based treatments.[12]

Breast Concerns

Breast development (thelarche) begins in most girls between the ages of 8 and 13 years and is often the first sign of puberty. Breast concerns are not uncommon among adolescents; PCPs can offer reassurance following a normal examination as well as educate patients on basic breast anatomy.[13]

Asymmetric Breasts

Significant differences in breast size can cause distress for patients and their parents. A breast examination should be done to confirm normal findings and verify that the size difference is not due to a cyst or mass in the larger breast. Young adolescents with this concern can be reassured that asymmetry will often improve over time and that surgical intervention is not usually needed.

Mastalgia

Mild breast pain is common among young people. Many fear that this symptom is due to breast cancer. Reassure patients and families that breast cancer is extremely uncommon in adolescents; it can also be helpful to explain that this condition usually does not cause pain. History elucidates whether breast pain is cyclic or noncyclic, as well as other possible factors including new medications, trauma, type of bra, and breast growth. Examine the patient for fibrocystic changes, mastitis, cysts, and chest wall pain. Pregnancy testing should also be done.

Breast Cyst or Mass

Due to increased awareness of breast cancer, a palpable breast cyst or mass in an adolescent can be very alarming to the patient and family. Breast cancer is extremely rare in the adolescent population; however, all findings require evaluation and appropriate clinical follow-up. The first step is a careful history, assessing for history of trauma, previous thoracic (chest/back) irradiation, associated symptoms, and family history of breast cancer. The breast examination in many cases reveals normal physiologic tissue or fibrocystic changes. Breast ultrasound is indicated for masses that are persistent or worrisome due to physical findings such as large size (>5 cm), skin changes, solid, or fixed on the underlying tissue. If a discrete but nonsuspicious mass is found, it is reasonable to observe it for 1 to 2 months and have the patient return for a repeat breast examination.

Nipple Discharge

Adolescents can express a small amount of clear discharge from their nipples; however, spontaneous nipple discharge needs further evaluation. Common causes include mechanical stimulation and irritation from clothing. Galactorrhea, which is a milky white discharge from both nipples, can be caused by hormonal medication, certain tranquilizers, antidepressants, and antihypertensives, as well as hypothyroidism or a prolactin-secreting pituitary adenoma. When nipple discharge persists, consultation with an adolescent gynecologist or pediatric endocrinologist should be obtained. Laboratory evaluation and imaging may be indicated.

Gynecologic Concerns in Adolescents With Physical and Developmental Disabilities

Similar to their peers, adolescents with physical and developmental disabilities need reproductive health care.[14] Menstrual suppression or reduction is a common request from adolescents and their families due to concerns about hygiene, mood changes before or during the menstrual cycle, exacerbation of conditions such as seizures, as well as other concerns. Many teens with disabilities can consent to sexual activity and desire contraception. Furthermore, caregivers may request contraception because of concerns that sexual abuse might

occur. Safety of the teen's environment and abuse prevention should be discussed with all teens and their families. Studies show that rates of all types of abuse among children with disabilities is higher than their peers and teens with disabilities in romantic relationships are at greater risk for dating violence than are their peers without disabilities.[15]

PCPs who care for adolescents with disabilities are well equipped to provide appropriate counseling for menstrual management and contraception (Fig. 43.13). The US Medical Eligibility Criteria (USMEC), described later, helps guide providers as to relative and absolute contraindication for contraception for individuals with medical conditions. Table 43.7 lists hormonal therapies available

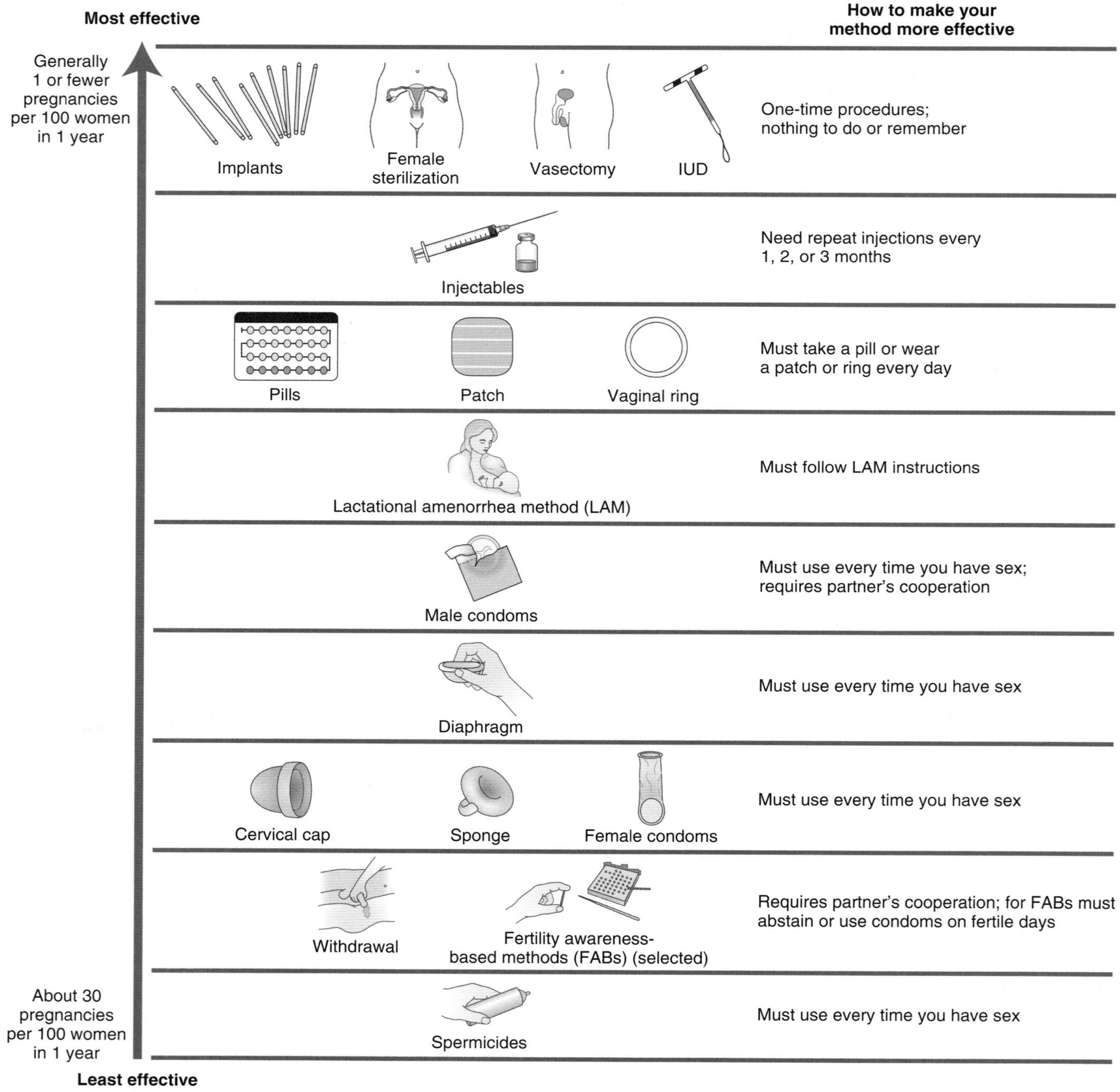

Most effective

Generally 1 or fewer pregnancies per 100 women in 1 year

| | | | | **How to make your method more effective** |

Implants — Female sterilization — Vasectomy — IUD → One-time procedures; nothing to do or remember

Injectables → Need repeat injections every 1, 2, or 3 months

Pills — Patch — Vaginal ring → Must take a pill or wear a patch or ring every day

Lactational amenorrhea method (LAM) → Must follow LAM instructions

Male condoms → Must use every time you have sex; requires partner's cooperation

Diaphragm → Must use every time you have sex

Cervical cap — Sponge — Female condoms → Must use every time you have sex

Withdrawal — Fertility awareness-based methods (FABs) (selected) → Requires partner's cooperation; for FABs must abstain or use condoms on fertile days

About 30 pregnancies per 100 women in 1 year

Spermicides → Must use every time you have sex

Least effective

• **Fig. 43.13** How Well Does Birth Control Work? *IUD*, Intrauterine device. (Modified from Association of Reproductive Health Professionals (ARHP): You decide tool kit: contraceptive efficacy tools. Adapted from World Health Organization. Comparing typical effectiveness of contraceptive methods. WHO: 2006.)

that can provide menstrual suppression. Combined OCP, skin patches, and vaginal rings can be used in extended or continuous dosing to reduce or eliminate menstrual periods. Amenorrhea will occur in 50% of patients after 1 year using continuous dosing. Breakthrough bleeding occurs most often in the first 3 months of use. When bleeding occurs with prolonged use, it can be managed with a 4-day break to allow for a withdrawal bleed and then restart. DMPA and amenorrhea will occur in 50% to 80% of patients after 1 year of use, but initial bleeding is very common. Concerns about weight gain and bone mineral density may limit its use. The levonorgestrel IUD 52 mg (Mirena, generic Liletta) is an excellent option for menstrual suppression as well as long-acting, highly effective contraception. There are very few medical contraindications to this IUD, and amenorrhea rates are 50% or higher at 1 year of use, with decreased flow in almost all users. Initial bleeding and spotting should be expected for first 3 to 6 months after IUD placement. The procedure for IUD insertion may require

anesthesia but can be coordinated with other procedures such as dental work. Oral progesterones are another option for menstrual suppression. Norethindrone acetate 5 mg is approved for the treatment of endometriosis and heavy menstrual bleeding; when given in continuous dosing, menstrual suppression is usually achieved.

Gynecologic Considerations in Nonbinary and Gender Diverse Adolescents

The care of nonbinary and gender diverse adolescents is reviewed in Chapter 7. Menstrual bleeding may be a source of gender dysphoria and menstrual management and suppression should be offered. Table 43.7 reviews options. Some individuals who do not identify as female may want to avoid combined hormonal methods (OCP, patch, ring) because they contain estrogen. All methods can be used concurrently with gender-affirming testosterone. Although

TABLE 43.7 Options for Menstrual Management and Suppression

Treatment	Advantages	Considerations
NSAIDs; most commonly ibuprofen and naproxen	Decrease blood flow and pain with periods Nonhormonal; can be used along with other methods Available OTC in pill and liquid forms	Can cause GI side effects Certain medical conditions may limit use
Combined hormonal contraception (methods that contain estrogen and progestin)	Can use in traditional, extended, or continuous dosing to have monthly, seasonal, or no scheduled periods Improve acne and hirsutism	All combined methods increase risk of DVT/VTE Avoid if known thrombophilia. Refer to USMEC for contraindications Antiepileptic enzyme-inducing drugs may reduce contraceptive efficacy
Oral contraceptive pills	Daily pill, can be crushed; chewable pill available	Pill needs to be taken same time each day
Patch	Apply to skin each week	Avoid if patient will remove patch
Ring	Insert into vagina each month	Requires insertion into vagina, which may not be acceptable
Oral progestins	Typically used in continuous fashion to suppress bleeding Do not contain estrogen; no increased risk DVT/VTE	Pill needs to be taken same time each day or breakthrough bleeding may occur
Norethindrone acetate 5 mg	Pill each day	Not an approved contraceptive
Medroxyprogesterone acetate 5–10 mg	Pill each day	Not an approved contraceptive
Progestin-only birth control pill (norethindrone 0.35 mg)	Pill each day	50% of users have breakthrough bleeding
Drospirenone progestin-only birth control pill	Pill each day	Novel progestin-only pill Brand name only available, which may create cost barrier
Depot medroxyprogesterone acetate (DMPA); injection every 12 weeks	Does not contain estrogen; no increased risk of DVT/VTE Option of SQ dosing in prefilled syringe for home use	Can be associated with decreased bone density and so may want to avoid when other risk factors present for bone concerns and other methods are acceptable May cause increase appetite and associated weight gain, especially in obese users
Subdermal implant: 4-mm flexible rod placed under the skin of the inner, upper arm	Excellent, long-acting contraception Easy to place and remove in office if patient is cooperative	Only 20% of users have amenorrhea so other methods should be considered if menstrual suppression is primary goal
Levonorgestrel-IUD: T-shaped device that sits inside the uterus and releases progestin; Mirena and Liletta effective for 7 years	FDA-approved treatment for menstrual bleeding and pain. Excellent contraception in addition to menstrual control Insertion under anesthesia can be offered	Insertion in the office may not be possible Misconceptions about safety may unfortunately limit use

DVT, Deep venous thrombosis; *FDA,* U.S. Food and Drug Administration; *GI,* gastrointestinal; *NSAID,* nonsteroidal antiinflammatory drug; *OTC,* over the counter; *USMEC,* US Medical Eligibility Criteria; *VTE,* venous thromboembolism.

testosterone may induce amenorrhea, it does not provide contraception; teens who have a vagina/uterus and are sexually active with a partner who has a penis and do not want to become pregnant will want to also use a contraceptive method.Sexual Health Sexual health is an essential aspect of routine preventive medical care for everyone, yet ongoing stigma prevents access for many, and particularly adolescents and young adults. As healthcare providers, PCPs who work with teens are powerful advocates for youth in the clinical setting as well as in the community. Key aspects of high-quality care include defining adolescent sexual development with a positive framework and relying on a strength-based approach to working with youth. How to complete a comprehensive adolescent interview that inquires about home, school, interests, safety, emotional and personal goals is reviewed in Chapter 13 and lays the groundwork for addressing sexual health topics. There are many key elements of sexual health; the following section addresses those aspects directly related to the gynecologic health of adolescents, specifically contraception and teen pregnancy as well as STI education, prevention, testing, and treatment.

Person-Centered and Teen-Centered Contraceptive Counseling

Person-centered contraceptive care is a framework that identifies the historic, systemic, community, and individual factors necessary to achieve equitable contraceptive coverage.[16]

Within the context of the provider-patient relationship, counseling should begin only after rapport is established and the adolescent has confirmed their interest in reviewing contraceptive methods. Patients should feel respected as a person, listened to regarding their preferences, and provided with enough information to make their own best decision.[17] Adolescents face significant barriers in obtaining contraception; PCPs should be familiar with all US Food and Drug Administration (FDA)-approved contraceptive options and know how their adolescent patients can access these methods including when confidentiality is necessary (Fig 43.14). Additional information on the sexual health interview is covered in Chapter 7, but central issues when contraception is discussed are highlighted here. Box 43.13 provides a summary of best practices in adolescent contraceptive counseling,

with a more in-depth discussion of several of these issues in the following paragraphs.

Address Confidentiality Concerns
Confidentiality is an essential component of adolescent health care and teens often forgo needed medical care unless confidentiality can be assured. Twenty states explicitly allow minors to consent to contraceptive services on their own, without the approval or consent of their parents. Other states allow minors to consent in certain circumstances, and four states have no explicit policy. Clinicians who provide health services to adolescents must be aware of the regulations in their state. The Guttmacher Institute[18] is a valuable resource to learn about state laws and policies related to minors' access to contraception. When necessary, providers should be aware of local resources for free and confidential reproductive health care. Examples may include Title X family planning clinics, community health centers, state and county public health clinics, school-based clinics, and private and/or nonprofit providers and organizations.

Rely on Good Resources
Many adolescents seek online resources on their own or when recommended by a health provider. Box 43.14 lists websites that present medically accurate, nonjudgmental health content in a format that is likely to appeal to teens and young adults. Given the volume of inaccurate information on the Internet, it is important

---

• BOX 43.13 Summary of Best Practices in Adolescent Contraceptive Counseling

- Start with rapport
  - Greet teens warmly and rely on a strength-based approach
- Address confidentiality concerns:
  - Take the time to do a one-on-one interview, even when the teen presents with her parent or partner.
  - Discuss confidentiality, privacy, limitations, and support conversations with family and friends.
  - Know your state laws and policies.
  - Develop and identify local resources for free and confidential reproductive health care.
- Use tools and techniques that reflect best practices:
  - Start the conversation by asking teens what matters to them in a birth control method.
  - Designed for young adults, with content and format for them.
  - Reflects best practices and current recommendations.
  - For teens that are interested in LARC, provide information on how and where to get it.
  - Address common myths and misperceptions about contraception.
  - Ask about opinions of friends and family members.
  - Educate teen on noncontraceptive benefits as well as possible common side effects.
  - Invest time in phone calls and return visits when needed to listen to concerns and provide reassurance.
- Follow updated clinical recommendations:
  - Use same-day start or "quick start" for all methods when possible.
  - Pelvic examination and testing not required before starting any method.
  - Multiple visits before or after starting a method are not required.
  - Do not unnecessarily restrict the use of contraception in teens with medical conditions. Instead, refer to USMEC.

LARC, Long-acting, reversible contraception; *STIs*, sexually transmitted infections; *USMEC*, US Medical Eligibility Criteria.

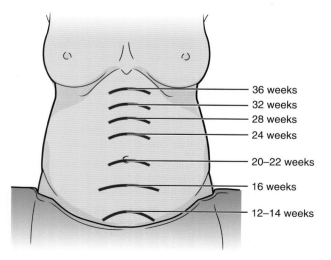

• **Fig. 43.14** Assessment of Gestation in Pregnancy by Uterine Size. (From Niedzwwiecki B, Pepper J, Weaver PA. *Kinn's Medical Assisting Fundamentals.* Elsevier; 2019.)

36 weeks
32 weeks
28 weeks
24 weeks
20–22 weeks
16 weeks
12–14 weeks

• BOX 43.14   Medically Accurate Websites on Sexual Health[a]

• BOX 43.14   Medically Accurate Websites on Sexual Health[a]

http://www.bedsider.org

An online birth control support network. No funding from pharmaceutical companies. Medical partners include the American College of Obstetricians and Gynecologists.

- Information and comparison of all contraceptive methods.
- Health clinic finder for birth control, abortion services, and on-line birth control (enter zip code).
- Can set up daily, weekly, monthly text message reminders.
- Can set up text and email reminders for next clinic appointment.

www.sexetc.org

From Answer, a national organization that provides and promotes access to comprehensive sexuality education for young people and the adults who teach them.

- Content is written for teens, by teens and reviewed by experts for accuracy.
- Information on birth control, STIs, relationships, LGBTQ and more.
- Action and advocacy section and live chat feature.

https://goaskalice.columbia.edu/ www.sexetc.org

Written and run by a team of health professionals and researchers at Columbia University.

- Sexual and reproductive health in questions and answer format.
- General health including alcohol and drugs, nutrition, relationships and more.

[a]These sites are directed to college-age teens and young adults.
STI, Sexually transmitted infection.

• BOX 43.15   Quick-Start Contraception

All methods of contraception can be quick started at any time during the menstrual cycle if pregnancy can be reasonably excluded. Criteria include any of the following:

- Has never had sexual intercourse before.
- Is currently using another effective method of contraception.
- Has regular monthly periods and is less than 7 days from the start of a normal period.
- Is less than 4 weeks postpartum or less than 7 days after spontaneous or induced abortion.
- Has not had unprotected sexual intercourse within the previous 2 weeks and has a negative pregnancy test today.

If unprotected sex in the previous 2 weeks but negative pregnancy test today, all methods can be quick started.

- Counsel that pregnancy test is not conclusive due to the chance of a luteal-phase pregnancy. However, if pregnancy does occur, contraceptive method does not cause harm. Starting method now is considered safe if desired by patient.
- Use backup method or no sex for 1 week.
- Return for repeat pregnancy test in 2 weeks.

for providers to highlight that these websites provide material that is written and reviewed by sexual health experts. This type of supplement to in-clinic conversations can allow teens and families to research options before and after their visits as well as provide ongoing support once a method is initiated.

Offer Ongoing Support

Effective contraceptive counseling includes ongoing support, education, and reassurance. When adolescents leave with a new contraceptive method, they must know how to contact the clinic with questions and concerns. Phone calls and follow-up visits should be encouraged and viewed as valued opportunities to provide additional support and education. Teens may need reassurance that an expected side effect, like breakthrough bleeding, is common and does not mean that the method is not working. An adolescent's decision to stop a method, including the request for long-acting, reversible contraception removal, should be addressed without delays.

Follow Updated Clinical Recommendations

Quick Start. All methods can be started on the same day if the provider can be reasonably sure a patient is not pregnant. "Quick start" (Box 43.15) refers to the practice of initiating a contraceptive method on the same day of the contraceptive visit, or on any day during the menstrual cycle. Multiple visits before or after starting a method should never be required. The general rule for most methods is to abstain or use a backup method for 7 days after starting a new method. If the adolescent had unprotected sexual intercourse in the previous 2 weeks before starting a method, they should still be offered quick start and advised to repeat a

pregnancy test in 2 weeks. Emergency contraception (EC) should be offered but never required.

No Tests Required Before Starting. For healthy adolescents, minimal to no testing should be required before starting birth control. Blood pressure should be assessed before initiating combined hormonal methods (OCPs, patch, ring), and initiation of an IUD requires a pelvic examination that, along with STI testing, if indicated, can be done at the time of insertion. Individuals with known medical problems might need additional evaluation and providers should rely on US Medical Eligibility Criterial (USMEC; see later) in these circumstances. There are no evidenced-based recommendations for follow-up testing or examinations once a method has been initiated. For users of combined hormonal contraception, routine assessment of blood pressure is recommended.

Prescribing Contraception in the Setting of Other Medical Conditions. Sometimes a provider's concern about the safety of birth control creates an unnecessary barrier to its initiation. The USMEC for Contraceptive Use was developed by the Centers for Disease Control and Prevention (CDC) and World Health Organization; it provides evidence-based guidance for safe contraceptive use in people with medical conditions and is an essential tool that allows PCPs to reduce barriers to contraceptive use. The USMEC, available free online and with a free smartphone application, is an evidence-based tool that is easy to use and can provide an immediate, direct answer to common clinical questions.[19] Box 43.16 describes common clinical scenarios where providers may have questions about contraceptive safety. USMEC presents evidence-based recommendations for safe use in these conditions as well as many others.

Contraceptive Methods

It is important for providers to have a working knowledge of all contraceptive methods. A brief overview of the advantages and potential challenges of the most effective and commonly prescribed methods is given in Table 43.8. In the following section, each contraceptive method is reviewed, including a description of the method and its mechanism of action, its advantages, counseling about what to expect with its use, and how to address common side effects.

BOX 43.16 Common Clinical Scenarios in Providing Contraception and US Medical Eligibility Criteria for Contraceptive Use

Sixteen-year-old with a **family history of breast cancer**. Both grandmother and mother of patient were diagnosed in their 40s, and mother of patient is worried that "hormones will cause cancer." *USMEC: All contraceptive methods, including OCPs, are safe to use and do not increase the risk of cancer. Of note, OCPs are known to decrease the risk of ovarian and uterine cancer.*

Fifteen-year-old with **previous pelvic inflammatory disease due to gonorrhea infection** requests an intrauterine device (IUD) for contraception. *USMEC: There are no restrictions for IUD use based on age, parity, history of sexually transmitted infections (STIs), history of pelvic inflammatory disease (PID), or prior ectopic pregnancy.*

Seventeen-year-old who is **obese** and has **major depression**. *USMEC: All contraceptive methods are safe to use in females with obesity and depressive disorders.*

Fourteen-year-old with **migraine headaches** *without* aura. *USMEC: All contraceptive methods are safe to use. Combined hormonal contraception (methods that contain estrogen) should be avoided in patients who have migraine WITH aura.*

Seventeen-year-old with **epilepsy,** currently on the anticonvulsant topiramate. *USMEC: All contraceptive methods are safe to use in females with epilepsy. However, combined hormonal contraception (CHC) should not be used in females on certain anticonvulsants like topiramate because of decreased contraceptive efficacy. (Medications to avoid with CHCs are listed at USMEC.)*

OCP, Oral contraceptive pill; *USMEC,* US Medical Eligibility Criteria for Contraceptive Use.

The Implant

The contraceptive implant is a single rod 4 cm in length and 2 mm in diameter; it is placed into the subdermal space of the upper inner nondominant arm. It consists of an ethylene vinyl acetate copolymer (latex free) that allows for the controlled release of etonogestrel (68 mg) over a period of 3 years, with contraceptive efficacy documented at 5 years. Etonogestrel is the main active metabolite of desogestrel, a progestin used in many OCPs. The implant is a progestin-only method. The currently available etonogestrel implant (Nexplanon) contains barium sulfate and is radiopaque.

The primary mechanism of action is suppression of ovulation; the progestin in the implant also thickens cervical mucus and induces atrophy of the endometrial lining. The implant is the most effective of any contraceptive option and the method of choice for many teens, particularly those ages 14 to 17 years. Insertion is quick and easy and does not require a pelvic examination. A teen can easily palpate the implant and be confident about its presence. Many teens prefer a method that requires no action on their part and is highly effective. The implant can be inserted at any time during the menstrual cycle using a quick start protocol. Users should be instructed to avoid sexual intercourse or use an alternative method for the first week. The implant can be placed immediately postpartum or following a spontaneous or induced abortion.

All PCPs who perform insertions and removals are required by the FDA to receive training from the manufacturer. The insertion procedure takes an average of 30 seconds and starts with the injection of a local anesthetic followed by device insertion. The application site is then dressed with a bandage and the patient can return immediately to usual activities. Infection site complications are rare and most commonly include local redness and bruising. The implant is palpable by the user but is very discreet,

TABLE 43.8 Advantages and Potential Challenges of Common Birth Control Methods

Advantages	Potential Challenges
Implant	
• Highest efficacy • High satisfaction and continuation • Simple and quick insertion • Discreet, immediate reversibility • Relief of dysmenorrhea	• Uterine bleeding, although not dangerous, may be frequent, unpredictable, and prolonged
Intrauterine Device (IUD)	
• Very high efficacy • Highest satisfaction and continuation of any method • Discreet, immediate reversibility • Levonorgestrel IUDs, treatment for bleeding, dysmenorrhea, anemia due to heavy bleeding • Safe for almost all teens, including those with complex medical conditions; no medication interactions	• Pelvic exam required for insertion • Copper IUD may increase bleeding and cramping and is relatively contraindicated in patients with heavy bleeding and/or severe dysmenorrhea
Depot Medroxyprogesterone Acetate (DMPA, "Depo")	
• High efficacy • Simple and quick injection; can be done in office or prescribed for self-injection at home • Discreet • Relief of dysmenorrhea and heavy bleeding • No medication interactions	• Possible increased appetite and associated weight gain not uncommon • Irregular bleeding common in first 3–9 months • Visit every 11–13 weeks
Combined Hormonal Contraception: Oral Contraceptive Pills (OCPs), Skin Patch, Vaginal Ring	
• Good efficacy when used correctly and consistently • Widespread familiarity • Many noncontraceptive benefits • User can start or stop at anytime • Immediate reversibility	• Remember each day (pills), week (patch), month (ring) • Visits to pharmacy for refills • Requires medication storage • Contain estrogen that may limit use in select medical conditions

given its location in the upper inner arm as well as its subdermal placement. It is helpful to reassure teens that the implant will not migrate and will not break. The procedure to remove the implant involves injection of a local anesthetic followed by a small incision for removal. If another implant is requested, the current implant is removed, and a new device placed via the same small incision.

Managing Common Expected Side Effects of the Implant. The contraceptive implant causes bleeding pattern changes that are unpredictable for its duration of use. About 25% of users will have little to no bleeding (amenorrhea) with other users experiencing occasional, frequent, or prolonged bleeding. There are no good models to predict bleeding patterns. Counseling and education about changes in bleeding patterns *before* receiving the implant increase satisfaction and continuation of the method.

When irregular or prolonged bleeding occurs, reassurance from the PCP is crucial and may be all that is necessary. With prolonged progestin exposure, the endometrium becomes atrophic, which can result in amenorrhea or spotting or frequent bleeding due to endometrial instability. For sexually active patients, STI and pregnancy testing may be indicated. For users who would like to use medication to treat bleeding, the CDC recommends NSAIDs for 5 to 7 days or (if medically eligible) as a first-line option. Other treatments include combined hormonal methods or estrogen alone for 10 to 20 days. Hormonal methods in addition to the implant can be continued longer if requested by the patient.

Intrauterine Devices

Five different IUDs are now available in the United States, all of which are safe and effective for teens and adult females who have not yet had children.

The copper-containing IUD is marketed under the name Paragard and has been approved by the FDA for 10 years, although contraceptive efficacy has been documented for 12 years. It is made of polyethylene with barium sulfate added to create x-ray visibility. Copper wire is wound around the vertical stem of the T-shaped device. Four IUDs contain the hormone levonorgestrel and include Liletta, Mirena, Kyleena, and Skyla. Mirena has been available in the United States since 2001 and in Europe a decade before that. The product consists of a T-shaped polyethylene frame with a vertical cylinder that slowly releases levonorgestrel directly into the endometrial cavity. Mirena is FDA-approved to use for 5 years, although its contraceptive efficacy has been documented for 7 years of use. Liletta®, a generic levonorgestrel IUD, is very similar to Mirena. Skyla and Kyleena are levonorgestrel IUDs that contain a lower dose of levonorgestrel and therefore are less likely to induce amenorrhea.

All IUDs produce a sterile foreign body reaction within the uterine cavity, which creates a hostile environment for sperm. The contraceptive effects of continuous IUD use occur before fertilization; therefore IUDs are not abortifacients. The copper IUD causes an increase in copper ions, enzymes, white blood cells, and prostaglandins in uterine and tubal fluids, which impair sperm function and prevent fertilization. Levonorgestrel IUDs have a local effect on the endometrium, causing the release of foreign body mediators, inhibiting sperm capacitation and survival, thickening cervical mucus, and suppressing the endometrium. Systemic absorption of levonorgestrel is low and most cycles are ovulatory. IUDs are very effective, with failure rates of less than 1%. The levonorgestrel IUDs have slightly lower failure rates than the copper IUD.

Advantages and Method Counseling. IUD users report higher satisfaction and continuation than users of any other contraceptive method. Satisfaction and continuation of the levonorgestrel IUD is higher than with the copper IUD. An IUD can be inserted at any time in a woman's menstrual cycle as long as the provider is reasonably sure she is not pregnant. Screening for chlamydia and gonorrhea is indicated at least annually for all sexually active teens and can be done at the same visit as insertion. If an STI is detected, treatment should occur with the IUD in place. An IUD can be inserted immediately following vaginal delivery or cesarean section. The procedure for IUD insertion includes a bimanual examination, speculum examination, measuring for uterine size, and placement of the IUD using a sterile, prepackaged applicator. IUD strings are cut to 3 cm in length, which allows them to curl up around the cervix so that they cannot be felt during intercourse. The pain experienced with IUD insertion is rated as tolerable by most, including adolescents and those who have not had children. After a detailed explanation of the insertion procedure, most patients clearly express their interest or noninterest in this method and the procedure required for insertion.

Managing Common Expected Side Effects of the Intrauterine Device. In the first days and weeks after IUD insertion, there may be bleeding and cramping related to the procedure itself. NSAIDs decrease bleeding and pain following insertion. Heavy bleeding, severe pain, nausea, vomiting, or fevers should be evaluated with a complete history and examination including a speculum examination to look for IUD strings and a bimanual examination to assess uterine tenderness. The risk of complications such as uterine perforation and infection is low but should be considered. There is a 5% risk of IUD expulsion, which is usually accompanied by increased cramping and bleeding. If the IUD strings are not visible, a pelvic ultrasound will confirm the intrauterine location. The patient must refrain from sex or use another effective method until the IUD location has been confirmed.

Users of the levonorgestrel IUD should expect unscheduled bleeding or spotting in the first 3 to 6 months of use; this bleeding is not harmful and decreases with continued use. Over time, many users experience only light menstrual bleeding or amenorrhea. Patients may need reassurance that amenorrhea is a safe, expected benefit of this IUD and that no treatment is needed. A pregnancy test can be done at any time if reassurance is needed, and some patients may request a pelvic examination to confirm that the IUD strings are present if they are unable to feel them on their own.

There is no evidence-based recommendation to have patients "check their strings" during IUD use. However, PCPs should be able to palpate and visualize IUD strings on pelvic examination. If strings are not visible, a pregnancy test should be done, followed by a pelvic ultrasound to confirm the intrauterine location of the IUD. Encourage patients to use another contraceptive method until the IUD location is confirmed. If the IUD is confirmed to be inside the uterus, no other treatment is needed.

Depot Medroxyprogesterone Acetate

DMPA (brand name Depo-Provera) is a progestin-only contraceptive. The most commonly used form is a 150-mg dose injected intramuscularly (deltoid or gluteus maximus) every 3 months. Another formulation of DMPA allows for a self-administered subcutaneous dose of 104 mg every 3 months. DMPA increases the circulating levels of progestin, which acts on the HPO axis to suppress ovulation. Progestin thins the lining of the endometrium and, over time, induces significant endometrial atrophy.

DMPA can be initiated in quick-start fashion. Patients who are at risk for an interval pregnancy due to recent unprotected intercourse should return in 2 to 4 weeks for a repeat pregnancy test. Repeat injections should be given at 11- to 13-week intervals. An injection can be given early when necessary (e.g., a patient is in clinic and this timing is more convenient than a return visit). The repeat injection can be given up to 2 weeks late (15 weeks from the last injection) without additional contraceptive protection or pregnancy testing.[20] If it has been more than 15 weeks from the last injection, the PCP should follow a quick-start protocol and give DMPA if pregnancy test is negative.

DMPA is safe in patients with medical contraindications to estrogen. Noncontraceptive benefits include improvements in dysmenorrhea and pain related to endometriosis, reduction of bleeding, and high rates of menstrual suppression with continued use. DMPA levels are not decreased by antiepileptics and there may be reduced seizure activity in some patients with epilepsy as well as reduced pain crises for individuals with sickle cell disease.

Side Effects. The main side effect of DMPA is irregular menstrual bleeding, which most patients will experience most commonly during the first 6 months of use and likely improves with method continuation. Amenorrhea occurs in most users after 1 year of use and occurs immediately for some. If bleeding becomes bothersome, a 5- to 7-day short-term treatment with NSAIDs or hormonal treatment with a combined hormonal contraceptive can be offered. Weight gain on DMPA is unpredictable and varies widely among users. Adolescents should be counseled about the possibility of increased appetite, which is thought to be the mechanism of weight gain. The package insert reports an average weight gain of 5 lb in the first year, although some may gain more and may do so quickly. Nutrition and counseling about lifestyle changes can be offered, but obesity and weight gain should never preclude use in an adolescent who feels that DMPA is their best contraceptive option. DMPA may have an effect on bone density that is reversible once the method is discontinued and may not be of clinical significance.[21] Experts do not recommend limiting the use of DMPA based on bone density concerns for those users who consider it their preferred option to prevent pregnancy.

Combined Hormonal Contraception

Combined hormonal contraception (CHC) contains both estrogen and progestin. This includes OCPs, the contraceptive patch, and the contraceptive ring. OCPs have been available in the United States since the 1960s and have been extensively studied. The levels of hormones contained in OCPs have decreased dramatically over the past 50 years as lower doses have been found to be efficacious, safer, and better tolerated. Although there are approximately 70 different combined OCPs available in the United States, differences in side effects are minimal. Furthermore, medical eligibility and counseling regarding risk should remain constant among all combined hormonal methods, including those labeled as containing very low doses. Examples of how pills differ are listed in Table 43.9. The major differences are in estrogen dose, progestin type, and packaging regimen of active and placebo pills. Best practices in prescribing CHC are listed in Box 43.17.

The transdermal contraceptive patch is a thin, beige adhesive patch that contains a progestin and ethinyl estradiol. It can be applied to the torso, buttocks, or upper arms and must be changed each week. The vaginal contraceptive ring is a soft, clear, flexible 54-mm-diameter ring that releases the progestins etonogestrel and ethinyl estradiol (EE). The ring is inserted by the user into the vagina and must be replaced monthly.

Mechanism of Action. The progestin component of combined hormonal methods provides the majority of its contraceptive efficacy by preventing ovulation via negative feedback on the HPO axis. The estrogen component is added to stabilize the endometrium and allow for better cycle control.

Managing Common Expected Side Effects

Missed Pills. OCP users who forget to take their pill should be advised to take it as soon as they remember. If a single pill is missed in a pill pack but taken within 24 hours of its usually scheduled time, contraceptive efficacy should not be affected. For the sake of simplicity and to avoid contraceptive failure, users who miss more than 1 pill in any given cycle should be advised to use

---

TABLE 43.9 Key Differences in Oral Contraceptive Pills

Variation	Detail	Comment
Amount of estrogen	Most OCPs contain 35 mcg or less, (low dose) "Very" low-dose pills contain 20 mcg or less	Current research does not support a difference in safety or efficacy among OCPs with <35 mcg EE Reasonable to try lower EE dose to manage side effects such as nausea or breast tenderness Lower EE pills may be associated with more breakthrough bleeding
Type of progestin	Several generations of progestins; examples: first: norethindrone second: levonorgestrel third: desogestrel, norgestimate fourth: drosperinone	Third- and fourth-generation progestin considered less androgenic Although certain progestins may confer a small, increased risk of venous thromboembolism, current evidence does not support recommending one pill over another based-on safety concerns Medical contraindications to CHC use apply to all types in this method category
Formulation	Monophasic: all active pills contain the same dose of estrogen and progestin Triphasic: dose of estrogen and progestin changes each week	Data do not support any advantage to triphasic formulations
Regimen	Traditional 21/7 (most common): 21 days of active pills + 7 days of placebo 24/4: 24 days active pills + 4 days of placebo	Bleeding occurs monthly due to hormonal withdrawal while placebo pills are being taken
	Extended 84/7 or other: With traditionally packaged pills write SIG: Take 1 active pill for 84 (4 packs) in a row then 7 days off Continuous: all pills active (no placebo breaks) With traditionally packaged pills write SIG: Take 1 active pill every day.	Bleeding occurs during placebo break every few months with extended use No scheduled bleeding with continuous use More likely to have unscheduled or "breakthrough bleeding," which will decrease with consistent use Breakthrough bleeding can be managed with a 4-day break from OCPs Any OCP can be used in extended or continuous fashion

CHC, Combined hormonal contraception; *EE*, ethinyl estradiol; *OCP*, oral contraceptive pill.

• BOX 43.17 Best Practice for Prescribing Combined Hormonal Contraception

Dispense	Provider writes to dispense a 3-month supply. Most insurance companies will dispense a 3-month supply; mail-order may be required
	Dispensing 13 months is ideal and the best option if insurance barriers can be overcome
Refills	Provide enough refills for at least 1 year
	Evidence does not support any requirements for follow-up after method initiation
Quick start	Teen should start method as soon as it is picked up
	No requirement for pelvic exam or pregnancy test
	Can return for a pregnancy test in 2 weeks if any possibility of interval pregnancy

---

• BOX 43.18 Approach to Counseling About Risk for Venous Thromboembolism/Stroke Before Initiating Combined Hormonal Contraception

1. Discuss that nonusers and users both risk VTE.
   - Healthy, non-OCP users: 1–4/10,000 women years
   - OCP users: 3–9/10,000 women years
   - Pregnancy: 5–20/10,000 women years
   - Postpartum: 40–65/10,000 women years
2. Do not use CHC if USMEC Category 3 and 4.
3. Overall risk very low, especially in healthy teens.
4. As with any treatment, benefits need to outweigh risks.

CHC, Combined hormonal contraception; *OCP,* oral contraceptive pill; *USMEC,* U.S. Medical Eligibility Criteria; *VTE,* venous thromboembolism.
From Committee on Gynecologic Practice. ACOG Committee Opinion Number 540: Risk of venous thromboembolism among users of drospirenone-containing oral contraceptive pills. *Obstet Gynecol.* 2012;120:1239-1243, reaffirmed 2020.

---

another form of contraception (such as condoms) or avoid sex until they have had at least 7 days of consistent pill use. Patients who have missed pills may have unscheduled bleeding. Finally, OCP users who are missing pills frequently should be asked if they are interested in learning about methods that do not rely on daily use.

Unexpected Bleeding. In the first 3 months of CHC use, unexpected bleeding is not uncommon and no treatment is needed. Providers should confirm that the user is taking the pill at the same time each day (or changing the patch or ring as directed) and reassure that bleeding resolves with continued and consistent use. Users of extended or continuous CHC should expect unscheduled bleeding especially in the first 4 months of use. Prolonged progestin exposure causes the endometrium lining to become thin, and instability may result in bleeding. Users can either continue the method, take a 4-day break to allow for a withdrawal bleed and enable the endometrium to stabilize, or try a 5-day course of NSAIDs.

Pill-Induced Amenorrhea. Some users of CHC experience amenorrhea during the hormone-free interval (that is, during the placebo pills of OCPs or the hormone-free week of patch or ring use). It is reasonable to obtain a urine pregnancy test to make sure that pregnancy has not occurred. Otherwise, no treatment is needed and the patient can be reassured that this is due to the progestin causing the endometrium to become atrophic. OCP users who prefer to have a monthly period can try switching to a different brand of pill.

Other Side Effects. CHC is well tolerated and causes minimal side effects. Breast pain and nausea may occur initially but usually resolve within the first few weeks of use. Switching to a different brand of OCP is always an option; trying a lower dose of estrogen (e.g., a pill that contains 20 mcg of EE or less) or a different progestin is reasonable. Some users may experience side effects that continue with use or are not attributable to the OCP. These include new-onset headaches, mood changes, and weight gain. Providers should evaluate patients for other causes of these symptoms as well as discuss different options for CHC or other methods.

Deep venous thrombosis (DVT) and stroke are rare with the use of CHC and can occur in healthy teens who are not on hormones. Patients who call with symptoms that are concerning for any serious medical condition should be evaluated immediately. Box 43.18 outlines the risk of venous thromboembolism (VTE) and/or stroke with use of CHC, which should be discussed with all users of these methods before initiation. Adolescents with

USMEC category 3 or 4 CHC contraindications should not use these methods.

Progestin-Only Pills

There are currently two types of progestin-only pills (POPs) available in the United States, one which has been available for decades, and one that is a novel formulation. POPs do not contain estrogen and are considered safe for individuals with an increased risk of thrombosis. The norethindrone POP (also called the "minipill") contains 0.35 mg of norethindrone and there are many generic versions available. The primary contraceptive mechanism of the norethindrone POPs is progestin-induced thickening of cervical mucus, which blocks sperm from entering the uterus. Norethindrone POPs do not consistently suppress ovulation and must be taken at the same time each day to be effective; 50% of users will have irregular bleeding, and some may have regular periods or amenorrhea. The novel POP containing drospirenone 4 mg works by preventing ovulation and there are noncontraceptive benefits due to the progestin effect on the endometrium. There is no generic formulation of the novel POP available, which may create cost barriers for some patients.

Emergency Contraception

Emergency contraception (EC) comprises methods of birth control used after unprotected intercourse that prevent pregnancy before it occurs. EC does not end a pregnancy and does not work if someone is already pregnant. The use of EC is time-sensitive, with better efficacy the sooner it is used after intercourse but can be used up to 5 days or 120 hours after unprotected sex. Some adolescents choose to obtain EC pills in advance to have them available for immediate use.

There are two types of pills and three types of IUDs available for EC in the Unites States (Box 43.19). The mechanism of action for EC pills is to delay or inhibit ovulation. Ulipristal acetate is a progesterone-receptor modulator that can be taken up to 5 days after the unprotected encounter with an effectiveness that ranges from 62% to 85%. Levonorgestrel is available over the counter, providing 74% effectiveness, and can be taken up to 72 hours (3 days) after unprotected intercourse. The IUDs that can be used as EC are 99% effective if inserted within 5 days of the unprotected encounter. The mechanism of action for IUDs is by preventing sperm from fertilizing an egg. Continued use of the IUD

Pills

Progestin-Only Emergency Contraceptive: Levonorgestrel 1.5 mg in One Dose
- Brand names: Plan B One-Step, Take Action, Next Choice One Dose, My Way
- Over the counter with unrestricted sale to any sex and any age person
- May not work if BMI is over 26

Ulipristal Acetate 30-mg Tablet
- Brand name: Ella
- Sold by prescription only regardless of age
- May be covered by insurance
- More effective than levonorgestrel ECPs; preferred option when possible
- May not work if BMI is over 35

IUDs
- Most effective option for EC (99% effective)
- Provides ongoing, highly effective contraception after inserted
- Several IUDs options: Paragard, Liletta, and Mirena

ECPs, Emergency contraceptive pills; *IUDs,* intrauterine device.

provides ongoing contraception by creating a hostile environment for sperm so that they do not travel into the tubes, where fertilization occurs.

There are no medical contraindications to oral EC and few contraindications to IUDs. Adolescents who use oral EC may experience irregular bleeding and should be counseled to do a pregnancy test in 2 weeks following its use.

Condoms

Condoms are the only methods of contraception that also provide protection against STIs. Male condoms are the most common form of contraception used. Condoms must be used consistently and correctly to be effective; most failures are due to incorrect and inconsistent use, resulting in a 15% or higher failure rate per year in most users. Adolescents benefit from learning how to obtain condoms and how to negotiate for their use as well as from a demonstration of correct condom use (Box 43.20). Condom use should be strongly encouraged and continued for STI prevention even if a more effective contraceptive method is started. Female condoms have not been studied as extensively but do offer protection from pregnancy and STIs and should be offered as an alternative if male condoms are not an option.

Coitus Interruptus and Other Less Effective Methods

Withdrawal (coitus interruptus) is a commonly used method of contraception but does have a failure rate of 27% each year with typical use. This method often fails because precum can contain active sperm and the partner may not be able to withdraw before ejaculation. Many teens may use withdrawal along with other contraceptive methods. Other less effective methods include spermicides or a sponge, diaphragm, cervical cap; these have fertility failure rates of 25% or higher per year.

Teen Pregnancy

Trends in Teen Pregnancy

Over the last several decades there has been a significant and continued decline in the U.S. teen pregnancy rate, largely attributable

• BOX 43.20 Condom Information

- There are no age or other restrictions on who can buy condoms.
- Carry a condom with you if sex is a possibility.
- Check the expiration date and make sure that the package is not damaged.
- Use a water-based lubricant (like KY jelly) and not petroleum jelly or oils.
- Unroll the condom on an erect penis.
- Withdraw when the penis is still erect, holding onto the base of the condom so it does not slip off.

to the increased use of contraception.[22] However, the United States rate remains the highest in the developed world, pointing to significant gaps in comprehensive sexual education and access to health care. PCPs play a central role in implementing practices and policies that improve reproductive health outcomes for teens including access to information, contraception, and support for those who are pregnant and/or parenting.

Diagnosis of Teen Pregnancy

Pregnancy testing should be done in any adolescent who is menarchal and has missed one or more periods. Though rare, pregnancies have been reported in pubertal girls who have not yet had their first period. Concerns about breast pain, nausea, vaginal bleeding, and pelvic pain all warrant pregnancy testing. Pregnancy can also present with fatigue, weight gain, and urinary frequency.

Urine hCG tests are sensitive and specific; they will detect pregnancy 14 to 17 days from sexual intercourse or at the time of the missed period in people with regular ovulatory cycles. False negatives occur with dilute urine or if testing is done too soon and hCG levels have not reached 100 mIU/mL. Serum hCG testing is not usually necessary but detects very low levels of hCG. In general, serum hCG results below 5 mIU/mg are considered negative.

When an adolescent presents with reports of a positive urine pregnancy test done at home, it is best to perform a urine pregnancy test in the clinic. Urine pregnancy kits can be misread, often because the control indicator is interpreted as a positive result. Teens who think that they may be pregnant should be seen quickly for pregnancy confirmation and counseling. If negative pregnancy results are obtained, the PCP should offer sexual health counseling, EC if it has been less than 5 days since the most recent unprotected intercourse, and contraception with a quick-start protocol if the teen is interested in birth control.

When pregnancy is diagnosed, an abdominal examination should be performed. The 12-week uterus is about the size of a grapefruit and can be palpated just above the pubic bone. The top of the uterus in a 20- to 22-week pregnancy is palpable at the umbilicus (see Fig. 43.14). A pelvic examination is needed to assess uterine size before 12 weeks; pelvic ultrasound is the most accurate way to date a pregnancy.

After Diagnosing Pregnancy

Before an in-depth conversation, PCPs should not make any assumptions about an individual's intentions or emotional response to pregnancy. The majority of teen pregnancies, but not all, are unintended. Disclosure of the result should occur with the adolescent alone. Sometimes the teen may insist that her partner or family member remain in the room. The provider must take into account respect for the teen's autonomy, the need for her privacy, safety, and any other factors known about the clinical situation. It is not necessary for the adolescent to make any decision about their intentions regarding the pregnancy at the time of diagnosis. The PCP and staff must remain supportive and unbiased. The teen should be allowed as much time as needed to understand the results. Most teens want to inform their parents or guardians; clinicians can play an instrumental role in facilitating this communication. Options counseling refers to the choices that individuals make regarding pregnancy: continue the pregnancy and raise the child, continue the pregnancy and make an adoption or kinship care plan, or end the pregnancy. Clinicians who do this work must be well versed in nonjudgmental, nondirective options counseling.

If the adolescent would like to continue the pregnancy, they should be seen by a prenatal provider within 1 to 2 weeks from diagnosis. Adolescent pregnancies are at higher risk for preterm delivery, low birth weight, and social and emotional concerns such as depression and partner violence. The teen should be strongly advised to avoid all alcohol, tobacco, marijuana, and other recreational drugs. Prescription medication should be reviewed, and any category X medications (e.g., isotretinoin and warfarin) should be stopped immediately. If the patient was using hormonal contraception, they should stop this medication and be reassured that it has not caused any harm. Additional referrals may be indicated to support other needs such as food and living arrangements during and after pregnancy.

If the adolescent is certain that they want to end the pregnancy, referral to a provider who performs abortions is made. Patients should be provided with reliable information on the local availability of abortion and other relevant information. When an adolescent expresses the desire to have an abortion, it is not appropriate for them to be referred to a crisis pregnancy center or pregnancy resource center that will not provide balanced counseling regarding options.

Preconceptual Counseling

Some adolescents seek to become pregnant, and some may be ambivalent about pregnancy and therefore do not use contraception. Ninety percent of adolescents become pregnant during a single year of sexual activity when no birth control method is used. Preconceptual counseling is recommended during the reproductive years and focuses on factors that result in better outcomes (Box 43.21).

Ectopic Pregnancy

An ectopic pregnancy is one that occurs when the fertilized egg implants outside of the uterine cavity, most commonly in the fallopian tube. Symptoms usually occur during the first few weeks of pregnancy when a teen may not even know they are pregnant; symptoms can include vaginal bleeding, pelvic and abdominal pain, and nausea and vomiting. If the ectopic pregnancy starts to rupture, there may be dizziness, fatigue, bloating, and referred pain in the shoulder, neck, or back. Adolescents who present with vaginal bleeding and abdominal pain should be assessed for pregnancy. If they are pregnant and having worrisome symptoms, an ultrasound should be performed to determine the location of the pregnancy; referral to the ED may be appropriate. Serial hCG levels that do not rise appropriately can be helpful in confirming the diagnosis. IUD users have a lower risk for ectopic pregnancy than individuals who do not use effective contraception; however, when a pregnancy does occur with an IUD in place, close to half of them are ectopic. Tubal pregnancy in an unstable patient is a medical emergency. Ruptured ectopic pregnancy is a significant cause of pregnancy-related mortality.[23]

• BOX 43.21 Preconceptual Counseling

- Make sure that vaccinations and STI screening are up to date.
- Start at least 400 mcg of folic acid each day.
- Stabilize medical conditions.
- Review use of all prescription and OTC medications.
- Learn about the patient's family history of medical conditions.
- Advise the patient to reach and maintain a healthy weight.
- Treat any mental health concerns.
- Stop using tobacco, alcohol, marijuana, and recreational drugs.
- Address partner violence if present.
- Discuss the importance of early prenatal care and discuss the option of the patient establishing a relationship with an obstetric provider if appropriate.

OTC, Over the counter; STI, sexually transmitted infection.

Sexually Transmitted Infections

STIs pass from one person to another during intimate physical contact and during sexual behaviors such as vaginal, oral, and anal sex. The most common and reportable STIs include chlamydia and gonorrhea. *STI* is a broader term that includes conditions that can cause infection but do not necessarily result in a disease process.

Sexually Transmitted Infection: Adolescent Health Disparity

Compared with other age groups, adolescents and young adults have disproportionately high rates of STIs. The CDC estimates that adolescents ages 15 to 24 account for over half of the 20 million new STIs in the United States each year. One in every four sexually active adolescent females has an STI such as chlamydia or HPV. Table 43.10 lists many of the factors that contribute to the high prevalence of STIs among young people and corresponding strategies that providers can adopt to address this health disparity. Discussing common myths about STIs (Table 43.11) with adolescent patients can be an effective way for clinicians to establish rapport as well as diminish fear and stigma regarding this topic.

Sexually Transmitted Infection: Prevention and Screening

The CDC's STI Treatment Guidelines are continually updated based on disease surveillance and should be consulted for up-to-date recommendations for prevention, screening, and treatment. The CDC website (www.cdc.gov) is the best way for providers to access this information when needed. Avoid referring to textbooks (including this one!) or handbooks that may contain older information.

PCPs are central to the prevention of STIs in the adolescent population (Box 43.22). STI prevention starts with appropriate vaccination, which is greatly influenced by the strength of the health provider's recommendation. Appropriate STI screening founded on evidence-based recommendations is a key strategy for prevention, as early treatment and risk reduction counseling results in improved outcomes. Table 43.12 outlines the screening recommendations for sexually active adolescents. Everyone should be tested for HIV at least once between ages 13 and 64 years. Females should be screened at least annually for gonorrhea and chlamydia. Additional STI testing is recommended if a teen is pregnant, symptoms are present, or if the patient falls into one of the CDC's special population categories, such as men who have sex with men.

TABLE 43.10 Factors That Lead to High Rates of Sexually Transmitted Infections Among Young People and Strategies to Address Them

Factors	Provider Strategy
Increased biologic susceptibility to infection due to cervical anatomy	• Follow age-based screening recommendations for annual GC/chlamydia testing: test all sexually active females annually until age 25 years • Teach how to use and to negotiate for condom use with every partner for oral, anal, and vaginal sex
Adolescent concerns about confidentiality and privacy	• Make it your regular practice to have a one-on-one interview with teens at each visit • Know the laws in your state. All states allow minors to consent to sexually transmitted infection (STI) services Go to www.gutmacher.org and learn about your state's laws and then share with your clinic team • Work with clinic schedulers, business managers to develop policies that follow state laws and allow for teen confidentiality • Understand how tests will be billed in your clinic and develop options to manage situations when confidentiality must be assured • Know and/or develop local resources for free and confidential testing when needed
Embarrassment about STIs	• Get comfortable talking about STIs and STI testing in a way that allows for questions and discussion. For example, talk about age-based screening in general, and common myths about STIs • During your confidential interview, establish rapport before taking a sexual history on all patients, not just those who ask for STI testing
Fear of testing method	• Urine testing for STIs is not painful or invasive • Pelvic exam (females) or urethral swab (males) is not needed for testing
Insurance coverage	• Help families and adolescents obtain coverage • Know local resources and/or offer free screening
Myths about STIs	• Address common myths and misperceptions when discussing STI testing and prevention (see Table 43.11)

TABLE 43.11 Common Sexually Transmitted Infections: Myths and Facts

Myth	Fact
"I can't have an STI if I've only had 1 partner," or "Only people that sleep around get STIs."	All sexually active adolescents should have testing for STIs based on screening recommendations and/or symptoms. It only takes one partner to get an STI
"You can tell if someone has a STI."	Over 70% of chlamydial and gonorrheal infections have no symptoms
"You can get a STI from a toilet seat."	No you can't. Intimate skin-to-skin contact is necessary for infection to occur
"You can't get a STI from oral sex."	Yes, you can. Chlamydia, gonorrhea, HPV, and herpes are transmitted by oral sex
"Using 2 condoms at once will prevent STIs better than using just 1"	One condom, used correctly, is best to prevent STIs Two condoms may increase friction and cause them to break or tear
"If the guy pulls out, this will prevent the spread of STIs."	Precum contains fluids that can spread infection. Some STIs can be spread via skin-to-skin contact alone
"HIV is a death sentence, so why bother getting tested?"	With regular treatment, HIV-infected people can live normal, healthy lives and have children that are HIV-negative. Knowing your HIV status is the only way to prevent spread of disease to people you care about PrEP is highly effective at preventing HIV acquisition and should be offered to anyone at risk
"I'm not gay so I don't need an HIV test."	HIV infection is also spread through penis-vagina
"I've already had PID and STIs. I can't get them again, and it doesn't matter anyway."	Repeat gonorrhea and chlamydia infections are common. You are not immune after having an infection. With each infection, there is a risk of serious complications
"My birth control will also protect me from STIs."	Except for condoms, birth control methods do not protect from STIs
"I hate condoms and never have one to use. There is nothing that works for me to prevent STIs."	Risk reduction makes a difference. Start using condoms some of the time. Bring condoms with you when going out. Get frequent STI testing so any infection is treated quickly. If you are at risk for HIV, learn more about PrEP

HPV, Human papillomavirus; *PID,* pelvic inflammatory disease; *PrEP,* preexposure prevention; *STI,* sexually transmitted infection.

Common Sexually Transmitted Infections

Although most people with STIs are asymptomatic, it is important for providers to recognize the symptoms of common STIs and test when indicated. Chlamydia and gonorrhea are the most common reportable STIs, and annual screening for them is indicated. Testing is also recommended in patients who present with genitourinary or gynecologic symptoms and report sexual activity, or when sexual abuse or sexual activity is suspected. Concerns about vaginal discharge and appropriate testing are discussed in Table 43.4.

Genital herpes causes a small, painful herpetic ulcer (Fig. 43.15). Primary herpes simplex virus (HSV) infection, when recognized, is often preceded by flu-like symptoms as well as multiple painful lesions that cause intense external dysuria and swelling. A single small painful lesion may be due to a recurrent HSV outbreak. Test lesions for HSV with a type-specific PCR test; serology can be done later if helpful but may not reveal antibodies to HSV until several weeks following infection. NSGUs, discussed earlier, also cause exquisitely painful vulvar ulcers, but the lesions are often larger than those due to herpes and PCR testing of the NSGU lesion will be negative for HSV.

1. Accurate risk assessment and education and counseling of persons at risk regarding ways to avoid STIs through changes in sexual behaviors and use of recommended prevention services.
2. Preexposure vaccination for vaccine preventable STIs (HPV, Hepatitis B, and Hepatitis A).
3. Identification of asymptomatically infected persons and persons with symptoms associated with STIs.
4. Effective diagnosis, treatment, counseling, and follow-up of infected persons.
5. Evaluation, treatment, and counseling of sex partners of persons who are infected with an STI (expedited partner therapy).

HPV, Human papilloma virus.
From Centers for Disease Control and Prevention. Sexually Transmitted Infections Treatment Guidelines, 2021. https://www.cdc.gov/std/treatment-guidelines/STI-Guidelines-2021.pdf.

TABLE 43.12 Routine Sexually Transmitted Infection Screening Recommendations for Sexually Active Populations

Population	Recommendation
Adolescent females	• Annual testing for chlamydia and gonorrhea until age 25 years and/or when presenting for STI evaluation and/or GU/GYN symptoms • RPR (for syphilis) and HIV if another STI detected • HIV testing at least once • Other screening may be indicated if also another special population such as IV drug use, corrections, sex work, or partners include MSM
Adolescent males	• Test for chlamydia and gonorrhea if: high prevalence community, seen at teen clinic, STI clinic, or correctional facility; and/or presenting for STI evaluation and/or GU symptoms • HIV test at least once • Young men who have sex with men should have testing per MSM recommendations
Pregnant females	• HIV, syphilis, hepatitis B, hepatitis C; chlamydia and gonorrhea if less than age 25 years
MSM (men who have sex with men)	• Annual testing for HIV, syphilis, chlamydia, and gonorrhea (pharyngeal, rectal, and/or urethral, depending on site of sexual contact), hepatitis B, hepatitis C; consider screening for HSV-2
WSW (women who have sex with women)	Same as adolescent female
Transgender and nonbinary people	Follow screening guidelines based on current anatomy and sexual behaviors

GU/GYN, Genitourinary/gynecologic; *HSV,* herpes simplex virus; *RPR,* rapid plasma reagin.
From CDC STI Treatment Guidelines 2021 at https://www.cdc.gov/std/treatment-guidelines/.

Treatment and Counseling

Treatment for common STIs is generally straightforward and effective and should be in accordance with current CDC recommendations found at www.cdc.gov (Table 43.13). When possible, onsite and directly observed single-dose therapy allows for maximum adherence and increases the opportunity for counseling. Ongoing care must be supportive of teens with regard to their medical, emotional, and social situation. General counseling topics that can be reviewed with adolescents who are receiving treatment for an STI are listed in Box 43.23.

Partner notification and treatment is a necessary step when a reportable infection is diagnosed. Time spent counseling on the importance of notification and providing patients with written information about the infection increases the rate of partner notification and treatment. If a sexual partner decides to see their own provider for treatment, presumptive treatment for the corresponding infection should be delivered, along with appropriate counseling and screening as indicated.

Expedited partner therapy is an effective strategy to prevent reinfection, transmission of new infections, and prevention of PID and other complications. It should be routinely offered to patients with chlamydia or gonorrhea infection when requested. (Box 43.24).

• Discuss how medications will be obtained as well as detailed instructions for use.
• Discuss the need for partner treatment and notification when appropriate.
• Offer expedited partner therapy (EPT) if there is infection with gonorrhea/chlamydia. All partners in the previous 60 days should be treated, or the most recent partner if no contact in >60 days.
• No sexual contact until 7 days after patient *and* partner have been treated.
• Review consistent and correct condom use to prevent future infections.
• Review current contraceptive method when appropriate.
• Screen for syphilis, HIV, and other STIs when indicated.
• Schedule a follow-up visit in 3 months to test for reinfection.

STIs, Sexually transmitted infections.
From Centers for Disease Control and Prevention. Sexually Transmitted Infections Treatment Guidelines, 2021. https://www.cdc.gov/std/treatment-guidelines/STI-Guidelines-2021.pdf

• Effective treatment of chlamydia and gonorrhea includes treatment of sex partners to prevent reinfection, transmission of new infections, and prevention of PID and other complications.
• EPT allows the clinician to provide a prescription for the sex partner or partners of the infected patients without an exam or visit.
• Encouraged by most state public health departments, visit https://www.cdc.gov/std/ept/default.htm to check for updated information on your state.

EPT, Expedited partner therapy; *PID,* pelvic inflammatory disease.

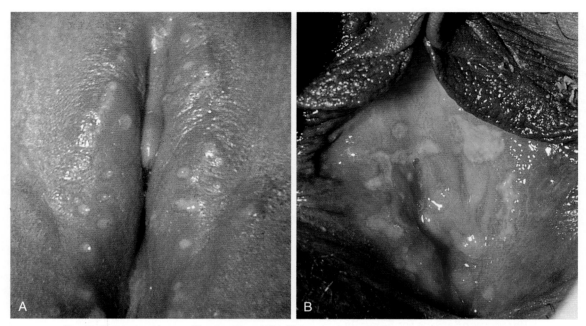

• **Fig. 43.15** Primary Herpes Simplex Virus With Vulvar Lesions. (A) Prepubertal child with numerous vesicular lesions, a few of which have ulcerated over perineum. (B) Full-blown ulcerative phase of herpetic vulvovaginitis in an adolescent. (From Montano GT, Torres OA. Pediatric and adolescent gynecology. In: *Zitelli and Davis' Atlas of Pediatric Physical Diagnosis,* 8th ed. Elsevier; 2023.)

TABLE 43.13 Overview of Common Sexually Transmitted Infections

Infection	Test	Symptoms/Sequelae	Treatment and Specific Follow-up
Chlamydia			
Most common reportable infection in the United States Largest burden of infection in females below age 25 years	Nucleic acid amplification test (NAAT) via urine sample, vaginal, endocervical, rectal, or oropharyngeal swab Vaginal and rectal swabs can be self-collected High specificity and high sensitivity	Majority of infections (75%) cause no symptoms In males, may cause dysuria, urethritis, proctitis, pharyngitis In females, may cause dysuria, vaginal discharge, vaginitis, cervicitis, postcoital bleeding, breakthrough bleeding, painful intercourse, and pelvic pain Sequelae of infection in females include PID, ectopic pregnancy, and infertility due to tubal disease	Doxycycline 100 mg orally bid for 7 days; alternative is azithromycin 1 g orally but no longer preferred treatment due to concerns about unrecognized anorectal infection that may not be cured with this option Treat all sex partners in previous 60 days If no sexual contact in >60 days, treat most recent partner Retesting at <3 weeks can lead to false positive result; re-treat if concerns about med compliance or reinfection Retest males and females treated for chlamydia in 3 months (due to risk of reinfection)
Gonorrhea			
Second most common reported infection in the United States Infections often concentrate in specific geographic locations and communities			Single 500 mg intramuscular dose of ceftriaxone for uncomplicated gonorrhea. Treatment for coinfection with *Chlamydia trachomatis* with oral doxycycline (100 mg twice daily for 7 days) should be administered when chlamydial infection has not been excluded Treat all sex partners in previous 60 days If no sexual contact in >60 days, treat the most recent partner Symptoms that persist after treatment should be evaluated by NAAT and culture with antimicrobial susceptibility due to concerns about resistant organisms. Contact local public health department for guidance when needed Retest for gonorrhea at 3 months (due to risk of reinfection)

Overview of Common Sexually Transmitted Infections—Cont'd

Infection	Test	Symptoms/Sequelae	Treatment and Specific Follow-up
Trichomoniasis			
Most common nonviral STI, but infection not reportable in the United States Untreated infections may last months to years	Testing should be done when a sexually active teen seeks care for vaginal discharge Screening in asymptomatic patients may be considered in high-prevalence settings and is recommended in females with HIV NAAT testing (or microscopy when not available) of vaginal/urethral secretions NAAT tests are 3–5 times more sensitive than microscopy Testing of rectal and oral sites not recommended	The majority of infections (70–85%) cause no or minimal symptoms In females, may cause diffuse, malodorous, or yellow-green discharge with or without vulvar irritation In males, may cause urethritis, epididymitis, or prostatitis Infection with trich is associated with an increased risk for PID and HIV acquisition	For females: Metronidazole 500 mg 2 times/day for 7 days For males: Metronidazole 2 g orally in a single dose Alternative treatment for anyone: Tinidazole 2 g orally in a single dose Sex partners should be referred for treatment. EPT can be offered but has not been proven to reduce reinfection rate Testing for chlamydia, gonorrhea, syphilis, and HIV should be performed when trich is detected Females who have been treated for trich should be retested at 3 months (due to risk of reinfection)
Syphilis			
Systemic disease caused by *Treponema pallidum*	Screening recommended in pregnant females, MSM, and HIV-infected individuals, and anyone diagnosed with an STI Diagnostic testing when patients have signs and symptoms of infection Serologic nontreponemal (RPR) and treponemal tests (FTA-ABS) can be used for initial screening	Primary infection: painless ulcer or chancre Secondary: skin rash, lymphadenopathy Latent infection are those lacking clinical manifestations	Penicillin G, administered parentally, is the preferred drug for treatment in all stages of disease See CDC STI treatment guidelines[a] and consult infection disease experts as needed All persons with infection should be screened for HIV Partners in previous 90 days preceding diagnosis should be treated presumptively. Partners previous to last 90 days should be screened for infection The rate of congenital syphilis has dramatically increased in the United States since 2021. All pregnant females should be screened at their first prenatal visit
Genital Herpes			
Lifelong viral infection. Most people with infection are unaware of it Most cases of recurrent genital herpes are due to HSV-2, but HSV-1 can cause genital lesions	Testing should be type-specific to differentiate between HSV-1 and HSV-2 infection given different prognoses for recurrent disease and viral shedding Polymerase chain reaction (PCR) test of the herpetic lesion is the test of choice in the acute setting Serologic testing weeks after infection can be helpful to guide counseling. Presence of HSV-2 antibodies strongly suggests anogenital infection Presence of HSV-1 antibodies alone may reflect oral HSV infection acquired in childhood, or genital HSV-1 General screening not recommended	Primary infection can present as flu-like illness in addition to multiple, extremely painful vesicles on the genital area Presenting complaint may be dysuria, tingling, burning, or itching: physical exam crucial for diagnosis Recurrent infections produce a single lesion and may have a prodrome	Many options: First clinical episode: Acyclovir 400 mg PO tid for 7–10 days or valacyclovir 1 g PO bid for 7–10 days Recurrent episode: Acyclovir 800 mg bid for 5 days or valacyclovir 1 g PO qd for 5 days Suppressive therapy: Acyclovir 400 mg bid daily or valacyclovir 1 g PO daily Many patients with HSV-2 opt for suppressive therapy to reduce shedding and transmission of infection as well as to reduce recurrences by 70–80%. Safety and efficacy of therapy are well established Asymptomatic sex partners should be offered serologic testing
HIV			
1.2 million people in the United States have HIV; 16% are unaware of the infection	All persons who seek evaluation and treatment for STIs should be screened for HIV All persons aged 13–64 should be screened for HIV at least once Additional consent forms for testing is not recommended Serologic testing for HIV-1 and HIV-2. Rapid tests are also available	Begins as brief, acute viral syndrome and transitions into chronic illnesses and immunodeficiency (AIDS)	Treatment is lifesaving and prevents spread of infection Partners need counseling and should be offered preexposure prevention (PrEP) to prevent infection Refer to Chapter 35 for a complete discussion of HIV infection Anyone who is at risk for HIV should be offered PrEP to reduce their risk of infection

[a]Check https://www.cdc.gov/std/treatment-guidelines for updates.

CDC, Centers for Disease Control and Prevention; *EPT*, expedited partner therapy; *FTA-ABS*, fluorescent treponemal antibody absorption; *HSV*, herpes simplex virus; *MSM*, men who have sex with men; *PID*, pelvic inflammatory disease; *RPR*, rapid plasma regain; *STI*, sexually transmitted infection.

Pelvic Inflammatory Disease

PID is an infection of the reproductive organs. It is most commonly caused by chlamydia and gonorrhea but can be caused by other infections. There is no simple test for PID and many episodes are subclinical and go unrecognized. The CDC recommends presumptive treatment for sexually active young females if they experience pelvic or lower abdominal pain when no other cause of pain can be identified.[24] Box 43.25 outlines clinical criteria for the diagnosis of PID and treatment guidelines. Females with PID should also be tested for syphilis and HIV. IUD users who are diagnosed with PID can be reassured that treatment will be effective and there is no reason for IUD removal.

• BOX 43.25 Pelvic Inflammatory Disease (PID) Overview

Diagnosis

- Presumptive PID if one or more present on pelvic exam in sexually active adolescent without other explanation for pain:
  - Cervical motion tenderness
  - Uterine tenderness
  - Adnexal tenderness
- Increased specificity of PID diagnosis if one or more present:
  - Oral temperature >101°F (38.3°C)
  - Mucopurulent cervical discharge or cervical friability
  - Abundant white blood cells in vaginal discharge microscopy
  - Elevated erythrocyte sedimentation rate, elevated C-reactive protein
  - Positive gonorrhea and/or chlamydia

Management

- Test for pregnancy, gonorrhea and chlamydia, HIV; other STIs if additional symptoms
- Treat partner(s) if gonorrhea/chlamydia detected
- Counsel to avoid sexual contact until patient and partner have completed treatment
- See patients within 72 h (3 days) to confirm response to treatment
- If gonorrhea/chlamydia detected, test for reinfection in 3 months
- Most patients can be treated on an outpatient basis. Decision to hospitalize for treatment is based on clinical judgment and often advised if any of the following:
  - Surgical emergency (i.e., appendicitis) cannot be reasonably excluded
  - Presence of tubo-ovarian abscess
  - Pregnancy
  - Severe illness, nausea, vomiting, high fever
  - Unable to tolerate or follow outpatient regimen
  - No response to oral therapy
- Antimicrobial treatment (always check for updates at www.cdc.gov)
  - Inpatient: Cefotetan 2 g IV q12h, PLUS doxycycline 100 mg PO or IV q12h, *plus* metronidazole 500 mg PO or IV q12h. See www.cdc.gov for alternative parental options.
  - Outpatient: Ceftriaxone 500 mg IM in a single dose, *plus* doxycycline 100 mg PO bid for 14 days with metronidazole 500 mg PO bid for 14 days. See www.cdc.gov for alternative parenteral options.

PID, Pelvic inflammatory disease; *STI*, sexually transmitted infection.

References

1. American College of Obstetricians and Gynecologists. Vaginitis in nonpregnant patients. ACOG practice bulletin No. 215. *Obstet Gynecol.* 2020;135:e1–e17.
2. Fontham ETH, Wolf AMD, Church TR, et al. Cervical cancer screening for individuals at average risk: 2020 guideline update from the American Cancer Society. *CA Cancer J Clin.* 2020;70(5):321–346.
3. Breuner CC, Mattson G. Committee on Adolescence, Committee on psychosocial aspects of child and family health: sexuality education for children and adolescents. *Pediatrics.* 2022;138(2).
4. Christi J, Alaniz VI, Appiah L, et al. Vulvar aphthous ulcer in an adolescent with COVID-19. *J Pediatr Adolesc Gynecol.* 2021;S1083–3188(21):00122–00124.
5. Brodie K, Alaniz V, Buyers E, et al. Study of adolescent female genitalia: what is normal? *J Pediatr Adolesc Gynecol.* 2019;32(1):27–31.
6. American College of Obstetricians and Gynecologists. ACOG Committee Opinion No. 795. Elective female genital cosmetic surgery. *Obstet Gynecol.* 2020;135:e36–e42.
7. American College of Obstetricians and Gynecologists, Committee Opinion No. 605. Primary ovarian insufficiency in adolescents and young women. *Obstet Gynecol.* 2021;123:193–197.
8. Teede H, Misso M, Costello M, et al. International Evidence-Based Guideline for the Assessment and Management of Polycystic Ovary Syndrome 2018. International PCOS Network.
9. American College of Obstetricians and Gynecologists. ACOG Committee Opinion No. 728. Müllerian agenesis: diagnosis, management, and treatment. *Obstet Gynecol.* 2018;131:e35–e42.
10. Stoffel NU, Zeder C, Brittenham GM, et al. Iron absorption from supplements is greater with alternate day than with consecutive day dosing in iron-deficient anemic women. *Haematologica.* 2021;105(5):1232–1239.
11. American College of Obstetricians and Gynecologists. ACOG Committee Opinion No. 760. Dysmenorrhea and endometriosis in the adolescent. *Obstet Gynecol.* 2018;132(6):1517–1518.
12. Yonkers KA, Simoni MK. Premenstrual disorders. *Am J Obstet Gynecol.* 2018;218(1):68–74.
13. Mareti E, Vatopoulou A, Spyropoulou GA, et al. Breast disorders in adolescence: a review of the literature. *Breast Care.* 2021;16(2):149–155.
14. Committee Opinion on Adolescent Health Care Opinion No. 668. Menstrual manipulation for adolescents with physical and developmental disabilities. *Obstet Gynecol.* 2021;128(2).
15. Amborski AM, Bussières EL, Vaillancourt-Morel MP. Sexual violence against persons with disabilities: a meta-analysis. *Trauma Violence Abuse.* 2021:1–14. Sage.
16. Holt K, Reed R, Crear-Perry J. Beyond same-day long-acting reversible contraceptive access: a person-centered framework for advancing high-quality, equitable contraceptive care. *Am J Obstet Gynecol.* 2020;222(4S):S878.e1–S878.e6.
17. Dehlendorf C, et al. Development of a patient-reported measure of the interpersonal quality of family planning care. 2018;97(1):34–40.
18. The Guttmacher Institute. www.guttmacher.org.
19. Center for Disease Control and Prevention. *Summary Chart of U.S. Medical Eligibility Criteria for Contraceptive Use;* 2020. https://www.cdc.gov/reproductivehealth/contraception/pdf/summary-chart-us-medical-eligibility-criteria_508tagged.pdf.

20. Center for Disease Control and Prevention. *Reproductive Health: Injectables*; 2021. https://www.cdc.gov/reproductivehealth/contraception/mmwr/spr/injectables.html.

21. Committee on Adolescent Health Care, Committee on Gynecologic Practice. ACOG Opinion 602. *Depot Medroxyprogesterone Acetate and Bone Effects*; 2020. https://www.acog.org/clinical/clinical-guidance/committee-opinion/articles/2014/06/depot-medroxyprogesterone-acetate-and-bone-effects.

22. Osterman MJK, Hamilton BE, Martin JA, et al. National vital statistics system births: final data for 2020 by division of vital statistics. U.S. Department of health and humans services, centers for disease control and prevention, national center for health statistics. *Natl Vital Stat Rep*. 2022;70(17). https://www.cdc.gov/nchs/data/nvsr/nvsr70/nvsr70-17.pdf.

23. Committee on Adolescent Health Care, Long-Acting Reversible Contraception Work Group 735. *Adolescents and Long-Acting Reversible Contraception: Implants and Intrauterine Devices*; 2021. https://www.acog.org/clinical/clinical-guidance/committee-opinion/articles/2018/05/adolescents-and-long-acting-reversible-contraception-implants-and-intrauterine-devices.

24. Center for Disease Control and Prevention. Sexually Transmitted Infections Treatment Guidelines. https://www.cdc.gov/std/treatment-guidelines/STI-Guidelines-2021.pdf.

Appendix A

Height and Ratio Measurements

Accurate serial height measurements documented over time on the appropriate growth chart are key tools in the evaluation of growth across the pediatric lifespan. Inaccurate measurement may result in failure to detect growth disorders or inappropriate referrals for typical growing children. The desired tool to measure height accurately is a wall-mounted, well-calibrated ruler with an attached horizontal measuring bar fixed at 90 degrees (e.g., a stadiometer). The child should stand erect, with the back of the head, back, buttocks area, and heels touching the vertical bar of the stadiometer; the horizontal measuring bar is lowered to the child's head to obtain the measurement. The child/teen is asked to remove any footwear and/or head ornaments before noting the measurement. The child should be asked to take a deep breath and stand as tall as possible. A deep breath straightens the spine and allows more accurate and consistent measurements.

A portable laser height meter was tested in comparison to a stadiometer in a 2020 study; it revealed reproducibility within and between different operators along with acceptable accuracy when compared to a stadiometer.[1] This device may prove to be useful in patients when standing height cannot be obtained or in the evaluation of remote populations when the use of a stadiometer may be difficult.

An alternative to standing height measures in children is the **sitting height** (Fig. A.1), which is measured from the vertex (top-most point of the head) to the sitting surface. The stadiometer is placed on a stool at a sufficient height to allow the participant's legs to form a 90-degree angle with the ground. The **crown rump height** (Fig. A.2) is used for younger children or those who are not able to stand. Sitting height and leg length (standing height minus sitting height) measurements are indicators of proportionality and can be used to evaluate children with disordered growth; however, population-specific reference data are required to interpret these growth measurements.

Arm span is an additional measure from the middle fingertip of both hands when stretching out both arms horizontally. The ratio of one's arm span to height is generally 1:1, meaning that a person's arm span is about equal to their height. It is an important tool in anthropometric measurements, especially in cases where direct measurement of stature is not possible or in the assessment of short-limbed short stature (or long-limbed high height) resulting from growth hormone deficiency, chromosomal disorders (e.g., Turner syndrome, Marfan syndrome), or skeletal dysplasia (e.g., achondroplasia, hypochondroplasia, rickets).

There are a number of ways to measure arm span. For teens and older children, the easiest method is by doubling the distance between the sternal notch and the tip of the middle finger of an extended arm. A second method, which is better for younger children, is to position the participant's back against the wall with arms spread against the wall at shoulder level and parallel to the floor with the palms facing forward. A steel measuring tape is used

to measure the distance from the tip of the middle finger on one hand across the chest to the tip of the middle finger on other hand. Infants need to be laid down on a flat surface.

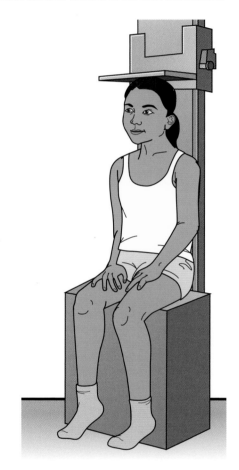

• **Fig. A.1** Sitting Height Measurement.

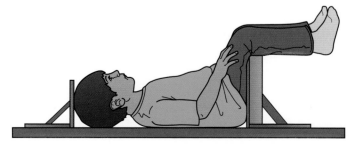

• **Fig. A.2** Crown to Rump Measurement.

References

1. Sørensen GVB, Riis J, Danielsen MB, et al. Reliability and agreement of a novel portable laser height metre. *PLoS One.* 2020;15(4):e0231449.
2. Hawkes CP, Mostoufi-Moab S, McCormack SE, Grimberg A, Zemel BS. Sitting Height to Standing Height Ratio Reference Charts for Children in the United States. *J Pediatr.* 2020;226:221–227.

Index

Page numbers followed by *t* indicate table, by *f* figure, and by *b* box.